P9-DCV-576

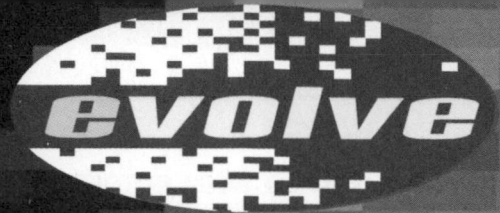

The Latest *Evolution* in Learning.

Evolve provides online access to free learning resources and activities designed specifically for the textbook you are using in your class. The resources will provide you with information that enhances the material covered in the book and much more.

Visit the Web address listed below to start your learning evolution today!

▶▶ *LOGIN: http://evolve.elsevier.com/Lewis/medsurg*

Evolve Online Courseware for the new 6th edition of *Medical-Surgical Nursing*: *Assessment and Management of Clinical Problems* offers the following features:

- **Web Links** to places of interest on the web specific to your classroom needs
- **Concept map creator** and examples of concept maps
- **Content updates** with the latest related news and research findings from the authors
- **Links to Related Products** to see what else Elsevier Science has to offer in a specific field of interest
- **And more. . .**

Think outside the book... evolve.

CD-ROM included with every copy of *Medical-Surgical Nursing*, 6th edition features:

- **40 Case Studies** followed by interactive learning activities*
- **Glossary** of key terms and definitions
- **40 *Patient and Family Instruction Guides*** in English and Spanish*
- **List of nursing diagnoses**
- **Laboratory values reference**

*Cross-referenced in the book with this symbol:

About the Authors

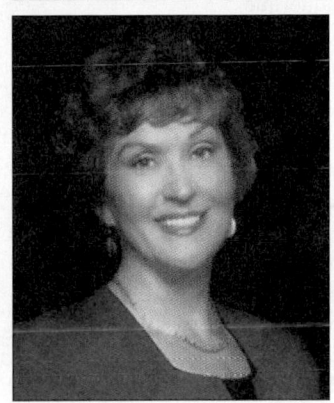

SHARON MANTIK LEWIS, RN, PhD, FAAN

Sharon Lewis received her Bachelor of Science in nursing from the University of Wisconsin-Madison, Master of Science in nursing with a minor in biological sciences from the University of Colorado-Denver, and PhD in immunology from the Department of Pathology at the University of New Mexico School of Medicine. She had a 2-year postdoctoral fellowship from the National Kidney Foundation. Her more than 30 years of teaching experience include inservice education and teaching in associate degree, baccalaureate, master's degree, and doctoral programs in Maryland, Illinois, Wisconsin, New Mexico, and Texas. Favorite teaching areas are pathophysiology, immunology, and renal failure. She has been actively involved in clinical research for the past 20 years, investigating altered immune responses in various disorders. Her current research focus is on the newly emerging field of psychoneuroimmunology. At this time she is using biofeedback and immune parameters to study the effects of relaxation therapy for caregivers of Alzheimer's patients. Her free time is spent playing tennis, landscaping, and gardening.

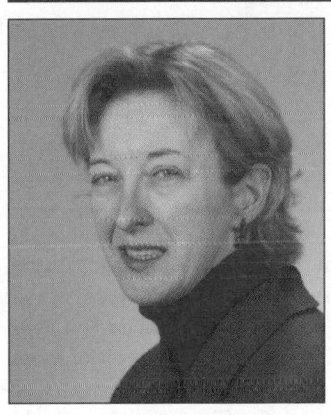

MARGARET McLEAN HEITKEMPER, RN, PhD, FAAN

Margaret Heitkemper is Professor and Chairperson, Department of Biobehavioral Nursing and Health Systems, and Adjunct Professor, Division of Gastroenterology, at the School of Medicine at the University of Washington. She is also Director of the National Institutes of Health–National Institute for Nursing Research–funded Center for Women's Health Research at the University of Washington. In the spring of 2001, Dr. Heitkemper was appointed the John and Marguerite Corbally Endowed Professor for Public Service. Dr. Heitkemper received her Bachelor of Science in nursing from Seattle University, her Master of Science in gerontologic nursing from the University of Washington, and her doctorate in Physiology and Biophysics from the University of Illinois at the Medical Center, Chicago. She has been on faculty at the University of Washington since 1981 and has been the recipient of three School of Nursing and one university-wide Excellence in Teaching awards. In addition, she has served as a Scientific Advisory Board member for two pharmaceutical companies and the Medical Advisory Board of *Woman's Day* magazine, and in 2002 received the Distinguished Nutrition Support Nurse Award from the American Society for Parenteral and Enteral Nutrition (ASPEN).

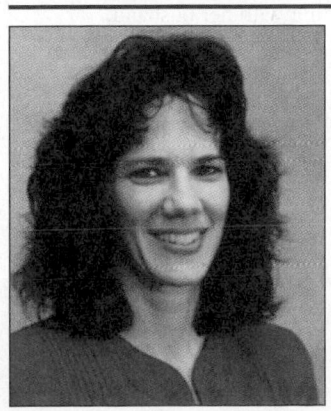

SHANNON RUFF DIRKSEN, RN, PhD

Shannon Dirksen received her Bachelor of Science in nursing from Arizona State University and her Master of Science and doctorate in nursing from the University of Arizona. In her 16 years of teaching at the graduate and undergraduate levels, she has taught at Edith Cowan University (Western Australia), Intercollegiate College of Nursing–Washington State University, University of New Mexico, and Arizona State University. She currently teaches nursing research and management and leadership. For the past 18 years, she has been actively involved in oncology research, focusing on survivorship well-being in white and Hispanic patients who have melanoma and breast cancer. She is the primary author of the *Clinical Companion to Medical-Surgical Nursing,* which accompanies this book.

PATRICIA GRABER O'BRIEN, RNCS, MA, MSN

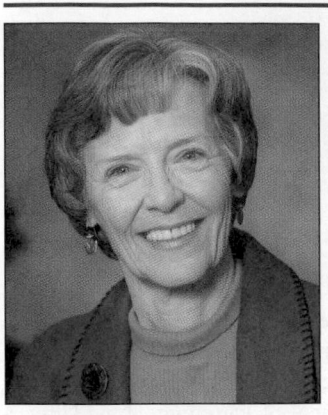

Patricia O'Brien received her Bachelor of Science in nursing from the University of Kansas, Master of Arts in adult education from the University of New Mexico, and Master of Science in nursing with majors in medical-surgical nursing and nursing administration from the University of Texas at El Paso. During her nursing career, she has worked in medical-surgical nursing and home health care, but most of her experience is in nursing education. She is a certified clinical nurse specialist in medical-surgical nursing. She has directed and taught in nursing programs of all levels of basic nursing preparation for more than 30 years. Her primary interests in teaching include nursing process, pharmacology, and metabolic problems. She formally retired from Albuquerque Technical-Vocational Institute, a community college, in 1993, and continues to teach part-time in the College of Nursing at the University of New Mexico. She is also employed part-time as a clinical research coordinator at Lovelace Scientific Resources in Albuquerque.

JEAN FORET GIDDENS, RN, PhD, CS

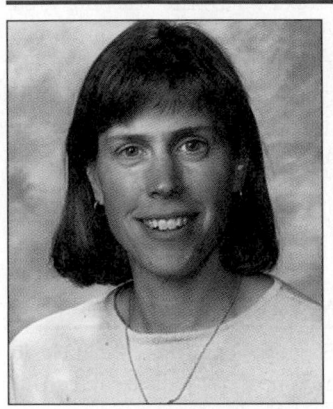

Jean Giddens received a Bachelor of Science in nursing from the University of Kansas, a Master of Science in nursing from the University of Texas at El Paso, and a PhD in Education and Human Resource Studies from Colorado State University. She is a certified clinical specialist in medical-surgical nursing. She has been involved in nursing education since 1984. She currently teaches nursing at the University of New Mexico, and also has taught in several other nursing programs, including Mesa State College in Grand Junction, Colorado, the University of Texas at El Paso, and Eastern New Mexico University at Roswell. Her content areas in nursing education include medical-surgical nursing, health assessment, nursing process, nursing fundamentals, and nursing pharmacology.

LINDA BUCHER, RN, DNSc

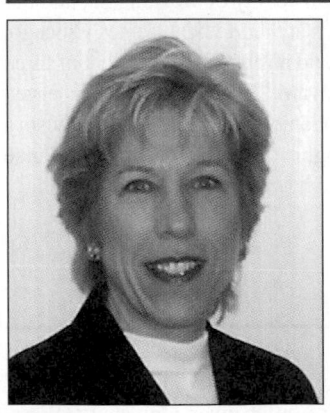

Linda Bucher received her Bachelor of Science in nursing from Thomas Jefferson University in Philadelphia, her Master of Science in adult health and illness from the University of Pennsylvania in Philadelphia, and her DNSc in nursing from Widener University in Chester, Pennsylvania. Her 22 years of teaching experience has spanned inservice and patient education, and teaching in associate, baccalaureate, and graduate nursing programs in New Jersey, Pennsylvania, and Delaware. Her preferred teaching areas include cardiopulmonary and emergency nursing and research. Currently, she holds a joint appointment as a Nursing Research Facilitator for Christiana Care Health Services and associate professor at the University of Delaware, both in Newark, Delaware. She maintains her practice by working per diem as an emergency nurse, is an active member of the American Association of Critical Care Nurses, and enjoys working as a volunteer nurse for Operation Smile. In her free time, she enjoys traveling in Europe and skiing with her husband.

Medical-Surgical Nursing

Assessment and Management of Clinical Problems

Make the MOST out of your study time... Get these companion resources today!

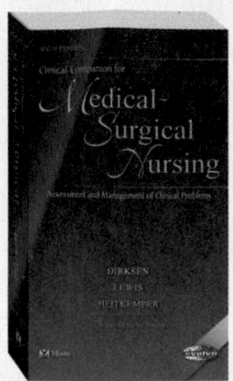

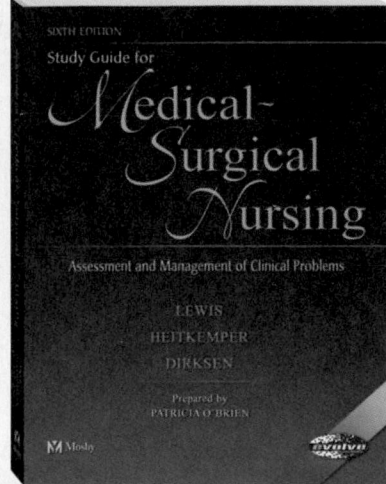

Clinical Companion for Medical-Surgical Nursing

Shannon Ruff Dirksen, RN, PhD; Sharon Mantik Lewis, RN, PhD, FAAN; and Margaret McLean Heitkemper, RN, PhD, FAAN

Thoroughly revised, this best-selling reference includes approximately 200 medical-surgical conditions and procedures in a concise, alphabetical format. This reference contains the information nurses need to know – in a format that's easy to use in clinical settings. The attractive and functional two-color design highlights key information for quick, easy reference. This new 3rd edition features expanded patient teaching information, and additional illustrations and tables.

July 2003 • Approx. 768 pp. • 0-323-01896-3

Study Guide for Medical Surgical Nursing

Patricia Graber O'Brien, RN, CS, BSN, MSN, MA

Thoroughly revised to reflect the new 6th edition of the text, the study guide includes a wide variety of exercises and activities – including fill-in-the-blank worksheets, anatomy and physiology review, true-false questions, critical thinking activities, crossword puzzles, case studies, matching, word scrambles, and multiple-choice questions. Answers for all exercises are included in the back to facilitate self-study with rationales provided for the multiple-choice questions.

June 2003 • Approx. 624 pp. • 0-323-01855-6

Your success is "virtually" guaranteed with VCE!

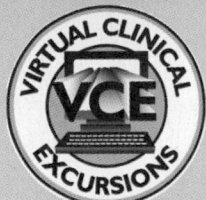

Virtual Clinical Excursions for Lewis: Medical-Surgical Nursing: Assessment and Management of Clinical Problems, 6th Edition

Have a real-world hospital experience without leaving the classroom or computer! These groundbreaking, new workbooks and CD-ROMs bring learning to life in two different multi-floor "virtual" hospital settings! Each lesson in Virtual Clinical Excursions has a core textbook reading assignment with corresponding CD-ROM and workbook activities. Each workbook acts as a map – guiding you through the CD-ROM as you care for patients in the virtual hospital. Each virtual hospital visit allows you to access realistic information resources essential to patient care and contains built-in testing of clinical knowledge with NCLEX-RN-type questions.

There's nothing like it in your Nursing Education!

VCE Version 1
June 2003 • Workbook and CD-ROM for Windows™ and Macintosh© • 0-323-02693-1

VCE Version 2
October 2003 • Workbook and CD-ROM for Windows™ and Macintosh© • 0-323-02692-3

Now you can choose between two different hospital settings — both with a wide range of patients and disorders!

For more information or to order....

Visit your local health sciences bookstore.
Call toll-free 1-800-545-2522.
Visit our website at www.elsevierhealth.com

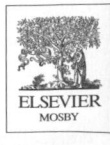

NMX-578

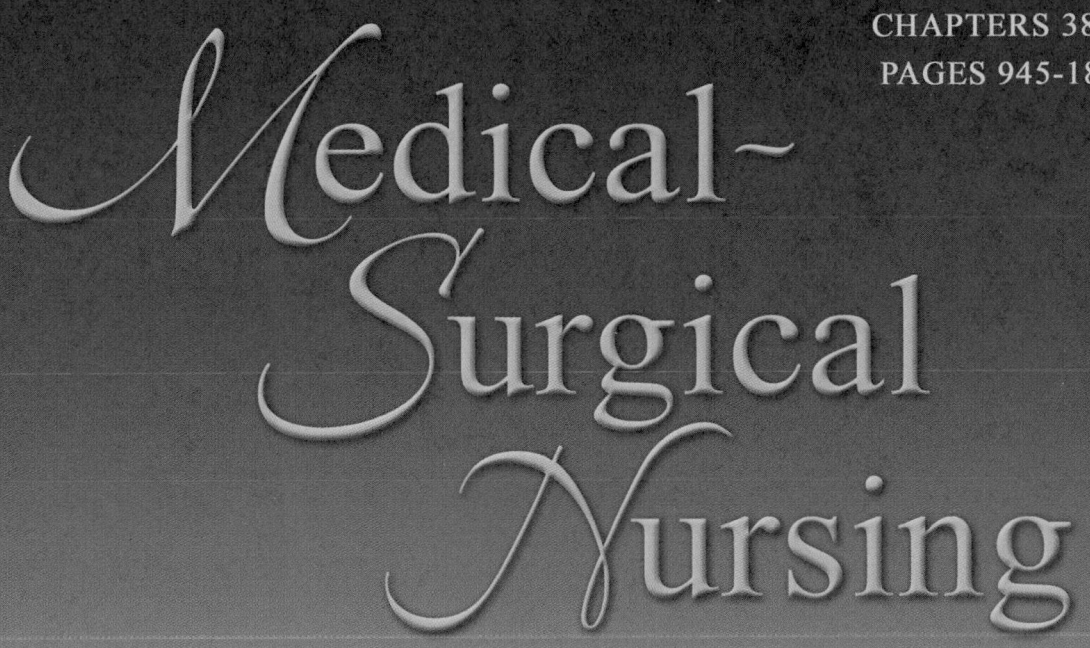

Medical~ Surgical Nursing

Assessment and Management of Clinical Problems

SHARON MANTIK LEWIS, RN, PhD, FAAN

Professor, Schools of Nursing and Medicine
Castella Distinguished Professor of Nursing
University of Texas Health Science Center;
Clinical Nurse Scientist
Geriatric Research, Education, and Clinical Center
South Texas Veterans Health Care System
San Antonio, Texas

MARGARET McLEAN HEITKEMPER, RN, PhD, FAAN

Professor, Biobehavioral Nursing and Health Systems
Corbally Professor for Public Service, School of Nursing;
Adjunct Professor, Division of Gastroenterology
School of Medicine
University of Washington
Seattle, Washington

SHANNON RUFF DIRKSEN, RN, PhD

Associate Professor
College of Nursing
Arizona State University
Tempe, Arizona

SECTION EDITORS

Patricia Graber O'Brien, RNCS, MA, MSN
Instructor, College of Nursing
University of New Mexico;
Clinical Research Coordinator
Lovelace Scientific Resources
Albuquerque, New Mexico

Jean Foret Giddens, RN, PhD, CS
Associate Professor
College of Nursing
University of New Mexico
Albuquerque, New Mexico

Linda Bucher, RN, DNSc
Associate Professor
College of Health and Nursing Sciences
University of Delaware
Newark, Delaware

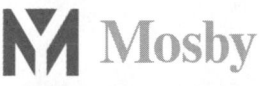

Mosby

An Affiliate of Elsevier Science

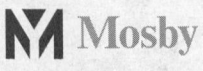

Mosby

An Affiliate of Elsevier Science

11830 Westline Industrial Drive
St. Louis, Missouri 63146

MEDICAL-SURGICAL NURSING: ASSESSMENT
AND MANAGEMENT OF CLINICAL PROBLEMS,
6th edition

Copyright © 2004, Mosby, Inc. All rights reserved.

ISBN 0-323-01611-1

NOTICE

Nursing is an ever-changing field. Standard safety precautions must be followed, but as new research and clinical experience broaden our knowledge, changes in treatment and drug therapy may become necessary or appropriate. Readers are advised to check the most current product information provided by the manufacturer of each drug to be administered to verify the recommended dose, the method and duration of administration, and contraindications. It is the responsibility of the licensed prescriber, relying on experience and knowledge of the patient, to determine dosages and the best treatment for each individual patient. Neither the publisher nor the editor assumes any liability for any injury and/or damage to persons or property arising from this publication.

Previous editions copyrighted 1983, 1987, 1992, 1996, 2000

International Standard Book Number
0-323-01611-1

Executive Vice President, Nursing and Health Professions: Sally Schrefer
Executive Publisher: Robin Carter
Senior Developmental Editor: Kristin Geen
Editorial Assistant: Jamie Randall
Publishing Services Manager: Catherine Albright Jackson
Senior Project Manager: Mary Stueck
Design Coordinator: Teresa McBryan Breckwoldt
Cover Art: Studio Montage

Printed in the United States of America

Last digit is the print number: 9 8 7 6 5 4 3 2 1

Contributors

Richard B. Arbour, RN, MSN, CCRN, CNRN
Staff Nurse, Medical Intensive Care Unit
Albert Einstein Medical Center
Philadelphia, Pennsylvania

Elizabeth A. Ayello, RN, PhD, CS, CWOCN, FAAN
Clinical Associate Professor and Director of Adult Nursing
   Science
Senior Advisor, The John A. Hartford Institute for Geriatric
   Nursing
The Steinhardt School of Education
Division of Nursing, New York University
New York, New York

Catherine M. Bender, RN, PhD
Assistant Professor, School of Nursing
University of Pittsburgh
Pittsburgh, Pennsylvania

Donna Zimmaro Bliss, RN, PhD, CCRN, FAAN
Associate Professor, School of Nursing
University of Minnesota
Minneapolis, Minnesota

Lucy Bradley-Springer, RN, PhD, ACRN
Director, Mountain Plains AIDS Education and Training
   Center;
Associate Professor of Medicine
University of Colorado Health Sciences Center
Denver, Colorado

Catherine E. Brown, RN, CRNH
Education and Research Associate
Hospice of the Valley
Phoenix, Arizona

Linda Bucher, RN, DNSc
Associate Professor, College of Health and Nursing Sciences
University of Delaware
Newark, Delaware

Maria A. Connolly, RN, DNSc, CCRN
Dean, College of Nursing and Allied Health
University of St. Francis
Joliet, Illinois

Elizabeth A. Crago, RN, MSN
Project Director, Research Associate
University of Pittsburgh School of Nursing
Pittsburgh, Pennsylvania

Janet T. Crimlisk, RNCS, MS, ANP
Clinical Nurse Specialist
Boston Medical Center
Boston, Massachusetts

Anne Croghan, RN, MN, ARNP
Nurse Practitioner
VA Puget Sound Health Care System
Seattle, Washington

Shannon Ruff Dirksen, RN, PhD
Associate Professor, College of Nursing
Arizona State University
Tempe, Arizona

Laura Dulski, RNC, MSN, CS
Senior Clinical Nurse
New Life Family Center
Rush Presbyterian–St. Luke's Medical Center
Chicago, Illinois

Sheila A. Dunn, RN, MSN, C-ANP
Adult Nurse Practitioner, Primary Care
Belleville Veterans Clinic
Belleville, Illinois

Mary Ersek, RN, PhD
Research Scientist, Pain Research Department
Swedish Medical Center
Seattle, Washington

Hatice Y. Foell, RN, ARNP, MSN
Congestive Heart Failure Disease Management Program
Health First Heart Institute
Melbourne, Florida

Jean Foret Giddens, RN, PhD, CS
Associate Professor, College of Nursing
University of New Mexico
Albuquerque, New Mexico

Nancy J. Girard, RN, PhD, FAAN
Associate Professor and Chair
Acute Nursing Care Department
University of Texas Health Science Center
San Antonio, Texas

D. Patricia Gray, RN, PhD
Associate Professor and Chair
Department of Adult Health
Virginia Commonwealth University
Richmond, Virginia

Mikel Gray, RN, PhD, CUNP, CCCN, FAAN
Professor and Nurse Practitioner
Department of Urology
University of Virginia
Charlottesville, Virginia

Peggi Guenter, RN, PhD, CNSN
Managing Editor for Special Projects
American Society for Parenteral and Enteral Nutrition
Havertown, PA

Debra A. Hagler, RN, MS, CS, CCRN
Clinical Associate Professor, College of Nursing
Arizona State University
Tempe, Arizona

Lissi Hansen, RN, PhD
Postdoctoral Fellow, John A. Hartford Foundation
Department of Biobehavioral Nursing and Health Systems
University of Washington
Seattle, Washington

Margaret McLean Heitkemper, RN, PhD, FAAN
Professor, Biobehavioral Nursing and Health Systems
School of Nursing;
Adjunct Professor, Division of Gastroenterology
School of Medicine
University of Washington
Seattle, Washington

Marcia J. Hill, RN, MSN
Senior Research Nurse
M.D. Anderson Cancer Center
Houston, Texas

Mary Jo Holechek, RN, MS, CRNP, CNN
Transplant Nurse Practitioner, Transplant Office
Johns Hopkins Hospital
Baltimore, Maryland

Mary Ann House-Fancher, RN, MSN, ARNP
Nurse Practitioner, Department of Cardiothoracic Surgery
Health First Heart Institute
Melbourne, Florida

Carolyn I. Johns, RN, MS, CANP
Adult Nurse Practitioner, Cardiology
Lovelace Health Systems
Albuquerque, New Mexico

Kathleen J. Jones, RN, MS, ANP
Adult Nurse Practitioner
Hematology-Oncology Clinic
Walter Reed Army Medical Center
Washington, D.C.

Duck-Hee Kang, RN, PhD
Associate Professor, School of Nursing
University of Alabama at Birmingham
Birmingham, Alabama

Mary E. Kerr, RN, PhD, FAAN
Associate Professor, School of Nursing
Director for Center for Nursing Research
University of Pittsburgh
Pittsburgh, Pennsylvania

Catherine Kirkness, RN, PhD, CNN(C)
Research Assistant Professor
Department of Biobehavioral Nursing and Health Systems
University of Washington
Seattle, Washington

Cynthia J. Knipe, RN
Administrative Director
Wishard Health Services
Indianapolis, Indiana

Cathleen E. Kunkler, RN, BSN, ONC, CNA
Clinical Faculty Practical Nursing Program
Northern Tier Career Center
Towanda, Pennsylvania

Nancy Stoetzner Kupper, RN, MSN
Associate Professor
Tarrant County Junior College
Fort Worth, Texas

Barbara S. Levine, RN, PhD, CRNP, CS
Gerontological Nurse Consultant
BSL Consulting Services
Wayne, Pennsylvania

Sharon Mantik Lewis, RN, PhD, FAAN
Professor, Schools of Nursing and Medicine
University of Texas Health Science Center;
Clinical Nurse Scientist
Geriatric Research, Education, and Clinical Center
South Texas Veterans Health Care System
San Antonio, Texas

Carol O. Long, RN, PhD
Director of Professional Services
Carrigan's Health Care Services
Phoenix, Arizona;
Faculty Associate, Gerontology Program
Arizona State University
Tempe, Arizona

Kathleen T. Lucke, RN, PhD
Assistant Professor, School of Nursing
University of Texas Health Science Center
San Antonio, Texas

Nancy J. MacMullen, RN, APN, CCNS, PhD
University Professor
Governors State University
University Park, Illinois

Lisa B. Malick, RNC, MS, OCN
Assistant Professor
The Community College of Baltimore County
Baltimore, Maryland

Linda Griego Martinez, RN, MSN, CS, CCRN
Cardiology Care Manager
Presbyterian Heart Group
Albuquerque, New Mexico

Dee Ann F. Mitchell, RN, PhD
Professor, Nursing Department
Tarrant County College
Fort Worth, Texas

Patricia Graber O'Brien, RNCS, MA, MSN
Instructor, College of Nursing
University of New Mexico;
Clinical Research Coordinator
Lovelace Scientific Resources
Albuquerque, New Mexico

Judith M. Ozuna, RN, MN, ARNP, CNRN
Clinical Nurse Specialist in Neurology
VA Puget Sound Health Care System
Seattle, Washington

JoAnne K. Phillips, RN, MSN, CCRN, CCNS
Clinical Nurse Specialist, Surgical Critical Care
Hospital of the University of Pennsylvania
Philadelphia, Pennsylvania

Carmencita M. Poe, RN, EdD
Clinical Nurse Manager, Oncology/Medical-Surgical Nursing
Bon Secours De Paul Medical Center
Norfolk, Virginia

Kathleen A. Pollard, RN, MSN, CHPN
Education and Research Associate
Hospice of the Valley
Phoenix, Arizona

Anita Ralstin, RN, MS, CS, CNP
New Mexico Heart Institute
Albuquerque, New Mexico

Kathleen Rich, RN, MS, CCNS
Critical Care Clinical Specialist
The Methodist Hospitals, Inc.
Gary, Indiana

Dottie Roberts, RN, C, MSN, MACI, ONC
Medical-Surgical Clinical Nurse Specialist
Palmetto Health Baptist Medical Center
Columbia, South Carolina

Margaret Rosenzweig, RN, PhD, CRNP, AOCN
Assistant Professor, School of Nursing
University of Pittsburgh
Pittsburgh, Pennsylvania

Lynda Sawchuk, RN, ARNP, CWOCN
Enterostomal Therapy Nurse
Virginia Mason Medical Center
Seattle, Washington

Susan Semb, RN, MSN, CDE
Health Educator
Kaiser Permanente Health Education Department
San Diego, California

Anita Shoup, RN, MSN, CNOR
Clinical Nurse Consultant
Regent Medical
Edmonds, Washington

Debra J. Smith, RN, MSN, CCRN
Instructor, College of Nursing
University of New Mexico
Albuquerque, New Mexico

Sarah C. Smith, RN, MA, CRNO
Educational Associate
University of Iowa Health Care
Iowa City, Iowa

Cheryl Ross Staats, RN, MSN, CS
Assistant Professor, School of Nursing
University of Texas Health Science Center
San Antonio, Texas

Kathleen R. Stevens, RN, EdD, FAAN
Professor and Director
Academic Center of Evidence-Based Practice
University of Texas Health Science Center
San Antonio, Texas

Barbara Van de Castle, RN, APRN, MSN, BC
Instructor
Johns Hopkins University School of Nursing
Baltimore, Maryland

Catherine Warms, RN, PhD
Postdoctoral Research Fellow
Department of Biobehavioral Nursing and Health Care Systems
University of Washington
Seattle, Washington

Barbara G. White, RN, MS
Clinical Associate Professor, College of Nursing
Arizona State University
Tempe, Arizona

Mary E. Wilbur, RN, MSN
Continuum of Care Manager
Medical University of South Carolina
Charleston, South Carolina

Deidre D. Wipke-Tevis, RNC, PhD
Assistant Professor, Sinclair School of Nursing
University of Missouri
Columbia, Missouri

Linda Witek-Janusek, RN, PhD
Professor of Nursing, Marcella Niehoff School of Nursing
Loyola University of Chicago
Maywood, Illinois

Reviewers

Elizabeth Alden, RNC, BSN, CDE
Albuquerque, New Mexico

Margaret M. Andrews, RN, PhD, CTN
Rochester, New York

Anne M. Aquila, RN, MSN, CS
New Haven, Connecticut

Mary S. Baird, RN, MN, CNRN, ARNP
Olympia, Washington

Valerie O'Toole Baker, RN, MSN, CS
Erie, Pennsylvania

Christine A. Balt, RN, MS, CS, ACRN
Indianapolis, Indiana

Ellen Barker, RN, MSN, CNRN
Greenville, Delaware

Joanne M. Bartram, RN, MS, CFNP
Albuquerque, New Mexico

Mary Ellen Beebe, RN, MSN, CEN
Cleveland, Wisconsin

Viola G. Benavente, RN, MSN, CNS
San Antonio, Texas

Jean K. Berry, RN, PhD, CS
Chicago, Illinois

Patricia A. Blissitt, RN, PhD, CCRN, CNRN, CCM, CS
Seattle, Washington

Peter Bonner, MA, MS
Placitas, New Mexico

Heather Boyd-Monk, SRN, BSN, CRNO
Philadelphia, Pennsylvania

Elisabeth G. Bradley, RN, APN, CCRN
Newark, Delaware

Elizabeth J. Bridges, RN, PhD, CCNS
San Antonio, Texas

Vanessa Briones, RN, BSN
San Antonio, Texas

Karen R. Bruni, RN, MSN, NP, CVN
Albany, New York

Erica Camarillo, RN, BSN
San Antonio, Texas

Janis L. Carelock, RN, MSN, CCRN, CNS
Austin, Texas

Sharon G. Childs, RN, MS, CRNP-CS, CEN, ONC
Baltimore, Maryland

Phyllis Christiansen, RN, MN, ARNP
Seattle, Washington

Terry Cicero, RN, MN, CCRN
Seattle, Washington

Dorothy Hendel Clough, RN, PhD
Albuquerque, New Mexico

Margaret F. Cramer, RN, MSN
Manheim, Pennsylvania

Rebecca Crane-Okada, RN, PhD, AOCN
Santa Monica, California

Karen A. Crisfulla, RN, MSN, CCRN
Mount Laurel, New Jersey

Anne Croghan, RN, MN, ARNP
Seattle, Washington

Patricia Cryer, RN, MS, MSN, CENP
Tyler, Texas

Barbara I. Damron, RN, PhD
Santa Fe, New Mexico

Yvonne M. D'Arcy, RN, ARNP, MS, C-CS
Baltimore, Maryland

Angela J. DiSabatino, RN, MS
Newark, Delaware

Sheila A. Dunn, RN, MSN, C-ANP
Belleville, Illinois

Brenda Elliff, RN, MPA, ONC, CCM, LNCC
Coeur d'Alene, Idaho

Rebecca Fix, RN, CNP
Grand Rapids, Minnesota

John J. Gallagher, RN, MSN, CCNS, CCRN, CEN, RRT
Upland, Pennsylvania

Beverly Gay, RN, MSN, CCRN
Richmond, Virginia

Nancy J. Girard, RN, PhD, FAAN
San Antonio, Texas

Susan K. Goebel, RNC, MS, WHNP, SANE
Grand Junction, Colorado

Karen Goff, RN, BSN
Atlanta, Georgia

Judy L. Goodhart, RN, MSN
Grand Junction, Colorado

Rebecca B. Griffin, RN, MS
Waco, Texas

M. Susan Grinslade, RN, PhD(c)
San Antonio, Texas

Catherine M. Harris, RNCS, PhD
San Antonio, Texas

Sherry Garrett Hendrickson, RN, PhD, CNS
Austin, Texas

Marcia J. Hill, RN, MSN
Houston, Texas

Roxana Huebscher, RN, PhD, FNPC, HNC, CMT
Oshkosh, Wisconsin

Monica Jarrett, RN, PhD
Seattle, Washington

Janene Council Jeffery, RN, MSN, CDE
Austin, Texas

Vicki Y. Johnson, RN, PhD, FN, CUCNS
Birmingham, Alabama

Karla Jones, RN, MS
Ontario, Oregon

Duck-Hee Kang, RN, PhD
Birmingham, Alabama

Tamara M. Kear, RN, MSN, CNN
Wilmington, Delaware

Michelle Kelly, RN, BSc, MN
Sydney, Australia

Mary Jean Klein, RN, MS
Houston, Texas

Judy A. Knighton, RN, MScN
Sharon, Ontario, Canada

JoAnne Konick-McMahan, RN, MSN, CCRN
Philadelphia, Pennsylvania

Cathleen E. Kunkler, RN, BSN, ONC, CNA
Towanda, Pennsylvania

Ann L. Lambeth, RN, MSN
Grand Junction, Colorado

Helen L. Lamothe, RN, BSN, PHN, ONC
Golden, Colorado

Linda Laskowski-Jones, RN, MS, CS, CCRN, CEN
Newark, Delaware

Natasha Leskovsek, RN, MBA, JD
Washington, D.C.

Barbara S. Levine, RN, PhD, CRNP, CS
Wayne, Pennsylvania

Patricia A. Loflin, RN, MSN, FNP
Albuquerque, New Mexico

Kathy Lopez-Bushnell, EdD, MPH, RNC (FNP), COHNS
Albuquerque, New Mexico

Kathleen T. Lucke, RN, PhD
San Antonio, Texas

Jane A. Madden, RN, MSN
St. Louis, Missouri

Lisa B. Malick, RNC, MS, OCN
Baltimore, Maryland

Linda Griego Martinez, RN, MSN, CS, CCRN
Albuquerque, New Mexico

Katheryn Ellen McCash, RNC, MSN
Albuquerque, New Mexico

Holly Fadness McFarland, RN, MSN, CNN
Greenville, North Carolina

Lora McGuire, RN, MS
Joliet, Illinois

Laura Wild McIntosh, RN, MSN, CRNA
New Brunswick, New Jersey

Mary Ann Siciliano McLaughlin, RN, MSN
Magnolia, New Jersey

Mary Merchant, RN, MSN, FNP
Charleston, South Carolina

Debra A. Morgan, RN, EdD
Wichita Falls, Texas

Joseph J. Napolitano, RN, MPH, MSN, APRN
Allentown, Pennsylvania

Leslie Neal, RN, C, PhD, CRRN
Arlington, Virginia

Barbara Owens, RN, PhD(c)
San Antonio, Texas

Carmencita M. Poe, RN, EdD
Norfolk, Virginia

Kathleen A. Pollard, RN, MSN, CHPN
Phoenix, Arizona

Virginia Printz-Feddersen, RN, CNS,
  MSN, RNC, CNRN, CNOR
Albuquerque, New Mexico

Maureen P. Reilly, RN, PhD, CRNA
San Antonio, Texas

Patsy Ruppert Rider, RN, MSN, CNS
Austin, Texas

Dottie Roberts, RN, C, MSN, MACI, ONC
Columbia, South Carolina

Sandra Rome, RN, MN, OCN
Torrance, California

Dana Rosdahl, RN-C, PhD(c), FNP
Tempe, Arizona

Lucinda W. Rossoll, RN, BSN, BA, CCRN, CEN
Lebannon, New Hampshire

Bette A. Schans, PhD, RT(R)
Grand Junction, Colorado

Marilee Schmelzer, RN, PhD
Arlington, Texas

Susan Semb, RN, MSN, CDE
San Diego, California

Susan M. Shea, RN, MSN, CDE
Galveston, Texas

Geoff F. Shuster, RN, DNSc
Albuquerque, New Mexico

Elaine A. Slabinski, RN, MS
Wilkes-Barre, Pennsylvania

Elizabeth Speakman, RN, EdD
Philadelphia, Pennsylvania

Cheryl Ross Staats, RN, MSN, CS
San Antonio, Texas

Alissa D. Stanley, RN, BSN
San Antonio, Texas

Linda L. Steele, RN, PhD, ANP
Charlotte, North Carolina

David Tilton, RN, BSN, ACLS, BCLSI
Gig Harbor, Washington

Martha S. Tingen, RN, PhD, ANP, CS
Augusta, Georgia

Donna Tomky, RN, MS, APRN, C-ANP, CDE
Albuquerque, New Mexico

Suzanne Michele Vanet, RN, C, BSN
Clarksburg, West Virginia

Barbara Velsor-Friedrich, RN, PhD
Chicago, Illinois

Marianne G. Walston, RN, MSN
Suffolk, Virginia

Barbara G. White, RN, MS
Tempe, Arizona

Jennifer Whitley, RN, MSN, CNOR
Decatur, Alabama

Joyce S. Willens, RN, PhD
Villanova, Pennsylvania

Deidre D. Wipke-Tevis, RNC, PhD
Columbia, Missouri

To the profession of nursing
and
to the important people in our lives

Preface

The sixth edition of *Medical-Surgical Nursing: Assessment and Management of Clinical Problems* has been thoroughly revised to incorporate the most recent medical-surgical nursing information in an attractive, easy-to-use format. More than just a textbook, this is a comprehensive resource containing essential information that students need to prepare for lectures, classroom activities, examinations, clinical assignments, and comprehensive care of patients. In addition to the readable writing style and full-color illustrations, the text includes many special features to help students learn the medical-surgical nursing content, including patient and family teaching, gerontology, collaborative care, cultural and ethnic considerations, nutrition, home care, evidence-based practice, nursing research, and much more.

The comprehensive and accurate content, special features, attractive layout, and student-friendly writing style combine to make this the number one medical-surgical nursing textbook used in more nursing schools around the country than any other medical-surgical nursing textbook.

The strengths of the first five editions have been retained, including the use of the nursing process as an organizational theme for nursing management. Numerous new features have been added to address some of the rapid changes in practice. Contributors have been selected for their acknowledged excellence in specific content areas; one or more specialists in the subject area have thoroughly reviewed each chapter to increase accuracy. The editors have undertaken final rewriting and editing to achieve internal consistency. All efforts were directed toward building on the strengths of the previous edition while preparing an even more effective new edition.

ORGANIZATION

Content is organized into two major divisions. The first division, Section One (Chapters 1 through 11), discusses general concepts related to adult patients. The second division, Sections Two through Twelve (Chapters 12 through 67), presents nursing assessment and nursing management of medical-surgical problems.

The various body systems are grouped to reflect their interrelated functions. Each section is organized around two central themes: assessment and management. Chapters dealing with assessment of a body system include a discussion of the following:

1. A brief review of anatomy and physiology, focusing on information that will promote understanding of nursing care
2. Health history and noninvasive physical assessment skills to expand the knowledge base on which decisions are made
3. Common diagnostic studies, expected results, and related nursing responsibilities to provide easily accessible information

Management chapters focus on the pathophysiology, clinical manifestations, diagnostic study results, collaborative care, and nursing management of various diseases and disorders. The nursing management sections are organized into assessment, nursing diagnoses, planning, implementation, and evaluation. To emphasize the importance of patient care in various clinical settings, nursing implementation of all major health problems is organized by the following levels of care:

1. Health Promotion
2. Acute Intervention
3. Ambulatory and Home Care

CLASSIC FEATURES

- **Patient and family teaching** is an ongoing theme throughout the text. Coverage includes a separate chapter (Chapter 4: Patient and Family Teaching) and more than 75 Patient and Family Teaching Guides throughout the text.
- **Home care/community-based care** is also emphasized in this edition. Coverage includes a separate chapter (Chapter 6: Community-Based Nursing and Home Care) and special Ambulatory and Home Care headings in Nursing Implementation sections.
- **Collaborative care** is highlighted in special Collaborative Care sections in all management chapters and more than 85 Collaborative Care tables throughout the text.
- **Gerontology coverage** includes Chapter 5: Older Adults, and appears throughout the text under Gerontologic Considerations headings and in Gerontologic Differences in Assessment and Effects of Aging tables.
- **Nutrition** is highlighted throughout the book. Nutritional Therapy tables summarize nutritional interventions for patients with various health problems.
- **Nursing management** is presented in a consistent and comprehensive format, with headings for Health Promotion, Acute Intervention, and Ambulatory and Home Care. In addition, **more than 60 Nursing Care Plans** appear in management chapters. These are thoroughly updated to incorporate current NANDA nursing diagnoses and defining characteristics, expected patient outcomes, specific nursing interventions with rationales, and collaborative problems.
- A separate chapter on **complementary and alternative therapy** addresses timely issues in today's health care settings related to nontraditional therapies.
- **Nursing research** encourages application of research into clinical practice. Nursing Research boxes appear throughout the text. Nursing Research Issues at the end of management chapters present possible research questions to be used for research studies.
- **Cultural and ethnic considerations** information is integrated into the text and appears in special boxes highlighting risk factors and other important issues related to the nursing care of various ethnic groups.

- **Ethical Dilemmas boxes** promote critical thinking for timely and sensitive issues that nursing students may deal with in clinical practice.
- **Emergency Management tables** outline the emergency treatment of health problems most likely to require emergency intervention.
- **Common Assessment Abnormalities tables** in assessment chapters alert the nurse to frequently encountered abnormalities and their possible etiologies.
- **Nursing Assessment tables** summarize the key subjective and objective data related to common diseases. Subjective data are organized by functional health patterns.
- **Health History tables** in assessment chapters present key questions to ask patients related to a specific disease or disorder.
- Student-friendly pedagogy includes:
  - **Learning Objectives** and **Key Terms** at the beginning of each chapter help students identify the key content for that body system or disorder.
  - **Review Questions** at the end of each chapter, which are matched to the learning objectives, help students learn the important points in the chapter. Answers are provided in an appendix so that the review questions serve as a self-study tool.
  - **Critical Thinking Exercises** appearing at the end of nursing management chapters include Case Studies with Critical Thinking Questions for clinical application as well as Nursing Research Issues.
  - **Resources** at the end of each chapter contain information about nursing and health care organizations that provide patient teaching and disease and disorder information. Resources include Internet sites to help students find current information online.

NEW FEATURES

- **Six new and expanded chapters:**
  - Culturally Competent Care (Chapter 2)
  - End-of-Life Care (Chapter 10)
  - Addictive Behaviors (Chapter 11)
  - Genetics and Altered Immune Responses (Chapter 13)
  - Nursing Management: Alzheimer's Disease and Dementia (Chapter 58)
  - Nursing Management: Musculoskeletal Trauma and Orthopedic Surgery (Chapter 61)
- **Complementary and Alternative Therapies boxes** expand on the information presented in Chapter 7, and summarize what nurses need to know about nontraditional therapies such as herbal remedies, acupuncture, and biofeedback.
- Selected nursing care plans incorporate **NIC (Nursing Interventions Classification) and NOC (Nursing Outcomes Classification)** to show how NIC, NOC, and NANDA nursing diagnoses can be linked.
- **Evidence-Based Practice boxes** present the use of evidence (results from research) to improve patient outcomes and the implications for nursing practice.
- A special **Culturally Competent Care heading** in selected Nursing Management sections highlights expanded cultural and ethnic content as it relates to specific diseases and disorders.
- **Genetics in Clinical Practice boxes** highlight the genetic basis, genetic testing, and clinical implications for genetic disorders that affect adults.

ANCILLARY PACKAGE

Learning Supplements for the Student

- The **Student CD-ROM** packaged with this text contains the following valuable learning aids:
  - **Forty disorder monographs,** including disorder overview, case study, and a variety of interactive learning activities, provide immediate feedback. This special icon 🔖 appears in the text to designate content areas where students are encouraged to use their CD-ROM for further self-study.
  - **Glossary** of key terms and definitions, available as one comprehensive glossary and organized by chapter
  - **Patient and Family Instruction handouts** in both English and Spanish to be printed and distributed to patients
- The **Virtual Clinical Excursions** CD-ROM and workbook to accompany this text is an exciting learning tool that sends students into the virtual clinical setting to "visit" patients, access charts, make assessments, monitor daily changes, formulate nursing diagnoses, plan interventions, and much more. This "hands-on" approach is ideal for learning communication, documentation, assessment, critical thinking, and other essential skills.
- The *Clinical Companion to Medical-Surgical Nursing,* **3rd edition,** presents approximately 200 common medical-surgical conditions and procedures in a concise, alphabetical format for quick clinical reference. Designed for portability, this popular reference includes the essential, need-to-know information for medical-surgical nursing practice. An attractive and functional two-color design highlights key information for quick, easy reference. This edition features expanded patient and family teaching content, as well as additional illustrations and tables to enhance usefulness and visual appeal.
- The **Study Guide** contains extensive review and testing material that has been thoroughly updated to reflect the revision of the textbook. It features a wide variety of clinically relevant exercises and activities, including fill-in-the-blank worksheets, anatomy identification review, true-false questions, critical thinking activities, crossword puzzles, case studies, matching exercises, word scrambles, and multiple-choice questions in NCLEX format. Answers to all questions are included in the back to provide students with immediate feedback as they study.
- The **Evolve website** 🔖 is available at *http://evolve.elsevier.com/Lewis/medsurg/* and features the following valuable learning aids:
  - Concept map creator and examples of concept maps
  - Glossary of key terms and definitions, available as one comprehensive glossary and organized by chapter
  - Patient and Family Instruction handouts in both English and Spanish that can be printed and distributed to patients
  - Content updates from the authors
  - WebLinks for each chapter
  - Chapter summaries
  - Case studies from the text with questions and the capability for students to submit answers to instructors online

Teaching Supplements for the Instructor

- The **Instructor's Resource Kit** remains the most comprehensive set of instructor's materials available, containing:
  - Suggested lecture strategies for each chapter, including teaching/learning objectives, chapter outlines, classroom strategies, and

collaborative/active learning activities with critical thinking questions

- A test bank with approximately 1500 questions with coded answers and text references (also available on CD-ROM in computerized format)
- The **Electronic Image Collection** contains more than 400 full-color images from the text for use in lectures and to import into PowerPoint.
- New to this edition are over 1600 **PowerPoint text slides** organized by diseases and disorders.

ACKNOWLEDGMENTS

The editors are especially grateful to many people at Elsevier who assisted with this major revision effort. In particular, we wish to thank the team of Robin Carter, Kristin Geen, Catherine Albright Jackson, Mary Stueck, and Teresa McBryan Breckwoldt. In addition, we want to thank the marketing team of Janet Blanner, Bob Boehringer, and Angel Magasano.

Our persevering typists have earned our special thanks and include Erica Camarillo, Vanessa Briones, and Jennifer Hale. Alissa Stanley and Barbara Owens worked diligently as research assistants. Barbara Van de Castle provided invaluable assistance as a consultant on nursing diagnoses and revision of the nursing care plans. Kathy Lucke assisted with a major revision of the ethical dilemmas boxes. Pat O'Brien's creative and conscientious work on the Study Guide, Student CD-ROM, Test Bank, Instructor's Resource Kit, and Evolve website was a tremendous asset. A special thanks goes to Peter Bonner who assisted with many details related to the production of the book.

We are particularly indebted to the nurses and student nurses who have put their faith in our book to assist them on their path to excellence. The increasing use of this book throughout the United States, Canada, Australia, and other parts of the world has been gratifying. We appreciate the many users who have shared their comments and suggestions on the previous editions.

We also wish to thank our contributors and reviewers for their assistance with the revision process. We sincerely hope that this book will assist both students and clinicians in practicing truly professional nursing.

Sharon Lewis
Margaret Heitkemper
Shannon Dirksen
Patricia O'Brien
Jean Giddens
Linda Bucher

Reference Guide for Student CD-ROM

The Student CD-ROM provided with this text contains the following features:
- **Glossary** of key terms and definitions
- **40 Case Studies** followed by interactive learning activities
- **40 Patient and Family Instruction guides** in both English and Spanish
- **List of nursing diagnoses**
- **Laboratory values reference**

This special icon 🖭 appears in the text to designate related study content on the CD-ROM.

CASE STUDIES

Abdominal Aortic Aneurysm
Acute Pancreatitis
Addison's Disease
Alzheimer's Disease
Asthma
Benign Prostatic Hyperplasia (BPH)
Bladder Cancer with Urinary Diversion
Breast Cancer
Burns
Cataract Surgery
Cholelithiasis/Cholecystitis
Chronic Myelogenous Leukemia
Chronic Obstructive Pulmonary Disease (COPD)
Chronic Peripheral Arterial Disease
Cushing Syndrome
Cystic Fibrosis
Endometrial Cancer
Glomerulonephritis and Chronic Renal Failure
Head Injury
Human Immunodeficiency Virus (HIV) Infection and Acquired Immunodeficiency Syndrome (AIDS)
Hypertensive Heart Disease
Hyperthyroidism
Kidney Transplant
Lung Cancer
Musculoskeletal Trauma
Myocardial Infarction (MI)
Oral Cancer
Parkinson's Disease and Hip Fracture
Peptic Ulcer Disease
Postnecrotic Cirrhosis
Pressure Ulcers
Pulmonary Embolism
Rheumatic Fever and Heart Disease
Rheumatoid Arthritis
Seizures
Sickle Cell Anemia
Spinal Cord Injury
Stroke
Type 2 Diabetes Mellitus
Ulcerative Colitis

PATIENT AND FAMILY INSTRUCTION GUIDES

Acute or Chronic Sinusitis
Back Exercises
Bowel Management after Spinal Cord Injury
Anticoagulant Therapy
Autonomic Dysreflexia
Care after a Hip Replacement
Care after an Amputation
Changing Your Ileal Conduit Appliance
Colostomy Irrigation
Congestive Heart Failure
Corticosteroid Therapy
Decreasing Risk Factors for Coronary Artery Disease
Early Warning Signs of Alzheimer's Disease
Exercise Guidelines after Myocardial Infarction
Exercise Guidelines for Patients with Diabetes Mellitus
Foot Care for Patients with Diabetes or Peripheral Vascular Disease
Head Injury
Headache Management
Home Oxygen Use
How to Reduce Symptoms of Allergic Rhinitis
How to Use a Dry Powder Inhaler (DPI)
How to Use a Peak Flow Meter
Insulin Administration
Joint Protection and Energy Conservation
Low Back Problems
Management of Diabetes Mellitus
Managing Alzheimer's Disease
Managing Constipation
Prevention of Musculoskeletal Problems in the Older Adult
The Proper Use of Injection Equipment
Protection of Small Joints
The Right Way to Use Antibiotics
Self-Monitoring of Blood Glucose (SMGB)
Signs and Symptoms That Patients with HIV Need to Report
Skin Care for Patients with Spinal Cord Injuries
Smoking and Tobacco Use Cessation
Testicular Self-Examination
Urinary Tract Infection
Use of Antiretroviral Drugs
Warning Signs of Stroke

Detailed Contents

 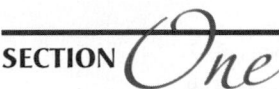
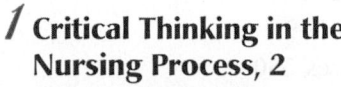

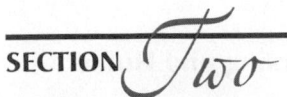

SECTION *Two*
Pathophysiologic Mechanisms of Disease

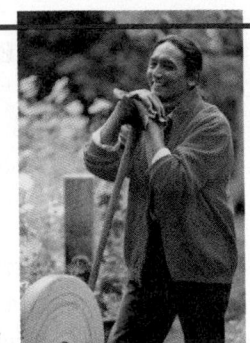

SECTION *Three*
Perioperative Care

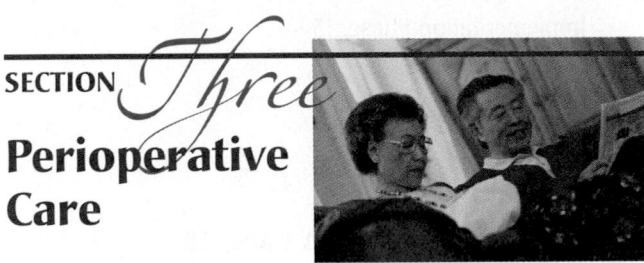

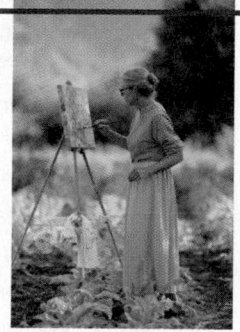
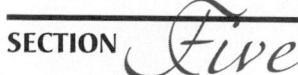
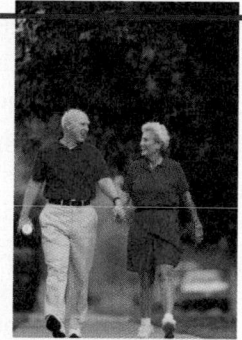

SECTION *Six*
Problems of Oxygenation: Transport

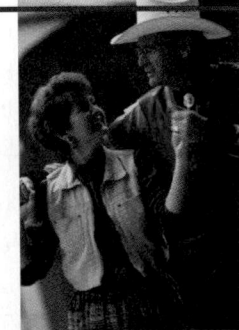

SECTION *Seven*
Problems of Oxygenation: Perfusion

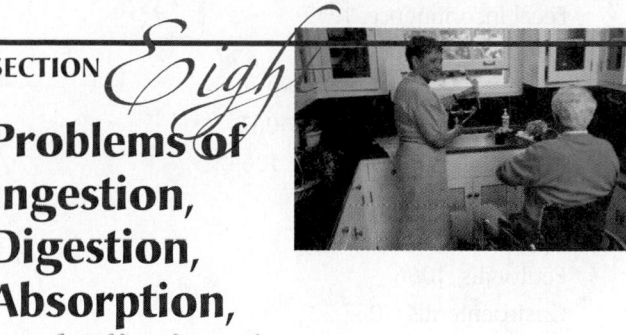

SECTION *Eight*
Problems of Ingestion, Digestion, Absorption, and Elimination

SECTION *Nine*

Problems of Urinary Function

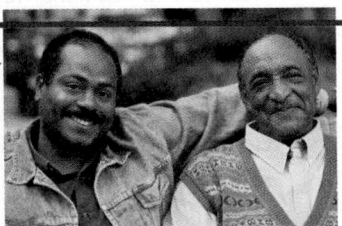

SECTION *Ten*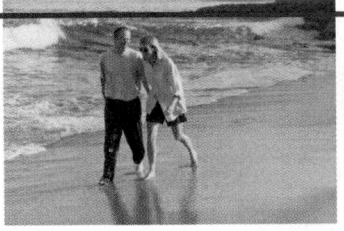

Problems Related to Regulatory Mechanisms

SECTION 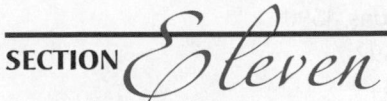 *Eleven*

Problems Related to Movement and Coordination

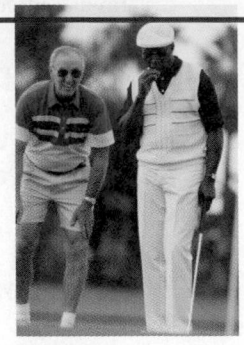

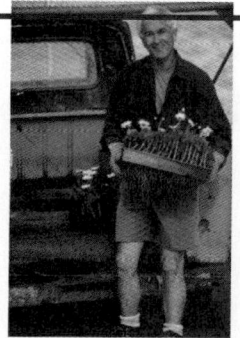

Problems of Ingestion, Digestion, Absorption, and Elimination

SECTION OUTLINE

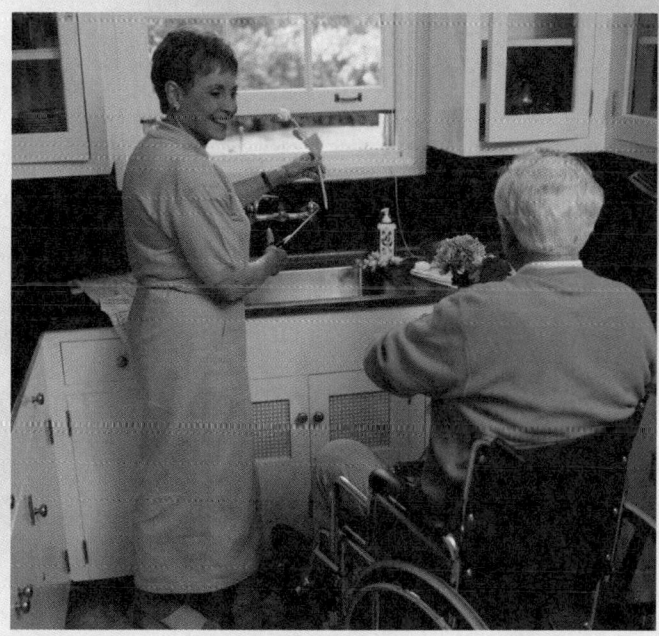

CHAPTER 38

NURSING ASSESSMENT
Gastrointestinal System

Anne Croghan

LEARNING OBJECTIVES

1. Describe the structures and functions of the organs of the gastrointestinal tract.
2. Describe the structures and functions of the liver, gallbladder, biliary tract, and pancreas.
3. Explain the processes of ingestion, digestion, absorption, and elimination.
4. Explain the processes of biliary metabolism, bile production, and bile excretion.
5. Describe age-related changes in the gastrointestinal system and differences in assessment findings.

6. Identify the significant subjective and objective data related to the gastrointestinal system that should be obtained from a patient.
7. Describe the appropriate techniques used in the physical assessment of the gastrointestinal system.
8. Differentiate normal from common abnormal findings of a physical assessment of the gastrointestinal system.
9. Describe the purpose, significance of results, and nursing responsibilities related to diagnostic studies of the gastrointestinal system.

KEY TERMS

absorption, p. 948
bilirubin, p. 952
borborygmi (Table 38-11), p. 960
cheilosis (Table 38-11), p. 960
defecation, p. 951
deglutition, p. 948
digestion, p. 948
endoscopy, p. 965
hematemesis (Table 38-11), p. 960
hepatocytes, p. 951

ingestion, p. 947
Kupffer cells, p. 951
melena (Table 38-11), p. 961
pyorrhea (Table 38-11), p. 960
pyrosis (Table 38-11), p. 960
steatorrhea (Table 38-11), p. 961
tenesmus (Table 38-11), p. 961
Valsalva maneuver, p. 951
villi, p. 948

The main function of the gastrointestinal (GI) system is to supply nutrients to body cells. This is accomplished through the processes of *ingestion* (taking in food), *digestion* (breakdown of food), and *absorption* (transfer of food products into circulation). *Elimination* is the process of excreting the waste products of digestion.

The GI system (also called the digestive system) consists of the GI tract and its associated organs and glands. Included in the GI tract are the mouth, esophagus, stomach, small intestine, large intestine, rectum, and anus. The associated organs are the liver, pancreas, and gallbladder (Fig. 38-1).

Factors outside the GI tract can influence its functioning. Both psychologic and emotional factors, such as stress and anxiety, influence GI functioning in many people. Stress may be manifested as anorexia, epigastric and abdominal pain, or diarrhea. However, GI problems should never be attributed solely to psychologic factors. Organic and psychologically based problems can exist independently or concurrently. Physical factors, such as dietary intake, ingestion of alcohol and caffeine-containing prod-

ucts, cigarette smoking, and fatigue, may also affect GI function. Some organic diseases of the GI system, such as peptic ulcer disease and ulcerative colitis, may be aggravated by stress.

STRUCTURES AND FUNCTIONS OF THE GASTROINTESTINAL SYSTEM

The GI tract is a tube approximately 30 feet (9 m) long extending from the mouth to the anus. The entire tract is composed of four common layers. From the inside to the outside, these layers are (1) mucosa, (2) submucosa, (3) muscle, and (4) serosa (Fig. 38-2). In the esophagus the outer coat is fibrous tissue rather than serosa. The muscular coat consists of two layers: the circular (inner) and the longitudinal (outer).

The GI tract is innervated by the parasympathetic and the sympathetic branches of the autonomic nervous system. The parasympathetic system is mainly excitatory, and the sympathetic system is mainly inhibitory. For example, peristalsis is increased by parasympathetic stimulation and decreased by sympathetic stimulation. Sensory information is relayed via both sympathetic and parasympathetic afferent fibers.

The GI tract also has its own nervous system: the enteric, or intrinsic, nervous system. The enteric nervous system is composed of two nerve layers that lie between the mucosa and the circular muscle layer and the circular and longitudinal muscle layers. These neurons contribute to the coordination of GI motor and secretory activities. The enteric nervous system is also known as the "gut brain." It contains numerous neurons (about as many as the spinal cord) and has the ability to control movement and secretion of the GI tract.

The GI tract and accessory organs receive approximately 25% to 30% of the cardiac output. Circulation in the GI system is unique in that venous blood draining the GI tract organs empties into the portal vein, which then perfuses the liver. The upper portion of the GI tract receives its blood supply from the splanchnic artery. The small intestine receives its blood supply from branches of the hepatic and superior mesenteric arteries. The large intestine receives its blood supply mainly from the superior and inferior

Reviewed by Phyllis Christiansen, RN, MN, ARNP, Adult and Geriatric Nurse Practitioner, University of Washington, Seattle, Wash.

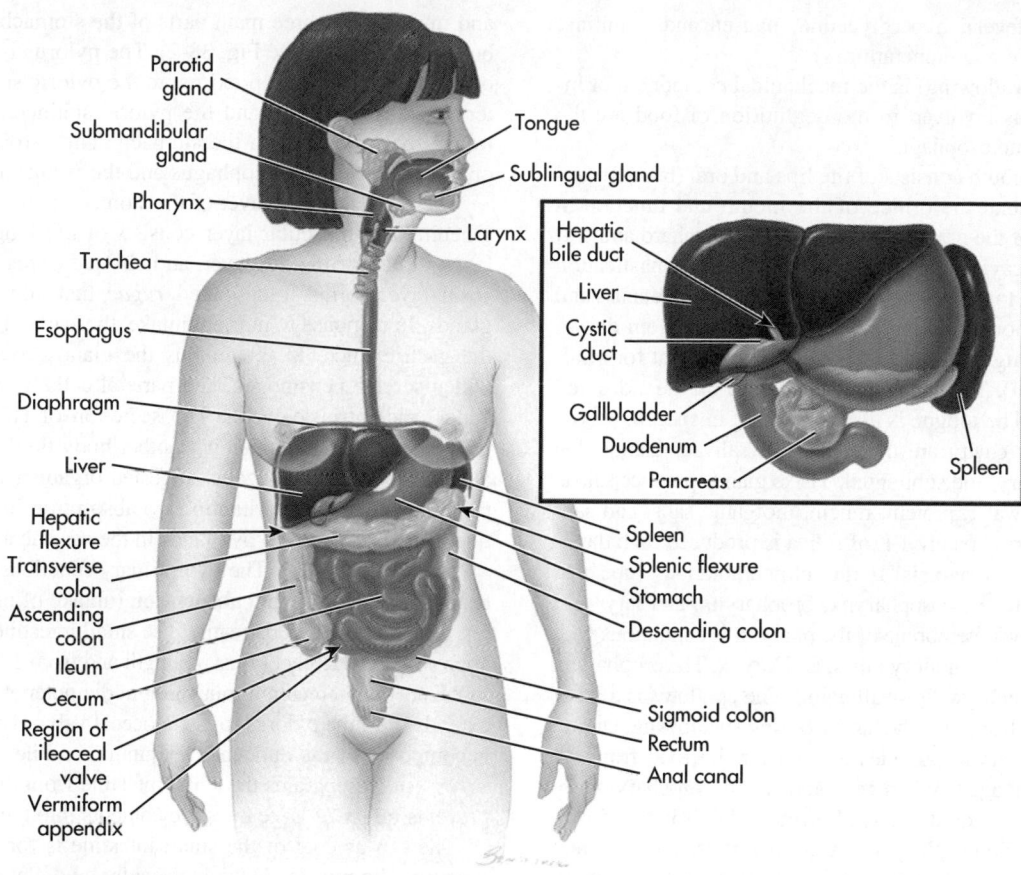

FIG. 38-1 Location of organs of the gastrointestinal system.

mesenteric arteries. Because such a large percentage of the cardiac output perfuses these organs, the GI tract is a major source from which blood flow can be diverted during exercise or stress.

The two types of movement of the GI tract are mixing (segmentation) and propulsion (peristalsis). The secretions of the GI system consist of enzymes and hormones for digestion, mucus to provide protection and lubrication, and water and electrolytes.

The abdominal organs are almost completely covered by the peritoneum. The two layers of the peritoneum are the *parietal,* which lines the abdominal cavity wall, and the *visceral,* which covers the abdominal organs. The peritoneal cavity is the potential space between the parietal and visceral layers. The two folds of the peritoneum are the mesentery and omentum. The mesentery attaches the small intestine and part of the large intestine to the posterior abdominal wall and contains blood and lymph vessels. The lesser omentum goes from the lesser curvature of the stomach and upper duodenum to the liver, and the greater omentum hangs from the stomach over the intestines like an apron. The omentum contains fat and lymph nodes.

The primary functions of the GI system are (1) ingestion and propulsion (movement) of food, (2) digestion, (3) absorption, and (4) elimination. Each part of the GI system performs different activities to accomplish these functions.

Ingestion and Propulsion of Food

Ingestion is the intake of food. A person's appetite or desire to ingest food is a significant factor in how much food is eaten. Multiple factors are involved in the control of appetite. An ap-

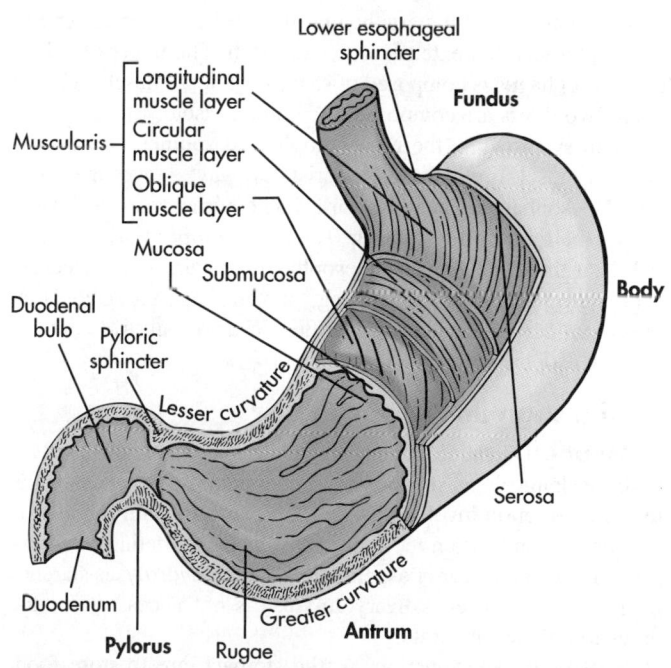

FIG. 38-2 Parts of the stomach.

petite center is located in the hypothalamus. It is directly or indirectly stimulated by hypoglycemia, an empty stomach, decrease in body temperature, and input from higher brain centers. The sight, smell, and taste of food frequently stimulate appetite. Appetite may be inhibited by stomach distention, illness (especially accompanied by fever), hyperglycemia, nausea and vomiting, and certain drugs (e.g., amphetamines).

Deglutition (swallowing) is the mechanical component of ingestion. The organs involved in the deglutition of food are the mouth, pharynx, and esophagus.

Mouth. The mouth consists of the lips and oral (buccal) cavity. The lips surround the orifice of the mouth and function in speech. The roof of the oral cavity is formed by the hard and soft palates. The oral cavity contains the teeth, used in mastication (chewing), and the tongue. The tongue is a solid muscle mass and assists in mastication by keeping food between the teeth during chewing and moving the food to the back of the throat for swallowing (deglutition). Taste receptors are found on the sides and tip of the tongue. The tongue is also important in speech.

Within the oral cavity are three pairs of salivary glands: the parotid, submaxillary, and sublingual. These glands produce saliva, which consists of water, protein, mucin, inorganic salts, and salivary amylase. Approximately 1 L of saliva is produced each day.

Pharynx. The pharynx is a musculomembranous tube that may be divided into the nasopharynx, oropharynx, and laryngeal pharynx. The mucous membrane of the pharynx is continuous with the nasal cavity, mouth, auditory tubes, and larynx. The oropharynx secretes mucus, which aids in swallowing. The epiglottis is a lid of fibrocartilage that closes over the larynx during swallowing. During ingestion the oropharynx provides a route for the food from the mouth to the esophagus. When receptors in the oropharynx are stimulated by food or liquid, the swallowing reflex is initiated.

Esophagus. The esophagus is a hollow, muscular tube that receives food from the pharynx and moves it to the stomach by peristaltic contractions. It is 9.2 to 10 inches (23 to 25 cm) long and 0.8 inch (2 cm) in diameter. The esophagus is located in the thoracic cavity, and it starts behind the trachea at the lower end of the pharynx and extends to the stomach. The upper one third of the esophagus is composed of striated skeletal muscle, and the distal two thirds are composed of smooth muscle.

With swallowing, the upper esophageal sphincter (cricopharyngeal muscle) relaxes and a peristaltic wave moves the bolus into the esophagus. The muscular layers contract (peristalsis) and propel the food to the stomach. The *lower esophageal sphincter* (LES) at the distal end of the esophagus remains contracted except during swallowing, belching, or vomiting. The LES is an important barrier that prevents reflux of acidic gastric contents into the esophagus.

Digestion and Absorption

Mouth. Digestion begins in the mouth. **Digestion** involves both mechanical (mastication) and chemical digestion. Saliva is the first secretion involved in digestion, and its main function is to lubricate and soften the food mass, thus facilitating swallowing. Saliva contains amylase (ptyalin), which hydrolyzes starches to maltose. However, salivary amylase is not necessary for the digestion of carbohydrates.

Stomach. The functions of the stomach are to store food, mix the food with gastric secretions, and empty contents into the small intestine at a rate at which digestion can occur. The stomach absorbs only small amounts of water, alcohol, electrolytes, and certain drugs.

The stomach lies obliquely in the epigastric, umbilical, and left hypochondriac regions of the abdomen (see Fig. 38-7 later in chapter). The shape and position of the stomach change based on the degree of gastric distention. It always contains gastric fluid

and mucus. The three main parts of the stomach are the fundus, body, and antrum (see Fig. 38-2). The pylorus is a small portion of the antrum that lies proximal to the pyloric sphincter. Sphincter muscles (the LES and the pyloric sphincter) guard the entrance to and exit from the stomach. The cardiac orifice is the opening between the esophagus and the stomach.

The serous (outer) layer of the stomach is formed by the peritoneum. The muscular layer consists of the longitudinal (outer) layer, circular (middle) layer, and oblique (inner) layer. The mucosal layer forms folds called *rugae* that contain many small glands. In response to nutrient intake, these glands secrete most of the gastric juice. In the fundus the glands contain chief cells, which secrete pepsinogen, and parietal cells, which secrete HCl, water, and intrinsic factor. The secretion of HCl makes gastric juice acidic in comparison with other body fluids. This acidic pH aids in the protection against ingested organisms. Intrinsic factor promotes cobalamin (vitamin B_{12}) absorption in the small intestine. Mucus is secreted by glands in the cardiac and pyloric areas.

Small Intestine. The two primary functions of the small intestine are digestion and **absorption** (uptake of nutrients from the gut lumen to the bloodstream). The small intestine is a coiled tube approximately 23 feet (7 m) in length and from 1 to 1.1 inches (2.5 to 2.8 cm) in diameter, diminishing in diameter at the lower end. It extends from the pylorus to the ileocecal valve. The small intestine is composed of the duodenum, jejunum, and ileum. The ileocecal valve, which separates the small intestine from the large intestine, prevents reflux of large intestine contents into the small intestine.

The serous coat of the small intestine is formed by the peritoneum. The mucosa is thick, vascular, and glandular. The circular folds in the mucous and submucous layers provide a greater surface area for digestion and absorption.

The functional units of the small intestine are villi. They are present in the entire small intestine. **Villi** are minute, fingerlike projections in the mucous membrane. They contain goblet cells that secrete mucus and epithelial cells that produce the intestinal digestive enzymes. The epithelial cells on the villi also have *microvilli,* which compose the brush border. Thus the presence of villi and microvilli greatly increases the surface area for absorption.

The digestive enzymes on the brush border of the microvilli chemically break down nutrients so that they can be absorbed. The villi are surrounded by the crypts of Lieberkühn, which contain the base columnar cells that are the stem cells for the other epithelial cell types. Brunner's glands in the submucosa of the duodenum secrete mucus.

Physiology of Digestion. *Digestion* is the physical and chemical breakdown of food into absorbable substances. Digestion in the GI tract is facilitated by the timely movement of food through the various organs and the secretion of specific enzymes. These enzymes break down foodstuffs to particles of appropriate size for absorption (Table 38-1).

The process of digestion begins in the mouth, where the food is chewed, mechanically broken down, and mixed with saliva. The saliva lubricates the food. In addition, salivary amylase begins the breakdown of starch. Salivary gland secretion is stimulated by chewing movements and the sight, smell, thought, and taste of food. The food is swallowed and passes into the esophagus, where peristaltic waves propel it to the stomach. No digestion or absorption occurs in the esophagus.

In the stomach the digestion of proteins begins with the release of pepsinogen from chief cells. The acidic environment of the stomach results in the conversion of pepsinogen to its active form, pepsin. Pepsin begins the initial breakdown of proteins. In the stomach there is minimal digestion of starches and fats. The food is mixed with gastric secretions, which are under neural and hormonal control (Tables 38-2 and 38-3). The stomach also serves as a reservoir for food, which is slowly expelled into the small intestine. The length of time that food remains in the stom-ach depends on the composition of the food, but average meals remain from 3 to 4 hours.

Digestion is completed in the small intestine, where carbohy-drates are hydrolyzed to monosaccharides, fats to glycerol and fatty acids, and proteins to amino acids. The physical presence of *chyme* (food mixed with gastric secretions), along with its chem-

TABLE 38-1   Gastrointestinal Secretions Related to Digestion

LOCATION	DAILY AMOUNT (ML)	SECRETIONS/ENZYMES	ACTION
Salivary glands	1000-1500	Salivary amylase (ptyalin)	Initiation of starch digestion
Stomach	2500	Pepsinogen	Protein digestion
		HCl	Protein digestion
		Lipase	Fat digestion
		Intrinsic factor	Essential for cobalamin absorption in ileum
Small intestine	3000	Enterokinase	Activation of trypsinogen to trypsin
		Amylase	Carbohydrate digestion
		Peptidases	Protein digestion
		Aminopeptidase	Protein digestion
		Maltase	Maltose to 2 glucose molecules
		Sucrase	Sucrose to glucose and fructose
		Lactase	Lactose to glucose and galactose
		Lipase	Fat digestion
Pancreas	700	Trypsinogen	Protein digestion
		Chymotrypsin	Protein digestion
		Amylase	Starch to disaccharides
		Lipase	Fat digestion
Liver and gallbladder	1000	Bile	Emulsification of fats and aid in absorption of fatty acids and fat-soluble vitamins (A, D, E, K)

TABLE 38-2   Phases of Gastric Secretion

PHASE	STIMULUS TO SECRETION	SECRETION
Cephalic (nervous)	Sight, smell, taste of food (before food enters stomach); initiated in the CNS and mediated by the vagus nerve	HCl, pepsinogen, mucus
Gastric (hormonal and nervous)	Food in antrum of stomach, vagal stimulation	Release of gastrin hormone from antrum into circulation to stimulate gastric secretions and motility
Intestinal (hormonal)	Presence of chyme in small intestine	Acidic chyme (pH <2): release of secretin, gastric inhibitory polypeptide, cholecystokinin into circulation to decrease acid secretion
		Chyme (pH >3): release of duodenal gastrin to increase acid secretion

CNS, Central nervous system.

TABLE 38-3   Major Hormones Controlling Gastrointestinal Secretion and Motility

HORMONE	SOURCE	ACTIVATING STIMULI	FUNCTION
Gastrin	Gastric and duodenal mucosa	Stomach distention, partially digested proteins in pylorus	Gastric acid secretion, increased motility, maintenance of lower esophageal sphincter tone
Secretin	Duodenal mucosa	Acid entering small intestine	Inhibition of gastric motility and acid secretion, stimulation of pancreatic bicarbonate secretion
Cholecystokinin	Duodenal mucosa	Fatty acids and amino acids in small intestine	Contraction of gallbladder and relaxation of sphincter of Oddi, allowing increased flow of bile into duodenum; release of pancreatic digestive enzymes
Gastric inhibitory peptide	Duodenal mucosa	Fatty acids and lipids in the small intestine	Inhibition of gastric acid secretion and gastric motility

ical nature in the small intestine, stimulates motility and secretion. Secretions involved in digestion include enzymes from the pancreas, bile from the liver (see Table 38-1), and intestinal secretions from glands in the small intestine. Both secretion and motility are under neural and hormonal control.

When food enters the stomach and small intestine, hormones are released into the bloodstream (see Table 38-3). The hormone secretin stimulates the pancreas to secrete fluid with a high concentration of bicarbonate. This alkaline secretion enters the duodenum and neutralizes acid in the chyme. The duodenal mucosa also secretes mucus to protect against the HCl. In response to the presence of chyme, the hormone cholecystokinin (CCK), produced by the duodenal mucosa, enters the bloodstream and stimulates contraction of the gallbladder and relaxation of the sphincter of Oddi. These actions permit bile to flow from the common bile duct into the duodenum. Bile is necessary for the digestion of fats. CCK also stimulates the pancreas to synthesize and secrete enzymes for enzymatic digestion of carbohydrates, fats, and proteins.

Enzymes present on the brush border of the microvilli complete the digestion process. These enzymes hydrolyze disaccharides to monosaccharides and peptides to amino acids for absorption.

Absorption is the transfer of the end products of digestion across the intestinal wall to the circulation. Most absorption occurs in the small intestine. The surface area of the small intestine is greatly increased by its circular folds, villi, and microvilli. The movement of the villi enables the end products of digestion to come in contact with the absorbing membrane. Monosaccharides (from carbohydrates), fatty acids (from fats), amino acids (from proteins), water, electrolytes, and vitamins are absorbed.

Elimination

Large Intestine. The large intestine is a hollow, muscular tube approximately 5 to 6 feet (1.5 to 2 m) long and 2 inches (5 cm) in diameter. The four parts of the large intestine are (1) the cecum and appendix, a narrow tube at the end of the cecum; (2) the colon (ascending colon on the right side, transverse colon across the abdomen, descending colon on the left side, and the sigmoid colon); (3) the rectum; and (4) the anus, the terminal portion of the large intestine (Fig. 38-3).

The most important function of the large intestine is the absorption of water and electrolytes. It also forms feces and serves as a reservoir for the fecal mass until defecation occurs. Feces are composed of water (75%), bacteria, unabsorbed minerals, undigested foodstuffs, bile pigments, and desquamated epithelial cells. The large intestine secretes mucus, which acts as a lubricant and protects the mucosa.

Microorganisms in the colon are responsible for the breakdown of proteins not digested or absorbed in the small intestine. These amino acids are deaminated by the bacteria, leaving ammonia, which is carried to the liver and converted to urea. Bacteria in the colon also synthesize vitamin K and some of the B vitamins. Bacteria also play a part in the production of flatus.

The movements of the large intestine are usually slow. When the circular muscles contract, they produce a kneading action

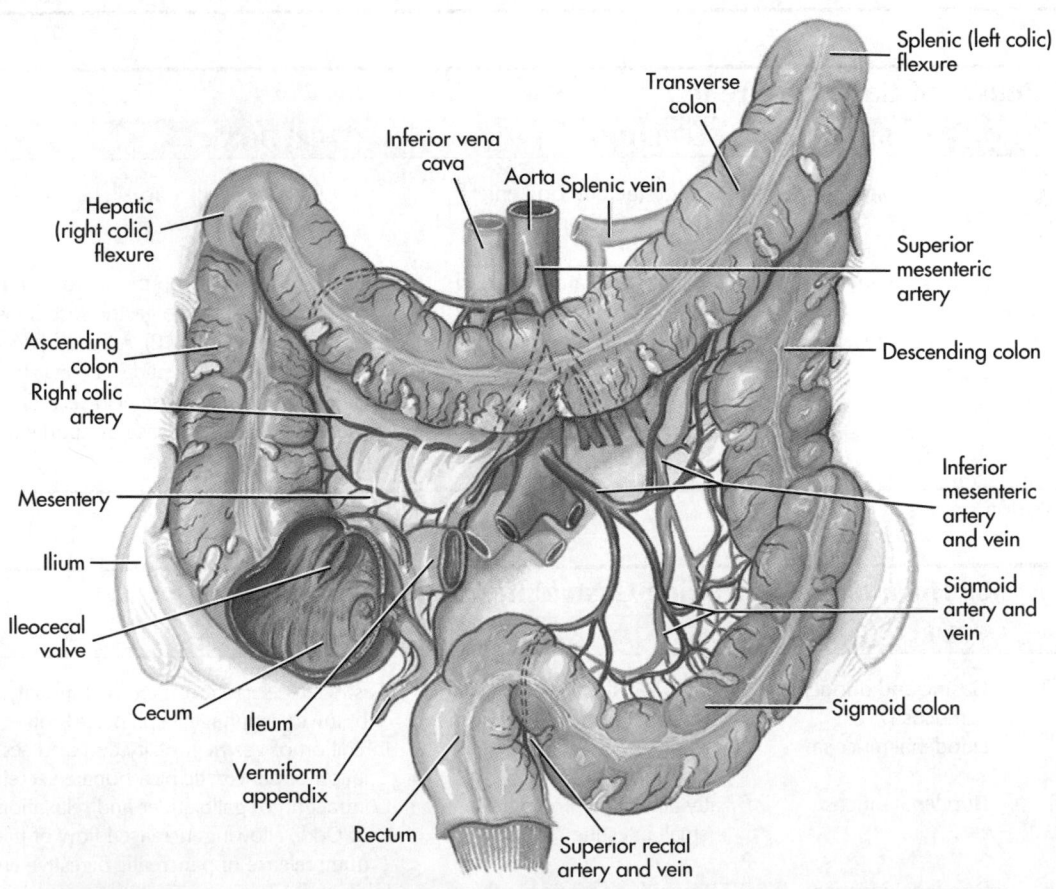

FIG. 38-3 Anatomic locations of the large intestine.

termed *haustral churning*. Propulsive (mass movements) peristalsis also occurs. When food enters the stomach and duodenum, the gastrocolic and duodenocolic reflexes are initiated, resulting in peristalsis in the colon. These reflexes are more active after the first daily meal and frequently result in bowel evacuation.

Defecation is a reflex action involving voluntary and involuntary control. Feces in the rectum stimulate sensory nerve endings that produce the desire to defecate. The reflex center for defecation is in the sacral portion of the spinal cord (parasympathetic nerve fibers). These fibers produce contraction of the rectum and relaxation of the internal anal sphincter. Defecation is controlled voluntarily by relaxing the external anal sphincter when the desire to defecate is felt. An acceptable environment for defecation is usually necessary or the urge to defecate will be ignored. If defecation is suppressed over long periods, problems can occur, such as constipation or stool impaction.

Defecation can be facilitated by the **Valsalva maneuver.** This maneuver involves contraction of the chest muscles on a closed glottis with simultaneous contraction of the abdominal muscles. These actions result in increased intraabdominal pressure. The Valsalva maneuver may be contraindicated in the patient with a head injury, eye surgery, cardiac problems, hemorrhoids, abdominal surgery, or liver cirrhosis with portal hypertension.

Constipation is common in the older adult and is due to many factors, including slower peristalsis, inactivity, decreased dietary fiber, decreased fluids, depression, constipating medications, and laxative abuse.[1] (Constipation is discussed in Chapter 41.)

Liver, Biliary Tract, and Pancreas

Liver. The liver is the largest internal organ in the body, weighing approximately 3 lb (1.37 kg) in the adult. It lies in the right hypochondriac and epigastric regions (see Fig. 38-7 later in chapter). Most of the liver is enclosed in peritoneum. It has a fibrous capsule that divides it into right and left lobes (Fig. 38-4).

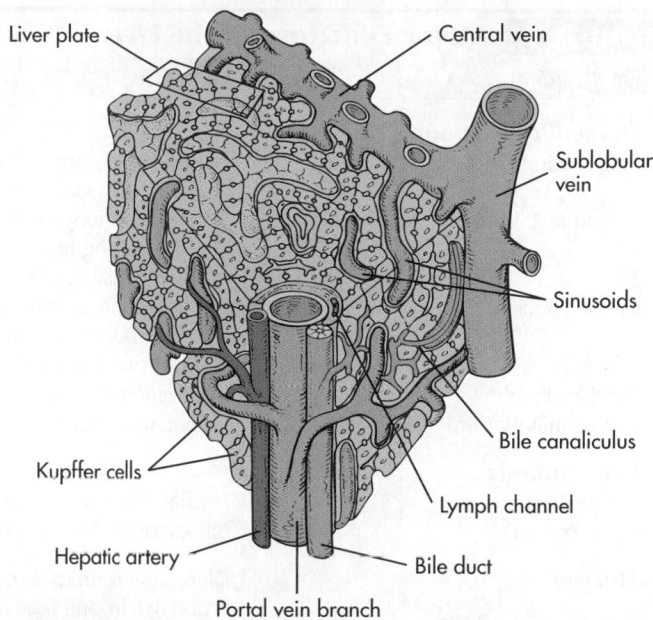

Microscopic structure of liver lobule.

The functional units of the liver are lobules (Fig. 38-5). The lobule consists of rows of hepatic cells (**hepatocytes**) arranged around a central vein. The capillaries (sinusoids) are located between the rows of hepatocytes and are lined with **Kupffer cells,** which carry out phagocytic activity (removal of bacteria and toxins from the blood). Interlobular bile ducts form from bile capillaries (canaliculi). The hepatic cells secrete bile into the canaliculi.

The nerve supply to the liver is from the left vagus and sympathetic celiac plexus. About one third of the blood supply comes from the hepatic artery (branch of the celiac artery), and two thirds come from the portal vein.

The portal circulatory system (enterohepatic) brings blood to the liver from the stomach, intestines, spleen, and pancreas. This blood enters the liver through the portal vein. The portal vein carries absorbed products of digestion directly to the liver. In the liver the portal vein branches and comes in contact with each lobule. The blood in the sinusoids is a mixture of arterial and venous blood.

The liver is essential for life. It functions in the manufacture, storage, transformation, and excretion of a number of substances involved in metabolism. The functions of the liver are numerous but can be classified into four main areas, as identified in Table 38-4.

Biliary Tract. The biliary tract consists of the gallbladder and the duct system. The gallbladder is a pear-shaped sac located below the liver. The function of the gallbladder is to concentrate and store bile. It can hold approximately 45 ml of bile.

Bile is produced by the hepatic cells and secreted into the biliary canaliculi of the lobules. Bile then drains into the interlobular bile ducts, which unite into the two main left and right hepatic ducts. The hepatic ducts merge with the cystic duct from the gallbladder to form the common bile duct (see Fig. 38-4). Most bile is stored and concentrated in the gallbladder. It is then released into the cystic duct and moves down the common bile duct to enter the duodenum at the ampulla of Vater. In the intestines, most of the bilirubin is reduced to stercobilinogen and urobilinogen by bacterial action. Stercobilinogen accounts for the brown color of stool. A small amount of conjugated bilirubin is reabsorbed by the blood.

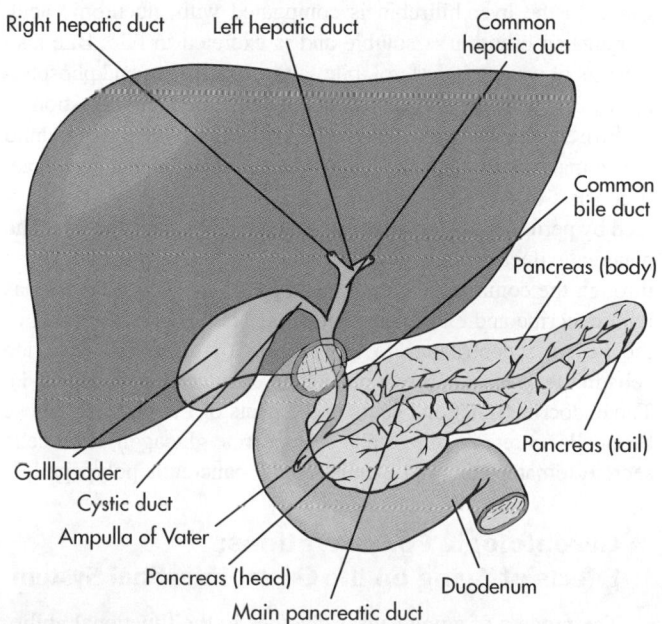

Gross structure of the liver, gallbladder, and pancreas and the duct system.

TABLE 38-4	Major Functions of the Liver
FUNCTION	**DESCRIPTION**
Metabolic Functions	
Carbohydrate metabolism	Glycogenesis (conversion of glucose to glycogen), glycogenolysis (process of breaking down glycogen to glucose), gluconeogenesis (formation of glucose from amino acids and fatty acids)
Protein metabolism	Synthesis of nonessential amino acids, synthesis of plasma proteins (except γ-globulin), synthesis of clotting factors, urea formation from NH_3 (NH_3 formed from deamination of amino acids by action of bacteria on proteins in colon)
Fat metabolism	Synthesis of lipoproteins, breakdown of triglycerides into fatty acids and glycerol, formation of ketone bodies, synthesis of fatty acids from amino acids and glucose, synthesis and breakdown of cholesterol
Detoxification	Inactivation of drugs and harmful substances and excretion of their breakdown products
Steroid metabolism	Conjugation and excretion of gonadal and adrenal steroid hormones
Bile Synthesis	
Bile production	Formation of bile, containing bile salts, bile pigments (mainly bilirubin), and cholesterol
Bile excretion	Bile excretion by liver about 1 L/day
Storage	Glucose in form of glycogen; vitamins, including fat soluble (A, D, E, K) and water soluble (B_1, B_2, cobalamin, and folic acid); fatty acids; minerals (iron and copper); amino acids in form of albumin and β-globulins
Mononuclear Phagocyte System	
Kupffer cells	Breakdown of old RBCs, WBCs, bacteria, and other particles; breakdown of hemoglobin from old RBCs to bilirubin and biliverdin

RBC, Red blood cell; *WBC*, white blood cell.

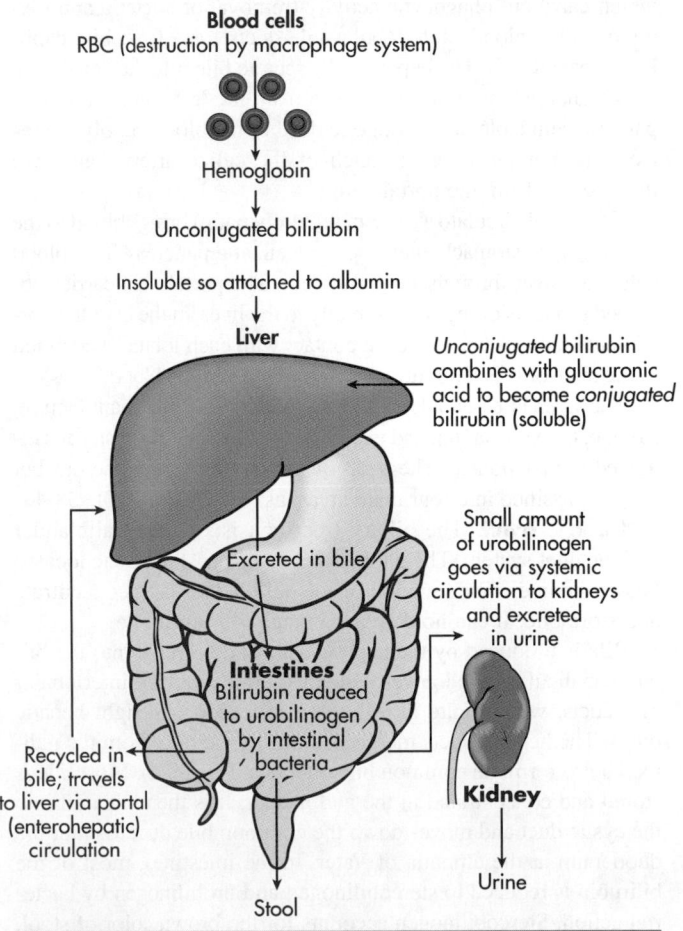

FIG. 38-6 Bilirubin metabolism and conjugation.

Some urobilinogen is reabsorbed by the blood and returned to the liver through the portal circulation (enterohepatic) and excreted in the bile. An insignificant amount of urobilinogen is excreted in the urine.[2] The sphincter of Oddi keeps the ampulla closed except when stimulated by the presence of food in the GI tract.

Bilirubin metabolism. Bilirubin, a pigment derived from the breakdown of hemoglobin, is constantly produced (Fig. 38-6). Because it is insoluble in water, it is bound to albumin for its transport to the liver. This form of bilirubin is referred to as unconjugated. In the liver bilirubin is conjugated with glucuronic acid. Conjugated bilirubin is soluble and is excreted in bile. Bile also consists of water, cholesterol, bile salts, electrolytes, and phospholipids. Bile salts are needed for fat emulsification and digestion.

Pancreas. The pancreas is a long, slender gland lying behind the stomach and in front of the first and second lumbar vertebrae. It consists of a head, body, and tail. The anterior surface is covered by peritoneum. The pancreas contains lobes and lobules. The pancreatic duct extends along the gland and enters the duodenum through the common bile duct (see Fig. 38-4). The pancreas has both exocrine and endocrine functions. The exocrine function of the pancreas contributes to the process of digestion. Exocrine cells in the pancreas secrete pancreatic enzymes (see Table 38-1). The endocrine function occurs in the islets of Langerhans, whose beta cells secrete insulin; alpha cells secrete glucagon; delta cells secrete somatostatin; and F cells secrete pancreatic polypeptide.

■ Gerontologic Considerations: Effects of Aging on the Gastrointestinal System

The process of aging causes changes in the functional ability of the GI system, although less than in other organ systems (Table 38-5). Tooth enamel and dentin wear down and make the

TABLE 38-5   *Gerontologic Differences in Assessment*   Gastrointestinal System

CHANGES	DIFFERENCES IN ASSESSMENT FINDINGS
Mouth	
Loss of teeth	Presence of dentures, difficulty chewing
Decreased taste buds, decreased sense of smell	Diminished sense of taste (especially salty and sweet)
Decreased volume of saliva	Dry oral mucosa
Atrophy of gingival tissue	Poor-fitting dentures
Esophagus	
Decreased tone and motility	Complaints of pyrosis (heartburn), dysphagia, eructation
Abdominal Wall	
Thinner and less taut	More visible peristalsis, easier palpation of organs
Decrease in number and sensitivity of sensory receptors	Less sensitivity to surface pain
Stomach	
Decreased acid secretion, atrophy of gastric mucosa	Food intolerances, signs of anemia as result of cobalamin mal-absorption
Small Intestines	
Decreased secretion of most digestive enzymes, decreased motility	Complaints of indigestion
Liver	
Decreased size and lowered in position	Easier palpation
Large Intestine, Anus, Rectum	
Decreased anal sphincter tone and nerve supply to rectal area	Fecal incontinence
Decreased muscular tone, decreased motility	Flatulence, abdominal distention, relaxed perineal musculature
Increase in transit time	Constipation, fecal impaction

teeth susceptible to cavities. Periodontal disease can lead to the loss of teeth. Taste buds decrease, the sense of smell diminishes, and salivary secretions diminish, all of which can lead to a decrease in appetite and make eating less pleasurable.

Age-related changes in the esophagus include delayed emptying resulting from smooth muscle weakness and an incompetent lower esophageal sphincter.[1] Motility of the GI system decreases with age, but secretion and absorption are affected to a lesser extent. The elderly patient often experiences a decrease in HCl secretion (hypochlorhydria), delayed gastric emptying, and constipation. With chronic atrophic gastritis there is a decrease in the number of parietal cells and subsequent reduction in the amount of acid and intrinsic factor secreted.

The liver size decreases after 50 years of age, but results of liver function tests remain within normal ranges. Enzyme changes in the liver that are age-related decrease the ability of the liver to metabolize drugs and hormones. The size of the pancreas is unaffected by aging but does undergo structural changes such as fibrosis, fatty acid deposits, and atrophy. Aging does not cause changes in the structure and function of the gallbladder and bile ducts. However, with aging there is an increase in the incidence of gallstones.[3]

The economic inability to purchase food supplies may affect nutritional intake, especially in the older adult. Economic constraints may also reduce the number of fresh fruits and vegetables consumed and thus the amount of fiber. A reduction in dietary fiber, along with reduced fluid intake and decreased physical activity, contributes to constipation. Age-related changes in the GI

system and differences in assessment findings are presented in Table 38-5.

ASSESSMENT OF THE GASTROINTESTINAL SYSTEM

Subjective Data

Important Health Information

Past health history. Information should be gathered from the patient about the history or existence of the following problems related to GI functioning: abdominal pain, nausea and vomiting, diarrhea, constipation, abdominal distention, jaundice, anemia, heartburn, dyspepsia, changes in appetite, hematemesis, food intolerance or allergies, indigestion, excessive gas, bloating, melena, hemorrhoids, or rectal bleeding. In addition, the patient should be asked about the history or existence of diseases such as gastritis, hepatitis, colitis, gallbladder disease, peptic ulcer, cancer, or hernias, especially hiatal hernias.

The patient should be questioned about weight history. Any unexplained or unplanned weight loss or weight gain within the past 12 months should be explored in detail. A history of chronic dieting and repeated weight loss and gain should be documented.

Medications. The health history should include an assessment of the patient's past and current use of medications. This is an important part of the assessment, particularly in relation to liver problems. It should include over-the-counter drugs, prescription drugs, and herbal products and nutritional supplements (see Complementary and Alternative Therapies box in Chapter 3 on p. 34). Many

TABLE 38-6	Potentially Hepatotoxic Chemicals and Drugs

acetaminophen
alcohol
anabolic steroids
arsenic
carbon tetrachloride
chloroform
gold compounds
halothane
isoniazid (INH)
6-mercaptopurine (6-MP)
mercury
methotrexate
phosphorus
propylthiouracil
sulfonamides
thiazide diuretics

TABLE 38-7	Surgeries of the Gastrointestinal System	
SURGICAL PROCEDURE	**DESCRIPTION**	
Antrectomy	Removal of antrum portion of stomach	
Cecostomy	Opening into cecum	
Cholecystectomy	Removal of gallbladder	
Cholecystostomy	Opening into gallbladder	
Choledochojejunostomy	Opening between common bile duct and jejunum	
Choledocholithotomy	Opening into common bile duct for removal of stones	
Colostomy	Opening into colon	
Esophagoenterostomy	Removal of portion of esophagus with segment of colon attached to remaining portion	
Esophagogastrostomy	Removal of esophagus and anastomosis of remaining portion to stomach	
Gastrectomy	Removal of stomach	
Gastrostomy	Opening into stomach	
Glossectomy	Removal of tongue	
Hemiglossectomy	Removal of half of tongue	
Ileostomy	Opening into ileum	
Mandibulectomy	Removal of mandible	
Pyloroplasty	Enlargement and repair of pyloric sphincter area	
Vagotomy	Resection of branch of vagus nerve	

chemicals and drugs are potentially hepatotoxic (Table 38-6). Antibiotics can cause changes in the normal bacterial composition in the GI tract, resulting in diarrhea. The nurse should ask the patient if laxatives or antacids are taken, including the kind and frequency.

The nurse should assess the patient's use of over-the-counter pain medications. Chronic high doses of acetaminophen and nonsteroidal antiinflammatory drugs (NSAIDs) can be hepatotoxic. Chronic NSAID use can also predispose a person to upper GI bleeding.

The use of prescription or over-the-counter appetite suppressants should be noted. The names of drugs and frequency and duration of use are also important.

Surgery or other treatments. Information should be obtained about hospitalizations for any problems related to the GI system. Data should also be obtained related to any abdominal or rectal surgery, including the year, reason for surgery, postoperative course, and possible blood transfusions. Terms related to surgery of the GI system are presented in Table 38-7.

Functional Health Patterns. Key questions to ask a patient with a GI problem are presented in Table 38-8.

Health perception–health management pattern. The nurse should ask about the patient's health practices related to the GI system, such as maintenance of normal body weight, attention to proper dental care, maintenance of adequate nutrition, and effective elimination habits.

The patient should be asked about recent foreign travel with possible exposure to hepatitis, parasitic, or bacterial infestation. Past history of receiving hepatitis A and/or hepatitis B vaccination should be documented.

The patient should be assessed in relation to certain habits that directly affect GI functioning. The consumption of alcohol in large quantities has detrimental effects on the mucosa of the stomach and also increases the secretion of HCl and pepsinogen. Chronic alcohol exposure causes fatty infiltration of the liver and can cause damage leading to cirrhosis. The nurse should obtain a history of cigarette smoking. Nicotine is irritating to the entire GI tract mucosa. Cigarette smoking is related to various GI cancers (especially mouth and esophageal cancers), esophagitis, and ulcers. Smoking will also delay the healing of ulcers.

Nutritional-metabolic pattern. A thorough nutritional assessment is essential. A dietary history should be taken and compared with the food pyramid (see Fig. 39-1). The nurse should ask open-ended questions that will allow the patient to express beliefs and feelings about the diet. The nurse may need to ask the patient to do a 24-hour dietary recall to analyze the adequacy of the diet. The nurse should assist the patient in recalling the preceding day's food intake, including early morning and nighttime intake. The nurse should find out about the intake of snacks, liquids, and vitamin supplements. The nurse must then evaluate the diet in terms of the recommended groups and servings on the food pyramid and try to determine whether the 24-hour recall is typical of the patient's usual eating habits. If weekend eating habits vary greatly, the nurse should obtain a separate weekend diet history and assess the patient's intake for both quality and quantity of food.

The nurse should ask the patient about the use of sugar and salt substitutes, use of caffeine, and amount of fluid and fiber intake. The patient should be questioned about any changes in appetite, food tolerance, and weight. Anorexia and weight loss may indicate the presence of cancer. The nurse should ask the patient about allergies to any food and determine what GI symptoms such allergic responses cause. The patient should be asked about dietary intolerances including lactose and gluten.

Elimination pattern. A detailed account of the patient's bowel elimination pattern should be elicited. The frequency, time of day, and usual consistency of stool should be noted. The use

TABLE 38-8	Health History
	Gastrointestinal System

Health Perception–Health Management Pattern
- Describe any measures used to treat GI symptoms such as diarrhea or vomiting.
- Do you smoke?* Do you drink alcohol?*
- Are you exposed to any chemicals on a regular basis?* Have you been exposed in the past?*
- Have you recently traveled outside the United States?*

Nutritional-Metabolic Pattern
- Describe your usual daily food and fluid intake.
- Do you take any supplemental vitamins or minerals?*
- Have you experienced any changes in appetite or food tolerance?*
- Has there been a weight change in the past?*
- Are you allergic to any foods?*

Elimination Pattern
- Describe the frequency and time of day you have bowel movements. What is the consistency of the bowel movement?
- Do you use laxatives or enemas?* If so, how often?
- Have there been any recent changes in your bowel pattern?*
- Describe any skin problems caused by GI problems.
- Do you need any assistive equipment, such as ostomy equipment?

Activity-Exercise Pattern
- Do you have limitations in mobility that make it difficult for you to procure and prepare food?*
- Are you able to feed yourself?
- Do you have any GI symptoms, such as vomiting or diarrhea, that affect your activity?*
- Do you have any difficulty accessing a toilet when needed?*
- Is a safe and comfortable environment for elimination available?

Sleep-Rest Pattern
- Do you experience any difficulty sleeping because of a GI problem?*
- Are you awakened by symptoms such as gas or esophageal burning?*

Cognitive-Perceptual Pattern
- Have you experienced any change in taste or smell that has affected your appetite?*
- Do you have any heat or cold sensitivity that affects eating?*
- Does pain interfere with food preparation, appetite, or chewing?*
- Do pain medications cause constipation or appetite suppression?*

Self-Perception–Self-Concept Pattern
- Describe any changes in your weight that have affected how you feel about yourself.
- Have you had any changes in normal elimination that have affected how you feel about yourself?*
- Have any symptoms of GI disease caused physical changes that are a problem for you?*

Role-Relationship Pattern
- Describe the impact of any GI problem on your usual roles and relationships.
- Have any changes in elimination affected your relationships?*
- Do you live alone? Describe how your family or others assist you with your GI problems.

Sexuality-Reproductive Pattern
- Describe the effect of your GI problem on your sexual activity.

Coping–Stress Tolerance Pattern
- Do you experience GI symptoms in response to stressful or emotional situations?
- Describe how you deal with any GI symptoms that result.

Value-Belief Pattern
- Describe any culturally specific health beliefs regarding food and food preparation that may influence the treatment of this GI problem.

*If yes, describe.

---

of laxatives and enemas, including type, frequency, and results, should be documented. Any recent change in bowel patterns should be investigated.

The amount and type of fluid and fiber intake should be determined because they have an important effect on the frequency and consistency of stools. Inadequate intake of fiber can be associated with constipation. Analysis of fluid intake and output could indicate the presence of a urinary problem and the possibility of fluid retention.

Food allergies can cause lesions, pruritus, and edema. Diarrhea can result in redness, irritation, and pain in the perianal area. External drainage systems such as an ileostomy or ileal conduit can cause local skin irritation. The possible association between a skin problem and a GI problem should be investigated.

Activity-exercise pattern. The patient's ambulatory status should be assessed to determine if the patient is capable of securing and preparing food. If the patient is unable to do these tasks, it should be determined if family or an outside agency is meeting this need. Any limitation in the patient's ability to feed self independently should be noted. Any difficulty accessing a safe environment of elimination should be assessed. Use of and access to elimination supplies should be assessed, such as a commode or ostomy supplies. Activity and exercise may affect GI motility. Immobility is a risk factor for constipation.

Sleep-rest pattern. Many food-related events can interrupt and interfere with the quality of sleep. Nausea, vomiting, diarrhea, indigestion, bloating, and hunger can produce sleep problems and should be investigated. The patient should be asked if GI symptoms affect sleep or rest. For example, a patient with a hiatal hernia may be awakened because of burning pain; sleep may be improved by elevating the head of the bed for this patient.

A patient often has a bedtime ritual that involves the use of a particular food or beverage. Milk is known to induce sleep through the effect of the serotonin precursor L-tryptophan. Herbal teas and melatonin are often sleep inducing. Individual routines should be noted and complied with whenever possible to avoid sleeplessness. Hunger can prevent sleep and should be relieved by a light, easily digested snack unless contraindicated.

Cognitive-perceptual pattern. Decreases in sensory adequacy can result in problems related to the acquisition, preparation, and ingestion of food. Changes in taste or smell can affect appetite and eating pleasure. Vertigo can make shopping and standing at a stove difficult and dangerous. Heat or cold sensitivity could make certain foods painful to eat. Problems in expressive communication could make it difficult and frustrating for the patient to make personal desires and preferences known. The nurse should assess the patient in this pattern to judge the effect of deficiencies on adequate nutritional intake. If the patient has been diagnosed as having a GI disorder, the nurse should ask questions to determine the patient's understanding of the illness and its treatment.

Pain is another area that requires careful assessment related to its effect on the GI system and nutrition. Relevant behaviors associated with chronic pain include avoidance of activity, fatigue, and disruption of eating patterns. The possible effects of narcotic pain medication related to constipation, nausea, sedation, and appetite suppression should be assessed.

Self-perception–self-concept pattern. Many GI and nutritional problems can have serious effects on the patient's self-perception. Overweight and underweight persons often have problems related to self-esteem and body image. Repeated attempts to achieve a personally acceptable weight can be discouraging and depressing for the patient. The manner in which a person recounts a weight history can alert the nurse to potential problems in this area.

Another potentially problematic area is the need for external devices to manage elimination, such as a colostomy or an ileostomy. The patient's willingness to engage in self-care and to discuss this situation should provide the nurse with valuable information related to body image and self-esteem.

The altered physical changes often associated with advanced liver disease can be problematic for the patient. Jaundice and ascites cause significant changes in external appearance. The patient's attitude toward these changes should be assessed.

Role-relationship pattern. Problems related to the GI system such as cirrhosis, alcoholism, hepatitis, ostomies, obesity, and carcinoma can have a major impact on the patient's ability to maintain usual roles and relationships. A chronic illness may necessitate leaving a job or reducing the number of hours worked. Changes in body image and self-esteem can affect relationships. The availability of and satisfaction with support should be determined. It is important that the nurse be aware of these possible consequences and assess for their presence.

Sexuality-reproductive pattern. Changes related to sexuality and reproductive status can result from problems of the GI system. For example, obesity, jaundice, anorexia, and ascites could decrease the acceptance of a potential sexual partner. The presence of an ostomy could affect the patient's confidence related to sexual activity. Chronic alcoholism could discourage a meaningful relationship that could develop into a sexual relationship. Sensitive questioning by the nurse could determine the presence of potential problems.

Anorexia can affect the reproductive status of a female patient. Alcoholism can affect the reproductive status of both men and women. A poor nutritional intake before and during pregnancy can result in a low-birth-weight infant.

Coping–stress tolerance pattern. The nurse should try to determine what is a stressor for the patient and what coping mechanisms the patient uses to function with these stressors. GI symptoms such as epigastric pain, nausea, and diarrhea develop in many people in response to stressful or emotional situations. Some GI problems such as peptic ulcers and irritable bowel syndrome are aggravated by stress.

Value-belief pattern. The patient's spiritual and cultural beliefs regarding food and food preparation should be assessed. Whenever possible, these preferences should be respected by the health care provider. In addition, it should be determined if any value or belief could interfere with planned interventions. For example, if the patient with anemia is a vegetarian, the prescription of a high-meat diet would be met with patient resistance. Thoughtful assessment and consideration of the patient's beliefs and values will usually increase patient compliance and satisfaction.

Objective Data

In addition to collecting subjective data related to a diet history and functional health patterns, objective data related to a nutritional assessment should be collected. Anthropometric measurements (height, weight, skinfold thickness) and blood studies such as serum protein, albumin, and hemoglobin are examples of important objective data related to the GI system. A physical examination also adds valuable information.

Physical Examination

Mouth

Inspection. The lips should be inspected for symmetry, color, and size. They should be observed for abnormalities such as pallor or cyanosis, cracking, ulcers, or fissures. The dorsum (top) of the tongue should have a thin white coating; the undersurface should be smooth. The nurse should observe for any lesions. Using a tongue blade, the nurse should inspect the buccal mucosa and note the color, any areas of pigmentation, and any lesions. Dark-skinned individuals normally have patchy areas of pigmentation. In assessing the teeth and gums, the nurse should look for caries; loose teeth; abnormal shape and position of teeth; and swelling, bleeding, discoloration, or inflammation of the gingivae. Any distinctive breath odor should be noted.

The pharynx is inspected by tilting the patient's head back and depressing the tongue with a tongue blade. The tonsils, uvula, soft palate, and anterior and posterior pillars should be observed. The nurse should have the patient say "ah." The uvula and soft palate should rise and remain in the midline.

Palpation. The nurse should palpate any suspicious areas in the mouth. Ulcers, nodules, indurations, and areas of tenderness should be palpated.

The mouth of the older adult requires careful assessment. Particular attention should be given to dentures (e.g., fit, condition), ability to swallow, the tongue, and lesions. The patient who has dentures must remove the dentures during an oral examination to allow for good visualization and palpation of the area.

Abdomen. Two systems are used to anatomically describe the surface of the abdomen. One system divides the abdomen into four quadrants by a perpendicular line from the sternum to the pubic bone and a horizontal line across the abdomen at the umbilicus (Fig. 38-7, *A*, and Table 38-9). The other system divides the abdomen into nine regions (Fig. 38-7, *B*), but only the epigastric, umbilical, and suprapubic or hypogastric regions are commonly addressed.

For the abdominal examination, good lighting should shine across the abdomen. The patient should be in the supine position

rounded [convex], concave, protuberant, distention), observable masses (hernias or other masses), and movement (pulsations and peristalsis). A normal aortic pulsation may be seen in the epigastric area. The nurse should look across the abdomen tangentially (across the abdomen in a line) for peristalsis. Peristalsis is not normally visible in an adult but may be visible in a thin person.

Auscultation. During examination of the abdomen, auscultation is done before percussion and palpation because these latter procedures may alter the bowel sounds. Auscultation of the abdomen includes listening for increased or decreased bowel sounds and vascular sounds. The diaphragm of the stethoscope is used to auscultate bowel sounds because they are relatively high pitched. The bell of the stethoscope is used to detect lower-pitched sounds. Normal bowel sounds occur 5 to 35 times per minute and sound like high-pitched clicks or gurgles.[4] Before auscultation, warming the stethoscope in the hands helps prevent abdominal muscle contraction. The nurse should listen in the epigastrium and in all four quadrants. The nurse should listen for bowel sounds for 2 to 5 minutes. Bowel sounds cannot be described as absent until no sound is heard for 5 minutes (in each quadrant).[5] The frequency and intensity of bowel sounds will vary, depending on the phase of digestion. Normally they will sound relatively high pitched and gurgling. Loud gurgles indicate hyperperistalsis and are termed *borborygmi* (stomach growling). The bowel sounds will be more high pitched (rushes and tinkling) when the intestines are under tension, such as in intestinal obstruction. The nurse should listen for decreased or absent bowel sounds. Terms used to describe bowel sounds include *present, absent, increased, decreased, high pitched, tinkling, gurgling,* and *rushing.* Normally no aortic bruits should be heard. A bruit, best heard with the bell of the stethoscope, is a swishing or buzzing sound and indicates turbulent blood flow.

Percussion. The purpose of percussion of the abdomen is to determine the presence of fluid, distention, and masses. Sound waves vary according to the density of underlying tissues; the presence of air produces a higher-pitched, hollow sound termed *tympany*; the presence of fluid or masses produces a short, high-pitched sound with little resonance termed *dullness.* The nurse should lightly percuss all four quadrants of the abdomen and assess the distribution of tympany and dullness. Tympany is the predominant percussion sound of the abdomen.

To percuss the liver, the nurse should start below the umbilicus in the right midclavicular line and percuss lightly upward until dullness is heard, thus determining the lower border of liver dullness. After the lower border of the liver has been determined, the nurse should start at the nipple line in the right midclavicular

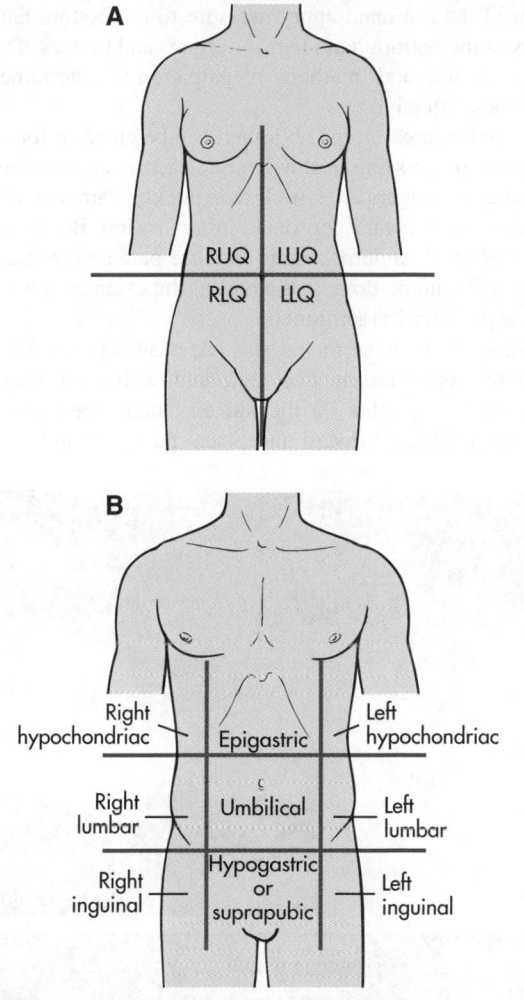

FIG. 38-7 A, Abdominal quadrants. B, Abdominal regions.

and as relaxed as possible. To help relax the abdominal muscles, the patient should slightly flex the knees and the head of the bed should be raised slightly. The patient should have an empty bladder. The examiner should use warm hands when doing the abdominal examination to avoid eliciting muscle guarding. The patient should be asked to breathe slowly through the mouth.

Inspection. The nurse should assess the abdomen for skin changes (color, texture, scars, striae, dilated veins, rashes, and lesions), umbilicus (location and contour), symmetry, contour (flat,

TABLE 38-9   Abdominal Structures in Regions of the Abdomen

RIGHT UPPER QUADRANT	LEFT UPPER QUADRANT	RIGHT LOWER QUADRANT	LEFT LOWER QUADRANT
Liver and gallbladder	Left lobe of liver	Lower pole of right kidney	Lower pole of left kidney
Pylorus	Spleen	Cecum and appendix	Sigmoid flexure
Duodenum	Stomach	Portion of ascending colon	Portion of descending colon
Head of pancreas	Body of pancreas	Bladder (if distended)	Bladder (if distended)
Right adrenal gland	Left adrenal gland	Right ovary and salpinx	Left ovary and salpinx
Portion of right kidney	Portion of left kidney	Uterus (if enlarged)	Uterus (if enlarged)
Hepatic flexure of colon	Splenic flexure of colon	Right spermatic cord	Left spermatic cord
Portion of ascending and transverse colon	Portion of transverse and descending colon	Right ureter	Left ureter

line and percuss downward between ribs to the area of dullness indicating the upper border of the liver. The height or vertical space between the two areas should be measured to determine the size of the liver. The normal range of liver height in the right midclavicular line is 2.4 to 5 inches (6 to 12 cm).

Palpation. *Light palpation* is used to detect tenderness or cutaneous hypersensitivity, muscular resistance, masses, and swelling. It also helps the patient to relax for deeper palpation. The nurse should keep fingers together and press gently with the pads of the fingertips, depressing the abdominal wall about 0.4 inch (1 cm). Smooth movements should be used and all quadrants palpated (Fig. 38-8, *A*).

Deep palpation is used to delineate abdominal organs and masses (Fig. 38-8, *B*). The palmar surfaces of the fingers should be used to press more deeply. Again, all quadrants should be palpated. When palpating masses, the nurse should note the location, size, shape, and presence of tenderness. The patient's facial expression should be observed during these maneuvers because it will provide nonverbal cues of discomfort or pain.

An alternative method for deep abdominal palpation is the two-hand method. One hand is placed on top of the other. The fingers of the top hand apply pressure to the bottom hand. The fingers of the bottom hand feel for organs and masses. The nurse should practice both methods of palpation to determine which one is most effective.[6]

A problem area on the abdomen can be checked for rebound tenderness by pressing in slowly and firmly over the painful site. The palpating fingers are withdrawn quickly. Pain on withdrawal of the fingers indicates peritoneal inflammation. Because assessing for rebound tenderness may produce pain and severe muscle spasm, it should be done at the end of the examination and only by an experienced practitioner.

To palpate the liver, the nurse's left hand is placed behind the patient to support the right eleventh and twelfth ribs (Fig. 38-9). The patient may relax on the nurse's hand. The nurse should press the left hand forward and place the right hand on the pa-

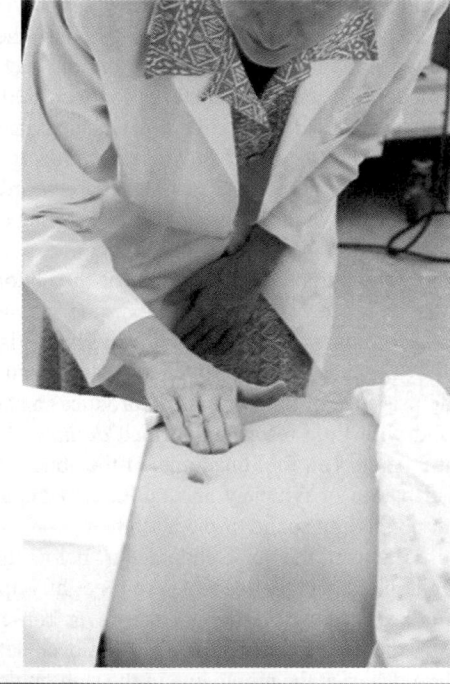
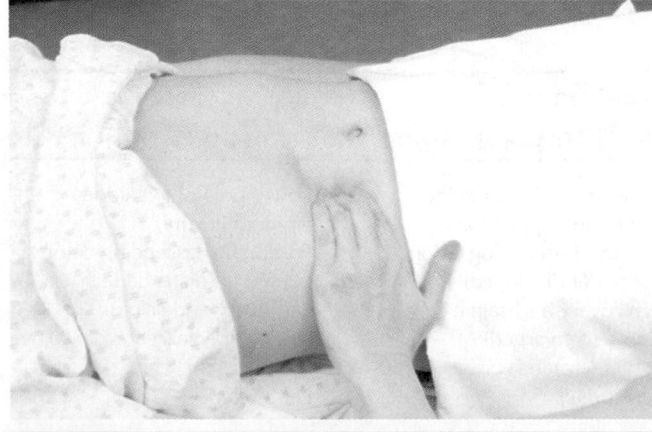

FIG. 38-8   A, Technique for light palpation of the abdomen. B, Technique for deep palpation.

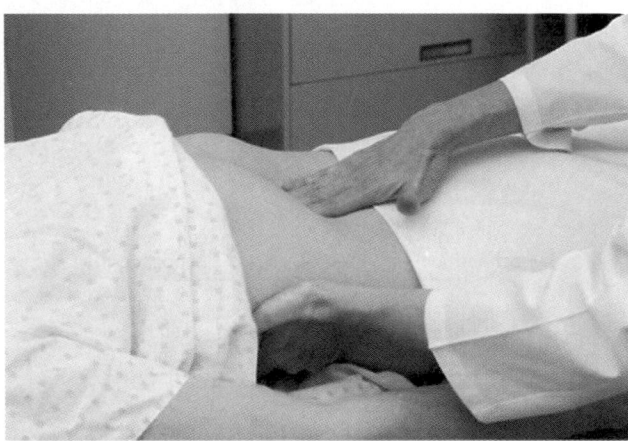
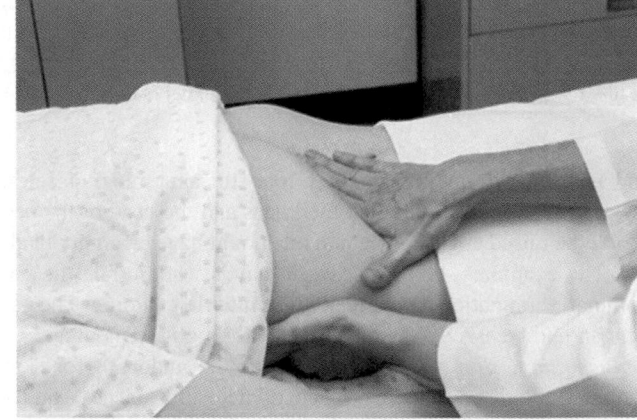
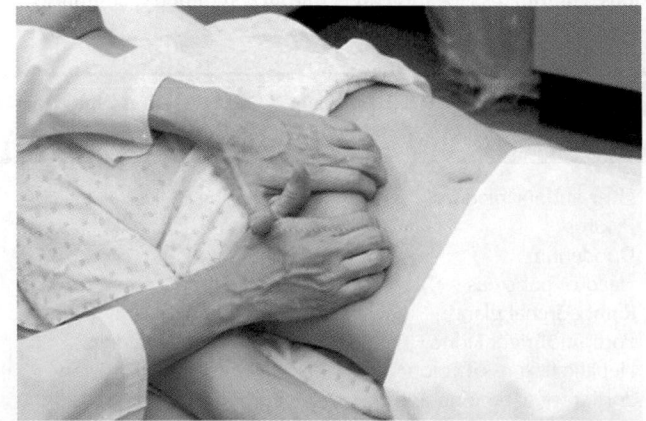

FIG. 38-9   A, Technique for liver palpation. B, Alternative technique. C, Palpation of liver with fingers hooked over the costal region.

tient's right abdomen lateral to the rectus muscle. The fingertips should be below the lower border of liver dullness and pointed toward the right costal margin. The nurse should gently press in and up. The patient should take a deep breath with the abdomen so that the liver drops and is in a better position to be palpated. The nurse should try to feel the liver edge as it comes down to the fingertips. During inspiration the liver edge should feel firm, sharp, and smooth. The surface and contour and any tenderness should be described.

To palpate the spleen, the nurse moves to the left side of the patient. The nurse places the right hand under the patient and supports and presses the patient's left lower rib cage forward. The left hand is placed below the left costal margin and presses it in toward the spleen. The nurse should ask the patient to breathe deeply. The tip or edge of an enlarged spleen will be felt by the fingertips. The spleen is normally not palpable. If it is palpable, the nurse should not continue because manual compression of an enlarged spleen may cause it to rupture.

The standard approach for examining the abdomen can be used on the older adult.[7] Palpation is important because it may reveal a tumor. The abdomen may be thinner and more lax unless the patient is obese. If the patient has chronic obstructive pulmonary disease, large lungs, or a low diaphragm, the liver may be palpated 0.4 to 0.8 inch (1 to 2 cm) below the right costal margin.

Rectum and anus. The perianal and anal area should be inspected for color, texture, lumps, rashes, scars, erythema, fissures, and external hemorrhoids. Any lumps or unusual areas should be palpated with a gloved hand.

For the digital examination of the rectum the gloved, lubricated index finger is placed against the anus while the patient strains (Valsalva maneuver). Then, as the sphincter relaxes, the finger is inserted. The finger is pointed toward the umbilicus. The nurse should try to get the patient to relax. The finger is inserted into the rectum as far as possible, and all surfaces are palpated. Nodules, tenderness, or any irregularities should be assessed. A sample of stool can be removed with the gloved finger and should be checked for occult blood.

Recording of the normal physical assessment of the GI system is found in Table 38-10. Gerontologic differences in the GI system and differences in assessment findings are described in Table 38-5. Common assessment abnormalities are presented in Table 38-11.

DIAGNOSTIC STUDIES OF THE GASTROINTESTINAL SYSTEM

Diagnostic studies provide important information to the nurse in monitoring the patient's condition and planning appropriate interventions. These studies are considered to be objective data. Table 38-12 presents diagnostic studies common to the GI system. For most diagnostic studies, nurses should make sure a signed consent form for the procedure has been completed and is in the medical record. It is the responsibility of the health care provider doing the procedure to explain the procedure and obtain the written consent. However, nurses play an important role in educating patients regarding the procedures. When preparing the patient it is important to ask about any known allergies to drugs or contrast medium.

Many of the diagnostic procedures of the GI system require measures to cleanse the GI tract, as well as the ingestion or injection of a contrast medium or a radiopaque tracer. Often the pa-

TABLE 38-10	Normal Physical Assessment of the Gastrointestinal System

Mouth
Moist and pink lips
Pink and moist buccal mucosa and gingivae without plaques or lesions
Teeth in good repair
Protrusion of tongue in midline without deviation or fasciculations
Pink uvula in midline, soft palate, tonsils, and posterior pharynx
Swallows smoothly without coughing or gagging

Abdomen
Flat without masses or scars
No abdominal tenderness
No bruises
Bowel sounds in all quadrants
Nonpalpable liver and spleen
Liver 10 cm in right midclavicular line
Generalized tympany

Anus
Absence of lesions, fissures, and hemorrhoids
Good sphincter tone
Rectal walls smooth/soft
No masses
Stool soft, brown, and heme negative

tient has a series of GI diagnostic tests done. The nurse must monitor the patient closely to ensure adequate hydration and nutrition during the testing period. Some diagnostic studies of the GI system are especially difficult and uncomfortable for the older adult. It may be necessary to individualize and make adjustments. It is particularly important to prevent diarrhea from bowel-cleansing procedures and dehydration from prolonged fluid restriction.[8]

Many radiologic studies use either barium sulfate or meglumine diatrizoate (Gastrografin) as a contrast medium. Barium sulfate is more effective for visualizing mucosal detail. Gastrografin is water soluble and rapidly absorbed, so it is preferred when a perforation is suspected. Spillage of barium into the peritoneal cavity can result in peritonitis. Under other circumstances in a person at high risk for aspiration, water-soluble media are contraindicated and barium is preferred.

Radiologic Studies

Upper Gastrointestinal Series. A barium swallow allows examination of the esophagus after swallowing a thick barium solution. An upper GI series with small bowel follow-through provides visualization of the esophagus, stomach, and small intestine by means of fluoroscopy and x-ray examination. The procedure consists of the patient swallowing contrast medium (a thick barium solution) and then assuming different positions on the x-ray table. The movement of the contrast medium is observed with fluoroscopy, and several x-rays are taken (see Table 38-12). A barium swallow is used to identify esophageal, stomach, and small intestine disorders such as esophageal strictures, varices, polyps, tumors, hiatal hernia, foreign bodies, and peptic ulcers in the stomach or duodenum (Fig. 38-10).

Text continued on p. 965

TABLE 38-11	*C*ommon Assessment Abnormalities Gastrointestinal System	
FINDING	**DESCRIPTION**	**POSSIBLE ETIOLOGY AND SIGNIFICANCE**
Mouth		
Ulcer, plaque on lips or in mouth	Sore or lesion	Carcinoma, viral infections
Cheilosis	Softening, fissuring, and cracking of lips at angles of mouth	Riboflavin deficiency
Cheilitis	Inflammation of lips (usually lower) with fissuring, scaling, crusting	Often unknown
Geographic tongue	Scattered red, smooth (loss of papillae) areas on dorsum of tongue	Unknown
Smooth tongue	Red, slick appearance	Cobalamin deficiency
Leukoplakia	Thickened white patches	Premalignant lesion
Pyorrhea	Recessed gums, purulent pockets	Periodontitis
Herpes simplex	Benign vesicular lesion	Herpesvirus
Candidiasis	White, curdlike lesions surrounded by erythematous mucosa	*Candida albicans*
Glossitis	Reddened, ulcerated, swollen tongue	Exposure to streptococci, irritation, injury, vitamin B deficiencies, anemia
Acute marginal gingivitis	Friable, edematous, painful, bleeding gingivae	Irritation from ill-fitting dentures, calcium deposits on teeth, food impaction
Esophagus and Stomach		
Dysphagia	Difficulty in swallowing, sensation of food sticking in esophagus	Esophageal problems, cancer of esophagus
Hematemesis	Vomiting of blood	Esophageal varices, bleeding peptic ulcer
Pyrosis	Heartburn, burning in epigastric or substernal area	Hiatal hernia, esophagitis, incompetent lower esophageal sphincter
Dyspepsia	Burning or indigestion	Peptic ulcer, gallbladder disease
Odynophagia	Painful swallowing	Cancer of esophagus, esophagitis
Eructation	Belching	Gallbladder disease
Nausea and vomiting	Feeling of impending vomiting, expulsion of gastric contents through mouth	GI infections, common manifestation of many GI diseases; stress, fear, and pathologic conditions
Abdomen		
Distention	Excessive gas accumulation, enlarged abdomen; generalized tympany	Obstruction, paralytic ileus
Ascites	Accumulated fluid within abdominal cavity; eversion of umbilicus (usually)	Peritoneal inflammation, congestive heart failure, metastatic carcinoma, cirrhosis
Bruit	Humming or swishing sound heard through stethoscope over vessel	Partial arterial obstruction (narrowing of vessel), turbulent flow (aneurysm)
Hyperresonance	Loud, tinkling rushes	Intestinal obstruction
Borborygmi	Waves of loud, gurgling sounds	Hyperactive bowel as result of eating
Absent bowel sounds	No auscultation of bowel sounds	Peritonitis, paralytic ileus, obstruction
Absence of liver dullness	Tympany on percussion	Air from viscus (e.g., perforated ulcer)
Masses	Lump on palpation	Tumors, cysts
Rebound tenderness	Sudden pain when fingers withdrawn quickly	Peritoneal inflammation, appendicitis
Nodular liver	Enlarged, hard liver with irregular edge or surface	Cirrhosis, carcinoma
Hepatomegaly	Enlargement of liver, liver edge >1-2 cm below costal margin	Metastatic carcinoma, hepatitis, venous congestion
Splenomegaly	Enlargement of spleen	Chronic leukemia, hemolytic states, portal hypertension, some infections
Hernia	Bulge or nodule in abdomen, usually appearing on straining	Inguinal (in inguinal canal), femoral (in femoral canal), umbilical (herniation of umbilicus), or incisional (defect in muscles after surgery)

TABLE 38-11   Common Assessment Abnormalities — Gastrointestinal System—cont'd

FINDING	DESCRIPTION	POSSIBLE ETIOLOGY AND SIGNIFICANCE
Rectum and Anus		
Hemorrhoids	Thrombosed veins in rectum and anus (internal or external)	Portal hypertension, chronic constipation, prolonged sitting or standing, pregnancy
Mass	Firm, nodular edge	Tumor, carcinoma
Pilonidal cyst	Opening of sinus tract, cyst in midline just above coccyx	Probably congenital
Fissure	Ulceration in anal canal	Straining, irritation
Melena	Abnormal, black, tarry stool containing digested blood	Cancer, bleeding in upper GI tract from ulcers, varices
Tenesmus	Painful and ineffective straining at stool	Ulcerative colitis, diarrhea secondary to GI infection such as food poisoning
Steatorrhea	Fatty, frothy, foul-smelling stool	Chronic pancreatitis, biliary obstruction, malabsorption problems

TABLE 38-12   Diagnostic Studies — Gastrointestinal System

STUDY	DESCRIPTION AND PURPOSE	NURSING RESPONSIBILITY
Radiologic		
Upper Gastrointestinal (GI) or Barium Swallow	X-ray study with fluoroscopy with contrast medium. Study is used to diagnose structural abnormalities of the esophagus, stomach, and duodenal bulb.	Explain procedure to patient and that patient will need to drink contrast medium and assume various positions on x-ray table. Keep patient NPO for 8-12 hr before procedure. Tell patient to avoid smoking after midnight the night before the study. After x-ray, take measures to prevent contrast medium impaction (fluids, laxatives). Tell patient that stool may be white up to 72 hr after test.
Small Bowel Series	Contrast medium is ingested and films taken q20min until medium reaches terminal ileum.	Same as for upper GI.
Lower GI or Barium Enema	Fluoroscopic x-ray examination of colon uses contrast medium, which is administered rectally (enema). Double-contrast or air-contrast barium enema is test of choice. Air is infused after barium is evacuated.	Before the procedure, administer laxatives and enemas until colon is clear of stool evening before procedure. Administer clear liquid diet evening before procedure. Keep patient NPO for 8 hr before test. Instruct patient about being given barium by enema. Explain that cramping and urge to defecate may occur during procedure and that patient may be placed in various positions on tilt table. After the procedure, give fluids, laxatives, or suppositories to assist in expelling barium. Observe stool for passage of contrast medium.
Ultrasound	Noninvasive procedure uses high-frequency sound waves (ultrasound waves), which are passed into body structures and recorded as they are reflected (bounded). A conductive gel (lubricant jelly) is applied to the skin and a transducer is placed on the area.	
▪ Abdominal ultrasound	Study detects abdominal masses (tumors and cysts) and is also used to assess ascites.	Instruct patient to be NPO 8-12 hr before ultrasound. Air or gas can reduce quality of images. Food intake can cause gallbladder contraction, resulting in suboptimal study.

NPO, Nothing by mouth.

Continued

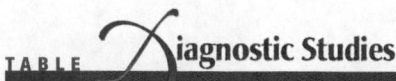

TABLE 38-12   Diagnostic Studies
Gastrointestinal System—cont'd

STUDY	DESCRIPTION AND PURPOSE	NURSING RESPONSIBILITY
Radiologic—cont'd		
Ultrasound—cont'd		
• Hepatobiliary ultrasound	Study detects subphrenic abscesses, cysts, tumors, and cirrhosis and is used to visualize biliary ducts.	Same as Abdominal ultrasound.
• Gallbladder (GB) ultrasound	Study detects gallstones (high degree of accuracy) and can be used for a patient with jaundice or allergic reaction to GB contrast media.	Same as Abdominal ultrasound.
Computed Tomography (CT)	Noninvasive radiologic examination combines special x-ray machine used for CT (exposures at different depths) with computer. Study detects mainly biliary tract, liver, and pancreatic disorders. Use of contrast medium accentuates density differences and helps detect biliary problems.	Explain procedures to patient. Determine sensitivity to iodine if contrast material used.
Magnetic Resonance Imaging (MRI)	Noninvasive procedure using radiofrequency waves and a magnetic field. Procedure is used to detect hepatic metastases and sources of GI bleeding and to stage colorectal cancer.	Keep patient NPO for 6 hr before procedure. Explain procedure to patient. Contraindicated in patient with metal implants (e.g., pacemaker) or who is pregnant.
Cholangiography		
• Percutaneous transhepatic cholangiogram (PTC)	After local anesthesia, liver is entered with long needle (under fluoroscopy), bile duct is entered, bile withdrawn, and radiopaque contrast medium injected. Fluoroscopy is used to determine filling of hepatic and biliary ducts.	Observe patient for signs of hemorrhage or bile leakage. Assess patient's medication for possible contraindications, precautions, or complications with the use of contrast medium.
• Surgical cholangiogram	Study is performed during surgery on biliary structures, such as GB. Contrast medium is injected into common bile duct.	Explain to patient that anesthetic will be used. Assess patient's medication for possible contraindications, precautions, or complications with the use of contrast medium.
• Magnetic resonance cholangiopancreatography (MRCP)	Noninvasive study uses MRI technology to obtain images of biliary and pancreatic ducts.	Same as MRI.
Nuclear Imaging Scans (Scintigraphy)	Purpose is to show size, shape, and position of organ. Functional disorders and structural defects may be identified. Radionuclide (radioactive isotope) is injected IV and a counter (scanning) device picks up radioactive emission, which is recorded on paper. Only tracer doses of radioactive isotopes are used.	Tell patient that substances contain only traces of radioactivity and pose little to no danger. Schedule no more than one radionuclide test on the same day. Explain to patient need to lie flat during scanning.
• Gastric emptying studies	Radionuclide study is used to assess ability of stomach to empty solids or liquids. In solid-emptying study, cooked egg white containing Tc-99m is eaten. In liquid-emptying study, orange juice with Tc-99m is drunk. Sequential images from gamma camera are recorded q2min for up to 60 min. Study is used in patients with emptying disorders from peptic ulcer, ulcer surgery, diabetes, or gastric malignancies.	Same as above.
• Hepatobiliary scintigraphy (HIDA)	Patient is given IV injection of Tc-99m and positioned under camera to record distribution of tracer in the liver, biliary tree, gallbladder, and proximal small bowel. Useful for identifying diffuse hepatic disease (such as cirrhosis or neoplasm), as well as to confirm acute cholecystitis.	Same as above.
• Scintigraphy of GI bleeding	Tc-99m–labeled sulfur colloid or Tc-99m labeling of the patient's own red blood cells (RBCs) can accurately determine the site of active GI blood loss. The sulfur colloid or the patient's RBCs are injected, and images of the abdomen are obtained at intermittent intervals.	Same as above.

IV, Intravenous.

TABLE 38-12 Diagnostic Studies — Gastrointestinal System—cont'd

STUDY	DESCRIPTION AND PURPOSE	NURSING RESPONSIBILITY
Endoscopic		
Upper GI Endoscopy • Esophagogastroduodenoscopy (EGD)	Technique directly visualizes mucosal lining of esophagus, stomach, and duodenum with flexible, fiberoptic endoscope. Test may use video imaging to visualize stomach motility. Inflammations, ulcerations, tumors, or varices, or Mallory-Weiss tear may be detected.	Before the procedure, keep patient NPO for 8 hr. Make sure signed consent is on chart. Give preoperative medication if ordered (diazepam, midazolam, or meperidine). Explain to patient that local anesthetic may be sprayed on throat before insertion of scope and that patient will be sedated during the procedure. After the procedure, keep patient NPO until gag reflex returns. Gently tickle back of throat to determine reflex. Use warm saline gargles for relief of sore throat. Check temperature q15–30min for 1-2 hr (sudden temperature spike is sign of perforation).
Colonoscopy	Study directly visualizes entire colon up to ileocecal valve with flexible fiberoptic scope. Patient's position is changed frequently during procedure to assist with advancement of scope to cecum. Test is used to diagnose inflammatory bowel disease, detect tumors, and dilate strictures. Procedure allows for removal of colonic polyps without laparotomy.	Before the procedure, keep patient on clear liquids 1-3 days and NPO for 8 hr. Administer laxatives 1-3 days before and enemas night before. Explain to patient same information regarding insertion of scope as for sigmoidoscopy. Explain to patient that sedation will be given. Administer alternate preparation of 1 gal of Golytely or Colyte evening before (8-oz glass q10min). On morning of procedure, allow clear liquids. After the procedure, be aware that patient may experience abdominal cramps caused by stimulation of peristalsis because the patient's bowel is constantly inflated with air during procedure. Observe for rectal bleeding and signs of perforation (e.g., malaise, abdominal distention, tenesmus). Check vital signs.
Proctosigmoidoscopy	Study directly visualizes rectum and sigmoid colon with lighted endoscope. It is usually done with rigid metal scope but may be done with flexible endoscope. Sometimes special table is used to tilt patient into knee-chest position. Test may detect tumors, polyps, inflammatory and infectious diseases, fissures, hemorrhoids.	Administer enemas evening before and morning of procedure. Be aware that patient may have clear liquids day before or that no dietary restrictions may be necessary. Explain to patient knee-chest position (unless patient is older or very ill), need to take deep breaths during insertion of scope, and possible urge to defecate as scope is passed. Encourage patient to relax—let abdomen go limp. Observe for rectal bleeding after polypectomy or biopsy.
Endoscopic Retrograde Cholangiopancreatography (ERCP)	Fiberoptic endoscope (using fluoroscopy) is inserted through the oral cavity into descending duodenum, then common bile and pancreatic ducts are cannulated. Contrast medium is injected into ducts and allows for direct visualization of structures. Technique can also be used to retrieve a gallstone from distal common bile duct, dilate strictures, obtain biopsy of tumors, diagnose pseudocysts.	Before the procedure, explain procedure to patient, including patient role. Keep patient NPO 8 hr before procedure. Ensure consent form signed. Administer sedation immediately before and during procedure. Administer antibiotics if ordered. After the procedure, check vital signs. Check for signs of perforation or infection. Be aware that pancreatitis is most common complication. Check for return of gag reflex.
Endoscopic Ultrasound	Combined use of endoscopy and ultrasound using an ultrasound transducer attached to an endoscope. Enables visualization of the esophagus, stomach, intestine, liver, and pancreas.	Similar to upper GI endoscopy.

Continued

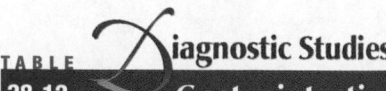

TABLE 38-12

Diagnostic Studies
Gastrointestinal System—cont'd

STUDY	DESCRIPTION AND PURPOSE	NURSING RESPONSIBILITY
Endoscopic—cont'd		
Peritoneoscopy (Laparoscopy)	Peritoneal cavity and contents are visualized with laparoscope. Biopsy specimen may also be taken. Done under general anesthesia in operating room. Double-puncture peritoneoscopy permits better visualization of abdominal cavity, especially liver. Technique can eliminate need for exploratory laparotomy in many patients.	Make sure signed permit is on chart. Keep patient NPO 8 hr before study. Administer preoperative sedative medication. Ensure that bladder and bowel are emptied. Instruct patient that local anesthetic is used before scope insertion. Observe for possible complications of bleeding and bowel perforation after the procedure.
Blood Chemistries		
▪ Serum amylase	Study measures secretion of amylase by pancreas and is important in diagnosing acute pancreatitis. Level of amylase peaks in 24 hr and then drops to normal in 48-72 hr. Depending on method, *normal finding* is 0-130 U/L (0-2.17 μkat/L).	Obtain blood sample in acute attack of pancreatitis. Explain procedure to patient.
▪ Serum lipase	Study measures secretion of lipase by pancreas. Level stays elevated longer than serum amylase. *Normal finding* is 0-160 U/L (0-2.66 μkat/L).	Explain procedure to patient.
Liver Biopsy	Percutaneous procedure uses needle inserted between sixth and seventh or eighth and ninth intercostal spaces on the right side to obtain specimen of hepatic tissue. Often done using ultrasound or CT guidance.	Before the procedure, check patient's coagulation status (prothrombin time, clotting or bleeding time). Ensure that patient's blood is typed and crossmatched. Take vital signs as baseline data. Explain holding of breath after expiration when needle is inserted. Ensure that informed consent has been signed. After the procedure, check vital signs to detect internal bleeding q15min × 2, q30min × 4, q1hr × 4. Keep patient lying on right side for minimum of 2 hr to splint puncture site. Keep patient in bed in flat position for 12-14 hr. Assess patient for complications such as bile peritonitis, shock, pneumothorax.
Miscellaneous Tests		
▪ Gastric analysis	Purpose is to analyze gastric contents for acidity and volume. NG tube is inserted, and gastric contents are aspirated. Contents are analyzed mainly for HCl, but pH, pepsin, and electrolytes may be determined. Histalog and pentagastrin may be used to stimulate HCl secretion. Exfoliative cytology may be done to determine whether malignant cells are present. With fasting, *normal acidity* is 2.5 mEq/L (2.5 mmol/L) and *normal volume* is 62 ml/hr; 30 min after Histalog or pentagastrin administration, *normal acidity* is 1.5 mEq/L (1.5 mmol/L) and *normal volume* is 110 ml/hr.	Keep patient NPO for 8-12 hr. Explain insertion of NG tube. Withhold drugs affecting gastric secretions 24-48 hr before test. Ensure no smoking morning of test (nicotine increases gastric secretion).
▪ Fecal analysis	Form, consistency, and color are noted. Specimen examined for mucus, blood, pus, parasites, and fat content. Tests for occult blood (guaiac test, Hemoccult, Hematest) are done.	Observe patient's stools. Collect stool specimens. Check stools for blood with Hemoccult or Hematest. Keep diet free of red meat for 24-48 hr before guaiac test.

NG, Nasogastric.

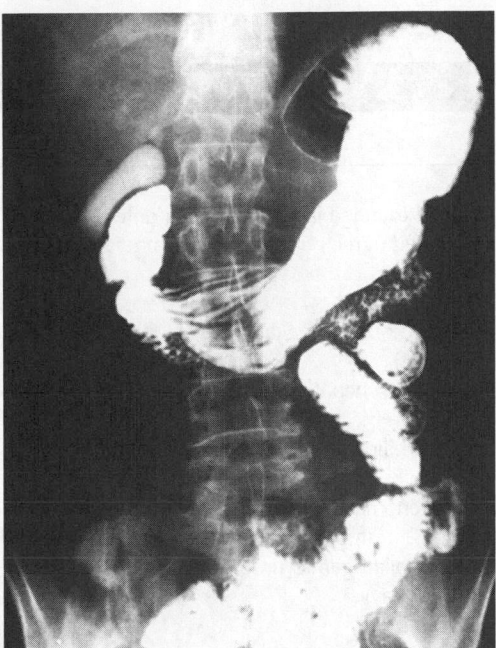

FIG. 38-10 Upper gastrointestinal tract x-ray.

Lower Gastrointestinal Series. The purpose of a lower GI series (barium enema) x-ray examination is to observe by means of fluoroscopy the filling of the colon with contrast medium and to observe by x-ray the filled colon. This procedure identifies polyps, tumors, and other lesions in the colon. It consists of administering an enema of contrast medium to the patient. The air-contrast barium enema provides better visualization of an inflammatory bowel disease, polyps, and tumors (Fig. 38-11). Because it requires the patient to retain the barium, it is not tolerated as well in an older or immobile patient.

Abdominal Ultrasound. Ultrasonography is used to show the size and configuration of organs. It is the diagnostic procedure of choice for detecting cholelithiasis (gallstones). Ultrasound is also used for detecting appendicitis, acute cholecystitis, and other changes in abdominal organs (see Table 38-12).

Endoscopy

Endoscopy refers to the direct visualization of a body structure through a lighted fiberoptic instrument (scope). The GI structures that can be examined by endoscopy include the esophagus, stomach, duodenum, colon, and, with the aid of fluoroscopy and x-rays, the pancreas and biliary tree. The pancreatic, hepatic, and common bile ducts can be visualized with side-viewing flexible endoscopes. This procedure is called *endoscopic retrograde cholangiopancreatography* (ERCP).[9]

The endoscope is an instrument channel through which biopsy forceps and cytology brushes may be passed. Cameras may be attached and video and still pictures taken. Endoscopy of the GI tract is often done in combination with biopsy and cytologic studies. The major complication of GI endoscopy is perforation through the structure being scoped. This complication is decreased with the use of the flexible fiberoptic scopes. All endoscopic procedures require informed, written consent. Specific endoscopy procedures are discussed in Table 38-12. In addition to diagnostic procedures, many invasive and therapeutic procedures may be done with endoscopes. These include procedures

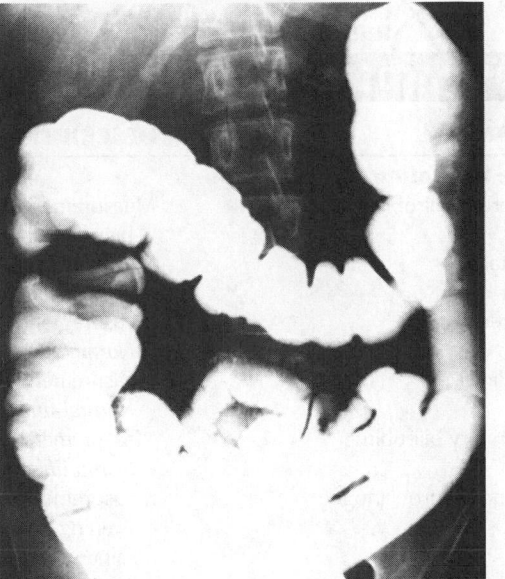

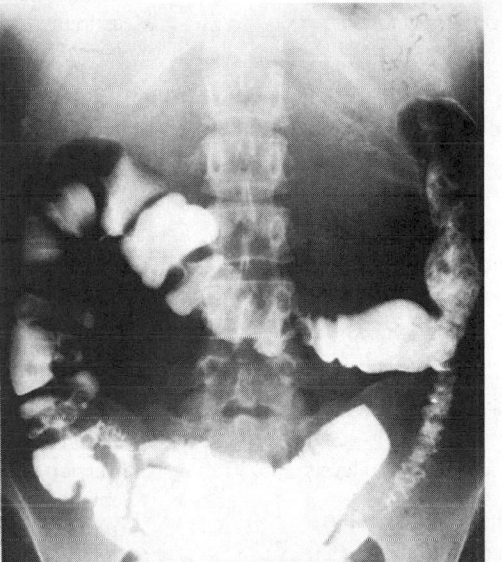

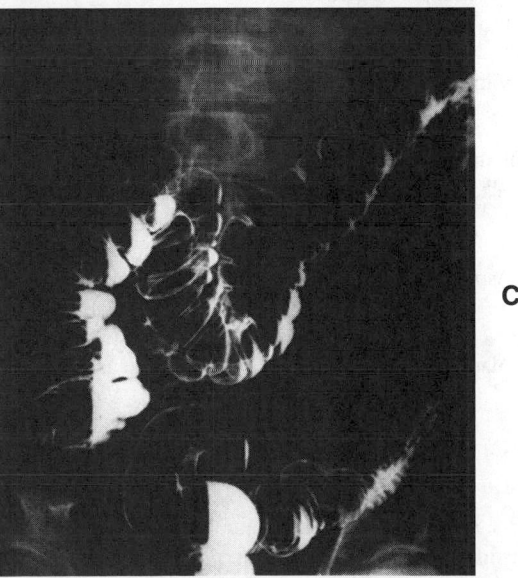

FIG. 38-11 Barium enema x-ray. A, Colon filled with barium. B, Colon after evacuation of barium. C, Air-contrast study of colon.

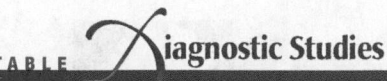

TABLE
38-13 **Diagnostic Studies**
Liver Function Tests

TEST	DESCRIPTION AND PURPOSE
Bile Formation and Excretion	
▪ Serum bilirubin	Measurement of ability of liver to conjugate and excrete bilirubin, allowing differentiation between unconjugated (indirect) and conjugated (direct) bilirubin in plasma
Total	Measurement of direct and indirect total bilirubin *Normal finding* of 0.2-1.3 mg/dl (3.4-22 μmol/L)
Direct	Measurement of conjugated bilirubin; elevation in obstructive jaundice *Normal finding* of 0.1-0.3 mg/dl (1.7-5.1 μmol/L)
Indirect	Measurement of unconjugated bilirubin; elevation in hepatocellular and hemolytic conditions *Normal finding* of 0.1-1 mg/dl (1.7-17 μmol/L)
▪ Urinary bilirubin	Measurement of urinary excretion of conjugated bilirubin *Normal finding* of 0
▪ Urinary urobilinogen	Measurement of urinary excretion of urobilinogen; maximum excretion midafternoon to early evening, collection of total urinary output for 2 hr in afternoon, sent to laboratory in dark container immediately because of oxidation of urobilinogen to urobilin on exposure to air *Normal finding* of 0.5-4 mg/day (0.8-6.8 μmol/day)
▪ Fecal urobilinogen	Measurement of fecal urobilinogen in stool specimen *Normal finding* of 30-220 mg/100 g stool (55-372 μmol/100 g of stool)
Dye Excretion Tests (Detoxification)	
▪ Indocyanine green	Determination of liver's ability to take up and excrete dye given IV, drawing of blood samples every 5 min for 20-30 min *Normal finding* of 500-800 ml/m² of body surface/min
Protein Metabolism	
▪ Serum protein levels	Measurement of serum proteins that are manufactured by the liver; measurement of albumin, *normal finding* of 3.5-5 g/dl (35-50 g/L); measurement of globulin, *normal finding* of 2-3.5 g/dl (20-35 g/L) *Normal total protein* of 6-8 g/dl (60-80 g/L) *Normal A/G ratio* of 1.5:1-2.5:1
▪ α-Fetoprotein	Indication of hepatic cancer *Normal finding* of <25 ng/ml (<25 μg/L)
▪ Blood ammonia levels	Conversion of ammonia to urea normally occurs in the liver; elevation can result in hepatic encephalopathy secondary to liver cirrhosis *Normal finding* of 30-70 μg/dl (17.6-41.1 μmol/L)
Hemostatic Functions	
▪ Prothrombin	Determination of prothrombin activity *Normal finding* of 12-15 sec
▪ Vitamin K production	Determination of response of liver to vitamin K, checking of prothrombin time necessary 24 hr after injection of vitamin K
Serum Enzyme Tests	
▪ Alkaline phosphatase (ALP)	Originating in bone and liver. Serum levels rise when excretion is impaired as a result of obstruction in the biliary tract. *Normal finding* of 30-120 U/L (0.5-2 μkat/L), depending on method and age
▪ Aspartate aminotransferase (AST)	Elevation in liver damage and inflammation *Normal finding* of 7-40 U/L (0.12-0.67 μkat/L)
▪ Alanine aminotransferase (ALT)	Elevation in liver damage and inflammation *Normal finding* of 5-36 U/L (0.08-0.6 μkat/L)
▪ γ-Glutamyl transpeptidase (GGT)	Present in biliary tract (not in skeletal muscle or cardiac), increase in hepatitis and alcoholic liver disease. More sensitive for liver dysfunction than ALP. *Normal finding* of 0-30 U/L (0-0.5 μkat/L)
Lipid Metabolism	
▪ Serum cholesterol	Synthesis and excretion by liver, increase in biliary obstruction, decrease in extensive liver disease and malnutrition *Normal finding* of 140-200 mg/dl (3.6-5.2 mmol/L), varying with age

such as polypectomy, sclerosis of varices, laser treatment, cauterization of bleeding sites, papillotomy, common bile duct stone removal, and balloon dilations. Many endoscopic procedures require intravenous short-acting sedation.

Endoscopic Ultrasound. Endoscopic ultrasound (EUS) is a relatively new endoscopic technique that provides highly accurate images of esophagus, GI tract, pancreas, and liver. EUS provides high-resolution imaging of the GI tract by its unique ability to differentiate the histologic layers of the GI tract wall. It is most often used for preoperative staging of esophageal, gastric, pancreatic, and colorectal cancers. It can also be used to detect gallstones.

Capsule Endoscopy. Capsule endoscopy is a new technique that uses a disposable video camera capsule swallowed by the patient. The image of the intestine is captured by the video camera and transmitted by radiofrequency. This procedure is particularly useful in visualization of the small bowel not within reach of standard upper and lower endoscopy. It allows more access to the small bowel for patients with an obscure source of GI bleeding. This technology may be particularly helpful in discovering the cause of GI bleeding when results of standard upper endoscopy and colonoscopy are negative.

Liver Biopsy

The purpose of a liver biopsy is to obtain hepatic tissue to be used in establishing a diagnosis such as fibrosis, cirrhosis, hepatitis, and neoplasms. It may also be useful for following the progress of liver disease.

The two types of liver biopsy are open and closed. The *open method* involves making an incision and removing a wedge of tissue. It is done in the operating room with the patient under general anesthesia, often concurrently with another surgical procedure. The *closed,* or *needle, biopsy* is a percutaneous procedure in which the site is infiltrated with a local anesthetic and a needle is inserted between the sixth and seventh or eighth and ninth intercostal spaces on the right side. The patient lies supine with the right arm over the head. The patient should be instructed to expire fully and not breathe while the needle is inserted (see Table 38-12). Nursing assessment before and after a liver biopsy is important.

Liver Function Studies

Liver function tests are usually described separately from other GI diagnostic studies. Liver function tests are laboratory (blood) studies that reflect hepatic disease. Table 38-13 describes some common liver function tests.

REVIEW QUESTIONS

The number of the question corresponds to the same-numbered objective at the beginning of the chapter.

1. A patient is admitted to the hospital with a diagnosis of diarrhea with dehydration. The nurse recognizes that increased peristalsis resulting in diarrhea can be related to
   a. sympathetic inhibition.
   b. mixing and propulsion.
   c. sympathetic stimulation.
   d. parasympathetic stimulation.

2. A patient has an elevated blood level of indirect (unconjugated) bilirubin. One cause of this finding is that
   a. the gallbladder is unable to contract to release stored bile.
   b. bilirubin is not being conjugated and excreted into the bile by the liver.
   c. the Kupffer cells in the liver are unable to remove bilirubin from the blood.
   d. there is an obstruction in the biliary tract preventing flow of bile into the small intestine.

3. As gastric contents move into the small intestine the bowel is normally protected from the acidity of gastric contents by the
   a. inhibition of secretin release.
   b. release of bicarbonate by the pancreas.
   c. release of pancreatic digestive enzymes.
   d. release of gastrin by the duodenal mucosa.

4. A patient is jaundiced and her stools are clay colored (gray). This is most likely related to
   a. decreased bile flow into the intestine.
   b. increased production of urobilinogen.
   c. increased production of cholecystokinin.
   d. increased bile and bilirubin in the blood.

5. An 80-year-old man states that although he adds a lot of salt to his food it still does not have much taste. The nurse's response is based on the knowledge that the older adult
   a. should not experience changes in taste.
   b. has a loss of taste buds, especially for sweet and salt.
   c. has some loss of taste but no difficulty chewing food.
   d. loses the sense of taste because the ability to smell is decreased.

6. When assessing the health promotion–health maintenance pattern as related to GI function, an appropriate question by the nurse is
   a. "What is your usual bowel elimination pattern?"
   b. "What percentage of your income is spent on food?"
   c. "Have you traveled to a foreign country in the last year?"
   d. "Do you have diarrhea when you are under a lot of stress?"

7. During an examination of the abdomen the nurse should
   a. position the patient in the supine position with the bed flat and knees straight.
   b. listen in the epigastrium and all four quadrants for 2 to 5 minutes for bowel sounds.
   c. use the following order of techniques: inspection, palpation, percussion, auscultation.
   d. describe bowel sounds as absent if no sound is heard in the lower right quadrant after 2 minutes.

8. A normal physical assessment finding of the GI system is
   a. tympany on percussion of the abdomen.
   b. liver edge 2 to 4 cm below the costal margin.
   c. finding of a firm, nodular edge on the rectal examination.
   d. easy palpation of the spleen edges with moderate pressure.

9. In preparing a patient for a colonoscopy the nurse explains that
   a. a signed permit is not necessary.
   b. sedation may be used during the procedure.
   c. only one cleansing enema is necessary for preparation.
   d. a light meal should be eaten the day before the procedure.

REFERENCES

1. Eliopoulos C: *Gerontological nursing*, ed 5, Philadelphia, 2000, Lippincott.
2. Porth CM: *Pathophysiology concepts of altered health states*, ed 6, Philadelphia, 2002, Lippincott.
3. Burke MM, Walsh MB: *Gerontologic nursing: wholistic care of the older adult*, ed 2, St Louis, 1997, Mosby.
4. Bickley LS et al: *Bates' guide to physical examination and history taking*, ed 7, Philadelphia, 1999, Lippincott.
5. Seidel HM et al: *Mosby's guide to physical examination*, ed 5, St Louis, 2003, Mosby.
6. Barkausus VH, Baumann LC, Darling-Fisher CS: *Health and physical assessment*, ed 3, St Louis, 2002, Mosby.
7. Ebersole P, Hess P: *Toward healthy aging*, ed 6, St Louis, 2001, Mosby.
8. Feldman M et al: *Sleisenger and Fordtran's gastrointestinal and liver disease: pathophysiology/diagnosis/management*, ed 6, Philadelphia, 1998, Saunders.
9. Domkowski, K: *Gastroenterology nursing: a core curriculum*, ed 2, St Louis, 1998, Mosby.

RESOURCES

Resources for this chapter are listed in Chapter 39 on page 1002, Chapter 40 on page 1051, Chapter 41 on page 1103, and Chapter 42 on page 1149.

CHAPTER *39*

NURSING MANAGEMENT
Nutritional Problems

Peggi Guenter

LEARNING OBJECTIVES

1. Describe the essential components of a nutritionally sound diet and their importance to good health.
2. Describe possible adverse interactions between drugs and various foods.
3. Describe the common etiologic factors, clinical manifestations, and management of malnutrition.
4. Explain the indications for use, complications, and nursing management of tube feedings.
5. Describe the types of feeding tubes and related nursing management.
6. Define the indications, complications, and nursing management related to the use of parenteral nutrition.
7. Discuss the etiologies, complications, and collaborative care of obesity.
8. Describe the nursing management related to conservative and surgical therapies for obesity.
9. Compare the etiologic factors, clinical manifestations, and nursing management of eating disorders.

KEY TERMS

anorexia nervosa, p. 999
body mass index, p. 991
bulimia nervosa, p. 999
kwashiorkor, p. 973
lipectomy, p. 995
malabsorption syndrome, p. 973
malnutrition, p. 972
marasmus, p. 973
morbid obesity, p. 991

nutrition, p. 969
obesity, p. 991
overnutrition, p. 972
parenteral nutrition, p. 987
protein-calorie malnutrition, p. 972
total parenteral nutrition, p. 987
tube feeding, p. 982
undernutrition, p. 972

CULTURAL & ETHNIC CONSIDERATIONS
Nutritional Problems

- Incidence of obesity is higher among African American women compared with white women.
- Anorexia nervosa is most common among women from middle and upper-middle classes.
- Anorexia nervosa and bulimia have a higher incidence among whites than among African Americans and Asian Americans.
- Lactase deficiency has a higher incidence among African Americans and Asians than among whites.

This chapter focuses on problems related to nutrition. The primary nutritional problems discussed are malnutrition, obesity, and eating disorders.

NUTRITIONAL PROBLEMS

Nutritional problems can occur in all age groups, cultures, ethnic groups, and socioeconomic classes. Intelligence and wealth do not necessarily preclude the development of poor nutritional habits. The nurse in the roles of caregiver, teacher, and resource person can have a strong influence on the nutritional practices of patients and their families. Together with the physician, the registered dietitian, and the pharmacist, the nurse is in an excellent position to assess the dietary practices of the patient and provide important information, as well as provide nutritional resources within and outside the institutional setting.

The nutritional status of a person or a family may be influenced by many factors. Attitudes toward the importance of food and eating habits are established early. Cultural or religious preferences and requirements are frequently reflected in dietary intake. The financial status of a family or an individual can determine the type and amount of nutritionally sound food that can be purchased. Findings support that generally the lower the socioeconomic status, the poorer the nutritional state.[1] The availability of food sources also contributes to the individual's nutritional status.

NORMAL NUTRITION

Nutrition is the process by which the body uses food for energy, growth, and maintenance and repair of body tissues. Good nutrition in the absence of any underlying disease process results from the ingestion of a balanced diet. The United States Department of Agriculture (USDA) has adopted the Food Guide Pyramid, which consists of food groups that are presented in proportions appropriate for a healthy diet. Fig. 39-1 and Table 39-1 show these food groups with the recommended daily requirements and examples of common sources. The essential components of the basic food groups are carbohydrates, fats, proteins, vitamins, and minerals.

Carbohydrates, the body's primary source of energy, yield approximately 4 kilocalories per gram. (Kilocalorie is the correct unit to designate caloric intake and expenditure. However, calorie is more commonly used.) Carbohydrates are either simple or complex. Simple carbohydrates come in two forms: *monosaccharides* (e.g., glucose and fructose), which are found in fruits and honey, and *disaccharides* (e.g., sucrose, maltose, and lac-

Reviewed by Karen Goff, RN, BSN, Case Manager, GI Services, Saint Joseph's Hospital of Atlanta, Atlanta, Ga.

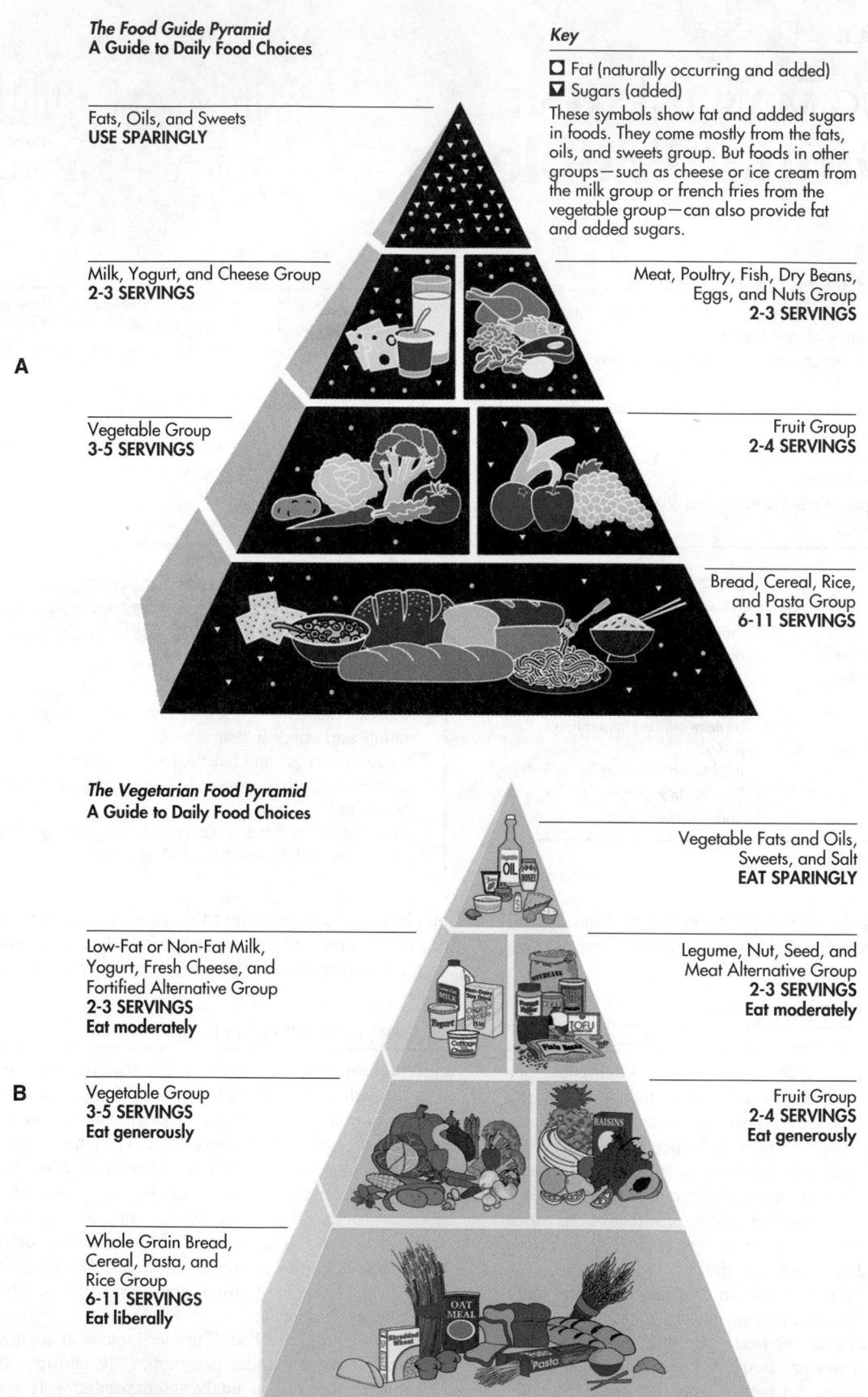

The Food Guide Pyramid
A Guide to Daily Food Choices

Key

☐ Fat (naturally occurring and added)
▽ Sugars (added)

These symbols show fat and added sugars in foods. They come mostly from the fats, oils, and sweets group. But foods in other groups—such as cheese or ice cream from the milk group or french fries from the vegetable group—can also provide fat and added sugars.

Fats, Oils, and Sweets
USE SPARINGLY

Milk, Yogurt, and Cheese Group
2-3 SERVINGS

Meat, Poultry, Fish, Dry Beans, Eggs, and Nuts Group
2-3 SERVINGS

A

Vegetable Group
3-5 SERVINGS

Fruit Group
2-4 SERVINGS

Bread, Cereal, Rice, and Pasta Group
6-11 SERVINGS

The Vegetarian Food Pyramid
A Guide to Daily Food Choices

Vegetable Fats and Oils, Sweets, and Salt
EAT SPARINGLY

Low-Fat or Non-Fat Milk, Yogurt, Fresh Cheese, and Fortified Alternative Group
2-3 SERVINGS
Eat moderately

Legume, Nut, Seed, and Meat Alternative Group
2-3 SERVINGS
Eat moderately

B

Vegetable Group
3-5 SERVINGS
Eat generously

Fruit Group
2-4 SERVINGS
Eat generously

Whole Grain Bread, Cereal, Pasta, and Rice Group
6-11 SERVINGS
Eat liberally

FIG. 39-1 **A,** Food guide pyramid: a guide to daily food choices and number of servings. **B,** Vegetarian food guide pyramid.

TABLE 39-1	Pyramid Food Groups and Recommended Number of Servings			
GROUP	**NUTRIENTS PROVIDED**	**NUMBER OF SERVINGS DAILY**	**SERVING SIZE**
• Bread, cereal, rice, pasta	Thiamine, niacin, iron, protein	6-11	1 slice of bread 1 oz ready-to-eat cereal ½ cup of cooked cereal, rice, or pasta
• Vegetable	Vitamins A and C, folic acid	3-5	1 cup of raw leafy vegetables ½ cup of other vegetables, cooked or raw ¾ cup of vegetable juice
• Fruit	Vitamins A and C	2-4	1 medium apple, banana, or orange ½ cup of chopped, cooked, or canned fruit ¾ cup of fruit juice
• Milk, yogurt, cheese	Calcium, protein, riboflavin, vitamin B_6, and cobalamin	2-3	1 cup of milk or yogurt 1½ oz of natural cheese 2 oz of processed cheese
• Meat, poultry, fish, dry beans, eggs, nuts	Protein, niacin, thiamine, iron, zinc, cobalamin, folic acid	2-3	2-3 oz of cooked lean meat, poultry, or fish ½ cup of cooked dry beans, 1 egg, or 2 tbs of peanut butter (count as 1 oz lean meat)

tose), which are found in such substances as table sugar, malted cereal, and milk, respectively. Complex carbohydrates or polysaccharides commonly appear in the diet as starches, such as cereal grains, potatoes, and legumes. Carbohydrates are the chief protein-sparing ingredient in a nutritionally sound diet and compose approximately 47% of the daily caloric needs of the body. The National Research Council recommends that at least half of the body's energy needs should come from carbohydrates, especially complex carbohydrates.[2]

Approximately 36% of the daily caloric intake in current American diets is derived from fat.[2] This level is considerably higher than that found in many other societies and is a cause for concern. The Food and Nutrition Board's Committee on Diet and Health recommends that people reduce their fat intake to 30% of their total daily caloric intake.[3] One gram of fat yields 9 calories. Fats are stored in adipose tissue and in the abdominal cavity. Besides being a major source of energy, fats act as insulation, which reduces loss of body heat in cold environments and provides padding and protection for vital organs. Fats also act as carriers of essential fatty acids and fat-soluble vitamins. Fats provide a feeling of satiety after eating, partly from the flavor added and partly from their slow rate of digestion, which delays hunger. The daily caloric requirements of a person are influenced by body build, age, gender, and physical activity. Adjustments in caloric intake are necessary depending on changes in health status and daily activity level. An average adult requires an estimated 20 to 35 calories per kilogram of body weight per day, leaning toward the higher end if the person is critically ill or very active and the lower end if the person is sedentary.[4]

Proteins, another essential component of a well-balanced diet, are obtained from both animal and plant sources. Ideally, proteins provide 15% to 20% of daily caloric needs.[3] The recommended daily protein intake is 0.8 to 1 g/kg of body weight. One gram of protein yields 4 calories. Proteins are complex nitrogenous organic compounds, of which amino acids are the fundamental units of structure. The 22 amino acids can be classified as essential and nonessential. The body is capable of synthesizing nonessential

TABLE 39-2	Good Sources of Protein	
COMPLETE PROTEINS	**INCOMPLETE PROTEINS**
Milk and milk products (e.g., cheese)	Grains (e.g., corn)
Eggs	Legumes (e.g., navy beans, soybeans, peas)
Fish	Nuts (e.g., peanuts)
Meats	Seeds (e.g., sesame seeds, sunflower seeds)
Poultry	

amino acids if an adequate supply of protein is available. However, the nine essential amino acids cannot be synthesized, and their availability depends totally on dietary sources. Protein sources containing all the essential amino acids are called *complete proteins*. Proteins that lack one or more of the essential amino acids are called *incomplete proteins*. Table 39-2 lists good sources of protein. Proteins are essential for tissue growth, repair, and maintenance; body regulatory functions; and energy production.

Vitamins are organic compounds required in small amounts by the body for normal metabolism. Vitamins function primarily in enzyme reactions that facilitate the metabolism of amino acids, fats, and carbohydrates. The body must rely on a dietary source to meet requirements for some vitamins, such as cobalamin (vitamin B_{12}). Vitamins are divided into two categories: water-soluble vitamins (vitamin C and the B-complex vitamins) and fat-soluble vitamins (vitamins A, D, E, and K).

Mineral salts (e.g., magnesium, iron, calcium) make up approximately 4% of the total body weight. When minerals are present in minute amounts, they are referred to as trace elements. Minerals required in amounts greater than 100 mg per day are called major minerals. Table 39-3 lists the major minerals and trace elements. Minerals are necessary for the body to build tissues, regulate body fluids, and assist in various body functions. Some minerals are stored in a manner similar to that of the fat-

TABLE 39-3	Major Minerals and Trace Elements	
MAJOR MINERALS	**TRACE ELEMENTS**	
Calcium	Chromium	
Chloride	Copper	
Magnesium	Fluoride	
Phosphorus	Iodine	
Potassium	Iron	
Sodium	Manganese	
Sulfur	Molybdenum	
	Selenium	
	Zinc	

TABLE 39-4	**Nutritional Therapy** Foods High in Iron*	
FOOD		**SELECTED SERVING SIZE**
Breads, Cereals, and Grain Products		
Farina, regular or quick cooked (enriched)		⅔ cup
Oatmeal, instant, fortified, prepared (enriched)		⅔ cup
Ready-to-eat cereals, fortified (enriched)		1 oz
Meat, Poultry, Fish, and Alternatives		
Beef liver, braised		3 oz
Pork liver, braised		3 oz
Chicken or turkey liver, braised		½ cup diced
Clams: steamed, boiled, or canned (drained)		3 oz
Oysters: baked, broiled, steamed, or canned (undrained)		3 oz
Soybeans, cooked		½ cup

*These foods provide 25% to 39% of the recommended dietary allowance (RDA) of iron.

soluble vitamins and can be toxic if taken in excess amounts. The amount of minerals needed in the daily diet varies greatly from a few micrograms of trace minerals to 1 g or more of the major minerals, such as calcium, phosphorus, and sodium. A well-balanced diet can usually meet the daily requirements of needed minerals. However, deficiency states can occur.

SPECIAL DIETS

Vegetarian Diet

The common element among all vegetarians is the exclusion of red meat from the diet. Vegetarians have a variety of reasons for following this dietary practice, including religious or cultural beliefs that it is a better way of attaining total health, respect for all living beings, ethical-ecologic ideals, and economics. Many vegetarians are *vegans,* who are pure or total vegetarians and eat only plant food, and *lacto-ovo-vegetarians,* who eat plant foods and sometimes dairy products and eggs.

Vegetarians can have vitamin or protein deficiencies unless their diets are well-planned. Plant protein, although of a lesser quality than that of animal origin, fulfills most of the protein requirements. Combinations of vegetable protein foods (e.g., cornmeal, kidney beans) can increase the nutritional value. Lacto-ovo-vegetarians obtain additional protein sources from dairy products and eggs. Milk made from soybeans is an excellent protein source, especially for the true vegan. The primary deficiency of a strict vegan is lack of cobalamin (vitamin B$_{12}$). This vitamin can be obtained only from animal protein, special supplements, or foods that have been fortified with the vitamin. Vegans not using cobalamin supplements are susceptible to the development of megaloblastic anemia and the neurologic signs of cobalamin deficiency. Strict vegetarians and lacto-ovo-vegetarians are also at risk for iron deficiency. Iron-enriched foods or iron supplements are prescribed during pregnancy, early childhood, and adolescence and after major blood loss. Table 39-4 lists examples of foods high in iron. Other deficiencies that may be present in a vegan diet include calcium, zinc, vitamins A and D, and protein.

MALNUTRITION

Malnutrition is an excess, deficit, or imbalance in the essential components of a balanced diet (Fig. 39-2). Terms such as undernutrition and overnutrition are also used to describe malnutrition. **Undernutrition** describes a state of poor nourishment as a result of inadequate diet or diseases that interfere with normal appetite and assimilation of ingested food. **Overnutrition** refers to the ingestion of more food than is required for body needs, as in obesity. An example of nutrient imbalance is a vitamin deficiency state such as *rickets,* a bone disorder caused by inadequate vitamin D. *Scurvy* is a condition characterized by weakness, anemia, and oral ulcerations that is associated with inadequate vitamin C intake.

Malnutrition is most prevalent in developing countries in which adequate food sources do not exist, the inhabitants are not well educated about their nutritional needs, and economic conditions often preclude the purchase of a balanced diet. Undernutrition does exist in the United States, and it is usually found in individuals or groups from the lower socioeconomic class or in individuals who have chronic or acute illnesses. Malnutrition is common in hospitalized patients, with an incidence of 30% to 55%.[5] The prevalence of elderly long-term care residents who can be found to have protein-calorie malnutrition ranges from 23% to 85%.[6]

Types of Malnutrition

Protein-Calorie Malnutrition. Protein-calorie malnutrition (PCM) is the most common form of undernutrition and can result from either primary or secondary factors. Primary PCM is present when nutritional needs are not met as a result of poor eat-

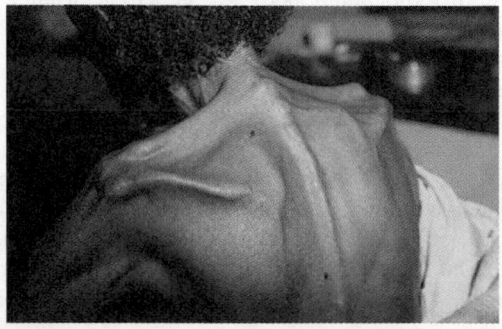

FIG. 39-2 Patient with malnutrition.

ing habits. Secondary PCM is the result of an alteration or defect in ingestion, digestion, absorption, or metabolism. In this type of malnutrition, tissue needs are not met even though the dietary intake would be satisfactory under normal conditions. Secondary malnutrition may occur as a result of gastrointestinal (GI) obstruction, surgical procedure, cancer, malabsorption syndromes, drugs, or infectious diseases.

PCM may also be due to the ingestion of foods deficient in protein. In addition to decreased quantities of protein, the diet is generally low in necessary vitamins and minerals. Most malnourished ill patients have this type of combined PCM.

Marasmus and Kwashiorkor. **Marasmus** is the result of a concomitant deficiency of both caloric and protein intake leading to generalized loss of body fat and muscle. Patients generally appear "wasted," or emaciated, but may have normal serum protein levels. **Kwashiorkor** is caused by a deficiency of protein intake that is superimposed on a catabolic stress event, such as a GI obstruction, a surgical procedure, cancer, a malabsorption syndrome, or an infectious disease. These patients may appear well nourished but have very low serum protein levels.

Etiology and Pathophysiology

Starvation Process. Knowledge of the phases of the starvation process is essential to better understand the physiologic changes that occur in PCM. Initially, the body selectively uses carbohydrates (glycogen) rather than fat and protein to meet metabolic needs. These carbohydrate stores, found in the liver and muscles, are minimal and may be totally depleted within 18 hours. During this early phase of starvation, the only use of protein is in its obligatory participation in cellular metabolism. However, once carbohydrate stores are depleted, protein begins to be converted to glucose for energy. Alanine and glutamine are the first amino acids to be used by the liver for the formation of glucose in a process termed *gluconeogenesis*. The resulting available plasma glucose allows the metabolic processes to continue. With these amino acids being used as energy sources, the person may be in negative nitrogen balance (greater nitrogen excretion). However, within 5 to 9 days, body fat is fully mobilized to supply much of the needed energy.

In prolonged starvation up to 97% of calories are provided by fat, and protein is conserved. Depletion of fat stores depends on the amount available, but fat stores are generally used up in 4 to 6 weeks. Once fat stores are used, body proteins, including those in internal organs and plasma, can no longer be spared and rapidly decrease because they are the only remaining body source of energy available.

If the malnourished patient has surgery, experiences bodily trauma, or has an infection, the stress response with concomitant increase in energy expenditure is superimposed on the starvation response. These body insults cause an increase in the metabolic rate, with a subsequent increase in energy requirements. Protein stores are no longer spared and are used with increasing frequency for body energy because of the increased metabolic energy needs.

As the protein depletion continues, liver function is impaired, and synthesis of proteins is diminished. The plasma oncotic pressure is decreased because of decreased protein synthesis. A major function of plasma proteins, primarily of albumin, is the maintenance of the osmotic pressure of the blood. Because of this decreased pressure, a shift in body fluids occurs from the vascular space into the interstitial compartment. As protein ingestion decreases and body stores are depleted, albumin eventu-

ally leaks into the interstitial space along with the fluid. Edema becomes clinically observable. Often the edema present in the face and legs of the patient masks the muscle wasting that occurs.

As the total blood volume is reduced, the skin appears dry and wrinkled. Along with the shift of fluids to the interstitial space, ions also move. Sodium (a predominant extracellular ion) is found in increased amounts within the cell, and potassium (a predominant intracellular ion) and magnesium are shifted to the extracellular space. The sodium-potassium exchange pump has high energy needs, using 20% to 50% of all calories ingested. When the diet is extremely deficient in calories and essential proteins, the pump will fail, leaving sodium inside the cell (along with water), and the cell will expand.

The liver is the body organ that loses the most mass during protein deprivation. It gradually becomes infiltrated with fat secondary to decreased synthesis of lipoproteins. Immediate restoration to a diet of protein and other necessary constituents must be instituted, or death will rapidly ensue.

Causes of Malnutrition. Many factors contribute to the development of malnutrition, including socioeconomic status, cultural influences, psychologic disorders, medical conditions, and medical treatments. Table 39-5 lists conditions that increase the risk of malnutrition. Because individuals and families from the lower socioeconomic class spend a greater percentage of their income on food, there is a tendency to seek out cheaper foods as the cost of food increases. These foods may not provide adequate or balanced nutrition. In contrast, some lower-income persons may prefer to select foods that are more expensive but only marginally nutritious because of their prestige value. The nurse and the registered dietitian can assist their patients in making food choices that meet nutritional requirements while staying within their limited resources.

Patients with physical illnesses. Regardless of the cause of the illness, the sick person has increased nutritional needs. Pathologic conditions are frequently aggravated by undernutrition, and an existing deficiency state is likely to become more severe during illness. Malnutrition is not an uncommon consequence of illness, surgery, injury, or hospitalization. Anorexia, nausea, vomiting, diarrhea, abdominal distention, and abdominal cramping may accompany diseases of the GI system. Any combination of these symptoms interferes with normal food consumption and metabolism. In addition, a patient may restrict the dietary intake to a few foods or fluids that may not be nutritionally sound out of fear of aggravating the already disturbed GI function.

Malabsorption syndrome is defined as the impaired absorption of nutrients from the GI tract. It may result from decreased amounts of necessary enzymes or a reduced bowel surface area

TABLE 39-5	Conditions That Increase the Risk for Malnutrition

- Chronic alcoholism
- Decreased mobility that limits access to food or its preparation
- Nutrient losses from malabsorption, dialysis, fistulas, or wounds
- Drugs with antinutrient or catabolic properties, such as corticosteroids and oral antibiotics
- Extreme need for nutrients because of hypermetabolism or stresses such as infection, burns, trauma, or fever
- No oral intake and/or receiving standard intravenous solutions (5% dextrose) for 10 days or for 5 days in older adults

and can quickly lead to a deficiency state. Many drugs may have undesirable GI side effects, as well as alter normal digestive and absorptive processes. For example, antibiotics change the normal flora of the intestines, decreasing the body's ability to synthesize biotin.

Fever accompanies many illnesses, injuries, and infections, with a concomitant increase in the body's basal metabolic rate (BMR). Each degree of temperature increase on the Fahrenheit scale raises the BMR by about 7%.[7] Without an increase in the amount of calories ingested in the diet, body protein stores will be used to supply calories, and protein depletion can become a problem.

The hospitalized patient, especially the older adult, is at risk of becoming malnourished. Prolonged illness, major surgery, sepsis, draining wounds, burns, hemorrhage, fractures, and immobilization can all contribute to malnutrition. The nurse must assume responsibility, along with the health care provider and the dietitian, for meeting the patient's nutritional needs. The nurse must also be knowledgeable of the requirements of a patient who is not overtly ill but who is undergoing diagnostic studies. This patient may be nutritionally fit on entering the hospital but can develop nutritional problems because of the dietary restrictions imposed by multiple diagnostic studies.

Incomplete diets. Vitamin deficiencies are rare in most of the developed countries of the world. When vitamin deficiencies are present, several vitamins are usually involved rather than a single vitamin deficiency. The recommended dietary allowances or Dietary Reference Intakes (DRIs) for essential vitamins and minerals can be obtained by eating a diet consisting of foods from the basic five food groups. DRIs from the Food and Nutrition Board have a safety margin because the levels exceed minimum daily requirements for most people.[8] When vitamin imbalances do occur, they are usually found among persons with a pattern of alcohol and drug abuse, persons who are chronically ill, and individuals who follow poor dietary practices. Followers of fad diets or poorly planned vegetarian diets are also subject to a potential deficiency state. Clinical manifestations of vitamin imbalances are most commonly exhibited as neurologic manifestations (Table 39-6). In the growing child, the central nervous system (CNS) is primarily involved, whereas the peripheral nervous system is most affected in the adult.

Food-drug interactions. When health conditions require drug therapy, drug and food interactions may not be explored before starting a prescription. Adverse interactions can include incompatibilities, altered drug effectiveness, and impaired nutritional status. Table 39-7 outlines examples of common drug

TABLE 39-6   Recommended Dietary Vitamin Allowances and Manifestations of Imbalance

VITAMIN	RDA	MANIFESTATIONS OF OVERDOSE	MANIFESTATIONS OF DEFICIENCIES
Fat Soluble			
A	Men: 1000 μg/retinol equivalents* Women: 800 μg/retinol equivalents	Hair loss, dry skin; headaches; dry mucous membranes; liver damage; bone and joint pain; blurred vision; nausea and vomiting	Dry, scaly skin; increased susceptibility to infection; night blindness; anorexia; eye irritation; xerosis (dry skin); keratinization of respiratory and GI mucosa; bladder stones; anemia; retarded growth
D	Adults: 5-10 μg of cholecalciferol†	Deposits of calcium and phosphorus in soft tissue; kidney and heart damage; bone fragility; constipation; anorexia, nausea, vomiting; headache	Muscular weakness; excessive sweating; diarrhea and other GI disturbances; bone pain; active rickets; healed rickets; osteomalacia
E	Men: 10 mg Women: 8 mg	Relatively nontoxic	Neurologic defects
K	Men: 70-80 μg Women: 60-65 μg	Anemia	Defective blood coagulation
Water Soluble			
B₁	Men: 1.2-1.5 mg Women: 1-1.1 mg	Not stored in body, therefore overdose does not occur	Loss of appetite; fatigue; nervous irritability; constipation; paresthesias; insomnia
B₆	Men: 1.7-2 mg Women: 1.4-1.6 mg	Not stored in body, therefore overdose does not occur	Seizures; dermatitis; anemia; neuropathy with motor weakness; anorexia
Cobalamin (B₁₂)	Adults: 2-10 μg	Not stored in body, therefore overdose does not occur	Megaloblastic anemia; inadequate myelin synthesis; anorexia; glossitis; sore mouth and tongue; pallor; neurologic problems such as depression and dizziness; weight loss; nausea; constipation
C	Adults: 50-60 mg	Not stored in body, therefore overdose does not occur	Bleeding gums; loose teeth; easy bruising; poor wound healing; scurvy; dry, itchy skin
Folic acid	Men: 200 μg Women: 180 μg	Not stored in body, therefore overdose does not occur	Impaired cell division and protein synthesis; megaloblastic anemia; anorexia; fatigue; sore tongue; diarrhea; forgetfulness

*1 Retinol equivalent = 10 IU vitamin A activity from β-carotene or 3.33 IU vitamin A activity from retinol.
†1 μg of cholecalciferol = 40 IU vitamin D.
GI, Gastrointestinal; *RDA,* recommended dietary allowance.

TABLE 39-7	Common Drug and Food/Nutrient Interactions	
DRUG CATEGORY/DRUG	**FOOD/NUTRIENT**	**DRUG-FOOD EFFECTS OR CAUTIONS**
Anticoagulants	Dietary vitamin K (e.g., green leafy vegetables, green tea, dairy products/meats)	Decrease or loss of anticoagulant effect
Antiseizure agents • phenytoin (Dilantin)	Folic acid	Long-term drug use may increase folic acid requirement
Antidepressants • trazodone (Desyrel)	Food	Food slows drug absorption
• Tricyclic antidepressants	Riboflavin	Riboflavin requirements may increase with amitriptyline (Elavil) or imipramine (Tofranil)
Antidiabetic agents • glyburide (Micronase, DiaBeta)	High-fat diet	Drug should not be taken with high-fat diet
Antithyroid agents • methimazole (Tapazole)	Food	Foods may inconsistently alter bioavailability of methimazole
Barbiturates • phenobarbital • mephobarbital (Mebaral)	Folic acid	Drugs may increase folic acid requirements; long-term therapy may require vitamin D supplements for osteomalacia
β-Adrenergic blockers • labetalol (Normodyne) • metaproterenol (Alupent) • carteolol (Cartrol) • sotalol (Betapace)	Food	Bioavailability of these drugs may be enhanced when taken with food
Bronchodilators • theophylline • oxtriphylline (Choledyl)	High-carbohydrate, low-protein diets	↓ Drug elimination
• dyphylline (Lufyllin)	Caffeine-containing foods and fluids	Caffeine may increase CNS stimulant effects of xanthine-derivative bronchodilators
cholestyramine (Questran)	Fat-soluble vitamins	Drug may interfere with their absorption
Corticosteroids (prolonged therapy)	Salt seasonings	May require decreased sodium and/or potassium supplementation intake
erythropoietin	Folic acid and/or cobalamin	Nutrient deficiencies may reduce/delay drug response
etidronate (Didronel)	Foods, fluids, or drugs high in calcium	May prevent drug absorption
furazolidone (Furoxone)	Food and fluids containing tyramine (e.g., aged cheese, smoked or pickled meats or poultry, fermented meat, overripe fruit, beer, wine, liqueurs)	MAO-inhibiting effects may last at least 2 wk after stopping drug. Dietary restrictions need to continue for at least 2 wk after MAO inhibitors discontinued if received large doses or prolonged therapy
isoniazid (INH)	Cheese (e.g., Swiss) or fish (e.g., tuna, skipjack)	Concurrent ingestion may lead to redness or itching, HR changes, sweating, chills or clammy feeling, headache or light-headedness; thought to be related to altered metabolism of tyramine in foods
Phenothiazines	Riboflavin	Drugs may increase riboflavin requirements
procarbazine (Matulane)	Food and fluids containing tyramine or other high-pressor amines (e.g., aged cheese, smoked or pickled meats or poultry, fermented meat, overripe fruit, beer, wine, liqueurs)	When used concurrently, may cause sudden and severe hypertensive reactions; dietary restrictions need to continue for at least 2 wk after MAO inhibitors discontinued
selegiline (Eldepryl)	Food and fluids containing tyramine (e.g., aged cheese, smoked or pickled meats or poultry, fermented meat, overripe fruit, beer, wine, liqueurs)	When used concurrently, may cause sudden and severe hypertensive reactions; dietary restrictions need to continue for at least 2 wk after MAO inhibitors discontinued
ticlopidine (Ticlid)	Food	Drug absorption increased when taken after a meal
zafirlukast (Accolate)	High-fat and high-protein meal	When taken concurrently, drug bioavailability reduced by about 40%
Zinc supplements	Foods	Many foods (e.g., fiber, milk casein) impair zinc absorption

CNS, Central nervous system; *HR,* heart rate; *MAO,* monoamine oxidase.

and food/nutrient interactions. As members of the health team, nurses have a responsibility for monitoring and preventing potential interactions for patients while in the hospital and at home.

Clinical Manifestations. The adult who is deprived of adequate protein and calories will have many of the clinical manifestations presented in Table 39-8. The most obvious clinical signs on physical examination are apparent in the skin, eyes, mouth, muscles, and CNS. The speed at which the protein deficiency develops depends on the quantity and quality of the protein intake, caloric value, illness, and the age of the person.

Clinical manifestations of malnutrition are the result of numerous interactions occurring at the cellular level. As protein intake is severely reduced, the muscles, which make up the largest reservoir of protein in the body, become wasted and flabby, leading to weakness, fatigability, and decreased endurance. There is decreased protein available for repair, and as a result, wound healing may be delayed. Malnutrition in the hospitalized patient may result in delayed recovery and prolonged hospitalization. The person is more susceptible to all types of infections. Both humoral and cell-mediated immunity are deficient in PCM. There is a decrease in leukocytes in the peripheral blood. Phagocytosis is altered as a result of the lack of energy (adenosine triphosphate [ATP]) necessary to drive the process. Most malnourished persons are anemic. Anemia resulting from PCM is usually caused by nutritional deficiencies in iron and folic acid, the necessary building blocks for red blood cells (RBCs).

The severity of complications from malnutrition ranges from mild to emaciation and death. Major complications center around

TABLE 39-8	Manifestations of Protein-Calorie Malnutrition	
BODY SYSTEM	**SUBCLINICAL MANIFESTATIONS**	**CLINICAL MANIFESTATIONS**
Integumentary	Slowed tissue turnover rate, surface temperature 1°-2° F cooler	Brittle nails, ↓ tone and elasticity of skin, xeroderma (dry skin), pigment changes (brown-gray), erythematous seborrheic dermatitis, scrotal dermatitis
Visual	Night blindness	Hair: easy loss of hair, color changes, lack of luster
		Blood vessel growth in cornea, Bitot's spots (gray keratinized epithelium on conjunctiva), dryness of conjunctiva and cornea, pale to red conjunctiva
Gastrointestinal		
Mouth and lips	Reduction in saliva production	Cheilosis (crusting and ulceration at angle of mouth)
Tongue	Mucosa more permeable to bacteria	Raw and beefy red, edematous and smooth, atrophy or hypertrophy of papillae
Teeth	Improper development, delayed eruption	Caries, loose teeth, discolored enamel
Gingivae		Periodontal disease, tendency to bleed easily, receding, pale, and soft
Stomach	↓ Gastric secretion, delayed gastric emptying	Constant hunger, ↑ incidence of ulcers
Intestines	↓ Motility and absorption, normal flora causing infection from ↑ permeability of mucosa	Diarrhea and flatulence, protruding abdomen, ↑ incidence of parasitic diseases
Liver-biliary	Fatty liver, ↓ absorption of fat-soluble vitamins	Hepatomegaly
Cardiovascular	↓ Cardiac output, ↓ hemoglobin, shift in heart position, ↑ risk of thrombophlebitis	↓ Blood pressure and pulse, slight cyanosis, anemia, body edema
Endocrine	↓ Insulin production	Thyroid enlargement, polydipsia, polyuria, ↑ sensitivity to cold
Immunologic	↓ Lymphocyte proliferation, ↓ albumin levels, ↓ antibody production, diminished febrile response to infection	↑ Number of infections, ↓ response to delayed hypersensitivity skin tests
Musculoskeletal	↓ Growth rate, ↓ body stature with chronic PCM, ↓ muscle mass	Prominence of bony structures such as face, clavicle, scapula, ribs, iliac crests, and spinal vertebrae due to subcutaneous tissue loss; weak and spindly arms and legs, flat buttocks, weak and flabby muscles; ↓ physical activity and ability to work; severe weight loss
Neurologic	Loss of ambition, feeling of being tired	Depression, confusion, ↓ reflexes in legs and ankles, ↓ position sense, ↓ vibratory sense, paresthesias of hands and feet, syncope, motor weakness
Renal	Negative nitrogen balance, ↓ BUN and creatinine levels	Nocturia, ↓ urinary output
Reproductive	↓ Gonadotropin levels	Amenorrhea, impotence, atrophied breasts
Respiratory	Pulmonary edema, ↓ strength of respiratory muscles	↑ Susceptibility to respiratory infection, ↓ respiratory rate, ↓ vital capacity

BUN, Blood urea nitrogen; *PCM*, protein-calorie malnutrition.

delayed wound healing and increased susceptibility to infection from decreased immune function.

Diagnostic Studies

History and physical examination. A diet history of foods eaten over the past week will reveal a great deal about the patient's dietary habits and knowledge of good nutrition. In addition to the height, weight, and vital signs, the patient's physical state should be thoroughly assessed and documented. Each body system should be assessed. Table 39-9 summarizes the assessment and findings of the patient with malnutrition.

The diagnosis of PCM can be determined by a variety of laboratory studies used in conjunction with the physical examination. Serum albumin is somewhat useful in the diagnosis of malnutrition. The degree of protein depletion can be identified with the use of the scale in Table 39-10. Serum albumin has a half-life of approximately 20 to 22 days. In the absence of marked fluid loss, such as from hemorrhage or burns, the serum albumin value lags behind actual protein changes by more than 2 weeks and

TABLE 39-10	Serum Albumin and Prealbumin Levels
Albumin	
Normal value	3.8-4.5 g/dl (38-45 g/L)
Mild depletion	3.0-3.7 g/dl (30-37 g/L)
Moderate depletion	2.5-2.9 g/dl (25-29 g/L)
Severe depletion	<2.5 g/dl (<25 g/L)
Prealbumin	
Normal value	20 mg/dl (200 mg/L)
Mild depletion	10-15 mg/dl (100-150 mg/L)
Moderate depletion	5-10 mg/dl (50-100 mg/L)
Severe depletion	<5 mg/dl (<50 mg/L)

TABLE 39-9	Nursing Assessment Malnutrition

Subjective Data

Important Health Information

Past health history: Severe burns, major trauma, hemorrhage, draining wounds, bone fractures with prolonged immobility, chronic renal or liver disease, cancer, malabsorption syndrome, GI obstruction, infectious diseases (TB, AIDS)

Medications: Corticosteroids, chemotherapeutic agents, diet pills

Surgery or other treatments: Recent surgery, radiation

Functional Health Patterns

Health perception–health management: Alcohol or drug abuse; malaise, apathy

Nutritional-metabolic: Increase or decrease in weight, weight problems; increase or decrease in appetite, typical dietary intake; food preferences and aversions; food allergies or intolerance; ill-fitting or absent dentures; dry mouth, difficulty in chewing or swallowing; bloating or gas; ↑ sensitivity to cold; delayed wound healing

Elimination: Constipation, diarrhea, nocturia, decreased urinary output

Activity-exercise: Increase or decrease in activity patterns; weakness, fatigue, decreased endurance

Cognitive-perceptual: Pain in mouth; paresthesias; loss of position and vibratory sense

Role-relationship: Change in family (e.g., loss of a spouse); financial resources

Sexual-reproductive: Amenorrhea, impotence, decreased libido

Objective Data

General

Listless, cachectic; underweight for height

Integumentary

Dry, brittle, sparse hair with color changes and lack of luster, alopecia; dry, scaly lips, fever blisters, angular crusts and lesions at corners of mouth (cheilosis); brittle, ridged nails; decreased tone and elasticity of skin; cool, rough, dry, scaly skin with brown-gray pigment changes; reddened, scaly dermatitis, scrotal dermatitis; slight cyanosis; peripheral edema

Eyes

Pale or red conjunctivae, gray keratinized epithelium on conjunctiva (Bitot's spots); dryness and dull appearance of conjunctiva and cornea, soft cornea; blood vessel growth in cornea; redness and fissuring of eyelid corners

Respiratory

Decreased respiratory rate, ↓ vital capacity, crackles, weak cough

Cardiovascular

Increase or decrease in heart rate, ↓ BP, arrhythmias

Gastrointestinal

Swollen, smooth, raw, beefy red tongue (glossitis), hypertrophic or atrophic papillae; dental caries, absent or loose teeth, discolored tooth enamel; spongy, pale, receded gums with a tendency to bleed easily, periodontal disease; ulcerations, white patches or plaques, redness, swelling of oral mucosa; distended, tympanic abdomen; ascites, hepatomegaly, decreased bowel sounds; steatorrhea

Neurologic

Decreased or loss of reflexes, tremor; inattention, irritability, confusion, syncope

Musculoskeletal

Decreased muscle mass with poor tone, "wasted" appearance; bowlegs, knock-knees, beaded ribs, chest deformity, prominent bony structures

Possible Findings

↓ Hemoglobin and hematocrit; ↓ MCV, MCH, or MCHC (iron deficiency); ↑ MCV or MHC (folic acid or cobalamin deficiency); altered serum electrolyte levels, especially hyperkalemia; ↓ BUN and creatinine; ↓ serum albumin, transferrin, and prealbumin; ↓ lymphocytes; ↑ liver enzymes; ↓ serum vitamin levels

AIDS, Acquired immunodeficiency syndrome; *BUN,* blood urea nitrogen; *GI,* gastrointestinal; *MCH,* mean corpuscular hemoglobin; *MCHC,* mean corpuscular hemoglobin concentration; *MCV,* mean corpuscular volume; *TB,* tuberculosis.

therefore is not a good indicator of acute changes in nutritional status. Prealbumin, a protein synthesized by liver, has a half-life of 2 days and is a better indicator of recent or current nutritional status.[9] Serum transferrin level is another indicator of protein status. Transferrin, a protein synthesized by the liver and used to transport iron, decreases during states of protein deficiency.

Serum electrolyte levels reflect changes taking place between the intracellular and the extracellular spaces. The serum potassium level is often elevated. The RBC count and the hemoglobin level indicate the presence and degree of anemia. The total lymphocyte count decreases during malnutrition states. The total lymphocyte count is calculated by multiplying the percent of lymphocytes times the total white blood cell (WBC) count. Liver enzyme levels, a reflection of liver function, may be elevated during malnutrition. Serum levels of both fat-soluble and water-soluble vitamins are usually diminished in malnutrition. The lowered levels of the fat-soluble vitamins correlate with the clinical signs of *steatorrhea* (fatty stools).

Anthropometric measurements. Anthropometric measurements, which include gross measures of fat and muscle contents, may be ordered. These measurements tend to be most beneficial in evaluating long-term effects of malnutrition or responses to nutritional interventions. They consist of measures of skinfold thickness at various sites, which is an indicator of subcutaneous fat stores, and midarm muscle circumference, an indicator of protein stores. These measurements are then compared with standards for healthy persons of the same age and gender. Training and practice are required to perform these measurements accurately and reliably. To provide information on the patient's nutritional status in response to treatment, serial measurements are needed. Sites most reflective of body fat are those over the biceps and the triceps, below the scapula, above the iliac crest, and over the upper thigh. Both skinfold thickness and mid-arm muscle circumference measurements are decreased in chronic PCM and acute protein malnutrition. These measurements may also be influenced by shifts in hydration status. The exact relationship of the midarm circumference measure to body composition of functional protein, both muscle and nonmuscle, remains to be established.

NURSING MANAGEMENT
MALNUTRITION

■ Nursing Assessment

Across all settings of care delivery, the nurse must be aware of the nutritional status of the patient. The recording of the patient's height and weight is an important component of this assessment. The patient's current weight relative to usual body weight and ideal body weight, such as that listed in the Metropolitan Life Insurance tables (Table 39-11), is determined. The percent change in body weight over time provides information on the degree of weight loss. In addition, the nurse should get a record of the complete diet history from the patient or the family. The patient's nutritional state may not be the reason medical assistance was sought. However, it may well be a major factor in the outcome and perhaps the underlying reason for illness. The registered dietitian, pharmacist, and physician should also be involved in the assessment and planning of care. However, the nurse, as the first-line health care professional dealing with the patient, should take the initiative in determining the severity of any nutritional problems.

TABLE 39-11	**Desirable Weights for Men and Women***		
	FRAME SIZE		
HEIGHT	**SMALL**	**MEDIUM**	**LARGE**
Men			
5'2"	128-134	131-141	138-150
5'3"	130-136	133-143	140-153
5'4"	132-138	135-145	142-156
5'5"	134-140	137-148	144-160
5'6"	136-142	139-151	146-164
5'7"	138-145	142-154	149-168
5'8"	140-148	145-157	152-172
5'9"	142-151	148-160	155-176
5'10"	144-154	151-163	158-180
5'11"	146-157	154-166	161-184
6'	149-160	157-170	164-188
6'1"	152-164	160-174	168-192
6'2"	155-168	164-178	172-197
6'3"	158-172	167-182	176-202
6'4"	162-176	171-187	181-207
Women			
4'10"	102-111	109-121	118-131
4'11"	103-113	111-123	120-134
5'	104-115	113-126	122-137
5'1"	106-118	115-129	125-140
5'2"	108-121	118-132	128-143
5'3"	111-124	121-135	131-147
5'4"	114-127	124-138	134-151
5'5"	117-130	127-141	137-155
5'6"	120-133	130-144	140-159
5'7"	123-136	133-147	143-163
5'8"	126-139	136-150	146-167
5'9"	129-142	139-153	149-170
5'10"	132-145	142-156	152-173
5'11"	135-148	145-159	155-176
6'	138-151	148-162	158-179

*From 1983 Metropolitan Life Insurance Company weight tables by height and size of frame for people aged 25 to 59, in 1-inch shoes and wearing 5 lb of indoor clothing for men or 3 lb for women.

In many institutions (acute and long-term care) and in home care, the nurse is responsible for nutritional screening. Nutritional screening identifies individuals who are malnourished or at risk for malnutrition. The purpose of the nutrition screening is to determine if a more detailed nutrition assessment is necessary.[9-12] Table 39-12 provides an example of a nursing nutrition screening tool.[11] In long-term care, the Minimum Data Set (MDS) form queries the health care team on a number of items related to nutritional status.[12] In home care, the Outcome and Assessment Information Set (OASIS) prompts the nurse to collect myriad information on diet, oral intake, dental health, swallowing difficulties, and any needs for meal assistance. If nutritional problems are identified, a referral to a dietitian is suggested.

If the nutrition screening identifies an individual at nutritional risk, a full nutrition assessment is most often warranted. A nutrition assessment is a comprehensive approach to defining nutrition status that uses medical, nutrition, and medication histories; physical examination; anthropometric measurements; and laboratory data.[9]

TABLE 39-12 Admission Nutrition Screening Tool

A. Diagnosis

If the patient has at least *one* of the following diagnoses, circle and proceed to section E to consider the patient AT NUTRITIONAL RISK and stop here.

- Anorexia nervosa/bulimia nervosa
- Malabsorption (celiac sprue, ulcerative colitis, Crohn's disease, short bowel syndrome)
- Multiple trauma (closed head injury, penetrating trauma, multiple fractures)
- Pressure ulcers
- Major gastrointestinal surgery within the past year
- Cachexia (temporal wasting, muscle wasting, cancer, cardiac)
- Coma
- Diabetes
- End-stage liver disease
- End-stage renal disease
- Nonhealing wounds

B. Nutrition Intake History

If the patient has at least *one* of the following symptoms, circle and proceed to section E to consider the patient AT NUTRITIONAL RISK and stop here.

- Diarrhea (>500 ml × 2 days)
- Vomiting (>5 days)
- Reduced intake (<½ normal intake for >5 days)

C. Ideal Body Weight Standards

Compare the patient's current weight for height to the ideal body weight chart.

If at <80% of ideal body weight, proceed to section E to consider the patient AT NUTRITIONAL RISK and stop here.

D. Weight History

Any recent unplanned weight loss? No ___ Yes ___
   Amount (lb or kg) _____
   If yes, within the past _____ weeks or _____ months
   Current weight (lb or kg) _____
   Usual weight (lb or kg) _____
   Height (ft, in, or cm) _____
Find percentage of weight loss:

$$\frac{\text{Usual wt} - \text{Current wt}}{\text{Usual wt}} \times 100 = \underline{\hspace{1cm}} \% \text{ wt loss}$$

Compare the % wt loss with the chart below and circle appropriate value

Length of Time	Significant (%)	Severe (%)
1 week	1-2	>2
2-3 weeks	2-3	>3
1 month	4-5	>5
3 months	7-8	>8
5+ months	10	>10

If the patient has experienced a significant or severe weight loss, proceed to section E and consider the patient AT NUTRITIONAL RISK

E. Nurse Assessment

Using the above criteria, what is this patient's nutritional risk? (circle one)

LOW NUTRITIONAL RISK   AT NUTRITIONAL RISK

Adapted from Kovacevich DS et al: Nutrition risk classification: a valid and reproducible tool for nurses, *Nutr Clin Practice* 12:20-25, 1997.

■ Nursing Diagnoses

Nursing diagnoses for the patient with malnutrition include, but are not limited to, the following:

- Imbalanced nutrition: less than body requirements *related to* decreased access, ingestion, digestion, or absorption of food or to anorexia
- Self-care deficit (feeding) *related to* decreased strength and endurance, fatigue, and apathy
- Constipation or diarrhea *related to* poor eating patterns, immobility, or medication effects
- Deficient fluid volume *related to* factors affecting access to or absorption of fluids
- Risk for impaired skin integrity *related to* poor nutritional state
- Noncompliance *related to* alteration in perception, lack of motivation, or incompatibility of regimen with lifestyle or resources
- Activity intolerance *related to* weakness, fatigue, and inadequate caloric intake or iron stores

■ Planning

The overall goals are that the patient with malnutrition will (1) achieve weight gain, (2) consume a specified number of calories per day (with a diet individualized for the patient), and (3) have no adverse consequences related to malnutrition or nutrition therapies.

■ Nursing Implementation

Health Promotion. The nurse is in a good position to teach and reinforce healthy eating habits with individuals and groups of persons throughout their life span. The gap between perceived importance of nutrition and care in selecting foods has widened. To assist in these efforts are the Food and Drug Administration (FDA)–mandated food labels that are now on all packaged foods. The Dietary Guidelines for Americans offers key recommendations for improving nutrition that are useful points for a teaching program (Table 39-13).[13]

Acute Intervention. The nurse must assess the patient's nutritional state, as well as focus on the other physical problems of the patient. The nurse must become more aware of who is at risk, why, and how to intervene appropriately. In states of increased stress, such as surgery, severe trauma, and sepsis, more calories and protein are needed. Wound healing requires increased protein synthesis. When fever is present, the metabolic rate is increased

TABLE 39-13 Patient & Family Teaching Guide — Good Nutrition

The following recommendations apply to most people:

- Eat a variety of foods
- Choose a diet moderate in sugars
- Choose a diet moderate in salt and sodium
- If you drink alcoholic beverages, do so in moderation
- Choose a diet low in fat, unsaturated fat, and cholesterol
- Choose a diet with plenty of grain products, vegetables, and fruits
- Balance the food you eat with physical activity to maintain or improve your weight

and nitrogen loss is accelerated. Despite the return of body temperature to normal, the rate of protein breakdown and resynthesis may be accelerated for several weeks. After major surgery, several weeks of increased protein and calorie intake are needed to promote healing and replenish body stores.

The nurse must have a thorough understanding of nutritional support and the rationale for recording the daily weight, intake, and output. Daily weights can give an ongoing record of body weight gain or loss. However, rapid gains and losses are usually the result of shifts in fluid balance. The body weight, in conjunction with accurate recording of food and fluid intake, provides a clearer picture of the patient's fluid and nutritional state. To obtain an accurate weight, the nurse should weigh the patient at the same time each day, on the same scale, with the same type or amount of clothing, and preferably with the bladder recently emptied.

The protein and calorie intake required in the malnourished patient depends on the cause of the malnutrition, the treatment being employed, and other stressors affecting the patient. If the patient is able to take food by mouth, a daily calorie count and diet diary can be obtained to give an accurate record of food intake. The nurse and the dietitian working with the patient and family can assist in the selection of high-calorie and high-protein foods (unless medically contraindicated). Preparation of foods preferred by the patient enhances the daily intake. Discussion with the patient and family about foods that should be eaten to provide high-protein, high-calorie content is important. The family can be encouraged to bring the patient's favorite foods from home while the patient is still hospitalized. Table 39-14 gives an example of a high-calorie, high-protein diet.

The undernourished patient usually needs to have between-meal supplements. These may consist of items prepared in the dietary department or commercially prepared products. Eating these items between meals increases the total daily intake and provides extra calories, proteins, fluids, and nutrients. In addition, multiple small feedings improve the tolerance for food intake by distributing the amount more evenly throughout the day. If the patient is unable to consume enough nutrition with a high-calorie, high-protein diet, nutrition supplements can be added.

TABLE 39-14 **Nutritional Therapy**

High-Calorie, High-Protein Diet

General Principles
1. A normal diet is supplemented with larger portions to increase the protein and caloric content. It is used for patients with hypermetabolism, burns, excessive stress, and cancer.
2. It is important to eat regularly and not to skip meals or snacks.

MEAL	PROTEIN (G)	SAMPLE MENU PLAN 1	SAMPLE MENU PLAN 2	MENU PLAN 3
Breakfast				
Fruit	2	Large orange juice	Large apple juice	½ grapefruit
Starch, fat		1 toast with butter or jelly	Flour tortilla with butter	Biscuits and gravy
Starch, protein supplement	4	Cream of wheat with 2 tbs skim milk powder	Atole with 2 tbs skim milk powder	Grits with 2 tbs margarine
2 meat	14	2 poached eggs	2 fried eggs	Omelet with 2 eggs
Milk, protein supplement	10	High-protein milk shake (2 tbs skim milk powder added)	High-protein milk shake	High-protein milk shake
Lunch				
4 meat	28	Cheeseburger on bun with double meat patty, lettuce, tomato	2 burritos with extra cheese, meat	Split pea soup with ham hocks
4 starches	8			Grilled cheese sandwich
Vegetable	2		Lettuce and tomato salad with dressing	Watermelon wedge
4 fats		French fried potatoes	Biscochitos	Sugar cookies
Milk, protein supplement	10	High-protein milk shake	High-protein milk shake	High-protein milk shake
Dinner				
4 meat	28	Spaghetti with 4 oz meat sauce, Parmesan cheese	2 tamales with red chili sauce	4 oz fried chicken
3 starches	6			Sweet potato
Vegetable	2	Green beans with 2 tbs margarine	Spanish rice	Mustard greens with 2 tbs butter
7 fats		Bread with butter Tapioca pudding	Peas with 2 tbs butter Custard	Biscuit Vanilla ice cream
Milk, protein supplement	10	High-protein milk shake	High-protein milk shake	High-protein milk shake
Snack				
Milk	8	Fruit yogurt	Cottage cheese with fruit	½ sandwich with peanut butter
Fruit				Banana
TOTAL	132			

Elemental diets are liquid products (e.g., Peptamen) that can be used as dietary supplements or complete meal replacements. They contain glucose, peptides, essential fatty acids, vitamins, and minerals, and can be fed orally or enterally. They require minimal digestion and are easily absorbed in the small intestine.

If the patient is still unable to take in enough calories, tube feedings may be considered. Total parenteral nutrition (TPN) may be initiated if enteral feedings are not feasible.

Ambulatory and Home Care. With shortened hospital stays, many patients are discharged on a therapeutic diet. Discharge preparation for both the patient and the family is important. They must be carefully instructed on the cause of the undernourished state and ways to avoid the problem in the future. The patient must be made aware that undernourishment, whatever the cause, can recur and that adhering to a diet high in protein and calories for a few weeks cannot fully restore a normal nutritional state. Many months are needed to reach this goal. Diet instruction is usually carried out by the dietitian, but it is important for the nurse to assess the patient's understanding and reinforce the information whenever possible. The patient's ability to comply with the dietary instructions must be examined in light of past eating habits, religious and ethnic preferences, age, income, other resources, and state of health.

Unless the patient and the family can be convinced of the necessity for dietary change and have the resources to effect change, it is likely that no long-term benefits will be achieved. Ways should be found in which the patient can become actively involved in the recovery. The need for continuous follow-up care must be strongly emphasized if rehabilitation is to be accomplished and maintained.

The nurse is in an ideal position to determine the need for nutritious meals and snacks after discharge from the hospital. In addition, it is important to consider the availability and acceptability of community resources that provide meals. Such aspects can be integrated into discharge planning and follow-up home visits by the nurse.

Keeping a diet diary or a calorie count for 3 days at a time is one way to analyze and reinforce healthful eating patterns. These records are also helpful to the health care team in the follow-up care. Self-assessment of progress can be encouraged by having the patient weighed once or twice a week and keeping a weight record.

■ Evaluation

The expected outcomes are that the patient who is malnourished will
- achieve and maintain optimal body weight
- consume a well-balanced diet
- experience no adverse outcomes related to malnutrition

■ Gerontologic Considerations: Malnutrition

Older adults are at risk for malnutrition with many factors influencing their nutritional intake (Table 39-15). Many of these factors may occur at the same time, thus further increasing the risk of malnutrition. The unique nutritional requirements of an older adult are often overlooked. As a person grows older there are decreases in lean body mass (the metabolically active tissue), basal metabolic rate, and physical activity. Combined, these factors decrease the caloric needs for energy. The older person frequently reduces the consumption of needed protein, vitamins, and minerals and may take in "empty calories," such as candy and pastries. As a group,

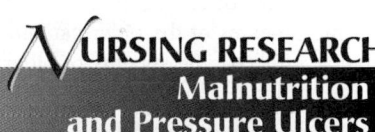

TABLE 39-15 Gerontologic Differences in Assessment: Factors Affecting Nutritional Intake in Older Adults

Physical Factors
Age
Anorexia
Decreased number of taste buds
Dental problems
Food intolerances
Health status
Physical disability
Prescribed diets
Prescribed or over-the-counter drugs

Psychosocial Factors
Importance of food in the past
Loneliness or loss
Mental awareness
Social isolation

Socioeconomic Factors
Available time for food preparation and eating
Availability of desired foods
Availability of transportation to food stores
Education level and nutritional knowledge
Food fads
Income level
Lack of food preparation equipment

NURSING RESEARCH
Malnutrition and Pressure Ulcers

Citation Guenter P et al: Survey of nutritional status in newly hospitalized patients with stage III or stage IV pressure ulcers, *Adv Skin Wound Care* 13:164, 2000.

Purpose To examine the relationship between nutritional status and pressure ulcers in patients newly admitted to an acute care facility.

Methods Newly admitted non-ICU patients (n = 120) with stage III or stage IV pressure ulcers were included in the study. Measures included demographic characteristics, weight, serum prealbumin and albumin levels, nutritional intake, and type of pressure ulcer.

Results and Conclusions The majority of patients were elderly; had a stage III sacral pressure ulcer, low prealbumin levels, and inadequate nutritional intake; and were below their usual weight. Patients admitted into acute care facilities with pressure ulcers are often malnourished, and aggressive nutritional therapy may be indicated.

Implications for Nursing Practice The nurse plays an important role in identifying patients at risk for malnutrition. The presence of pressure ulcers or delays in wound healing are important signs that nutritional intake may not be adequate. Older patients are particularly at risk for malnutrition and its adverse consequences.

ICU, Intensive care unit.

older adults may be less well informed about what constitutes a well-balanced diet.

When these factors are added to already existing medical problems, it is easy to see why poor dietary practices develop. In addition, poor dentition, ill-fitting dentures, anorexia, multiple losses affecting the social setting of meals, low income, and medical conditions involving the GI tract contribute to the type and amount of foods that are eaten. The nurse, working with the dietitian, must be aware of common medical and psychosocial factors in the older adult and should incorporate interventions for overcoming these problems in the plan of care.

Some of the physiologic changes associated with aging affect the nutritional status of older adults. The following changes are of particular interest:

1. Changes in the oral cavity (e.g., change in bite surfaces of the teeth, periodontal disease, drying of the mucous membrane of the mouth and tongue, poorly fitting dentures, decreased muscle strength for chewing, decreased number of taste buds, decreased saliva production)
2. Changes in digestion and motility (e.g., decreased absorption of cobalamin, vitamin A, and folic acid and decreased GI motility)
3. Changes in the endocrine system (e.g., decreased tolerance to glucose)
4. Changes in the musculoskeletal system (e.g., decreased bone density, degenerative joint changes)
5. Decrease in vision and hearing (e.g., procurement and preparation of food are more difficult)

Certain illnesses that are more prevalent in the older population are considered to be diet related. These include atherosclerosis, osteoporosis, diabetes mellitus, and diverticulosis. Multiple drugs are often required to treat these and other common chronic illnesses of the older patient. These drugs often have an adverse effect on the appetite of older adults, increasing the possibility of inadequate intake caused by anorexia.

To date, with the exception of calories, it has not been determined that older adults have different requirements for specific nutrients from those of middle-aged adults. Generally, caloric intake should decrease with age because of the progressive loss of lean body mass and a decrease in the basal metabolic rate. Therefore fewer calories are needed to meet metabolic needs. Unless caloric intake is decreased by careful attention to food intake, or energy expenditure is increased through greater physical activity and exercise, obesity will result.

Socioeconomic factors are important variables when assessing the nutritional status of an older adult. Because more than one third of older adults have incomes below the poverty level, obtaining adequate and nutritious food can be an ongoing problem. In many cases the older person cannot afford to purchase meat, fresh vegetables, and fruits that provide many necessary nutrients.

Lifestyle changes such as retirement or relocation to a nursing home can have a significant impact on the eating habits of the older adult. Other important considerations that should be assessed include the ethnic background, previous dietary practices, food preferences, knowledge of proper diet, availability and accessibility of food stores, transportation, and health status. Problems related to any or all of these areas can alert the nurse to the possibility of a nutritional problem.

Malnutrition can occur in an older person even though the caloric requirements decrease with age. If malnutrition is present, few malnourished older persons are able to ingest enough food to correct the malnourished state. Special strategies, such as adaptive devices (e.g., large-handled eating utensils), often are helpful in increasing dietary intake. Some older persons may require nutritional support therapies until their strength and general health are improved.

Many community nutritional programs are available to the older person to make mealtime a pleasant, social event. Improving the social setting of a meal often improves the dietary intake. Home-delivered meals and meal sites in a central location are popular meal alternatives for many older adults. The use of food stamps is another alternative that allows low-income households, regardless of age, to buy more food of a greater variety.

TYPES OF SPECIALIZED NUTRITION SUPPORT

Oral Feeding

High-calorie oral supplements may be used in the patient whose nutritional intake is deficient. This may include milk shakes, puddings, or commercially available products (e.g., Ensure, Sustacal). Research suggests that ingestion of these beverages may have a role in improving the nutritional status of elderly patients.[14] These supplements should not be used as meal substitutes but between meals as snacks. In some long-term care facilities, these beverages are used instead of water with oral medication administration to increase caloric intake.

Tube Feeding

Tube feeding refers to the administration of a nutritionally balanced liquefied food or formula through a tube inserted into the stomach, duodenum, or jejunum. Tube feedings may be ordered for the patient who has a functioning GI tract but is unable to take any or enough oral nourishment. Specific indications for tube feeding include those persons with anorexia, orofacial fractures, head and neck cancer, neurologic or psychiatric conditions that prevent oral intake, and extensive burns and those who are receiving chemotherapy or radiation therapy. Tube feedings are considered to be easily administered, safer, more physiologically efficient, and definitely less expensive than parenteral nutrition. They are used to provide nutrients by way of the GI tract either alone or as a supplement to oral or parenteral nutrition.

Common delivery options are continuous infusion by pump, intermittent by gravity, intermittent bolus by syringe, and cyclic feedings by infusion pump. Continuous infusion is most often used with critically ill patients and feedings into the small intestine. Intermittent feeding may be preferred as the patient improves or is receiving such feedings at home.[15]

A nasogastric (NG) tube is most commonly used for short-term feeding problems. If the feedings are necessary for an extended time, other means of feeding may be used, such as an esophagostomy tube, a gastrostomy tube (placed surgically, endoscopically, or radiologically), or a jejunostomy tube that empties directly into the jejunum. Transpyloric (nasointestinal) tube placement or placement into the jejunum is used when physiologic conditions warrant feeding the patient below the pyloric sphincter. (Fig. 39-3 shows the locations of commonly used enteral feeding tubes.)

Nasogastric and Nasointestinal Tubes. Feeding tubes made of polyurethane or silicone materials have added to the comfort level of the patient over extended periods. These tubes are long, small in diameter, soft, and flexible, thereby decreasing the risk of mucosal damage from prolonged placement. The older

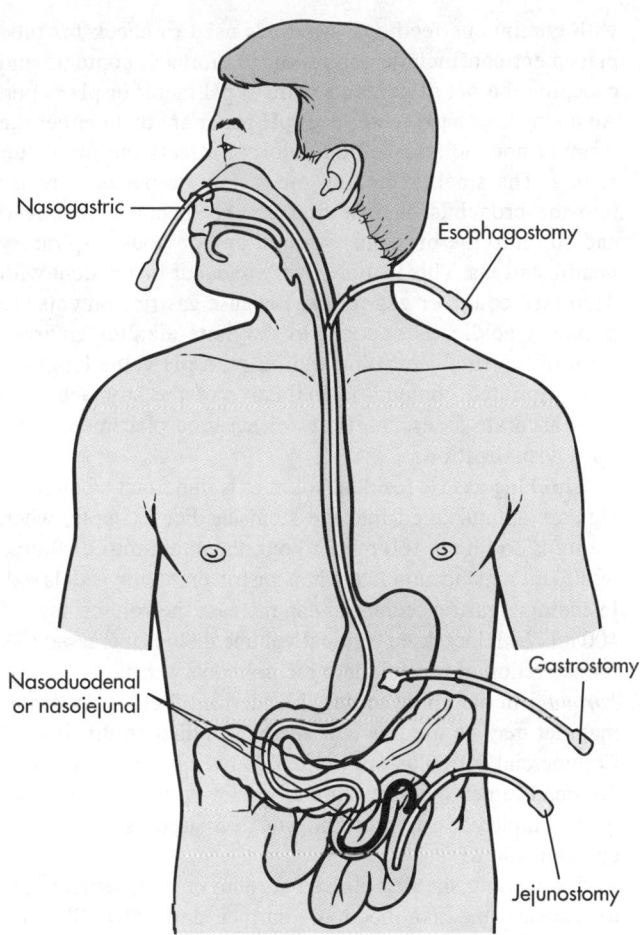

FIG. 39-3 Common enteral feeding tube placement locations.

Nasogastric
Esophagostomy
Nasoduodenal or nasojejunal
Gastrostomy
Jejunostomy

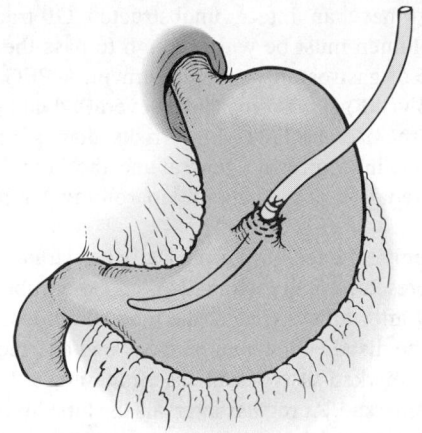

FIG. 39-4 Placement of a gastrostomy tube.

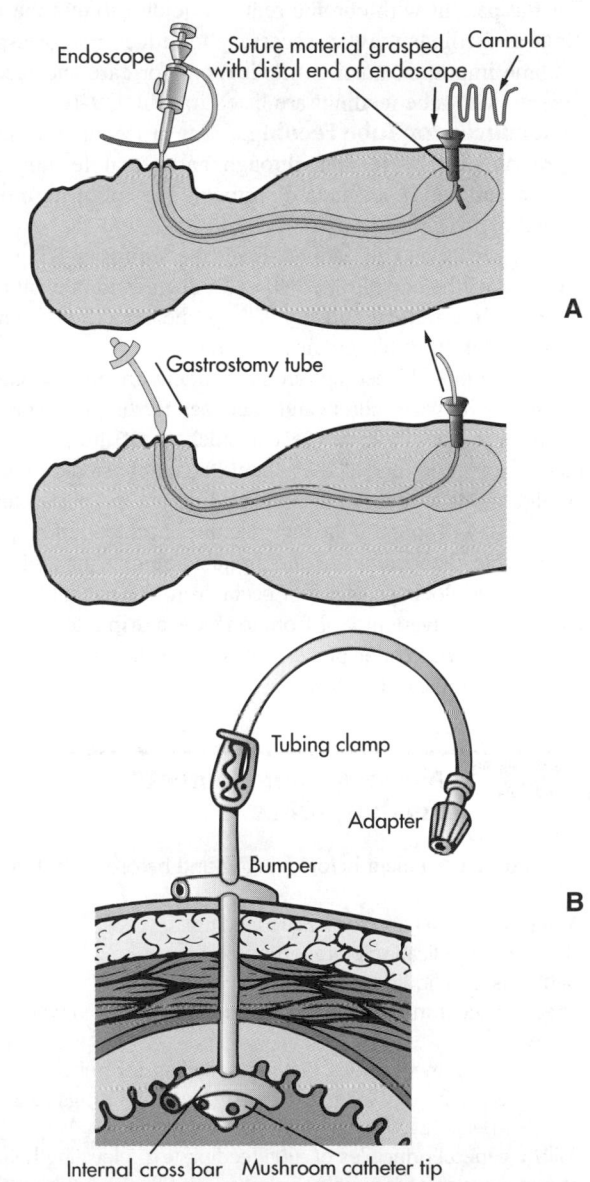

FIG. 39-5 Percutaneous endoscopic gastrostomy. **A,** Gastrostomy tube placement via percutaneous endoscopy. Using endoscopy, a gastrostomy tube is inserted through the esophagus into the stomach and then pulled through a stab wound made in the abdominal wall. **B,** A retention disk and bumper secure the tube.

tubes made of rubber or polyvinyl chloride tend to stiffen with time. Polyurethane and silicone tubes are radiopaque, making their position readily identified by x-ray. Many of these tubes also have weighted tips, allowing for easier passage of the tube through the pylorus into the duodenum. Placement into the intestine theoretically decreases the likelihood of regurgitation of contents into the esophagus and subsequent aspiration. With the use of a stylet, these tubes can be placed in a comatose patient because the ability to swallow is not essential during insertion.

Although the smaller feeding tubes have many advantages over wider-lumen tubes, such as the standard decompression NG tube, there are some disadvantages. Because of the small diameter, these tubes are more easily clogged when feedings are thick and are more difficult to use for checking residual volumes. They are particularly prone to obstruction when oral drugs have not been thoroughly crushed and dissolved in water before administration. They can become dislodged by vomiting or coughing and can also become knotted or kinked in the GI tract. Failure to flush the tubing after both drug administration and residual volume determinations can result in tube clogging. When the tube becomes clogged, it may necessitate removal and insertion of a new tube, adding to cost and patient discomfort.

Gastrostomy and Jejunostomy. A gastrostomy tube may be used for a patient who requires tube feedings over an extended time (Fig. 39-4). Gastrostomy tubes can be placed surgically, radiologically, or endoscopically. See Fig. 39-5 for the placement procedure of a percutaneous endoscopic gastrostomy (PEG). The patient must have an intact, unobstructed GI tract, and the esophageal lumen must be wide enough to pass the endoscope for this type of gastrostomy tube placement. A PEG and a radiologically placed gastrostomy have several advantages. These procedures themselves have fewer risks than surgical placement. Because it requires no general anesthesia and only minimum or no sedation of the patient, laparotomy can be done at a lower cost.

Gastrostomy tube feedings can usually be started when bowel sounds are present, usually within 24 hours after tube placement. Immediately after tube insertion, the tube length from the insertion site to the distal end should be measured and recorded. The tube is then marked at the skin insertion site, although many tubes are premarked. At regular intervals the tube insertion length should be rechecked. The tube is most often connected to a pump for continuous feeding. Water may be infused within 2 hours after placement.

For the patient with chronic reflux, a jejunostomy tube with continuous feedings may be necessary to reduce risk of aspiration. Some important nursing implications for care and feeding of patients with tube feedings are listed in Table 39-16.

Procedures for Tube Feedings. The procedure for the administration of tube feeding through an enteral feeding tube should be outlined in a standard protocol. The following principles apply:

1. *Patient position.* The patient should be sitting or lying with the head of the bed elevated 30 to 45 degrees to prevent aspiration. If intermittent delivery is used, the head should remain elevated for 30 to 60 minutes after feeding.
2. *Patency of tube.* If feedings are intermittent, the tube should be irrigated with water before and after each feeding to ensure that the tube is patent and to prevent blockage of the tube. If the feedings are continuous, they should be administered by using an electric or a battery-operated feeding pump with a built-in alarm that will sound if the tube becomes occluded. If no pump is available, the feedings require frequent monitoring of the drip rate so that blockage does not occur from the patient lying on the tubing inadvertently or from too slow a drip rate.
3. *Tube position.* Proper placement of the tube in the stomach should be checked before each feeding or every 8 hours

---

TABLE 39-16 Nursing Management: Feeding Tubes

- Check tube placement before feeding and before each drug administration.
- Assess for bowel sounds before feeding.
- Use liquid medications rather than pills.
  Dilute viscous liquid medications.
  Check to see if medications are intended to be taken with meals.
  Avoid adding medications to enteral feeding formula.
- If it is necessary to use tablets, be sure to crush drugs to a fine powder to avoid clogging feeding tubes.
- Follow general principles of tube feeding (e.g., elevating head of bed, checking for residual volumes, and flushing tube with water).
- Assess regularly for complications (e.g., aspiration, diarrhea, abdominal distention, hyperglycemia, constipation, and fecal impaction).

---

with continuous feedings. Methods used to check for tube placement can include aspiration of stomach contents and checking the pH of contents using a pH meter or pH paper. Advantages of a pH meter over pH paper are that neither the formula nor the added food coloring affects the pH meter results. The smaller feeding tubes may be passed directly into the bronchus on insertion or may become dislodged and slip into the bronchus without any obvious respiratory manifestations. This is more likely to occur in a patient with decreased cough or gag reflex. Because gastric contents are primarily acidic, as opposed to the more alkaline environment of the small intestine and lungs, a pH value less than 5 on aspirated contents is indicative of the stomach. The most accurate assessment for correct tube placement is by x-ray visualization.

Checking gastric residual volumes is important when feedings are administered into the stomach. For example, when the infusion rate is 100 ml per hour, the total infused volume of 400 ml may accumulate when gastric emptying is delayed. In addition, gastric secretions can increase the volume beyond 400 ml. With increased residual volume there is increased risk for aspiration of formula into the pulmonary tract.

4. *Formula.* In the home setting, blenderized foods from a normal diet may be used as tube feedings, although this is rare. Commercial formulas are preferable over blenderized foods for small-lumen tubes because of the lower risk of tube clogging, completeness of nutrition, and decreased risk of formula contamination.

The feeding should be given at room or body temperature to decrease the likelihood of diarrhea and other GI complaints. The pleasurable aspects of eating, such as smelling, seeing, tasting, and chewing the food, are frequently denied the tube-fed patient. If the clinical condition permits, the patient may be allowed to smell, taste, and even chew small amounts of food before the feeding, and then the chewed food must be spit out. The patient may hesitate to do this because it is not esthetic, but it stimulates salivary and gastric secretions and provides the pleasurable sensations associated with oral intake. Before initiating the feeding, the nurse should aspirate gastric contents and measure the amount. If the volume is greater than 200 ml and there are clinical signs of intolerance, including nausea or increase in abdominal girth, the next feeding is held for 1 hour and then the residual volume is rechecked. The aspirate should be reinstilled.[16]

5. *Administration of feeding.* Feedings are administered either by gravity drip method or by feeding pump. Applying pressure to force the feeding can damage the tube. The feeding rate or volume is increased gradually for 24 to 48 hours to minimize side effects, such as nausea or diarrhea. If intermittent feedings are ordered, the volume is usually 200 to 500 ml per feeding. It is important to remember that the patient still needs water, and this may be administered with flush water or as additional boluses of water as tolerated.

6. *General nursing considerations.* The patient should be weighed daily or several times a week, and accurate intake and output records should be maintained. These measures provide information on weight gain or loss, as well as tolerance of the feedings. Initially blood glucose checks to assess glucose tolerance are performed at the bedside. An older patient who has baseline glucose intolerance is particularly at risk for hyperglycemia.

Feedings that have been opened and not refrigerated or feedings that have been infusing longer than 8 hours should be discarded to prevent the administration of possible contaminated feedings. Feedings should be labeled with the date and time they are initially used. If a pump is used, pump tubing should be changed every 24 hours or per manufacturer's guidelines. See NCP 39-1 for care of the patient receiving enteral nutrition.

Complications Related to Tubes and Feedings. The types of problems encountered in patients receiving tube feedings and corrective measures are presented in Table 39-17. When commercial products are used, the concentration, flavor, osmolarity, and amounts of protein, sodium, and fat vary according to the manufacturer. Most commercial formulas are lactose free. The concentrations range from 1 to 2 kcal/ml, with most between 1 and 1.5 kcal/ml.

NURSING CARE PLAN 39-1

Patient Receiving Enteral Nutrition

EXPECTED PATIENT OUTCOMES	NURSING INTERVENTIONS and *RATIONALES*
NURSING DIAGNOSIS	**Imbalanced nutrition: less than body requirements** *related to* enteral feeding problems *as manifested by* body weight less than ideal, diarrhea, abdominal distention.
▪ Stable or gain in weight ▪ No diarrhea or abdominal distention	▪ Monitor weight and compare with baseline *to make adjustments as needed in calorie intake.* ▪ Progress the patient slowly from clear liquids to blenderized foods *to prevent gastric distention.* ▪ Gradually add high-calorie foods to patient's blenderized foods *to maintain body weight while preventing distention.*
NURSING DIAGNOSIS	**Impaired skin integrity** *related to* enzymatic action of gastric juices that may leak around tube *as manifested by* red, irritated tissue around the tube.*
▪ No skin breakdown around tube ▪ Daily inspections of skin performed and any problems reported	▪ Assess skin daily for signs of irritation *so that early treatment is provided.* ▪ Wash skin around the tube with soap and water daily; apply a protective skin barrier such as zinc oxide or petrolatum or a Stomahesive wafer *to maintain skin integrity.* ▪ Teach patient and family to assess and provide care *to ensure involvement in self-care and early detection of problems.*
NURSING DIAGNOSIS	**Disturbed body image** *related to* presence of feeding tube *as manifested by* refusal to participate in own feeding, verbalization of fear of rejection by family and friends, avoidance of social activities associated with food and eating.
▪ Participation in self-care related to feedings ▪ Verbalization of acceptance of enteral feeding	▪ Encourage patient to express feelings about the enteral feedings *to increase the patient's self-awareness.* ▪ Provide information about the tube, feedings, purpose, and patient progress *so that the patient makes decisions based on correct information.* ▪ Acknowledge the patient's fears *to establish a trusting nurse-patient relationship.*
NURSING DIAGNOSIS	**Risk for deficient fluid volume** *related to* diarrhea or inadequate fluid intake.
▪ No signs of fluid volume deficit ▪ Adequate fluid intake	▪ Monitor patient for poor skin turgor, decreased blood pressure, tachycardia, decreased urine output, and dry mucous membranes *to identify signs of fluid volume deficit.* ▪ Provide adequate fluid intake, including water, as determined by intake records. ▪ Monitor urine output for osmotic diuresis, *which may occur secondary to high glucose load of feedings or too rapid infusion.* ▪ Identify possible cause of diarrhea *so that appropriate treatment is started.*
NURSING DIAGNOSIS	**Ineffective therapeutic regimen management** *related to* care required for skin around tubing and tube feedings *as manifested by* questioning about self-care.
▪ Demonstration of skin care and tube feeding before discharge	▪ Assess the patient's home environment and lifestyle *to make teaching relevant to individual requirements.* ▪ Provide detailed information about how to prepare the formula and how to manage the tube feeding *to facilitate self-care.* ▪ Use return demonstration technique *to validate patient's and family's learning of the necessary skills.*
NURSING DIAGNOSIS	**Risk for aspiration** *related to* enteral tube with tube feedings.
▪ No aspiration Able to describe measures to prevent aspiration	▪ During feeding have the patient's head elevated at least 30 degrees; remain in this position 30 minutes after feeding *to prevent aspiration.* ▪ Aspirate gastric contents before feeding *to validate gastric emptying.* ▪ Reinstill the residual gastric contents *to prevent excessive fluid and electrolyte losses.*

*This applies to feeding tubes that have been inserted through the skin.

TABLE 39-17 Common Problems of Patients Receiving Tube Feedings

PROBLEMS AND POSSIBLE CAUSES	CORRECTIVE MEASURES
Vomiting and/or Aspiration	
• Improper placement of tube	Replace tube in proper position. Check tube position before beginning feeding and every 8 hr if continuous feedings.
• Delayed gastric emptying, increased residual volume	Hold feeding 1 hr; then if residual volume is less than previous rate, resume feeding.
• Potential for aspiration	Keep head of bed elevated to 30- to 45-degree angle. Have patient sit up on side of bed or in chair. Encourage ambulation unless contraindicated.
• Contamination of formula	Refrigerate unused formula and record date opened. Discard outdated formula every 24 hr. Discard formula left standing for longer than manufacturer's guidelines: 8-12 hr for ready-to-feed formulas (cans) or 4 hr for reconstituted formula. Use closed system to prevent contamination.
Diarrhea	
• Feeding too fast, hypertonic formula, or medications	Decrease rate of feeding. Change to continuous drip feedings. Check for drugs that may cause diarrhea (e.g., antibiotics).
• Lactose intolerance	Consult health care provider for change in formula to lactose-free solution.
• Contamination of formula or tubing	Change tubing every 24 hr. Hang 8-hr formula at a time. Do not exceed manufacturer's guidelines.
• Low-fiber formula	Change to formula with more fiber.
• Tube moving distally	Properly secure tube before beginning feeding. Check before each feeding or at least every 24 hr if continuous feedings.
Constipation	
• Formula components	Consult health care provider for change in formula to one with more fiber content. Obtain laxative order.
• Poor fluid intake	Increase fluid intake if not contraindicated. Give free water, as well as formula. Give total fluid intake of 30 ml/kg body weight.
• Drugs	Check for drugs that may be constipating.
• Impaction	Perform rectal examinations to check and manually remove feces if present.
Dehydration	
• Excessive diarrhea, vomiting	Decrease rate or change formula. Check drugs that patient is receiving, especially antibiotics. Take care to prevent bacterial contamination of formula and equipment.
• Poor fluid intake	Increase intake and check amount and number of feedings. Increase amount of intake if appropriate.
• High protein formula	Change formula.
• Hyperosmotic diuresis	Check blood glucose levels frequently. Change formula.

The osmolality of the solution is determined by the number and size of particles in solution. With regard to feeding formulas, the more hydrolyzed or broken down the nutrients, the greater the osmolality. Many tube feeding formulas are isotonic, although some are hypertonic. The more calorically dense the formula, the less water it contains. Protein content greater than 16% can lead to dehydration unless the patient is given supplemental fluids or is sufficiently alert to request additional fluids. The nurse must be aware of this potential problem and must provide extra fluids through the feeding tube or, if permitted, by mouth. Tube feedings with high sodium content are contraindicated in the patient with cardiovascular problems, such as congestive heart failure. High fat content is not advocated for a patient with short bowel syndrome or ileocecal resections because of impaired fat absorption.

The dietitian can be of considerable assistance to the nursing staff. When close consultation with the nursing staff occurs, existing problems with tube feedings can be quickly and efficiently addressed and resolved. Some institutions have nutrition support teams composed of a physician, nurse, dietitian, and pharmacist whose function is to oversee the nutrition support of select inpatients and outpatients.

In patients receiving gastrostomy or jejunostomy feeding, the nurse should be alert to two possible problems: (1) skin irritation and (2) pulling out of the tube. Skin care around the tube site is important because the action of the digestive juices is irritating to the skin. The skin around the feeding tube should be assessed daily for signs of redness and maceration. To keep the skin clean and dry, initially it should be rinsed with sterile water and dried. Once the site has healed, it can be washed with mild soap and water. A protective ointment (zinc oxide, petroleum gauze) or a skin barrier (Karaya, Stomahesive) may be used on the skin around the tube. A small dressing may be placed around the tube until the site is healed and must be changed promptly if it gets wet. Other types of drain or tube pouches may be used if there is a problem with skin irritation, and an enterostomal therapist can be of great assistance to the nurse if these issues arise. The patient and family members can be taught how to care for the feeding tube. Teaching should include skin care, care of the tube, and complete information about feeding administration and potential complications.[17]

■ Gerontologic Considerations: Enteral Nutrition

Enteral nutrition strategies, including NG, nasointestinal, and gastrostomy feedings, are often used in the older patient to improve nutritional status. Because of physiologic changes associated with aging, the older adult is more vulnerable to complications associated with these interventions, especially fluid and electrolyte imbalances. Complications such as diarrhea can leave the patient dehydrated. Decreased thirst perception or impaired cognitive function decreases the ability of the patient to seek additional fluids.

With aging there is decreased ability to handle glucose loads (glucose intolerance). As a result, the older patient may be more susceptible to problems of hyperglycemia in response to the high carbohydrate load of some enteral feeding formulas. If the older adult has compromised cardiovascular function (e.g., congestive heart failure), there will be a decreased ability to handle large volumes of formula. In this situation the use of more concentrated formulas may be warranted. The older adult also is at increased risk for aspiration caused by gastroesophageal reflux disease, hiatal hernia, or diminished gag reflex. Physical mobility, fine motor movement, and visual system changes associated with aging may contribute to difficulties in managing enteral nutrition equipment at home. In addition, age-related changes such as a decrease in lean muscle mass influence the reliability of measures used for nutritional assessment.

Total Parenteral Nutrition

When the GI tract cannot be used for the ingestion, digestion, and absorption of essential nutrients, TPN may be substituted. **Parenteral nutrition** refers to the administration of nutrients by a route (e.g., bloodstream) other than the GI tract. **Total parenteral nutrition** is the delivery of a nutritionally adequate hypertonic solution consisting of glucose, protein hydrolysates, minerals, and vitamins using an intravenous (IV) route. TPN has become a relatively safe and practical method of delivering total nutritional needs. The goal of using TPN is to meet the patient's nutritional needs and to allow growth of new body tissue. Regular IV solutions of 5% dextrose (5 g dextrose/100 ml) in water (D5W) or 5% dextrose in lactated Ringer's solution (D5LR) contain no protein and have approximately 170 calories per liter. The normal adult requires a minimum of 1200 to 1500 calories per day to carry out normal physiologic functions. Patients who sustain severe injury, surgery, or burns and those who are malnourished as a result of medical treatment or disease processes have greatly increased nutritional needs. The volume of regular dextrose solutions needed to meet these high caloric requirements could exceed the capacity of the cardiovascular system. Table 39-18 lists common indications for the use of TPN.

Composition. Commercially prepared TPN base solutions are available for both central and peripheral use. These base solutions contain dextrose and protein in the form of amino acids. The pharmacy adds the prescribed electrolytes (e.g., sodium, potassium, chloride, calcium, magnesium, and phosphate), vitamins, and trace elements (e.g., zinc, copper, chromium, and manganese) to customize the solution for the patient. A three-in-one

TABLE 39-18	Common Indications for Total Parenteral Nutrition

- Chronic diarrhea and vomiting
- Complicated surgery or trauma
- Gastrointestinal obstruction
- Gastrointestinal tract anomalies and fistulae
- Hypermetabolic states (sepsis, fractures)
- Intractable diarrhea
- Malnutrition
- Pancreatitis
- Severe anorexia nervosa
- Severe malabsorption
- Short bowel syndrome

or total nutrient admixture containing an IV fat emulsion, dextrose, and amino acids has become widely used, especially in the home setting.

Calories. Calories in TPN are supplied primarily by carbohydrates in the form of dextrose and by fat in the form of fat emulsion. The administration of between 100 and 150 g of dextrose (1 g provides approximately 3.4 calories, as opposed to oral carbohydrates, which provide 4 calories) daily has a protein-sparing effect. Adequate nonprotein calories in the form of glucose and lipids must be provided to allow metabolism of amino acids for wound healing and not as energy. However, overfeeding can lead to metabolic complications. To minimize these problems, an energy intake of 25 to 30 calories per kilogram per day in a nonobese patient is often recommended. Providing both lipid and carbohydrate components meets the energy requirement while minimizing problems of overfeeding. The FDA has approved the use of 10%, 20%, and 30% fat emulsion solutions. These lipid emulsions provide approximately 1 calorie per milliliter (10% solution) or 2 calories per milliliter (20% solution). The contents of fat emulsion are primarily soybean or safflower triglycerides with egg phospholipids added as an emulsifier. In practice, the conservative approach is IV-administered fat emulsions providing not more than 30% of the total energy to minimize possible immunosuppressive effects of linoleic acid. The maximum fat emulsion amount should not exceed a dose of 2.5 g/kg per day[18] and should be administered slowly over 12 to 24 hours. Nausea, vomiting, and elevated temperature have been reported, especially when lipids are infused quickly. The administration of fat emulsion is contraindicated in the patient with a disturbance in fat metabolism. It should also be used with caution in the patient who is in danger of fat embolism (e.g., fractured femur) and the patient with an allergy to eggs.

Protein. The normal healthy person of average body size needs approximately 45 to 65 g of protein daily. Protein should be provided at the rate of 1 to 1.5 g/kg per day depending on the patient's needs. In a nutritionally depleted patient under the stress of illness or surgery, requirements can exceed 150 g per day to ensure a positive nitrogen balance. In the most recent guidelines, protein intake levels of 1.5 to 2 g/kg per day are suggested for most patients with moderate to severe stress.[4]

Electrolytes. The assessment of individual requirements should take place daily at the beginning of therapy and then several times a week as the treatment progresses. The following are ranges for average daily electrolyte requirements for adult patients without renal or hepatic impairment:

Sodium: 1 to 2 mEq/kg
Potassium: 1 to 2 mEq/kg
Chloride: As needed to maintain acid-base balance
Magnesium: 8 to 20 mEq
Calcium: 10 to 15 mEq
Phosphate: 20 to 40 mmol

The exact amount needed depends on the patient's health problem and on electrolyte levels as determined by blood testing.

Trace elements. Zinc, copper, chromium, manganese, selenium, molybdenum, and iodine supplements may be added according to the patient's condition and needs. Levels of these elements are monitored in the patient receiving TPN. The health care provider may order additional amounts of these elements to be added to the solutions according to the patient's requirements.

Vitamins. The daily addition of a multivitamin preparation to the TPN generally meets the vitamin requirements. If multivitamin infusion is used, the cobalamin (vitamin B_{12}) requirement may be met without the need for supplemental injections. It may be necessary for the physician to order vitamin K separately because it is currently not included in the multivitamin preparation.

Methods of Administration. Parenteral nutrition may be administered by central or peripheral veins. *Central parenteral nutrition* is given through a catheter whose tip lies in the superior vena cava. The central venous catheter often originates at the subclavian or jugular vein. More recently, single- or double-lumen peripherally inserted central catheters (PICCs) are being placed, usually into the basilic or cephalic vein and then advanced into the central circulation. Such catheters are made of soft, flexible material (silicon, polymer) and are 20 to 24 inches long. Ease of placement, cost, and limited complications make this an attractive alternative to a subclavian vein catheter. Central TPN is indicated when long-term parenteral support is necessary or when the patient has high protein and caloric requirements.

Peripheral parenteral nutrition (PPN) is administered through a peripherally inserted catheter or vascular access device, which uses a large peripheral vein. PPN is used when (1) nutritional support is needed for only a short time, (2) protein and caloric requirements are not high, (3) the risk of a central catheter is too great, or (4) parenteral nutrition is used to supplement inadequate oral intake. Both central and peripheral parenteral nutrition are used in a patient who is not a candidate for enteral support.

Central and peripheral parenteral nutrition differ in tonicity, which is measured in milliosmoles (mOsm; the concentration of particles in a fluid). Blood is isotonic and measures approximately 280 mOsm/L. The standard IV solutions of D_5W and normal saline are essentially isotonic. Central TPN solutions are hypertonic, measuring at least 1600 mOsm/L. The high glucose content ranges from 20% to 50%. Central TPN must be infused in a large central vein so that rapid dilution can occur. The use of a peripheral vein for central TPN would cause irritation and thrombophlebitis. Nutrients can be infused using smaller volumes than PPN. PPN is hypertonic (using as much as 20% glucose), but less so than central TPN, and can be safely administered through a large peripheral vein, although phlebitis can occur. Another potential complication of PPN is fluid overload.

All TPN solutions should be prepared by a pharmacist or a trained technician using strict aseptic techniques under a laminar flow hood. Nothing should be added to parenteral nutrition solutions after they are prepared in the pharmacy. The danger of drug incompatibilities and contamination is high. The fewer the personnel involved in the preparation and administration of TPN, the lower the risk of infection for the patient. In most hospitals the health care provider must order the TPN solution daily. In this way the solution and additives can be adjusted to the patient's current needs. Each TPN solution label indicates the nutrient content, all additives, the time mixed, and the date and time of expiration. In general, solutions are good for 24 hours and must be refrigerated until a half hour before use.

Catheter Placement. The central placement of the catheter into a large main vein for TPN is performed by the physician or a specially trained advanced practice nurse. The vein most commonly used is the subclavian, although the innominate or the jugular vein may be used. The procedure is the same as for the insertion of a central venous pressure line and should be done under strict aseptic conditions.

A standard isotonic IV solution is infused through the central line until x-ray confirms proper placement of the catheter tip in the superior vena cava and not in the jugular vein. The catheter insertion site is covered with a sterile dressing. The date is marked on the dressing.

Placement of a PICC catheter is done under sterile conditions, often by a specially trained nurse. A baseline measurement of the upper arm circumference is recommended. A tourniquet is then placed around the upper arm near the axilla to allow examination of the antecubital fossa and selection of a vein. If possible, the patient should be supine with the arm straight and at a 90-degree angle. Preparation of the insertion site should be done according to institutional policy. The sterile catheter is cut to the predetermined length, depending on the vein selected.

A local anesthetic is usually used at the insertion site. This site should be cleaned, protected, and maintained according to institutional policy. As with the centrally placed line, a chest x-ray is needed to verify proper tip placement before administering any TPN solution. Proper placement of a catheter for central TPN is illustrated in Fig. 39-6. Complications frequently

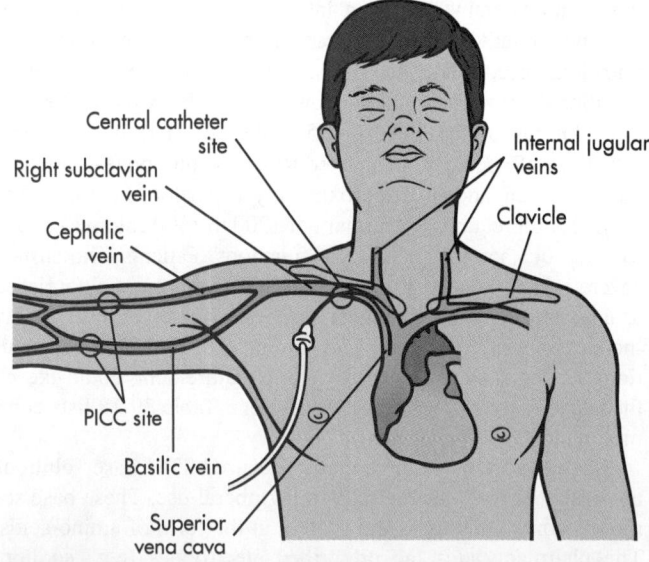

FIG. 39-6 Placement of a catheter for total parenteral nutrition using subclavian vein. Peripherally inserted central catheters (PICC) are inserted using the basilic or cephalic vein.

TABLE 39-19	Complications of Total Parenteral Nutrition

Infection
Fungus
Gram-positive bacteria
Gram-negative bacteria

Metabolic Problems
Hyperglycemia; hypoglycemia; and hyperosmolar, hyper-
   glycemic state
Prerenal azotemia
Essential fatty acid deficiency
Electrolyte and vitamin excesses and deficiencies
Trace mineral deficiencies
Hyperlipidemia

Mechanical Problems
Insertion
   Air embolus
   Pneumothorax, hemothorax, and hydrothorax
   Hemorrhage
Dislodgement
Thrombosis of great vein
Phlebitis

associated with catheter placement are hemorrhage, hydrothorax and pneumothorax, hemothorax, air embolus, and venous thrombosis. Once established for TPN, a single-lumen central catheter should not be used for the administration of blood or antibiotics, the drawing of blood samples, or the monitoring of central venous pressure.

Administration of Solution. Because TPN solutions are excellent media for microbial growth, it is essential that proper aseptic techniques be followed. The FDA recommends that a 0.22-micron Millipore filter be placed on parenteral solutions not containing fat emulsion and a 1.2-micron filter placed on solutions containing fat emulsion.[18] Filters and IV tubing are changed every 24 hours. The tubing and the filter should be clearly labeled with the date and the time they are put into use. Complications of TPN can be divided into three categories: (1) infection, (2) metabolic, and (3) mechanical. The major complications of each category are presented in Table 39-19.

NURSING MANAGEMENT
TOTAL PARENTERAL NUTRITION

Vital signs should be monitored every 4 to 8 hours in the patient receiving TPN. Daily weights give an indication of the patient's hydration status as therapy progresses. Body weight is considered the sum of the changes in protein, fat, and water. On a daily basis, body water fluctuates more than protein or fat. Analysis must be made of whether gains or losses in weight are caused by fluid gained from edema, fluid lost through diuresis, or actual increase or decrease in tissue weight. Blood levels of glucose, electrolytes, and urea nitrogen; a complete blood count; and hepatic enzyme studies are followed 3 times per week until stable and then weekly as the patient's condition warrants. Assessment of these important values assists the nurse in evaluat-

ing the patient's tolerance of parenteral nutrition. A nursing care plan for the patient receiving parenteral nutrition is presented on page 990.

Dressings covering the catheter site are changed according to institutional protocol, ranging from every other day to once a week. Some institutions have specially trained nurses from the IV team or the nutritional support team who are responsible for these dressing changes, whereas others have the staff nurse do the dressing changes after special instruction. The procedure for changing the dressing is similar to that followed after catheter insertion. The institutional routine should be followed with respect to the appropriate use of solutions for the dressing change. The site is carefully observed for signs of inflammation and infection. Phlebitis can readily occur in the vein as a result of the hypertonic infusion, and the area can become infected. The patient receiving parenteral nutrition may be immunosuppressed and thus more susceptible to opportunistic infections. In this patient, signs of inflammation or infection can be subtle, if present at all. Many patients receiving TPN are receiving chemotherapy, corticosteroids, or antibiotics, which can mask signs of infection.

If sutures are used to anchor the catheter, they may become infected. If an infection is suspected during dressing change, a culture specimen of the site and drainage should be sent for analysis, and the health care provider should be notified immediately. The use of an occlusive dressing protects the wound from contamination.

Hyperglycemia is a metabolic complication of parenteral nutrition. At the beginning of TPN therapy, the solution is infused at a gradually increasing rate for 24 to 48 hours. This allows the pancreas to adapt to the increased amount of glucose in the circulation by producing more insulin. Blood glucose levels should be checked at the bedside every 4 to 6 hours with a glucose-testing meter (see Chapter 47). Some increase in the blood glucose level is expected during the first few days after TPN is started. A sliding scale dose of insulin may be ordered to keep the glucose level below 150 mg/dl (8.34 mmol/L).[19]

The nurse must be made aware that speeding or slowing the infusion rate is contraindicated. Speeding up the rate results in a large amount of glucose entering the circulation. Endogenous insulin levels often are not adequate to handle this increase in glucose, and a hyperglycemic state results. Conversely, slowing the rate may result in a hypoglycemic state because it takes time for the pancreatic islet cells to adjust to a reduced glucose level. Checking the amount infused and the rate every 30 minutes to 1 hour is recommended. An infusion pump must be used during administration of TPN so that the infusion rate can be maintained, and an alarm will sound if the tubing becomes obstructed. Even though an infusion pump is being used, the nurse should periodically check the volume infused because pump malfunctions can alter the rate.

Before setting up and administering TPN, the nurse must check the label and ingredients in the solution to see that they are what the health care provider ordered. Solutions must also be examined for signs of contamination, such as a cloudy appearance. If contamination is suspected, the solution should be returned promptly to the pharmacy for replacement. It is the nurse's responsibility to ensure that the TPN solution is discontinued and replaced with a new solution if the bag is not empty at the end of 24 hours. At room temperature, the solution is an excellent medium for microorganism growth.

NURSING CARE PLAN 39-2

Patient Receiving Total Parenteral Nutrition

EXPECTED PATIENT OUTCOMES	NURSING INTERVENTIONS and *RATIONALES*
NURSING DIAGNOSIS	**Risk for infection** *related to* placement of a central venous access catheter, inadequate aseptic practices, and decreased defense mechanisms.
• No manifestations of infection • Normal body temperature	• Use protocols for infusion of solution and tubing and filter changes; change occlusive dressing over catheter site according to institutional policy *to minimize the possibility of infection.* • Observe for signs of inflammation and infection; monitor vital signs q4hr *to ensure early detection of infection.*
NURSING DIAGNOSIS	**Anxiety** *related to* inability to ingest food and fluids; lack of knowledge regarding catheter position; benefits and management of TPN *as manifested by* restlessness and apprehension; frequent questioning regarding care of catheter and TPN line.
• Statement of rationale for and demonstration of care of TPN line	• Instruct patient on rationale and benefits of TPN and care of line *because knowledge and facts may reduce anxiety.* • Illustrate catheter position by drawings and pictures *to increase patient understanding.*

COLLABORATIVE PROBLEMS

NURSING GOALS	NURSING INTERVENTIONS and *RATIONALES*
POTENTIAL COMPLICATIONS	**Hyperglycemia, hypoglycemia, and electrolyte imbalances.**
• Monitor blood glucose and serum electrolytes • Report deviations from acceptable parameters • Carry out medical and nursing interventions	• Monitor for signs of hyperglycemia such as thirst, polyuria, confusion, elevated blood glucose, blurred vision, dizziness, nausea and vomiting, and dehydration to plan appropriate treatment. • Monitor for signs of hypoglycemia such as sweating, hunger, weakness, and tremors *to ensure early intervention.* • Monitor serum electrolyte levels daily *to identify and treat complications early.* • Check for symptoms of hyperkalemia (e.g., muscle weakness, flaccid paralysis, cardiac arrhythmias, abdominal cramps, diarrhea) and hypokalemia (e.g., general weakness, decreased muscle tone, weak or irregular pulse, low blood pressure, shallow respirations, abdominal distention, and ileus).* • Maintain accurate infusion rate *to control the amount of glucose administered and prevent fluctuations in blood glucose levels.* • Never increase or decrease flow rate by more than 10% *to prevent fluctuations in blood glucose levels.* • Never stop TPN abruptly unless it is replaced by another glucose source *to prevent hypoglycemia.*

*Other manifestations of electrolyte imbalances are discussed in Chapter 16.

Sometimes fat emulsions are infused separately from the parenteral nutrition solution. The preferred delivery method is a continuous low volume, such as 20% lipids delivered over 12 hours, depending on patient needs. Adverse reactions that can occur are allergic manifestations, dyspnea, cyanosis, fever, flushing, phlebitis, chest and back pain, and pain at the IV site. A major benefit derived from IV fat administration is that a large number of calories can be provided in a relatively small amount of fluid. This is especially beneficial when the patient is at risk for fluid overload.

Catheter-related infection and septicemia can occur in patients receiving TPN through both peripherally and centrally placed lines. Local manifestations of infection include erythema, tenderness, and exudate at the catheter insertion site. Systemically the patient may have fever, chills, nausea, vomiting, and malaise. If no other causes can be identified, a catheter-related infection is suspected. Because of the risk of infection, catheters with antibiotic or antiseptic surfaces may be used. To diagnose the presence of infection and to determine the causative organism, cultures are performed of the catheter tip if the catheter has been removed or of the blood in the catheter if still in place. Blood cultures are drawn simultaneously from the catheter and a peripheral vein. A chest x-ray is taken to detect changes in pulmonary status. The current TPN solution with tubing and filter should also be cultured and replaced with an entirely new setup. When the catheter tip is the source of infection, antibiotic therapy may not be necessary because removal of the catheter can eliminate the problem.[20] A new central line may be immediately established or replaced by a peripheral route. It is important that a glucose source be maintained to prevent rebound hypoglycemia.

The same precautions should be followed in weaning from TPN as when therapy is being initiated. The flow rate must be gradually decreased for 1 to 2 hours, while oral intake is increased. If an emergency situation precludes a slow weaning process, other dextrose- or glucose-containing nutrients should be administered. When the catheter is removed, the dressing should be changed daily until the wound heals. Oral nourishment should be encouraged, and a careful record of intake should be maintained. Recording of body weight and laboratory analysis of serum electrolyte and glucose levels may continue.

■ Home Nutrition Support

Home parenteral or enteral nutrition is an accepted mode of nutritional therapy for the person who does not require hospitalization but who benefits from continued nutritional support. Some patients have been successfully treated at home for many months and even years. It is important for the nurse to educate the patient or the family about catheter or tube care, proper technique in mixing and handling of the solutions and tubing, and side effects.

Home nutrition therapies are expensive. For patients to be reimbursed for expenses, there are specific criteria that must be met. The nurse should have the discharge planning personnel involved early in the admission to help plan for such issues. Home nutrition support may also be a burden on the patient and caregivers and may affect quality of life. The nurse should make the family aware of support groups such as the OLEY Foundation (see resources at end of chapter for information) who provide peer support and advocacy.[4]

OBESITY

Obesity is as an abnormal increase in the proportion of fat cells, mainly in the viscera and subcutaneous tissues of the body. Obesity has reached epidemic proportions in our society. In the United States obesity is the most common nutritional problem. Recent data document that over 50% of adults are overweight, 15% are obese, 5% are seriously obese, and 3% have clinically severe obesity.[21]

The calculated **body mass index** (BMI) is a common clinical index of obesity or altered body fat distribution. A well-accepted scale has been developed to calculate BMI by gender using weight-to-height ratios[22] (see Chapter 38, Fig. 38-6). Individuals with a BMI of 25 to 29.9 kg/m^2 are classified as being overweight, those with values of 30 kg/m^2 or more are classified as obese, and those with a BMI of more than 40 kg/m^2 have clinically severe obesity.

The waist-to-hip ratio is another way to define obesity. This ratio is a method of describing the distribution of both subcutaneous and intraabdominal adipose tissue. The waist measurement is divided by the hip measurement to calculate the ratio. A number greater than 1 in men and 0.8 in women indicates overweight. This ratio increases with age and excessive weight.[22] When body weight exceeds 100% of the ideal body weight, it is classified as **morbid obesity.**

In obese persons a variety of problems occur at a rate higher than the expected rate. These include hypertension, hyperlipidemia, type 2 diabetes mellitus, degenerative joint disease, gout, insulin resistance with hyperinsulinemia, respiratory problems, cardiovascular disease, gallbladder disease, non-alcoholic fatty liver disease, stroke, and some kinds of cancer (e.g., breast, colon).[23] Several of these conditions improve if weight loss occurs.

Etiology and Pathophysiology

Many factors have been investigated in an effort to identify the critical elements in the development and maintenance of obesity. Once obesity is present, the number of calories consumed must exceed the energy expended for the condition to continue. However, there is debate about processes leading to obesity.

When assessing the obese patient, the nurse should consider several different types of questions, such as the following:

1. What is the psychologic importance of food to the patient?
2. Is the patient's food intake influenced by hunger?
3. Do the taste and appearance of food or other physical factors in the environment stimulate the patient to eat?
4. Is an emotional problem stimulating the patient to eat?
5. Are any stressors influencing the patient's eating patterns?
6. Do members of the patient's family have a tendency to be overweight?

The nurse must recognize that environmental and genetic factors are important. The children of obese parents tend to be obese. Obesity tends to affect several persons within a family. One biologic component related to obesity is leptin. Leptin is a hormone that mediates the expression of a host of neuropeptides regulating energy intake and expenditure.[24,25] Much more research is needed in this area of biologic and genetic etiologies. Environmental factors play a role in the development of obesity. These include sedentary lifestyle, plentiful food in the household, and socioeconomic status.

The emotional component of the tendency to overeat is powerful. People use food for many reasons, including comfort and reward. Some people are triggered by specific foods to continue eating beyond satiety. The social component of eating develops early in life when food is associated with pleasure and fun at such events as birthday parties, Thanksgiving, and religious holidays. All of these factors must be included when considering the etiology of obesity.

Diagnostic Studies

The majority of obese persons have *primary obesity,* that is, excess calorie intake for the body's metabolic demands. Others have *secondary obesity,* which can result from various congenital anomalies, chromosomal anomalies, metabolic problems, or CNS lesions and disorders. The first step in the treatment process is to determine whether any physical conditions are present. A thorough history and physical examination are necessary and will reveal the extent and duration of the obese state.

The current approach to determining the presence of obesity is the BMI discussed earlier in this chapter. The BMI is not dependent on frame size. Because the BMI value rises with age, it has been suggested that age-specific guidelines for older adults be established. The way to determine BMI is to measure height without shoes and weight with minimal clothing. The weight (expressed in kilograms) is divided by the height squared (expressed in meters). Normal BMI is 20 to 24.9[26] (see Fig. 39-7).

More sophisticated measures of obesity use densitometry, dual photon absorption, magnetic resonance imaging, and ultrasonography. However, such measures are generally used only for research purposes.

Collaborative Conservative Care

The health care provider should explore genetic and endocrine factors such as hypothyroidism, hypothalamic tumors, Cushing syndrome, hypogonadism in men, or polycystic ovarian disease in women. Laboratory tests of liver function, fasting glucose level, triglyceride level, and low- and high-density lipoprotein cholesterol levels assist in evaluating the cause and effects of obesity.

When no organic cause can be found for obesity, it should be considered a chronic, complex illness. Any supervised plan of

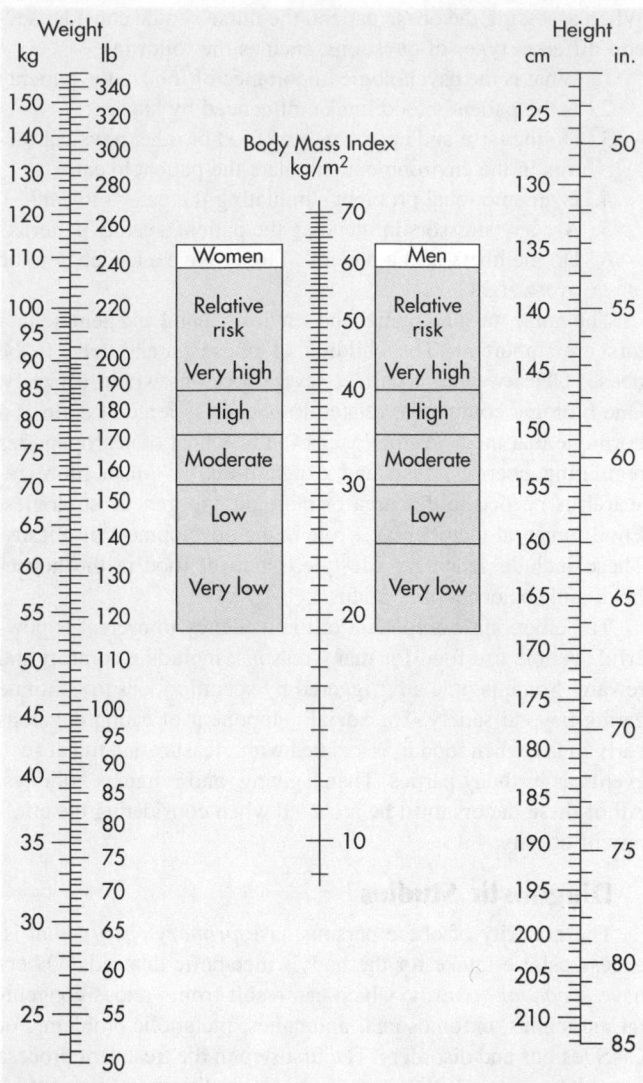

FIG. 39-7 Nomogram for determining body mass index (BMI). To use this nomogram, place a rule or other edge between the column for height and the column for weight connecting an individual's numbers for these two variables. Read the BMI in kg/m² where the straight line crosses the middle lines when the height and weight are connected. Overweight: BMI of 25 to 29.9 kg/m²; obesity: BMI of 30 kg/m² or more. Heights and weights are without shoes or clothes. Relative risk for health problems associated with obesity is shown.

care should be directed at (1) successful weight loss, requiring a short-term energy deficit, and (2) successful weight control, requiring long-term behavior changes. These are two different processes. A multipronged approach ought to be used with attention to multiple factors including dietary intake, physical activity, behavioral-cognitive modification, and perhaps drug therapy. Focusing on more than one aspect will likely give better balance to weight-loss and weight-control efforts.

Nutritional Therapy. Restricted food intake is a cornerstone for any weight loss or maintenance program. A good weight loss plan should contain foods from the basic food groups. Diets may be classified as low calorie (800 to 1200 calories per day) or very low calorie (less than 800 calories per day). Persons on low- and very low-calorie diets need frequent professional monitoring because the severe energy restriction places them at risk for mul-

*E*VIDENCE-BASED PRACTICE
Diet and Mortality Risk in Women

Clinical Problem
Is quality of diet associated with risk for mortality in women?

Best Clinical Practice
- Diet quality was assessed in 42,254 women over a 1-year period. Data were adjusted for age, race, education level, body mass index, smoking status, alcohol use, energy intake, hormone use, physical activity, and history of cancer, heart disease, or diabetes.
- Analyses showed an association between quality of diet (including fruits, vegetables, whole grains, low-fat dairy products, and lean meats) and risk of death from all causes, all types of cancer, coronary artery disease, and stroke.

Implications for Nursing Practice
Consumption of foods that are recommended in current dietary guidelines, including fruits, vegetables, whole grains, low-fat dairy products, and lean meats and poultry, can help decrease the risk for mortality in women.
Reference for Evidence
Kant AK et al: A prospective study of diet quality and mortality in women, *JAMA* 283:2109, 2000.

tiple nutrient deficiencies. A diet that includes adequate amounts of fruits and vegetables provides enough bulk to prevent constipation and meets daily vitamin A and vitamin C requirements. Lean meat, fish, and eggs provide sufficient protein, as well as the B-complex vitamins. Table 39-20 contains a sample 1200-calorie reducing diet.

The only effective method of treating primary obesity is to restrict dietary intake so that it is below energy requirements. It is rare to find an overweight person who has not at some time attempted to lose weight. Some have met with limited and temporary success, and others have met only with failure. It is likely that the majority of these persons attempted weight loss by trying out at least one of the many fad diets that offer the enticement to eat and get slim. In general, fad diets claim weight loss quickly, easily, and inexpensively. Although it is true that initially weight is lost, it is not fat but body water that is lost. The normal fat cell is composed of approximately 80% fat, 18% water, and 2% protein. It is also a storage area for small amounts of glycogen. Glycogen is known to bind with water. When reducing diets severely restrict carbohydrates, the body's glycogen stores become depleted within a few days. It is only when the glycogen pool is almost depleted that protein and adipose tissues are burned to release energy for bodily functions. An obese patient must understand that following a well-balanced, low-calorie diet is an essential part of weight loss.

The degree of success of any reducing diet depends in part on the amount of weight to be lost. A moderately obese person will obviously attain the goal more easily than will a massively obese person. Perhaps because men have a higher percentage of lean body mass, men are able to lose weight more quickly than women. Women have a higher percentage of body fat, which is metabolically less active than muscle tissue.

Motivation is an essential ingredient for successful achievement of weight loss. The obese patient must see the need for weight loss and weight control and the advantages that will oc-

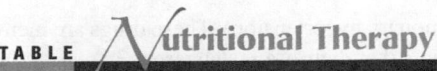

TABLE 39-20	Nutritional Therapy
	1200-Calorie-Restricted Weight-Reduction Diet*

General Principles
1. Eat regularly. Do not skip meals.
2. Measure foods to determine the correct portion size.
3. Avoid concentrated sweets, such as sugar, candy, honey, pies, cakes, cookies, and regular sodas.
4. Reduce fat intake by baking, broiling, or steaming foods.
5. Maintain a regular exercise program for successful weight loss.

MEAL	EXCHANGES	MEAL PLAN 1	MEAL PLAN 2	MEAL PLAN 3
Breakfast	1 meat	1 scrambled egg	1 hard-boiled egg	1 oz ham
	2 bread	1 slice toast	1 flour tortilla	2 griddle cakes with diet syrup
		¾ cup dry cereal (unsweetened)	½ cup Cream of Wheat	
	1 fruit	½ small banana	⅓ cup orange juice	⅓ cup pineapple juice
	1 fat	1 tsp margarine	1 slice bacon	1 tsp margarine
	1 dairy	1 cup low-fat milk	1 cup low-fat milk	1 cup low-fat milk
	Beverage	Coffee	Coffee	Coffee
Lunch	2 meat	1 slice bologna	Cheese enchiladas (made with 2 oz cheese, 2 corn tortillas, chili sauce)	2 oz baked breaded pork chop
		1 slice cheese		
	2 bread	2 slices bread		1 corn muffin
	Vegetable	Lettuce, pickles	Tomato wedges	Spinach
	1 fruit	Fresh grapes (12)	2 canned peach halves (packed in water)	Fresh orange
	Beverage	Diet soda	Artificially sweetened lemonade	Unsweetened iced tea
Dinner	2 meat	1 oz roast beef	Chili con carne (made with ½ cup ground beef, ½ cup pinto beans, and chili powder)	2 oz baked chicken
	1 bread	Baked potato with 1 tsp margarine†		Corn on the cob with 1 tsp margarine
	Vegetable	Cooked carrots	Tossed salad and 1 tbs salad dressing†	Okra
	1 fruit	¾ cup strawberries	Fresh apple	Fruit cocktail (packed in water)
	1 milk	1 cup low-fat milk	1 cup low-fat milk	1 cup low-fat milk

*For 1000 calories, omit 1 fruit exchange and change low-fat milk to skim milk. For 1500 calories, add 1 meat, 1 fruit, and 2 fat exchanges; change low-fat milk to whole milk. For 1800 calories, add 2 bread, 3 meat, 3 fat, and 1 fruit exchanges; change low-fat milk to whole milk.

†One extra fat exchange allowed for each cup of 2% low-fat milk; 2 extra fat exchanges allowed for each cup of skim milk.

cur. The nurse can assist by helping the patient track eating patterns by keeping a diet diary. A frank discussion of eating habits helps the patient realize that often eating is the result of bad habits picked up with time and not of hunger. The bad habits must be changed, or weight loss will be only temporary.

Setting a realistic goal, such as losing 1 to 2 pounds per week, must be mutually agreed on at the outset. Trying to lose too much too fast usually results in a sense of frustration and failure for the patient. The nurse can help the patient understand that losing large amounts of weight in a short period causes skin and underlying tissue to lose elasticity and tone and become unsightly folds of flabby tissue. Slower weight loss offers better cosmetic results. Inevitably, the patient reaches plateau periods during which no weight is lost. These plateaus may last from several days to several weeks. It is especially important for the patient to realize that these are normal occurrences during weight reduction, so that discouragement, frustration, and giving up of the prescribed dietary plan are prevented. A weekly check of body weight is a good method of monitoring progress. Daily weighing is not recommended because of the frequent fluctuations resulting from retained water (including urine) and elimination of feces. The patient should be instructed to record the weight at the same time of the day, wearing the same type of clothing.

There is no firm agreement on the number of meals to be eaten when a person is on a diet. Some nutritionists advocate several small meals per day because the body's metabolic rate is temporarily increased immediately after eating. When several small meals a day are ingested, more calories are used. There seems to be general agreement that consumption of most of the daily caloric intake at a large evening meal results in less weight loss than when the calories are evenly distributed throughout the day.

When a person is first starting on a weight-reduction program, food portions should be weighed to stay within the dietary guidelines. After a time, weighing may not be necessary because the patient can make more accurate judgments of size and weight. A list of permitted foods serves as a good reference and permits an occasional meal to be eaten at a restaurant. The patient who carefully follows the prescribed diet may not need to take vitamin supplements. Appropriate fluid intake should be encouraged. Alcoholic beverages are usually not permitted on a reducing diet because they increase the caloric intake and are low in nutritional value.

Exercise. Exercise is an essential part of a weight-control program. There is no evidence that increased activity promotes an increase in appetite or leads to dietary excess. In fact, exercise frequently has the opposite effect. The addition of exercise produces more weight loss than does dieting alone. Exercise has a favorable effect on body fat distribution, with a reduction in waist-to-hip ratio with increased exercise. Exercise is especially important in maintaining weight loss in overweight persons. Overweight men and women who are active and fit have lower rates of morbidity and mortality than overweight persons who are sedentary and unfit. Therefore exercise is of benefit to overweight persons even if it does not make them lean.

Behavior-Cognitive Modification. For successful long-term weight loss management, behavior modification or cognitive therapy should be integrated into the management plan. Useful basic techniques include (1) self-monitoring, (2) stimulus control, and (3) rewards. Self-monitoring can focus on a record that shows what and when foods are eaten, as well as how the person was feeling when the foods were consumed. Stimulus control is aimed at separating events that trigger eating from the act of eating. Rewards may be used as incentive for weight loss. Short- and long-term goals are useful benchmarks for earning rewards. It is important that the reward for a specified weight loss not be associated with food, such as dinner out or a favorite treat. Reward items do not have to have a monetary component. For example, time for a hot bath or an hour of pleasure reading would be an enjoyable reward for many people. People may participate in group or individual sessions, or both, as they work toward their goals.

Drug Therapy. Drugs have been used in the treatment of obesity but only as adjuncts to a good diet and exercise program. Drugs approved for weight loss can be classified into two categories: (1) those that decrease food intake by reducing appetite or increasing satiety (sense of feeling full after eating) and (2) those that decrease nutrient absorption. Drugs that increase energy expenditure (e.g., ephedrine) are not FDA approved for weight loss in the United States at this time.

Appetite-suppressing drugs. Appetite suppressants reduce food intake through noradrenergic (drugs that mimic norepinephrine) or serotonergic mechanisms in the CNS. Noradrenergic agents include phentermine (Adipex-P, Fastin), diethylpropion (Tenuate, Tepanil), phendimetrazine (Bontril, Plegine), and benzphetamine (Didrex). Amphetamines are not recommended because of their abuse potential. Benzphetamine and phendimetrazine are also classified as Schedule III drugs by the Drug Enforcement Administration because of their potential for abuse. These drugs are recommended for short-term use (i.e., less than 12 weeks) in the management of obesity. Adverse effects of these drugs include palpitations, tachycardia, overstimulation, restlessness, dizziness, insomnia, weakness, and fatigue.[24,25]

Serotonergic drugs act to either increase the release of serotonin or decrease its uptake, thus reducing its metabolism. Fenfluramine (Pondimin) and dexfenfluramine (Redux) were the first drugs in this class. However, in 1997 these drugs were withdrawn from the market because of reported adverse effects (e.g., valvu-

lar heart disease, pulmonary hypertension). These drugs are mentioned to advise patients that their use is dangerous.[24]

Mixed noradrenergic-serotonergic agents are also used in weight management. Sibutramine (Meridia) inhibits both serotonin and norepinephrine uptake, thus increasing their levels in the CNS. Sibutramine along with a reduced-calorie diet has been shown to reduce body weight. Unlike fenfluramine it does not stimulate the release of serotonin, which is thought to be associated with adverse side effects.[25] Side effects include increased blood pressure and heart rate, dry mouth, headache, insomnia, and constipation. Other selective serotonin-reuptake inhibitors that are approved for the management of depression and other psychiatric conditions may have a short-term effect on weight loss, but the effect does not appear to last over time.[25]

Nutrient absorption–blocking drugs. Orlistat (Xenical), a drug that was developed for weight loss and maintenance, works by blocking fat breakdown and absorption in the intestine. It inhibits the action of intestinal lipases. The undigested fat is excreted in the feces. Though this drug has a high safety profile, some fat-soluble vitamin levels may drop and may need to be supplemented.[25,26] Side effects include increased intestinal gas (flatulence), fecal urgency, fecal incontinence, and steatorrhea.

Because drugs will not cure obesity without substantial changes in food intake and increased physical activity, weight gain will occur when short-term drug therapy is stopped. Supervised long-term drug therapy with safe compounds can contribute to weight management, as well as loss. As with any pharmacologic treatment, there are side effects. Careful evaluation for the presence of other medical conditions can help determine which drugs, if any, would be advisable for a given patient.

The role of the nurse in relation to drug therapy should center on teaching the patient about proper administration and side effects and how the drugs fit into the larger weight loss plan. The modification of dosage without consultation with the physician or the nurse can have detrimental effects. The nurse should reemphasize that the diet and exercise regimens are the cornerstones of permanent weight loss. Drugs may be helpful, but they do not help the patient change eating behavior. The purchase of over-the-counter diet aids should be discouraged.

Even with a comprehensive action plan, there is a high rate of weight regain among all age groups. For successful management of obesity, it helps if obesity is viewed as a chronic condition that necessitates day-to-day attention to maintain weight loss.

Collaborative Surgical Care

Many different types of surgical techniques have been described for treating obesity. These techniques can be classified as physical or mechanical (e.g., lipectomy) or nutrient intake limiting (e.g., gastric bypass, banding gastroplasty). For a patient to be selected for any of the operations for morbid obesity, the following criteria are considered:

1. Gross obesity for 5 years
2. Failure to reduce weight with other forms of therapy
3. Body weight 100% above the ideal for age, gender, and height
4. No serious endocrine problem causing the obesity
5. Absence of other medical conditions (liver disease, alcoholism, cardiovascular or pulmonary disease, inflammatory bowel disease, cancer)
6. Psychiatric and social stability and willingness to cooperate with long-term follow-up

7. Availability of a team of health care providers (nurses, physicians, dietitians) to provide immediate and long-term care

8. Presence of a high-risk condition (degenerative joint disease) that weight loss would ameliorate

Lipectomy. **Lipectomy** (adipectomy) is performed to remove unsightly flabby folds of adipose tissue. The patient who chooses lipectomy does so for cosmetic reasons. In some patients, up to 15% of the total fat cells can be removed from the breasts, abdomen, and lumbar and femoral areas. There is no evidence that a regeneration of adipose tissue occurs at the surgical sites. However, it must be emphasized to the patient that surgical removal does not prevent obesity from recurring, especially if lifetime eating habits remain the same. Although body image and self-esteem may be enhanced by such procedures, these operations are not without complications. The dangerous effects of anesthesia and the potential for poor wound healing in the obese patient cannot be overemphasized. It is more useful for the majority of patients contemplating a lipectomy to be instructed in preventive health measures, such as slow weight reduction to maintain and preserve tissue integrity, the value of exercise, and behavior-modification techniques.

Liposuction. Another surgical procedure is *liposuction,* or suction-assisted lipectomy. The current use is for cosmetic purposes and not for weight reduction. This surgical intervention helps improve facial appearance or body contours. A good candidate for this type of surgery is one who has achieved weight reduction but who has excess fat under the chin, along the jawline, in the nasolabial folds, over the abdomen, or around the waist and upper thighs. The procedure is relatively free of major complications. A long, hollow, stainless steel cannula is inserted through a small incision over the fatty tissue to be suctioned. The purpose of this type of surgery is to improve body appearance, thereby enhancing body image and self-concept. It is not usually recommended for the older person because the skin is less elastic and will not accommodate the new underlying shape.

Gastrointestinal Surgeries. Surgical approaches within the GI tract have been directed toward either limiting food intake or producing malabsorption. Many different types of GI surgery have been tried for severe obesity and rejected primarily because of complications or because they were not effective. However, two nutrient intake–limiting procedures currently used are vertical banded gastroplasty and Roux-en-Y gastric bypass[27] (Table 39-21 and Fig. 39-8).

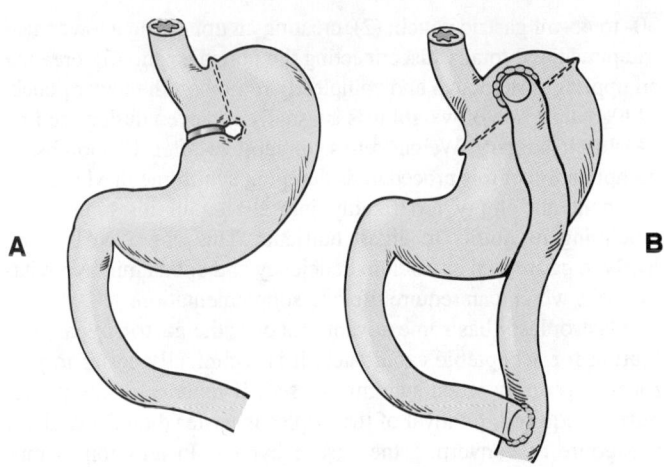

FIG. 39-8 Two gastrointestinal surgical procedures for limiting nutrient intake are currently being used in the treatment of morbid obesity. **A,** Vertical banded gastroplasty consists of constructing a small pouch with a restricted outlet along the lesser curvature of the stomach. This outlet may be externally reinforced to prevent disruption or dilation. **B,** Roux-en-Y gastric bypass procedure involves constructing a proximal gastric pouch whose outlet is a Y-shaped limb of small bowel.

Vertical banded gastroplasty. *Vertical banded gastroplasty* is the most frequently used procedure to produce weight loss in obese people. This approach leads to physical restriction of food intake. In vertical banded gastroplasty, the stomach is partitioned into a small (usually about 30 ml) upper portion along the lesser curvature of the stomach. This small pouch drastically limits capacity. In addition, the stoma opening to the rest of the stomach is banded to delay emptying of solid food from the proximal pouch. This procedure has achieved considerable success in management of weight loss. Problems associated with this gastric restriction operation include intractable vomiting from too rapid intake of solids, distention of the wall of the proximal pouch, rupture of the staple line, and erosion of the band into the stomach.

Gastric bypass. The Roux-en-Y surgical procedure is the most commonly used gastric bypass surgery. In this procedure, the stomach size is decreased with a gastric pouch anastomosis emptying directly into the jejunum. Variations of this procedure include (1) stapling the stomach without transection to create a small,

TABLE 39-21   Surgical Interventions for Morbid Obesity

PROCEDURE	METHOD OF WEIGHT LOSS	ANATOMIC CHANGES	ADVANTAGES	RISKS
▪ Roux-en-Y gastric bypass*	Reduced gastric capacity Some malabsorption	Gastric pouch and gastrojejunostomy	Large weight loss	Staple line dehiscence; iron, calcium, cobalamin deficiency; dumping syndrome with dietary intake of refined carbohydrates
▪ Vertical banded gastroplasty*	Reduced gastric capacity	Small gastric pouch along lesser stomach curvature	Easy to perform procedure (e.g., no anastomosis necessary); more normal anatomy and physiology maintained	Less weight loss than gastric bypass; disrupted staple line; dilated pouch; erosion at band into stomach (rare); potential for maladaptive eating (e.g., ingestion of calorically dense food)

*See Fig. 39-8.

30- to 45-ml gastric pouch; (2) creating an upper and a lower gastric pouch and totally disconnecting the pouches; and (3) creating an upper gastric pouch and completely removing the lower pouch. The greatest rate of weight loss is usually achieved during the first year after surgery. Weight tends to stabilize after 18 months. A complication of this procedure is dumping syndrome in which gastric contents empty too rapidly into the small intestine, overwhelming its ability to digest nutrients. This operation is more likely to cause iron or calcium deficiency and cobalamin hypovitaminosis, which can require lifelong supplementation.

Gastroplasty has some advantages over the gastric bypass operation for acceptable candidates. It is technically easier to perform, especially when stapling is used. If reversal of the procedure is required, removal of the staples is easier than the difficult procedure of converting the gastric bypass. In addition, symptoms of the dumping syndrome and malabsorption are eliminated. However, the weight loss record is often disappointing.[27]

An early surgery that led to malabsorption was the jejunoileal bypass. This procedure resulted in excellent weight loss. However, because of frequent serious health-related complications, including electrolyte imbalance, osteoporosis, bypass enteritis, and liver failure, this surgery is no longer performed. Many patients had surgical procedures done to reverse the bypass. A group of patients may still have a malabsorptive biliopancreatic diversion procedure performed. Weight loss is superior to the gastric bypass, but metabolic and nutritional disturbances remain with this technique.[27]

NURSING MANAGEMENT
OBESE PATIENT

■ Nursing Assessment

The nurse, working closely with the other members of the health care team, plays a major role in the planning and management of the obese patient. To be effective, the nurse must be aware of perceptions of and beliefs about obesity. If a health care provider associates this condition with lack of will power and gluttony, the patient can experience shame in a setting that claims to be a caring one. By being sensitive when asking specific and leading questions, the nurse can often obtain information that the patient may withhold out of embarrassment or shyness or because of being a poor historian. Information that can assist the nurse in understanding an obese patient and provide a basis for intervention is presented in Table 39-22. The nurse must provide acceptable reasons for such personally intrusive questions, respond to the patient's concerns about diagnostic tests, and interpret test outcomes. The patient's answers to questions must be treated with respect, understanding, and a nonjudgmental attitude.

Measurements used with the obese person may include skinfold thickness, height, weight, and BMI. *Android obesity,* in which fat is distributed over the abdomen and upper body (neck, arms, and shoulders), is associated with a greater cardiovascular risk of hypertension, type 2 diabetes mellitus, dyslipidemia, ischemic heart disease, stroke, and death. The nurse should emphasize the importance of vigorous treatment of this type of obesity. The patient should be informed that *gynecoid obesity* (fat distribution over hips) carries a better prognosis but may be more difficult to treat.

As part of the initial nursing physical assessment, each body system should be examined with particular attention to the organ system in which the patient has expressed a problem or concern. Providing specific documentation on these areas assists the physician with a more in-depth history and physical examination.

■ Nursing Diagnoses

Nursing diagnoses for the patient with obesity include, but are not limited to, the following:

1. Imbalanced nutrition: more than body requirements *related to* excessive intake in relation to metabolic need and decreased activity
2. Impaired physical mobility *related to* excessive body weight

TABLE 39-22	Nursing Assessment Obese Patient
Subjective Data	*Role-relationship:* Change in financial status or family; personal, social, and financial resources to support a reducing diet
Important Health Information	*Sexuality-reproductive:* Menstrual irregularity, heavy menstrual flow in women, infertility; effect of obesity on sexual activity
Past health history: Time of obesity onset; diseases related to metabolism and obesity such as hypertension, cardiovascular problems, stroke, cancer, chronic joint pain, respiratory problems, diabetes mellitus, cholelithiasis	**Objective Data**
Medications: Thyroid preparations, use of diet pills	**General**
Surgery or other treatments: Weight-reduction procedures	Body mass index ≥30 kg/m²; waist-to-hip ratio greater than 0.8 (women) or 1 (men), body weight 20% above ideal for height and frame, triceps skinfold greater than 25 (women) or 15 (men)
Functional Health Patterns	**Respiratory**
Health perception–health management: Family history of obesity; perception of problem; methods of weight loss attempted	Hypoventilation
Nutritional-metabolic: Amount and frequency of eating; overeating in response to boredom, stress, specific times or activities	**Cardiovascular**
Elimination: Constipation	Hypertension
Activity-exercise: Typical physical activity; drowsiness, somnolence; dyspnea on exertion, orthopnea, paroxysmal nocturnal dyspnea	**Musculoskeletal**
Sleep-rest: Sleep apnea	Decreased joint mobility
Cognitive-perceptual: Feelings of rejection, isolation, guilt, or shame; meaning or value of food; compliance with prescribed reducing diets, degree of long-term commitment to a weight-loss program	**Possible Findings**
	Elevated serum glucose, cholesterol, triglycerides; polycythemia

3. Social isolation *related to* alterations in physical appearance and perceived unattractiveness

4. Impaired skin integrity *related to* alterations in nutritional state (obesity), immobility, excess moisture, and multiple skinfolds

5. Ineffective breathing pattern *related to* decreased lung expansion from obesity

6. Noncompliance *related to* alteration in perception or lack of motivation

7. Disturbed body image *related to* deviation from usual or expected body size and inability to lose or retain weight loss

▪ Planning

The overall goals are that the obese patient will (1) achieve weight loss to a specified level, (2) maintain weight loss at a specified level, (3) modify eating levels, and (4) participate in a regular physical activity program.

▪ Nursing Implementation

Health Promotion. In collaboration with the dietitian, the nurse is in a prime position to participate in formal and informal health and nutritional teaching activities. Targeting groups in the work setting is one way health promotion activities can be conducted and reinforced. Group competition within the work environment has been reported to offer moderate success for participants. Interrelated key factors are group support coupled with competition.

Acute Intervention. Special considerations are necessary in the care of the patient who is admitted to the hospital for surgical treatment of obesity, especially the morbidly obese. Most nursing units are not prepared to meet the needs of a patient who is often too large for a typical hospital or recovery room bed or who has arms that even a large-size blood pressure cuff will not fit. To eliminate embarrassment for the patient and frustration for the staff, plans for these special needs should be made before the patient's admission. Oversized blood pressure cuffs should be ready for use when the patient arrives. A private room may be necessary for privacy of the patient and to accommodate the bed and sitting arrangements. A strongly reinforced trapeze bar should be placed over the bed to facilitate movement and positioning. In some cases a specially constructed chair may have to be built and beds joined together to allow the patient to sit and sleep in comfort.

A care-planning conference should be a priority so that even simple nursing care measures do not become impossible tasks. Consideration should be given to questions such as how the patient will be weighed, how the patient will be transported throughout the hospital, and how simple physical assessment strategies may have to be adjusted to accommodate the morbidly obese patient. Anticipation of the need to use the hospital's meat or freight scales saves time and energy later for both the staff and the patient. Another need is a wheelchair with removable arms that is large enough to safely accommodate the patient and that will pass easily through doorways.

Strategies for bathing, turning, and ambulating the patient, including the number of extra people needed to carry out these measures, are invaluable when the actual need arises. Special gowns are also needed for the patient. Routine physical assessment strategies do not work well with a morbidly obese female patient who has numerous layers of skinfolds covering the chest and abdomen in addition to huge, pendulous breasts obscuring the area to be assessed. Without identifying alternatives or unique methods of dealing with this problem, assessment of respiratory status and bowel sounds or even wound inspection could be awkward for the nurse and embarrassing for the patient.

Wound infection is one of the most common complications after surgery. Because of the many layers of flabby skinfolds, especially in the abdominal area, preoperative skin preparation is important. Frequently the patient is instructed to take several showers a day for a few days before admission to the hospital. Careful cleansing with soap and warm water of the abdominal area from the breasts to below the waist is emphasized.

The patient must be instructed in the proper coughing technique, deep breathing, and methods of turning and positioning to prevent pulmonary complications after surgery. The use of a spirometer may be introduced before surgery. Because most obese patients breathe shallowly, use of the spirometer helps prevent and alleviate postoperative lung congestion. Practicing these strategies preoperatively can aid in performing them correctly postoperatively.

All patients admitted for major gastric surgery procedures have an NG tube inserted during surgery and attached to low suction after surgery. Allowing the patient to see a typical tube and explaining why it is necessary is a good method of involving the patient in the plan of care. The patient should know that oral nourishment will be impossible for a few days after the surgery and that IV fluids will be the main source of intake.

Early ambulation is essential for the obese patient. It is important that the patient know that it is usually necessary to get out of bed soon after surgery and with increasing frequency thereafter, generally 3 to 4 times each day. The dangers of thrombophlebitis and measures to counteract its development are a routine part of preoperative teaching. The patient should know that elastic stockings, elastic compression stockings, or elastic wraps will be applied to the legs and that active and passive range-of-motion exercises will be a frequent part of daily care. Low-dose heparin often will be ordered. (General preoperative nursing care is discussed in Chapter 17.)

The patient experiences considerable abdominal pain after surgery. Administration of pain medications should be given as frequently as necessary during the immediate postoperative period. If pain medication is not given by patient-controlled analgesia, the nurse must remember that intramuscular medications must be given with an extra-long needle, such as a spinal needle, so that the medication is administered into the muscle and not into the adipose or subcutaneous tissue, which will delay absorption. Keeping the head of the bed elevated at a 30-degree angle at all times facilitates ventilatory efforts. Encouraging and assisting the patient to turn, cough, and deep breathe at least every 1 to 2 hours minimizes the risk for atelectasis and pneumonia. Frequent mouth and nose care also helps breathing efforts because the NG tube is inserted through one nostril.

Position changes and range-of-motion exercises are instituted immediately after surgery and carried out every 1 to 2 hours. Ambulatory efforts generally are begun on the evening of surgery. For patient safety, the nurse should enlist the assistance of other staff members during these initial efforts, while encouraging the patient to help.

The abdominal wound requires frequent observation for the amount and type of drainage, condition of the sutures, and signs of infection. The incision must be protected against undue straining that accompanies turning and coughing. Wound dehiscence and wound healing are potential problems for all obese patients. Monitoring the vital signs assists in identifying problems such as infection.

It is important that the NG tube be kept patent and in the correct position. Vomiting is common following gastric procedures. If tube patency is blocked or the tube requires repositioning, the physician should be notified at once. The upper gastric pouch is small, and irrigating the tube with too much solution or manipulating tube position can lead to disruption of the anastomosis or staple line. In most cases the NG tube can be removed in approximately 48 hours, or when bowel sounds have resumed.

Skin care should be carried out several times each shift. Perspiration may be excessive at times. The many layers of skin should be kept clean and dry so that this source of irritation is eliminated. For the patient who has an indwelling catheter, perineal care is important so that a urinary tract infection can be prevented.

Clear liquids are given orally when tolerance is established. The amount offered at first is necessarily limited to approximately 1 ounce, which is to be sipped slowly. More solid types of food are given to the patient who has had gastric surgery as progress is made through the postoperative recovery period.

Ambulatory and Home Care. The patient who has undergone major surgical treatment for obesity has not, in the past, been successful in following or maintaining a prescribed diet. Now the patient is forced to reduce the oral intake as a result of the anatomic changes brought about by the operation. This patient finds that adherence to a reduced intake is necessary because of the concern for abdominal distention, cramping abdominal pain, and perhaps diarrhea.

Weight loss is considerable during the first 6 to 12 months. It is during this time that the patient must learn to adjust intake sufficiently to maintain a stable weight. Although behavior modification was not an intended outcome when these surgical procedures were devised, it becomes an unexpected secondary gain. The diet generally prescribed should be high in protein and low in carbohydrates, fat, and roughage and consist of six small feedings daily. Fluids should not be ingested with the meal, and in some cases, fluids should be restricted to less than 1000 ml per day. Fluids and foods high in carbohydrate tend to promote diarrhea and symptoms of the dumping syndrome. Generally, calorically dense foods (foods high in fat) should be avoided to permit more nutritionally sound food to be consumed.

Proper diet must be clearly understood by the patient. Late complications can be anticipated after gastric bypass or gastroplasty, including anemia, vitamin deficiencies, diarrhea, and psychiatric problems. Failure to lose weight or loss of too much weight may be caused by the surgical formation of too large a stomach pouch or of an outlet that is much too small, respectively. Peptic ulcer formation, dumping syndrome, and small bowel obstruction may be seen late in the recovery and rehabilitative stage.

Long-term follow-up care must be stressed, in part because of complications late in the recovery period. The patient must be encouraged to adhere strictly to the prescribed diet and to keep the care provider informed of any changes in physical or emotional condition. Some patients have been known to overeat when they return home and gain rather than lose weight.

The nurse must anticipate and recognize several potential psychologic problems after surgery. Some patients express guilt feelings concerning the fact that the only way they could lose weight was by surgical means rather than by the "sheer willpower" of reduced dietary intake. The nurse should be ready to provide support so that this patient does not dwell on negative feelings.

Many morbidly obese patients who blamed their feelings of social inferiority or inadequacies on their appearance before bypass surgery may suffer from episodes of depression. By 6 to 8 months after surgery, considerable weight loss has occurred, and they are able to see clearly how much their appearance has changed. Massive weight loss often leaves the patient with large quantities of flabby skin that can result in problems related to altered body image. Reconstructive surgery at least 1 full year after the initial surgery may alleviate this situation. Reduction of the breasts, upper arms, thighs, and excess abdominal skinfolds are possible solutions. Discussion of this possible outcome with the patient before surgery and again during the rehabilitation phase of recovery helps facilitate the patient's adjustment to a new body image and social reintegration.

Physical activity. Once a physical activity program has been outlined for the patient, the nurse can reinforce instruction and help individualize it to the patient's time schedule and physical limitations. The nurse should point out that engaging in weekend exercise only or in spurts of strenuous activity is not advantageous and can actually be dangerous. Joining a health club can be one mechanism of getting exercise. Walking, swimming, and cycling are sensible forms of exercise and have long-term benefits. The combination of a good reducing diet and an increased physical activity program can have profound effects on the patient's achievement of weight loss. When large muscles are involved in the exercise program, a primary benefit is cardiovascular conditioning.

Many psychologic benefits can be derived from an increased physical activity program. Reduction in tension and stress, better-quality sleep and rest, decreased desire to eat excessively, increased stamina and energy, improved self-concept and self-confidence, better attitudes toward work and play, and increased optimism about the future can be achieved.

Cognitive-behavior modification. The person who is on any type of restrictive dietary program is often encouraged to join a group of other obese persons who are receiving professional counseling to help them modify their eating habits. The assumption behind behavior modification is that obesity is a learned disorder caused by overeating and that the critical difference between an obese person and a nonobese person is in the cues that stimulate eating behavior. Therefore most behavior-modification programs de-emphasize the diet and focus on how and when the person eats. Participants often are taught to restrict their eating to designated meals and to increase the amount of physical activity in their lives. Persons who have undergone behavior therapy are more successful in maintaining their losses over an extended time than those who do not participate in such training.

Many self-help groups are available to the person who wants to learn more about successful dieting and who likes the support of others having the same problems and experiences. Take Off Pounds Sensibly (TOPS) is the oldest nonprofit organization of this type. Behavioral modification is an integral part of the program, along with nutrition education. Weight Watchers International, Inc., is probably the most successful commercial weight-reduction enterprise. Weight Watchers offers a food plan that is nutritionally balanced and practical to follow, and it has used behavior-modification techniques since 1974. There has been a proliferation of commercial weight-reduction centers across the nation. Many of these programs are staffed by nurses or dietitians, or both, and require an initial physical examination by a care provider before a candidate is accepted for weight reduction. These weight-reduction centers are costly and therefore are cost prohibitive for those with limited financial resources. Many of these programs also offer special prepackaged foods and supplements that must be purchased as part of the weight-reduction plan. Only these prescribed foods and drinks are to be consumed until an agreed-on amount of weight is lost. The patient is encouraged to buy the same type of foods for the maintenance phase of the program, lasting from 6 months to 1 year. Behavior-modification training is incorporated within these programs as well.

Regardless of the commercial products used, successful weight loss and control are limited and require individualized programs consisting of restricted caloric intake, behavior modification, and exercise. Although persons who follow this type of program are likely to lose weight, once they leave the program the weight is usually regained because they tend to resume previous eating behaviors and return to the foods previously eaten.

A new concept of influencing health behavior and better employee health has occurred recently. Programs on health teaching and maintenance have been started at places of employment. The rationale for such programs is that better health repays the cost of the programs through improved work performance, decreased absenteeism, and eventually less hospitalization. Weight-reduction and hypertension-reduction programs have been instituted and are popular with employees.

■ Evaluation

The expected outcomes are that the obese patient will
- experience long-term weight loss
- have improvement in obesity-related comorbidities
- integrate healthy practices into daily routines
- monitor for adverse side effects of surgical therapy
- have an improved self-image

EATING DISORDERS

Eating disorders are primarily psychiatric disorders. However, there are a number of nutritional problems associated with these disorders that require the nurse to implement a nutritional plan of care. According to the American Dietetic Association, over 5 million Americans suffer from eating disorders. It primarily affects young women. It is estimated that 6% of those with severe eating disorders will die, and only 50% report being cured.[28]

Anorexia Nervosa

Anorexia nervosa is characterized by a self-imposed weight loss, endocrine dysfunction, and a distorted psychopathologic attitude toward weight and eating.[29] Anorexia nervosa clinically manifests as abnormal weight loss, deliberate self-starvation, intense fear of gaining weight, *lanugo* (soft, downy hair covering the body except the palms and soles), refusal to eat, continuous dieting, hair loss, sensitivity to cold, compulsive exercise, absent or irregular menstruation, dry skin, and constipation. Diagnostic studies often show iron deficiency anemia and an elevated blood urea nitrogen level that is reflective of marked intravascular volume depletion and prerenal azotemia. Lack of potassium in the diet and loss of potassium in the urine lead to potassium deficiency. Manifestations of potassium deficiency include muscle weakness, cardiac arrhythmias, and renal failure. If the eating pattern is permitted to continue for a prolonged time, body wasting and signs of severe malnutrition are evident.

Multidisciplinary treatment must involve a combination of nutritional support and psychiatric care. Hospitalization may be necessary if there are severe physical complications that cannot be managed in an outpatient therapy program. Nutritional replenishment must be closely supervised to ensure consistent and ongoing weight gains. The use of tube or parenteral feedings may be necessary. Improved nutrition, however, is not a cure for anorexia nervosa. The underlying psychiatric problem must be addressed by identification of the disturbed patterns of individual and family interactions, followed by individual and family counseling.

Bulimia Nervosa

Bulimia nervosa is a disorder characterized by frequent binge eating and self-induced vomiting associated with loss of control over eating and a persistent concern with body image.[29] These individuals may have normal weight for height, or their weight may fluctuate with bingeing and purging. They may also abuse laxatives, diuretics, exercise, or diet drugs. They may have signs of frequent vomiting, such as macerated knuckles, swollen salivary glands, broken blood vessels in the eyes, and dental problems.

Bulimia is increasing in incidence and may be even more prevalent than anorexia nervosa. Female college students seem to be most susceptible to this syndrome. The cause remains unclear but is thought to be similar to that of anorexia nervosa. Substance abuse, anxiety, affective disorders, and personality disturbances have been reported among persons with bulimia.

The patient with bulimia, similar to the one with anorexia nervosa, goes to great lengths to conceal abnormal eating habits. As the behavior persists, many problems associated with the condition become increasingly hard to deal with effectively. As with anorexia, a treatment combination of psychologic counseling and diet therapy is essential. Education and emotional support for the patient and family are vital. Support groups such as the National Association of Anorexia Nervosa and Associated Disorders (see resources for information) are extremely helpful to those affected by these disorders.

■ Culturally Competent Care: Nutrition

People have unique cultural heritages that may affect eating customs and nutritional status. Culture along with personal preferences, socioeconomic status, and religious preferences can influence food choices. Each culture has its own beliefs and behaviors related to food and the role that food plays in the etiology and treatment of disease. In addition, culture can dictate what food is considered edible, as well as how it is prepared and when it is eaten. There are a wide array of cultural influences on diet ranging from what foods are selected to when meals are eaten and how and who prepares them. For example, some religions require periods of fasting.

The nurse should include cultural and ethnic considerations when assessing the patient's diet history and implementing interventions that require dietary changes. At the same time, the nurse needs to avoid *cultural stereotyping* by making assumptions or generalizations about diet based on the individual's cultural background. For example, not all Jewish patients eat only kosher foods.

It is important to know whether the patients eats "traditional foods" associated with the culture. If traditional foods are eaten, the nurse should assess for their impact on health. For example, "soul foods," which include traditional foods eaten by some African Americans, tend to be high in fat, cholesterol, and sodium. Traditional foods eaten by some Asian Americans may be high in fiber and low in fat and cholesterol but also low in calcium content because of the lack of milk products.

Consideration of cultural beliefs is very important when planning dietary changes and monitoring acceptance of dietary changes. For example, perception of body weight and size may also be influenced by culture. Thus the nurse needs to ask the patient or family about how culture affects dietary choices and weight maintenance. In some cultures an overweight person may be seen as a sign of success. Thus the nurse would have a challenging time trying to convince that person to lose weight. ■

Teaching related to dietary restrictions and recommended dietary changes should involve the patient's family. In many situations it is a family member who does the grocery shopping and cooking.

CRITICAL THINKING EXERCISES

Case Study
Obesity
Patient Profile. Mrs. Estella Rodriguez is a 60-year-old Hispanic woman who is 5 feet 4 inches tall and weighs 190 pounds.
Subjective Data
- Reports gradual weight gain during past 40 years
- Spends most of her free time watching television
- Reports health problems related to type 2 diabetes mellitus, shortness of breath, hypertension, chest pressure, and osteoarthritis
- Had knee replacement surgery at age 56 for osteoarthritis
Objective Data
Physical Examination
- Has obese, nontender, soft abdomen
- BP is 150/90
Laboratory Results
- Fasting blood glucose: 250 mg/dl (13.9 mmol/L)
- Total cholesterol: 205 mg/dl (5.3 mmol/L)
- Triglyceride: 298 mg/dl (3.36 mmol/L)
- HDL cholesterol: 31 mg/dl (0.8 mmol/L)

CRITICAL THINKING QUESTIONS
1. What are Mrs. Rodriguez's obesity risk factors?
2. What is her estimated BMI?
3. Of the possible complications of obesity, which ones does Mrs. Rodriguez have? What are contributing factors to her developing type 2 diabetes mellitus, cardiovascular disease manifestations, and osteoarthritis?

4. What would you, as the nurse, include in a successful weight loss and weight management program for Mrs. Rodriguez?
5. Is Mrs. Rodriguez a candidate for surgical intervention for obesity? If so, why? If not, why not?
6. Based on the assessment data presented, write one or more appropriate nursing diagnoses. Are there any collaborative problems?

Nursing Research Issues
1. What nursing interventions can be used to reduce diarrhea associated with tube feedings?
2. What happens to serum calcium and bone density in vegetarian patients over time?
3. What is the effect of surgical procedures for obesity on the quality of life or on functional abilities?
4. Does early enteral feeding reduce the risk of sepsis in critically ill patients?
5. Are there valid and reliable bedside methods for determining nasogastric (NG) and nasointestinal tube placement?
6. What are the ways to reduce the risk of catheter sepsis in a patient receiving TPN?

REVIEW QUESTIONS

The number of the question corresponds to the same-numbered objective at the beginning of the chapter.

1. The nurse identifies a need for dietary teaching for the patient whose daily intake of food groups consists of
   a. 2 to 4 servings of the fruit group.
   b. 2 to 3 servings of the milk, yogurt, and cheese group.
   c. 4 to 5 servings of the bread, cereal, rice, and pasta group.
   d. 2 to 3 servings of the meat, poultry, fish, beans, egg, and nut group.

2. In general, nutrient or food interactions with drugs can result in all of the following except
   a. enhancing drug absorption.
   b. decreasing drug bioavailability.
   c. increasing a nutrient requirement.
   d. all of the above options can happen.

3. During the first 24 hours of starvation, the order in which the body obtains substrate for energy is
   a. glycogen, skeletal protein.
   b. visceral protein, fat stores, glycogen.
   c. fat stores, skeletal protein, visceral protein.
   d. liver protein, muscle protein, visceral protein.

4. An elderly patient with a recent stroke is exhibiting signs of severe dysphagia. The optimal form of nutrition support at this time would be
   a. TPN.
   b. regular diet.
   c. nasoenteric tube feedings.
   d. nothing by mouth (NPO) until dysphagia resolves.

5. A nutritionally stressed patient weighing 60 kg is NPO and receiving TPN. In evaluating the patient's nutritional intake, the nurse calculates that the daily TPN solution should provide
   a. 40 g fat.
   b. 80 g protein.
   c. 20 calories per kilogram.
   d. 1000 calories from carbohydrate.

6. One advantage of a percutaneous endoscopic gastrostomy tube placement relative to NG feedings for the patient receiving long-term enteral nutrition is that
   a. it increases patient comfort.
   b. it eliminates the risk of aspiration.
   c. feedings can be initiated before bowel sounds are present.
   d. more calories can be delivered compared with NG feeding.

7. The obesity aspect that is most often associated with cardiovascular health problems is
   a. primary obesity.
   b. secondary obesity.
   c. gynoid fat distribution.
   d. android fat distribution.

8. A morbidly obese patient has undergone Roux-en-Y gastric bypass surgery. In planning postoperative care, the nurse anticipates that the patient
   a. may have severe diarrhea early in the postoperative period.
   b. will require nasogastric suction until healing of the site occurs.
   c. will not be allowed to ambulate for 5 to 7 days postoperatively.
   d. may have only liquids orally, and in very limited amounts, during the early postoperative period.

9. The nurse recognizes that the major goal of treatment for a patient with anorexia nervosa is being met when the patient
   a. demonstrates a rapid weight gain.
   b. consumes the required daily intake of nutrients.
   c. commits to long-term individual and family counseling.
   d. verbalizes feelings regarding self-image and fears of becoming obese.

REFERENCES

1. Fiscella K et al: Does patient educational level affect office visits to family physicians? *J Natl Med Assoc* 94:157, 2002.
2. Lutz CA, Przytulski KR: *Nutrition and diet therapy,* ed 3, Philadelphia, 2001, FA Davis.
3. Frazao E: America's eating habits: changes and consequences, *Agriculture Information Bulletin* No. 750, May 1999.
4. ASPEN Board of Directors: Guidelines for the use of parenteral and enteral nutrition in adult and pediatric patients: 2001 revision, *J Parenter Enteral Nutr* 26 (suppl 1):1SA, 2002.
5. Shopbell JM, Hopkins B, Shronts EP: Nutrition screening and assessment. In Gottschlich MM, editor: *The science and practice of nutrition support,* Dubuque, Iowa, 2001, Kendall/Hunt.
6. Thomas DR et al: Nutritional management in long-term care: development of a clinical guideline, *J Gerontol Med Sci* 55A:M725, 2000.
7. Wilmore DW: *The metabolic management of the critically ill,* New York, 1977, Plenum Publishing.
8. Institute of Medicine, Food, and Nutrition Board: *Dietary reference intakes: vitamin A, vitamin K, arsenic, boron, chromium, copper, iodine, iron, manganese, molybdenum, nickel, silicon, vanadium, and zinc,* Washington DC, 2001, National Academy Press.
9. American Dietetic Association: ADA's definition for nutrition screening and assessment, *J Am Diet Assoc* 94:838, 1994.
10. Project of the American Academy of Family Physicians, The American Dietetic Association, and National Council on Aging: *Nutrition intervention manual for professional caring for older Americans,* Washington DC, 1994, Nutrition Screening Initiative.
*11. Kovacevich DS et al: Nutrition risk classification: a reproducible and valid tool for nurses, *Nutr Clin Pract* 12:20, 1997.
*12. Keller JJ, Hirdes JP: Using the minimum data set to determine the prevalence of nutrition problems in an Ontario population of chronic care patients, *Can J Diet Pract Res* 61:165, 2000.
13. US Dept of Agriculture and US Dept of Health and Human Services: *Dietary guidelines for Americans,* ed 4, Home and garden bulletin. No. 232. Washington DC, 1995, US Government Publishing Office.
*14. Keele AM et al: Two phase randomized controlled clinical trial of postoperative oral dietary supplements in surgical patients, *Gut* 40:393, 1997.
15. Guenter P: Tube feeding administration. In Guenter P, Silkroski M, editors: *Tube feeding: practical guidelines and nursing protocols,* Gaithersburg, Md, 2001, Aspen.

*Nursing research–based reference.

16. Edwards SJ, Metheny NA: Measurement of gastric residual volume: state of the science, *MedSurg Nurs* 9:125, 2000.
17. Guenter P: Nursing care of patients with enteral feeding devices. In Guenter P, Silkroski M, editors: *Tube feeding: practical guidelines and nursing protocols*, Gaithersburg, Md, 2001, Aspen.
18. National Advisory Group on Standards and Practice Guidelines for Parenteral Nutrition: Safe practices for parenteral nutrition formulations, *JPEN* 22:49, 1998.
19. Shuster MH: Parenteral nutrition. In Hennessey KA, Orr ME, editors: *Nutrition support nursing core curriculum*, ed 3, Silver Spring, Md, 1996, Aspen.
20. Krzywda EA, Andris DA, Edmiston CE: Catheter infections: diagnosis, etiology, treatment, and prevention. *Nutr Clin Pract* 14:178, 1999.
21. Flegal KM et al: Overweight and obesity in the United States: prevalence and trends 1960-1994, *Int J Obes Relat Metab Disord* 22:39, 1998.
22. Bray G: Obesity: part 1—pathogenesis, *West J Med* 149:431, 1988.
23. Dwyer J: Medical evaluation and class of obesity. In Blackburn GL, Kanders BS, editors: *Obesity pathophysiology, psychology and treatment*, New York, 1994, Chapman & Hall.
24. Apovian CM: Medical management of obesity and the role of pharmacotherapy: an update, *Nutr Clin Pract* 15:5, 2000.
25. Yanovski SZ, Yanovski JA: Drug therapy: obesity, *N Engl J Med* 346:591, 2002.
26. Pi-Sunyer FX: Obesity. In Shils ME, Olsen JA, Ross CA, editors: *Modern nutrition in health and disease*, ed 9, Baltimore, 1999, Williams & Wilkins.
27. Shikora SA: Surgical treatment for severe obesity: the state-of-the-art for the new millennium, *Nutr Clin Pract* 15:13, 2000.
28. American Dietetic Association: Position of the ADA: Nutrition intervention in the treatment of anorexia nervosa, bulimia nervosa, and eating disorders not otherwise specified, *J Am Diet Assoc* 101:810, 2001.
29. Muse DM, Lucas AR: Behavioral disorders affecting food intake: anorexia nervosa, bulimia nervosa and other psychiatric conditions. In Shils ME, Olsen JA, Ross CA, editors: *Modern nutrition in health and disease*, ed 9, Baltimore, 1999, Williams & Wilkins.

RESOURCES

Academy for Eating Disorders
6728 Old McLean Village Drive
McLean, VA 22101
703-556-9222
Fax: 703-556-8729
www.aedweb.org/

American Dietetic Association
216 West Jackson Blvd.
Chicago, IL 60606-6995
800-877-1600
312-899-0040
www.eatright.org

American Society for Bariatric Surgery
7328 West University Avenue, Suite F
Gainesville, FL 32607
352-331-4900
Fax: 352-331-4975
www.asbs.org

American Society for Parenteral and Enteral Nutrition
8630 Fenton Street, Suite 412
Silver Spring, MD 20910
800-727-4567
301-587-6315
Fax: 301-587-2365
www.nutritioncare.org

Council for Nutrition Clinical Strategies in Long-Term Care
Programs in Medicine
3415 West Chester Pike
Newtown Square, PA 19073

FDA Center for Food Safety and Applied Nutrition (CFSAN)
5100 Paint Branch Parkway
College Park, MD 20740-3835
www.cfsan.fda.gov

Healthy People 2010
Office of Disease Prevention and Health Promotion
Hubert H. Humphrey Building, Room 738G
200 Independence Avenue SW
Washington, DC 20201
Fax: 202-205-9478
www.health.gov/healthypeople/

National Association of Anorexia Nervosa and Associated Disorders (ANAD)
PO Box 7
Highland Park, IL 60035
847-831-3438
Fax: 847-433-4632
www.anad.org/

National Center for Complementary and Alternative Medicine (NCCAM)
National Institutes of Health
Bethesda, MD 20892
http://nccam.nih.gov

National Eating Disorder Information Centre
CW 1-211, 200 Elizabeth Street
M5G 2C4
Toronto, Canada
866-NEDIC-20
416-340-4156
Fax: 416-340-4736
E-mail: nedic@uhn.on.ca
www.nedic.ca/

National Eating Disorders Association
603 Stewart Street, Suite 803
Seattle, WA 98101
800-931-3327
206-382-3587
Fax: 206-829-8501
www.nationaleatingdisorders.org

OLEY Foundation
214 Hun Memorial, A-28
Albany Medical Center
Albany, NY 12208-3478
800-776-OLEY
518-262-5079
Fax: 518-262-5528
http://c4isr.com/oley/

Overeaters Anonymous Headquarters
PO Box 44020
Rio Rancho, NM 87174-4020
505-891-2664
Fax: 505-891-4320
www.overeatersanonymous.org/

For additional Internet resources, see the website for this book at *http://evolve.elsevier.com/Lewis/medsurg/*.

CHAPTER 40

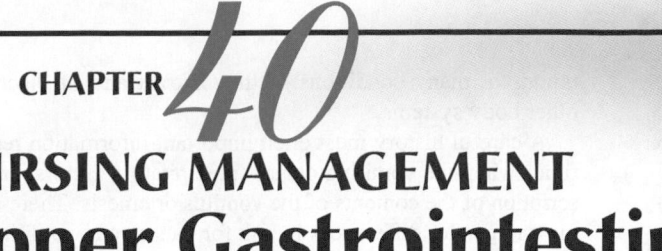

NURSING MANAGEMENT
Upper Gastrointestinal Problems

Margaret McLean Heitkemper

LEARNING OBJECTIVES

1. Describe the etiology, complications, collaborative care, and nursing management of nausea and vomiting.
2. Describe the etiology, clinical manifestations, and treatment of common oral inflammations and infections.
3. Describe the etiology, clinical manifestations, complications, collaborative care, and nursing management of oral cancer.
4. Explain the types, pathophysiology, clinical manifestations, complications, and collaborative care including surgical therapy and nursing management of gastroesophageal reflux disease and hiatal hernia.
5. Describe the pathophysiology, clinical manifestations, complications, and collaborative care of esophageal cancer, diverticula, achalasia, and esophageal strictures.
6. Differentiate between acute and chronic gastritis, including the etiology, pathophysiology, collaborative care, and nursing management.
7. Explain the common etiology, clinical manifestations, collaborative care, and nursing management of upper gastrointestinal bleeding.
8. Compare and contrast gastric and duodenal ulcers, including etiology and pathophysiology, clinical manifestations, complications, collaborative care, and nursing management.
9. Describe the clinical manifestations, collaborative care, and nursing management of gastric cancer.
10. Identify the common types of food poisoning and the nursing responsibilities related to food poisoning.

KEY TERMS

achalasia, p. 1019
Barrett's esophagus, p. 1012
dysphagia, p. 1009
esophageal cancer, p. 1017
esophageal diverticula, p. 1019
esophagitis, p. 1012
gastric cancer, p. 1044
gastritis, p. 1020
gastroesophageal reflux disease, p. 1011

hiatal hernia, p. 1015
leukoplakia, p. 1009
Mallory-Weiss tear, p. 1023
nausea, p. 1003
peptic ulcer disease, p. 1028
physiologic stress ulcers, p. 1031
vomiting, p. 1003

NAUSEA AND VOMITING

Nausea and vomiting are the most common manifestations of gastrointestinal (GI) diseases. **Nausea** is a feeling of discomfort in the epigastrium with a conscious desire to vomit. **Vomiting** is the forceful ejection of partially digested food and secretions *(emesis)* from the upper GI tract. Vomiting is a complex act that requires the coordinated activities of several structures: closure of the glottis, deep inspiration with contraction of the diaphragm in the inspiratory position, closure of the pylorus, relaxation of the stomach and lower esophageal sphincter, and contraction of the abdominal muscles with increasing intraabdominal pressure. These simultaneous activities force the stomach contents up through the esophagus, into the pharynx, and out the mouth. Although nausea and vomiting can occur independently, they are usually closely related and usually treated as one problem.

Etiology and Pathophysiology

Nausea and vomiting are found in a wide variety of GI disorders, as well as in conditions that are unrelated to GI disease. These include pregnancy, infectious diseases, central nervous system (CNS) disorders (e.g., meningitis, CNS tumor), cardiovascular problems (e.g., myocardial infarction, congestive heart failure), metabolic disorders (e.g., Addison's disease, uremia), side effects of drugs (e.g., narcotics, digitalis), and psychologic factors (e.g., stress, fear).

Generally, nausea occurs before vomiting and is characterized by contraction of the duodenum and by slowing of gastric motility and emptying. A single episode of nausea accompanied by vomiting may not be significant. However, if vomiting occurs several times, it is important that the cause be identified.

A vomiting center in the brainstem coordinates the multiple components involved in vomiting. This center receives input from various stimuli. Neural impulses reach the vomiting center via afferent pathways through branches of the autonomic nervous system. Visceral receptors for these afferent fibers are located in the GI tract, kidneys, heart, and uterus. When stimulated, these receptors relay information to the vomiting center, which then initiates the vomiting reflex (Fig. 40-1).

In addition, the chemoreceptor trigger zone (CTZ) located on the floor of the fourth ventricle in the brain responds to chemical stimuli of drugs and toxins. The CTZ also plays a role in vomiting when it is due to labyrinthine stimulation (e.g., motion sickness). Once stimulated, the CTZ transmits impulses directly to the vomiting center.

Vomiting also can occur when the GI tract becomes overly irritated, excited, or distended. It can be a protective mechanism to rid the body of spoiled or irritating foods and liquids. Immediately

Reviewed by Marilee Schmelzer, RN, PhD, Associate Professor, University of Texas at Arlington, Arlington, Tex.

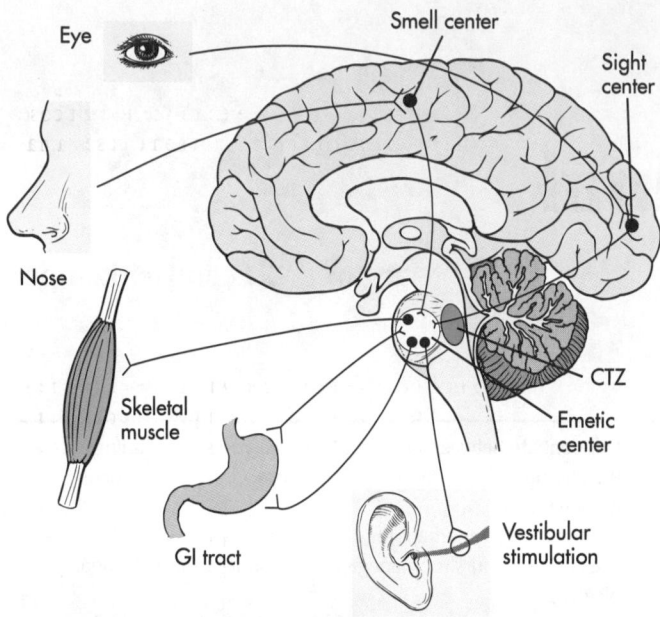

FIG. 40-1 Stimuli involved in the act of vomiting. *CTZ*, Chemoreceptor trigger zone; *GI*, gastrointestinal.

before the act of vomiting, the person becomes aware of the need to vomit. The autonomic nervous system is activated, resulting in both parasympathetic and sympathetic nervous system stimulation. Sympathetic activation produces tachycardia, tachypnea, and diaphoresis. Parasympathetic stimulation causes relaxation of the lower esophageal (cardiac) sphincter, an increase in gastric motility, and a pronounced increase in salivation. These manifestations are experienced immediately before vomiting.

Clinical Manifestations

Nausea is a subjective complaint. *Anorexia* (lack of appetite) usually accompanies nausea and is brought on by unpleasant stimulation involving any of the five senses. When nausea and vomiting are prolonged, dehydration can rapidly occur. In addition to water, essential electrolytes (e.g., potassium, sodium, chloride, hydrogen) are also lost. As vomiting persists, there may be severe electrolyte imbalances, loss of extracellular fluid volume, decreased plasma volume, and eventually circulatory failure. Metabolic alkalosis can result from loss of gastric hydrochloric acid (HCl). Metabolic acidosis can occur because of the loss of bicarbonate when contents from the small intestine are vomited. However, metabolic acidosis as a result of severe vomiting is less common than metabolic alkalosis. Weight loss resulting from fluid loss is evident in a short time when vomiting is severe.

The threat of pulmonary aspiration is a concern when vomiting occurs in the patient who is elderly, is unconscious, or has other conditions that impair the gag reflex. The patient who cannot adequately manage self-care should be put in a semi-Fowler's or side-lying position to prevent aspiration.

Collaborative Care

The goals of collaborative care are to determine and treat the underlying cause of the nausea and vomiting and to provide symptomatic relief of nausea and vomiting. Determining the cause is often difficult because nausea and vomiting are manifes-

tations of many conditions of the GI tract and of disorders of other body systems.

A careful history must elicit important information regarding times when the vomiting occurs, precipitating factors, and a description of the contents of the vomitus or emesis. There are ethnic and gender differences in risk for nausea and vomiting associated with both surgical procedures and motion sickness.[1] Asian Americans, Middle Easterners, and African Americans are more likely to experience nausea and vomiting than whites. Women are more likely than men to experience nausea and vomiting.

In all patients, differentiation must be made between vomiting, regurgitation, and projectile vomiting. *Regurgitation* is a process in which partially digested food is slowly brought up from the stomach. Retching or vomiting seldom precedes it. *Projectile vomiting* is a very forceful expulsion of stomach contents without nausea and is characteristic of CNS tumors.

The presence of fecal odor and bile after prolonged vomiting indicates intestinal obstruction below the level of the pylorus. The presence of bile in the emesis may suggest obstruction below the ampulla of Vater or bile reflux gastritis. The presence of partially digested food several hours after a meal is indicative of gastric outlet obstruction or delay in gastric emptying.

The color of the emesis aids in determining the presence and source of bleeding. Vomitus with a "coffee ground" appearance is associated with bleeding in the stomach, where blood changes to dark brown as a result of its interaction with gastric acid. Bright red blood indicates active bleeding, which is suggestive of a tear in the mucosal lining of the lower esophagus or fundus of stomach, bleeding gastric or duodenal ulcer or neoplasm, or bleeding esophageal varices.

The time of day at which the vomiting occurs is often helpful in determining the cause. Early morning vomiting is a frequent occurrence in pregnancy. Emotional stressors with no evident pathologic disorder may elicit vomiting during or immediately after the ingestion of a meal.

Drug Therapy. The use of drugs in the treatment of nausea and vomiting depends on the cause of the problem. Many different drugs can be used (Table 40-1). Because the cause cannot always be readily determined, drugs must be used with caution. The use of antiemetics before the cause of the vomiting is established can mask the underlying disease process and delay diagnosis and treatment. Many of the antiemetic drugs act on the CNS at the level of the CTZ. In general, they block the neurochemicals that appear to trigger nausea and vomiting.

Drugs that control nausea and vomiting include antimuscarinics (e.g., scopolamine), antihistamines (e.g., diphenhydramine [Benadryl]), and phenothiazines (e.g., chlorpromazine [Thorazine], prochlorperazine [Compazine]). Because many of these drugs have anticholinergic actions, they are contraindicated for the patient with glaucoma, prostatic hyperplasia, pyloric or bladder neck obstruction, or biliary obstruction. They share many common side effects, which include dry mouth, hypotension, sedative effects, rashes, and GI disturbances such as constipation. Consultation with a pharmacist may be indicated before administering these drugs to the patient with multiple medical problems.

Other drugs with antiemetic properties include metoclopramide (Reglan) and domperidone (Motilium). These drugs act both centrally and peripherally on dopamine receptors. Peripherally they enhance the release of acetylcholine, resulting in increased gastric emptying. Because of this effect, these drugs are

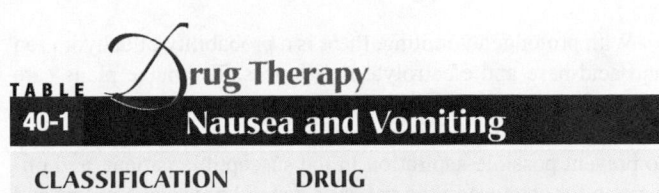

CLASSIFICATION	DRUG
Antiemetic and antipsychotic	chlorpromazine (Thorazine)
	haloperidol (Haldol)
	perphenazine (Trilafon)
	prochlorperazine (Compazine)
	promazine (Sparine)
	trifluoperazine (Stelazine)
	triflupromazine (Vesprin)
Antihistamine	buclizine (Bucladin-S)
	cyclizine (Marezine)
	dimenhydrinate (Dramamine)
	diphenhydramine (Benadryl)
	hydroxyzine (Vistaril)
	meclizine (Antivert, Bonine)
	promethazine (Phenergan)
Prokinetic	domperidone (Motilium)
	metoclopramide (Reglan)
Serotonin antagonist	dolasetron (Anzemet)
	granisetron (Kytril)
	ondansetron (Zofran)
Antimuscarinic	scopolamine transdermal (Transderm-Scop)
Others	benzquinamide (Emete-Con)
	dexamethasone (Decadron)
	diphenidol (Vontrol)
	dronabinol (Marinol)
	thiethylperazine (Torecan)
	trimethobenzamide (Tigan)

considered *prokinetics*. However, about 10% to 20% of patients taking metoclopramide experience CNS side effects ranging from anxiety to hallucinations. Extrapyramidal side effects including tremor and dyskinesias similar to Parkinson's disease may also occur. Domperidone does not cross the blood-brain barrier, resulting in fewer side effects compared with metoclopramide.

Antagonists to specific serotonin (5-HT) receptors have been found to act both centrally and peripherally to reduce nausea and vomiting. In particular, antagonists to the 5-HT$_3$ receptors are effective in reducing cancer chemotherapy–induced vomiting, vomiting caused by total body radiation, GI motility disturbances, carcinoid syndrome, and nausea and vomiting related to migraine headache and anxiety. Serotonin antagonists including ondansetron (Zofran), granisetron (Kytril), and dolasetron (Anzemet) act centrally in the vomiting center, as well as peripherally to enhance gastric emptying.

Dexamethasone (Decadron) is used in the management of cancer chemotherapy–induced emesis, usually in combination with other antiemetics. Dexamethasone alone or in combination with ondansetron reduces both acute and delayed chemotherapy-induced nausea and vomiting. Dronabinol (Marinol) is an orally active cannabinoid. It can be used alone or in combination with other antiemetics for the prevention of chemotherapy-induced emesis. Because of the potential for abuse, as well as CNS side effects including drowsiness and sedation, this drug is used when other therapies are ineffective.

Nutritional Therapy. The patient with severe vomiting requires intravenous (IV) fluid therapy with electrolyte and glucose replacement until able to tolerate oral intake. In some cases a nasogastric (NG) tube and suction are used to decompress the stomach. Once the symptoms have subsided, oral nourishment beginning with clear liquids is started. Extremely hot or cold liquids are not usually well tolerated. Carbonated beverages at room temperature and with the carbonation gone and warm tea are more easily tolerated. The addition of dry toast or crackers may alleviate the feeling of nausea and help prevent vomiting. Although broth and Gatorade have been used widely for the patient with severe vomiting, these substances are high in sodium and should be administered with caution. Water is the initial fluid of choice for rehydration by mouth.

As the patient's condition improves, a diet high in carbohydrates and low in fatty foods should be provided. Items such as a baked potato, plain gelatin, cereal with milk and sugar, and hard candy may be added. Foods that are known to be poorly tolerated include coffee, spicy foods, and highly acidic foods. Food should be eaten slowly and in small amounts to prevent overdistention of the stomach. When solid foods have been reintroduced, fluids should be taken between meals rather than with meals. It is advised that the patient remain quietly relaxed for approximately 1 hour after meals. A dietitian may be consulted regarding appropriate foods that have nutritional value and are well tolerated by the patient during the recovery process.

NURSING MANAGEMENT
NAUSEA AND VOMITING

■ **Nursing Assessment**

Each patient with a history of prolonged and persistent nausea or vomiting requires a thorough nursing assessment before a specific plan of care is developed. Although the conditions associated with nausea and vomiting are numerous, the nurse should have a basic understanding of the more common conditions and should be able to identify the patient who is at high risk. Knowledge of the physiologic mechanisms involved in nausea and vomiting and the demonstration of a genuine regard for the patient are essential. Table 40-2 presents subjective and objective data that should be obtained from a patient with nausea and vomiting, regardless of the underlying cause.

COMPLEMENTARY & ALTERNATIVE THERAPIES
Ginger

Clinical Uses
Dyspepsia, nausea and vomiting, and motion sickness.

Effects
Analgesic and sedative effects. Reduction of GI motility. May also decrease the effects of acid-inhibiting drugs. Overdoses can cause CNS depression and cardiac arrhythmias.

Nursing Implications
Should not be taken if using anticoagulant therapy, digoxin, or hypoglycemic agents. Should not be used if patient has gallstones or heart failure.

CNS, Central nervous system; *GI,* gastrointestinal.

TABLE 40-2	**Nursing Assessment** **Nausea and Vomiting**

Subjective Data
Important Health Information
Past health history: GI disorders, chronic indigestion, food allergies, pregnancy, infection, CNS disorders, recent travel, bulimia, metabolic disorders, cancer, cardiovascular disease, renal disease
Medications: Use of antiemetics, digitalis, opiates, ferrous sulfate, aspirin, aminophylline, alcohol, antibiotics; general anesthesia; chemotherapy
Surgery or other treatments: Recent surgery
Functional Health Patterns
Nutritional-metabolic: Amount, frequency, character, and color of vomitus; dry heaves; anorexia; weight loss
Activity-exercise: Weakness, fatigue
Cognitive-perceptual: Abdominal tenderness or pain
Coping-stress tolerance: Stress, fear

Objective Data
General
Lethargy, sunken eyeballs
Integumentary
Pallor, dry mucous membranes, poor skin turgor
Gastrointestinal
Amount, frequency, character (e.g., projectile), content (undigested food, blood, bile, feces), and color of vomitus (red, "coffee ground," green-yellow)
Urinary
Decreased output, concentrated urine
Possible Findings
Altered serum electrolytes (especially hypokalemia), metabolic alkalosis, abnormal upper GI findings on endoscopy or abdominal x-rays

CNS, Central nervous system; *GI,* gastrointestinal.

■ Nursing Diagnoses

Nursing diagnoses for the patient with nausea and vomiting may include, but are not limited to, those presented in NCP 40-1.

■ Planning

The overall goals are that the patient with nausea and vomiting will (1) experience minimal or no nausea and vomiting, (2) have normal electrolyte levels and hydration status, and (3) return to a normal pattern of fluid balance and nutrient intake.

■ Nursing Implementation

Acute Intervention. The majority of individuals with nausea and vomiting can be managed at home. However, when nausea and vomiting persist regardless of home treatment strategies, hospitalization may be necessary for diagnosis of the underlying problem. Until a diagnosis is confirmed, the patient is kept on nothing-by-mouth (NPO) status and given IV fluids. An NG tube connected to suction may be necessary for the patient with persistent vomiting, as well as for the patient in whom the possible diagnosis may be bowel obstruction or paralytic ileus. Keeping the stomach empty reduces the stimulus to vomit. The NG tube should be stabilized to eliminate its movement in the nose and back of the throat because this can stimulate nausea and vomiting.

With prolonged vomiting, there is a probability of dehydration and acid-base and electrolyte imbalances. The nurse plans care that includes accurate recording of intake and output, monitoring vital signs, assessing for signs of dehydration, proper positioning to prevent possible aspiration in the susceptible patient, and observing for changes in the patient's general physical comfort and mentation. The nurse takes responsibility for providing physical and emotional support; maintaining a quiet, odor-free environment; and giving explanations regarding any diagnostic tests or procedures performed.

Patients who are hospitalized for other health problems may be prone to episodes of nausea and vomiting. These individuals include the postoperative patient who is recovering from the effects of a surgical procedure, anesthesia, and pain. Nausea and vomiting are common side effects in the cancer patient receiving chemotherapeutic drugs. (Nursing care of the cancer patient is found in Chapter 15.)

Ambulatory and Home Care. The patient and family may need instructions on (1) how to deal successfully with the unpleasant sensations of nausea, (2) methods of preventing nausea and vomiting, and (3) strategies to maintain fluid and nutritional intake. The occurrence of nausea or vomiting may be minimized if measures are taken to keep the immediate environment quiet, free of noxious odors, and well ventilated. The avoidance of sudden changes of position and unnecessary activity is also helpful. Use of relaxation techniques, frequent rest periods, and diversional tactics help prevent nausea and vomiting or facilitate a more rapid recovery from their effects. Cleansing the face and hands with a cool washcloth and mouth care between episodes increase the person's comfort level. When the symptoms occur, all foods and drugs should be stopped until the acute phase is past.

If a medication is suspected as the cause, the health care provider should be notified immediately so that either the dosage can be altered or a new drug can be prescribed. The patient should be reminded that stopping the drug without consulting the health care provider may eliminate the immediate cause of the nausea and vomiting but that omission of the prescribed drug may have detrimental effects on health or the disease state.

When food is identified as the precipitating cause of nausea and vomiting, the nurse should help the patient solve the problem. What food was it? When was it eaten? Has this food caused problems in the past? Is anyone else in the family sick?

When the patient believes some foods and fluids can be tolerated, the nurse might suggest that it would be helpful to begin with clear liquids or warm cola beverages, Gatorade, tea or broth, dry crackers or toast, and then plain gelatin. Bland foods, such as pasta, rice, and cooked chicken, are generally well tolerated in small amounts. An antiemetic drug should be taken only if prescribed by the health care provider. Taking over-the-counter (OTC) drugs for relief of symptoms may make the condition worse.

■ Evaluation

The expected outcomes are that the patient with nausea and vomiting will
- be comfortable with minimal or no nausea and vomiting
- maintain body weight
- have electrolyte levels within normal range
- be able to maintain adequate intake of fluids and nutrients

NURSING CARE PLAN 40-1

Patient with Nausea and Vomiting

EXPECTED PATIENT OUTCOMES	NURSING INTERVENTIONS and *RATIONALES*
NURSING DIAGNOSIS	**Nausea** *related to* multiple etiologies *as manifested by* episodes of nausea and vomiting
▪ Minimal or no nausea ▪ Verbalization of satisfaction with care	▪ Assess duration, frequency, and nature of nausea and vomiting and aggravating and alleviating factors *to plan appropriate interventions.* ▪ Remove visual stimuli and source of odors *to avoid precipitating triggers of nausea and/or vomiting.* ▪ Provide mouth care; change soiled gown and linens *to ensure patient comfort.* ▪ Maintain quiet environment, restrict visitors, and avoid unnecessary procedures or activities *to minimize triggers of vomiting.* ▪ Administer antiemetic as ordered. ▪ Instruct patient to take several deep breaths; prevent sudden changes in position; keep head of bed elevated *to decrease stimulation of the vomiting center.* ▪ Instruct patient to avoid foods and beverages *that stimulate nausea and vomiting.*
NURSING DIAGNOSIS	**Deficient fluid volume** *related to* prolonged vomiting and inability to ingest, digest, or absorb food and fluids *as manifested by* decreased urine output and increased urine concentration, increased pulse rate, hypotension (postural), decreased intake, decreased skin turgor, dry skin and mucous membranes
▪ No signs of dehydration	▪ Assess for signs of dehydration *to plan appropriate care.* ▪ Administer and monitor amount and type of IV fluid *to maintain fluid and electrolyte balance.* ▪ Administer antiemetic as prescribed. ▪ Provide small amounts of clear liquids when vomiting stops *to maintain hydration.* ▪ Record amount and frequency of vomitus; maintain accurate intake and output records; weigh daily in acute phase *to monitor fluid balance accurately.* ▪ Monitor laboratory results of serum sodium, potassium, chloride, and bicarbonate *as indicators of electrolyte balance.*
NURSING DIAGNOSIS	**Imbalanced nutrition: less than body requirements** *related to* nausea and vomiting *as manifested by* lack of interest in or aversion to food, perceived or actual inability to ingest food, weight loss
▪ Gradual return to usual weight and eating habits	▪ Assess patient's interest in food, ability to ingest food, and weight *to determine if a problem is present.* ▪ Assure patient that appetite will return when nausea and vomiting are controlled. ▪ Maintain IV feedings or total parenteral nutrition until oral intake is possible *to provide necessary fluids, electrolytes, calories, and protein intake.* ▪ Instruct patient to resume eating cautiously with bland, nonirritating foods in small amounts *to avoid irritating the stomach and initiating recurrence of nausea and vomiting.*

▪ Gerontologic Considerations: Nausea and Vomiting

The older patient experiencing nausea and vomiting requires careful assessment and monitoring, particularly during periods of fluid loss and subsequent rehydration therapy. Older patients are more likely to have cardiac or renal insufficiency that places them at greater risk for life-threatening fluid and electrolyte imbalances. In addition, excessive replacement of fluid and electrolytes may result in adverse consequences for the elderly person who has congestive heart failure or renal disease. Finally, the older adult with a decreased level of consciousness may be at high risk for aspiration of vomitus. Close monitoring of the patient's physical status and level of consciousness during episodes of vomiting must be a primary concern for the nurse.

In addition, the elderly are particularly susceptible to the CNS side effects of antiemetic drugs; these drugs may produce confusion. Dosages should be reduced and efficacy closely evaluated. Safety precautions also should be instituted for these patients. ▪

ORAL INFLAMMATIONS AND INFECTIONS

Oral infections and inflammations may be specific mouth diseases, or they may occur in the presence of some systemic diseases such as leukemia or vitamin deficiency. When oral inflammations and infections are present, they can severely impair the ingestion of food and fluids. Common inflammations and infections of the oral cavity are presented in Table 40-3. The patient who is immunosuppressed (e.g., patient with acquired immunodeficiency syndrome or receiving chemotherapy) is most susceptible to oral infections. Patients receiving corticosteroid inhalant treatment for asthma are at risk for oral infections, especially candidiasis.

Oral infections may predispose to infections in other body organs. For example, the oral cavity can be considered a potential reservoir for respiratory pathogens. In addition, oral pathogens have also been associated with heart disease.

An important element in reducing oral infections and inflammation is good oral hygiene. Management of oral infections and inflammation is focused on identification of the cause, elimination of infection, provision of comfort measures, and maintenance of nutritional intake.

ORAL CANCER

Oral (or oropharyngeal) cancer may occur on the lips or anywhere within the mouth (e.g., tongue, floor of the mouth, buccal mucosa, hard palate, soft palate, pharyngeal walls, and tonsils). Oral cancer is diagnosed in 30,100 Americans annually, and it is estimated that 7800 persons a year die from the disease.[2] It is more common after 40 years of age, with 60 years being the average age at onset. Oral cancer occurs in all ethnic groups. It is more common in men (male-to-female ratio of 2:1). Squamous cell carcinoma is the most common oral malignant tumor (more than 90%). Mortality rates have been decreasing since the early 1980s. The 5-year survival for all stages of cancer of the oral cavity and pharynx combined is 53%, and the 10-year rate is 43%.[2]

TABLE 40-3   Infections and Inflammation of the Mouth

CONDITION	ETIOLOGY	CLINICAL MANIFESTATIONS	TREATMENT
Gingivitis	Neglected oral hygiene, malocclusion, missing or irregular teeth, faulty dentistry, eating of soft rather than fibrous foods	Inflamed gingivae and interdental papillae; bleeding during toothbrushing; development of pus; formation of abscess with loosening of teeth (periodontitis)	Prevention through health teaching, dental care, gingival massage, professional cleaning of teeth, fibrous foods, conscientious brushing habits with flossing
Vincent's infection (acute necrotizing ulcerative gingivitis, trench mouth)	Fusiform bacteria; Vincent spirochetes; predisposing factors of stress, excessive fatigue, poor oral hygiene, nutritional deficiencies (B and C vitamins)	Painful, bleeding gingivae; eroding necrotic lesions of interdental papillae; ulcerations that bleed; increased saliva with metallic taste; fetid mouth odor; anorexia, fever, and general malaise	Rest (physical and mental); avoidance of smoking and alcoholic beverages; soft, nutritious diet; correct oral hygiene habits; topical applications of antibiotics; mouth irrigations with hydrogen peroxide and saline solutions
Oral candidiasis (moniliasis or thrush)	*Candida albicans* (a yeastlike fungus), debilitation, prolonged high-dose antibiotic or corticosteroid therapy	Pearly, bluish white "milk-curd" membranous lesions on mucosa of mouth and larynx; sore mouth; yeasty halitosis	Nystatin or amphotericin B as oral suspension or buccal tablets, good oral hygiene
Herpes simplex (cold sore, fever blister)	Herpes simplex virus, type I or II; predisposing factors of upper respiratory infections, excessive exposure to sunlight, food allergies, emotional tension, onset of menstruation	Lip lesions, mouth lesions, vesicle formation (single or clustered), shallow, painful ulcers	Spirits of camphor, corticosteroid cream, mild antiseptic mouthwash, viscous lidocaine; removal or control of predisposing factors, antiviral agents (e.g., acyclovir [Zovirax], penciclovir [Denavir])
Aphthous stomatitis (canker sore)	Recurrent and chronic form of infection secondary to systemic disease, trauma, stress, or unknown causes	Ulcers of mouth and lips, causing extreme pain; ulcers surrounded by erythematous base	Corticosteroids (topical or systemic), tetracycline oral suspension
Parotitis (inflammation of parotid gland, surgical mumps)	Usually *Staphylococcus* species, *Streptococcus* species occasionally, debilitation and dehydration with poor oral hygiene, NPO status for an extended time	Pain in area of gland and ear, absence of salivation, purulent exudate from gland, erythema, ulcers	Antibiotics, mouthwashes, warm compresses; preventive measures such as chewing gum, sucking on hard candy (lemon drops), adequate fluid intake
Stomatitis (inflammation of mouth)	Trauma; pathogens; irritants (tobacco, alcohol); renal, liver, and hematologic diseases; side effect of many cancer chemotherapy drugs and radiation	Excessive salivation, halitosis, sore mouth	Removal or treatment of cause, oral hygiene with soothing solutions, topical medications; soft bland diet

Most of the oral malignant lesions occur on the lower lip in men. Other common sites are the lateral border and undersurface of the tongue, the labial commissure, and the buccal mucosa. Carcinoma of the lip has the most favorable prognosis of any of the oral tumors. This is probably because lip lesions are more apparent to the patient than other oral lesions and are usually diagnosed earlier.

Etiology and Pathophysiology

Although the definitive cause of oral cancer is unknown, there are a number of predisposing factors (Table 40-4). Factors that influence the development of oral cancer include tobacco use (e.g., cigar, cigarette, pipe, snuff), excessive alcohol intake, and chronic irritation such as from a jagged tooth or poor dental care. A positive history of tobacco and alcohol use, in the past or currently, is the most significant etiologic factor in oral cancer.[2] Constant overexposure to ultraviolet radiation from the sun is also a factor in the development of cancer of the lip. Irritation from the pipe stem resting on the lip is a factor in pipe smokers.

Clinical Manifestations

The common manifestations of oral cancer are leukoplakia, erythroplakia, ulcerations, a sore that bleeds easily and does not heal, and a rough area (felt with the tongue). **Leukoplakia,** called "white patch" or "smoker's patch," is often considered a precancerous lesion, although less than 5% of these lesions actually transform into malignant cells. It is a whitish patch on the mucosa of the mouth or tongue. The patch becomes *keratinized* (hard and leathery) and is sometimes described as hyperkeratosis. Leukoplakia is the result of chronic irritation, especially from smoking. *Erythroplasia* (erythroplakia), which is seen as a red velvety patch on the mouth or tongue, is also considered a precancerous lesion. Areas of erythroplakia have a 90% chance of becoming malignant. Later symptoms of oral cancer are pain, **dysphagia** (difficulty swallowing), and difficulty in moving the jaw (e.g., chewing and speaking).

Cancer of the lip usually appears as an indurated, painless ulcer on the lip. The first sign of carcinoma of the tongue is an ulcer or area of thickening. Soreness or pain of the tongue may occur, especially when eating hot or highly seasoned foods. Cancerous lesions are most likely to develop in the proximal half of the tongue. Some patients experience limitation of movement of the tongue. Later symptoms of cancer of the tongue include increased salivation, slurred speech, dysphagia, toothache, and earache. Approximately 30% of patients with oral cancer have an asymptomatic neck mass.

Diagnostic Studies

Biopsy of the suspected lesion with cytologic examination is the best definitive diagnostic study for oral cancer. Oral exfoliative cytology involves scraping the suspicious lesion and spreading this scraping on a slide. Unlike biopsy, a negative cytologic smear does not reliably rule out the possibility of a malignant condition, but it may be used as an initial screening test. The toluidine blue test may also be used as a screening test for oral cancer. Toluidine blue is applied topically to stain an area, and cancer cells preferentially take up the dye. However, the definitive diagnosis of cancer is based on biopsy and histology.[3]

Collaborative Care

Collaborative care of oral carcinoma usually consists of surgery, radiation, chemotherapy, or a combination of these (Table 40-5).

TABLE 40-5	*C*ollaborative Care Oral Cancer

Diagnostic
History and physical examination
Biopsy
Oral exfoliative cytology
Toluidine blue test
CT and MRI scans

Collaborative Therapy*
Surgery
  Surgical excision of the tumor
  Radical neck dissection
Radiation (internal or external)
Combined surgical resection with radiation
Chemotherapy

*Any of the following approaches may be used, depending on the primary lesion and the extent of metastasis.
CT, Computed tomography; *MRI*, magnetic resonance imaging.

TABLE 40-4 Types and Characteristics of Oral Cancer

LOCATION	PREDISPOSING FACTORS	CLINICAL MANIFESTATIONS	TREATMENT
• Lip	Constant overexposure to sun, ruddy and fair complexion, recurrent herpetic lesions, irritation from pipe stem, syphilis, immunosuppression	Indurated, painless ulcer	Surgical excision, radiation
• Tongue	Tobacco, alcohol, chronic irritation, syphilis	Ulcer or area of thickening; soreness or pain; increased salivation, slurred speech, dysphagia, toothache, earache (later signs)	Surgery (hemiglossectomy or glossectomy), radiation
• Oral cavity	Poor oral hygiene, tobacco usage (pipe and cigar smoking, snuff, chewing tobacco), chronic alcohol intake, chronic irritation (jagged tooth, ill-fitting prosthesis, chemical or mechanical irritants)	Leukoplakia; erythroplakia; ulcerations; sore spot; rough area; pain, dysphagia, difficulty in chewing and speaking (later signs)	Surgery (mandibulectomy, radical neck dissection, resections of buccal mucosa), internal and external radiation

Surgical Therapy. Surgery remains the most effective treatment, especially for removing the central core of the tumor. Many of the operations are radical procedures involving extensive resections. Various surgical procedures may be performed, depending on the location and extent of the tumor. Some examples are partial *mandibulectomy* (removal of the mandible), *hemiglossectomy* (removal of half of the tongue), *glossectomy* (removal of the tongue), resections of the buccal mucosa and floor of the mouth, and radical neck dissection. Composite resections, which are combinations of the various surgical procedures, may be performed.

Because cancers of the oral cavity metastasize early to the cervical lymph nodes, a radical neck dissection is commonly performed. It includes wide excision of the involved primary lesion with removal of the regional lymph nodes, the deep cervical lymph nodes, and their lymphatic channels. In addition, the following structures may also be removed or transected (depending on the extent of the primary lesion): sternocleidomastoid muscle and other closely associated muscles, internal jugular vein, mandible, submaxillary gland, part of the thyroid and parathyroid glands, and spinal accessory nerve. A tracheostomy is commonly performed along with the radical neck dissection. Drainage tubes are inserted into the surgical area and connected to suction to remove fluid and blood.

Nonsurgical Therapy. Chemotherapy and radiation therapy are used together when the lesions are more advanced or involve several structures of the oral cavity. Chemotherapy may also be used when surgery and radiation therapy fail or as the initial therapy for smaller tumors. Chemotherapeutic agents used include 5-fluorouracil (5-FU), cyclophosphamide (Cytoxan), bleomycin (Blenoxane), vinblastine (Velban), hydroxyurea (Hydrea), and cisplatin (Platinol) (see Chapter 15).

Palliative treatment may be the best management when the prognosis is poor, the cancer is inoperable, or the patient decides against surgery. Palliation aims to treat the symptoms and make the patient more comfortable. If it becomes difficult for the patient to swallow, a gastrostomy may be performed to allow for adequate nutritional intake (see Gastrostomy in Chapter 39). Analgesic medication should be given freely to this patient. Frequent suctioning of the oral cavity becomes necessary when swallowing becomes difficult. (Other nursing measures for the terminally ill patient are discussed in Chapter 15.)

Nutritional Therapy. Because of depression, alcoholism, or presurgery radiation treatment, patients may be malnourished even before surgery. After radical neck surgery, the patient may be unable to take in nutrients through the normal route of ingestion because of swelling, location of sutures, or difficulty with swallowing. Parenteral fluids will be given for the first 24 to 48 hours. After this time, tube feedings are usually given via an NG or nasointestinal tube that was placed during surgery. Sometimes a temporary feeding gastrostomy may be used. (NG and gastrostomy feedings are described in Chapter 39.) Cervical esophagostomy and pharyngostomy have also been used. The nurse must observe for tolerance of the feedings and adjust the amount, time, and formula if nausea, vomiting, diarrhea, or distention occurs. The patient is instructed about the tube feedings. When the patient can swallow, small amounts of water are given. Close observation for choking is essential. Suctioning may be necessary to prevent aspiration.

NURSING MANAGEMENT
ORAL CANCER

■ Nursing Assessment

Subjective and objective data that should be obtained from a patient with oral cancer are presented in Table 40-6.

■ Nursing Diagnoses

Nursing diagnoses for the patient with oral cancer may include, but are not limited to, the following:

- Imbalanced nutrition: less than body requirements *related to* oral pain, difficulty chewing and swallowing, surgical resection, and radiation treatment
- Chronic pain *related to* the tumor and surgical radiation
- Anxiety *related to* diagnosis of cancer, uncertain future, potential for disfiguring surgery, potential for recurrence, and prognosis
- Ineffective coping *related to* body image change
- Ineffective health maintenance *related to* lack of knowledge of disease process and therapeutic regimen and unavailability of a support system

■ Planning

The overall goals are that the patient with carcinoma of the oral cavity will (1) have a patent airway, (2) be able to communicate, (3) have adequate nutritional intake to promote wound healing, and (4) have relief of pain and discomfort.

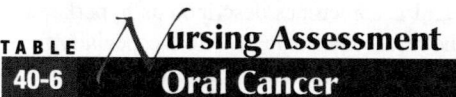

TABLE 40-6	Nursing Assessment Oral Cancer

Subjective Data

Important Health Information

Past health history: Recurrent oral herpetic lesions, syphilis, exposure to sunlight

Medications: Immunosuppressants

Surgery or other treatments: Removal of prior tumors or lesions

Functional Health Patterns

Health perception–health management: Use of alcohol and tobacco, pipe smoking; poor oral hygiene

Nutritional-metabolic: Reductions in oral intake, weight loss; difficulty in chewing food; increased salivation; intolerance to certain foods or temperatures of food

Cognitive-perceptual: Mouth or tongue soreness or pain, toothache, earache, neck stiffness, dysphagia, difficulty speaking

Objective Data

Integumentary

Indurated, painless ulcer on lip; painless neck mass

Gastrointestinal

Areas of thickening or roughness, ulcers, leukoplakia, or erythroplakia on the tongue or oral mucosa; limited movement of the tongue; increased salivation, drooling; slurred speech; foul breath odor

Possible Findings

Positive exfoliative smear cytology (microscopic examination of cells removed by scraping); positive biopsy

■ Nursing Implementation

Health Promotion. The nurse has a significant role in early detection and treatment of oral cancer. The nurse needs to provide the patient with information regarding predisposing factors, such as constant overexposure to the sun, tobacco, and other irritants. Smoking and the long-term use of smokeless tobacco are the major risk factors for oral cancer. A patient identified as a smoker should be informed about smoking cessation programs available in the community. (Smoking cessation is discussed in Chapter 11 and Tables 11-13 and 11-14).

It is important that adolescents and teenagers be informed about the danger of using snuff, or chewing tobacco. In addition, oral cancers have an increased chance of recurrence if risk factors are not reduced. The nurse should also teach correct oral hygiene and dental care and encourage the patient to seek preventive dental care. Risk factors should be identified. Because early detection of oral cancer is important, the patient should be taught to examine the mouth and to recognize danger signals of oral cancer. If any of these signals are present, the patient should be instructed to visit a health care provider. Danger signals include unexplained pain or soreness in the mouth, unusual bleeding from the oral cavity, dysphagia, and swelling or lump in the neck.

Any individual with an ulcerative lesion that does not heal within 2 to 3 weeks should be referred to a health care provider, and a biopsy of the lesion should probably be performed. The nurse should inspect the patient's oral cavity to detect suspicious lesions.

Acute Intervention. Preoperative care for the patient who is to have a radical neck dissection involves consideration of the patient's physical and psychosocial needs. Physical preparation is the same as for any major surgery, with special emphasis on oral hygiene. Thorough assessment of alcohol intake should be done, and measures to assess and treat withdrawal if it is a problem should be implemented early. Explanations and emotional support are of special significance and should include postoperative measures relating to communication and feeding. The surgical procedure should be explained to the patient, and the nurse should make sure that the patient understands the information. Radical neck dissection and related nursing management are discussed in Chapter 26 and NCP 26-2.

■ Evaluation

The expected outcomes are that the patient with oral cancer will

- have no respiratory complications
- be able to communicate
- participate in regular follow-up examinations
- maintain an adequate nutritional intake to promote wound healing
- experience minimal pain and discomfort with eating, drinking, and talking

Esophageal Disorders

GASTROESOPHAGEAL REFLUX DISEASE

Etiology and Pathophysiology

Gastroesophageal reflux disease (GERD) is not a disease but a syndrome. The term *GERD* is defined as any clinically significant symptomatic condition or histopathologic alter-

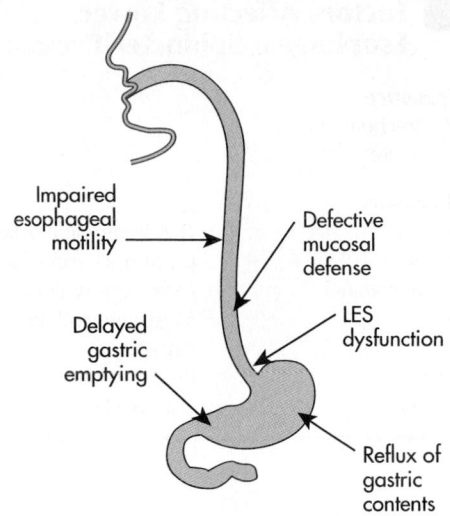

FIG. 40-2 Factors involved in the pathogenesis of gastroesophageal reflux disease (GERD). *LES,* Lower esophageal sphincter.

ation presumed to be secondary to reflux of gastric contents into the lower esophagus. Approximately 5% to 7% of the world's population experience GERD. More than 60 million Americans periodically experience symptoms of gastroesophageal reflux, and approximately 17.5 million (or 7%) experience daily symptoms.[4]

There is no one single cause of GERD. Several factors or combination of factors can be involved (Fig. 40-2). It results when the defenses of the lower esophagus are overwhelmed by the reflux of stomach acidic contents into the esophagus. Predisposing conditions include hiatal hernia, incompetent lower esophageal sphincter (LES), decreased esophageal clearance (ability to clear liquids or food from the esophagus into the stomach) resulting from impaired esophageal motility, and decreased gastric emptying. The acidic gastric secretions that reflux up into the lower esophagus result in esophageal irritation and inflammation (esophagitis). In addition, the presence of the gastric enzyme pepsin and intestinal enzymes (e.g., trypsin) and bile salts are also corrosive to the esophageal mucosa. The degree of inflammation depends on the amount and composition of gastric reflux and on the ability of the esophagus to clear the acidic contents.

One of the primary factors in GERD is an incompetent LES. An incompetent LES results in a decrease in pressure in the distal portion of the esophagus. As a result, gastric contents are able to move from an area of higher pressure (stomach) to an area of lower pressure (esophagus) when the patient is in a supine position or has an increase in intraabdominal pressure. Decreased LES pressure can be due to certain foods (e.g., caffeine, chocolate) and drugs (e.g., anticholinergics). A common cause of GERD is a hiatal hernia, which is discussed in the next section.

Clinical Manifestations

The symptoms of GERD vary from individual to individual. Heartburn *(pyrosis)* from gastroesophageal reflux is the most common clinical manifestation. It is caused by irritation of the esophagus by the gastric secretions. Heartburn is described as a

TABLE 40-7	Factors Affecting Lower Esophageal Sphincter Pressure

Increase Pressure
bethanechol (Urecholine)
metoclopramide (Reglan)

Decrease Pressure

Alcohol	β-Adrenergic blockers
Anticholinergics	Calcium channel blockers
Chocolate (theobromine)	Diazepam (Valium)
Fatty foods	Morphine sulfate
Nicotine	Nitrates
Peppermint, spearmint	Progesterone
Tea, coffee (caffeine)	Theophylline

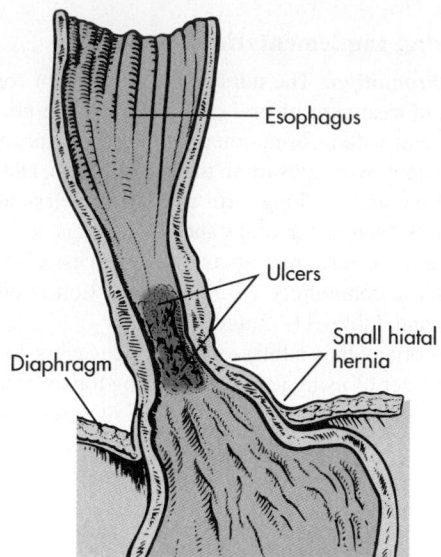

FIG. 40-3 Esophagitis with esophageal ulcerations.

burning, tight sensation that is felt intermittently beneath the lower sternum and spreads upward to the throat or jaw. The majority of individuals have mild symptoms including heartburn after a meal that occurs about once a week with no evidence of mucosal damage. However, the persistence of mild symptoms for a period of 5 years or more or symptoms associated with difficulty swallowing should be evaluated. In addition, heartburn that occurs more frequently than once a week, becomes more severe, or occurs at night and wakes a person from sleep may be a sign of a more serious condition, and consultation with a health care provider is advised.[5]

Heartburn may occur following ingestion of food or drugs that decrease the LES pressure or are directly irritating to the esophageal mucosa (Table 40-7). Heartburn is relieved with milk, alkaline substances, or water. An individual with GERD may also report respiratory symptoms including wheezing, coughing, and dyspnea. Otolaryngologic symptoms include hoarseness, sore throat, a globus sensation (sense of a lump in the throat), and choking. *Regurgitation* (effortless return of food or gastric contents from the stomach into esophagus or mouth) is a fairly common manifestation of GERD. It is often described as hot, bitter, or sour liquid coming into the throat or mouth. Gastric symptoms including early satiety, postmeal bloating, nausea, and vomiting are related to delayed gastric emptying.

Complications

Complications of GERD are related to the direct local effects of gastric acid on the esophageal mucosa. **Esophagitis** (inflammation of the esophagus) is a frequent complication of GERD. Other risk factors for esophagitis include hiatal hernia, chemical irritation from lye or physical irritants such as smoking, cold or hot liquids, and excessive alcoholic intake. Trauma to the esophagus may also produce inflammation. Esophagitis with esophageal ulcerations is shown in Fig. 40-3.

Repeated exposure may cause scar tissue formation and decreased distensibility *(esophageal stricture)* of the esophagus. This may result in dysphagia.

Another complication of GERD is **Barrett's esophagus** (esophageal metaplasia). Barrett's esophagus is considered a precancerous lesion, which places the patient at risk for esophageal cancer. In Barrett's esophagus there is replacement of the normal squamous

epithelium of the esophagus with columnar epithelium. These cell changes are thought to be related to chronic reflux esophagitis. Signs and symptoms of Barrett's esophagus can range from none to mild to bleeding and perforation. Because patients with Barrett's esophagus are at higher risk for adenocarcinoma, they may need to be monitored on a regular basis (every 1 to 3 years) by endoscopy and biopsy.

Respiratory complications of GERD include bronchospasm, laryngospasm, and cricopharyngeal spasm. These complications are due to irritation of the upper airway by gastric secretions. With GERD there is also the potential for pneumonia as a result of aspiration of gastric contents into the respiratory system. Dental erosion, especially in the posterior teeth, may result from acid reflux into the mouth.

Diagnostic Studies

Diagnostic studies are performed to determine the cause of the GERD (e.g., hiatal hernia) (Table 40-8). Barium swallow is done to determine if there is protrusion of the upper part of the stomach (called the *gastric fundus*). Endoscopy is useful in assessing the competence of the LES and the extent of inflammation (if present), potential scarring, and strictures. Biopsy and cytologic specimens can be taken to differentiate carcinoma of the stomach or esophagus from Barrett's esophagus. Esophageal manometric studies are performed to measure pressure in the esophagus, as well as in the LES. The determination of pH using specially designed probes in the laboratory or using ambulatory monitoring systems may demonstrate the presence of acid in the normally alkaline esophagus. Radionuclide tests may also be performed to detect reflux of gastric contents and the rate of esophageal clearance.

Because of the cost and discomfort of diagnostic procedures, it has been suggested that high-dose proton pump inhibitor (PPI) treatment (explained under Drug Therapy) for a short period (2 weeks) can be used as a first step in the diagnosis of GERD.[6] In patients with GERD, PPI treatment should result in a marked reduction or elimination of symptoms.[7]

TABLE 40-8	Collaborative Care
	Gastroesophageal Reflux Disease (GERD) and Hiatal Hernia

Diagnostic

History and physical examination
Upper GI endoscopy with biopsy and cytologic analysis
Barium swallow
Motility (manometry) studies
pH monitoring (laboratory or 24 hr ambulatory)

Collaborative Therapy

Conservative

Elevation of head of bed on 4- to 6-inch blocks
High-protein, low-fat diet with avoidance of foods that decrease LES pressure or irritate acid-sensitive esophagus
Antacids
Antisecretory agents
  H₂-receptor blockers*
  Proton pump inhibitors*
Prokinetic drug therapy*
Cholinergic drugs

Surgical

Nissen fundoplication
Toupet fundoplication
Hill gastropexy
Belsey fundoplication

Endoscopic

Stretta device

*See Table 40-9.
LES, Lower esophageal sphincter.

Collaborative Care

Most patients with GERD can be successfully managed by lifestyle modifications and drug therapy. These are long-term approaches requiring patient teaching and compliance with therapies. When these therapies are ineffective, surgery is an option (see Table 40-8).

Lifestyle Modifications. The patient with GERD is taught to avoid factors that aggravate symptoms. Particular attention is given to diet and drugs that may affect the LES, acid secretion, or gastric emptying. Patients who smoke are encouraged to stop. Cigarette smoking has been associated with decreased acid clearance from the lower esophagus.[8]

Nutritional Therapy. Diet does not cause GERD, but food can aggravate symptoms. No specific diet is necessary, but foods that cause reflux should be avoided. Fatty foods stimulate the release of cholecystokinin, a hormone from the duodenum that decreases LES pressure. High-fat foods also decrease the rate of gastric emptying. Foods that decrease LES pressure, such as chocolate, peppermint, coffee, and tea (see Table 40-7), should be avoided because they predispose to reflux. Milk products should be avoided, especially at bedtime, because milk increases gastric acid secretion. Small, frequent meals are advised to prevent overdistention of the stomach. The patient should avoid late evening meals and nocturnal snacking. Fluids should be taken between rather than with meals to reduce gastric distention. Certain foods (e.g., tomato-based products, orange juice) may irritate the acid-sensitive esophagus and may need to be avoided. To reduce intraabdominal pressure, weight reduction is recommended if the patient is overweight.

Drug Therapy. Drug therapy for GERD is focused on improving LES function, increasing esophageal clearance, decreasing volume and acidity of reflux, and protecting the esophageal mucosa (Table 40-9). There are two approaches to drug therapy. The first is the "step-up" approach, which means starting with antacids and OTC histamine-2 receptor (H₂R) blockers and increasing to prescription H₂R blockers and, finally, PPIs. The "step-down" approach involves starting with a PPI and over time titrating down to prescription H₂R blockers and, finally, OTC H₂R blockers and antacids.

Antacids produce quick but short-lived relief of heartburn. They act by neutralizing HCl. They should be taken 1 to 3 hours after meals and at bedtime. OTC antacids with or without alginic acid (e.g., Gaviscon) may be useful in patients with mild, intermittent heartburn. The alginic acid reacts with sodium bicarbonate and forms a viscous solution that floats to the surface of the gastric contents and coats the esophagus, acting as a mechanical barrier to reflux. However, in patients with moderate to severe or frequent symptoms or patients with documented esophagitis, these regimens are not effective in relieving symptoms or healing erosive lesions.

Antisecretory agents decrease the secretion of HCl acid by the stomach. H₂R blockers (e.g., cimetidine [Tagamet], ranitidine [Zantac], famotidine [Pepcid], nizatidine [Axid]) are available in OTC and prescription formulations. OTC preparations (e.g., Pepcid AC, Tagamet HB, Zantac 75, Axid AR) have lower drug dosages compared with prescription drugs (e.g., Zantac 75 has 75 mg compared with 150 mg in prescription Zantac). Some formulations include an H₂R plus antacid combinations. For example, Pepcid Complete includes famotidine, calcium carbonate, and magnesium hydroxide. In prescription doses, H₂R blockers reduce symptoms and promote esophageal healing in approximately 50% of patients. Patients frequently relapse (i.e., GERD symptoms return) with discontinuance of the drug.

PPIs such as omeprazole (Prilosec), esomeprazole (Nexium), pantoprazole (Protonix), lansoprazole (Prevacid), and rabeprazole (Aciphex) also decrease stomach HCl acid secretion. These agents act by inhibiting the proton pump mechanism responsible for the secretion of H⁺ ions. PPIs promote esophageal healing in approximately 80% to 90% of patients but are more expensive than H₂R blockers. PPIs may also be beneficial in decreasing the incidence of esophageal strictures, a complication of chronic GERD.

Another drug that may be used to treat GERD is sucralfate (Carafate), an antiulcer drug used for its cytoprotective properties. Cholinergic drugs, such as bethanechol (Urecholine), may be used to increase LES pressure, improve esophageal emptying in the supine position, and increase gastric emptying. However, the value of current cholinergic agents is limited because they also stimulate HCl acid secretion. Prokinetic (motility-enhancing) drugs such as metoclopramide (Reglan) promote gastric emptying and reduce the risk of gastric acid reflux (see Table 40-9).

Surgical Therapy. Surgical therapy (antireflux surgery) may be necessary if long-term conservative therapy fails; if a hiatal hernia is present; or if complications, such as esophageal stricture and stenosis (narrowing), chronic esophagitis, and

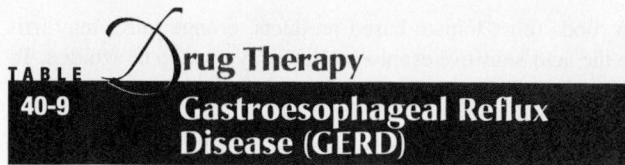

TABLE 40-9	*Drug Therapy* Gastroesophageal Reflux Disease (GERD)	
MECHANISM OF ACTION	**EXAMPLES**
Increase LES Pressure Cholinergic	bethanecol (Urecholine)
Promotility Prokinetic	metoclopramide (Reglan)
Acid Neutralizing Antacids	Gelusil, Maalox, Mylanta
Antisecretory H₂-receptor blockers	cimetidine (Tagamet) famotidine (Pepcid) nizatidine (Axid) ranitidine (Zantac)
Proton pump inhibitors (PPIs)	esomeprazole (Nexium) lansoprazole (Prevacid) omeprazole (Prilosec) pantoprazole (Protonix) rabeprazole (Aciphex)
Cytoprotective Alginic acid–antacid Acid-protective	Gaviscon sucralfate (Carafate)

LES, Lower esophageal sphincter.

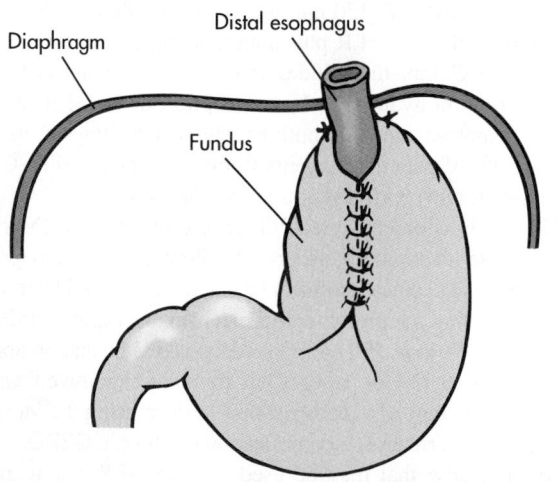

FIG. 40-4 Nissen fundoplication for repair of hiatal hernia. Fundus of stomach is wrapped around distal esophagus and sutured to itself.

bleeding, exist. Most surgical procedures are performed laparoscopically. The objective of surgical interventions for GERD is to reduce reflux of gastric contents by enhancing the integrity of the LES. Surgical interventions for GERD are called *antireflux* procedures. In these procedures the fundus of the stomach is wrapped around the lower portion of the esophagus in varying positions.

The Nissen fundoplication is shown in Fig. 40-4. Laparoscopically performed Nissen and Toupet fundoplications have

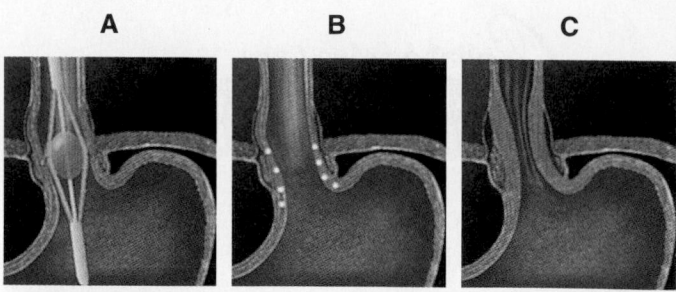

FIG. 40-5 Stretta procedure used to treat GERD. **A,** Catheter positioned. **B,** Multiple sites treated with radiofrequency energy. **C,** Remodeling occurs with collagen formation.

become the standard antireflux surgeries.[9] The use of laparoscopic antireflux surgery for GERD has reduced complications, overall morbidity, and the cost of hospitalization compared with a thoracic or open abdominal approach.

Endoscopic Therapy. Recently the Food and Drug Administration approved the use of the Stretta device, which is a balloon-tipped four-needle catheter that delivers radiofrequency energy to the smooth muscle of the gastroesophageal junction for the management of GERD[10] (Fig. 40-5). The radiofrequency energy induces collagen contraction, which helps to form a barrier against acid reflux. This procedure can be performed endoscopically under conscious sedation. The Stretta procedure can be used in patients who have breakthrough symptoms while receiving drug therapy, are intolerant to drug therapy, are candidates for antireflux surgery but desire a less invasive option, or are not surgical candidates because of comorbidities. At this time, the long-term benefit of this approach remains to be determined.

NURSING MANAGEMENT
GASTROESOPHAGEAL REFLUX DISEASE

Patients with GERD must avoid factors that cause reflux. A patient teaching guide is provided in Table 40-10. The patient who is a smoker should stop smoking. Smoking causes an almost immediate drop in LES pressure and decreases the ability to clear acid from the esophagus. The patient may need to be referred to other members of the health care team or to community resources for assistance in stopping smoking. (See Chapter 11 for additional information related to smoking cessation.) Substances that decrease LES pressure and tone should be avoided (see Table 40-7). If stress seems to cause symptoms, measures to cope with stress should be discussed. (See Chapter 8 for stress management techniques.) The patient should also be taught possible side effects of drugs.

Nursing care for the patient who is having acute symptoms consists mainly of encouraging the patient to follow the necessary regimen. The nurse should ensure that the head of the bed is elevated to approximately 30 degrees (usually on 4- to 6-inch blocks) and that the patient does not lie down during the first 2 to 3 hours after eating. Teaching the patient to avoid food and activities that cause reflux is important (e.g., late-night eating should be avoided). The patient may be taking drugs to relieve heartburn, so the nurse must observe for side effects, as well as

Patient & Family Teaching Guide
Prevention of Gastroesophageal Reflux Disease (GERD)

The following are teaching guidelines for the patient and family:
1. Explain the rationale for a high-protein, low-fat diet.
2. Encourage the patient to eat small, frequent meals to prevent gastric distention.
3. Explain the rationale for avoiding alcohol, smoking (causes an almost immediate, marked decrease in LES pressure), and beverages that contain caffeine.
4. Teach the patient not to lie down for 2 to 3 hours after eating, wear tight clothing around the waist, or bend over (especially after eating).
5. Encourage the patient to sleep with head of bed elevated on 4- to 6-inch blocks (gravity fosters esophageal emptying).
6. Teach information regarding drugs, including rationale for their use and common side effects.
7. Discuss strategies for weight reduction if appropriate.
8. Encourage patient and family to share concerns about lifestyle changes and living with a chronic problem.

evaluate their effectiveness. Even when symptoms are brought under control, the patient may need to continue drugs because the underlying problem is still present. Because of the link between GERD and metaplastic changes in the lower esophagus (Barrett's esophagus), patients are instructed to see their health care provider if symptoms persist.

The nurse needs to observe for and instruct the patient about side effects of the drugs being taken. Side effects with H_2R blockers and PPIs are rare. Antacids have minimal side effects. Antacids that contain aluminum tend to cause constipation, whereas those that contain magnesium tend to cause diarrhea. Several of the antacids are combinations of aluminum and magnesium designed to minimize these side effects. If the patient is taking bethanechol, side effects to observe for include urinary urgency, increased salivation, abdominal cramping with diarrhea, nausea, vomiting, and hypotension. Such side effects often limit the effectiveness of cholinergic agents in the treatment of GERD. Side effects of metoclopramide include restlessness, anxiety, insomnia, and hallucinations. Side effects of sucralfate include drowsiness, dizziness, nausea, vomiting, constipation, urticaria, and rash.

Postoperative care focuses on concerns related to prevention of respiratory complications, maintenance of fluid and electrolyte balance, and prevention of infection. If a thoracic approach is used, a chest tube is inserted. Assessment and management related to closed chest drainage are important (see Chapter 27).

If an open abdominal incision is used, respiratory complications can occur in a patient because of the high abdominal incision. Respiratory assessment should include respiratory rate and rhythm, pulse rate and rhythm, and signs of pneumothorax (e.g., dyspnea, chest pain, cyanosis). Deep breathing is essential to fully expand the lungs.

The patient receives IV fluids and electrolytes until the return of peristalsis. Care should be taken to maintain patency of the NG tube (if present) to prevent the need to reinsert the tube. It is dangerous to attempt to replace the tube because of the possibility of perforation of the surgical repair. Immediately after the surgical procedure, the patient cannot voluntarily vomit or belch, and this may cause the bloating and abdominal discomfort. When peristalsis returns, only fluids are given initially. Solids are added gradually so that the stomach is not overdistended. The nurse must maintain an accurate recording of intake and output and observe for fluid and electrolyte imbalances (see Chapter 16). (Care of the patient undergoing a laparotomy procedure is described in NCP 41-2 on p. 1063.)

After surgical therapy, there should be no symptoms of gastric reflux. However, the recurrence rate may range from 10% to 30% over a 20-year period following surgery. The patient should be instructed to report symptoms such as heartburn and regurgitation. Such problems may be temporary and resolve with time. In the first month after surgery the patient may report mild dysphagia caused by edema, but it should resolve.[5] The patient should report persistent dysphagia, epigastric fullness, and bloating. A normal diet is gradually resumed. The patient should avoid foods that are gas forming and should try to prevent gastric distention. Food should be chewed thoroughly.

HIATAL HERNIA

Hiatal hernia is herniation of a portion of the stomach into the esophagus through an opening, or hiatus, in the diaphragm. It is also referred to as diaphragmatic hernia and esophageal hernia. The incidence of hiatal hernia is difficult to determine. However, it is the most common abnormality found on x-ray examination of the upper GI tract. Hiatal hernias are common in older adults and occur more often in women than in men.

Types

Hiatal hernias are classified into the following two types (Fig. 40-6):
1. *Sliding:* The junction of the stomach and esophagus is above the hiatus of the diaphragm, and a part of the stomach slides through the hiatal opening in the diaphragm. The stomach "slides" into the thoracic cavity when the patient is supine and usually goes back into the abdominal cavity when the patient is standing upright. This is the most common type of hiatal hernia.
2. *Paraesophageal or rolling:* The esophagogastric junction remains in the normal position, but the fundus and the greater curvature of the stomach roll up through the diaphragm, forming a pocket alongside the esophagus.

Etiology and Pathophysiology

The actual cause of hiatal hernia is unknown. Many factors contribute to the development of hiatal hernia. Structural changes, such as weakening of the muscles in the diaphragm around the esophagogastric opening, are usually contributing factors. Factors that increase intraabdominal pressure, including obesity, pregnancy, ascites, tumors, tight corsets, intense physical exertion, and heavy lifting on a continual basis, may also predispose to development of a hiatal hernia. Other predisposing factors are increased age, trauma, poor nutrition, and a forced recumbent position, as when a prolonged illness confines the person to bed. In some cases, congenital weakness is a contributing factor.

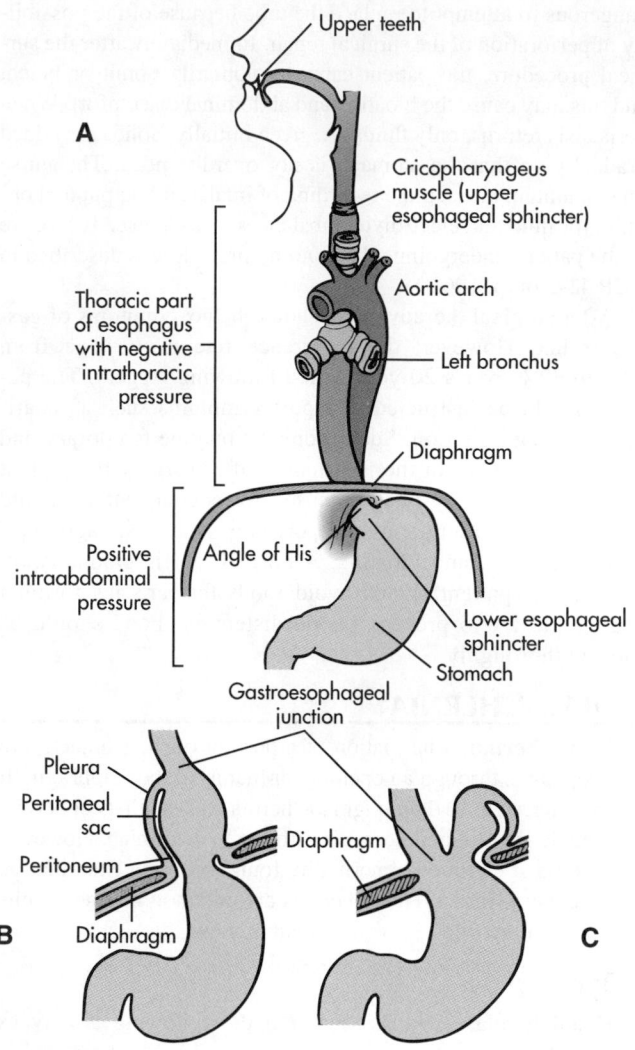

FIG. 40-6 A, Normal esophagus. B, Sliding hiatal hernia. C, Rolling or paraesophageal hernia.

Clinical Manifestations

Persons with hiatal hernia may be asymptomatic. When present, the signs and symptoms of hiatal hernia are similar to those described for GERD. Heartburn, especially after a meal or after lying supine, is a common symptom. Patients may complain of dysphagia. Frequently the symptoms of hiatal hernia mimic gallbladder disease, peptic ulcer disease, and angina. However, some patients with hiatal hernia have no symptoms. Reflux and discomfort are also associated with position, occurring soon or several hours after lying down. Bending over may cause a severe burning pain, which is usually relieved by sitting or standing. Other common precipitating factors of pain include large meals, alcohol, and smoking. Nocturnal symptoms of heartburn are common, especially if the person has eaten before going to sleep.

Complications

Complications that may occur with hiatal hernia include GERD, hemorrhage from erosion, stenosis (narrowing of the esophagus), ulcerations of the herniated portion of the stomach, strangulation of the hernia, and regurgitation with tracheal aspiration. Patients with a history of hiatal hernia are more at risk for hospitalization for respiratory disease.[11]

Diagnostic Studies

A barium swallow is an important diagnostic measure that may show the protrusion of gastric mucosa through the esophageal hiatus in the patient with hiatal hernia. Endoscopic visualization of the lower esophagus provides information on the degree of mucosal inflammation or other abnormalities. Other tests are similar to those described in Table 40-8.

NURSING *and* COLLABORATIVE MANAGEMENT HIATAL HERNIA

■ Conservative Therapy

Conservative therapy of hiatal hernia is similar to that described under GERD, including lifestyle modifications (e.g., reduction of intraabdominal pressure by eliminating constricting garments, avoiding lifting and straining, eliminating alcohol and smoking, elevating the head of the bed), and the use of antacids and antisecretory agents (PPIs, H₂R blockers). Elevation of the bed on 4- to 6-inch blocks assists gravity in maintaining the stomach in the abdominal cavity and also helps prevent reflux and tracheal aspiration. If overweight, the patient should be encouraged to lose weight.

■ Surgical Therapy

The objective of surgical interventions for hiatal hernia is to reduce reflux by enhancing the integrity of the LES. There are four slightly varied procedures: the Nissen fundoplication, the Toupet fundoplication or technique, the Hill gastropexy, and the Belsey fundoplication. These surgical procedures are all variations of fundoplication, which involves "wrapping" the fundus of the stomach around the lower portion of the esophagus in varying positions. These procedures reduce the hernia, provide an acceptable LES pressure, and prevent movement of the gastroesophageal junction. The Nissen fundoplication is shown in Fig. 40-4. Similar to GERD, laparoscopically performed Nissen and Toupet techniques have become the standard antireflux surgeries for hiatal hernia.[9] A thoracic or open abdominal approach may also be used in selected cases.

■ Gerontologic Considerations: GERD and Hiatal Hernia

The incidence of both GERD and hiatal hernia increases with age. It is associated with weakening of the diaphragm, obesity, kyphosis, and use of corsets or other factors that increase intraabdominal pressure. Some older adults with hiatal hernia are asymptomatic. The first indications may include esophageal bleeding secondary to esophagitis or respiratory complications (e.g., aspiration pneumonia) related to aspiration of gastric contents. The LES may become less competent with aging in some individuals.

The clinical course and management of GERD and hiatal hernia in the older adult are similar to that for the younger adult. With the increased use of laparoscopic procedures, surgical risks have been reduced. However, an older adult with cardiovascular and pulmonary problems may not be a good candidate for surgical intervention. In addition, changes in lifestyle, including elimination of dietary factors, such as caffeine-containing beverages and chocolate, and elevating the head of the bed on blocks, may be more difficult for the older adult.

ESOPHAGEAL CANCER

Esophageal cancer (a rare malignant neoplasm of the esophagus) is unique in its geographic distribution. There are parts of Asia in which the rate of esophageal cancer is extremely high, whereas in Western societies the incidence is relatively low. For example, esophageal cancer is the second most common type of cancer in China. In the United States in 2002 there were 13,100 cases of esophageal cancer (9800 were men) and 12,600 Americans died from esophageal cancer. Because esophageal cancer is rarely diagnosed in early stages, the 5-year survival rate is 12%.[2]

Estimates of the percentage of esophageal cancer that are adenocarcinomas range from 30% to 70% with the remainder being squamous cell. The incidence of squamous cell esophageal cancer is currently decreasing in the United States, whereas the incidence of adenocarcinoma of the distal esophagus is increasing.[2] In the last 30 years, the incidence of adenocarcinoma has increased sevenfold.[12] Adenocarcinomas arise from the glands lining the esophagus and resemble cancers of the stomach and small intestine. The incidence of esophageal cancer increases with age. There is a higher incidence of esophageal cancer in African Americans relative to whites. The incidence of esophageal cancer is also higher in Alaska Native men and women compared with whites.

One risk factor for esophageal adenocarcinoma is Barrett's esophagus. At this time, it is estimated that 1 of 200 cases of Barrett's esophagus will progress to esophageal cancer. Barrett's esophagus is described earlier under GERD.

Etiology and Pathophysiology

The cause of esophageal cancer is unknown. Two important risk factors are smoking and excessive alcohol intake. Diets that are low in fruits and vegetables and certain minerals and vitamins may increase the risk of this cancer. Lye that is found in strong cleaners like drain cleaners can burn and destroy esophageal cells. As a result, a person who has swallowed lye has a higher risk of squamous cell cancer. A patient with a history of *achalasia,* a condition in which there is delayed emptying of the lower esophagus, is also at greater risk for squamous cell cancer. Other risk factors include exposure to asbestos and metal.[2]

The majority of esophageal tumors are located in the middle and lower portions of the esophagus. The malignant tumor usually appears as an ulcerated lesion and has often advanced by the time the patient experiences symptoms. The tumor may penetrate the muscular layer and even extend outside the wall of the esophagus. Obstruction of the esophagus occurs in the later stages.

Clinical Manifestations

The onset of symptoms is usually late in relation to the extent of the tumor. Progressive dysphagia is the most common symptom and may be expressed as a substernal feeling (globus sensation) as if food is not passing. Initially the dysphagia occurs only with meat, then with soft foods, and eventually with liquids.

Pain develops late and is described as occurring in the substernal, epigastric, or back areas and usually increases with swallowing. The pain may radiate to the neck, jaw, ears, and shoulders. If the tumor is in the upper third of the esophagus, symptoms such as sore throat, choking, and hoarseness may occur. Weight loss is fairly common. When esophageal stenosis is severe, regurgitation of blood-flecked esophageal contents is common.

Complications

Hemorrhage may occur if the cancer erodes through the esophagus and into the aorta. Esophageal perforation with fistula formation into the lung or trachea sometimes develops. The tumor may enlarge enough to cause esophageal obstruction. There is spread via the lymph system, with the liver and lung being common sites of metastasis.

Diagnostic Studies

Barium swallow with fluoroscopy may demonstrate a narrowing of the esophagus at the site of the tumor (Table 40-11). Sometimes a crater is visible. Endoscopy with biopsy is necessary to make a definitive diagnosis of carcinoma by identification of malignant cells. Endoscopic ultrasonography is an important tool used to stage esophageal cancer. A bronchoscopic examination may be performed to detect malignant involvement of the lung. Computed tomography (CT) scanning and magnetic resonance imaging (MRI) are also used to assess the extent of the disease.

Collaborative Care

The treatment of esophageal cancer depends on the location of the tumor and whether invasion or metastasis has occurred (see Table 40-11). Esophageal cancer has a poor prognosis, mainly because it is not usually diagnosed until the disease is advanced. The best results may be obtained with a combination of surgery, chemotherapy, and radiation.

The types of surgical procedures that can be performed are (1) removal of part or all of the esophagus *(esophagectomy)* with use of a Dacron graft to replace the resected part, (2) resection of a portion of the esophagus and anastomosis of the remaining portion to the stomach *(esophagogastrostomy),* and (3) resection of a portion of the esophagus and anastomosis of a segment of colon to the remaining portion *(esophagoenterostomy).* The surgical approaches may be thoracic or both abdominal and thoracic.

TABLE 40-11 Collaborative Care — Esophageal Cancer

Diagnostic
History and physical examination
Endoscopy of esophagus with biopsy
Barium swallow
Endoscopic ultrasonography
Bronchoscopy
CT and MRI

Collaborative Therapy
Surgical resection
Esophagectomy
Esophagogastrostomy
Esophagoenterostomy
Radiation
Chemotherapy
Palliative
    Dilation
    Stent or prosthesis
    Laser therapy
    Gastrostomy

Surgery may not be performed if the patient is an older adult or in poor physical health.

Chemotherapeutic agents cisplatin (Platinol), paclitaxel (Taxol), and 5-FU in combination with radiation before and/or after surgery are currently used.[13] If the tumor is in the cervical section (upper third) of the esophagus, radiation is usually indicated. A tumor in the lower third of the esophagus is usually resected surgically.

Palliative therapy consists of restoration of the swallowing function and maintenance of nutrition and hydration. Dilation, stent placement, or both can relieve obstruction. Dilation is done with various types of dilators (e.g., Celestin tube). Dilation often relieves dysphagia and allows for improved nutrition. Placement of a stent or prosthesis may help when dilation is no longer effective. The prostheses are composed of silicone rubber or nylon-reinforced latex tubes with distal and proximal collars. The prosthesis is placed in the esophagus so that food and fluids can pass through the stenotic segment of the esophagus. The prosthesis can be placed endoscopically.

Endoscopic laser therapy or vaporization of the tumor may be used in combination with dilation. Obstruction recurs as the tumor grows, but laser therapy can be repeated. Sometimes these procedures are combined with radiation therapy. Other measures for palliation include gastrostomy or esophagostomy tube placements for nutrition support and pain management.

Nutritional Therapy. After esophageal surgery, parenteral fluids are given. When fluids are allowed after bowel sounds have returned, 30 to 60 ml of water are given hourly, with gradual progression to small, frequent bland meals. The patient should be in an upright position to prevent regurgitation of the fluid. The patient is observed for signs of intolerance to the feeding or leakage of the feeding into the mediastinum. Symptoms that indicate leakage are pain, increased temperature, and dyspnea. Symptoms of food intolerance include vomiting and abdominal distention. A gastrostomy may be performed for the purpose of feeding the patient. (Gastrostomy and tube feedings are discussed in Chapter 39.)

NURSING MANAGEMENT
ESOPHAGEAL CANCER

■ Nursing Assessment

The patient should be asked about any history of GERD, hiatal hernia, achalasia, or Barrett's esophagus. The patient is also questioned regarding tobacco and alcohol use. The patient should be assessed for progressive dysphagia and *odynophagia* (burning, squeezing pain while swallowing). The nurse should question the patient regarding the type of substances ingested that cause dysphagia, such as meat, soft foods, and liquids. The patient is also assessed for pain (substernal, epigastric, or back areas), choking, heartburn, hoarseness, cough, anorexia, weight loss, and regurgitation (sometimes bloody).

■ Nursing Diagnoses

Nursing diagnoses for the patient with esophageal cancer include, but are not limited to, the following:

- Imbalanced nutrition: less than body requirements *related to* dysphagia, odynophagia, weakness, chemotherapy, and radiation therapy
- Chronic pain *related to* the tumor
- Deficient fluid volume *related to* inadequate intake

- Risk for aspiration *related to* impaired esophageal function
- Anxiety *related to* diagnosis of cancer, uncertain future, and poor prognosis
- Anticipatory grieving *related to* diagnosis of life-threatening malignancy
- Ineffective health maintenance *related to* lack of knowledge of disease process and therapeutic regimen, unavailability of a support system, and chronic debilitating disease

■ Planning

The overall goals are that the patient with esophageal cancer will (1) have relief of symptoms including pain and dysphagia, (2) achieve optimal nutritional intake, (3) understand the prognosis of the disease, and (4) experience a quality of life appropriate to disease progression.

■ Nursing Implementation

Health Promotion. Patients with diagnosed GERD and hiatal hernia need to be counseled regarding regular follow-up evaluation. Health counseling should focus on elimination of smoking and excessive alcohol intake, as well as other risk factors for GERD. Maintenance of good oral hygiene and dietary habits (intake of fresh fruits and vegetables) may also be helpful.

Patients diagnosed with Barrett's esophagus need to be monitored because this is considered a premalignant condition. Early diagnosis of esophageal tumors is important but difficult because the onset of symptoms is usually late. Patients are encouraged to seek medical attention for any esophageal problems, especially dysphagia. Patients who are at risk for esophageal adenocarcinoma, such as those with evidence of Barrett's esophagus and a diagnosis of achalasia (discussed later under Other Esophageal Disorders), may need regular endoscopic screening with biopsy and cytologic study.

Acute Intervention

Preoperative care. In addition to general preoperative teaching and preparation, particular attention to the patient's nutritional needs and oral care is important. Many patients are poorly nourished because of the inability to ingest adequate amounts of food and fluids before surgery. A high-calorie, high-protein diet is recommended. It may have to be in liquid form. Some patients may need IV fluid replacement or total parenteral nutrition. The patient and/or family member is instructed on how to keep an intake and output record and assess for signs of fluid and electrolyte imbalance. Some treatment protocols necessitate preoperative radiation and chemotherapy.

Meticulous oral care is essential. The mouth, including tongue, gingivae, and teeth or dentures, must be cleaned thoroughly. It may be necessary to use swabs or a gauze pad and to really scrub the mouth, including the tongue. Milk of magnesia with mineral oil may be used to remove crust formation. A mixture of mouthwash, ice, and water makes a refreshing rinse for the patient.

Teaching should include information about chest tubes (if a thoracic approach is used), IV lines, NG tube, gastrostomy feeding, turning, coughing, and deep breathing. (General preoperative care is presented in Chapter 17.)

Postoperative care. The patient usually has an NG tube in place, and there may be bloody drainage for 8 to 12 hours. The drainage gradually changes to greenish yellow. Assessment of the drainage, maintenance of the tube, and oral and nasal care are nursing responsibilities. The NG tube should not be repositioned or reinserted without consulting with the surgeon.

Because of the location of the incision and the general condition of the patient, special emphasis must be placed on prevention of respiratory complications. Turning and deep breathing should be done every 2 hours. Use of an incentive spirometer helps to prevent respiratory complications.

The patient should be positioned in a semi-Fowler's or Fowler's position to prevent reflux and aspiration of gastric secretions. When the patient can drink fluids or eat, the upright position should be maintained for at least 2 hours after eating to assist the movement of food through the GI tract.

Ambulatory and Home Care. Many patients require long-term follow-up care after surgery for esophageal cancer. The patient may undergo chemotherapy and radiation treatment following surgery. The patient needs encouragement and assistance in maintaining adequate nutrition. The patient may need a permanent feeding gastrostomy. The patient usually has fears and anxieties about a diagnosis of cancer. The nurse should know what the health care provider has told the patient regarding the prognosis and then provide appropriate counseling.

Referral to a home health nurse may be necessary for continued care of the patient (e.g., gastrostomy teaching, follow-up wound care). (See Chapter 10 for management of the terminally ill patient and Chapter 15 for the cancer patient.)

■ Evaluation

The expected outcomes are that the patient with esophageal cancer will

- maintain a patent airway
- have relief of pain
- be able to swallow comfortably
- consume adequate nutritional intake
- understand the prognosis of the disease
- experience quality of life appropriate to disease progression

OTHER ESOPHAGEAL DISORDERS

Esophageal Diverticula

Esophageal diverticula are saclike outpouchings of one or more layers of the esophagus. They occur in three main areas: (1) above the upper esophageal sphincter *(Zenker's diverticulum),* which is the most common location; (2) near the esophageal midpoint (traction diverticulum); and (3) above the LES (epiphrenic diverticulum) (Fig. 40-7). Pharyngeal pouches (Zenker's diverticula) occur most commonly in elderly patients (over 70 years), and typical symptoms include dysphagia, regurgitation, chronic cough, aspiration, and weight loss.[14] Traction diverticulum may not cause signs and symptoms. The patient frequently complains of tasting sour food and smelling a foul odor caused by the stagnant food. Complications include malnutrition, aspiration, and perforation. A diagnosis is easily established by barium studies.

There is no specific treatment for diverticula. Some patients find they can empty the pocket of food that collects by applying pressure at a point on the neck. The diet may have to be limited to foods that pass more readily (e.g., blenderized foods). Treatment of the diverticulum may be necessary if nutrition becomes disrupted. Treatment is surgical via an endoscopic or external cervical approach and should include a cricopharyngeal myotomy. Open approaches have been associated with significant

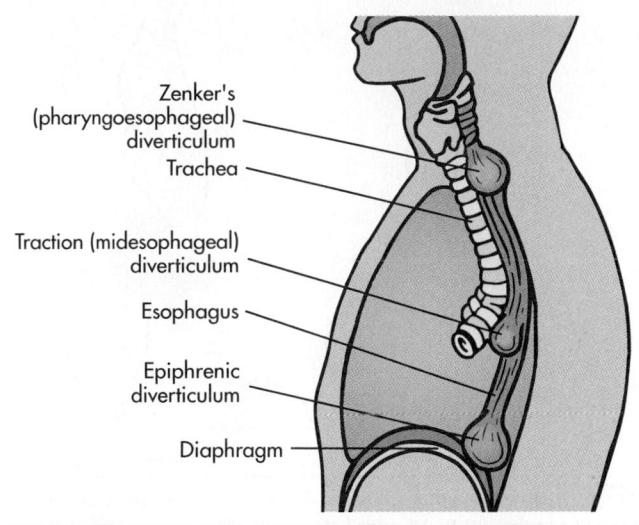

FIG. 40-7 Possible sites for the occurrence of esophageal diverticula. These hollow outpouchings may occur just above the upper esophageal sphincter (Zenker's, the most common type of pulsion diverticulum), near the midpoint of the esophagus (traction), and just above the lower esophageal sphincter (epiphrenic).

morbidity because the majority of patients are elderly and often have general medical problems. Treatment by endoscopic stapling diverticulotomy has become increasingly popular with its distinct advantages related to decreased complications, although long-term results are not yet available.[14]

Esophageal Strictures

The most common causes of esophageal strictures are strong acids or alkalis that have been ingested and reflux of gastric juices. Trauma such as throat lacerations and gunshot wounds may also lead to strictures as a result of scar formation (collagen deposition) from healing. The strictures usually develop over a long time. Strictures can be dilated endoscopically using *bougies* (dilating instruments). Another technique is balloon dilation, which is done under endoscopy and does not require fluoroscopy. Surgical excision with anastomosis is sometimes necessary. The patient may have a temporary or permanent gastrostomy.

Achalasia

In **achalasia** (cardiospasm), peristalsis of the lower two thirds (smooth muscle) of the esophagus is absent. Pressure in the LES is increased, along with incomplete relaxation of the LES. Obstruction of the esophagus at or near the diaphragm occurs. Food and fluid accumulate in the lower esophagus. The result of this condition is dilation of the lower esophagus (Fig. 40-8). The altered peristalsis is a result of impairment of the neurons that innervate the lower esophagus. There is a selective loss of inhibitory neurons, resulting in unopposed excitation of the LES. Achalasia affects all ages and both genders. The course of the disease is chronic.

Dysphagia (difficulty swallowing) is the most common symptom and occurs with both liquids and solids. Patients may report a globus sensation (a lump in the throat). Substernal chest pain (similar to the pain of angina) occurs during or immediately after a meal. *Halitosis* (foul-smelling breath) and the inability to eructate (belch) are other symptoms. Another common symptom is re-

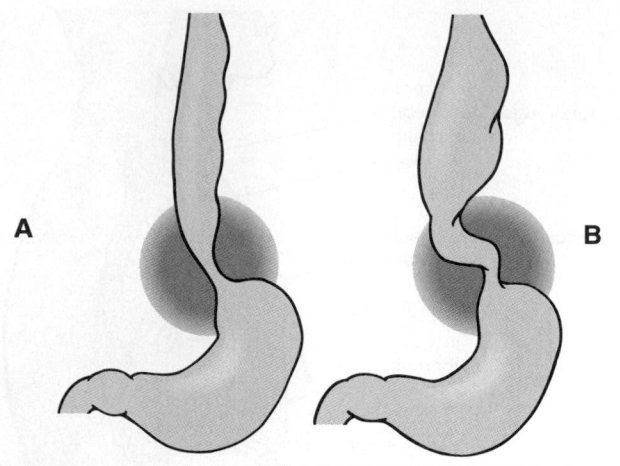

FIG. 40-8 Esophageal achalasia. A, Early stage, showing tapering of lower esophagus. B, Advanced stage, showing dilated, tortuous esophagus.

gurgitation of sour-tasting food and liquids, especially when the patient is in a horizontal position. Patients with achalasia also report symptoms (e.g., heartburn) of GERD. Weight loss is typical.

Diagnosis usually involves radiologic studies, manometric studies of the lower esophagus, and endoscopy. The exact cause of achalasia is not known, so treatment is focused on symptom management. Treatment consists of dilation, surgery, and use of drugs. All these therapies are directed at relieving the stasis caused by the increased LES pressure, nonrelaxing LES, and aperistaltic esophagus. Symptomatic treatment consists of a semisoft bland diet, eating slowly and drinking fluid with meals, and sleeping with the head elevated.

Esophageal dilation *(bougienage)* is an effective treatment measure for many patients. Pneumatic dilation of the LES with a balloon-tipped dilator passed orally is usually used. A variety of different dilators are available for this procedure. All depend on forcible expansion of a balloon in the LES (Fig. 40-9). The force-

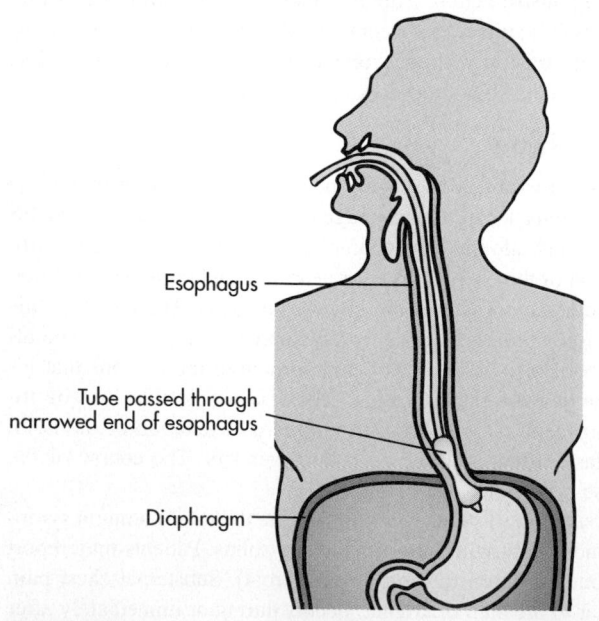

Esophagus

Tube passed through narrowed end of esophagus

Diaphragm

FIG. 40-9 Pneumatic dilation attempts to treat achalasia by maintaining an adequate lumen and decreasing lower esophageal sphincter (LES) tone.

ful dilation does not restore normal esophageal motility, but it does provide for emptying of the esophagus into the stomach.

Surgical intervention may become necessary. An esophagomyotomy may be performed. In this procedure the muscle fibers that enclose the narrowed area of the esophagus are divided. This allows the mucosa to pouch out through the division in the muscle layer so that food can be swallowed without obstruction.

A similar procedure is Heller myotomy (cardiomyotomy), which disrupts the LES and reduces LES pressure. An antireflux procedure is often done with the myotomy. This procedure can be performed laparoscopically, reducing the potential for postoperative complications.[15]

Drug therapy is used to manage early achalasia when there is no significant esophageal dilation. Drug therapy is used as a short-term measure and is considered as an alternative only in patients unfit to undergo pneumatic dilation or surgery. Endoscopic injection of botulinum toxin (Botox) into the LES is gaining acceptance.[16] It works by inhibiting the release of acetylcholine from nerve endings, thereby promoting relaxation of the smooth muscle. This treatment does not carry the risk of perforation that can occur with pneumatic dilation. However, symptomatic improvement with botulinum toxin only lasts a few months. Therefore either repeated injections are required or the patient must be switched to other therapy. There may be, however, subsets of patients, such as elderly patients or those with multiple medical problems who are poor candidates for more invasive procedures, for whom Botox injection is the preferred approach. Other classes of drugs used in the management of achalasia include anticholinergics, calcium channel blockers (e.g., nifedipine [Procardia]), and long-acting nitrates, which act by relaxing the smooth muscle.

Esophageal Varices

Esophageal varices are dilated, tortuous veins occurring in the lower portion of the esophagus as a result of portal hypertension. Esophageal varices are a common complication of liver cirrhosis and are discussed in Chapter 42.

Disorders of the Stomach and Upper Small Intestine

GASTRITIS

Types

Gastritis, an inflammation of the gastric mucosa, is one of the most common problems affecting the stomach. Gastritis may be acute or chronic and may be diffuse or localized. Chronic gastritis has been further divided into three subtypes including (1) autoimmune, which involves the body and fundus of the stomach; (2) diffuse antral, which primarily affects the antrum; and (3) multifocal, which is diffuse throughout the stomach. Presently, the causes of gastritis and its relationship to other gastric disorders, such as *Helicobacter pylori* infection and gastric cancer, are the focus of ongoing research.

Etiology and Pathophysiology

Gastritis occurs as the result of a breakdown in the normal gastric mucosal barrier. This mucosal barrier normally protects the stomach tissue from autodigestion by HCl acid and the proteolytic enzyme pepsin. When the barrier is broken, HCl acid can diffuse back into the mucosa. The acid back diffusion results in

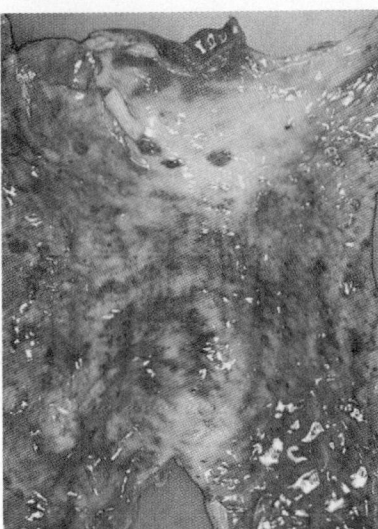

FIG. 40-10 Acute erosive gastritis is shown in the opened stomach. The mucosa appears hyperemic, and the foci of superficial ulceration are manifest as scattered, small, red areas termed erosions.

TABLE 40-12	Causes of Gastritis

Drugs
Aspirin
Corticosteroid drugs
Nonsteroidal antiinflammatory drugs

Diet
Alcohol
Spicy, irritating food

Microrganisms
Helicobacter pylori
Salmonella
Staphylococcus organisms

Environmental Factors
Radiation
Smoking

Pathophysiologic Conditions
Burns
Large hiatal hernia
Physiologic stress
Reflux of bile and pancreatic secretions
Renal failure (uremia)
Sepsis
Shock

Other Factors
Endoscopic procedures
Nasogastric suction
Psychologic stress

tissue edema, disruption of capillary walls with loss of plasma into the gastric lumen, and possible hemorrhage (Fig. 40-10).

Causes of gastritis are listed in Table 40-12. Drugs such as aspirin, nonsteroidal antiinflammatory drugs (NSAIDs), and digitalis have direct irritating effects on the gastric mucosa. For example, the ingestion of even small amounts of aspirin by the susceptible person is known to result in asymptomatic GI bleeding manifested by positive stool tests for occult blood. In addition, corticosteroids and NSAIDs are known to inhibit the synthesis of prostaglandins that are protective to the gastric mucosa. This leaves the gastric mucosa more susceptible to mucosal damage. NSAID-related gastritis is associated with many of the older drugs, including piroxicam (Feldene), naproxen (Naprosyn), sulindac (Clinoril), indomethacin (Indocin), diclofenac (Voltaren), and ibuprofen (Motrin, Advil). The use of cyclooxygenase-2 (COX-2) inhibitors (e.g., celecoxib [Celebrex], rofecoxib [Vioxx], valdecoxib [Bextra]) has been associated with fewer GI side effects as compared to nonselective NSAIDs. However, even these agents are associated with an increased risk of upper GI inflammation and bleeding. Risk factors for NSAID-induced gastritis include being female, being over the age of 60, and taking other ulcerogenic drugs including corticosteroids and anticoagulants (warfarin [Coumadin]).[17]

Dietary indiscretions can also result in acute gastritis. After an alcoholic drinking binge, acute damage to the gastric mucosa can range from local destruction of superficial epithelial cells to desquamation and destruction of the mucosa, with mucosal congestion, edema, and hemorrhage. Prolonged damage induced by repeated alcohol abuse can result in chronic gastritis. Eating large quantities of spicy, irritating foods and metabolic conditions such as uremia can also cause acute gastritis.

An important causative factor in chronic gastritis, in particular, diffuse antral and multifocal, is *H. pylori* infection. *H. pylori*–associated gastritis is a common problem in adults, many of whom do not have symptoms of gastritis. It is currently thought that *H. pylori* infection is acquired in childhood and is able to survive in the hostile environment of the gastric lumen. For reasons not clearly understood, *H. pylori* is capable of promoting the breakdown of the gastric mucosal barrier, given certain "triggers" or conditions. Thus, given time, *H. pylori* will eventually have a destructive effect on its host environment. This is consistent with the finding that the incidence of chronic gastritis increases with age. However, studies also have shown that not all persons infected with *H. pylori* go on to develop chronic gastritis or peptic ulcer disease. Thus a combination of factors may be at work to "turn on" the virulent process by which *H. pylori* damage the gastric mucosal barrier. The role of *H. pylori* in ulcer development is discussed in greater detail on pp. 1030-1031.

Autoimmune atrophic gastritis is a form of chronic gastritis that affects both the fundus and body of the stomach and is associated with an increased risk of gastric cancer. Approximately 30% of patients with *H. pylori* infection are also found to have antigastric antibodies. Thus there may be a link between the host's response to the presence of *H. pylori* and the development of autoimmune chronic gastritis.

Although not as common, other causes of chronic gastritis have been identified. Bacterial, viral, and fungal infections including *Mycobacterium,* cytomegalovirus, and syphilis are associated with chronic gastritis. Gastritis can occur from reflux of bile salts from the duodenum into the stomach as a result of anatomic changes following surgical procedures such as gastroduodenostomy and gastrojejunostomy. Prolonged vomiting may also cause reflux of bile salts. Intense emotional responses and CNS lesions may also produce inflammation of the mucosal lining as a result of hypersecretion of HCl acid or corticosteroids (Cushing syndrome).

Progressive gastric mucosal atrophy from chronic alterations in the protective mucosal barrier causes the chief and parietal cells to die eventually. With the decrease in the number of acid-secreting parietal cells and atrophy of the gastric mucosa, *hypochlorhydria* (decreased acid secretion) or *achlorhydria* (lack of acid secretion) occurs.

Clinical Manifestations

The symptoms of acute gastritis include anorexia, nausea and vomiting, epigastric tenderness, and a feeling of fullness. Hemorrhage is commonly associated with alcohol abuse and at times may be the only symptom. Acute gastritis is self-limiting, lasting from a few hours to a few days, with complete healing of the mucosa expected.

The manifestations of chronic gastritis are similar to those described for acute gastritis. Some patients have no symptoms directly associated with the gastric lesion. However, when the acid-secreting cells are lost or do not function as a result of atrophy, the source of intrinsic factor is also lost. The loss of *intrinsic factor,* a substance secreted by the gastric mucosa that is essential for the absorption of cobalamin (vitamin B_{12}) in the terminal ileum, ultimately results in cobalamin deficiency. With time, the body's storage of cobalamin in the liver is depleted, and a deficiency state exists. Lack of this important vitamin, which is essential for the growth and maturation of red blood cells (RBCs), results in the development of anemia and neurologic complications. (Cobalamin deficiency anemia is discussed in Chapter 30.)

Diagnostic Studies

Diagnosis of acute gastritis is most often based on a history of drug and alcohol use. The diagnosis of chronic gastritis may be delayed or completely missed because the symptoms are nonspecific. Endoscopic examination with biopsy is necessary to obtain a definitive diagnosis. Breath, urine, serum, or gastric tissue biopsy tests are available for the determination of *H. pylori.* These tests are described under Peptic Ulcer Disease. Radiologic studies are not helpful because the superficial mucosa is generally involved, and changes will not show clearly on x-ray. A complete blood count (CBC) may demonstrate the presence of anemia from blood loss or lack of intrinsic factor. Stools are tested for the presence of occult blood. A gastric analysis, although currently not used as much, demonstrates the amount of HCl acid present, with achlorhydria being a common sign of severe atrophic gastritis. Serum tests for antibodies to parietal cells and intrinsic factor may be performed. Tissue biopsy with cytologic examination is necessary to rule out gastric carcinoma.

NURSING and COLLABORATIVE MANAGEMENT GASTRITIS

■ Acute Gastritis

Eliminating the cause and preventing or avoiding it in the future are generally all that is needed to treat acute gastritis. The plan of care is supportive and similar to that described for nausea and vomiting. If vomiting accompanies acute gastritis, bed rest, NPO status, and IV fluids may be prescribed. Dehydration can occur rapidly in acute gastritis with vomiting. Fluids and electrolytes lost through vomiting and, occasionally, diarrhea are replaced. Antiemetics are given for nausea and vomiting (see Table 40-1). In severe cases of acute gastritis an NG tube may be used,

either for lavage of the precipitating agent from the stomach or in conjunction with suction to keep the stomach empty and free of noxious stimuli. Clear liquids are resumed when acute symptoms have subsided, with gradual reintroduction of solid, bland foods.

If hemorrhage is considered likely, frequent checking of vital signs and testing the vomitus for blood are indicated. All of the management strategies discussed in the section on upper GI bleeding also apply to the patient with severe gastritis.

Drug therapy is focused on reducing irritation of the gastric mucosa and providing symptomatic relief. Antacids are beneficial in the relief of abdominal discomfort by raising intragastric pH to above 6. H_2R blockers (e.g., ranitidine [Zantac], cimetidine [Tagamet]) or PPIs (e.g., omeprazole [Prilosec], lansoprazole [Prevacid]) may be used to reduce gastric HCl acid secretion. An agent that contains an H_2R blocker plus bismuth (ranitidine bismuth citrate [Tritec]) has been shown to reduce bleeding and promote healing of erosive gastritis. It is essential that the nurse have knowledge of the action and therapeutic effects of PPIs and H_2R blockers to teach the patient and to monitor the effects of the drugs.

■ Chronic Gastritis

The treatment of chronic gastritis focuses on evaluating and eliminating the specific cause (e.g., cessation of alcohol intake, abstinence from drugs, *H. pylori* eradication). Currently, antibiotic and antisecretory agent combinations are used to eradicate infection with *H. pylori* (Table 40-13). For the patient with pernicious anemia, regular injections of cobalamin are needed (see Chapter 30). Discussion of the continued need for this essential vitamin must be included in the plan of care.

The patient undergoing treatment for chronic gastritis may have to adapt to many lifestyle changes and adopt a strict adherence to a drug regimen. A nonirritating diet consisting of six small feedings a day and the use of an antacid after meals may help provide symptomatic relief. Smoking is contraindicated in

TABLE 40-13	Drug Therapy *Helicobacter pylori* Infection		
TREATMENT		**DURATION**	**ERADICATION RATE**
Triple Drug Therapy Proton pump inhibitor* or ranitidine bismuth citrate (Tritec) amoxicillin clarithromycin (Biaxin)		7 days	>90%
Dual Therapy ranitidine bismuth citrate (Tritec) clarithromycin (Biaxin)		7 days	>90%
Quadruple Therapy Proton pump inhibitor* bismuth tetracycline metronidazole (Flagyl)		14 days	60%-80%

*See Table 40-9.

all forms of gastritis. An interdisciplinary team approach in which the physician, nurse, dietitian, and pharmacist provide consistent information and support may increase the patient's success in making these alterations. Because the incidence of gastric cancer is higher in the patient who has a history of chronic gastritis, especially atrophic gastritis, close medical follow-up should be stressed.

UPPER GASTROINTESTINAL BLEEDING

In the United States there are approximately 150,000 to 200,000 hospital admissions each year for upper GI bleeding.[18,19] Despite advances in intensive care, hemodynamic monitoring, and endoscopy, there has been little change in the mortality rate for upper GI bleeding, which has remained approximately 6% to 10% for the past 40 years. This is due in part to the greater incidence of upper GI bleeding in older adults, especially women, related to the use of NSAIDs.

Etiology and Pathophysiology

Although the most serious loss of blood from the upper GI tract is characterized by a sudden onset, insidious occult bleeding can also be a major problem. The severity of bleeding depends on whether the origin is venous, capillary, or arterial. (Types of upper GI bleeding are presented in Table 40-14.) Bleeding from an arterial source is profuse, and the blood is bright red. The bright red color indicates that the blood has not been in contact with the stomach's acid secretions. In contrast, "coffee ground" vomitus reveals that the blood and other contents have been in the stomach for some time and have been changed by contact with gastric secretions. A massive upper GI hemorrhage is generally defined as a loss of more than 1500 ml of blood or a loss of 25% of intravascular blood volume. *Melena* (black, tarry stools) indicates slow bleeding from an upper GI source. The longer the passage of blood through the intestines, the darker the color of the stool as a result of the degradation of hemoglobin and the release of iron.

Discovering the cause of the bleeding is not always an easy task. A variety of areas in the GI tract may be involved, and there may be many different reasons for the blood loss. Table 40-15 lists the common causes of bleeding. Although systemic diseases (e.g., leukemia, blood dyscrasias) that interfere with normal

TABLE 40-14	Types of Upper Gastrointestinal Bleeding
TYPE	**CLINICAL MANIFESTATIONS**
Obvious bleeding	
• Hematemesis	Bloody vomitus appearing as fresh, bright red blood or "coffee ground" appearance (dark, grainy digested blood)
• Melena	Black, tarry stools (often foul smelling) caused by digestion of blood in the GI tract. The black appearance is from the presence of iron
Occult bleeding	Small amounts of blood in gastric secretions, vomitus, or stools not apparent by appearance; detectable by guaiac test

TABLE 40-15	Common Causes of Upper Gastrointestinal Bleeding
Drug Induced	
Corticosteroids	
Nonsteroidal antiinflammatory drugs	
Salicylates	
Esophagus	
Esophageal varices	
Esophagitis	
Mallory-Weiss tear	
Stomach and Duodenum	
Gastric cancer	
Hemorrhagic gastritis	
Peptic ulcer disease	
Polyps	
Stress ulcer	
Systemic Diseases	
Blood dyscrasias (e.g., leukemia, aplastic anemia)	
Renal failure (uremia)	

blood clotting must be considered whenever upper GI bleeding occurs, the most common sites are the esophagus, stomach, and duodenum.

Esophageal Origin. Bleeding from an esophageal source is most likely the result of chronic esophagitis, bleeding from a tear in the mucosa near the esophagogastric junction (Mallory-Weiss tear), or esophageal varices. Chronic esophagitis can be caused by the ingestion of chemicals, including drugs irritating to the mucosa. Alcohol and smoking are known irritants of the esophageal mucosa. GERD with or without a hiatal hernia can lead to chronic irritation and erosion. A **Mallory-Weiss tear** is usually caused by severe retching and vomiting. This tear occurs in the esophageal mucosa at the junction of the esophagus and stomach and results in severe bleeding.

Esophageal varices usually occur secondary to cirrhosis of the liver. Branches of the vena cava and the azygos vein from the systemic circulation converge with the smaller vessels of the lower esophagus. These vessels are inelastic and become engorged and tortuous because of increased pressure exerted on them secondary to portal hypertension. Anything that may increase the pressure (e.g., coughing, sneezing, trauma) or cause mechanical irritation (e.g., vomiting, irritation, erosion) may result in sudden, massive bleeding. (Esophageal varices are discussed in Chapter 42.)

Stomach and Duodenal Origin. Bleeding ulcers account for the majority of cases of upper GI bleeding.[20] Erosion of a blood vessel by an ulcer located in the stomach or duodenum must always be considered as a possible cause of upper GI bleeding. A gastric ulcer may penetrate the left gastric artery, and a duodenal ulcer may penetrate the superior pancreaticoduodenal artery. Most bleeding ulcers are related to the presence of *H. pylori* or drug use.[21]

Acute gastritis produced by ingestion of drugs or alcohol or the reflux of bile from the small intestine can result in bleeding. Drugs, either prescribed by the health care provider or OTC, are a major cause of upper GI bleeding. For example, the patient who regularly takes aspirin or aspirin-containing compounds may be at risk for bleeding episodes. Aspirin, NSAIDs (e.g., ibuprofen), and corticosteroids can cause irritation and disruption of the gastric mucosal barrier. Aspirin-containing products are sold without prescriptions as OTC drugs. It is not unusual for a patient to deny the use of aspirin yet be self-medicating with aspirin-containing drugs, such as Alka-Seltzer, Bufferin, and Excedrin. A careful history of all commonly used drugs is therefore necessary whenever upper GI bleeding is suspected.

Physiologic stress ulcers, which may occur after severe burn, trauma, or major surgery, erode more superficial blood vessels than does a peptic ulcer. In one study, mucosal injury was found to be present in 70% of patients in an intensive care unit.[18] The combination of hypoperfusion and gastric irritants (HCl and pepsin) likely contributes to this mucosal damage. Gastric cancer can also result in upper GI bleeding. Gastric cancer can be the cause of a steady blood loss as it grows and ulcerates through the mucosa and blood vessels located in its path.

Emergency Assessment and Management

Although approximately 80% to 85% of patients who have massive hemorrhage spontaneously stop bleeding, the cause must be identified and treatment initiated immediately. Although a complete history of events leading to the bleeding episode is important in discovering the cause of the blood loss, it should be deferred until emergency care has been initiated. The immediate physical examination must include a systemic evaluation of the patient's condition with emphasis on blood pressure, rate and character of pulse, peripheral perfusion with capillary refill, and observation for the presence or absence of neck vein distention. Vital signs should be monitored every 15 to 30 minutes. Signs and symptoms of shock must be evaluated, and treatment should be started as soon as possible (see Chapter 65). The patient's respiratory status is carefully assessed, along with a thorough abdominal examination. The presence or absence of bowel sounds should be assessed and noted. A tense, rigid, boardlike abdomen may indicate a perforation and peritonitis.

Once the immediate interventions have begun, the patient or family should answer the following questions. Is there a history of previous bleeding episodes? Has weight loss been a recent problem? Has the patient received blood transfusions in the past, and were there any transfusion reactions? Is there a religious preference that prohibits the use of blood or blood products? Are there any other illnesses that may contribute to bleeding or interfere with treatment (e.g., congestive heart failure, diabetes mellitus)?

Laboratory studies are ordered, including a CBC, blood urea nitrogen (BUN), serum electrolytes, blood glucose, prothrombin time, liver enzymes, arterial blood gases (ABGs), and a type and crossmatch for possible blood transfusions. All vomitus and stools should be tested for the presence of gross and occult blood. A urinalysis provides information on the presence of blood in the urine, and the specific gravity gives an immediate indication of the patient's hydration status.

IV lines, preferably two, with a 16- or 18-gauge needle should be established for fluid and blood replacement. The type and amount of fluids infused are dictated by physical and laboratory findings. It is generally best to begin with an isotonic crystalloid solution (e.g., lactated Ringer's solution). Whole blood, packed RBCs, and fresh frozen plasma may be used for replacement of lost volume in massive hemorrhage. Because of the potential for fluid overload and immunologic reactions, packed RBCs are often preferred over whole blood. (The use of blood transfusions and volume expanders is discussed in Chapter 30.) The hemoglobin and hematocrit values are not of immediate assistance in estimating the degree of blood loss, but they provide a baseline for guiding further treatment. The initial hematocrit may be normal and may not reflect the loss until 4 to 6 hours after fluid replacement has taken place, since initially the loss of plasma and RBCs is equal. When upper GI bleeding is less profuse, infusion of isotonic saline solution followed by packed RBCs permits restoration of the hematocrit more quickly and does not create complications related to fluid volume overload. The use of supplemental oxygen delivered by face mask or nasal cannula may help increase blood oxygen saturation.

For most patients who are bleeding profusely, an indwelling urinary catheter is inserted so that urine volume can be accurately assessed hourly. A central venous pressure line may be inserted so that the patient's fluid volume status can be monitored easily. When a history of valvular heart disease, coronary artery disease, or congestive heart failure is elicited or when pulmonary edema is a factor, the use of a pulmonary artery catheter may be necessary to monitor the patient.

Most endoscopists advocate endoscopy without prior lavage to avoid delays in treatment. However, others prefer an NG tube to be placed and lavage with room temperature water or saline to be initiated before endoscopy. In this case a large tube passed through the mouth may be more beneficial than a small one passed through the nose. Passage through the mouth is easier, but no tube should ever be advanced against resistance because of the likelihood of damaging the gastric mucosa or causing perforation. Aspiration of stomach contents through a large-bore tube such as an Ewald tube facilitates the removal of clots from the stomach and alleviates the patient's need to vomit. Gastric lavage with water or saline may be initiated to ensure that blood will not interfere with emergency endoscopic visualization of the gastric mucosa. If used, the usual procedure for gastric lavage is to instill approximately 50 to 100 ml of tap water or saline solution each time, leave it in place for several minutes, and then allow drainage by gravity or low suction. This procedure may be repeated every 30 to 45 minutes.

Diagnostic Studies

In addition to using endoscopic procedures to stop bleeding, these procedures also allow direct visualization of the bleeding site. Endoscopy is quite accurate in identifying the specific source of the bleeding. When a skilled practitioner performs the procedure, bleeding from severe gastritis can be easily distinguished from that of a gastric or duodenal ulcer.

Angiography is used in diagnosing upper GI bleeding only when endoscopy cannot be done. It is an invasive procedure requiring preparation and setup time and may not be appropriate for a high-risk, unstable patient. In this procedure a catheter is placed into the left gastric or superior mesenteric artery and advanced until the site of bleeding is discovered.

Barium contrast studies are of little value in the identification of major bleeding sites during the acute phase of treatment. After the acute bleeding phase, barium studies can document an actual lesion but cannot verify that it is the bleeding source.

Collaborative Care

Endoscopic Therapy. The goal of endoscopic hemostasis is to coagulate or thrombose the bleeding artery and then reduce the necessity of a surgical procedure. This procedure has proven useful in stopping the bleeding of gastritis, Mallory-Weiss tear, esophageal and gastric varices, bleeding peptic ulcers, and polyps. Several techniques are used, including (1) thermal (heat) probe, (2) multipolar and bipolar electrocoagulation probe, and (3) neodymium:yttrium-aluminum-garnet (Nd:YAG) laser. Multipolar electrocoagulation and thermal probe are the two most commonly used procedures. The heat probe coagulates tissue by directly applying a heating element to the bleeding site. Overall, endoscopic therapy is more effective than medical management alone in reducing bleeding episodes.[18]

Surgical Therapy. Surgical intervention is indicated when bleeding continues regardless of the therapy provided and when the site of the bleeding has been identified. A high percentage of patients are known to have another massive hemorrhage within 5 years after the first bleeding episode. Some physicians regard surgical therapy as necessary when the patient continues to bleed after rapid transfusion of up to 2000 ml of whole blood or remains in shock after 24 hours. The site of the hemorrhage determines the choice of operation. In addition, the surgeon must consider the age of the patient because mortality rates increase considerably over the age of 60 years. It is essential that the operation be performed as soon as the need has been established.

Drug Therapy. During the acute phase, drugs are used to decrease bleeding, decrease HCl acid secretion, and neutralize the HCl acid that is present. Drug therapy to decrease bleeding is administered during endoscopy. Injection therapy with absolute alcohol (ethanol) or epinephrine (1:10,000 dilution) is effective for acute hemostasis. These agents produce tissue edema and, ultimately, pressure on the source of bleeding. To prevent rebleed-

ing, injection therapy is often combined with other therapies (e.g., thermocoagulation or laser treatment). A *sclerosant* (an agent that produces inflammation and results in fibrosis of the tissues) such as ethanolamine (Ethamolin) or morrhuate (Scleromate) may be used, especially if the cause of bleeding is esophageal varices.

For variceal bleeding, vasopressin (Pitressin), which is posterior pituitary extract, can be used to produce vasoconstriction. It is used to treat upper GI bleeding in those patients who do not respond to other therapies and are poor surgical risks. It is administered systemically through a vein or intraarterially at the local site of actual bleeding. Side effects of intravenously administered vasopressin include decreased myocardial contractility and decreased coronary blood flow. The patient undergoing vasopressin therapy must be closely monitored for its myocardial, visceral, and peripheral ischemic side effects. Vasopressin should be used with caution in the patient with a known history of vascular disease.

Efforts are made to reduce acid secretion because the acidic environment can alter platelet function, as well as interfere with clot stabilization. H_2R blockers (e.g., cimetidine [Tagamet]) or PPIs (e.g., pantoprazole [Protonix]) are administered intravenously to decrease acid secretion. Table 40-16 reviews the mechanism of action of H_2R blockers and PPIs. Although these drugs have no proven ability to control active bleeding, they have become part of standard treatment protocols.

In patients with upper GI bleeding, early administration of the somatostatin analog octreotide (Sandostatin) may be used. The drug reduces splanchnic blood flow, as well as acid secretion. This drug is given in IV boluses up to 5 to 6 days after the initiation of bleeding.

Antacids have long been known to neutralize HCl acid and continue to be used as an adjunct therapy for peptic ulcer disease. Because antacids neutralize HCl acid and increase the pH of gas-

TABLE 40-16	Drug Therapy Gastrointestinal Bleeding		
DRUG	**SOURCE OF GI BLEEDING**	**MECHANISM OF ACTION**
Antacids*	Duodenal ulcer, gastric ulcer, acute gastritis (corrosive, erosive, and hemorrhagic)	Neutralizes acid and maintains gastric pH above 5.5; elevated pH inhibits activation of pepsinogen
H_2-receptor blockers cimetidine (Tagamet) famotidine (Pepcid) nizatidine (Axid) ranitidine (Zantac)	Duodenal ulcer, gastric ulcer, esophagitis, acute gastritis (especially hemorrhagic)	Inhibits action of histamine at H_2-receptors on parietal cells and decreases HCl acid secretion
Proton pump inhibitors omeprazole (Prilosec) esomeprazole (Nexium) lansoprazole (Prevacid) pantoprazole (Protonix)	—	Inhibits the cellular pump, which is necessary for secretion of HCl acid
vasopressin (Pitressin)	Acute gastritis (corrosive, erosive, and hemorrhagic), esophageal varices	Causes vasoconstriction and increases smooth muscle activity of the GI tract; reduces pressure in the portal circulation and arrests bleeding
octreotide (Sandostatin)	Upper gastrointestinal bleeding, esophageal varices	Somatostatin analog that decreases splanchnic blood flow; decreases HCl acid secretion via decrease in release of gastrin

*See Table 40-21.

tric contents to above 5, there is inhibition of the conversion of pepsinogen to its active form pepsin. The most frequently used antacid preparations are magnesium hydroxide, magnesium trisilicate, aluminum hydroxide, calcium carbonate, and sodium bicarbonate (see Table 40-21 later in this chapter). Aluminum hydroxide and magnesium trisilicate are the most useful because they are nonabsorbable. Calcium carbonate and sodium bicarbonate are absorbable, and prolonged use can lead to systemic alkalosis.

Sedatives to control agitation and restlessness should be administered cautiously. They make accurate assessment of the patient's condition more difficult. Anticholinergic drugs are contraindicated in acute upper GI bleeding episodes.

NURSING MANAGEMENT
UPPER GASTROINTESTINAL BLEEDING

■ Nursing Assessment

As the nurse begins care of the patient admitted with upper GI bleeding, a thorough and accurate nursing assessment is an essential first step. Subjective and objective data that should be obtained from the patient or significant others are presented in Table 40-17.

The patient experiencing upper GI bleeding may not be able to provide specific information about the cause of the bleeding until the immediate physical needs are met. An immediate nursing assessment is performed while getting the patient ready for initial treatment. The assessment includes the patient's level of consciousness, vital signs, appearance of neck veins, skin color, and capillary refill. The abdomen is checked for distention, guarding, and peristalsis. Immediate determination of vital signs indicates whether the patient is in shock from blood loss and also provides a baseline blood pressure and pulse by which to monitor the progress of treatment. Signs and symptoms of shock include low blood pressure; rapid, weak pulse; increased thirst; cold, clammy skin; and restlessness. Vital signs are monitored every 15 to 30 minutes, and the health care provider should be informed of any significant changes.

When obtaining vital signs, the nurse considers the patient's age and physical condition. Taking the blood pressure and pulse with the patient lying down and then sitting will indicate postural changes that occur after acute blood loss. The older the patient, the more changes in vital signs should be expected.

■ Nursing Diagnoses

Nursing diagnoses for the patient with upper GI bleeding include, but are not limited to, the following:

- Deficient fluid volume *related to* acute loss of blood, as well as gastric secretions
- Ineffective tissue perfusion *related to* loss of circulatory volume
- Anxiety *related to* upper GI bleeding, hospitalization, uncertain outcome, source of bleeding
- Ineffective coping *related to* situational crisis and personal vulnerability
- Risk of aspiration *related to* active bleeding and altered level of consciousness
- Decreased cardiac output *related to* loss of blood

■ Planning

The overall goals are that the patient with upper GI bleeding will (1) have no further GI bleeding, (2) have the cause of the bleeding identified and treated, (3) experience a return to a nor-

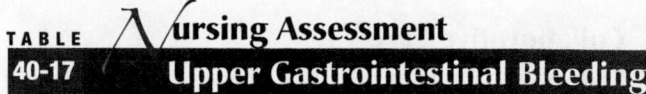

TABLE 40-17	Nursing Assessment Upper Gastrointestinal Bleeding

Subjective Data

Important Health Information

Past health history: Precipitating events before bleeding episode, previous bleeding episodes and treatment, peptic ulcer disease, esophageal varices, esophagitis, acute and chronic gastritis, stress ulcers

Medications: Use of aspirin, nonsteroidal antiinflammatory drugs, corticosteroids, anticoagulants

Functional Health Patterns

Health perception–health management: Family history of bleeding, smoking, alcohol use

Nutritional-metabolic: Nausea, vomiting, weight loss; thirst

Elimination: Diarrhea; black, tarry stools; decreased urinary output; sweating

Activity-exercise: Weakness, dizziness, fainting

Cognitive-perceptual: Epigastric pain, abdominal cramps

Coping–stress tolerance: Acute or chronic stressors

Objective Data

General

Fever

Integumentary

Clammy, cool, pale skin; pale mucous membranes, nailbeds, and conjunctivae; spider angiomas; jaundice; peripheral edema

Respiratory

Rapid, shallow respirations

Cardiovascular

Tachycardia, weak pulse, orthostatic hypotension, slow capillary refill

Gastrointestinal

Red or "coffee ground" vomitus; tense, rigid abdomen, ascites; hypoactive or hyperactive bowel sounds; black, tarry stools

Urinary

Decreased urinary output, concentrated urine

Neurologic

Agitation, restlessness; decreasing level of consciousness

Possible Findings

↓ Hematocrit and hemoglobin; hematuria; guaiac-positive stools, emesis, or gastric aspirate; ↓ levels of clotting factors; ↑ liver enzymes; abnormal upper GI studies or endoscopy results

mal hemodynamic state, and (4) experience minimal or no symptoms of pain or anxiety.

■ Nursing Implementation

Health Promotion. Although not all cases of upper GI bleeding can be anticipated and prevented, the nurse shares responsibility with the health care provider in trying to identify the patient who is at high risk. The patient with a history of chronic gastritis or peptic ulcer disease should always be considered in the high-risk category because of the increased incidence of bleeding associated with chronic irritation or chronic ulcers. The patient who has had one major bleeding episode is more likely to have another bleed. The patient is instructed to avoid gastric irritants such as alcohol and smoking, to prevent or decrease stress-inducing situations at home or at work, and to take only prescribed medications. OTC drugs can be harmful because they may contain ingredients (e.g., aspirin) that have potentially irritating effects on the mucosa. The patient is instructed in the methods of testing vomitus or stools for the presence of occult blood. Positive results should be promptly reported to the health care provider or the nurse.

The patient who requires regular administration of ulcerogenic drugs, such as aspirin, corticosteroids, or NSAIDs, needs instruction regarding the potential adverse effects that these agents may have on the GI mucosa. These drugs are avoided if at all possible. However, if aspirin must be prescribed, enteric-coated tablets can be substituted for regular tablets. Taking the drugs with meals or snacks lessens the potential irritating effects. For patients who must take NSAIDs, a change to a preparation with less GI toxicity may be considered. Cyclooxygenase-2 (COX-2) inhibitors (e.g., rofecoxib [Vioxx], celecoxib [Celebrex], valdecoxib [Bextra]) have less of an effect on the production of tissue prostaglandins and are associated with fewer GI side effects.[22] The co-administration of an NSAID with a PPI can reduce bleeding risk. For the patient at risk for gastric ulcers because of NSAID use, misoprostol (Cytotec) may also be prescribed. This prostaglandin analog inhibits acid secretion and reduces upper GI bleeding episodes associated with NSAID use. However, the drug has several important side effects, including uterine cramping in women and diarrhea. Because of its effects on the uterus, it is contraindicated in women of childbearing age.

When the nurse is working with the patient who has a history of liver cirrhosis with esophageal varices, the instructions must be specific regarding the importance of avoiding known irritants, such as alcohol and smoking. The prompt treatment of an upper respiratory tract infection should be stressed. Severe coughing or sneezing can create increased pressure on the already fragile varices and may result in massive hemorrhage.

The patient who is known to have blood dyscrasias (e.g., aplastic anemia) or liver dysfunction or who is taking cancer chemotherapeutic drugs has a potential bleeding problem because of altered hemostasis caused by a decrease in clotting factors and platelets. When these patients also have a history of ulcer disease, gastritis, varices, or drug and alcohol abuse, they should be carefully instructed regarding their disease process and drugs, and they should be closely observed for bleeding.

Acute Intervention. The patient should be approached in a calm and assured manner to help decrease the level of anxiety. Caution should be used before administering sedatives for restlessness because it is one of the warning signs of shock and may be masked by the drugs.

Once an infusion has been started, the IV line must be maintained for fluid or blood replacement. An accurate intake and output record is essential so that the patient's hydration status can be assessed. Urine output should be measured hourly. A rate of at least 0.5 ml/kg per hour indicates adequate renal perfusion. Lesser amounts may indicate renal ischemia secondary to loss of blood volume. Urine specific gravity should be measured because it gives additional information regarding the patient's hydration status. Consistent readings greater than 1.025 (normal is 1.005 to 1.025) indicate that the urine is extremely concentrated and that there is probably a low blood volume. The health care provider must be kept informed of these important parameters so that the IV solutions can be increased or decreased accordingly. If the patient has a central venous pressure line or pulmonary artery catheter in place, readings should be recorded every 1 to 2 hours. Hemodynamic monitoring provides an accurate and quick assessment of blood flow and pressure within the cardiovascular system (see Chapter 64).

The older adult or the patient with a history of cardiovascular problems should be observed closely for signs of fluid overload. However, the threat of volume overload and pulmonary edema must be a constant concern in all patients who are receiving large amounts of IV fluids within a short time. Therefore auscultation of breath sounds and close observation of respiratory effort are important. Electrocardiographic (ECG) monitoring can also be used to evaluate cardiac function.

Foods such as beets or even swallowed mouthwash can give vomitus a bloody appearance. Unless the contents of the vomitus are checked for occult blood, false information may be recorded. Swallowed blood from a nosebleed must also be accurately noted to avoid misdiagnosis of an upper GI bleeding episode. When an NG tube is inserted, the nurse must pay special attention to keeping it in proper position and observing the aspirate for blood.

The majority of upper GI bleeding episodes cease spontaneously, even without intervention. Although the use of room temperature, cool, or iced gastric lavage is used in some institutions, its effectiveness is of questionable value. Water has the advantage of being able to break up large clots more easily than saline solution, is less expensive, and is always available. A disadvantage of tap water is that it may create more electrolyte imbalances than would an isotonic saline solution.

When lavage is used, approximately 50 to 100 ml of fluid is instilled at a time into the stomach. The lavage fluid may be aspirated from the stomach or drained by gravity. When aspiration is the method used, it is important not to aspirate if resistance is felt. The tip of the NG tube may be up against the gastric mucosal lining. The constant pressure from attempts to aspirate the lavage fluid may cause erosion of the mucosa. When resistance is a factor, the nurse should use gravity as the alternative method of gastric drainage. Close monitoring of vital signs, especially in the patient with cardiovascular disease, is important because arrhythmias may occur. Keeping the patient warm and the head of the bed elevated provides comfort and prevents possible aspiration problems.

The nurse caring for a patient with upper GI bleeding should be well informed as to what constitutes blood in the stools. Black, tarry stools are not usually associated with a brisk hemorrhage but are indicative of the presence of bleeding of prolonged duration. Bright red blood in the stool is usually from a source in the lower bowel. Menses and bleeding hemorrhoids should be ruled out as possible sources of blood in the stools. When vomitus contains blood but the stool contains no gross or occult blood, the hemorrhage is considered to have been of short duration.

Monitoring the patient's laboratory studies enables the nurse to estimate the effectiveness of therapy. The hemoglobin and hematocrit are usually evaluated about every 4 to 6 hours if the patient is actively bleeding. At first the hematocrit level may not accurately reflect the amount of blood lost or the amount of blood replaced and will appear falsely high or low. The patient's BUN level is assessed. It is generally elevated with a significant hemorrhage because blood proteins are broken down by GI tract bacteria. However, renal disease may also result in an elevated BUN level. Many patients receive oxygen by mask or nasally to ensure that the circulating blood has an adequate oxygen content.

When oral nourishment is begun, the patient is observed for symptoms of nausea and vomiting and a recurrence of bleeding.

Feedings initially consist of clear fluids or milk and are given hourly until tolerance is determined. These feedings help neutralize the gastric secretions and assist in the mucosal repair. Gradual introduction of foods follows if the patient exhibits no signs of discomfort.

The patient in whom hemorrhage was the result of chronic alcohol abuse requires close observation for the beginning of delirium tremens as withdrawal from alcohol takes place. Symptoms indicating the beginning of delirium tremens are agitation, uncontrolled shaking, sweating, and vivid hallucinations. (Alcohol withdrawal is discussed in Chapter 11.)

Ambulatory and Home Care. The patient and family must be taught how to avoid future bleeding episodes. Ulcer disease, drug or alcohol abuse, and liver and respiratory diseases can all result in upper GI bleeding. The patient and family must be made aware of the consequences of noncompliance with diet and drug therapy. It must be emphasized that no drugs (especially aspirin, NSAIDs) other than those prescribed by the health care provider should be taken. Smoking and alcohol should be eliminated because they are sources of irritation and interfere with tissue repair. The need for long-term follow-up care may be necessary because of the possibility of another bleeding episode. The patient and family should be instructed on what to do if an acute hemorrhage occurs in the future.

■ Evaluation

The expected outcomes are that the patient with upper GI bleeding will

- have no upper GI bleeding
- maintain normal fluid volume
- experience a return to a normal hemodynamic state
- experience absence or tolerable levels of pain and is comfortable
- understand potential etiologic factors and make appropriate lifestyle modifications

PEPTIC ULCER DISEASE

Peptic ulcer disease is a condition characterized by erosion of the GI mucosa resulting from the digestive action of HCl acid and pepsin. Any portion of the GI tract that comes into contact with gastric secretions is susceptible to ulcer development, including the lower esophagus, stomach, duodenum, and margin of gastrojejunal anastomosis after surgical procedures. It is estimated that approximately 10% of men and 4% of women in the United States will have ulcers during their lifetimes.

Types

Peptic ulcers can be classified as acute or chronic, depending on the degree and duration of mucosal involvement (Fig. 40-11), and gastric or duodenal, according to the location. The *acute ulcer* (see Fig. 40-11) is associated with superficial erosion and minimal inflammation. It is of short duration and resolves quickly when the cause is identified and removed. A chronic ulcer (Fig. 40-12) is one of long duration, eroding through the muscular wall with the formation of fibrous tissue. It is present continuously for many months or intermittently throughout the person's lifetime. A chronic ulcer is at least four times as common as acute erosion.

Gastric and duodenal ulcers, although defined as peptic ulcers, are different in their etiology and incidence (Table 40-18). Generally, the treatment of all types of ulcers is quite similar.

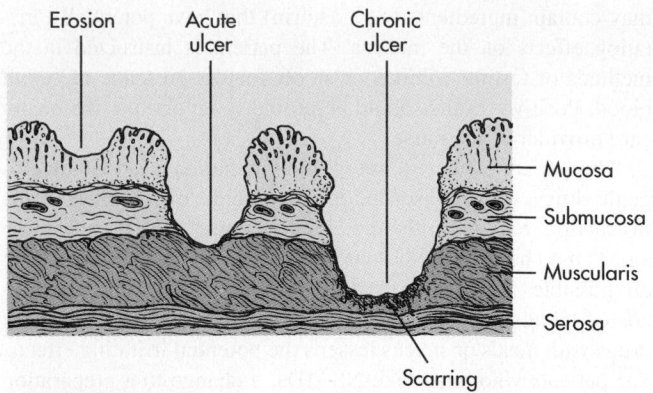

FIG. 40-11 Peptic ulcers, including an erosion, acute ulcer, and chronic ulcer. Both the acute and chronic ulcer may penetrate the entire wall of the stomach.

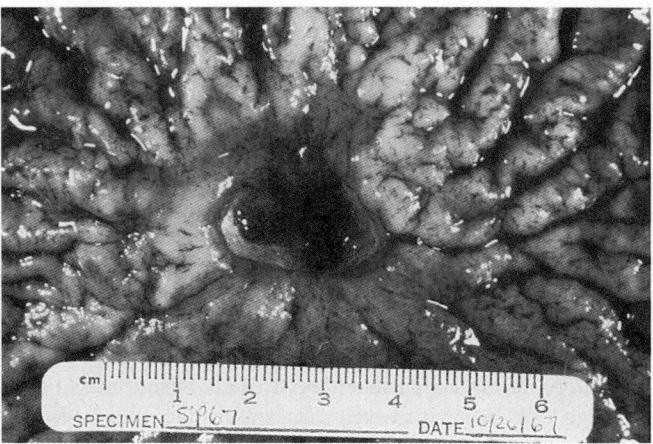

FIG. 40-12 Photograph of a chronic peptic ulcer located in the lesser curvature of stomach.

Etiology and Pathophysiology

Peptic ulcers develop only in the presence of an acid environment. It has been well established that the patient with pernicious anemia and achlorhydria rarely has gastric ulcers. An excess of gastric acid may not be necessary for ulcer development. The typical person with a gastric ulcer has normal to less than normal gastric acidity compared with the person with a duodenal ulcer. However, some intraluminal acid does seem to be essential for a gastric ulcer to occur.

Pepsinogen, the precursor of pepsin, is activated to pepsin in the presence of HCl acid and a pH of 2 to 3. The secretion of HCl acid by the parietal cells has a pH of 0.8. After mixing with the stomach contents, the pH reaches 2 to 3, a highly favorable range of acidity for pepsin activity. When the stomach acid level is neutralized by the presence of food or antacids or acid secretion is blocked by drugs, the pH is increased to 3.5 or more. At a pH of 3.5 or more, pepsin has little or no proteolytic activity.

The stomach is normally protected from autodigestion by the gastric mucosal barrier. The GI tract has a high cell turnover rate, and the surface mucosa of the stomach is renewed about every 3 days. As a result of this high turnover rate, the mucosa can continually repair itself except in extreme instances when the cell breakdown surpasses the cell renewal rate. Normally, water, electrolytes, and water-soluble substances (e.g., glucose) can easily

TABLE 40-18 Comparison of Gastric and Duodenal Ulcers		
	GASTRIC ULCERS	**DUODENAL ULCERS**
Lesion	Superficial; smooth margins; round, oval, or cone shaped	Penetrating (associated with deformity of duodenal bulb from healing of recurrent ulcers)
Location of lesion	Predominantly antrum, also in body and fundus of stomach	First 1-2 cm of duodenum
Gastric secretion	Normal to decreased	Increased
Incidence	• Greater in women • Peak age 50-60 yr • More common in persons of lower socioeconomic status and in unskilled laborers • Increased with smoking, drug, and alcohol use • Increased with incompetent pyloric sphincter and bile reflux • Increased with stress ulcers after severe burns, head trauma, and major surgery	• Greater in men, but increasing in women, especially postmenopausal • Peak age 35-45 yr • Associated with psychologic stress • Increased with smoking, drug, and alcohol use • Associated with other diseases (e.g., chronic obstructive pulmonary disease, pancreatic disease, hyperparathyroidism, Zollinger-Ellison syndrome, chronic renal failure)
Clinical manifestations	• Burning or gaseous pressure in high left epigastrium and back and upper abdomen • Pain 1-2 hr after meals; if penetrating ulcer, aggravation of discomfort with food • Occasional nausea and vomiting, weight loss	• Burning, cramping, pressurelike pain across mid-epigastrium and upper abdomen; back pain with posterior ulcers • Pain 2-4 hr after meals and midmorning, midafternoon, middle of night, periodic and episodic • Pain relief with antacids and food; occasional nausea and vomiting
Recurrence rate	High	High
Complications	Hemorrhage, perforation, outlet obstruction, intractability	Hemorrhage, perforation, obstruction

pass through the barrier. However, the mucosal barrier prevents the back diffusion of acid from the gastric lumen through the mucosal layers to the underlying tissue.

Under specific circumstances the mucosal barrier can be impaired and back diffusion of acid can occur (Fig. 40-13). When the barrier is broken, HCl acid freely enters the mucosa and injury to the tissues occurs. This results in cellular destruction and inflammation. Histamine is released from the damaged mucosa, resulting in vasodilation and increased capillary permeability. The released histamine is then capable of stimulating further secretion of acid and pepsin.

As described in the section on gastritis, a variety of agents are known to destroy the mucosal barrier. By generating ammonia in the mucous layer, *H. pylori* may create a condition of chronic inflammation, rendering the mucosa especially vulnerable to other noxious substances. Ulcerogenic drugs, such as aspirin and NSAIDs, inhibit synthesis of prostaglandins and cause abnormal permeability. Corticosteroids have the ability to decrease the rate of mucosal cell renewal and thereby decrease its protective effects. Lipid-soluble cytotoxic drugs can pass through the barrier and destroy it.

When the mucosal barrier is disrupted, there is a compensatory increase in blood flow (Fig. 40-14). This phenomenon can occur in several ways. Prostaglandin-like substances and histamine act as vasodilators, thus increasing capillary blood flow. As blood flow increases within the affected mucosa, hydrogen ions are rapidly removed from the area, buffers are delivered to help neutralize the hydrogen ions present, nutrients necessary for cell function arrive, and the rate of mucosal cell replication increases. When the increase is sufficient to dilute, buffer, and remove the excess hydrogen ions, tissue damage may be minimal or may result in no injury at all. When blood flow is not sufficient to carry out these events, tissue injury results. Fig. 40-14 shows a repre-

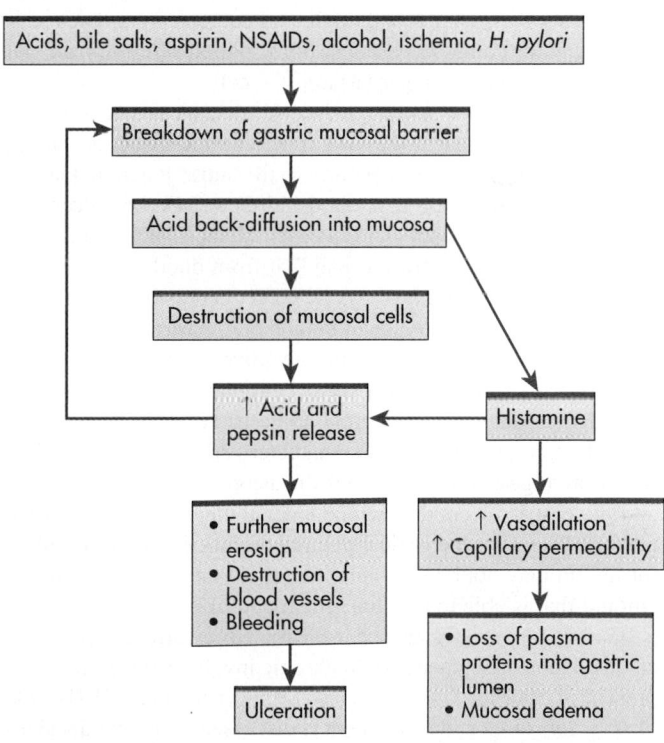

FIG. 40-13 Disruption of gastric mucosa and pathophysiologic consequences of back-diffusion of acids.

sentation of the interrelationship between the mucosal blood flow and disruption of the gastric mucosal barrier.

There are two mechanisms that protect against damage. First, mucus is secreted by superficial mucous cells and forms a layer that can entrap or slow the diffusion of hydrogen ions across the

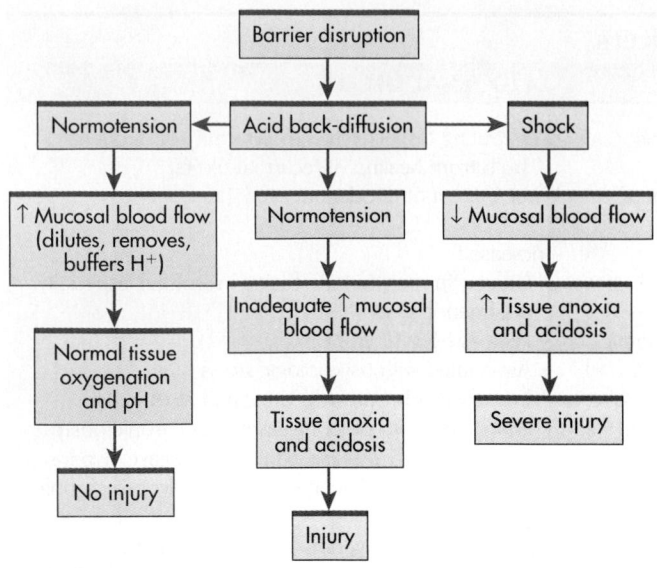

FIG. 40-14 Relationship between mucosal blood flow and disruption of the gastric mucosal barrier.

mucosal barrier in the stomach. Second, bicarbonate is secreted by the gastric and duodenal mucosa, and this helps neutralize HCl acid in the lumen of the GI tract.

Increased vagal nerve stimulation from a variety of causes (e.g., emotions) results in hypersecretion of HCl acid. Increased concentrations of HCl acid can alter the mucosal barrier. Duodenal ulcers are associated with high acid content. It has been suggested that the continual response of the parietal cells to maximal stimulation results in hyperplasia of the cells.

Gastric Ulcers. Although gastric ulcers can occur in any portion of the stomach, they are most commonly found on the lesser curvature in close proximity to the antral junction. Gastric ulcers are less common than duodenal ulcers. Gastric ulcers are more prevalent in women and in older adults. The mortality rate from gastric ulcers is greater than that from duodenal ulcers because the peak incidence of gastric ulcers occurs in persons over 50 years of age. Contrary to common belief, gastric ulcers are not more prevalent among those in executive or managerial positions. Persons from the lower socioeconomic class and manual or unskilled workers are more prone to gastric ulcers.

Although gastric ulcers are characterized by a normal to low secretion of gastric acid, the back diffusion of acid is greater with chronic gastric ulcers than with duodenal ulcers or in the healthy person. Therefore the critical pathologic process in gastric ulcer formation may not be the amount of acid that is secreted but the amount that is able to penetrate the mucosal barrier.

Gastric ulcers have also been attributed to various factors that can lead to acute episodes or to chronic involvement. *H. pylori* is present in 50% to 70% of patients with gastric ulcers.[22] The role of *H. pylori* in ulcer development is discussed under duodenal ulcers. It is thought that destruction of the gastric mucosa by noxious agents such as drugs or smoking may be enhanced by the presence of *H. pylori*, which further promotes gastric mucosal destruction.

Drugs can cause acute gastric ulcers and in some cases can lead to the development of chronic ulcers. The drugs most often implicated include aspirin, corticosteroids, NSAIDs (e.g., ibuprofen), and reserpine (Serpasil). It is estimated that 1% to 3% of patients taking NSAIDs for 1 year experience serious GI complications, including gastritis, gastric ulcer, upper GI hemorrhage, or perforation. It is estimated that approximately 10 million Americans use NSAIDs, and 100,000 to 300,000 GI adverse events associated with NSAID use are reported each year.[21] Other known causative factors of gastric ulcer formation are chronic alcohol abuse, chronic gastritis, and bile reflux gastritis from an incompetent pyloric sphincter. Cigarette smoking is positively linked with gastric ulcers. Nicotine seems to enhance reflux of duodenal contents into the antrum of the stomach. The ingestion of hot, rough, or spicy foods has been suggested as a causative factor, but there is no evidence to substantiate this claim.

Duodenal Ulcers. Duodenal ulcers account for about 80% of all peptic ulcers. Although duodenal ulcers still affect more men than women, the incidence of duodenal ulcers has followed a downward trend in men and a steady increase in women. The explanation for this change has not been clearly identified. Duodenal ulcers may occur at any age, but the incidence is especially high between the ages of 35 and 45 years. Duodenal ulcers can develop in anyone, regardless of occupation or socioeconomic group.

The development of duodenal ulcers is associated with a high HCl acid secretion. Several diseases have been identified with a high risk of duodenal ulcer development, including chronic obstructive pulmonary disease, cirrhosis of the liver, chronic pancreatitis, hyperparathyroidism, chronic renal failure, and the Zollinger-Ellison syndrome. (*Zollinger-Ellison syndrome* is a rare condition characterized by severe peptic ulceration, gastric acid hypersecretion, elevated serum gastrin levels, and gastrinoma of the pancreas or duodenum.) It is possible that the treatments used for these conditions may also promote ulcer development. Alcohol ingestion and heavy smoking habits are also associated with duodenal ulcer formation because both are known stimulants of acid secretion.

Although many factors are thought to contribute to the formation of duodenal ulcers, *H. pylori* has been identified as playing a key role. *H. pylori* is found in approximately 90% to 95% of patients with duodenal ulcers.[22] However, a clear-cut direct causal relationship between *H. pylori* and duodenal ulcer formation has not yet been proven. Not all individuals with evidence of *H. pylori* go on to develop ulcers, suggesting that additional factors are needed to produce these conditions. *H. pylori* survives in the human upper GI tract for a long time as a result of its ability to move in mucus and attach to mucosal cells. In addition, it secretes a substance called *urease,* which buffers the area around the bacterium and protects it from destruction in an acidic environment.

Infection with *H. pylori* is highest in underdeveloped countries and in persons of low socioeconomic status. Although the routes of transmission are largely unknown, it is thought that infection occurs during childhood via transmission from family members to the child, possibly through a fecal-oral and/or oral-oral route. In the United States and Canada, persons born before 1940 have a significantly higher risk of carrying *H. pylori* than persons in younger age groups. This enhanced prevalence in older persons has been attributed to the presence of crowded living conditions and poor sanitation practices, which were more common in the first half of the last century.

Research into a genetic cause for ulcers has shown that some members of the same family are more prone to develop gastric or duodenal ulcers. Supporting a genetic etiology is the fact that persons with blood group O have an increased incidence of duodenal ulcers. This may be related to increased susceptibility to *H. pylori.* Evidence is not complete, however, and the ulcer development could just as well be due to the sharing of the same environment.

Physiologic Stress Ulcers. **Physiologic stress ulcers** are acute ulcers that develop following a major physiologic insult such as trauma or surgery. A physiologic stress ulcer is a form of erosive gastritis. It is believed that the gastric mucosa of the body of the stomach undergoes a period of transient ischemia in association with hypotension, severe injury, extensive burns, and complicated surgery. The ischemia is due to decreased capillary blood flow or shunting of blood away from the GI tract so that blood flow bypasses the gastric mucosa. This occurs as a compensatory mechanism in hypotension or shock. The decrease in blood flow produces an imbalance between the destructive properties of HCl acid and pepsin and protective factors of the stomach's mucosal barrier, especially in the fundic portion, resulting in ulceration. Multiple superficial erosions result, and these may bleed. Risk factors for development of stress ulcer bleeding are respiratory failure and coagulopathy. These patients should receive prophylaxis with antisecretory agents. The diagnosis of stress gastritis is made on endoscopy, and treatment is with aggressive reduction of gastric acid secretions using H_2R blockers or PPIs.

Clinical Manifestations

It is common for the person with gastric or duodenal ulcers to have no pain or other symptoms. The gastric and duodenal mucosas are not rich in sensory pain fibers, which may account for this phenomenon. When pain does occur with duodenal ulcer, it is described as "burning" or "cramplike." It is most often located in the midepigastric region beneath the xiphoid process. The pain associated with gastric ulcers is located high in the epigastrium and occurs spontaneously about 1 to 2 hours after meals. The pain is described as "burning" or "gaseous." The pain can occur when the stomach is empty or when food has been ingested. If the ulcer has eroded through the gastric mucosa, food tends to aggravate rather than alleviate the pain. Some persons do not experience any pain until the presence of the ulcer is demonstrated through a serious complication such as hemorrhage or perforation.

Ulcers located on the posterior aspect of the duodenum can be manifested by back pain. The pain usually occurs 2 to 4 hours after meals. It is relieved by antacids alone or in combination with an H_2R blocker and sometimes by foods that neutralize and dilute the HCl acid. A characteristic of duodenal ulcer is its tendency to occur continuously for a few weeks or months and then disappear for a time, only to recur some months later. Some patients claim their symptoms worsen in the spring and fall of the year, thus strengthening the concept of a seasonal trend in occurrence.

Complications

The three major complications of chronic peptic ulcer disease are hemorrhage, perforation, and gastric outlet obstruction. All are considered emergency situations and are initially treated conservatively. However, surgery may become necessary at any time during the course of the therapy.

Hemorrhage. Hemorrhage is the most common complication of peptic ulcer disease. It develops from erosion of the granulation tissue found at the base of the ulcer during healing or from erosion of the ulcer through a major blood vessel. Duodenal ulcers account for a greater percentage of upper GI bleeding episodes than gastric ulcers.

Perforation. Perforation is considered the most lethal complication of peptic ulcer. Perforation is commonly seen in large penetrating duodenal ulcers that have not healed and are located on the posterior mucosal wall (Fig. 40-15). Perforated gastric ulcers are most often located on the lesser curvature of the stomach. Even though duodenal ulcers are more prevalent and perforate more frequently, mortality rates associated with perforation of gastric ulcers are higher. The older age of the patient with gastric ulcers, who often has other concurrent medical problems, is thought to be the crucial factor in the higher mortality rates.

Perforation of a peptic ulcer occurs when the ulcer penetrates the serosal surface, with spillage of either gastric or duodenal contents into the peritoneal cavity. The size of the perforation is directly proportional to the length of time the patient has had the ulcer. The larger the perforation, the longer the history of the ulcer. Small perforations seal themselves and result in a cessation of symptoms; larger perforations require immediate surgical closure. Spontaneous sealing occurs as a result of large amounts of fibrin being produced in response to the perforation. This leads to fibrinous fusion of the duodenum or gastric curvature to adjacent tissue, mainly the liver.

The clinical manifestations of perforation are characterized by their sudden and dramatic onset. The patient experiences sudden, severe upper abdominal pain that quickly spreads throughout the abdomen. The visceral and parietal layers of the peritoneum have an abundance of pain receptors, and this contributes to the abrupt, intense pain experienced. There may be shoulder pain if the spillage causes irritation to the phrenic nerve. The abdominal muscles contract, appearing rigid and boardlike as they attempt to protect the abdomen from further injury. The patient's respirations become shallow and rapid. Bowel sounds are usually absent. Nausea and vomiting may occur but are generally absent. Many patients report a history of ulcer disease or recent symptoms of indigestion.

The contents entering the peritoneal cavity from the stomach or duodenum contain a variety of ingredients that include air, saliva, food particles, HCl acid, pepsin, bacteria, bile, and pancreatic fluid and enzymes. Bacterial peritonitis may occur within

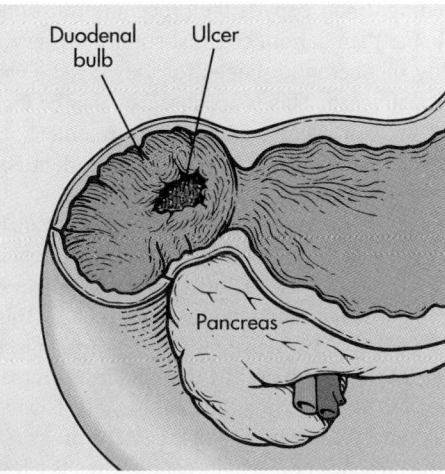

FIG. 40-15 Duodenal ulcer of the posterior wall penetrating into the head of the pancreas, resulting in walled-off perforation.

6 to 12 hours. The intensity of the peritonitis is proportional to the amount and duration of the spillage through the perforation. It is difficult to determine from the sudden onset of symptoms whether gastric or duodenal ulcer is the cause because the clinical characteristics of intestinal perforation are the same (see Chapter 41).

Gastric Outlet Obstruction. Ulcers located in the antrum and the prepyloric and pyloric areas of the stomach and the duodenum can predispose to gastric outlet obstruction. In the early phase of obstruction (often referred to as the compensated phase), gastric emptying is normal to near normal. Over time, increased contractile force needed to empty the stomach results in hypertrophy of the stomach wall. After long-standing obstruction the stomach enters the decompensated phase, which results in dilation and atony. The obstruction is not totally due to fibrous scar tissue because active ulcer formation is associated with edema, inflammation, and pylorospasm, all of which contribute to the narrowing of the pylorus.

The patient with gastric outlet obstruction generally has a long history of ulcer pain. Ulcerlike pain of short duration or complete absence of pain is more indicative of a malignant obstruction. The pain progresses to a more generalized upper abdominal discomfort that becomes worse toward the end of the day as the stomach fills and dilates. Relief may be obtained by belching or by self-induced vomiting. Vomiting is common and often projectile. The vomitus contains food particles that were ingested many hours or even a day or two before the vomiting episode. There is often an offensive odor if the contents have been dormant in the stomach for a time. The patient who vomits frequently will be anorectic, with evident weight loss, and will complain of thirst and an unpleasant taste in the mouth. Constipation is a common complaint that usually results from dehydration and lack of roughage in the diet.

The patient with gastric outlet obstruction may show a swelling in the upper abdomen indicating dilation of the stomach. Loud peristalsis can be heard, and visible peristaltic waves are often observed passing across the abdomen from left to right. If the stomach is grossly dilated, it is possible to palpate it as well.

Diagnostic Studies

The diagnostic measures used to determine the presence and location of a peptic ulcer are similar to those used for acute upper GI bleeding. Endoscopy is the procedure most often used. It is more reliable than barium contrast studies because of the maneuverability of fiberoptic scopes for viewing the entire gastric and duodenal mucosa. This procedure can also be used to determine the degree of ulcer healing after treatment. During endoscopy, tissue specimens can be obtained for identification of *H. pylori* and to rule out gastric cancer.

There are currently several diagnostic tests available to confirm *H. pylori* infection. These are classified as noninvasive and invasive. Noninvasive tests include serum or whole blood antibody tests, in particular, immunoglobulin G (IgG). This test is approximately 90% to 95% sensitive for *H. pylori* infection. However, because of the length of time that IgG levels remain elevated in the blood after the infection, the serologic tests will not distinguish active from recently treated disease. The urea breath test can determine the presence of active infection. Urea is a by-product of the metabolism of *H. pylori* bacteria. Invasive tests involve biopsy of the stomach and include the rapid urease test, as well as other

histologic markers of infection. These tests have greater sensitivity and specificity but involve an endoscopic procedure.[22]

Barium contrast studies, although widely used, are not accurate in identifying shallow, superficial ulcers because of failure of the barium to properly fill the ulcer crater. X-ray studies are also ineffective in differentiating a peptic ulcer from a malignant tumor. In addition, x-rays do not as readily demonstrate the degree of healing that can be visually determined with the endoscope. Barium studies are of benefit in the diagnosis of gastric outlet obstruction. Barium normally should pass from the stomach within 2 hours, but with gastric outlet obstruction, 50% of the barium remains on follow-up films up to 6 hours later.

Gastric analysis has questionable value in the diagnosis of peptic ulcer disease because in many patients gastric secretions are normal in amount and composition. However, it can provide important data in (1) identifying a possible gastrinoma (Zollinger-Ellison syndrome), (2) determining the degree of gastric hyperacidity, and (3) evaluating the results of therapy such as vagotomy and antisecretory drug therapy. Gastric analysis procedure is described in Table 38-12.

Laboratory analyses, including a CBC, urinalysis, liver enzyme studies, serum amylase determination, and stool examination, should be performed. A CBC may indicate the presence of anemia secondary to bleeding from the ulcer. Liver enzyme studies help determine any liver problems, such as cirrhosis, that may complicate the treatment of the ulcer. Urine and stool are routinely tested for the presence of blood. A serum amylase determination is frequently ordered to provide information on pancreatic function in patients in whom posterior penetration of the pancreas is suspected.

Collaborative Care: Conservative Therapy

When the patient's clinical manifestations and health history suggest the diagnosis of peptic ulcer disease and diagnostic studies confirm it, a medical regimen is instituted (Table 40-19). The regimen consists of adequate rest, dietary modifications, drug therapy, elimination of smoking, and long-term follow-up care. The aim of the treatment program is to decrease the degree of gastric acidity, enhance mucosal defense mechanisms, and minimize the harmful effects on the mucosa.

Patients are generally treated in ambulatory care clinics. The healing of a peptic ulcer requires many weeks of therapy. Pain disappears after 3 to 6 days, but ulcer healing is much slower. Complete healing may take 3 to 9 weeks, depending on ulcer size and the treatment regimen employed. Healing of the ulcer should be assessed by means of x-rays or endoscopic examination. Barium contrast films provide a rough estimate of the degree of ulcer healing. However, it should be noted that endoscopic examination is the only accurate method to monitor for ulcer healing.

Adequate rest, both physical and emotional, is important in the treatment process. A quiet, calm environment at home or on the job is not easy to achieve and may require some modifications in the patient's daily routine. The benefits derived from the elimination or reduction of stressors help decrease the stimulus for overproduction of HCl acid. Moderation in daily activity is essential.

Aspirin and nonselective NSAIDs with GI side effects may be discontinued or NSAIDs that are COX-2 inhibitors are used.[23] When aspirin or nonselective NSAIDs must be continued, enteric-coated preparations or co-administration with a PPI or misoprostol (Cytotec) should be considered.

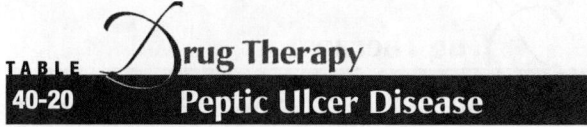

TABLE 40-19 Collaborative Care
Peptic Ulcer Disease

Diagnostic
History and physical examination
Upper GI endoscopy with biopsy
H. pylori testing of breath, urine, blood, tissue
Upper GI barium contrast study
Complete blood count
Urinalysis
Liver enzymes
Serum electrolytes

Collaborative Therapy
Conservative Therapy
Adequate rest
Bland diet (six small meals a day)
Cessation of smoking
Drug therapy
　H_2-receptor blockers (see Table 40-20)
　Proton pump inhibitors (see Table 40-20)
　Antibiotics for *H. pylori* (see Table 40-13)
　Antacids (see Table 40-21)
　Anticholinergics
　Cytoprotective drugs
Stress reduction
Acute Exacerbation without Complications
NPO
NG suction
Adequate rest
Cessation of smoking
IV fluid replacement
Drug therapy
　H_2-receptor blockers
　Proton pump inhibitors
　Antacids
　Anticholinergics
　Sedatives
Acute Exacerbation with Complications (Hemorrhage, Perforation, Obstruction)
NPO
NG suction
Bed rest
IV fluid replacement (lactated Ringer's solution)
Blood transfusions
Stomach lavage (possible)
Surgical Therapy
Perforation—simple closure with omentum graft
Gastric outlet obstruction—pyloroplasty and vagotomy
Ulcer removal/reduction
　Billroth I and II
　Vagotomy and pyloroplasty

GI, Gastrointestinal; IV, intravenous; NG, nasogastric; NPO, nothing by mouth.

TABLE 40-20 Drug Therapy
Peptic Ulcer Disease

Antisecretory
H_2-receptor blockers
　cimetidine (Tagamet)
　ranitidine (Zantac)
　famotidine (Pepcid)
　nizatidine (Axid)
Proton pump inhibitors
　omeprazole (Prilosec)
　lansoprazole (Prevacid)
　esomeprazole (Nexium)
　pantoprazole (Protonix)
Anticholinergics

Antisecretory and Cytoprotective
misoprostol (Cytotec)

Cytoprotective
sucralfate (Carafate)
bismuth subsalicylate (Pepto-Bismol)

Neutralizing
Antacids*

Antibiotics for *H. pylori*
amoxicillin
metronidazole (Flagyl)
tetracycline
clarithromycin (Biaxin)

Others
Tricyclic antidepressants
　imipramine (Tofranil)
　doxepin (Sinequan)

*See Table 40-21.

dered, and the expected benefits. Strict adherence to the prescribed regimen of drugs is important. Drug therapy includes the use of antacids, H_2R blockers, PPIs, antibiotics, antacids, anticholinergics, and cytoprotective therapy (Tables 40-19 through 40-22).

Because recurrence of peptic ulcer is frequent, interruption or discontinuation of therapy can have detrimental results. The patient must be encouraged to comply with therapy and continue with follow-up care for at least 1 year. If changes in lifestyle are part of the prescribed therapy, they should be maintained. Antacids, H_2R blockers, and PPIs may be stopped after the ulcer has healed or may be prescribed in the form of low-dose maintenance therapy. No other drugs, unless prescribed by the health care provider, should be taken because they may have an ulcerogenic effect. Finally, the patient and family should be told what to do in the event that pain and discomfort recur or blood is noted in the vomitus or stools.

Histamine-2 receptor blockers. H_2R blockers, cimetidine (Tagamet), ranitidine (Zantac), famotidine (Pepcid), and nizatidine (Axid), are frequently used in the management of peptic ulcer disease. These drugs block the action of histamine on the H_2 receptors and thus reduce HCl acid secretion. This decreases the conversion of pepsinogen to pepsin, and accelerates ulcer heal-

Smoking has an irritating effect on the mucosa, increases gastric motility, and delays mucosal healing. It should be eliminated completely or severely reduced. The combination of adequate rest and abstinence from smoking accelerates ulcer healing.

Drug Therapy. Drugs are a vital part of therapy. The patient must be well informed about each drug prescribed, why it is or-

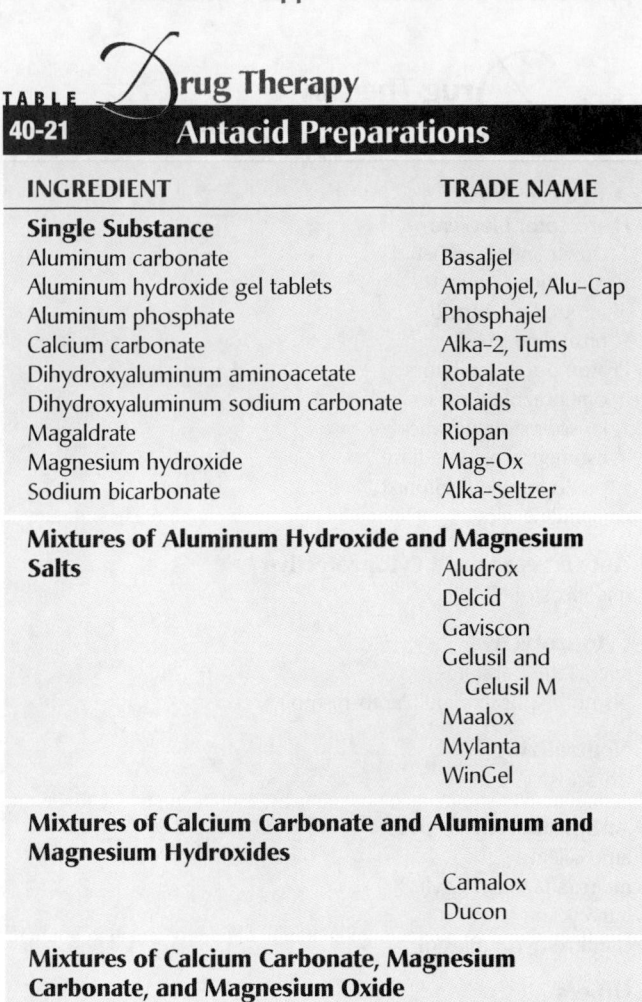

TABLE 40-21 — Drug Therapy: Antacid Preparations

INGREDIENT	TRADE NAME
Single Substance	
Aluminum carbonate	Basaljel
Aluminum hydroxide gel tablets	Amphojel, Alu-Cap
Aluminum phosphate	Phosphajel
Calcium carbonate	Alka-2, Tums
Dihydroxyaluminum aminoacetate	Robalate
Dihydroxyaluminum sodium carbonate	Rolaids
Magaldrate	Riopan
Magnesium hydroxide	Mag-Ox
Sodium bicarbonate	Alka-Seltzer
Mixtures of Aluminum Hydroxide and Magnesium Salts	Aludrox
	Delcid
	Gaviscon
	Gelusil and Gelusil M
	Maalox
	Mylanta
	WinGel
Mixtures of Calcium Carbonate and Aluminum and Magnesium Hydroxides	Camalox
	Ducon
Mixtures of Calcium Carbonate, Magnesium Carbonate, and Magnesium Oxide	Alkets

TABLE 40-22 — Drug Therapy: Side Effects of Antacid Therapy

ANTACID	REACTIONS
Aluminum hydroxide gels	Constipation, phosphorus depletion with chronic use
Calcium carbonate	Constipation or diarrhea, hypercalcemia, milk-alkali syndrome, renal calculi
Magnesium preparations	Diarrhea, hypermagnesemia
Sodium preparations	Milk-alkali syndrome if used with large amounts of calcium; used with caution in patients on sodium restrictions

ing. (Antihistamine drugs used to treat allergies are H_1R blockers and have no effect on gastric acid secretion.)

H_2R blocker drugs may be administered orally or intravenously. Depending on the specific drug, therapeutic effects last up to 12 hours. However, the onset of action (i.e., symptom relief) is longer than antacids. H_2R blockers have demonstrated capabilities in the healing of gastric and duodenal ulcers. Famotidine, ranitidine, and nizatidine have longer half-lives than cimetidine, thus requiring fewer doses and providing nocturnal HCl acid suppression. More side effects are associated with cimetidine. These include granulocytopenia, gynecomastia, diarrhea, fatigue, dizziness, rash, and mental confusion in the older adult. However, the rate of these side effects is low. Famotidine and nizatidine are considered more potent at reduced dosage levels as compared with cimetidine, and side effects are minimal. There are OTC forms of H_2R blockers currently available. Such preparations are at a lower dose than drugs that are prescribed. H_2Rs are used in combination with antibiotics to treat ulcers related to *H. pylori*.

Proton pump inhibitors. PPIs, such as omeprazole (Prilosec), lansoprazole (Prevacid), pantoprazole (Protonix), and esomeprazole (Nexium), block the ATPase enzyme that is important for the secretion of HCl acid. These agents are more effective than H_2R blockers in reducing gastric acid secretion and promoting ulcer healing. PPIs are also used in combination with antibiotics to treat ulcers caused by *H. pylori*.

Antibiotic therapy. Antibiotics to eradicate *H. pylori* infection are prescribed. The treatment of *H. pylori* is the most important element of treating ulcer disease in patients positive for *H. pylori*. When *H. pylori* is present, ulcer recurrence rates with H_2R blockers alone can be as high as 75% to 90%, whereas with antibiotic treatment the recurrence rate may be less than 10%. Antibiotic therapy for *H. pylori* is shown in Table 40-13.

Once the presence of *H. pylori* has been determined, antibiotic treatment is instituted. The regimen of choice is based on the antibiotic susceptibility of the *H. pylori* organism, patient compliance, side effects, and costs. Most drug regimens involve treatment for 7 to 14 days. No single agents have been effective in eliminating *H. pylori* (see Table 40-13). Bismuth subsalicylate (Pepto-Bismol) or bismuth combined with an H_2R (Tritec) is used as part of one therapy to facilitate healing. Bismuth is nonabsorbable and causes black stools.

Antacids. Antacids are used as adjunct therapy for peptic ulcer disease. They increase gastric pH by neutralizing the acid. As a result, the acid content of chyme reaching the duodenum is reduced. In addition, some antacids, such as aluminum hydroxide, can bind to bile salts, thus decreasing the detrimental effects of bile on the gastric mucosa. Patients who are vulnerable for physiologic stress ulcer formation may be treated prophylactically with antacids along with an antisecretory agent.

Antacids consist of systemic and nonsystemic types. Systemic antacids, such as sodium bicarbonate, are extremely soluble and are absorbed into the circulation. Their long-term use can lead to systemic alkalosis; therefore they are rarely used in ulcer treatment. The nonsystemic antacids are insoluble and poorly absorbed. The common commercial nonsystemic antacids consist of magnesium hydroxide or aluminum hydroxide as single preparations or in various combinations (see Table 40-21).

The antacid preparation may be in liquid or tablet form. A large number of tablets may be required to equal the same dose of a liquid preparation. Because the tablets are chewable, some of the drug is left coating the teeth and gingivae instead of the stomach.

The neutralizing effects of antacids taken on an empty stomach last only 20 to 30 minutes because they are quickly evacuated. When antacids are taken after meals, the effects may last as long as 3 to 4 hours. Therapy recommending frequent dosing (e.g., hourly) often results in poor compliance.

After the acute phase of bleeding has diminished, antacids are generally administered hourly, either orally or through the NG tube. If the tube is in place, the stomach contents should be aspirated and tested periodically for pH level. If pH is less than 5, intermittent suction may be used, or the frequency or dosage of the antacid may be increased.

The type and dosage of antacid prescribed depends on side effects (see Table 40-22), as well as potential drug interactions. Preparations high in sodium (e.g., Titralac) should be used with caution in older adults and in the patient with liver cirrhosis, hypertension, congestive heart failure, and renal disease. Magnesium preparations should not be prescribed for the patient with renal failure because of the risk of magnesium toxicity. The most frequent side effect experienced with magnesium antacids is diarrhea. Aluminum hydroxide causes constipation. An antacid combination of aluminum and magnesium salts seems to lessen the side effects of both.

Antacids have the capacity to interact unfavorably with some drugs. They can enhance the absorption of drugs such as dicumarol and amphetamines. The action of digitalis preparations can be potentiated when taken in combination with calcium or magnesium antacids. In some instances, antacids may decrease the absorption rates of prescribed drugs, such as tetracycline. Therefore it is important to inform the health care provider of any drugs that are being taken before antacid therapy is begun.

Anticholinergic drugs. Anticholinergic drugs are only occasionally ordered in the treatment of peptic ulcer disease. These drugs decrease cholinergic (vagal) stimulation of HCl acid. There is divided opinion concerning their efficacy in preventing recurrences and their therapeutic effectiveness in alleviating symptoms and preventing complications. Because of their tendency to decrease gastric motility, they should not be used for gastric ulcers in which stasis of secretions increases the patient's pain and discomfort. Anticholinergics are associated with a high number of side effects, such as dry mouth and skin, flushing, thirst, tachycardia, dilated pupils, blurred vision, and urine retention. Anticholinergics must be prescribed with caution in the patient with narrow-angle glaucoma, benign prostatic hyperplasia, and gastric outlet obstruction.

Cytoprotective drug therapy. Sucralfate (Carafate) is used for the short-term treatment of ulcers. It has proven to be cytoprotective of the esophagus, stomach, and duodenum. Its ability to accelerate ulcer healing is thought to be a result of the formation of an ulcer-adherent complex covering the ulcer and thereby protecting it from erosion caused by pepsin, acid, and bile salts. Sucralfate does not have acid-neutralizing capabilities. Its action is most effective at a low pH, and it should be given at least 30 minutes before or after an antacid. Adverse side effects are minimal. However, it does bind with cimetidine, digoxin, warfarin (Coumadin), phenytoin (Dilantin), and tetracycline, causing reduced bioavailability of these drugs.

Misoprostol (Cytotec) is a synthetic prostaglandin analog. It has protective and some antisecretory effects on gastric mucosa. Misoprostol is the only drug approved in the United States for the prevention of gastric ulcers induced by NSAIDs and aspirin. A major advantage of misoprostol is that it does not interfere with the therapeutic effects of aspirin and NSAIDs. Persons who require chronic NSAID therapy, such as those with osteoarthritis, may benefit from the use of misoprostol. All NSAIDs, even COX-2 inhibitors, impair ulcer healing.

Other drugs. Tricyclic antidepressants (e.g., imipramine [Tofranil], doxepin [Sinequan]) and serotonin reuptake inhibitors may be prescribed for patients with ulcer disease. Antidepressants may contribute to overall pain relief through their effects on afferent pain fiber transmission. In addition, tricyclic antidepressants have, to varying degrees, some anticholinergic properties, which results in reduced acid secretion.

Nutritional Therapy. Dietary modifications may be necessary so that foods and beverages irritating to the patient can be avoided or eliminated. A nonirritating or bland diet consisting of six small meals a day may be recommended for the patient during the symptomatic phase. However, there is considerable controversy over the actual therapeutic benefits derived from a bland diet because the rationale is not supported by scientific evidence. Each patient should be instructed to eat and drink foods and fluids that do not cause any distressing symptoms. Alcohol and caffeine-containing products should be eliminated because of their irritating effects.

Dietary instructions should include a sample diet with a list of foods that usually cause distress and should therefore be eliminated from the diet. Foods known to irritate the gastric mucosa include hot, spicy foods and pepper, alcohol, carbonated beverages, tea, coffee, and broth (meat extract). These foods also have limited buffering ability in addition to stimulating gastric acid secretion. Foods high in roughage, such as raw fruit, salads, and vegetables, may irritate an inflamed mucosa. If these foods are well chewed, this seems to be less of a problem.

Protein is considered the best neutralizing food, but it also stimulates gastric secretions. Carbohydrates and fats are the least stimulating to HCl acid secretion, but they do not neutralize well. The patient must determine a suitable combination of these essential nutrients without causing undue distress.

Historically, milk was an essential part of ulcer therapy until it was learned that milk proteins and calcium stimulate gastric acid production. For this reason, milk as part of diet therapy for ulcers was out of favor for a time. However, milk is again used as part of the diet plan because it can neutralize gastric acidity and contains prostaglandins and growth factors, both of which may protect the GI mucosa from injury.

Therapy Related to Complications of Peptic Ulcer Disease

Acute exacerbation. The patient with an acute exacerbation of peptic ulcer can usually be treated with the same regimen used for conservative therapy. However, the situation is considered more serious because of the possible complications of perforation, hemorrhage, and gastric outlet obstruction.

An acute exacerbation is frequently accompanied by bleeding, increased pain and discomfort, and nausea and vomiting. If the patient experiences recurrent vomiting or gastric outlet obstruction, an NG tube is placed into the stomach with intermittent suction for about 24 to 48 hours.

If there is a history of an incompetent pyloric sphincter allowing reflux of duodenal contents into the stomach, an NG tube will remove intestinal contents from the stomach. This period of stomach rest eliminates any causative factors that may have precipitated the acute exacerbation and permits the resolution of edema and inflammation of the mucosa. Fluids and electrolytes are replaced by IV infusion until the patient is able to tolerate oral feedings without distress.

Management is similar to that described for upper GI bleeding. Blood or blood products may be administered. Careful monitoring of the vital signs, intake and output, laboratory studies, and signs of impending shock are important during this acute episode.

Endoscopic evaluation is performed to reveal the degree of inflammation or bleeding, as well as the ulcer location. It is important to ascertain the presence of a prepyloric or pyloric ulcer that can cause gastric outlet obstruction. When endoscopic examination reveals no major problems and the patient's physical condition stabilizes, the plan of care for the patient should follow the same regimen of diet, activity, and drugs used in conservative therapy. A 5-year follow-up program is recommended after acute exacerbation. An increase in the healing rate is achieved after conservative treatment, but the treatment plan cannot prevent the scar formation that can result in gastric outlet obstruction.

Perforation. The immediate focus of management of a patient with a perforation is to stop the spillage of gastric or duodenal contents into the peritoneal cavity and restore blood volume. An NG tube is inserted into the stomach to provide continuous aspiration and gastric decompression to halt spillage through the perforation. Although duodenal aspiration is not achieved as promptly, placement of the tube as near to the perforation site as possible facilitates decompression.

Circulating blood volume must be replaced with lactated Ringer's and albumin solutions. These solutions substitute for the fluids lost from the vascular and interstitial space as the peritonitis develops. Blood replacement in the form of packed RBCs may be necessary. Unless contraindicated, a central venous pressure line and an indwelling urinary catheter should be inserted and monitored hourly. The patient with a history of cardiac disease requires ECG monitoring or placement of a pulmonary artery catheter for more accurate assessment of left ventricular function. Broad-spectrum antibiotic therapy should be started immediately to treat bacterial peritonitis. Administration of pain medications provides comfort.

The operative procedure involving the least risk to the patient is simple oversewing of the perforation and reinforcement of the area with a graft of omentum. The excess gastric contents are suctioned from the peritoneal cavity during the surgical procedure. There is controversy regarding the need for more definitive surgical treatment of a perforated ulcer than can be achieved with simple closure. Other types of surgical procedures depend on the location of the peptic ulcer and the surgeon's preference. If cure of the ulcer is the ultimate goal, the surgical procedures may include gastric resection or vagotomy and pyloroplasty.

Gastric outlet obstruction. The aim of therapy for obstruction is to decompress the stomach, correct any existing fluid and electrolyte imbalances, and improve the patient's general state of health. An NG tube is inserted into the stomach and attached to continuous suction to remove excess fluids and undigested food particles. With continuous decompression for several days, the stomach has the opportunity to regain its normal muscle tone, the ulcer can begin healing, and the inflammation and edema will subside.

The tube is clamped after several days of suction, and gastric residue is measured periodically. The frequency and amount of time the tube remains clamped are proportional to the amount of aspirate obtained and the comfort level of the patient. A method commonly followed is to clamp the tube overnight for approximately 8 to 12 hours and to measure the gastric residue in the morning. When the aspirate falls below 200 ml, it is considered

to be within a normal range and the patient can begin oral intake of clear liquids. Initially, oral fluids are begun at 30 ml per hour and then gradually increased in amount. The patient must be watched carefully for signs of distress or vomiting. As the amount of gastric residue decreases, solid foods are added and the tube is removed.

IV fluids and electrolytes are administered according to the degree of dehydration, vomiting, and electrolyte imbalance indicated by laboratory studies. Pain relief results from the decompression measures, and analgesics are usually not necessary. Antacids and antisecretory drug therapy (i.e., H_2R blockers, PPIs) are an integral part of treatment if the obstruction has been determined on endoscopic examination to be the result of an active ulcer. Pyloric obstruction may be treated nonsurgically by balloon dilations performed through the endoscope. Surgical intervention may be necessary to remove scar tissue.

NURSING MANAGEMENT
PEPTIC ULCER DISEASE

■ Nursing Assessment

Subjective and objective data that should be obtained from a patient with peptic ulcer disease are presented in Table 40-23.

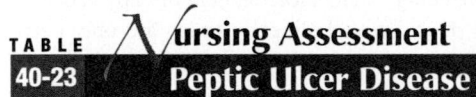

TABLE 40-23	Nursing Assessment — Peptic Ulcer Disease

Subjective Data
Important Health Information
Past health history: Chronic renal failure, pancreatic disease, chronic obstructive pulmonary disease, serious illness or trauma, hyperparathyroidism, cirrhosis of the liver, Zollinger-Ellison syndrome
Medications: Use of aspirin, corticosteroids, nonsteroidal anti-inflammatory drugs
Surgery or other treatments: Complicated or prolonged surgery
Functional Health Patterns
Health perception–health management: Chronic alcohol abuse, smoking, caffeine use; family history of peptic ulcer disease
Nutritional-metabolic: Weight loss, anorexia; nausea and vomiting, hematemesis; dyspepsia, heartburn, belching
Elimination: Black, tarry stools
Cognitive–perceptual: Duodenal ulcers—burning, midepigastric or back pain occurring 2 to 4 hours after meals and relieved by food; nocturnal pain common; Gastric ulcers—high epigastric pain occurring 1 to 2 hours after meals; pain may be precipitated or aggravated by food
Coping-stress tolerance: Acute or chronic stress

Objective Data
General
Anxiety, irritability
Gastrointestinal
Epigastric tenderness
Possible Findings
Anemia; guaiac-positive stools; gastric analysis indicating high gastric acid secretion; positive blood, urine, breath, or stool tests for *H. pylori*; abnormal upper gastrointestinal endoscopic and barium studies

■ Nursing Diagnoses

Nursing diagnoses related to peptic ulcer disease may include, but are not limited to, those presented in NCP 40-2.

■ Planning

Overall goals are that the patient with peptic ulcer disease will (1) comply with the prescribed therapeutic regimen, (2) experience a reduction or absence of discomfort related to peptic ulcer disease, (3) exhibit no signs of GI complications related to the ulcerative process, (4) have complete healing of the peptic ulcer, and (5) make appropriate lifestyle changes to prevent recurrence.

■ Nursing Implementation

Health Promotion. Nurses need to be involved in identifying patients at risk for ulcer development. Early detection and treatment of ulcers are important aspects of reducing morbidity associated with ulcers. Patients who are taking ulcerogenic drugs such as aspirin and NSAIDs are at risk for ulcer development. Patients need to be encouraged to take these drugs with food or milk. Patients should be taught to report symptoms related to gastric irritation, including epigastric pain, to their health care provider.

Acute Intervention. During the acute exacerbation of an ulcer, the patient generally complains of increased pain and nausea and vomiting, and some may have evidence of bleeding. Initially many patients attempt to cope with the symptoms at home before seeking medical assistance.

During this acute phase the patient may be maintained on NPO status for a few days, have an NG tube inserted and connected to intermittent suction, and have fluids replaced intravenously. The rationale for this therapy must be conveyed to the anxious patient and family. They must understand that the advantages far outweigh any temporary discomfort imposed by the presence of the tube. Regular mouth care alleviates the dry mouth. Cleansing and lubrication of the nares facilitate breathing and decrease soreness. Gastric contents may be analyzed for pH, blood, bile, or other irritating substances. When the stomach is kept empty of gastric secretions, the ulcer pain diminishes and ulcer healing begins. Usually this form of intervention is effective.

Because the patient is on NPO status, IV fluids are ordered. The type and amount administered are directly related to the fluid lost; the manifestations exhibited by the patient; and the results of the hemoglobin, hematocrit, and electrolyte determinations. The nurse should be aware of any other current health problem that could be adversely affected by the type of fluid used or the rate of the infusion. Repeated monitoring of these parameters provides information on the hydration status and the effectiveness of treatment. Vital signs are initially taken at least hourly so that shock can be detected and treated.

Physical and emotional rest are conducive to ulcer healing. The patient's immediate environment should be quiet and restful. The use of a mild sedative or tranquilizer has beneficial effects when the patient is anxious and apprehensive. The nurse must use good judgment before sedating a person who is becoming increasingly restless. There is danger that the drug will mask the signs of shock secondary to upper GI bleeding.

If the patient's condition improves without progression of symptoms (e.g., increased pain, vomiting, and hemorrhage), the regimen outlined for conservative therapy is followed. However, complications such as hemorrhage, perforation, and obstruction can occur.

Hemorrhage. Changes in the vital signs and an increase in the amount and redness of the aspirate often signal massive upper GI bleeding. When there is an increased amount of blood in the gastric contents, the patient's pain is often decreased because the blood helps to neutralize the acidic gastric contents. It is important to maintain the patency of the NG tube so that blood clots do not obstruct the tube. If the tube becomes blocked, the patient can develop abdominal distention. Similar interventions to those described for upper GI bleeding on pp. 1025-1026 are used. The nurse needs to monitor the results of the hemoglobin and hematocrit determinations.

Perforation. When there is sudden, severe abdominal pain unrelated in intensity and location to the pain that brought the patient to the hospital, the nurse must recognize the possibility of ulcer perforation. When any person with an ulcer, particularly a chronic duodenal ulcer, demonstrates these manifestations, perforation should be suspected and the health care provider notified immediately.

Perforation is indicated by a rigid, boardlike abdomen; severe generalized abdominal and shoulder pain; drawing up of the knees; and shallow, grunting respirations. The bowel sounds that may have been previously normal or hyperactive may diminish and become absent.

Vital signs are important parameters and should be promptly taken and recorded every 15 to 30 minutes. The nurse should temporarily stop all oral or NG drugs and feedings until the health care provider can be notified and a definitive diagnosis made. If perforation does exist, anything taken internally can add to the spillage into the peritoneal cavity and increase discomfort. If IV fluids are being administered at the time of the perforation, the rate should be maintained or increased to replace the depleted plasma volume.

When perforation is confirmed, the nurse should ensure that any known patient allergies have been recorded on the chart. This is important because antibiotic therapy is usually started, and careful observation for allergic reactions must be made. When the perforation fails to seal spontaneously, surgical closure is necessary and is performed as soon as possible. There is often little time to prepare the patient and family thoroughly for the surgical intervention, yet some instructions can be carried out while the immediate therapy is begun. If major reconstructive surgery is anticipated, the patient and family may question the need when the problem is only a small hole.

Gastric outlet obstruction. Gastric outlet obstruction can occur at any time and is most likely to occur in the patient whose ulcer is located close to the pylorus. Because the onset of symptoms is usually gradual, the condition is not generally as serious an emergency as hemorrhage or perforation. Relief of symptoms may be achieved by constant NG aspiration of stomach contents. This allows edema and inflammation to subside and then permits normal flow of gastric contents through the pylorus.

Obstruction can also occur during the treatment of an acute episode of peptic ulcer exacerbation. If these symptoms are experienced while the patient is still on NPO status, the patency of the NG tube should be suspected. Regular irrigation of the tube with a saline solution facilitates proper functioning. It may be helpful to reposition the patient from side to side so that the tube tip is not constantly lying against the mucosal surface.

NURSING CARE PLAN 40-2

Patient with Peptic Ulcer Disease

EXPECTED PATIENT OUTCOMES	NURSING INTERVENTIONS and *RATIONALES*

CONSERVATIVE MANAGEMENT

NURSING DIAGNOSIS   **Acute pain** *related to* increased gastric secretions, decreased mucosal protection, and ingestion of gastric irritants *as manifested by* burning cramplike pain in epigastrium and abdomen; pain onset 1 to 2 hr after meals with gastric ulcer; pain onset 2 to 4 hr after meals (midmorning, midafternoon) and middle of night with duodenal ulcer.

- Verbalization of satisfaction with pain control

- Determine pain characteristics from verbal description and physical assessment data *so that appropriate interventions can be planned.*
- Administer antacids, H_2-receptor blockers, proton pump inhibitors, anticholinergics, and cytoprotective agents as ordered *to reduce pain.*
- Teach patient to avoid smoking and ingesting spicy, hot or cold foods, coffee, tea and cola drinks, and alcoholic beverages *to prevent irritation and increasing acid production.*
- Teach patient stress reduction *as relaxation results in decreased acid production and reduction in pain.*

NURSING DIAGNOSIS   **Ineffective therapeutic regimen management** *related to* lack of knowledge of long-term management of peptic ulcer disease and consequences of not following treatment plan and unwillingness to modify lifestyle *as manifested by* frequent questions about home care, incorrect responses to questions about peptic ulcer disease, noncompliance with medical regimen.

- Verbalization of plan to modify lifestyle and incorporate therapeutic regimen into lifestyle

- Explain peptic ulcer disease process at patient's level *to foster understanding.*
- Help patient identify stressors and initiate modifications in daily routine *as stress causes hypersecretion of HCl acid and pepsin, which can alter the mucosal barrier.*
- Discuss diet plan and assist with implementation at home and in work setting.
- Explain rationale for the elimination of alcohol, spicy foods, coffee, tea, and colas from diet; explain the harmful effects of smoking *as these agents increase acid production and directly irritate gastric mucosa.*
- Provide information on actions and side effects of drug therapy *to ensure safe self-administration.*
- Inform patient what to do if symptoms related to ulcers recur *to ensure early initiation of treatment.*

EXACERBATION MANAGEMENT

NURSING DIAGNOSIS   **Acute pain** *related to* exacerbation of disease process and inadequate comfort measures *as manifested by* verbalization of increase in pain, nonverbal indicators of pain (e.g., moaning, crying, doubling up).

- Expression of satisfaction with pain management

- Encourage bed rest or light activity *to conserve energy and promote comfort.*
- Provide quiet, relaxed environment and limit visitors *to decrease stress and other factors that increase acid secretion.*
- Administer medications as ordered *to relieve pain.*

NURSING DIAGNOSIS   **Nausea** *related to* acute exacerbation of disease process *as manifested by* episodes of nausea and/or vomiting (See NCP 40-1).

When oral feedings have been resumed and symptoms of obstruction are observed, the health care provider should be promptly informed. Generally, all that is necessary to treat the problem is to resume gastric aspiration so that the edema and inflammation resulting from the acute episode have time to resolve. IV fluids with electrolyte replacement keep the patient hydrated during this period. The NG tube can be clamped and gastric fluids can be aspirated to check for retention. It is important to maintain accurate intake and output records, especially of the gastric aspirate. The patient should be kept aware of why these symptoms are being experienced. In some instances in which treatment is not successful, surgery may be performed after the acute phase has passed.

Ambulatory and Home Care. The patient in whom peptic ulcer disease has been diagnosed has specific needs that must be met to prevent and avoid recurrence or complications. General instructions should cover aspects of the disease process itself, drugs, possible changes in lifestyle (including diet), and regular follow-up care. Table 40-24 provides a patient and family teaching guide for the patient with peptic ulcer disease.

Knowing the cause of the ulcer and understanding the disease process may motivate the patient to become more involved in care and increase compliance with therapy. The patient must understand the dietary modifications and why they are important for recovery and health maintenance. The nurse and the dietitian should elicit a dietary history from the patient and plan for ways that dietary modifications can be easily incorporated into the patient's home and work setting. The patient who is following a diet prescribed for another illness needs to know how to balance the two so that neither condition is harmed by dietary interventions.

NURSING CARE PLAN 40-2

Patient with Peptic Ulcer Disease—cont'd

COLLABORATIVE PROBLEMS

NURSING GOALS	NURSING INTERVENTIONS AND RATIONALES
POTENTIAL COMPLICATION	**Hemorrhage** secondary to eroded mucosal tissue.
▪ Monitor for signs of hemorrhage ▪ Carry out medical and nursing interventions if hemorrhage occurs	▪ Assess for evidence of hematemesis, bright red or melena stool, abdominal pain or discomfort, symptoms of shock (e.g., decreased blood pressure; cool, clammy skin; dyspnea; tachycardia; decreased urine output) *to plan appropriate interventions.* ▪ If ulcer is actively bleeding, observe NG tube aspirate or emesis for amount and color *to assess degree of bleeding.* ▪ Take vital signs every 15 to 30 minutes *to determine patient's hemodynamic status and as indicators of shock.* ▪ Maintain IV infusion line *to provide ready access for blood and fluid replacement.* ▪ If RBC transfusion is given, observe for transfusion reaction *so that appropriate actions can be taken immediately.* ▪ Monitor hematocrit and hemoglobin *as indicators of severity of hemorrhage and need for fluid and blood replacement.* ▪ Record intake and output *to monitor fluid balance.* ▪ Reassure patient and family to decrease their anxiety. ▪ Remain calm and confident in plan of care *to foster calm and confidence in patient and family.* ▪ Prepare patient for possible endoscopy or surgery.
POTENTIAL COMPLICATION	**Perforation of GI mucosa** secondary to impaired mucosal tissue integrity.
▪ Monitor for signs of perforation ▪ Carry out appropriate medical and nursing interventions	▪ Observe for manifestations of perforation (e.g., sudden, severe abdominal pain; rigid, boardlike abdomen; radiating pain to shoulders; increasing distention; decreasing bowel sounds) *to ensure early recognition and intervention.* ▪ Take vital signs every 15 to 30 minutes *to determine patient's hemodynamic status and as indicators of shock.* ▪ Maintain NG tube to suction *to provide continuous aspiration and gastric decompression to prevent further leakage of gastric fluid through the perforation.* ▪ Administer pain medication *to promote comfort and reduce anxiety.* ▪ Prepare patient for emergency diagnostic tests and possible surgery *to foster timely intervention.*

The patient does not always give the health care provider accurate information regarding habitual use of alcohol or cigarettes. The nurse should provide useful information about the detrimental effects of alcohol and cigarettes on ulcer disease and ulcer healing.

The nurse should teach the patient about prescribed drugs, including their actions, side effects, and inherent dangers if omitted for any reason. The patient should know why OTC drugs (e.g., aspirin) should not be taken unless approved by the health care provider. Because antacids and some H₂R blockers may be bought without a prescription, the patient must be informed that interchanging brands without checking with the health care provider or nurse can lead to harmful side effects.

Efforts should be made to obtain more information about the patient's psychosocial status. Knowledge of lifestyle, occupation, and coping behaviors can be helpful to the plan of care. The patient may be reluctant to talk about personal subjects, the stress experienced at home or on the job, the usual methods of coping, or dependence on drugs or alcohol. Unfortunately, the patient does not often see the relationship between lifestyle or occupation and ulcer disease. It is important to listen for subtle clues

from the patient's statements and to observe for behaviors that broaden this database.

The need for long-term follow-up care must be stressed. Because successful treatment is frequently followed by a recurrence of the ulcer disease, the patient should be encouraged to seek immediate intervention if symptoms of the disease come back. The patient who has recurrence of ulcer disease following initial healing must learn to live with a disease that is chronic. The patient may be angry and frustrated, especially if the prescribed mode of therapy has been faithfully followed yet has failed to prevent the recurrence or extension of the disease process.

Unfortunately, many patients do not comply with the plan of care originally designed, and they experience repeated exacerbations. Patients quickly learn that they often experience no discomfort when they omit prescribed drugs or indulge in occasional dietary indiscretions. Consequently, they make no or little alteration in lifestyle. After an acute exacerbation the patient is often more amenable to following the plan of care and open to suggestions for changes in lifestyle. Changes, such as smoking cessation and alcohol abstinence, are difficult for many people and may be met with resistance. The patient may fare better from

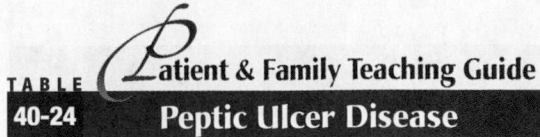

TABLE 40-24   Patient & Family Teaching Guide

Peptic Ulcer Disease

The following are teaching guidelines for the patient and family:

1. Explain dietary modifications, including avoidance of foods that cause epigastric distress. This may include black pepper, spicy foods, and acidic foods. Small frequent meals are better tolerated than large meals.
2. Explain the rationale for avoiding cigarettes. In addition to promoting ulcer development, smoking will delay ulcer healing.
3. Encourage the need to reduce or eliminate alcohol ingestion.
4. Explain the rationale for avoiding OTC drugs unless approved by the patient's care provider. Many preparations contain ingredients, such as aspirin, that should not be taken unless approved by the health care provider. Check with the care provider regarding the use of nonsteroidal antiinflammatory drugs.
5. Explain the rationale for not interchanging brands of antacids and H_2-receptor blockers that can be purchased OTC without checking with the health care provider. This can lead to harmful side effects.
6. Teach the need to take all medications as prescribed. This includes both antisecretory and antibiotic drugs. Failure to take medications as prescribed can result in relapse.
7. Explain the importance of reporting any of the following:
   - Increased nausea and/or vomiting
   - Increase in epigastric pain
   - Bloody emesis or tarry stools
8. Explain the relationship between symptoms and stress. Stress-reducing activities or relaxation strategies are encouraged.
9. Encourage patient and family to share concerns about lifestyle changes and living with a chronic illness.

OTC, Over-the-counter.

a reduction in his or her use of these substances rather than from total elimination. Although alcohol and smoking are known to interfere with ulcer healing, they frequently serve as coping mechanisms. From the patient's point of view, the distress caused by their total elimination may outweigh the benefits to be gained from abstention. The goal, however, should always be total cessation. A patient with chronic ulcers must be aware of the complications that may result from the disease, the clinical manifestations indicating their presence, and what to do until the health care provider can be seen.

■ Evaluation

Expected outcomes for the patient with a peptic ulcer disease are addressed in NCP 40-2.

Collaborative Therapy: Surgical Therapy for Peptic Ulcer Disease

Less than 20% of patients with ulcers need surgical intervention. Because there is a high recurrence rate for both duodenal and gastric ulcers and complications increase with the duration of the ulcer, many health care providers believe that surgery is

necessary after therapy has been tried and has proven unsuccessful. The following criteria are used as general indications for surgical intervention:

- Intractability: failure of the ulcer to heal or recurrence of the ulcer after therapy
- History of hemorrhage or increased risk of bleeding during treatment
- Prepyloric or pyloric ulcers (both have high recurrence rates)
- Concurrent condition, such as severe burns, trauma, or sepsis
- Multiple ulcer sites
- Drug-induced ulcers, especially when withdrawal from the drug may put the person at risk
- Possible existence of a malignant ulcer
- Obstruction

A variety of surgical procedures are used to treat ulcer disease. They usually involve a partial gastrectomy, vagotomy, or pyloroplasty. Partial gastrectomy with removal of the distal two thirds of the stomach and anastomosis of the gastric stump to the duodenum is called a *gastroduodenostomy* or *Billroth I* operation (Fig. 40-16). Partial gastrectomy with removal of the distal two thirds of the stomach and anastomosis of the gastric stump to the jejunum is called a *gastrojejunostomy* or *Billroth II* operation. In both procedures the antrum and the pylorus are removed. Because the duodenum is bypassed, the Billroth II operation is the preferred surgical procedure to prevent recurrence of duodenal ulcers.

Vagotomy is the severing of the vagus nerve, either totally (truncal) or selectively at some point in its innervation to the stomach. In a truncal vagotomy both the anterior and posterior trunks are severed. *Selective vagotomy* consists of cutting the nerve at a particular branch of the vagus nerve, resulting in denervation of only a portion of the stomach, such as the antrum or the parietal cell mass.

Pyloroplasty consists of surgical enlargement of the pyloric sphincter to facilitate the easy passage of contents from the stomach. It is most commonly done after vagotomy or to enlarge an opening that has been constricted from scar tissue. A vagotomy decreases gastric motility and, subsequently, gastric emptying. A pyloroplasty accompanying vagotomy increases gastric emptying.

The combination of a Billroth I or II procedure with vagotomy has the advantage of eliminating the ulcer and the stimulus for acid secretion. Surgical removal of the antrum results in removal of the source of gastrin secretion. (Gastrin normally stimulates parietal and chief cells.) Vagotomy eliminates the stimulus of HCl acid and gastrin hormone secretion caused by vagal stimulation.

Postoperative Complications. The most common postoperative complications from peptic ulcer surgery are (1) dumping syndrome, (2) postprandial hypoglycemia, and (3) bile reflux gastritis.

Dumping syndrome. *Dumping syndrome* is the direct result of surgical removal of a large portion of the stomach and the pyloric sphincter. These changes drastically reduce the reservoir capacity of the stomach. Although dumping syndrome is more commonly experienced after a Billroth II procedure, it can occur after any gastric reconstruction and vagotomy.

Dumping syndrome is associated with meals having a hyperosmolar composition. Normally, gastric chyme enters the small intestine in small amounts, and shifts in fluid from the extracellular space are minimal. After surgery, however, the stomach no longer has control over the amount of gastric chyme entering the

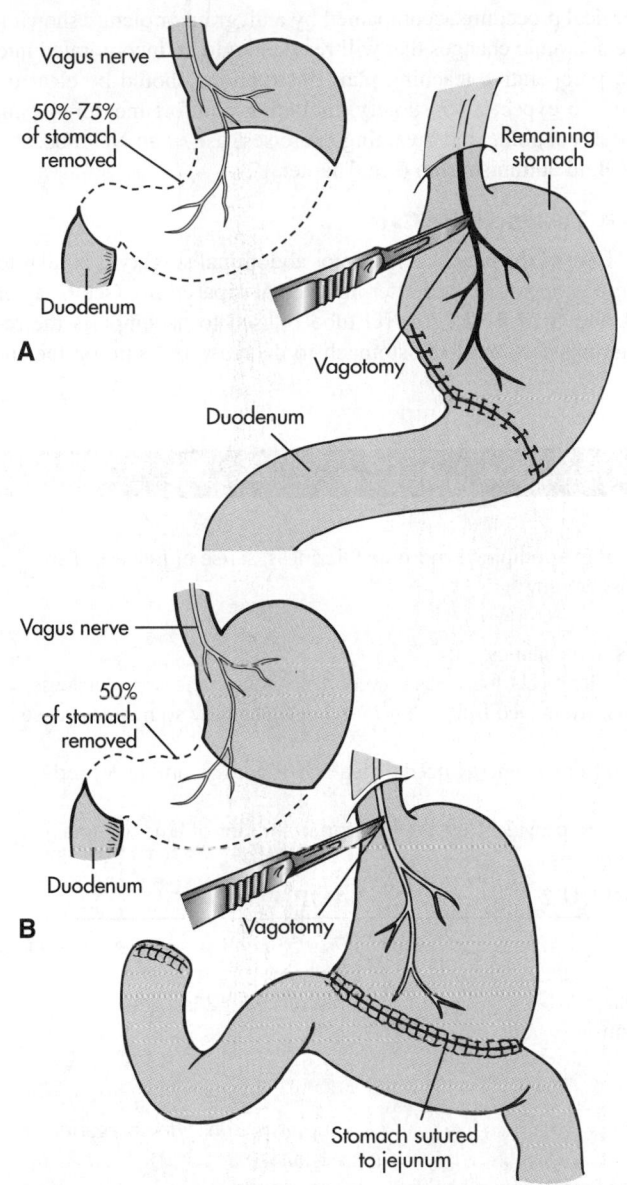

FIG. 40-16 A, Billroth I procedure (subtotal gastric resection with gastroduodenostomy anastomosis). B, Billroth II procedure (subtotal gastric resection with gastrojejunostomy anastomosis).

small intestine. Consequently, a large bolus of hypertonic fluid enters the intestine and results in fluid being drawn into the bowel lumen. This creates a decrease in plasma volume. A secondary consequence of this fluid shift is distention of the bowel lumen, which stimulates intestinal motility and the urge to defecate.

Approximately one third to one half of patients experience dumping syndrome after peptic ulcer surgery. The onset of symptoms occurs at the end of a meal or within 15 to 30 minutes after eating. The patient usually describes feelings of generalized weakness, sweating, palpitations, and dizziness. These symptoms are attributed to the sudden decrease in plasma volume. The patient complains of abdominal cramps, borborygmi (audible abdominal sounds produced by hyperactive intestinal peristalsis), and the urge to defecate. These manifestations usually last for no longer than an hour after meals.

Postprandial hypoglycemia. *Postprandial hypoglycemia* is considered a variant of the dumping syndrome because it is the result of uncontrolled gastric emptying of a bolus of fluid high in carbohydrate into the small intestine. The bolus of concentrated carbohydrate results in hyperglycemia and the release of excessive amounts of insulin into the circulation. A secondary hypoglycemia then occurs, with symptoms appearing about 2 hours after meals. The symptoms experienced are the ones observed in any hypoglycemic reaction and include sweating, weakness, mental confusion, palpitations, tachycardia, and anxiety.

Bile reflux gastritis. Gastric surgery that involves the pylorus, either reconstruction or removal, can result in reflux alkaline gastritis. Prolonged contact of bile, especially bile salts, causes damage to the gastric mucosa. Chronic gastritis of this form may result in the back diffusion of hydrogen ions through the gastric mucosa. Paradoxically, peptic ulcer may recur after surgical treatment that was intended as a cure.

The symptoms associated with reflux alkaline gastritis are continuous epigastric distress that increases after meals. Vomiting relieves the distress but only temporarily. The administration of cholestyramine (Questran), either before or with meals, has met with success. Cholestyramine binds with the bile salts that are the source of irritation in this condition. Aluminum hydroxide antacids have also been used in the treatment of this condition.

Nutritional Therapy. Discharge planning and instruction should be started as soon as the immediate postoperative period is successfully passed. Dietary instructions may be given by the dietitian and reinforced by the nursing staff. Because the stomach's reservoir has been greatly diminished after gastric resection, the meal size must be reduced accordingly. The patient should be advised to eliminate drinking fluids with meals. Dry foods with a low-carbohydrate content and moderate protein and fat content are better tolerated initially. These dietary changes, with the incorporation of a short rest period after each meal, reduce the likelihood of dumping syndrome. Reassurance that following these dietary measures will result in cessation of these symptoms within a few months is essential to long-term compliance.

Postprandial hypoglycemic reaction can be avoided if these dietary instructions are followed. The immediate ingestion of sugared fluids or candy relieves the hypoglycemic symptoms. The treatment of this type of hypoglycemia is similar to that of dumping syndrome. To avoid similar occurrences the patient should be instructed to limit the amount of sugar consumed with each meal and to eat small, frequent meals with moderate amounts of protein and fat. Although only a small percentage of patients experience bile reflux gastritis, the patient must be cautioned to notify the health care provider of any continuous epigastric distress after meals that is similar to that felt before surgery.

With regard to dumping syndrome, the symptoms are self-limiting and often disappear within several months to a year after surgery. Interventions prescribed for the patient are diet instruction, rest, and reassurance. The diet should consist of small dry feedings daily that are low in carbohydrate, are restricted in refined sugars, and contain moderate amounts of protein and fat. Sample menu plans are presented in Table 40-25. Fluids should be taken between meals but not with the meal, and the patient should plan rest periods of at least 30 minutes after each meal. The recumbent position is the most beneficial if the patient can arrange it. Reassuring the patient that the unpleasant symptoms are usually of short duration is helpful in gaining cooperation. A small percentage of patients experience long-term problems and may require further reconstructive surgery.

NURSING MANAGEMENT
SURGICAL THERAPY FOR PEPTIC ULCER DISEASE

■ Preoperative Care

When surgery is planned with the goal of curing the ulcer disease, the surgeon should provide necessary information about the procedure and the expected outcome so that the patient can make an informed decision. The nurse can help the patient and family by clarifying and interpreting their questions. A discussion of the surgical procedure accompanied by a diagram or picture showing the anatomic changes that will result should be incorporated into the preoperative teaching plan. Instructions should be clear on what to expect after surgery, including comfort measures, pain relief, coughing and breathing exercises, use of an NG tube, and IV fluid administration (see Chapter 17).

■ Postoperative Care

Care of the patient after major abdominal surgery is similar to the postoperative care after abdominal laparotomy (see Chapter 41 and NCP 41-2). An NG tube is used to decompress the remaining portion of the stomach to decrease pressure on the su-

TABLE 40-25 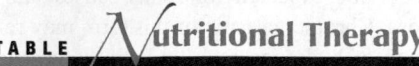 **Nutritional Therapy**
Postgastrectomy Dumping Syndrome

Purpose
To slow the rapid passage of food into the intestine; to control symptoms of the dumping syndrome (dizziness, sense of fullness, diarrhea, tachycardia), which sometimes occur following a partial or total gastrectomy

Diet Principles
1. Meals are divided into six small feedings to avoid overloading intestines at mealtimes.
2. Fluids should not be taken with meals but at least 30–45 minutes before or after meals; this helps prevent distention or a feeling of fullness.
3. Concentrated sweets (e.g., honey, sugar, jelly, jam, candies, sweet pastries, sweetened fruit) are avoided because they sometimes cause dizziness, diarrhea, and a sense of fullness.
4. Protein and fats are increased to promote rebuilding of body tissues and to meet energy needs. Meat, cheese, eggs, and milk products are specific foods to increase in the diet.
5. Amount of time these restrictions should be followed varies. The health care provider decides the proper amount of time to remain on this prescribed diet according to the patient's clinical condition and progress.

EXCHANGES	SAMPLE MENU 1	SAMPLE MENU 2	SAMPLE MENU 3
Breakfast			
1 meat	1 poached egg	1 fried egg	1 oz ham
1 starch	1 slice toast	1 corn tortilla	2 biscuits with 2 tsp gravy
Fat	2 sausage	2 slices bacon	
	Margarine	Margarine	
10 AM snack			
1 starch	¾ cup dry cereal	½ cup atole	½ cup grits with 2 tbs margarine
½ cup milk	½ cup milk	½ cup milk	added
1 fruit	½ fresh banana	2 unsweetened canned peach halves	⅓ cantaloupe
	Sugar substitute	Sugar substitute	½ cup buttermilk
Lunch			
2 meat	Grilled cheese sandwich with 2 oz	1 burrito with 1 oz meat, 1 oz	2 oz fried fish
2 starch	cheese, lettuce	cheese, ½ cup pinto beans,	½ cup buttered rice
1 vegetable	2 unsweetened pear halves	1 flour tortilla	½ cup mustard greens
1 fruit		½ diet gelatin dessert with fruit	1 fresh apple
Fat		cocktail added	1 slice bread
2 PM snack			
1 meat or substitute	½ cup plain yogurt	½ cup cottage cheese	2 tsp peanut butter
1 starch	2 graham crackers	5 soda crackers	1 slice bread
Dinner			
2 meat	2 oz tomato meatloaf	2 tamales	2 oz fried pork chop
1 starch	½ cup mashed potatoes with	½ cup buttered corn	½ cup black-eyed peas
Vegetable	gravy	1 fresh orange	½ cup buttered carrots
1 fruit	½ cup buttered green beans		1 fresh plum
Fat	½ cup unsweetened apple sauce		
8 PM snack			
1 meat	½ sandwich with 1 slice bread,	1 corn tortilla with 1 oz melted	½ sandwich with 1 slice bread,
1 starch	1 oz roast beef, lettuce,	cheese and green chili	1 slice salami, lettuce,
Vegetable	mayonnaise		mayonnaise
Fat			

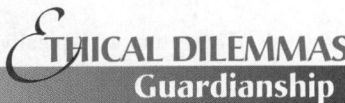

ture line and to allow for resolution of edema and inflammation resulting from surgical trauma.

The gastric aspirate must be carefully observed for color, amount, and odor during the immediate postoperative period. The color of the aspirate is expected to be bright red at first, with a gradual darkening within the first 24 hours after surgery. Normally the color changes to yellow-green within 36 to 48 hours. If the tube becomes clogged during this period, the health care provider may order periodic gentle irrigations with normal saline solution. It is essential that the NG suction is working and that the tube remains patent so that accumulated gastric secretions do not put a strain on the anastomosis. This can lead to distention of the remaining portion of the stomach and result in (1) rupture of the sutures, (2) leakage of gastric contents into the peritoneal cavity, (3) hemorrhage, and (4) possible abscess formation. If the

tube must be replaced or repositioned, the health care provider must be called to perform this task because of the danger of perforating the gastric mucosa or disrupting the suture line.

The nurse observes the patient for signs of decreased peristalsis and lower abdominal discomfort that may indicate impending intestinal obstruction. Accurate intake and output records must be kept. Vital signs are monitored and recorded every 4 hours.

The patient is kept comfortable and free of pain by the administration of the prescribed drugs and by frequent changes in position. The incision is relatively high in the epigastrium and may interfere with deep-breathing and coughing measures. Splinting the area with a pillow while gently and persistently encouraging the patient to put forth the best efforts possible helps prevent pulmonary complications. Splinting also protects the abdominal suture line from rupturing during coughing. The dressing must be observed for signs of bleeding or odor and drainage indicative of an infection. Ambulation is encouraged and is increased daily.

While the NG tube is connected to suction, IV therapy is maintained. Potassium and vitamin supplements are added to the infusion until oral feedings are resumed. Before the NG tube is removed, the patient is started on oral feedings of clear liquids to determine the tolerance level. The stomach is aspirated within 1 or 2 hours to assess the amount remaining and its color and consistency. When fluids are well tolerated, the tube is removed and fluids are increased in frequency with a slow progression to regular foods. The regimen of six small meals a day is begun.

Pernicious anemia is a long-term complication of total gastrectomy and may occur after partial gastrectomy. Pernicious anemia is caused by the loss of intrinsic factor, which is produced by the parietal cells. Depending on the amount of parietal cell mass removed in surgery, the patient may eventually require regular injections of cobalamin (vitamin B_{12}). (Cobalamin deficiency and pernicious anemia are discussed in Chapter 30.)

Peptic ulcer disease is a chronic problem, and ulcers can recur especially at the site of the anastomosis. Adequate rest, nutrition, and avoidance of known irritants and stressors are keys to complete recovery. Avoiding the use of drugs not prescribed by the health care provider is reemphasized, along with restrictions on smoking and alcohol use. If the patient is willing to make these kinds of adjustment in lifestyle, a successful rehabilitation is more likely.

■ Gerontologic Considerations:
Peptic Ulcer Disease

The incidence of peptic ulcers and, in particular, gastric ulcers in patients over 60 years of age is increasing. This is related to the increased use of NSAIDs. In the elderly patient, pain may not be the first symptom associated with an ulcer. For some patients the first manifestation may be frank gastric bleeding (e.g., hematemesis, melena) or a decrease in hematocrit. The morbidity and mortality rates associated with gastric ulcers in the elderly patient are higher than those for younger adults because of concomitant health problems (e.g., cardiovascular, pulmonary) and a decreased ability to withstand hypovolemia.

The treatment and management of ulcers in older adults are similar to that in younger adults. An emphasis is placed on prevention of both gastritis and peptic ulcers. This includes teaching the patient to take NSAIDs and other gastric-irritating drugs with food, milk, or antacids. The patient may be treated with antisecretory agents (i.e., PPIs or H$_2$R blockers). The patient should be instructed to avoid irritating substances, such as alcohol and smoking, and to report abdominal pain or discomfort to his or her health care provider.

GASTRIC CANCER

Gastric cancer is an adenocarcinoma of the stomach wall. The rate of gastric cancer has been steadily declining in the United States since the 1930s. However, it still accounts for more than 12,400 deaths and 21,600 new cancer cases annually.[1] Worldwide gastric adenocarcinoma is the second most common malignant growth. Gastric cancer is more prevalent in men of the lower socioeconomic class, primarily those living in urban areas. Gastric or stomach cancer is typically at an advanced stage when diagnosed and is not usually amenable to surgical resection. Only 10% to 20% of patients develop disease confined to the stomach. The five-year survival rate is 75% in patients with early stages of gastric cancer and less than 30% in those with advanced disease.

Etiology and Pathophysiology

Many factors have been implicated in the development of gastric cancer, yet no single causative agent has been identified. It is believed that a diet of smoked, highly salted, or spiced foods may have a carcinogenic effect. At the same time there appears to be a negative association between fresh fruits and the development of gastric cancer. A genetic etiology has been postulated because of the greater than normal occurrence of stomach cancer in immediate family members. However, at the present time there is no universally accepted genetic basis for gastric cancer.

Gastric carcinogenesis probably begins with a nonspecific mucosal injury as a result of aging, autoimmunity, or repeated exposure to irritants such as bile, antiinflammatory agents, or alcohol. Nutritional or other undetermined genetic deficiencies may impede mucosal repair, resulting in chronic gastritis and subsequent proliferation of *H. pylori*. Infection with *H. pylori*, especially at an early age, is considered a definite risk factor for gastric cancer. It is possible that *H. pylori* and resulting metabolic changes can induce a sequence of transitions from dysplasia to carcinoma in situ.

Other predisposing factors associated with a high incidence of gastric cancer are atrophic gastritis, pernicious anemia, adenomatous polyps, hyperplastic polyps, and achlorhydria. The relationship between chronic gastric ulcers and the development of gastric cancer is still controversial. Malignant transformation of a benign chronic ulcer does occur but accounts for less than 5% of all gastric cancers. It is known that the person with achlorhydria or pernicious anemia is more likely to develop gastric cancer than is the person with normal gastric acid production.

Gastric cancers often spread to adjacent organs before any distressing symptoms occur. The tumor may grow to large dimensions without obstructing the lumen of the stomach simply because the lumen itself is so large. The mean interval from onset of symptoms to consultation with a health care provider may be as long as 6 months. This long delay is largely attributed to the vague, intermittent abdominal distress experienced by the patient. Unfortunately, most healthy persons at one time or another experience these symptoms as a result of dietary indiscretions, nervous tension, and anxiety.

Gastric cancer can occur in any portion of the stomach. Tumors located at the cardia and fundus are associated with a poor prognosis. These tumors typically infiltrate rapidly to the surrounding tissue, regional lymph nodes, and liver. The patient with tumor growth along the lesser curvature has a better survival rate. Adenocarcinomas account for more than 95% of the cancers, and sarcomas (comprising lymphomas and leiomyomas) make up the rest.

The tumor growth is insidious and follows a pattern of continuous infiltration. Gastric cancer may spread by direct extension along the mucosal surface and infiltrate through the stomach wall. The rich lymphatic plexuses in the stomach facilitate distant metastasis. Seeding of tumor cells into the peritoneal cavity may occur late in the course of the disease. Evidence of spread to the peritoneal cavity is manifested by ascites and by spread to the ovaries.

Clinical Manifestations

The clinical manifestations exhibited by persons with gastric cancer can be categorized by signs and symptoms of anemia, peptic ulcer disease, or indigestion. Anemia is a common occurrence with stomach cancer. It is caused by chronic blood loss as the lesion erodes through the mucosa or as a direct result of pernicious anemia, which develops when intrinsic factor is lost. The person appears pale and weak and complains of fatigue, weakness, dizziness, and, in extreme cases, shortness of breath. The stool may be positive for occult blood.

The symptoms of gastric cancer are sometimes identical to those of peptic ulcer disease. The pain and discomfort may be alleviated by belching and by the use of antacids, antisecretory agents, and diet modifications. Manifestations related to indigestion include vague epigastric fullness with feelings of early satiety after meals. Weight loss, dysphagia, and constipation frequently accompany epigastric distress. When nausea, vomiting, and hematemesis occur, they may indicate gastric outlet obstruction or may be a warning of impending hemorrhage.

With more advanced disease, the physical examination may reveal that the patient is pale and lethargic if anemia is present. When the appetite has been poor and weight loss has been considerable, the patient may appear cachectic. A mass can often be detected beneath the abdominal wall and is seen to move with each inspiration. On palpation the mass may be felt in the epigastrium. Masses that are predominantly in the antrum of the stomach are generally found to the left of the midline. Masses located to the right of midline usually tend to be metastases to the liver or indicate involvement of the perigastric lymph nodes. Supraclavicular lymph nodes that are hard and enlarged and located on the left side are suggestive of metastasis via the thoracic duct from the stomach lesion. The presence of ascites is a poor prognostic sign.

Diagnostic Studies

The diagnostic studies for gastric cancer are presented in Table 40-26. Upper GI barium studies may demonstrate alterations in gastric contractility and emptying. On x-ray examination the malignant ulcer crater is more irregular around the edges and more elevated than the craters found with benign peptic ulcers. Barium studies do not always detect small lesions of the cardia and fundus.

Endoscopic examination of the stomach remains the best diagnostic tool. Lesions that go undetected on x-ray can be more easily viewed and a biopsy performed when endoscopy is used.

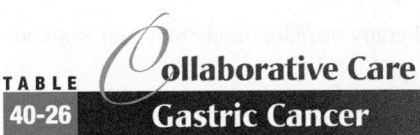

TABLE 40-26   Collaborative Care

Gastric Cancer

Diagnostic
History and physical examination
Upper GI barium study
Endoscopy and biopsy
Exfoliative cytology
Endoscopic ultrasonography
Upper GI barium study
Complete blood count
Urinalysis
Stool examination
Liver enzymes
Serum amylase
Tumor markers
　Carcinoembryonic antigen (CEA)
　Carbohydrate antigen (CA) 19-9

Collaborative Therapy
Surgery
Subtotal gastrectomy–Billroth I or II procedure
Total gastrectomy with esophagojejunostomy
Adjuvant therapy
Radiation therapy
Chemotherapy
Combination radiation therapy and chemotherapy

GI, Gastrointestinal.

The stomach can be distended with air during the procedure so that the mucosal folds can be stretched. Fixation of the mucosa is indicative of malignancy.

Blood chemistry studies assist in the determination of anemia and its severity. Elevations in liver enzymes and serum amylase levels may indicate liver and pancreatic involvement. Stool examination provides evidence of occult or gross bleeding.

Several tumor markers are often present in patients with gastric cancer. These include carcinoembryonic antigen (CEA) and carbohydrate antigen (CA) 19-9.[24] Serum tests for these markers are commonly performed before surgery for gastric cancer. Studies have shown that serum levels of these markers are correlated with the degree of invasion, liver metastasis, and cure rate.[24] Serum markers are not used as the only diagnostic tools for gastric cancer because elevations may be related to other factors such as smoking and the presence of benign lesions. (CEA and other tumor markers are discussed in Chapter 15.)

Collaborative Care

When the diagnosis of gastric cancer has been confirmed, the treatment of choice is surgical removal of the tumor. The preoperative management of the patient with gastric cancer focuses on the correction of nutritional deficits, treatment of anemia, and replacement of blood volume.

Transfusions of packed RBCs correct the anemia. If a gastric lesion has been located at or near the pylorus and is causing gastric outlet obstruction, gastric decompression may be necessary before surgery. When the tumor has extended into the transverse colon and partial colon resection is also required, special preparation of the bowel is necessary. This preparation may include a low-residue diet, enemas to cleanse the bowel, and the use of antibiotics to reduce the intestinal bacteria. Correction of malnutrition is important if surgery is planned. Malnutrition is associated with increased postoperative complications and mortality rates.

Surgical Therapy. The surgical intervention used in the treatment of gastric cancer may be the same surgical procedures used for peptic ulcer disease. Surgical resection is curative in less than 40% of cases of gastric cancer.[25] The location and extent of the lesion, the patient's physical condition, and preference of the surgeon determine the specific surgery employed. When metastasis is widespread at the time of diagnosis, surgical intervention may be only palliative.

The surgical aim is to remove as much of the stomach as necessary to remove the tumor and a margin of normal tissue. When the lesion is located in the cardia or high in the fundus, a total gastrectomy with esophagojejunostomy is performed. This procedure involves anastomosis of the lower end of the esophagus to the jejunum (Fig. 40-17). Lesions located in the antrum or the pyloric region are generally treated by either a Billroth I or Billroth II procedure. When metastasis has occurred to adjacent organs, such as the spleen, ovaries, or bowel, the surgical procedures must be modified and extended as necessary.

The chance of a complete cure by surgical means is decreased considerably when the lymph nodes are involved. Survival rates are considerably shortened when organs adjacent to the stomach show evidence of invasion at the time of surgery.

Adjuvant Therapy. Surgery is the only definitive means of achieving a cure. However, when the patient cannot physically withstand a surgical procedure or when surgical cure is not feasible, radiation or chemotherapy alone or in combination may be used. Neither radiation therapy nor chemotherapeutic agents have been very successful when used as the primary mode of treatment. Because the radiosensitivity of gastric cancers is low, radiation therapy has proven to be of little value. When radiation

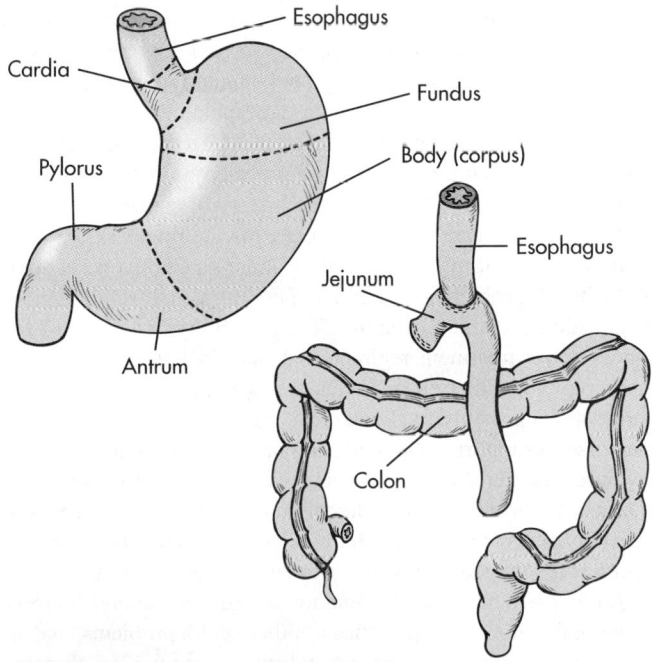

FIG. 40-17 Total gastrectomy for gastric cancer (total gastrectomy with esophagojejunostomy).

is used as a palliative measure, the tumor mass can be decreased, with temporary relief of the cardia or pyloric obstruction.

The combination of chemotherapy and radiation is now being used for patients who are at high risk for disease recurrence following surgery. Until recently, single-agent chemotherapy for gastric cancer has proven to be of little value. Agents that have been identified as having some effect on gastric cancer are 5-FU, BCNU, methyl-CCNU, and doxorubicin (Adriamycin). Combination of radiation and chemotherapy involving 5-FU and leucovorin following surgical resection increases survival. Additional therapies including intraperitoneal administration of chemotherapeutic agents are undergoing evaluation. The role of biologic therapy is still under investigation for use in gastric cancer. (These therapies are discussed in Chapter 15.)

NURSING MANAGEMENT
GASTRIC CANCER

■ Nursing Assessment

The assessment of a person with possible gastric cancer is similar to that done for peptic ulcer disease (see Table 40-23). Important data to be obtained from the patient and the family should include a nutritional assessment, a psychosocial history, the patient's perceptions of the health problem and need for hospitalization, and the physical examination of the patient.

The nutritional assessment must elicit information regarding appetite and changes in eating patterns over the previous 6 months. It is necessary to determine the patient's normal weight and any changes that may have occurred in the past few months. Unexplained weight loss is common in many types of cancer before diagnosis. A history of vague symptoms of dyspepsia, early satiety, feeling full after consuming even a small amount of food, or reporting symptoms of gas pain should help the nurse differentiate these typical gastric cancer symptoms from those of peptic ulcer. The nurse should determine whether pain is present, where and when it occurs, and how it is relieved. When the pain has been controlled with ingestion of foods, fluids, or antacids for a period of time but now continues or worsens regardless of interventions, gastric cancer may be the underlying cause.

Psychosocial and demographic data include age, present or previous occupation, and financial status. Gastric cancer can occur at any age, but the risk is more prevalent in men in the fifth to the sixth decade of life. A family history of cancer, especially gastric cancer, puts a person at greater than normal risk.

It is important to determine the patient's personal perception of the health problem and method of coping with hospitalization, diagnostic tests, and procedures. The possibility of a diagnosis of cancer and a treatment regimen that may include surgery, chemotherapy, or radiation treatment forecast a prolonged stressful period and a possibly fatal outcome. Therefore it is important for the nurse to support the patient and family if tests result in an unfavorable diagnosis and complex treatment interventions are planned. If surgery is probable, the nurse should assess what the patient expects from surgery (cure or palliation) and how that patient has responded to any previous surgical procedures.

A complete physical examination reveals the patient's current functional abilities, the presence of other health problems, and an estimate of how well the patient may respond to therapy. Cachexia may be evident if the nutritional state has been compromised for an extended time. A malnourished patient does not

respond well to chemotherapy or radiation therapy and is a poor surgical risk.

■ Nursing Diagnoses

Nursing diagnoses for the patient with gastric cancer include, but are not limited to, the following:

- Imbalanced nutrition: less than body requirements *related to* inability to ingest, digest, or absorb nutrients
- Activity intolerance *related to* generalized weakness, abdominal discomfort, and nutritional deficits
- Anxiety *related to* lack of knowledge of diagnostic tests, unknown diagnostic outcome, disease process, and therapeutic regimen
- Acute pain *related to* underlying disease process and side effects of surgery, chemotherapy, or radiation therapy
- Anticipatory grieving *related to* perceived unfavorable diagnosis and impending death

■ Planning

The overall goals are that the patient with gastric cancer will (1) experience minimal discomfort, (2) achieve optimal nutritional status, and (3) maintain a degree of spiritual and psychologic well-being appropriate to the disease stage.

■ Nursing Implementation

Health Promotion. The nursing role in the early detection of cancer of the stomach is focused primarily on identification of the patient at risk because of specific disorders such as pernicious anemia and achlorhydria. The nurse should be aware of symptoms associated with gastric cancer, method of spread, and the significant findings on physical examination. The nurse should understand that the cure rate is often quite dismal because symptoms arise late in the course of the disease process, are vague, and often mimic other conditions, such as peptic ulcer disease.

The nurse must be alert to problems suggesting gastric cancer, such as poor appetite, weight loss, fatigue, and persistent gastric distress. If any of these manifestations are present, medical attention should be obtained and the necessary diagnostic tests performed.

In addition, any patient with a positive family history of gastric cancer should be encouraged to undergo diagnostic evaluation if manifestations of anemia, peptic ulcer, or vague epigastric distress are present. It is important that the nurse recognize the possible existence of stomach cancer in a patient who is treated for peptic ulcer and who fails to have relief after 3 weeks of prescribed therapy. The ulcer, if it is benign, should show signs of healing on x-ray examination.

Acute Intervention

Preoperative care. When the diagnostic tests confirm the presence of a malignancy, the patient and the family generally react with shock, disbelief, and depression, regardless of how thoroughly they may have been prepared for this possible outcome. Throughout this period the nurse must give emotional and physical support, provide information, clarify test results, and maintain a positive attitude with respect to the patient's immediate recovery and long-term survival.

On admission to the hospital, the patient may be in poor physical condition. Surgery may have to be delayed while the patient becomes more physically able to withstand the strain of major surgery. A positive nutritional state enhances wound healing, as well as the ability to withstand infection and other possible postoperative complications. Often the patient is better able to tolerate several small meals a day rather than three regular meals. The diet may be supplemented by a variety of commercial liquid supplements (see Chapter 39) and vitamins. The nurse is challenged to find innovative ways of persuading the patient to eat when lack of appetite and state of mind make eating difficult and unrewarding. Getting the patient's family to assist with meals and encourage intake may be beneficial. If the patient is unable to ingest oral feedings, it may be necessary to provide for nutritional needs with tube feedings or parenteral nutrition.

If needed, blood replacement and fluid volume restoration may be carried out in the preoperative period. Because anemia is usually present, packed RBCs may be administered. Close observation for reactions to the transfusions is important. Monitoring the hemoglobin and hematocrit levels provides information on the progress of therapy.

The preoperative teaching plan before gastric surgery for cancer is much the same as that for peptic ulcer surgery (see the previous section, Surgical Therapy for Peptic Ulcer Disease).

Postoperative care. Postoperative care of the patient with gastric carcinoma is similar to that following a Billroth I or II procedure (see the previous section, Surgical Therapy for Peptic Ulcer Disease). When the surgical intervention has involved a total gastrectomy, the plan of care is somewhat different. The operation performed usually requires some resecting of the lower esophagus along with the removal of the entire stomach and anastomosis of the esophagus to the jejunum. The chest cavity must be entered, and drainage is accomplished by the insertion of chest tubes. (Chest surgery and drainage tubes are discussed in Chapter 27.) After total gastrectomy, the NG tube does not drain a large quantity of secretions because removal of the stomach has eliminated the reservoir capacity. The NG tube is removed after several days, when intestinal peristalsis has resumed. Small amounts of clear fluid may then be started. The patient requires close observation for signs of leakage of the fluids at the anastomosis as evidenced by an elevation in the temperature and increasing dyspnea. When fluids are well tolerated without distress, the amount may be increased along with the addition of some solid foods.

As a consequence of a total gastrectomy, a patient experiences the symptoms of the dumping syndrome. Unfortunately, weight loss is very common, and poor nutritional intake often contributes. Postoperative wound healing may be impaired because of inadequate dietary intake. This necessitates the IV or oral replacement of vitamins C, D, K, and the B complex vitamins and intramuscular administration of cobalamin. Because these vitamins (with the exception of cobalamin) are absorbed primarily in the upper part of the small intestine, they must be replaced because the duodenum has been bypassed in the surgical procedure.

A patient who has had a Billroth I or II operative procedure should receive the same postoperative care as someone who has had peptic ulcer surgery. This patient is also subject to the same type of postoperative complications such as the dumping syndrome and postprandial hypoglycemia.

The patient with advanced malignant disease can be offered only palliative treatment. The chemotherapy agent found most useful for controlling symptoms of gastric cancer is 5-FU. When this drug or any of the combination drugs is prescribed, the nurse

must have current information regarding the action and side effects of the drugs. The patient should be made aware of the potential benefits and hazards that can result from the chemotherapy. (The care of the patient receiving chemotherapy is discussed in detail in Chapter 15.)

Radiation therapy can be used as an adjuvant to surgery or for palliation. A patient is generally quite fearful of radiation and may develop many misconceptions regarding its value and dangers. To reassure the patient and ensure completion of the designated number of treatments, the nurse must provide detailed instruction. Because most therapy is completed on an outpatient basis, the nurse should assess the patient's knowledge of radiation, care of the skin, the need for good nutrition and fluid intake during therapy, and the appropriate use of antiemetic drugs. (Specific care of the patient receiving radiation therapy is discussed in Chapter 15.)

Ambulatory and Home Care. Before the patient is discharged, the need for teaching should be reviewed. Most dietary measures useful after peptic ulcer surgery are applicable after surgery for gastric carcinoma. Plans should be made for the relief of pain, including comfort measures and the judicious use of analgesics. Wound care, if needed, must be taught to the primary caregiver in the home situation. Dressings, special equipment, or special services may be required for the patient's continued care at home. A list of community agencies that are available for assistance can be provided before the patient goes home. The services of the American Cancer Society are especially helpful.

When treatment in the form of chemotherapy or radiation therapy is to be continued after discharge, a referral to the home health nurse may be beneficial. The home health nurse can assist with recovery, determine the degree of patient compliance, and be a sympathetic health care provider with whom the patient can consult.

Long-term follow-up must be stressed. The patient must be encouraged to comply with the prescribed dietary and drug regimens, to keep appointments for chemotherapy administration or radiation treatments, and to keep the physician informed of changes in physical condition. (Long-term management of the cancer patient is discussed in Chapter 15.)

■ Evaluation

Expected outcomes are that the patient with gastric cancer will

- experience no or minimal discomfort, pain, or nausea
- achieve optimal nutritional status
- maintain a degree of psychologic well-being appropriate to the disease stage

FOOD POISONING

Food poisoning is a nonspecific term that describes acute GI symptoms such as nausea, vomiting, diarrhea, and colicky abdominal pain caused by the intake of contaminated food. Food most commonly causes illness if it is contaminated with microorganisms or their products. The GI tract is frequently the portal of entry for the microorganisms. The epidemiology of foodborne illness is changing. There are new organisms, and many have spread worldwide. The two main types of food poisoning are (1) acute gastroenteritis from bacteria and (2) neurologic symptoms from botulism. The most common bacterial food poisonings are presented in Table 40-27.

TABLE 40-27 Bacterial Food Poisoning

TYPE	CAUSATIVE AGENT	SOURCES	ONSET OF SYMPTOMS	MANIFESTATIONS	TREATMENT	PREVENTION
Staphylococcal	Toxin from *Staphylococcus aureus*	Meat, bakery products, cream fillings, salad dressings, milk; skin and respiratory tract of food handlers	30 min–7 hr	Vomiting, nausea, abdominal cramping, diarrhea	Symptomatic, fluid and electrolyte replacement, antiemetics	Immediate refrigeration of foods, monitoring of food handlers
Clostridial	*Clostridium perfringens*	Meat or poultry dishes cooked at lower temperature (stew or pot pie), re-warmed meat dishes, gravies, improperly canned vegetables	8–24 hr	Diarrhea, nausea, abdominal cramps, vomiting (rare); midepigastrium pain	Symptomatic, fluid replacement	Correct preparation of meat dishes, serving of food immediately after cooking or rapid cooling of food
Salmonella	*Salmonella typhimurium* (grows in gut)	Improperly cooked poultry, pork, beef, lamb, and eggs	8 hr–several days	Nausea and vomiting, diarrhea, abdominal cramps, fever and chills	Symptomatic, fluid and electrolyte replacement	Correct preparation of food
Botulism	Toxin from *Clostridium botulinum*, ingested toxin absorbed from gut and blocks acetylcholine at neuromuscular junction	Improperly canned or pre-served food, home-preserved vegetables (most common), preserved fruits and fish, canned commercial products	12–36 hr	GI symptoms of nausea, vomiting, abdominal pain, constipation, distention. Central nervous system symptoms of headache, dizziness, muscular incoordination, weakness, inability to talk or swallow, diplopia, breathing difficulties, paralysis, delirium, coma	Maintenance of ventilation, polyvalent antitoxin, guanidine hydrochloric acid (enhances acetylcholine release)	Correct processing of canned foods, boiling of suspected canned foods for 15 min before serving
Escherichia coli	*E. coli* serotype 0157:H7	Contaminated beef, pork, milk, cheese, fish	Varies by strain: 8 hr–1 wk	Bloody stools, hemolytic uremic syndrome, abdominal cramping, profuse diarrhea	Symptomatic, fluid and electrolyte replacement	Correct preparation of food

Poisonous chemicals, such as mercury, arsenic, zinc, and potassium chlorate, may contaminate foods. Poisoning can also occur from ingestion of poisonous plants (e.g., certain mushroom species).

Prevention of occurrence is the focus of interventions. Teaching should include correct food preparation and cleanliness, adequate cooking, and refrigeration. If the patient is hospitalized, care focuses on correction of fluid and electrolyte imbalance from diarrhea and vomiting. With botulism, additional assessment and care relative to neurologic symptoms are indicated (see Chapter 59).

Escherichia coli 0157:H7 Poisoning

Of recent importance is the increase in number of cases of hemorrhagic colitis caused by the presence of the bacterial strain *Escherichia coli 0157:H7*. Widespread outbreaks in the United States, Canada, and Japan have increased the public's awareness of this organism. Poisoning with *E. coli* 0157:H7 can be life threatening, particularly in the very young and the elderly. *E. coli* 0157:H7 is found primarily in undercooked meats, such as hamburger, roast beef, ham, and turkey. However, other sources include cheese sandwiches, apple cider, and unpasteurized milk. *E. coli* 0157:H7 can also be transmitted from person to person, particularly in settings such as nursing homes and day care centers. *E. coli* 0157:H7 may be responsible for 0.6% to 2.4% of all nonbloody diarrhea and 15% to 36% of all cases of bloody diarrhea.

The clinical manifestations of *E. coli* 0157:H7 vary from mild diarrhea to bloody diarrhea and systemic complications, including hemolytic uremia and thrombocytopenic purpura and even death. The diarrhea may start out as watery but may progress to bloody. Treatment involves supportive care to maintain intravascular volume. Other therapies may include dialysis and plasmapheresis. The use of antibiotics remains controversial.

CRITICAL THINKING EXERCISES

Case Study
Hiatal Hernia
Patient Profile. Mary, a 63-year-old white elementary school teacher, has had a sliding hiatal hernia for 10 years. Mary is admitted to the hospital for a hiatal hernia repair.

Subjective Data
- Reports increasing heartburn, especially at night
- Is currently on a bland diet and taking antacids
- Complains of substernal pain and heartburn
- Reports some problems with regurgitation

Objective Data
Physical Examination
- 5 feet 2 inches tall and weighs 195 pounds

Diagnostic Study
- Barium swallow and an endoscopy revealed a large sliding hiatal hernia.

Collaborative Care
- Mary had a Nissen fundoplication through a laparoscopic approach.

CRITICAL THINKING QUESTIONS

1. Explain the pathophysiology of a hiatal hernia. What is the difference between a sliding and a paraesophageal hiatal hernia?
2. What are the characteristic symptoms of a hiatal hernia? Which of these did Mary have?
3. Describe a Nissen fundoplication procedure. What is the objective of this surgical procedure? Why was a laparoscopic approach used?
4. What are potential postoperative complications, and what nursing measures prevent them?
5. What should be included in a teaching plan for Mary?
6. Based on the assessment data presented, write one or more nursing diagnoses. Are there any collaborative problems?

Nursing Research Issues

1. What are the most effective topical methods to relieve pain related to stomatitis secondary to infection?
2. Are dietary interventions successful in improving symptoms in the patient with gastroesophageal reflux disease?
3. What are optimal strategies to promote multiple lifestyle changes in a patient with peptic ulcer disease?
4. What are environmental manipulations that could be used to promote decreased nausea in patients receiving chemotherapy?
5. What sensory stimuli in the environment, including sight, smell, and sound, could promote optimal nutrient intake in the chemotherapy patient who is experiencing nausea?
6. What is the most effective way to obtain a nutritional assessment from a patient with gastric carcinoma?

REVIEW QUESTIONS

The number of the question corresponds to the same-numbered objective at the beginning of the chapter.

1. Mrs. Jones calls to tell you that her elderly mother, who is 85 years of age, has been nauseated all day and has vomited twice. Before you hang up and telephone the health care provider to communicate your assessment data, you instruct Mrs. Jones to
   a. administer antispasmodic drugs and observe skin turgor.
   b. give her mother sips of water and elevate the head of her bed to prevent aspiration.
   c. offer her mother a high-protein liquid supplement to drink to maintain her nutritional needs.
   d. offer her mother large quantities of Gatorade to drink because elderly people are at risk for sodium depletion.

2. The nurse explains to the patient with Vincent's infection that treatment will include
   a. smallpox vaccinations.
   b. viscous lidocaine rinses.
   c. amphotericin B suspension.
   d. topical application of antibiotics.

3. The nurse is involved in health promotion related to oral cancer. Teaching of adolescents regarding behaviors that put them at risk for oral cancer includes
   a. avoiding use of perfumed lip gloss.
   b. discouraging use of chewing gum.
   c. avoiding use of smokeless tobacco.
   d. discouraging drinking of carbonated beverages.

4. The nurse explains to the patient with gastroesophageal reflux disease that this disorder
   a. results in acid erosion and ulceration of the esophagus caused by the frequent vomiting.
   b. will require surgical wrapping or repair of the pyloric sphincter to control the symptoms.
   c. is the protrusion of a portion of the stomach into the esophagus through an opening in the diaphragm.
   d. often involves relaxation of the lower esophageal sphincter, allowing stomach contents to back up into the esophagus.

5. A patient who has undergone an esophagectomy for esophageal cancer develops increasing pain, fever, and dyspnea when a full liquid diet is started postoperatively. The nurse recognizes that these symptoms are most indicative of
   a. an intolerance to the feedings.
   b. extension of the tumor into the aorta.
   c. leakage of fluid or foods into the mediastinum.
   d. esophageal perforation with fistula formation into the lung.

6. The pernicious anemia that may accompany gastritis is due to which of the following?
   a. Chronic autoimmune destruction of cobalamin stores in the body
   b. Progressive gastric atrophy from chronic breakage in the mucosal barrier and blood loss
   c. A lack of intrinsic factor normally produced by acid-secreting cells of the gastric mucosa
   d. Hyperchlorhydria resulting from an increase in acid-secreting parietal cells and degradation of RBCs

7. Your teaching plan for the patient being discharged following an acute episode of GI bleeding will include information concerning the importance of
   a. taking only drugs prescribed by the health care provider.
   b. avoiding taking aspirin with acidic beverages such as orange juice.
   c. taking all drugs 1 hour before mealtime to prevent further bleeding.
   d. reading all OTC drug labels to avoid those containing stearic acid and calcium.

8. You are teaching your patient and her family about possible causative factors for peptic ulcers. You explain that ulcer formation is
   a. caused by a stressful lifestyle and other acid-producing factors such as *C. pylori.*
   b. inherited within families and reinforced by bacterial spread of *Staphylococcus aureus* in childhood.
   c. promoted by factors that tend to cause oversecretion of acid, such as excess dietary fats, smoking, and *B. pylori.*
   d. promoted by a combination of possible factors that may result in erosion of the gastric mucosa, including certain drugs and alcohol.

9. An optimal teaching plan for an outpatient with gastric carcinoma receiving radiation therapy should include information about
   a. cancer support groups, alopecia, and stomatitis.
   b. avitaminosis, ostomy care, and community resources.
   c. prosthetic devices, skin conductance, and grief counseling.
   d. wound and skin care, nutrition, drugs, and community resources.

10. Several patients are seen at an urgent care center with symptoms of nausea, vomiting, and diarrhea that began 2 hours ago while attending a large family reunion potluck dinner. The nurse questions the patients specifically about foods they ingested containing
    a. beef.
    b. meat and milk.
    c. poultry and eggs.
    d. home-preserved vegetables.

REFERENCES

1. McLauchlan R et al: Ethnic variation in fluorescein angiography induced nausea and vomiting, *Eye* 15(Pt 2):159, 2001.
2. American Cancer Society: *Cancer facts and figures 2001,* Atlanta, Ga, 2001, American Cancer Society.
3. Handlers JP: Diagnosis and management of oral soft-tissue lesions: the use of biopsy, toluidine blue staining, and brush biopsy, *J Calif Dent Assoc* 29:602, 2001.
4. Bjorkman DJ: Community issues in gastroesophageal reflux disease: what we know and what we do not know, *Am J Gastroenterol* 96(8 suppl):S34, 2001.
5. Richter JE: Noncardiac (unexplained) chest pain, *Curr Treat Options Gastroenterol* 3:329, 2000.
6. Fass R et al: Clinical and economic assessment of the omeprazole test in patients with symptoms suggestive of gastroesophageal reflux disease, *Arch Intern Med* 159:2161, 1999.
7. Kaynard A, Flora K: Gastroesophageal reflux disease: control of symptoms, prevention of complications, *Postgrad Med* 110:42, 2001.
8. Smit CF et al: Effect of cigarette smoking on gastropharyngeal and gastroesophageal reflux, *Ann Otol Rhinol Laryngol* 110:190, 2001.
9. Livingston CD et al: Laparoscopic hiatal hernia repair in patients with poor esophageal motility or paraesophageal herniation, *Am Surg* 67:987, 2001.
10. Richards WO et al: Initial experience with the Stretta procedure for the treatment of gastroesophageal reflux disease, *J Laparoendosc Adv Surg Tech* 11:267, 2001.
11. Ruhl CE, Sonnenberg A, Everhart JE: Hospitalization with respiratory disease following hiatal hernia and reflux esophagitis in a prospective, population-based study, *Ann Epidemiol* 11:477, 2001.
12. Bollschweiler E et al: Demographic variations in the rising incidence of esophageal adenocarcinoma in white males, *Cancer* 92:549, 2001.
13. Ajani JA et al: A three-step strategy of induction chemotherapy then chemoradiation followed by surgery in patients with potentially resectable carcinoma of the esophagus or gastroesophageal junction, *Cancer* 92:279, 2001.
14. Siddiq MA, Sood S, Strachan D: Pharyngeal pouch (Zenker's diverticulum), *Postgrad Med J* 77:506, 2001.
15. Diener U et al: Laparoscopic Heller myotomy relieves dysphagia in patients with achalasia and low LES pressure following pneumatic dilatation, *Surg Endosc* 15:687, 2001.
16. Bruley des Varannes S, Scarpignato C: Current trends in the management of achalasia, *Dig Liver Dis* 33:266, 2001.
17. Huang JP, Hunt RH: Treatment of acute gastric and duodenal ulcers. In MM Wolfe, editor: *Therapy of digestive diseases*, Philadelphia, 2000, WB Saunders.
18. Yacyshyn BR, Thomson A: Critical review of acid suppression in nonvariceal, acute, upper gastrointestinal bleeding, *Dig Dis* 18:117, 2000.
19. Lichtenstein DR: Nonvariceal upper GI hemorrhage. In MM Wolfe, editor: *Therapy of digestive diseases*, Philadelphia, 2000, WB Saunders.
20. Chan HL et al: Is non-*Helicobacter pylori,* non-NSAID peptic ulcer a common cause of upper GI bleeding? A prospective study of 977 patients, *Gastrointest Endosc* 53:438, 2001.
21. Fennerty MB: NSAID-related gastrointestinal injury: evidence-based approach to a preventable complication, *Postgrad Med* 110:87, 2001.
22. Knigge KL: The role of *H pylori* in gastrointestinal disease: a guide to identification and eradication, *Postgrad Med* 110:71, 2001.
23. Giercksky KE, Haglund U, Rask-Madsen J: Selective inhibitors of COX-2—are they safe for the stomach? *Scand J Gastroenterol* 35:1121, 2000.
24. Ishigami S et al: Clinical importance of preoperative carcinoembryonic antigen and carbohydrate antigen 19-9 levels in gastric cancer, *J Clin Gastroenterol* 32:41, 2001.
25. Macdonald JS et al: Chemoradiotherapy after surgery compared with surgery alone for adenocarcinoma of the stomach or gastroesophageal junction, *N Engl J Med* 345:725, 2001.

RESOURCES

American College of Gastroenterology
4900 B South 31st Street
Arlington, VA 22206
703-820-7400
Fax: 703-931-4520
www.acg.gi.org/

American Gastroenterological Association
7910 Woodmont Avenue, 7th Floor
Bethesda, MD 20814
301-654-2055
Fax: 301-652-3890
www.gastro.org/

American Society for Gastrointestinal Endoscopy
1520 Kensington Road, Suite 202
Oak Brook, IL 60523
630-573-0600
Fax: 630-573-0691
www.asge.org/

Digestive Disease National Coalition
711 2nd Street, NE, Suite 200
Washington, DC 20002
202-544-7497
Fax: 202-546-7105
www.ddnc.org/

Digestive Health Resource Center
www.gastro.org/public/digestinfo.html

National Digestive Diseases Information Clearinghouse
2 Information Way
Bethesda, MD 20892-3570
800-891-5389 or 301-654-3810
Fax: 301-907-8906
www.niddk.nih.gov/health/digest/nddic.htm

National Heartburn Alliance
877-471-2081
www.heartburnalliance.org/

National Institute of Diabetes & Digestive & Kidney Diseases (NIDDK)
Building 31, Room 9A-52
Bethesda, MD 20892
301-496-5877
www.niddk.nih.gov/index.htm

Society of Gastroenterology Nurses and Associates (SGNA)
401 North Michigan Avenue
Chicago, IL 60611-4267
800-245-7462 or 312-321-5165
Fax: 312-527-6658
www.sgna.org

For additional Internet resources, see the website for this book at *http://evolve.elsevier.com/Lewis/medsurg/.*

CHAPTER *41*

NURSING MANAGEMENT
Lower Gastrointestinal Problems

Donna Zimmaro Bliss
Lynda Sawchuk

LEARNING OBJECTIVES

1. Explain the common etiologies, collaborative care, and nursing management of diarrhea, fecal incontinence, and constipation.
2. Describe common causes of acute abdominal pain and nursing management of the patient following an exploratory laparotomy.
3. Describe the collaborative care and nursing management of acute appendicitis, peritonitis, and gastroenteritis.
4. Compare and contrast ulcerative colitis and Crohn's disease, including pathophysiology, clinical manifestations, complications, collaborative care, and nursing management.
5. Differentiate among mechanical, neurogenic, and vascular bowel obstructions, including causes, collaborative care, and nursing management.
6. Describe the clinical manifestations and collaborative management of colorectal cancer.
7. Explain the anatomic and physiologic changes and nursing management of the patient with an ileostomy and colostomy.
8. Differentiate between diverticulosis and diverticulitis, including clinical manifestations, collaborative care, and nursing management.
9. Compare and contrast the types of hernias, including etiology and surgical and nursing management.
10. Describe the types of malabsorption syndrome and collaborative care of sprue syndrome, lactase deficiency, and short bowel syndrome.
11. Describe the types, clinical manifestations, collaborative care, and nursing management of anorectal conditions.

KEY TERMS

anal fissure, p. 1100	intestinal obstruction, p. 1078
anal fistula, p. 1101	irritable bowel syndrome, p. 1064
appendicitis, p. 1064	lactase deficiency, p. 1098
constipation, p. 1057	nontropical sprue, p. 1097
Crohn's disease, p. 1076	ostomy, p. 1087
diarrhea, p. 1052	paralytic (adynamic) ileus, p. 1078
diverticulum, p. 1093	peritonitis, p. 1066
fecal impaction, p. 1056	pilonidal sinus, p. 1101
fecal incontinence, p. 1055	pseudoobstruction, p. 1078
gastroenteritis, p. 1067	short bowel syndrome, p. 1098
hemorrhoids, p. 1099	steatorrhea, p. 1096
hernia, p. 1095	ulcerative colitis, p. 1068
inflammatory bowel disease, p. 1067	Valsalva maneuver, p. 1057

DIARRHEA

Diarrhea—the frequent passage of loose, watery stools—is not a disease but a symptom. The term *diarrhea* may mean different things to different patients. It is commonly used to denote an increase in stool frequency or volume and an increase in the looseness of stool.

Etiology and Pathophysiology

Causes of diarrhea can be divided into the general classifications of decreased fluid absorption, increased fluid secretion, motility disturbances, or a combination of these (Table 41-1). Causes of acute infectious diarrhea are listed in Table 41-2.

Clinical Manifestations

Diarrhea may be acute or chronic. Acute diarrhea most commonly results from infection. Bacterial or viral infection of the intestine may result in explosive watery diarrhea, *tenesmus* (spasmodic contraction of anal sphincter with pain and persistent desire to defecate), and abdominal cramping pain. Perianal skin irritation may also develop. Systemic manifestations include fever, nausea, vomiting, and malaise. Leukocytes, blood, and mucus may be present in the stool, depending on the causative agent (see Table 41-2). Acute diarrhea is often self-limiting in the adult. Symptoms continue until the irritant or causative agent is excreted. The mucous membrane lining of the gastrointestinal (GI) tract is composed of epithelial cells, which regenerate following the inflammatory response.

Diarrhea is considered chronic when it persists for at least 2 weeks or when it subsides and returns more than 2 to 4 weeks after the initial episode. Severe diarrhea may be debilitating and life threatening. A patient may have severe dehydration (water and sodium loss) and electrolyte disturbances (e.g., hypokalemia). Malabsorption and malnutrition are also sequelae of chronic diarrhea. Throughout the world, diarrhea is one of the major causes of death.

Diagnostic Studies

Accurate diagnosis and management require a thorough history, physical examination, and, when indicated, laboratory tests. A history of travel, medication use, diet, previous surgery, interpersonal contacts, and family history should be obtained. Blood tests may identify anemia, elevated white blood cell (WBC) count, iron and folate deficiencies, elevated liver enzyme levels, and electrolyte disturbances. Stools may be examined for the

Reviewed by Marilee Schmelzer, RN, PhD, Associate Professor, University of Texas at Arlington, Arlington, Tex.

presence of blood, mucus, WBCs, and parasites. Stool cultures help to identify infectious organisms.

In a patient with chronic diarrhea, measurement of stool electrolytes, pH, and osmolality may help determine whether the diarrhea is related to decreased fluid absorption or increased fluid secretion (secretory diarrhea). Measurement of stool fat and undigested muscle fibers may indicate fat and protein malabsorption conditions, including pancreatic insufficiency. Elevated serum levels of GI hormones such as vasoactive intestinal polypeptide and gastrin may be present in some patients with secretory diarrhea. Endoscopy may be used to examine the mucosa and to obtain specimens via biopsy for examination. Upper and lower radiologic studies with barium contrast may be helpful in detecting mucosal disease, as well as structural abnormalities.

Collaborative Care

The treatment of diarrhea is based on the cause and is aimed at replacing fluid and electrolytes and decreasing the number, volume, and frequency of stools. Oral solutions containing glucose and electrolytes (e.g., Gatorade, Pedialyte) may be sufficient to replace losses from mild diarrhea. In situations of severe diarrhea, parenteral administration of fluids, electrolytes, vitamins, and nutrition is warranted.

Once the cause of the diarrhea has been determined, antidiarrheal agents may be given to coat and protect mucous membranes, absorb irritating substances, inhibit GI motility, decrease intestinal secretions, and decrease central nervous system stimulation of the GI tract (Table 41-3). Antiperistaltic agents are not given to a patient who has infectious diarrheal syndromes because of the potential of prolonging exposure to the infectious agent. Regardless of the cause of diarrhea, antidiarrheal drugs should not be given for a prolonged time.

Antibiotics are reserved for treating specific bacterial organisms. Antibiotics can cause diarrhea by altering the normal bowel flora. Patients receiving antibiotics (e.g., clindamycin [Cleocin]) are susceptible to *Clostridium difficile (C. difficile)* infection. Health care workers who do not adhere to infection control precautions can transmit *C. difficile* from patient to patient. Some

TABLE 41-1   Causes of Diarrhea

Decreased Fluid Absorption

Oral intake of poorly absorbable solutes (e.g., laxatives)
Maldigestion and malabsorption
Mucosal damage: tropical sprue, celiac disease, Crohn's disease, radiation injury, ulcerative colitis, ischemic bowel disease
Pancreatic insufficiency
Intestinal enzyme deficiencies (e.g., lactase)
Bile salt deficiency
Decreased surface area (e.g., intestinal resection)

Increased Fluid Secretion

Infectious: bacterial endotoxins (e.g., *Cholera, Escherichia coli, Shigella, Salmonella, Staphylococcus, Clostridium difficile*, viral agents [rotavirus], and parasitic agents [*Giardia lamblia*])
Drugs: laxatives, antibiotics, suspensions or elixirs containing sorbitol (e.g., valproic acid syrup [Depakene])
Foods: candy, gum, and mints containing sorbitol
Hormonal: vasoactive intestinal polypeptide secretion from adenoma of the pancreas; gastrin secretion caused by Zollinger-Ellison syndrome; calcitonin secretion from carcinoma of the thyroid
Tumor: Villous adenoma

Motility Disturbances

Irritable bowel syndrome: ↑ visceral sensitivity and transit
Diabetic enteropathy: ↑ transit secondary to peripheral neuropathy
Gastrectomy: ↑ transit as a result of dumping syndrome

TABLE 41-2   Causes of Acute Infectious Diarrhea

	ONSET	DURATION	SYMPTOMS AND SIGNS
Viral			
Rotavirus, Norwalk	18-24 hr	24-48 hr	Explosive, watery diarrhea; nausea; vomiting; abdominal cramps
Bacterial			
Escherichia coli	4-24 hr	3-4 days	Four or five loose stools per day, nausea, malaise, low-grade fever
Enterohemorrhagic *E. coli* (0157:H7)	4-24 hr	4-9 days	Bloody diarrhea, severe cramping, fever
Shigella	24 hr	7 days	Watery stools containing blood and mucus, tenesmus, urgency, severe cramping, fever
Salmonella	6-48 hr	2-5 days	Watery diarrhea, nausea, vomiting, abdominal cramps, fever
Campylobacter species	24 hr	<7 days	Profuse, watery diarrhea; malaise, nausea, abdominal cramps, low-grade fever
Clostridium perfringens	8-12 hr	24 hr	Watery diarrhea, abdominal cramps, vomiting
Clostridium difficile	4-9 days after start of antibiotics	24 hr	Associated with antibiotic treatment; symptoms range from mild, watery diarrhea to severe abdominal pain, fever, leukocytosis, leukocytes in stool
Parasitic			
Giardia lamblia	1-3 wk	Few days to 3 months	Sudden onset; malodorous, explosive, watery diarrhea; flatulence, epigastric pain and cramping, nausea
Entamoeba histolytica	4 days	Weeks to months	Frequent soft stools with blood and mucus (in severe cases, watery stools), flatulence, distention, abdominal cramps, fever, leukocytes in stool
Cryptosporidium	2-10 days	1-6 months	Watery diarrhea, nausea, vomiting, abdominal cramps, weight loss in AIDS

AIDS, Acquired immunodeficiency syndrome.

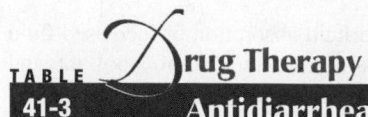

TABLE 41-3　Drug Therapy: Antidiarrheal Drugs

TYPE	MECHANISM OF ACTION	EXAMPLES
Demulcent	Soothes, coats, and protects mucous membranes	bismuth subsalicylate* (Pepto-Bismol); calcium polycarbophil (Mitrolan-OTC); activated charcoal; kaolin,[†] pectin, hyoscyamine sulfate, and hyoscine hydrobromide (Donnagel)*[†]; Donnagel and opium (Donnagel-PG)*[†]
Anticholinergic	Inhibits GI motility	Donnagel,*[†] Donnagel-PG,*[†] diphenoxylate with atropine sulfate (Lomotil, Colonaid), loperamide (Imodium)[†‡]
Antisecretory	Decreases intestinal secretion	octreotide (Sandostatin), a synthetic analog of somatostatin
Narcotic	Decreases CNS stimulation of GI tract motility and secretion; directly inhibits GI motility	camphorated tincture of opium (paregoric); Donnagel-PG[†]; paregoric, pectin, and kaolin (Parepectolin)[†]; tincture of opium, homatropine methylbromide, and pectin (Dia-Quel liquid OTC)[§]

*Also inhibits bacterial activity.
[†]Also absorbent, which contributes to the adhesiveness of the stool.
[‡]Has cholinergic and noncholinergic actions.
[§]Also an anticholinergic
CNS, Central nervous system; GI, gastrointestinal.

strains of *C. difficile* release a toxin that causes mucosal damage, resulting in cramping, pain, and diarrhea that may be bloody. *C. difficile* infection can also result in pseudomembranous enterocolitis and intestinal perforation.[1] Vancomycin (Vancocin) or metronidazole (Flagyl) is used to treat *C. difficile*.

NURSING MANAGEMENT
ACUTE INFECTIOUS DIARRHEA

■ Nursing Assessment

Nursing assessment should begin with a thorough history and physical examination (Table 41-4). The patient should be asked to describe the stool pattern and associated symptoms. Questions should focus on the duration, frequency, character, and consistency of stool. A medication history should include use of antibi-

otics, laxatives, and other drugs known to cause diarrhea. Recent travel, stress, and health and family illnesses should be discussed. Dietary history should include questions about eating habits, appetite, and food intolerances, especially milk and dairy products, and food preparation practices.

Physical examination begins with obtaining vital signs, height, and weight. The patient's skin should be inspected for decreased turgor, dryness, and areas of breakdown. The abdomen should be inspected for distention, auscultated for bowel sounds, and palpated for tenderness.

■ Nursing Diagnoses

Nursing diagnoses for the patient with acute infectious diarrhea may include, but are not limited to, those presented in NCP 41-1 on the facing page.

TABLE 41-4　Nursing Assessment: Diarrhea

Subjective Data
Important Health Information
Past health history: Recent travel, infections, stress; diverticulitis or malabsorption; metabolic disorders; inflammatory bowel disease; irritable bowel syndrome
Medications: Use of laxatives, magnesium-containing antacids, sorbitol-containing suspensions or elixirs, antibiotics, methyldopa, digitalis, colchicine; OTC antidiarrheal medications
Surgery or other treatments: Stomach or bowel surgery, radiation
Functional Health Patterns
Health perception–health management: Chronic laxative abuse, malaise
Nutritional-metabolic: Ingestion of coarse and spicy foods, food intolerances; anorexia, nausea, vomiting; weight loss; thirst
Elimination: Increased stool frequency, volume, and looseness; change in color and character of stools; abdominal bloating; decreased urinary output
Cognitive-perceptual: Abdominal tenderness, abdominal pain and cramping; tenesmus

Objective Data
General
Lethargy, sunken eyeballs, fever, malnutrition
Integumentary
Pallor, dry mucous membranes, poor skin turgor, perianal irritation
Gastrointestinal
Frequent soft to liquid stools that may alternate with constipation; altered stool color; abdominal distention, hyperactive bowel sounds; presence of pus, blood, mucus, or fat in stools; fecal impaction
Urinary Tract
Decreased output, concentrated urine
Possible Findings
Abnormal serum electrolyte levels; anemia; leukocytosis; eosinophilia, hypoalbuminemia; positive stool cultures; presence of ova, parasites, leukocytes, blood, or fat in stool; abnormal sigmoidoscopic or colonoscopic findings; abnormal lower GI series

GI, Gastrointestinal; OTC, over-the-counter.

NURSING CARE PLAN 41-1

Patient with Acute Infectious Diarrhea

EXPECTED PATIENT OUTCOMES	NURSING INTERVENTIONS and *RATIONALES*
NURSING DIAGNOSIS	**Diarrhea** *related to* acute infectious process *as manifested by* frequent loose, watery stools
• Normal bowel elimination • Afebrile	• Monitor frequency, amount, color, and consistency of stools *to determine severity of diarrhea and need for intervention.* • Follow hospital procedure for infection control precautions; use strict medical asepsis when handling bedpan, linens, or patient *to prevent spread of infection.* • Administer antiinfective and antidiarrheal medications as ordered *to treat bacterial infection and relieve diarrhea.*
NURSING DIAGNOSIS	**Deficient fluid volume** *related to* excessive fluid loss and decreased fluid intake secondary to diarrhea *as manifested by* dry skin and mucous membranes, poor skin turgor, hypotension, tachycardia, decreased urine output, electrolyte imbalances
• Normal vital signs • Normal skin turgor • Moist mucous membranes • Urine output >0.5 ml/kg/hr • Normal serum electrolytes	• Assess for skin turgor changes, sunken eyes, rapid pulse, and anorexia *as indicators of fluid volume deficit.* • Monitor intake and output *to determine fluid balance.* • Monitor serum sodium and potassium levels *so that abnormalities can be reported to the health care provider.* • Monitor vital signs q4hr *because changes can indicate hypovolemia.* • Weigh patient daily *to monitor fluid loss.* • Administer IV fluids as ordered and increase intake of fluids as tolerated to at least 3000 ml/day *to replace fluids and electrolytes lost in stools.* • Assess mouth for dryness and note patient's complaints of thirst *because dry mucous membranes and thirst are indicators of dehydration.* • If patient is not vomiting, administer oral fluids, such as Gatorade or Pedialyte, *to replace electrolytes lost in stools.*
NURSING DIAGNOSIS	**Impaired skin integrity** *related to* contact with diarrheal stools and inadequate perianal hygiene *as manifested by* redness, irritation, swelling, possible ulceration of skin, pain during defecation and urination
• No evidence of skin breakdown in perianal area	• Assess skin of perianal area *to plan appropriate interventions.* • Cleanse area with warm water after each bowel movement, rinse well, and dry with a soft towel *to prevent skin breakdown and promote patient comfort.* • Apply ointment (e.g., A and D, zinc oxide) *to protect skin and promote healing.* • Use an anesthetic ointment or spray foam *to decrease local discomfort.*

■ Planning

The overall goals are that the patient with diarrhea will (1) not transmit the microorganism causing the infectious diarrhea, (2) cease having diarrhea and resume normal bowel patterns, (3) have normal fluid and electrolyte and acid-base balance, (4) have normal nutritional intake, and (5) have no perianal skin breakdown.

■ Nursing Implementation

Adherence to infection control precautions for infectious diseases (see Table 12-19) is important because some cases of acute diarrhea are infectious. All cases of acute diarrhea should be considered infectious until the cause is determined. The use of precautions is effective in reducing the spread of infectious diarrhea.

Hand washing is the most important measure in preventing the transfer of microorganisms. Hands should be washed before and after contact with each patient and when body fluids of any kind are handled. The patient should be taught the principles of hygiene, infection control precautions, and the potential dangers of an illness that is infectious to themselves and others. Proper handling, cooking, and storage of food should be discussed with the patient suspected of having infectious diarrhea.

FECAL INCONTINENCE

Etiology and Pathophysiology

Fecal incontinence, or the involuntary passage of stool, may be due to multiple causes (Table 41-5). It is important to have an understanding of normal fecal continence to understand fecal incontinence. Normally, fecal contents pass from the sigmoid colon into the rectum, causing rectal distention. Sensory (stretch) receptors in the muscles surrounding the rectum provide the sensation of rectal filling. This causes a reflex relaxation of the internal anal sphincter and contraction of the external anal sphincter. Sensory receptors in the epithelium of the anal canal can usually distinguish among solid, liquid, and gas. The combination of contraction of the abdominal muscles, relaxation of the pelvic muscles, squatting (which straightens the anorectal angle), and voluntary relaxation of the external anal sphincter allows for

TABLE 41-5	Causes of Fecal Incontinence

Traumatic
Anorectal surgery
Fistulectomy
Hemorrhoidectomy
Postabdominal surgery

Neurologic
Degenerative diseases
Dementia
Diabetes mellitus (secondary to neuropathic changes)
Multiple sclerosis
Spinal cord injuries
Spinal cord tumor
Stroke

Inflammatory
Infection
Radiation
Trauma

Other
Diarrhea
Fecal impaction
Loss of rectal elasticity

Pelvic Floor Dysfunction
Medications
Rectal prolapse

Functional
Physical or mobility impairments affecting toileting ability

elimination of feces. Therefore motor (contraction of muscles) or sensory (ability to perceive presence of stool or to experience the urge to defecate) problems or their combination can result in fecal incontinence. In addition, fecal incontinence can be secondary to **fecal impaction,** which is an accumulation of hardened feces in the rectum or sigmoid colon that the individual is unable to move. Fecal incontinence caused by fecal impaction is a common problem in older adults.

Diagnostic Studies and Collaborative Care

The diagnosis and effective management of fecal incontinence require a thorough health history and physical examination with appropriate diagnostic studies. In all cases a rectal examination should be performed, followed by examination with a flexible sigmoidoscope. Fecal impaction, internal prolapse, increased perineal descent, and rectocele may be identified by rectal examination. If the impaction is higher in the colon, an abdominal x-ray may be helpful. Flexible sigmoidoscopy may identify inflammation, tumors, fissures, and other sigmoid-rectum pathologic conditions. Other studies may include barium enema, colonoscopy, and anorectal manometry.

Treatment of incontinence depends on the underlying cause. If fecal incontinence is related to noninfectious diarrhea, antidiarrheal agents may be prescribed. For example, loperamide (Imodium) may be useful in reducing diarrhea and increasing sphincter tone.

Fecal impaction usually resolves after manual disimpaction and cleansing enemas. To prevent recurrence, a high-fiber diet (see Table 41-9 later in this chapter), along with increased fluid intake, should be given unless contraindicated. Dietary fiber supplements or bulk-forming laxatives (e.g., psyllium in Metamucil) can improve continence by increasing stool bulk, firming consistency, and promoting sensation of rectal filling.[2] Perianal pouching or disposable pads or briefs provide containment of stool, protect skin, and promote comfort and dignity.

Biofeedback therapy is aimed at improving awareness of rectal sensation and coordination of the internal and external anal sphincters and increasing the strength of contraction of the external sphincter.[3] Biofeedback training requires adequate mental status and motivation to learn. Components of biofeedback include education, reinforcement, and concentration. It is a safe, painless, and inexpensive treatment for fecal incontinence. (Biofeedback is discussed further in Chapter 7.)

Surgery (e.g., sphincter repair procedures) should be considered only when conservative treatment fails, in cases of full-thickness prolapse, and when the sphincter needs repair.

NURSING MANAGEMENT
FECAL INCONTINENCE

■ Nursing Assessment

Fecal incontinence is not only an embarrassment to the patient but also a potential hazard to normal skin integrity. An assessment of the patient's general condition is necessary to identify the best alternative for managing the patient with fecal incontinence. The health care provider should identify normal bowel habits and current symptoms, including stool frequency and consistency. Information about the passage of blood or mucus, pain during defecation, and a feeling of incomplete evacuation is sought. The health care provider determines whether the patient has defecation urgency and is aware of leaking stool. The coexistence of urinary incontinence should be determined.[4]

A neurologic assessment that includes evaluation of mental status can be helpful in identifying the most effective treatment for the patient. Assessment should also include history of multiple or traumatic childbirths, previous anorectal surgery, and injury.

■ Nursing Diagnoses

Nursing diagnoses for the patient with fecal incontinence include, but are not limited to, the following:

- Bowel incontinence *related to* inability to control bowel function
- Toileting self-care deficit *related to* inability to manage bowel evacuation voluntarily
- Risk for situational low self-esteem *related to* inability to control bowel movements
- Risk for impaired skin integrity *related to* incontinence of stool
- Social isolation *related to* inability to control bowel functions

■ Planning

The overall goals are that the patient with fecal incontinence will (1) have normal bowel control, (2) maintain perianal skin integrity, and (3) not suffer any self-esteem problems related to problems with bowel control.

■ Nursing Implementation

Prevention and treatment of fecal incontinence may be managed by implementing a bowel training program. Bowel training is effective in many patients because once the bowel is empty the rectum does not fill until the next day. The lack of stool in the rectum reduces the likelihood of incontinence. The patient should be put on a bedpan, assisted to a bedside commode, or walked to the bathroom at a regular time daily to assist with reestablishment of bowel regularity. A good time to establish this pattern is within 30 minutes after breakfast. Most individuals experience an urge to defecate following the first meal of the day because of the gastrocolic reflex. If the usual bowel habits differ from this pattern, efforts should be made to adhere to the patient's individual timing.

If these techniques are ineffective in reestablishing bowel regularity, a bisacodyl (Dulcolax), glycerin suppository, or a small phosphate enema may be administered 15 to 30 minutes before the usual evacuation time. These preparations stimulate the anorectal reflex and often can be discontinued when a regular pattern is reestablished.

Maintenance of skin integrity is of utmost importance, especially in the bedridden and older adult patient. Nursing management may necessitate the use of drainage tubes or catheters, incontinence briefs, and meticulous skin care. Rectal tubes and catheters are usually not recommended because their use for an extended period may decrease responsiveness of the rectal sphincter and cause ulceration of the rectal mucosa. Use of incontinence briefs may be helpful in maintaining skin integrity if changed frequently, but this can be demeaning and humiliating to the patient. Meticulous cleaning after each stool is required. Washing, rinsing, thorough drying, and application of a protective barrier are essential to the maintenance of skin integrity. Because the patient may have several stools each day, maintaining skin integrity is a time-consuming task for the nurse and the family.

Perianal pouching is an alternative in the management of fecal incontinence. Pouching provides skin protection and fecal containment, as well as comfort and dignity. Because odor is often a problem, deodorant sprays and room deodorizers may be used. For the patient who is ambulatory, a regular chair or special commode wheelchair may be used. Regardless of the patient's mobility, the nurse must make sure the skin is clean, odorless, and intact.

CONSTIPATION

Constipation is a decrease in frequency of bowel movements from what is "normal" for the individual; hard, difficult-to-pass stools; a decrease in stool volume; and retention of feces in the rectum. Normal bowel elimination may vary from three times a day to once every 3 days.[4] Because of this variability, it is important to determine the severity of constipation on the basis of the patient's normal pattern of elimination. It is important to remember that changes in bowel habits may also indicate bowel obstruction produced by a tumor.

Etiology and Pathophysiology

Often constipation may be due to insufficient dietary fiber, inadequate fluid intake, medications, and lack of exercise. If proper preventive measures are subsequently taken, constipation should

TABLE 41-6	Causes of Constipation
Colonic Disorders	**Systemic Disorders**
Luminal or extraluminal obstructing lesions	***Metabolic/Endocrine***
Inflammatory strictures	Diabetes mellitus
Volvulus	Hypothyroidism
Intussusception	Pregnancy
Irritable bowel syndrome	Hypercalcemia/ hyperparathyroidism
Diverticular disease	Pheochromocytoma
Rectocele	***Collagen Vascular Disease***
	Systemic sclerosis (scleroderma)
Drug Induced	Amyloidosis
Antacids (calcium and aluminum)	***Neurologic Disorders***
Antidepressants	Hirschsprung's megacolon
Anticholinergics	Neurofibromatosis
Antipsychotics	Autonomic neuropathy (secondary to diabetes mellitus)
Antihypertensives	
Barium sulfate	Multiple sclerosis
Iron supplements	Parkinson's disease
Bismuth	Spinal cord lesions or injury
Calcium supplements	Stroke
Laxative abuse	

not recur. Constipation may also be due to sociocultural beliefs, environmental constraints, ignoring the urge to defecate, chronic laxative abuse, and multiple organic causes (Table 41-6). Changes in diet, mealtime, or daily routines are a few environmental factors that may cause constipation. Depression and stress can also result in constipation. For many patients with constipation, however, it is not possible to identify the underlying cause.[5]

Some patients believe that they are constipated if they do not have a daily bowel movement. This can result in chronic laxative use and subsequent cathartic colon syndrome. In this condition, the colon becomes dilated and *atonic* (lacking muscle tone).

Ignoring the urge to defecate for a period of time causes the muscles and mucosa in the rectal area to become insensitive to the presence of feces. In addition, the prolonged retention of feces in the rectum results in drying of stool because of the absorption of water. The harder and drier the feces, the more difficult it is to expel.

Clinical Manifestations

The clinical presentation of constipation may vary from a chronic discomfort to an acute event mimicking an "acute abdomen." Other clinical manifestations are presented in Table 41-7. Hemorrhoids are the most common complication of chronic constipation. They result from venous engorgement caused by repeated Valsalva maneuvers (straining) and venous compression from hard impacted stool.

Valsalva maneuver, which occurs during straining to pass a hardened stool, may cause serious problems in patients with congestive heart failure, cerebral edema, hypertension, and coronary artery disease. During straining, the patient takes a deep inspiration, the breath is held, and the glottis closes and traps the air. The abdominal muscles contract and try to push against the colon. Increases in intraabdominal pressure and in-

TABLE 41-7 Clinical Manifestations of Constipation

Abdominal distention/bloating
Abdominal pain
Anorexia
Decreased frequency of bowel movements
Hard, dry stool
Headache
Increased flatulence
Increased rectal pressure
Nausea
Palpable mass
Stone or rock-shaped stool
Stool with blood
Straining
Tenesmus

trathoracic pressure occur, reducing venous return to the heart. The heart slows temporarily (bradycardia), the cardiac output is decreased, and there is a transient drop in arterial pressure. When the patient relaxes, there is decreased thoracic pressure and a sudden flow of blood into the heart, causing distention and an increase in heart rate. Immediately the arterial pressure rises momentarily. These changes may be fatal for the patient who

cannot compensate for sudden overload of blood flow returning to the heart.

Diverticulosis is another potential complication of chronic constipation. This is a relatively common complication in an older adult. Diverticula or outpouchings of the colon wall are thought to be due to the increased intraluminal pressure needed to expel hard stool. Diverticulosis and diverticulitis are described later in this chapter.

In the presence of *obstipation,* or fecal impaction secondary to constipation, colonic perforation may occur. Perforation, which is life threatening, causes abdominal pain, nausea, vomiting, fever, and an elevated WBC count. An abdominal x-ray shows the presence of free air, which is diagnostic of perforation. Rectal mucosal ulcers may also occur as a result of stool stasis or straining. These complications are most common in older patients.

Diagnostic Studies and Collaborative Care

A thorough history and physical examination should be performed so that the underlying cause of constipation can be identified and treatment started. Abdominal x-rays, barium enema, colonoscopy, sigmoidoscopy, and anorectal manometry may be helpful in the diagnosis. Most cases of constipation can be managed with diet therapy including fiber and fluids and an exercise program. Laxatives (Table 41-8) should always be used cautiously because with chronic overuse they may become a cause of constipation. A stepwise approach for laxative use that pro-

TABLE 41-8 Drug Therapy Cathartic Agents

CATEGORY	MECHANISMS OF ACTION	EXAMPLE	ONSET OF ACTION	COMMENTS
• Bulk forming	Absorbs water; increases bulk, thereby stimulating peristalsis	Metamucil, Perdiem, Konsyl, Hydrocil, Citrucel, FiberCon	Usually within 24 hr	Contraindicated in patients with abdominal pain, nausea, and vomiting and in patients suspected of having appendicitis, biliary tract obstruction, or acute hepatitis; must be taken with fluids
• Stool softeners and lubricants	Lubricate intestinal tract and soften feces, making hard stools easier to pass; do not affect peristalsis	Mineral oil, dioctyl sodium, sulfosuccinate, Colace, Peri-Colace, Doxidan	Softeners up to 72 hr, lubricants up to 8 hr	Can block absorption of fat-soluble vitamins such as vitamin K, which may increase risk of bleeding in patients on anticoagulants
• Saline and osmotic solutions	Cause retention of fluid in intestinal lumen caused by osmotic effect	Magnesium salts: magnesium citrate, Milk of Magnesia; Sodium phosphates: Fleet enema, Phospho-Soda; Lactulose; Polyethylene glycol saline solutions; Go-Lytely, Colyte	15 min to 3 hr	Magnesium-containing products may cause hypermagnesemia in patients with renal insufficiency
• Stimulants	Increase peristalsis by irritating colon wall and stimulating enteric nerves	Antraquinone drugs: cascara sagrada, senna; Phenolphthalein drugs: Ex-Lax, Correctol, Feen-a-Mint, bisacodyl, Dulcolax	Usually within 12 hr	Cause melanosis coli (brown or black pigmentation of colon); are most widely abused laxatives; should not be used in patients with impaction or obstipation

gresses from bulk-forming fiber preparations to stimulants is recommended, depending on the acuteness of the constipation episode.[6] Enemas are fast acting and are beneficial in the immediate treatment of constipation, but they should be limited in their use for long-term treatment of constipation. Soapsuds enemas should be avoided because they may lead to inflammation of colon mucosa. Excessive hypotonic enemas with tap water can cause water excess, and sodium phosphate enemas have been associated with electrolyte imbalances. Oil-retention enemas may be used to soften fecal impactions. Biofeedback therapy may benefit patients who are constipated as a result of *anismus* (uncoordinated contraction of the anal sphincter during straining).[7]

For the patient in whom perceived constipation is related to rigid beliefs regarding bowel function, the nurse should initiate a discussion about these beliefs with the patient. Appropriate information on normal bowel function needs to be given and discussed along with the adverse consequences of excessive use of laxatives and enemas.

A patient with severe constipation related to bowel motility or mechanical disorders may require more intensive treatment. Diagnostic studies such as anorectal manometry, GI tract transit studies, and sigmoidoscopic rectal biopsies should be performed before treatment. In a patient with unrelenting constipation, a subtotal colectomy with ileorectal anastomosis is the procedure of choice.

Nutritional Therapy. Diet is an important factor in the prevention of constipation. Many patients experience an improvement in their symptoms when they simply increase their intake of dietary fiber and fluids.[8] Dietary fiber is found in two forms: insoluble and soluble in water. Both are contained in most foods, but some foods are higher in soluble fiber (Table 41-9).

Insoluble fiber, which is found in higher concentrations in whole wheat and bran, remains essentially unchanged by the time it reaches the colon. Soluble fibers form gel-like substances that add viscosity to the digested contents, causing decreased gastric emptying and increased transit in the small intestine. When these fibers are fermented, they increase stool bulk, promoting defecation and sequestering fluid, which softens stools. Soluble fiber is found in oat bran, fruits, vegetables, and psyllium. Patients should be told that initially fiber will increase gas production but that this effect decreases with time.

The diet should also include a fluid intake of at least 3000 ml per day, unless contraindicated by cardiac or renal disease. Increasing fiber intake without increasing fluids may predispose the patient to impaction or obstruction. The nurse should encourage the selection of foods that the patient likes, is able to prepare, and can afford. The patient's understanding of the diet and the importance of dietary fiber is important to ensure compliance.

NURSING MANAGEMENT
CONSTIPATION

■ Nursing Assessment

Subjective and objective data that should be obtained from a patient with constipation are presented in Table 41-10.

■ Nursing Diagnoses

Nursing diagnosis for the patient with constipation includes, but is not limited to, the following:
- Constipation *related to* inadequate intake of dietary fiber and fluid and decreased physical activity

TABLE 41-9 Nutritional Therapy — High-Fiber Foods*

	FIBER PER SERVING (G)	SIZE OF SERVING	CALORIES PER SERVING
Vegetables			
Asparagus	3.5	½ cup	18
Beans			
Navy	8.4	½ cup	80
Kidney	9.7	½ cup	94
Lima	8.3	½ cup	63
Pinto	8.9	½ cup	78
String	2.1	½ cup	18
Broccoli	3.5	½ cup	18
Carrots, raw	1.8	½ cup	15
Corn	2.6	½ medium ear	72
Peas, canned	6.7	½ cup	63
Potatoes			
Baked	1.9	½ medium	72
Sweet	2.1	½ medium	79
Squash			
Acorn	7.0	1 cup	82
Tomato, raw	1.5	1 small	18
Fruits			
Apple	2.0	½ large	42
Banana	1.5	½ medium	48
Blackberries	6.7	¾ cup	40
Orange	1.6	1 small	35
Peach	2.3	1 medium	38
Pear	2.0	½ medium	44
Raspberries	9.2	1 cup	42
Strawberries	3.1	1 cup	45
Grain Products			
Bread			
Rye	0.8	1 slice	62
White	0.7	1 slice	64
Whole wheat	1.3	1 slice	59
Cereal			
All Bran (100%)	8.4	⅓ cup	70
Corn Flakes	2.6	¾ cup	70
Shredded Wheat	2.8	1 biscuit	70
Crackers			
Graham	1.4	2 squares	53
Popcorn	3.0	3 cups	62
Rice			
Brown	1.6	⅓ cup	72
White	0.5	⅓ cup	76

*Recommended for patients with diverticulosis, irritable bowel syndrome, constipation, hemorrhoids, colon cancer, atherosclerosis, hyperlipidemia, and diabetes mellitus.

■ Planning

The overall goals are that the patient with constipation will (1) increase dietary intake of fiber and fluids; (2) have the passage of soft, formed stools; and (3) not have any complications, such as bleeding hemorrhoids.

TABLE 41-10	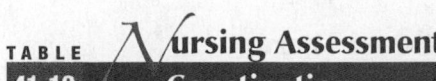 Nursing Assessment Constipation

Subjective Data

Important Health Information*

Past health history: Colorectal disease, neurologic dysfunction, bowel obstruction, environmental changes, cancer, irritable bowel syndrome

Medications: Use of aluminum and calcium antacids, anticholinergics, antidepressants, antihistamines, antipsychotics, diuretics, narcotics, iron, laxatives, enemas

Functional Health Patterns

Health perception–health management: Chronic laxative or enema abuse; rigid beliefs regarding bowel function; malaise

Nutritional-metabolic: Changes in diet or mealtime; inadequate fiber and fluid intake; anorexia, nausea

Elimination: Change in usual elimination patterns; hard, difficult-to-pass stool, decrease in frequency and amount of stools; flatus, abdominal distention; tenesmus, rectal pressure; fecal incontinence (if impacted)

Activity-exercise: Change in daily activity routines; immobility; sedentary lifestyle

Cognitive-perceptual: Dizziness, headache, anorectal pain; abdominal pain on defecation

Coping–stress tolerance: Acute or chronic stress

Objective Data

General

Lethargy

Integumentary

Anorectal fissures, hemorrhoids, abscesses

Gastrointestinal

Abdominal distention; hypoactive or absent bowel sounds; palpable abdominal mass; fecal impaction; small, hard, dry stool; stool with blood

Possible Findings

Guaiac-positive stools; abdominal x-ray demonstrating stool in lower colon

*See Table 41-6.

■ Nursing Implementation

Nursing management should be based on the patient's symptoms (see Table 41-7) and the assessment of the patient (see Table 41-10). An important role of the nurse is teaching the patient the importance of dietary measures to prevent constipation. A patient and family teaching guide for constipation is presented in Table 41-11. Emphasis should be placed on maintenance of a high-fiber diet, increasing fluid intake, and a regular exercise program. The patient should be taught to establish a regular time to defecate and not to suppress the urge to defecate. In many persons the urge to defecate occurs after breakfast because of the stimulation of the gastrocolic reflex. The patient should be discouraged from using laxatives and enemas to achieve fecal elimination.

Proper position is important when defecating. For a patient in bed, the bedpan should be placed and the head of the bed should be elevated as high as the patient can tolerate. For the person who can sit on a toilet, a footstool may be placed in front of the toilet. Placing the feet on the footstool promotes flexion of the thighs, which assists in defecation.

The patient with poor muscle tone should be encouraged to exercise the abdominal muscles and can be taught to contract the abdominal muscles several times a day. Sit-ups and straight leg raises can also be used to improve abdominal muscle tone.

TABLE 41-11	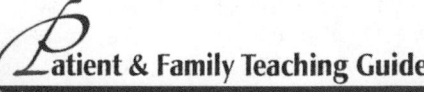 Patient & Family Teaching Guide Constipation

The following are teaching guidelines for the patient and family:

1. **Eat dietary fiber**
   Eat 20 to 30 g of fiber per day. Gradually increase the amount of fiber eaten over 1 to 2 weeks. Fiber softens hard stools and adds bulk to stool, promoting evacuation.
   - Foods high in fiber: raw vegetables and fruits, beans, breakfast cereals (All Bran, oatmeal)
   - Fiber supplements: Metamucil, Citrucel, FiberCon

2. **Drink fluids**
   Drink 3 quarts per day. Drink water or fruit juices; avoid caffeinated coffee, tea, and cola. Fluid softens hard stools; caffeine stimulates fluid loss through urination.

3. **Exercise regularly**
   Walk, swim, or bike at least 3 times per week. Contract and relax abdominal muscles when standing or by doing sit-ups to strengthen muscles and prevent straining. Exercise stimulates bowel motility and moves stool through the intestine.

4. **Establish a regular time to defecate**
   First thing in the morning or after the first meal of the day is a good time because people often have the urge to defecate at this time.

5. **Do not delay defecation**
   Respond to the urge to have a bowel movement as soon as possible. Delaying defecation results in hard stools and a decreased "urge" to defecate. Water is absorbed from stool by the intestine over time. The intestine becomes less sensitive to the presence of stool in the rectum.

6. **Record your bowel elimination pattern**
   Develop a habit of recording when you have a bowel movement on your calendar. Regular monitoring of bowel movement will assist in early identification of a problem.

7. **Avoid laxatives and enemas**
   Do not overuse laxatives and enemas because they can actually cause constipation. The normal motility of the bowel is interrupted, and bowel movements slow or stop.

ACUTE ABDOMINAL PAIN

Etiology and Pathophysiology

The causes of an acute onset of abdominal pain are varied (Table 41-12).

Clinical Manifestations

Pain is the most common presenting symptom. The patient may also complain of abdominal tenderness, vomiting, diarrhea, constipation, flatulence, fatigue, fever, and an increase in abdominal girth.

TABLE 41-12 Causes of Acute Abdominal Pain	
Abdominal penetrating trauma	Pancreatitis
Acute ischemic bowel injury	Pelvic inflammatory disease
Appendicitis	Peptic ulcer
Bowel obstruction with perforation or necrosis	Perforated gastrointestinal malignancy
Cholecystitis	Peritonitis
Crohn's disease	Ruptured abdominal aneurysm
Diverticulitis with peritonitis	Ruptured ectopic pregnancy
Foreign body perforation	Ruptured ovarian cyst
Gastritis	Ulcerative colitis
Gastroenteritis	Uterine rupture
Mesenteric adenitis	Volvulus

Diagnostic Studies and Collaborative Management

Many disorders must be ruled out before a diagnosis is confirmed. Diagnosis begins with a complete history and physical examination. Physical examination should include a rectal and pelvic examination. A complete blood count (CBC), urinalysis, abdominal x-ray, and an electrocardiogram are done initially. Pregnancy tests should be performed in women of childbearing age who have acute abdominal pain to rule out ectopic pregnancy. The findings of these studies may provide some information about the cause of the acute abdomen.

Emergency management of the patient with acute abdominal pain is presented in Table 41-13. The goal of management is to identify and treat the cause. The health care provider attempts to make a differential diagnosis when the patient is seen with an acute abdomen because many causes of abdominal pain do not require surgery (see Table 41-12). It was previously thought that pain medication should be withheld because analgesics might obscure progression of clinical manifestations and impede diagnosis. Appropriate pain management that does not result in altered consciousness (e.g., ketorolac [Toradol]) can decrease diffuse pain and abdominal rigidity and help localize the pain. This can lead to earlier diagnosis and treatment.[9]

In addition to being a therapeutic measure, surgery can also be diagnostic. Operative exploration is usually done after a careful examination of the patient and is justified when "look and see" is better than "wait and see." The surgical procedure is an *ex-*

TABLE 41-13 Emergency Management Acute Abdominal Pain

ETIOLOGY	ASSESSMENT FINDINGS	INTERVENTIONS
Inflammation Appendicitis Cholecystitis Crohn's disease Gastritis Pancreatitis Pyelonephritis Ulcerative colitis	**Abdominal/Gastrointestinal Findings** • Diffuse, localized, dull, burning, or sharp abdominal pain or tenderness • Rebound tenderness • Abdominal distention • Abdominal rigidity • Nausea and vomiting • Diarrhea • Hematemesis • Melena	**Initial** • Ensure patent airway. • Administer oxygen via nasal cannula or non-rebreather mask. • Establish IV access with large-bore catheter and infuse warm normal saline or lactated Ringer's solution. Insert additional large-bore catheter if shock present. • Obtain blood for CBC and electrolytes. • Anticipate order for amylase level, pregnancy tests, clotting studies, and type and crossmatch as appropriate. • Insert indwelling urinary catheter. • Obtain urinalysis. • Insert NG tube as needed.
Vascular Problems Ruptured aortic aneurysm Mesenteric vascular occlusion	**Hypovolemic Shock** • ↓ Blood pressure • ↓ Pulse pressure • Tachycardia • Cool, clammy skin • ↓ Level of consciousness	
Gynecologic Problems Pelvic inflammatory disease Ruptured ectopic pregnancy Ruptured ovarian cyst		**Ongoing Monitoring** • Monitor vital signs, level of consciousness, O_2 saturation, and intake/output. • Assess quality and amount of pain. • Assess amount and character of emesis. • Anticipate surgical intervention. • Keep NPO.
Infectious Disease *Giardia* *Salmonella*		
Other Obstruction or perforation of abdominal organ Gastrointestinal bleeding Trauma		

CBC, Complete blood count; *IV,* intravenous; *NG,* nasogastric; *NPO,* nothing by mouth.

ploratory laparotomy, in which an opening is made through the abdominal wall into the peritoneal cavity to determine the cause of acute abdominal pain. If the cause of the acute abdomen can be surgically removed (e.g., inflamed appendix) or surgically repaired (e.g., ruptured abdominal aneurysm), surgery is considered definitive therapy.

NURSING MANAGEMENT
ACUTE ABDOMINAL PAIN

■ Nursing Assessment

Vital signs should be taken immediately. Blood pressure and pulse rate should be obtained to determine hypovolemic changes. An elevated temperature may indicate an inflammatory or infectious process. The abdomen should be inspected for distention, masses, abnormal pulsation, rashes, scars, and pigmentation changes. Bowel sounds should be auscultated. Bowel sounds that are diminished or absent in a quadrant may indicate a complete bowel obstruction, acute peritonitis, or paralytic ileus. Palpation should be gentle.

A thorough assessment of the patient's symptoms should be made to determine the onset, location, intensity, duration, frequency, and character of pain. The nurse should determine whether the pain has spread or moved to new locations (quadrants), as well as what makes the pain worse or better. It should also be determined whether the pain is associated with other symptoms, such as nausea, vomiting, changes in bowel and bladder habits, or vaginal discharge in women. Assessment of vomiting should include the amount, color, consistency, and odor of the vomitus. Bowel patterns and habits should also be assessed carefully.

■ Nursing Diagnoses

Nursing diagnoses for the patient with acute abdominal pain include, but are not limited to, the following:

- Acute pain *related to* inflammation of the peritoneum and abdominal distention
- Risk for deficient fluid volume *related to* collection of fluid in peritoneal cavity secondary to inflammation or infection
- Imbalanced nutrition: less than body requirements *related to* anorexia, nausea, and vomiting
- Anxiety *related to* uncertainty of cause or outcome of condition and pain

■ Planning

The overall goals are that the patient with acute abdominal pain will have (1) resolution of inflammation, (2) relief of abdominal pain, (3) freedom from complications (especially hypovolemic shock), and (4) normal nutritional status.

■ Nursing Implementation

Nursing interventions are based on the diagnosis and medical or surgical management of the patient. General care for the patient involves management of fluid and electrolyte imbalances, pain, and anxiety.

Acute Intervention

Preoperative care. Emergency preparation of the patient with acute abdominal pain is usually limited to a CBC, typing and crossmatching of blood, and clotting studies. Catheterization, preparation of the abdominal skin, and the passage of a nasogas-

tric (NG) tube may be done in the emergency department or operating room. (General care of the preoperative patient is discussed in Chapter 17.)

Postoperative care. Postoperative care depends on the type of surgical procedure performed. The increased use of laparoscopic procedures has reduced the risk of postoperative complications related to wound care and altered GI motility. These procedures generally result in shorter hospital stays.

A general nursing care plan for the postoperative patient is presented in Chapter 19. Nursing care for the patient following a laparotomy is presented in NCP 41-2.

An NG tube may or may not be present in the patient returning from surgery. If present, the NG tube is connected to suction as ordered. The purpose of the NG tube is to empty the stomach of secretions and gas to prevent gastric dilation. GI peristaltic activity is often impaired because of the manipulative procedures of the surgery and anesthesia. Low intermittent suctioning is ordered to prevent trauma to the gastric mucosa.

If the upper GI tract has been entered, drainage from the NG tube may be dark brown to dark red for the first 12 hours. Later it should be light yellowish brown, or it may have a greenish tinge because of the presence of bile. If a dark red color continues or if bright red blood is observed, the health care provider should be notified at once of the possibility of hemorrhage. "Coffee ground" granules in the drainage are due to the presence of small amounts of blood that have been chemically acted on by gastric secretions.

The NG tube is checked frequently for patency. The tube may become obstructed with mucus, sediment, or blood clots. An order is usually written to irrigate the tube with 20 to 30 ml of normal saline solution if needed. Repositioning the tube may facilitate drainage.

An accurate record of intake and output, including emesis and gastric drainage, is essential. The nurse assesses serum electrolyte values and acid-base balance because prolonged gastric suctioning can result in loss of sodium, chloride, potassium, water, and hydrochloric acid.

The NG tube is removed when intestinal peristalsis returns, usually 24 to 72 hours after surgery. Motility of the stomach normally returns within 24 to 48 hours. Motility of the small intestine usually resumes within 24 hours, whereas return of large intestine motility may take as long as 3 to 5 days. Peristaltic activity is assessed by auscultation for bowel sounds.

Mouth care and nasal care are essential. The patient tends to breathe through the mouth while the NG tube is in place. In addition, increased nasal secretions and crusting result from mechanical stimulation of the NG tube.

Parenteral fluids are administered to provide the patient with fluids and electrolytes until bowel sounds return. Occasionally, ice chips may be ordered because they aid in the flow of saliva and prevent a dry mouth. When bowel sounds return, fluids and food are increased gradually. The diet may be supplemented with multivitamins and iron.

Nausea and vomiting are not uncommon after abdominal surgery. These problems are often self-limiting. Observation is important in determining the cause. Antiemetics such as promethazine (Phenergan), ondansetron (Zofran), prochlorperazine (Compazine), or trimethobenzamide (Tigan) may be ordered.

Abdominal distention and gas pains are also common after surgery; these are due to swallowed air and impaired peristalsis

NURSING CARE PLAN 41-2

Patient Following Laparotomy

EXPECTED PATIENT OUTCOMES	NURSING INTERVENTIONS and *RATIONALES*
NURSING DIAGNOSIS	**Acute pain** *related to* surgical incision and inadequate pain control measures *as manifested by* complaints of pain, body posturing, unwillingness to move in bed or to ambulate
▪ Satisfactory level of pain control	▪ Assess for pain and give pain medication every 3 to 4 hr as ordered for first 72 hr *to treat pain appropriately.* ▪ Splint incision with pillows during coughing, deep breathing, and moving *to relieve pain while performing these activities.* ▪ Position patient comfortably *to relieve pain.*
NURSING DIAGNOSIS	**Nausea** *related to* decreased GI motility, GI distention, and narcotics *as manifested by* nausea, vomiting, lack of or diminished bowel sounds, abdominal distention
▪ Relief of nausea and vomiting.	▪ Administer antiemetic medications (as ordered) *to relieve nausea and vomiting.* ▪ Assess response to pain medications *to determine if this is a possible cause of nausea and vomiting.* ▪ Maintain patency of NG tube (if present) *to prevent accumulation of gastric secretions and subsequent vomiting.* ▪ Assess for bowel sounds and abdominal distention *to determine return of peristalsis.* ▪ Keep patient on NPO status until bowel sounds return *to prevent vomiting.* ▪ Limit unpleasant sights, smells, and stimuli *to prevent initiating episodes of nausea and vomiting.*
NURSING DIAGNOSIS	**Constipation** *related to* immobility, pain, medication, and decreased GI motility *as manifested by* decreased or absent bowel sounds, abdominal pain, abdominal distention, inability to pass flatus or stool
▪ Normal bowel sounds within 72 hr after surgery ▪ Soft, formed bowel movement within 4 days	▪ Assess abdomen for distention and bowel sounds every 8 hours *to determine need for intervention.* ▪ Administer stool softener (if ordered) *to soften fecal mass or promote elimination.* ▪ Encourage frequent position changes and ambulation as tolerated *to increase peristalsis.* ▪ Encourage increased fluid intake as tolerated *to soften fecal material.*

*General nursing care for the postoperative patient is presented in the NCP 19-1 in Chapter 19 on pp. 402-403.

resulting from immobility, manipulation of abdominal contents during surgery, and side effects of anesthesia. The pain can be so uncomfortable that drugs to stimulate peristalsis, such as bethanechol (Urecholine) or neostigmine methylsulfate (Prostigmin), may be given. A rectal tube or moist heat on the abdomen may be effective in relieving distention. The health care provider should be informed of abdominal distention and rigidity. Gradually, as intestinal activity increases, distention and gas pains decrease.

Ambulatory and Home Care. Preparation for discharge begins when the patient returns from the operating room. Instructions to the patient and the family should include any modifications in activity, care of the incision, diet, and drug therapy. Small, frequent meals high in calories should be taken initially, with a gradual increase in intake of food as tolerated.

Normal activities should be resumed gradually, with planned rest periods. The patient should be aware of possible complications after surgery and should notify the health care provider immediately if vomiting, pain, weight loss, incisional drainage, or changes in bowel function occur.

▪ Evaluation

The expected outcomes are that the patient with acute abdominal pain will have (1) resolution of the cause of the acute abdominal pain; (2) relief of abdominal pain and discomfort; (3) freedom from complications (especially hypovolemic shock

and septicemia); and (4) normal fluid, electrolyte, and nutritional status.

Chronic Abdominal Pain

Chronic abdominal pain may originate from abdominal structures or may be referred from a site with the same or a similar nerve supply. Some common causes are irritable bowel syndrome (IBS), peptic ulcer disease, diverticulitis, chronic pancreatitis, hepatitis, cholecystitis, pelvic inflammatory disease, and vascular insufficiency.

Diagnosis of chronic abdominal pain presents a challenge. Assessment should begin with a thorough history and identification of the specific pain pattern. Character and severity of pain, location, duration, and onset should be determined. The assessment should also include the relationship of pain to meals, defecation, and activity and factors that increase or decrease the pain. Chronic abdominal pain is often described as dull, aching, or diffuse.

Endoscopy, computed tomography (CT) scans, magnetic resonance imaging, laparoscopy, and radiologic barium studies have decreased the need for exploratory laparotomy. Treatment for chronic abdominal pain is comprehensive and directed toward palliation of symptoms using analgesics and antiemetics, as well as psychologic or behavioral therapies (e.g., relaxation therapies).

IRRITABLE BOWEL SYNDROME

Irritable bowel syndrome (IBS) is a symptom complex characterized by intermittent and recurrent abdominal pain associated with an alteration in bowel function (diarrhea or constipation). Other symptoms commonly found include abdominal distention, excessive flatulence, bloating, urge to defecate, urgency, and sensation of incomplete evacuation. IBS is a common problem affecting approximately 15% to 20% of the population in the United States.[10] In western societies, approximately 2 to 3 times as many women as men seek health care services for IBS. Stress, psychologic factors, and specific food intolerances have been identified as major factors that precipitate IBS symptoms.

The key to accurate diagnosis is a thorough history and physical examination. Emphasis should be on symptoms, past health history (including psychosocial aspects such as physical or sexual abuse), family history, and drug and dietary history. Diagnostic tests should be selectively used to rule out more serious life-threatening disorders with symptoms similar to those of IBS, such as colorectal cancer, peptic ulcer disease, inflammatory bowel disease, and malabsorption disorders. Symptom-based criteria for IBS have been standardized and are referred to as the Rome criteria.[10]

The health care provider should establish a trusting relationship with the patient at the onset of treatment. The patient should be encouraged to verbalize concerns and anxiety. A diet containing at least 20 g per day of dietary fiber should be initiated (see Table 41-9). This may also include the addition of psyllium-containing products (e.g., Metamucil).

The patient whose primary symptoms are abdominal distention and increased flatulence should be advised to eliminate common gas-producing foods such as broccoli and cabbage from the diet and to substitute yogurt for milk products if there is lactose intolerance. Anticholinergic agents, such as dicyclomine (Bentyl), may be helpful if taken before meals to alleviate the pain associated with ingestion of food. Alosetron (Lotronex) is used to treat IBS that causes diarrhea and severe pain in women who have failed other therapies. Its use must be monitored closely because of side effects. Tegaserod (Zelnorm) recently has been approved to treat women with IBS whose primary bowel symptom is constipation. It increases the movement of stools through the colon. Other therapies include relaxation and stress management techniques, acupuncture, and Chinese herbs although no single therapy has been found to be effective for all patients with IBS.

ABDOMINAL TRAUMA

Etiology and Pathophysiology

Injuries to the abdominal area most often occur as a result of blunt trauma (e.g., motor vehicle accident) or penetration injuries, primarily gunshot wounds or stab wounds to the abdomen. Blunt trauma is most common. Regardless of whether it is a blunt or penetration injury, the result is often the same damage to or alteration of the internal organs.

Common injuries of the abdomen include lacerated liver, ruptured spleen, pancreatic trauma, mesenteric artery tears, diaphragmatic rupture, urinary bladder rupture, great vessel tears, renal injury, and stomach or intestinal rupture. These injuries may result in massive blood loss and hypovolemic shock. Surgery must be performed as early as possible to repair the damaged organs and to stop the bleeding. Common sequelae of intraabdominal trauma are peritonitis and sepsis, particularly when the bowel is perforated.

Clinical Manifestations

Clinical manifestations of abdominal trauma are (1) guarding and splinting of the abdominal wall; (2) a hard, distended abdomen (indicating intraabdominal bleeding); (3) decreased or absent bowel sounds; (4) contusions, abrasions, or bruising over the abdomen; (5) abdominal pain; (6) pain over the scapula caused by irritation of the phrenic nerve by free blood in the abdomen; (7) hematemesis or hematuria; and (8) signs of hypovolemic shock (Table 41-14). An ecchymotic discoloration around the umbilicus (Cullen sign) can indicate intraabdominal or retroperitoneal hemorrhage.

Intraabdominal injuries are often associated with low rib fractures, fractured femur, fractured pelvis, and thoracic injury. If any of these injuries are present, the patient should be observed for abdominal trauma.

Diagnostic Studies

Specific diagnostic procedures include CBC, urinalysis, x-ray of the abdomen, CT scan, and peritoneal lavage. In peritoneal lavage the abdomen below the umbilicus is locally anesthetized, and a large angiocatheter or peritoneal dialysis catheter is inserted into the abdomen. A syringe is attached to the catheter, and an attempt is made to gently aspirate any blood. If less than 10 ml of blood is aspirated, a liter of saline solution is then infused into the abdomen and drained. The fluid is observed for gross abnormalities, especially blood, and is sent to the laboratory for microscopic evaluation. Positive findings may include (1) red blood cell count greater than $100,000/\mu l$; (2) WBC count greater than $500/\mu l$; (3) high amylase level; and (4) presence of bacteria, bile, or fecal material. If the results are positive, immediate surgery is indicated. If the results are negative, continued observation of the patient is warranted. An impaled object should never be removed until skilled care is available. Removal may cause further injury and bleeding.

NURSING *and* COLLABORATIVE MANAGEMENT ABDOMINAL TRAUMA

Emergency management of abdominal trauma focuses on establishing a patent airway and adequate breathing, fluid replacement, and prevention of hypovolemic shock (see Table 41-14). IV lines are inserted, and volume expanders or blood is given if the patient is hypotensive. An NG tube is inserted to decompress the stomach and prevent the aspiration of vomitus.

Regardless of the mechanism of injury, physical evidence of abdominal trauma in a patient who is hemodynamically unstable mandates immediate laparotomy. In other cases the indications for laparotomy must be correlated with the mechanism of injury. For example, if an individual has a gunshot wound or impaled object, surgery is usually indicated. If surgery is performed, the postoperative nursing care is similar to the care of the patient after laparotomy (see NCP 41-2).

Inflammatory Disorders

APPENDICITIS

Appendicitis is an inflammation of the appendix, a narrow blind tube that extends from the inferior part of the cecum. Appendicitis occurs in 7% to 12% of the world's population. Peak incidence is between the ages of 11 and 19 years, and males in this age group are afflicted more often than females.[11]

TABLE 41-14 Emergency Management

Abdominal Trauma

ETIOLOGY	ASSESSMENT FINDINGS	INTERVENTIONS
Blunt Falls Motor vehicle collisions Pedestrian event Assault with blunt object Crush injuries Explosions **Penetrating** Knife Gunshot wounds Other missiles	**Hypovolemic Shock** • ↓ Level of consciousness • Tachypnea • Tachycardia • ↓ Blood pressure • ↓ Pulse pressure **Surface Findings** • Abrasions or ecchymoses on abdominal wall, flank, or peritoneum • Open wounds: lacerations, eviscerations, puncture wounds, gunshot wounds • Impaled object • Healed incisions or old scars **Abdominal/Gastrointestinal Findings** • Nausea and vomiting • Bloody urine • Abdominal distention • Abdominal rigidity • Abdominal pain with palpation • Rebound tenderness • Pain radiation to shoulder and back	**Initial** • Ensure patent airway. • Administer O_2 via non-rebreather mask. • Control external bleeding with direct pressure or sterile pressure dressing. • Establish IV access with two large-bore catheters and infuse warm normal saline or lactated Ringer's solution. • Obtain blood for type and crossmatch and CBC. • Remove clothing. • Stabilize impaled objects with bulky dressing—*do not remove*. • Cover protruding organs or tissue with sterile, saline dressing. • Insert indwelling urinary catheter if there is no blood at the meatus, pelvic fracture, or boggy prostate. • Obtain urine for urinalysis. • Insert NG tube if no evidence of facial trauma. • Anticipate diagnostic peritoneal lavage. **Ongoing Monitoring** • Monitor vital signs, level of consciousness, O_2 saturation, and urine output. • Maintain patient warmth using blankets, warm IV fluids, or warm humidified oxygen.

CBC, Complete blood count; *IV*, intravenous, *NG*, nasogastric.

Etiology and Pathophysiology

The most common causes of appendicitis are obstruction of the lumen by a *fecalith* (accumulated feces) (Fig. 41-1), foreign bodies, tumor of the cecum or appendix, or intramural thickening caused by hypergrowth of lymphoid tissue. Obstruction results in distention, venous engorgement, and the accumulation of mucus and bacteria, which can lead to gangrene and perforation.[10]

Clinical Manifestations

Appendicitis typically begins with periumbilical pain, followed by anorexia, nausea, and vomiting. The pain is persistent and continuous, eventually shifting to the right lower quadrant and localizing at McBurney's point (located halfway between the umbilicus and the right iliac crest). Further assessment of the patient reveals localized tenderness, rebound tenderness, and muscle guarding. The patient usually prefers to lie still, often with the right leg flexed. Low-grade fever may or may not be present, and coughing aggravates pain. Rovsing's sign may be elicited by palpation of the left lower quadrant, causing pain to be felt in the right lower quadrant. Complications of acute appendicitis are perforation, peritonitis, and abscesses.

Diagnostic Studies and Collaborative Care

Examination of the patient includes a complete history and physical examination (particularly palpation of the abdomen) and a differential WBC count. A urinalysis may be done to rule

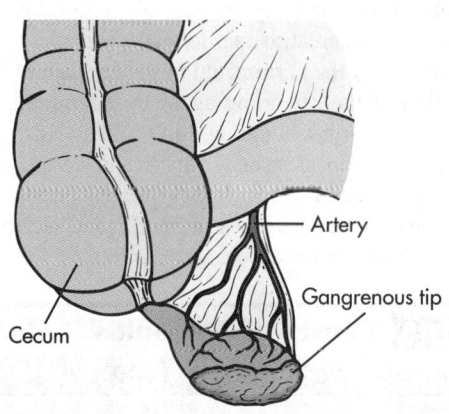

FIG. 41-1 In appendicitis the blood supply of the appendix is impaired by inflammation and bacterial infection in the wall of the appendix, which may result in gangrene.

out genitourinary conditions that mimic the manifestations of appendicitis.

The treatment of appendicitis is immediate surgical removal (appendectomy) if the inflammation is localized. If the appendix has ruptured and there is evidence of peritonitis or an abscess, conservative treatment, consisting of antibiotic therapy and parenteral fluids, may be used to prevent sepsis and dehydration for 6 to 8 hours before an appendectomy is performed.

NURSING MANAGEMENT
APPENDICITIS

The patient with abdominal pain is encouraged to see a health care provider and to avoid self-treatment, particularly the use of laxatives and enemas. The increased peristalsis from them may cause perforation of the appendix. Until the patient is seen by a health care provider, nothing should be taken by mouth (NPO) to ensure that the stomach is empty in the event that surgery is needed. An ice bag may be applied to the right lower quadrant to decrease the flow of blood to the area and impede the inflammatory process. Heat is never used because it may cause the appendix to rupture. Surgery is usually performed as soon as a diagnosis is made.

Postoperative nursing management is similar to postoperative care of the patient after laparotomy (see NCP 41-2). In addition, the patient should be observed for evidence of peritonitis. Ambulation begins the day of surgery or the first postoperative day. The diet is advanced as tolerated. The patient is usually discharged on the first or second postoperative day, and normal activities are resumed 2 to 3 weeks after surgery.

PERITONITIS
Etiology and Pathophysiology

Peritonitis results from a localized or generalized inflammatory process of the peritoneum. Causes of peritonitis are listed in Table 41-15. Peritonitis may appear in acute and chronic forms, and trauma or rupture of an organ containing chemical irritants or bacteria (which are released into the peritoneal cavity) may cause it. Examples of a chemical peritonitis include peptic ulcer perforation and ruptured ectopic pregnancy. A chemical peritonitis is commonly followed by bacterial invasion. Bacterial peritonitis can be caused by a traumatic injury (e.g., gunshot wound, ruptured appendix), or it can be secondary to other diseases or conditions (e.g., pancreatitis, peritoneal dialysis).

The response of the peritoneum to the leakage of GI contents is localization of the offending agent by attempting to "wall it off" by exuding fibrin-containing fluids and swelling. Adhesions may form. These adhesions may shrink and disappear when the infection is eliminated. Normally, peritoneal injuries heal without formation of adhesions unless other factors, such as infection, ischemia, or foreign substances, are present.

Clinical Manifestations

Abdominal pain is the most common symptom of peritonitis.[9] A universal sign of peritonitis is tenderness over the involved area. Rebound tenderness, muscular rigidity, and spasm are other major signs of irritation of the peritoneum. Abdominal distention or ascites, fever, tachycardia, tachypnea, nausea, vomiting, and altered bowel habits may also be present. These manifestations vary, depending on severity and acuteness of the underlying cause. Complications of peritonitis include hypovolemic shock, septicemia, intraabdominal abscess formation, paralytic ileus, and organ failure.

Diagnostic Studies

A CBC is done to determine elevations in WBC and hemoconcentration (Table 41-16). Peritoneal aspiration may be performed and the fluid analyzed for blood, bile, pus, bacteria, fungus, and amylase content. An x-ray of the abdomen may show dilated loops of bowel consistent with paralytic ileus, free air if perforation has occurred, or air and fluid levels if an obstruction is present. Ultrasound and CT scans may be useful in identifying the presence of ascites and abscesses. *Peritoneoscopy* (an endoscope is placed through a stab wound in the abdomen to inspect the peritoneum) may be helpful in the patient without ascites. Direct examination of the peritoneum can be obtained, along with biopsy specimens for diagnosis.

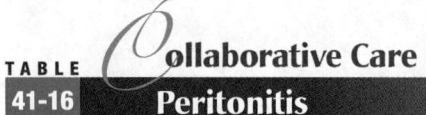

| TABLE 41-16 | Collaborative Care — Peritonitis |

Diagnostic
History and physical examination
CBC
Serum electrolytes
Abdominal x-ray
Abdominal paracentesis and culture of fluid
CT scan or ultrasound
Peritoneoscopy

Collaborative Therapy
Preoperative or Nonoperative
NPO status
Fluid replacement
Antibiotic therapy
NG suction
Analgesics
Preparation for surgery to include the above and total parenteral nutrition

Postoperative
NPO status
NG tube to low-intermittent suction
Semi-Fowler's position
IV fluids with electrolyte replacement
Total parenteral nutrition as needed
Antibiotic therapy
Blood transfusions as needed
Sedatives and narcotics

CBC, Complete blood count; *CT,* computed tomography; *IV,* intravenous; *NG,* nasogastric; *NPO,* nothing by mouth.

| TABLE 41-15 | Causes of Peritonitis |

PRIMARY	SECONDARY
Blood-borne organisms	Appendicitis with rupture
Genital tract organisms	Blunt or penetrating trauma to abdominal organs
Cirrhosis with ascites	Diverticulitis with rupture
	Ischemic bowel disorders
	Obstruction in the gastrointestinal tract
	Pancreatitis
	Perforated peptic ulcer
	Peritoneal dialysis
	Postoperative (breakage of anastomosis)

Collaborative Care

The goals of management of peritonitis are to identify and eliminate the cause, combat infection, and prevent complications. Patients with milder cases of peritonitis or those who are poor surgical risks may be managed nonsurgically. Treatment consists of antibiotics, NG suction, analgesics, and IV fluid administration. Patients who require surgery need preoperative preparation as previously described. Those patients may be placed on total parenteral nutrition (TPN) because of increased nutritional requirements.

NURSING MANAGEMENT
PERITONITIS

■ Nursing Assessment

Assessment of the patient's pain, including the location, is important and may help in determining the cause of peritonitis. The patient should be assessed for the presence and quality of bowel sounds, increasing abdominal distention, abdominal guarding, nausea, fever, and manifestations of hypovolemic shock.

■ Nursing Diagnoses

Nursing diagnoses for the patient with peritonitis include, but are not limited to, the following:
- Acute pain *related to* inflammation of the peritoneum and abdominal distention
- Risk for deficient fluid volume *related to* collection of fluid in peritoneal cavity secondary to trauma, infection, or ischemia
- Imbalanced nutrition: less than body requirements *related to* anorexia, nausea, and vomiting
- Anxiety *related to* uncertainty of cause or outcome of condition and pain

■ Planning

The overall goals are that the patient with peritonitis will have (1) resolution of inflammation, (2) relief of abdominal pain, (3) freedom from complications (especially hypovolemic shock), and (4) normal nutritional status.

■ Nursing Implementation

The patient with peritonitis is extremely ill and needs skilled supportive care. The patient is monitored for pain and response to analgesic therapy. The patient may be positioned with knees flexed to increase comfort. The nurse should provide rest and a quiet environment. Sedatives may be given to allay anxiety.

Accurate monitoring of fluid intake and output and electrolyte status is necessary to determine replacement therapy. Vital signs are monitored frequently. Antiemetics may be administered to decrease nausea and vomiting and further fluid losses. The patient is on NPO status and may have an NG tube in place to decrease gastric distention.

If the patient has an open surgical procedure, drains are inserted to remove purulent drainage and excessive fluid. Postoperative care of the patient is similar to the care of the patient with an exploratory laparotomy (see NCP 41-2).

GASTROENTERITIS

Gastroenteritis is an inflammation of the mucosa of the stomach and small intestine. Clinical manifestations include nausea, vomiting, diarrhea, abdominal cramping, and distention. Fever, increased WBC, and blood or mucus in the stool may be

present. Causative agents are varied (see Table 41-2). Most cases are self-limiting and do not require hospitalization. However, older adults and chronically ill patients may be unable to consume sufficient fluids orally to compensate for fluid loss. Until vomiting has ceased, the patient should be on NPO status. If dehydration has occurred, IV replacement of fluids may be necessary. As soon as tolerated, fluids containing glucose and electrolytes (e.g., Pedialyte) should be given. If the causative agent is identified, appropriate antibiotic, antimicrobial, or antiinfective drugs are given.

NURSING MANAGEMENT
GASTROENTERITIS

Accurate monitoring of intake and output is important for successful replacement of lost fluid. Strict medical asepsis and infection control precautions should be instituted when indicated. The patient should be instructed in the importance of proper food handling and preparation of food to prevent infections such as salmonellosis and trichinosis (see Chapter 40, Table 40-27).

Symptomatic nursing care is given for nausea, vomiting, and diarrhea. The importance of rest and increased fluid intake should be stressed. The nurse should assess complaints of pain, vomiting, and diarrhea because gastroenteritis is often confused with appendicitis. To allay the patient's apprehension, the nurse should explain that gastroenteritis usually runs an acute course with no sequelae.

Inflammatory Bowel Disease

Crohn's disease and ulcerative colitis are immunologically related disorders that are referred to as **inflammatory bowel disease** (IBD). These disorders are characterized by chronic, recurrent inflammation of the intestinal tract. For both conditions, the clinical manifestations are varied, with long periods of remission interspersed with episodes of acute inflammation. Both diseases can be debilitating.

Although there has been extensive research on the etiology of IBD, the cause of both ulcerative colitis and Crohn's disease remains unknown. Possible causes include (1) an infectious agent (e.g., virus, bacteria) because IBD produces mucosal changes in the colon similar to those of infectious diarrhea, although no consistent pathogen has been identified; (2) an autoimmune reaction from the presence of other immune-related disorders, such as systemic lupus erythematosus, ankylosing spondylitis, and erythema nodosum in patients with IBD; (3) food allergies (al-

CULTURAL & ETHNIC CONSIDERATIONS
Colon Disorders

- Inflammatory bowel disease (IBD) is more common among whites than African Americans and Asian Americans.
- IBD is more common among Jewish people and those of middle European origin.
- Colorectal cancer is higher in the United States and Canada than in Japan, Finland, or Africa.
- Incidence of colorectal cancer is declining in the United States except for African American men.

though this has not been substantiated); and (4) heredity. Both Crohn's disease and ulcerative colitis occur more commonly in families. It is likely that more than one of the above factors may be involved in the pathogenesis of IBS. For example, a patient who is genetically susceptible to IBD may develop active IBD after a viral GI infection. Studies of identical twins and siblings with IBS support that there is a genetic predisposition to IBD.[12]

ULCERATIVE COLITIS

Ulcerative colitis is characterized by inflammation and ulceration of the colon and rectum. It may occur at any age but peaks between the ages of 15 and 25 years. There is a second, smaller peak onset between 60 and 80 years of age. Ulcerative colitis equally affects both sexes.[13] It is more common in Jewish and upper-middle-class urban populations.

Etiology and Pathophysiology

The inflammation of ulcerative colitis is diffuse and involves the mucosa and submucosa, with alternate periods of exacerbations and remissions (Table 41-17). The disease usually begins in the rectum and sigmoid colon and spreads up the colon in a continuous pattern.

The mucosa of the colon is hyperemic and edematous in the affected area (Fig. 41-2). Multiple abscesses develop in the crypts of Lieberkühn (intestinal glands). As the disease advances, the abscesses break through the crypts into the submucosa, leaving ulcerations. These ulcerations also destroy the mucosal epithelium, causing bleeding and diarrhea. Losses of fluid and electrolytes occur because of the decreased mucosal surface area for absorption. Breakdown of cells results in protein loss through the stool. Areas of inflamed mucosa form pseudopolyps, tonguelike

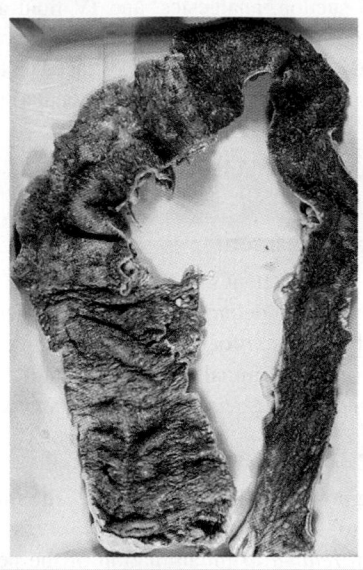

FIG. 41-2 Acute ulcerative colitis. Colitis with extensive mucosal ulceration involving the entire colon.

TABLE 41-17 Comparison of Ulcerative Colitis and Crohn's Disease

CHARACTERISTIC	ULCERATIVE COLITIS	CROHN'S DISEASE
Clinical		
Usual age at onset	Young to middle age	Young
Diarrhea	Common	Common
Abdominal cramping pain	Possible	Common
Fever (intermittent)	During acute attacks	Common
Weight loss	Common	Severe
Rectal bleeding	Common	Infrequent
Tenesmus	Severe	Rare
Malabsorption and nutritional deficiencies	Minimal incidence	Common
Pathologic		
Location	Starts distally and spreads in a continuous pattern up the colon	Occurs anywhere along GI tract in characteristic skip lesions; most frequent site is terminal ileum
Distribution	Continuous	Segmental
Depth of involvement	Mucosa and submucosa	Entire thickness of bowel wall (transmural)
Granulomas	Absent	Common
Cobblestoning of mucosa	Rare	Common
Pseudopolyps	Common	Rare
Small bowel involvement	Minimal	Common
Complications		
Fistulas	Rare	Common
Strictures	Rare	Common
Anal abscesses	Rare	Common
Perforation	Common	Common
Toxic megacolon	Common	Rare
Carcinoma	Increased incidence after 10 yr of disease	Slightly greater than general population
Recurrence after surgery	Cure with colectomy	40% to 60% or more recurrence after segmental resections of small or large intestine

projections into the bowel lumen. Granulation tissue develops, and the mucosa musculature becomes thickened, shortening the colon.

Although the precipitating factors involved in ulcerative colitis are poorly understood, it is clear that once initiated the inflammatory response is involved. Specific proinflammatory cytokines such as tumor necrosis factor-alpha (TNF-α) have been implicated in promoting this inflammatory response.

Clinical Manifestations

Ulcerative colitis may appear as an acute fulminating crisis or, more commonly, as a chronic disorder with mild to severe acute exacerbations that occur at unpredictable intervals over many years. The major symptoms of ulcerative colitis are bloody diarrhea and abdominal pain. Pain may vary from the mild lower abdominal cramping associated with diarrhea to the severe, constant abdominal pain that may be associated with acute perforations. With mild disease, diarrhea may consist of one or two semiformed stools containing small amounts of blood per day. The patient may have no other systemic manifestations. In moderate ulcerative colitis there is increased stool output (four to five stools per day), increased bleeding, and systemic symptoms (fever, malaise, anorexia). In severe cases, diarrhea is bloody, contains mucus, and occurs 10 to 20 times a day. In addition, fever, weight loss greater than 10% of total body weight, anemia, tachycardia, and dehydration are present. Acute fulminant colitis is present in only 6% to 10% of patients with severe ulcerative colitis.[14]

Complications

Complications of ulcerative colitis may be classified into those that are intestinal and those that are extraintestinal. Intestinal complications of ulcerative colitis include hemorrhage, strictures, perforation, toxic megacolon, and colonic dilation. Hemorrhage is a result of inflamed, ulcerated mucosa and is usually controlled with conservative therapy. Massive hemorrhage is unusual and requires emergency surgery. Strictures are less common in ulcerative colitis than in Crohn's disease and are seen most often in patients with severe, long-standing disease. *Toxic megacolon* (dilation and paralysis of the colon) occurs in approximately 5% of patients with ulcerative colitis.[14] Colonic dilation, most often in the transverse colon, occurs as a result of severe acute inflammation of the entire colon wall. Perforation is most often associated with toxic megacolon but may occur alone. Most cases of perforation occur in the left side of the colon.

A patient who has had ulcerative colitis for more than 10 years is at greater risk of colorectal cancer. The risk of cancer depends on age at onset, duration, and extent of disease. The patient should be periodically screened with colonoscopy. During this procedure, biopsy specimens should be taken every 10 cm throughout the entire colon.

Extraintestinal complications may be directly related to the colitis and small intestinal pathologic conditions (malabsorption), or they may be nonspecific complications mediated by a disturbance in the immune system (Table 41-18). Colitis-related complications are associated with active inflammation and often respond to treatment of the underlying bowel disease. These manifestations can involve the joints, skin, mouth, and eyes, as well as disturbances of the hematologic system including anemia, leukocytosis, and thrombocytosis.[14] Skin lesions such as

TABLE 41-18	Extraintestinal Complications of Ulcerative Colitis
Colitis Related	
Joints	
Peripheral arthritis (colitic)	
Ankylosing spondylitis	
Sacroiliitis	
Finger clubbing	
Skin	
Erythema nodosum	
Pyoderma gangrenosum	
Mouth	
Aphthous ulcers	
Eye	
Conjunctivitis	
Uveitis	
Episcleritis	
Related to Small Bowel Pathology	
Malabsorption	
Gallstones	
Kidney stones	
Nonspecific	
Liver disease—primary sclerosing cholangitis	
Osteoporosis	
Amyloidosis	
Peptic ulcer disease	

erythema nodosum and pyoderma gangrenosum are among the most frequently seen extraintestinal manifestations. Uveitis is the most common eye problem. Hepatobiliary disease may accompany ulcerative colitis.[15]

Diagnostic Studies

Several studies are appropriate for diagnosis of ulcerative colitis (Table 41-19). Blood studies should include a CBC, serum electrolyte levels, and serum protein levels. A CBC typically shows iron deficiency anemia from blood loss. An elevated WBC count may indicate toxic megacolon or perforation. Decreases in serum electrolytes, such as sodium, potassium, chloride, bicarbonate, and magnesium, are due to fluid and electrolyte losses from diarrhea and vomiting. Hypoalbuminemia is present with severe disease and is due to protein loss from the bowel. The stool should be examined for blood, pus, and mucus. Stool cultures should be obtained to rule out infectious causes of inflammation.

Examinations with a sigmoidoscope and a colonoscope allow direct examination of the mucosa of the large intestine. Using a sigmoidoscope the health care provider can view the rectum, the sigmoid colon, and the descending colon. The colonoscope allows for examination of the entire large intestine. The extent of inflammation, ulcerations, pseudopolyps, strictures, and lesions may be identified. Biopsy specimens should be taken for definitive diagnosis.

A double-contrast barium enema may show areas of granular inflammation with ulcerations. The colon may appear narrow and shortened, and pseudopolyps may be present. A double-contrast study (in which air is introduced into the bowel after the expul-

TABLE 41-19   Collaborative Care
Ulcerative Colitis

Diagnostic
History and physical examination
Colonoscopy
Sigmoidoscopy
Barium enema
CBC
Testing of stool for occult blood
Culture and sensitivity testing of stool

Collaborative Therapy
Mild and Moderate Disease
Low-roughage diet and no milk or milk products
Antimicrobial therapy*
5-Aminosalicylates*
Corticosteroids*
Anticholinergic therapy*
Antidiarrheal agents*
Severe (Fulminant) Disease
IV fluids with electrolytes
Blood transfusions
NPO status
NG tube to low suction
Antimicrobial therapy*
Immunosuppressants*
Immunomodulators*
Corticosteroids*
Parenteral nutritional therapy
Surgery if no improvement (colon resection with ileostomy)

*See Table 41-20.
CBC, Complete blood count; *IV,* intravenous; *NG,* nasogastric; *NPO,* nothing by mouth.

sion of barium) is effective in detecting mucosal abnormalities in ulcerative colitis.

Collaborative Care

The goals of treatment are to (1) rest the bowel, (2) control the inflammation, (3) combat infection, (4) correct malnutrition, (5) alleviate stress, and (6) provide symptomatic relief using drug therapy. The mainstays of drug therapy are sulfasalazine (Azulfidine) and corticosteroids. Hospitalization is indicated if the patient fails to respond to corticosteroid therapy or if complications are suspected.

Drug Therapy. Drug therapy is an extremely important aspect of treatment[15] (Table 41-20). Sulfasalazine, a combination of sulfapyridine and 5-aminosalicylic acid (5-ASA), is the principal drug used. It is effective in the maintenance of clinical remission and in the treatment of mild to moderately severe attacks. After remission is obtained, therapy is continued with a gradual reduction over several months. The maintenance dose is usually continued for at least 1 year.

During active disease, 5-ASA (the active form of sulfasalazine) and 4-ASA, given as retention enemas, are effective in the treatment of left-sided ulcerative colitis and proctitis. Topical salicylate therapy is the treatment of choice in patients with localized disease. 5-ASA (mesalamine [Rowasa]) can also be administered orally. The acrylic-coated tablets provide delivery of the drug more distally in the intestine.

Corticosteroids are of proven benefit in the management of active ulcerative colitis. Oral prednisone or prednisolone is effective in treatment of mild to moderate disease without systemic manifestations. If remission is not achieved, the patient requires hospitalization and IV corticosteroid therapy. The patient is placed on a regimen of bowel rest. Fluids and electrolytes are administered intravenously. For *proctitis* (inflammation of the rectum and anus), hydrocortisone enemas, rectal foams, or suppositories are effective in the treatment of inflammation. Rectal foams are usually administered in 5-ml volumes and are generally preferred over enemas because of the ease of administration. However, enemas are the preferred choice if the disease spreads beyond the sigmoid colon. Retention enemas have been shown to deliver drugs into the descending colon and beyond in patients with active disease. Although corticosteroids are reported to bring remission in 60% to 89% of cases, they do not necessarily prolong remission.[16] The patient taking corticosteroids needs to be monitored for signs of Cushing syndrome, hypertension, hirsutism, and mood swings.

Immunosuppressive drugs (e.g., 6-mercaptopurine [6-MP]) have been used in severe cases of ulcerative colitis when a patient has failed to respond to any of the usual drugs and before surgery is considered. Side effects of 6-MP, including bone marrow suppression and increased risk of infection, necessitate that it be used cautiously in these patients. Patients receiving this drug need to maintain an adequate fluid intake of 1800 to 2400 ml to reduce the risk of nephrotoxicity. The drug should be taken with food and milk to reduce gastric irritation. Cyclosporine (discussed in Chapter 13) and methotrexate have been evaluated for their effectiveness in the treatment of severe ulcerative colitis that is unresponsive to corticosteroid treatment. Although the monoclonal antibody against TNF-α (infliximab [Remicade]) is used more often in Crohn's disease, it has been used in patients with refractory ulcerative colitis.

Epidemiologic studies showing a low incidence of ulcerative colitis among smokers has led to investigation of nicotine transdermal patches or delayed-release nicotine capsules to induce remission.[16] For distal ulcerative colitis, rectal enemas containing short-chain fatty acids have been evaluated for their antiinflammatory effects. Short-chain fatty acids are important fuels supporting colonic cell function and are naturally produced from fiber fermentation.[17]

Surgical Therapy. Approximately 80% to 85% of patients with ulcerative colitis go into remission with conservative therapy and nursing management, but 15% to 20% require surgery. Surgery is indicated if (1) the patient fails to respond to treatment; (2) exacerbations are frequent and debilitating; (3) massive bleeding, perforation, strictures, or obstruction occur; (4) tissue changes that suggest that dysplasia is occurring; or (5) carcinoma develops.

Surgical procedures used to treat chronic ulcerative colitis include (1) total proctocolectomy with permanent ileostomy, (2) total proctocolectomy with continent ileostomy (Kock pouch), and (3) total colectomy with rectal mucosal stripping and ileoanal reservoir.

Total proctocolectomy with permanent ileostomy. *Total proctocolectomy with a permanent ileostomy* is a one-stage operation involving the removal of the colon, rectum, and anus with closure of the anus. The end of the terminal ileum is brought out through the abdominal wall and forms a stoma, or ostomy. The stoma is usually placed in the right lower quadrant below the belt line.

TABLE 41-20 Drug Therapy — Inflammatory Bowel Disease

CATEGORY	ACTION	EXAMPLES
Antimicrobial	Prevent or treat secondary infection	metronidazole (Flagyl)
5-Aminosalicylates (5-ASA)	Decrease GI inflammation*	*Systemic:* sulfasalazine (Azulfidine), mesalamine (Rowasa), olsalazine (Dipentum), balsalazide (Colazal); *Rectal suppository:* mesalamine (Canasa)
Corticosteroids	Decrease inflammation	*Systemic:* corticosteroids (cortisone, prednisone, budesonide [Entocort]); *Enemas:* hydrocortisone (Cortenema); *Rectal suppository:* Cortifoam
Anticholinergics	Decrease GI motility and secretions and relieve smooth muscle spasms†	methantheline bromide (Banthine), propantheline (Pro-Banthine), oxyphencyclimine (Daricon)
Sedatives	Reduce anxiety and restlessness	diazepam (Valium), flurazepam (Dalmane)
Antidiarrheal	Decrease GI motility†	diphenoxylate (Lomotil)
Immunosuppressants	Suppress immune response	azathioprine (Imuran), cyclosporine
Immunomodulators	Inhibit the cytokine tumor necrosis factor–alpha (TNF-α)	infliximab (Remicade)
	Block lymphocyte adhesion to blood vessel walls and subsequent migration into tissues	natalizumab (Antegren)
Hematinics and vitamins	Correct iron deficiency anemia and promote healing	oral ferrous sulfate, ferrous gluconate; iron dextran injection (Imferon), cobalamin, zinc

*Mechanism of action unknown, possibly antimicrobial, as well as antiinflammatory.
†Used with caution during severe disease because of potential to produce toxic megacolon.
CNS, Central nervous system; GI, gastrointestinal.

Total proctocolectomy with continent ileostomy. *Total proctocolectomy with continent ileostomy* (Kock pouch) is a variation from the traditional ileostomy (Fig. 41-3). This method eliminates the need for the patient to wear an external pouch over the stoma. The stoma is usually covered with a cap or dressing in case of mucous leakage. This procedure is considered curative for ulcerative colitis but has a higher complication rate than the traditional ileostomy.

In this procedure an internal pouch in the distal segment of the ileum is made surgically, the intestine is split, a fold is made, and a one-way nipple valve is created and sutured into place on the abdomen. The pouch acts as a reservoir and is drained at regular intervals by insertion of a catheter. During surgery, a catheter is inserted into the pouch to allow suture lines to heal and to allow fixation of scar tissue around the valve to prevent slippage. Postoperative irrigations are performed every 2 to 4 hours to rinse mucus from the pouch. The catheter may stay in place for up to 3 to 4 weeks. Once the catheter is removed, insertion of a catheter to remove contents begins every 2 hours and is gradually decreased until it is needed only 3 to 6 times a day. The patient eventually determines the frequency by the changes in sensation of pressure in the pouch. A continuous leakage of fluid is prevented by the one-way valve created at the internal end of the ileum from the stoma to the ileal pouch. Pressure created when the pouch fills with feces forces the valve to close. The majority of complications that arise are a result of valve failure, which has been reported to be as high as 40%.

The primary late complications of the procedure include pouchitis, fistula development, and nipple valve extrusion. These complications affect function by increasing intubation frequency and compromising pouch continence. Manifestations of pouchitis are increased stool frequency, *hematochezia* (passage of blood), urgency, abdominal cramping, and, occasionally, fever, malaise, and pelvic pain.[18] The lining appears red and inflamed, and the biopsy result shows nonspecific inflammation. Patients usually respond to treatment with metronidazole (Flagyl). Patients who require repeated treatment or whose inflammation is unresponsive to therapy are considered to have chronic pouchitis.

Total colectomy and ileal anal reservoir. A more widely performed procedure involves total colectomy and ileoanal anastomosis with the formation of an ileal anal reservoir (Fig. 41-4). The ileoanal surgical procedure is usually a combination of two procedures performed approximately 8 to 12 weeks apart. The initial procedure includes colectomy, rectal mucosectomy, ileal reservoir construction, ileoanal anastomosis, and temporary ileostomy. The second surgery involves closure of the ileostomy, which functionalizes the reservoir. Adaptation of the reservoir occurs over the next 3 to 6 months, which usually results in the ability to control and have decreased numbers of bowel movements over a 24-hour period.

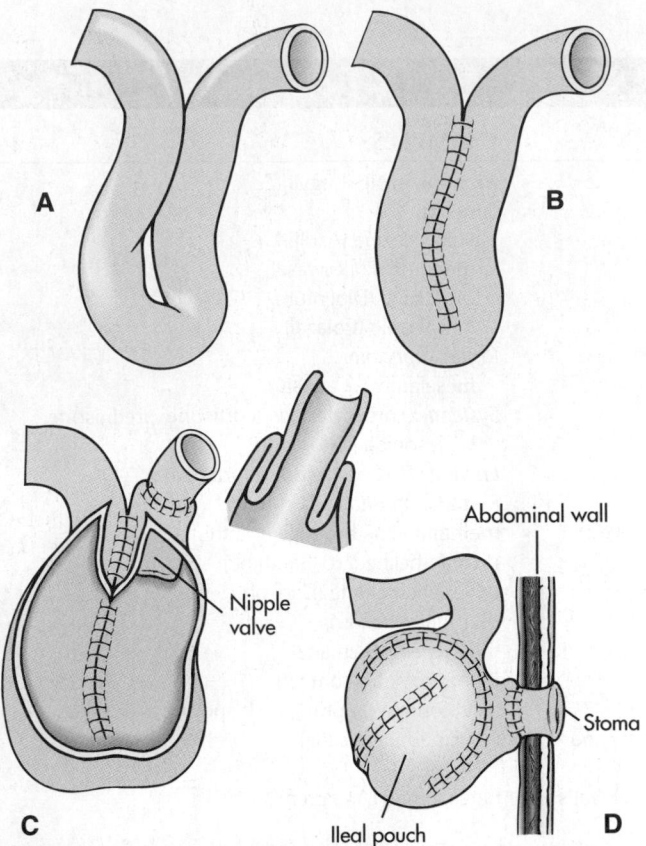

FIG. 41-3 Surgical formation of continent ileostomy (Kock pouch). A, Loop of terminal ileum. B, Both limbs sutured together and incised in a U *shape*. C, Pouch created with nipple valve. D, Pouch sutured to abdominal wall.

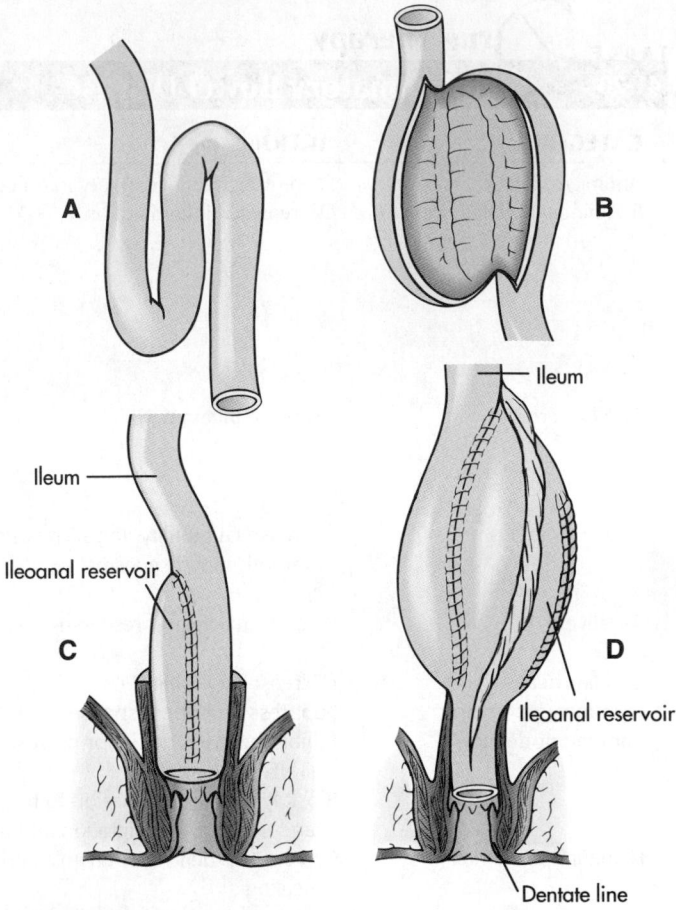

FIG. 41-4 Ileoanal reservoir. A, Formation of a reservoir. B, Posterior suture lines completed. C, J-shaped configuration for ileoanal reservoir. D, S-shaped configuration for ileoanal reservoir.

Patient selection criteria include absence of colorectal cancer, small intestine free of disease (e.g., Crohn's disease), competent anorectal sphincter, and physical status adequate to permit lengthy surgery. In addition, the patient needs to be motivated and capable of understanding self-care instructions.

Postoperative care. Postoperative care following surgical procedures to treat ulcerative colitis includes routine observations for patients who have had abdominal surgery. Stoma viability, mucocutaneous juncture (the area where the mucous membrane of the bowel interfaces with the skin), and peristomal skin integrity must be monitored. Because a more proximal portion of the bowel is used to create the ileostomy, output initially may be as high as 1500 to 2000 ml per 24 hours. The patient must be observed for signs of hemorrhage, abdominal abscess, small bowel obstruction, dehydration, and other related complications. If an NG tube is used, it will be removed when bowel function returns and oral intake is instituted. Drainage of serosanguineous fluid from the abdominal drain site may vary from 100 to 150 ml per 24 hours. The drain is usually removed within 4 days of surgery. The urinary catheter is removed 2 to 5 days after surgery. Systemic antibiotics are discontinued within 24 hours of the operation, and corticosteroids, if used, are tapered.

Transient incontinence of mucus is a result of intraoperative manipulation of the anal canal. The patient should be reassured before the operation regarding this potential transient problem. Kegel exercises are recommended later on (several weeks postopera-

tively) to strengthen the pelvic floor and sphincter muscles. They are not recommended in the immediate postoperative period. Perianal skin care must be implemented to protect the epidermis from mucous drainage and maceration. The patient should be instructed to gently rinse the skin with water and dry thoroughly. A moisture barrier ointment may be used, and a perineal pad may be required.

The most frequent type of ileostomy that is constructed is a loop. This often presents a pouching challenge because it retracts or drains inferiorly, resulting in effluent contact with the skin and predisposing to a denuded epidermis. An enterostomal therapy (ET) nurse should help with these challenging problems. Self-care instructions should be reviewed and written information provided before discharge. Stoma care is presented later in this chapter (see p. 1089).

Nutritional Therapy. An important component in the treatment of ulcerative colitis is diet. The dietitian is an important member of the team and should be consulted regarding dietary recommendations. The goals of diet management are to provide adequate nutrition without exacerbating symptoms, to correct and prevent malnutrition, to replace fluid and electrolyte losses, and to prevent weight loss. The diet for each patient must be individualized.

Traditionally during the acute phase the patient may be on NPO status. When food is permitted, a high-calorie, high-protein, low-residue diet with vitamin and iron supplements is frequently prescribed. (A low-residue diet is presented in Table 41-21.) Special dietary restrictions are not usually necessary. Some health care providers allow the patient to eat anything that does not

TABLE 41-21	Nutritional Therapy
	Low-Residue Diet

Purpose
Low-residue diet provides foods low in fiber, which will result in a reduced amount of fecal material in the lower intestinal tract.

General Principles
1. This diet eliminates foods that are indigestible or stimulating to the intestinal tract to reduce the amount of residue in the colon. Foods should be included or excluded according to the following list.
2. Hot and cold foods should be eaten slowly.
3. Milk products are limited to 2 cups daily. For a more restricted-residue diet, milk should be eliminated.

FOOD	FOODS INCLUDED	FOODS EXCLUDED
Beverages	Carbonated drinks, coffee, tea, cocoa, strained fruit juices	Alcohol, fruit juices with pulp
Bread	White bread, rolls, rusk, melba toast, crackers	Bread and crackers containing whole grain flour or bran; any hot breads such as biscuits, muffins, waffles, or pancakes
Cereals	Cooked, refined, or strained cereals: Cream of Wheat, Cream of Rice, farina, grits, dry cereals without bran, noodles, spaghetti, and macaroni	Whole grain cereals; cereals containing bran, nuts, and raisins; Shredded Wheat
Meat	Lean, tender ground beef, lamb, pork, veal or fish, broiled, stewed, or baked; canned tuna or salmon; shellfish; crisp bacon, chicken or turkey without skin; liver; creamy peanut butter	Fried, smoked, pickled, or cured meats, highly seasoned ham, fried fish, luncheon meats
Egg	All but fried	Fried or uncooked eggs
Cheese	Milk, cheese (American, cheddar), cottage cheese	All other cheeses
Milk	Limit to 1-2 cups (if tolerated), including that used in cooking; plain yogurt	Fruit yogurt
Fats	Butter, margarine, cream, oil, crisp bacon, mayonnaise, plain gravy	Any other; rich or spiced gravies
Soup	Cream and vegetable soups made from foods allowed and with milk allowed, bouillon, broth; strained vegetable juices	Cream and vegetable soups from foods not allowed (peas and dried beans)
Vegetables	Tender carrots, beets, or asparagus; strained vegetables; potatoes without skins; vegetable juices	Raw vegetables, all vegetables not strained, dried beans, peas, and legumes
Fruits	Strained fruit juices, ripe bananas, applesauce, pears, peaches, peeled apricots, Napoleon cherries, baked apple (no skin)	Raw fruits, fruits with skins, seeds
Desserts	Plain desserts (custards and puddings, plain ice cream for milk allowance), sherbet, plain gelatin desserts, angel food cake, sponge cake, plain butter cake, plain cookies	Nuts, coconut, raisins, rich desserts (pies, rich cakes, cobblers)
Condiments	Allspice, cinnamon, mace, paprika, salt, ground thyme, sugar, vinegar, lemon juice	All others

BREAKFAST	LUNCH	DINNER
Sample Menu Plan		
½ cup applesauce	Roast beef sandwich on 2 slices white bread (no lettuce or tomato)	Baked chicken
½ cup Cream of Wheat		Mashed potato
Scrambled egg	1 tbs mayonnaise	Cooked carrots
White toast	2 sugar cookies	White bread
Butter or jelly	Canned peach halves	Butter
1 cup milk	Coffee	Angel food cake
Coffee		1 cup milk
		Coffee

cause symptoms. Cold foods, high-residue foods (whole-wheat bread, cereal with bran, nuts, raw fruit), and smoking increase GI motility and should be avoided. Fish oil preparations have been evaluated for their ability to reduce inflammation in active ulcerative colitis. However, their palatability has been low.[17]

Often enteral supplements and parenteral nutrition are necessary. Patients with systemic manifestations, significant fluid and electrolyte losses, or malabsorption may need parenteral nutrition or enteral feedings, such as elemental diets. Elemental diets are high in calories and nutrients, lactose free, and absorbed in the proximal small intestine, which allows the more distal bowel to rest.

Parenteral nutrition allows for a positive nitrogen balance while resting the bowel. Vitamins, minerals, electrolytes, and other important nutrients (e.g., glucose, amino acids) can be administered to promote healing and correct nutritional deficiencies. (TPN is discussed in Chapter 39.)

Supplemental iron (ferrous sulfate or ferrous gluconate) may be necessary to prevent or treat iron deficiency anemia resulting from chronic blood loss. Parenteral iron may be needed for patients who cannot tolerate oral iron. Iron dextran (Imferon) intramuscularly by Z-track or intravenously may be necessary if anemia is severe. In patients receiving long-term sulfasalazine therapy, folic acid deficiency may develop, and supplementation may be necessary. Potassium supplements may be necessary if corticosteroid therapy is used because retention of sodium and loss of potassium can result in hypokalemia and subsequent toxic megacolon. Zinc deficiency can result from severe or chronic diarrhea, and supplementation may be necessary.

NURSING MANAGEMENT
ULCERATIVE COLITIS

■ Nursing Assessment

Subjective and objective data that should be obtained from a patient with ulcerative colitis are presented in Table 41-22.

■ Nursing Diagnoses

Nursing diagnoses for the patient with ulcerative colitis include, but are not limited to, those presented in NCP 41-3.

■ Planning

The overall goals are that the patient with ulcerative colitis will (1) experience a decrease in number and severity of acute exacerbations, (2) maintain normal fluid and electrolyte balance, (3) be free from pain or discomfort, (4) comply with medical regimens, and (5) maintain nutritional balance.

■ Nursing Implementation

During the acute phase, attention is focused on hemodynamic stability, pain control, fluid and electrolyte balance, and nutritional support. Accurate intake and output records must be maintained. The number and appearance of stools are monitored. Nursing care of the patient with ulcerative colitis is directed toward an intensive therapeutic and supportive program (see NCP 41-3). It is important that the nurse establishes a good working relationship and encourages the patient to talk about self and daily activities. Honesty, patience, and understanding are crucial in the relationship with the patient. An explanation of all procedures and treatment is necessary and may allay some apprehension.

Psychotherapy may be indicated if the patient is experiencing emotional problems, but the nurse must recognize that the patient's behavior may result from factors other than emotional ones. Any person who has 10 to 20 bowel movements a day and has rectal discomfort may be anxious, frustrated, discouraged, and depressed. Along with other team members, the nurse can assist the patient to accept the chronic condition and to have an optimistic view with the possibility of cure after surgery. The nurse may find that inadequate coping mechanisms in the patient with ulcerative colitis are due to early onset of the disease (often at 10 to 15 years of age), which may have interfered with usual growth, development, and maturation.

Restricted physical activity and possibly bed rest may be ordered if the patient has a severe exacerbation. Nursing interventions to prevent complications of immobility should be instituted. A sedative or tranquilizer may be prescribed to ensure rest. Teaching related to treatment, drugs, diet, diagnostic tests, and the disease and its management is important.

Rest is important in the management of ulcerative colitis. Patients may lose much sleep because of frequent episodes of diarrhea and abdominal pain. Nutritional deficiencies and anemia leave the patient feeling weak and listless. Activities should be scheduled around rest periods. The nurse should also set limits and follow through because the patient can be demanding. The patient needs to know and understand that the nurse wants to help and does not consider the care repugnant.

Until diarrhea is controlled, the patient must be kept clean, dry, and free of odor. A bedpan and wipes should be kept within reach of the patient. The bedpan should be emptied as soon as possible. A deodorizer should be placed in the room. Antidiarrheal agents should be administered as ordered. If the patient has continuous diarrhea, the ET nurse may give helpful suggestions. Meticulous perianal skin care using plain water (no harsh soap) is necessary to treat and prevent skin breakdown. Dibucaine (Nupercainal), witch

TABLE 41-22	Nursing Assessment Ulcerative Colitis	
Subjective Data	**Objective Data**
Important Health Information	**General**
Past health history: Infection, autoimmune disorders	Intermittent fever; emaciated appearance
Medications: Use of antidiarrheal medications	**Integumentary**
Functional Health Patterns	Pale skin with poor turgor, dry mucous membranes; rash, nodules, or blisters; anorectal irritation
Health perception–health management: Family history of ulcerative colitis; fatigue, malaise	**Gastrointestinal**
Nutritional-metabolic: Nausea, vomiting; anorexia; weight loss	Abdominal distention, hyperactive bowel sounds
Elimination: Frequent bloody stools containing mucus and pus	**Cardiovascular**
Cognitive-perceptual: Lower abdominal pain (worse before defecation), cramping, tenesmus	Tachycardia, hypotension
	Possible Findings
	Anemia; leukocytosis; electrolyte imbalance; hypoalbuminemia; vitamin and trace metal deficiencies; guaiac-positive stool; abnormal sigmoidoscopic, colonoscopic, and barium enema findings

NURSING CARE PLAN 41-3

Patient with Ulcerative Colitis

EXPECTED PATIENT OUTCOMES	NURSING INTERVENTIONS and *RATIONALES*
NURSING DIAGNOSIS	**Diarrhea** *related to* irritated bowel and intestinal hyperactivity *as manifested by* frequent diarrheal stools (>10 per day).
• Fewer, firmer stools	• Monitor frequency and character of stools *to evaluate effectiveness of therapy and dietary restrictions.* • Maintain food and fluid restrictions *to rest bowel during exacerbations.* • Teach patient to avoid smoking, caffeine, and foods or fluids that *are irritating to bowel or cause increased motility.*
NURSING DIAGNOSIS	**Anxiety** *related to* possible social embarrassment, unfamiliar environment, diagnostic tests, and treatment *as manifested by* expression of concerns about effect of disease on social relationships, questions about disease and treatment.
• Decreased anxiety	• Monitor for signs of anxiety *to plan appropriate interventions.* • Encourage open discussion of feelings about diagnosis *to demonstrate acceptance and concern for patient and allow verbalization of concerns.* • Explain disease treatments, diagnostic tests, and drugs *because understanding may reduce anxiety.* • Provide privacy *to reduce embarrassment and anxiety associated with frequent bowel movements.*
NURSING DIAGNOSIS	**Imbalanced nutrition: less than body requirements** *related to* decreased intake, decreased absorption, and increased nutrient loss through diarrhea *as manifested by* anorexia, weight loss, weakness, lethargy, anemia.
• Maintenance of body weight within normal range • Adequate nutritional intake • Increased strength and activity tolerance	• Assess for signs of malnutrition (e.g., hair loss, fatigue) *to direct plan for treating the problem.* • Record daily weights *to evaluate nutritional status and response to treatment.* • Perform ongoing calorie counts *to determine adequacy of caloric intake.* • Administer IV fluids and TPN as ordered *to allow for a positive nitrogen balance while resting the bowel.* • Give and instruct patient on high-caloric, nonspicy, caffeine-free, low-residue diet with small, frequent feedings *to reduce discomfort associated with eating.* • Administer nutritional supplements (as ordered) *to provide additional calories, protein, and fluid.*
NURSING DIAGNOSIS	**Impaired skin integrity** *related to* diarrhea and altered nutritional status *as manifested by* erythema of perianal area, discomfort around perianal area during and after evacuation.
• No evidence of skin breakdown in the perianal area	• Assess skin for signs of breakdown *to ensure early intervention.* • Cleanse perianal area after each bowel movement with mild soap and warm water and dry thoroughly *to remove bacteria, provide comfort, and stimulate circulation to treat and prevent skin breakdown.* • Provide sitz baths for comfort and hygiene and apply protective ointment. • Instruct patient and family on proper skin care techniques *to enable them to participate fully in treatment plan.*
NURSING DIAGNOSIS	**Ineffective coping** *related to* chronic disease, lifestyle changes, stress, and pain *as manifested by* inability to express feelings and concerns; display of dependent, attention-getting behavior.
• Development of healthy coping behaviors	• Identify ineffective behaviors and institute plan *to assist patient in learning more effective behaviors.* • Encourage patient's expression of feelings *to provide support as patient explores areas of concern and add to patient's feelings of self-worth.* • Offer reassurance and psychologic support *to demonstrate caring and concern.* • Know limitations and refer to counseling when appropriate *because more intensive treatment may be required to deal with specific stress/problem areas.*
NURSING DIAGNOSIS	**Ineffective therapeutic regimen management** *related to* lack of knowledge of course of disease, appropriate lifestyle adjustments, and nutritional and drug therapy *as manifested by* questioning about disease and treatment, poor decisions about activities of daily living.
• Able to repeat correct information about disease and treatment	• Provide information about the disease *to ensure that patient has adequate knowledge about the disease and treatment.* • Refer to dietitian if complex dietary changes are necessary *to provide patient with expert counseling.* • Teach about the relationships of stress to the disease *because stress may stimulate hyperreactivity of the colon in susceptible persons.* • Teach stress-reduction techniques *to assist patient in developing positive ways to reduce stress.* • Recommend regular colorectal cancer screening *because of increased risk of cancer.*

hazel, or other soothing compresses or prescribed ointment and sitz baths may reduce irritation and relieve discomfort of the anus.

■ Evaluation

The expected outcomes for the patient with ulcerative colitis are presented in NCP 41-3.

CROHN'S DISEASE

Crohn's disease is a chronic, nonspecific inflammatory bowel disorder of unknown origin that can affect any part of the GI tract from the mouth to the anus. It was once thought to be a disease specific to the small intestine and was called regional enteritis.

Crohn's disease may occur at any age but occurs most often between the ages of 15 and 30 years. When it occurs in older adults, the morbidity and mortality rates are higher because of other chronic problems that may be present. Both genders are affected, with a slightly higher incidence in women. Similar to ulcerative colitis, it occurs more often in Jewish and upper-middle-class urban populations. The incidence of Crohn's disease is slightly lower than that of ulcerative colitis.

Etiology and Pathophysiology

Crohn's disease is characterized by inflammation of segments of the GI tract. It can affect any part of the GI tract but is most often seen in the terminal ileum, jejunum, and colon. Involvement of the esophagus, stomach, and duodenum is rare. The inflammation involves all layers of the bowel wall (i.e., transmural). Areas of involvement are usually discontinuous *skip lesions,* with segments of normal bowel occurring between diseased portions (see Table 41-17). Typically, ulcerations are deep and longitudinal and penetrate between islands of inflamed edematous mucosa, causing the classic cobblestone appearance (Fig. 41-5). Thickening of the bowel wall occurs, as well as narrowing of the lumen with stricture development. The areas of inflammation can extend through all layers of the bowel wall. Abscesses or fistula tracts that communicate with other loops of bowel, skin, bladder, rectum, or vagina may develop. Histologically, granulomas are present in 50% of patients and may be located in any layer of the bowel wall.

TNF-α may be directly related to the pathogenesis of Crohn's disease. Levels of TNF-α are elevated in the stools of patients with Crohn's disease and correlate with disease activity. Treatment with the TNF-α blocker (discussed later under

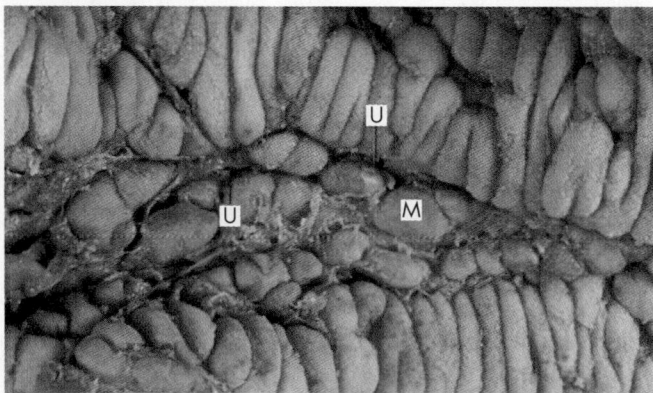

FIG. 41-5 Crohn's disease. The mucosa in Crohn's disease demonstrates a cobblestone pattern as a result of fissured ulcers *(U)* with intervening areas of edematous mucosa *(M).*

Drug Therapy) decreases endoscopic and histologic disease activity in Crohn's colitis.[19] Other proinflammatory cytokines may also be involved in the pathophysiology of Crohn's disease (e.g., interleukin-1 [IL-1], interleukin-6 [IL-6]).

Clinical Manifestations

The manifestations depend largely on the anatomic site of involvement, extent of the disease process, and presence or absence of complications. The onset of Crohn's disease is usually insidious, with nonspecific complaints such as diarrhea, fatigue, abdominal pain, weight loss, and fever. Early diagnosis may be more difficult than for ulcerative colitis. The principal manifestations of Crohn's disease are diarrhea and abdominal pain. Diarrhea is usually nonbloody and is a result of the inflammatory process or malabsorption. Pain may be severe and intermittent or constant, depending on the cause. Other manifestations include abdominal cramping and tenderness, abdominal distention, fever, and fatigue. Similar to ulcerative colitis, extraintestinal complications may be directly related to the GI inflammation and small intestinal pathologic conditions (malabsorption), or they may be nonspecific complications mediated by a disturbance in the immune system. Extraintestinal manifestations, such as arthritis and finger clubbing, may precede the onset of bowel disease. As the disease progresses, there is weight loss, malnutrition, dehydration, electrolyte imbalances, anemia, increased peristalsis, and pain around the umbilicus and right lower quadrant.

Crohn's disease is a chronic disorder with unpredictable periods of recurrence and remission. Attacks are intermittent, usually recurring over a period of several weeks to months, with diarrhea and abdominal pain subsiding spontaneously.

Complications

Complications, both GI and extragastrointestinal, are common in Crohn's disease. Scar tissue from the inflammation narrows the lumen of the intestine and may cause strictures and obstruction, a frequent complication. Fistulas are a cardinal feature and may develop between segments of bowel. Cutaneous fistulas, common in the perianal area, and rectovaginal fistulas also occur. Fistulas communicating with the urinary tract may cause urinary tract infections. Inflammation of the intestines may involve all layers, predisposing the patient to perforation and the formation of intraabdominal abscesses and peritonitis.

Impaired absorption causing various nutritional abnormalities may occur as a result of damage to areas of the intestinal mucosa. Fat malabsorption causes a deficiency in the fat-soluble vitamins (A, D, E, and K). The patient may have an intolerance to gluten (a protein found in barley, rye, and wheat).

Systemic complications are similar to those of ulcerative colitis and include arthritis, liver disease, cholelithiasis (especially with ileal involvement), ankylosing spondylitis, pyoderma gangrenosum, erythema nodosum, and uveitis. Renal disorders are common, especially nephrolithiasis (kidney stones) secondary to increased oxalate absorption.

Diagnostic Studies

Diagnosis of Crohn's disease can be made by means of a thorough history and physical examination to establish clinical signs and symptoms, barium studies, and endoscopy with biopsy (Table 41-23). Laboratory studies may determine electrolyte disturbances and the presence of anemia. Barium studies are useful in determining location and extent of the disease and may reveal classic findings, such as stricturing of the ileum (string sign), cobblestoning of the mucosa, fistulas, and areas of abnormal and normal mucosa. Endoscopic studies, such as colonoscopy and sigmoidoscopy, are useful in detecting such early mucosal changes as patchy inflammation, small ulcerations, and skip areas that may not be seen radiologically. Biopsies may be performed to determine the presence of *granulomas* (chronic inflammatory lesions). Barium studies are performed to determine the degree of ileal involvement. Upper GI barium studies are done to diagnose upper gastroduodenal disease.

Collaborative Care

The goal of collaborative care is to control the inflammatory process, relieve symptoms, correct metabolic and nutritional problems, and promote healing. Drug therapy and nutritional support are the mainstays of treatment. Balloon dilation of strictures may be effective in relieving symptoms in some patients. This is usually performed through a colonoscope or under fluoroscopic guidance. Strictures most often dilated are those in the colon or small bowel.

Drug Therapy. Drug therapy for Crohn's disease is presented in Table 41-20. Sulfasalazine is effective when the disease involves the large intestine but is much less effective when only the small intestine is involved. Corticosteroid therapy is effective in reducing inflammation and suppressing disease. The dosage and the route of administration depend on the severity of the illness and the area involved. Once clinical symptoms subside, the dosage should be tapered. Immunosuppressive agents (6-MP, azathioprine) may be tried if repeated trials with corticosteroids fail. Patients require close monitoring because of the serious side effects of these drugs. Metronidazole (Flagyl) is useful in treating Crohn's disease of the perianal area. Marked exacerbations have been reported when the drug is stopped. In patients with Crohn's disease in remission, fish oil preparations have been

evaluated for their ability to prevent recurrence of inflammation; however, their palatability has been low.

Biologic drug therapies of Crohn's disease include monoclonal antibodies to TNF-α (infliximab [Remicade]) and to a leukocyte adhesion molecule (natalizumab [Antegren]). Infliximab (by blocking the action of TNF-α) has been shown to reduce the degree of inflammation in patients who are refractory to other drug therapies. However, not all patients with Crohn's disease respond to infliximab. Natalizumab, on the other hand, works by interrupting the movement of lymphocytes into the endothelial layer of the gut wall. By reducing the migration of lymphocytes, the inflammatory process can be decreased.

Nutritional Therapy. Elemental diets and parenteral nutrition may be used in the patient with Crohn's disease (see Chapter 39). Parenteral nutrition may be given to patients with severe disease, small bowel fistulas, or short bowel syndrome (described later in this chapter). It is given before and after surgery to promote wound healing, reduce complications, and hasten recovery. The elemental diet provides a high-calorie, high-nitrogen, fat-free, no-residue substrate that is absorbed in the proximal small bowel. This diet can be given to most patients with Crohn's disease, even during acute exacerbations.

The diet should otherwise be low in residue, roughage, and fat but high in calories and protein. It may be difficult to maintain adequate absorption during periods of disease exacerbation and even during periods of remission. Milk and milk products may have to be excluded from the diet. Lactose, the primary disaccharide found in milk, may not be adequately digested because of the inability of the damaged intestinal mucosa to produce sufficient amounts of lactase. High-fat diets are poorly tolerated because of the loss of absorbing mucosa and altered bile salt metabolism and absorption.

Vitamin deficiencies may develop as a result of malabsorption. Cobalamin (vitamin B_{12}) injections every month may be needed because of the inability of the terminal ileum (if affected) to absorb this vitamin.

Surgical Therapy. Surgery is used in patients with severe symptoms that are unresponsive to therapy and in those with life-threatening complications. The majority of patients with Crohn's disease eventually require surgery at least once in the course of their disease. Indications for surgery are outlined in Table 41-24. Unlike ulcerative colitis, which can be cured by total proctocolectomy, Crohn's disease is not cured by surgery. The recurrence rate after surgery is high. The surgical procedure depends on the affected area and the condition of the patient. Conservative intestinal resection with anastomosis of healthy bowel is the procedure of choice.

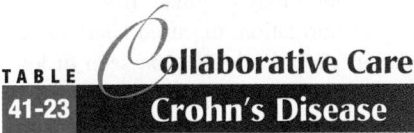

TABLE 41-23	Collaborative Care — Crohn's Disease
Diagnostic	
History and physical examination	
CBC	
Serum chemistries	
Testing of stool for occult blood	
Radiologic studies with barium contrast	
Sigmoidoscopy and colonoscopy with biopsy	
Collaborative Therapy	
High-calorie, high-vitamin, high-protein, low-residue, milk-free diet	
Antimicrobial agents*	
Corticosteroid drugs*	
Immunosuppressants*	
Immunomodulators*	
Supplementary parenteral nutrition	
Elemental diet	
Physical and emotional rest	
Surgery†	

*See Table 41-20.
†See Table 41-24.
CBC, Complete blood count.

TABLE 41-24	Indications for Surgical Therapy of Crohn's Disease
• Drainage of abdominal abscess	
• Failure to respond to conservative therapy	
• Fistulas	
• Inability to decrease corticosteroids	
• Intestinal obstruction	
• Massive hemorrhage	
• Perforation	
• Secondary hydronephrosis	
• Severe anorectal disease	
• Suspicion of carcinoma	

NURSING MANAGEMENT
CROHN'S DISEASE

Care of the patient is similar to that of the patient with ulcerative colitis (see NCP 41-3 and p. 1075). As the patient's condition improves, the nurse should allow for more self-care, provide frequent rest periods, and advise the patient of the importance of rest and avoidance or control of emotional stress. Initially this may be difficult for the patient when told the nature of the disease and the limitations of the treatment. Patients who have perianal fistulas or abscesses may need special skin care. Postoperative care should be the same as for exploratory laparotomy (see pp. 1062-1063).

In the majority of patients with Crohn's disease the course is chronic and intermittent, regardless of the site of involvement. The patient and significant others may need help in setting realistic short-term and long-term goals. Teaching is important and should include (1) the importance of rest and diet management, (2) perianal care, (3) action and side effects of drugs, (4) symptoms of recurrence of disease, (5) when to seek medical care, and (6) use of diversional activities to reduce stress.

■ Gerontologic Considerations: Inflammatory Bowel Disease

Although inflammatory bowel diseases (i.e., ulcerative colitis and Crohn's disease) are considered diseases of young adults, a second peak in the distribution of these inflammatory conditions occurs around the age of 70 years. The pathogenesis, natural history, and clinical course of ulcerative colitis and Crohn's disease in older adults are similar to those observed in younger patients. However, the distribution of the inflammation appears to be somewhat different. In the older patient with ulcerative colitis, the distal colon (proctitis) is usually involved. In the older patient with Crohn's disease, the colon rather than the small intestine tends to be involved. There is less recurrence of Crohn's disease in older patients treated with surgical resection. The degree of inflammation associated with both conditions tends to be less in the older adult than in the younger patient.

Collaborative care of the older patient with one of these conditions is similar to care of the younger patient. However, because of increased risk of cardiovascular and pulmonary complications, older adults tend to have increased morbidity associated with surgical procedures.

In addition to Crohn's disease and ulcerative colitis, older adults are also vulnerable to inflammation of the colon (colitis) from medication use and systemic vascular disease. Drugs such as nonsteroidal antiinflammatory drugs (NSAIDs), digitalis, vasopressin, estrogen, and allopurinol (Zyloprim) have been associated with colitis development in the elderly patient. Colitis may also be secondary to ischemic bowel disease related to atherosclerosis and congestive heart failure.

Inflammation of the colon as a result of Crohn's disease or ulcerative colitis results in diarrhea, which may be bloody. The loss of fluid and electrolytes and possibly blood may leave the older adult more vulnerable to problems related to volume depletion and dehydration. This may be particularly problematic in the patient with diminished renal and cardiovascular function. Thus nursing management is focused on careful assessment of fluid and electrolyte status and evaluation of the replacement therapies.

INTESTINAL OBSTRUCTION

Intestinal obstruction occurs when intestinal contents cannot pass through the GI tract, and it requires prompt treatment. The obstruction may be partial or complete. The causes of intestinal obstruction can be classified as mechanical or nonmechanical.

Types of Intestinal Obstruction

Mechanical. *Mechanical obstruction* may be caused by an occlusion of the lumen of the intestinal tract. Most intestinal obstructions occur in the small intestine, most often in the ileum. Mechanical obstruction accounts for 90% of all intestinal obstructions[20] (Fig. 41-6). Adhesions account for 50%, hernias for 15%, and neoplasms for 15% of obstructions of the small intestine. Adhesions can develop after abdominal surgery. Obstruction can occur within days of surgery or years later. Carcinoma is the most common cause of large bowel obstruction, followed by volvulus and diverticular disease.

Nonmechanical. A *nonmechanical obstruction* may result from a neuromuscular or vascular disorder. **Paralytic (adynamic) ileus** (lack of intestinal peristalsis) is the most common form of nonmechanical obstruction. It occurs to some degree after any abdominal surgery. Other causes of paralytic ileus include inflammatory responses (e.g., acute pancreatitis, acute appendicitis), electrolyte abnormalities, and thoracic or lumbar spinal fractures.

Pseudoobstruction is an apparent mechanical obstruction of the intestine without demonstration of obstruction by radiologic methods. Collagen vascular diseases and neurologic and endocrine disorders may cause pseudoobstruction, but mostly it is found to be idiopathic.

Vascular obstructions are rare and are due to an interference with the blood supply to a portion of the intestines. The most common causes are emboli and atherosclerosis of the mesenteric arteries. The celiac, inferior, and superior mesenteric arteries supply blood to the bowel. Emboli may originate from thrombi in patients with chronic atrial fibrillation, diseased heart valves, and prosthetic valves. Venous thrombosis may be seen in low-blood-flow states, such as heart failure and shock.

Etiology and Pathophysiology

Normally 6 to 8 L of fluid enters the small bowel daily. Most of the fluid is absorbed before it reaches the colon. Approximately 75% of intestinal gas is swallowed air. Bacterial metabolism produces methane and hydrogen gases. Fluid, gas, and intestinal contents accumulate proximal to the intestinal obstruction. This causes distention, and the distal bowel may collapse. The distention reduces the absorption of fluids and stimulates intestinal secretions. As the fluid increases, so does the pressure in the lumen of the bowel. The increased pressure leads to an increase in capillary permeability and extravasation of fluids and electrolytes into the peritoneal cavity. Edema, congestion, and necrosis from impaired blood supply and possible rupture of the bowel may occur. The retention of fluid in the intestine and peritoneal cavity can lead to a severe reduction in circulating blood volume and result in hypotension and hypovolemic shock.

The electrolyte-rich fluids, which are normally absorbed in the bowel, are retained in the bowel and subsequently lost into the peritoneal cavity. The location of the obstruction determines the extent of fluid, electrolyte, and acid-base imbalances. If the ob-

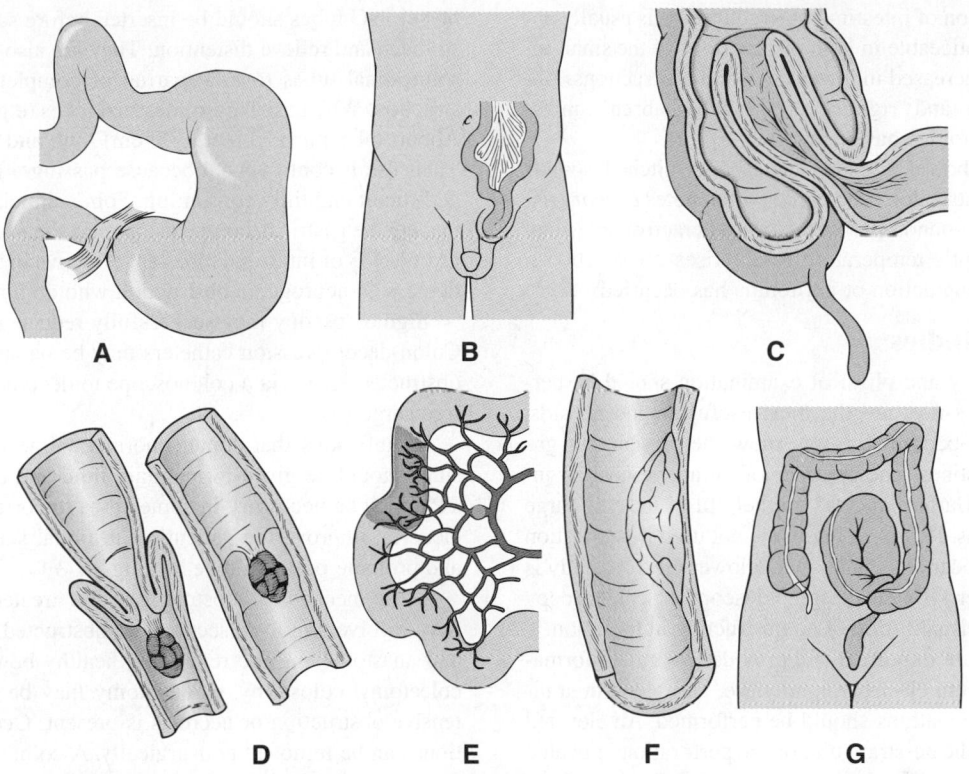

FIG. 41-6 Bowel obstructions. A, Adhesions. B, Strangulated inguinal hernia. C, Ileocecal intussusception. D, Intussusception from polyps. E, Mesenteric occlusion. F, Neoplasm. G, Volvulus of the sigmoid colon.

struction is high, as in the pylorus, metabolic alkalosis may result from the loss of hydrochloric acid from the stomach through vomiting or NG intubation.

When the obstruction is located in the small bowel, dehydration occurs rapidly. Dehydration and electrolyte imbalances do not occur early in large bowel obstruction. If the obstruction is below the proximal colon, most GI fluids have been absorbed before reaching the point of the obstruction. Solid fecal material accumulates until symptoms of discomfort appear. Reverse peristalsis may cause vomiting of fecal material very late in the bowel obstruction.

Simple obstructions of the intestine involve blockage of the lumen in one spot. A closed-loop obstruction occurs when the lumen is blocked in two different spots (e.g., *volvulus*). This results in an isolated segment of bowel and obstruction proximal to that segment. Strangulation and gangrene are likely to develop if treatment is not immediate. A strangulated obstruction occurs when the circulation to the obstructed intestine is impaired. This is the most dangerous form of obstruction because it may lead to necrosis of the intestine *(incarcerated)*. Volvulus, hernias, or adhesions are the most common causes.

Clinical Manifestations

The clinical manifestations of intestinal obstruction vary, depending on the location of the obstruction, and include nausea, vomiting, abdominal pain, distention, inability to pass flatus, and obstipation (Table 41-25). Obstruction located high in the small intestine produces rapid-onset, sometimes projectile vomiting with bile-containing vomitus. Vomiting from more distal obstructions of the small intestine is more gradual in onset. The

TABLE 41-25 Clinical Manifestations of Small and Large Intestinal Obstructions

CLINICAL MANIFESTATION	SMALL INTESTINE	LARGE INTESTINE
Onset	Rapid	Gradual
Vomiting	Frequent and copious	Rare
Pain	Colicky, cramplike, intermittent	Low-grade, cramping abdominal pain
Bowel movement	Feces for a short time	Absolute constipation
Abdominal distention	Minimally increased	Greatly increased

vomitus may be orange-brown and foul smelling because of bacterial overgrowth. Vomiting may be entirely absent in large bowel obstruction if the ileocecal valve is competent; otherwise, the patient may eventually vomit fecal material.

Vomiting usually relieves abdominal pain in high intestinal obstructions. Persistent, colicky abdominal pain is seen with lower intestinal obstruction. A characteristic sign of mechanical obstruction is pain that comes and goes in waves. This is due to intestinal peristalsis trying to move bowel contents past the obstructed area. In contrast, paralytic ileus produces a more constant generalized discomfort. Strangulation causes severe, constant pain that is rapid in onset. Abdominal distention is a common manifestation of intestinal obstructions. It is usually absent or minimally noticeable in high obstructions of the small intestine and greatly increased in lower intestinal obstructions. Abdominal tenderness and rigidity are usually absent unless strangulation or peritonitis has occurred.

Auscultation of bowel sounds reveals high-pitched sounds above the area of obstruction. The patient often notes *borborygmi* (audible abdominal sounds produced by hyperactive intestinal motility). The patient's temperature rarely rises above 100° F (37.8° C) unless strangulation or peritonitis has occurred.

Diagnostic Studies

A thorough history and physical examination should be performed. Abdominal x-rays are the most useful diagnostic aids. Upright and lateral abdominal x-rays show the presence of gas and fluid in the intestines. The presence of intraperitoneal air indicates perforation. Barium enemas are helpful in locating large intestinal obstructions. However, barium is not used if perforation is suspected. If the location is unknown, a lower GI tract study is done before an upper GI series. Sigmoidoscopy or colonoscopy may provide direct visualization of an obstruction in the colon.

Laboratory tests are important and provide essential information. A CBC and serum electrolyte, amylase, and blood urea nitrogen (BUN) determinations should be performed. An elevated WBC count may indicate strangulation or perforation; elevated hematocrit values may reflect hemoconcentration. Decreased hemoglobin and hematocrit values may indicate bleeding from a neoplasm or strangulation with necrosis. Serum electrolytes should be monitored frequently. They provide essential information on the patient's fluid and electrolyte balance. Serum sodium, potassium, and chloride concentrations are decreased in small bowel obstruction. The BUN value may be increased because of dehydration. The stool should be checked for occult blood.

Collaborative Care

Treatment is directed toward decompression of the intestine by removal of gas and fluid, correction and maintenance of fluid and electrolyte balance, and relief or removal of the obstruction. NG or intestinal tubes (Fig. 41-7) may be used to decompress the bowel. NG tubes should be inserted before surgery to empty the stomach and relieve distention. They are also used instead of nasointestinal tubes to treat partial or complete small bowel obstruction. When used, nasointestinal tubes (e.g., Cantor or Miller-Abbott tubes) are 10 feet (300 cm) long and mercury weighted. Their use is controversial because passing a long intestinal tube is difficult and time consuming. Some clinicians believe there is inadequate gastric decompression once the tube is in the small intestine. NG or intestinal tubes are effective in the treatment of patients with neurogenic obstruction who do not require surgery.

Sigmoidoscopy may successfully reduce a sigmoid volvulus. Colon-decompression catheters may be passed through partially obstructed areas via a colonoscope to decompress the bowel before surgery.

IV infusions that contain normal saline solution and potassium should be given to maintain fluid and electrolyte balance. TPN may be necessary in some cases to correct nutritional deficiencies, improve the patient's nutritional status before surgery, and promote postoperative healing.

Most mechanical obstructions are treated surgically. They may involve simply resecting the obstructed segment of bowel and anastomosing the remaining healthy bowel. Partial or total colectomy, colostomy, or ileostomy may be required when extensive obstruction or necrosis is present. Occasionally obstructions can be removed nonsurgically. A colonoscope can be used to remove polyps, dilate strictures, and remove and destroy tumors with a laser.

NURSING MANAGEMENT INTESTINAL OBSTRUCTION

■ Nursing Assessment

Intestinal obstruction is a potentially life-threatening condition. Nursing assessment must begin with a detailed patient history and physical examination. The type and location of obstruction usually cause characteristic symptoms. The nurse should determine the location, duration, intensity, and frequency of abdominal pain and whether abdominal tenderness or rigidity is present. Onset, frequency, color, odor, and amount of vomitus

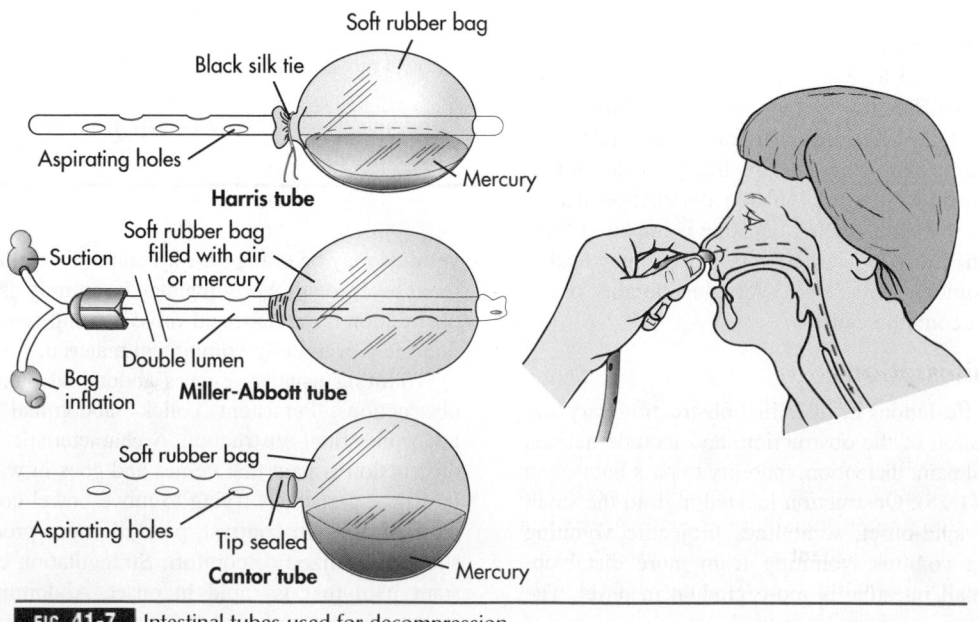

FIG. 41-7 Intestinal tubes used for decompression.

should be recorded. Bowel function, including passage of flatus, should be determined. The nurse auscultates for bowel sounds and documents the character and location; inspects the abdomen for scars, palpable masses, and distention; and observes for muscle guarding and tenderness.

■ Nursing Diagnoses

Nursing diagnoses for the patient with intestinal obstructions include, but are not limited to, the following:

- Acute pain *related to* abdominal distention and increased peristalsis
- Deficient fluid volume *related to* decrease in intestinal fluid absorption and loss of fluids secondary to vomiting
- Imbalanced nutrition: less than body requirements *related to* intestinal obstruction and vomiting

■ Planning

The overall goals are that the patient with an intestinal obstruction will have (1) relief of the obstruction and return to normal bowel function, (2) minimal to no discomfort, and (3) normal fluid and electrolyte status.

■ Nursing Implementation

The patient should be monitored closely for signs of dehydration and electrolyte imbalance. A strict intake and output record should be maintained. All vomitus and tube drainage should be included. IV fluids should be administered as ordered. Serum electrolyte levels should be monitored closely. A patient with a high obstruction is more likely to have metabolic alkalosis; a patient with a low obstruction is at greater risk of metabolic acidosis. The patient is often restless and constantly changes position to relieve the pain. Analgesics may be withheld until the obstruction is diagnosed because they may mask other signs and symptoms and decrease intestinal motility. The nurse should provide comfort measures, promote a restful environment, and keep distractions and visitors to a minimum. Nursing care of the patient after surgery for an intestinal obstruction is similar to care of the patient after a laparotomy (see NCP 41-2 and p. 1063).

Care of Nasogastric and Nasointestinal Tubes. Although the health care provider usually inserts intestinal tubes, the nurse assists with the procedure. Insertion is easier if the patient relaxes, takes deep breaths, and swallows when instructed. If insertion of the tube to the small intestine is desired, the patient may be instructed or positioned to lie on the right side to facilitate tube passage through the pylorus. In some situations a prokinetic drug such as metoclopramide (Reglan) may be used to facilitate tube movement.

Once the tube is in place, mouth care is extremely important. Vomiting leaves a terrible taste in the patient's mouth, and fecal odor may be present. When an NG or nasointestinal tube is in place, the patient breathes through the mouth, drying the mouth and lips. The nurse should encourage and assist the patient to brush the teeth frequently. Mouthwash and water for the patient to use in rinsing the mouth and petroleum jelly or water-soluble lubricant for the lips should be provided at the bedside.

The patient's nose should be checked for signs of irritation from the NG or nasointestinal tube. This area should be cleaned and dried daily with application of a water-soluble lubricant and retaping of the tube. NG and intestinal tubes should be checked every 4 hours for patency. The patient may be placed on a schedule to clamp the tube for 1 hour out of every 3 hours or for 3 out of every 4 hours before removal of the tube.

POLYPS OF THE LARGE INTESTINE

Colonic polyps arise from the mucosal surface of the colon and project into the lumen. They may be *sessile* (flat, broad based, and attached directly to the intestinal wall) or *pedunculated* (attached to the intestinal wall by a thin stalk). Polyps tend to be sessile when small and become pedunculated as they enlarge, especially if they are in the left or descending colon (Fig. 41-8). They may be found anywhere in the large intestine but are most commonly found in the rectosigmoid area. Although most polyps are asymptomatic, rectal bleeding or occult blood in the stool are the most common manifestations.

Types of Polyps

The most common types of polyp are hyperplastic and adenomatous. *Hyperplastic polyps* originate from the epithelium and are nonneoplastic growths. They rarely grow larger than 5 mm in size and never cause clinical symptoms. Other benign (nonneoplastic) polyps include inflammatory polyps, lipomas, and juvenile polyps (Table 41-26).

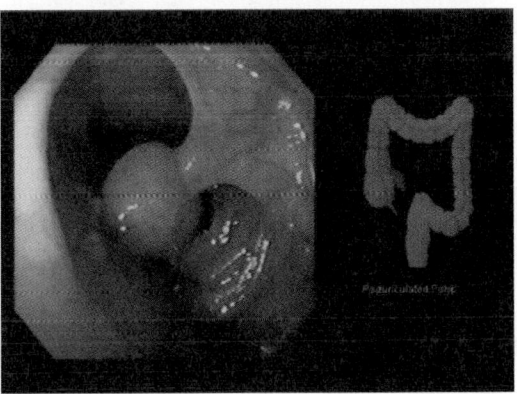

FIG. 41-8 Endoscopic image of pedunculated polyp in descending colon.

TABLE 41-26 Types of Polyps of the Large Intestine

Neoplastic
Epithelial polyps (adenomatous)
  Tubular adenoma
  Tubular villous adenoma
  Villous adenoma
Hereditary polyposis syndromes (adenomatous polyposis syndrome)
  Familial adenomatous polyposis

Nonneoplastic
Epithelial polyps (hyperplastic)
Hereditary polyposis syndromes
  Familial juvenile polyposis
Inflammatory polyps
  Pseudopolyps
  Benign lymphoid polyp
Submucosal
  Lipomas
  Leiomyomas
  Fibromas

Adenomatous polyps are characterized by neoplastic changes in the epithelium. They are closely linked to colorectal adenocarcinoma. Structurally, there are three types, with tubular adenomas being the most prevalent. The risk of cancer in the polyp increases with polyp size and villous structure. Villous adenomas have a higher risk of turning cancerous than tubular adenomas. Removing adenomatous polyps has been reported to decrease the occurrence of subsequent colorectal cancer by 90%.[21]

Although there are several polyposis syndromes, they are relatively rare. Of these, *familial adenomatous polyposis (FAP)* is the most common (see the Genetics in Clinical Practice box below. This disorder is characterized by multiple polyps that at times number in the thousands and that are located in the large intestine and sometimes in other areas of the GI tract. Patients with a history of FAP have a lifetime risk of developing colorectal cancer that approaches 100%. They also develop cancer at an earlier age (i.e., 40 years of age) than patients with non-FAP colorectal cancer. For children of patients with FAP, screening must be initiated at puberty and then conducted annually. There is a 50% risk for these children to develop FAP. When there is indication of disease, total colectomy with ileostomy is the treatment of choice.[22]

Diagnostic Studies and Collaborative Care

Barium enema, sigmoidoscopy, and colonoscopy are used to diagnose polyps. All polyps are considered abnormal and should be removed. In patients whose polyps are identified through barium enema, removal (polypectomy) should be done through a colonoscope or a sigmoidoscope. If the polyp is not removable, a biopsy specimen should be taken for tissue examination. Surgery is not indicated unless carcinoma is present or certain cases of polyposis syndromes warrant it. The patient should be observed for rectal bleeding, fever, severe abdominal pain, and abdominal distention, which may indicate hemorrhage or perforation.

COLORECTAL CANCER

Colorectal cancer is the third most common cause of cancer death in the United States. Colorectal cancer in the United States accounts for an estimated 56,600 deaths each year. In 2002, there were approximately 148,300 new cases of colorectal cancer in the United States. Colorectal cancer may occur at any age but is most prevalent over the age of 50 years. The 5-year survival rate is 90% for early, localized colorectal cancers and 64% for cancer that has spread to adjacent organs and lymph nodes.[23]

The incidence of colorectal cancer at specific sites varies (Fig. 41-9). In both sexes, the incidence of right colon cancers has increased and cancers in the rectum have decreased. The highest percentages of colorectal cancers in the United States are currently located in the rectum, ascending colon, and sigmoid colon. Approximately 20% of colorectal cancers are within reach of the examining finger, and 50% are within reach of the sigmoidoscope.

Etiology and Pathophysiology

The causes of colorectal cancer remain unclear. Groups at high risk of colorectal cancer have been identified (Table 41-27). For at least 6% of patients who develop colorectal cancer there is a clear genetic predisposition (see the Genetics in Clinical Practice boxes at left and on p. 1083). Age is a risk factor in both men and women. The risk for development in the general population increases slightly after the age of 40 years and then rises rapidly in the following decades. Diet, especially the high-calorie, high-fat Western diet, has been associated with development of colorectal cancer.

Adenocarcinoma is the most common type of colorectal cancer. Most colorectal cancers appear to arise from adenomatous polyps. All tumors tend to spread through the walls of the intestine and into the lymphatic system. Tumors commonly spread to

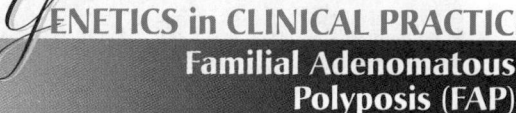

GENETICS in CLINICAL PRACTICE
Familial Adenomatous Polyposis (FAP)

Genetic Basis
- Autosomal dominant disorder
- Mutation in adenomatous polyposis coli (APC) gene located on chromosome 5

Incidence
- 1 in 5000-7500 people
- Men and women affected equally

Genetic Testing
- DNA testing available to detect APC gene mutation

Clinical Implications
- FAP is characterized by the presence of colorectal polyps (usually >1000).
- Polyps are not present at birth but appear during adolescence and early adulthood.
- FAP accounts for at least 1% of all colorectal cancers.
- If untreated, FAP almost always results in the development of colon cancer before the age of 40.
- With FAP, there is also increased incidence of gastric and small intestinal polyps.
- Many deaths related to FAP could be prevented with early and aggressive monitoring and treatment including frequent colonoscopies and total colectomy.
- Individuals with a family history of FAP could benefit from genetic counseling and teaching.

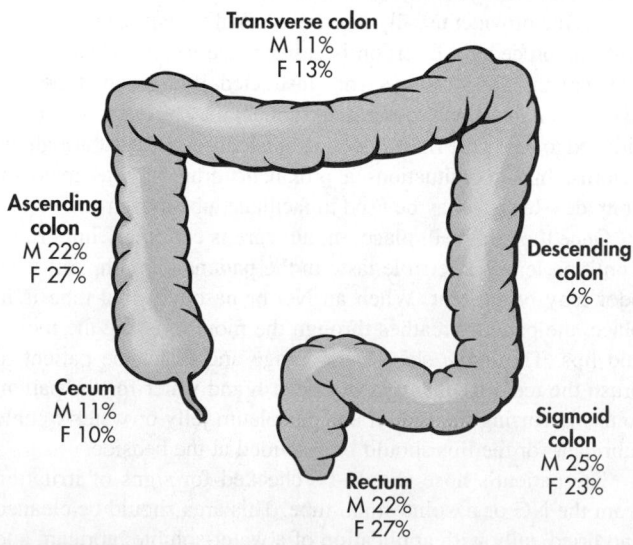

FIG. 41-9 Incidence of cancer. Approximately one half of all colon cancers occur in the rectosigmoid area. Percentages are listed for males (M) and females (F).

Transverse colon
M 11%
F 13%

Ascending colon
M 22%
F 27%

Descending colon
6%

Cecum
M 11%
F 10%

Sigmoid colon
M 25%
F 23%

Rectum
M 22%
F 27%

TABLE 41-27 Risk Factors for Colorectal Cancer

- Age >50 years
- Familial polyposis
- Colorectal polyps
- Chronic inflammatory bowel disease
- Family history of colorectal cancer or adenomas
- Previous history of colorectal cancer
- History of ovarian or breast cancer (women)
- High-fat and/or low-fiber diet (controversial)

𝒢ENETICS in CLINICAL PRACTICE
Hereditary Nonpolyposis Colorectal Cancer (HNPCC)

Genetic Basis
- Autosomal dominant disorder
- Mutations in genes that error-check DNA (repair genes)

Incidence
- 1 in 500 to 2000 people

Genetic Testing
- DNA testing available

Clinical Implications
- HNPCC accounts for 5% of all colorectal cancers.
- Individuals with gene mutation have 80% to 90% lifetime risk of developing colorectal cancer.
- Average age of diagnosis is in the mid-40s.
- Cancer arises from single colorectal lesion in absence of polyposis.
- Cancers tend to occur on right side of colon.
- HNPCC is less aggressive, and survival rates are longer than colon cancers that develop without known risk factors.
- Persons with gene mutation are also at high risk of developing other cancers, including uterine, ovarian, ureter, pancreas, stomach, and small intestinal cancer.
- Individuals with known gene mutations should be monitored with colonoscopy every year. Examination by pelvic ultrasound and endometrial biopsy should also be considered for women.

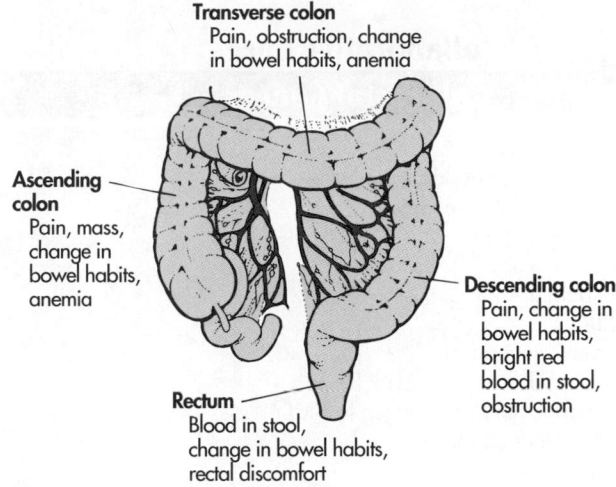

FIG. 41-10 Signs and symptoms of colorectal cancer by location of primary lesion.

nal pain may be present. Iron deficiency anemia and occult bleeding dictate further investigation. Weakness and fatigue result from anemia.

Diagnostic Studies

A thorough history with close attention to family history should be obtained, and a physical examination should be performed initially (Table 41-28). The digital rectal examination is the most important aspect of the physical examination because many rectal cancers are within reach of the finger. In the asymptomatic person who is 50 years or older with no risk factors (other than age), fecal occult blood testing once a year and flexible sigmoidoscopy every 5 years beginning at age 50 are important aspects of the examination.[24] (Screening options for colorectal cancer are presented in Table 15-7.) If colorectal cancer is suspected, examinations with the flexible sigmoidoscope and a double-contrast barium enema (in combination) are often performed. Colonoscopy is the gold standard for colorectal cancer screening. If not used as the primary screening method, it is the procedure of choice if a questionable lesion is seen on barium enema or sigmoidoscopy. Other procedures include endorectal ultrasonography and a CT scan of the abdomen and pelvis to localize the lesion or determine its size. Synchronous lesions may be present at other sites in the colon, and tissue diagnosis may be made by brushing or biopsy during the procedure.

Fecal occult blood tests have been used for over 30 years to screen for colorectal cancer and continue to be widely used in North America. Patients need to be taught to abstain from red meat and NSAIDs before testing to avoid false positives. Newer, more sensitive stool tests are undergoing clinical evaluation. These include the presence of cancer cell markers (e.g., neoplasm specific DNA alterations).[25]

Laboratory studies should include a CBC to check for anemia, clotting studies, and liver function tests. A CT scan of the abdomen may be helpful in detecting liver metastases, retroperitoneal and pelvic disease, and depth of penetration of tumor into the bowel wall. A CT scan should be done before surgery. Liver function tests are performed to determine liver metastases.

A carcinoembryonic antigen (CEA) test is often performed, although it is not specific for colorectal cancer. A normal level of

the liver because the venous blood flow from the colorectal tumor is through the portal vein.

Clinical Manifestations

Clinical manifestations of colorectal cancer are usually nonspecific or do not appear until the disease is advanced. Cancer on the right side of the colon gives rise to clinical manifestations that are different from those on the left side of the colon.[24] Rectal bleeding, the most common symptom of colorectal cancer, is most often seen with left-sided lesions. Other commonly seen manifestations of left-sided lesions include alternating constipation and diarrhea, change in stool caliber (narrow, ribbonlike), and sensation of incomplete evacuation. Obstruction symptoms appear earlier with left-sided lesions because of the smaller lumen size (Fig. 41-10).

Cancers of the right side of the colon are usually asymptomatic. Vague abdominal discomfort or crampy, colicky abdomi-

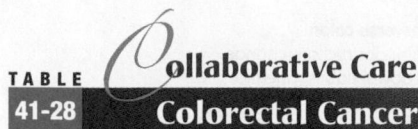

TABLE 41-28 Collaborative Care Colorectal Cancer

Diagnostic
History and physical examination
Digital rectal examination
Sigmoidoscopy
Colonoscopy
Barium enema
CBC
Liver function tests
Testing of stool for occult blood
Carcinoembryonic antigen test (CEA)
CT scan of abdomen
Ultrasound

Collaborative Therapy
Surgery
  Right hemicolectomy
  Left hemicolectomy
  Abdominal-perineal resection
  Laparoscopic colectomy
Radiation
Chemotherapy
  5-fluorouracil (5-FU)
  leucovorin (Wellcovorin)
  leucovorin-modulated 5-FU (Orzel)
  irinotecan (Camptosar)
  capecitabine (Xeloda)
  levamisole (Ergamisol)
  oxaliplatin (Eloxatin)
  raltitrexed (Tomudex)

CBC, Complete blood count.

TABLE 41-29 Dukes' Staging System for Colorectal Cancer

CLASSIFICATION	DESCRIPTION
A	Negative nodes, limitation of lesion to mucosa
B_1	Negative nodes, extension of lesion through mucosa but still within bowel wall
B_2	Negative nodes, extension through entire bowel wall
C_1	Positive nodes, limitation of lesion to bowel wall
C_2	Positive nodes, extension of lesion through entire bowel wall
D	Presence of distant, unresectable metastases

CEA does not exclude the possibility of a malignant condition. This test is used most effectively in following the progress of a patient after surgery. Return to normal of a previously elevated CEA indicates successful removal of the tumor. In contrast, persistent postoperative elevated or increasing CEA levels suggest residual tumor or tumor spread.

TABLE 41-30 Tumor–Node–Metastasis (TNM) Classification of Colorectal Cancer

T	PRIMARY TUMOR
T_X	Primary tumor cannot be assessed
T_0	No evidence of primary tumor
T_{is}	Carcinoma in situ
T_1	Tumor invades submucosa
T_2	Tumor invades muscularis propria
T_3	Tumor invades through the muscularis propria into the subserosa or into nonperitonealized pericolic or perirectal tissues
T_4	Tumor perforates the visceral peritoneum or directly invades other organs or structures

N	REGIONAL LYMPH NODE INVOLVEMENT
N_X	Regional lymph node cannot be assessed
N_0	No regional lymph node metastasis
N_1	Metastasis in one to three pericolic or perirectal lymph nodes
N_2	Metastasis in four or more pericolic or perirectal lymph nodes
N_3	Metastasis in any lymph node along the course of a named vascular trunk

M	DISTANT METASTASIS
M_X	Presence of distant metastasis cannot be assessed
M_0	No distant metastasis
M_1	Distant metastasis

STAGE	TNM		
0	T_{is}	N_0	M_0
IA	T_1	N_0	M_0
IB	T_2	N_0	M_0
II	T_1	N_2	M_0
	T_2	N_1	M_0
	T_3	N_0	M_0
IIIA	T_2	N_2	M_0
	T_3	N_{1-2}	M_0
IIIB	T_4	N_{0-1}	M_0
IV	T_4	N_2	M_0
	T_{1-4}	N_{0-2}	M_1

Collaborative Care

Prognosis and treatment correlate with pathologic staging of the disease. Several methods of staging are currently being used. The most widely known is Dukes' classification (Table 41-29). Surgical removal of the primary lesion is the treatment for Dukes' stages A, B, and C. The 5-year survival rate for Dukes' stage A is 90% to 100%, compared with less than 15% for Dukes' stage D.

Another classification system for colorectal cancer is the TNM system (Table 41-30), which is based on pathologic assessment and includes data from the history and physical examination and presurgical endoscopic and laboratory evaluations. Colorectal cancer can also be divided into stages, with stage 0 representing cancer in situ, stage I corresponding to Dukes' A and B_1, stage II corresponding to B_2, stage III corresponding to C_1 and C_2, and stage IV corresponding to Dukes' D.

Several noninvasive procedures may be performed through a colonoscope to effectively treat certain types of colorectal cancer.

Endoscopic polypectomy is a highly effective and safe procedure. Adequate treatment can be obtained if the resected margin of the polyp is free of cancer, the cancer is well differentiated, and there is no apparent lymphatic or blood vessel involvement. Laser therapy may be used to ablate nonresectable tumors. This is usually used only as palliative therapy in patients with obstructive symptoms.

Surgical Therapy. Surgery is the only curative treatment of colorectal cancer. The location and extent of the cancer determine the type of surgery performed. Success of surgery depends on resection of the tumor with an adequate margin of healthy bowel and resection of the regional lymph nodes.

Right hemicolectomy is performed when the cancer is located in the cecum, ascending colon, hepatic flexure, or transverse colon to the right of the middle colic artery. A portion of the terminal ileum, the ileocecal valve, and the appendix are removed, and an ileotransverse anastomosis is performed. A left hemicolectomy involves resection of the left transverse colon, the splenic flexure, the descending colon, the sigmoid colon, and the upper portion of the rectum.

Clear margins are most difficult to obtain with rectal carcinoma. Location of the rectal lesion determines the surgical procedure to be performed. There must be enough rectum left to ensure a secure anastomosis, or an abdominal-perineal resection is indicated. Abdominal-perineal resection is most often performed when the cancer is located within 5 cm of the anus.

In the abdominal-perineal resection, an abdominal incision is made, and the proximal sigmoid is brought through the abdominal wall in a permanent colostomy. The distal sigmoid, rectum, and anus are removed through a perineal incision. The perineal wound may be closed around a drain or left open with packing to allow healing by granulation. Complications that can occur are delayed wound healing, hemorrhage, persistent perineal sinus tracts, infections, and urinary tract and sexual dysfunctions.

Low anterior resection may be indicated for tumors of the rectosigmoid and the mid-to-upper rectum. The use of EEA (end-to-end anastomosis) staplers has allowed lower and more secure anastomoses. The stapler is passed through the anus, where the colon is stapled to the rectum. This technique has made it possible to resect lesions as low as 5 cm from the anus.

Sphincter-sparing procedures are being performed on the patient who is a poor operative risk and for the patient with early disease. The number of these procedures may increase with continued early detection and surveillance. In these procedures a local resection is performed, and the anal sphincters are left intact.

Laparoscopic colectomy is being evaluated for its effectiveness in eliminating cancer and improving survival. Potential benefits are faster return of bowel function, fewer incisional infections, shortened hospital stay, and improved cosmetic appearance.[26]

Chemotherapy and Radiation Therapy. Chemotherapy is recommended when a patient has positive lymph nodes at the time of surgery or has metastatic disease. Chemotherapy is used both as an adjuvant therapy following colon resection and as primary treatment for nonresectable colorectal cancer.[27] At present, the combination of 5-fluorouracil (5-FU) plus leucovorin and irinotecan (Camptosar) is approved as first-line chemotherapy for patients with metastatic colorectal cancer. Additional treatment protocols include the use of 5-FU and levamisole (Ergamisol) with or without leucovorin (Wellcovorin). For patients who are not considered appropriate candidates for this triple therapy, either leucovorin-modulated 5-FU (Orzel) or capecitabine (Xeloda) is used as an acceptable alternative first-line treatment. New agents being examined for adjuvant therapy of colorectal cancer include oxaliplatin (Eloxatin), raltitrexed (Tomudex), and monoclonal antibodies.[27]

Radiation may be used postoperatively as an adjuvant to colon resection and chemotherapy or as a palliative measure for patients with advanced lesions. As a palliative measure, its primary objective is to reduce tumor size and provide symptomatic relief. (For discussion on radiation therapy, see Chapter 15.)

NURSING MANAGEMENT
COLORECTAL CANCER

■ Nursing Assessment

Subjective and objective data that should be obtained from a patient with colorectal cancer are presented in Table 41-31.

■ Nursing Diagnoses

Nursing diagnoses for the patient with cancer of the colon or rectum include, but are not limited to, the following:

- Diarrhea or constipation *related to* altered bowel elimination patterns
- Acute pain *related to* difficulty in passing stools because of partial or complete obstruction from tumor
- Fear *related to* diagnosis of colorectal cancer, surgical or therapeutic interventions, and possible terminal illness
- Ineffective coping *related to* diagnosis of cancer and side effects of treatment

TABLE 41-31 Nursing Assessment Colorectal Cancer

Subjective Data
Important Health Information
Past health history: Previous breast or ovarian cancer, familial polyposis, villous adenoma, adenomatous polyps, inflammatory bowel disease
Medications: Use of any medications affecting bowel function (e.g., cathartics, antidiarrheal drugs)
Functional Health Patterns
Health perception–health management: Family history of colorectal, breast, or ovarian cancer; weakness, fatigue
Nutritional-metabolic: High-calorie, high-fat, low-fiber diet; anorexia, weight loss; nausea and vomiting
Elimination: Change in bowel habits; alternating diarrhea and constipation, defecation urgency; rectal bleeding; mucoid stools; black, tarry stools; increased flatus, decrease in stool caliber; feelings of incomplete evacuation
Cognitive-perceptual: Abdominal and low back pain, tenesmus

Objective Data
General
Pallor, cachexia, lymphadenopathy (later signs)
Gastrointestinal
Palpable abdominal mass, distention, ascites, and hepatomegaly (liver metastasis)
Possible Findings
Anemia; guaiac-positive stools, palpable mass on digital rectal examination; positive sigmoidoscopy, colonoscopy, barium enema, or CT scan; positive biopsy

NURSING RESEARCH
Demands of Colorectal Cancer

Citation   Klemm P, Miller MA, Fernsler J: Demands of illness in people treated for colorectal cancer, *Oncol Nurs Forum* 27:633, 2000.

Purpose   To describe the most common and intense demands of illness in patients with colorectal cancer.

Methods   Patients who were treated for colorectal cancer were recruited through online computer postings. Patients (n = 121) were mailed Demands of Illness Inventory and demographic questionnaires that were returned to the investigators. Respondents were from 35 states and 5 countries.

Results and Conclusions   Overall the greatest demands reported were related to psychosocial and existential concerns. The demands of illness were greatest in the personal meaning domain with 93% of patients reporting that they thought about the value of life and how long they might live and 83% reported uncertainty. Younger patients (<45 years of age) reported more demands than older patients. Time since treatment, perception of illness, and activity level all influenced the demands of illness scores.

Implications for Nursing Practice   Patients with colorectal cancer experience a number of physical and psychologic challenges, especially the younger patients. Nurses need to address these concerns with patients, as well as provide interventions to reduce the psychologic distress associated with the diagnosis and treatment of colorectal cancer.

■ Planning

The overall goals are that the patient with colorectal cancer will have (1) normal bowel elimination patterns, (2) quality of life appropriate to disease progression, (3) relief of pain, and (4) feelings of comfort and well-being.

■ Nursing Implementation

Health Promotion. The current recommendations from the American Cancer Society for colorectal cancer screening in patients who are not at high risk include annual digital rectal examination beginning at the age of 50 years. Starting at the age of 50 years, fecal testing for occult blood should be done every year, and flexible sigmoidoscopy should be performed every 5 years. Positive findings should be followed with colonoscopy or double-contrast barium enema.[24]

Screening for high-risk patients should begin before age 50, usually beginning with colonoscopy and continuing at more frequent intervals that vary according to risk factors.[24] Participation in early cancer screening is effective in decreasing mortality, but barriers exist, including lack of information and fear of diagnosis.[28]

Recent epidemiology studies reported that use of NSAIDs (e.g., sulindac [Clinoril], ibuprofen [Motrin])[29] or long-term use of aspirin (four to six tablets per day)[30] may reduce the risk of colorectal cancer.

Acute Intervention

Preoperative care. Acute nursing care for the patient with a colon resection is similar to care of the patient having a laparotomy (see NCP 41-2). In addition to general preoperative teaching and ostomy care instructions, the patient undergoing abdominal-perineal resection should be informed of the extent of the surgical procedure and the amount of care necessary to facilitate complete wound healing. The patient should be taught side-to-side positioning and made to understand that short walks are better than sitting. The nurse should teach and assist the patient in proper positioning for taking a sitz bath. The patient may not know that the sitz bath and positioning are sources of comfort. The patient may experience phantom rectal sensation because the sympathetic nerves responsible for rectal control are not severed during the surgery. The nurse must be astute in distinguishing phantom sensations from perineal abscess pain.

Postoperative care. After an abdominal-perineal resection, there are two wounds, and a stoma is surgically constructed in the left lower quadrant. There is an abdominal incision through which the colon is resected, and an incision is made in the perineum. The management of a perineal incision differs depending on the type of wound. Three techniques are used: (1) packing of the entire open wound, (2) partial closure with Penrose drains for open drainage, and (3) primary closure of the perineal wound with closed-suction drainage of the pelvic cavity. The type of management of the perineal wound is individualized. The open and packed method is used in patients with extensive surgery or uncontrollable bleeding in the pelvic wound. When infection or contamination is minimal, a partial closure with drains is used. Wound sites connected to low intermittent suction or a Jackson-Pratt or Hemovac suction placed in the perineal wound is commonly used to provide drainage of the operative site during the

EVIDENCE-BASED PRACTICE
Follow-up for Patients with Colorectal Cancer

Clinical Problem

Does intensive follow-up of patients with nonmetastatic colorectal cancer improve survival?

Best Clinical Practice

- Considerable controversy exists about how often patients should be seen and what tests should be performed after surgery for colorectal cancer in patients with no evidence of metastatic disease at the time of surgery.
- Results of a review of five randomized controlled clinical trials suggest there is an overall survival benefit for intensifying the follow-up of patients, including visits to health care provider and diagnostic studies (e.g., liver imaging).
- Ongoing clinical trials will investigate the best combination and frequency of clinical visits, blood tests, endoscopic procedures, and other diagnostic tests to maximize the outcomes for these patients.

Implication for Nursing Practice

Patients may assume their surgery was "curative" and not feel the necessity to return for periodic follow-up evaluations. It is very important that nurses emphasize the value of follow-up visits to a health care provider after surgery for colorectal cancer.

Reference for Evidence

Jeffery GM, Hickey BE, Hider P: Follow-up strategies for patients treated for non-metastatic colorectal cancer, *Cochrane Database of Systematic Reviews,* Issue 2, 2002.

early postoperative period. This usually remains until drainage is less than 50 ml per 24 hours, which occurs after approximately 3 to 5 days.

A patient who has open and packed wounds requires meticulous postoperative care. During the immediate postoperative period the perineal dressing is reinforced and changed frequently because drainage can be profuse for several hours after surgery. All drainage is carefully assessed for amount, color, and consistency. The drainage is usually serosanguineous.

The packing is usually left in place for 2 to 3 days. Packing the pelvic cavity for prolonged periods may result in sepsis and rigidity of the cavity wall and thus impede the healing process. The nurse should examine the wound regularly and record bleeding, excessive drainage, and unusual odor. The perineal wound is usually irrigated with a normal saline solution when the dressings are changed. Dressings are changed several times a day, and aseptic technique is always used.

If the wound is partially closed and drains are in place, the nurse assesses the incision for suture integrity and signs and symptoms of wound inflammation and infection. The drainage is examined for amount, color, and characteristics. When the primary closure technique is used, the catheters are left in place for approximately 3 to 5 days, and during this time the drainage is examined and observations recorded. The area around the catheter is observed for signs of inflammation and kept clean and dry. The nurse should observe for signs of edema, erythema, drainage around the suture line, fever, and elevated WBC count. If the perineal wound was not closed, warm sitz baths at 100.4° to 106° F (38° to 41° C) for 10 to 20 minutes three to four times a day assist in tissue debridement, provide comfort, and increase circulation to the area. Moist heat causes vasodilation, which allows more oxygen to flow to the affected area. Sitz baths of more than 20 minutes may result in too much vasodilation, causing congestion and discomfort.

The patient may complain of pain and itching in and around the wound. There is no physiologic explanation of sensations that are felt, but a careful examination should be made to rule out delayed wound healing. Antipruritic agents and sitz baths are usually ordered. Use of a pressure-reducing chair cushion provides comfort when sitting. Sitting on a toilet for prolonged periods is discouraged until the perineal wound is well healed.

Sexual dysfunction is a possible complication of an abdominal-perineal resection and should be included in the plan of care. Although the effect of the procedure depends on the technique used, the surgeon should discuss the subject intelligently and tactfully, with follow-up as necessary by other members of the health care team. The nurse should understand that erection, ejaculation, and orgasm involve different nerve pathways and that a dysfunction of one does not mean total sexual dysfunction. The ET nurse is an important member of the team and can often provide correct and factual information concerning sexual dysfunction resulting from an abdominal-perineal resection.

Ambulatory and Home Care. Psychologic support for the patient and family is important. The recovery period is long, and the possibility of recurrence of cancer is always present. The overall 5-year survival rate for all patients undergoing resection for colorectal cancer is less than 50%. This presents a problem for the patient and health care providers because of the often painful, debilitating, and demoralizing manifestations produced by the recurrent disease and the lack of any effective palliative

therapy. Chemotherapy may be used as an adjuvant measure for the patient with evidence of local or distant metastasis. (The special needs of the cancer patient are discussed in Chapter 15.)

The perineal wound may not be completely healed before discharge. After discharge the health care provider, the home health nurse, and the ET nurse in an outpatient clinic usually see the patient. The wound is usually irrigated and debrided. The skin around the wound should be assessed for loose hair. Shaving may be necessary to prevent the development of a chronic draining sinus. The nurse should report the drainage because it may also indicate the presence of a foreign body, fistula, or rectal tissue not removed during surgery. The patient and significant others are taught management of the wound and the procedure to take a sitz bath at home. The patient and the family should be aware of all community services available for assistance.

■ Evaluation

The expected outcomes for the patient with colorectal cancer are that the patient will have
- minimal alterations in bowel elimination patterns
- relief of pain
- balanced nutritional intake
- quality of life appropriate to disease progression
- feelings of comfort and well-being

OSTOMY SURGERY

Types

An **ostomy** is a surgical procedure in which an opening is made to allow the passage of intestinal contents from the bowel to an incision or stoma. The stoma, which is the opening on the surface of the abdomen, is created when the intestine is brought through the abdominal wall and sutured to the skin. It may be permanent or temporary. Fecal matter is diverted through the stoma to the outside of the abdominal wall.

An *ileostomy* is an opening from the ileum through the abdominal wall and is also referred to as a conventional or Brooke ileostomy (Fig. 41-11). It is most commonly used in surgical treatment of ulcerative colitis, Crohn's disease, and familial polyposis.

A *cecostomy* is an opening between the cecum and the abdominal wall. Both cecostomies and ascending colostomies are uncommon. They are usually temporary and most often are used for fecal diversion before surgery or for palliation.

A *colostomy* is an opening between the colon and the abdominal wall. The proximal end of the colon is sutured to the skin. Locations for colostomies are shown in Fig. 41-11. A temporary colostomy is usually performed to protect an end-to-end anastomosis after a bowel resection or is an emergency measure following bowel obstruction (e.g., malignant tumor), abdominal trauma (e.g., gunshot wound), or a perforated diverticulum. Temporary colostomies are usually located in the transverse colon. Loop colostomy (Fig. 41-12) and double-barrel colostomy (see Fig. 41-11) are most commonly performed as temporary colostomies, but they may be permanent. A comparison of colostomies and ileostomy is shown in Table 41-32.

Surgical Therapy

End stoma. An end stoma is surgically constructed by dividing the bowel and bringing out the proximal end as a single stoma. The distal portion of the GI tract is surgically removed, or the distal segment is oversewn and left in the abdominal cavity with its

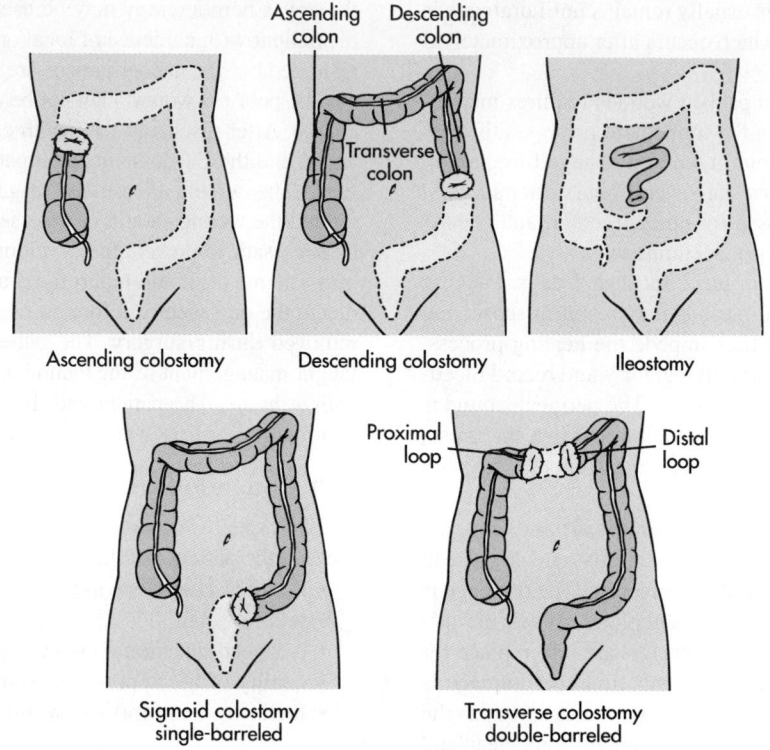

FIG. 41-11 Types of ostomies.

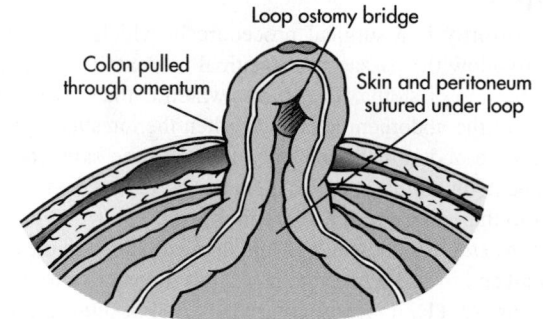

FIG. 41-12 Loop colostomy.

mesentery intact. An end colostomy or ileostomy is then constructed. When the distal bowel is oversewn rather than removed, the procedure is known as a Hartmann's pouch (Fig. 41-13). If the distal bowel is removed, the stoma is permanent; if the distal bowel remains intact and oversewn, the potential exists for the bowel to be reanastomosed and the stoma to be closed (referred to as a *takedown*).

Loop stoma. A loop stoma is constructed by bringing a loop of bowel to the abdominal surface and then opening the anterior wall of the bowel to provide fecal diversion. This results in one stoma with a proximal and distal opening and an intact posterior

TABLE 41-32 Comparison of Colostomies and Ileostomy

	COLOSTOMY			ILEOSTOMY
	ASCENDING	**TRANSVERSE**	**SIGMOID**	
Stool consistency	Semiliquid	Semiliquid to semiformed	Formed	Liquid to semiliquid
Fluid requirement	Increased	Possibly increased	No change	Increased
Bowel regulation	No	Uncommon	Yes (if there is a history of a regular bowel pattern)	No
Pouch and skin barriers	Yes	Yes	Dependent on regulation	Yes
Irrigation	No	No	Possible every 24–48 hr (if patient meets criteria)	No
Indications for surgery	Perforating diverticulitis in lower colon; trauma; inoperable tumors of colon, rectum, or pelvis; rectovaginal fistula	Same as for ascending; birth defect	Cancer of the rectum or rectosigmoidal area; perforating diverticulum; trauma	Ulcerative colitis, Crohn's disease, diseased or injured colon, birth defect, familial polyposis, trauma, cancer

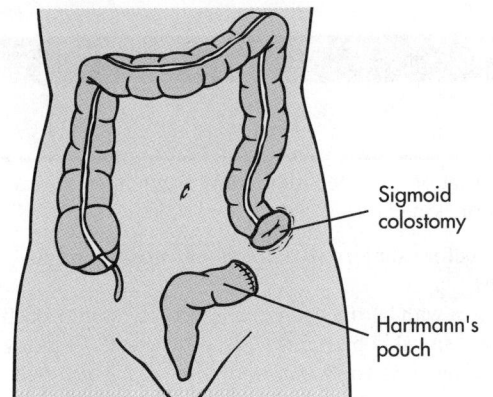

FIG. 41-13 Sigmoid colostomy. Distal bowel is oversewn and left in place to create Hartmann's pouch.

wall that separates the two openings. The loop of bowel is frequently held in place with a plastic rod for 7 to 10 days after surgery to prevent it from slipping back into the abdominal cavity (see Fig. 41-12). A loop stoma is usually temporary.

Double-barrel stoma. When the bowel is divided, both the proximal and distal ends are brought through the abdominal wall as two separate stomas (see Fig. 41-11). The proximal one is the functioning stoma; the distal, nonfunctioning stoma is referred to as the mucus fistula. The double-barrel stoma is usually temporary.

Kock pouch. As described previously in this chapter (see pp. 1071-1072), the *Kock pouch* is a continent ileostomy, which is a variation from the traditional ileostomy (see Fig. 41-3).

Ileoanal reservoir. As previously described in this chapter (pp. 1071-1072), this procedure involves total colectomy and ileoanal anastomosis with the formation of an ileal reservoir (see Fig. 41-4).

NURSING MANAGEMENT OSTOMY SURGERY

■ Preoperative Care

It is important to review the information the patient has received from the health care provider. Psychologic preparation is very important. The family and the patient usually have many questions concerning the procedures. If available, an ET nurse should visit with the patient and the family. The nurse or ET nurse must determine the patient's ability to perform self-care, identify support systems, and determine potential adverse factors that could be modified to facilitate learning during rehabilitation. Preoperative assessment must be comprehensive and include physical, psychologic, social, cultural, and educational components. Assessment is ongoing, including both the patient and family. The ET nurse marks the stoma site before surgery. An improperly placed stoma complicates rehabilitation by increasing time and expense of pouch change routine. It can also contribute to skin irritation and poor adaptation. The patient and the family should understand the extent of surgery, the type of stoma, and its care.

If the patient desires a referral and the health care provider agrees, a trained ostomy visitor from the United Ostomy Association can provide meaningful psychologic support. The patient has the opportunity to see a person who has adjusted well and who has experienced some of the same feelings and concerns. The family will also benefit from the visit.

Bowel preparation before surgery decreases the chance of a postoperative infection by cleansing the bowel of feces and bacteria. Orally administered osmotic lavages (e.g., Go-Lytely) have shortened the classic 72-hour preparation with clear liquids, cathartics, and enemas. IV and oral antibiotics are given. Nonabsorbable neomycin and erythromycin are given orally to decrease the number of intracolonic bacteria.

■ Colostomy Care

Postoperative nursing care should focus on assessing the stoma, protecting the skin, selecting the pouch, and assisting the patient to adapt psychologically to a changed body. Nursing care for the patient with a colostomy is presented in NCP 41-4.

The stoma should be pink. A dusky blue stoma indicates ischemia, and a brown-black stoma indicates necrosis. The nurse should assess and document stoma color every 8 hours. There is mild to moderate swelling of the stoma the first 2 to 3 weeks after surgery (Table 41-33). A skin barrier should be applied to protect the peristomal skin surrounding the stoma. Solid skin barriers include Stomahesive (Convatec), Coloplast, and Hollister skin barriers. The skin should be washed with mild soap, rinsed with warm water, and dried thoroughly before the barrier is applied.

TABLE 41-33	Characteristics of Stoma
CHARACTERISTIC	**DESCRIPTION OR CAUSE**
Color*	
Rose to brick red	Viable stoma mucosa
Pale	May indicate anemia
Blanching, dark red to purple	Indicates inadequate blood supply to the stoma or bowel from adhesions, low flow state, or excessive tension on the bowel at the time of construction
Edema†	
Mild to moderate edema	Normal in the initial postoperative period
	Trauma to the stoma
	Any medical condition that results in edema
Moderate to severe edema	Obstruction of the stoma
	Allergic reaction to food
	Gastroenteritis
Bleeding	
Small amount	Oozing from the stoma mucosa when touched is normal because of its high vascularity
Moderate to large amount‡	Moderate to large amount‡ of bleeding from the stoma mucosa could indicate coagulation factor deficiency; stomal varices secondary to portal hypertension
	Moderate to large amount from intestinal stoma opening could indicate lower gastrointestinal bleeding

*Sustained color changes must be reported to surgeon.
†Closely observe and report to the surgeon and adjust the stoma opening size in the pouch.
‡Report moderate to large amounts of bleeding to surgeon.

NURSING CARE PLAN 41-4

Patient with a Colostomy/Ileostomy

EXPECTED PATIENT OUTCOMES	NURSING INTERVENTIONS and *RATIONALES*
NURSING DIAGNOSIS	**Risk for impaired skin integrity** *related to* irritation from fecal drainage around peristomal area, irritation of appliance, and lack of knowledge of skin care.
▪ Normal skin integrity ▪ Intact pouch seal	▪ Have enterostomal therapy nurse see patient before surgery *to mark stoma site in area free of creases and folds for better seal of the pouch.* ▪ After surgery, assess peristomal skin for erythema with burning and itching, poorly fitting pouch with leakage, lack of adequate skin care, and failure to use skin barrier *to initiate treatment if indicated.* ▪ During pouch change, assess skin for signs of breakdown *to initiate treatment if indicated.* ▪ Clean area with mild soap and water, rinse, and dry thoroughly *to prevent irritation from intestinal contents or pouch adhesive.* ▪ Apply skin barrier *to protect skin and prevent direct contact with intestinal contents.* ▪ Teach patient proper skin and appliance care *to ensure proper technique for long-term care.* ▪ Plan for outpatient or home visit *for continued teaching and monitoring.* ▪ Empty pouch when it is one third to one half full or inflated with gas *to prevent the pouch from leaking.*
NURSING DIAGNOSIS	**Disturbed body image** *related to* presence of ostomy and malodor *as manifested by* verbalization of embarrassment or shame caused by malodor or presence of stoma.
▪ Adjustment to altered body image ▪ Satisfactory plan for control of odor	▪ Assess patient's attitude toward ostomy *to determine if problem is present* and, if indicated, *plan appropriate intervention.* ▪ Instruct patient on measures for odor control, use of odor-proof pouch, pouch deodorants, use of room deodorants when pouch is emptied, and avoidance of foods that are known to increase odor *to minimize embarrassing odors from drainage.* ▪ Discuss normal emotional response to stoma and encourage patient to express feelings *to assist patient in adjusting to change in body.* ▪ Provide patient with information on local United Ostomy Association *to offer patient and family an opportunity for education and support.* ▪ Prepare patient to do own stoma and appliance care *to increase independence and enhance self-esteem/image.*
NURSING DIAGNOSIS	**Imbalanced nutrition: less than body requirements** *related to* lack of knowledge of appropriate foods and decreased appetite *as manifested by* weight loss, vitamin and mineral deficiencies, inability to tolerate certain foods.
▪ Adequate dietary intake to maintain weight at optimum level	▪ Assess nutritional intake *to determine need for intervention.* ▪ Gradually introduce foods one at a time *to identify individual foods that may be problematic* and begin with low-residue diet, *which is usually well-tolerated.* ▪ Teach patient to chew food slowly and thoroughly *to facilitate digestion and prevent gas.* ▪ Give list of foods (high roughage) that have potential for obstruction to ileostomy patients *so that patient has a ready source for reference.* ▪ Arrange visit with dietitian if indicated.
NURSING DIAGNOSIS	**Ineffective sexuality patterns** *related to* perceived loss of sexual appeal and possibility of accidental seepage of fecal material during sexual activity *as manifested by* verbalization of concern about intimate relations with spouse or significant other.
▪ Confidence in ability to resume previous sexual activity	▪ Assess patient's attitude about impact of ostomy on sexual functioning *to determine if a problem exists and if there is a need to plan interventions.* ▪ Encourage discussion of meaning of sexuality to patient and significant other *to allow patient opportunity to discuss sensitive topic in a nonthreatening situation.* ▪ Discuss ways to avoid seepage and conceal stoma and/or appliance during intimate relations *to decrease fear of embarrassment or withdrawal from intimate situations because of anxiety over "accidents."* ▪ If appropriate, arrange visit with person of same sex and condition *to discuss sexual concerns and share potential solutions; to provide an opportunity to ask questions; and to get practical, realistic answers from a supportive, understanding other.* ▪ Encourage use of perfumes or fragrant body oils during sexual activity *to decrease fear of having an offensive body odor.*

NURSING CARE PLAN 41-4

Patient with a Colostomy/Ileostomy—cont'd

EXPECTED PATIENT OUTCOMES	NURSING INTERVENTIONS and *RATIONALES*
NURSING DIAGNOSIS	**Risk for deficient fluid volume** *related to* excess fluid loss from ileostomy or diarrhea with a colostomy and inadequate oral intake.
• Normal serum electrolytes • Normal vital signs • Good skin turgor • Urine output >0.5 ml/kg/hr	• Assess for signs of weakness, poor skin turgor, sunken eyes, hypotension, tachycardia, hypokalemia, hyponatremia, oliguria *to determine presence of fluid volume deficit and, if present, plan appropriate interventions.* • Record intake and output and include ileostomy drainage *to have an accurate record of fluid balance.* • Ensure fluid intake of at least 3000 ml/day in the initial postoperative period *to prevent dehydration.* • Instruct patient to maintain high fluid intake and to increase it during very hot weather, when patient is perspiring excessively, and during episodes of diarrhea *to ensure adequate fluid intake in various situations.* • Monitor serum electrolytes *to detect any imbalances.* • Instruct patient on signs and symptoms of sodium, potassium, and fluid deficits *to ensure early reporting and correction of underlying problem.*

With an open-ended, transparent, plastic, odor-proof pouch, it is easy to protect the skin and to observe and collect the drainage. The pouch must fit snugly to prevent leakage around the stoma. The size of the stoma is determined with a stoma-measuring card. Although the pouch is applied after surgery, the colostomy functions when peristalsis has been adequately restored. When a temporary colostomy is performed and the stoma is opened in the operating room with no bowel preparation being done previously, the stoma functions immediately.

The volume, color, and consistency of the drainage are recorded. Each time the pouch is changed, the condition of the skin is observed for irritation. A pouch should never be placed directly on irritated skin without the use of a skin barrier.

A colostomy in the ascending and transverse colon has semiliquid stools. The patient needs to be instructed to use a drainable pouch. A colostomy in the sigmoid or descending colon has semiformed or formed stools and can sometimes be regulated by the irrigation method. The patient may or may not wear a drainage pouch. A nondrainable pouch should have a gas filter.

For most patients with colostomies, there are few, if any, dietary restrictions. A well-balanced diet and adequate fluid intake are important. The patient's medical and surgical history must be considered when individualizing dietary instructions. Table 41-34 lists foods and their effects on stoma output.

Colostomy Irrigations. Colostomy irrigations are intended to regulate bowel function, treat constipation, or prepare the bowel for surgery. When done to achieve a regular bowel pattern, the irrigations stimulate the bowel to function at a specific time every day or every other day. If control is achieved, there should be little or no spillage between irrigations. The patient who establishes regularity may need to wear only a pad or small pouch over the stoma. The patient who cannot or chooses not to establish regularity by irrigations must wear a pouch at all times. The procedure for colostomy irrigation is presented in Table 41-35.

All equipment should be assembled before the irrigation. A commercially obtained irrigation set usually has all the equipment needed. The nurse should encourage the patient to watch

TABLE 41-34   Nutritional Therapy

Effects of Food on Stoma Output

Odor Producing*	Diarrhea Causing*
Eggs	Alcohol
Garlic	Beer
Onions	Cabbage family
Fish	Spinach
Asparagus	Green beans
Cabbage	Coffee
Broccoli	Spicy foods
Alcohol	Fruits (raw)
Gas Forming*	**Potential Obstruction in Ileostomy†**
Beans	Nuts
Cabbage family	Raisins
Onions	Popcorn
Beer	Seeds
Carbonated beverages	Vegetables (raw)
Cheeses (strong)	Celery
Sprouts	Corn

*The effect of food on stoma output is individual. Patients are not discouraged from eating the above-listed foods and beverages.
†Patients are encouraged to chew high-roughage food well and initially limit the amount, and to drink increased amounts of fluids.

the procedure and should explain each step to the patient. The cone tip on the tubing controls the depth of insertion and prevents the water from coming out from the stoma and not going into the colon. If resistance is met, force should not be used because perforation of the intestine can result. However, this is unlikely when using a stoma cone. A hard plastic catheter is not recommended because of the risk of intestinal perforation. The procedure should not be rushed; the patient should feel relaxed. The patient or family member must be instructed in the procedure and

TABLE 41-35 — Patient & Family Teaching Guide: Colostomy Irrigation

Equipment
Lubricant

Irrigation set (1000- to 2000-ml container, tubing with irrigating stoma cone, clamp)

Irrigating sleeve with adhesive or belt

Toilet tissue to clean around the stoma

Disposal sack for soiled dressing

Procedure
1. Place 500 to 1000 ml of lukewarm water (not to exceed 105° F [40.5° C]) in container. The volume is titrated for the individual; use enough irrigant to distend the bowel but not enough to cause cramping pain. Most adults use 500 to 1000 ml of water.
2. Ensure comfortable position. Patient may sit in chair in front of toilet or on the toilet if the perineal wound is healed.
3. Clear tubing of all air by flushing it with fluid.
4. Hang container on hook or IV pole (18 to 24 inches) above stoma (about shoulder height).
5. Apply irrigating sleeve and place bottom end in toilet bowl.
6. Lubricate stoma cone, insert cone tip gently into the stoma, and hold tip securely in place.
7. Allow irrigation solution to flow in steadily for 5 to 10 minutes.
8. If cramping occurs, stop the flow of solution for a few seconds, leaving the cone in place.
9. Clamp the tubing and remove irrigating cone when the desired amount of irrigant has been delivered or when the patient senses colonic distention.
10. Allow 30 to 45 minutes for the solution and feces to be expelled. Initial evacuation is usually complete in 10 to 15 minutes. Close off the irrigating sleeve at the bottom to allow ambulation.
11. Clean, rinse, and dry peristomal skin well.
12. Replace the colostomy drainage pouch or desired stoma covering.
13. Wash and rinse all equipment and hang to dry.

TABLE 41-36 — Patient & Family Teaching Guide: Ostomy Self-Care

The following are guidelines to include for patient and family teaching:

1. Explain the following principles of ostomy and pouch care
   - Apply and change pouch to collect intestinal drainage.
   - Empty pouch before it is one-third full to prevent leakage.
   - Cleanse skin and use skin barriers and deodorizers to prevent skin breakdown and malodor.
   - Irrigate colostomy to regulate bowel elimination (optional).
   - Explain how to contact the enterostomal therapy nurse with questions.
   - Explain how to obtain additional supplies.
2. Teach the following dietary and fluid intake guidelines
   - Identify a well-balanced diet and dietary supplements to prevent nutritional deficiencies.
   - Identify foods to avoid to reduce diarrhea, gas, or obstruction (with ileostomy).
   - Drink at least 3000 ml/day of fluid to prevent dehydration (unless contraindicated).
   - Increase fluid intake during hot weather, excessive perspiration, and diarrhea to replace losses and prevent dehydration.
   - Explain how to contact registered dietitian with questions.
3. Describe potential resources to assist with emotional and psychologic adjustment
   - Identify persons available to provide emotional support.
   - Identify community resources for psychologic counseling.
   - Contact United Ostomy Association for information or peer support.
   - Inform that treatment for potential depression is available if needed.
4. Explain the importance of follow-up care

   Report signs and symptoms of:
   - Fluid and electrolyte deficits
   - Fever
   - Diarrhea
   - Skin irritation
   - Other stoma problems, including a change in appearance of the stoma or its function, a change in the peristomal area, tenderness, erythema, or pain

must be able to demonstrate the ability to irrigate before being independent. This can be done in the outpatient setting.

The patient should be able to perform a pouch change, care for skin, control odor, care for the stoma, and identify signs and symptoms of complications. The patient should know the importance of fluids and food in the diet, have names and addresses of the United Ostomy Association, and know when to seek medical care. Home care and outpatient follow-up by an ET nurse is highly recommended. Patients should be discharged with written instructions for pouch change, teaching literature relevant to the type of stoma they have, a list of equipment they use, a list of equipment retailers (including names and phone numbers), outpatient follow-up appointments with the surgeon and ET nurse, and the phone numbers of the surgeon and nurse. The patient and family teaching guidelines are included in Table 41-36.

■ Ileostomy Care

Care of the ileostomy is presented in NCP 41-4. An ileostomy stoma protrusion of at least 1 to 1.5 cm makes care easier. When the stoma is flat, seepage occurs, resulting in altered skin integrity. Drainage is frequent and extremely irritating to the skin. Regularity cannot be established. A pouch must be worn at all times. An open-ended, drainable pouch is worn by the patient so that drainage can be emptied when one-third full. The drainable pouch is usually worn for 4 to 7 days before being changed as long as leakage does not occur around the stoma. If pouch leakage occurs, the pouch should be promptly removed, the skin should be cleansed, and a new pouch placed. A solid skin barrier should always be used. A transparent pouch should be used in the initial postoperative period to facilitate assessment of stoma viability and ease of pouch application by the patient.

Immediately after surgery, intake and output must be accurately monitored. The patient should be observed for signs and symptoms of fluid and electrolyte imbalance, particularly potassium, sodium, and fluid deficits. In the first 24 to 48 hours after surgery the amount of drainage from the stoma may be negligible. A person with an ileostomy has lost the absorptive functions provided by the colon, as well as the delay feature provided by the ileocecal valve. Once peristalsis returns, the patient may experience a period of high-volume output of 1000 to 1800 ml per day. Later on, the average amount can be 800 ml daily because the proximal small bowel adapts. If the small bowel has been shortened as a result of surgical resections, the drainage from the ileostomy may be greater. The patient must understand the importance of fluid and electrolyte balance.

The patient should be instructed to drink at least 2 to 3 L of fluid daily; more may be necessary when diarrhea occurs and when perspiration is increased. Diarrhea from an ileostomy produces acidosis from the loss of bicarbonate. The health care provider may instruct the patient to take an electrolyte solution at home (e.g., 1 teaspoon of salt and 1 teaspoon of baking soda in 1 quart of water). Fluids rich in electrolytes should be encouraged.

Usually a low-roughage diet is ordered initially. Fiber-containing foods are reintroduced gradually. Later there are no dietary restrictions. It is important to limit the amount of high-roughage foods (e.g., popcorn), chew them well, and accompany them with fluids. The goal for the patient is a return to a normal, presurgical diet.

The stoma may bleed easily when it is touched because it has a high vascular supply. The patient should be told that minimal oozing of blood is normal. If the terminal ileum has been removed, the patient may need cobalamin (vitamin B_{12}) injections.

■ Adaptation to an Ostomy

Adaptation to the ostomy is a gradual process. The patient experiences a grief reaction to the loss of a body part and an alteration in body image. Each person uses different coping mechanisms. The adjustment period for the person depends on the individual. Psychologic support during the grieving process is needed. There are concerns about body image, sexual activity, family responsibilities, and changes in lifestyle. The patient may become resentful and have fears of odor or soiling. Supportive measures by nurses include helping the patient acquire knowledge, providing or recommending support services, and identifying coping mechanisms that are effective. The nurse provides support by responding to the physiologic needs of stoma care and the psychosocial needs of self-esteem.

The patient should not be forced to learn to care for the stoma. The nurse should watch for clues that the patient is ready. Teaching at the appropriate time is an important part of the care and can contribute to a smooth adjustment process.

Activities of daily living are resumed within 6 to 8 weeks. Heavy lifting should be avoided. The patient's physical condition determines when sports may be resumed. Bathing and swimming are not prohibited. Water does not harm the stoma.

■ Sexual Dysfunction after Ostomy Surgery

Discussion of sexuality and sexual function must be incorporated in the plan of care. The nurse can help the patient understand that sexual function or sexual activity may be affected, but sexuality does not have to be altered.

Pelvic surgery can disrupt nerve and vascular supply to the genitals. Radiation, chemotherapy, and medications can also alter sexual function. Hormones and overall physical health of the patient influence desire. Certain pain medications and antiemetics can lower the sex drive. Generalized fatigue caused by illness can also influence desire. By communicating this information to patients, they can plan sexual activity around a drug schedule and energy levels. Any pelvic surgery that removes the rectum has the potential of damaging the parasympathetic nerve plexus. Erection in men depends on the parasympathetic nerves that control blood flow and vascular supply to the pelvis and the pudendal nerves that transmit sensory responses from the genital area. Nerve-sparing surgical techniques are used when possible to preserve sexual function. Radiation therapy to the pelvis can reduce blood vascularity to the pelvis by causing scarring in the small blood vessels. A woman's sexual functioning after healing includes expansion and lubrication of the vagina. Pelvic surgery usually does not affect a woman's arousal unless part of or the entire vagina is removed. Radiation therapy can affect vaginal expansion and lubrication.

Muscular contraction and genital pleasure that occur during orgasm are not disrupted by pelvic surgery. If the sympathetic nerves in the presacral area are damaged, the male mechanism of emission can be disrupted. This can occur in an abdominal-perineal resection. Orgasms can occur in both men and women who have had stoma surgery, although other aspects of the sexual response may be affected.

The psychologic impact of the stoma and how it affects the patient's body image and self-esteem must be discussed. Emotional factors can contribute to sexual problems. A life-threatening illness can override concerns about sexual function. The nurse can assist a patient to identify ways of coping with depression and anxiety resulting from illness, surgery, or postoperative problems.

The social impact of the stoma is interrelated with the psychologic, physical, and sexual aspects. Concerns of people with stomas include the ability to resume sexual activity, altering clothing styles, the effect on daily activities, sleeping while wearing a pouch, passing gas, the presence of odor, cleanliness, and deciding when or if to tell others about the stoma. The fear of rejection from a partner or the fear that others will not find them desirable as a sexual partner can be a concern. The nurse should encourage open communication about feelings and should realize that the patient needs time to adjust to the pouch and to body changes before feeling secure in his or her sexual functioning.

Although pregnancy is possible, the health care provider may recommend a limited number of pregnancies on the basis of the patient's physical condition. The person with an ostomy who becomes pregnant should have regular medical care.

DIVERTICULOSIS AND DIVERTICULITIS

A **diverticulum** is a saccular dilation or outpouching of the mucosa through the circular smooth muscle of the intestinal wall. Clinically, diverticular disease occurs in two forms: diverticulosis and diverticulitis. Multiple noninflamed diverticula are present with *diverticulosis*. The patient is most often free of symptoms but may have some abdominal discomfort. In *diverticulitis*, inflammation of the diverticula occurs (Fig. 41-14). Diverticula may occur at any point within the GI tract but are most commonly found in the sigmoid colon.

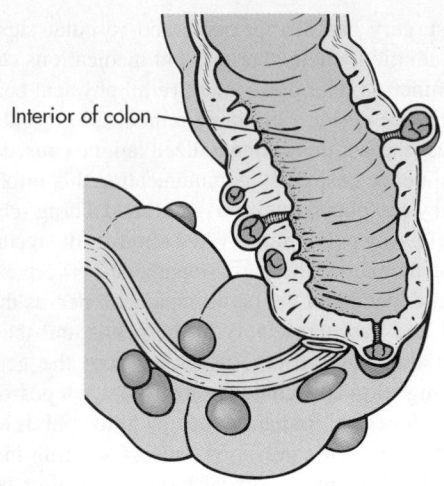

FIG. 41-14 Diverticula are outpouchings of the colon. When they become inflamed, the condition is diverticulitis. The inflammatory process can spread to the surrounding area in the intestine.

Etiology and Pathophysiology

Diverticular disease is a common GI disorder that affects 5% of the population by the age of 40 years and 50% by the age of 80 years.[31] It affects men and women equally, but men seem to have a higher complication rate. Although it affects almost 30 million Americans, most are asymptomatic.

There is no known cause of diverticular disease, but deficiency in dietary fiber has been associated with it. The disease is more prevalent in Western populations that consume diets low in fiber and high in refined carbohydrates, and it is virtually unknown in areas of the world, such as rural Africa, where high-fiber diets are consumed.

When diverticula form, the smooth muscle of the colon wall becomes thickened (Fig. 41-15). Lack of dietary fiber slows transit time, and more water is absorbed from the stool, making it more difficult to pass through the lumen. Decreased bulk of the stool, combined with a more narrowed lumen in the sigmoid colon, causes high intraluminal pressures. These factors are believed to contribute to the formation of diverticula.

The cause of diverticulitis is related to the retention of stool and bacteria in the diverticulum, forming a hardened mass called a *fecalith*. This causes inflammation and usually small perfora-

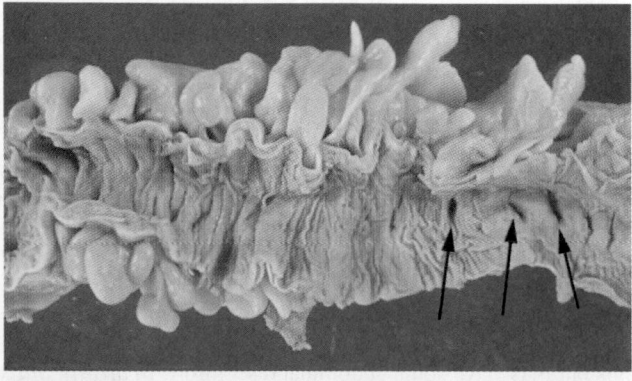

FIG. 41-15 In diverticular disease, the outpouches *(arrows)* of mucosa appear as slitlike openings from the mucosal surface of the open bowel.

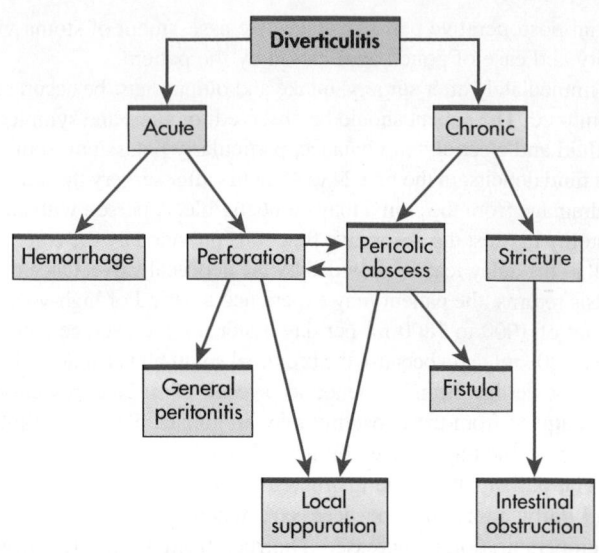

FIG. 41-16 Complications of diverticulitis.

tions. Inflammation of the diverticulum spreads to the surrounding area in the intestines (Fig. 41-16), causing the tissue to become edematous. Abscesses may form, or complete perforation with peritonitis may occur.

Clinical Manifestations

The majority of patients with diverticulosis have no symptoms. Those with symptoms typically have crampy abdominal pain located in the left lower quadrant that is usually relieved by passage of flatus or bowel movement. Alternating constipation and diarrhea may be present.

Approximately 15% of patients with diverticulosis progress to acute diverticulitis. In patients with diverticulitis, abdominal pain is localized over the involved area of the colon. A tender, left lower quadrant mass may be felt on palpation of the abdomen. Fever, chills, nausea, anorexia, and elevated WBC may be present. Elderly patients with diverticulitis are frequently afebrile, with a normal WBC, and little, if any, abdominal tenderness.

Complications of diverticulitis include perforation with peritonitis, abscess and fistula formation, bowel obstruction, ureteral obstruction, and bleeding. Bleeding is a common complication of diverticulitis and is manifested by *hematochezia* (maroon stools). Bleeding usually stops spontaneously.

Diagnostic Studies

A CT scan with oral contrast is the test of choice for diverticulitis.[31] A CBC, urinalysis, and fecal occult blood test should be performed (Table 41-37). A barium enema is used to determine narrowing or obstruction of the colonic lumen. A colonoscopy may be performed to rule out possible hidden polyps or lesions. A patient with acute diverticulitis should not have a barium enema or colonoscopy because of the possibility of perforation and peritonitis.

NURSING *and* COLLABORATIVE MANAGEMENT
DIVERTICULOSIS AND DIVERTICULITIS

Uncomplicated diverticular disease is treated with a high-fiber diet (see Table 41-9) and bulk laxatives, such as psyllium hydrophilic mucilloid (Metamucil). Anticholinergic drugs such as

TABLE 41-37   Collaborative Care — Diverticulosis and Diverticulitis

Diagnostic
History and physical examination
Testing of stool for occult blood
Barium enema
Sigmoidoscopy
Colonoscopy
CBC
Urinalysis
Blood culture

Collaborative Therapy
Ambulatory and Home Care
High-residue diet
Dietary fiber supplements
Stool softeners
Anticholinergics
Mineral oil
Bed rest
Clear liquid diet
Oral antibiotics
Bulk laxatives
Acute Care: Diverticulitis
Antibiotics
NPO status
IV fluids
Possible colon resection for obstruction or hemorrhage
Bed rest
NG suction

CBC, Complete blood count; *IV,* intravenous; *NG,* nasogastric; *NPO,* nothing by mouth.

dicyclomine (Bentyl) and Donnatal may be used to relieve discomfort from spasm of the bowel (see Table 41-37).

Fluids should be increased because fibers retain water, thus decreasing the amount absorbed by the body. If the patient is obese, a reduction in weight is needed. Increased intraabdominal pressure should be avoided because it may precipitate an attack. Factors that increase intraabdominal pressure are straining at stool, vomiting, bending, lifting, and tight, restrictive clothing.

In acute diverticulitis, the goal of treatment is to allow the colon to rest and the inflammation to subside. The patient is kept on NPO status and bed rest and is given parenteral fluids. An NG tube may be necessary. The patient should be observed for signs of possible peritonitis. In acute diverticulitis, broad-spectrum antibiotic therapy is required. The WBC count is monitored.

When the acute attack subsides, oral fluids progressing to a semisolid diet are allowed. Ambulation is also permitted. At this stage the patient should be observed for a recurrent attack. If the patient has a bowel resection or colostomy, the nursing care is the same as for these procedures.

Approximately 30% of patients with acute diverticulitis require surgical intervention. Patients with complicated diverticular disease often require surgery. Surgical intervention is necessary to drain abscesses or to resect an obstructing inflammatory mass. The usual surgical procedures involve resection of the involved colon with a temporary diverting colostomy. The colostomy is reanastomosed after the colon is healed.

The patient should be provided with a full explanation of the condition. The better the patient understands the disease process and adheres to the prescribed regimen, the less likely the exacerbation of the disease and the onset of complications.

HERNIAS

A **hernia** is a protrusion of a viscus through an abnormal opening or a weakened area in the wall of the cavity in which it is normally contained. A hernia may occur in any part of the body, but it usually occurs within the abdominal cavity. If the hernia can be placed back into the abdominal cavity, it is known as *reducible.* The hernia can be reduced by manipulation, or it can occur without manipulation when the person lies down. If the hernia cannot be placed back into the abdominal cavity, it is known as *irreducible,* or incarcerated. In this situation the intestinal flow may be obstructed. When the hernia is irreducible and the intestinal flow and blood supply are obstructed, the hernia is strangulated. The result is an acute intestinal obstruction.

Types

The *inguinal hernia* is the most common type of hernia and occurs at the point of weakness in the abdominal wall where the spermatic cord in men and the round ligament in women emerge (Fig. 41-17). When the protrusion escapes through the inguinal ring and follows the spermatic cord or the round ligament, it is termed an *indirect* hernia. When it escapes through the posterior inguinal wall, it is a *direct* hernia. An inguinal hernia is more common in men.

A femoral hernia occurs when there is a protrusion through the femoral ring into the femoral canal. It occurs below the inguinal (Poupart's) ligament as a bulge. It becomes strangulated easily and occurs more often in women. The umbilical hernia occurs when the rectus muscle is weak or the umbilical opening fails to close after birth.

Ventral, or incisional, hernia is due to weakness of the abdominal wall at the site of a previous incision. It is found most commonly in patients who are obese, who have had multiple surgical procedures in the same area, and who have had inadequate wound healing because of poor nutrition or infection.

Clinical Manifestations

A hernia commonly occurs over the involved area when the patient stands or strains. There may be some discomfort as a result of tension. Severe pain is caused if the hernia becomes strangulated. In this situation, the clinical manifestations of a bowel obstruction, such as vomiting, crampy abdominal pain, and distention, are found.

NURSING *and* COLLABORATIVE MANAGEMENT HERNIAS

Diagnosis is based on history and physical examination findings. Surgery is the treatment of choice for hernias to prevent the possible complication of strangulation. The surgical repair of a hernia is known as a *herniorrhaphy.* The reinforcement of the weakened area with wire, fascia, or mesh is known as a *hernioplasty.* When there is strangulation, necrosis and gangrene may develop if immediate care is not given. A bowel resection of the involved area or a temporary colostomy may be needed to treat a strangulated hernia.

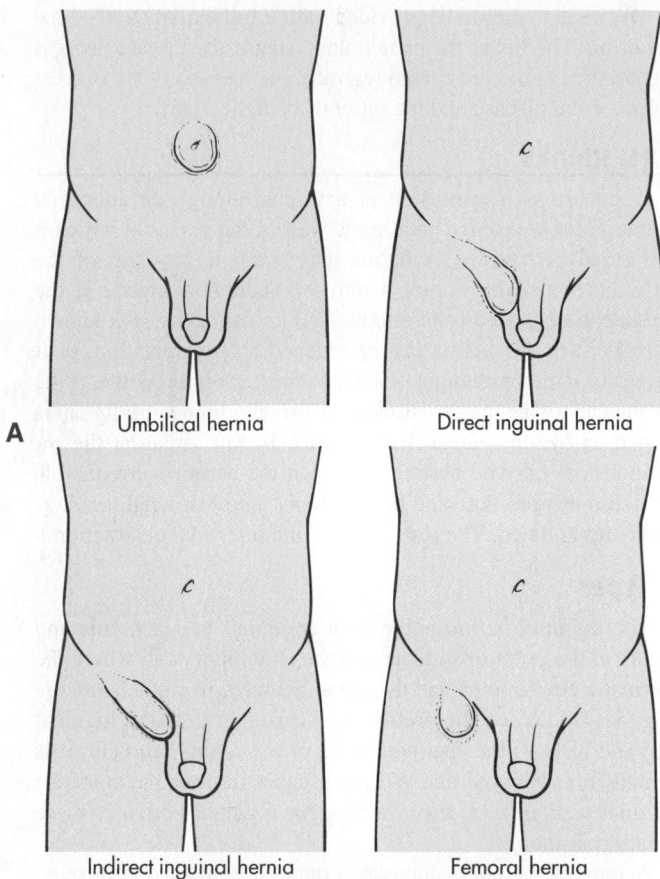

A, Umbilical hernia   Direct inguinal hernia

Indirect inguinal hernia   Femoral hernia

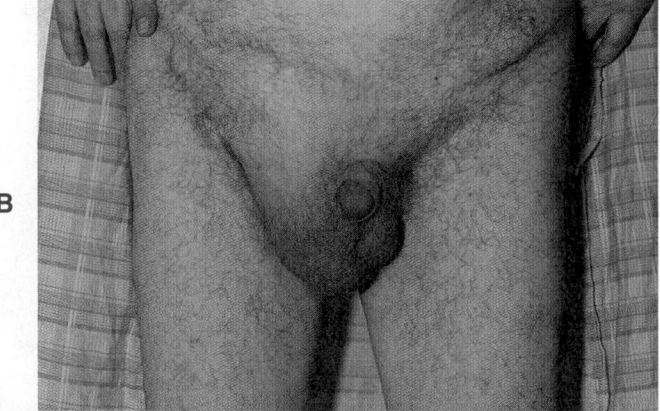

B

FIG. 41-17 A, Types of hernias. B, Indirect inguinal hernia.

Some patients with hernias wear a *truss,* a pad placed over the hernia and held in place with a belt. The truss is worn to keep the hernia from protruding. If a patient wears a truss, the nurse should check for skin irritation caused by the continual rubbing of the truss.

After a hernia repair, the patient may have difficulty voiding. Therefore the nurse should observe for a distended bladder. An accurate intake and output record is important. Scrotal edema is a painful complication after an inguinal hernia repair. A scrotal support with application of an ice bag may help relieve pain and edema. Coughing is not encouraged, but deep breathing and turning should be done. If the patient needs to cough or sneeze, the incision should be splinted during coughing, and sneezing should be done with the mouth open.

After discharge the patient may be restricted from heavy lifting for 6 to 8 weeks. Some surgeons do not put any limitations on physical activities.

Malabsorption Syndrome

Malabsorption results from impaired absorption of fats, carbohydrates, proteins, minerals, and vitamins. The stomach, small intestine, liver, and pancreas regulate normal digestion and absorption. Digestive enzymes ordinarily break down nutrients so that absorption can take place through the intestinal mucosa and nutrients can get into the bloodstream. If there is an interruption in this process at any point, malabsorption may occur. Several problems can cause malabsorption (Table 41-38). They can be classified into malabsorptions caused by (1) biochemical or enzyme deficiencies, (2) bacterial proliferation, (3) disruption of small intestine mucosa, (4) disturbed lymphatic and vascular circulation, or (5) surface area loss. Lactose intolerance is the most common malabsorption disorder, followed by inflammatory bowel disease, nontropical (celiac) and tropical sprue, and cystic fibrosis.

The most common clinical manifestation of malabsorption is **steatorrhea** (bulky, foul-smelling, yellow-gray, greasy stools with puttylike consistency). Bulky, foul-smelling stools that float in water and are difficult to flush are characteristic of steatorrhea (Table 41-39). However, steatorrhea does not occur with lactose intolerance.

Screening tests available for malabsorption include qualitative examination of stool for fat (Sudan stain), a 72-hour stool

TABLE 41-38	Common Causes of Malabsorption

Biochemical or Enzyme Deficiencies
Lactase deficiency
Biliary tract obstruction
Pancreatic insufficiency
   Cystic fibrosis
   Chronic pancreatitis
   Zollinger-Ellison syndrome

Bacterial Proliferation
Tropical sprue
Parasitic infection

Small Intestinal Mucosal Disruption
Celiac disease
Whipple's disease
Crohn's disease

Disturbed Lymphatic and Vascular Circulation
Lymphoma
Ischemia
Lymphangiectasia
Heart failure

Surface Area Loss
Billroth II gastrectomy
Short bowel syndrome
Distal ileal resection, disease, or bypass

TABLE 41-39   Clinical Manifestations of Malabsorption

MANIFESTATIONS	PATHOPHYSIOLOGY
Gastrointestinal	
Weight loss	Malabsorption of fat, carbohydrates, and protein leading to loss of calories; marked reduction in caloric intake or increased use of calories
Diarrhea	Impaired absorption of water, sodium, fatty acids, bile, or carbohydrates
Flatulence	Bacterial fermentation of unabsorbed carbohydrates
Steatorrhea	Undigested and unabsorbed fat
Glossitis, cheilosis, stomatitis	Deficiency of iron, riboflavin, cobalamin, folic acid, and other vitamins
Hematologic	
Anemia	Impaired absorption of iron, cobalamin, and folic acid
Hemorrhagic tendency	Vitamin C deficiency
	Vitamin K deficiency inhibiting production of clotting factors II, VII, IX, and X
Musculoskeletal	
Bone pain	Osteoporosis from impaired calcium absorption
	Osteomalacia secondary to hypocalcemia, hypophosphatemia, inadequate vitamin D
Tetany	Hypocalcemia, hypomagnesemia
Weakness, muscle cramps	Anemia, electrolyte depletion (especially potassium)
Muscle wasting	Protein malabsorption
Neurologic	
Altered mental status	Dehydration
Paresthesias	Cobalamin deficiency
Peripheral neuropathy	Cobalamin deficiency
Night blindness	Thiamine deficiency
	Vitamin A deficiency
Integumentary	
Bruising	Vitamin K deficiency
Dermatitis	Fatty acid deficiency, zinc deficiency, niacin and other vitamin deficiencies
Brittle nails	Iron deficiency
Hair thinning and loss	Protein deficiency
Cardiovascular	
Hypotension	Dehydration
Tachycardia	Hypovolemia, anemia
Peripheral edema	Protein malabsorption, protein loss in diarrhea

collection for quantitative measurement of fecal fat, and the D-xylose absorption-excretion test, which is a good screening test for carbohydrate absorption (see Table 38-12). Other diagnostic studies include three different kinds of breath tests: (1) the bile acid breath test, which is used to evaluate bile salt malabsorption or malabsorption from bacterial overgrowth; (2) the triolein breath test, which measures carbon dioxide excretion after ingestion of a radioactive triglyceride; and (3) the excretion of breath hydrogen after ingestion of lactose, which is a sensitive, specific, and noninvasive test for detection of lactase deficiency. The rationale for the hydrogen breath test is that undigested lactose, which when metabolized by bacteria in the colon produces an increase in hydrogen production, is excreted via the lungs.

A pancreatic secretion test may be performed to rule out pancreatic insufficiency. Endoscopy may be used to obtain a small bowel biopsy specimen for diagnosis. Radiologic studies of the esophagus, stomach, and small intestine may be indicated. A small bowel barium enema is often performed to identify abnormal mucosal patterns.

Laboratory studies that are frequently ordered include a CBC, determination of prothrombin time, serum vitamin A and carotene levels, serum electrolytes, cholesterol, and calcium.

SPRUE

Two closely related malabsorption conditions are nontropical sprue and tropical sprue. Tropical and nontropical sprue are found in adults. **Nontropical sprue** is most commonly referred to as celiac sprue (especially in children) but is also called adult celiac disease and gluten-induced enteropathy.

Etiology and Pathophysiology

In celiac disease there is marked atrophy and flattening of the villi. As a result, absorption within the small intestine is reduced. The proposed reason for the injury to the villi is a hypersensitivity response initiated by gluten and *gliadin* (a breakdown product of gluten). *Gluten* is a protein found in wheat, rye, barley, and oats. The hypersensitivity leads to an inflammatory response of the mucosa.

Tropical sprue is a chronic disorder acquired in endemic tropical areas. The exact cause is unknown, but the disorder has been linked to an infectious agent. Folate deficiency is also believed to play a role in the development of this disease. Clinically, it resembles nontropical sprue.

Clinical Manifestations

A patient may become symptomatic at any age with celiac sprue, but the incidence peaks in childhood when gluten is first introduced and then during the fourth and fifth decades.[32] Symptoms include steatorrhea, diarrhea, weight loss, abdominal distention, and excessive flatulence. There may also be signs of multiple vitamin deficiencies (e.g., glossitis, cheilosis).

Diagnostic Studies and Collaborative Care

Diagnosis of sprue may be made by stool content analyses or intestinal biopsy. Barium enema may demonstrate abnormalities, including obliteration of intestinal folds. Treatment of sprue syndrome is based on the underlying cause. In nontropical sprue, a gluten-free diet usually leads to clinical recovery. Wheat, barley, oats, and rye products should be avoided. Soybean flours may be used. Foods must be scrutinized for the gluten content. Additives such as hydrolyzed vegetable proteins are often derived from cereal grains, including wheat. For those patients who are unresponsive to dietary exclusion therapy (gluten-free diet), corticosteroids may be used to treat nontropical sprue. The basis for this treatment is that the inflammatory response is mediated by an immunologic response.

Tropical sprue is treated with broad-spectrum antibiotics (e.g., tetracycline) in conjunction with folic acid therapy. The patient who responds to this therapy and achieves a remission is usually maintained on folic acid.

LACTASE DEFICIENCY

Lactase deficiency is a condition in which the lactase enzyme is deficient or absent. *Lactase* is the enzyme that breaks down lactose into two simple sugars—glucose and galactose. Although primary lactase deficiency seems to be hereditary, milk intolerance may not become clinically evident until late adolescence or early adulthood. About 5% of the adult population has primary lactase deficiency. The highest incidence is found in African Americans, Native Americans, Mexican Americans, Asian Americans, and persons of Jewish descent. Acquired lactase deficiency is often seen in other GI diseases in which the mucosa has been damaged, including ulcerative colitis, Crohn's disease, gastroenteritis, and tropical and nontropical sprue.

Clinical Manifestations

The symptoms of lactose intolerance include bloating, flatulence, crampy abdominal pain, and diarrhea. They may occur within a half hour to several hours after drinking a glass of milk or ingesting a milk product. The diarrhea of lactose intolerance results from fluid secretion into the small intestines, responding to the osmotic action of undigested lactose.

NURSING and COLLABORATIVE MANAGEMENT LACTASE DEFICIENCY

Many lactose-intolerant persons are aware of their milk intolerance and avoid milk. A lactose intolerance test can be performed to rule out milk allergies. The patient is given 50 g of lactose orally. Blood samples are drawn before the consumption of lactose and at 15-, 30-, 60-, and 90-minute intervals. Failure of the blood glucose level to increase more than 20 mg/dl is suggestive of lactase deficiency. Results of the hydrogen breath test after ingestion of lactose are abnormal.

Treatment consists of eliminating lactose from the diet by avoiding milk and milk products. A lactose-free diet is given initially and is gradually advanced to a low-lactose diet as tolerated by the patient. The objective of care is to teach the importance of adherence to the diet. Many lactose-intolerant persons may not exhibit symptoms if lactose is taken in small amounts. In some persons, lactose may be tolerated better if taken with meals.

The patient needs to be aware that milk, ice cream, cottage cheese, and cheese have a high lactose content. If the milk has been fermented (e.g., cultured buttermilk, yogurt, sour cream), the patient with low lactase levels may tolerate it better.

Lactase enzyme (Lactaid) is available commercially as an over-the-counter (OTC) product. It is mixed with milk and breaks down the lactose before the milk is ingested.

SHORT BOWEL SYNDROME

Short bowel syndrome (SBS) results from extensive resection of the small intestine. Rapid intestinal transit, impaired digestive and absorption processes, and fluid and electrolyte losses characterize the syndrome. In adults, resection of the small intestine may be necessary for bowel infarction because of vascular thrombosis or insufficiency, abdominal trauma, cancer, radiation enteritis, or Crohn's disease.

The length and portions of small bowel resected are associated with the number and severity of symptoms. Resections of up to 50% of the small intestine cause little disturbance of bowel function, especially if the terminal ileum and ileocecal valve remain intact. After large resections, the remaining intestine undergoes adaptive changes that are more pronounced in the ileum. The villi and crypts increase in size, and absorptive capacity of the remaining intestine increases. Intestinal adaptation is enhanced by the presence of food, fiber, bile, and pancreatic secretions in the lumen and continues for up to 2 years. Resection of the ileum, ileocecal valve, or colon results in a rapid intestinal transit, decreasing absorption time. Ileal resection causes malabsorption of cobalamin, bile salts, and fat, resulting in steatorrhea.

Clinical Manifestations

The predominant manifestations of SBS are diarrhea or steatorrhea.[33] There may be signs of malnutrition and multiple vitamin and mineral deficiencies (e.g., weight loss, cobalamin and zinc deficiency, hypocalcemia). The patient may develop lactase deficiency and bacterial overgrowth. Oxalate kidney stones may form from increased colonic absorption of oxalate.

Collaborative Care

The overall goals are that the patient with SBS will have fluid and electrolyte balance, normal nutritional status, and control of diarrhea. In the period immediately following massive bowel resection, patients receive TPN to replace fluid, electrolyte, and nutrient losses and to rest the bowel. Hypersecretion of gastric acid, for which the cause is unknown, is reduced by proton pump inhibitors (e.g., omeprazole [Prilosec]).

A diet high in carbohydrate and low in fat is recommended. A high-carbohydrate, low-fat diet supplemented with soluble fiber, pectin, the amino acid glutamine, and parenteral growth hormone improves nutrient absorption, decreases stool output, and enables patients to wean off parenteral nutrition.[33] The patient with SBS is encouraged to eat at least six meals per day to increase the time of contact between food and the intestine. Oral intake can be supplemented with elemental nutrient formulas and tube feeding during the night. For patients with severe malabsorption, TPN may be reinstituted. Oral supplements of calcium, zinc, and multivitamins are typically recommended.

Narcotic antidiarrheal drugs are the most effective in decreasing intestinal motility (see Table 41-3). For patients with limited ileal resections (<100 cm), cholestyramine (Questran) reduces diarrhea resulting from unabsorbed bile acids and increases their excretion in feces. Bile acids stimulate intestinal fluid secretion and reduce colonic fluid absorption.

Anorectal Problems

HEMORRHOIDS

Hemorrhoids are dilated hemorrhoidal veins. They may be *internal* (occurring above the internal sphincter) or *external* (occurring outside the external sphincter) (Fig. 41-18). Symptoms of hemorrhoids, including bleeding, pruritus, prolapse, and pain, are common in all age groups. In affected persons, hemorrhoids appear periodically, depending on amount of anorectal pressure.

Etiology and Pathophysiology

Hemorrhoids are thought to develop as a result of shearing forces during defecation. This force damages supporting muscles. When supporting tissues in the anal canal weaken, usually as a result of straining at defecation, venules become dilated. In addition, blood flow through the veins of the hemorrhoidal

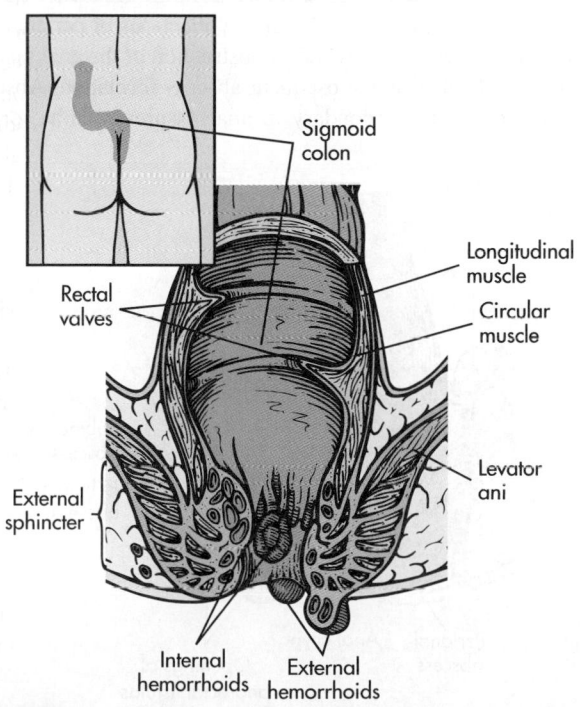

FIG. 41-18 Anatomic structures of the rectum and anus with external and internal hemorrhoids.

plexus is impaired. An intravascular clot in the venule results in a thrombosed external hemorrhoid. They are the most common cause of bleeding with defecation. The amount of blood lost at one time may be small but may lead to iron deficiency anemia over time.

Hemorrhoids may be precipitated by many factors, including pregnancy, prolonged constipation, straining in an effort to defecate, heavy lifting, prolonged standing and sitting, and portal hypertension (as found in cirrhosis).

Clinical Manifestations

The patient with internal hemorrhoids may be asymptomatic. However, when internal hemorrhoids become constricted, the patient will report pain. Internal hemorrhoids can bleed, resulting in blood on toilet paper after defecation or blood on the outside of stool. The patient may report a chronic, dull aching discomfort, particularly when the hemorrhoids have prolapsed.

External hemorrhoids are reddish blue and seldom bleed or cause pain unless a vein ruptures. If the blood clots in external hemorrhoids, they become inflamed and painful and are said to be thrombosed. External hemorrhoids cause intermittent pain, pain on palpation, itching, and burning. Patients also report bleeding associated with defecation. Constipation or diarrhea can aggravate these symptoms.

Diagnostic Studies and Collaborative Care

Internal hemorrhoids are diagnosed by digital examination, anoscopy, or sigmoidoscopy. External hemorrhoids can be diagnosed by visual inspection and digital examination. Therapy should be directed toward the causes and the patient's symptoms. A high-fiber diet and increased fluid intake prevent constipation and reduce straining, which allows engorgement of the veins to subside. Ointments such as Nupercainal; creams, suppositories, and impregnated pads that contain antiinflammatory agents (e.g., hydrocortisone); or astringents and anesthetics (e.g., witch hazel, pramoxine, benzocaine) may be used to shrink the mucous membranes and relieve discomfort. Stool softeners may be ordered to keep the stools soft, and sitz baths may be ordered to relieve pain.

Application of ice packs for a few hours, followed by warm packs, may be used for thrombosed external hemorrhoids. Another conservative treatment involves use of a sclerosing solution such as 5% phenol in oil, or a combined solution of quinine and urea may be injected into the submucosal tissue surrounding the hemorrhoids, causing a fibrosing and shrinking of the supporting tissues. Topical nitroglycerin has been shown to be effective in reducing acute hemorrhoidal thrombosis.

For internal hemorrhoids, one of four nonsurgical approaches (band ligation, infrared coagulation, cryotherapy, laser treatment) can be used. The first is *band ligation*. Through an anoscope the hemorrhoid is identified and then ligated with a rubber band. The constrictive effect impairs circulation, and the tissue becomes necrotic, separates, and sloughs off. There is some local discomfort with this procedure, but no anesthetic is required. Aspirin or propoxyphene (Darvon) is usually given for discomfort. *Infrared coagulation* can be used to treat bleeding internal hemorrhoids. In this procedure, either infrared or electrical current produces local inflammation. *Cryotherapy* involves rapid freezing of the hemorrhoid. Because this method can result in acute pain, it is used less often. Finally, *laser treatment* can be used to treat internal hemorrhoids. This procedure involves expensive equipment and tends to be more costly compared with band ligation and coagulation therapies.

A *hemorrhoidectomy* is the surgical excision of hemorrhoids. Surgery is indicated when there is prolapse, excessive pain or bleeding, or large hemorrhoids. In general, hemorrhoidectomy is reserved for patients with severe symptoms related to multiple thrombosed hemorrhoids or marked protrusion. Surgical removal may be done by cautery, clamp, or excision. One surgical approach is to leave the area open so that healing takes place by secondary intention. In another approach the hemorrhoids are removed, the tissue is sutured, and healing takes place by primary-intention wound healing.

NURSING MANAGEMENT
HEMORRHOIDS

Conservative nursing management for the patient with hemorrhoids includes teaching measures to prevent constipation, avoidance of prolonged standing or sitting, proper use of OTC drugs available for hemorrhoidal symptoms, and the need to seek medical care for severe symptoms of hemorrhoids (e.g., excessive pain and bleeding, prolapsed hemorrhoids) when necessary. Sitz baths (15 to 20 minutes) two to three times each day for 7 to 10 days may be helpful to reduce discomfort and swelling associated with hemorrhoids.

Pain caused by sphincter spasm is a common problem after a hemorrhoidectomy. The nurse must be aware that although the procedure is minor, the pain is severe. Narcotics are usually given initially. Postoperatively, topical nitroglycerin preparations may be used to decrease pain and subsequent narcotic use.[34]

Sitz baths are started 1 to 2 days after surgery. A warm sitz bath provides comfort and keeps the anal area clean. A sponge ring in the sitz bath helps relieve pressure on the area. Initially the patient should not be left alone because of the possibility of weakness or fainting.

Packing may be inserted into the rectum to absorb drainage. A T-binder may hold the dressing in place. If packing is inserted, it usually is removed on the first or second postoperative day. The nurse should assess for rectal bleeding. The patient may be embarrassed when the dressing is changed, and privacy should be provided. The patient usually dreads the first bowel movement and often resists the urge to defecate. Pain medication may be given before the bowel movement to reduce discomfort.

A stool softener such as docusate (Colace) is usually ordered for the first few postoperative days. If the patient does not have a bowel movement within 2 to 3 days, an oil-retention enema is given.

Patients are taught the importance of diet, care of the anal area, symptoms of complications (especially bleeding), and avoidance of constipation and straining. Sitz baths are recommended for 1 to 2 weeks. The health care provider may order a stool softener to be taken for a time. Hemorrhoids may recur. Occasionally, anal strictures develop and dilation is necessary. Regular checkups are important in the prevention of any further problems.

ANAL FISSURE

An **anal fissure** is a skin ulcer or a crack in the lining of the anal wall that is caused by trauma, local infection, or inflammation. Fissures are considered either primary or secondary based

on their etiology. Primary fissures usually occur as a result of local trauma associated with defecation. When there is high pressure in the internal anal sphincter, it can result in ischemia, which can lead to fissuring. Thus conditions that promote constipation are likely to be associated with fissure development. Secondary fissures are due to a variety of conditions, including inflammatory bowel disease (Crohn's disease, ulcerative colitis), prior anal surgery, infection (syphilis, tuberculosis, chlamydia, gonorrhea, herpes simplex virus), and human immunodeficiency virus infection.

The most common clinical manifestations are painful spasms of the anal sphincter and severe, burning pain during defecation. Some bleeding may occur, and constipation results because of fear of pain associated with bowel movements.

Anal fissures are diagnosed through physical examination. Treatment of anal fissures is directed at correcting the underlying conditions, such as hard stools. Most acute fissures require 2 to 4 weeks to heal. Conservative treatment consists of bowel regulation with mineral oil and stool softeners. Warm sitz baths (15 to 20 minutes, 3 times a day) and anal anesthetic suppositories (Anusol) are also ordered. The application of nitroglycerin topical ointment before and immediately after a bowel movement can reduce pain. More recently, injection of botulinum toxin (Botox), which results in reversible paralysis of the internal anal sphincter, has been performed to promote fissure healing.[34] This treatment is transient (i.e., effects last approximately 6 weeks) and invasive. Side effects of Botox include transient incontinence and perianal thrombosis.

For chronic fissures, other invasive procedures may be needed. These include coagulation therapy or surgical treatment (sphincterotomy). Surgical treatment involves excision of the fissure. Postoperative nursing care is the same as the care for the patient who has had a hemorrhoidectomy.

ANORECTAL ABSCESS

Anorectal abscesses are undrained collections of perianal pus (Fig. 41-19). They are the result of obstruction of the anal glands, leading to infection and subsequent abscess formation. Abscess formation can occur secondary to anal fissures, trauma, or in-

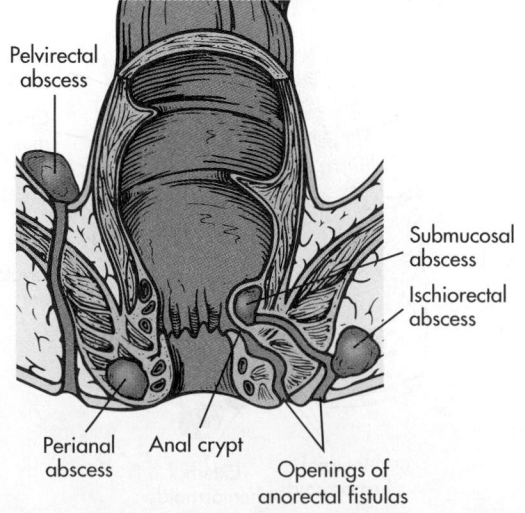

FIG. 41-19 Common sites of anorectal abscesses and fistula formation.

flammatory bowel disease. The most common causative organisms are *Escherichia coli*, staphylococci, and streptococci. Clinical manifestations include local pain and swelling, foul-smelling drainage, tenderness, and elevated temperature. Sepsis can occur as a complication. Anorectal abscesses are diagnosed by rectal examination.

Surgical therapy consists of drainage of abscesses. If packing is used, it should be impregnated with petroleum jelly, and the area should be allowed to heal by granulation. The packing is changed every day, and moist, hot compresses are applied to the area. Care must be taken to avoid soiling the dressing during urination or defecation. A low-residue diet is given. The patient may leave the hospital with the area open. Discharge teaching should include wound care, the importance of sitz baths, thorough cleaning after bowel movements, and follow-up visits to a health care provider.

ANAL FISTULA

An **anal fistula** is an abnormal tunnel leading out from the anus or rectum. It may extend to the outside of the skin, vagina, or buttocks. Anal fistulas are a complication of Crohn's disease. This condition often precedes an anorectal abscess.

Feces may enter the fistula and cause an infection. There may be persistent, blood-stained, purulent discharge or stool leakage from the fistula. The patient may have to wear a pad to prevent staining of clothes.

Surgical therapy involves a fistulotomy or a fistulectomy. In a *fistulotomy* the fistula is opened, and healthy tissue is allowed to granulate. A *fistulectomy* is an excision of the entire fistulous tract. Gauze packing is inserted, and the wound is allowed to heal by granulation. Care is the same as that given after a hemorrhoidectomy.

PILONIDAL SINUS

A **pilonidal sinus** is a small tract under the skin between the buttocks in the sacrococcygeal area. It is thought to be of congenital origin. It may have several openings and is lined with epithelium and hair, thus given the name *pilonidal* ("a nest of hair").

The skin is moist, and movement of the buttocks causes the short, wiry hair to penetrate the skin. The irritated skin becomes infected and forms a pilonidal cyst or abscess. There are no symptoms unless there is an infection. If it becomes infected, the patient complains of pain and swelling at the base of the spine.

The formed abscess requires incision and drainage. The wound may be closed or left open to heal by secondary intention. The wound is packed, and sitz baths are ordered.

Nursing care includes hot, moist heat applications when an abscess is present. The patient is usually more comfortable lying on the abdomen or side. The patient should be instructed to avoid contaminating the dressing when urinating or defecating and to avoid straining whenever possible.

CRITICAL THINKING EXERCISES

Case Study
Colorectal Cancer

Patient Profile. Joseph Sandoval, a 58-year-old Native American, is from a Pueblo tribe in northern New Mexico. Mr. Sandoval's wife and family drove 50 miles to take him to the Indian Health Service Hospital because of his deteriorating health.

Subjective Data
- Complains of bright red bleeding during a bowel movement
- Family states that he has become thinner over the past several months and has little appetite
- Describes feeling weak and being easily fatigued; he appears ill
- Complains of abdominal pain and a feeling of fullness
- Bowel pattern has episodes of constipation followed by diarrhea
- No prior screening for colorectal cancer; family history of colorectal cancer is unknown

Objective Data
Physical Examination
- Temperature: 100.4° F (38° C)
- Heart rate is 100 beats/min; BP is 120/74 mm Hg
- Weight: 140 lb (63.6 kg); height: 5 feet 9 inches (172.5 cm)
- Mild palpation over transverse and descending colon elicits pain
- Digital rectal exam revealed a mass

Laboratory Tests
- Double-contrast barium enema showed two medium-sized tumors
- Hct: 26%
- Hb: 9 g/dl (90 g/L)

CRITICAL THINKING QUESTIONS
1. What are the signs and symptoms of colorectal cancer that Mr. Sandoval manifests?
2. What is the significance of Mr. Sandoval's tachycardia?
3. What types of diagnostic information are available from a colonoscopy versus a double-contrast barium enema?
4. What nursing interventions are indicated for Mr. Sandoval at this stage of his illness?
5. What is a culturally sensitive way for the nurse to support Mr. Sandoval and his family in making decisions about his continued health care?
6. Based on the assessment data, write one or more nursing diagnoses. Are there any collaborative problems?

Nursing Research Issues
1. What are the primary problems related to sexuality and sexual function in patients with an ostomy?
2. Are the psychologic responses and coping strategies of younger patients receiving an ostomy different from those of older patients?
3. What can a nurse do to help improve the self-image of patients with ostomies?
4. Do psychosocial factors have a significant role in the exacerbation of IBD?
5. Which sources of dietary fiber are most effective in treating fecal incontinence and IBS?

REVIEW QUESTIONS

The number of the question corresponds to the same-numbered objective at the beginning of the chapter.

1. The appropriate collaborative therapy for the patient with acute diarrhea caused by rotavirus is to
   a. increase fluid intake.
   b. administer an antibiotic.
   c. administer antimotility drugs.
   d. quarantine the patient to prevent spread of the virus.

2. During the assessment of a patient with acute abdominal pain, the nurse should
   a. perform deep palpation before auscultation.
   b. obtain blood pressure and pulse rate to determine hypervolemic changes.
   c. auscultate bowel sounds because hyperactive bowel sounds suggest paralytic ileus.
   d. measure body temperature because an elevated temperature may indicate an inflammatory or infectious process.

3. The nurse would increase the comfort of the patient with appendicitis by
   a. having the patient lie prone.
   b. flexing the patient's right knee.
   c. sitting the patient upright in a chair.
   d. turning the patient onto his or her left side.

4. In planning care for the patient with Crohn's disease, the nurse recognizes that a major difference between ulcerative colitis and Crohn's disease is that Crohn's disease
   a. frequently results in toxic megacolon.
   b. causes fewer nutritional deficiencies than does ulcerative colitis.
   c. often recurs after surgery, whereas ulcerative colitis is curable with a colectomy.
   d. is manifested by rectal bleeding and anemia more frequently than is ulcerative colitis.

5. The nurse performs a detailed assessment of the abdomen of a patient with a possible bowel obstruction, knowing that a manifestation of an obstruction in the large intestine is
   a. a largely distended abdomen.
   b. diarrhea that is loose or liquid.
   c. persistent, colicky abdominal pain.
   d. profuse vomiting that relieves abdominal pain.

6. A patient with metastatic colorectal cancer is scheduled for both chemotherapy and radiation therapy. Patient teaching regarding these therapies for this patient would include an explanation that
   a. chemotherapy can be used to cure colorectal cancer.
   b. radiation is routinely used as adjuvant therapy following surgery.
   c. both chemotherapy and radiation can be used as palliative treatments.
   d. the patient should expect few if any side effects from chemotherapeutic agents.

7. The nurse explains to the patient undergoing ostomy surgery that the procedure that maintains the most normal functioning of the bowel is
   a. a sigmoid colostomy.
   b. a transverse colostomy.
   c. a descending colostomy.
   d. an ascending colostomy.

8. In contrast to diverticulitis, the patient with diverticulosis
   a. has rectal bleeding.
   b. often has no symptoms.
   c. has localized crampy pain.
   d. frequently develops peritonitis.

9. A nursing intervention that is most appropriate to decrease postoperative edema and pain following an inguinal herniorrhaphy is
   a. applying a truss to the hernia site.
   b. allowing the patient to stand to void.
   c. supporting the incision during routine coughing.
   d. elevating the scrotum with a support or small pillow.

10. The nurse determines that the goals of dietary teaching have been met when the patient with nontropical sprue selects from the menu
    a. scrambled eggs and sausage.
    b. buckwheat pancakes with syrup.
    c. oatmeal, skim milk, and orange juice.
    d. yogurt, strawberries, and rye toast with butter.

11. Which of the following should a patient be taught after a hemorrhoidectomy?
    a. Do not use the Valsalva maneuver.
    b. Eat a low-fiber diet to rest the colon.
    c. Administer oil-retention enema to empty the colon.
    d. Use prescribed pain medication before a bowel movement.

REFERENCES

1. Miller MA et al: Morbidity, mortality, and healthcare burden of nosocomial *Clostridium difficile*-associated diarrhea in Canadian hospitals, *Infect Control Hosp Epidemiol* 23:137, 2002.
*2. Bliss DZ et al: Supplementation with dietary fiber improves fecal incontinence, *Nurs Res* 50:203, 2001.
3. Cooper ZR, Rose S: Fecal incontinence: a clinical approach, *M Sinai J Med* 67:96, 2000.
4. Norton C, Chelvanayagam S: A nursing assessment tool for adults with fecal incontinence, *J WOCN* 27: 279, 2000.
5. Camilleri M et al: Insights into the pathology and mechanisms of constipation, irritable bowel syndrome, and diverticulosis in older people, *JAGS* 48:1142, 2000.

*6. Hinrichs M, Huseboe J: Research-based protocol: management of constipation, *J Gerontol Nurs* 27:17, 2001.
7. Thompson WG: Constipation: a physiological approach, *Can J Gastroenterol* 14:155D, 2000.
8. Muller-Lissner S: General geriatrics and gastroenterology: constipation and faecal incontinence, *Best Pract Res Clin Gastroenterol* 16:115, 2002.
9. Wolfe JM et al: Analgesic administration to patients with an acute abdomen: a survey, *Am J Emerg Med* 18:250, 2000.
10. Heitkemper M, Jarrett M: It's not all in your head: irritable bowel syndrome, *AJN* 101:26, 2001.
11. Gauf CL: Diagnosing appendicitis across the life span, *J Am Acad Nurse Pract* 12:129, 2000.
12. van Heel DA et al: Inflammatory bowel disease: progress toward a gene, *Can J Gastroenterol* 14:207, 2000.
13. Andres PG, Friedman LS: Epidemiology and the natural course of inflammatory bowel disease, *Gastroenterol Clin North Am* 28:255, 1999.

*Nursing research–based reference.

14. Worley J: Diagnosis and management of inflammatory bowel disease, *J Am Acad Nurs Pract* 11:23, 1999.
15. Hugot JP et al: Etiology of the inflammatory bowel diseases, *Int J Colorect Dis* 14:2, 1999.
16. Guslandi M: Nicotine treatment for ulcerative colitis, *J Clin Pharmacol* 48:481, 1999.
17. Wachtershauser A, Stein J: Rationale for the luminal provision of butyrate in intestinal diseases, *Eur J Nutr* 39:164, 2000.
18. Collins J, Corless CL, Deveney K: Pouchitis, *Clin Perspect Gastroent* 5:156, 2002.
19. Sandborn WJ: Transcending conventional therapies: the role of biologic and other novel therapies, *Inflamm Bowel* (Suppl 1):S9, 2001.
20. McCloy C et al: The etiology of intestinal obstruction in patients without prior laparotomy or hernia, *Am Surg* 64:19, 1998.
21. Bond JH: Clinical evidence for the adenoma-carcinoma sequence, and the management of patients with colorectal adenomas, *Semin Gastrointest Dis* 11:176, 2000.
22. Read TE, Kodner IJ: Colorectal cancer: risk factors and recommendations for early detection, *Am Fam Physician* 59:3083, 1999.
23. American Cancer Society: *Cancer facts and figures 2002*, Atlanta, 2002, American Cancer Society.
24. Pontieri-Lewis V: Colorectal cancer: prevention and screening, *Medsurg Nurs* 9:9, 2000.
25. Ahlquist DA, Shuber AP: Stool screening for colorectal cancer: evolution from occult blood to molecular markers, *Clin Chim Acta* 315:157, 2002.
26. Gibson M et al: Laparoscopic colon resections: a five-year retrospective review, *Am Surg* 66:245, 2000.
27. Royce ME, Hoff PM, Pazdur R: Progress in colorectal cancer chemotherapy: how far have we come, how far to go? *Drugs Aging* 17:201, 2000.
28. Beeker C et al: Colorectal cancer screening in older men and women: qualitative research findings and implications for intervention, *J Community Health* 25:263, 2000.
29. Moran EM: Epidemiological and clinical aspects of nonsteroidal antiinflammatory drugs and cancer risks, *J Environ Pathol Toxicol Oncol* 2:193, 2002.
30. Reddy BS, Rao CV: Novel approaches for colon cancer prevention by cyclooxygenase-2 inhibitors, *J Environ Pathol Toxicol Oncol* 2:155, 2002.
31. Carter JJ, Whelan RL: Evaluation and medical management of diverticular disease, *Sem Colon Rectal Surg* 11:196, 2000.
32. Green PHR et al: Characteristics of adult celiac disease in the USA: results of a national survey, *Am J Gastroenterol* 96:126, 2001.
33. Lord LM et al: Management of the patient with short bowel syndrome, *AACN Clin Iss* 11:604, 2000.
34. Lysy J et al: Topical nitrates potentiate the effect of botulinum toxin in the treatment of patients with refractory anal fissure, *Gut* 48:221, 2001.

RESOURCES

American Cancer Society
1599 Clifton Road NE
Atlanta, GA 30329
800-ACS-2345
www.cancer.org

American Gastroenterological Association
7910 Woodmont Avenue, Seventh Floor
Bethesda, MD 20814
301-654-2055
Fax: 301-654-5920
www.gastro.org

American Society for Gastrointestinal Endoscopy (ASGE)
1520 Kensington Road, Suite 202
Oak Brook, IL 60523
630-573-0600
Fax: 630-573-0691
www.asge.org

Crohn's & Colitis Foundation of America (CCFA)
386 Park Avenue South, 17th Floor
New York, NY 10016
800-932-2423
Fax: 212-779-4098
E-mail: info@ccfa.org
www.ccfa.org

Crohn's & Colitis Foundation of Canada (CCFC)
60 St. Clair Avenue East, Suite 600
Toronto, ON
M4T 1N5 Canada
800-387-1479 or 416-920-5035
Fax: 416-929-0364
www.ccfc.ca

International Ostomy Association
c/o British Colostomy Association
15 Station Road
Reading Berks
RG1 1LG England
44 1189 391537
Fax: 44 1189 569095
www.ostomyinternational.org

Society of Gastroenterology Nurses and Associates
401 North Michigan Avenue
Chicago, IL 60611-4267
800-245-7462 or 312-321-5165
Fax: 312-527-6658
www.sgna.org

United Ostomy Association (UOA)
19772 MacArthur Boulevard, Suite 200
Irvine, CA 92612-2405
800-826-0826
www.uoa.org

Wound, Ostomy and Continence Nurses Society
WOCN National Office
4700 West Lake Avenue
Glenview, IL 60025
888-224-WOCN or 866-615-8560
Fax: 866-615-8560
www.wocn.org

For additional Internet resources, see the website for this book at *http://evolve.elsevier.com/Lewis/medsurg/.*

CHAPTER *42*

NURSING MANAGEMENT
Liver, Biliary Tract, and Pancreas Problems

Margaret McLean Heitkemper

LEARNING OBJECTIVES

1. Define jaundice and describe signs and symptoms that may occur with the different types of jaundice.
2. Differentiate among the types of viral hepatitis, including etiology, pathophysiology, clinical manifestations, complications, and collaborative care.
3. Describe the nursing management of the patient with viral hepatitis.
4. Explain the etiology, pathophysiology, clinical manifestations, complications, and collaborative care of the patient with cirrhosis of the liver.
5. Describe the nursing management of the patient with cirrhosis.
6. Describe the clinical manifestations and management of liver cancer.

7. Describe the pathophysiology, clinical manifestations, complications, and collaborative care of acute and chronic pancreatitis.
8. Describe the nursing management of the patient with pancreatitis.
9. Explain the clinical manifestations and collaborative care of the patient with pancreatic cancer.
10. Explain the pathophysiology, clinical manifestations, complications, and collaborative care, including surgical therapy, of gallbladder disorders.
11. Describe the nursing management of the patient undergoing conservative or surgical treatment of cholecystitis and cholelithiasis.

KEY TERMS

acute pancreatitis, p. 1133	fulminant viral hepatitis, p. 1109
ascites, p. 1118	hepatic encephalopathy, p. 1120
asterixis, p. 1120	hepatitis, p. 1105
cholecystitis, p. 1141	hepatorenal syndrome, p. 1120
cholelithiasis, p. 1141	jaundice, p. 1104
chronic pancreatitis, p. 1138	paracentesis, p. 1121
cirrhosis, p. 1116	portal hypertension, p. 1118
esophageal varices, p. 1118	pseudocyst, p. 1134
fetor hepaticus, p. 1120	spider angiomas, p. 1117
fulminant hepatic failure, p. 1131	

JAUNDICE

Jaundice, a yellowish discoloration of body tissues, results from an alteration in normal bilirubin metabolism or flow of bile into the hepatic or biliary duct systems. It is a symptom rather than a disease. Jaundice results when the concentration of bilirubin in the blood becomes abnormally increased. The bilirubin level has to be approximately 3 times the normal levels (2 to 3 mg/dl [34 to 51 mol/L]) for jaundice to occur. Jaundice can usually first be detected in the sclera and skin (Fig. 42-1).

Most of the body's bilirubin is formed from the breakdown of hemoglobin (from erythrocytes) by macrophages (see Fig. 38-6). This unconjugated (indirect) bilirubin is released into the circulation bound to albumin and is not water soluble. Because it is not water soluble and cannot be filtered in the kidneys, unconju-

gated bilirubin is not excreted in the urine. In the liver the unconjugated bilirubin is conjugated with glucuronic acid to form conjugated (direct) bilirubin, which is water soluble. Conjugated bilirubin is secreted into bile, which flows through the hepatic and biliary duct system into the small intestine. In the large intestine, bilirubin is converted to stercobilinogen and urobilinogen by bacterial action. Stercobilinogen gives the characteristic brown color to feces. Some urobilinogen is reabsorbed into the portal circulation and returned to the liver. Normally a very small amount of urobilinogen is excreted in urine.

The three types of jaundice are classified as hemolytic, hepatocellular, and obstructive. Diagnostic findings associated with these types of jaundice are shown in Table 42-1.

Hemolytic Jaundice

Hemolytic (prehepatic) jaundice is due to an increased breakdown of red blood cells (RBCs), which produces an increased amount of unconjugated bilirubin in the blood (Table 42-1). The liver is unable to handle this increased load. Causes of hemolytic jaundice include blood transfusion reactions, sickle cell crisis, and hemolytic anemia.

Hepatocellular Jaundice

Hepatocellular (hepatic) jaundice results from the liver's altered ability to take up bilirubin from the blood or to conjugate or excrete it. Initially both unconjugated and conjugated bilirubin serum levels are increased (see Table 42-1). In hepatocellular disease the hepatocytes are damaged and leak bilirubin, thus increasing levels of conjugated bilirubin. In severe disease, both unconjugated and conjugated bilirubin are elevated as a result of both the inability of hepatocytes to conjugate bilirubin

---

Reviewed by Anne Croghan, RN, MN, ARNP, Nurse Practitioner, Hepatology, VA Puget Sound Health Care System, Seattle, Wash.

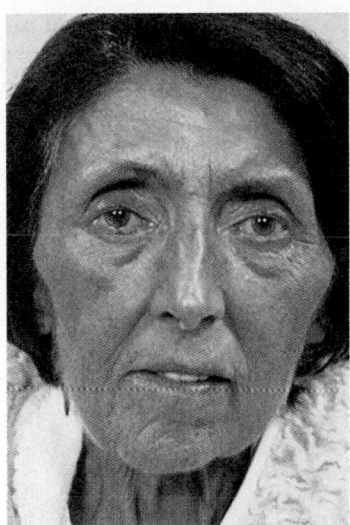

FIG. 42-1 Severe jaundice.

TABLE 42-1 **Diagnostic Findings in Jaundice**

	Hemolytic	Hepatocellular	Obstructive
Serum bilirubin			
Unconjugated (indirect)	↑	↑	Somewhat ↑
Conjugated (direct)	Normal	↑↓	Moderately ↑
Urine bilirubin	Negative	↑	↑
Urobilinogen			
Stool	↑	Normal to ↓	↓
Urine	↑	Normal to ↑	↓

and continued cell leaking of conjugated bilirubin. As the number of unhealthy hepatocytes increases, the ability to conjugate bilirubin will eventually decrease. Because conjugated bilirubin is water soluble, it is excreted in the urine. The most common causes of hepatocellular jaundice are hepatitis, cirrhosis, and hepatic carcinoma.

Obstructive Jaundice

Obstructive (posthepatic) jaundice is due to impeded or obstructed flow of bile through the liver or biliary duct system. The obstruction may be intrahepatic or extrahepatic. Intrahepatic obstructions are due to swelling or fibrosis of the liver's canaliculi and bile ducts. This can be caused by damage from liver tumors, hepatitis, or cirrhosis. Causes of extrahepatic obstruction include common bile duct obstruction from a stone, sclerosing cholangitis, and carcinoma of the head of the pancreas. Laboratory findings show an elevation of both unconjugated and conjugated bilirubin and urine bilirubin (see Table 42-1). Because bilirubin does not enter the intestines, there is decreased to no fecal or urinary urobilinogen. With complete obstruction, the stools are clay colored.

Disorders of the Liver

HEPATITIS

Hepatitis is an inflammation of the liver. Acute viral hepatitis is the most common cause of hepatitis. The types of infectious viral hepatitis are A, B, C, D, E, and G. Hepatitis may also be caused by drugs (including alcohol), chemicals (see Table 38-6), and autoimmune liver disease. Rarely, hepatitis is caused by bacteria, such as streptococci, salmonellae, and *Escherichia coli.*

Viral hepatitis is a major public health concern in the United States. Approximately 152,000 cases of hepatitis A occur annually in the United States, and 10 million, worldwide.[1] It is nearly universal during childhood in developing countries. Worldwide, nearly 300 million people are infected with the hepatitis B virus (HBV). Of these approximately 50% to 75% have active viral replication or chronic active infection. There are an estimated 80,000 new cases of hepatitis B annually in the United States.[1] In the 1990s the incidence of hepatitis B decreased overall because of the widespread use of the HBV vaccine. Today, the highest rate of the disease occurs in those 20 to 49 years of age. Currently, 1.25 million Americans are chronically infected with HBV, 20% to 30% of whom acquired the infection in childhood.[1-3]

Worldwide, approximately 170 million people are infected with hepatitis C virus (HCV). In the United States it is estimated that 4 million individuals (1.8% of the population) have been exposed, with 3 million of them chronically infected.[4] Of these nearly 50% are not aware of their infection.[1] Currently, an estimated 25,000 new cases are diagnosed annually.[1] HCV accounts for 45% of all cases of chronic viral hepatitis, and it is the most common liver disease in the United States.[1] Approximately 20% of patients with chronic HCV will progress to cirrhosis within 20 years. It is estimated that 8000 to 10,000 individuals in the United States die each year from complications of end-stage liver disease secondary to chronic HCV.[2,5] The characterization of the virus and the introduction of transfusion blood and blood product testing along with safer needle-using practices by injecting drug users has resulted in a drop in new cases since the late 1980s. However, because of the 15- to 20-year delay between infection and the clinical appearance of liver damage, it is likely that the long-term effects of HCV infection will pose important health care challenges for the next 20 years.[5-7]

Coinfection of HCV and human immunodeficiency virus (HIV) is increasing. Approximately 40% of HIV-infected patients also have HCV. This high rate of coinfection is primarily related

CULTURAL & ETHNIC CONSIDERATIONS
Disorders of the Liver, Pancreas, and Gallbladder

- Mortality from cirrhosis occurs more frequently among African Americans than in other ethnic groups.
- Primary hepatic cancer has a higher incidence among African Americans, Asian Americans, and Eskimos than whites.
- Pancreatic cancer occurs more frequently among African Americans and Asian Americans than whites.
- Whites and Native Americans have a higher incidence of gallbladder disease than African Americans or Asian Americans.

to intravenous (IV) drug use. The presence of both HIV and HCV places the patient at greater risk for end-stage liver disease.

Etiology

Viral hepatitis can be caused by one of five major viruses: A, B, C, D, and E. Hepatitis G has recently been described. Other viruses known to produce liver inflammation and damage include cytomegalovirus, Epstein-Barr virus, herpesvirus, coxsackie-virus, and rubella virus.

The only definitive way to distinguish among the various forms of viral hepatitis is by the presence of the antigens and antigenic subtypes and the subsequent development of antibodies to them. Outbreaks of hepatitis are consistently caused by hepatitis A virus (HAV). Approximately 50% of acute viral hepatitis cases in adults in the United States are hepatitis B, 20% are hepatitis C, and 30% are hepatitis A.[1] Infection with each virus provides immunity to that virus (homologous immunity). However, the patient can still develop another type of viral hepatitis. Characteristics of hepatitis viruses are summarized in Table 42-2.

Hepatitis A Virus. HAV is an RNA virus that is transmitted through the fecal-oral route. It frequently occurs in small outbreaks caused by fecal contamination of food or drinking water. It is found in feces 2 or more weeks before the onset of symptoms and up to 1 week after the onset of jaundice (Fig. 42-2). It is present in the blood only briefly. Anti-HAV (antibody to HAV) immunoglobulin M (IgM) appears in the serum as the stool becomes negative for the virus. Detection of IgM anti-HAV indicates acute hepatitis, and IgG anti-HAV is an indicator of past infection. The presence of IgG antibody provides lifelong immunity.

The mode of transmission of HAV is predominantly fecal-oral (mainly by ingestion of food or liquid infected with the virus) and rarely parenteral. Poor hygiene, crowded situations, and poor san-

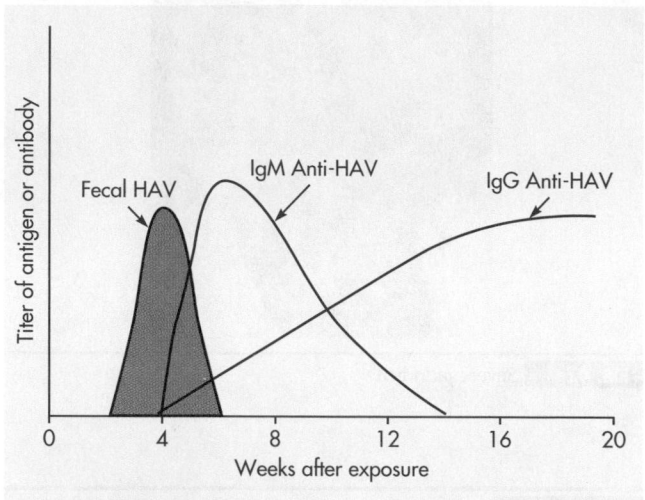

FIG. 42-2 Serologic events of a typical patient infected with hepatitis A virus (HAV). Elevated alanine aminotransferase (ALT) levels are present by 4 weeks, and jaundice appears by about 5 weeks after exposure to the virus.

TABLE 42-2	**Characteristics of Hepatitis Viruses**			
	INCUBATION PERIOD	**MODE OF TRANSMISSION**	**SOURCES OF INFECTION AND SPREAD OF DISEASE**	**INFECTIVITY**
Hepatitis A virus (HAV)	15–50 days (average 28)	Fecal–oral (fecal contamination and oral ingestion)	Crowded conditions; poor personal hygiene; poor sanitation; contaminated food, milk, water, and shellfish; persons with subclinical infections; infected food handlers; sexual contact	Most infectious during 2 weeks before onset of symptoms; infectious until 1–2 weeks after symptoms start
Hepatitis B virus (HBV)	45–180 days (average 56–96)	Percutaneous (parenteral)/permucosal exposure to blood or blood products Sexual contact Perinatal transmission	Contaminated needles, syringes, and blood products; sexual activity with infected partners; asymptomatic carriers Tattoo/body piercing, bites	Before and after symptoms appear; infectious for 4–6 months; in carriers continues for patient's lifetime
Hepatitis C virus (HCV)	14–180 days (average 56)	Percutaneous (parenteral)/permucosal exposure to blood or blood products High-risk sexual contact Perinatal contact	Blood and blood products, needles and syringes, sexual activity with infected partners	1–2 weeks before symptoms; continues during clinical course; 75%–85% go on to develop chronic hepatitis
Hepatitis D virus (HDV)	2–26 weeks HBV must precede HDV; chronic carriers of HBV are always at risk	Can cause infection only together with HBV; routes of transmission same as for HBV	Same as HBV	Blood is infectious at all stages of HDV infection
Hepatitis E virus (HEV)	15–64 days (average 26–42 days in different epidemics)	Fecal–oral Outbreaks associated with contaminated water supply in developing countries	Contaminated water; poor sanitation; found in Asia, Africa, and Mexico; not common in the United States and Canada	Not known; may be similar to HAV

itary conditions are all factors related to hepatitis A. Transmission occurs between family members, institutionalized individuals, children in day care centers, and from common-source outbreaks. The disease occurs more frequently in underdeveloped countries. Food-borne hepatitis A outbreaks are usually due to contamination of food during preparation by an infected food handler.

There is no chronic carrier state for HAV. The virus is present in feces during the incubation period, so it can be carried and transmitted by persons who have undetectable, subclinical infections. The greatest risk of transmission occurs before clinical symptoms are apparent. It can also be transmitted by patients with *anicteric* (nonjaundice) hepatitis A.

Hepatitis B Virus. HBV is a DNA virus that is transmitted by percutaneous (e.g., IV drug use, accidental needle-stick punctures) or permucosal exposure to infectious blood, blood products, or other body fluids (e.g., semen, vaginal secretions, saliva). Transmission occurs when infected blood or other body fluids enter the body of a person who is not immune to the virus. Perinatal transmission from mother to infant can occur. Approximately 90% of infants infected at birth go on to develop chronic hepatitis B.[1] In persons who have HBV, hepatitis B surface antigen (HBsAg) has been detected in almost every body fluid, including vaginal secretions, menstrual fluids, semen, saliva, respiratory secretions, tears, gastric juice, synovial fluid, and cerebrospinal fluid. Infected semen and saliva contain much lower concentrations of HBV than blood, but the virus can be transmitted via these secretions. If gastrointestinal (GI) bleeding occurs, feces can be contaminated with the virus from the blood. There is no evidence that urine, feces (without GI bleeding), breast milk, tears, and sweat are infective. In 20% to 30% of patients with acute hepatitis B, there are no readily identifiable risk factors.

Hepatitis B is a sexually transmitted disease. Approximately 30% of HBV cases are related to heterosexual activity (e.g., unprotected sex with an infected person). Male homosexuals (especially those practicing unprotected anal intercourse) are at risk for HBV infection. Although there is a much lower risk of transmission, kissing and sharing of food items may spread the virus via saliva. Other at-risk individuals include those who have household contacts with chronically infected persons, hemodialysis patients, and health care and public safety workers. The HBV can live on a dry surface for at least 7 days. HBV is much more infectious than HIV.

HBV is a complex structure with three distinct antigens: the surface antigen (HBsAg), the core antigen (HBcAg), and the e antigen (HBeAg). The persistence of HBsAg in the serum for 6 to 12 months or longer after infection with the virus indicates a carrier state of hepatitis B. Each antigen has a corresponding antibody that may be elicited during acute viral hepatitis B. These antibodies can be detected in the serum of persons with prior exposure to the antigenic virus (Fig. 42-3). The presence of hepatitis B surface antibody (anti-HBs or HBsAB) indicates immunity from the HBV vaccine or from past HBV infection.

From 2% to 10% of adults who become infected with HBV become chronic HBV carriers and may transmit the virus.[1] The HBsAg level remains detectable in chronic carriers (HBsAg positive on at least two occasions at least 6 months apart). With chronic carrier states, liver enzyme values may be normal or elevated. Patients with chronic HBV may have a normal liver, low-grade disease, or severe liver disease. They are also at higher risk of developing hepatocellular carcinoma.

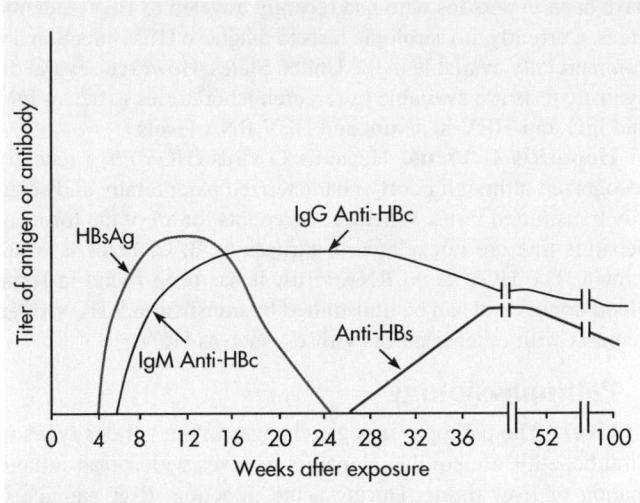

FIG. 42-3 Clinical and serologic events of a typical patient infected with acute hepatitis B virus (HBV). Elevated alanine aminotransferase (ALT) levels are present by about 8 weeks, and jaundice appears by about 10 weeks after exposure to the virus. *HBc,* Hepatitis B core antigen; *HBsAg,* hepatitis B surface antigen.

Hepatitis C Virus. HCV is an RNA virus that is primarily transmitted percutaneously. The major risk factor for infection is direct percutaneous exposure, such as injecting drugs, transfusion of infected blood products, hemodialysis, high-risk sexual behavior (e.g., unprotected sex, multiple partners), organ transplants, and exposure to blood and blood products by health care workers. In the United States IV drug use is the most common method of transmission, accounting for approximately 60% of all cases, and in Canada this number approaches 90%.[8-10] In the United States, approximately 20% of all cases are thought to be due to sexual transmission and another 10% to occupational exposure, hemodialysis, and perinatal transmission. However, 10% of patients with HCV cannot identify a source. A reliable antibody test for HCV was not widely available before 1992, so any patients given blood or blood products before then are at risk for chronic HCV infection and should be tested. Additional data are needed regarding the risks of body piercings, tattooing, and intranasal (e.g., cocaine) drug use in the transmission of HCV.

Hepatitis D Virus. Hepatitis D virus (HDV), also called *delta virus,* is a defective single-stranded RNA virus that cannot survive on its own. HDV requires the helper function of HBV to replicate. The importance of HDV relates to its clinical virulence. HDV infection can be acquired as a coinfection with HBV, often resulting in a superinfection; that is, patients with HBV-HDV coinfection may have more severe acute disease and a greater risk of fulminant hepatitis (2% to 20%) compared with those infected with HBV alone. However, in HBV patients coinfected with HDV, chronic HBV is less likely to develop. HDV is transmitted percutaneously, similar to HBV. However, the risk of transmission via sexual activity is much less.[1]

Hepatitis E Virus. Hepatitis E virus (HEV) is an RNA virus that is transmitted by the fecal-oral route. The most common mode of transmission is drinking contaminated water. Hepatitis E occurs primarily in developing countries. There have been reported epidemics in India, Asia, Mexico, and Africa. Only a few cases have been reported in the United States, and these cases have been in persons who had recently traveled to HEV-endemic areas. Currently, no serologic tests to diagnose HEV infection are commercially available in the United States. However, several diagnostic tests are available in research laboratories to detect IgM and IgG anti-HEV in serum and HEV RNA levels.[1]

Hepatitis G Virus. Hepatitis G virus (HGV) is a recently recognized although poorly characterized parenterally and sexually transmitted virus. Whether it accounts for all of the forms of hepatitis that are not related to viruses A, B, C, D, or E is not known. The HGV is an RNA virus. It has been found in some blood donors and can be transmitted by transfusion.[11] HGV often coexists with other hepatitis viruses, such as HCV.

Pathophysiology

Liver. The pathophysiologic changes in the various types of viral hepatitis are similar. Hepatitis involves widespread inflammation of liver tissue. During acute infection, liver damage is mediated by cytotoxic cytokines and natural killer cells that cause lysis of infected hepatocytes. Liver cell damage results in hepatic cell necrosis. There is proliferation and enlargement of the Kupffer cells. Inflammation of the periportal areas may interrupt bile flow. Cholestasis may occur. The liver cells can regenerate in an orderly manner, and if no complications occur, they should resume their normal appearance and function.

Systemic Effects. The antigen-antibody complexes between the virus and its corresponding antibody form a circulating immune complex in the early phases of hepatitis. The circulating immune complexes activate the complement system (see Chapter 13). The clinical manifestations of this activation are rash, angioedema, arthritis, fever, and malaise. *Cryoglobulinemia* (abnormal proteins found in the blood), glomerulonephritis, and vasculitis have also been found secondary to immune complex activation.

Clinical Manifestations

A large number of patients have no symptoms. For example, 30% of patients with acute HBV and 80% of patients with acute HCV will be asymptomatic. The clinical manifestations of viral hepatitis may be classified into three phases: (1) preicteric or prodromal phase, (2) icteric phase, and (3) posticteric or convalescent phase (Table 42-3).

Preicteric Phase. The preicteric phase precedes jaundice and lasts from 1 to 21 days. This is the period of maximal infectivity for hepatitis A. Hepatitis B patients who are HBsAg positive and patients with HCV can be infective for years. GI symptoms include anorexia, nausea, abdominal (right upper quadrant) discomfort, and sometimes vomiting, constipation, or diarrhea. The anorexia is frequently severe and may be due to cytokines or other chemicals produced by the infected liver. The patient may find food repugnant and, if a smoker, may have a distaste for cigarettes. There is also a decreased sense of smell. Weight loss occurs during the preicteric phase. Other symptoms during this phase are malaise, headache, low-grade fever, arthralgias, and skin rashes. Physical examination reveals hepatomegaly, lymphadenopathy, and sometimes splenomegaly.

Icteric Phase. The icteric phase lasts 2 to 4 weeks and is characterized by jaundice. Jaundice results when bilirubin diffuses into the tissues. The urine may darken because of excess bilirubin being excreted by the kidneys. If conjugated bilirubin cannot flow out of the liver because of obstruction or inflamma-

TABLE 42-3	Clinical Manifestations of the Phases of Hepatitis	
PREICTERIC	**ICTERIC**	**POSTICTERIC**
Anorexia	Jaundice	Malaise
Nausea, vomiting	Pruritus	Easy fatigability
Right upper quadrant discomfort	Dark urine	Hepatomegaly
	Bilirubinuria	
	Light stools	
Constipation or diarrhea	Fatigue	
Decreased sense of taste and smell	Continued hepatomegaly with tenderness	
Malaise	Weight loss	
Headache		
Fever		
Arthralgias		
Urticaria		
Hepatomegaly		
Splenomegaly		
Weight loss		

tion of the bile ducts, the stools will be light or clay colored. Pruritus sometimes accompanies the jaundice, especially if cholestasis is present. The pruritus occurs as a result of the accumulation of bile salts beneath the skin.

When jaundice occurs, the fever usually subsides. The GI symptoms usually remain, and some fatigue may continue. The liver is usually enlarged and tender.

Posticteric Phase. The convalescent stage of the posticteric phase begins as jaundice is disappearing and lasts weeks to months, with an average of 2 to 4 months. During this period the patient's major complaint is malaise and easy fatigability. Hepatomegaly remains for several weeks, but splenomegaly subsides during this period. Relapses may occur, and the disappearance of jaundice does not mean the patient has totally recovered.

General Considerations. Not all patients with viral hepatitis have jaundice. This is termed *anicteric hepatitis*. A high percentage of persons with HAV are anicteric and do not have symptoms.

There is some slight variation in manifestations between the types of hepatitis. In hepatitis A the onset is more acute, and the symptoms are usually mild, flulike manifestations. In hepatitis B the onset is more insidious, and the symptoms are usually more severe, but there may be fewer GI symptoms. In hepatitis C the majority of cases are asymptomatic or mild. However, HCV has a high rate of persistence and can induce chronic liver disease.

Complications

Most patients with acute viral hepatitis recover completely with no complications. The overall mortality rate for acute hepatitis is less than 1%. The mortality rate is higher in older adults and those with underlying debilitating illnesses (including chronic liver disease). Complications that can occur include fulminant hepatic failure, chronic hepatitis, cirrhosis of the liver, and hepatocellular carcinoma.

HAV infection can cause fulminant hepatic failure but does not cause chronic hepatitis. HBV can also cause fulminant hepatic failure and results in chronic infection in approximately 10% of those infected. Chronic HBV is identified by the persistence of HBsAg for longer than 6 months. Patients with chronic HBV are evaluated by assessment of liver function tests, HBV DNA (which measures the level of circulating HBV), and the presence of HBeAg and anti-HBe. A liver biopsy may be required to assess for the degree of inflammation and the presence and degree of fibrosis. Fibrosis may progress to cirrhosis in some patients. Chronic hepatitis B is a risk factor for the development of hepatocellular carcinoma.

It is not known what factors contribute to the persistence of the virus in some patients. Chronic HBV is more likely to develop in infants born to infected mothers and those who acquire the infection as children (e.g., before the age of 5) compared with those who acquire the virus over the age of 5. Alterations in the patient's cellular immune response may be important in the development of the chronic HBsAg carrier state and consequent progression from acute hepatitis B to chronic active hepatitis. These immune system alterations may explain why the patient with chronic renal failure who is undergoing dialysis when hepatitis B develops is more at risk for chronic hepatitis. (Persons with chronic renal failure are known to have a depressed cellular immune response.)

There is a greater risk for HCV infection to become chronic compared with HBV. Approximately 75% to 85% of patients who acquire HCV will go on to develop chronic infection.[2] Approximately 20% of patients with HCV will develop cirrhosis over 20 to 30 years; of these, 20% will develop liver failure. The prognosis of chronic HCV has greatly increased the demand for liver transplants. Risk factors for progression to cirrhosis include male gender, heavy alcohol consumption, and excess iron deposition in the liver. Steatorrhea, obesity, and diabetes mellitus are also risk factors for the progression of HCV to chronic liver disease. Patients who have cirrhosis caused by HCV are at risk for hepatocellular carcinoma.

Fulminant Hepatitis. **Fulminant viral hepatitis** is a clinical syndrome that results in severe impairment or necrosis of liver cells and potential liver failure. Fulminant viral hepatitis develops in a small percentage of patients. The disorder may occur as a complication of hepatitis B, particularly hepatitis B accompanied by infection with delta virus (HDV). Fulminant hepatitis occurs much less frequently with HCV. Toxic reactions to drugs and congenital metabolic disorders may also cause fulminant hepatitis and liver failure. Hepatocellular failure with death usually occurs.

Diagnostic Studies

Tests for the different types of viral hepatitis are presented in Table 42-4. In viral hepatitis many of the liver function tests show significant abnormalities. The common abnormalities are identified in Table 42-5.

Several tests are available to determine the presence of HCV. Unlike HAV and HBV, antibodies to hepatitis C are not protective and may be an indicator of chronic disease. For the patient who has a positive anti-HCV test by enzyme immunoassay, or if the HCV is suspected and there is a false positive antibody test (approximately 90% of patients with HCV are positive for anti-HCV), more sensitive testing is required. The HCV recombinant immunoblot assay is a more sensitive antibody test. To detect active disease (the presence of circulating HCV), HCV RNA polymerase chain reaction (PCR) is performed. This may be particularly helpful in the immunocompromised patient (e.g., patient with HIV) whose antibody production is very low (below the detection level of the antibody tests). In addition, this test may be helpful in identifying the presence of the virus in exposed individuals (e.g., health care workers) before the development of antibodies. However, HCV RNA PCR testing is not done as the initial testing for HCV infection.

For those patients who test positive for HCV, genotyping of the virus may also be done. Genotyping does not influence the type of treatment but may be used to guide length of treatment.

TABLE 42-4	Tests for Viral Hepatitis	
VIRUS	**TESTS**	**SIGNIFICANCE**
A	Anti-HAV IgM	Acute infection
	Anti-HAV IgG	Previous infection and long-term immunity
B	HBsAg (hepatitis B surface antigen)	Current infection (but not necessarily acute)*
		Positive in chronic carriers
	Anti-HBs (antibody to surface antigen)	Indicates previous infection with hepatitis B or immunization
		Marker of response to vaccine
	HBeAg (hepatitis B e antigen)	Indicates high infectivity; present in acute, active infection
	Anti-HBe (antibody to e antigen)	Indicates previous infection
	HBcAg (hepatitis B core antigen)	Ongoing infection with hepatitis B
	Anti-HBc IgM	Acute infection*
	Anti-HBc IgG (antibody to HB core antigen)	Indicates previous infection or ongoing infection with hepatitis B
		Does not appear after vaccination
	HBV DNA	Indicates active ongoing viral replication
		Best indicator of viral replication
C	Anti-HCV (antibody to hepatitis C)	Marker for acute or chronic infection with HCV
	Enzyme immunoassay (EIA)	Used in initial screening for HCV
	Recombinant immunoblot assay (RIBA)	More sensitive antibody test
	HCV RNA (RNA polymerase chain reaction [PCR] assay)	Indicates active ongoing viral replication
D	Anti-HDV	Present in past or current infection with hepatitis D

*If positive HBsAg and anti-HBc IgM, it indicates the presence of acute infection.
A, Hepatitis A virus (HAV); *B*, hepatitis B virus (HBV); *C*, hepatitis C virus (HCV); *D*, hepatitis D virus (HDV); *DNA*, deoxyribonucleic acid; *RNA*, ribonucleic acid.

TABLE 42-5	**Diagnostic Findings in Acute Hepatitis**	
TEST	**ABNORMAL FINDING**	**ETIOLOGY**
Transaminases (aminotransferases)		
Aspartate aminotransferase (AST)	Elevation in preicteric phase; decrease as jaundice disappears	Liver cell injury
Alanine aminotransferase (ALT)	Elevation in preicteric phase; decrease as jaundice disappears	Liver cell injury
γ-Glutamyl transpeptidase (GGT)	Elevation	Liver cell injury
Alkaline phosphatase	Some elevation	Impaired excretory function of the liver
Serum proteins		
γ-Globulin	Normal or increased	Impaired clearance of the liver
Albumin	Normal or decreased	Liver damage
Serum bilirubin (total)	Elevation to about 8-15 mg/dl (137-257 μmol/L)	Liver cell damage
Urinary bilirubin	Elevation	Conjugated hyperbilirubinemia
Urinary urobilinogen	Elevation 2-5 days before jaundice	Diminished reabsorption of urobilinogen
Prothrombin time	Prolonged	Decreased absorption of vitamin K in intestine with decreased production of prothrombin by liver

Genotype 1, the most common form in the United States, Canada, and other Western countries, is more resistant to treatment than genotypes 2 through 6.[6]

Physical assessment reveals hepatic tenderness, hepatomegaly, and splenomegaly. The liver is palpable. A liver biopsy is not indicated in acute hepatitis unless the diagnosis is in doubt. In chronic persistent hepatitis a liver biopsy may be performed to assess the degree of liver damage.

Patients with chronic HBV and HCV may undergo liver biopsy. Biopsy of liver tissue allows for histologic examination of liver cells and characterization of the degree of inflammation, fibrosis, or cirrhosis that may be present.[12] A patient who has a bleeding disorder may not be an appropriate candidate for biopsy because of the risk of bleeding.

Collaborative Care

There is no specific treatment or therapy for acute viral hepatitis. Most patients can be managed at home. Emphasis is on measures to rest the body and assist the liver in regenerating (Table 42-6). Adequate nutrients and rest seem to be most beneficial for healing and liver cell (*hepatocyte*) regeneration. Dietary emphasis is on a well-balanced diet that the patient can tolerate. Rest reduces the metabolic demands on the liver and promotes cell regeneration. Bed rest may be indicated while the patient is symptomatic. The degree of rest ordered depends on the severity of symptoms, but usually alternating periods of activity and rest are adequate. Counseling should include the importance of avoiding alcohol and notification of possible contacts for testing and prophylaxis, if indicated.

Drug Therapy. There are no specific drug therapies for the treatment of acute viral hepatitis. Supportive drug therapy may include antiemetics, such as dimenhydrinate (Dramamine) or trimethobenzamide (Tigan). Phenothiazines should not be used because of their possible cholestatic and hepatotoxic effects. If the patient requires a sedative or hypnotic drug, diphenhydramine (Benadryl) or chloral hydrate may be used.

Chronic hepatitis B. Drug therapy for chronic HBV is focused on decreasing the viral load, decreasing the rate of disease progression, and decreasing the rate of drug-resistant HBV. At the moment, several drugs are useful in suppressing viral activity

TABLE 42-6	***Collaborative Care*** **Viral Hepatitis**

Diagnostic
History and physical examination
Liver function studies
  Alanine aminotransferase (ALT)
  Aspartate aminotransferase (AST)
Hepatitis testing
  Anti-HAV—IgM and IgG
  HBsAg (HBeAg in some cases)
  Anti-HBs
  Anti-HBc—IgM and IgG
  HBV DNA
  Anti-HCV
  HCV RNA
  Anti-HDV

Collaborative Therapy
Acute and Chronic
High-calorie, high-protein, high-carbohydrate, low-fat diet
Vitamin supplements
Rest—degree of strictness varies
Avoid alcohol intake and drugs detoxified by the liver
Chronic HBV and HCV
α-Interferon (Peg-Intron, Pegasys)
Antiviral agents (lamivudine [Epivir], ribavirin [Rebetol])

DNA, Deoxyribonucleic acid; *HAV*, hepatitis A virus; *HB*, hepatitis B; *HBV*, hepatitis B virus; *HCV*, hepatitis C virus; *HDV*, hepatitis D virus; *RNA*, ribonucleic acid.

and decreasing viral load in patients with chronic HBV. However, the percentage of patients seroconverting (developing antibodies against the virus) remains relatively low.

Lamivudine (Epivir, 3TC), a reverse transcriptase inhibitor, is used to treat chronic HBV. This drug taken orally for 1 year has beneficial effects in terms of reducing viral load, decreasing liver damage, and decreasing liver enzymes in approximately two thirds of patients.[13,14] However, seroconversion occurs in less than 20% of patients. When lamivudine is stopped, the majority of patients (except those who have seroconverted)

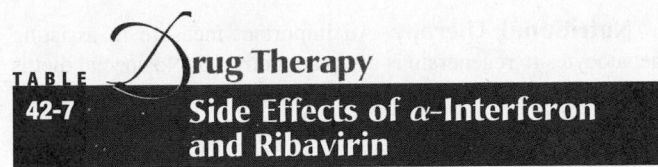

TABLE 42-7 Drug Therapy: Side Effects of α-Interferon and Ribavirin

α-Interferon

Flulike Symptoms
Arthralgia
Asthenia (loss of strength)
Fatigue
Headache
Myalgia
Nausea/anorexia

Other Effects
Anemia
Decline in platelet and neutrophil counts
Depression
Hair loss (alopecia)
Insomnia
Rash
Thyroid dysfunction
Weight loss

Less Common Effects
Diarrhea
Peripheral neuropathy
Retinopathy
Seizures
Vasculitis

Ribavirin
Anemia (hemolytic)
Anorexia
Cough
Dyspnea
Insomnia
Pruritus
Rash
Teratogenicity (interferes with normal fetal development)

have HBV DNA and inflammation levels that return to pretreatment levels. Approximately 20% to 30% of patients develop resistance to the drug. Lamivudine has been used along with HBV immunoglobulin to reduce viral activity in patients who have a liver transplant for HBV. Other drugs in this class undergoing investigation include famciclovir (Famvir) and ganciclovir (Cytovene).[13]

α-Interferon is an important drug in the treatment of chronic HBV. A 4-month course of treatment with α-interferon results in a significant reduction of serum HBV DNA levels, normalization of alanine aminotransferase (ALT) level, and loss of HBV antigen (HBeAg) in 30% to 40% of those treated.[11] In addition, the development of cirrhosis and hepatocellular cancer appears to be decreased in those who receive α-interferon treatment. α-Interferon treatment is associated with a number of side effects (Table 42-7). These side effects are dose related and tend to decrease in severity with continued treatment.

Adefovir dipivoxil (Hepsera) can be used for the treatment of chronic HBV in patients with active viral replication and either elevations of serum ALT or AST, or histologically active disease. Hepsera slows the progression of chronic HBV by interfering with viral replication.

Chronic hepatitis C. Drug therapy is directed at reducing the viral load, decreasing progression of the disease, and promoting seroconversion. Treatment for HCV includes monotherapy with α-interferon alone or the combination of ribavirin (Rebetol) and α-interferon. Approximately 40% to 50% of patients will initially respond to α-interferon alone (monotherapy) with a decrease in HCV RNA levels. However, approximately 50% of these patients will relapse in 6 months, indicating that α-interferon monotherapy is effective in less than 25% of patients with chronic HCV. Currently there are pegylated formulas of α-interferon (e.g., Peg-Intron, Pegasys) that allow for once weekly administration as opposed to three injections weekly. In these formulations polyethylene glycol is attached to the interferon, providing a protective barrier against its breakdown. With pegylated forms of α-interferon, the blood levels of the drug remain sustained over a longer period and provide more constant suppression of HCV.[15]

Ribavirin, given in combination with α-interferon, has a synergistic effect and has been used to reduce the rate of relapse following α-interferon therapy for HCV. Combination therapy (α-interferon plus ribavirin) has been shown to be more effective than monotherapy in the treatment of HCV.[16] Patients who have advanced fibrosis or cirrhosis can be treated with drug therapy as long as liver decompensation (e.g., ascites, esophageal hemorrhage, jaundice, wasting, encephalopathy) is not present. Ribavirin has a number of side effects, as shown in Table 42-7.

An increasing number of patients with HIV also have HCV. Patients who have stable HIV and relatively intact immune systems (CD4+ counts >200) are treated for HCV with the goal of eradicating HCV and enhancing quality of life. However, for those with advanced liver disease, the goal of HCV treatment is to delay disease progress.

The drug treatment of HIV in patients with coexisting HCV requires close attention to liver function. Treatment of HCV in patients with HIV requires close attention to lymphocyte and white and red blood cell counts. HCV treatment with ribavirin and α-interferon may reduce CD4+ counts, increase leukopenia, and increase the patient's risk for anemia (ribavirin effects). Drug interactions may also occur in patients being treated for both HIV and HCV. Depending on the degree of liver damage associated with HCV, drug therapy for HIV may need to be altered because of the decreased ability of the liver to metabolize the drugs.

Prevention

Hepatitis A. Both hepatitis A vaccine and immune globulin (IG) are used for prevention of hepatitis A. The vaccine is used for preexposure prophylaxis, and IG can be used either before or after exposure. IG provides temporary (6 to 8 weeks) passive immunity and is effective for preventing hepatitis A if given within 1 to 2 weeks after exposure. IG is recommended for persons who do not have anti-HAV antibodies and are exposed to hepatitis A from close (household, day care center) contact with persons who have HAV or food-borne exposure.[17] Because patients with hepatitis A are most infectious just before the onset of symptoms, those exposed through household contact or food-borne outbreaks should be given IG within 1 to 2 weeks of exposure. Although IG may not prevent infection in all persons, it may modify the illness to a subclinical infection. It may also be used as a prophylactic measure for travelers to countries that have a high incidence of hepatitis A.

There are currently several forms of the hepatitis A vaccine, including Havrix, Vaqta, and Avaxim. Active immunization is an important and effective means of controlling hepatitis A from a public health perspective. Primary immunization consists of a single dose administered intramuscularly in the deltoid muscle. A booster is recommended any time between 6 and 12 months after the initiation of the primary dose to ensure adequate antibody titers and long-term protection. However, a primary immunization provides immunity within 30 days after a single dose. The vaccine may be administered concomitantly with IG, although the ultimate antibody titer obtained is likely to be lower than if the vaccine is given alone.

Twinrix, a combined HAV and HBV vaccine, is available for persons over the age of 18 years.[18] The primary immunization consists of three doses, given on a 0-, 1-, and 6-month schedule, the same schedule as that used for the single HBV vaccine. Twinrix may be given to high-risk individuals, including patients with chronic liver disease, users of illicit injectable drugs, men who have sex with men, and persons with clotting factor disorders who receive therapeutic blood products. The side effects of the vaccine are mild and are usually limited to soreness and redness at the injection site.

Hepatitis B. Immunization with hepatitis B vaccine is the most effective method of preventing HBV infection. Recommendations from the Centers for Disease Control and Prevention (CDC) Immunization Practices Advisory Committee include making hepatitis B vaccine a part of routine vaccination schedules for all newborns and adolescents.

In addition to immunizing newborns and adolescents, it is important to vaccinate adults in the major risk groups, such as IV drug users and household members living with a hepatitis B carrier. It is hoped that universal vaccination will lead to eventual prevention and control of hepatitis B.

Hepatitis B vaccine is produced through recombinant DNA technology (see Fig. 13-15). The vaccines are Recombivax HB and Engerix-B. The vaccine is given in a series of three intramuscular injections in the deltoid muscle. The second dose is administered within 1 month of the first one, and the third one within 6 months of the first. The vaccine is greater than 95% effective. Successful vaccination should result in Anti-HBs titers of 10 mIU/ml or greater. However, it has not been definitely determined what level of antibody is required to provide protection. Therefore it remains to be determined how frequently boosters (additional doses) are necessary. Only minor adverse reactions have been reported with vaccination, including transient fever and soreness at the injection site. The vaccine is not contraindicated in pregnancy.

For postexposure prophylaxis, the vaccine and hepatitis B immune globulin (HBIG) are used. HBIG contains antibodies to HBV and confers temporary passive immunity. HBIG is prepared from plasma of donors with a high titer of anti-HBs and is expensive. HBIG is recommended for postexposure prophylaxis in cases of needle stick, mucous membrane contact, or sexual exposure and for infants born to mothers who are positive for HBsAg. It should be given after exposure, preferably within 24 hours. The vaccine series should also be started.

Hepatitis C. Currently there are no products to prevent HCV. However, several vaccines are in development. The CDC does not recommend IG or antiviral agents such as α-interferon for postexposure prophylaxis (e.g., needle-stick exposure from an infected patient) for HCV infection. Following an acute exposure (e.g., needle stick), the person (i.e., the source) should have anti-HCV testing done.[19] For the person exposed to HCV, baseline anti-HCV and ALT levels should be measured. Follow-up testing should be done at 4 to 6 months for anti-HCV and ALT activity. Testing for HCV RNA may be performed at 4 to 6 weeks. It is not known if antiviral therapy initiated after exposure has any positive effect.

Nutritional Therapy. An important measure in assisting hepatocytes to regenerate is adequate nutrition. No special diet is required in the treatment of viral hepatitis. However, a diet high in carbohydrates and proteins with low fat content is usually recommended. Adequate calories are important because the patient usually loses weight. If fat content is poorly tolerated because of decreased bile production, it should be reduced. Basically, the specific foods in the diet are dictated by the patient. Vitamin supplements, particularly B-complex vitamins and vitamin K, are frequently used. If anorexia, nausea, and vomiting are severe, IV solutions of glucose or supplemental tube feedings may be used. Fluid and electrolyte balance must be maintained.

NURSING MANAGEMENT
HEPATITIS

■ Nursing Assessment

Subjective and objective data that should be obtained from a person with hepatitis are presented in Table 42-8.

TABLE 42-8	Nursing Assessment Hepatitis

Subjective Data
Important Health Information
Past health history: Hemophilia; exposure to infected persons; ingestion of contaminated food or water; exposure to benzene, carbon tetrachloride, or other hepatotoxic agents; crowded, unsanitary living conditions; exposure to contaminated needles; recent travel; organ transplant recipient; exposure to new drug regimens
Medications: Use and misuse of acetaminophen, phenytoin, halothane, methyldopa

Functional Health Patterns
Health perception–health management: IV drug and alcohol abuse; malaise, distaste for cigarettes (in smokers), high-risk sexual behaviors
Nutritional-metabolic: Weight loss, anorexia, nausea, vomiting; feeling of fullness in right upper quadrant
Elimination: Dark urine; light-colored stools, constipation or diarrhea; skin rashes, hives
Activity-exercise: Fatigue, arthralgias, myalgias
Cognitive-perceptual: Right upper quadrant pain and liver tenderness, headache; pruritus
Role-relationship: Exposure as health care worker, chronic care institution resident, incarceration

Objective Data
General
Low-grade fever, lethargy, lymphadenopathy
Integumentary
Rash, angioedema, jaundice, icteric sclera, injection sites
Gastrointestinal
Hepatomegaly, splenomegaly
Possible Findings
Abnormal liver enzyme studies; ↑ serum total bilirubin, hypoalbuminemia, anemia, bilirubin in urine and increased urobilinogen, prolonged prothrombin time, positive tests for hepatitis including anti-HAV IgM, anti-HAV IgG, HBsAg, HBeAg, HBcAg, anti-HBc IgM, HBV DNA, anti-HCV, HCV RNA, anti-HDV; abnormal liver scan; positive liver biopsy

DNA, Deoxyribonucleic acid; *HAV,* hepatitis A virus; *HB,* hepatitis B; *HBV,* hepatitis B virus; *HCV,* hepatitis C virus; *HDV,* hepatitis D virus; *RNA,* ribonucleic acid.

Nursing Diagnoses

Nursing diagnoses for the patient with hepatitis may include, but are not limited to, those presented in NCP 42-1.

Planning

The overall goals are that the patient with viral hepatitis will (1) have relief of discomfort, (2) be able to resume normal activities, and (3) return to normal liver function without complications.

Nursing Implementation

Health Promotion. Viral hepatitis is a community health problem. The nurse must assume a significant role in the control and prevention of this disease. It is helpful to first understand the epidemiology of the different types of viral hepatitis before considering appropriate control measures.

Hepatitis A. Vaccination is the best protection against HAV. Vaccination is recommended for persons 2 years of age and older who travel to areas with increased rates of hepatitis A, men who have sex with men, injecting and noninjecting drug users, per-

sons with clotting factor disorders (e.g., hemophilia), persons with chronic liver disease, and children living in regions of the United States with consistently increased rates of hepatitis A.

Outbreaks of viral hepatitis are usually due to HAV. In the United States there is usually one major outbreak per decade, the last being in 1995.[1] Preventive measures include personal and environmental hygiene and health education to promote good sanitation (Table 42-9). Hand washing is essential and is probably the most important precaution. Health teaching should include careful hand washing after bowel movements and before eating. When hepatitis A occurs in a food handler, IG should be administered to all other food handlers at the establishment. Patrons may also need to be given IG.

Isolation is not required for hepatitis A. For a patient with hepatitis A, infection control precautions should be used (see Table 12-19). A private room is indicated if the patient is incontinent of stool or has poor personal hygiene.

Hepatitis B. The use of the hepatitis B vaccine is the best means of protection. Control and prevention of hepatitis B also focus on identification of possible exposure via percutaneous and sexual transmission (see Table 42-9). The nurse must be aware of

NURSING CARE PLAN 42-1

Patient with Acute Viral Hepatitis

EXPECTED PATIENT OUTCOMES	NURSING INTERVENTIONS and *RATIONALES*
NURSING DIAGNOSIS	**Imbalanced nutrition: less than body requirements** *related to* anorexia, nausea, and reduced metabolism of nutrients by liver *as manifested by* inadequate food intake; perceived inability to ingest food.
• Adequate nutritional intake • Progression toward or maintenance of normal body weight	• Collaborate with health care provider, dietitian, and family to provide appropriate diet *so the proper nutritional requirements can be provided.* • Assess patient's appetite and adequacy of intake *so appropriate interventions can be planned.* • Offer frequent small meals, provide oral care before *meals to enhance patient's dietary intake.* • Allow patient to choose food items; serve high-carbohydrate and high-protein foods at time of day the patient feels most like eating *to increase likelihood of adequate intake.* • Provide attractively served meals in pleasant surroundings *to stimulate patient's appetite.* • Take weight daily on same scale, at same time, with same clothing *to monitor weight loss secondary to poor appetite.*
NURSING DIAGNOSIS	**Activity intolerance** *related to* fatigue and weakness *as manifested by* verbal report of fatigue or weakness, altered response to activity (as measured by BP, pulse, respiratory rate).
• Increased tolerance for activity	• Provide rest periods. • Increase patient's activity gradually as allowed and tolerated *so previous activity pattern can be resumed.* • Conserve patient's strength by careful monitoring of activity *to prevent increasing weakness and fatigue.* • Teach patient to monitor and control activities that provoke fatigue *so patient can be an active participant in plan.*
NURSING DIAGNOSIS	**Ineffective therapeutic regimen management** *related to* lack of knowledge of follow-up care *as manifested by* frequent questions about transmission of disease, activities allowed, and general follow-up care.
• Verbalization of understanding of follow-up care • Able to explain methods of transmission and methods of preventing transmission to others	• Teach patient basic facts about illness, modes of transmission, diet, activities allowed, avoidance of alcohol, and need for follow-up care *so appropriate follow-up care will be planned and carried out.* • Teach patient to watch for and report signs of complications such as muscle cramps, bleeding gums or stools, worsening of symptoms *to enable prompt intervention.* Emphasize the importance of adequate rest *to enable liver to repair itself and to prevent relapse.* • Teach use of infection control precautions *to reduce risk of cross-contamination.*

TABLE 42-9 Preventive Measures for Viral Hepatitis	
HEPATITIS A	**HEPATITIS B AND C**

General Measures
Hand washing
Proper personal hygiene
Environmental sanitation
Control and screening (signs, symptoms) of food handlers
Serologic screening while carrying virus
Active immunization: HAV vaccine to anyone over age 2
 	
Use of Immune Globulin
Early administration (1-2 wk after exposure) to those exposed
Prophylaxis for travelers to areas where hepatitis A is common if not vaccinated with HAV vaccine
	Percutaneous Transmission
	Screening of donated blood
	  B—HBsAg
	  C—anti-HCV
	Use of disposable needles and syringes
	
	Sexual Transmission
	Acute exposure: HBIG administration to sexual partner of HBsAg-positive person
	Administer hepatitis B vaccine series to uninfected sexual partners
	Use condoms for sexual intercourse
	
	General Measures
	Hand washing
	Avoid sharing toothbrushes and razors
	HBIG administration for one-time exposure (needle stick, contact of mucous membranes with infectious material)
	Active immunization: HBV vaccine

the individuals at high risk of contracting hepatitis B and teach methods to reduce risks. These include patients receiving frequent transfusions or hemodialysis, workers in hemodialysis units and laboratories where blood is handled, IV drug users, persons with multiple sexual partners, prisoners, and household members and sexual partners of HBV carriers.[1,19]

Good hygienic practices, including hand washing and the use of gloves when expecting contact with blood, are important. A condom is advised for sexual intercourse, and the partner should be vaccinated. Razors, toothbrushes, and other personal items should not be shared. Close contacts of the patient with hepatitis B who are HBsAg negative and antibody negative should be vaccinated.

According to CDC guidelines, infection control precautions should be followed for the patient with hepatitis B. This includes the use of disposable needles and syringes, which should be disposed of in puncture-resistant disposal units without recapping, bending, or breaking. (See Table 12-19 for various types of infection control precautions.)

Hepatitis C. There is no vaccine currently available. The primary measures to prevent HCV transmission are screening of blood, organ, and tissue donors; use of infection control precautions; and modification of high-risk behavior. Similar to HBV prevention, the nurse should identify individuals at high risk for contracting HCV and teach methods to reduce risks. Individuals at risk include those who use IV drugs (or have ever used, even once many years ago), patients who received blood or blood products before 1992, patients who are or have been on hemodialysis, workers in hemodialysis units and laboratories in which blood is handled, persons with multiple sexual partners, prisoners, and sexual partners of individuals with HCV. Infection with HCV often coexists with HIV infection.

The use of gloves when expecting contact with blood is important. A condom is advised for sexual intercourse with an individual with HCV. Razors, toothbrushes, and other personal items should not be shared. Preventive and control measures for hepatitis A, B and C are summarized in Table 42-9.

Acute Intervention

Jaundice. The nurse should assess for the degree of jaundice. In light-skinned persons the jaundice is usually observed first in the sclera of the eyes and later in the skin. In dark-skinned persons, jaundice is observed in the hard palate of the mouth and inner canthus of the eyes. Ictotest reagent tablets may be used to detect urinary bilirubin. The urine may have a dark brown or brownish red color because of the presence of bilirubin. Comfort measures to relieve pruritus (if present), headache, and arthralgias are helpful (see NCP 42-1).

Ensuring that the patient receives adequate nutrients is not always easy. The anorexia and extreme distaste for food cause nutritional problems. Dietary assessment must be considered. The nurse should try to determine whether there is something that appeals to the patient in spite of the anorexia. Small, frequent meals may be preferable to three large ones and may also help prevent nausea. Often, a patient with hepatitis finds that anorexia is not as severe in the morning, so it is easier to eat a good breakfast than a large dinner. Measures to stimulate the appetite, such as mouth care, antiemetics, and attractively served meals in pleasant surroundings, should be included in the nursing care plan. Other measures that may be tried to counteract the anorexia are carbonated beverages and avoidance of very hot or very cold foods. Adequate fluid intake (2500 to 3000 ml per day) is important.

Rest. Rest is essential and is an important factor in promoting liver cell regeneration. The nurse must assess the patient's response to the rest and activity plan and modify it accordingly. If the patient is on strict bed rest, measures to prevent respiratory and circulatory complications should be initiated. Assessment of the liver function tests and symptoms should continue as a guide to activity.

Psychologic and emotional rest is as essential as physical rest. Strict bed rest may produce anxiety and extreme restlessness in some patients and may be more damaging than reasonable ambulation. Diversional activities, such as reading and hobbies (e.g., knitting, stamp collecting), may help the patient.

Ambulatory and Home Care. Most patients with viral hepatitis will be cared for at home, so the nurse must assess the patient's knowledge of nutrition and provide the necessary dietary teaching. Rest and adequate nutrition are especially important until studies show that liver function has returned to normal. The patient must be cautioned about overexertion and the need to follow the physician's advice about when it is safe to return to work. The nurse must also teach the patient and family about preventive measures and how to prevent transmission to other family members. The patient should know what symptoms should be reported to the health care provider.

The patient should be assessed for any manifestations indicative of complications. Bleeding tendencies with increasing prothrombin time values, symptoms of encephalopathy, or abnormal liver function tests indicate problems, and the patient should be assessed and treated promptly.

The patient should be instructed to have regular follow-up for at least 1 year after the diagnosis of hepatitis. Because relapses are fairly common with hepatitis B and C, the patient should be instructed about the symptoms of recurrence and the need for follow-up evaluations. All patients with chronic HBV or HCV should avoid alcohol.

A patient who remains positive for HBsAg is a chronic carrier and should never be a blood donor. A patient who tests positive for the HCV antibody should also not donate blood. The patient with HBV and HCV should also be instructed to use a condom when engaging in sexual intercourse.

The patient who is receiving α-interferon for the treatment of hepatitis B or C requires education regarding this drug. α-Interferon is administered intramuscularly or subcutaneously, and thus the patient or family member needs to be taught how to administer the drug. There are numerous side effects with the therapy, including flulike symptoms (e.g., fever, malaise, fatigue, chills). The physician may recommend that acetaminophen be administered 30 to 60 minutes before injection to reduce these symptoms. Other significant side effects include thrombocytopenia, neutropenia, psychologic disturbances (e.g., mood swings, depression), and limited alopecia (see Table 42-7).

(Additional information on α-interferon is presented in Chapters 13 and 15.)

■ Evaluation

Expected outcomes for the patient with hepatitis are addressed in NCP 42-1.

Control of Hepatitis in Health Care Personnel

Hepatitis A. Hepatitis A is rarely transmitted from patients to health care personnel. When this does occur, it is associated with patients with undiagnosed hepatitis A who are treated for other problems. Usually these patients are incontinent of feces. The use of infection control precautions should prevent transmission of HAV to health care personnel.

Hepatitis B. Health care workers may be exposed to HBV from needle sticks or blood contamination to mucous membranes or nonintact skin. If a health care worker is exposed to HBV through a needle stick and does not receive the vaccine, there is a 6% to 30% chance of infection with hepatitis B.[1] Vaccination is the most effective method to prevent HBV in health care workers. Employers are required by the Occupational Safety and Health Administration to provide free HBV immunization to employees at risk for infection.

The principal mode of transmission of HBV for health care personnel is parenteral. Examples of parenteral transmission include accidental needle sticks and, rarely, transfusion of contaminated blood or blood products. Because all blood and blood products are tested for HBV and anti-HCV, there is diminishing risk of this latter mode of transmission. Other forms of transmission include contamination of fresh cutaneous scratches or abrasions, burns, and contamination of mucosal surfaces with infective blood, blood products, saliva, or semen.

Hepatitis C. Transmission is usually due to percutaneous needle exposure or other blood exposure and undetected parenteral transmission. Measures to prevent transmission of the viruses from patients to health care personnel are presented in Table 42-10. Very rarely do health care workers infect patient contacts.

TABLE 42-10	Measures to Prevent Transmission of Hepatitis Viruses from Patients to Health Care Personnel*	
HEPATITIS A	**HEPATITIS B**	**HEPATITIS C**
Always maintain good personal hygiene.	Use infection control precautions.†	Use infection control precautions.†
Wash hands after contact with a patient or removal of gloves.	Wash hands.	Wash hands.
	Reduce contact with blood or blood-containing secretions.	Reduce contact with blood or blood-contaminated secretions.
Use infection control precautions.†	Handle the blood of patients as potentially infective.	Handle the blood of patients as potentially infective.
	Dispose of needles properly.	Dispose of needles properly.
	Administer HBV vaccine to all health care personnel.	Use needleless IV access devices when available.
	Use needleless IV access devices when available.	

*A suggested guideline for general practice to prevent the nurse from contracting viral hepatitis from diagnosed and undiagnosed patients and carriers is for the nurse to wear disposable gloves, goggles, gowns (sometimes) when fecal or blood contamination is likely in handling (1) soiled bedpans, urinals, and catheters and (2) patient's bed linens soiled by body excreta or secretions.
†See Table 12-19.
IV, Intravenous.

TOXIC AND DRUG-INDUCED HEPATITIS

Liver injury and death may occur after the inhalation, parenteral injection, or ingestion of certain chemical substances (see Table 38-6). The two major types of chemical hepatotoxicity are toxic and drug-induced hepatitis. Agents producing toxic hepatitis are generally systemic poisons (e.g., carbon tetrachloride, gold compounds) or are converted in the liver to toxic metabolites (e.g., acetaminophen). Liver necrosis generally occurs within 2 to 3 days of acute exposure to a toxic substance.

Idiosyncratic drug reactions produce drug-induced hepatitis. Such agents as halothane (Fluothane), isoniazid (INH), chlorothiazides (e.g., Diuril), methotrexate, and methyldopa (Aldomet) may produce idiosyncratic reactions because of patient susceptibility (metabolic reactivity) to these agents or immunologically mediated hypersensitivity responses. Liver injury may occur at any time during or shortly after exposure. Some responses occur 2 to 5 weeks after exposure.

Older patients are particularly vulnerable to drug-induced hepatitis. This is due to several factors, including increased use of prescription and over-the-counter drugs, which can lead to drug interactions and potential drug toxicity. Age-related decreases in liver function caused by decreased liver blood flow and enzyme activity result in decreased drug metabolism. In addition, with aging there is a decreased ability of the liver to recover from drug-induced injury.

Toxic and drug-induced hepatitis are similar to viral hepatitis in the pathophysiologic changes in the liver and the clinical manifestations. The usual presenting clinical findings are anorexia, nausea, vomiting, hepatomegaly, splenomegaly, and abnormal liver function studies. Treatment is largely supportive as in acute viral hepatitis. Recovery may be rapid if the hepatotoxin is identified and removed. Liver transplantation may be necessary.

AUTOIMMUNE HEPATITIS

Chronic hepatitis may also occur in a number of patients who have no known risk factors for the development of viral hepatitis. This form of hepatitis is idiopathic; that is, the cause is unknown. However, because many of these patients often have a number of systemic problems, including glomerulonephritis and arthritis, the disease is thought to be autoimmune. The presenting signs and symptoms are variable and similar to viral hepatitis. Laboratory tests (elevation of liver enzymes) reveal liver inflammation without evidence of viral antigens. The majority (70% to 80%) of patients who are diagnosed with autoimmune hepatitis are women. The course of the disease is also variable, with the majority of the patients exhibiting chronic active hepatitis.

Unlike viral hepatitis, autoimmune hepatitis (in which there is evidence of necrosis and cirrhosis) is treated with corticosteroids or other immunosuppressive agents. Daily treatment with methylprednisolone alone or in combination with azathioprine (Imuran) will induce remission in approximately 80% of patients. If these drugs do not work, other immunosuppressive therapies (e.g., cyclosporine, tacrolimus [Prograf], or mycophenolate mofetil [CellCept]) are initiated. Liver transplant is indicated for liver failure.

CIRRHOSIS OF THE LIVER

Cirrhosis is a chronic progressive disease of the liver characterized by extensive degeneration and destruction of the liver parenchymal cells (Fig. 42-4). The liver cells attempt to regenerate, but the regenerative process is disorganized, resulting in ab-

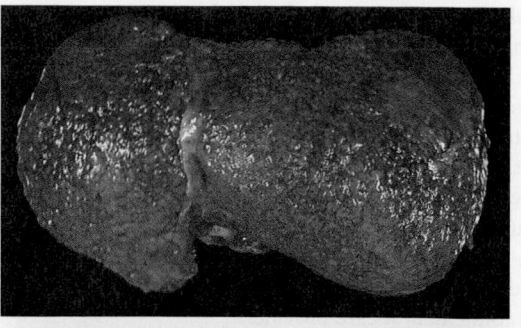

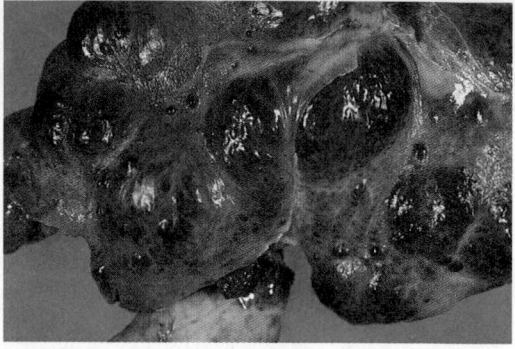

FIG. 42-4 Cirrhosis. **A,** Micronodular cirrhosis. **B,** Macronodular cirrhosis.

normal blood vessel and bile duct relationships from the fibrosis. The overgrowth of new and fibrous connective tissue distorts the liver's normal lobular structure, resulting in lobules of irregular size and shape with impeded vascular flow. Cirrhosis may have an insidious, prolonged course.

Cirrhosis is ranked as the ninth leading cause of death in the United States and the fourth leading cause of death in persons between 35 and 54 years of age. The highest incidence occurs between the ages of 40 and 60, and it is twice as common in men as in women. Excessive alcohol ingestion is the single most common cause of cirrhosis.

Etiology and Pathophysiology

The four types of cirrhosis, in order of incidence, are as follows:
1. *Alcoholic* (previously called *Laënnec's*) *cirrhosis,* also called *portal* or *nutritional cirrhosis,* is usually associated with alcohol abuse. The first change in the liver from excessive alcohol intake is an accumulation of fat in the liver cells. Uncomplicated fatty changes in the liver are potentially reversible if the person stops drinking alcohol. If the alcohol abuse continues, widespread scar formation occurs throughout the liver.
2. *Postnecrotic cirrhosis* is a complication of viral, toxic, or idiopathic (autoimmune) hepatitis. Broad bands of scar tissue form within the liver.
3. *Biliary cirrhosis* is associated with chronic biliary obstruction and infection. There is diffuse fibrosis of the liver with jaundice as the main feature.
4. *Cardiac cirrhosis* results from long-standing, severe right-sided heart failure in patients with cor pulmonale, constrictive pericarditis, and tricuspid insufficiency.

In cirrhosis, cell necrosis occurs, and the destroyed liver cells are replaced by scar tissue. The normal lobular architecture becomes nodular. Eventually, irregular, disorganized regeneration;

poor cellular nutrition; and hypoxia caused by inadequate blood flow and scar tissue result in decreased functioning of the liver.

The specific cause of cirrhosis may not be determined in all patients. It is known that cirrhosis occurs with greatest frequency among alcoholics.[20] There continues to be some controversy as to whether the cause is the alcohol or the malnutrition that frequently coexists with chronic ingestion of alcohol. A common problem in alcoholics is protein malnutrition. There have been cases of nutritional cirrhosis resulting from extreme dieting or malnutrition. It is believed that the combined impact of malnutrition and alcohol is especially damaging to hepatocytes. Alcohol alone has a direct hepatotoxic effect. It is known to produce necrosis of cells and fatty infiltration. Some persons seem to have a predisposition to cirrhosis, regardless of their dietary or alcohol intake.

Approximately 20% of patients with chronic hepatitis C and 10% to 20% of those with chronic hepatitis B will develop cirrhosis. Chronic inflammation and cell necrosis result in fibrosis and, ultimately, cirrhosis. The combination of chronic hepatitis and alcohol ingestion is synergistic in terms of accelerating liver damage.

Clinical Manifestations

Early Manifestations. The onset of cirrhosis is usually insidious. Occasionally there is an abrupt onset of symptoms. GI disturbances are common early symptoms and include anorexia, dyspepsia, flatulence, nausea and vomiting, and change in bowel habits (diarrhea or constipation). These symptoms occur as a result of the liver's altered metabolism of carbohydrates, fats, and proteins. The patient may complain of abdominal pain described as a dull, heavy feeling in the right upper quadrant or epigastrium. The pain may be due to swelling and stretching of the liver capsule, spasm of the biliary ducts, and intermittent vascular spasm. Other early manifestations are fever, lassitude, slight weight loss, and enlargement of the liver and spleen. The liver is palpable in many patients with cirrhosis.

Later Manifestations. Later symptoms may be severe and result from liver failure and portal hypertension. Jaundice, peripheral edema, and ascites develop gradually. Other late symptoms include skin lesions, hematologic disorders, endocrine disturbances, and peripheral neuropathies (Fig. 42-5). In the advanced stages the liver becomes small and nodular.

Jaundice. Jaundice results from the functional derangement of liver cells and compression of bile ducts by connective tissue overgrowth. Jaundice occurs as a result of the decreased ability to conjugate and excrete bilirubin (hepatocellular jaundice). The jaundice may be minimal or severe, depending on the degree of liver damage. If obstruction of the biliary tract occurs, obstructive jaundice may also occur and is usually accompanied by pruritus. The pruritus is due to an accumulation of bile salts underneath the skin.

Skin lesions. Various skin manifestations are commonly seen in cirrhosis. **Spider angiomas** (*telangiectasia* or *spider nevi*) are small, dilated blood vessels with a bright red center point and spi-

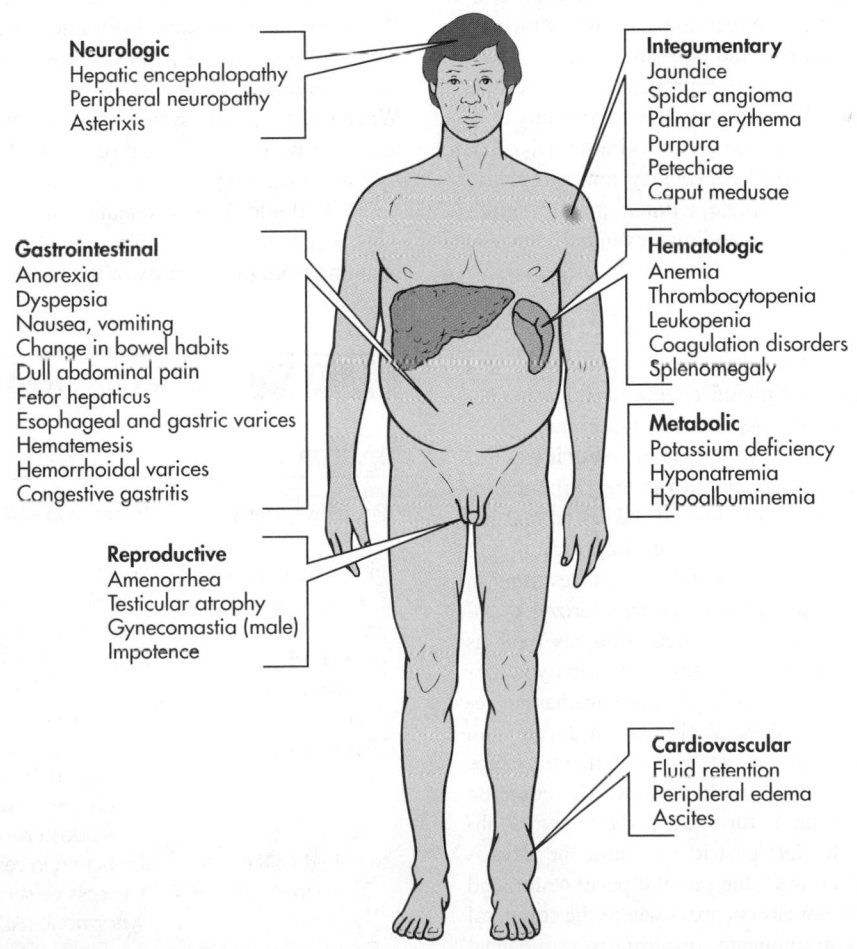

Neurologic
Hepatic encephalopathy
Peripheral neuropathy
Asterixis

Integumentary
Jaundice
Spider angioma
Palmar erythema
Purpura
Petechiae
Caput medusae

Gastrointestinal
Anorexia
Dyspepsia
Nausea, vomiting
Change in bowel habits
Dull abdominal pain
Fetor hepaticus
Esophageal and gastric varices
Hematemesis
Hemorrhoidal varices
Congestive gastritis

Hematologic
Anemia
Thrombocytopenia
Leukopenia
Coagulation disorders
Splenomegaly

Metabolic
Potassium deficiency
Hyponatremia
Hypoalbuminemia

Reproductive
Amenorrhea
Testicular atrophy
Gynecomastia (male)
Impotence

Cardiovascular
Fluid retention
Peripheral edema
Ascites

FIG. 42-5 Systemic clinical manifestations of liver cirrhosis.

derlike branches. They occur on the nose, cheeks, upper trunk, neck, and shoulders. *Palmar erythema* (a red area that blanches with pressure) is located on the palms of the hands. Both of these lesions are attributed to an increase in circulating estrogen as a result of the damaged liver's inability to metabolize steroid hormones.

Hematologic problems. Hematologic problems include thrombocytopenia, leukopenia, anemia, and coagulation disorders. Thrombocytopenia, leukopenia, and anemia are probably caused by the splenomegaly. Splenomegaly results from backup of blood from the portal vein into the spleen. Overactivity of the enlarged spleen results in increased removal of blood cells from circulation. The anemia is also due to inadequate RBC production and survival. Other factors involved in the anemia relate to poor diet, poor absorption of folic acid, and bleeding from varices.

The coagulation problems result from the liver's inability to produce prothrombin and other factors essential for blood clotting. Coagulation problems are manifested by hemorrhagic phenomena or bleeding tendencies, such as epistaxis, purpura, petechiae, easy bruising, gingival bleeding, and heavy menstrual bleeding.

Endocrine disturbances. Several signs and symptoms relating to the metabolism and inactivation of adrenocortical hormones, estrogen, and testosterone occur in cirrhosis. Normally the liver metabolizes these hormones. When the damaged liver is unable to do this, various manifestations occur. In men, gynecomastia, loss of axillary and pubic hair, testicular atrophy, and impotence with loss of libido may occur as a result of estrogen accumulation. In younger women amenorrhea may occur, and in older females there may be vaginal bleeding. The liver fails to metabolize aldosterone adequately, resulting in hyperaldosteronism with subsequent sodium and water retention and potassium loss.

Peripheral neuropathy. Peripheral neuropathy is a common finding in alcoholic cirrhosis. It is probably due to a dietary deficiency of thiamine, folic acid, and cobalamin (vitamin B_{12}). The neuropathy usually results in mixed nervous system symptoms, but sensory symptoms may predominate. Clinical manifestations of cirrhosis of the liver are numerous and may eventually involve the total body (see Fig. 42-5).

Complications

Major complications of cirrhosis are portal hypertension with resultant esophageal varices, peripheral edema and ascites, hepatic encephalopathy (coma), and hepatorenal syndrome.

Portal Hypertension and Esophageal Varices. Because of the structural changes in the liver from the cirrhotic process, there is compression and destruction of the portal and hepatic veins and sinusoids. These changes result in obstruction to the normal flow of blood through the portal system, resulting in portal hypertension. **Portal hypertension** is characterized by increased venous pressure in the portal circulation, as well as splenomegaly, large collateral veins, ascites, systemic hypertension, and esophageal varices. Many pathophysiologic changes result from portal hypertension. Collateral circulation develops in an attempt to reduce this high portal pressure and also to reduce the increased plasma volume and lymphatic flow. The common areas where the collateral channels form are in the lower esophagus (the anastomosis of the left gastric vein and the azygos veins), the anterior abdominal wall, the parietal peritoneum, and the rectum. Varicosities may develop in areas where the collateral and systemic circulations communicate, resulting in esophageal

and gastric varices, *caput medusae* (ring of varices around the umbilicus), and hemorrhoids.

Esophageal varices are a complex of tortuous veins at the lower end of the esophagus, enlarged and swollen as a result of portal hypertension. Esophageal varices are a common complication of cirrhosis, occurring in two thirds to three fourths of patients with cirrhosis. These collateral vessels contain little elastic tissue and are quite fragile. They tolerate the high pressure poorly, and the result is distended veins that bleed easily. Large varices are more likely to bleed.

Bleeding esophageal varices are the most life-threatening complication of cirrhosis. Approximately 30% to 50% of patients with cirrhosis die within 6 weeks of their first esophageal bleed.[21] The varices rupture and bleed in response to ulceration and irritation. Factors producing ulceration and irritation include alcohol ingestion; swallowing of poorly masticated food; ingestion of coarse food; acid regurgitation from the stomach; and increased intraabdominal pressure caused by nausea, vomiting, straining at stool, coughing, sneezing, or lifting heavy objects. The patient may have melena or hematemesis. There may be slow oozing or massive hemorrhage. Massive hemorrhage is a medical emergency.

Peripheral Edema and Ascites. Peripheral edema sometimes precedes ascites, but in some patients its development coincides with or occurs after ascites. Edema results from decreased colloidal oncotic pressure from impaired liver synthesis of albumin and increased portocaval pressure from portal hypertension. Peripheral edema occurs as ankle and presacral edema.

Ascites is the accumulation of serous fluid in the peritoneal or abdominal cavity. It is a common manifestation of cirrhosis. When the blood pressure is elevated in the liver, as occurs in cirrhosis, proteins move from the blood vessels via the larger pores of the sinusoids (capillaries) into the lymph space (Fig. 42-6). When the lymphatic system is unable to carry off the excess proteins and water, they leak through the liver capsule into the peritoneal cavity. The osmotic pressure of the proteins pulls additional fluid into the peritoneal cavity (Table 42-11).

A second mechanism of ascites formation is hypoalbuminemia resulting from the inability of the liver to synthesize albumin. The

TABLE 42-11   Factors Involved in the Development of Ascites

FACTOR	MECHANISM
Portal hypertension	Increase in resistance of blood flow through liver
Increased flow of hepatic lymph	Weeping of protein-rich lymph from surface of cirrhotic liver, intrahepatic blockage of lymph channels
Decreased serum colloidal oncotic pressure	Impairment of liver synthesis of albumin, loss of albumin into peritoneal cavity
Hyperaldosteronism	Increase in aldosterone secretion stimulated by decreased renal blood flow; impairment of liver metabolism of aldosterone
Impaired water excretion	Reduction in renal vascular flow and excessive serum levels of antidiuretic hormone (ADH)

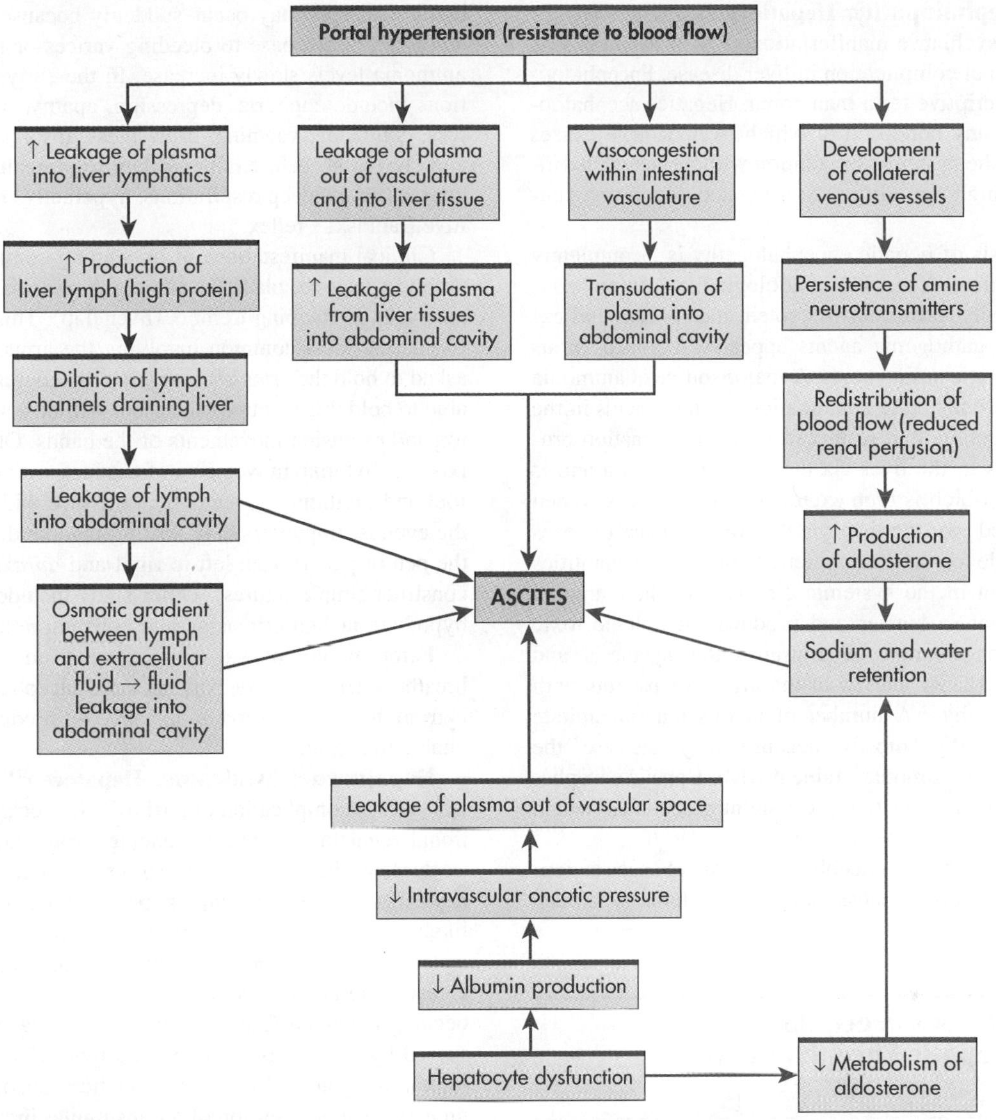

Portal hypertension (resistance to blood flow)

↑ Leakage of plasma into liver lymphatics

Leakage of plasma out of vasculature and into liver tissue

Vasocongestion within intestinal vasculature

Development of collateral venous vessels

↑ Production of liver lymph (high protein)

↑ Leakage of plasma from liver tissues into abdominal cavity

Transudation of plasma into abdominal cavity

Persistence of amine neurotransmitters

Dilation of lymph channels draining liver

Redistribution of blood flow (reduced renal perfusion)

Leakage of lymph into abdominal cavity

ASCITES

↑ Production of aldosterone

Osmotic gradient between lymph and extracellular fluid → fluid leakage into abdominal cavity

Sodium and water retention

Leakage of plasma out of vascular space

↓ Intravascular oncotic pressure

↓ Albumin production

Hepatocyte dysfunction

↓ Metabolism of aldosterone

FIG. 42-6 Mechanisms for development of ascites.

hypoalbuminemia results in decreased colloidal oncotic pressure. A third mechanism of ascites, hyperaldosteronism, results when aldosterone is not metabolized by damaged hepatocytes. The increased level of aldosterone causes increased sodium reabsorption by the renal tubules. This retention of sodium, as well as an increase in antidiuretic hormone, causes additional water retention in these patients. Because of edema formation there is decreased intravascular volume and, subsequently, decreased renal blood flow and glomerular filtration.

Ascites is manifested by abdominal distention with weight gain (Fig. 42-7). If the ascites is severe, the umbilicus may be everted. Abdominal striae with distended abdominal wall veins may be present. The patient has signs of dehydration (e.g., dry tongue and skin, sunken eyeballs, muscle weakness). There is also a decrease in urinary output. Hypokalemia is common and is due to an excessive loss of potassium because of the effects of aldosterone. Low potassium levels can also result from diuretic therapy used to treat the ascites.

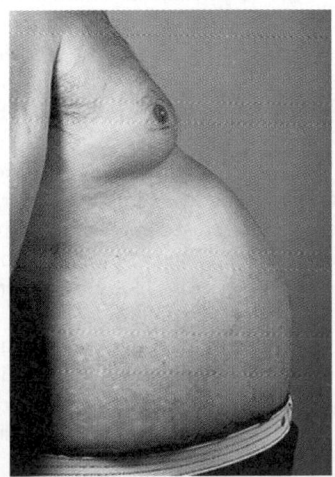

FIG. 42-7 Ascites and gynecomastia associated with cirrhosis of the liver. Photograph was taken after a paracentesis was performed.

Hepatic Encephalopathy. **Hepatic encephalopathy,** or coma, is a neuropsychiatric manifestation of liver damage. It is considered a terminal complication in liver disease. Encephalopathy is a more descriptive term than coma. Hepatic encephalopathy can occur in any condition in which liver damage causes ammonia to enter the systemic circulation without liver detoxification. There is a high mortality rate associated with hepatic encephalopathy.

The pathogenesis of hepatic encephalopathy is incompletely understood at this time. A number of etiologic factors may be involved. It is basically a disorder of protein metabolism and excretion. The main pathogenic agents appear to be nitrogenous ammonia and aromatic amino acids. A major source of ammonia is the bacterial and enzymatic deamination of amino acids in the intestines. The ammonia that results from this deamination process normally goes to the liver via the portal circulation and is converted to urea, which is then excreted by the kidneys. When the blood is shunted past the liver via the collateral anastomoses or the liver is unable to convert ammonia to urea, large quantities of ammonia remain in the systemic circulation. The ammonia crosses the blood-brain barrier and produces neurologic toxic manifestations. For example, neurotransmitter synthesis and degradation are markedly altered in the brains of patients with hepatic encephalopathy.[22] A number of factors may precipitate hepatic encephalopathy, mostly because they increase the amount of circulating ammonia (Table 42-12). Hepatic encephalopathy is also an outcome of surgical shunt procedures, which are used to reduce portal hypertension.[23]

Clinical manifestations of encephalopathy are changes in neurologic and mental responsiveness, ranging from lethargy to deep coma. Changes may occur suddenly because of an increase in ammonia in response to bleeding varices or gradually as blood ammonia levels slowly increase. In the early stages, manifestations include euphoria, depression, apathy, irritability, memory loss, confusion, yawning, drowsiness, insomnia, agitation, slow and slurred speech, emotional lability, impaired judgment, hiccups, slow and deep respirations, hyperactive reflexes, and a positive Babinski's reflex.

Clinical manifestations of impending coma include disorientation as to time, place, or person. A characteristic symptom is **asterixis,** or flapping tremors (liver flap). This may take several forms, the most common involving the arms and hands. When asked to hold the arms and hands stretched out, the patient is unable to hold this position, and there will be a series of rapid flexion and extension movements of the hands. Other signs of asterixis are rhythmic movements of the legs with dorsiflexion of the foot and rhythmic movements in the face with strong closure of the eyelids. Impairments in writing involve difficulty in moving the pen or pencil from left to right and *apraxia* (the inability to construct simple figures). Other signs include hyperventilation, hypothermia, and grimacing and grasping reflexes.

Fetor hepaticus—a musty, sweet odor of the patient's breath—occurs in some patients with encephalopathy. This odor is from the accumulation of digestive by-products that the liver is unable to degrade.

Hepatorenal Syndrome. **Hepatorenal syndrome** (HRS) is a serious complication of cirrhosis. It is characterized by functional renal failure with advancing azotemia, oliguria, and intractable ascites. There is no structural abnormality of the kidneys. The etiology is complex, but the final common pathway is likely to be that portal hypertension along with liver decompensation results in splanchnic and systemic vasodilation and decreased arterial blood volume. As a result, renal vasoconstriction occurs, and renal failure occurs. This renal failure can be reversed by liver transplantation. Current efforts are underway to look at the potential use of splanchnic vasoconstrictors and volume expanders, insertion of a transjugular intrahepatic portosystemic shunt radiologically, and improved forms of dialysis to manage this severe complication. In the patient with cirrhosis, HRS frequently follows diuretic therapy, GI hemorrhage, or paracentesis.[24]

Diagnostic Studies

In cirrhosis there are abnormalities in most of the liver function studies. Enzyme levels, including alkaline phosphatase, aspartate aminotransferase (AST) (serum glutamic-oxaloacetic transaminase [SGOT]), alanine aminotransferase (ALT) (serum glutamate pyruvate transaminase [SGPT]), and γ-glutamyl transferase (GGT), are elevated because of the release of these enzymes from damaged liver cells. Protein metabolism tests show decreased total protein, decreased albumin, and increased globulin levels. The liver does not synthesize γ-globulins but does synthesize albumin. γ-Globulins (antibodies) are produced by B lymphocytes. The globulin level often increases in cirrhosis and indicates increased synthesis or decreased removal. Fat metabolism abnormalities are reflected by decreased cholesterol levels. The prothrombin time is prolonged, and bilirubin metabolism is altered (Table 42-13). Liver biopsy may be performed to identify liver cell changes and alterations in the lobular structure. Differential analysis of ascitic fluid may be helpful in establishing a diagnosis.

FACTOR	MECHANISM
GI hemorrhage	Increase in ammonia in GI tract
Constipation	Increase in ammonia from bacterial action on feces
Hypokalemia	Potassium ions are needed by brain to metabolize ammonia
Hypovolemia	Increase in blood ammonia by causing hepatic hypoxia; impairment of cerebral, hepatic, and renal function because of decreased blood flow
Infection	Increase in catabolism, increase in cerebral sensitivity to toxins
Cerebral depressants (e.g., narcotics)	No detoxification by liver, causing increase in cerebral depression
Metabolic alkalosis	Facilitation of transport of ammonia across blood-brain barrier, increase in renal production of ammonia
Paracentesis	Loss of sodium and potassium ions, decrease in blood volume
Dehydration	Potentiation of ammonia toxicity
Increased metabolism	Increase in workload of liver
Uremia (renal failure)	Retention of nitrogenous metabolites

TABLE 42-12   Factors Precipitating Hepatic Encephalopathy

GI, Gastrointestinal.

TABLE 42-13	Bilirubin Metabolism Abnormalities in Cirrhosis*	
TYPE	**FINDING**	
Serum bilirubin		
Unconjugated	↑	
Conjugated	↑↓	
Urine bilirubin	↑	
Urobilinogen		
Stool	Normal, ↓	
Urine	Normal, ↑	

*Bilirubin metabolism abnormalities occurring with hepatocellular jaundice, the most frequent type of jaundice with cirrhosis.

Collaborative Care

Rest. Although there is no specific therapy for cirrhosis, certain measures can be taken to promote liver cell regeneration and prevent or treat complications (Table 42-14). Rest is significant in reducing metabolic demands of the liver and allowing for recovery of liver cells. At various times during the progress of cirrhosis, the rest may have to take the form of complete bed rest.

Ascites. Management of ascites is focused on sodium restriction, diuretics, and fluid removal. The amount of sodium restriction is based on the degree of ascites. Initially the patient may be encouraged to limit sodium intake to 2 g per day. Patients with severe ascites may need to restrict their sodium intake to 250 to 500 mg per day. Very low sodium intake can result in reduced nutritional intake and subsequent problems associated with malnutrition. The patient is usually not on restricted fluids unless severe ascites develops. There should be accurate assessment and control of fluid and electrolyte balance. Bed rest initially produces diuresis, which increases fluid excretion. Salt-poor albumin may be used to help maintain intravascular volume and adequate urinary output by increasing plasma colloid osmotic pressure.

Diuretic therapy is an important part of management. Often a combination of drugs that work at multiple sites in the nephron is more effective. Spironolactone (Aldactone) is an effective diuretic, even in patients with severe sodium retention. Spironolactone is an antagonist of aldosterone and is potassium sparing. Other potassium-sparing diuretics include amiloride (Midamor) and triamterene (Dyrenium). A high-potency loop diuretic, such as furosemide (Lasix), is frequently used in combination with a potassium-sparing drug. Chlorothiazide (Diuril) or hydrochlorothiazide (HydroDiuril) may also be used, but the thiazide diuretics are not as potent as the loop diuretics.

A **paracentesis** (needle puncture of the abdominal cavity) may be performed to remove ascitic fluid. However, it is reserved for the patient with impaired respiration or abdominal pain caused by severe ascites. It is only a temporary measure because the fluid tends to reaccumulate.

Peritoneovenous shunt. *Peritoneovenous shunt* is a surgical procedure that provides continuous reinfusion of ascitic fluid into the venous system. One type, the LaVeen peritoneovenous shunt, consists of a tube and a one-way valve. The tube runs from the abdominal cavity through the peritoneum, under the subcutaneous tissue, and into the jugular vein or superior vena cava (Fig. 42-8). The valve opens when the pressure in the peritoneal cavity is 3 to 5 cm H_2O higher than that in the superior vena cava. This allows the ascitic fluid to flow into the venous system. The patient's inspiration increases the intraperitoneal pressure, causing the valve to open. This shunting of the ascitic fluid causes an improvement

TABLE 42-14	Collaborative Care — Cirrhosis of the Liver	
Diagnostic	**Ascites**
History and physical examination	Administration of 3000-calorie, high-carbohydrate, protein
Liver function studies	(depends on stage), low fat diet, low sodium for ascites
Liver biopsy (percutaneous needle)	Diuretics
Esophagogastroduodenoscopy	spironolactone (Aldactone)
Angiography (percutaneous transhepatic portography)	amiloride (Midamor)
Liver scan	triamterene (Dyrenium)
Liver ultrasound	furosemide (Lasix)
Serum electrolytes	Paracentesis (if indicated)
Prothrombin time	Peritoneovenous shunt (if indicated)
Serum albumin	**Esophageal Varices**
CBC	β-Adrenergic blockers
Testing of stool for occult blood	vasopressin (Pitressin)
Upper GI barium swallow	Endoscopic sclerotherapy or ligation
Collaborative Therapy	Balloon tamponade
Conservative Therapy	octreotide (Sandostatin)
Administration of B-complex vitamins	Surgical shunting procedure
Rest	Transjugular intrahepatic portosystemic shunt (TIPS)
Avoidance of alcohol and aspirin	**Hepatic Encephalopathy**
	Antibiotics to decrease bacterial flora in GI tract
	lactulose (Cephulac)

CBC, Complete blood count; *GI,* gastrointestinal.

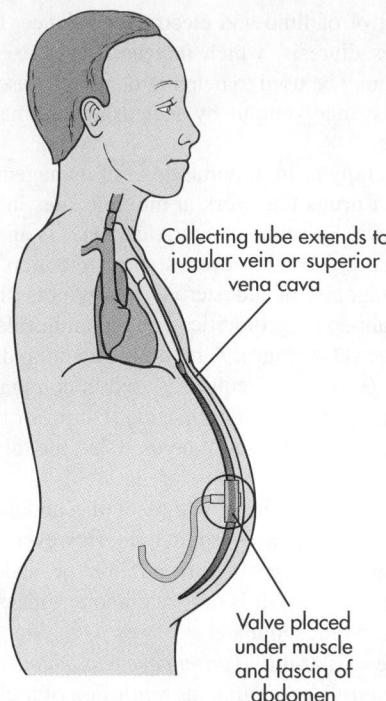

Collecting tube extends to jugular vein or superior vena cava

Valve placed under muscle and fascia of abdomen

FIG. 42-8   Peritoneovenous shunt.

in hemodynamic factors and increases sodium and fluid excretion. Urine output is also increased.

Peritoneovenous shunt is not a first-line therapy for ascites because of the number of complications associated with it, including thrombosis formation at the venous tip of the shunt, infection, fluid overload, disseminated intravascular coagulopathy, variceal hemorrhage, and shunt occlusion. In addition, peritoneovenous shunts do not improve patient survival rates. Transjugular intrahepatic portosystemic shunt (TIPS) (discussed later in this section) is used increasingly to alleviate ascites.

Esophageal Varices. The main therapeutic goal related to esophageal varices is avoidance of bleeding and hemorrhage. Risk factors for esophageal bleeding include variceal size, decreased wall thickness, and degree of liver dysfunction. The patient who has esophageal varices should avoid ingesting alcohol, aspirin, and irritating foods. Upper respiratory infections should be treated promptly, and coughing should be controlled. For patients who have not bled from esophageal varices, prophylactic treatment with nonselective β-blockers (e.g., propranolol [Inderal]) has been shown to reduce the risk of bleeding, as well as bleeding-related deaths.[25]

Management of bleeding esophageal varices includes emergency, therapeutic, and prophylactic interventions. Management, which involves a combination of drug and endoscopic therapy, is more successful than either approach alone.[25] Drug therapy may include octreotide (Sandostatin), vasopressin (VP), nitroglycerin (NTG), and β-adrenergic blockers. Endoscopic therapies include sclerotherapy, ligation of varices, and shunt therapy.

When esophageal variceal bleeding occurs, the first step is to stabilize the patient and manage the airway. IV therapy is initiated and may include administration of blood products. The diagnosis of esophageal variceal bleeding is made by endoscopic examination as soon as possible. At the time of endoscopy, sclerotherapy

or banding of the varices may be performed. The main goal of drug therapy is to stop bleeding so that treatment measures can be done. The initial measures to stop the bleeding include IV administration of VP, which produces vasoconstriction of the splanchnic arterial bed, decreases portal blood flow, and decreases portal hypertension. It has many side effects, including decreased coronary blood flow and heart rate and increased blood pressure. Current drug therapy in some institutions is a combination of VP and NTG. The NTG reduces the detrimental effects of the VP while enhancing its beneficial effect. VP should be avoided or used cautiously in the older adult because of the risk of cardiac ischemia.[26]

Endoscopic sclerotherapy is a treatment method for both acute and chronic bleeding varices in many institutions. The sclerosing agent, introduced via endoscopy, thromboses and obliterates the distended veins.

Another procedure for managing acute variceal bleeding is endoscopic ligation or banding of the varices. A small rubber band (elastic O-ring) is slipped around the base of the varix. Endoscopic variceal ligation can be done using clips instead of the O-rings (endoscopic clipping). Endoscopic ligation is as effective as endoscopic sclerotherapy with fewer complications. A combination of endoscopic sclerotherapy and ligation may be used and seems to be more effective than either treatment alone.

Balloon tamponade may be used in patients with brisk esophageal or gastric variceal hemorrhage that cannot be controlled on initial endoscopy. Balloon tamponade controls the hemorrhage by mechanical compression of the varices. The Minnesota or Sengstaken-Blakemore tube is used for this purpose (Fig. 42-9). These tubes have two balloons: gastric and esophageal. The Sengstaken-Blakemore tube has three lumens: one for the gastric balloon, one for the esophageal balloon, and one for gastric aspiration. The Minnesota tube has an esophageal aspiration port. When inflated, the gastric and esophageal balloons put mechanical compression on the varices. The gastric balloon anchors the tube in position and also applies pressure to any bleeding gastric varices.

Supportive measures during an acute variceal bleed include administration of fresh frozen plasma and packed RBCs, vitamin K (AquaMEPHYTON), and histamine (H_2)–receptor blockers such as cimetidine (Tagamet). Lactulose (Cephulac) and neomycin administration may be started to prevent hepatic encephalopathy from breakdown of blood and the release of ammonia in the intestine.

Long-term management. Long-term management of patients who have had an episode of bleeding includes β-adrenergic blockers, repeated sclerotherapy, endoscopic ligation, and portosystemic shunts. There is a high incidence of recurrent bleeding with a high mortality risk with each bleeding episode, so continued therapy is necessary. Repeated endoscopic sclerotherapy and ligation are commonly used.

Propranolol (Inderal), a β-adrenergic blocker, can be given orally to prevent recurrent GI bleeding. It reduces portal venous pressure. This effect is due to reduced cardiac output and, possibly, constriction of splanchnic vessels. However, because it reduces hepatic blood flow, it can enhance the possibility of hepatic encephalopathy.

Shunting procedures. Surgical and nonsurgical methods of shunting blood away from the esophageal varices are available. Shunting procedures tend to be used more after a second major bleeding episode than an initial bleeding episode. *Transjugular intrahepatic portosystemic shunt (TIPS)* is a nonsurgical procedure

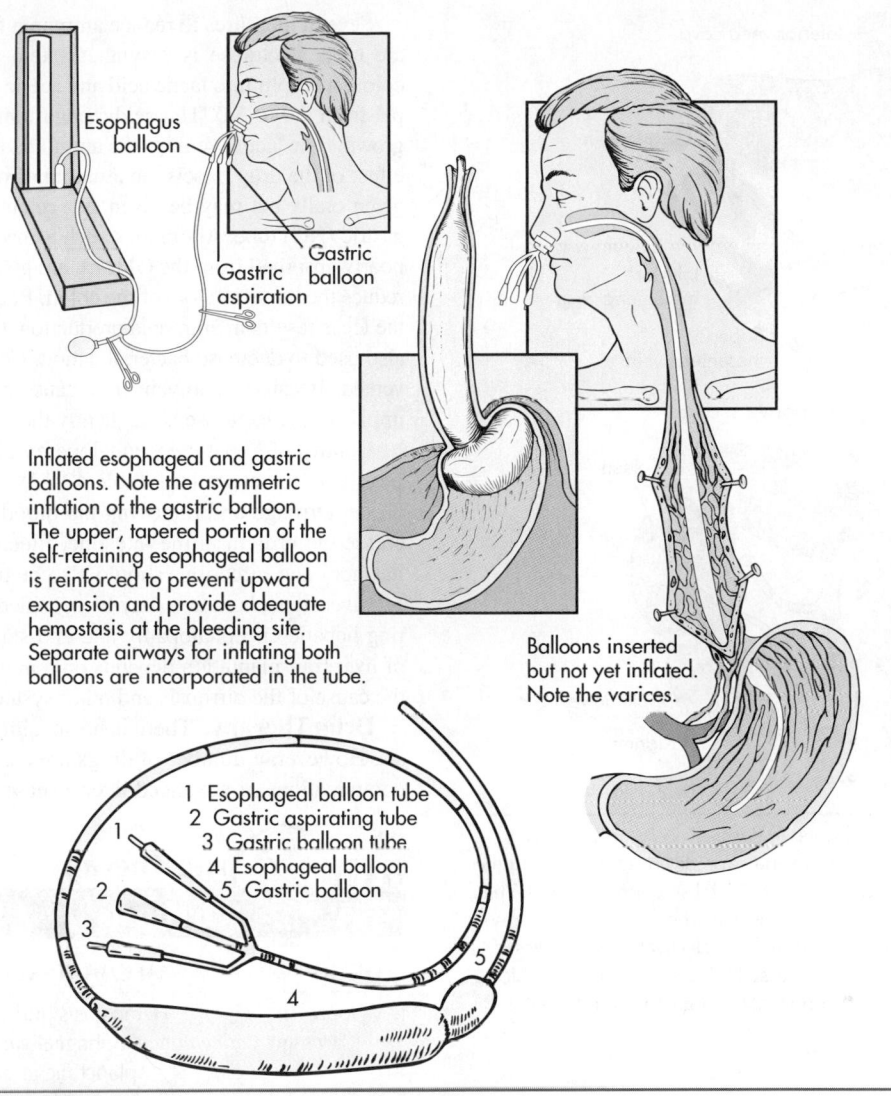

Inflated esophageal and gastric balloons. Note the asymmetric inflation of the gastric balloon. The upper, tapered portion of the self-retaining esophageal balloon is reinforced to prevent upward expansion and provide adequate hemostasis at the bleeding site. Separate airways for inflating both balloons are incorporated in the tube.

Balloons inserted but not yet inflated. Note the varices.

1 Esophageal balloon tube
2 Gastric aspirating tube
3 Gastric balloon tube
4 Esophageal balloon
5 Gastric balloon

FIG. 42-9 Esophageal tamponade accomplished with Sengstaken-Blakemore tube.

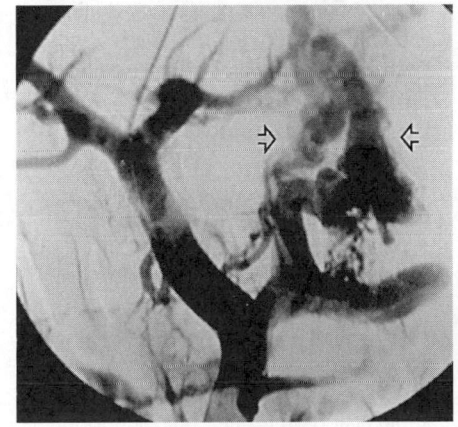

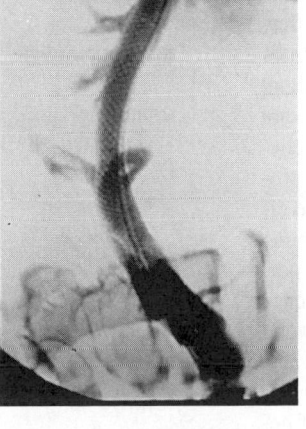

A

B

FIG. 42-10 Total portal diversion after transjugular intrahepatic portosystemic shunt (TIPS). **A,** Portal venogram before TIPS shows filling of large esophageal varices *(arrows).* **B,** After insertion of a TIPS, flow to varices is eliminated. Intrahepatic portal vein flow is now reversed, with the direction of intrahepatic flow toward the TIPS.

in which a tract (shunt) between the systemic and portal venous systems is created to redirect portal blood flow (Fig. 42-10). A catheter is placed in the jugular vein and then threaded through the superior and inferior vena cava to the hepatic vein. The wall of the hepatic vein is punctured and the catheter is directed to the portal vein. Stents are positioned along the passageway, overlapping in the liver tissue and extending into both veins.

This procedure reduces portal venous pressure and decompresses the varices, thus controlling bleeding. This procedure does not interfere with future liver transplantation. Limitations of the

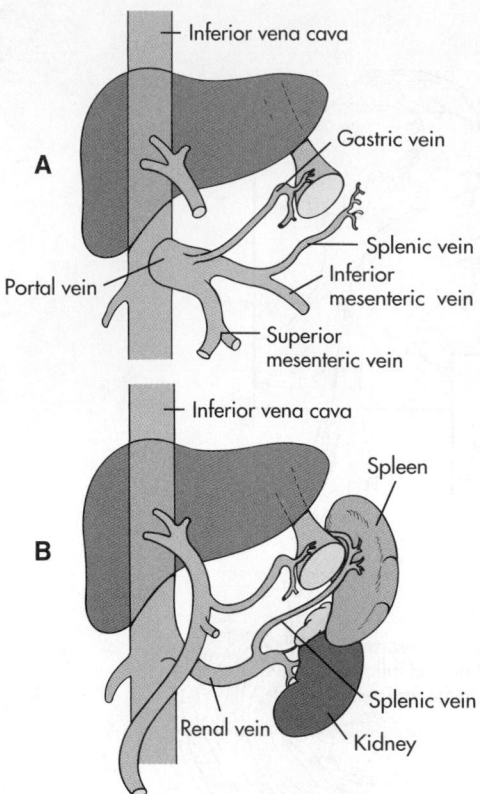

FIG. 42-11 Portosystemic shunts. **A,** Portacaval shunt. The portal vein is anastomosed to the inferior vena cava, diverting blood from the portal vein to the systemic circulation. **B,** Distal splenorenal shunt. The splenic vein is anastomosed to the renal vein. The portal venous flow remains intact while esophageal varices are selectively decompressed. (The short gastric veins are decompressed.) The spleen conducts blood from the high pressure of the esophageal and gastric varices to the low-pressure renal vein.

TIPS procedure include the increased risk of hepatic encephalopathy and stenosis of the stent.

Various surgical shunting procedures may be used to decrease portal hypertension by diverting some of the portal blood flow while at the same time allowing adequate liver perfusion. Currently, the surgical shunts most commonly used are the portacaval shunt and the distal splenorenal shunt (Fig. 42-11). Surgical shunts are more likely to be used in emergency situations. Although a prophylactic portacaval shunt decreases bleeding episodes, it does not prolong life. Patients die of hepatic encephalopathy caused by the diversion of the ammonia past the liver and into the systemic circulation. The distal splenorenal shunt (Warren shunt) leaves portal venous flow intact (see Fig. 42-11), so it has a lower incidence of hepatic encephalopathy. However, with time the flow of blood through the liver decreases. Similar to TIPS, surgical stents are also prone to occlusion, necessitating angiography and stent dilation.

Hepatic Encephalopathy. The goal of management of hepatic encephalopathy is the reduction of ammonia formation. This consists mainly of protein restriction and reduction of ammonia formation in the intestines. The degree of protein restriction is determined by the severity of mental change. The protein restriction may range from 0 to 40 g per day. With improvement of mental function, dietary protein content is increased gradually over days.

Several measures to reduce ammonia formation in the intestines are used. Lactulose is a synthetic keto-analog of lactose. In the colon, it is split into lactic acid and acetic acid, which decreases the pH from 7.0 to 5.0. The acidic environment discourages bacterial growth. The lactulose traps the ammonia in the gut, and the laxative effect of the drug expels the ammonia from the colon. It is usually given orally but may be given as a retention enema or via a nasogastric (NG) tube. Antibiotics such as neomycin sulfate, which are poorly absorbed from the GI tract, are given orally or rectally. They reduce the bacterial flora of the colon. Bacterial action on protein in the feces results in ammonia production. Cathartics and enemas are also used to decrease bacterial action. Constipation should be prevented. Because neomycin may cause renal toxicity and hearing impairments, lactulose is frequently the preferred drug.

Control of hepatic encephalopathy also involves treatment of precipitating causes (see Table 42-12). This involves controlling GI hemorrhage and removing the blood from the GI tract to decrease the protein in the intestine. Electrolyte and acid-base imbalances and infections should also be treated.

Liver transplantation may be considered in patients with recurring hepatic encephalopathy and end-stage liver disease. The use of liver transplantation depends on a number of factors, including the cause of the cirrhosis and other systemic medical problems.[27]

Drug Therapy. There is no specific drug therapy for cirrhosis. However, a number of drugs are used to treat symptoms and complications of advanced liver disease (Table 42-15).

TABLE 42-15	Drug Therapy — Cirrhosis
DRUG	**MECHANISM OF ACTION**
vasopressin (Pitressin)	Hemostasis and control of bleeding in esophageal varices, constriction of splanchnic arterial bed
propranolol (Inderal)	Reduction of portal venous pressure, reduction of esophageal varices bleeding
lactulose (Cephulac)	Acidification of feces in bowel and trapping of ammonia, causing its elimination in feces
neomycin sulfate	Decrease in bacterial flora, decreasing formation of ammonia
cimetidine (Tagamet)	Decrease in gastric acidity
Diuretics	
spironolactone (Aldactone)	Blocking of action of aldosterone, potassium sparing
amiloride (Midamor)	Inhibits reabsorption of sodium and secretion of potassium
chlorothiazide (Diuril)	Thiazide that acts on proximal tubule to decrease reabsorption of sodium and water
furosemide (Lasix)	Rapid action on distal tubule and loop of Henle to prevent reabsorption of sodium and water
triamterene (Dyrenium)	Inhibits reabsorption of sodium and secretion of potassium
magnesium sulfate	Magnesium replacement; hypomagnesemia occurs with liver dysfunction
Vitamin K	Correction of clotting abnormalities

Nutritional Therapy. The diet for the patient with cirrhosis without complications is high in calories (3000 kcal per day) with high carbohydrate content and moderate to low fat levels. The amount of protein varies depending on the degree of liver damage and the potential for encephalopathy. When the patient is symptomatic (e.g., ascites, edema, mental changes), a low-protein diet is indicated. When there is reduced risk of encephalopathy, 1.5 g of protein per kilogram of body weight may be ordered to maintain plasma osmotic balance and promote liver cell regeneration. Foods high in protein include meat, fish, poultry, eggs, and dairy products. High-protein nourishment in the form of eggnogs, milkshakes, or protein supplements may be used, particularly for the patient who is malnourished. Vitamin supplements are usually given.

The patient with hepatic encephalopathy is on a very-low-protein to no-protein diet (Table 42-16). Foods allowed include toast, cereal, rice, tea, fruit juices, and hard candies. Sufficient carbohydrate intake must be provided to maintain an intake of 1500 to 2000 calories to prevent hypoglycemia and catabolism. Glucose polymer (Polycose) is protein free and can be used as a source of

---

TABLE **Nutritional Therapy**
42-16   **Low-Protein Diet for Hepatic Failure***

General Principles
Limit protein to 20 g per day at onset of severe hepatic failure.
Protein must be from protein sources with high biologic value.
Diet must be high in calories.
Fat is limited only to prevent early satiety.
Protein is increased in diet by 10-g increments as tolerated without causing signs and symptoms of hepatic encephalopathy.
Sodium is also usually restricted, as well as fluid when edema and ascites are present.

MEAL	MENU PLAN 1	MENU PLAN 2	MENU PLAN 3
Breakfast			
1 fruit, calorie supplement	½ cup grape juice with 2 tbs Polycose powder[†]	¼ cup cranberry juice with 2 tbs Polycose powder	¼ cup prune juice with 2 tbs Polycose powder
1 low-protein bread	French toast made with low-protein bread, 1 egg, 3 tsp salt-free butter and syrup	Low-protein toast with 3 tsp salt-free butter and 2 tsp jelly	Low-protein toast with 3 tsp salt-free butter
1 egg (protein)		1-egg omelet with 3 tsp salt-free butter	1 egg fried in 3 tsp salt-free butter
Fat, calorie supplement	¼ cup milk	¼ cup milk	¼ cup milk
¼ cup milk (2 g protein)			
Snack			
Calorie supplement	Jelly beans	Hard candy	Sugar mints
Lunch			
2 starch (4 g protein)	¼ cup half and half	¼ cup half and half	¼ cup half and half
1 vegetable (2 g protein)	½ cup Cream of Wheat with 3 tsp salt-free butter	½ cup cornmeal (atole) with 3 tsp salt-free butter	½ cup grits with 3 tsp salt-free butter
1 fruit, calorie supplement	Applesauce with whipped topping or Lipomul[‡]	Small guacamole salad	Cucumbers in sour cream
Fat, calorie supplement	Small tossed salad with 3 tbs oil and vinegar[§]	Gelatin with whipped topping or Lipomul	Peaches with whipped topping or Lipomul
	Peas with 3 tsp salt-free butter	Corn with 3 tsp salt-free butter	Sweet potatoes with brown sugar and 3 tsp salt-free butter
Snack			
Calorie supplement	Low-protein cookies	Low-protein bread cubes with whipped cream and strawberries	Popsicles made with Polycose
Dinner			
1 starch (2 g protein)	½ baked potato	½ cup fried potatoes with 1 tsp melted salt-free butter	½ cup mashed potatoes
1 vegetable (2 g protein)	3 tsp salt-free butter	½ cup zucchini with 3 tsp salt-free butter	½ cup fried okra
1 low-protein bread	Low-protein bread	Low-protein toast with 3 tsp salt-free butter and 2 tsp marmalade	Low-protein toast with 3 tsp salt-free butter and 2 tsp jam
¼ cup milk (2 g protein)	¼ cup sour cream	¼ cup milk	¼ cup milk
Fat, calorie supplement	½ cup green beans with 3 tsp salt-free butter and 2 tsp jelly		
	¼ cup milk		

*The diet plan contains approximately 20 g protein.
†Polycose is a brand-name product made by Ross Laboratories.
‡Lipomul is a fat emulsion made by Upjohn.
§Crisp food should be avoided because of the possibility of esophageal varices.

calories. It can be given orally or via NG tube. A patient with alcoholic cirrhosis frequently has protein-calorie malnutrition. For the patient with protein malnutrition, enteral formulas such as Travasorb Hepatic or Hepatic-Aid may be used. These supplements contain protein from branched-chain amino acids that are metabolized by the muscles. They provide protein but put less burden on the liver. TPN or tube feedings may be required.

The patient with ascites and edema is on a low-sodium diet. The degree of sodium restriction varies depending on the patient's condition. The patient needs instruction regarding the degree of restriction. Table salt is the most common source of sodium. Sodium is also present in baking soda and baking powder. Foods that are high in sodium content include canned soups and vegetables, salted snacks such as potato chips, nuts, smoked meats and fish, crackers, breads, olives, pickles, ketchup, and beer.

Sodium is also present in many over-the-counter drugs (e.g., antacids). However, most antacids are now lower in sodium than previously. Carbonated beverages tend to be high in sodium, and low-sodium and sodium-free carbonated drinks are available. The patient should be advised to read labels. Foods high in protein usually have large amounts of sodium. Alternative protein supplements that are low in sodium may have to be used. The patient and the family need assistance to make the diet more palatable by the use of seasonings such as garlic, parsley, onion, lemon juice, and spices.

NURSING MANAGEMENT
CIRRHOSIS

■ Nursing Assessment

Subjective and objective data that should be obtained from an individual with cirrhosis are presented in Table 42-17.

■ Nursing Diagnoses

Nursing diagnoses for the patient with cirrhosis include, but are not limited to, those presented in NCP 42-2.

■ Planning

The overall goals are that the patient with cirrhosis will (1) have relief of discomfort, (2) have minimal to no complications (ascites, esophageal varices, hepatic encephalopathy), and (3) return to as normal a lifestyle as possible.

■ Nursing Implementation

Health Promotion. The common etiologies of cirrhosis are alcohol, malnutrition, hepatitis, biliary obstruction, and right-sided heart failure. Prevention and early treatment of cirrhosis must focus on the primary cause. Alcoholism must be treated. Patients should be urged to avoid alcohol ingestion, and their efforts should be supported. Adequate nutrition, especially for the alcoholic and other individuals at risk for cirrhosis, is essential to promote liver regeneration. Acute hepatitis must be identified and treated early so that it does not progress to chronic hepatitis. Biliary disease must be treated so that the stones do not cause obstruction and infection. The underlying cause (e.g., chronic lung disease) of right-sided heart failure must be treated so that the heart failure does not lead to cirrhosis.

Acute Intervention. The focus of nursing care for the patient with cirrhosis is on conserving the patient's strength (see NCP 42-2). Rest enables the liver to restore itself. Complete bed rest may not always be necessary. When the patient requires complete bed rest, measures to prevent pneumonia, thromboembolic problems, and pressure ulcers should be taken. The activity and rest schedule may be modified according to

TABLE 42-17	Nursing Assessment Cirrhosis
Subjective Data	**Objective Data**
Important Health Information	**General**
Past health history: Previous viral, toxic, or idiopathic hepatitis; chronic biliary obstruction and infection; severe right-sided heart failure	Fever, cachexia, wasting of extremities
	Integumentary
Medications: Adverse reaction to any medication; use of anticoagulants, aspirin, acetaminophen	Icteric sclera, jaundice, petechiae, ecchymoses, spider angiomas, palmar erythema, alopecia, loss of axillary and pubic hair, peripheral edema
Functional Health Patterns	**Respiratory**
Health perception–health management: Chronic alcoholism; weakness, fatigue	Shallow, rapid respirations, epistaxis
Nutritional-metabolic: Anorexia, weight loss, dyspepsia, nausea and vomiting; gingival bleeding	**Gastrointestinal**
	Abdominal distention, ascites, distended abdominal wall veins, palpable liver and spleen, foul breath; hematemesis; black, tarry stools; hemorrhoids
Elimination: Dark urine, decreased urinary output; light-colored or black stools, flatulence, change in bowel habits; dry, yellow skin, bruising	**Neurologic**
	Altered mentation, asterixis
Cognitive-perceptual: Dull, right upper quadrant or epigastric pain; numbness, tingling of extremities; pruritus	**Reproductive**
Sexuality-reproductive: Impotence, amenorrhea	Gynecomastia and testicular atrophy (men), impotence (men), loss of libido (men and women), amenorrhea or heavy menstrual bleeding (women)
	Possible Findings
	Anemia, thrombocytopenia; leukopenia; ↓ serum albumin, ↓ potassium; abnormal liver function studies; ↑ coagulation studies, ammonia, and bilirubin levels; abnormal abdominal ultrasound and liver scan; positive liver biopsy

NURSING CARE PLAN 42-2

Patient with Cirrhosis

EXPECTED PATIENT OUTCOMES	NURSING INTERVENTIONS and *RATIONALES*
NURSING DIAGNOSIS	**Imbalanced nutrition: less than body requirements** *related to* anorexia, impaired use and storage of nutrients, nausea, and loss of nutrients from vomiting *as manifested by* lack of interest in food, aversion to eating, reported inadequate food intake.
• Adequate intake of nutrients • Maintenance of normal body weight	• Monitor weight *to evaluate nitrogen balance.* • Provide oral care before meals *to remove foul tastes and improve taste of food.* • Administer antiemetics as ordered *to relieve vomiting.* • Provide small, frequent meals with nourishments *to prevent feeling of fullness and maintain nutritional status.* • Determine food preferences and allow these whenever possible *to increase nutritional appeal for patient since a low- or no-protein diet is unpalatable.*
NURSING DIAGNOSIS	**Impaired skin integrity** *related to* edema, ascites, and pruritus *as manifested by* complaints of itching; areas of excoriation caused by scratching; taut, shiny skin over edematous areas; areas of skin breakdown.
• Maintenance of skin integrity • Relief of pruritus	• Restrict sodium intake as ordered *to prevent additional fluid retention.* • Restrict fluids if ordered *to reduce fluid retention.* • Administer prescribed diuretics *to prevent fluid retention and promote diuresis.* • Monitor intake and output *to maintain necessary fluid restrictions and assess renal function.* • Assess location and extent of edema by weighing patient at the same time each day, taking daily measurements of extremities and of abdominal girth (same location each time) *to determine patient's response to treatment.* • Provide meticulous skin care *as edematous tissues are easily traumatized and subject to breakdown.* • Reposition patient at least q2hr *to relieve pressure over bony prominences.* • Elevate edematous areas *to promote venous drainage.* • Have patient use pressure-relieving devices, such as alternating-air pressure or egg crate mattress *to reduce the risk of skin breakdown from prolonged pressure.* • Clip patient's nails short and keep clean *to prevent excoriation caused by pruritus secondary to deposit of bile salts on skin.* • Administer antipruritic medication as ordered *to relieve itching.* • Provide diversions and distractions *to assist patient in coping with the discomfort of itching and edema.*
NURSING DIAGNOSIS	**Ineffective breathing pattern** *related to* pressure on diaphragm and reduced lung volume secondary to ascites *as manifested by* dyspnea, cyanosis, cough, changes in pulse or respiratory rate, depth, or pattern.
• Able to breathe with minimal difficulty • Effective breathing pattern • Absence of cyanosis and other signs and symptoms of hypoxia	• Place patient in semi-Fowler's or Fowler's position; support the arms and chest with pillows *to facilitate breathing by relieving pressure on diaphragm.* • Auscultate chest for crackles *to identify collection of fluid in lungs.* • Assess respiratory rate and rhythm *to identify increasing dyspnea.*
NURSING DIAGNOSIS	**Risk for injury** *related to* diminished sensory perception secondary to peripheral neuropathy.
• No injury caused by decreased sensory perception	• Assess for numbness and tingling of lower extremities, decreased sensation in lower extremities *to determine risk of injury.* • Prevent excess stimulation or trauma to extremities *because patient may not be able to detect harmful stimuli.* • Do not use restrictive bed linens *because they reduce circulation and place pressure on edematous tissue.* • Instruct patient to avoid tight clothing *because it impedes circulation.* • Use care with heat and cold applications *because patient's ability to perceive temperature is impaired.* • Assist with ambulation *to assess patient's ability to safely ambulate and to prevent injury.*

Continued

NURSING CARE PLAN 42-2

Patient with Cirrhosis—cont'd

EXPECTED PATIENT OUTCOMES	NURSING INTERVENTIONS and *RATIONALES*
NURSING DIAGNOSIS	**Risk for infection** *related to* leukopenia and increased susceptibility to environmental pathogens.
▪ No signs or symptoms of infections	▪ Use appropriate infection control measures. ▪ Assess patient for evidence of risk factors, including leukopenia, altered immune response, and altered circulation *to ensure early identification of infection.* ▪ Monitor patient's temperature every 2 to 4 hours *because fever is an indicator of infection.* ▪ Observe for any local and systemic manifestations of infection *to enable early diagnosis and treatment.* ▪ Protect patient from others with infections *to reduce the risk of infection secondary to decreased resistance.* ▪ Monitor white blood cell count *to assess patient's response to treatment.*

COLLABORATIVE PROBLEMS

NURSING GOALS	NURSING INTERVENTIONS and *RATIONALES*
POTENTIAL COMPLICATION	**Hepatic encephalopathy** *related to* increased formation of ammonia and aromatic amino acids.
▪ Monitor for signs of hepatic encephalopathy ▪ Report deviation from acceptable parameters ▪ Carry out appropriate medical and nursing interventions	▪ Monitor for encephalopathy by assessing patient's general behavior, orientation to time and place, speech, blood pH, and ammonia levels *because liver is unable to convert accumulating ammonia to urea for renal excretion.* ▪ Encourage fluids (if not restricted) and give laxatives and enemas as ordered *to decrease production of ammonia.* ▪ Provide low-protein or no-protein diet as ordered *because ammonia (a breakdown product of protein) is responsible for mental changes.*
POTENTIAL COMPLICATION	**Hemorrhage** *related to* bleeding tendency secondary to altered clotting factors and rupture of esophageal or gastric varices.
▪ Monitor for signs of hemorrhage ▪ Initiate appropriate medical and nursing interventions	▪ Limit physical activity *because exercise produces ammonia as a by-product of metabolism.* ▪ Monitor for hemorrhage by assessing for epistaxis, purpura, petechiae, easy bruising, gingival bleeding, heavy menstrual bleeding, hematuria, melena *because liver disease results in impaired synthesis of clotting factors.* ▪ Provide gentle nursing care *to minimize the risk of tissue trauma.* ▪ Observe for bleeding from body orifices, urine, and stool *to detect bleeding early and allow prompt intervention.* ▪ Use smallest-gauge needle possible when giving injection and apply gentle but prolonged pressure after injection *to minimize risk of bleeding into tissue.* ▪ Advise use of soft-bristle toothbrush and avoidance of irritating food *to reduce trauma because mucous membranes have increased risk of injury as a result of high vascularity.* ▪ Teach patient to avoid straining at stool, vigorous blowing of nose, and coughing *to reduce risk of hemorrhage from these areas.* ▪ Observe for bruising on the forearms, axillae, and skin. ▪ Monitor laboratory results (hematocrit, hemoglobin, and prothrombin time) *as indicators of anemia, active bleeding, or impending complications.*

signs of clinical improvement (e.g., decreasing jaundice, improvement in liver function studies). Major concerns of the nurse in determining appropriate nursing care measures to meet the need for rest involve regulation of the physical, emotional, and social climate.

Anorexia, nausea and vomiting, pressure from ascites, and poor eating habits all create problems in maintaining an adequate intake of nutrients. The nursing measures relating to nutrition for patients with hepatitis also apply here. Oral hygiene before meals may improve the patient's taste sensation. Between-meal nourishments should be available so that they can be provided at times when the patient can best tolerate them. Food preferences should be provided whenever possible. The reason for any dietary restrictions should be explained to the patient and family.

Nursing assessment and care should include the patient's physiologic response to cirrhosis. Is jaundice present? Where is it observed—sclera, skin, hard palate? What is the progression of jaundice? If the jaundice is accompanied by pruritus, measures to relieve itching should be carried out. Cholestyramine (Questran) may be ordered to help relieve the pruritus. The color of the urine and stools should be noted. With jaundice the urine is often dark brown and foamy when shaken. The stool is gray or tan.

Edema and ascites are frequent manifestations of cirrhosis and require nursing assessments and interventions. Accurate calculation and recordings of intake and output, daily weights, and measurements of extremities and abdominal girth help in the ongoing assessment of the location and extent of the edema. If the patient can assume a kneeling position when abdominal girth measurement is taken, the abdominal fluid will go to the most dependent part of the abdomen. This gives the best measurement of abdominal girth. For many patients, girth must be measured in the standing or lying position. Where the measurements are taken should be recorded and should be a part of the nursing care plan.

When a paracentesis is done, the nurse must have the patient void immediately before the procedure to prevent puncture of the bladder. The patient should sit on the side of the bed or be placed in high-Fowler's position. Following the procedure the nurse should monitor for hypovolemia and electrolyte imbalances and check the dressing for bleeding and leakage.

Dyspnea is a frequent problem for the patient with ascites. A semi-Fowler's or Fowler's position allows for maximal respiratory efficiency. Pillows can be used to support the arms and chest and may increase the patient's comfort and ability to breathe.

Meticulous skin care is essential because the edematous tissues are subject to breakdown. An alternating–air pressure mattress or other special mattress should be used. A turning schedule (minimum of every 2 hours) must be adhered to rigidly. The abdomen may be supported with pillows. If the abdomen is taut, cleansing must be done very gently. This patient tends to move very little because of the abdominal discomfort and dyspnea. Therefore range-of-motion exercises are helpful, and measures such as coughing and deep breathing to prevent respiratory problems should be implemented. The lower extremities may be elevated. If scrotal edema is present, a scrotal support provides some comfort.

When the patient is taking diuretics, the serum levels of sodium, potassium, chloride, and bicarbonate should be monitored. The patient should be observed for signs of fluid and electrolyte imbalance, especially hypokalemia. Hypokalemia may be manifested by cardiac arrhythmias, hypotension, tachycardia, and generalized muscle weakness. Water excess is manifested by muscle cramping, weakness, lethargy, and confusion.

Observations and nursing care in relation to hematologic disorders (bleeding tendencies, anemia, increased susceptibility to infection) are the same as for the patient with advanced liver disease (see NCP 42-2).

The nurse must assess the patient's response to altered body image resulting from jaundice, spider angiomas, palmar erythema, ascites, and gynecomastia. The patient may experience a great deal of anxiety regarding these changes. The nurse should explain these phenomena and should be a supportive listener. Nursing care with concern and warmth regardless of physical changes helps the patient maintain self-esteem.

Bleeding esophageal varices. If the patient has esophageal varices in addition to cirrhosis, the nurse must observe for any signs of bleeding from the varices, such as hematemesis and melena. If hematemesis occurs, the nurse should assess the patient for hemorrhage, call the physician, and be ready to assist with whatever treatment is used to control the bleeding. The patient will be admitted to the intensive care unit (ICU). The patient's airway must be maintained. To stop the bleeding the physician may perform sclerotherapy or ligation procedures.

Balloon tamponade is not used as first-line therapy for bleeding esophageal varices. However, it is used in those patients who have refractory bleeding that is unresponsive to sclerotherapy or ligation. When balloon tamponade is used, the initial nursing task related to insertion of the tube is to explain the use of the tube and how it will be inserted. The balloons should be checked for patency. It is usually the physician's responsibility to insert the tube. It may be inserted via the nose or the mouth (see Fig. 42-9). Then the gastric balloon is inflated with approximately 250 ml of air, and the tube is retracted until resistance (gastroesophageal junction) is felt. The tube is secured by placement of a piece of sponge or foam rubber at the nostrils (nasal cuff). For continued bleeding the esophageal balloon is then inflated. A sphygmomanometer is used to measure and maintain the desired pressure at 20 to 40 mm Hg. The position of the balloons is verified by x-ray.

Sometimes saline lavage is used to remove blood from the stomach. (Nursing care of upper GI bleeding is discussed in Chapter 40.) This helps prevent the blood from degrading to ammonia, leading to encephalopathy. The esophageal balloon should be deflated every 8 to 12 hours to avoid necrosis. Each lumen must be labeled to avoid confusion. The NG lumen may be connected to suction to remove blood and keep the stomach empty to reduce the risk of aspiration. The most common complication of balloon tamponade therapy is aspiration pneumonia.

Nursing care includes monitoring for complications of rupture or erosion of the esophagus, regurgitation and aspiration of gastric contents, and occlusion of the airway by the balloon. If the gastric balloon breaks or is deflated, the esophageal balloon will slip upward, obstructing the airway and causing asphyxiation. If this happens, the nurse must cut the tube or deflate the esophageal balloon. Scissors should be kept at the bedside. Regurgitation can be minimized by oral and pharyngeal suctioning and by keeping the patient in a semi-Fowler's position.

The patient is unable to swallow saliva because of the inflated esophageal balloon occluding the esophagus. With the Minnesota tube, which has an esophageal aspiration lumen, this problem can be alleviated. The nurse should encourage the patient to expectorate and should provide an emesis basin and tissues. Frequent oral and nasal care provides relief from the taste of blood and irritation from mouth breathing.

Hepatic encephalopathy. The focus of nursing care of the patient with hepatic encephalopathy is on sustaining life and assisting with measures to reduce the formation of ammonia. The nurse should assess (1) the patient's level of responsiveness (e.g., reflexes, pupillary reactions, orientation), (2) sensory and motor abnormalities (e.g., hyperreflexia, asterixis, motor coordination), (3) fluid and electrolyte imbalances, (4) acid-base imbalances, and (5) the effect of treatment measures.

The neurologic status, including an exact description of the patient's behavior, should be assessed and recorded at least every 2 hours. Care of the patient with neurologic problems should be based on the severity of the encephalopathy.

Nursing measures to prevent constipation should be instituted to decrease ammonia production. Drugs, laxatives, and enemas should be given as ordered. Encouragement of fluids may also help if not contraindicated. The patient should not strain at stool because this may cause bleeding of hemorrhoidal varices. Any GI bleeding may worsen the coma. The patient who is taking lactulose should be assessed for diarrhea and excessive fluid and electrolyte losses. Some physicians have diarrhea as a goal because diarrhea increases ammonia expulsion from the colon. Because lactulose can cause severe purging, the nurse should observe the patient for excessive fluid and electrolyte losses.

Factors that are known to precipitate coma should be controlled as much as possible. Because exercise produces ammonia as a by-product of metabolism, the physical activity of the patient must be limited. Hypokalemia should be controlled.

The patient is on either a very low-protein or a no-protein diet, neither of which is very palatable. Vegetable protein is better tolerated than meat protein. Foods and fluids high in carbohydrate should be given because the liver is not synthesizing and storing glucose. The patient may require tube feedings if an adequate diet cannot be ingested.

Ambulatory and Home Care. The patient with cirrhosis may be faced with a prolonged course and the possibility of serious, life-threatening problems and complications. The nurse should be a resource person in helping the patient achieve the highest level of wellness. The patient and the family need to understand the importance of continuous health care and medical supervision. They should be taught symptoms of complications and when to seek medical attention. Patients with cirrhosis should avoid activities that place them at risk for contracting viral hepatitis.

Measures to achieve and maintain a remission should be encouraged. These include proper diet, rest, avoidance of potentially hepatotoxic over-the-counter drugs such as acetaminophen, and abstinence from alcohol. Abstinence from alcohol is important and results in improvement in most patients. The nurse must realize the difficulty this poses for some patients. The nurse's own attitude regarding the patient whose cirrhosis is attributed to alcohol abuse should be explored. Care should be given without rejection and moralizing. The alcoholic patient should be treated with a caring attitude (see Chapter 11).

Cirrhosis is a chronic disease. The patient is affected not only physically but also psychologically, socially, and economically. Major adjustments may be required to make lifestyle changes, especially if alcohol abuse is the primary etiologic factor. The nurse should provide information regarding community support programs, such as Alcoholics Anonymous, for help with alcohol abuse.

Adequate explanations, along with written instructions, related to fluid or dietary restrictions should be given to the patient and the family (Table 42-18). Other health teaching should include instruction about adequate rest periods, how to detect early signs of complications, skin care, drug therapy precautions, observation for bleeding, and protection from infection. Counseling information regarding sexual problems may be needed. Referral to a community or home health nurse may be helpful to ensure adequate patient compliance with prescribed therapy. The emphasis of home care for the patient with cirrhosis should be on helping the patient maintain the highest level of wellness possible and initiate and maintain necessary lifestyle changes.

■ Evaluation

Expected outcomes for the patient with cirrhosis are addressed in NCP 42-2.

ETHICAL DILEMMAS
Rationing

Situation
A 43-year-old patient with cirrhosis of the liver is frequently admitted to the hospital. She has been told that her continued drinking will inevitably lead to her death. Now she has been admitted for GI bleeding and needs blood transfusions. She has a rare blood type, and it is frequently difficult to get compatible blood. Should the nurse call an ethics consultation?

Important Points for Consideration
- Rationing or the distribution of scarce resources is a difficult ethical problem. The needs of an individual patient or group of patients are weighed against the needs of many patients who may have a greater chance of recovery and the availability of the needed resources.
- Because alcoholism has a behavioral component, health care providers sometimes view these patients as noncompliant and not deserving of aggressive treatment.
- Whether blood transfusions at this point will alter the course of the patient's disease, extend her life, or improve the quality of her life are important questions to determine if this treatment is medically futile.
- Triage is the basis for rationing decisions. The amount of blood supply available, the number of people needing the blood, and the degree to which their condition can be effectively treated by blood transfusions should provide the justification for treatment decisions.
- An ethics consultation could assist in determining who would receive the greatest benefit from the scarce resource, rather than a health care provider deciding for a particular patient.

Critical Thinking Questions
1. What are your feelings about patients with disorders such as substance abuse, which have a behavioral component? Are these patients deserving of aggressive treatment?
2. How would you proceed to make a decision in this case? Would you request an ethics committee consult?

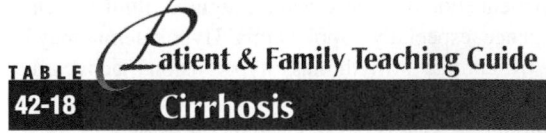

TABLE	Patient & Family Teaching Guide
42-18	**Cirrhosis**

1. Explain to the patient and family the importance of continuous health care so that they understand that cirrhosis is a chronic illness.
2. Teach the patient and family symptoms of complications and when to seek medical attention to enable prompt treatment of complications.
3. Teach proper diet because a low-protein, high-carbohydrate diet is usually indicated and can be difficult to follow.
4. Teach the patient to avoid potentially hepatotoxic over-the-counter drugs because the diseased liver is unable to metabolize these drugs.
5. Encourage abstinence from alcohol because continued use of alcohol will increase the risk of liver complications.
6. Instruct the patient to avoid aspirin and control coughing to prevent hemorrhage when esophageal or gastric varices are present.
7. Teach the patient to avoid spicy and rough foods and activities that increase portal pressure, such as straining at stool, coughing, sneezing, and retching and vomiting because hemorrhage is a danger as a result of the inability of the liver to produce clotting factors.

FULMINANT HEPATIC FAILURE

Fulminant hepatic failure is a clinical syndrome characterized by severe impairment of liver function associated with hepatic encephalopathy. In fulminant hepatic failure the encephalopathy occurs within 8 weeks of the first symptoms. The most common cause is viral hepatitis, in particular HBV, but it may also occur with HAV and less frequently with HCV.

Drugs are the second most common cause of fulminant hepatic failure. Acetaminophen in combination with alcohol is a common offending agent. Persons who abuse alcohol are particularly susceptible to detrimental effects of acetaminophen on the liver. Other drugs include isoniazid (INH), halothane (Fluothane), sulfa-containing drugs, and nonsteroidal antiinflammatory drugs.

The patient has jaundice and signs of encephalopathy. Laboratory tests reveal elevated liver function tests, prolonged prothrombin time, and increased bilirubin. Depending on the degree of liver failure, treatment may involve liver transplantation.

LIVER CANCER

Primary liver cancer (originating in the liver) is rare. In 2002 in the United States there were 16,600 new cases of liver cancer and 14,100 deaths related to liver cancer.[28] Of these, the majority occur in males. Hepatocellular carcinoma is the most common primary liver cancer. The remaining primary tumors are cholangiomas or bile duct carcinomas. A high percentage of patients with primary cell carcinoma have cirrhosis of the liver. Hepatocellular carcinoma is often associated with chronic liver diseases including chronic hepatitis B or C. Metastatic carcinoma of the liver is more common than primary carcinoma. The liver is a common site of metastatic growth because of its high rate of blood flow and extensive capillary network. Cancer cells in other parts of the body are commonly carried to the liver via the portal circulation.

The malignant cells cause the liver to be enlarged and misshapen. Hemorrhage and necrosis in the liver are common (Fig. 42-12). Lesions may be singular or numerous and nodular or diffusely spread over the entire liver. Some tumors infiltrate into other organs such as the gallbladder or into the peritoneum or diaphragm. Primary liver tumors commonly metastasize to the lung.

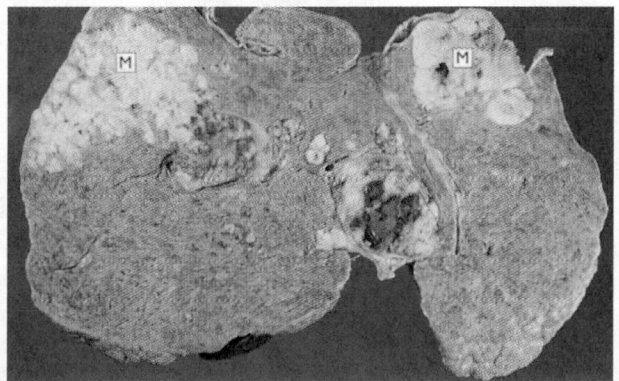

FIG. 42-12 Hepatocellular carcinoma. Macroscopically, hepatocellular carcinoma may be single or multifocal. They usually develop in a liver already affected by cirrhosis. Tumor appears as an abnormal mass (M) within the liver.

Clinical Manifestations and Diagnostic Studies

It is difficult to diagnose liver cancer. It is particularly difficult to differentiate it from cirrhosis in its early stages because many of the clinical manifestations (e.g., hepatomegaly, weight loss, peripheral edema, ascites, portal hypertension) are similar. Other common manifestations include dull abdominal pain in the epigastric or right upper quadrant region, jaundice, anorexia, nausea and vomiting, and extreme weakness. Patients frequently have pulmonary emboli. Tests used to assist in the diagnosis are a liver scan, computed tomography (CT), magnetic resonance imaging, hepatic arteriography, endoscopic retrograde cholangiopancreatography (ERCP), and a liver biopsy. The test for α-fetoprotein (AFP) may be positive in hepatocellular carcinoma. AFP is elevated in approximately 70% of patients with hepatocellular carcinoma and helps to distinguish primary cancer from metastatic cancer. (AFP is discussed in Chapter 15.)

NURSING *and* COLLABORATIVE MANAGEMENT
LIVER CANCER

Treatment of liver cancer is largely palliative. Overall the management is similar to liver cirrhosis. Surgical excision (lobectomy) is sometimes performed if the tumor is localized to one portion of the liver. Only 30% to 40% of patients have surgically resectable disease. Usually surgery is not feasible because the cancer is too far advanced when it is detected. Surgical excision of the entire tumor offers the best chance for cure of liver cancer. Other treatment options are ablation with radiofrequency, cryosurgery, or alcohol injection, and chemotherapy and/or chemoembolization.

In *radiofrequency* treatment electrical energy is used to create heat in a specific location for a limited amount of time. The end result is destruction of liver tumors. This procedure can be done percutaneously, laparoscopically, or through an open incision. This therapy, while not ideal for all patients, can be used both for tumors that are considered resectable as well as for palliative purposes. Complications are not common but can include infection, bleeding, arrhythmias, and skin burn.

Cryosurgery is another procedure used for patients whose tumors are considered unresectable but who do not have signs of metastasis. Cryosurgery involves an open surgical approach. Cryoprobes are placed directly into the liver, and liquid nitrogen/argon gas flows through the probe and freezes the liver tissue. The tissue in the area surrounding the probe is destroyed. Cryosurgery is not used for metastatic liver disease.

Percutaneous ethanol injection (PEI) is used to treat unresectable liver cancer that has not metastasized outside the liver. This is an outpatient procedure in which a catheter is guided to the liver using ultrasound. Ethanol is injected for six to eight treatments over a 3- to 4-week period, with two to three injections each week. The most common side effect is transient pain following the procedure. Other, less frequent adverse events include intraperitoneal hemorrhage, hepatic insufficiency, bile duct necrosis, hepatic infarction, and transient hypotension.

Chemotherapy is used for patients with hepatocellular cancer who are not likely to benefit from other procedures (e.g., surgery, transplantation, ablation). A variety of chemotherapeutic agents (e.g., 5-fluorouracil [5-FU] and leucovorin) administered either systemically or regionally has been used to treat liver cancer.

Other chemotherapeutic drugs include raltitrexed (Tomudex) and experimental drugs. However, the overall response has been poor. Regional chemotherapy includes portal vein or hepatic artery perfusion with 5-FU or other chemotherapeutic agents. Chemotherapy delivered directly to the liver is referred to as hepatic arterial infusion therapy. With the patient under general anesthesia, a catheter is placed in the hepatic artery and a pump is implanted percutaneously for administration of chemotherapy. Systemic chemotherapy may also be given along with hepatic administration.

Chemoembolization is a minimally invasive procedure frequently performed in the interventional radiology department. In this procedure a catheter is placed in the arteries to the tumor and an embolic agent is administered, often mixed with a chemotherapeutic agent(s). The embolic agent reduces the blood supply, thus allowing greater exposure of liver cells to the chemotherapy drugs.

Liver transplantation is an option for patients with liver cancer that has not spread beyond the liver. However, there is a limited availability of organs.

Nursing intervention for the patient with liver cancer focuses on keeping the patient as comfortable as possible. Because this patient manifests the same problems as any patient with advanced liver disease, the nursing interventions discussed for cirrhosis of the liver apply. (See Chapter 15 for care of the patient with cancer.)

The prognosis for patients with liver cancer is poor. The cancer grows rapidly, and death may occur within 4 to 7 months as a result of hepatic encephalopathy or massive blood loss from GI bleeding.

LIVER TRANSPLANTATION

The first human liver transplant was performed in 1963 at the University of Colorado by Thomas Starzl. Liver transplantation has become a practical therapeutic option for many people with irreversible liver disease. It improves the quality of life for end-stage liver patients and is an accepted treatment modality for these patients. Indications for liver transplantation include congenital biliary abnormalities, inborn errors of metabolism, hepatic malignancy (confined to the liver), sclerosing cholangitis, and chronic end-stage liver disease. Liver disease related to chronic viral hepatitis is the leading indication for liver transplantation.[27] Liver transplants are not recommended for the patient with widespread malignant disease.

The major postoperative complications are rejection and infection. Rejection is not as major a problem as it is in kidney transplants. The liver seems to be less susceptible to rejection than the kidney. Cyclosporine is an effective immunosuppressant drug. The use of cyclosporine has been a major factor in the success rates of liver transplantation. The mechanism of action and side effects of cyclosporine are discussed in Chapter 13 and Table 13-17. It does not cause bone marrow suppression and does not impede wound healing. Other immunosuppressants used include azathioprine (Imuran), corticosteroids, tacrolimus (Prograf), and the monoclonal antibody OKT3 (see Table 13-17). Newer agents including the interleukin-2 receptor antagonists basiliximab (Simulect) and daclizumab (Zenapax) are being used in combination with other immunosuppressive agents to reduce rejection. Other factors in the improved success rate are advances in surgical techniques, better selection of potential recipients, and improved management of the underlying liver disease before surgery.

Patients who have liver disease secondary to viral hepatitis often experience reinfection of the transplanted liver with hepatitis B or C. HCV recurrence as evidence by histologic damage is almost universal after transplant. Approximately 20% to 30% of patients will develop cirrhosis of the transplanted liver by the fifth year posttransplant.[27] Antiviral therapy for HCV initiated posttransplant even before the development of histologic evidence of recurrence has failed to alter this recurrence pattern.[27]

The patient who has had a liver transplant requires competent and highly skilled nursing care, either in an ICU or in some other specialized unit. Postoperative nursing care includes assessing neurologic status; monitoring for signs of hemorrhage; preventing pulmonary complications; monitoring drainage, electrolyte levels, and urinary output; and monitoring for signs and symptoms of infection and rejection. Common respiratory problems are pneumonia, atelectasis, and pleural effusions. The nurse should have the patient use measures such as coughing, deep breathing, incentive spirometry, and repositioning to prevent these complications. Drainage from the Jackson-Pratt drain, NG tube, and T tube should be measured, and the color and consistency of drainage noted. A critical aspect of nursing care following liver transplantation is monitoring for infection. The first 2 months after the surgery are critical. Infection can be viral, fungal, or bacterial. Fever may be the only sign of infection. Emotional support and teaching the patient and family are essential.

NURSING RESEARCH

Physical Activity and Liver Transplant

Citation Painter P et al: Physical activity and health-related quality of life in liver transplant recipients, *Liver Transpl* 7:213, 2001.

Purpose This study was conducted to determine the relationship between physical activity and health-related quality of life in patients following a liver transplant.

Methods The Medical Outcomes Study Short Form-36 (SF-36) Health Status Questionnaire was sent to patients who were 5 years or more posttransplantation. Data obtained related to coexisting medical problems and participation in regular physical activity. Regression analyses were performed.

Results and Conclusions Patients who participated in regular physical activity had significantly higher scores on all physical scales and the physical component scale. The regression model, which included age, sex, time posttransplantation, retransplantation, recurrence of hepatitis C, number of comorbid conditions, and physical activity participation, showed that the number of comorbid conditions and participation in physical activity were significant independent contributors to the physical functioning scale. This study indicates that physical activity is related to quality of life following liver transplant.

Implications for Nursing Practice There are many positive benefits of physical activity for patients following a liver transplant. These patients should be encouraged to engage in physical activity for the potential benefits related to their cardiovascular health and to enhance their overall physical functioning.

Disorders of the Pancreas

ACUTE PANCREATITIS

Acute pancreatitis is an acute inflammatory process of the pancreas. The degree of inflammation varies from mild edema to severe hemorrhagic necrosis. Acute pancreatitis is most common in middle-aged men and women, but it affects more men than women. The severity of the disease varies according to the extent of pancreatic destruction. Some patients recover completely, others have recurring attacks, and chronic pancreatitis develops in others. Acute pancreatitis can be life threatening.

Etiology and Pathophysiology

Many factors can cause injury to the pancreas. The primary etiologic factors are biliary tract disease and alcoholism. In the United States the most common cause is alcoholism, followed by gallbladder disease. Other, less common causes of acute pancreatitis include trauma (postsurgical, abdominal), viral infections (mumps, coxsackievirus B), penetrating duodenal ulcer, cysts, abscesses, cystic fibrosis, Kaposi's sarcoma, certain drugs (corticosteroids, thiazide diuretics, oral contraceptives, sulfonamides, nonsteroidal antiinflammatory drugs), and metabolic disorders (hyperparathyroidism, hyperlipidemia, renal failure). Pancreatitis may occur after surgical procedures on the pancreas, stomach, duodenum, or biliary tract. Pancreatitis can also occur after ERCP. In some cases the cause is not known (idiopathic).

The most common pathogenic mechanism is believed to be autodigestion of the pancreas (Fig. 42-13). The etiologic factors cause injury to pancreatic cells or activation of the pancreatic enzymes in the pancreas rather than in the intestine. It is not clear how the activation of pancreatic enzymes occurs. One possible cause is believed to be the reflux of bile acids into the pancreatic ducts through an open or distended sphincter of Oddi. This reflux may occur because of gallstones impacted at the ampulla of Vater, atony and edema of the sphincter, or obstruction of pancreatic ducts and pancreatic ischemia.

Trypsinogen is an inactive proteolytic enzyme produced by the pancreas. Normally it is released into the small intestine via the pancreatic duct. In the intestine it is activated to trypsin by enterokinase. Normally, trypsin inhibitors in the pancreas and plasma bind and inactivate any trypsin that is inadvertently produced. In pancreatitis, activated trypsin is present in the pancreas.

This enzyme can digest the pancreas and can activate other proteolytic enzymes such as elastase and phospholipase A.

Elastase and phospholipase A play a major role in autodigestion of the pancreas. Elastase causes hemorrhage by producing dissolution of the elastic fibers of blood vessels. Phospholipase A is probably activated by trypsin and bile acids and causes fat necrosis.

It is not entirely clear how alcohol causes acute pancreatitis. One theory is that it stimulates secretion and excess production of hydrochloric acid. A decrease in the gastric pH results in the release of the hormone secretin from the intestinal mucosa. This hormone then stimulates pancreatic secretions. Alcohol may also cause regurgitation of duodenal contents into the pancreatic duct, resulting in inflammation.

The pathophysiologic involvement of acute pancreatitis ranges from *edematous pancreatitis* (which is mild and self-limiting) to *necrotizing pancreatitis* (in which the degree of necrosis correlates with the severity of manifestations) (Fig. 42-14).

Clinical Manifestations

Abdominal pain is the predominant symptom of acute pancreatitis. The pain is usually located in the left upper quadrant, but it may be in the midepigastrium. It commonly radiates to the back because of the retroperitoneal location of the pancreas. The pain has a sudden onset and is described as severe, deep, piercing, and continuous or steady. It is aggravated by eating and frequently has its onset when the patient is recumbent; it is not relieved by vomiting. The pain may be accompanied by flushing,

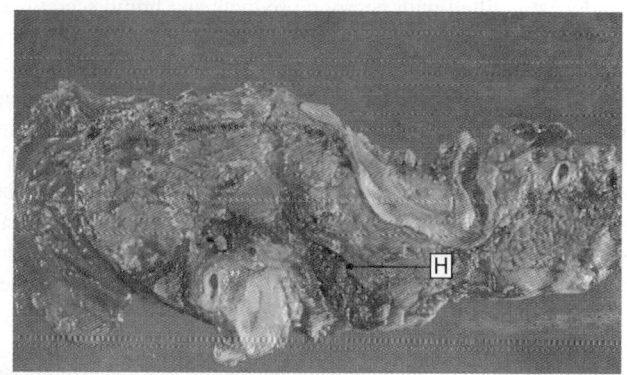

FIG. 42-14 In acute pancreatitis, the pancreas appears edematous and is commonly hemorrhagic *(H).*

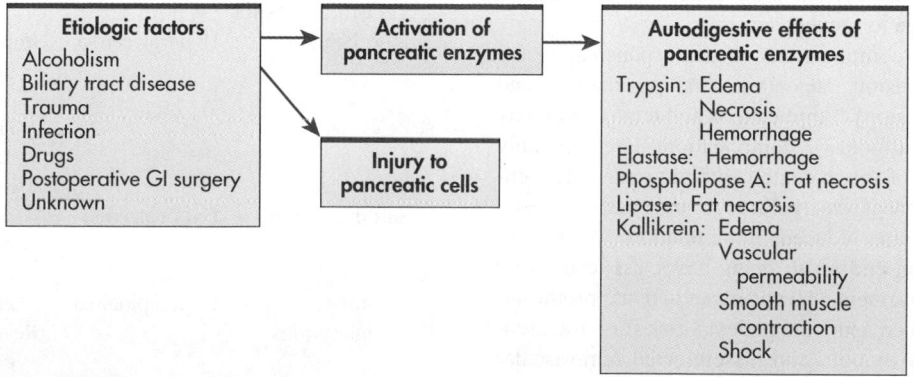

FIG. 42-13 Pathogenic process of acute pancreatitis. *GI,* Gastrointestinal.

cyanosis, and dyspnea. The patient may assume various positions involving flexion of the spine in an attempt to relieve the severe pain. The pain is due to distention of the pancreas, peritoneal irritation, and obstruction of the biliary tract.

Other manifestations of acute pancreatitis include nausea and vomiting, low-grade fever, leukocytosis, hypotension, tachycardia, and jaundice. Abdominal tenderness with muscle guarding is common. Bowel sounds may be decreased or absent. Ileus may occur and causes marked abdominal distention. The lungs are frequently involved, with crackles present. Intravascular damage from circulating trypsin may cause areas of cyanosis or greenish to yellow-brown discoloration of the abdominal wall. Other areas of ecchymoses are the flanks (*Grey Turner spots or sign,* a bluish flank discoloration) and the periumbilical area (*Cullen's sign,* a bluish periumbilical discoloration). These result from seepage of blood-stained exudate from the pancreas and may occur in severe cases.

Shock may occur because of hemorrhage into the pancreas or toxemia from the activated pancreatic enzymes. The increased formation of kinin peptides (activated by trypsin), such as kallikrein and bradykinin, causes vasodilation, increased capillary permeability, and altered vasomotor tone. Hypovolemia also occurs as a result of exudation of blood and plasma proteins into the retroperitoneal space (massive fluid shifts).

Complications

Two significant local complications of acute pancreatitis are pseudocyst and abscess. A pancreatic **pseudocyst** is a cavity continuous with or surrounding the outside of the pancreas. The pseudocyst is filled with necrotic products and liquid secretions, such as plasma, pancreatic enzymes, and inflammatory exudates. As pancreatic enzymes escape from the pseudocyst, the serosal surfaces next to the pancreas become inflamed, with subsequent formation of granulation tissue leading to encapsulation of the exudate. Manifestations of pseudocyst are abdominal pain, palpable epigastric mass, nausea, vomiting, and anorexia. The serum amylase level frequently remains elevated. These cysts usually resolve spontaneously within a few weeks but may perforate, causing peritonitis, or rupture into the stomach or duodenum. Treatment consists of an internal drainage procedure with an anastomosis between the pancreatic duct and the jejunum.

A pancreatic abscess is a large fluid-containing cavity within the pancreas. It results from extensive necrosis in the pancreas. It may become infected or perforate into adjacent organs. Manifestations of an abscess include upper abdominal pain, abdominal mass, high fever, and leukocytosis. Pancreatic abscesses require prompt surgical drainage to prevent sepsis.

The main systemic complications of acute pancreatitis are pulmonary (pleural effusion, atelectasis, and pneumonia) and cardiovascular (hypotension) complications and tetany caused by hypocalcemia. The pulmonary complications are probably caused by the passage of the exudate containing pancreatic enzymes from the peritoneal cavity through transdiaphragmatic lymph channels. Enzyme-induced inflammation of the diaphragm occurs with an end result being atelectasis caused by reduced diaphragm movement.[29] Trypsin can activate prothrombin and plasminogen, increasing the patient's risk for intravascular thrombi, pulmonary emboli, and disseminated intravascular coagulation.[29] When hypocalcemia occurs, it is a sign of severe disease. It is due in part to the combining of calcium and fatty acids during fat necrosis. The exact mechanisms of how or why hypocalcemia occurs are not well understood.

Diagnostic Studies

The primary diagnostic tests for acute pancreatitis are serum amylase and lipase and urinary amylase levels (Table 42-19). The serum amylase level is the criterion most commonly used. It may be elevated to levels greater than 200 U/L (3.34 μkat/L). The serum amylase is usually elevated early and remains elevated for 24 to 72 hours.

The serum lipase is also elevated in acute pancreatitis and is a helpful complementary test because other disorders (e.g., mumps, cerebral trauma, renal transplantation) may also cause an increase in serum amylase. The serum lipase level may be especially useful in patients with alcohol-induced acute pancreatitis.[30]

There is an increase in urinary amylase, which may persist several days beyond the elevation of serum amylase. Urinary amylase may be increased to more than 3600 U per day. Normally a timed collection (e.g., a 2-hour collection) is a more dependable measure than a randomly collected urinary specimen. The renal amylase-creatinine clearance test estimates the amount of blood cleared of amylase by the kidney per minute. The finding that the renal clearance of amylase is higher than the creatinine clearance in acute pancreatitis has led to the suggestion that the amylase-creatinine clearance ratio is a more specific test than urinary amylase levels alone. A new urinary test strip that uses trypsinogen-2 is being investigated for its use in diagnosing acute pancreatitis.[30]

Other laboratory abnormalities include hyperglycemia, hyperlipidemia, and hypocalcemia (see Table 42-19). There is a high incidence of hyperlipidemia with recurrent pancreatitis.

TABLE 42-19 Diagnostic Studies: Acute Pancreatitis

LABORATORY TEST	ABNORMAL FINDING	ETIOLOGY
Primary Tests		
Serum amylase	Increased (>200 U/L [3.34 μkat/L])	Pancreatic cell injury
Serum lipase	Elevated	Pancreatic cell injury
Urinary amylase	Elevated	Pancreatic cell injury
Secondary Tests		
Blood glucose	Hyperglycemia	Impairment of carbohydrate metabolism due to β-cell damage and decrease in insulin secretion and increase in glucagon release
Serum calcium	Hypocalcemia	Saponification of calcium by fatty acids in areas of fat necrosis
Serum triglycerides	Hyperlipidemia	Release of free fatty acids by lipase

Diagnostic evaluation of acute pancreatitis is also directed at determining the cause. An abdominal ultrasound, x-ray, or CT can be used to identify pancreatic problems. The CT scan can also determine the presence of pseudocysts and abscesses. ERCP is the definitive diagnostic test for gallstones, pancreatic cysts, and abscesses. Endoscopic ultrasound and magnetic resonance cholangiopancreatography are being used with greater frequency. A combination of laboratory studies and ERCP is usually used to help make the diagnosis.

Collaborative Care

Objectives of collaborative care for acute pancreatitis include (1) relief of pain; (2) prevention or alleviation of shock; (3) reduction of pancreatic secretions; (4) control of fluid and electrolyte imbalance; (5) prevention or treatment of infections; and (6) removal of the precipitating cause, if possible (Table 42-20).

Conservative Therapy. Treatment is principally focused on supportive care including aggressive hydration, pain management, management of metabolic complications, and minimizing pancreatic stimulation. A primary consideration in the treatment of acute pancreatitis is the relief and control of pain. Meperidine (Demerol) was once the preferred pain medication because it causes less spasm of the smooth muscles of the ducts than morphine. However, IV morphine may be used because of its longer half-life. Pain medications may be combined with an antispasmodic. However, atropine-like drugs should be avoided when paralytic ileus is present because they may contribute to the problem. Other medications that relax smooth muscles (spasmolytics), such as nitroglycerin or papaverine, may be used.

If shock is present, blood volume replacements are used. Plasma or plasma volume expanders such as dextran or albumin may be given. Fluid and electrolyte imbalances are corrected with lactated Ringer's solution or other electrolyte solutions. Central venous pressure readings may be used to assist in determination of fluid replacement requirements. Vasoactive drugs such as dopamine (Intropin) may be used to increase systemic vascular resistance in patients with ongoing hypotension.

It is important to reduce or suppress pancreatic enzymes to decrease stimulation of the pancreas and allow it to rest. This is accomplished in several ways. First, the patient is allowed to take nothing by mouth (NPO). Second, NG suction may be used to reduce vomiting and gastric distention and to prevent gastric acidic contents from entering the duodenum. These measures suppress pancreatic secretion. Certain drugs may also be used for this purpose (Tables 42-20 and 42-21).

The inflamed and necrotic pancreatic tissue is a good medium for bacterial growth. Therefore it is important to prevent infections. There is some controversy about the prophylactic use of antibiotics. It is important to monitor the patient closely so that antibiotic therapy can be instituted early if infection occurs.

Peritoneal lavage or dialysis has been used to remove the kinin and phospholipase A–containing exudate from the peritoneal cavity. This has proved beneficial in some cases of severe acute pancreatitis. It prevents early death but has little effect on overall mortality rate.

Surgical Therapy. When the acute pancreatitis is related to the presence of gallstones, an urgent ERCP plus endoscopic sphincterotomy may be performed. This may be followed by laparoscopic cholecystectomy to reduce the potential for recurrence. Surgical intervention may also be indicated when the diagnosis is uncertain and in patients who do not respond to conservative therapy. Surgery is necessary for an abscess, acute pseudocyst, and severe peritonitis. Percutaneous drainage of a pseudocyst can be performed, and a drainage tube is left in place.

Drug Therapy. Several different drugs may be used in the treatment of both acute and chronic pancreatitis (see Table 42-21). A number of drugs are used in an effort to suppress pancreatic secretion, but these drugs have not proved effective in the management of pancreatitis.

Nutritional Therapy. Initially the patient with acute pancreatitis is on NPO status to reduce pancreatic secretion. When food is allowed, small, frequent feedings are given. The diet is usually high in carbohydrate content because that is the least stimulating to the exocrine portion of the pancreas. The diet is bland, with no stimulants (e.g., caffeine) or alcohol. Supplemental fat-soluble vitamins may be given. The patient may require enteral feeding via jejunal feeding tube. If severe nutritional deficiencies exist, total parenteral nutrition (TPN) may be used (see Chapter 39).

NURSING MANAGEMENT
ACUTE PANCREATITIS

■ **Nursing Assessment**

Subjective and objective data that should be obtained from a person with acute pancreatitis are presented in Table 42-22.

TABLE 42-20	**Collaborative Care** **Acute Pancreatitis**

Diagnostic
History and physical examination
Serum amylase
Serum lipase
Two-hour urinary amylase and renal amylase clearance
Blood glucose
Serum calcium
Triglycerides
Flat plate of the abdomen
Abdominal ultrasound
Endoscopic ultrasound
CT scan of the pancreas
Magnetic resonance cholangiopancreatography
ERCP
Chest x-rays

Collaborative Therapy
Pain medication (meperidine, morphine)
NPO with NG tube to suction
Albumin (if shock present)
IV calcium gluconate (10%) (if tetany present)
Lactated Ringer's solution
cimetidine (Tagamet) or omeprazole (Prilosec)
Antibiotics (if necrotizing pancreatitis)

CT, Computed tomography; *ERCP*, endoscopic retrograde cholangiopancreatography; *IV*, intravenous; *NG*, nasogastric; *NPO*, nothing by mouth.

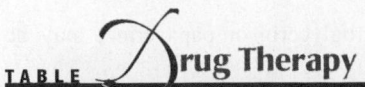

TABLE 42-21 **Drug Therapy**
Acute and Chronic Pancreatitis

DRUG	MECHANISM OF ACTION
Acute Pancreatitis	
meperidine (Demerol), morphine	Relief of pain
nitroglycerin or papaverine	Relaxation of smooth muscles and relief of pain
Antispasmodics (e.g., dicyclomine [Bentyl], propantheline bromide [Pro-Banthine])	Decrease of vagal stimulation, motility, pancreatic outflow (inhibition of volume and concentration of bicarbonate and enzymatic secretion); contraindicated in paralytic ileus
Carbonic anhydrase inhibitor (acetazolamide [Diamox])	Reduction in volume and bicarbonate concentration of pancreatic secretion
Antacids	Neutralization of gastric HCl secretion and subsequent decrease in secretin, which stimulates production and secretion of pancreatic secretions
Histamine H_2-receptor antagonists (cimetidine [Tagamet], ranitidine [Zantac]); proton pump inhibitors (omeprazole [Prevacid])	Decrease in HCl secretion (HCl stimulates pancreatic activity)
Chronic Pancreatitis	
pancreatin (Viokase), pancrelipase (Cotazym)	Replacement therapy for pancreatic enzymes
Insulin	Treatment for diabetes mellitus if it occurs or for hyperglycemia

HCl, Hydrochloric acid.

TABLE 42-22 **Nursing Assessment**
Acute Pancreatitis

Subjective Data	Objective Data
Important Health Information	**General**
Past health history: Biliary tract disease, alcohol use, abdominal trauma, duodenal ulcers, infection, metabolic disorders	Restlessness, anxiety, low-grade fever
	Integumentary
Medications: Use of thiazides, nonsteroidal antiinflammatory drugs	Flushing, diaphoresis, discoloration of abdomen and flanks, cyanosis, jaundice; decreased skin turgor, dry mucous membranes
Surgery or other treatments: Surgical procedures on the pancreas, stomach, duodenum, or biliary tract; endoscopic retrograde cholangiopancreatography	**Respiratory**
	Tachypnea, basilar crackles
Functional Health Patterns	**Cardiovascular**
Health perception–health management: Alcohol abuse; weakness	Tachycardia, hypotension
Nutritional-metabolic: Nausea and vomiting; anorexia	**Gastrointestinal**
Activity-exercise: Dyspnea	Abdominal distention, tenderness, and muscle guarding; diminished bowel sounds
Cognitive-perceptual: Severe midepigastric or left upper quadrant pain that may radiate to the back, aggravated by food and alcohol intake and unrelieved by vomiting	**Possible Findings**
	↑ Serum amylase and lipase, leukocytosis, hyperglycemia, ↑ urine amylase, hyperlipidemia, hypocalcemia, abnormal ultrasound and CT scans of pancreas, abnormal ERCP

CT, Computed tomography; *ERCP,* endoscopic retrograde cholangiopancreatogram.

■ Nursing Diagnoses

Nursing diagnoses for the patient with acute pancreatitis may include, but are not limited to, those presented in NCP 42-3.

■ Planning

The overall goals are that the patient with acute pancreatitis will have (1) relief of pain, (2) normal fluid and electrolyte balance, (3) minimal to no complications, and (4) no recurrent attacks.

■ Nursing Implementation

Health Promotion. The major factors involved in health promotion are assessment of the patient for predisposing and etiologic factors of pancreatitis and encouragement of early treatment of these factors to prevent occurrence of acute pancreatitis. The nurse should encourage the early diagnosis and treatment of biliary tract disease, such as cholelithiasis. The patient should be encouraged to eliminate alcohol intake, especially if there have been

NURSING CARE PLAN 42-3

Patient with Acute Pancreatitis

EXPECTED PATIENT OUTCOMES	NURSING INTERVENTIONS and *RATIONALES*
NURSING DIAGNOSIS	**Acute pain** *related to* distention of pancreas, peritoneal irritation, obstruction of biliary tract, and ineffective pain and comfort measures *as manifested by* communication of pain descriptors, guarding behavior, behaviors indicative of pain (e.g., moaning), diaphoresis, changes in blood pressure, pulse, and respiratory rate.
▪ Minimal to no pain	▪ Assess degree and nature of pain *to plan appropriate interventions.* ▪ Give ordered analgesic and antispasmodic medications before pain gets too severe *to ensure more effective relief of pain.* ▪ Ascertain how long the medication provides relief *to adjust pain medication administration to provide ongoing relief of pain.* ▪ Provide comfort measures, such as positioning patient comfortably with frequent changes in position and diversional activities *to assist in reducing the restlessness that usually accompanies the pain and to demonstrate caring behaviors by the nurse.*
NURSING DIAGNOSIS	**Deficient fluid volume** *related to* nausea, vomiting, NG suction, and restricted oral intake *as manifested by* thirst, increased fluid output, altered intake, dry skin and mucous membranes, decreased skin turgor, decreased oral intake.
▪ Normal skin turgor ▪ Moist mucous membranes ▪ Stable weight ▪ Normal serum electrolyte levels	▪ Give antiemetics as ordered *to reduce fluid loss by preventing vomiting.* ▪ Measure and describe emesis *as indicators of replacement needs and effectiveness of treatment.* ▪ Observe for manifestations of electrolyte imbalances such as confusion, irritability, tachycardia, nausea, vomiting, muscle cramps, and tetany caused by loss of chloride, sodium, potassium, and calcium *so that appropriate replacements can be started promptly.*
NURSING DIAGNOSIS	**Imbalanced nutrition: less than body requirements** *related to* anorexia, dietary restrictions, nausea, loss of nutrients from vomiting, and impaired digestion resulting in decreased use of nutrients *as manifested by* weight loss, weakness, fatigue, weight below normal for height and age.
▪ Weight appropriate for height ▪ No further weight loss ▪ Normal stool	▪ Monitor weight and laboratory values *as indicators of patient's response to treatment.* ▪ Observe stools for steatorrhea, *which may develop from incomplete digestion of fats.* ▪ Administer nasointestinal tube feedings or total parenteral nutrition (if severe pancreatitis) if ordered *to provide carbohydrates, lipids, and amino acids to prevent negative nitrogen balance.* ▪ Implement measures to reduce pain and nausea *to increase patient's desire to eat.* ▪ Provide oral care before and after meals *to decrease foul taste and odor that inhibit appetite.* ▪ If oral intake is allowed, provide small portions of high-carbohydrate, low-fat foods *to decrease stimulation of pancreas.*
NURSING DIAGNOSIS	**Ineffective therapeutic regimen management** *related to* lack of knowledge of preventive measures, diet restrictions, restriction of alcohol intake, and follow-up care *as manifested by* verbalization of the problem, request for information, inaccurate follow-through on instructions.
▪ Verbalization of understanding of condition or disease process and treatment ▪ Initiation of lifestyle changes ▪ Participation in treatment regimen	▪ Teach patient to (1) abstain from alcohol *to prevent the patient from experiencing future attacks of acute pancreatitis and development of chronic pancreatitis,* (2) restrict fats and avoid rich and stimulating foods *to decrease stimulation of the pancreas and allow it to rest,* (3) use more carbohydrates in diet *because these are less stimulating to pancreas,* and (4) correctly measure blood glucose levels and observe for steatorrhea *because high blood glucose and fatty stools indicate destruction of pancreatic tissue or loss of viable pancreatic tissue.* ▪ Assess patient's understanding of prescribed regimen; provide details on follow-up care *to increase likelihood of successful convalescence and to minimize the possibility of recurrence.* ▪ Suggest follow-up if alcohol use problematic *because continued use of alcohol will result in additional attacks of acute pancreatitis and eventual chronic pancreatitis.*

any previous episodes of pancreatitis. Attacks of pancreatitis become milder or disappear with the discontinuance of alcohol use.

Acute Intervention. During the acute phase, it is important to monitor vital signs. Hemodynamic stability may be compromised by hypotension, fever, and tachypnea, which may result in fluid volume deficit. IV fluids are ordered, and the response to

therapy is monitored. A vital part of the nursing care plan for this patient is observation for electrolyte imbalances. Frequent vomiting, along with gastric suction, may result in decreased chloride, sodium, and potassium levels.

Respiratory failure may develop in the patient with severe acute pancreatitis. It is important that respiratory function be assessed (e.g., lung sounds). If acute respiratory distress syndrome develops, the patient may require intubation and mechanical ventilatory support.

Because hypocalcemia can also occur, the nurse must observe for symptoms of tetany, such as jerking, irritability, and muscular twitching. Numbness or tingling around the lips and in the fingers is an early indicator of hypocalcemia. The patient should be assessed for a positive Chvostek or Trousseau sign (see Chapter 16). Calcium gluconate (as ordered) should be given to treat symptomatic hypocalcemia. In addition, hypomagnesemia may develop, necessitating the observation of serum magnesium levels.

Because abdominal pain is a prominent symptom of pancreatitis, a major focus of nursing care is the relief of pain (see NCP 42-3). Giving the prescribed medications before the pain becomes too severe makes the medication more effective. Morphine or meperidine may be used for pain relief. The nurse should ascertain how long the pain medication provides relief. Measures such as comfortable positioning, frequent changes in position, and relief of nausea and vomiting assist in reducing the restlessness that usually accompanies the pain. Some patients experience lessened pain by assuming positions that flex the trunk and draw the knees up to the abdomen. A side-lying position with the head elevated 45 degrees decreases tension on the abdomen and may help ease the pain. It is important to control the pain and restlessness because they increase body metabolism and subsequent stimulation of pancreatic secretions.

Nursing measures for the patient who is on NPO status or has an NG tube should be employed. Frequent oral and nasal care to relieve the dryness of the mouth and nose is comforting to the patient. Oral care is essential to prevent parotitis. If the patient is taking anticholinergics to decrease GI secretions, there will be additional dryness of the mouth caused by the side effects of the drug. If the patient is taking antacids to suppress secretions, they should be sipped slowly or inserted in the NG tube. The nurse must regularly assess the functioning of the suction.

The patient with acute pancreatitis is susceptible to infections. The nurse should observe for fever and other manifestations of infection. Respiratory infections are common because the retroperitoneal fluid raises the diaphragm, which causes the patient to take shallow, guarded abdominal breaths. Measures to prevent respiratory infections include turning, coughing, deep breathing, and assuming a semi-Fowler's position.

Other important assessments are observation for signs of paralytic ileus, renal failure, and mental changes. Determination of the blood glucose level should be done to assess damage to the β-cells of the islets of Langerhans in the pancreas.

After pancreatic surgery the patient may require special wound care for an anastomotic leak or a fistula. Measures to prevent skin irritation should be used. These include skin barriers such as Stomahesive, Karaya paste, or Colly-Seel; pouching; and drains. In addition to protecting the skin, pouching also provides a more accurate determination of fluid and electrolyte losses and increases patient comfort. Sterile pouching systems are available. The nurse may want to consult with a clinical specialist or an enterostomal therapy nurse, if available.

Ambulatory and Home Care. After acute pancreatitis, most patients will need home care follow-up. The patient may have lost physical reserve and muscle strength. Physical therapy may be needed. Continued care to prevent infection and detect any complications is important. Because frequent doses of narcotics may be required for this patient during the acute stage, follow-up for assessment of possible narcotic addiction may be indicated. This is a more likely problem with chronic pancreatitis than in the patient with acute pancreatitis. Counseling regarding abstinence from alcohol is important to prevent the patient from experiencing future attacks of acute pancreatitis and development of chronic pancreatitis. Beverages with caffeine should not be consumed. Because smoking and stressful situations can overstimulate the pancreas, they should be avoided.

Dietary teaching should include restriction of fats because they stimulate the secretion of cholecystokinin, which then stimulates the pancreas. Carbohydrates are less stimulating to the pancreas, so they should be encouraged. The patient should be instructed to avoid crash dieting and bingeing because they can precipitate attacks.

The patient and the family should be given instructions regarding the recognition and reporting of symptoms of infection, diabetes mellitus, or steatorrhea (foul-smelling, frothy stools). These changes indicate possible destruction of pancreatic tissue. The nurse should make sure the patient fully understands the prescribed regimen. Each aspect must be explained. The importance of taking the required medications and following the recommended diet should be stressed.

■ Evaluation

Expected outcomes for the patient with acute pancreatitis are presented in NCP 42-3.

CHRONIC PANCREATITIS

Chronic pancreatitis is progressive destruction of the pancreas with fibrotic replacement of pancreatic tissue. Strictures and calcifications may also occur in the pancreas.

Etiology and Pathophysiology

There are several types of chronic pancreatitis, but they all have a common underlying pathophysiologic disorder. The two major types are *chronic obstructive pancreatitis* and *chronic calcifying pancreatitis*. Chronic pancreatitis may follow acute pancreatitis, but it may also occur in the absence of any history of an acute condition.

Chronic obstructive pancreatitis is associated with biliary disease. The most common cause is inflammation of the sphincter of Oddi associated with cholelithiasis. Cancer of the ampulla of Vater, duodenum, or pancreas can also cause this type of chronic pancreatitis.

In chronic calcifying pancreatitis there is inflammation and sclerosis, mainly in the head of the pancreas and around the pancreatic duct. This type of chronic pancreatitis is the most common form. It is also called alcohol-induced pancreatitis. Increases in heavy social drinking have produced a higher incidence in countries in which the disease was previously considered rare. In the United States, chronic pancreatitis is found almost exclusively in alcoholics. As with cirrhosis there seems to be a metabolic abnormality that predisposes a person who drinks to the direct toxic effect of the alcohol on the pancreas.

In chronic calcifying pancreatitis the ducts are obstructed with protein precipitates. These precipitates block the pancreatic duct and eventually calcify. This is followed by fibrosis and glandular atrophy. Pseudocysts and abscesses commonly develop.

Clinical Manifestations

As with acute pancreatitis, a major manifestation of chronic pancreatitis is abdominal pain. The patient may have episodes of acute pain, but it usually is chronic (recurrent attacks at intervals of months or years). The attacks may become more and more frequent until they are almost constant, or they may diminish as the pancreatic fibrosis develops. The pain is located in the same areas as in acute pancreatitis but is usually described as a heavy, gnawing feeling or sometimes as burning and cramplike. The pain is not relieved with food or antacids.

Other clinical manifestations include symptoms of pancreatic insufficiency, including malabsorption with weight loss, constipation, mild jaundice with dark urine, steatorrhea, and diabetes mellitus. The steatorrhea may become severe, with voluminous, foul, fatty stools. Urine and stool may be frothy. Some abdominal tenderness may be present.

Diagnostic Studies

In chronic pancreatitis the levels of serum amylase and lipase may be elevated slightly or not at all, depending on the degree of pancreatic fibrosis. Increased serum bilirubin and increased alkaline phosphatase levels may be present. There is usually mild leukocytosis and an elevated sedimentation rate.

The secretin stimulation test is used to assess pancreatic function. In the normal pancreas secretin stimulates HCO_3^- secretion. In the stimulation test secretin is given intravenously, and gastric-duodenal secretions are collected with a double-lumen tube for separate gastric and duodenal aspiration. In chronic pancreatitis there is reduced volume of secretions and reduced bicarbonate concentration (less than 90 mEq/L). Normally, secretin stimulates the production of pancreatic fluid high in bicarbonate content.

Other abnormal diagnostic findings are hyperglycemia and fatty stools (steatorrhea). Stools are examined for fecal fat content. Arteriography and x-rays may demonstrate fibrosis and calcification.

ERCP involves cannulation and visualization of the pancreatic and common bile ducts through an endoscope that is inserted into the esophagus and then into the duodenum. The common bile duct and the pancreatic duct are then cannulated. Contrast dye can be injected into the ducts for visualization. Changes in the pancreatic ductal system, such as gross dilation and microcysts, can be visualized through the use of ERCP.

Imaging studies such as CT, MRI, transabdominal ultrasound, and endoscopic ultrasound are useful in patients with chronic pancreatitis. Transabdominal ultrasonography, CT, and MRI show a variety of changes including calcifications, ductal dilation, pseudocysts, and pancreatic enlargement.

Collaborative Care

When the patient with chronic pancreatitis is experiencing an acute attack, the therapy is identical to that for acute pancreatitis. At other times the focus is on prevention of further attacks, relief of pain, and control of pancreatic exocrine and endocrine insufficiency. It sometimes takes large, frequent doses of analgesics to relieve the pain.

Diet, pancreatic enzyme replacement, and control of the diabetes are measures used to control the pancreatic insufficiency. The diet is bland, low in fat, and high in carbohydrate. The patient does not tolerate fatty, rich, and stimulating foods, and these should be avoided to decrease pancreatic secretions and demands on the pancreas. Alcohol must be totally eliminated.

Pancreatic enzymes such as pancreatin (Viokase) and pancrelipase (Cotazym) contain amylase, lipase, and trypsin and are used to replace the deficient pancreatic enzymes. They are usually enteric coated to prevent their breakdown or inactivation by gastric acid. Bile salts are sometimes given to facilitate the absorption of the fat-soluble vitamins (A, D, E, and K) and prevent further fat loss. If diabetes develops, it is controlled with insulin or oral hypoglycemic agents. Acid-neutralizing (e.g., antacids) and acid-inhibiting drugs (e.g., H_2-receptor blockers, proton pump inhibitors, anticholinergics) may be given to decrease hydrochloric acid but have little overall effect on the outcome of the disease.

Treatment of chronic pancreatitis sometimes requires surgery. When biliary disease is present or if obstruction or pseudocyst develops, surgery may be indicated. Surgical procedures can divert bile flow or relieve ductal obstruction. A choledochojejunostomy diverts bile around the ampulla of Vater, where there may be spasm or hypertrophy of the sphincter. In this procedure the common bile duct is anastomosed into the jejunum. If the pancreatic sphincter is fibrotic, a sphincterotomy enlarges it. Pancreatic drainage procedures relieve ductal obstruction. One type is the Roux-en-Y pancreatojejunostomy, in which the pancreatic duct is opened and an anastomosis is made with the jejunum.

NURSING MANAGEMENT
CHRONIC PANCREATITIS

Except during an acute episode, the focus of nursing management is on chronic care and health promotion. The patient should be instructed to take measures to prevent further attacks. Dietary control, along with consistency of other treatment measures, such as taking pancreatic enzymes, is essential. The pancreatic extracts are usually given with meals or can be given with a snack. The nurse should observe the patient's stools for steatorrhea to help determine the effectiveness of the enzymes. The patient and the family need instructions regarding observation of stools.

If diabetes has developed, the patient will need instruction regarding testing of blood glucose levels and drugs (see Chapter 47). The nurse should make sure that the patient who is taking antacids takes them as ordered to control gastric acidity. Antacids should be taken after meals.

Alcohol must be avoided, and the patient may need assistance with this problem. If the patient has developed a dependence on alcohol, referral to other agencies or resources may be necessary (see Chapter 11).

PANCREATIC CANCER

In the United States in 2002 30,300 people were diagnosed with pancreatic cancer and 29,700 died of pancreatic cancer. It is the fourth leading cause of death from cancer in the United States and Canada. The risk increases with age, with the peak incidence occurring between 65 and 80 years of age.[28]

Most of the pancreatic tumors are adenocarcinomas originating from the epithelium of the ductal system. More than half the tumors occur in the head of the pancreas. As the tumor grows, the common bile duct becomes obstructed, and obstructive jaundice develops. Tumors starting in the body or tail often remain silent until their growth is advanced. The majority of cancers have metastasized at the time of diagnosis. The signs and symptoms of pancreatic cancer are often similar to chronic pancreatitis. The prognosis of a patient with cancer of the pancreas is poor. The majority of patients die within 5 to 12 months of the initial diagnosis, and the 5-year survival rate is only about 10%.[31] The prognosis is related to the location of the tumor.

Etiology and Pathophysiology

The cause of pancreatic cancer remains unknown. There may be some relationship among cancer, diabetes mellitus, and chronic pancreatitis. However, it is not clear whether the cancer follows these diseases or whether these diseases occur as a result of pancreatic cancer. It is known that pancreatic cancer can be induced with chemicals such as nitrosoureas. Major risk factors seem to be cigarette smoking, high-fat diet, diabetes, and exposure to chemicals such as benzidine and coke. The most firmly established risk factor is cigarette smoking. Pancreatic cancer develops twice as often in persons with a history of heavy cigarette use (more than two packs a day) than in nonsmokers. The carcinogens from the tobacco probably reach the pancreatic ducts by bile reflux or via the bloodstream. Another risk factor is the Western diet, particularly the high-fat content. High consumption of meat has also been implicated.

Clinical Manifestations

Common manifestations of pancreatic cancer include abdominal pain (dull, aching), anorexia, rapid and progressive weight loss, nausea, and jaundice. Pain is common and is related to the location of malignancy. Extreme, unrelenting pain is related to extension of the cancer into the retroperitoneal tissues and nerve plexuses. The pain is frequently located in the upper abdomen or left hypochondrium and often radiates to the back. It is commonly related to eating, and it also occurs at night. Weight loss is due to poor digestion and absorption caused by lack of digestive enzymes from the pancreas.

Diagnostic Studies

Better diagnostic measures are needed for detection of pancreatic cancer because most of the current methods detect only advanced stages. Transabdominal ultrasound and CT are the most commonly used diagnostic imaging techniques for pancreatic diseases including cancer. CT scan is often the initial study and provides information on metastasis and vascular involvement. ERCP is the "gold standard" for visualization of the pancreatic duct and biliary system.[31] When ERCP is used, pancreatic secretions, as well as tissue, can be collected for analysis of different tumor markers. Endoluminal ultrasound involves imaging the pancreas with the use of an endoscope positioned in the stomach and duodenum. This procedure also allows for fine needle aspiration of the tumor.

Tumor markers are used both for establishing the diagnosis of pancreatic adenocarcinoma and for monitoring the response to treatment. CA19-9 is most frequently increased in pancreatic cancer but may also be elevated in gallbladder cancer, as well as in benign conditions such as acute and chronic pancreatitis, hepatitis, and biliary obstruction.[31] Carcinoembryonic antigen (CEA) is a protein expressed in the colon during embryonic development and is used as a tumor marker in pancreatic cancer. However, CEA is best known as a tumor marker for colon cancer and is less specific for pancreatic cancer.

Collaborative Care

Surgery provides the most effective treatment of cancer of the pancreas. The classic surgery is a *radical pancreaticoduodenectomy*, or *Whipple's procedure* (Fig. 42-15). This entails resection of the proximal pancreas (proximal pancreatectomy), the adjoining duodenum (duodenectomy), the distal portion of the stomach (partial gastrectomy), and the distal segment of the common bile duct. An anastomosis of the pancreatic duct, common bile duct, and stomach to the jejunum is done. A total pancreatectomy is performed in some institutions for cancers of the head of the pancreas. Sometimes a simple bypass procedure, such as a cholecystojejunostomy to relieve biliary obstruction, may be used as a palliative measure. Some surgeons suggest a more radical resection, such as a total pancreaticoduodenectomy with splenectomy. Biliary stents (e.g., Cotton-Leung stent) can be used as a palliative measure when tumors compress the bile duct.

Radiation therapy alters survival rates little but is effective for pain relief. External radiation is usually used, but implantation of internal radiation seeds into the tumor has also been used. The current role of chemotherapy in pancreatic cancer is limited. Chemotherapy usually consists of 5-FU and gemcitabine (Gemzar) either alone or in combination.[32,33] However, response rates are below 15% with minor effects on overall survival. Because of the aggressive nature of pancreatic cancer, current emphasis of new experimental chemotherapy is also focused on clinical benefits including reductions in pain. Several oral formulations of 5-FU, such as capecitabine (Xeloda) and eniluracil with 5-FU, have been developed to simulate long-term continuous infusion. Response rates of these formulations are comparable to those of 5-FU continuous infusion and 5-FU bolus injections. Combinations of drugs such as 5-FU and carmustine (BCNU) produce a better response than single chemotherapeutic agents. Gemcitabine is currently a main treatment for pancreatic

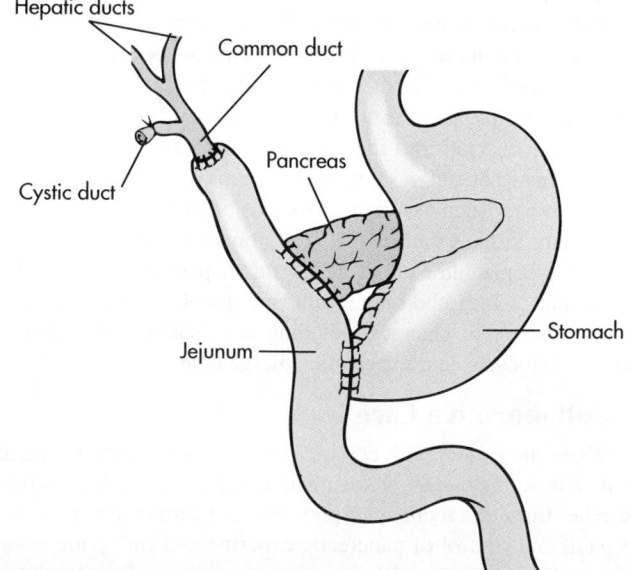

FIG. 42-15 Whipple procedure or radical pancreaticoduodenectomy. This surgical procedure involves resection of the proximal pancreas, adjoining duodenum, distal portion of the stomach, and distal portion of the common bile duct. An anastomosis of the pancreatic duct, common bile duct, and stomach to the jejunum is done.

cancer that has metastasized. Adjuvant therapy, which uses surgical resection, radiation, and chemotherapy, is believed by some to be the most effective way to manage cancer of the pancreas.

NURSING MANAGEMENT
PANCREATIC CANCER

Because the patient with pancreatic cancer has many of the same problems as the patient with pancreatitis, nursing care includes the same measures (see NCP 42-3). The nurse should provide symptomatic and supportive nursing care. Medications and comfort measures to relieve pain should be provided before the patient reaches the peak of pain. Psychologic support is essential, especially during times of anxiety or depression, which seem to occur frequently in these patients.

Adequate nutrition is an important part of the nursing care plan. Frequent and supplemental feedings may be necessary. Measures to stimulate the appetite as much as possible and to overcome anorexia, nausea, and vomiting should be included in the nursing care. Because bleeding can result from impaired vitamin K production, the nurse should assess for bleeding from body orifices and mucous membranes. If the patient is undergoing radiation therapy, the nurse must observe for adverse reactions, such as anorexia, nausea, vomiting, and skin irritation.

The prognosis for a patient with pancreatic cancer is not good. A significant component of the nursing care is helping the patient and the family or significant others through the grieving process.

Disorders of the Biliary Tract

CHOLELITHIASIS AND CHOLECYSTITIS

The most common disorder of the biliary system is **cholelithiasis** (stones in the gallbladder) (Figs. 42-16 and 42-17). **Cholecystitis** (inflammation of the gallbladder) is usually associated with cholelithiasis. The stones may be lodged in the neck of the gallbladder or in the cystic duct. Cholecystitis may be acute or chronic. These conditions usually occur together.

Gallbladder disease is a common health problem in the United States. It is estimated that 8% to 10% of the adults in the United States have cholelithiasis. The actual number is not known because many persons are asymptomatic with stones. *Cholecystec-* *tomy* (removal of the gallbladder) ranks among the most common surgical procedures performed in the United States. The incidence of cholelithiasis is higher in women, multiparous women, and persons over 40 years of age. Postmenopausal women on estrogen therapy are at somewhat greater risk of having gallbladder disease than are women who are taking birth control pills. Oral contraceptives alter the character of bile, resulting in increased cholesterol saturation. Other factors that seem to increase the occurrence of gallbladder disease are a sedentary lifestyle, a familial tendency, and obesity. Obesity causes increased secretion of cholesterol in bile. Gallbladder disease is more common in whites than in Asian Americans and African Americans. There is an especially high incidence in the Native American population, particularly in the Navajo and Pima tribes.

Etiology and Pathophysiology

Cholecystitis. Cholecystitis is most commonly associated with obstruction caused by gallstones or biliary sludge. When cholecystitis occurs in the absence of obstruction (acalculous cholecystitis), it is most often in older adults and in patients who have trauma, extensive burns, or recent surgery. Acalculous cholecystitis can also occur as a result of prolonged immobility and fasting, prolonged total parenteral nutrition, and diabetes mellitus. Bacteria reaching the gallbladder via the vascular or lymphatic route, or chemical irritants in the bile can also produce cholecystitis. *Escherichia coli* is the most common bacteria involved. Streptococci and salmonellae are also common causative bacteria. Other etiologic factors include adhesions, neoplasms, anesthesia, and narcotics.[34]

Inflammation is the major pathophysiologic condition and may be confined to the mucous lining or involve the entire wall of the gallbladder. During an acute attack of cholecystitis the gallbladder is edematous and hyperemic. It may be distended with bile or pus. The cystic duct is also involved and may become occluded. The wall of the gallbladder becomes scarred after an acute attack. Decreased functioning occurs if large amounts of tissue are fibrosed.

Cholelithiasis. The actual cause of gallstones is unknown. Basically, cholelithiasis develops when the balance that keeps cholesterol, bile salts, and calcium in solution is altered so that precipitation of these substances occurs. Conditions that upset this balance include infection and disturbances in the metabolism

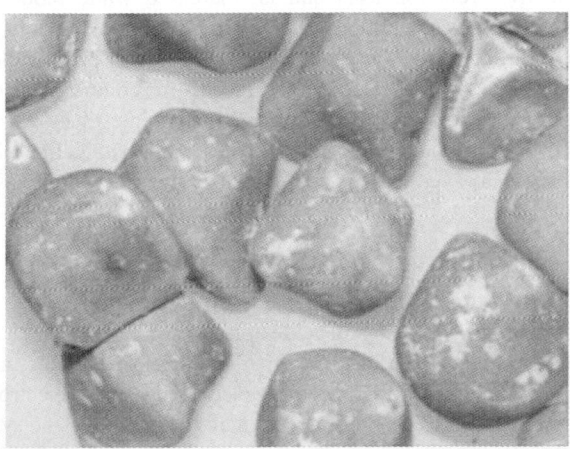

FIG. 42-16 Gallstones.

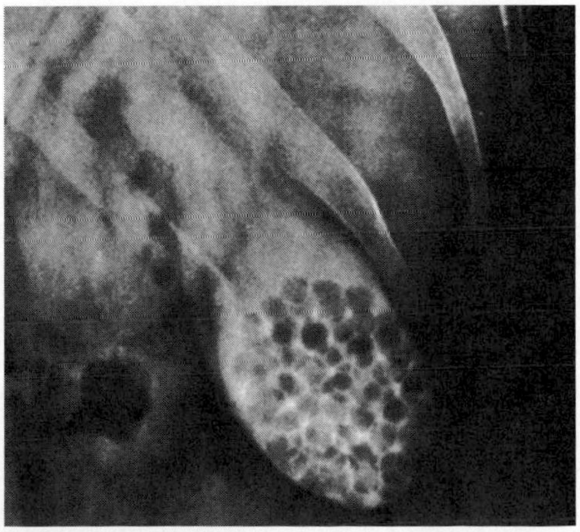

FIG. 42-17 X-ray of a gallbladder with gallstones.

of cholesterol. It is known that in patients with cholelithiasis the bile secreted by the liver is supersaturated with cholesterol (lithogenic bile). The bile in the gallbladder also becomes supersaturated with cholesterol. Whenever bile is supersaturated with cholesterol, precipitation of cholesterol will occur.

A high percentage of gallstones are precipitates of cholesterol. Other components of bile that precipitate into stones are bile salts, bilirubin, calcium, and protein. The stones sometimes have a mixed consistency. Mixed cholesterol stones, which are predominantly cholesterol, are the most common gallstones.

The changes in the composition of bile are probably significant in the formation of gallstones. Stasis of bile leads to progression of the supersaturation and changes in the chemical composition of the bile. Immobility, pregnancy, and inflammatory or obstructive lesions of the biliary system decrease bile flow. Hormonal factors during pregnancy may cause delayed emptying of the gallbladder.

The stones may remain in the gallbladder or migrate to the cystic duct or to the common bile duct. They cause pain as they pass through the ducts, and they may lodge in the ducts and produce an obstruction. Small stones are more likely to move into a duct and cause obstruction. Table 42-23 depicts the changes and manifestations that occur when the stones obstruct the common bile duct. If the blockage occurs in the cystic duct, the bile can continue to flow into the duodenum directly from the liver. However, when the bile in the gallbladder cannot escape, this stasis of bile may lead to cholecystitis.

Clinical Manifestations

Manifestations of cholecystitis vary from indigestion to moderate to severe pain, fever, and jaundice. Initial symptoms of acute cholecystitis include indigestion and pain and tenderness in the right upper quadrant, which may be referred to the right shoulder and scapula. The pain may be acute and be accompanied by nausea and vomiting, restlessness, and diaphoresis. Manifestations of inflammation include leukocytosis and fever. Physical findings include right upper quadrant tenderness and abdominal rigidity. Symptoms of chronic cholecystitis include a history of fat intolerance, dyspepsia, heartburn, and flatulence.

Cholelithiasis may produce severe symptoms or none at all. Many patients have "silent cholelithiasis." The severity of symptoms depends on whether the stones are stationary or mobile and whether obstruction is present. When a stone is lodged in the ducts or when stones are moving through the ducts, spasms may result. The gallbladder spasms occur in response to the stone. This sometimes produces severe pain, which is termed *biliary colic* even though the pain is rarely colicky; it is more often steady. The pain can be excruciating and accompanied by tachycardia, diaphoresis, and prostration. The severe pain may last up to an hour, and when it subsides there is residual tenderness in the right upper quadrant. The attacks of pain frequently occur 3 to 6 hours after a heavy meal or when the patient assumes a recumbent position. When total obstruction occurs, symptoms related to bile blockage are manifested (see Table 42-23).

Complications

Complications of cholecystitis include subphrenic abscess, pancreatitis, *cholangitis* (inflammation of biliary ducts), biliary cirrhosis, fistulas, and rupture of the gallbladder, which can produce bile peritonitis.

Many of the same complications can occur from cholelithiasis, including cholangitis, biliary cirrhosis, carcinoma, and peritonitis. *Choledocholithiasis* (stone in the common bile duct) may occur, producing symptoms of obstruction.

Diagnostic Studies

Ultrasonography is probably the best means of diagnosing gallstones (see Table 38-12). It is 90% to 95% accurate in detecting stones. It is especially useful for patients with jaundice (because it does not depend on liver function) and for patients who are allergic to contrast medium. ERCP allows for visualization of the gallbladder, cystic duct, common hepatic duct, and common bile duct. Bile taken during ERCP is sent for culture to identify any possible infecting organism.

Percutaneous transhepatic cholangiography may be used to diagnose obstructive jaundice and to locate stones within the bile ducts. Laboratory tests may demonstrate abnormalities in some of the liver function tests and an increased white blood cell (WBC) count as a result of inflammation. Both the direct and indirect bilirubin levels are elevated, as is the urinary bilirubin level if there is an obstructive process present. If the common bile duct is obstructed, no bilirubin will reach the small intestine to be converted to urobilinogen. Serum enzymes, such as alkaline phosphatase, ALT, and AST, may be elevated. The serum amylase is increased if there is pancreatic involvement.

Collaborative Care

Conservative Therapy

Cholecystitis. During an acute episode of cholecystitis the focus of treatment is on control of pain, control of possible infection with antibiotics, and maintenance of fluid and electrolyte balance (Table 42-24). Treatment is mainly supportive and symptomatic. If nausea and vomiting are severe, gastric decompression may be used to prevent further gallbladder stimulation. An-

TABLE 42-23	Clinical Manifestations Caused by Obstructed Bile Flow
CLINICAL MANIFESTATION	**ETIOLOGY**
Obstructive jaundice	No bile flow into duodenum
Dark amber urine, which foams when shaken	Soluble bilirubin in urine
No urobilinogen in urine	No bilirubin reaching small intestine to be converted to urobilinogen
Clay-colored stools	Same as above
Pruritus	Deposition of bile salts in skin tissues
Intolerance for fatty foods (nausea, sensation of fullness, anorexia)	No bile in small intestine for fat digestion
Bleeding tendencies	Lack of or decreased absorption of vitamin K, resulting in decreased production of prothrombin
Steatorrhea	No bile salts in duodenum, preventing fat emulsion and digestion

TABLE 42-24	*C*ollaborative Care Cholelithiasis and Acute Cholecystitis

Diagnostic
History and physical examination
Ultrasound
Liver function studies
WBC count
Serum bilirubin
ERCP

Collaborative Therapy
Conservative Therapy
IV fluid
NPO with NG tube, later progressing to low-fat diet
Antiemetics
Analgesics (e.g., meperidine)
Fat-soluble vitamins (A, D, E, and K)
Anticholinergics (antispasmodics)
Antibiotics (for secondary infection)
ERCP with sphincterotomy (papillotomy)
Extracorporeal shock-wave lithotripsy
Dissolution Therapy
ursodeoxycholic acid (UDCA)
ursodiol (Actigall)
chenodeoxycholic acid (CDCA)
Surgical Therapy*
Laparoscopic cholecystectomy
Incisional cholecystectomy

*See Table 42-25.
ERCP, Endoscopic retrograde cholangiopancreatography; IV, intravenous; NG, nasogastric; NPO, nothing by mouth; WBC, white blood cell.

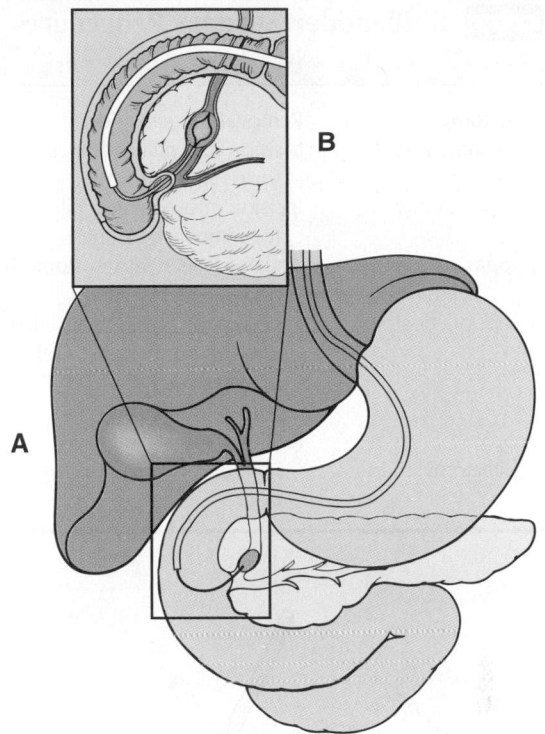

FIG. 42-18 **A,** During endoscopic sphincterotomy, an endoscope is advanced through the mouth and stomach until its tip sits in the duodenum opposite the common bile duct. **B,** After widening the duct mouth by incising the sphincter muscle, the physician advances a basket attachment into the duct and snags the stone.

ticholinergics to decrease secretions (which prevents biliary contraction) and counteract smooth muscle spasms may be administered. Analgesics are given to decrease the pain.

Cholelithiasis. There are two nonsurgical approaches for biliary stone removal. Most patients are treated by means of ERCP. Standard ERCP techniques will clear stones from the biliary tree in approximately 90% of patients. This procedure allows for visualization of the biliary system, as well as the placement of stents and sphincterotomy (papillotomy) if warranted. Endoscopic sphincterotomy is especially effective in removing common bile duct stones (Fig. 42-18). The endoscope is passed to the duodenum. With an electrodiathermy knife attached to the endoscope, the sphincter of Oddi is widened by incision of the sphincter muscle (sphincterotomy). A basket is used to retrieve the stone. The stone may be removed in the basket, but more commonly it is left in the duodenum and will be passed naturally in the stool.

If the stone is too large to pass through the duct, the endoscopist can crush the stone (mechanical lithotripsy). The limitation of this procedure is ERCP-induced acute pancreatitis. In approximately 10% of patients, nonstandard management, including peroral or percutaneous mechanical, electrohydraulic, or laser lithotripsy, will be needed. Other options for cholelithiasis include cholesterol solvents such as methyl tertiary terbutyl ether (MTBE), oral drugs that dissolve stones, endoscopic sphincterotomy, extracorporeal shock-wave lithotripsy (ESWL), and surgery. A direct-contact dissolving agent such as MTBE can be instilled into the gallbladder via a percutaneous catheter. MTBE dissolves cholesterol stones within hours. The gallstones may recur. Oral bile acids are also used to dissolve stones.

In ESWL a biliary lithotriptor uses high-energy shock waves to disintegrate gallstones. The patient must have a functioning gallbladder. An ultrasound scan is first done to locate the stones and to determine where to direct the shock waves. The shock waves are directed through the abdomen as a water-filled cushion is pressed against the area. It usually takes 1 to 2 hours to disintegrate the stones. After they are broken up, the fragments pass through the common bile duct and into the small intestine. There has been mixed success with ESWL.

Supportive treatment, similar to that given for cholecystitis, may also be necessary. If the stones cause an obstruction, additional treatment consists of replacement of fat-soluble vitamins, administration of bile salts to facilitate digestion and vitamin absorption, and a low-fat diet.

Surgical Therapy. Surgical intervention for cholelithiasis is often indicated and may consist of any one of several procedures (Table 42-25). The procedure of choice for most patients is still a cholecystectomy. This is a safe procedure with minimal morbidity, and it requires only a brief hospitalization. One procedure is removal of the gallbladder through a right subcostal incision. A T tube is inserted into the common bile duct during surgery when a common bile duct exploration is part of the surgical procedure (Fig. 42-19). This ensures patency of the duct until the edema produced by the trauma of exploring and probing the duct has sub-

TABLE 42-25	Gallbladder Surgery Procedures
NAME	**DESCRIPTION**
Cholecystectomy	Removal of gallbladder
Cholecystostomy (usually an emergency)	Incision into gallbladder (usually for removal of stones)
Choledocholithotomy	Incision into common bile duct for removal of stones
Cholecystogastrostomy	Anastomosis between stomach and gallbladder
Cholecystoduodenostomy	Anastomosis between gallbladder and duodenum to relieve obstruction at distal end of common bile duct
Laparoscopic cholecystectomy	Removal of gallbladder via laparoscopy using a dissecting laser

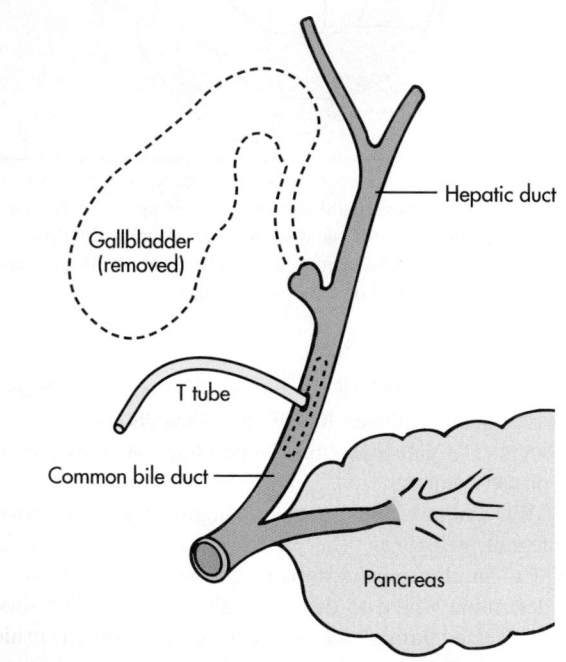

Hepatic duct

Gallbladder (removed)

T tube

Common bile duct

Pancreas

FIG. 42-19 Placement of T tube. Dotted lines indicate parts removed.

sided. It also allows the excess bile to drain while the small intestine is adjusting to receiving a continuous flow of bile.

The *laparoscopic cholecystectomy* has become the treatment of choice for cholecystectomy. Currently, approximately 92% of all cholecystectomies are performed laparoscopically. In this procedure the gallbladder is removed through one of four small punctures in the abdomen. A 1 cm puncture is made slightly above the umbilicus, and the surgeon inflates the abdominal cavity with 3 to 4 L of CO_2 to improve visibility. A laparoscope, which has a camera attached, is then inserted into the abdomen. Two additional punctures are made just below the ribs, one on the right anterior axillary line and the other on the right midclavicular line. These punctures are used for insertion of grasping forceps. A dissection laser is inserted into the fourth puncture, which is made just right of the midsection. (The incision sites

may vary.) Using closed-circuit monitors to view the abdominal cavity, the surgeon retracts and dissects the gallbladder and removes it with grasping forceps.

This procedure is relatively minor with few complications. Most patients experience minimal postoperative pain and are discharged the day of surgery or the day after. In most cases they are able to resume normal activities and return to work within 1 week.

Advantages of the laparoscopic cholecystectomy include decreased postoperative pain, shorter hospital stay, and earlier return to work and full activity. The main complication is injury to the common bile duct. There are few contraindications to laparoscopic cholecystectomy. The primary ones are peritonitis, cholangitis, gangrene or perforation of the gallbladder, portal hypertension, and serious bleeding disorders.

Transhepatic Biliary Catheter. The transhepatic biliary catheter can be used preoperatively in biliary obstruction and in hepatic dysfunction secondary to obstructive jaundice. It can also be inserted when inoperable liver, pancreatic, or bile duct carcinoma obstructs bile flow. The catheter is inserted under fluoroscopy and involves percutaneous insertion across the liver parenchyma into the common bile duct and duodenum. It decompresses obstructed extrahepatic bile ducts so that bile can flow freely. After insertion, the catheter is connected to a drainage bag. The skin around the catheter insertion site has to be cleansed daily with an antiseptic. It is important to observe for bile leakage at the insertion site. Depending on the reason the catheter was inserted, the patient may be discharged with it in place.

Drug Therapy. The most common drugs used in the treatment of gallbladder disease are analgesics, anticholinergics (antispasmodics), fat-soluble vitamins, and bile salts. Meperidine (Demerol) is used if a narcotic analgesic is required. This causes less spasm in the ducts than opiates such as morphine. Anticholinergics such as atropine and other antispasmodics may be used to relax the smooth muscle and decrease ductal tone.

If the patient has chronic gallbladder disease or any biliary tract obstruction, fat-soluble vitamins (A, D, E, and K) will probably be given. Bile salts may be administered to facilitate digestion and vitamin absorption.

For treatment of pruritus, cholestyramine (Questran) may provide relief. This is a resin that binds bile salts in the intestine, increasing their excretion in the feces. Cholestyramine is administered in powder form and should be mixed with milk or juice. Side effects include nausea, vomiting, diarrhea or constipation, and skin reactions.

Medical dissolution therapy is recommended for patients with small radiolucent stones who are mildly symptomatic and are poor surgical risks. Ursodeoxycholic acid (UDCA), ursodiol (Actigall), and chenodeoxycholic acid (CDCA, chenodiol, Chenix) may be used to dissolve the stones. The main side effects of CDCA are cramps and diarrhea, but these are usually not severe. A more serious side effect is hepatotoxicity. UDCA has fewer side effects than CDCA. Dissolution therapy may take anywhere from 6 months to 2 years for dissolution of the stones, and low-dose therapy is recommended to prevent recurrence. The drugs to dissolve the gallstones are not used as much currently because of high use of laparoscopic cholecystectomy and ERCP.

Nutritional Therapy. The major dietary modification for a patient with cholelithiasis and cholecystitis is a low-fat diet (see Table 33-4). If obesity is a problem, a reduced-calorie diet is indicated. The low-fat diet decreases stimulation of the gallbladder.

Foods that are avoided include dairy products such as whole milk, cream, butter, whole milk cheese, and ice cream; fried foods; rich pastries; gravies; and nuts. Many patients have fewer problems if they eat smaller, more frequent meals.

After a laparoscopic cholecystectomy the patient is instructed to have liquids for the rest of the day and eat light meals for a few days. If an incisional cholecystectomy is done, the patient will progress from liquids to a bland diet once bowel sounds have returned. The amount of fat in the postoperative diet depends on the patient's tolerance of fat. A low-fat diet may be helpful if the flow of bile is reduced (usually only in the early postoperative period) or if the patient is overweight. Sometimes the patient is instructed to restrict fats for 4 to 6 weeks. Otherwise, no special dietary instructions are needed other than to eat nutritious meals and avoid excessive fat intake.

NURSING MANAGEMENT
GALLBLADDER DISEASE

■ Nursing Assessment

Subjective and objective data that should be obtained from a person with gallbladder disease are presented in Table 42-26.

■ Nursing Diagnoses

Nursing diagnoses for the patient with gallbladder disease treated surgically include, but are not limited to, the following:
- acute pain *related to* surgical procedure
- ineffective therapeutic regimen management *related to* lack of knowledge of diet and postoperative management

■ Planning

The overall goals are that the patient with gallbladder disease will have (1) relief of pain and discomfort, (2) no complications postoperatively, and (3) no recurrent attacks of cholecystitis or cholelithiasis.

■ Nursing Implementation

Health Promotion. The nurse should assume responsibility for recognition of predisposing factors of gallbladder disease in general health screening. Ethnic groups in which the disease is

more common, such as Native Americans, should be taught initial manifestations and instructed to seek medical care if these manifestations occur. The patient with chronic cholecystitis does not have acute symptoms and may not seek help until jaundice and biliary obstruction occur. Earlier detection in these patients is beneficial so that they can be managed with a low-fat diet and monitored more closely.

Acute Intervention. Nursing objectives for the patient undergoing conservative therapy include relieving pain, relieving nausea and vomiting, providing comfort and emotional support, maintaining fluid and electrolyte balance and nutrition, making accurate assessments for effectiveness of treatment, and observing for complications.

The patient with acute cholecystitis or cholelithiasis is frequently experiencing severe pain. The medications ordered to relieve the pain should be given as required by the patient and before the pain becomes more severe. The nurse should assess what medications relieve the pain and how much medication is required. Observations for side effects of the medications must be part of the continued assessment. Nursing comfort measures,

TABLE 42-26	Nursing Assessment — Cholecystitis or Cholelithiasis	

Subjective Data	Objective Data
Important Health Information	**General**
Past health history: Obesity, multiparity, infection, cancer, extensive fasting, pregnancy	Fever, restlessness
Medications: Use of estrogen or oral contraceptives	**Integumentary**
Surgery or other treatments: Previous abdominal surgery	Jaundice, icteric sclera; diaphoresis
Functional Health Patterns	**Respiratory**
Health perception–health management: Positive family history; sedentary lifestyle	Tachypnea, splinting during respirations
Nutritional-metabolic: Weight loss, anorexia; indigestion, fat intolerance, nausea and vomiting, dyspepsia; chills	**Cardiovascular**
	Tachycardia
Elimination: Clay-colored stools, steatorrhea, flatulence; dark urine	**Gastrointestinal**
	Palpable gallbladder, abdominal guarding and distention
Cognitive-perceptual: Moderate to severe pain in right upper quadrant that may radiate to the back or scapula; pruritus	**Possible Findings**
	↑ Serum liver enzymes and bilirubin, absence of urobilinogen in urine, ↑ urinary bilirubin; leukocytosis, abnormal gallbladder ultrasound

such as a clean bed, comfortable positioning, and oral care, are appropriate.

Some patients have more severe nausea and vomiting than others. For these patients it may be necessary to use gastric decompression. The elimination of intake of food and fluids also prevents further stimulation of the gallbladder. Oral hygiene, care of nares, accurate intake and output measurements, and maintenance of suction should be a part of the nursing care plan for this patient. For patients with less severe nausea and vomiting, antiemetics are usually adequate. When the patient is vomiting, comfort measures such as frequent mouth rinses should be provided. Any vomitus should be immediately removed from the patient's view.

If pruritus occurs with jaundice, measures to relieve itching are necessary. Such measures include baking soda or Alpha Keri baths; lotions, such as those containing calamine; antihistamines; soft, old linen; and control of the temperature (not too hot and not too cold). The patient's nails should be kept short and clean. Patients should be taught to rub with their knuckles rather than scratch with their nails when they cannot resist scratching.

A significant portion of the nursing care plan for this patient centers on accurate assessment of progression of the symptoms and development of complications. The nurse must be knowledgeable of and observe for signs of obstruction of the ducts by stones. These include jaundice; clay-colored stools; dark, foamy urine; steatorrhea; fever; and increased WBC count.

When symptoms of obstruction are present (see Table 42-23), the nurse must be aware of the possibility of bleeding as a result of decreased prothrombin production. Common sites to observe for bleeding are the mucous membranes of the mouth, nose, gingivae, and injection sites. If injections are given, a small-gauge needle should be used and gentle pressure applied after the injection. The nurse should know the patient's prothrombin time and use this as a guide in the assessment process.

Assessment for infections includes monitoring of vital signs. A temperature elevation with chills and jaundice may indicate choledocholithiasis.

Nursing care of the patient after endoscopic papillotomy includes assessment to detect complications such as pancreatitis, perforation, infection, and bleeding. The patient's vital signs should be monitored. Abdominal pain and fever may indicate pancreatitis. The patient should be on bed rest for several hours and should have nothing by mouth until the gag reflex returns.

Postoperative care. Postoperative nursing care following a laparoscopic cholecystectomy includes monitoring for complications such as bleeding, making the patient comfortable, and preparing the patient for discharge. A common postoperative problem is referred pain to the shoulder because of the CO_2 that was not released or absorbed by the body. The CO_2 can irritate the phrenic nerve and the diaphragm, causing some difficulty breathing. Placing the patient in Sims' position (left side with right knee flexed) helps move the gas pocket away from the diaphragm. Deep breathing should be encouraged, along with movement and ambulation. There is usually minimal pain that can be relieved by narcotic analgesics such as oxycodone (Oxycontin) or codeine. The patient is allowed clear liquids and can walk to the bathroom to void. Many patients go home the same day, but some will stay overnight.

Postoperative nursing care for incisional cholecystectomy focuses on adequate ventilation and prevention of respiratory com-

---

TABLE 42-27 Patient & Family Teaching Guide

Postoperative Laparoscopic Cholecystectomy

1. Instruct patient to remove the bandages on the puncture site the day after surgery and bathe or shower.
2. Explain the need to report the following signs and symptoms:
   - Redness, swelling, bile-colored drainage or pus from any incision
   - Severe abdominal pain, nausea, vomiting, fever, chills
3. Explain that normal activities can be resumed gradually.
4. Instruct that returning to work can occur within 1 week of surgery.
5. Instruct to resume usual diet; may need to be a low-fat diet for several weeks following surgery.

---

plications. Other nursing care is the same as general postoperative nursing care (see Chapter 19).

If the patient has a T tube (see Fig. 42-19), part of the nursing care plan is related to maintaining bile drainage and observation of the T-tube functioning and drainage. The T tube is connected to a closed gravity drainage system. If the Penrose or Jackson-Pratt drain or the T tube is draining large amounts, it is helpful to use a sterile pouching system to protect the skin.

Ambulatory and Home Care. When the patient has conservative therapy, long-term nursing management depends on symptoms and on whether surgical intervention is being planned. Dietary teaching is usually necessary. The diet is usually low in fat, and sometimes a weight-reduction diet is also recommended. The patient may need to take fat-soluble vitamin supplements. The nurse should provide instructions regarding observations that the patient should make indicating obstruction (stool and urine changes, jaundice, and pruritus). Continued health care is important, and its significance should be explained and stressed.

The patient who undergoes a laparoscopic cholecystectomy is discharged soon after the surgery, so home care is important. Teaching is essential (Table 42-27).

After an open-incision cholecystectomy, the patient may be discharged as soon as 2 to 3 days. The patient should be instructed to avoid heavy lifting for 4 to 6 weeks. Usual sexual activities, including intercourse, can be resumed as soon as the patient feels ready unless given other instructions by the physician.

Sometimes the patient is required to remain on a low-fat diet for 4 to 6 weeks. If so, a dietary teaching plan is necessary. A weight-reduction program may be helpful if the patient is overweight. Most patients tolerate a regular diet with no difficulties but should avoid excessive fats.

■ Evaluation

The overall expected outcomes are that the patient with gallbladder disease will
- appear comfortable and verbalize pain relief
- verbalize knowledge of activity level and dietary restrictions

GALLBLADDER CANCER

Primary cancer of the gallbladder is uncommon. The majority of gallbladder carcinomas are adenocarcinomas. There seems to be a definite relationship between cancer of the gallbladder and chronic cholecystitis and cholelithiasis. The early symptoms of carcinoma of the gallbladder are insidious and are similar to those of chronic cholecystitis and cholelithiasis, which makes diagnosis difficult. Later symptoms are usually those of biliary obstruction.

Diagnosis and staging of gallbladder cancer is done using endoscopic ultrasound, transabdominal ultrasound, CT, MRI, and/or MR cholangiopancreatography. Unfortunately, gallbladder cancer often presents with advanced disease.[35] When found early, surgery can be curative. Several factors influence successful surgical outcomes, including the depth of cancer invasion, extent of liver involvement, presence of venous or lymphatic invasion, and lymph node metastasis. Extended cholecystectomy with lymph node dissection has improved the outcomes for patients with gallbladder cancer. When surgery is not an option, endoscopic stenting of the biliary tree to reduce obstructive jaundice may be warranted. Adjuvant therapies including radiation therapy and chemotherapy may be used depending on the disease state. Overall cancer of the gallbladder has a poor prognosis.

Nursing management involves supportive care with special attention to nutrition, hydration, skin care, and pain relief. Many of the nursing care measures used for patients with cholecystitis and cholelithiasis are frequently applied, as well as nursing care measures for the patient with cancer (see Chapter 15).

CRITICAL THINKING EXERCISES

Case Study
Cirrhosis of the Liver
Patient Profile. Mr. Begay is a 55-year-old Native American man admitted with a diagnosis of cirrhosis of the liver.

Subjective Data
- Has had cirrhosis for 12 years
- Acknowledges that he had been drinking heavily for 20 years but has been sober for the past 2 years
- Complains of anorexia, nausea, and abdominal discomfort

Objective Data
Physical Examination
- Thin and malnourished
- Has moderate ascites
- Has jaundice of sclera and skin
- Has 4+ pitting edema of the lower extremities
- Liver and spleen are palpable

Laboratory Values
- Total bilirubin: 15 mg/dl (257 mmol/L)
- Serum ammonia: 220 mg/dl (122 mmol/L)
- AST: 190 U/L (3.2 μkat/L)
- ALT: 210 U/L (3.5 μkat/L)

CRITICAL THINKING QUESTIONS
1. What are possible causes of cirrhosis? What type of cirrhosis does Mr. Begay probably have?
2. Describe the pathophysiologic changes that occur in the liver as cirrhosis develops.
3. List Mr. Begay's clinical manifestations of liver failure. For each manifestation, explain the pathophysiologic basis.
4. Explain the significance of the results of his laboratory values.
5. If Mr. Begay begins to manifest signs and symptoms of hepatic encephalopathy, what would you monitor? What measures should be instituted to control or decrease the ammonia level?
6. Mr. Begay was being closely observed for the possibility of gastrointestinal bleeding. Why is this considered a possible complication?
7. In the early stages of cirrhosis, what can be done to control the disease?
8. Based on the assessment data presented, write one or more nursing diagnoses. Are there any collaborative problems?

Nursing Research Issues
1. What is the most effective way to assess jaundice in a dark-skinned person?
2. What are the most significant psychosocial problems experienced by a patient with viral hepatitis?
3. What are the best ways to treat pruritus associated with jaundice in patients with hepatitis?
4. What is the quality of life for a patient after a liver transplant?
5. Can nutritional support improve outcomes in patients with alcohol-related cirrhosis?
6. What support resources are needed by the family of a patient with pancreatic cancer?

REVIEW QUESTIONS

The number of the question corresponds to the same-numbered objective at the beginning of the chapter.

1. During assessment of a patient with obstructive jaundice the nurse would expect to find
   a. clay-colored stools.
   b. dark urine and stools.
   c. pyrexia and severe pruritus.
   d. elevated urinary urobilinogen.

2. A patient with hepatitis A is in the prodromal (pre-icteric) phase. The nurse plans care for the patient based on the knowledge that
   a. pruritus is a common problem with jaundice in this phase.
   b. the patient is most likely to transmit the disease during this phase.
   c. gastrointestinal symptoms are not as severe in hepatitis A as they are in hepatitis B.
   d. extrahepatic manifestations of glomerulonephritis and polyarteritis are common in this phase.

3. A patient with hepatitis B is being discharged in 2 days. The nurse includes in the discharge teaching plan instructions to
   a. avoid alcohol for 3 weeks.
   b. use a condom during sexual intercourse.
   c. have family members get an injection of immunoglobulin.
   d. follow a low-protein, moderate-carbohydrate, moderate-fat diet.

4. The patient with advanced cirrhosis asks the nurse why his abdomen is so swollen. The nurse's response to the patient is based on the knowledge that
   a. a lack of clotting factors promotes the collection of blood in the abdominal cavity.
   b. portal hypertension and hypoalbuminemia cause a fluid shift into the peritoneal space.
   c. decreased peristalsis in the GI tract contributes to gas formation and distention of the bowel.
   d. bile salts in the blood irritate the peritoneal membranes, causing edema and pocketing of fluid.

5. When caring for a patient with hepatic encephalopathy, the nurse may give enemas, provide a low-protein diet, and limit physical activity. These measures are done to
   a. promote fluid loss.
   b. decrease portal pressure.
   c. eliminate potassium ions.
   d. decrease the production of ammonia.

6. In planning care for a patient with metastatic cancer of the liver, the nurse includes interventions that
   a. focus primarily on symptomatic and comfort measures.
   b. reassure the patient that chemotherapy offers a good prognosis for recovery.
   c. promote the patient's confidence that surgical excision of the tumor will be successful.
   d. provide information necessary for the patient to make decisions regarding liver transplantation.

7. The nurse explains to the patient with acute pancreatitis that the most common pathogenic mechanism of the disorder is
   a. cellular disorganization.
   b. overproduction of enzymes.
   c. lack of secretion of enzymes.
   d. autodigestion of the pancreas.

8. Nursing management of the patient with acute pancreatitis includes
   a. checking for signs of hypercalcemia.
   b. observing stools for signs of steatorrhea.
   c. providing a diet low in carbohydrates with moderate fat.
   d. monitoring for infection, particularly respiratory infection.

9. A patient with pancreatic cancer is admitted to the hospital for evaluation for treatment. The patient asks the nurse to explain the Whipple procedure the surgeon has described. The nurse's explanation includes the information that a Whipple procedure involves
   a. creating a bypass around the obstruction caused by the tumor by joining the gallbladder to the jejunum.
   b. resection of the entire pancreas and the distal portion of the stomach, with anastomosis of the common bile duct and stomach into the duodenum.
   c. removal of part of the pancreas, part of the stomach, the duodenum, and the gallbladder, with joining of the pancreatic duct, common bile duct, and stomach into the jejunum.
   d. radical removal of the pancreas, duodenum, and spleen, attaching the stomach to the jejunum, which requires oral supplementation of pancreatic digestive enzymes and insulin replacement therapy.

10. The nursing management of the patient with cholecystitis associated with cholelithiasis is based on the knowledge that
    a. a low-fat diet is recommended.
    b. gallstones once removed tend not to recur.
    c. meperidine is to be avoided in the management of pain.
    d. the disorder can be successfully treated with oral bile salts that dissolve gallstones.

11. Teaching in relation to home management following a laparoscopic cholecystectomy should include
    a. keeping the bandages on the puncture sites for 48 hours.
    b. reporting any bile-colored drainage or pus from any incision.
    c. using over-the-counter antiemetics if nausea and vomiting occur.
    d. emptying and measuring the contents of the bile bag from the T tube every day.

REFERENCES

1. National Center for Infection Control: Hepatitis. Available at *www.cdc.gov/ncidod/diseases/hepatitis*. Site last accessed December 28, 2002.
2. Alter MJ et al: The epidemiology of hepatitis C. In Liang TJ, Hoofnagle JH, editors: *Hepatitis C*, Boston, 2000, Academic Press.
3. Wasley A, Alter MJ: Epidemiology of hepatitis C: geographic differences and temporal trends, *Semin Liver Dis* 20:1, 2000.
4. Rehermann B: Immunopathogenesis of hepatitis C. In Liang TJ, Hoofnagle JH, editors: *Hepatitis C*, Boston 2000, Academic Press.
5. Wong JB et al: Estimating future hepatitis C morbidity, mortality, and costs in the United States, *Am J Public Health* 90:1562, 2000.
6. Williams I: Epidemiology of hepatitis C in the United States, *Am J Med* 27:2S, 1999.
7. Goldman M, Spurll G: Hepatitis C lookback, *Curr Opin Hematol* 7:392, 2000.
8. Patrick DM et al: Public health and hepatitis C, *Can J Public Health* 91(suppl 1):S18, 2000.
9. Thorpe LE et al: Hepatitis C virus infection: prevalence, risk factors, and prevention opportunities among young injection drug users in Chicago, 1997-1999, *J Infect Dis* 182:1588, 2000.
10. Diaz T et al: Several factors associated with prevalent hepatitis C virus infection differ among young adult injection drug users in lower and upper Manhattan, New York City, *Am J Public Health* 91:23, 2001.
11. Giulivi A et al: Prevalence of GBV-C/hepatitis G virus viremia and anti-E2 in Canadian blood donors, *Vox Sang* 79:201, 2000.
12. Dougherty AS, Dreher HM: Hepatitis C: current treatment strategies for an emerging epidemic, *Medsurg Nurs* 10:9, 2001.
13. Torresi J, Locarnini S: Antiviral chemotherapy for the treatment of hepatitis B virus infections, *Gastroenterology* 118:S83, 2000.
14. Dienstag JL et al: Lamivudine as initial treatment for chronic hepatitis B in the United States, *N Engl J Med* 341:1256, 1999.
15. Perry CM, Jarvis B: Peginterferon-alpha-2a (40kD): a review of its use in the management of chronic hepatitis C, *Drugs* 61:2263, 2001.
16. Wilkinson T: Hepatitis C virus: prospects for future therapies, *Curr Opin Investig Drugs* 2:1516, 2001.
17. Prevention of hepatitis A through active or passive immunization: recommendations of the Advisory Committee on Immunization Practices, *MMWR Morb Mortal Wkly Rep* 48(RR12):1, 1999.
18. FDA approval for a combined hepatitis A and B vaccine, *MMWR Morb Mortal Wkly Rep* 50:806, 2001.
19. Beltrami EM et al: Risk and management of bloodborne infections in health-care workers, *Clin Microbiol Rev* 13:385, 2000.
20. Riley TR, Bhatti AM: Preventive strategies in chronic liver disease: alcohol, vaccines, toxic medications and supplements, diet and exercise, *Am Fam Physician* 64:1555, 2001.
21. McCormick PA, O'Keefe C: Improving prognosis following a first variceal haemorrhage over four decades, *Gut* 49:682, 2001.
22. Butterworth RF: Neurotransmitter dysfunction in hepatic encephalopathy: new approaches and new findings, *Metab Brain Dis* 16.55, 2001.
23. Klempnaue J, Schrem H: Review: surgical shunts and encephalopathy, *Metab Brain Dis* 16:21, 2001.
24. Wong F, Blendis L: New challenge of hepatorenal syndrome: prevention and treatment, *Hepatology* 34:1242, 2001.
25. Brandenburger LA et al: Variceal hemorrhage, *Curr Treat Options Gastroenterol* 5:73, 2002.
26. Anand BS: Drug treatment of the complications of cirrhosis in the older adult, *Drugs Aging* 18:575, 2001.
27. Rosen HR: Hepatitis B and C in the liver transplant recipient: current understanding and treatment, *Liver Transpl* 7(11 suppl 1):S87, 2001.
28. American Cancer Society: *Facts and figures 2002*, Atlanta, Ga, 2002. Available at *www.cancer.org*. (accessed Dec 28, 2002).
29. Cole L: Unraveling the mystery of acute pancreatitis, *Nursing* 31:58, 2001.
30. Smotkin J, Tenner S: Laboratory diagnostic tests in acute pancreatitis, *J Clin Gastroenterol* 34:459, 2002.
31. Brand R: The diagnosis of pancreatic cancer, *Cancer J* 7:287, 2001.
32. Kozuch P, Grossbard ML, Barzdins A: Irinotecan combined with gemcitabine, 5-fluorouracil, leucovorin, and cisplatin (G-FLIP) is an effective and noncrossresistant treatment for chemotherapy refractory metastatic pancreatic cancer, *Oncologist* 6:488, 2001.
33. Heinemann V: Gemcitabine-based combination treatment of pancreatic cancer, *Semin Oncol* 29:25, 2002.
34. Farrar JA: Acute cholecystitis, *Am J Nurs* 101:35, 2001.
35. Dawes LG: Gallbladder cancer, *Cancer Treat Res* 109:145, 2001.

RESOURCES

American Association for the Study of Liver Diseases (AASLD)
1729 King Street, Suite 200
Alexandria, VA 22314
703-299-9766
Fax: 703-299-9622
www.aasld.org

American Gastroenterological Association
7910 Woodmont Avenue, Seventh Floor
Bethesda, MD 20814
301-654-2055
Fax: 301-652-3890
www.gastro.org

American Liver Foundation
75 Maiden Lane, Suite 603
New York, NY 10038
800-GO-LIVER (465-4837)
www.liverfoundation.org

United Ostomy Association
19772 MacArthur Boulevard, Suite 200
Irvine, CA 92612-2405
800-826-0826
www.uoa.org

For additional Internet resources, see the website for this book at *http://evolve.elsevier.com/Lewis/medsurg/*.

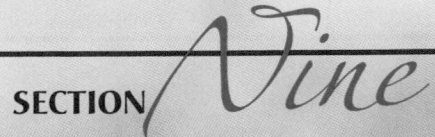

Problems of Urinary Function

SECTION OUTLINE

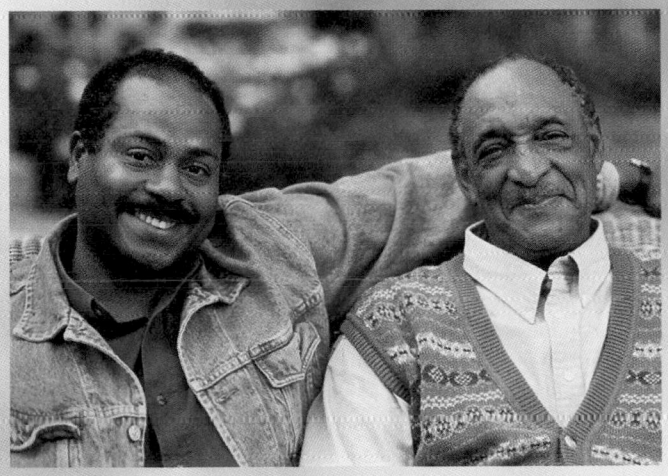

CHAPTER *43*

NURSING ASSESSMENT
Urinary System

Mikel Gray

LEARNING OBJECTIVES

1. Describe the anatomic location and functions of the kidneys, ureters, bladder, and urethra.
2. Explain the physiologic events involved in the formation and passage of urine from glomerular filtration to voiding.
3. Identify the significant subjective and objective data related to the urinary system that should be obtained from a patient.
4. Describe age-related changes in the urinary system and differences in assessment findings.
5. Describe the appropriate techniques used in the physical assessment of the urinary system.
6. Differentiate normal from common abnormal findings of a physical assessment of the urinary system.
7. Describe the purpose, significance of results, and nursing responsibilities related to diagnostic studies of the urinary system.
8. Describe the normal physical and chemical characteristics of urine.

KEY TERMS

costovertebral angle, p. 1161	intravenous pyelogram, p. 1167
creatinine, p. 1166	nephron, p. 1152
cystometrogram, p. 1170	renal arteriogram, p. 1168
cystoscopy, p. 1169	renal biopsy, p. 1169
glomerular filtration rate, p. 1154	retrograde pyelogram, p. 1167
glomerulus, p. 1153	urinalysis, p. 1162

"Bones can break, muscles can atrophy, glands can loaf, even the brain can go to sleep without immediate danger to survival. But should the kidneys fail . . . neither bone, muscle, gland, nor brain could carry on."[1] This statement underlines the importance of kidneys to our lives. Adequate functioning of the kidneys is essential to the maintenance of a healthy body. If there is complete kidney failure and treatment is not given, death is inevitable.

The kidneys are the principal organs of the urinary system. In addition to the two kidneys, the urinary system consists of two ureters, a urinary bladder, and a urethra (Fig. 43-1). The other organs can be thought of as storage and drainage channels for the urine after it is formed by the kidneys.

The primary functions of the kidneys are (1) to regulate the volume and composition of extracellular fluid (ECF) and (2) excrete waste products from the body. Additional functions of the kidneys include blood pressure control, erythropoietin production, vitamin D activation, and acid-base balance regulation.

STRUCTURES AND FUNCTIONS OF THE URINARY SYSTEM

Kidneys

Macrostructure. The paired kidneys are bean-shaped organs that are retroperitoneal (behind the peritoneum) on either side of the vertebral column at about the level of the twelfth thoracic (T12) vertebra to the third lumbar (L3) vertebra. Each kidney weighs 4 to 6 ounces (115 to 175 g) and is about 5 inches (12 cm) long. The right kidney, with the liver above it, is lower than the left. The right kidney is at the level of the twelfth rib. An adrenal gland lies on top of each kidney.

Each kidney is surrounded by a considerable amount of fat and connective tissue that serves to support and maintain its position. The surface of the kidney is covered by a thin, smooth layer of fibrous membrane called the *capsule.* These structures protect the kidney and serve as a shock absorber should the kidney be subjected to a sudden force from a blunt object striking the abdomen or back. The *hilus* on the medial side of the kidney serves as the entry site for the renal artery and nerves, as well as the exit site for the renal vein and ureter.

On a longitudinal section of the kidney (Fig. 43-2), the parenchyma (actual tissue) of the kidney can be visualized. The outer layer is termed the *cortex,* and the inner layer is called the *medulla.* The medulla consists of a number of pyramids. The apices of these pyramids are called *papillae,* through which urine passes to enter the calyces. The minor calyces widen and merge to form major calyces, which form a funnel-shaped sac called the *renal pelvis.* The minor and major calyces transport urine to the renal pelvis in preparation for transportation to the bladder via the ureter. The pelvis of the kidney can store a small volume of urine (3 to 5 ml).

Microstructure. The functional unit of the kidney is termed the **nephron.** Each kidney has more than 1 million nephrons. A nephron is composed of a glomerulus, Bowman's capsule, and tubular system. The tubular system consists of the proximal convoluted tubule, the loop of Henle, and the distal convoluted tubule (Fig. 43-3). Several nephrons converge into a collecting duct, which eventually merges into a pyramid and empties via the papilla into a minor calyx.

The glomeruli, Bowman's capsule, proximal tubule, and distal tubule are located in the cortex of the kidney. The loop of Henle and the collecting ducts are located in the medulla.

Blood Supply. A blood supply of about 1200 ml per minute, which is 20% to 25% of the cardiac output, flows to the two kidneys. Blood reaches the kidneys via the renal artery, which arises from the aorta and enters the kidney through the hilus. The renal artery divides into secondary branches and then into still smaller branches,

Reviewed by Vicki Y. Johnson, RN, PhD, FN, CUCNS, Assistant Professor, University of Alabama, School of Nursing, Birmingham, Ala.

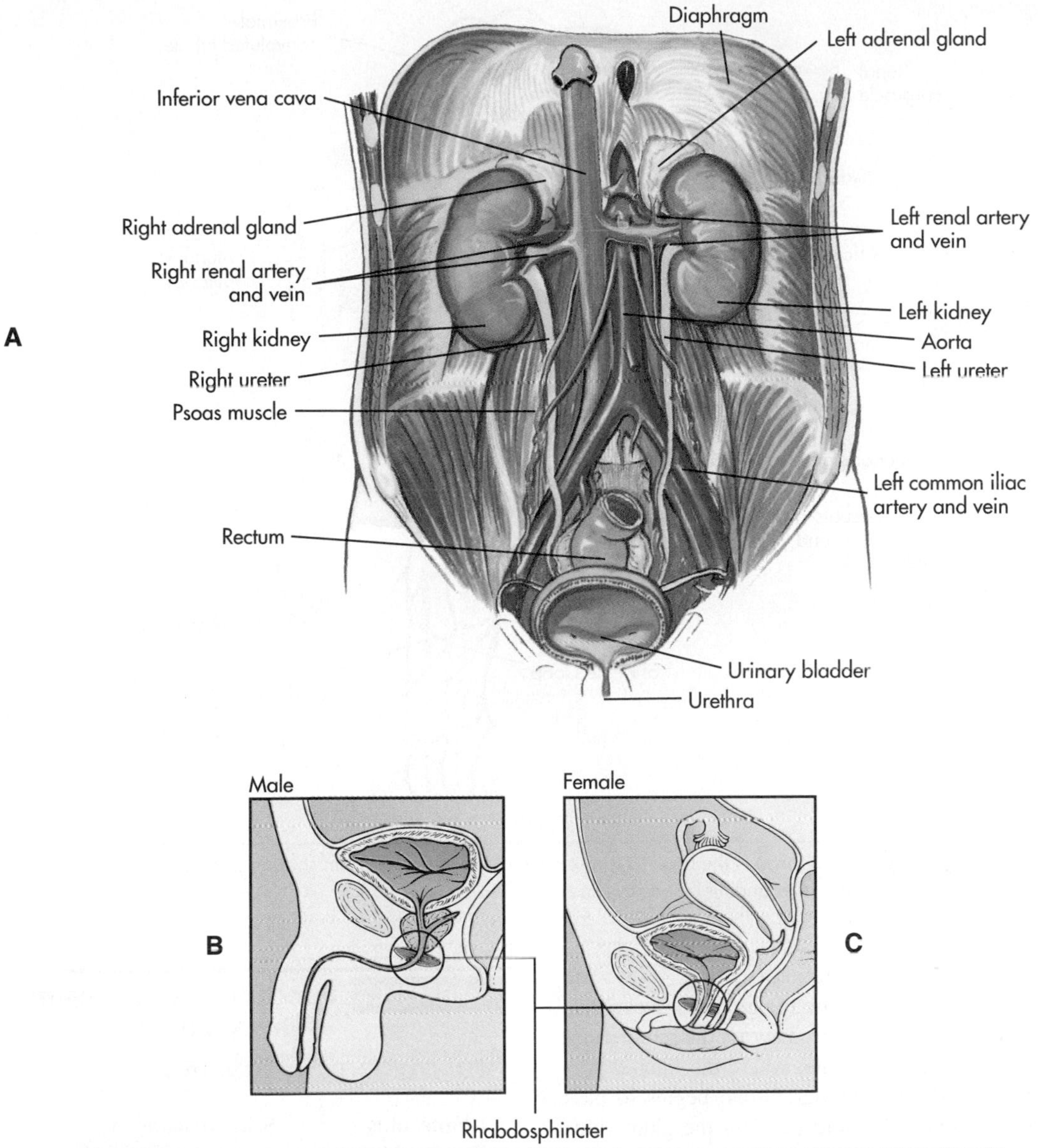

Diaphragm

Left adrenal gland

Inferior vena cava

Right adrenal gland

Right renal artery and vein

Left renal artery and vein

Right kidney

Left kidney

Right ureter

Aorta

Psoas muscle

Left ureter

Rectum

Left common iliac artery and vein

A

Urinary bladder

Urethra

Male

Female

B

C

Rhabdosphincter

FIG. 43-1 Organs of the urinary system. **A,** Upper urinary tract in relation to other anatomic structures. **B,** Male urethra in relation to other pelvic structures. **C,** Female urethra.

each of which eventually forms an afferent arteriole. The afferent arteriole divides into a capillary network termed the *glomerulus,* which is a tuft of up to 50 capillaries (see Fig. 43-3). The capillaries of the glomerulus eventually unite in the efferent arteriole. This arteriole splits to form a capillary network called the peritubular capillaries, which, as the name suggests, surround the tubular system. All peritubular capillaries eventually drain into the venous system. The renal vein empties into the inferior vena cava.

Physiology of Urine Formation. The process of urine formation is extremely complex. It represents the outcome of a multistep process of filtration, reabsorption, secretion, and excretion of water, electrolytes, and metabolic waste products. Although urine formation is the result of this process, the primary function of the kidneys is to filter the blood and maintain the body's internal homeostasis.[2]

Glomerular function. Urine formation starts at the glomerulus, where blood is filtered. The **glomerulus,** which is a semi-

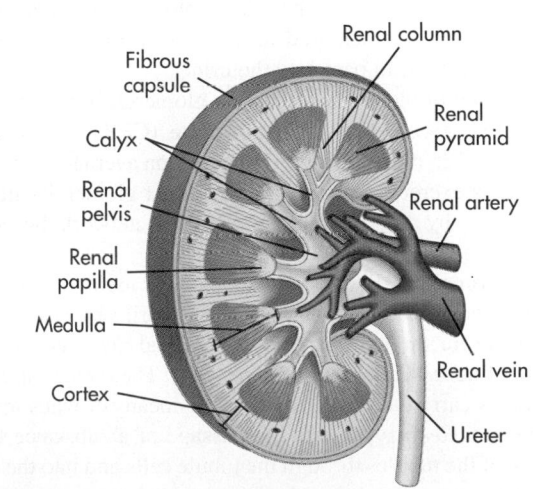

Fibrous capsule

Renal column

Renal pyramid

Calyx

Renal pelvis

Renal artery

Renal papilla

Medulla

Renal vein

Cortex

Ureter

FIG. 43-2 Longitudinal section of the kidney.

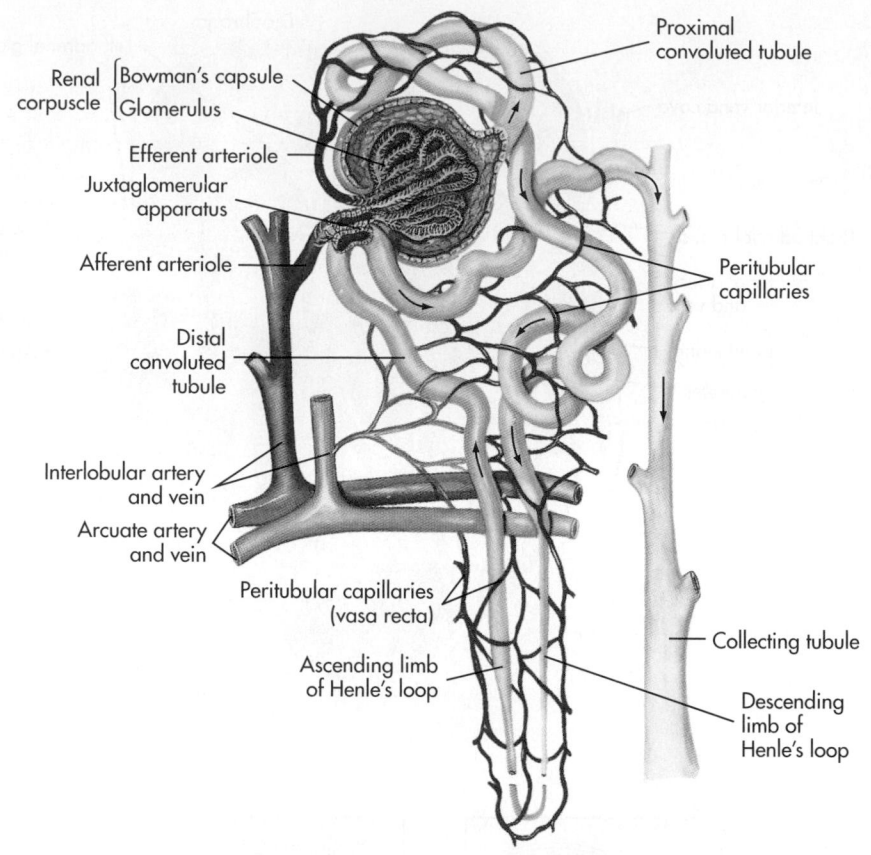

FIG. 43-3   The nephron is the basic functional unit of the kidney. This illustration of a single nephron unit also shows the surrounding blood vessels.

permeable membrane, allows for filtration (see Fig. 43-3). The hydrostatic pressure of the blood within the glomerular capillaries causes a portion of blood to be filtered across the semipermeable membrane into Bowman's capsule, where the filtered portion of the blood called the glomerular filtrate begins to pass down to the tubule. Filtration is more rapid in the glomerulus than in ordinary tissue capillaries because of the porosity of the glomerular membrane. The ultrafiltrate is similar in composition to blood except that it lacks blood cells, platelets, and large plasma proteins. Under normal conditions the capillary pores are too small to allow the loss of these large blood components. Capillary permeability is increased in many renal diseases, permitting plasma proteins to pass into the urine.

The amount of blood filtered by the glomeruli in a given time is termed the **glomerular filtration rate** (GFR). The normal GFR is about 125 ml per minute. However, on average, only 1 ml per minute is excreted as urine because most glomerular filtrate is reabsorbed by the peritubular capillary network before it reaches the end of the collecting duct.

Tubular function. Because the glomerular membrane is a selective filtration membrane that filters primarily by size, provision is made for the reabsorption of essential materials and the excretion of nonessential ones (Table 43-1). The tubules and collecting ducts carry out these functions by means of reabsorption and secretion. *Reabsorption* is the passage of a substance from the lumen of the tubules through the tubule cells and into the capillaries. This process involves both active and passive transport. Tubular *secretion* is the passage of a substance from the capillaries through the tubular cells into the lumen of the tubule. Reab-

TABLE 43-1	**Functions of the Segments of the Nephron**
COMPONENT	**FUNCTION**
Glomerulus	Selective filtration
Proximal tubule	Reabsorption of 80% of electrolytes and water; reabsorption of all glucose and amino acids; reabsorption of HCO_3^-; secretion of H^+ and creatinine
Loop of Henle	Reabsorption of Na^+ and Cl^- in ascending limb; reabsorption of water in descending loop; concentration of filtrate
Distal tubule	Secretion of K^+, H^+, ammonia; reabsorption of water (regulated by ADH); reabsorption of HCO_3^-; regulation of Ca^{2+} and PO_4^{2-} by parathyroid hormone, regulation of Na^+ and K^+ by aldosterone
Collecting duct	Reabsorption of water (ADH required)

ADH, Antidiuretic hormone; Ca^{2+}, calcium; Cl^-, chloride; H^+, hydrogen; HCO_3^-, bicarbonate; K^+, potassium; Na^+, sodium; PO_4^{2-}, phosphate.

sorption and secretion occur along the entire length of the tubule, causing numerous changes in the composition of the glomerular filtrate as it moves through the tubules.

In the proximal convoluted tubule, about 80% of the electrolytes are reabsorbed. Normally, all the glucose, amino acids, and small proteins are reabsorbed. For the most part, reabsorption occurs by active transport. Hydrogen ions (H$^+$) and creatinine are secreted into the filtrate.[3]

The loop of Henle is important in conserving water and thus concentrating the filtrate. In the loop of Henle, reabsorption continues. The descending loop is permeable to water and moderately permeable to sodium, urea, and other solutes. In the ascending limb, chloride ions (Cl$^-$) are actively reabsorbed, followed passively by sodium ions (Na$^+$). About 25% of the filtered sodium is reabsorbed here.

Two important functions of the distal convoluted tubules are final regulation of water balance and acid-base balance. Antidiuretic hormone (ADH), released by the posterior pituitary gland, is required for water reabsorption. The stimuli for ADH release are increased serum osmolality and decreased blood volume. ADH makes the distal convoluted tubules and the collecting ducts permeable to water, allowing it to be reabsorbed into the peritubular capillaries and to be eventually returned to circulation. In the absence of ADH the tubules are practically impermeable to water, and any water in the tubules leaves the body as urine.

In the presence of aldosterone (released from the adrenal cortex) acting on the distal tubule, reabsorption of Na$^+$ and water occurs. In exchange for Na$^+$, potassium ions (K$^+$) are excreted. The secretion of aldosterone is influenced by both circulating blood volume and plasma concentrations of Na$^+$ and K$^+$.

Acid-base regulation involves reabsorbing and conserving most of the bicarbonate (HCO$_3^-$) and secreting excess H$^+$. The distal tubule functions in different ways to maintain the pH of ECF within a range of 7.35 to 7.45 (see Chapter 16).

Atrial natriuretic factor (ANF) is a hormone secreted from cells in the right atrium when right atrial blood pressure increases. ANF inhibits the secretion and effect of ADH and results in a large volume of dilute urine (see Chapter 46).

Parathyroid hormone is released from the parathyroid gland in response to low serum calcium levels. It causes increased tubular reabsorption of calcium ions (Ca^{2+}) and decreased tubular reabsorption of phosphate ions (PO$_4^{2-}$). Therefore serum Ca^{2+} levels are increased.

The basic function of nephrons is to clean or clear blood plasma of unnecessary substances. After the glomerulus has filtered the blood, the tubules separate the unwanted from the wanted portions of tubular fluid. The necessary portions are returned to the blood, and the unnecessary portions pass into urine.

Other Functions of the Kidney. In addition to their function in regulating the volume and composition of ECF, the kidneys also have other vital functions, including the production of erythropoietin, production and secretion of renin, and activation of vitamin D.

Erythropoietin is produced and released in response to hypoxia and decreased renal blood flow. Erythropoietin stimulates the production of red blood cells (RBCs) in the bone marrow. A deficiency of erythropoietin leads to anemia in renal failure.

Vitamin D is a hormone that can be obtained in the diet or synthesized by the action of ultraviolet radiation on cholesterol in the skin. These forms of vitamin D are inactive and require two more steps to become metabolically active. The first step in activation occurs in the liver. The second step occurs in the kidneys. Active vitamin D is essential for the absorption of calcium from the gastrointestinal (GI) tract. The patient with renal failure has a deficiency of the active metabolite of vitamin D and manifests problems of altered calcium and phosphate balance (see Chapter 45).

Renin is important in the regulation of blood pressure. Renin is released from the *juxtaglomerular apparatus* of the nephron (Fig. 43-4). Renin is released in response to decreased arterial blood pressure, renal ischemia, ECF depletion, increased norepinephrine, and increased urinary Na$^+$ concentration. Renin catalyzes the splitting of the plasma protein angiotensinogen (from the liver) into angiotensin I, which is subsequently converted to angiotensin II by a converting enzyme made in the lungs. Angiotensin II stimulates the release of aldosterone from the adrenal cortex, which causes Na$^+$ and water retention, leading to an increased ECF volume. Angiotensin II also causes increased peripheral vasoconstriction. The increase in ECF and vasoconstriction causes an elevation in blood pressure, which should inhibit renin release. Excessive renin production caused by impaired re-

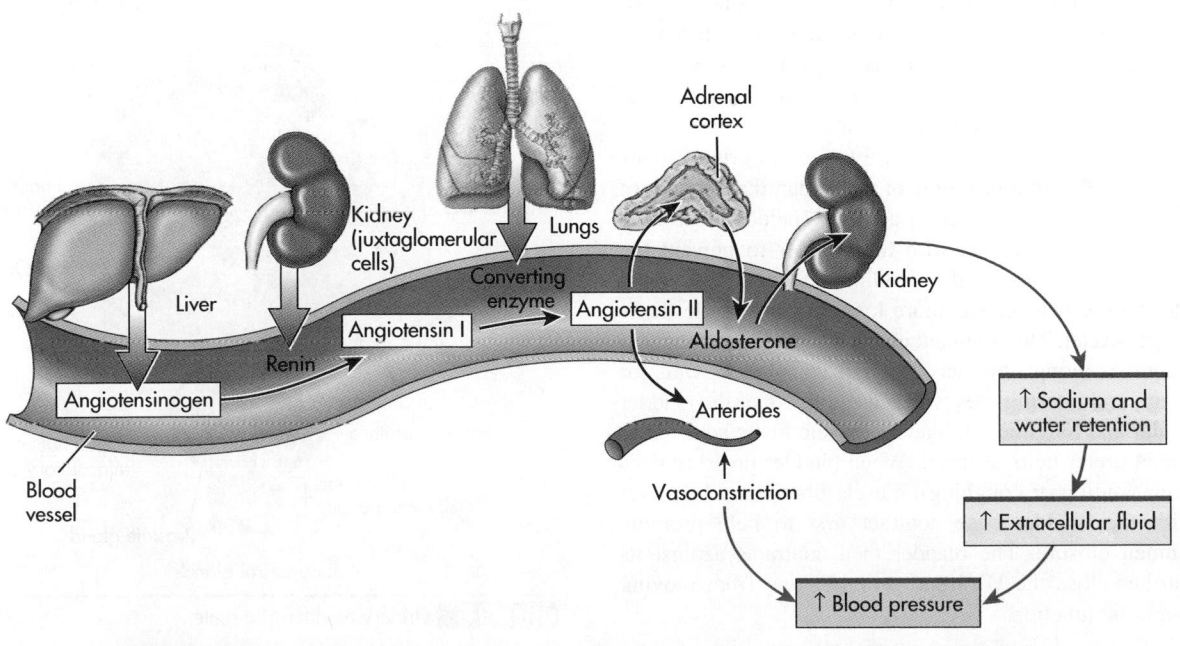

FIG. 43-4 Renin-angiotensin-aldosterone system.

nal perfusion may be a contributing factor in the etiology of hypertension (see Chapters 32 and 45).

Prostaglandins (PGs) are synthesized by most body tissues from the precursor, arachidonic acid, in response to appropriate stimuli. PGs, which are involved in the regulation of cell function and host defenses, exert their influence primarily on cells or tissues that are close to the site where they are synthesized. (See Chapter 12 and Fig. 12-7 for a more detailed discussion of PGs.)

In the kidney, PG synthesis (primarily PGE_2 and PGI_2) occurs primarily in the medulla. These PGs have a vasodilating action in addition to increasing renal blood flow and promoting Na^+ excretion. They counteract the vasoconstrictor effect of substances such as angiotensin and norepinephrine. Renal PGs may have a systemic effect in lowering blood pressure by decreasing systemic vascular resistance.[4]

The significance of these PGs is related to the role of the kidneys in causing hypertension. In renal failure with a loss of functioning tissue, these renal vasodilator factors are also lost. This may be one factor that contributes to the common finding of hypertension in renal failure (see Chapter 45).

Ureters

The ureters are tubes approximately 10 to 12 inches (25 to 35 cm) long and 0.08 to 0.3 inch (0.2 to 0.8 cm) in diameter that carry urine from the renal pelvis to the bladder (see Fig. 43-1). The narrow area where the ureter joins the renal pelvis is termed the *ureteropelvic junction.* After coursing down along the psoas muscle, the ureter crosses over the pelvic brim and iliac artery and inserts into the base of the bladder at the *ureterovesical junction* (UVJ). The ureteral lumen is narrowest at these junctions; consequently, they are often the sites of urinary stone (calculi) obstruction. Because the lumen of the ureter is narrow, it can be easily occluded internally (e.g., calculi) or externally (e.g., tumors, adhesions, inflammation).

Sympathetic and parasympathetic nerves, along with the vascular supply, surround the mucosal lining of the ureter. Circular and longitudinal smooth muscle fibers are arranged in a meshlike outer layer and contract to promote the peristaltic one-way flow of urine. These muscle contractions can be affected by distention and neurologic, endocrine, and pharmacologic factors. Stimulation of these nerves during passage of a stone or clot may cause acute, severe pain termed *renal colic.*

Because the renal pelvis holds only 3 to 5 ml of urine, kidney damage can result from a backflow of more than that amount of urine. The UVJ relies on the ureter's angle of bladder penetration and muscle fiber attachments with the bladder to prevent the backflow of urine *(reflux)* and ascending infection. The distal ureter entering the bladder has more longitudinal muscle fibers than the upper ureter. This segment enters the bladder laterally at its base, courses along obliquely through the bladder wall for about 1.5 cm, and intermingles with muscle fibers of the bladder base. Circular and longitudinal bladder muscle fibers adjacent to the imbedded ureter help secure it. When bladder pressure rises (e.g., during voiding or coughing), muscle fibers that the ureter shares with the bladder base contract first to help promote ureteral lumen closure. The bladder then contracts against its base to further close the UVJ and prevent urine from moving back through the junction.

Bladder

The urinary bladder is a distensible organ positioned behind the symphysis pubis and anterior to the vagina and rectum (Fig. 43-5). Its primary functions are to serve as a reservoir for urine and to help the body eliminate waste products. Normal adult urine output is approximately 1500 ml per day, which varies with food and fluid intake. The volume of urine produced at night is less than half of that formed during the day because of hormonal influences (e.g., ADH). This diurnal pattern of urination is normal. Most people urinate five to six times during the day and occasionally at night.

The triangular area formed by the two ureteral openings and the bladder neck at the base of the bladder is termed the *trigone.* It is affixed to the pelvis by many ligaments, and it does not change its shape during bladder filling or emptying. The bladder muscle, termed the *detrusor,* is composed of layers of intertwined smooth muscle fibers and is capable of considerable distention during bladder filling and contraction during emptying. It is affixed to the abdominal wall by an umbilical ligament. Consequently, as the bladder fills, it rises toward the umbilicus. The dome, anterior, and lateral aspects of the bladder expand and contract. When the bladder is empty, it appears as multiple folds within the pelvis.

On the average, 200 to 250 ml of urine in the bladder causes moderate distention and the urge to urinate. When the quantity of urine reaches about 400 to 600 ml, the person feels uncomfortable. Bladder capacity varies with the individual, usually ranging from 600 to 1000 ml. Evacuation of urine is termed *urination, micturition,* or *voiding.*

The bladder has the same mucosal lining as that of the renal pelvis, ureter, and bladder neck. It is called transitional cell epithelium or urothelium and is unique to the urinary tract. Transitional cell epithelium is resistant to absorption of urine. Therefore urinary wastes produced by the kidneys do not leak out of the urinary system after they leave the kidneys. Microscopically, transitional cell epithelium is several cells deep. These cells

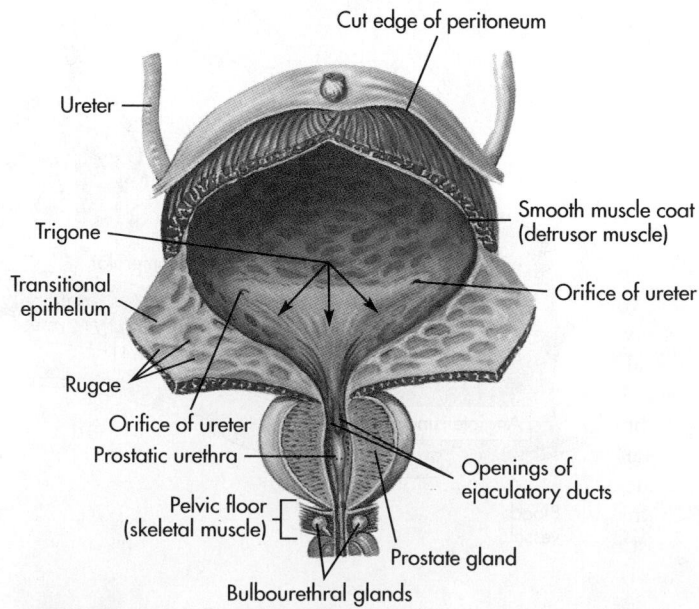

FIG. 43-5 Urinary bladder of a male.

stretch out in the bladder to only a few cells deep as it accommodates filling. As the bladder empties, the epithelium resumes its multicellular layer formation.

Because the lining is the same, transitional cell tumors that occur in one section of the urinary tract can easily metastasize to other urinary tract areas. Malignant cells may move down from upper urinary tract tumors and imbed in the bladder, or large bladder tumors can invade the ureter. Tumor recurrence within the bladder is common. Intact urothelium also has phagocytic properties, although the exact mechanism is unknown.

Urethra

The urethra is a small muscular tube that leads from the bladder neck to the external meatus. Its primary function is to serve as a conduit for urine to the bladder and then to the outside of the body.

The urothelium and submucosal layers are the same as that of the bladder. Smooth muscle fibers extend from the bladder neck down into the urethra and are further supported by circular smooth muscle fibers around the urethra. Special C-shaped striated muscle fibers (the rhabdosphincter, or external sphincter) surround a portion of the urethra and voluntarily contract and prevent leaking when bladder pressure increases.

The female urethra is 1 to 2 inches (3 to 5 cm) long and lies behind the symphysis pubis but anterior to the vagina (see Fig. 43-1, C). The rhabdosphincter encircles the middle third of the urethra. The short urethra is a contributing factor to the increased incidence of urinary tract infections in women.

The male urethra, which is about 8 to 10 inches (20 to 25 cm) long, originates at the bladder neck and extends the length of the penis (see Fig. 43-1, B). It is often separated into three parts. The prostatic urethra extends from the bladder neck through the prostate to the urogenital diaphragm. The membranous urethra passes through the urogenital diaphragm. The rhabdosphincter encircles this portion. Because of the concentrated muscular support, this short portion is not as expandable; consequently, stricture formation in this area after instrumentation is common. The penile urethra continues through the corpus spongiosum, a cavernous penile body, from the urogenital diaphragm to a distal dilated area, the fossa navicularis, before terminating at the meatus.

Urethrovesical Unit Function

Together, the bladder, urethra, and pelvic floor muscles form what is called the urethrovesical unit. Normal voluntary control of this unit is defined as *continence*. Various areas of the brain send stimulating and inhibiting impulses to the thoracolumbar (T11 to L2) and sacral (S2 to S4) areas of the spinal cord to control voiding. Distention of the bladder stimulates stretch receptors within the bladder wall. Impulses are transmitted to the sacral spinal cord and then to the brain, causing a desire to urinate. If the time to void is not appropriate, inhibitor impulses in the brain are stimulated and transmitted back to the thoracolumbar and sacral nerves innervating the bladder. In a coordinated fashion, the detrusor accommodates to the pressure (does not contract) while the sphincter and pelvic floor muscles tighten to resist bladder pressure. If voiding is appropriate, cerebral inhibition is voluntarily suppressed, and impulses are transmitted via the spinal cord for the bladder neck, sphincter, and pelvic floor muscles to relax and for the bladder to contract. The sphincter

closes and the detrusor muscle relaxes when the bladder is empty.

Any disease or trauma that affects function of the brain, spinal cord, or nerves that directly innervate the bladder, bladder neck, external sphincter, or pelvic floor can affect bladder function. These conditions include diabetes mellitus, paraplegia, and tetraplegia (quadriplegia). Drugs affecting nerve transmission also can affect bladder function.

■ Gerontologic Considerations: Effects of Aging on the Urinary System

Anatomic changes in the aging kidney include a 20% to 30% decrease in size and weight between the ages of 30 and 90 years. This loss in renal mass is predominantly in the cortex. The aging nephron fails as a unit because glomerular and tubular function appears to decrease at the same rate. By the seventh decade of life, 30% to 50% of glomeruli have lost their function. Despite losing this original kidney volume, older individuals maintain body fluid homeostasis unless they encounter diseases or other physiologic stressors.[5]

Blood flow to and within the kidneys also decreases. There is no evidence that atherosclerotic vascular disease is primarily responsible for the age-related changes in the kidneys.

Physiologic changes in the aging kidney include decreased renal blood flow, decreased GFR, and decreased ability to conserve Na^+, dilute or concentrate urine, and excrete an acid load. Under normal conditions, the aging kidney is able to maintain homeostasis, but after abrupt changes in blood volume, acid load, or other insults, the kidney may not be able to function effectively because much of its renal reserve has been lost.[6]

Physiologic changes also occur in the aging bladder and urethra. Estrogen receptors exist in the female urethra, bladder, vagina, and pelvic floor. As estrogen levels decrease with age, tissues become less elastic, thin, and less vascular. Periurethral striated muscle fibers and muscles supporting the bladder relax. Consequently, older women are more prone to urethral irritation, urethral and bladder infections, and urinary incontinence.

Men's prostates enlarge as they age, and because the prostate surrounds the proximal urethra, increasing prostate size may affect urinary patterns in men, causing hesitancy, retention, slow stream, and bladder infections.

Constipation, a complaint often expressed by the elderly, can also affect urination. Partial urethral obstruction may occur because of the rectum's close proximity to the urethra.

Age-related changes in the urinary system and differences in assessment findings are presented in Table 43-2. ■

ASSESSMENT OF THE URINARY SYSTEM

Subjective Data

Important Health Information

Past health history. The patient should be questioned about the presence or history of diseases that are known to be related to renal or other urologic problems. Some of these diseases are hypertension, diabetes mellitus, gout and other metabolic problems, connective tissue disorders (e.g., systemic lupus erythematosus, systemic sclerosis [scleroderma]), skin or upper respiratory infections of streptococcal origin, tuberculosis, viral hepatitis, con-

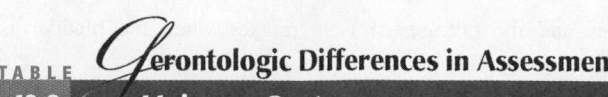

TABLE 43-2 Gerontologic Differences in Assessment — Urinary System

CHANGES	DIFFERENCES IN ASSESSMENT FINDINGS
Kidney	
↓ Amount of renal tissue	Less palpable
↓ Number of nephrons and renal blood vessels; thickened basement membrane of Bowman's capsule and glomeruli	↓ Creatinine clearance, ↑ BUN level
↓ Function of loop of Henle and tubules	Alterations in drug excretion; nocturia; loss of normal diurnal excretory pattern because of ↓ ability to concentrate urine; less concentrated urine
Ureter, Bladder, and Urethra	
↓ Elasticity and muscle tone	Palpable bladder after urination because of retention
Weakening of urinary sphincter	Stress incontinence (especially during Valsalva maneuver), dribbling of urine after urination
↓ Bladder capacity and sensory receptors	Frequency, urgency, nocturia, overflow incontinence
Estrogen deficiency leading to thin, dry vaginal tissue	Stress or overactive bladder, dysuria
↑ Prevalence of unstable bladder contractions	Overactive bladder
Prostatic enlargement	Hesitancy, frequency, urgency, nocturia, straining to urinate, retention, dribbling

BUN, Blood urea nitrogen.

TABLE 43-3 Potentially Nephrotoxic Agents

ANTIBIOTICS	OTHER AGENTS
amikacin (Amikin)	captopril (Capoten)
amphotericin B	cimetidine (Tagamet)
bacitracin	cisplatin (Platinol)
Cephalosporins	cocaine
gentamicin	Contrast medium
kanamycin	cyclosporine
neomycin	Ethylene glycol
polymyxin B	Gold
streptomycin	Heavy metals
Sulfonamides	Heroin
tobramycin (Nebcin)	lithium
vancomycin	methotrexate
	Nitrosoureas (e.g., carmustine)
	Nonsteroidal antiinflammatory drugs (e.g., ibuprofen, indomethacin)
	phenacetin
	quinine
	rifampin
	Salicylate (large quantities)

genital disorders, neurologic conditions (e.g., stroke, back injury), or trauma. Specific urinary problems such as cancer, infections, benign prostatic hyperplasia, and calculi should be noted.

Medications. An assessment of the patient's current and past use of medications is important. This should include over-the-counter drugs, as well as prescription medications and herbs. Drugs affect the urinary tract in several ways. Many drugs are known to be nephrotoxic (Table 43-3). Certain drugs may alter the quantity and character of urine output (e.g., diuretics). Numerous drugs such as phenazopyridine (Pyridium) and nitrofurantoin (Macrodantin) change its color. Anticoagulants may cause hematuria. Many antidepressants, calcium channel blockers, antihistamines, and drugs used for neurologic and musculoskeletal disorders affect the ability of the bladder or sphincter to contract or relax normally.

Surgery or other treatments. The patient should also be questioned about any previous hospitalizations related to renal or urologic diseases and all urinary problems during past pregnancies. The duration, severity, and patient's perception of any problem and its treatment should be elicited. Past surgeries, particularly pelvic surgeries, or urinary tract instrumentation should be documented. Information should be obtained from the patient about any radiation or chemotherapy treatment for cancer.

Functional Health Patterns. Key questions to ask a patient with problems related to the urinary system are listed in Table 43-4.

Health perception–health management pattern. The nurse should ask about the patient's general health, particularly when disease affecting the kidneys is suspected. Sometimes responses such as "feeling tired all of the time," changes in weight or appetite, excess thirst, fluid retention, and complaints of headache, pruritus, or blurred vision may be related to abnormal kidney function. Similarly, the elderly patient may report malaise and nonlocalized abdominal discomfort as the only symptoms of a urinary tract infection.[7]

An occupational history should be taken. Exposure to certain chemicals can affect the kidneys and urinary tract system. Phenol and ethylene glycol are examples of nephrotoxic chemicals. Aromatic amines and certain organic chemicals may increase the risk of bladder cancers. Textile workers, painters, hairdressers, and industrial workers have a high incidence of bladder tumors.

TABLE 43-4	Health History
	Urinary System

Health Perception–Health Management Pattern
- How is your energy level compared with a year ago?
- Do you notice any visual changes?*
- Have you ever smoked? If yes, how many packs per day?

Nutritional–Metabolic Pattern
- How is your appetite?
- Has your weight changed over the past year?*
- Do you take vitamin or mineral supplements?*
- How much and what kinds of fluids do you drink daily?
- How many dairy products or meat do you eat?
- Do you drink coffee? Colas?
- Do you eat chocolate?
- Do you spice your food heavily?*

Elimination Pattern
- Are you able to sit through a 2-hour meeting or ride in a car for 2 hours without urinating? Do you awaken at night with the desire to urinate? If so, how many times does this occur during an average night?
- Do you ever notice blood in your urine?* If so, at what point in the urination does it occur?
- Do you find it difficult to postpone urination when you feel the urge to urinate?*
- Do you ever leak urine? If so, what causes urine leakage? Do you leak when you cough, walk, run, or lift a heavy object? Do you leak if you are unable to reach a toilet right away? Do you ever find that you have leaked without awareness of doing so?
- Do you use special devices or supplies for urine elimination or control?*
- Do you ever have pain when you urinate?* If so, where is the pain?
- Do you use special devices or supplies for urine elimination or control?*
- How often do you move your bowels? Do you ever experience constipation (hardened stools that are difficult to pass or a sensation that you are unable to completely evacuate your bowels)?
- Do you frequently experience diarrhea (high-volume, loose watery stools)? Do you ever have problems controlling your bowels? If so, do you have problems controlling the passage of gas? Watery or liquid stool? Solid stool?

Activity-Exercise Pattern
- Have you noticed any changes in your ability to do your usual daily activities?*
- Do certain activities aggravate your urinary problem?*
- Has your urinary problem caused you to alter or stop any activity or exercise?*
- Do you require assistance in moving or getting to the bathroom?*

Cognitive-Perceptual Pattern
- Describe any pain you have in relation to urination.

Self-Perception–Self-Concept Pattern
- How does your urinary problem make you feel about yourself?
- Do you perceive your body differently since you have developed a urinary problem?

Role-Relationship Pattern
- Does your urinary problem interfere with your relationships with family or friends?*
- Has your urinary problem caused a change in your job status or affected your ability to carry out job-related responsibilities?*

Sexuality-Reproductive Pattern
- Has your urinary problem caused any change in your sexual pleasure or performance?*
- Do you have hygiene problems related to sexual activities that cause you concern?*

Coping–Stress Tolerance Pattern
- Do you feel able to manage the problems associated with your urinary problem? If not, explain.
- What strategies are you using to cope with your urinary problem?

Values-Beliefs Pattern
- Has your present illness affected your belief system?*
- Are your treatment decisions related to your urinary problem in conflict with your value system?*

*If yes, describe.

A smoking history should be obtained. Cigarette smoking is a major factor in the risk for bladder cancer. Tumors occur four times more frequently in cigarette smokers than in nonsmokers.

Places where a patient has lived may be important information to obtain. It has been shown that persons living in certain parts of the United States (Great Lakes, Southwest, Southeast) have a higher than normal incidence of urinary calculi. This may be caused by the higher mineral content of the soil and water. A person living in Middle Eastern countries or Africa can acquire certain parasites that can cause cystitis or bladder cancer.

The presence of certain renal or urologic problems in a family history increases the likelihood of similar problems occur-

ring in the patient. The nurse should ask about family members who have had any of the diseases referred to in the past health history, as well as polycystic renal disease and congenital urinary tract abnormalities, such as Alport syndrome (congenital nephritis).

Nutritional-metabolic pattern. The usual quantity and types of fluid a patient drinks are important information related to urinary tract disease. Dehydration may contribute to urinary infections, calculi formation, and renal failure. Large intake of particular foods, such as dairy products or foods high in proteins, may also lead to calculi formation. Coffee, alcohol, carbonated beverages, or spicy foods often aggravate urinary inflammatory diseases. An unexplained weight gain may be the result of fluid retention secondary to a renal problem. Anorexia, nausea, and vomiting can dramatically affect fluid status and require careful assessment. Information on vitamin and mineral supplements and herbal therapies should be obtained. The patient may not think of these supplements and therapies when listing over-the-counter drugs; supplements are often considered part of nutritional intake.

Elimination pattern. Questions about urine elimination patterns are the cornerstone of the health history in the patient with a lower urinary tract disorder. This line of inquiry begins with a question of how the patient manages urine elimination. The majority of patients eliminate urine by spontaneous voiding, and they should be asked about daytime (diurnal) voiding frequency and the frequency of nocturia. Patients should also be queried about additional bothersome lower urinary tract symptoms, including urgency, incontinence, or urinary retention. Table 43-5 lists some of the common clinical manifestations of urinary tract disorders. Changes in the color and appearance of urine are often significant and should be evaluated. If blood is visible in the urine, it should be determined if it occurs at the beginning, throughout, or at the end of urination.

Bowel function should also be investigated. Problems with fecal incontinence may signal neurologic causes for bladder problems because of shared nerve pathways. Constipation and fecal impaction can partially obstruct the urethra, causing inadequate bladder emptying, overflow incontinence, and infection.

TABLE 43-5   Clinical Manifestations of Disorders of the Urinary System

General Manifestations

Fatigue	Itching
Headaches	Excess thirst
Blurred vision	Chills
Elevated blood pressure	Change in body weight
Anorexia	Change in mentation
Nausea and vomiting	

Related to Urinary System

Pain	*Changes in Urine Output*
Dysuria	Polyuria
Flank or costovertebral angle	Oliguria
Groin	Anuria
Suprapubic	*Changes in Urine*
Changes in Patterns	*Composition*
of Urination	Hematuria
Frequency	Pyuria
Nocturia	Concentrated
Dysuria	Dilute
Hesitancy of stream	Color (red, brown, yellowish
Change in stream	green)
Overactive bladder	*Edema*
Urgency	Facial (periorbital)
Retention	Ankle
Incontinence	Ascites
Stress incontinence	Anasarca
Dribbling	Sacral

The nurse should find out the patient's method of handling a urinary problem. A patient may already be using a catheter or collection device. Sometimes a patient has to assume a particular position to urinate or perform such maneuvers as pressing on the lower abdomen (Credé method), straining (Valsalva maneuver), or stretching the rectum to empty the bladder.

Activity-exercise pattern. The patient's level of activity should be assessed. A sedentary person is more likely than an active individual to have stasis of urine, which can predispose to infection and calculi. Demineralization of bones in a person with limited physical activity causes increased urine calcium precipitation.

An active person may find that increasing activity aggravates the urinary problem. The patient who has had prostate surgery or who has weakened pelvic floor muscles may leak urine when attempting particular activities such as running. Some men may develop chronic inflammatory prostatitis or epididymitis after heavy lifting or long-distance driving.

Sleep-rest pattern. Nocturia is a common and a particularly bothersome lower urinary tract symptom that often leads to sleep deprivation, daytime sleepiness, and fatigue. It occurs in multiple disorders affecting the lower urinary tract, including urinary incontinence, urinary retention, and interstitial cystitis. Nocturia also may be attributable to polyuria owing to renal disease, poorly controlled diabetes mellitus, alcoholism, excessive fluid intake, or obstructive sleep apnea. When asking about nocturia, it is helpful to determine whether it is the desire to urinate that causes the person to arise from sleep or whether pain or some other symptom interrupts sleep and the person urinates as a matter of habit before returning to bed. Up to one episode of nocturia is considered normal in younger adults, and up to two episodes are acceptable among adults age 65 years or older. Sleep problems associated with a urinary disorder should be documented. The older adult may awaken many times during the night to urinate and may need to be assured that this may be normal. However, a complete assessment should be made to rule out any problem.

Cognitive-perceptual pattern. Level of mobility, visual acuity, and dexterity are important factors to determine for a patient with urologic problems when managing his or her own care at home, particularly when urine retention or incontinence is a problem. It should be determined if the patient is alert, able to understand instructions, and can recall the instructions when necessary.

If urinary incontinence is present, a thorough history of the problem should be elicited to assist in determining the type of incontinence. It is important to document what the patient has previously tried to manage the problem. Incontinence is a distressing problem and calls for great sensitivity on the part of the nurse if accurate information is to be obtained.

Pain is a frequent symptom of urinary tract disease. Types of pain associated with renal and urologic problems include dysuria, groin pain, costovertebral pain, and suprapubic pain. If present, the location, character, and duration should be assessed. The absence of pain when other urinary symptoms exist is also significant. Many urinary tract tumors are painless in the early stages.

Self-perception–self-concept pattern. Problems associated with the urinary system, such as incontinence, urinary diversion procedures, and chronic fatigue, can result in loss of self-esteem and a negative body image. Sensitive questioning may elicit cues to problems in this area.

Role-relationship pattern. Urinary problems can affect many aspects of a person's life, including the ability to work and relationships with others. These factors will have important implications on future treatment and management. The nurse must be aware of cues from the patient.

Urinary system problems may be serious enough to cause problems in job-related and social situations. Chronic dialysis therapy often makes regular employment or full-time homemaking difficult. Also, concurrent poor health and negative body image can seriously alter existing roles. The nurse should assess this area to plan appropriate interventions.

Sexuality-reproductive pattern. The patient should be questioned about the effect of a renal or urologic problem on her or his sexual patterns and satisfaction. Problems related to personal hygiene and fatigue can seriously affect a sexual relationship. Although urinary incontinence is not directly associated with sexual dysfunction, it often has a devastating effect on self-esteem and social and intimate relationships. Counseling of both the patient and partner may be indicated.

Objective Data
Physical Examination
Inspection. The nurse should assess for changes in the following:

Skin: pallor, yellow-gray cast, excoriations, changes in turgor, bruises, texture (e.g., rough, dry skin)

Mouth: stomatitis, ammonia breath odor

Face and extremities: generalized edema, peripheral edema, bladder distention, masses, enlarged kidneys

Abdomen: skin changes described earlier, as well as striae, abdominal contour for midline mass in lower abdomen (may indicate urinary retention) or unilateral mass (occasionally seen in adult, indicating enlargement of one or both kidneys from large tumor or polycystic kidney)

Weight: weight gain secondary to edema; weight loss and muscle wasting in renal failure

General state of health: fatigue, lethargy, and diminished alertness

Palpation. The kidneys are posterior organs protected by the abdominal organs, the ribs, and the heavy back muscles. A landmark useful in locating the kidneys is the **costovertebral angle** (CVA) formed by the rib cage and the vertebral column. The normal-sized left kidney is rarely palpable because the spleen lies directly on top of it. Occasionally the lower pole of the right kidney is palpable.

To palpate the right kidney, the examiner's left hand is placed behind and supports the patient's right side between the rib cage and the iliac crest (Fig. 43-6). The right flank is elevated with the left hand, and the right hand is used to palpate deeply for the right kidney. The lower pole of the right kidney may be felt as a smooth, rounded mass that descends on inspiration. If the kidney is palpable, its size, contour, and tenderness should be noted. Kidney enlargement is suggestive of neoplasm or other serious renal pathologic conditions.

The urinary bladder is normally not palpable unless it is distended with urine. If the bladder is full, it may be felt as a smooth, round, firm organ and is sensitive to palpation.

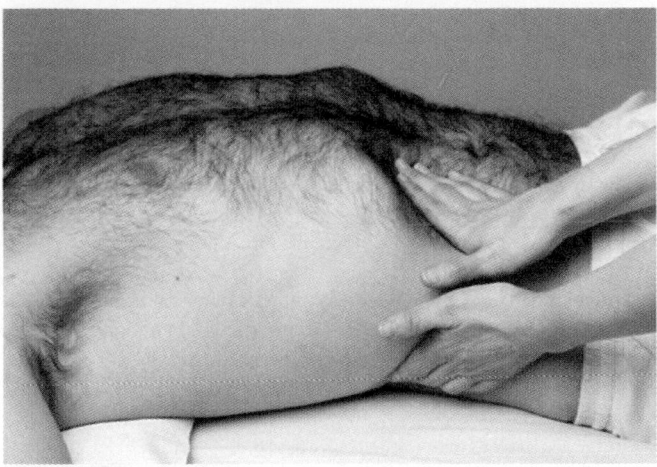

FIG. 43-6   Palpating the right kidney.

TABLE 43-6   Normal Physical Assessment of the Urinary System

No costovertebral angle tenderness
Nonpalpable kidney and bladder
No palpable masses

Percussion. Tenderness in the flank area may be detected by fist percussion. This technique is performed by striking the fist (kidney punch) of one hand against the dorsal surface of the other hand, which is placed flat along the posterior CVA margin. Normally a firm blow in the flank area should not elicit pain. If CVA tenderness and pain are present, it may indicate a kidney infection or polycystic kidney disease.

Normally a bladder is not percussible until it contains 150 ml of urine. If the bladder is full, dullness is heard above the symphysis pubis. A distended bladder may be percussed as high as the umbilicus.

Auscultation. The diaphragm of the stethoscope may be used to auscultate over both CVAs and in the upper abdominal quadrants. With this technique, the abdominal aorta and renal arteries are auscultated for a bruit (an abnormal murmur), which indicates impaired blood flow to the kidneys.

Table 43-6 shows how to record the normal physical assessment findings of the urinary system. Table 43-7 presents common assessment abnormalities of the urinary system. Normally, assessment findings may vary in the older adult. Table 43-2 shows the age-related changes in the urinary system and differences in assessment findings.

DIAGNOSTIC STUDIES OF THE URINARY SYSTEM

Table 43-8 discusses diagnostic studies common to the urinary system. Diagnostic studies are important in locating and understanding problems of the urinary system. The accuracy of the results is influenced by (1) adherence to the proper procedures related to the study and (2) cooperation of the patient in restrict-

TABLE 43-7 Common Assessment Abnormalities
Urinary System

FINDING	DESCRIPTION	POSSIBLE ETIOLOGY AND SIGNIFICANCE
Dysuria	Painful or difficult urination	Sign of urinary tract infection and interstitial cystitis and wide variety of pathologic conditions
Frequency	Increased incidence of urinating	Acutely inflamed bladder, retention with overflow, excess fluid intake
Enuresis	Involuntary nocturnal urinating	Symptomatic of lower urinary tract disorder
Hesitancy	Delay or difficulty in initiating urination	Partial urethral obstruction
Urgency	Strong desire to urinate	Inflammatory lesions in bladder or urethra, acute bacterial infections
Hematuria	Blood in the urine	Cancer of genitourinary tract, blood dyscrasias, renal disease, urinary tract infection, stones in kidney or ureter, medications (anticoagulants)
Burning on urination	Stinging pain in urethral area	Urethral irritation, urinary tract infection
Pneumaturia	Passage of urine containing gas	Fistula connections between bowel and bladder, gas-forming urinary tract infections
Retention	Inability to urinate, even though bladder contains excessive amount of urine	Finding after pelvic surgery, childbirth, catheter removal; urethral stricture or obstruction; neurogenic bladder; postanesthesia
Pain	Presence over suprapubic area (related to bladder), urethral pain (irritation of bladder neck), flank (CVA) pain	Infection, urinary retention, foreign body in urinary tract, urethritis, pyelonephritis, renal colic or stones
Incontinence	Inability to voluntarily control discharge of urine	Neurogenic bladder, bladder infection, injury to external sphincter
Stress incontinence	Involuntary urination with increased pressure (sneezing or coughing)	Weakness of sphincter control
Nocturia	Frequency of urination at night	Renal disease with impaired concentrating ability, bladder obstruction, congestive heart failure, diabetes mellitus, finding after renal transplant
Polyuria	Large volume of urine in a given time	Diabetes mellitus, diabetes insipidus, chronic renal failure, diuretics, excess fluid intake
Anuria	Technically no urination (24-hr urine output <100 ml)	Acute renal failure, end-stage renal disease, bilateral ureteral obstruction
Oliguria	Diminished amount of urine in a given time (24-hr urine output of 100-400 ml)	Severe dehydration, shock, transfusion reaction, kidney disease, end-stage renal disease

CVA, Costovertebral angle.

ing fluids, collecting urine specimens, lying quietly on the examination table, or following other instructions.

Many radiologic studies require the use of a bowel preparation the evening before the study to clear the lower GI tract of feces and flatus. Because the kidneys lie in a retroperitoneal location, the contents of the colon may obstruct visualization of the urinary tract. If a bowel preparation is not properly done, the study may be unsuccessful and have to be rescheduled. Commonly used bowel preparations include enemas, castor oil, magnesium citrate, and bisacodyl (Dulcolax) tablets or suppositories. Some bowel preparations, such as magnesium citrate and Fleet enema, are contraindicated in the patient with renal failure. Magnesium cannot be excreted by patients with renal failure (see Chapter 45).

When a patient has repeated diagnostic studies on consecutive days, it is important to prevent dehydration. It is not uncommon to have a patient take nothing by mouth (NPO) after midnight, spend all morning in the x-ray department, be too tired to eat, sleep all afternoon, and be on NPO status after midnight again because of studies scheduled for the next day. Severe dehydration, especially in a diabetic, debilitated, or older patient, may lead to acute renal failure. The nurse is responsible for ensuring that a patient undergoing diagnostic studies is properly hydrated and given adequate nourishment between studies. The nurse should also check with the health care provider regarding the insulin dose for the diabetic patient who is NPO.

Urine Studies

Urinalysis. In evaluating disorders of the urinary tract, one of the first studies done is a **urinalysis** (Tables 43-8 and 43-9). This test may provide information about possible abnormalities, indicate what further studies need to be done, and supply information on the progression of a diagnosed disorder.

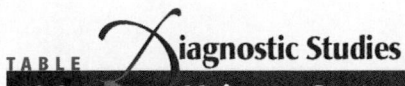

TABLE 43-8 **Diagnostic Studies**

Urinary System

STUDY	DESCRIPTION AND PURPOSE	NURSING RESPONSIBILITY
Urine Studies		
• Urinalysis	Study is a general examination of urine to establish baseline information or provide data to establish a tentative diagnosis and determine whether further studies are to be ordered (see Table 43-9).	Try to obtain first urinated morning specimen. Ensure that specimen is examined within 1 hr of urinating. Wash perineal area if soiled with menses or fecal material.
• Creatinine clearance	Creatinine is a waste product of protein breakdown (primarily body muscle mass). Clearance of creatinine by the kidney approximates the GFR. *Normal finding* is 85-135 ml/min.	Collect 24-hr urine specimen. Discard first urination when test is started. Save urine from all subsequent urinations for 24 hr. Instruct patient to urinate at end of 24 hr and add specimen to collection. Ensure that serum creatinine is determined during 24-hr period.
• Urine culture ("clean catch," "midstream")	Study is done to confirm suspected urinary tract infection and identify causative organisms. *Normally,* bladder is sterile, but urethra contains bacteria and a few WBCs. If properly collected, stored, and handled: <10,000 organisms/ml usually indicates no infection; 10,000-100,000/ml is usually not diagnostic, and test may have to be repeated; >100,000/ml indicates infection.	Use sterile container for collection of urine. Touch only outside of container. For women, separate labia with one hand and clean meatus with other hand, using at least three sponges (saturated with cleansing solution) in a front-to-back motion. For men, retract foreskin (if present) and cleanse glans with at least three cleansing sponges. After cleaning, instruct patient to start urinating and then continue voiding in sterile container. (The initial voided urine flushes out most contaminants in the urethra and perineal area.) Catheterization may be needed if patient is unable to cooperate with this procedure.
• Concentration test	Study evaluates renal concentration ability. Concentration is measured by specific gravity readings. *Normal finding* is 1.020-1.035.	Instruct patient to fast after given time in evening (in usual procedure). Collect three urine specimens at hourly intervals in morning.
• Residual urine	Study determines amount of urine left in bladder after urinating. Finding may be abnormal in problems with bladder innervation, sphincter impairment, BPH, or urethral strictures. *Normal finding* is ≤50 ml urine (increases with age).	If residual urine test is ordered, catheterize patient immediately after urinating or use bladder ultrasound equipment. If a large amount of residual urine is obtained, health care provider may want catheter left in bladder.
• Protein determination Dipstick (Albustix, Combistix)	Test detects protein (primarily albumin) in urine. *Normal finding* is 0-trace.	Dip end of stick in urine and read result by comparison with color chart on label as directed. Grading is from 0 to 4+. Interpret with caution. A positive result may not indicate significant proteinuria; some medications may give false-positive readings.
Quantitative test for protein	A 12- or 24-hr collection gives a more accurate indication of the amount of protein in urine. Persistent proteinuria usually indicates glomerular renal disease. *Normal finding* is <150 mg/24 hr (<0.15 g/24 hr), consisting mainly of albumin.	Perform 12- or 24-hr urine collection.
• Urine cytology	Study is used to identify changes in cellular structure indicative of malignancy, especially bladder cancer.	Obtain urine and send immediately to lab. The first morning specimen should *not* be used.
Blood Chemistries		
• BUN	Study is most commonly used to identify presence of renal problems. Concentration of urea in blood is regulated by rate at which kidney excretes urea. *Normal finding* is 10-30 mg/dl (1.8-7.1 mmol/L).	Be aware that when interpreting BUN, nonrenal factors may cause increase (e.g., rapid cell destruction from infections, fever, GI bleeding, trauma, athletic activity and excessive muscle breakdown, corticosteroid therapy).
• Creatinine	Study is more reliable than BUN as a determinant of renal function. Creatinine is end product of muscle and protein metabolism and is liberated at a constant rate. *Normal finding* is 0.5-1.5 mg/dl (44-133 µmol/L). Results are higher in men.	Explain test and watch for postpuncture bleeding.
• BUN/creatinine ratio	*Normal finding* is 10:1.	

BPH, Benign prostatic hyperplasia; *BUN,* blood urea nitrogen; *GI,* gastrointestinal; *GFR,* glomerular filtration rate; *WBC,* white blood cell.

Continued

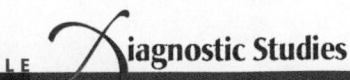

TABLE 43-8	Diagnostic Studies	
Urinary System—cont'd		
STUDY	**DESCRIPTION AND PURPOSE**	**NURSING RESPONSIBILITY**
Blood Chemistries—cont'd		
• Uric acid	Study is used as a screening test primarily for disorders of purine metabolism but can indicate kidney disease as well. Values depend on renal function and rate of purine metabolism and dietary intake of food rich in purines. *Normal finding* is 2.5-5.5 mg/dl (149-327 μmol/L) for women and 4.5-6.5 mg/dl (268-387 μmol/L) for men.	Explain test and watch for postpuncture bleeding.
• Sodium (Na^+)	Sodium is main extracellular electrolyte determining blood volume. Usually, values stay within normal range until late stages of renal failure. *Normal finding* is 135-145 mEq/L (135-145 mmol/L).	Explain test and watch for postpuncture bleeding.
• Potassium (K^+)	Kidneys are responsible for excreting majority of body's potassium. In renal disease, K^+ determinations are critical because K^+ is one of the first electrolytes to become abnormal. Elevated K^+ levels of >6 mEq/L can lead to muscle weakness and cardiac arrhythmias. *Normal finding* is 3.5-5.5 mEq/L (3.5-5.5 mmol/L).	Explain test and watch for postpuncture bleeding.
• Calcium (Ca^{2+})	Calcium is main mineral in bone and aids in muscle contraction, neurotransmission, and clotting. In renal disease, decreased reabsorption of Ca^{2+} leads to renal osteodystrophy. *Normal finding* is 9-11 mg/dl (4.5-5.5 mEq/L, 2.25-2.74 mmol/L).	Explain test and watch for postpuncture bleeding.
• Phosphorus	Phosphorus balance is inversely related to Ca^{2+} balance. In renal disease, phosphorus levels are elevated because the kidney is the primary excretory organ. *Normal finding* is 2.8-4.5 mg/dl (0.95-1.45 mmol/L)	Explain test and watch for postpuncture bleeding.
• Bicarbonate (HCO_3^-)	Most patients in renal failure have metabolic acidosis and low serum HCO_3^- levels. *Normal finding* is 20-30 mEq/L (20-30 mmol/L).	Explain test and watch for postpuncture bleeding.
Radiologic Procedures		
• Kidneys, ureters, bladder (KUB)	Study involves x-ray examination of abdomen and pelvis and delineates size, shape, and position of kidneys.	Perform bowel preparation (if ordered).
• Intravenous pyelogram (IVP)	X-ray examination visualizes urinary tract after IV injection of contrast material.	Evening before procedure, give cathartic or enema to empty colon of feces and gas. Keep patient on NPO status 8 hr before procedure. Before procedure, assess patient for iodine sensitivity to avoid anaphylactic reaction. Inform patient that procedure involves lying on table and having serial x-rays taken. After procedure, force fluids (if permitted) to flush out contrast material.
• Nephrotomogram	X-ray is taken with rotating tubes. Test delineates segments of the kidney at different levels. Multiple exposures are taken to visualize specific sections of the kidney after IV injection of contrast material.	Explain procedure and prepare patient as for IVP.
• Retrograde pyelogram	X-ray of urinary tract is taken after injection of contrast material into kidneys. Cystoscope is inserted, and ureteral catheters are inserted through it into renal pelvis. Contrast material is injected through catheters.	Prepare patient as for IVP. Inform patient that pain may be experienced from distention of pelvis and discomfort from cystoscope. Inform patient that anesthesia may be given for procedure.
• Renal arteriogram (angiogram)	Study is performed by injecting contrast material into renal artery via catheter inserted into femoral artery. Purpose is to visualize renal blood vessels.	Prepare patient evening before procedure by giving cathartic or enema. Before injection of contrast material, test for iodine sensitivity. After procedure, check insertion site for bleeding and take peripheral pulses in involved leg every 30-60 min to detect occluded blood flow.

NPO, Nothing by mouth.

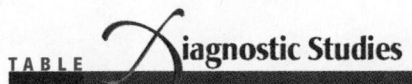

TABLE 43-8

Diagnostic Studies
Urinary System—cont'd

STUDY	DESCRIPTION AND PURPOSE	NURSING RESPONSIBILITY
Radiologic Procedures—cont'd		
• Renal ultrasound	Small external ultrasound probe is placed on patient's skin. Conductive gel is applied to the skin. Noninvasive procedure involves passing sound waves into body structures and recording images as they are reflected back. Computer interprets tissue density based on sound waves and displays it in picture form. Study is most valuable in detection of renal or perirenal masses, differential diagnosis of renal cysts, solid masses, and identification of obstructions. It can be used safely in patients with renal failure.	Explain procedure to patient.
• CT scan	Study provides excellent visualization of kidneys. Kidney size can be evaluated; tumors, abscesses, suprarenal masses (e.g., adrenal tumors, pheochromocytomas), and obstructions can be detected. Advantage of CT over ultrasound is its ability to distinguish subtle differences in density. Use of IV-administered contrast media during CT accentuates density of renal tissue and helps differentiate masses.	Explain procedure to patient. Ask patient about iodine sensitivity.
• MRI	Computer-generated films rely on radiofrequency waves and alteration in magnetic field. Useful for visualization of kidneys. Not proven useful for detecting urinary calculi or calcified tumors.	Explain procedure to patient. Have patient remove all metal objects. Patients with a history of claustrophobia may need to be sedated.
• Cystogram	Contrast material is instilled into bladder via cystoscope or catheter. Purpose is to visualize bladder and evaluate vesicoureteral reflux.	Explain procedure to patient. If done via cystoscope, follow nursing care related to cystoscopy.
Renal Radionuclide Imaging		
• Renal scan	Radioactive isotopes are injected IV. Radiation detector probes are placed over kidney, and scintillation counter monitors radioactive material in kidney. Purpose is to show blood flow, glomerular filtration, tubular function, and excretion. Radioisotope distribution in kidney is scanned and mapped. Test is useful in showing location, size, and shape of kidney and, in general, assessing blood perfusion and its ability to secrete urine. Abscesses, cysts, and tumors may appear as cold spots because of presence of nonfunctioning tissue.	Requires no dietary or activity restriction. Inform patient that no pain or discomfort should be felt during test.
Renal Biopsy	Technique is usually done as a skin (percutaneous) biopsy through needle insertion into lower lobe of kidney. Can be performed with CT or ultrasound guidance. Purpose is to obtain renal tissue for examination to determine type of renal disease or to follow progress of renal disease.	Before procedure, ascertain coagulation status through patient history, medication history, CBC, hematocrit, prothrombin time, and bleeding and clotting time. Type and crossmatch patient for blood. Ensure consent form is signed. After procedure, apply pressure dressing to biopsy site and check frequently for bleeding. Take vital signs frequently. Observe urine for gross bleeding. Determine microscopic bleeding by use of dipstick. Assess patient for flank pain. Monitor hematocrit levels.

CBC, Complete blood count; *CT,* computed tomography; *MRI,* magnetic resonance imaging.

Continued

TABLE 43-8   Diagnostic Studies   Urinary System—cont'd

STUDY	DESCRIPTION AND PURPOSE	NURSING RESPONSIBILITY
Endoscopy ▪ Cystoscopy	Study involves use of tubular lighted scope to inspect bladder. Lithotomy position is used. It may be done using local or general anesthesia, depending on needs and condition of patient.	Before procedure, force fluids or give IV fluids if general anethesia is to be used. Ensure consent form is signed. Explain procedure to patient. Give preoperative medication. After procedure, explain that burning on urination, pink-tinged urine, and urinary frequency are expected effects after cystoscopy. Do not let patient walk alone immediately after procedure because orthostatic hypotension may occur. Offer warm sitz baths, heat, mild analgesics to relieve discomfort.
Urodynamics ▪ Cystometrogram	Study involves insertion of catheter and instillation of water or saline solution into bladder. Measurements of pressure exerted against bladder wall are recorded. Purpose is to evaluate bladder tone, sensations of filling, and bladder (detrusor) stability.	Explain procedure to patient. Observe patient for manifestations of urinary infection after procedure.

For a routine urinalysis, a specimen may be collected at any time of the day. However, it is best to obtain the first specimen urinated in the morning. This concentrated specimen is more likely to contain abnormal constituents if they are present in the urine. The specimen should be examined within 1 hour of urinating. If it is not, bacteria multiply rapidly, RBCs hemolyze, casts (molds of renal tubules) disintegrate, and the urine becomes alkaline as a result of urea-splitting bacteria. If it is not possible to send the specimen to the laboratory immediately, it should be refrigerated. However, to obtain the best results, the nurse should coordinate specimen collection with routine laboratory hours.

Multiple reagent strips (also called urine dipsticks) are commonly used by laboratories and in outpatient settings to provide chemical analysis of urine along with a microscopic interpretation. The results of a urinalysis usually include a description of the appearance, specific gravity (mass and density), pH, glucose, ketones, and protein in the urine and a microscopic examination of urine sediment for white blood cells (WBCs), RBCs, crystals, and casts (see Table 43-9).

Composite Urine Collections. Composite urine specimens are collected over a period that may range from 2 to 24 hours. The purpose of a composite specimen is to examine or measure specific components, such as electrolytes, glucose, protein, 17-ketosteroids, catecholamines, creatinine, and minerals. These specimens may have to be refrigerated, or preservatives may have to be added to the container used for collecting urine.

For collection of a composite urine specimen, the patient is instructed to urinate and discard this first urine specimen. This time is noted as the start of the test. All urine from subsequent urinations is saved in a container for the designated period. Finally, at the end of the period, the patient is asked to urinate, and this urine is added to the container. Incomplete collections do not provide valid results. Reminding the patient to save all urine during the study period is critical.

Creatinine Clearance. One of the most common composite indicators used to analyze urinary system disorders is creatinine clearance. **Creatinine** is a waste product produced by muscle breakdown. Urinary excretion of creatinine is a measure of the amount of active muscle tissue in the body, not of body weight. Therefore people with larger muscle mass have higher values. Because almost all creatinine in the blood is normally excreted by the kidneys, creatinine clearance is the most accurate indicator of renal function. The result of a creatinine clearance test closely approximates that of the GFR.[8] A blood specimen for serum creatinine determination should be obtained during the period of urine collection. Creatinine clearance is calculated as follows:

$$\text{Creatinine clearance (ml/min)} = \frac{\text{Urine creatinine (mg/ml)} \times \text{Urine volume (ml/min)}}{\text{Serum creatinine (mg/ml)}}$$

Creatinine levels remain remarkably constant for each person because they are not significantly affected by protein ingestion, muscular exercise, water intake, or rate of urine production. Normal creatinine clearance values range from 85 to 135 ml per minute. After age 40, the creatinine clearance rate decreases at a rate of about 1 ml per minute per year.

Urine Cytology. Urine can be checked for abnormal cellular structures that occur with bladder cancer. Specimens may be obtained by voiding, catheterization, or bladder irrigation (bladder washing). The first morning's voided specimen should not be used because epithelial cells may change in appearance in urine held in the bladder overnight. As with urinalysis, the specimen should be fresh or brought to the lab within the hour. An alcohol-based fixative is then added to preserve the cellular structure. Urine cytology is used for detection of and following the prognosis of bladder cancer.

Radiologic Studies (See Table 43-8)

Kidney, Ureter, and Bladder Film. The kidney, ureter, and bladder (KUB) film is an abdominal view taken without using a contrast medium to show the renal outline, psoas shadow, and the bladder, if full. Radiopaque stones and foreign bodies can

TABLE 43-9	**Urinalysis Findings**	
TEST	**NORMAL**	**ABNORMAL FINDING AND SIGNIFICANCE**
Color	Amber yellow	• Dark, smoky color suggests hematuria. Yellow-brown to olive green indicates excessive bilirubin. Orange-red or orange-brown caused by phenazopyridine (Pyridium). Cloudiness of freshly voided urine indicates infection. Colorless urine indicates excessive fluid intake, renal disease, or diabetes insipidus.
Smell	Aromatic	• On standing, urine becomes more ammonia-like in smell. In urinary tract infections, urine smells unpleasant.
Protein	0-150 mg/24 hr 0-18 mg/dl	• Persistent proteinuria is characteristic of acute and chronic renal disease, especially involving glomeruli. In absence of disease, positive reading may be caused by high-protein diet, strenuous exercise, dehydration, fever, or emotional stress. Vaginal secretions may contaminate urine specimen and give positive reading.
Glucose	None	• Glycosuria indicates diabetes mellitus or low renal threshold for glucose reabsorption (if blood glucose level is normal). Small amounts may be found after glucose loading (e.g., glucose tolerance test).
Ketones	None	• Altered carbohydrate and fat metabolism indicates diabetes mellitus and starvation. Findings can also be seen in dehydration, vomiting, and severe diarrhea.
Bilirubin	None	• Presence of bilirubinuria is as significant as jaundice in detection of liver disorders. Bilirubin may appear in urine before jaundice becomes visible or may be present in persons with hepatic disorders who do not have recognizable jaundice.*
Specific gravity	1.003-1.030	• Specific gravity of morning urine specimen reflects maximum concentrating ability of kidney and is 1.025-1.030. Low specific gravity indicates dilute urine and possibly excessive diuresis. High specific gravity indicates dehydration. If it becomes fixed at about 1.010, this indicates renal inability to concentrate urine, suggesting that kidney is progressing to end-stage renal disease.
Osmolality	300-1300 mOsm/kg (300-1300 mmol/kg)	• Measurement is a more accurate method than specific gravity for determining diluting and concentrating ability of kidneys. Deviations from normal indicate tubular dysfunction. Findings indicate if kidney has lost ability to concentrate or dilute urine. (Not part of routine urinalysis.)
pH	4.0-8.0 (average, 6.0)	• If >8.0, finding may be the result of standing of urine or urinary tract infections because bacteria decompose urea to form ammonia. If <4.0, may indicate respiratory or metabolic acidosis.
RBC	0-4/hpf	• Bleeding in urinary tract is caused by calculi, cystitis, neoplasm, glomerulonephritis, tuberculosis, kidney biopsy, or trauma.
WBC	0-5/hpf	• Increased number of WBCs in urine (pyuria) indicates urinary tract infection or inflammation.
Casts	None-occasional hyaline	• Casts are molds of the renal tubules and may contain protein, WBCs, RBCs, or bacteria. Noncellular casts are hyaline in appearance, and a few may be found in normal urine. Casts indicate renal dysfunction or upper urinary tract infections.
Culture for organisms	No organisms in bladder, $<10^4$ organisms/ml result of normal urethral flora	• Bacteria counts $>10^5$/ml indicate urinary tract infection. Organisms most commonly found in urinary tract infections are *Escherichia coli*, enterococci, *Klebsiella*, *Proteus*, and streptococci.

*See Chapter 42 for further discussion.
hpf, High-powered field.

be seen on this x-ray. The form, size, and position of the kidneys can also be seen. Abscesses, tumors, and cysts may distort anatomic relationships on the KUB. Sometimes nephrotomograms (sectional views that focus on a single plane of the kidney) are ordered at the same time as the KUB x-ray to maximize visualization of the kidneys.

Intravenous Pyelogram. The **intravenous pyelogram** (IVP), or excretory urogram, allows visualization of the urinary tract. The presence, position, size, and shape of the kidneys, ureters, and bladder can be evaluated. Cysts, tumors, lesions, and obstructions cause a distortion in the normal appearance of these structures.

The procedure consists of injecting an intravenous dose of contrast material, which circulates in the blood and is excreted by the kidneys into the urine. During injection, the patient may experience warmth, a flushed face, and a salty taste. After injection, films are taken sequentially. The sequencing of films is planned

so that contrast excretion can be followed from the cortex of the kidney to the bladder. The presence of bladder atony or outlet obstruction also can be detected by a film taken after urination, which shows the residual volume of urine in the bladder.

The patient with significantly decreased renal function should not have an IVP because the contrast material will not be properly excreted by the kidneys. Contrast medium can also be nephrotoxic and can worsen renal function.

Retrograde Pyelogram. A **retrograde pyelogram** is an x-ray visualization of the kidneys, ureter, and bladder after direct injection of a contrast material into the kidney via a ureteral catheter introduced through a cystoscope. It may be done if an IVP does not visualize the urinary tract or if the patient is allergic to the contrast material or has decreased renal function. The dangers associated with a retrograde pyelogram are similar to those related to cystoscopy, including the risk of infection and the use of anesthesia.

Antegrade Pyelogram. Sometimes an antegrade pyelogram is done to evaluate the upper urinary tract when there is allergy to contrast media or decreased renal function and when abnormalities prevent passage of a ureteral catheter. Contrast media may be injected percutaneously into the renal pelvis or via a nephrostomy tube that is already in place (also called a nephrostogram) when determining tube function or ureteral integrity after trauma or surgery. Complications of an antegrade pyelogram include hematuria, infection, and hematoma.

Renal Ultrasound. A renal ultrasound uses high-frequency waves to image the kidneys, ureter, and bladder. Because radiation exposure is avoided, a number of images can be obtained, and repeat studies over a brief period of time can be done. Images can be obtained from both the prone and supine positions. A bowel preparation is not required for a renal ultrasound.

Computed Tomography Scan. Computed tomography (CT) scan of the abdomen and pelvis may be done to detect tumors and possible metastases. The CT scan can differentiate these from cysts or abscesses. Contrast material may be used to help visualize urinary structures more clearly in the computer-generated images. The patient is instructed to lie very still during the procedure while the machine takes precise transaxial images. Sedation may be required if the patient is unable to cooperate.

Renal Arteriogram. The purpose of a **renal arteriogram** (angiogram) is to visualize the renal blood vessels. The findings of an arteriogram can assist in diagnosing renal artery stenosis (Fig. 43-7), additional or missing renal blood vessels, and renovascular hypertension and can assist in differentiating between a

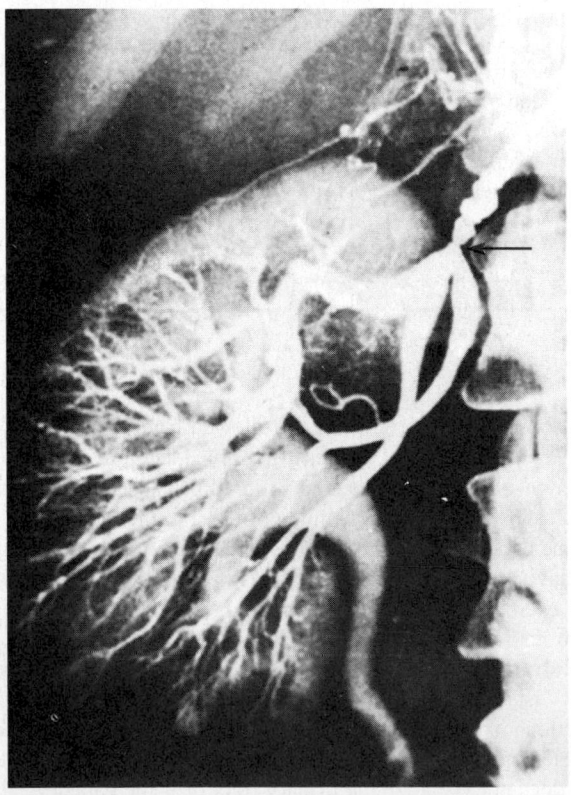

FIG. 43-7 Renal arteriogram showing stenosis of the right renal artery.

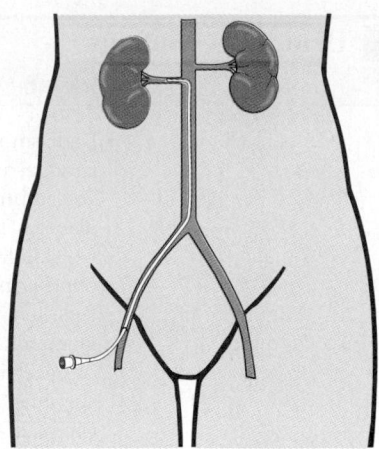

FIG. 43-8 Catheter insertion for a renal arteriogram.

renal cyst and a renal tumor. Renal arteriograms are also included in the workup of a potential renal transplant donor.

The patient is given a local anesthetic at the site of catheter insertion. A catheter is usually inserted into the femoral artery and passed up the aorta to the level of the renal arteries (Fig. 43-8). Contrast media is then injected to outline the renal blood supply, and x-rays are taken. The patient may experience a transient warm feeling along the course of the blood vessel when the contrast material is injected. As with all contrast studies, possible iodine and shellfish allergies should be determined before the study.

After the catheter is removed, a pressure dressing is placed over the femoral injection site. It is important to observe the site for bleeding. Bed rest is usually prescribed with the affected leg straight. Peripheral pulses in the involved leg should be taken at least every 30 to 60 minutes to detect occlusion of blood flow caused by a thrombus. Complications that may result from a renal arteriogram include thrombus, embolus, local inflammation, and hematoma. The patient with baseline renal insufficiency may experience a decrease in renal function secondary to the nephrotoxic contrast material.

Cystogram. The purpose of a cystogram is to outline and visualize the bladder and evaluate the UVJ for reflux. In addition to suspected vesicoureteral reflux, indications for a cystogram include a neurogenic bladder and recurrent urinary tract infections. A cystogram can also delineate abnormalities of the bladder, such as diverticula, calculi, and tumors. The procedure involves instillation of a contrast material into the bladder, which may be done via a cystoscope or catheter.

A *voiding cystourethrogram* (VCUG) is a voiding study of the bladder opening (bladder neck) and urethra. The bladder is filled with contrast material. During urination, films are taken to visualize the bladder and urethra. After urination, another film is taken to assess for residual urine. A VCUG can detect abnormalities of the lower urinary tract, urethral stenosis, bladder neck obstruction, and prostatic enlargement.[9]

Urethrogram. A urethrogram is similar to a cystogram. Contrast material is injected retrograde into the urethra to identify strictures, diverticula, or other urethral pathologic conditions. When urethral trauma is suspected, a urethrogram is done before catheterization.

Loopogram. A loopogram is used to detect obstructions, anastomotic leaks, stones, reflux, and other uropathologic features when a patient has a urinary pouch or ileal conduit. Because urinary diversions are created with bowel, there is risk of contrast absorption. The patient should be closely monitored for reactions to the contrast media.

Renal Radionuclide Imaging. Renal scans involving the use of radionuclides are useful in evaluating the anatomic structures, perfusion, and function of the kidneys. The results reveal the difference between the two kidneys with respect to blood flow, tubular function, and excretion. A normal scan shows symmetric functioning of both kidneys. Normally the distribution of activity is recorded throughout the kidneys. A lesion (e.g., a tumor) is indicated by the absence of radioactivity in the involved area and the appearance of the resultant defect on the scan. This study is particularly useful in detecting renal vascular disease, acute renal failure, and upper urinary tract obstruction. It is also useful in monitoring the function of a transplanted kidney.

Renal Biopsy. The purpose of a **renal biopsy** is to determine the nature and extent of renal disease. This information can be used in establishing a diagnosis or following the progression of renal disease. Biopsy material can be obtained through an open biopsy or a closed percutaneous needle biopsy. An open biopsy is rarely performed because it requires a surgical procedure with anesthesia. A percutaneous needle biopsy is more commonly done.

Absolute contraindications to a percutaneous renal biopsy are bleeding disorders, the presence of a single kidney, and uncontrolled hypertension. Relative contraindications include suspected renal infection, hydronephrosis, and possible vascular lesions. The patient who is going to have a biopsy done should not be taking aspirin or warfarin (Coumadin) before the procedure.

The procedure consists of having the patient lie prone with a pillow or sandbag to elevate the abdomen and kidneys. The position of the kidney is marked on the body using CT, IVP, or ultrasound guidance. Local anesthesia is used, and a biopsy needle is inserted into the kidney just below the twelfth rib. The patient is instructed to hold his or her breath while the biopsy specimen is being taken.

After the procedure, a pressure dressing is applied, and the patient is kept prone for 30 to 60 minutes. Usually bed rest is prescribed for 24 hours. Vital signs should be taken every 5 to 10 minutes during the first hour and then with decreasing frequency, if no problems are noted. The biopsy site should be inspected frequently for bleeding. Serial urine specimens should be assessed for gross and microscopic hematuria. A dipstick can be used to test for bleeding, even when hematuria is not obvious. The physician may order all urine sent for laboratory analysis to detect possible hematuria. The patient should also be assessed for flank pain, hypotension, decreasing hematocrit, and temperature elevation. The patient should be observed for chills, urinary frequency, and dysuria.

Complications of a renal biopsy include renal hemorrhage, hematoma, and infection. Even if no complications occur, the patient should be instructed to avoid lifting heavy objects for 5 to 7 days. The patient should be instructed not to take any anticoagulant drugs until permission is given by the physician who performed the biopsy.

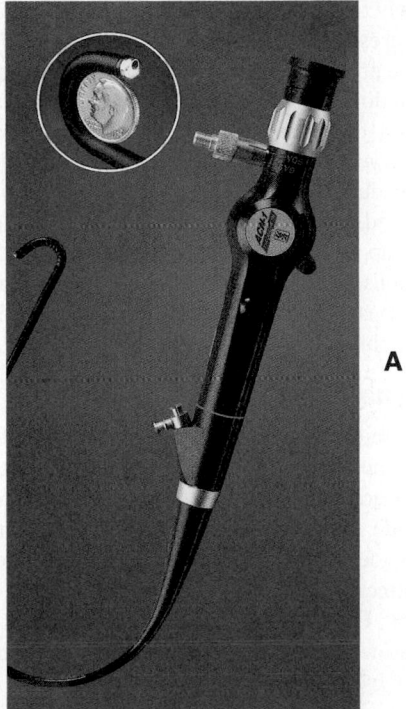

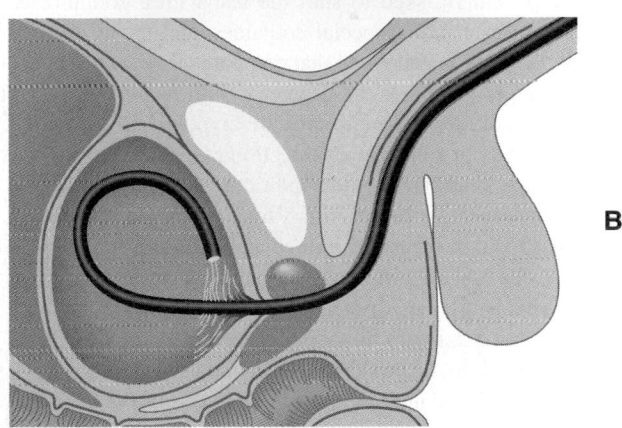

FIG. 43-9 Cystoscopic examination of the bladder in a man. A, Flexible Cysto Nephroscope B, Scope inserted into bladder.

Endoscopy

Cystoscopy. The main purpose of **cystoscopy** is to inspect the interior of the bladder with a tubular lighted scope called a cystoscope (Fig. 43-9). Cystoscopes can be used to insert ureteral catheters, remove calculi, obtain biopsy specimens of bladder lesions, and treat bleeding lesions. In most cases, bladder disorders can be determined by cystoscopic examination.

Cystoscopy is usually done in a cystoscopy room in the x-ray department, in urology clinics, or in the operating room. Most of the pain associated with cystoscopy results from spasms and contractions of bladder and sphincter. Relaxation and deep breathing by the patient may alleviate some of the bladder and sphincter spasms. A local anesthetic is instilled into the urethra before scope insertion. During the examination, saline solution is instilled slowly to distend the bladder. This allows better visualization but causes an urge to urinate.

After the procedure the patient can expect to have some burning on urination, blood-tinged urine, and urinary frequency from the irritation of scope insertion and manipulation. The nurse should observe for bright red bleeding, which is not normal. After the procedure the nurse is responsible for keeping the patient well hydrated, administering mild analgesics, providing sitz baths, and applying heat to decrease the patient's discomfort. Complications that may result from cystoscopy include urinary retention, urinary tract hemorrhage, bladder infection, and perforation of the bladder.

Urodynamics

Urodynamics is a set of tests that are designed to measure urinary tract function. Urodynamic tests study the storage of urine within the bladder and the flow of urine through the urinary tract to the outside of the body. A combination of techniques may be used to provide a detailed urinary incontinence assessment of urinary incontinence.[10]

Urinary Flow Study. The urinary flow study (uroflow) measures urine volume in a single voiding expelled in a period of time and is expressed as milliliters per second. As the patient voids, the stream pattern is depicted graphically on a printout.

The patient is asked to start the test with a comfortably full bladder, urinate into a special container, and try to empty completely. A graph is generated that compares flow rate to time. This test is used to (1) assess the degree of outflow obstruction caused by such conditions as benign prostatic hyperplasia or stricture, (2) assess bladder or sphincter dysfunction effects on voiding such as occurs with neuropathologic conditions, and (2) evaluate the effects of treatment for lower urinary tract problems. A residual urine volume should be measured immediately after a urinary flow study because this will help to identify the degree of chronic urinary retention that is often associated with abnormal flow patterns.

A normal maximum flow rate for men is about 20 to 25 ml per second and about 25 to 30 ml per second for women. However, the volume voided and the patient's age can affect the flow rate, so normal variations are common. Graphic displays can illustrate straining and intermittent flow patterns or other abnormal voiding disorders.

Cystometrogram. A **cystometrogram** evaluates the compliance (elastic property) and stability of the detrusor muscle of the bladder. It is a measurement of intravesical pressure during the course of bladder filling. It is usually ordered if a patient has incontinence or neurogenic bladder. The procedure consists of insertion of a specially designed catheter while the patient is in a supine position. If abdominal pressure is measured, a second tube is inserted into the rectum or vagina. This tube is typically attached to a small fluid-filled balloon to allow pressure recording. Saline or sterile water for irrigation or contrast used for a cystogram is infused into the bladder, and pressures are measured. During the infusion, the patient is asked about sensations of bladder filling, usually including the first desire (urge) to urinate, a strong desire to urinate, and perception of bladder fullness.

Sphincter Electromyography (EMG). An EMG is a recording of the electrical activity created when the nervous system stimulates motor units within a muscle. By placing needles, percutaneous wires, or patches near the urethra, the pelvic floor muscle activity can be assessed. During the filling cystometrogram, the sphincter EMG is used to identify voluntary pelvic floor muscle contractions and the response of these muscles to bladder filling, coughing, and other provocative maneuvers.

Voiding Pressure Flow Study. The voiding pressure flow study combines a urinary flow rate, cystometric pressures (intravesical, abdominal, and detrusor pressures), and a sphincter EMG for detailed evaluation of micturition. It is completed by assisting the patient to a specialized toilet and allowing the person to urinate while the various pressure tubes and EMG apparatus remain in place.

Videourodynamics. *Videourodynamics* is a combination of the filling cystometrogram, sphincter EMG, and/or urinary flow study with anatomic imaging of the lower urinary tract, typically via fluoroscopy. This combination is used in selected cases to identify an obstructive lesion and characterize anatomic changes in the bladder and lower urinary tract.

Whitaker Study. The Whitaker study is used to measure the pressure differential between the renal pelvis and the bladder. The presence of a ureteral obstruction can be assessed. Percutaneous access is gained to the renal pelvis by placing a catheter in the renal pelvis. A catheter is also placed in the bladder. Fluid is perfused through the percutaneous tube or needle at a rate of 10 ml per minute. Pressure data are then collected. These pressure measurements are combined with fluoroscopic imaging to identify the level of obstruction.

REVIEW QUESTIONS

The number of the question corresponds to the same-numbered objective at the beginning of the chapter.

1. A renal stone in the pelvis of the kidney will alter the function of the kidney by interfering with
   a. the structural support of the kidney.
   b. regulation of the concentration of urine.
   c. the entry and exit of blood vessels at the kidney.
   d. collection and drainage of urine from the kidney.

2. A patient with renal disease has oliguria and a creatinine clearance of 40 ml per minute. The nurse recognizes that these findings most directly reflect abnormal function of
   a. tubular secretion.
   b. glomerular filtration.
   c. capillary permeability.
   d. concentration of filtrate.

3. The nurse identifies a risk for urinary calculi in a patient who relates a past health history that includes
   a. measles.
   b. gastric ulcer.
   c. diabetes mellitus.
   d. hyperparathyroidism.

4. Normal changes associated with aging of the urinary system that the nurse expects to find include
   a. decreased levels of BUN.
   b. urine postvoiding residual.
   c. increased bladder capacity.
   d. more easily palpable kidneys.

5. During physical assessment of the urinary system, the nurse
   a. percusses the flank area with a firm blow.
   b. palpates an empty bladder as a small nodule.
   c. positions the patient prone to palpate the kidneys.
   d. uses auscultation to determine the level of urine in the bladder.

6. Normal findings expected by the nurse on physical assessment of the urinary system include
   a. nonpalpable left kidney.
   b. auscultation of renal artery bruit.
   c. CVA tenderness elicited by a kidney punch.
   d. palpable bladder to the level of the pubic symphysis.

7. An important nursing responsibility after an IVP is to
   a. assess the patient for flank pain.
   b. encourage extra oral fluid intake.
   c. observe urine for remaining contrast material.
   d. encourage ambulation 2 to 3 hours after the study.

8. On reading the urinalysis results of a dehydrated patient, the nurse would expect to find
   a. a pH of 8.4.
   b. RBC of 4/hpf.
   c. color: yellow, cloudy.
   d. specific gravity of 1.035.

REFERENCES

1. Smith HW: *Fish to philosopher,* Boston, 1953, Little, Brown.
2. Gray ML: Physiology of voiding. In Doughty DB, editor: *Urinary and fecal incontinence: nursing management,* St Louis, 2000, Mosby.
3. McCance KL, Huether SE: *Pathophysiology: the biologic basis for disease in adults and children,* ed 4, St Louis, 2002, Mosby.
4. Guyton AC: *Textbook of medical physiology,* Philadelphia, 2000, Saunders.
5. Hazzard WR: Aging kidneys in an aging population: how does this impact nephrology and nephrologists? *Geriatr Nephrol Urol* 9:177, 1999.
6. Muhlberg W, Platt D: Age-dependent changes of the kidneys: pharmacological implications, *Gerontology* 45:243, 1999.
7. Greenberg A: *Primer on kidney disease,* San Diego, 2001, Academic Press.
8. Manjunath G, Sarnak MJ, Levey AS: Estimating the glomerular filtration rate: dos and don'ts for assessing kidney function, *Postgrad Med* 110:55, 2001.
9. Gordon D, Groutz A: Evaluation of female lower urinary tract symptoms: overview and update, *Curr Opin Obstet Gynecol* 13:521, 2001.
10. Gray M: Urodynamics in the clinical management of urinary incontinence in men and women, *Topics in Geriatric Rehabilitation* 15:42, 2000.

RESOURCES

Resources for this chapter are listed in Chapter 44 on page 1209 and Chapter 45 on page 1246.

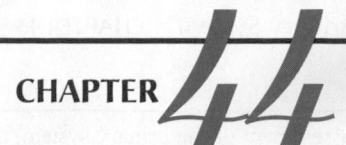

CHAPTER **44**

NURSING MANAGEMENT
Renal and Urologic Problems

Mikel Gray

LEARNING OBJECTIVES

1. Describe the pathophysiology, clinical manifestations, collaborative care, and drug therapy of cystitis, urethritis, and pyelonephritis.
2. Explain the nursing management of urinary tract infections.
3. Describe the immunologic mechanisms involved in glomerulonephritis.
4. Explain the clinical manifestations and nursing and collaborative management of acute poststreptococcal glomerulonephritis, Goodpasture syndrome, and chronic glomerulonephritis.
5. Describe the common causes, clinical manifestations, collaborative care, and nursing management of nephrotic syndrome.
6. Compare and contrast the etiology, clinical manifestations, collaborative care, and nursing management of various types of urinary calculi.
7. Explain the common causes and management of renal trauma, renal vascular problems, and hereditary renal problems.
8. Describe the mechanisms of renal involvement in metabolic and connective tissue disorders.
9. Describe the clinical manifestations and collaborative care of kidney and bladder cancer.
10. Describe the common causes and management of bladder dysfunctions.
11. Differentiate among ureteral, suprapubic, nephrostomy, and urethral catheters with regard to indications for use and nursing responsibilities.
12. Explain the nursing management of the patient undergoing nephrectomy or urinary diversion surgery.

KEY TERMS

calculus, p. 1186	nephrosclerosis, p. 1191
cystitis, p. 1173	nephrotic syndrome, p. 1183
glomerulonephritis, p. 1180	polycystic kidney disease, p. 1192
Goodpasture syndrome, p. 1182	pyelonephritis, p. 1173
hydronephrosis, p. 1184	renal artery stenosis, p. 1191
hydroureter, p. 1184	renal vein thrombosis, p. 1191
ileal conduit, p. 1203	stricture, p. 1189
interstitial cystitis, p. 1179	urethritis, p. 1173
lithotripsy, p. 1188	urinary incontinence, p. 1195
nephrolithiasis, p. 1185	urinary retention, p. 1195

Renal and urologic disorders encompass a wide spectrum of clinical problems. The diverse causes of these disorders may involve infectious, immunologic, obstructive, metabolic, collagen-vascular, traumatic, congenital, neoplastic, and neurologic mechanisms. This chapter discusses specific disorders of the kidneys, ureters, bladder, and urethra. Acute renal failure and chronic kidney disease are discussed in Chapter 45. Female reproductive problems are discussed in Chapter 52. Male genitourinary problems are discussed in Chapter 53.

Infectious and Inflammatory Disorders of the Urinary System

URINARY TRACT INFECTION

Urinary tract infections (UTIs) are the second most common bacterial disease. UTIs account for more than 8 million office visits per year. More than 100,000 people are hospitalized annu-

ally because of UTIs. More than 15% of patients who develop gram-negative bacteremia die, and one third of these are caused by bacterial infections originating in the urinary tract.[1]

Inflammation of the urinary tract may be attributable to a variety of disorders, but bacterial infection is by far the most common.[2] In the majority of healthy persons, the bladder and its contents are free from bacteria. Nevertheless, a minority of otherwise healthy individuals, including many young adult women and older women and men, have some bacteria colonizing the bladder. This condition is called *asymptomatic bacteriuria* and does not justify treatment. In contrast, an infection of the urinary system is diagnosed when bacterial invasion of the urinary tract occurs.

Escherichia coli (E. coli) (Table 44-1) is the most common pathogen leading to a UTI. Bacterial counts of 10^5 colony-forming units per milliliter (CFU/ml) or higher typically indicate a clinically significant UTI. However, counts as low as 10^2 to 10^3 CFU/ml in a person with signs and symptoms are indicative of UTI. Although fungal and parasitic infections may also cause UTIs, they are uncommon. UTIs from these causes are sometimes observed in patients who are immunosuppressed, have diabetes mellitus, or have undergone multiple courses of antibiotic

CULTURAL & ETHNIC CONSIDERATIONS
Urologic Disorders

- Urinary tract calculi are more common among whites than African Americans.
- Jewish men have a high incidence of uric acid stones.
- Bladder cancer has a higher incidence among white men than African American men.
- In all ethnic groups, bladder cancer affects men about three times more often than women.

Reviewed by Vicki Y. Johnson, RN, PhD, FN, CUCNS, Assistant Professor, University of Alabama, School of Nursing, Birmingham, Ala.

TABLE 44-1 Common Microorganisms Causing Urinary Tract Infections

*Escherichia coli**	*Proteus*
Enterococcus	*Pseudomonas*
Klebsiella	*Staphylococcus*
Enterobacter	*Candida*
Serratia	

*Causes about 80% of cases in persons who do not have urinary tract structural abnormalities or calculi.

therapy. They also may be seen in persons living in or having traveled to certain third world countries.

Classification

Several classification systems can be used for UTIs.[2,3] For example, a UTI can be broadly classified as an upper or lower UTI according to its location within the urinary system (Fig. 44-1). Infection of the upper urinary tract (involving the renal parenchyma, pelvis, and ureters) typically causes fever, chills, and flank pain, whereas a UTI confined to the lower urinary tract does not usually have systemic manifestations. Specific terms are used to further delineate the location of a UTI or inflammation. For example, **pyelonephritis** implies inflammation (usually due to infection) of the renal parenchyma and collecting system, **cystitis** indicates inflammation of the bladder wall, and **urethritis** means inflammation of the urethra.

Classifying a UTI as complicated or uncomplicated is also useful. *Uncomplicated* infections are those that occur in an otherwise normal urinary tract.[4] *Complicated* infections include those with coexisting presence of obstruction, stones, or catheters; existing di-

abetes or neurologic diseases; or an infection that is recurrent. The individual with a complicated infection is at risk for renal damage.

UTIs can also be classified according to their natural history. An *initial infection* (sometimes called a first or isolated infection) refers to an uncomplicated UTI in a person who has never had an infection or experiences one that is remote from any previous UTI (usually separated by a period of years). In contrast, a *recurrent UTI* is a reinfection in a person who experienced a previous infection that was successfully eradicated. If a recurrent UTI occurs because the original infection is not adequately eradicated, it is classified as unresolved bacteriuria or bacterial persistence. *Unresolved bacteriuria* occurs when bacteria are initially resistant to the antibiotic used to treat an infection, when the antibiotic agent fails to achieve adequate concentrations in the urine or bloodstream to kill bacteria, or when the drug is discontinued before the underlying bacteriuria is completely eradicated. *Bacterial persistence* also may occur when bacteria develop resistance to the antibiotic agent selected for treatment or when a foreign body in the urinary system serves as a harbor or anchor allowing bacteria to survive despite appropriate therapy.

Etiology and Pathophysiology

The urinary tract above the urethra is normally sterile. Several physiologic and mechanical defense mechanisms assist in maintaining sterility and preventing UTIs. These defenses include normal voiding with complete emptying of the bladder, normal antibacterial ability of the bladder mucosa and urine, ureterovesical junction competence, and peristaltic activity that propels urine toward the bladder. An alteration in any of these defense mechanisms increases the risk of contracting a UTI. Table 44-2 lists predisposing factors to UTIs.

TABLE 44-2 Predisposing Factors to Urinary Tract Infections

Factors Increasing Urinary Stasis
- Intrinsic obstruction (stone, tumor of urinary tract)
- Extrinsic obstruction (tumor, fibrosis compressing urinary tract)
- Urinary retention (including neurogenic bladder and low bladder wall compliance)

Foreign Bodies
- Urinary calculi
- Indwelling catheter
- Ureteral stent

Anatomic Factors
- Congenital defects leading to obstruction or urinary stasis
- Fistula (abnormal opening) exposing urinary stream to skin, vagina, or fecal stream
- Shorter female urethra

Factors Compromising Immune Response
- Human immunodeficiency virus infection
- Diabetes mellitus

Functional Disorders
- Constipation
- Voiding dysfunction with detrusor sphincter dyssynergia

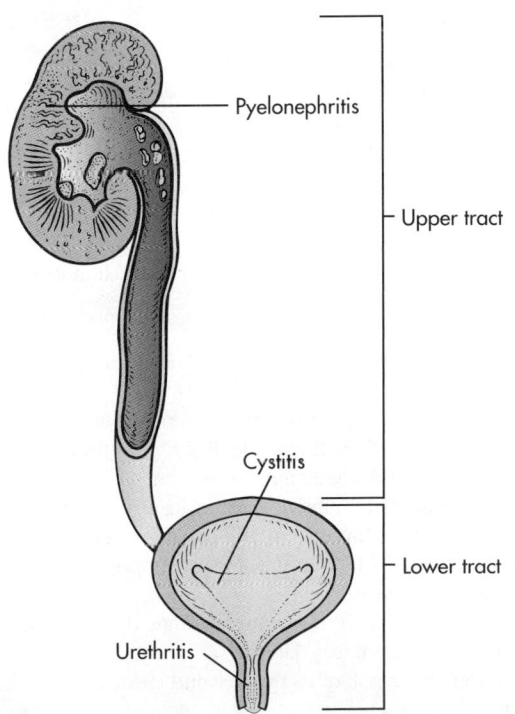

FIG. 44-1 Sites of infectious processes in the urinary tract.

The organisms that usually cause UTIs are introduced via the ascending route from the urethra. Other less common routes are via the bloodstream or lymphatic system. Most infections are due to gram-negative bacilli normally found in the gastrointestinal (GI) tract, although gram-positive organisms such as streptococci, enterococci, and *Staphylococcus saprophyticus* can also cause urinary infections. A common factor contributing to ascending infection is urologic instrumentation (e.g., catheterization, cystoscopic examinations). Instrumentation allows bacteria that are normally present at the opening of the urethra to enter the urethra or bladder. Sexual intercourse promotes "milking" of bacteria from the vagina and perineum and may cause minor urethral trauma that predisposes women to UTIs.

Rarely do UTIs result from a hematogenous route, where blood-borne bacteria secondarily invade the kidneys, ureters, or bladder from elsewhere in the body. For a kidney infection to occur from hematogenous transmission, there must be prior injury to the urinary tract, such as obstruction of the ureter, damage caused by stones, or renal scars.

An important source of UTIs is hospital-acquired, or *nosocomial,* infection. The cause of nosocomial infection is often *E. coli* and, less frequently, *Pseudomonas* organisms. Urologic instrumentation, particularly with an indwelling urinary catheter, is the most common predisposing factor.

Clinical Manifestations

Bothersome lower urinary tract symptoms are seen in UTIs of the upper urinary tracts, as well as those confined to the lower tract. These symptoms include dysuria, frequent urination (more often than every 2 hours), urgency, and suprapubic discomfort or pressure. The urine may contain grossly visible blood (hematuria) or sediment, giving it a cloudy appearance. Flank pain, chills, and the presence of a fever indicate an infection involving the upper urinary tract (pyelonephritis). It is important to remember that these symptoms, considered characteristic of a UTI, are often absent in older adults. Older adults tend to experience nonlocalized abdominal discomfort rather than dysuria and suprapubic pain.[2] In addition, they may have cognitive impairment.[4] Older adults are also less likely to experience a fever with infection of the upper urinary tract. Patients over age 80 years may experience a slight decline in temperature. People with significant bacteriuria may have no symptoms or may have nonspecific symptoms such as fatigue or anorexia.

Multiple factors may produce bothersome lower urinary tract symptoms similar to a UTI. For example, patients with bladder tumors or those receiving intravesical chemotherapy or pelvic radiation usually experience urinary frequency, urgency, and dysuria. Interstitial cystitis, a chronic inflammatory condition of unknown etiology, also produces bothersome urinary symptoms that are sometimes confused with a UTI. (Interstitial cystitis is discussed later in this chapter.)

Diagnostic Studies

Dipstick urinalysis should be obtained initially to identify the presence of nitrites (indicating bacteriuria), white blood cells (WBCs), and leukocyte esterase (an enzyme present in WBCs). These findings can be confirmed by microscopic urinalysis. Following confirmation of bacteriuria and pyuria, a urine culture may be obtained. A urine culture is indicated in complicated or nosocomial UTIs, persistent bacteria, or frequently recurring UTIs (more than two to three episodes per year). Urine also may be cultured when the infection is unresponsive to empiric therapy or the diagnosis is questionable.[5] A voided midstream technique yielding a clean-catch urine sample is preferred for obtaining a urine culture in most circumstances. (See Table 43-8 for an explanation of this technique.) However, a specimen obtained by catheterization or suprapubic needle aspiration provides more accurate results and may be necessary when an adequate clean-catch specimen cannot be readily obtained.

A urine culture is accompanied by *sensitivity testing* to determine the bacteria's susceptibility to a variety of antibiotic drugs. The results of this test allow the health care provider to select an antibiotic known to be capable of destroying the bacterial strain producing a UTI in a specific patient.

Imaging studies of the urinary tract are indicated in selected cases. For example, an intravenous pyelogram (IVP) or abdominal computed tomography (CT) scan may be obtained when obstruction of the urinary system is suspected of causing a UTI.

Collaborative Care and Drug Therapy

Once a UTI has been diagnosed, appropriate antimicrobial therapy is initiated. An antibiotic may be selected based on the health care provider's best judgment (empiric therapy) or the

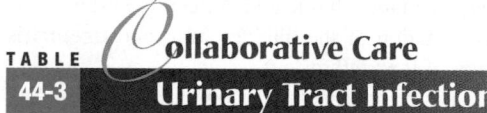

TABLE 44-3	Collaborative Care Urinary Tract Infection

Diagnostic
History and physical examination
Urinalysis
Urine for culture and sensitivity (if indicated)
Imaging studies of urinary tract (e.g., IVP, cystoscopy) (if indicated)

Collaborative Therapy
Uncomplicated UTI
Antibiotic: 1- to 3-day treatment regimen
  trimethoprim-sulfamethoxazole (Bactrim, Septra)
  nitrofurantoin (Macrodantin, Macrobid)
Adequate fluid intake
Urinary analgesic such as phenazopyridine (Pyridium) or combination agent (e.g., Urised)
Counseling about risk of recurrence and reduction of risk factors

Recurrent, Uncomplicated UTI
Repeat urinalysis and consideration of need for urine culture and sensitivity testing
Antibiotic: 3- to 5-day treatment regimen
  trimethoprim-sulfamethoxazole (Bactrim, Septra)
  nitrofurantoin (Macrodantin, Furadantin)
  Sensitivity-guided antibiotic (ampicillin, amoxicillin, first-generation cephalosporin, fluoroquinolone)
Consideration of 3- to 6-month trial of suppressive antibiotics
Adequate fluid intake
Urinary analgesic such as phenazopyridine (Pyridium) or combination agent (e.g., Urised)
Counseling about risk of recurrence and reduction of risk factors
Imaging study of urinary tract in selected cases

IVP, Intravenous pyelogram; *UTI,* urinary tract infection.

results of sensitivity testing. The collaborative care and drug therapy of cystitis are summarized in Table 44-3. Uncomplicated cystitis can be treated by a short-term course of antibiotics, typically for 1 to 3 days. In contrast, complicated UTIs require longer-term treatment, lasting 7 to 14 days or even longer.[6,7]

Trimethoprim-sulfamethoxazole (TMP-SMX) or nitrofurantoin (Macrodantin) is often used to empirically treat uncomplicated or initial UTIs. TMP-SMX has the advantages of being relatively inexpensive and is taken twice daily. Nitrofurantoin is normally given 3 to 4 times daily, but a long-acting preparation (Macrobid) is available that is taken twice daily. Ampicillin or amoxicillin are not frequently selected when empirically treating a noncomplicated UTI because they must be administered 3 to 4 times daily. In addition to these agents, the fluoroquinolones (including ciprofloxacin [Cipro], levofloxacin [Levaquin], norfloxacin [Noroxin], ofloxacin [Floxin], or gatifloxacin [Tequin]) may be used to treat complicated UTIs.

A number of over-the-counter (OTC) or prescription drugs may be used in combination with antibiotic agents to relieve the discomfort associated with a UTI. Phenazopyridine (Pyridium) is an OTC drug that provides a soothing effect on the urinary tract mucosa. It also stains the urine a reddish orange that may be mistaken for blood in the urine, and it may permanently stain underclothing. Although this drug is typically effective in relieving the transient acute discomfort associated with a UTI, patients should be advised to avoid long-term use of phenazopyridine because it can produce hemolytic anemia. Combination agents such as Urised (methenamine, phenylsalicylate, atropine, hyoscyamine) may also be used to relieve the pain associated with a UTI. The patient taking a combination agent such as Urised should be advised that preparations containing methylene blue are expected to tint the urine blue or green.

Prophylactic or *suppressive antibiotics* are sometimes administered to patients who experience repeated UTIs. A low dose of TMP-SMX, nitrofurantoin, or another antibiotic may be administered on a daily basis in an attempt to prevent recurring UTIs, or a single dose may be taken before an event likely to provoke a UTI, such as intercourse. However, although suppressive therapy is often effective on a short-term basis, this strategy is limited because of the risk of antibiotic resistance ultimately leading to breakthrough infections with increasingly virulent pathogens.[8]

NURSING MANAGEMENT
URINARY TRACT INFECTION

■ Nursing Assessment

Subjective and objective data that should be obtained from a patient with a UTI are presented in Table 44-4.

■ Nursing Diagnoses

Nursing diagnoses for the patient with a UTI may include, but are not limited to, those presented in NCP 44-1.

■ Planning

The overall goals are that the patient with a UTI will have (1) relief from bothersome lower urinary tract symptoms, (2) prevention of upper urinary tract involvement, and (3) prevention of recurrence.

■ Nursing Implementation

Health Promotion. Health promotion measures include recognizing individuals who are at risk for a UTI. Debilitated persons, older adults, patients with underlying diseases (e.g., cancer, human immunodeficiency virus [HIV], or diabetes mellitus) that compromise host immune responses, and patients treated with immunosuppressive drugs or corticosteroids are at high risk for UTIs. Especially for these individuals, health promotion activities can help decrease the frequency of infections and promote early detection of infection. Health promotion activities include teaching preventive measures, such as (1) emptying the bladder regularly and completely, (2) evacuating the bowel regularly, (3) wiping the perineal area from front to back after urination and defecation, and (4) drinking an adequate amount of liquid each day. The recommended daily liquid intake for the ambulatory adult is approximately 15 ml per pound of body weight per day. Thus a 150-pound person would require 2250 ml each day. Because the person will obtain approximately 20% of this fluid from food, this leaves 1800 ml obtained by drinking, or just over seven 8-ounce glasses of fluid. Although suppressive antibiotics are not generally recommended, daily intake of cranberry juice (consumed as pure juice, 8 ounces twice daily) or cranberry essence tablets may reduce the risk of certain UTIs.[9] In addition, it is important to teach the patient to seek early treatment once symptoms are identified.

TABLE 44-4	Nursing Assessment Urinary Tract Infection

Subjective Data

Important Health Information

Past health history: Previous urinary tract infections; urinary calculi, stasis, reflux, strictures, or retention; neurogenic bladder; pregnancy; prostatic hyperplasia; sexually transmitted disease; bladder cancer

Medications: Use of antibiotics, anticholinergics, antispasmodics

Surgery or other treatments: Recent urologic instrumentation (catheterization, cystoscopy, surgery)

Functional Health Patterns

Health perception–health management: Urinary hygiene practices; lassitude, malaise

Nutritional-metabolic: Nausea, vomiting, and anorexia; chills

Elimination: Urinary frequency, urgency, hesitancy; nocturia

Cognitive-perceptual: Suprapubic or low back pain, costovertebral tenderness; bladder spasms, dysuria, burning on urination

Objective Data

General

Fever

Urinary

Hematuria; cloudy, foul-smelling urine; tender, enlarged kidney

Possible Findings

Leukocytosis; urinalysis positive for bacteria, pyuria, RBCs, and WBCs; positive urine culture; IVP, CT scan, ultrasound, voiding cystourethrogram and cystoscopy demonstrating abnormalities of urinary tract

CT, Computed tomography; *IVP,* intravenous pyelogram; *RBCs,* red blood cells; *WBCs,* white blood cells.

NURSING CARE PLAN 44-1

Patient with a Urinary Tract Infection

NURSING DIAGNOSIS   **Acute pain** *related to* inflammation of mucosal tissue of urinary tract *as manifested by* pain on urination, flank pain, suprapubic pain, lower back pain, bladder spasms.

OUTCOMES—NOC	INTERVENTIONS—NIC and *RATIONALES*
Pain Control (1605)	*Pain Management (1400)*
▪ Uses nonanalgesic relief measures ____	▪ Perform a comprehensive assessment of pain to include location, characteristics, onset and duration, frequency, quality, intensity or severity, and precipitating factors *to establish history and baseline pain level.*
▪ Uses analgesics appropriately ____	▪ Provide the patient optimal pain relief by administering analgesics such as phenazopyridine (Pyridium) or combination agents (e.g., Urised) as ordered *to promote comfort.*
	▪ Alert patient that phenazopyridine will color urine orange and combination agents containing methylene blue will color urine blue or green *to prevent concern over unusual appearance of urine.*
Outcome Scale	▪ Teach the use of nonpharmacologic techniques (e.g., heating pad to suprapubic area or lower back, warm showers) during painful episodes along with other relief measures *to supplement pain medication and increase pain relief.*
1 = Never demonstrated	
2 = Rarely demonstrated	
3 = Sometimes demonstrated	
4 = Often demonstrated	
5 = Consistently demonstrated	

NURSING DIAGNOSIS   **Impaired urinary elimination** *related to* urinary tract infection (UTI) *as manifested by* bothersome urgency, daytime voiding frequency, nocturia, or hematuria and verbalization of concern over altered elimination pattern.

OUTCOMES—NOC	INTERVENTIONS—NIC and *RATIONALES*
Urinary Elimination (0503)	*Urinary Elimination Management (0590)*
▪ Elimination pattern IER ____	▪ Monitor urinary elimination including frequency, consistency, odor, volume, and color (as appropriate) *to assess elimination status.*
▪ Urine passes without urgency ____	▪ Obtain midstream voided specimen for culture and sensitivity (as appropriate) *to determine pathogen causing UTI or to monitor effectiveness of treatment.*
▪ Urine free of blood ____	▪ Administer antimicrobial drugs as ordered *to eliminate symptoms by inhibiting bacterial growth.*
▪ Digestion of adequate fluids ____	▪ Teach patient signs and symptoms of UTI *to monitor effectiveness of treatment and recognize symptoms of recurrence.*
Outcome Scale	▪ Encourage adequate fluid *to help prevent infection and dehydration.*
1 = Extremely compromised	
2 = Substantially compromised	
3 = Moderately compromised	
4 = Mildly compromised	
5 = Not compromised	

IER, In expected range.

The nurse can play a major role in the prevention of nosocomial infections. Avoidance of unnecessary catheterization and early removal of indwelling catheters are the most effective means for reducing nosocomial UTIs. All patients undergoing instrumentation of the urinary tract are at risk for developing a nosocomial UTI. Aseptic technique must always be followed during these procedures. Washing hands before and after contact with each patient and wearing gloves for care involving the urinary system are especially important. When a catheter has been inserted, special measures must be employed as explained in the section on urethral catheterization later in this chapter.

Routine and thorough perineal hygiene is important for all hospitalized patients, especially when a bedpan is used. Incontinent episodes should be avoided by answering the call light quickly or offering the bedpan or urinal at frequent intervals to the bedridden patient.

Acute Intervention. Acute intervention for a patient with a UTI includes ensuring adequate fluid intake if it is not contraindicated. It is sometimes difficult to get the patient to maintain an adequate fluid intake because the person may think it will worsen the discomfort and frequency associated with a UTI. The patient needs to be told that fluids will increase frequency of urination at first but will also dilute the urine, making the bladder less irritable. Fluids will help flush out bacteria before they have a chance to colonize in the bladder. Caffeine, alcohol, citrus juices, chocolate, and highly spiced foods or beverages should be avoided because they are potential bladder irritants.

Application of local heat to the suprapubic area or lower back may relieve the discomfort associated with a UTI. The patient can be advised to apply a heating pad (turned to its lowest setting) against the back or suprapubic area. A warm shower or sitting in a tub of warm water filled above the waist can also be effective in providing temporary relief.

The patient should be instructed about the prescribed drug therapy, including side effects. The nurse should emphasize the importance of taking the full course of antibiotics. Often patients stop antibiotic therapy once symptoms disappear. This practice can lead to inadequate treatment and recurrence of infection or to bacterial resistance to antibiotics. Sometimes a second drug or a reduced dose of drug is ordered after the initial course to suppress bacterial growth in certain patients susceptible to recurrent UTI. The patient should be instructed to watch for any changes in the color or consistency of the urine and a decrease in or cessation of symptoms as a sign of the effectiveness of therapy. The patient should be counseled that persistence of bothersome lower urinary tract symptoms beyond the antibiotic treatment course or the onset of flank pain or fever should be reported promptly to a health care provider.

Ambulatory and Home Care. Home care for the patient with a UTI should emphasize the patient's compliance with the drug regimen. The nurse's responsibility is to teach the patient about the need for ongoing care (Table 44-5). This includes taking antimicrobial drugs as ordered, maintaining adequate daily fluid intake, regular voiding (approximately every 2 to 4 hours), urinating after intercourse, and temporarily discontinuing the use of a diaphragm (if used).

The patient must understand the need for follow-up care with urine culture to determine if the infection has been adequately treated. Recurrent symptoms because of bacterial persistence or inadequate treatment typically occur within 1 to 2 weeks after completion of therapy. If the patient has been compliant, a relapse indicates the need for further evaluation.

■ Evaluation

The expected outcomes for the patient with a UTI are presented in NCP 44-1.

TABLE 44-5   *Patient & Family Teaching Guide*   Urinary Tract Infection

The following are important to teach to the patient with a UTI to prevent recurrence:

1. Explain importance of taking all antibiotics as prescribed. Symptoms may improve after 1 to 2 days of therapy, but organisms may still be present.
2. Instruct the patient on appropriate hygiene, including the following:
   a. Careful cleansing of perineal region
   b. Wiping from front to back after urinating
   c. Cleansing with soap and water after each bowel movement
3. Explain the importance of emptying the bladder before and after intercourse.
4. Instruct the patient to urinate regularly, approximately every 2 to 4 hours during the day.
5. Instruct the patient about the need to maintain adequate fluid intake (one-half ounce per pound of body weight per day).
6. Instruct the patient to avoid harsh soaps, bubble baths, powders, and sprays in the perineal area.
7. Advise the patient to report symptoms or signs of recurrent UTI (e.g., cloudy urine, pain on urination, urgency, frequency).

UTI, Urinary tract infection.

ACUTE PYELONEPHRITIS

Etiology and Pathophysiology

Pyelonephritis is an inflammation of the renal parenchyma and collecting system (including the renal pelvis). The most common cause is bacterial infection, but fungi, protozoa, or viruses sometimes infect the kidney.[10]

Urosepsis is a systemic infection arising from a urologic source. Its prompt diagnosis and effective treatment are critical because it can lead to septic shock and death in 15% of cases unless promptly eradicated. Septic shock is the outcome of unresolved bacteremia involving a gram-negative organism. (Septic shock is discussed in Chapter 65.)

Pyelonephritis usually begins with colonization and infection of the lower urinary tract via the ascending urethral route. Bacteria normally found in the intestinal tract, such as *E. coli, Proteus, Klebsiella,* or *Enterobacter* species, frequently cause pyelonephritis. A preexisting factor is often present, such as *vesicoureteral reflux* (retrograde or backward movement of urine from lower to upper urinary tract) or dysfunction of lower urinary tract function such as obstruction from benign prostatic hyperplasia, a stricture, or urinary stone.

Acute pyelonephritis commonly starts in the renal medulla and spreads to the adjacent cortex. Recurring episodes of pyelonephritis, especially in the presence of obstructive abnormalities, can lead to a scarred, poorly functioning kidney and a condition called *chronic pyelonephritis.*

Clinical Manifestations and Diagnostic Studies

The clinical manifestations of acute pyelonephritis vary from mild fatigue to the sudden onset of chills, fever, vomiting, malaise, flank pain, and the bothersome lower urinary tract symptoms characteristic of cystitis. *Costovertebral tenderness* is typically present on the affected side. The clinical manifestations usually subside within a few days, even without specific therapy, but bacteriuria and pyuria usually persist.

Urinalysis shows pyuria, bacteriuria, and varying degrees of hematuria. White blood cell (WBC) casts may be found in the urine, indicating involvement of the renal parenchyma. A complete blood count will show leukocytosis and a shift to the left with an increase in immature neutrophils (bands). Urine cultures must be obtained when pyelonephritis is suspected. In patients with more severe illness who are hospitalized, blood cultures are also obtained.

Imaging studies, such as an IVP or CT scan, requiring intravenous injection of contrast materials are usually not obtained in the early stages of pyelonephritis to prevent the possible spread of infection. Alternatively, ultrasonography of the urinary system may be obtained to identify anatomic abnormalities or the presence of an obstructing stone. Imaging studies are also used to assess for complications of pyelonephritis such as impaired renal function, scarring, chronic pyelonephritis, or abscesses.

Urosepsis is characterized by bacteriuria and bacteremia (presence of bacteria in blood). If bacteremia is a possibility, close observation and vital sign monitoring are essential. Prompt recognition and treatment of septic shock may prevent irreversible damage or death.

Collaborative Care and Drug Therapy

The diagnostic tests and collaborative therapy of acute pyelonephritis are summarized in Table 44-6. Patients with severe infections or complicating factors such as nausea and vomiting with dehydration require hospital admission.

The patient with mild symptoms may be treated as an outpatient with antibiotics for 14 to 21 days (see Table 44-6). Parenteral antibiotics are often given initially in the hospital to rapidly establish high serum and urinary drug levels. When initial treatment resolves acute symptoms and the patient is able to tolerate oral fluids and drugs, the person may be discharged on a regimen of oral antibiotics for an additional 14 to 21 days. Symptoms and signs typically improve or resolve within 48 to 72 hours after starting therapy.[11,12]

Relapses may be treated with a 6-week course of antibiotics. Reinfections may be treated as individual episodes of disease or managed with long-term antibiotic therapy. Antibiotic prophylaxis may also be used for recurrent infections. The effectiveness of therapy is evaluated in accordance with the presence or absence of bacterial growth on urine culture.

TABLE 44-6	Collaborative Care Acute Pyelonephritis

Diagnostic
History and physical examination
Urinalysis
Urine for culture and sensitivity
Ultrasound (initially), IVP, VCUG, radionuclide imaging, CT scan
CBC count with WBC differential
Blood culture (if bacteremia is suspected)
Palpation for flank pain

Collaborative Therapy
Mild Symptoms
Outpatient management or short hospitalization for IV antibiotics
- Empirically selected broad-spectrum antibiotics (ampicillin, vancomycin) combined with an aminoglycoside (e.g., tobramycin [Nebcin], gentamicin [Garamycin])
- Switch to sensitivity-guided therapy (when results available) for 14 to 21 days
  trimethoprim-sulfamethoxazole (Bactrim, Septra)
  Fluoroquinolones (ciprofloxacin [Cipro], ofloxacin [Floxin], norfloxacin [Noroxin], gatifloxacin [Tequin])
Adequate fluid intake
Nonsteroidal antiinflammatory drugs or antipyretic drugs
Urinary analgesics (e.g., phenazopyridine [Pyridium])
Follow-up urine culture and imaging studies
Severe Symptoms
Hospitalization
Parenteral antibiotics
- Empirically selected broad-spectrum antibiotics (e.g., ampicillin, vancomycin) combined with an aminoglycoside (e.g., tobramycin, gentamicin)
- Switch to sensitivity-guided antibiotic therapy when results of urine and blood culture are available
Oral antibiotics when patient tolerates oral intake; administer for 7 to 21 days
Adequate fluid intake (parenteral initially, switched to oral fluids as nausea, vomiting, and dehydration subside)
Nonsteroidal antiinflammatory or antipyretic drugs to reverse fever and relieve discomfort
Urinary analgesics (e.g., to relieve bothersome lower urinary tract symptoms)
Follow-up urine culture and imaging studies

CBC, Complete blood count; *CT,* computed tomography; *IVP,* intravenous pyelogram; *VCUG,* voiding cystourethrogram; *WBC,* white blood cell.

NURSING MANAGEMENT
ACUTE PYELONEPHRITIS

■ Nursing Assessment

Subjective and objective data that should be obtained from a patient with pyelonephritis are presented in Table 44-4.

■ Nursing Diagnoses

Nursing diagnoses for the patient with pyelonephritis include, but are not limited to, those for the patient with UTI (see NCP 44-1).

■ Planning

The overall goals are that the patient with pyelonephritis will have (1) relief of pain, (2) normal body temperature, (3) no complications, (4) normal renal function, and (5) no recurrence of symptoms.

■ Nursing Implementation

Health Promotion. Health promotion and maintenance measures are similar to those for cystitis (see p. 1175). In addition, it is important that the patient receive early treatment for cystitis to prevent ascending infections. Because the patient with structural abnormalities of the urinary tract is at high risk for infection, the need for regular medical care should be stressed to these patients.

Acute Intervention and Home Care. Nursing interventions vary depending on the severity of symptoms. These interventions include teaching the patient about the disease process with emphasis on (1) the need to continue drugs as prescribed, (2) the need for a follow-up urine culture to ensure proper management, and (3) identification of risk for recurrence or relapse (see Table 44-5 and NCP 44-1). In addition to antibiotic therapy, the patient should be encouraged to drink at least eight glasses of fluid every day, even after the infection has been treated. Rest is often indicated to increase patient comfort. The patient with frequent relapses or reinfections may be treated with long-term, low-dose antibiotics. Understanding the rationale for therapy is important to enhance patient compliance.

■ Evaluation

The expected outcomes for the patient with pyelonephritis are presented in NCP 44-1.

CHRONIC PYELONEPHRITIS

Chronic pyelonephritis is a term used to describe a kidney that has become shrunken and has lost function owing to scarring or fibrosis.[13] It usually occurs as the outcome of recurring infections involving the upper urinary tract. However, it also may occur in the absence of an existing infection and a recent or remote history of UTIs. Alternative terms used to describe this condition include *interstitial nephritis,* chronic atrophic pyelonephritis, or reflux nephropathy (when scarring occurs in the presence of vesicoureteral reflux).

Chronic pyelonephritis is diagnosed by radiologic imaging and histologic testing rather than clinical features. Imaging studies reveal a small, contracted kidney with a thinned parenchyma. The collecting system may be small or hydronephrotic. Pathologic analysis reveals loss of functioning nephrons, infiltration of the parenchyma with inflammatory cells, and fibrosis.

The level of renal function in chronic pyelonephritis varies, depending on whether one or both kidneys are affected, the magnitude of scarring, and the presence of coexisting infection. Chronic pyelonephritis often progresses to end-stage renal disease when both kidneys are involved, even if the underlying infection is successfully eradicated. (Nursing and collaborative management of the patient with chronic kidney disease is discussed in Chapter 45.)

URETHRITIS

Urethritis is an inflammation of the urethra. Causes of urethritis include a bacterial or viral infection, *Trichomonas* and monilial infection (especially in women), chlamydia, and gonorrhea (especially in men). Among men, the causes of urethritis are usually sexually transmitted. In men, purulent discharge usually indicates a gonococcal urethritis, whereas a clear discharge typically signifies a nongonococcal urethritis.[14] (Sexually transmitted diseases are discussed in Chapter 51). Urethritis also produces bothersome lower urinary tract symptoms, including dysuria and frequent urination, similar to those seen with cystitis.

In women, urethritis is difficult to diagnose. It frequently produces bothersome lower urinary tract symptoms as described previously, but urethral discharge may not be present. Cultures on split urine collections (taken at beginning of urine flow and then midstream) or any urethral discharge may confirm a diagnosis of urethral infection.

Treatment is based on identifying and treating the cause and providing symptomatic relief. Sulfamethoxazole with trimethoprim or nitrofurantoin are examples of drugs used for bacterial infections. Metronidazole (Flagyl) and clotrimazole (Mycelex) may be used for treating *Trichomonas.* Drugs such as nystatin (Mycostatin) or fluconazole (Diflucan) may be prescribed for monilial infections. In chlamydial infections, doxycycline (Vibramycin) may be used. Women with negative urine cultures and no pyuria do not usually respond to antibiotics. Hot sitz baths may temporarily relieve bothersome symptoms. The patient should be instructed to avoid the use of vaginal deodorant sprays, properly cleanse the perineal area after bowel movements and urination, and avoid intercourse until symptoms subside.

INTERSTITIAL CYSTITIS

Interstitial cystitis (IC) is a chronic, painful inflammatory disease of the bladder. It is thought to affect as many 700,000 Americans. The average age at onset is 40 years. The ratio of women to men with IC is 10-12:1. Although the etiology of IC remains unknown, probable contributing factors include chronic inflammation with mast cell invasion of the bladder wall (possibly provoked by an infection or an autoimmune disorder), defects of the glycosaminoglycan layer that protects the bladder mucosa from the irritating effects of urine exposure, abnormal constituents in the urine, dysfunction of the sympathetic innervation of the lower urinary tract, or a reflex sympathetic dystrophy.[15]

The two primary clinical manifestations that characterize IC include pain and bothersome lower urinary tract symptoms (e.g., frequency, urgency). The pain associated with IC is usually located in the suprapubic area but may involve the vagina, labia, or entire perineal region. It varies from moderate to severe in intensity and is exacerbated by bladder filling, postponing urination, physical exertion, pressure against the suprapubic area, dietary intake of certain foods, or emotional distress. The pain is transiently relieved by urination. Bothersome lower urinary tract symptoms are very similar to a UTI, and the condition is often misdiagnosed as a recurring or chronic UTI. The pain and bothersome voiding symptoms produced by IC remit and exacerbate over time. Some patients experience an onset of symptoms that disappears altogether after a period of weeks to months, whereas others have persistent symptoms over a period of months to years.

IC is a diagnosis of exclusion. The condition is suspected whenever a patient experiences symptoms of a UTI despite the absence of bacteriuria, pyuria, or a positive urine culture. A careful history and physical examination are necessary to exclude a variety of disorders that may produce somewhat similar symptoms, such as UTI or endometriosis. This evaluation must include at least one negative urine culture during a period of active symptoms. Cystoscopic examination may reveal a small bladder capacity and superficial ulcerations with bladder filling called *glomerulations,* but these findings are frequently absent and are not unique to IC. Criteria for diagnosing IC are presented in Table 44-7.

Collaborative Care and Drug Therapy

Because the etiology of IC is unknown, no single treatment has been identified that consistently reverses or relieves symptoms. Various therapies have been effective in alleviating or relieving bothersome symptoms in most patients.[15]

Dietary and lifestyle alterations are used to relieve pain and diminish voiding frequency and nocturia. Dietary alterations in-

---

TABLE 44-7   Clinical Criteria for the Diagnosis of Interstitial Cystitis

Inclusion Criteria
- Pain with bladder filling or postponing urination
- Bothersome urinary urgency
- Small bladder capacity on urodynamic testing
- Cystoscopic evidence of ulcerations or glomerulations (*not* specific to interstitial cystitis)

Exclusion Criteria
- Bladder capacity >350 ml on urodynamic testing
- Overactive bladder contractions on urodynamic testing
- Daytime voiding frequency <8 times per day
- Active genital herpes
- History of chemotherapy, particularly if treated with cyclophosphamide (Cytoxan)
- Tubercular cystitis
- History of pelvic radiation
- Bladder tumor

clude elimination of foods and beverages likely to exacerbate the symptoms. A diet low in acidic foods and avoiding beverages such as coffee, tea, and carbonated and alcoholic drinks can be helpful in reducing IC symptoms. Patients may be advised that an OTC dietary supplement called calcium glycerophosphate (Prelief) alkalinizes the urine and can provide relief from the irritating effects of certain foods. This agent may be particularly helpful when dining away from home where the patient has less control over the preparation of foods.

Two tricyclic antidepressants, amitriptyline (Elavil) and nortriptyline (Doxepin), are used to reduce the burning pain and urinary frequency. Pentosan (Elmiron) is a drug used to enhance the protective effects of the glycosaminoglycan layer of the bladder. It is thought to relieve pain associated with IC by reducing the irritative effects of urine on the bladder wall. Drugs that provide modest relief from IC symptoms in certain cases include nifedipine (Procardia), which is a calcium channel blocker. These drugs are effective over time (weeks to months), but they do not provide immediate relief that may be needed when a patient experiences an acute exacerbation of symptoms. In this case, a short course of opioid analgesics may be given.

Several agents may be instilled directly into the bladder through a small catheter. Dimethyl sulfoxide probably acts by desensitizing pain receptors in the bladder wall. Heparin and hyaluronic acid also may be instilled into the bladder to relieve IC symptoms. Like pentosan, they are thought to enhance the protective properties of the glycosaminoglycan layer of the bladder. These drugs are often administered with lidocaine, which rapidly desensitizes the bladder wall, rendering the patient better able to tolerate instillation of additional heparin or hyaluronic acid and providing transient relief from pain. Bacille Calmette-Guérin (BCG), an attenuated form of the *Mycobacterium bovis*, administered intravesically is now in clinical trials. The mechanism of action of BCG is unclear, but it may alleviate a possible autoimmune disorder provoking the chronic inflammation characteristic of the disorder.

Distention of the bladder during endoscopic examination relieves IC-related pain and voiding frequency, probably by temporarily disrupting sensory nerve endings in the bladder wall. Several surgical procedures have been used in an attempt to relieve severe, debilitating pain.[15] Urinary diversion is an approach that can be used when other measures fail. Unfortunately, some patients have reported pain within the urinary diversion, possibly indicating that components of the urine may contribute to IC in certain cases.

NURSING MANAGEMENT
INTERSTITIAL CYSTITIS

Assessment focuses on characterization of the pain associated with IC. The patient is asked about specific dietary or lifestyle factors known to exacerbate or alleviate pain and about the intensity of the pain. Objective data collection includes a bladder log or voiding diary kept over a period of at least 3 days to determine diurnal voiding frequency and patterns of nocturia. A simultaneous pain record may be useful.

Reassurance that IC is a real condition experienced by others and that it can be effectively treated may relieve the anxiety, anger, guilt, and frustration related to experiences of chronic pain and voiding dysfunction in the absence of a clear-cut diagnosis and treatment strategy. A UTI may occur during the course of IC management. A UTI is likely to produce an acute exacerbation of

bothersome lower urinary tract symptoms and urinary frequency, as well as dysuria (not typically associated with IC) and odorous urine, possibly with hematuria.

The patient also must be given instruction about the need to maintain good nutrition, particularly in light of the broad dietary restrictions often necessary to control IC-related pain. Specifically, the patient may be advised to take a multivitamin containing no more than the recommended dietary allowance for essential vitamins and to avoid high-potency vitamins because these formulations may irritate the bladder. The patient is also assisted to obtain information from the Interstitial Cystitis Association, which includes recipes and menus for a well-balanced diet that is specifically designed to avoid bladder-irritating foods and beverages.

Elimination of a variety of foods and beverages from the diet that are likely to irritate the bladder typically provides modest to profound relief from symptoms. Typical bladder irritants include caffeine, alcohol, citrus products, aged cheeses, nuts, foods containing vinegar, curries or hot peppers, and foods or beverages likely to lower urinary pH. In addition, the patient should be taught to self-use Prelief. The patient is advised to avoid clothing that creates suprapubic pressure, including pants with tight belts or restrictive waistlines.

Written educational materials concerning diet, coping with the need for frequent urination, and strategies for coping with the emotional burden of IC are available from the Interstitial Cystitis Association (www.ichelp.com). Providing such materials provides an excellent opportunity for the nurse to introduce the patient to the existence of this patient advocacy group and to participate in local support groups when desired.

RENAL TUBERCULOSIS

Renal tuberculosis (TB) is rarely a primary lesion. It is usually secondary to TB of the lung. In a small percentage of patients with pulmonary TB, the tubercle bacilli reach the kidneys via the bloodstream. Onset occurs 5 to 8 years after the primary infection. The patient is often asymptomatic when the kidney is initially infiltrated with bacilli. Sometimes the patient complains of fatigue and develops a low-grade fever. As the lesions ulcerate, infection descends to the bladder, and the patient experiences frequent urination, burning on voiding, and epididymitis (in men). Symptoms of a UTI are the first sign in the majority of patients with renal TB. Renal lesions may calcify as they heal. Infrequently, renal colic, lumbar and iliac pain, and hematuria may be present. A diagnosis is based on localization of tubercle bacilli in the urine and on IVP findings.[16]

Long-term complications of renal TB depend on the duration of the disease before treatment. Scarring of the renal parenchyma and the development of ureteral strictures occur. The earlier treatment is initiated, the less likely renal failure will develop. Reduced bladder volume may be irreversible in advanced disease. The patient may require long-term urologic follow-up. (Nursing and collaborative management for the patient with TB is discussed in Chapter 27.)

Immunologic Disorders of the Kidney
GLOMERULONEPHRITIS

Immunologic processes involving the urinary tract predominantly affect the renal glomerulus. The disease process results in **glomerulonephritis** (inflammation of the glomeruli), which affects both kidneys equally. Although the glomerulus is the primary site of inflammation, tubular, interstitial, and vascular changes also occur. Glomerulonephritis is divided into a number of classifications, which may describe (1) the extent of damage (diffuse or focal), (2) the initial cause of the disorder (systemic lupus erythematosus, systemic sclerosis [scleroderma], streptococcal infection), or (3) the extent of changes (minimal or widespread).

Etiology and Pathophysiology

Two types of antibody-induced injury can initiate glomerular damage. In the first type, the antibodies have specificity for antigens within the glomerular basement membrane (GBM). These are termed anti-GBM antibodies. Immunoglobulins and complement are deposited along the basement membrane. The mechanism that causes a person to develop antibodies against its GBM is not known. Production of autoantibodies (antibodies to one's own tissue) may be stimulated by a structural alteration in the GBM or by a reaction of the basement membrane with an exogenous agent (e.g., hydrocarbon, viruses).

In the second type of immune process, the antibodies react with circulating nonglomerular antigens and are randomly deposited as immune complexes along the GBM. On electron microscopy of renal tissue sections, the deposits appear "lumpy-bumpy." In this immune complex process, the antigens do not come from the glomeruli but from either endogenous circulating native deoxyribonucleic acid (DNA) or exogenous sources (e.g., bacteria, viruses, chemicals, drugs). Bacterial products appear to be important in poststreptococcal glomerulonephritis. Viral agents have been recognized in certain cases of glomerulonephritis that develop after hepatitis B or C and rubella (measles).

All forms of immune complex disease are characterized by an accumulation of antigen, antibody, and complement in the glomeruli, which can result in tissue injury. The immune complexes activate complement (see Chapters 12 and 13). Complement activation results in the release of chemotactic factors that attract polymorphonuclear leukocytes and causes the release of histamine and other inflammatory mediators. The end result of these processes is glomerular injury as a result of inflammation.

Clinical Manifestations

Clinical manifestations of glomerulonephritis include varying degrees of hematuria (ranging from microscopic to gross) and urinary excretion of various formed elements, including red blood cells (RBCs), WBCs, and casts. Proteinuria and elevated blood urea nitrogen (BUN) and serum creatinine levels are other manifestations. In most cases, recovery from the acute illness is complete. However, if progressive involvement occurs, the result is destruction of renal tissue and marked renal insufficiency.

The patient's history provides important information related to glomerulonephritis. It is necessary to assess exposure to drugs, immunizations, microbial infections, and viral infections such as hepatitis. It is also important to evaluate the patient for more generalized conditions involving immune disorders, such as systemic lupus erythematosus and systemic sclerosis.

ACUTE POSTSTREPTOCOCCAL GLOMERULONEPHRITIS

Acute poststreptococcal glomerulonephritis (APSGN) is most common in children and young adults, but all age groups can be affected. APSGN develops 5 to 21 days after an infection of the pharynx or skin (e.g., streptococcal sore throat, impetigo) by certain nephrotoxic strains of group A β-hemolytic streptococci. The person produces antibodies to the streptococcal antigen. Although the specific mechanism is not known, the antigen-antibody complexes are deposited in the glomeruli and activate complement.[17] Complement activation causes an inflammatory reaction to the injury. The response to the injury is also a decrease in the filtration of metabolic waste products from the blood and an increase in the permeability of the glomerulus to larger protein molecules.

Clinical Manifestations and Complications

The clinical manifestations of APSGN appear as a variety of signs and symptoms, which may include generalized body edema, hypertension, oliguria, hematuria with a smoky or rusty appearance, and proteinuria. Fluid retention occurs as a result of decreased glomerular filtration. The edema appears initially in low-pressure tissues, such as around the eyes (periorbital edema), but later progresses to involve the total body as ascites or peripheral edema in the legs. Smoky urine indicates bleeding in the upper urinary tract. The degree of proteinuria varies with the severity of the glomerulonephropathy. Hypertension primarily results from increased extracellular fluid volume. The patient with APSGN may have abdominal or flank pain. At times the patient has no symptoms, with the problem found on routine urinalysis.

More than 95% of patients with APSGN recover completely or improve rapidly with conservative management. Chronic glomerulonephritis develops in 5% to 15% of the affected persons, and irreversible renal failure occurs in less than 1% of patients.[17]

Diagnostic Studies

The diagnosis of APSGN is based on a complete history and physical examination and laboratory studies (Table 44-8) to determine the presence or history of a group A β-hemolytic streptococcus in a throat or skin lesion. An immune response to the streptococcus is often demonstrated by assessment of antistreptolysin O (ASO) titers. The finding of decreased complement components (especially C3 and CH50) indicates an immune-mediated response. A renal biopsy may be performed to confirm the presence of the disease.

TABLE 44-8 Collaborative Care Acute Glomerulonephritis
Diagnostic
History and physical examination
Urinalysis
CBC
BUN, serum creatinine, and albumin
Complement levels and ASO titer
Renal biopsy (if indicated)
Collaborative Therapy
Rest
Sodium and fluid restriction
Diuretics
Antihypertensive therapy
Adjustment of dietary protein intake to level of proteinuria and uremia

ASO, Antistreptolysin O; *BUN,* blood urea nitrogen; *CBC,* complete blood count.

Dipstick and urine sediment microscopy will reveal the presence of erythrocytes in significant numbers. Erythrocyte casts are highly suggestive of acute glomerulonephritis. Proteinuria may range from mild to severe. Screening blood tests include BUN and serum creatinine to assess the extent of renal impairment.

NURSING *and* COLLABORATIVE MANAGEMENT ACUTE POSTSTREPTOCOCCAL GLOMERULONEPHRITIS

The management of APSGN focuses on symptomatic relief (see Table 44-8). Rest is recommended until the signs of glomerular inflammation (proteinuria, hematuria) and hypertension subside. Edema is treated by restricting sodium and fluid intake and by administrating diuretics. Severe hypertension is treated with antihypertensive drugs. Dietary protein intake may be restricted if there is evidence of an increase in nitrogenous wastes (e.g., elevated BUN value). The restriction varies with the degree of proteinuria. (Low-protein, low-sodium, fluid-restricted diets are discussed in Chapter 45.)

Antibiotics should be given only if the streptococcal infection is still present. Corticosteroids and cytotoxic drugs have not been shown to be of value.

One of the most important ways to prevent the development of APSGN is to encourage early diagnosis and treatment of sore throats and skin lesions. If streptococci are found in the culture, treatment with appropriate antibiotic therapy (usually penicillin) is essential. The patient must be encouraged to take the full course of antibiotics to ensure that the bacteria have been eradicated. Good personal hygiene is an important factor in preventing the spread of cutaneous streptococcal infections.

GOODPASTURE SYNDROME

Goodpasture syndrome, an example of cytotoxic (type II) autoimmune disease, is characterized by the presence of circulating antibodies against GBM and alveolar basement membrane.[18] Although the primary target organ is the kidney, the lungs are also involved. The pathologic nature of the syndrome results when binding of the antibody causes an inflammatory reaction mediated by complement fixation and activation (see Chapters 12 and 13). The causative factors for development of autoantibody production are unknown, although type A influenza viruses, hydrocarbons, penicillamine, and unknown genetic factors may be involved.

Goodpasture syndrome is a rare disease that is seen mostly in young male smokers. The clinical manifestations include hemoptysis, pulmonary insufficiency, crackles, rhonchi, renal involvement with hematuria and renal failure, weakness, pallor, and anemia. Pulmonary hemorrhage usually occurs and may precede glomerular abnormalities by weeks or months. Abnormal diagnostic findings include low hematocrit and hemoglobin levels, elevated BUN and serum creatinine levels, hematuria, and proteinuria. Circulating serum anti-GBM antibodies parallel the activity of the renal disease and are diagnostic of this syndrome.

NURSING *and* COLLABORATIVE MANAGEMENT GOODPASTURE SYNDROME

Until recently, the prognosis for the patient with Goodpasture syndrome was poor.[19] Management consists of corticosteroids, immunosuppressive drugs (e.g., cyclophosphamide [Cytoxan],

azathioprine [Imuran]), plasmapheresis (see Chapter 13), and dialysis. Plasmapheresis removes the circulating anti-GBM antibodies, and immunosuppressive therapy inhibits further antibody production. Renal transplantation can be attempted after the circulating anti-GBM antibody titer decreases. Although recurrences may develop, the disease is not a contraindication to transplantation. In selected patients with severe pulmonary hemorrhage, bilateral nephrectomy has been helpful. The exact mechanism for improvement has not been determined.

Nursing management appropriate for a critically ill patient who is experiencing symptoms of acute renal failure and respiratory distress is instituted. Death is often secondary to hemorrhage in the lungs and respiratory failure. (Nursing interventions for a patient in acute renal failure are discussed in Chapter 45, and nursing interventions for a patient with respiratory failure are discussed in Chapter 66.) Because this syndrome is rare and primarily affects previously healthy young adults, support and understanding of the patient and family are of major importance. The patient and family need instructions concerning current therapy, drugs, and complications of the disease process.

RAPIDLY PROGRESSIVE GLOMERULONEPHRITIS

Rapidly progressive glomerulonephritis (RPGN) is glomerular disease associated with rapid, progressive loss of renal function over days to weeks. Renal failure may occur within weeks to months in contrast to chronic glomerulonephritis, which develops insidiously and progresses over many years. The manifestations of RPGN are hypertension, edema, proteinuria, hematuria, and RBC casts.

RPGN can occur in a variety of situations: (1) as a complication of inflammatory or infectious disease (e.g., APSGN), (2) as a complication of a multisystemic disease (e.g., systemic lupus erythematosus, Goodpasture syndrome), (3) as an idiopathic disease, or (4) in association with the use of certain drugs (e.g., penicillamine).

Treatment is directed toward correction of fluid overload, hypertension, uremia, and inflammatory injury to the kidney. Treatment includes corticosteroids, cytotoxic agents, and plasmapheresis. Dialysis therapy and transplantation are used as maintenance therapy for the patient with RPGN. Following renal transplantation, RPGN may recur.

CHRONIC GLOMERULONEPHRITIS

Chronic glomerulonephritis is a syndrome that reflects the end stage of glomerular inflammatory disease. Most types of glomerulonephritis and nephrotic syndrome can eventually lead to chronic glomerulonephritis.

The syndrome is characterized by proteinuria, hematuria, and the slow development of uremic syndrome (see Chapter 45) as a result of decreasing renal function. Chronic glomerulonephritis does not usually follow an acute course. It progresses insidiously toward renal failure over a few to as many as 30 years.

Chronic glomerulonephritis is often found coincidentally when an abnormality on a urinalysis or elevated blood pressure is detected. It is common to find that the patient has no recollection or history of acute nephritis or any renal problems. A renal biopsy may be performed to determine the exact cause and nature of the glomerulonephritis. However, ultrasound and CT scanning are generally preferred as diagnostic measures.

Treatment is supportive and symptomatic. Hypertension and UTIs should be treated vigorously. Protein and phosphate restrictions may slow the rate of progression of kidney disease. (Management of chronic kidney disease is discussed in Chapter 45.)

NEPHROTIC SYNDROME

Etiology and Clinical Manifestations

Nephrotic syndrome describes a clinical course that can be associated with a number of disease conditions. Some of the more common causes of nephrotic syndrome are listed in Table 44-9. In adults about one third of patients with nephrotic syndrome will have a systemic disease such as diabetes or systemic lupus erythematosus. The remainder will be categorized as having idiopathic nephrotic syndrome.[20]

The characteristic manifestations include peripheral edema, massive proteinuria, hyperlipidemia, and hypoalbuminemia. Characteristic blood chemistries include decreased serum albumin, decreased total serum protein, and elevated serum cholesterol. The increased glomerular membrane permeability found in nephrotic syndrome is responsible for the massive excretion of protein in the urine. This results in decreased serum protein and subsequent edema formation. Ascites and anasarca develop if there is severe hypoalbuminemia.

The diminished plasma oncotic pressure from the decreased serum proteins stimulates hepatic lipoprotein synthesis, which results in hyperlipidemia. Initially, cholesterol and low-density lipoproteins are elevated. Later the triglyceride level is also increased. Fat bodies (fatty casts) commonly appear in the urine.

Immune responses, both humoral and cellular, are altered in nephrotic syndrome. As a result, infection is an important cause of morbidity and mortality. Calcium and skeletal abnormalities may occur, including hypocalcemia, blunted calcemic response to parathyroid hormone, hyperparathyroidism, and osteomalacia.

TABLE 44-9   Causes of Nephrotic Syndrome
Primary Glomerular Disease
Membraneous proliferative glomerulonephritis
Primary nephrotic syndrome
Focal glomerulonephritis
Inherited nephrotic disease
Extrarenal Causes
Multisystem Disease
Systemic lupus erythematosus
Diabetes mellitus
Amyloidosis
Infections
Bacterial (streptococcal, syphilis)
Viral (hepatitis, human immunodeficiency virus infection)
Protozoal (malaria)
Neoplasms
Hodgkin's disease
Solid tumors of lungs, colon, stomach, breast
Leukemias
Allergens (e.g., bee sting, pollen)
Drugs
Penicillamine
Nonsteroidal antiinflammatory drugs
captopril (Capoten)
Heroin

With nephrotic proteinuria, loss of clotting factors can result in a relative hypercoagulable state. Hypercoagulability with thromboembolism is potentially the most serious complication of nephrotic syndrome. The renal vein is the site most commonly involved for thrombus formation. Pulmonary emboli occur in about 40% of nephrotic patients with thrombosis.

Collaborative Care

Treatment of nephrotic syndrome is symptomatic.[20] The goals are to relieve edema and cure or control the primary disease. Management of the edema includes the cautious use of angiotensin-converting enzyme inhibitors, nonsteroidal antiinflammatory drugs, and a low-sodium (2 to 3 g per day), low- to moderate-protein diet (0.5 to 0.6 kg per day). Dietary salt restrictions are a key to managing edema. In some individuals, thiazide or loop diuretics may be needed. If urine protein loss exceeds 10 g per 24 hours, additional dietary protein may be needed.

The treatment of hyperlipidemia is often unsuccessful. However, treatment with lipid-lowering agents, such as colestipol (Colestid) and lovastatin (Mevacor), may result in moderate decreases in serum cholesterol levels. If thrombosis is detected, anticoagulant therapy may be necessary for up to 6 months.

Corticosteroids and cyclophosphamide (Cytoxan) may be used for the treatment of severe cases of nephrotic syndrome. Prednisone has been effective to varying degrees in persons with lipoid nephrosis, membranous glomerulonephritis, proliferative glomerulonephritis, and lupus nephritis. Management of diabetes and treatment of edema are the only measures used for nephrotic syndrome related to diabetes.

NURSING MANAGEMENT
NEPHROTIC SYNDROME

A major nursing intervention for a patient with nephrotic syndrome is related to edema. It is important to assess the edema by weighing the patient daily, accurately recording intake and output, and measuring abdominal girth or extremity size. Comparing this information daily provides the nurse with a tool for assessing the effectiveness of treatment. The edematous skin must be cleaned carefully. Trauma should be avoided, and the effectiveness of diuretic therapy must be monitored.

The patient with nephrotic syndrome has the potential to become malnourished from the excessive loss of protein in the urine. Maintaining a low- to moderate-protein diet that is also low in sodium is not always easy. The patient is usually anorexic. Serving small, frequent meals in a pleasant setting may encourage better dietary intake.

Because the patient is susceptible to infection, measures should be taken to avoid exposure to persons with known infections. The person with nephrotic syndrome is often ashamed of an edematous appearance and needs support in dealing with an altered body image.

RENAL DISEASE AND ACQUIRED IMMUNODEFICIENCY SYNDROME

The patient with HIV infection can have a variety of renal manifestations, ranging from mild fluid and electrolyte abnormalities to progressive renal impairment resulting in end-stage renal disease. The incidence of renal disease associated with HIV infection is about 10% and is highest among IV drug users.

HIV-associated renal syndromes include the following:
1. *Proteinuria and nephrotic syndrome,* which occurs in about 10% of patients with HIV infection. It may be the initial sign of HIV infection in some persons.
2. *HIV-associated nephropathy,* which is characterized by proteinuria, progressive azotemia, absence of hypertension, large kidney size on renal imaging studies, and unusually rapid progression to end-stage renal disease.
3. *Acute renal failure,* which is most commonly seen in the patient with acquired immunodeficiency syndrome (AIDS) who is critically ill with HIV-related infection or malignancy. The natural cause of acute renal failure secondary to AIDS is similar to acute renal failure associated with other acute illnesses (see Chapter 45). Survival and recovery usually depend on the treatment of the primary cause of renal failure and support of renal function by dialysis. (HIV infection is discussed in Chapter 14.)

Obstructive Uropathies

Urinary obstruction refers to any anatomic or functional condition that blocks or impedes the flow of urine (Fig. 44-2). It may be congenital or acquired. Obstruction may be due to intrinsic causes such as anomalies, diverticula, tumors, or benign growth within the urinary tract; extrinsic causes such as tumors, adhesions, retroperitoneal fibrosis, or prolapsed adjacent organs; or functional causes as a result of neurologic or psychogenic factors. Some common intrinsic obstructions are narrowing of the ureteropelvic junction (UPJ), bladder neck contracture, benign prostatic hyperplasia, urethral stricture, and urethral meatal stenosis. Common extrinsic causes include pelvic and abdominal tumors or a prolapsed uterus. Examples

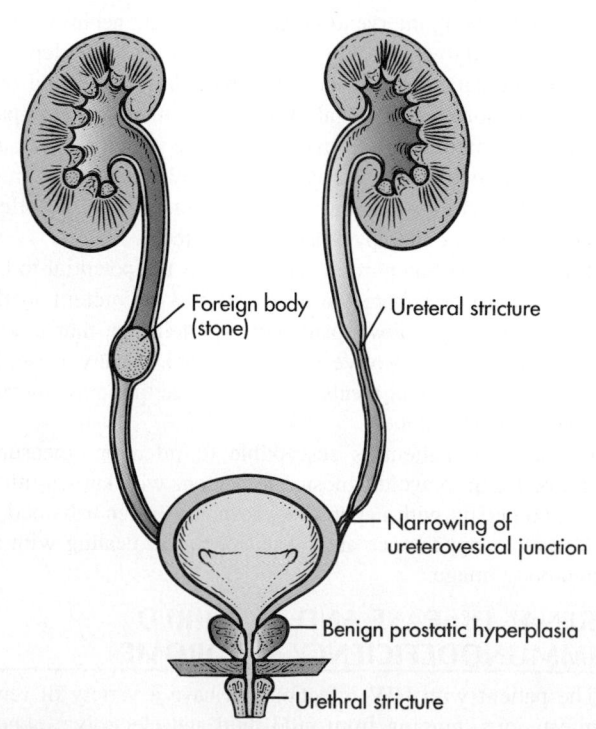

Foreign body (stone)

Ureteral stricture

Narrowing of ureterovesical junction

Benign prostatic hyperplasia

Urethral stricture

FIG. 44-2 Common causes of urinary tract obstruction.

of functional causes are neurogenic bladder and vesicosphincter dyssynergia (disturbance in muscle coordination) after spinal cord injury.

Damaging effects from urinary tract obstruction affect the system above the level of the obstruction. The severity of these effects depends on the location, duration of obstruction, amount of pressure or dilation, presence of urinary stasis, and whether infection is present. Infection increases the risk of irreversible damage.

Although obstruction distal to the prostate in men or the bladder neck in women causes mucosal scarring and a slower stream, it rarely results in major obstructive uropathy because the urethral wall pressure is less than that of the bladder neck and bladder. Urethral obstruction may contribute to outlet resistance and cause lower or upper urinary tract damage when other obstructive or dysfunctional factors are also present. For example, there is an increased risk of compromised renal function in the patient with a spinal cord injury with vesicosphincter dyssynergia.

When obstruction occurs at the level of the bladder neck or prostate, significant bladder changes can occur. Detrusor muscle fibers *hypertrophy* (increase in size) to contract harder to push urine out a narrower pathway. Over a long period, the detrusor loses its ability to compensate for this resistance. Muscle bundles separate and become less compliant. This separation is called *trabeculation.* Trabeculation is caused by the deposition of collagen in the bladder wall that separates the smooth muscle fascicles. Trabeculation may hasten the decompensation of the detrusor. The areas between these muscle bundles are called *cellules.* Because these areas have no muscle support, the bladder mucosa can herniate between detrusor muscle bundles, forming sacs that drain poorly, called *diverticula.* Residual urine can be very high in a noncompensating bladder.

Pressure increases during bladder filling or storage and can be transmitted to the ureter when *bladder outlet obstruction* is present. This pressure overcomes the normal peristaltic pressure and leads to *reflux* (a backflow of urine); ureteral dilation, kinking, and tortuosity; **hydroureter** (dilation of the renal pelvis); vesicoureteral reflux (backflow or backward movement of urine from the lower to upper urinary tracts); and **hydronephrosis** (dilation or enlargement of the renal pelves and calyces) (Fig. 44-3), and consequent chronic pyelonephritis and renal atrophy. If only one kidney is obstructed, the other kidney may try to compensate by hypertrophy, but the ureter will not be dilated on this contralateral side.

Partial obstruction may occur in the ureter or at the UPJ. If the pressure remains low or moderate, the kidney may continue to dilate with no noticeable loss of function. There is an increased risk of pyelonephritis because of urinary stasis and reflux. If only one kidney is involved and the other kidney is functioning, the patient may be free of symptoms. If both kidneys or only one functioning kidney is involved (e.g., if the patient has only one kidney), alterations in renal function (e.g., increased BUN or serum creatinine levels) are found. If the obstruction progresses, oliguria or anuria develops. Often episodes of oliguria are followed by polyuria if the obstruction is a stone that becomes dislodged. Treatment requires location and relief of the blockage. This can include insertion of a tube (e.g., urethral or ureteral), surgical correction of the disease process, or diversion of the urinary stream above the level of blockage.

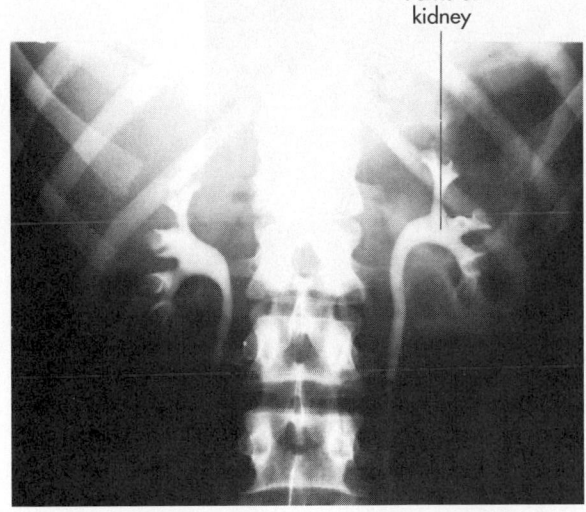

Pelvis of
kidney

A

Distended pelvis and
kidney secondary to
hydronephrosis

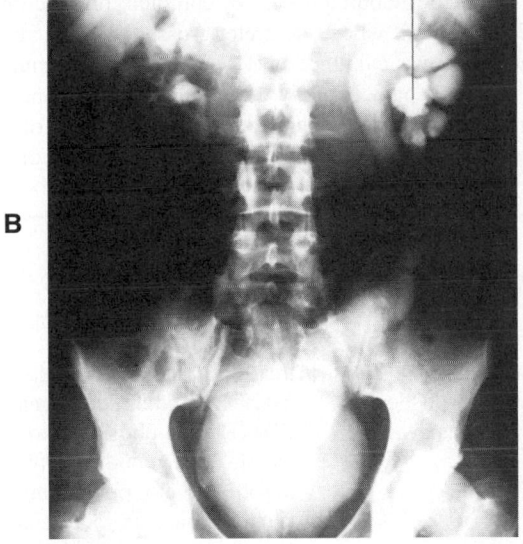

B

FIG. 44-3 A, Normal intravenous pyelogram (IVP). B, IVP showing
hydronephrosis and hydroureter.

URINARY TRACT CALCULI

Each year an estimated 500,000 people in the United States have **nephrolithiasis** (kidney stone disease). Many of these people require hospitalization. In the United States the incidence of urinary stone disease is highest in the Southeast and Southwest, followed by the Midwest. Except for struvite (magnesium-ammonium phosphate) stones associated with UTI, stone disorders are more common in men than in women.[21] The majority of patients are between 20 and 55 years of age. Stone formation is more frequent in whites than in African Americans. The incidence is also higher in persons with a family history of stone formation. Recurrence of stones can occur in up to 50% of patients.[22] There is seasonal variation, with stone formation occurring more often in the summer months, thus supporting the role of dehydration in this process. Stone formation

in the kidney also seems to increase in incidence as countries become more industrialized, whereas the incidence of bladder stones decreases.

Etiology and Pathophysiology

Many factors are involved in the incidence and type of stone formation, including metabolic, dietary, genetic, climatic, lifestyle, and occupational influences (Table 44-10). Many theories have been proposed to explain the formation of stones in the urinary tract. No single theory can account for stone formation in all cases. Crystals, when in a supersaturated concentration, can precipitate and unite to form a stone. Keeping urine dilute and free flowing reduces the risk of recurrent stone formation in many individuals. It is known that a mucoprotein is formed (the matrix for the stone) in the kidneys that form stones. Urinary pH, solute load, and inhibitors in the urine affect the formation of stones. The higher the pH, the less soluble are calcium and phosphate. The lower the pH, the less soluble are uric acid and cystine.

Other important factors in the development of stones include obstruction with urinary stasis and urinary infection with urea-splitting bacteria (e.g., *Proteus, Klebsiella, Pseudomonas,* and some species of staphylococci). These bacteria cause the urine to become alkaline and contribute to the formation of struvite (calcium-magnesium-ammonium phosphate) stones.[23] Infected stones, when they are entrapped in the kidney, may assume a staghorn configuration as they enlarge (Fig. 44-4). Infected stones are frequent in the patient with an external urinary diversion, long-term indwelling catheter, neurogenic bladder, or urinary retention. Genetic factors may also contribute to urine stone formation. Cystinuria is an autosomal recessive disorder. In this disorder there is a marked increased excretion of cystine.

TABLE 44-10	**Risk Factors for the Development of Urinary Tract Calculi**

Metabolic
Abnormalities that result in increased urine levels of calcium, oxaluric acid, uric acid, or citric acid

Climate
Warm climates that cause increased fluid loss, low urine volume, and increased solute concentration in urine

Diet
Large intake of dietary proteins that increases uric acid excretion
Excessive amounts of tea or fruit juices that elevate urinary oxalate level
Large intake of calcium and oxalate
Low fluid intake that increases urinary concentration

Genetic Factors
Family history of stone formation, cystinuria, gout, or renal acidosis

Lifestyle
Sedentary occupation, immobility

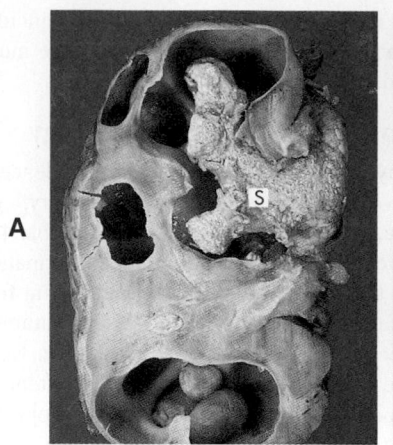
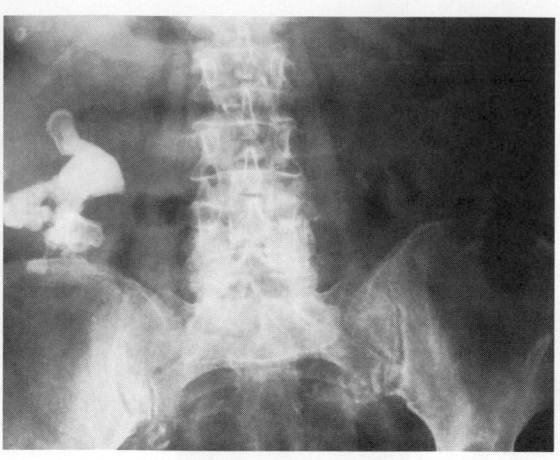

FIG. 44-4   A, Renal staghorn calculus. The renal pelvis is filled with a large calculus that is shaped to its contours, resembling the horn of a stag *(S).* B, Staghorn calculus as seen on an intravenous pyelogram (IVP).

Types

The term **calculus** refers to the stone, and *lithiasis* refers to stone formation. The five major categories of stones are (1) calcium phosphate, (2) calcium oxalate, (3) uric acid, (4) cystine, and (5) struvite (magnesium-ammonium phosphate) (Table 44-11). Stone composition may be mixed, although calcium stones are the most common. Calculi can be found in various locations in the urinary tract (Fig. 44-5).

Clinical Manifestations

Urinary stones cause clinical manifestations when they obstruct urinary flow. Common sites of complete obstruction are at the UPJ (the point where the ureter crosses the iliac vessels) and at the ureterovesical junction (UVJ). Symptoms include abdominal or flank pain (usually severe), hematuria, and renal colic. The pain may be associated with nausea and vomiting. The type of pain is determined by the location of the stone (see

TABLE 44-11   Types of Urinary Tract Calculi

URINARY STONE	INCIDENCE (%)	CHARACTERISTICS	PREDISPOSING FACTORS	THERAPEUTIC MEASURES
Calcium oxalate*	35-40	Small, often possible to get trapped in ureter; more frequent in men than in women	Idiopathic hypercalciuria, hyperoxaluria, independent of urinary pH, family history	Increase hydration. Reduce dietary oxalate.‡ Give thiazide diuretics. Give cellulose phosphate to chelate calcium and prevent GI absorption. Give potassium citrate to maintain alkaline urine. Give cholestyramine to bind oxalate. Give calcium lactate to precipitate oxalate in GI tract.
Calcium phosphate	8-10	Mixed stones (typically), with struvite or oxalate stones	Alkaline urine, primary hyperparathyroidism	Treat underlying causes and other stones.
Struvite (MgNH₄PO₄)	10-15	Three to four times as common in women than men, always in association with urinary tract infections, large staghorn type (usually)†	Urinary tract infections (usually *Proteus* organisms)	Administer antimicrobial agents, acetohydroxamic acid. Use surgical intervention to remove stone. Take measures to acidify urine.
Uric acid	5-8	Predominant in men, high incidence in Jewish men	Gout, acid urine, inherited condition	Reduce urinary concentration of uric acid. Alkalinize urine with potassium citrate. Administer allopurinol. Reduce dietary purines.‡
Cystine	1-2	Genetic autosomal recessive defect, defective absorption of cystine in GI tract and kidney, excess concentrations causing stone formation	Acid urine	Increase hydration. Give α-penicillamine and tiopronin to prevent cystine crystallization. Give potassium citrate to maintain alkaline urine.

*Calcium stones can exist as calcium oxalate, calcium phosphate, or a mixture of both. Calcium stones account for the majority of all stones.
†See Figure 44-4.
‡See Table 44-12.
GI, Gastrointestinal.

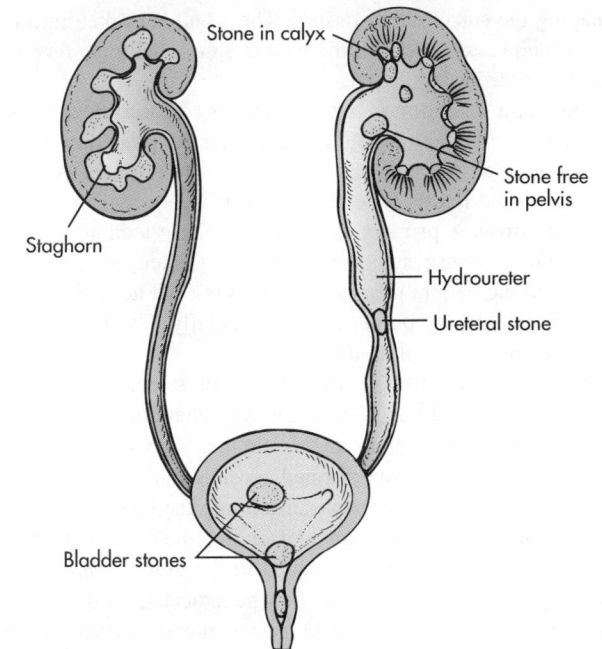

FIG. 44-5 Location of calculi in the urinary tract.

Fig. 44-5). If the stone is nonobstructing, pain may be absent. If the obstruction is in a calyx or at the UPJ, the patient may experience dull costovertebral flank pain or even colic. Pain resulting from the passage of a calculus down the ureter is intense and colicky. The patient may be in mild shock with cool, moist skin. As a stone nears the UVJ, pain will be felt in the lateral flank and sometimes down into the testicles, labia, or groin. Other clinical manifestations include the presence of urinary infection accompanied by fever, vomiting, nausea, and chills.

Diagnostic Studies

Diagnostic studies useful in the evaluation and management of renal lithiasis include urinalysis, urine culture, IVP, retrograde pyelogram, ultrasound, and cystoscopy. A plain film of the abdomen and renal ultrasound will identify larger, radiopaque stones. An IVP or retrograde pyelogram is used to localize the degree and site of obstruction or to confirm the presence of a radiolucent stone, such as a uric acid or cystine calculus (see Fig. 44-4, *B*). Ultrasonography can be used to identify a radiopaque or radiolucent calculus in the renal pelvis, calyx, or proximal ureter. It is less useful when attempting to locate stones trapped in the midureter. A CT scan may be used to differentiate a nonopaque stone from a tumor.

Retrieval and analysis of the stones are important in the diagnosis of the underlying problem contributing to stone formation. The patient's BUN and serum creatinine levels are also measured to assess renal function. A careful history, including previous stone formation, prescribed and OTC medications and dietary supplements, and family history of urinary calculi is useful. Measurement of urine pH is useful in the diagnosis of struvite stones and renal tubular acidosis (tendency to alkaline pH) and uric acid stones (tendency to acidic pH).[24]

Collaborative Care

Evaluation and management of a patient with renal lithiasis consist of two concurrent approaches. The first approach is directed toward management of the acute attack. This involves treating the symptoms of pain, infection, or obstruction as indicated for the individual patient. At frequent intervals, narcotics are typically required for relief of renal colic pain. Many stones pass spontaneously. However, stones larger than 4 mm are unlikely to pass through the ureter.

The second approach is directed toward evaluation of the cause of the stone formation and the prevention of further development of stones. Information to be obtained from the patient includes family history of stone formation, geographic residence, nutritional assessment including the intake of vitamins A and D, activity pattern (active or sedentary), history of periods of prolonged illness with immobilization or dehydration, and any history of disease or surgery involving the GI or genitourinary tract.

Therapy for people who are active stone formers requires a concerted management approach, with primary emphasis on teaching and on developing a therapeutic regimen with which the patient can comply. Adequate hydration, dietary sodium restrictions, dietary changes (Table 44-12), and the use of drugs minimize urinary stone formation. Various drugs are prescribed, depending on the specific problem underlying stone formation. These drugs prevent stone formation in various ways, including altering urine pH, preventing excessive urinary excretion of a substance, or correcting a primary disease (e.g., hyperparathyroidism).

Treatment of struvite stones requires control of infection. This may be difficult if the stone remains in place. In addition to antibiotics, acetohydroxamic acid may be used in the treatment of kidney infections that result in the continual formation of struvite stones. Acetohydroxamic acid, an inhibitor of the chemical action caused by the persistent bacteria, can be used effectively to retard struvite stone formation.[25] If the infection cannot be controlled, the stone may have to be removed surgically.

Indications for endourologic, lithotripsy, or open surgical stone removal include the following:

1. Stones too large for spontaneous passage
2. Stones associated with bacteriuria or symptomatic infection
3. Stones causing impaired renal function
4. Stones causing persistent pain, nausea, or ileus
5. Inability of patient to be treated medically
6. Patient with one kidney

TABLE 44-12	Nutritional Therapy Urinary Tract Calculi

The following is a list of foods high in purine, calcium, or oxalate content.

Purine
High: Sardines, herring, mussels, liver, kidney, goose, venison, meat soups, sweetbreads
Moderate: Chicken, salmon, crab, veal, mutton, bacon, pork, beef, ham

Calcium
Milk, cheese, ice cream, yogurt, sauces containing milk; all beans (except green beans), lentils; fish with fine bones (e.g., sardines, kippers, herring, salmon); dried fruits, nuts; chocolate, cocoa, Ovaltine

Oxalate
Spinach, rhubarb, asparagus, cabbage, tomatoes, beets, nuts, celery, parsley, runner beans; chocolate, cocoa, instant coffee, Ovaltine, tea; Worcestershire sauce

Endourologic Procedures. If the stone is located in the bladder, a cystoscopy is done to remove small stones. For large stones a *cystolitholapaxy* is done. In this procedure, large stones can be broken up with an instrument called a lithotrite (stone crusher). The bladder is then irrigated and the crushed stones washed out. A *cystoscopic lithotripsy* uses an ultrasonic lithotrite to pulverize stones. Complications associated with these cystoscopic procedures include hemorrhage, retained stone fragments, and infection.

Flexible *ureteroscopes,* inserted via a cystoscope, can be used to remove stones from the renal pelvis and upper urinary tract. Ultrasonic, laser, or electrohydraulic lithotripsy can be used in conjunction with the ureteroscope to pulverize and break the stone into fragments.

In *percutaneous nephrolithotomy* a nephroscope is inserted through a sinus tract from the skin into the kidney pelvis. Stones can be fragmented using ultrasound, electrohydraulic, or laser lithotripsy. The stone fragments are removed and the pelvis irrigated. A percutaneous nephrostomy tube is usually left in place to ensure that the ureter is not obstructed. Complications include bleeding, injury to adjacent structures, and infection.

Lithotripsy. Lithotripsy is a procedure used to eliminate calculi from the urinary tract. Lithotripsy techniques include percutaneous ultrasonic lithotripsy, electrohydraulic lithotripsy, laser lithotripsy, and extracorporeal shock-wave lithotripsy.[26] Extracorporeal shock-wave lithotripsy and laser lithotripsy are the most common. In *percutaneous ultrasonic lithotripsy* an ultrasonic probe is placed in the renal pelvis via a percutaneous nephroscope (inserted through a small incision in the flank) and is positioned against the stone. (The patient is given general or spinal anesthesia for this procedure.) The probe produces ultrasonic waves, which break the stone into sandlike particles. Percutaneous lithotripsy is not used as much as a primary approach to renal or upper ureteral stones unless the stone is large and other lithotripsy procedures have failed.

The *electrohydraulic lithotripsy* probe is also placed directly on a stone, but it breaks the stone into small fragments that are removed by forceps or by suction. A continuous saline irrigation flushes out the stone particles, and all outflow drainage is strained so that the particles can be analyzed. The calculi can also be removed by forceps or basket extraction. Complications are rare but include hemorrhage, sepsis, and abscess formation. Postoperatively, the patient usually complains of moderate to severe colicky pain. The first few voids are bright red; as the bleeding subsides, the urine becomes dark red or turns a smoky color. Antibiotics are usually given for 2 weeks to reduce the risk of infection.

Laser lithotripsy probes are used to fragment lower ureteral and large bladder stones. A holmium laser medium is preferred; it fragments stones but does not injure the surrounding tissue.

In *extracorporeal shock-wave lithotripsy,* a noninvasive procedure, the patient is anesthetized (spinal or general) and placed in a water bath. Anesthesia is necessary to keep the patient very still during the procedure. Some of the newer-generation lithotripters do not require submersion and use other means of initiating shock waves. The lithotripters are categorized as electrohydraulic, electromagnetic, and piezoelectric. The second-generation lithotripters use less power to fragment stones. Lower power reduces a patient's pain, but usually some sedation or analgesia is necessary.

Fluoroscopy or ultrasound is used to focus the lithotripter on the affected kidney, and a high-voltage spark generator produces high-energy acoustic shock waves that shatter the stone without damaging the surrounding tissues. The stone is broken into fine sand, which is excreted into the patient's urine within a few days after the procedure.

Hematuria is common after lithotripsy procedures. A self-retaining ureteral stent is often placed after the procedure to promote passage of this sand and to prevent obstruction caused by a buildup of sand in the ureter. The stent is removed 1 to 2 weeks after lithotripsy. A primary advantage of these techniques compared with open surgery is the decrease in the length of hospitalization and the patient's earlier return to normal activities. Additional treatment may be necessary, especially if a stone is large and in the mid or distal ureter.

Surgical Therapy. A small group of select patients need open surgical procedures, such as the very obese patient or the individual with complex abnormalities in the calyces or at the UPJ. The type of open surgery performed depends on the location of the stone. A *nephrolithotomy* is an incision into the kidney to remove a stone. A *pyelolithotomy* is an incision into the renal pelvis to remove a stone. If the stone is located in the ureter, a *ureterolithotomy* is performed. A *cystotomy* may be indicated for bladder calculi. For open surgery on the kidney or ureter, a flank incision directly below the diaphragm and across the side is usually the preferred surgical approach. Complications related to hemorrhage are the most common following these surgical procedures.

Nutritional Therapy. When managing an obstructing stone, the patient is advised to drink adequate fluids to avoid dehydration. Forcing fluids is avoided because this strategy has not proved effective in assisting the patient to spontaneously "pass" (excrete) the stone via the urine. In addition, forcing fluids may exacerbate the colic associated with this episode.

A high fluid intake (approximately 3000 ml per day) is recommended after an episode of urolithiasis to produce a urine output of at least 2 L per day. High urine output prevents supersaturation of minerals (i.e., dilutes the concentration) and flushes them out before the minerals have a chance to precipitate and form a stone. Increasing the fluid intake is especially important for the patient who is active in sports, lives in a dry climate, performs physical exercise, has a family history of stone formation, or works in an occupation that requires outdoor work or a great deal of physical activity that can lead to dehydration. Water is the preferred fluid, and consumption of colas, coffee, and tea should be limited because high intake of these beverages tends to increase rather than diminish the risk of recurring urinary calculi.[27]

Dietary intervention may be important in the management of urolithiasis. In the past, calcium restriction was routinely implemented for the patient with kidney stones. However, more recent research suggests that a high dietary calcium intake, which was previously thought to contribute to kidney stones, may actually lower the risk by reducing the urinary excretion of oxalate, a common factor in many stones.[28] Initial nutritional management should include limiting oxalate-rich foods and thereby reducing oxalate excretion. Foods high in calcium, oxalate, and purines are presented in Table 44-12.

NURSING MANAGEMENT
RENAL CALCULI

■ Nursing Assessment

Subjective and objective data that should be obtained from a patient with urinary tract lithiasis are presented in Table 44-13.

TABLE 44-13	Nursing Assessment
	Urinary Tract Calculi

Subjective Data

Important Health Information

Past health history: Recent or chronic UTI; bed rest; immobilization; previous urinary tract stones, obstruction, or kidney disease with urinary stasis; gout; prostatic hyperplasia; hyperparathyroidism

Medications: Prior use of medication for prevention of stones or treatment of UTI; allopurinol, analgesics

Surgery or other treatments: External urinary diversion, long-term indwelling urinary catheter

Functional Health Patterns

Health perception–health management: Family history of renal calculi; sedentary lifestyle

Nutritional-metabolic: Nausea, vomiting; dietary intake of purines, calcium, oxalates, phosphates; low fluid intake; chills

Elimination: Decreased urinary output, urinary urgency, frequency, feeling of bladder fullness

Cognitive-perceptual: Acute, severe, colicky pain in flank, back, abdomen, groin, or genitalia; burning on urination, dysuria, anxiety

Objective Data

General

Guarding, fever

Integumentary

Warm, flushed skin or pallor with cool, moist skin (mild shock)

Gastrointestinal

Abdominal distention, absence of bowel sounds

Urinary

Oliguria, hematuria, tenderness on palpation of renal areas, passage of stone or stones

Possible Findings

↑ BUN and serum creatinine levels; RBCs, WBCs, pyuria, crystals, casts, minerals, bacteria on urinalysis; ↑ uric acid, calcium, phosphorus, oxalate, or cystine values on 24-hr urine sample; calculi or anatomic changes on IVP or KUB x-ray; direct visualization of obstruction on cystoureteroscopy

BUN, Blood urea nitrogen; *IVP,* intravenous pyelogram; *KUB,* kidneys, ureters, bladder; *RBCs,* red blood cells; *UTI,* urinary tract infection; *WBCs,* white blood cells.

■ **Nursing Diagnoses**

Nursing diagnoses for the patient with urinary tract lithiasis include, but are not limited to, those presented in NCP 44-2.

■ **Planning**

The overall goals are that the patient with urinary tract calculi will have (1) relief of pain, (2) no urinary tract obstruction, and (3) an understanding of measures to prevent further recurrence of stones.

■ **Nursing Implementation**

A program to prevent stone recurrence always includes adequate fluid intake to produce a urine output of approximately 2 L per day, and it may include measures to alleviate metabolic or secondary risk factors. The nurse should consult with the health care provider concerning recommendations for fluid intake in a given patient. In the modestly active, ambulatory person, this re-

quires the patient to drink about 2000 to 2200 ml per day with the residual 20% to 30% of fluids gained through consumption of foods. The volume of fluids will be higher in the highly active patient who works outdoors or who regularly engages in demanding athletic activities. In contrast, fluid intake will be less for the very sedentary or immobile person. Preventive measures related to the person who is on bed rest or is relatively immobile for a prolonged time include maintaining an adequate fluid intake, turning the patient every 2 hours, and helping the patient to sit or stand, if possible, to maximize urinary flow.[29]

Additional preventive measures focus on reducing metabolic or secondary risk factors. For example, dietary restriction of purines may be helpful to the patient at risk for developing uric acid stones. Reduced intake of oxalates may be indicated in the person with recurring calcium oxalate calculi. The patient is taught the dosage, scheduling, and potential side effects of drugs used to reduce the risk of stone formation. Selected patients may be taught to self-monitor urinary pH, or they may be asked to measure urinary output.

Pain management and patient comfort are primary nursing responsibilities when managing an obstructing stone and renal colic (see NCP 44-2). It is important to ensure that the patient retrieves any spontaneously passed stones. All urine voided by the patient should be strained through gauze or a special urine strainer in an effort to detect the stone. The high fluid intake necessary for stone prevention is avoided, but consumption should be adequate to meet daily needs and avoid dehydration. Ambulation is generally encouraged to promote the movement of the stone from the upper to lower urinary tract, but the patient should not walk unattended when experiencing acute colic, particularly if opioid analgesics are being used.

■ **Evaluation**

The expected outcomes for the patient with urinary calculi are presented in NCP 44-2.

STRICTURES

A **stricture** is a narrowing of the lumen of the ureter or urethra.

Ureteral Strictures

Ureteral strictures can affect the entire length of the ureter, from the UPJ to UVJ.[30] These strictures are usually an unintended result of surgical intervention, usually secondary to adhesions or scar formation. Depending on its severity, ureteral obstruction can threaten the function of the kidney. Clinical manifestations of a ureteral stricture include mild to moderate colic; this pain may be of moderate to severe intensity if the patient consumes a large volume of fluids (such as alcohol) over a brief period. Infection is unusual unless a calculus or foreign object such as a stent or nephrostomy tube is present.

The discomfort and obstruction of a ureteral stricture may be temporarily bypassed by placing a stent under endoscopic control or by diverting urinary flow via a nephrostomy tube inserted into the renal pelvis of the affected kidney. Definitive correction requires dilation with a balloon or catheter. If the stricture is severe or recurs after initial balloon or catheter dilation, it may be incised under endoscopic control *(endoureterotomy).* In selected cases, an open surgical approach may be required to excise the stenotic area and reanastomose the ureter to the contralateral ureter *(ureteroureterostomy)* or to the renal pelvis. Alternatively,

NURSING CARE PLAN 44-2

Patient with Acute Renal Lithiasis

EXPECTED PATIENT OUTCOMES	NURSING INTERVENTIONS and *RATIONALES*
NURSING DIAGNOSIS	**Acute pain** *related to* irritation of stone and inadequate pain control or comfort measures *as manifested by* complaints of pain, facial grimacing, restlessness.
• Minimal or no pain • Decrease in pain and satisfaction with pain control	• Assess for pain location and severity *to plan appropriate interventions.* • Encourage fluid intake unless contraindicated *to promote passage of stone, dilute the urine, and reduce risk of additional stone formation.* • Administer pain medication as ordered *to promote comfort.* • Apply heat to flank area as needed *because heat reduces reflex muscle spasm and promotes comfort.*
NURSING DIAGNOSIS	**Anxiety** *related to* uncertain outcome and lack of knowledge regarding possible surgery *as manifested by* expressions of concern about future treatments.
• Relief of anxiety • Expression of confidence in treatment plan	• Assess cause and level of anxiety *to plan appropriate interventions.* • Explain surgical or nonsurgical procedure (include insertion of urethral catheters) *because accurate information often decreases anxiety and fosters control.* • Encourage patient to express feelings of anxiety, fear of surgery *to validate feelings and provide support.*
NURSING DIAGNOSIS	**Ineffective therapeutic regimen management** *related to* lack of knowledge about prevention of recurrence, diet, fluid requirements, and symptoms of recurrence *as manifested by* questions that indicate inadequate knowledge of disorder.
• Verbalization of correct self-care measures • Able to list symptoms of recurrence	• Instruct patient during initial hospital stay regarding increasing fluids unless contraindicated and diet restrictions and rationale *to prepare for home self-care.* • Inform patient about rationale, dose, frequency, and side effects of medication *to foster adherence to medication regimen.* • Tell patient to strain all urine through a urine strainer or piece of gauze (if necessary) *to determine if stones are passed* and to bring stone to physician for analysis. • Teach patient about symptoms of recurrence (e.g., hematuria, flank pain) *to ensure early reporting and initiation of treatment.*
NURSING DIAGNOSIS	**Impaired urinary elimination** *related to* trauma or blockage of ureters or urethra *as manifested by* decrease in urinary output, bloody urine.
• Free flow of urine • Minimal to no hematuria • Maintains balanced intake and output	• Monitor urine amount and character *to ensure patency in urinary system and that hematuria is not excessive.* • Encourage increased fluid intake *as increased hydration flushes bacteria and blood and may facilitate passage of stone fragments.*
NURSING DIAGNOSIS	**Risk for infection** *related to* introduction of bacteria following manipulations of the urinary tract and obstructed urinary flow.
• No urinary tract infections	• Assess for elevation in temperature; chills; cloudy, foul-smelling urine *as indicators of potential infection.* • Monitor vital signs and observe for fever *because abnormalities may indicate infection.* • Encourage high fluid intake unless contraindicated *because stones form more readily in concentrated urine and increased fluids help the stone fragments pass down urinary tract.*

distal ureteral strictures may be managed by a *ureteroneocystostomy* (reimplantation of the ureter into the bladder wall).

Urethral Stricture

A *urethral stricture* is the result of fibrosis or inflammation of the urethral lumen.[31] Causes of urethral strictures include trauma, urethritis (particularly following gonococcal infection), iatrogenic (following surgical intervention), or a congenital defect in the canalization of the urethra. Once the process of inflammation and fibrosis begins, the lumen of the urethra narrows, and its

compliance (ability to close or open in response to bladder filling or micturition) is compromised. Meatal stenosis, a narrowing of the urethral opening, is also common. A urethral stricture creates symptoms when it creates voiding dysfunction or bladder outlet obstruction.[32]

Clinical manifestations associated with a urethral stricture include a diminished force of the urinary stream, spraying, or a split urine stream. The patient may report feelings of incomplete bladder emptying with urinary frequency and nocturia. Moderate to severe obstruction of the bladder outlet may lead to acute urinary retention. The patient may report a history of urethritis, difficulty with placement of a urinary catheter, or trauma involving the penis or perineum. However, many patients are unable to recall any such events, thus leading to a diagnosis of an idiopathic stricture. A history of a UTI is not uncommon, particularly if the stricture involves the distal urethra.

Initial management of a stricture may be based on dilation. A metal instrument (urethral sound) may be placed, or a series of progressively enlarging stents can be placed into the urethra (filiforms and followers) to expand its lumen in a stepwise fashion. While initially successful, recurring stenosis is frequent. Recurrences may be managed by teaching the patient to repeatedly dilate the urethra by self-catheterization every few days. Alternatively, an endoscopic or open surgical procedure may be completed to provide a more durable solution to an obstructive urethral stricture. Shorter strictures may be managed by resection of the fibrotic area with primary reanastomosis. Longer strictures may require autotransplantation of a substitute segment such as a skin flap.

Renal Trauma

A continual increase in the incidence of traumatic renal injuries is related to an increase in the mechanization and speed of transportation and to the increase in violent crimes and injuries. The majority of incidents occur in men younger than 30 years of age. Blunt trauma is the most common cause. Injury to the kidney should be considered in multiple or sports injuries, traffic accidents, and falls. It is especially likely when the patient injures the abdomen, flank, or back. Penetrating injuries may result from violent encounters (e.g., gunshot or stabbing incidents) or from iatrogenic injuries.

Clinical findings include a history of trauma to the area of the kidneys. Gross or microscopic hematuria may be present. Diagnostic studies include urinalysis, IVP with cystography, ultrasound, CT, or magnetic resonance imaging (MRI) evaluation. Renal arteriography may also be used. Both the injured kidney and the noninvolved kidney should be evaluated to provide information for further management.

The severity of renal trauma depends on the extent of the injury. Treatments range from bed rest, fluids, and analgesia to surgical exploration and repair or nephrectomy.

Nursing interventions vary with the type and extent of associated injuries. Specific interventions related to renal trauma include ensuring increased fluid intake, providing comfort measures, monitoring intake and output, observing for hematuria, determining the presence of myoglobinuria, assessing the cardiovascular status, and monitoring potentially nephrotoxic antibiotics.

Renal Vascular Problems

Vascular problems involving the kidney include (1) nephrosclerosis, (2) renal artery stenosis, and (3) renal vein thrombosis.

NEPHROSCLEROSIS

Nephrosclerosis consists of sclerosis of the small arteries and arterioles of the kidney. There is decreased blood flow, which results in patchy necrosis of the renal parenchyma. Ischemic necrosis and destruction of glomeruli with subsequent fibrosis also occur.

Benign nephrosclerosis usually occurs in adults 30 to 50 years of age. It is caused by vascular changes resulting from hypertension and from the atherosclerosis process. Atherosclerotic vascular changes account for most of the loss of renal function associated with aging. There is a direct relation between the degree of nephrosclerosis and the severity of hypertension. The patient with benign nephrosclerosis may have normal renal function in the early stages. The only detectable abnormality may be hypertension.

Accelerated nephrosclerosis, or *malignant nephrosclerosis,* is associated with malignant hypertension, a complication of hypertension characterized by a sharp increase in BP with a diastolic pressure greater than 130 mm Hg. The patient is usually a young adult, with a male-to-female predominance of 2:1. Renal insufficiency progresses rapidly.

Treatment for benign nephrosclerosis is the same as that for essential hypertension (see Chapter 32). Malignant nephrosclerosis is treated with aggressive antihypertensive therapy (see Chapter 32). The availability and use of antihypertensives have improved the prognosis for the patient with benign and malignant nephrosclerosis. Renal dysfunction and renal failure (in some persons) constitute two of the major complications of hypertension. The prognosis for the patient with malignant hypertension is poor, with the major cause of death related to renal failure.

RENAL ARTERY STENOSIS

Renal artery stenosis is a partial occlusion of one or both renal arteries and their major branches. It can be due to atherosclerotic narrowing or fibromuscular hyperplasia. Renal artery stenosis accounts for 1% to 2% of all cases of hypertension.

When hypertension develops rather abruptly, renal artery stenosis should be considered as a possible cause, especially in the patient under 30 or over 50 years of age and in the patient with no familial history of hypertension. This contrasts with the age distribution for essential hypertension, which is 30 to 50 years of age. A renal arteriogram is the best diagnostic tool for identifying renal artery stenosis.

The goals of therapy are control of BP and restoration of perfusion to the kidney. Percutaneous transluminal renal angioplasty is the procedure of first choice, especially in older patients who are poor surgical risks. Surgical revascularization of the kidney is indicated when blood flow is decreased enough to cause renal ischemia or when evidence indicates that renovascular hypertension is present and surgical intervention may result in the patient becoming normotensive. The surgical procedure usually involves anastomoses between the kidney and another major artery, usually the splenic artery or aorta. In selected cases of unilateral renal involvement with high renin production, unilateral nephrectomy may be indicated.

RENAL VEIN THROMBOSIS

Renal vein thrombosis may occur unilaterally or bilaterally. Trauma, extrinsic compression (e.g., tumor, aortic aneurysm), renal cell carcinoma, pregnancy, contraceptive use, and nephrotic syndrome are associated with renal vein thrombosis.

The patient has symptoms of flank pain, hematuria, or fever or has nephrotic syndrome. Anticoagulation is important in treatment because there is a high incidence of pulmonary emboli. Corticosteroids may be used for the patient with nephrosis. Sur-

GENETICS in CLINICAL PRACTICE
Polycystic Kidney Disease

	ADULT	CHILD
Genetic basis	• Autosomal dominant	• Autosomal recessive
Incidence	• 1 in 500 to 1000	• 1 in 6000 to 40,000
Gene location	• Chromosomes 4 and 16	• Chromosome 6
Genetic testing	• DNA testing available	• DNA testing available
Age of onset	• Third to fourth decade of life	• Infancy or childhood
Clinical implications	• Multisystem involvement	• Up to 30% to 50% of affected newborns die shortly after birth
	• Systemic hypertension occurs in 60% to 80% of patients	
	• Families at risk should be screened	

gical thrombectomy may be performed instead of or along with anticoagulation.

Hereditary Renal Diseases

Hereditary renal diseases involve developmental abnormalities of the renal parenchyma. These abnormalities are either isolated or part of more complex malformation syndromes. The majority of inherited structural abnormalities are cystic. However, cysts may also develop as a result of obstructive uropathies, metabolic derangements, or neurologic diseases. Cysts may be evaluated to rule out any tumor content.

POLYCYSTIC KIDNEY DISEASE

Polycystic kidney disease (PKD) is one of the most common genetic diseases, affecting 600,000 people in the United States.[33] There are two forms of hereditary polycystic renal disease. It may be manifested in childhood or adulthood. The childhood form of PKD is a rare autosomal recessive disorder that is often rapidly progressive (see the Genetics in Clinical Practice box).

The adult form of PKD is an autosomal dominant disorder. It is latent for many years and is usually manifested between 30 and 40 years of age. However, PKD has also been found in newborns. It involves both kidneys and occurs in both men and women. The cortex and the medulla are filled with thin-walled cysts that are several millimeters to several centimeters in diameter (Fig. 44-6). The cysts enlarge and destroy surrounding tissue by compression. They are filled with fluid and may contain blood or pus.

Clinical Manifestations

In the patient with PKD, symptoms appear when the cysts begin to enlarge. A common early symptom of adult PKD is abdominal or flank pain, which is steady and dull or abrupt in onset, as well as episodic and colicky. This pain is often caused by bleeding into the cysts. On physical examination, palpable bilateral enlarged kidneys are often found (Fig. 44-7). Other clinical manifestations include hematuria (from rupture of cysts), UTI, and hypertension.

Diagnosis is based on clinical manifestations, family history, IVP, ultrasound, or CT scan. Usually the disease progresses to end-stage renal failure, although some individuals have relatively mild disease and die from unrelated problems. Loss of kidney function to the point of end-stage renal disease occurs by age 60 in 50% of patients.[33]

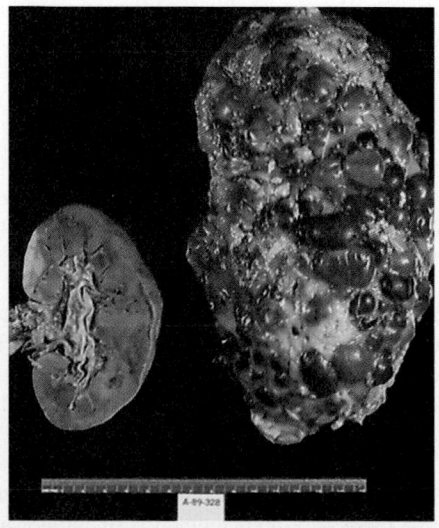

FIG. 44-6 Comparison of polycystic kidney with normal kidney.

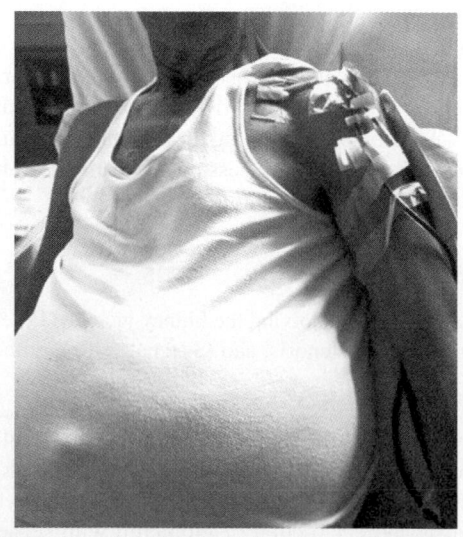

FIG. 44-7 Man with a 24–pound polycystic kidney.

Collaborative Care

There is no specific treatment for PKD. A major aim of treatment is to prevent infections of the urinary tract and/or to treat them with appropriate antibiotics if they occur. Nephrectomy may be necessary if pain, bleeding, or infection becomes a chronic, serious problem.

When the patient begins to experience progressive renal failure, the interventions are determined by the remaining renal function. Nursing measures are those used for management of end-stage renal disease (see Chapter 45). They include diet modification, fluid restriction, drugs (e.g., antihypertensives), assisting the patient to accept the chronic disease process, and assisting the patient and family to deal with financial concerns and other issues related to the hereditary nature of the disease.

The patient who has adult polycystic disease often has children by the time the disease is diagnosed. Each child of a parent with PKD has a 50% chance of having the disease. The patient will need appropriate counseling regarding plans for having more children. In addition, genetic counseling resources should be provided for the children.

MEDULLARY CYSTIC DISEASE

Medullary cystic disease is a hereditary disorder that occurs in two forms. The *autosomal recessive form* is associated with renal failure before age 20; the *autosomal dominant form* is associated with renal failure after age 20. Most cysts are located in the medulla. The kidneys are asymmetric in shape and are significantly scarred. There are defects in the concentration ability of the kidneys. Polyuria, progressive renal failure, severe anemia, metabolic acidosis, and poor sodium conservation are common. Hypertension can be a terminal event. Genetic counseling may be helpful in family planning. Treatment measures are those related to end-stage renal disease (see Chapter 45).

ALPORT SYNDROME

Alport syndrome is also known as *chronic hereditary nephritis*. Two forms of the disease exist: (1) classic Alport syndrome, which is inherited as a sex-linked disorder with hematuria, sensorineural deafness, and deformities of the anterior surface of the lens, and (2) nonclassical Alport syndrome, which is inherited as an autosomal trait that causes hematuria but not deafness or lens deformities.[34] Men are affected earlier and more severely than women. The disease is often diagnosed in the first decade of life. The basic defect is altered synthesis of the GBM. The patient most commonly has hematuria and progressive uremia. Treatment is supportive. Corticosteroids and cytotoxic drugs are not effective. The disease does not recur after kidney transplantation.

Renal Involvement in Metabolic and Connective Tissue Diseases

Various metabolic and connective tissue disease processes may have an effect on renal function. The pathophysiologic effects on the renal parenchyma are not always specific to each process. The clinical course of renal involvement is that of chronic progressive nephropathy, which can result in uremia and death. Management includes treatment of the primary disorder along with symptomatic relief of renal involvement. If renal involvement progresses to end-stage renal disease, management includes dialysis or transplantation (see Chapter 45). Nursing interventions include teaching the patient about the primary disease process, the renal involvement, and the resulting need to comply with dietary and fluid restrictions and drug regimens.

Diabetic nephropathy is the primary cause of end-stage renal failure in the United States. Diabetes mellitus may affect the kidneys in several ways. Microangiopathic changes in diabetes consist of diffuse glomerulosclerosis, involving thickening of the glomerular basement membrane (GBM), and nodular glomerulosclerosis (Kimmelstiel-Wilson syndrome), which is characterized by nodular lesions. Nodular glomerulosclerosis is reasonably specific for type 1 diabetes mellitus. The diabetic patient prone to glomerulonephropathy (e.g., the presence of trace proteinuria or retinopathy) requires careful monitoring of glucose levels and insulin requirements. (Diabetes mellitus is discussed in Chapter 47.)

Gout is a syndrome of acute attacks of arthritis caused by hyperuricemia (see Chapter 63). Monosodium urate crystals deposited in joints are responsible for the syndrome. Renal disease may develop as a result of damage caused by deposition of uric acid crystals in the renal interstitium and tubules.

Amyloidosis is a group of disorders manifested by impaired organ function from the infiltration of tissues with a hyaline substance (amyloid). The hyaline consists largely of protein. Kidney involvement is common in amyloidosis. Proteinuria is often the first clinical manifestation.

Systemic lupus erythematosus is a connective tissue disorder characterized by the involvement of several tissues and organs, particularly the joints, skin, and kidneys. (Systemic lupus erythematosus is discussed in Chapter 63). Clinical manifestations of lupus nephritis are similar to those of other forms of glomerulonephritis. Renal failure frequently occurs in systemic lupus erythematosus and has a poor prognosis.

Systemic sclerosis (scleroderma) is a disease of unknown etiology characterized by widespread alterations of connective tissue and by vascular lesions in many organs (see Chapter 63). In the kidney, vascular lesions are associated with fibrosis. An immune complex mechanism has been postulated as a possible etiologic factor. The severity of renal involvement varies. The patient who develops severe renal lesions has a poor prognosis.

Urinary Tract Tumors

KIDNEY CANCER

In 2002 in the United States 31,800 new cases of kidney cancer were diagnosed and 11,600 people died from kidney cancer.[35] Kidney cancers arise from the cortex or pelvis (and calyces). Tumors arising from both areas may be benign or malignant. However, malignant tumors are more frequent. Renal cell carcinoma (adenocarcinoma) is the most common type. Adenocarcinoma occurs twice as often in men as in women and is typically discovered when the person is 50 to 70 years old. Cigarette smoking is the most significant risk factor for the development of renal cell carcinoma. Other risk factors are obesity and the use of phenacetin-containing analgesics and exposure to asbestos, cadmium, and gasoline.[36]

TABLE 44-14   Robson's System of Staging Renal Carcinoma

STAGE	DESCRIPTION
I	Limitation to renal capsule
II	Spreading to perirenal fat but confined within fascia; includes metastasis to adrenal gland
III	Regional lymph node involvement, tumor thrombus in renal vein or vena cava, involvement of renal vein or vena cava
IV	Presence of distant metastases

There are no characteristic early symptoms. Generalized symptoms of weight loss, weakness, and anemia are the earliest manifestations. The classic manifestations of gross hematuria, flank pain, and a palpable mass are those of advanced disease. The most common sites of metastases include the lungs, liver, and long bones. Local extension of kidney cancer into the renal vein and vena cava is common. Renal cystic disease and renal-associated carcinomas may develop in the patient with end-stage renal disease who is receiving maintenance renal dialysis (see Chapter 45).

Several studies are used to diagnose kidney cancer. IVP with nephrotomography is the primary examination by which most masses are detected and evaluated. Ultrasounds have improved the ability to differentiate between a tumor and a cyst. Angiography, percutaneous needle aspiration, CT, and MRI are also used in the diagnosis of renal tumors. Small renal tumors are found earlier because of the increased use of CT scans and MRI. Radionuclide isotope scanning is used to detect metastases.

Robson's system of staging renal carcinoma is presented in Table 44-14. The treatment of choice is a radical nephrectomy. Radical nephrectomy is the removal of the kidney, adrenal gland, surrounding fascia, part of the ureter, and draining lymph nodes. Radiation therapy is used palliatively in inoperable cases and when there are metastases to bone or lungs. No effective chemotherapy is available for metastatic renal cell carcinoma. Biologic therapy, including α-interferon and interleukin-2 (IL-2), is most promising in the treatment of metastatic disease.[37,38] Side effects of IL-2 include capillary leakage syndrome, fever, chills, fatigue, and hypotension.

BLADDER CANCER

In 2002 there were about 56,500 new cases of bladder cancer and 12,600 deaths related to bladder cancer. Bladder cancer accounts for nearly 1 in every 20 cancers diagnosed in the United States.[35] The most frequent malignant tumor of the urinary tract is transitional cell carcinoma of the bladder. Most bladder tumors are papillomatous growths within the bladder. Cancer of the bladder is most common between the ages of 60 and 70 years and is at least three times as common in men as in women. Risk factors for bladder cancer include cigarette smoking, exposure to dyes used in the rubber and cable industries, and chronic abuse of phenacetin-containing analgesics. Women treated with radiation for cervical cancer and patients receiving cyclophosphamide (Cytoxan) also have increased risk, but the reason is unknown.

Individuals with chronic, recurrent stones (often bladder) and chronic lower urinary infections have an increased risk of squamous cell cancer of the bladder. Patients who have indwelling catheters for long periods can develop these chronic conditions.

Clinical Manifestations and Diagnostic Studies

Gross, painless hematuria (chronic or intermittent) is the most common clinical finding. Bladder irritability with dysuria, frequency, and urgency may also occur. When cancer is suspected, urine specimens for cytology can be obtained to determine the presence of neoplastic or atypical cells. Exfoliated cells from the epithelial surface of the bladder can readily be detected in voided specimens. Other recent urine tests assess for specific factors associated with bladder cancer, such as bladder tumor antigens. Bladder cancers can be detected using IVP, ultrasound, CT, or MRI. However, the presence of cancer is confirmed by cystoscopy and biopsy.

The clinical staging of carcinoma of the bladder is determined by the depth of invasion of the bladder wall and surrounding tissue. The Jewett-Strong-Marshall classification system broadly classifies bladder cancer as superficial (carcinoma in situ [CIS], O, A), invasive (B1, B2, C), or metastatic (D1 to D4) disease. Pathologic grading systems are also used to classify the malignant potential of tumor cells, indicating a scale from well-differentiated to anaplastic categories. Low-stage, low-grade bladder cancers are the most responsive to treatment and are more easily cured.

NURSING *and* COLLABORATIVE MANAGEMENT
BLADDER CANCER

Collaborative care of bladder cancer is outlined in Table 44-15.

■ Surgical Therapy

Surgical therapies include a variety of procedures. *Transurethral resection with fulguration* (electrocautery) is used for the diagnosis and treatment of superficial lesions with a low recurrence rate. This procedure is also used to control bleeding in the patient who is a poor operative risk or who has advanced tumors. With this technique the tumor mass is excised by means of a blade inserted through the cystoscope. The remaining portions of the tumor are cauterized.

A second technique, *laser photocoagulation,* is also used to treat superficial bladder cancers. This procedure can be repeated a number of times for recurrence. The advantages of laser include bloodless destruction of the lesion, minimal risk of perforation, and lack of need for a urinary catheter. The primary disadvantage is destruction of the tumor, so pathologic evaluation for grading and staging cannot be completed.

A third technique used is *open loop resection* (snaring of polyp types of lesion) *with fulguration.* It is used for the control of bleeding, for large superficial tumors, and for multiple lesions. Treatment of large lesions entails a segmental resection of the bladder *(segmental cystectomy).*

Postoperative management of the patient who has had any of these surgical procedures includes instructions to drink a large volume of fluid each day for the first week following the procedure and to avoid intake of alcoholic beverages. The patient is taught to self-monitor the urine. It is anticipated to be pink during the first several days after the procedure, but it should not be bright red or

TABLE 44-15	Collaborative Care Bladder Cancer

Diagnostic
History and physical examination
Urinalysis
Intravenous pyelogram
Cystoscopy with biopsy
Cytology studies
Ultrasound
CT scan

Collaborative Therapy
Surgical treatment
   Transurethral resection with fulguration
   Laser photocoagulation
   Open loop resection or fulguration
   Segmental cystectomy
   Radical cystectomy
Radiation
Intravesical immunotherapy
   Bacille Calmette-Guérin (BCG)
   α-Interferon
Intravesical chemotherapy
   thiotepa
   mitomycin (Mutamycin)
   doxorubicin (Adriamycin)
   valrubicin (Valstar)
Systemic chemotherapy

CT, Computed tomography.

contain blood clots. Approximately 7 to 10 days following tumor resection or ablation, the patient may observe dark red or rust-colored flecks in the urine. These are anticipated and represent scabs from the healing tumor resection sites. Opioid analgesics may be required for a brief period after the procedure, along with stool softeners. The patient can be encouraged to take a 15- to 20-minute sitz bath two to three times a day to promote muscle relaxation and to reduce the risk of urinary retention. The nurse should also help the patient and family cope with fears about cancer, surgery, and sexuality and should emphasize the importance of regular follow-up care. Frequent routine cystoscopies are required.

When the tumor is invasive or when it involves the trigone (the area where the ureters insert into the bladder) and the patient is free from metastasis beyond the pelvic area, a partial or radical cystectomy with urinary diversion is the treatment of choice (see the following section on urinary diversion). A *partial cystectomy* includes resection of that portion of the bladder wall containing the tumor, along with a margin of normal tissue. A *radical cystectomy* involves removal of the bladder, prostate, and seminal vesicles in men and the bladder, uterus, cervix, urethra, and ovaries in women.[39]

■ Radiation Therapy and Chemotherapy

Radiation therapy is used with cystectomy or as the primary therapy when the cancer is inoperable or when surgery is refused. Increasingly, radiation therapy is being combined with systemic chemotherapy. Sometimes combination systemic chemotherapy is used for bladder cancer, usually preoperatively or before radiation therapy, or is used to treat distant metastases.

Chemotherapy drugs used in treating invasive bladder cancer include cisplatin (Platinol), vinblastine (Velban), doxorubicin (Adriamycin), and methotrexate.

■ Intravesical Therapy

Chemotherapy with local instillation of chemotherapeutic or immune-stimulating agents can be delivered directly into the bladder by a urethral catheter. Protocols vary, but *intravesical* therapy is usually initiated at weekly intervals for 6 to 12 weeks. The chemotherapeutic agents are instilled directly into the patient's bladder and retained for about 2 hours. The patient's position may be changed every 15 minutes for maximum contact in all areas of the bladder, especially if the tumor occurred on the bladder dome. The use of maintenance therapy after the initial induction regimen may be beneficial.

BCG, a weakened strain of *Mycobacterium bovis,* is the treatment of choice for carcinoma in situ. BCG stimulates the immune system rather than acting directly on cancer cells in the bladder. When BCG fails, α-interferon in addition to BCG may be used. Other treatments that can be used when BCG fails include thiotepa, an alkylating agent, and valrubicin (Valstar), an antineoplastic antibiotic.

Most patients have irritative voiding symptoms and hemorrhagic cystitis following intravesical therapy. Thiotepa (when absorbed into circulation from the bladder wall) can significantly reduce WBC and platelet counts in some individuals. BCG may cause flulike symptoms, hematuria, or systemic infection. Other side effects usually associated with chemotherapy, such as nausea, vomiting, and hair loss, are not experienced with intravesical chemotherapy.

Nursing responsibilities include encouraging the patient to increase the daily fluid intake and to quit smoking, assessing the patient for secondary UTI, and stressing the need for routine urologic follow-up. The patient may have fears or concerns about sexual activity or bladder function that will need to be addressed.[40]

URINARY INCONTINENCE AND RETENTION

Urinary incontinence (UI) is defined as an uncontrolled loss of urine that is of sufficient magnitude to be a problem. Approximately 13 million people living in the United States suffer from UI. Among younger adults, UI affects far more women than men. Estimates of UI prevalence in working older women exceed 50%. In contrast, UI affects 2% to 9% of working older men.[41,42] Although the prevalence of incontinence is higher among older women and older men, it is not a natural consequence of aging. Although UI has traditionally been viewed as a social or hygienic problem, it is now known to affect quality of life, as well as contribute to serious health problems in older adults.[41]

Anything that interferes with bladder or urethral sphincter control can result in UI. Causes may be transient (e.g., caused by confusion or depression, infection, drugs, restricted mobility, or stool impaction). Congenital disorders that produce incontinence include exstrophy of the bladder, epispadias, spina bifida with myelomeningocele, and ectopic ureteral orifice. Acquired disorders are described in Table 44-16. Patients may have more than one type of incontinence.

Urinary retention is the inability to empty the bladder despite micturition or the accumulation of urine in the bladder because of an inability to urinate.[43] In certain cases, it is associated with dribbling urinary leakage called overflow UI. *Acute urinary retention* is the total inability to pass urine via micturition; it is a

TABLE 44-16   Acquired Disorders Causing Urinary Incontinence

TYPE AND DESCRIPTION	CAUSES	TREATMENT
Stress Incontinence* Sudden increase in intraabdominal pressure causes involuntary passage of urine. It can occur during coughing, heavy lifting, straining, or laughing.	Condition is found most commonly in women with relaxed pelvic musculature (frequently from obstetric complications or multiple pregnancies). Structures of the female urethra atrophy when estrogen decreases. Prostate surgery for benign prostatic hyperplasia or prostatic carcinoma.	Perineal muscle exercises (e.g., Kegel exercises), weight loss if patient is obese, insertion of vaginal pessary, estrogen vaginal creams, condom catheters or penile clamp, surgery Urethral inserts, patches, or bladder neck support devices to correct underlying problem
Urge Incontinence* Condition occurs randomly when involuntary urination is preceded by warning of few seconds to few minutes. Leakage is periodic but frequent. Nocturnal frequency and incontinence are common. Condition may appear with varying severity during psychologic stress.	Condition is caused by uncontrolled contraction or overactivity of detrusor muscle. Bladder escapes central inhibition and contracts reflexively. Conditions include central nervous system disorders (e.g., cerebrovascular disease, Alzheimer's disease, brain tumor, Parkinson's disease), bladder disorders (e.g., carcinoma in situ, radiation effects, interstitial cystitis), interference with spinal inhibitory pathways (e.g., malignant growth in spinal cord, spondylosis), and bladder outlet obstruction, as well as conditions of unknown etiology.	Treatment of underlying cause, instruction to have patient urinate more frequently or on time schedule, anticholinergic drugs (e.g., propantheline [Pro-Banthine]) imipramine (Tofranil) at bedtime, calcium channel blockers, condom catheters, vaginal estrogen creams
Overflow Incontinence Condition occurs when the pressure of urine in overfull bladder overcomes sphincter control. Leakage of small amounts of urine is frequent throughout the day and night. Urination may also occur frequently in small amounts. Bladder remains distended and is usually palpable.	Disorder is caused by outlet obstruction (prostatic hyperplasia, bladder neck obstruction, urethral stricture) or by underactive detrusor muscle caused by myogenic or neurogenic factors (e.g., herniated disk, diabetic neuropathy). It may also occur after anesthesia and surgery (especially procedures such as hemorrhoidectomy, herniorrhaphy, cystoscopy). Neurogenic bladder (flaccid type) is another cause.	Urinary catheterization to decompress bladder, implementation of Credé or Valsalva maneuver, α-adrenergic blocker (e.g., prazosin [Minipress]) to decrease outlet resistance, bethanechol (Urecholine) to enhance bladder contractions, intermittent catheterization, surgery to correct underlying problem
Reflex Incontinence Condition occurs when no warning or stress precedes periodic involuntary urination. Urination is frequent, is moderate in volume, and occurs equally during the day and night.	Spinal cord lesion above S2 interferes with central nervous system inhibition. Disorder results in detrusor hyperreflexia and interferes with pathways coordinating detrusor contraction and sphincter relaxation.	Treatment of underlying cause, bladder decompression to prevent ureteral reflux and hydronephrosis, intermittent self-catheterization, α-adrenergic blocker (e.g., prazosin [Minipress]) to relax internal sphincter, diazepam or baclofen to relax external sphincter, prophylactic antibiotics, surgical sphincterotomy
Incontinence After Trauma or Surgery Vesicovaginal or urethrovaginal fistula may occur in women. Alteration in continence control in men involves proximal urethral sphincter (bladder neck and prostatic urethra) and distal urethral sphincter (external striated muscle).	Fistulas may occur during pregnancy, after delivery of baby, as a result of hysterectomy or invasive cancer of cervix, or after radiation therapy. Incontinence is found as postoperative complication after transurethral, perineal, or retropubic prostatectomy.	Surgery to correct fistula, urinary diversion surgery to bypass urethra and bladder, external condom catheter, penile clamp, placement of artificial implantable sphincter
Functional Incontinence Loss of urine resulting from problems of patient mobility or environmental factors.	Elderly often have problems that affect balance and mobility.	Modifications of environment or care plan that facilitate regular, easy access to toilet and promote patient safety (e.g., better lighting, ambulatory assistance equipment, clothing alterations, timed voiding, different toileting equipment)

*Patients can have combination of stress and urge incontinence that is referred to as mixed incontinence.

medical emergency. *Chronic urinary retention* is defined as incomplete bladder emptying despite urination. The postvoid residual volumes in patients with chronic urinary retention vary widely; values of 150 to 200 ml or higher generally require further evaluation. Even smaller volumes may justify evaluation when they produce bothersome lower urinary tract symptoms or occur in a context of recurring UTIs.

Urinary retention is caused by two different dysfunctions of the urinary system: bladder outlet obstruction and deficient detrusor contraction strength. Obstruction leads to urinary retention when the blockage is sufficiently severe so that the bladder can no longer evacuate its contents despite a detrusor contraction. A common cause of obstruction in men is an enlarged prostate. Deficient detrusor contraction strength leads to urinary retention when the muscle is no longer able to contract with enough force or for a sufficient period of time to completely empty the bladder.

Common causes of deficient detrusor contraction strength are neurologic diseases affecting sacral segments 2, 3, and 4; longstanding diabetes mellitus; overdistention; chronic alcoholism; and drugs (e.g., anticholinergic drugs).

Diagnostic Studies

The basic evaluation for UI and urinary retention includes a focused history, physical assessment, and a bladder log or voiding record whenever possible. Information should be obtained on the onset of UI, factors that provoke urinary leakage, and associated conditions. The nurse should pay special attention to factors known to produce transient UI, particularly when a relatively sudden onset of urine loss is reported.[44] The physical examination begins with an assessment of general health and functional issues associated with urinary function, including mobility, dexterity, and cognitive function. A pelvic examination includes careful inspection of the perineal skin for signs of erosion or rashes related to UI. Local innervation and pelvic muscle strength should also be evaluated. Whenever possible, the patient is asked to keep a bladder log or voiding diary documenting the timing of urinations, episodes of urinary leakage, and frequency of nocturia for a period of 1 to 7 days. This record can be kept by nursing staff if the person is in an inpatient facility.

The urinalysis is used to identify possible factors contributing to transient UI or urinary retention (e.g., urinary infection, diabetes mellitus). A postvoid residual urine must be measured in the patient undergoing evaluation for urinary retention and UI. The postvoid residual volume is obtained by asking the patient to urinate, followed by catheterization within a relatively brief period (preferably 5 to 10 minutes). Alternatively, a bladder scan device can be used to estimate the residual volume. Although less accurate than the catheterized residual measurement, this technique avoids catheterization with its associated discomfort and risk of UTI. Urodynamic testing is indicated in selected cases of UI and urinary retention.[45] Imaging studies of the upper urinary tract (e.g., ultrasound, IVP) are obtained when retention or UI is associated with UTIs or when there is evidence of upper urinary tract involvement.

Collaborative Care: Urinary Incontinence

An estimated 80% of incontinence can be cured or significantly improved. Transient, reversible factors are corrected initially, followed by management of established UI (see Table 44-16). In general, less invasive treatments are attempted before more invasive methods (e.g., surgery) are used. Nevertheless, the choice of initial treatment is highly individualized and based on patient preference, the type and severity of UI, and associated anatomic defects.

Several behavioral therapies may be employed to improve urinary continence. Pelvic muscle training (Kegel exercises) is used to manage stress, urge, or mixed UI. Biofeedback is used to assist the patient to identify, isolate, contract, and relax the pelvic muscles (see the Complementary and Alternative Therapies box). Strength training is used to improve the efficiency of the sphincter. Neuromuscular education is used to teach patients how and when to contract the pelvic floor muscles to maximize continence. Bladder training or habit training involves rigidly scheduled toileting inter-

---

COMPLEMENTARY & ALTERNATIVE THERAPIES
Biofeedback for Urinary Incontinence

Clinical Uses
Kegel exercises help to strengthen the pelvic floor muscles. Biofeedback helps to isolate muscle groups in the pelvis.

Effects
Sensors for biofeedback are placed in the vagina or on the skin outside of the vagina. These sensors measure electrical signals produced when muscles contract. Biofeedback training develops an awareness of and control of the pelvic floor muscles.

Nursing Implications
If done correctly, pelvic floor exercise is effective treatment for mild to moderate urinary incontinence and other conditions related to pelvic floor weakness. Unfortunately, many women do not do these exercises correctly. Biofeedback is a tool to make sure that these exercises are done correctly. Most insurance companies cover the cost of biofeedback.

EVIDENCE-BASED PRACTICE
Pelvic Floor Muscle Training for Incontinence

Clinical Problem
Pelvic floor muscle training is a commonly recommended treatment for women with stress incontinence. Is pelvic floor muscle training effective for women with symptoms or urodynamic diagnoses of stress, urge, or mixed incontinence?

Best Clinical Practice
- Pelvic floor muscle training is an effective treatment for adult women with stress or mixed incontinence.
- Pelvic floor muscle training is better than no treatment or placebo treatments.
- Evidence for the effectiveness of pelvic floor muscle training for urge incontinence is inconclusive.

Nursing Implications
- Women who have problems with incontinence should be taught how to do Kegel exercises.
- It is important that patients learn the correct technique for pelvic floor muscle training to avoid squeezing the wrong muscles.
- It is recommended that Kegel exercises be done 5 minutes twice a day, once the correct technique has been established.

Reference for Evidence
Hay-Smith EJC et al: Pelvic floor muscle training for urinary incontinence in women. (Systematic review) Cochrane Incontinence Group, *Cochrane Database of Systematic Reviews*, issue 4, 2002.

vals designed to enhance bladder capacity and reduce the frequency and volume of urine loss. *Prompted toileting* is a behavioral technique used in patients with functional UI. In this case, the patient with impaired cognitive function is regularly reminded to urinate, assisted to the toilet, and offered praise for successful toileting.

Electrical stimulation of the pelvic floor muscles relies on very low-voltage and low-frequency pulses to stimulate muscle contraction and diminish overactive bladder contractions. It can be used as monotherapy for the treatment of urge or mixed UI or in conjunction with pelvic muscle training in the management of stress UI. Minimally invasive electrical stimulation uses a transvaginal or transrectal probe, or a device can be surgically implanted near the pelvic nerve roots.

Drug Therapy. Drug therapy varies according to the UI type (Table 44-17). Drugs have a very limited role in the management of stress UI. α-Adrenergic agonists can be used to increase urethral resistance at the level of the sphincter mechanism. Unfortunately, they exert a limited beneficial effect, and they are associated with adverse effects including exacerbation of hypertension and tachycardia. Drugs play a more central role in the management of urge or reflex UI. Antimuscarinic (also called anticholinergic or antispasmodic) drugs relax the bladder muscle and inhibit overactive detrusor contractions. Two preparations, long-acting tolterodine (Detrol LA) and oxybutynin in a releasing capsule (Ditropan XL) are preferred because of their efficacy and modest incidence of side effects compared with older antimuscarinic agents.

Surgical Therapy. Surgical techniques also vary according to the type of UI.[46,47] The Marshall-Marchetti procedure involves sus-

pending the urethra and bladder neck by suturing the anterior vaginal wall on each side to the periosteum of the pubic bones and lower rectum through an abdominal incision. The Pereyra procedure and subsequent modifications involve suspending the tissues adjacent to the bladder neck to the abdominal fascia, mainly through a transvaginal approach. Placement of a suburethral sling, using autologous fascia, cadaveric fascia, or a synthetic material, is also used to correct stress UI in women. An artificial urethral sphincter can be used in women or men with intrinsic sphincter deficiency and severe stress UI. Bolsters can also be implanted in men with stress UI to increase urethral resistance. This procedure is technically similar to the suburethral sling surgery often performed in women.

Alternatively, one of several bulking agents can be injected underneath the mucosa of the urethra to correct stress UI in women or men.[48] Bulking agents include glutaraldehyde cross-linked bovine collagen (GAX collagen), small silicone beads (Durasphere), or polytetrafluoroethylene (Teflon). Because of the risk of migration of Teflon particles, GAX collagen or Durasphere injections are most commonly used today. Although treatment with suburethral compounds avoids the risk associated with open surgery, reinjection after a period of several years is typically required.

NURSING MANAGEMENT
URINARY INCONTINENCE

The nurse must recognize both the physical and the emotional problems associated with UI. The patient's dignity, privacy, and feelings of self-worth must be maintained or enhanced. This often

TABLE 44-17	Drug Therapy Urinary Incontinence*	
DRUG CLASS AND MECHANISM OF ACTION	**DRUG**
Muscarinic Receptor Antagonists and Anticholinergics Reduce overactive bladder contractions	oxybutynin (Ditropan IR, Ditropan XL) tolterodine (Detrol IR, Detrol LA) hyoscyamine (Levsin, Levbid) dicyclomine (Bentyl) flavoxate (Urispas) propantheline (Pro-Banthine)
α-Adrenergic Antagonists Reduce urethral sphincter resistance to urinary outflow	doxazosin (Cardura) terazosin (Hytrin) tamsulosin (Flomax)
α-Adrenergic Agonists Increase urethral resistance	Phenylpropanolamine
Tricyclic Antidepressants Reduce sensory urgency and burning pain of interstitial cystitis Reduce overactive bladder contractions	imipramine (Tofranil) desipramine (Norpramin) nortriptyline (Aventyl)
Calcium Channel Blockers Reduces smooth muscle contraction strength May reduce burning pain of interstitial cystitis	nifedipine (Adalat) diltiazem (Cardizem) verapamil (Calan, Isoptin)
Hormone Replacement Therapy Local application reduces urethral irritation and increases host defenses against UTI	Premarin cream Estrace cream EST ring Vagifem

*The type of drug therapy depends on the type of incontinence.
UTI, Urinary tract infection.

includes a two-step approach comprising containment devices to manage existing urinary leakage and a definitive plan of management designed to reduce or resolve the factors leading to UI.

Management includes instructing the patient on consumption of an adequate volume of fluids and reduction or elimination of bladder irritants (particularly caffeine and alcohol) from the diet. The patient is advised to maintain a regular, flexible schedule of urination (usually every 2 to 3 hours while awake). In addition, patients are strongly advised to quit smoking because this habit increases the risk of stress incontinence. Patients should also be counseled about the relationship among constipation, UI, and urinary retention. Aggressive management of constipation, beginning with ensuring adequate fluid intake, increasing dietary fiber, light exercise, and judicious use of stool softeners, is recommended. (The management of constipation is discussed in Chapter 41.)

The nurse should assess strategies the patient uses to contain UI and offer advice concerning alternative devices when indicated. When attempting to manage UI, many women use feminine hygiene pads, and many men and women use household products such as rags, paper towels, or folded toilet tissue. Unfortunately, none of these products are adequately designed to wick urine away from the skin, prevent soiling of clothing, and reduce or eliminate odor. Instead, the nurse should share information on products specifically designed to contain urine. For example, patients with mild to moderate UI often benefit from incontinent pads containing Superabsorbent, a material specifically designed to absorb many times its weight in water. Patients with higher volume urine loss or those with double urinary and fecal incontinence may benefit from disposable or reusable incontinence briefs or pad/pant systems designed for more severe cases.

Several behavioral interventions are used in the management of UI. Habit training or prompted toileting are useful for patients with urge, mixed, and functional UI, respectively. Habit training uses the results of a voiding diary or bladder log to determine patterns of daytime voiding frequency. The patient and nurse then negotiate a goal for voiding frequency, usually ranging from 2 to 3 hours. The patient is taught to schedule rigidly during waking hours according to the baseline urinary frequency identified on the bladder log. At night the person is advised to urinate as normal if awakened from sleep with the desire to void. This interval is increased in a stepwise fashion to the goal negotiated with the nurse, usually over a period of 2 to 6 weeks. Habit training may be combined with pelvic muscle training, focusing on techniques such as urge suppression. Prompted toileting is indicated for patients with altered cognitive function and functional UI (usually coexisting with urge UI). In this case, caregivers are taught to remind the patient to toilet on a regular basis (usually every 2 to 3 hours), and the patient is assisted to the toilet and given praise for successful toileting. A trial of prompted toileting, in conjunction with a urologic evaluation, is used to predict the ultimate success of such a program.

In the hospital, nursing management includes maximizing toilet access. This assistance may take the form of offering the urinal or bedpan or assisting the patient to the bathroom every 2 to 3 hours or at scheduled times. The nurse ensures that patient toilets are accessible to patients and that adequate privacy occurs to allow effective urine elimination.

Collaborative Care: Urinary Retention

Behavioral therapies also may be used in the management of urinary retention.[49] Scheduled toileting and double voiding may be effective in chronic urinary retention with moderate postvoid

residual volumes. However, for acute or chronic urinary retention, catheterization may be required. Ideally, intermittent catheterization is used to manage urinary retention. It allows the patient to remain free of an indwelling catheter with its associated risk of UTI and urethral irritation. Despite these potential advantages, an indwelling catheter is preferred in certain cases (e.g., the patient who is unwilling or unable to perform intermittent catheterization). An indwelling catheter is also used when urethral obstruction renders intermittent catheterization uncomfortable or unfeasible.

Drug Therapy. Several drugs may be administered to promote bladder evacuation. For the patient with obstruction at the level of the bladder neck, an α-adrenergic blocker may be prescribed. These drugs relax the smooth muscle of the bladder neck, prostatic urethra, and possibly dual innervated rhabdosphincter, diminishing urethral resistance. Examples of α-adrenergic blocking agents are listed in Table 44-17. They are indicated in patients with benign prostatic hyperplasia, bladder neck dyssynergia, or detrusor sphincter dyssynergia. Finasteride (Proscar) is a 5-α-reductase enzyme inhibitor that reduces prostate size by inhibiting the conversion of testosterone to dihydrotestosterone. Finasteride is also useful for the hematuria that occasionally complicates symptomatic benign prostatic hyperplasia in older men. Bethanechol chloride (Urecholine) is sometimes prescribed to promote contractility in the weakened detrusor muscle.[50]

Surgical Therapy. Surgical interventions are often useful when managing urinary retention caused by obstruction. Transurethral or open surgical techniques are used to treat benign or malignant prostatic enlargement, bladder neck contracture, urethral strictures, or dyssynergia of the bladder neck in selected patients. Pelvic reconstruction using an abdominal or transvaginal approach can be used to correct bladder outlet obstruction in women with severe pelvic organ prolapse.

Unfortunately, surgery plays little role in the management of urinary retention caused by deficient detrusor contraction strength. Attempts to create a bladder stimulator (implanted device capable of stimulating micturition) have proved largely unsuccessful because of the difficulty achieving a coordinated detrusor contraction associated with pelvic muscle and striated sphincter relaxation.

NURSING MANAGEMENT
URINARY RETENTION

Acute urinary retention is a medical emergency that requires prompt recognition and bladder drainage. The nurse should insert a catheter (as prescribed) unless otherwise directed. A catheter with a retention balloon is used in anticipation of the need for an indwelling catheter.

The patient with acute urinary retention (as well as the patient predisposed to these episodes) should be taught strategies to minimize risk, including avoiding intake of large volumes of fluid over a brief period. Instead, the patient is advised to drink small volumes throughout the day. The patient is advised to warm up before attempting urination when chilled and to avoid large volumes of alcohol intake because it leads to polyuria and a diminished awareness of the need to urinate until the bladder is distended. A patient who is unable to urinate is advised to drink a cup of coffee or brewed tea containing caffeine to create or maximize urinary urgency and to sit in a tub of warm water or take a warm shower and attempt to urinate while in the bath tub or shower. The patient can be reassured that he or she can easily bathe immediately following bladder evacuation. If this does not lead to successful urination, the patient is advised to seek immediate care.

Patients with chronic urinary retention may be managed by behavioral methods, indwelling or intermittent catheterization, surgery, or drugs.[49] Scheduled toileting and double voiding are the primary behavioral interventions used for chronic retention. Scheduled toileting is used to reduce rather than expand bladder capacity. In this case, patients are asked to void every 3 to 4 hours regardless of the desire to urinate. This intervention is particularly useful in the patient with chronic overdistention, diabetes mellitus, or chronic alcoholism characterized by a large bladder capacity and diminished or delayed sensations of bladder filling and urgency. Double voiding is an attempt to maximize bladder evacuation. The patient is asked to urinate, sit on the toilet for 3 to 4 minutes, and urinate again before exiting the bathroom.

INSTRUMENTATION

Reasons for urinary catheterization are listed in Table 44-18. Two reasons that are not indications for catheterization are (1) routine acquisition of a urine specimen for laboratory analysis and (2) convenience of the nursing staff or the patient's family. The risks of nosocomial infection are too high to allow catheterization of a patient for the convenience of hospital personnel or family members. Catheterization for sterile urine specimens may occasionally be indicated when patients have a history of complicated urinary infection. These specimens have to be as free of contaminants as possible. A catheter should be the final means of providing the patient with a dry environment for prevention of skin breakdown and protection of dressings or skin lesions.

Urinary catheterization is commonly used in the management of the hospitalized patient. However, it is not without serious risks. The urinary tract is the most common site of nosocomial infections. Urinary catheterization is a major cause of UTIs. Scrupulous aseptic technique is mandatory when a urinary catheter is inserted. After insertion, maintenance and protection of the closed drainage system are major nursing responsibilities. Irrigation of the catheter should not be routinely performed.

TABLE 44-18 Indications for Urinary Catheterization

1. Relief of urinary retention caused by lower urinary tract obstruction, paralysis, or inability to void
2. Bladder decompression preoperatively and operatively for lower abdominal or pelvic surgery
3. Facilitation of surgical repair of urethra and surrounding structures
4. Splinting of ureters or urethra to facilitate healing after surgery or other trauma in area
5. Instillation of medications into bladder
6. Accurate measurement of urinary output in critically ill patient
7. Measurement of residual urine after urination
8. Study of anatomic structures of urinary system
9. Urodynamic testing
10. Collection of sterile urine sample in selected situations

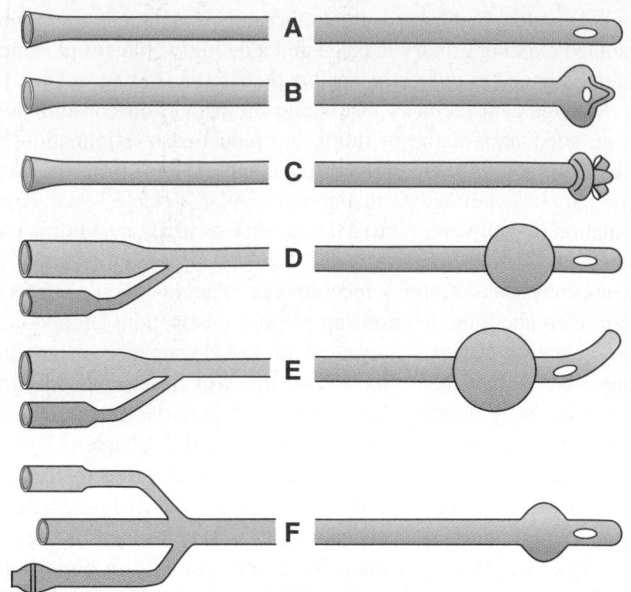

FIG. 44-8 Different types of commonly used catheters. A, Simple urethral catheter. B, Mushroom or Pezzar (can be used for suprapubic catheterization). C, Winged-tip or Malecot. D, Indwelling with inflated balloon. E, Indwelling with Coudé tip or Tiemann. F, Three-way indwelling (the third lumen is used for irrigation of the bladder).

While the patient has a catheter in place, nursing actions should include maintaining patency of the catheter, managing fluid intake, providing for the comfort and safety of the patient, and preventing infection. Attention should be given to the psychologic implications of urinary drainage. Concerns of the patient can include embarrassment related to exposure of the body, an altered body image, and fear concerning the care of the catheter that results in increased dependency.

Catheters vary in construction materials, tip shape (Fig. 44-8), and size of the lumen. Catheters are sized according to the French scale. Each French unit equals 0.33 mm of diameter. The diameter measured is the internal diameter of the catheter. The size used varies with the size of the individual and the purpose for catheterization. In women, urethral catheter sizes 12F to 14F are the most common; in men, sizes 14F to 16F are used. The primary problem resulting from too large a catheter is tissue erosion secondary to excessive pressure on the meatus or urethra. Four routes are used for urinary tract catheterization: urethral, ureteral, suprapubic, and via a nephrostomy tube.

Urethral Catheterization

The most common route of catheterization is insertion of the catheter through the external meatus into the urethra, past the internal sphincter, and into the bladder. Principles that should be considered in the management of the patient with a urethral catheter include the following:

1. The catheterized patient, particularly the person who is ambulatory, should receive appropriate instruction regarding catheter care.
2. A sterile, closed drainage system should always be used in short-term catheterization. The distal urinary catheter and the proximal drainage tube should not be disconnected except for necessary catheter irrigation. Unobstructed down-

hill flow must be maintained. The collecting bag should be emptied regularly and kept below the level of the bladder. A poorly functioning catheter should be replaced. The leg bag should not be used for the short-term patient in the hospital setting because the risk of bacterial infection is great when the catheter is disconnected and the drainage bags are exchanged.

3. Perineal care (one to two times per day and when necessary) should include cleaning of the meatus-catheter junction with soap and water. Following this, an antimicrobial ointment may be applied. Lotion or powder should not be used near the catheter. The catheter should be properly secured to the leg to prevent movement and urethral traction.

4. Sterile technique must be used whenever the collecting system is opened. Catheter irrigation is performed only when obstruction or blood clots are suspected or, in the case of long-term catheterization, to reduce sediment buildup. If frequent irrigations are necessary in short-term catheterization for catheter patency, a triple-lumen catheter may be preferable, permitting continuous irrigations within a closed system. Small volumes of urine for culture can be aspirated from the distal catheter by means of a sterile syringe and a 21-gauge needle after the drainage tubing is clamped. The puncture site must first be prepared with a tincture of iodine or alcohol solution. Many drainage systems are now equipped with a sampling port. Silicone or plastic catheters do not self-seal. Urine for chemical analysis (e.g., electrolytes) can be obtained from the drainage bag.

5. When the patient is catheterized for less than 2 weeks, routine catheter change is not necessary. For long-term use of an indwelling catheter, regular replacement is necessary. With long-term use of a catheter, a leg bag may be used. If the collection bag is reused, it should be washed in soap and water and rinsed thoroughly. When not reused immediately, it should be filled with ½ cup of vinegar and drained. The vinegar is effective against *Pseudomonas* and other organisms and eliminates odors.

Ureteral Catheters

The ureteral catheter is placed through the ureters into the renal pelvis. The catheter is inserted either (1) by being threaded up the urethra and bladder to the ureters under cystoscopic observation or (2) by surgical insertion through the abdominal wall into the ureters. The ureteral catheter is used after surgery to splint the ureters and to prevent them from being obstructed by edema. The urine volume from the ureteral catheter should be recorded separately from other urinary catheters. The patient is usually kept on bed rest while a ureteral catheter is in place until specific orders indicate that ambulation is permissible. The self-retaining ureteral catheter is often inserted after a lithotripsy procedure or when ureteral obstruction from adjacent tumors or fibrosis threatens renal function. The double-J ureteral catheter is often used and allows the patient to ambulate. One end coils up in the kidney pelvis, while the other coils in the bladder.

The placement of the ureteral catheter should be checked frequently, and tension on the catheter should be avoided. The catheter drains urine from the renal pelvis, which has a capacity of 3 to 5 ml. If the volume of urine in the renal pelvis increases, tissue damage to the pelvis will result from pressure. Therefore the ureteral catheter should not be clamped. If the physician orders irrigation of the ureteral catheter, strict aseptic technique is required. If output is decreased, the physician should be notified immediately. Drainage should be checked often (at least every 1 to 2 hours). It is normal for some urine to drain around the ureteral catheter into the bladder. Accurate recording of urine output from both the ureters and the urethral catheter is essential. Sometimes a ureteral catheter may be used as a stent and is not expected to drain. It is important to check with the physician as to the type of catheter and what to expect.

Suprapubic Catheters

Suprapubic catheterization is the simplest and oldest method of urinary diversion. The two methods of insertion of a suprapubic catheter into the bladder are (1) through a small incision in the abdominal wall and (2) by the use of a trocar. A suprapubic catheter is placed while the patient is under general anesthesia for another surgical procedure or at the bedside with a local anesthetic. The catheter may be sutured into place. The nursing responsibility includes taping the catheter to prevent dislodgment. The care of the tube and catheter is similar to that of the urethral catheter. A pectin-base skin barrier (e.g., Stomahesive) is effective around the insertion site in protecting the skin from breakdown.

The suprapubic catheter is used in temporary situations such as bladder, prostate, and urethral surgery. The suprapubic catheter is also used long term in selected patients (e.g., male tetraplegic (quadriplegic) patient who tends to form penoscrotal fistulas).

A suprapubic catheter is prone to poor drainage because of mechanical obstruction of the catheter tip by the bladder wall, sediment, and clots. Nursing interventions to ensure patency of the tube include (1) preventing tube kinking by coiling the excess tubing and maintaining gravity drainage, (2) having the patient turn from side to side, and (3) milking the tube. If these measures are not effective, the catheter is irrigated with sterile technique after a physician's order has been obtained.

If the patient experiences bladder spasms that are difficult to control, urinary leakage may result. Oxybutynin (Ditropan) or other oral antispasmodics or belladonna and opium (B&O) suppositories may be prescribed to decrease bladder spasms.

Nephrostomy Tubes

The nephrostomy tube (catheter) is inserted on a temporary basis to preserve renal function when a complete obstruction of the ureter is present. It is inserted directly into the pelvis of the kidney and attached to connecting tubing for closed drainage. The principle is the same as with the ureteral catheter; that is, the catheter should never be kinked, laid or leaned on, or clamped. If the patient complains of excessive pain in the area or if there is excessive drainage around the tube, the catheter should be checked for patency. If irrigation is ordered, strict aseptic technique is required. No more than 5 ml of sterile saline solution is gently instilled at one time to prevent overdistention of the kidney pelvis and renal damage. Infection and secondary stone formation are complications associated with the insertion of a nephrostomy tube.

Intermittent Catheterization

An alternative approach to a long-term indwelling catheter is intermittent catheterization.[51] It is being used with increasing frequency in conditions characterized by neurogenic bladder (e.g., spinal cord injuries, chronic neurologic diseases) or bladder outlet obstruction in men. This type of catheterization may also be used in the oliguric and anuric phases of acute renal failure to reduce the possibility of infection from an indwelling catheter. Intermittent catheterization is also used postoperatively, often after a surgical procedure for female incontinence or radioactive seed implantation into the prostate for cancer. The main goal of intermittent catheterization is to prevent urinary retention, stasis, and compromised blood supply to the bladder caused by prolonged pressure.

The technique consists of inserting a urethral catheter into the bladder every 3 to 5 hours. Some patients do intermittent catheterization only once or twice a day to measure residual urine and to ensure an empty bladder. Patients should be instructed to wash and rinse the catheter and their hands with soap and water before and after catheterization. Lubricant is necessary for men and may make catheterization more comfortable for women. The catheter may be inserted by the patient or the care provider. The bladder is emptied and the catheter is removed. The catheter can be dried and placed in a carrying pouch or purse or folded in a paper towel until it is next needed. The same catheter can be used for weeks at a time. In general, patients should change the catheter every 2 to 4 weeks.

In the hospital, sterile technique is used. For home care, a clean technique that includes good hand washing with soap and water is used. There has been no significant increase in infection with the use of an appropriate clean technique as compared with sterile technique. The patient is taught to observe for signs of UTI so that treatment can be instituted early. If indicated, some patients are placed on a regimen of prophylactic antibiotics.

Surgery of the Urinary Tract

RENAL AND URETERAL SURGERY

The most common indications for nephrectomy are a renal tumor, polycystic kidneys that are bleeding or severely infected, massive traumatic injury to the kidney, and the elective removal of a kidney from a donor. Surgery involving the ureters and kidneys is most commonly performed to remove calculi that become obstructive, correct congenital anomalies, and divert urine when necessary.

Preoperative Management

The basic needs of the patient undergoing renal and ureteral surgery are similar to those of any patient who experiences surgery (see Chapters 17 through 19). In addition, it is especially important preoperatively to ensure adequate fluid intake and a normal electrolyte balance. The patient should be told that there will probably be a flank incision on the affected side and that surgery will require a hyperextended, side-lying position. This position frequently causes the patient to experience muscle aches after surgery. If a nephrectomy is planned, the patient must be assured that one working kidney is sufficient to maintain normal renal function.

Postoperative Management

Specific postoperative needs of a patient are related to urine output, respiratory status, and abdominal distention.

Urine Output. In the immediate postoperative period, urine output should be determined at least every 1 to 2 hours. Drainage from various catheters should be recorded separately. The catheter or tube should not be clamped or irrigated without a specific order. The total urine output should be at least 0.5 ml/kg per hour. It is also important to assess for urine drainage on the dressing and to estimate the amount. Daily weighing of the patient is important. The same scale should be used and properly balanced, and the patient should wear similar clothing and dressings each time.

It is important to observe and monitor the color and consistency of urine. Urine with increased amounts of mucus, blood, or sediment may occlude the drainage tubing or catheter.

Respiratory Status. Renal surgery is often performed through a flank incision just below the diaphragm and often involves removal of the twelfth rib. Postoperatively, it is important to ensure adequate ventilation. The patient is often reluctant to turn, cough, and deep breathe because of the incisional pain. Adequate pain medication should be given to ensure the patient's comfort and ability to perform coughing and deep-breathing exercises. Frequently, additional respiratory devices such as an incentive spirometer are used every 2 hours while the patient is awake. In addition, early and frequent ambulation assists in maintaining adequate respiratory function.

Abdominal Distention. Abdominal distention is present to some degree in most patients who have had surgery on their kidneys or ureters. It is most commonly due to paralytic ileus caused by manipulation and compression of the bowel during surgery. Oral intake is restricted until bowel sounds are present (usually 24 to 48 hours after surgery). IV fluids are given until the patient can take oral fluids. Progression to a regular diet follows.

Laparoscopic Nephrectomy

Laparoscopic nephrectomy can be performed in selected situations to remove a diseased kidney. Laparoscopic nephrectomy can also be used to obtain a kidney from a living donor to be transplanted into a person with end-stage renal disease. In contrast to the open incision of about 7 inches (18 cm) required in a conventional nephrectomy, a laparoscopic nephrectomy is performed using five puncture sites. One incision is to view the kidney and another is to dissect it. The laparoscope contains a miniature camera so that the surgeons can watch what they are doing on a video monitor. Once dissected, the kidney is maneuvered into a nylon impermeable sack, and its contents can then be safely removed from the patient. Compared with conventional nephrectomy, the laparoscopic approach is less painful and requires no sutures or staples, involves a shorter hospital stay, and has a much faster recovery.

URINARY DIVERSION

Urinary diversion may be performed with and without cystectomy. Urinary diversion procedures are performed to treat cancer of the bladder, neurogenic bladder, congenital anomalies, strictures, trauma to the bladder, and chronic infections with deterioration of renal function. Numerous urinary diversion techniques and bladder substitutes are possible, including an incontinent urinary diversion, continent urinary diversion catheterized by patient, or an orthotopic bladder so that the patient voids urethrally.[52] Types of these surgical procedures are presented in Table 44-19 and Fig. 44-9.

TABLE 44-19 **Types of Urinary Diversion Surgery Requiring Collection Devices**

TYPE	DESCRIPTION	ADVANTAGES	DISADVANTAGES	SPECIAL CONSIDERATIONS
Ileal Conduit	Ureters are implanted into part of ileum or colon that has been resected from intestinal tract. Abdominal stoma is created.	Relatively good urine flow with few physiologic alterations	External appliance necessary to continually collect urine	Surgical procedure is more complex. Postoperative complications may be increased. Reabsorption of urea by ileum occurs. Meticulous attention is necessary to care for stoma and collecting device.
Cutaneous Ureterostomy	Ureters are excised from bladder and brought through abdominal wall, and stoma is created. Ureteral stomas may be created from both ureters, or ureters may be brought together and one stoma created.	No need for major surgery as required with ileal conduit	External appliance necessary because of continuous urine drainage; possibility of stricture or stenosis of small stoma	Periodic catheterizations may be required to dilate stomas to maintain patency.
Nephrostomy	Catheter is inserted into pelvis of kidney. Procedure may be done to one or both kidneys and may be temporary or permanent. It is most frequently done in advanced disease as palliative procedure.	No need for major surgery	High risk of renal infection; predisposition to calculus formation from catheter	Nephrostomy tube may have to be changed every month. Catheter must never be clamped.

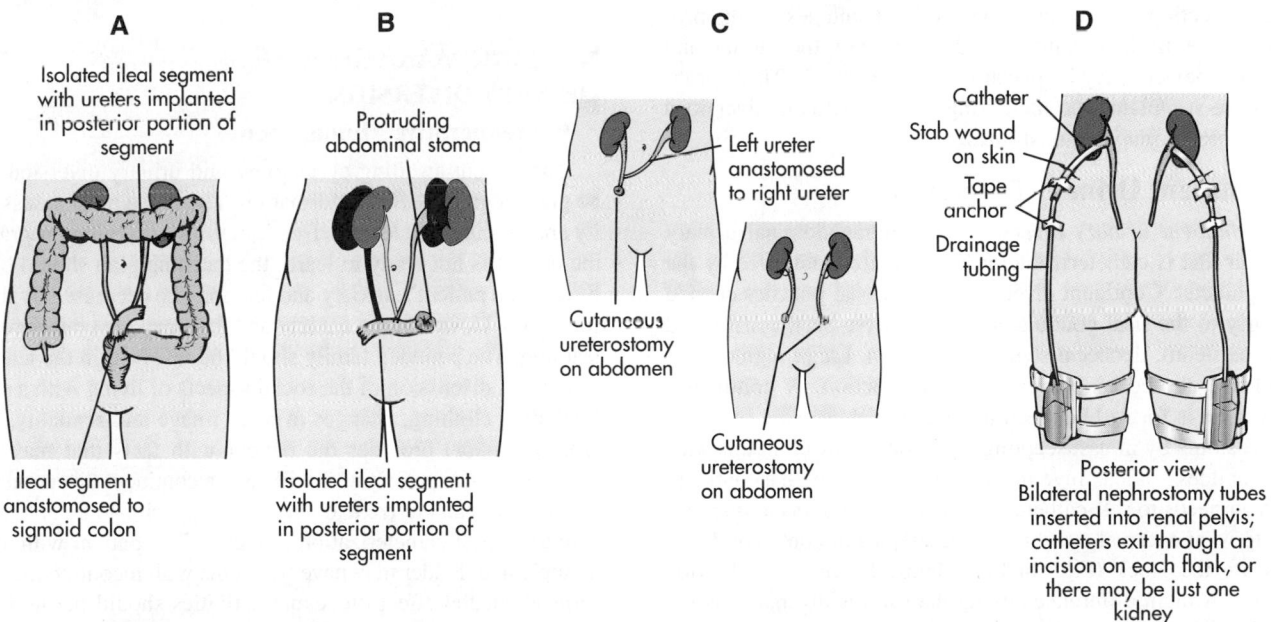

A
Isolated ileal segment with ureters implanted in posterior portion of segment

Ileal segment anastomosed to sigmoid colon

B
Protruding abdominal stoma

Isolated ileal segment with ureters implanted in posterior portion of segment

C
Left ureter anastomosed to right ureter

Cutaneous ureterostomy on abdomen

Cutaneous ureterostomy on abdomen

D
Catheter
Stab wound on skin
Tape anchor
Drainage tubing

Posterior view
Bilateral nephrostomy tubes inserted into renal pelvis; catheters exit through an incision on each flank, or there may be just one kidney

FIG. 44-9 Methods of urinary diversion. A, Ureteroileosigmoidostomy. B, Ileal loop (or ileal conduit). C, Ureterostomy (transcutaneous ureterostomy and bilateral cutaneous ureterostomies). D, Nephrostomy.

Incontinent Urinary Diversion

Incontinent urinary diversion is diversion to the skin, requiring an appliance. The simplest form is the cutaneous ureterostomy, but scarring and strictures of the ureter have led to the use of ileal or colonic conduits. The most commonly performed in-

continent urinary diversion procedure is the **ileal conduit** (ileal loop). In this procedure a 6- to 8-inch (15- to 20-cm) segment of the ileum is converted into a conduit for urinary drainage. The colon (colon conduit) can be used instead of the ileum. The ureters are anastomosed into one end of the conduit, and

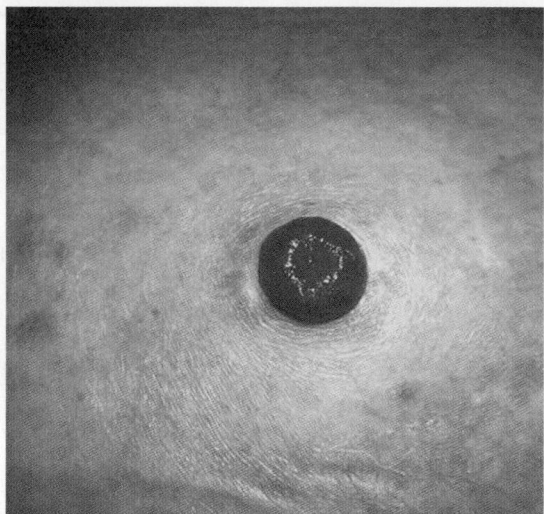

FIG. 44-10 Ideal urinary stoma. It is symmetric, has no skin breakdown, and protrudes about 1.5 cm; the mucosa is a healthy red, and the configuration is flat when the patient is upright and supine.

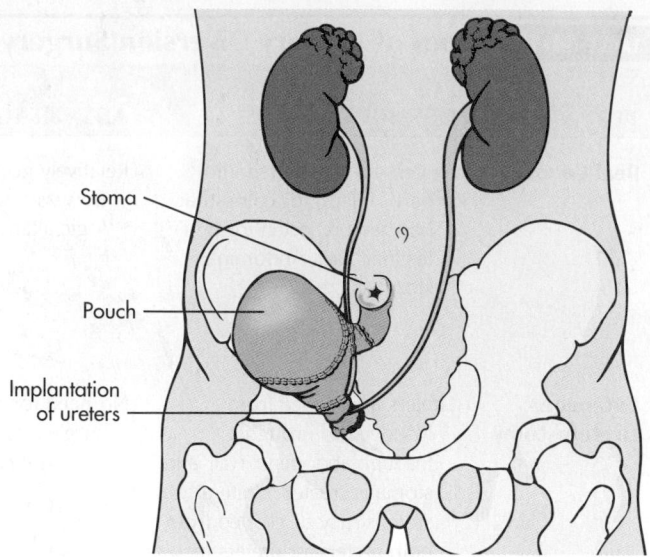

FIG. 44-11 Creation of a Kock pouch with implantation of ureters into one intussuscepted portion of the pouch and creation of a stoma with the other intussuscepted portion.

the other end of the bowel is brought out through the abdominal wall to form a stoma (Fig. 44-10). Although the segment of bowel remains supported by the mesentery, it is completely isolated from the intestinal tract. The bowel is anastomosed and continues to function normally. Because there is no valve and no voluntary control over the stoma, drops of urine flow from the stoma every few seconds, requiring the use of a permanent external collecting device. The visible stoma and the need for external collection devices are obvious disadvantages of this procedure. The lifelong care and dealing with the stoma and collection devices may be psychologically difficult. These problems have stimulated the increasing use of continent diversions and orthotopic bladder substitutes.

Continent Urinary Diversions

A *continent urinary diversion* is an intraabdominal urinary reservoir that is catheterizable or has an outlet controlled by the anal sphincter. Continent diversions are internal pouches created similarly to the ileal conduit. Reservoirs have been constructed from the ileum, ileocecal segment, or colon. Large segments of bowel are altered to prevent peristaltic action. A continence mechanism is formed between this large, low-pressure reservoir and the stoma by intussuscepting a portion of bowel. In this way, a patient does not leak involuntarily. The patient with a continent reservoir needs to self-catheterize every 4 to 6 hours but does not need to wear external attachments. Examples of continent diversions are the Kock (Fig. 44-11), Mainz, Indiana, and Florida pouches. A main difference among the various diversions is the segment of bowel used. For example, the Indiana pouch uses the right colon as a reservoir and has become a popular form of continent urinary diversion.

Orthotopic Bladder Substitution

Orthotopic bladder substitutes can be derived from various segments of the intestines. An isolated segment of the distal ileum is often preferred. Various procedures include the hemi-Kock pouch, Studer pouch, and the ileal W-neobladder. In these procedures the bowel is surgically reshaped to become a neobladder. The ureters and urethra are sutured into the neobladder. Orthotopic bladder substitution has been more commonly done in men because in women the urethra is usually removed when the bladder is resected.[53] The advantage of orthotopic bladder substitution is that it allows for natural micturition. Incontinence is a possible problem with this technique, and intermittent catheterization may be required.

NURSING MANAGEMENT
URINARY DIVERSION

■ Preoperative Management

The patient awaiting cystectomy and urinary diversion must be given a great deal of information. The nurse must assess ability and readiness to learn before initiating a teaching program. If the patient is not ready to learn, the teaching plan should be adjusted. The patient's anxiety and fear may be decreased by the information. However, the anxiety and fear may also interfere with learning. The patient's family should be involved in the teaching process. A discussion of the social aspects of living with a stoma (including clothing, changes in body image and sexuality, exercise, and odor) provides the patient with facts that may allay some fears. The patient who will have a continent diversion must be taught to catheterize and irrigate the pouch and be able to adhere to a strict catheterization schedule. The patient with an orthotopic neobladder may have problems with incontinence. Concerns about the effect on sexual activities should be discussed. The enterostomal therapy nurse should be involved in the preoperative phase of the patient's care. A visit from an ostomate or enterostomal therapy nurse can be helpful. Additional interventions are presented in NCP 44-3.

■ Postoperative Management

Nursing interventions during the postoperative period (see NCP 44-3 for care after an ileal conduit) should be planned to prevent surgical complications such as postoperative atelectasis and shock (see Chapter 19). After pelvic surgery, there is an in-

NURSING CARE PLAN 44-3

Patient with an Ileal Conduit

EXPECTED PATIENT OUTCOMES	NURSING INTERVENTIONS and *RATIONALES*
NURSING DIAGNOSIS	**Anxiety** *related to* effects of ileal conduit on lifestyle and relationships; lack of knowledge regarding surgical procedure, appliance, and its use *as manifested by* frequent questions about surgical procedure, restlessness, inability to sleep.
• Knowledgeable about preoperative, operative, and postoperative procedures, including both stoma and appliance	• Instruct patient in preoperative, operative, and postoperative procedures including diet, drugs, nasogastric tube, IVs, NPO status, pain management, turning, deep breathing, and leg exercises *to reduce anxiety and facilitate patient's progress through postoperative recovery.* • Demonstrate how to apply appliance and use equipment *because knowledge before surgery reduces patient's postoperative concerns.* • Answer questions honestly and provide emotional support *to reduce fear of the unknown and convey a caring attitude.* • Arrange for visit with person with an ileal conduit or with enterostomal therapy nurse *to provide patient with significant information related to ostomy care.*
NURSING DIAGNOSIS	**Risk for infection** *related to* surgical procedure, ureteral obstruction, chronic use of external appliance, and incorrect or inadequate stoma care.
• No urinary tract infection	• Assess patient for elevation in body temperature, pain in back or abdomen, bloody or cloudy urine, decrease in urinary output *to ensure early detection of UTI.* • Empty appliance q2-3hr or when one-third to one-half full of urine *to reduce risk of urinary reflux.* • Use bedside drainage bag at night *to prevent reflux of urine into conduit.* • Instruct patient about symptoms to be reported *as indicators of possible infection.*
NURSING DIAGNOSIS	**Disturbed body image** *related to* effects of change in body function on lifestyle or relationships *as manifested by* negative feelings about self, refusal to look at or touch stoma or participate in self-care, expression of concern about effect on family and lifestyle.
• Acceptance of changes in body image and function	• Encourage patient to share feelings *to provide opportunity to assist with issues and misconceptions and plan appropriate interventions.* • Demonstrate willingness to listen and answer questions *to convey interest in the patient's concerns and to provide needed information.* • Determine the need for additional support (e.g., psychiatric support, visit by an ostomate) *because these persons may provide new information and suggestion of ways to modify lifestyle.* • Encourage gradual involvement in self-care *because independence in self-care helps to improve self-esteem.*
NURSING DIAGNOSIS	**Ineffective therapeutic regimen management** *related to* lack of knowledge regarding stoma and appliance care *as manifested by* expression of concern about how to manage ileal conduit, frequent questions or inaccurate responses regarding stoma care.
• Able to change stoma bag and clean stoma • Able to maintain permanent appliance	• Demonstrate proper method of changing stoma bag and have patient give return demonstration *to teach correct care and evaluate learning.* • Teach measures such as high fluid intake, regular activity, and urine acidification *to prevent urinary calculi and infection.* • Teach practices such as proper stoma and pouch care; empty or change pouch when one-third to one-half full; avoid odor-producing foods such as onions, fish, eggs, cheese; drink cranberry juice or use a liquid appliance deodorant *to enable satisfactory self-care.*
NURSING DIAGNOSIS	**Risk for impaired skin integrity** *related to* ill-fitting appliance, inadequate hygiene, and lack of knowledge regarding stoma care.
• Intact, viable stoma • Clean and intact skin surrounding stoma	• Assess skin for improperly fitted appliance, reddened and irritated skin around stoma *to ensure prompt identification of the problem.* • Check appliance position *to prevent leakage of caustic drainage onto skin.* • Observe stoma for any bleeding or eroded areas *for early identification and treatment of complications.* • Cleanse stoma as ordered *to reduce encrustations and bacterial contact with the stoma and surrounding skin.* • Allow no tight clothing or binders over stoma *to enable unobstructed circulation of blood and flow of urine.*

IVs, Intravenous lines; *NPO,* nothing by mouth; *UTI,* urinary tract infection.

Continued

NURSING CARE PLAN 44-3

Patient with an Ileal Conduit—cont'd

EXPECTED PATIENT OUTCOMES	NURSING INTERVENTIONS and *RATIONALES*
NURSING DIAGNOSIS	**Ineffective sexuality patterns** *related to* perceived or actual effects of surgery on sexual activity *as manifested* by verbalizing concerns about sexuality and unwillingness to discuss sexual issues with partner.
• Satisfaction with sexual practices	• Assess patient's concerns related to sexuality such as future sexual functioning and lack of understanding by significant other *to determine presence and extent of problem.* • Provide accurate information related to sexual activity *so that patient will know the effect of this surgery on sexual activities and practices.*

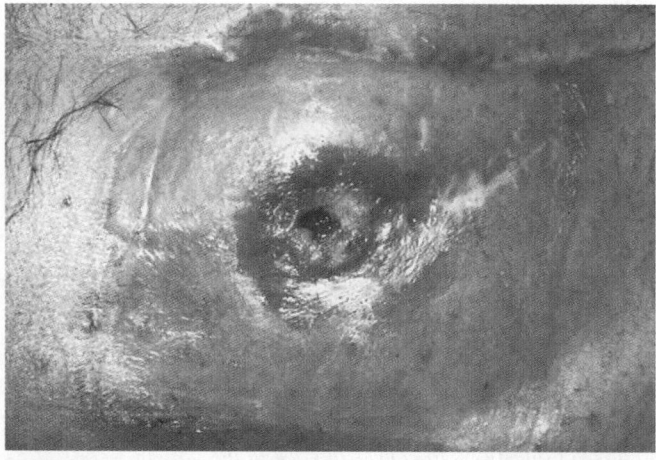

FIG. 44-12   Ammonia salt encrustation secondary to alkaline urine.

creased incidence of thrombophlebitis. With removal of part of the bowel, the incidence of paralytic ileus and small bowel obstruction is increased, the patient is NPO, and a nasogastric tube is necessary for 3 to 5 days.

Specific attention should be given to preventing injury to the stoma and maintaining urine output. Mucus is present in the urine because it is secreted by the intestines as a result of the irritating effect of the urine. The patient should be told that this is a normal occurrence. A high fluid intake is encouraged to "flush" the ileal conduit or continent diversion.

When an ileal conduit is created, the skin around the stoma requires meticulous care. Alkaline encrustations with dermatitis may occur when alkaline urine comes in contact with exposed skin (Fig. 44-12). Other common peristomal skin problems include yeast infections, product allergies, and shearing-effect excoriations. Changing appliances (pouches) is described in Table 44-20. A properly fitting appliance is essential to prevent

TABLE
44-20   *Patient & Family Teaching Guide*
Changing Ileal Conduit Appliances

Temporary Appliance
1. Cut hole in pouch to fit over stoma (pouch 3.2 mm [⅛ in] larger than stoma).
2. Remove old pouch.
3. Clean area gently and remove old adhesive.
4. Wash area with warm water.
5. Place wick (rolled-up 4 × 4–in pad) over stoma to keep area dry during rest of procedure.
6. Dry skin around stoma.
7. Apply tincture of benzoin or other skin protectant around stoma to area where pouch will be placed.
8. Apply pouch by first smoothing its edges toward side and lower portion of body.
9. Remove wick and complete application of bag.
10. If patient is usually in bed, apply bag so that it lies toward side of body.
11. If patient is ambulatory, apply bag so that it lies vertically.
12. Connect drainage tubing to pouch.
13. Keep drainage pouch on same side of bed as stoma.

Permanent Appliance*
1. Keep appliance in place for 2 to 14 days.
2. Change appliance when fluid intake has been restricted for several hours.
3. Have patient sit or stand in front of mirror.
4. Moisten edge of faceplate with adhesive solvent and gently remove.
5. Clean skin with adhesive solvent.
6. Wash skin with warm water. (Patient may shower.)
7. Dry skin and inspect.
8. Place wick (rolled-up 4 × 4–in pad) over stoma to keep skin free of urine.
9. Apply skin cement to faceplate and skin.
10. Place appliance over stoma.
11. Wash removed appliance with soap and lukewarm water; soak in distilled vinegar; rinse with lukewarm water and air dry.

*Many disposable appliances with self-adhesive backing are used as permanent appliances.

skin problems. The appliance should be about 0.1 inch (0.2 cm) larger than the stoma. It is normal for the stoma to shrink within the first few weeks after surgery. The urine is kept acidic to prevent alkaline encrustations.

Acceptance of the surgery and of alterations in body image is needed to ensure the patient's best adjustment. Concerns of the patient include fear that the stoma will be offensive to others and will interfere with sexual, personal, professional, and recreational activities. The patient should know that few activities, if any, will be restricted as a result of the urinary diversion.

Discharge planning after an ileal conduit includes teaching the patient symptoms of obstruction or infection and care of the ostomy. The patient with an ileal conduit is fitted for a permanent appliance 7 to 10 days after surgery and may need to be refitted at a later time, depending on the degree of stoma shrinkage. Appliances are made of a variety of products, including natural and synthetic rubbers, plastics, and metals. Most appliances have a faceplate that adheres to the skin, a collecting pouch, and an opening to drain the pouch. The faceplate may be secured to the skin with glues, adhesives, or adhering synthetic wafers. Some appliances do not require adhesives, but their design relies on pressure to keep the pouch in place. If improperly fitted or applied, the faceplate may cause skin problems (Fig. 44-13). The patient needs information on

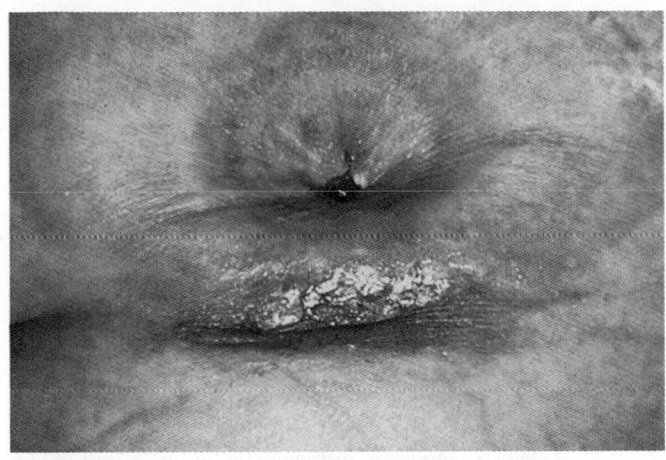

FIG. 44-13 Retracted urinary stoma with pressure sore from faceplate above stoma.

where to purchase supplies, emergency telephone numbers, location of ostomy clubs, and follow-up visits with an enterostomal therapist. Physician follow-up is imperative to monitor and correct homeostatic abnormalities and to prevent complications and renal function deterioration.

CRITICAL THINKING EXERCISES

Case Study
Urinary Tract Infection
Patient Profile. Suzanna, a 28-year-old Hispanic woman, was seen in the nurse practitioner's office for a history of painful, frequent urination.

Subjective Data
- Has had a history of painful, frequent urination with passage of small volumes of urine for 3 days
- Has had intermittent fever, chills, and back pain during these 3 days
- Was frightened when she saw blood in her urine
- Is anxious because her father died of kidney cancer

Objective Data
Physical Examination
- Complains of bilateral flank pain and abdominal tenderness to palpation
- Temperature is 100.4° F (38° C)

Diagnostic Study
- Urinalysis: pyuria and hematuria

CRITICAL THINKING QUESTIONS
1. What are the most common organisms that cause UTIs?
2. What factors predispose a patient to a UTI?
3. What is the difference between upper and lower UTIs?
4. What nursing interventions will help Suzanna cope with her symptoms?
5. What can the nurse do to help Suzanna prevent another UTI?
6. Based on the data presented, write one or more appropriate nursing diagnoses. Are there any collaborative problems?

Nursing Research Issues
1. In the patient with UTI, what are the most effective methods to ensure compliance with therapy and follow-up care?
2. What therapeutic measures are most effective in treating stress incontinence?
3. What are the differences in quality of life of the patient with an ileal conduit compared with the patient with a continent urinary diversion?
4. What are the most effective ways to manage pain following lithotripsy?
5. Does biofeedback improve the effectiveness of pelvic muscle exercises?

REVIEW QUESTIONS

The number of the question corresponds to the same-numbered objective at the beginning of the chapter.

1. In teaching a patient with pyelonephritis about the disorder, the nurse informs the patient that the organisms that cause pyelonephritis most commonly reach the kidneys through
   a. the bloodstream.
   b. the lymphatic system.
   c. a descending infection.
   d. an ascending infection.

2. The nurse teaches the female patient who has frequent UTIs that she should
   a. urinate after sexual intercourse.
   b. take tub baths with bubble bath.
   c. take prophylactic sulfonamides for the rest of her life.
   d. restrict fluid intake to prevent the need for frequent voiding.

3. The immunologic mechanisms involved in glomerulonephritis include
   a. tubular blocking by precipitates of bacteria and antibody reactions.
   b. deposition of immune complexes and complement along the GBM.
   c. thickening of the GBM from autoimmune microangiopathic changes.
   d. destruction of glomeruli by proteolytic enzymes contained in the GBM.

4. One of the most important roles of the nurse in relation to acute poststreptococcal glomerulonephritis is to
   a. promote early diagnosis and treatment of sore throats and skin lesions.
   b. encourage patients to request antibiotic therapy for all upper respiratory infections.
   c. teach patients with APSGN that long-term prophylactic antibiotic therapy is necessary to prevent recurrence.
   d. monitor patients for respiratory symptoms that indicate that the disease is affecting the alveolar basement membrane.

5. The edema that occurs in nephrotic syndrome is due to
   a. decreased aldosterone secretion from adrenal insufficiency.
   b. increased hydrostatic pressure caused by sodium retention.
   c. increased fluid retention caused by decreased glomerular filtration.
   d. decreased colloidal osmotic pressure caused by loss of serum albumin.

6. A patient is admitted to the hospital with severe renal colic caused by renal lithiasis. The nurse's first priority in management of the patient is to
   a. administer narcotics as prescribed.
   b. obtain supplies for straining all urine.
   c. encourage fluid intake of 3 to 4 L per day.
   d. keep the patient NPO in preparation for surgery.

7. The nurse recommends genetic counseling for the children of a patient with
   a. nephrotic syndrome.
   b. chronic pyelonephritis.
   c. malignant nephrosclerosis.
   d. adult-onset polycystic renal disease.

8. The nurse encourages strict diabetic control in the patient prone to diabetic nephropathy knowing that the renal tissue changes that may occur in this condition include
   a. uric acid calculi and nephrolithiasis.
   b. renal sugar-crystal calculi and cysts.
   c. lipid deposits in the glomeruli and nephrons.
   d. thickening of the GBM and glomerulosclerosis.

9. The nurse identifies a risk factor for kidney and bladder cancer in a patient who relates a history of
   a. aspirin use.
   b. tobacco use.
   c. chronic alcohol abuse.
   d. use of artificial sweeteners.

10. In planning nursing interventions to increase bladder control in the patient with urinary incontinence, the nurse includes
    a. restricting fluids to diminish the risk of urinary leakage.
    b. counseling the patient concerning choice of incontinence containment device.
    c. clamping and releasing a catheter to increase bladder tone.
    d. teaching the patient biofeedback mechanisms to suppress the urge to void.

11. A patient with a ureterolithotomy returns from surgery with a nephrostomy tube in place. Postoperative nursing care of the patient includes
    a. encouraging the patient to drink fruit juices and milk.
    b. forcing fluids of at least 2 to 3 L per day after nausea has subsided.
    c. notifying the physician if nephrostomy tube drainage is more than 30 ml per hour.
    d. irrigating the nephrostomy tube with 10 ml of normal saline solution as needed.

12. A patient has had a cystectomy and ileal conduit diversion performed. Four days postoperatively, mucous shreds are seen in the drainage bag. The nurse should
    a. notify the physician.
    b. notify the charge nurse.
    c. irrigate the drainage tube.
    d. chart it as a normal observation.

REFERENCES

1. Moore KN, Day RA, Albers M: Pathogenesis of urinary tract infections, *J Clin Nurs* 11:568, 2002.
2. Warren JW: Practice guidelines for the treatment of uncomplicated cystitis, *Curr Urol Rep* 2:326, 2001.
3. Bjerklund Johansen TE: Diagnosis and imaging in urinary tract infections, *Curr Opin Urol* 12:39, 2002.
4. Bostwick JM: The many faces of confusion: timing and collateral history often hold the key to diagnosis, *Postgrad Med* 108:60, 2000.
5. Graham JC, Galloway A: ACP best practice no 167: the laboratory diagnosis of urinary tract infection, *J Clin Pathol* 54:911, 2001.

6. Gupta K, Hooton TM, Stamm WE: Increasing antimicrobial resistance and the management of uncomplicated community-acquired urinary tract infections, *Ann Intern Med* 135:41, 2001.

7. Nicolle LE: A practical guide to antimicrobial management of complicated urinary tract infection, *Drugs Aging* 18:243, 2001.

8. Schaeffer AJ: Urinary tract infections: antimicrobial resistance, *Curr Opin Urol* 10:23, 2000.

9. Kontiokari T et al: Randomized trial of cranberry-lingonberry juice and Lactobacillus GG drink for the prevention of urinary tract infections in women, *BMJ* 322:1571, 2001.

10. Kincaid-Smith P: Acute pyelonephritis. In Brumfitt W, Hamilton-Miller JMT, Bailey RR, editors: *Urinary tract infection,* London, 1998, Chapman & Hall Medical.

11. Roberts JA: Management of pyelonephritis and upper urinary tract infections, *Urol Clin North Am* 26:753, 1999.

12. Nickel JC: The management of acute pyelonephritis in adults, *Can J Urol* 8(suppl 1):29, 2001.

13. Roberts JA: Management of pyelonephritis and upper urinary tract infections, *Urol Clin North Am* 26:753, 1999.

14. Nickel P, Naher H: Nongonococcal urethritis, *Curr Probl Dermatol* 24:97, 1996.

15. Gray M, Albo M, Hufstuttler S: Interstitial cystitis: a guide to recognition, evaluation and management for nurse practitioners, *J Wound Ostomy Continence Nurs* 29:93, 2002.

16. Eastwood JB, Corbishley CM, Grange JM: Tuberculosis and the kidney, *J Am Soc Nephro* 12:1307, 2001.

17. Watanabe T, Yoshizawa N: Recurrence of acute poststreptococcal glomerulonephritis, *Pediatr Nephrol* 16:598, 2001.

18. Turner AN: Goodpasture's disease, *Nephrol Dial Transplant* 16(suppl 6):52, 2001.

19. Salama AD et al: Goodpasture's disease, *Lancet* 358:917, 2001.

20. Schwarz A: New aspects of the treatment of nephrotic syndrome, *J Am Soc Nephrol* 12(suppl 17):S44, 2001.

21. Bushinsky DA. Kidney stones, *Adv Intern Med* 47:219, 2001.

22. Morton AR, Iliescu EA, Wilson JW: Nephrology: investigation and treatment of recurrent kidney stones, *CMAJ* 166:213, 2002.

23. Wilkinson H: Clinical investigation and management of patients with renal stones, *Ann Clin Biochem* 38:180, 2001.

24. Lindbloom EJ: What is the best test to diagnose urinary tract stones? *J Fam Pract* 50:657, 2001.

25. Blair B, Fabrizio M: Pharmacology for renal calculi, *Expert Opin Pharmacother* 1:435, 2000.

26. Painter D, Keeley FX: New concepts in the treatment of ureteral calculi, *Curr Opin Urol* 11:373, 2001.

27. Colussi G, et al: Medical prevention and treatment of urinary stones, *J Nephrol* 13(suppl 3):S65, 2000.

28. Jenkins AD: Calculus formation. In Gillenwater JY et al, editors: *Adult and pediatric urology,* ed 4, Philadelphia, 2002, Lippincott Williams & Wilkins.

29. Pearle MS: Prevention of nephrolithiasis, *Curr Opin Nephrol Hypertens* 10.203, 2001.

30. Clayman RV et al: Endourology of the upper urinary tract: noncalculous applications. In Gillenwater JY et al, editor: *Adult and pediatric urology,* ed 4, Philadelphia, 2002, Lippincott Williams & Wilkins.

31. Andrich DE, Mundy AR: Urethral strictures and their surgical management, *BJU Int* 86:571, 2000.

32. Valchanov K et al: An unusual cause of acute renal failure: urethral stricture in a female, *Nephron* 87:89, 2001.

33. Igarashi P, Somlo S: Genetics and pathogenesis of polycystic kidney disease, *J Am Soc Nephrol* 13:9, 2002.

34. Tachibana M: Alport syndrome, *Adv Otorhinolaryngol* 56:19, 2000.

35. American Cancer Society: *2002 Cancer facts and figures,* Atlanta, Ga, 2002, ACS.

36. Godley P, Kim SW: Renal cell carcinoma, *Curr Opin Oncol* 14:280, 2002.

37. Tian GG, Dawson NA: New agents for the treatment of renal cell carcinoma, *Expert Rev Anticancer Ther* 1:546, 2001.

38. Fishman M, Seigne J: Immunotherapy of metastatic renal cell cancer, *Cancer Control* 9:293, 2002.

39. Sarosdy MF, Machtens S: Advanced bladder cancer: where are we now and where are we going? *World J Urol* 20:143, 2002.

40. Roodhouse A: Management of bladder cancer: a nursing view, *Prof Nurse* 16:987, 2000.

41. Wells M: Meeting the needs of people with urinary incontinence, *Community Nurse* 6:35, 2000.

42. Miller JA: Urinary incontinence: a classification system and treatment protocols for the primary care provider, *J Am Acad Nurse Pract* 12:374, 2000.

43. Gray M: Urinary retention: management in the acute care setting (part 1), *Am J Nurs* 100:40, 2000.

44. Vickerman J: Thorough assessment of functional incontinence, *Nurs Times* 98:58, 2002.

45. Glazener CM, Lapitan MC: Urodynamic investigations for management of urinary incontinence in adults, *Cochrane Database Syst Rev* 3:CD003195, 2002.

46. Jarvis GJ: Surgery for urinary incontinence, *Best Pract Res Clin Obstet Gynecol* 14:315, 2000.

47. Leng WW, McGuire EJ: Reconstructive surgery for urinary incontinence, *Urol Clin North Am* 26:61, 1999.

48. Kershen RT, Atala A: New advances in injectable therapies for the treatment of incontinence and vesicoureteral reflux, *Urol Clin North Am* 26:81, 1999.

49. Gray M: Urinary retention: management in the acute care setting, part 2. *Am J Nurs* 100:36, 2000.

50. De Wachter S, Wyndaele JJ: Does bladder tone influence sensation of filling and electro-sensation in the bladder? A blind controlled study in young healthy volunteers using bethanechol, *J Urol* 165:802, 2001.

51. Hollander JB, Biokno AC: Clean intermittent catheterization: an update, *Infect Urol* 9:118, 1996.

52. Turner WH, Studer UE: Cystectomy and urinary diversion, *Semin Surg Oncol* 13:350, 1997.

53. Montie JE, Park JM: Orthotopic diversion in women, *Semin Urol Oncol* 15:184, 1997.

RESOURCES

American Urological Association
1120 North Charles Street
Baltimore, MD 21201
410-727-1100
Fax: 410-223-4370
www.auanet.org

Bladder Health Council
American Foundation for Urologic Disease
1128 North Charles Street
Baltimore, MD 21201
800-242-2383 or 410-727-2908
www.afud.org/education/bladder.html

National Association for Continence (NAFC)
PO Box 8310
Spartanburg, SC 29305-8310
800-BLADDER (252-3337) or 864-579-7900
Fax: 864-579-7902
www.nafc.org

Society of Urological Nurses and Associates
East Holly Avenue, Box 56
Pitman, NJ 08071-0056
888-TAP-SUNY or 856-256-2335
Fax: 856-589-7463
www.suna.org

United Ostomy Association
19772 MacArthur Boulevard, Suite 200
Irvine, CA 92612-2405
800-826-0826
www.uoa.org

Wound, Ostomy and Continence Nurses Society
4700 West Lake Avenue
Glenview, IL 60025
888-224-WOCN or 866-615-8560
Fax: 866-615-8560
www.wocn.org

Also see Resources for Chapter 45 on page 1246.

For additional Internet resources, see the website for this book at
http://evolve.elsevier.com/Lewis/medsurg.

CHAPTER 45

NURSING MANAGEMENT
Acute Renal Failure and Chronic Kidney Disease

Mary Jo Holechek

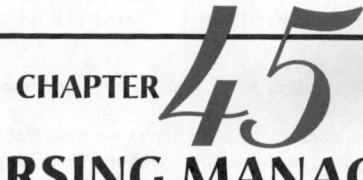

LEARNING OBJECTIVES

1. Differentiate between acute renal failure and chronic kidney disease.
2. Differentiate among the causes of prerenal, intrarenal, and postrenal acute renal failure.
3. Describe the clinical course of reversible acute renal failure.
4. Explain the collaborative care and nursing management of a patient with acute renal failure.
5. Describe the systemic manifestations of chronic kidney disease.
6. Explain the conservative collaborative care and the related nursing management of the patient with chronic kidney disease.
7. Differentiate between peritoneal dialysis and hemodialysis in terms of purpose, indications, advantages and disadvantages, and nursing responsibilities.
8. Describe common vascular access sites used for hemodialysis.
9. Compare dialysis and renal transplantation as methods of treatment for end-stage renal disease.
10. Describe the nursing management of patients in the preoperative, intraoperative, and postoperative stages of kidney transplantation.
11. Discuss the potential long-term problems of the patient with a kidney transplant.

KEY TERMS

acute renal failure, p. 1210	continuous renal replacement therapy, p. 1236
acute tubular necrosis, p. 1211	dialysis, p. 1228
arteriovenous grafts, p. 1232	end-stage renal disease, p. 1217
automated peritoneal dialysis, p. 1230	hemodialysis, p. 1228
azotemia, p. 1210	oliguria, p. 1212
chronic kidney disease, p. 1217	peritoneal dialysis, p. 1228
continuous ambulatory peritoneal dialysis, p. 1230	renal osteodystrophy, p. 1220
	uremia, p. 1210, 1218

Renal failure is the partial or complete impairment of kidney function. There is an inability to excrete metabolic waste products and water, as well as functional disturbances of all body systems. Renal failure is classified as acute or chronic. Acute renal failure (ARF) has a rapid onset. Although ARF is potentially reversible, the mortality rate for intrarenal ARF remains at about 50% despite advances in treatment over the last 30 years.[1]

Chronic kidney disease usually develops slowly over months to years and necessitates the initiation of dialysis or transplantation for long-term survival. The focus in chronic kidney disease has changed from treating a terminally ill patient to caring for a person with a manageable chronic disease that requires long-term care. The change in focus is a result of technical advances, improved surgical techniques, and more effective immunosuppressive therapy.

ACUTE RENAL FAILURE

Acute renal failure (ARF) is a clinical syndrome characterized by a rapid loss of renal function with progressive **azotemia** (an accumulation of nitrogenous waste products such as blood urea nitrogen [BUN]) and increasing levels of serum creatinine.

Uremia is the condition in which renal function declines to the point that symptoms develop in multiple body systems. ARF is often associated with oliguria, which is a decrease in urinary output to less than 400 ml per day. In about 50% of the cases there is normal or increased urinary output. Patients with oliguric ARF have a higher mortality rate.[2]

ARF usually develops over hours or days with progressive elevations of BUN, creatinine, and potassium with or without oliguria. Most commonly, ARF follows severe, prolonged hypotension or hypovolemia or exposure to a nephrotoxic agent.

Etiology and Pathophysiology

The causes of ARF are multiple and complex. They are categorized according to similar pathogenesis into prerenal, intrarenal (or intrinsic), and postrenal causes (Table 45-1).

Prerenal ARF is due to factors external to the kidneys that reduce renal blood flow and lead to decreased glomerular perfusion

CULTURAL & ETHNIC CONSIDERATIONS
Chronic Kidney Disease

- Chronic kidney disease has a disproportionate impact on minority populations, especially African Americans and Native Americans. A history of hypertension and diabetes mellitus is also more common in these high-risk groups.
- The rate of chronic kidney disease is six times higher among Native Americans with diabetes than among other ethnic groups with diabetes.
- The risk of chronic kidney disease as a complication of hypertension is significantly increased in African Americans.
- African Americans live longer and have better outcomes on chronic dialysis than whites.

TABLE 45-1	Common Causes of Acute Renal Failure	
PRERENAL	**INTRARENAL**	**POSTRENAL**

• Hypovolemia
  Dehydration
  Hemorrhage
  GI losses (diarrhea, vomiting)
  Excessive diuresis
  Hypoalbuminemia
  Burns
• Decreased cardiac output
  Cardiac arrhythmias
  Cardiogenic shock
  Congestive heart failure
  Myocardial infarction
  Pericardial tamponade
  Pulmonary edema
  Valvular heart disease
• Decreased peripheral vascular resistance
  Anaphylaxis
  Antihypertensive drugs
  Neurologic injury
  Septic shock
• Decreased renovascular blood flow
  Bilateral renal vein thrombosis
  Embolism
  Hepatorenal syndrome
  Renal artery thrombosis
	• Prolonged prerenal ischemia
	• Nephrotoxic injury
	  Drugs (aminoglycosides [gentamicin, amikacin], amphotericin B)
	  Radiocontrast agents
	  Hemolytic blood transfusion reaction
	  Severe crush injury
	  Chemical exposure (ethylene glycol, lead, arsenic, carbon tetrachloride)
	• Acute glomerulonephritis
	• Thrombotic disorders
	• Toxemia of pregnancy
	• Malignant hypertension
	• Systemic lupus erythematosus
	• Interstitial nephritis
	  Allergies (antibiotics [sulfonamides, rifampin], nonsteroidal antiinflammatory drugs, ACE inhibitors)
	  Infections (bacterial [acute pyelonephritis], viral [CMV], fungal [candidiasis])
		• Benign prostatic hyperplasia
		• Bladder cancer
		• Calculi formation
		• Neuromuscular disorders
		• Prostate cancer
		• Spinal cord disease
		• Strictures
		• Trauma (back, pelvis, perineum)

ACE, Angiotensin-converting enzyme; CMV, cytomegalovirus; GI, gastrointestinal.

and filtration. Hypovolemia, decreased cardiac output, decreased peripheral vascular resistance, and vascular obstruction all can decrease the effective circulating volume of the blood. Prerenal ARF can lead to intrarenal disease if renal ischemia is prolonged. Prerenal causes account for approximately 55% to 60% of all cases of ARF.[1]

Intrarenal causes include conditions that cause direct damage to the renal tissue (parenchyma), resulting in impaired nephron function. Intrarenal causes account for approximately 35% to 40% of all cases of ARF.[1] Intrarenal ARF is usually due to prolonged ischemia, nephrotoxins (e.g., aminoglycoside antibiotics, contrast media), hemoglobin released from hemolyzed red blood cells (RBCs), or myoglobin released from necrotic muscle cells. Nephrotoxins can cause obstruction of intrarenal structures by crystallization or actual damage to the epithelial cells of the tubules. Hemoglobin and myoglobin block the tubules and cause renal vasoconstriction. Primary renal diseases such as acute glomerulonephritis and systemic lupus erythematosus may also cause ARF.

Acute tubular necrosis (ATN) is a type of intrarenal ARF caused by ischemia, nephrotoxins, or pigments.[3] Ischemic and nephrotoxic ATN are responsible for 90% of intrarenal ARF cases.[1]

Postrenal causes involve mechanical obstruction of urinary outflow. As the flow of urine is obstructed, urine refluxes into the renal pelvis, impairing kidney function. The most common causes are benign prostatic hyperplasia, prostate cancer, calculi, trauma, and extrarenal tumors. Postrenal causes of ARF account for less than 5% of the cases.[3] Postrenal ARF is almost always treatable if identified before permanent kidney damage occurs.

The two most common causes of ARF are prolonged renal ischemia and nephrotoxic injury, which lead to ATN (Fig. 45-1). Severe renal ischemia causes a disruption in the basement membrane and patchy destruction of the tubular epithelium. Nephrotoxic agents cause necrosis of tubular epithelial cells, which slough off and plug the tubules. Nephrotoxic injury usually leaves the basement membrane intact. ATN is potentially reversible if the basement membrane is not destroyed and the tubular epithelium regenerates.

Possible pathologic processes involved in ATN include the following.

1. Hypovolemia and decreased renal blood flow stimulate renin release, which activates the renin-angiotensin-aldosterone system (see Fig. 43-4) and results in constriction of the peripheral arteries and the renal afferent arterioles. With decreased renal blood flow, there is decreased glomerular capillary pressure and glomerular filtration rate (GFR), as well as tubular dysfunction and, ultimately, oliguria.

2. Ischemia alters glomerular epithelial cells and decreases glomerular capillary permeability. This reduces the GFR, which significantly reduces blood flow and leads to tubular dysfunction.

3. When tubules are damaged, interstitial edema occurs, and necrotic epithelial cells accumulate in the tubules. The debris lowers the GFR by obstructing the tubules and increasing intratubular pressure.

4. Glomerular filtrate leaks back into plasma through holes in the damaged tubular membranes, which decreases intratubular fluid flow.

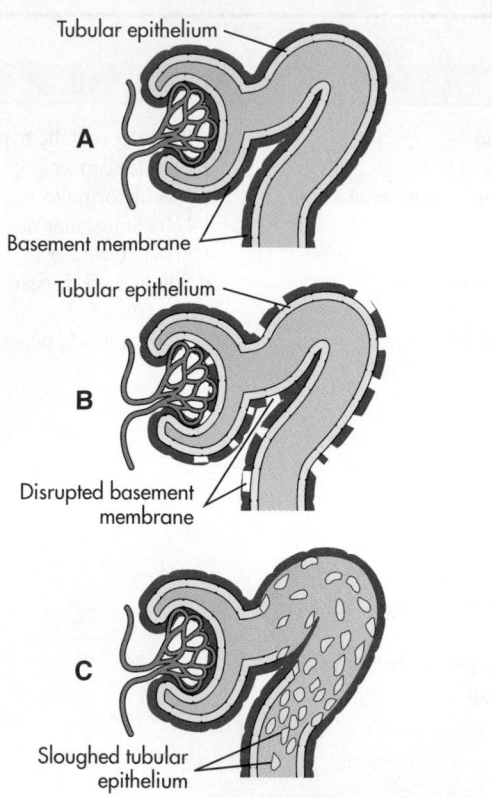

FIG. 45-1 Nephron destruction in acute renal failure. **A,** Normal nephron. **B,** Damage from renal ischemia results in patchy necrosis of the tubule. The lumen may also be blocked by casts. **C,** Damage from nephrotoxic agents.

Clinical Course

Prerenal and postrenal ARF resolve quickly with correction of the cause, but intrarenal disease with ATN has a prolonged course of recovery because actual parenchymal damage has occurred. Clinically, ARF may progress through four phases: initiating, oliguric, diuretic, and recovery. In some situations, the patient does not recover from ARF, and chronic kidney disease results.

Initiating Phase. This begins at the time of the insult and continues until the signs and symptoms become apparent. It can last hours to days.

Oliguric Phase. The most common initial manifestation of ARF is oliguria caused by a reduction in the GFR. **Oliguria** (<400 ml of urine in 24 hours) usually occurs within 1 to 7 days of the causative event. If the cause is ischemia, oliguria may occur within 24 hours. When nephrotoxic drugs are involved, the onset may be delayed for as long as a week. About 50% of the patients will not demonstrate oliguria, making the initial diagnosis more difficult.[3] The duration of the oliguric phase lasts on average about 10 to 14 days but can last months in some cases. The longer the oliguric phase lasts, the poorer the prognosis for recovery of complete renal function.

It is important to distinguish prerenal oliguria from the oliguria of intrarenal ARF. In prerenal oliguria there is no damage to the renal tissue. The oliguria is caused by a decrease in circulating blood volume (e.g., as a result of severe dehydration, decreased cardiac output, burns) and is usually reversible. With a decrease in circulating blood volume, autoregulatory mechanisms that increase angiotensin II, aldosterone, norepinephrine,

and antidiuretic hormone attempt to preserve blood flow to essential organs. Vasoconstriction occurs along with sodium and water retention. Prerenal oliguria is characterized by urine with a high specific gravity (>1.015) and a low sodium concentration (<10 to 20 mEq/L [10 to 20 mmol/L]).

In contrast, oliguria of intrarenal failure is characterized by urine with a normal specific gravity (1.010) and a high sodium concentration (>40 mEq/L [>40 mmol/L]), indicating that the injured tubules cannot respond to autoregulatory mechanisms. In addition, the oliguria of intrarenal failure caused by ATN from ischemia or toxins is characterized by the presence of tubular, RBC, and white blood cell (WBC) casts in the urine. The casts are formed from mucoprotein impressions of the necrotic renal tubular epithelial cells, which detach or slough into the tubules.

The manifestations of the oliguric phase are changes in urinary output, fluid and electrolyte abnormalities, and uremia. The nurse must be alert for the signs and symptoms of these changes.

Urinary changes. Urinary output decreases to less than 400 ml per 24 hours for about 50% of the patients. A urinalysis may show casts, RBCs, WBCs, a specific gravity fixed at around 1.010, and urine osmolality at about 300 mOsm/kg (300 mmol/kg). This is the same specific gravity and osmolality as for plasma, reflecting tubular damage with a loss of concentrating ability by the kidney. Proteinuria may be present if the renal failure is related to glomerular membrane dysfunction.

Fluid volume excess. When urinary output decreases, fluid retention occurs. The severity of the symptoms depends on the extent of the fluid overload. The neck veins may become distended with a bounding pulse. Edema and hypertension may develop. Fluid overload can eventually lead to congestive heart failure (CHF), pulmonary edema, and pericardial and pleural effusions.

Metabolic acidosis. In renal failure, the kidneys cannot synthesize ammonia, which is needed for hydrogen ion excretion, or excrete acid products of metabolism. The serum bicarbonate level decreases because bicarbonate is used up in buffering hydrogen ions. In addition, defective reabsorption and regeneration of bicarbonate occurs. The patient may develop Kussmaul respirations (rapid, deep respirations) to increase the excretion of carbon dioxide. Lethargy and stupor will occur if treatment is not started.

Sodium balance. Damaged tubules cannot conserve sodium. Consequently, the urinary excretion of sodium may increase, resulting in normal or below normal levels of serum sodium. Excessive intake of sodium should be avoided because it can lead to volume expansion, hypertension, and CHF. Uncontrolled hyponatremia or water excess can lead to cerebral edema.

Potassium excess. The serum potassium levels increase because the normal ability of the kidneys to excrete 80% to 90% of the body's potassium is impaired. If the ARF is caused by massive tissue trauma, the damaged cells release additional potassium into the extracellular fluid. Bleeding and blood transfusions cause cellular destruction, releasing more potassium into the extracellular fluid. Acidosis worsens hyperkalemia as hydrogen ions enter the cells and potassium is driven out of the cells into the extracellular fluid.

When potassium levels exceed 6 mEq/L (6 mmol/L) or arrhythmias are identified, treatment must be initiated immediately. Before clinical signs of hyperkalemia are apparent, the electrocardiogram (ECG) will show tall, peaked T waves; widening of the QRS complex; and ST depression. Progressive changes in the ECG, which are related to increasing potassium levels, are depicted in Fig. 16-14. The cardiac muscle is very intolerant of acute increases in potassium.

Hematologic disorders. Several hematologic disorders are seen in ARF. Anemia occurs because renal failure results in impaired erythropoietin production. The anemia may be compounded by platelet abnormalities that can lead to bleeding from multiple sources (intestines, brain). WBCs are also altered, causing immunodeficiency. This leaves the patient susceptible to numerous systemic and local infections. Infection is the major cause of death in ARF.[1]

Calcium deficit and phosphate excess. A low serum calcium level results from decreased gastrointestinal (GI) absorption of calcium. To absorb calcium from the GI tract, activated vitamin D must be present. Only functioning kidneys can activate vitamin D, allowing absorption to occur. When hypocalcemia occurs, the parathyroid gland secretes parathyroid hormone (PTH), which stimulates bone demineralization, thereby releasing calcium from the bones. Phosphate is released as well, worsening the hyperphosphatemia. Elevated serum phosphate levels are also a result of its decreased excretion by the kidneys. Normally plasma calcium is found ionized or free (physiologically active form) or bound to protein. In renal failure it is unusual for hypocalcemia to be symptomatic. The reason for this is that in the acidotic state associated with renal failure, more calcium is in the ionized form rather than bound to protein. However, a low ionized calcium level can lead to tetany.

Waste product accumulation. The kidneys are the primary excretory organs for urea, an end product of protein metabolism, and creatinine, an end product of endogenous muscle metabolism. The BUN and serum creatinine levels are elevated in kidney failure. An elevated BUN level must be interpreted with caution because dehydration, corticosteroids, and catabolism resulting from infections, fever, severe injury, or GI bleeding can also elevate BUN. The best serum indicator of renal failure is creatinine because it is not significantly altered by other factors. Measuring creatinine clearance with a 24-hour urine study or using radioactive tracer is the best method for assessing renal function. But clinically, serum creatinine is most commonly used.

Neurologic disorders. Neurologic changes can occur as the nitrogenous waste products accumulate in the brain and other nervous tissue. The symptoms can be as mild as fatigue and difficulty concentrating and escalate to seizures, stupor, and coma.

Eventually all body systems become involved in the acute uremic syndrome (Table 45-2). The extrarenal manifestations are generally similar to those found in the patient with chronic uremia (see Fig. 45-3 later in this chapter).

Diuretic Phase. The diuretic phase begins with a gradual increase in daily urine output to 1 to 3 L per day, but it may reach 3 to 5 L or more per day. Although urine output is increasing, the nephrons are still not fully functional. The high urine volume is caused by osmotic diuresis from the high urea concentration in the glomerular filtrate and the inability of the tubules to concentrate the urine. In this phase the kidneys have recovered their ability to excrete wastes, but not to concentrate the urine. Hypovolemia and hypotension can occur from massive fluid losses.

At this stage the uremia may still be severe, as reflected by low creatinine clearances, elevated serum creatinine and BUN levels, and persistent signs and symptoms. Because of the large losses of fluid and electrolytes, the patient must be monitored for hyponatremia, hypokalemia, and dehydration. The diuretic phase may last 1 to 3 weeks. Near the end of this phase the patient's

TABLE 45-2	Manifestations of Acute Renal Failure
BODY SYSTEM	**CLINICAL MANIFESTATIONS**
Urinary	↓ Urinary output
	Proteinuria
	Casts
	↓ Specific gravity
	↓ Osmolality
	↑ Urinary sodium
Cardiovascular	Volume overload
	Congestive heart failure
	Hypotension (early)
	Hypertension (after development of fluid overload)
	Pericarditis
	Pericardial effusion
	Arrhythmias
Respiratory	Pulmonary edema
	Kussmaul respirations
	Pleural effusions
Gastrointestinal	Nausea and vomiting
	Anorexia
	Stomatitis
	Bleeding
	Diarrhea
	Constipation
Hematologic	Anemia (development within 48 hr)
	↑ Susceptibility to infection
	Leukocytosis
	Defect in platelet functioning
Neurologic	Lethargy
	Seizures
	Asterixis
	Memory impairment
Metabolic	↑ BUN
	↑ Creatinine
	↓ Sodium
	↑ Potassium
	↓ pH
	↓ Bicarbonate
	↓ Calcium
	↑ Phosphate

BUN, Blood urea nitrogen.

acid base, electrolyte, and waste product (BUN, creatinine) values begin to normalize.

Recovery Phase. The recovery phase begins when the GFR increases, allowing the BUN and serum creatinine levels to plateau and then decrease. Although the major improvements occur in the first 1 to 2 weeks of this phase, renal function may take up to 12 months to stabilize.

The outcome of ARF is influenced by the patient's overall health, the severity of renal failure, and the number and type of complications. Some individuals do not recover and progress to chronic kidney disease. The older adult patient is less likely to recover full kidney function than the younger patient. Among the individuals who recover, the majority achieves clinically normal kidney function with no complications (e.g., hypertension).

Diagnostic Studies. A thorough history is essential for diagnosing the etiology of ARF. Prerenal causes should be considered when there is a history of dehydration, blood loss, or severe heart disease. Intrarenal causes may be suspected if the patient has been taking potentially nephrotoxic drugs or has a recent history of prolonged hypotension or hypovolemia. Postrenal ARF is suggested by a history of changes in urinary stream, stones, benign prostatic hyperplasia, or cancer of the bladder or prostate.

Urinalysis is an important diagnostic test. Urine sediment containing abundant cells, casts, or proteins suggests intrarenal disorders. The urine osmolality, sodium content, and specific gravity help to differentiate the three different types of ARF. Urine sediment may be normal in both prerenal and postrenal ARF. Hematuria, pyuria, and crystals may be seen with postrenal ARF.

To establish a diagnosis of ARF, other testing may be required. A renal ultrasound is often the first test done and provides information about anatomy and function. A renal scan can assess renal blood flow and the integrity of the collecting system. A computed tomography (CT) scan and magnetic resonance imaging can identify masses, collections, and vascular anomalies.

Collaborative Care

Because ARF is potentially reversible, the primary goals of treatment are to eliminate the cause, manage the signs and symptoms, and prevent complications while the kidneys recover (Table 45-3). The first step is to determine if there is adequate intravascular volume and cardiac output to ensure adequate perfusion of the kidneys. Diuretic therapy is often administered along with volume expanders to prevent fluid overload. Diuretic therapy usually includes loop diuretics (e.g., furosemide [Lasix]), bumetanide [Bumex]), or an osmotic diuretic (e.g., mannitol). If ARF is already established, forcing fluids and diuretics will not be effective and may, in fact, be harmful. Conservative therapy may be all that is necessary until renal function improves. The general trend is to initiate early and frequent dialysis to minimize symptoms and prevent complications.

Fluid intake must be closely monitored during the oliguric phase. The general rule for calculating the fluid restriction is to add all losses for the previous 24 hours (e.g., urine, diarrhea, emesis, blood) plus 600 ml for insensible losses (e.g., respiration, diaphoresis). For example, if a patient excreted 300 ml of urine on Tuesday with no other losses, the fluid restriction on Wednesday would be 900 ml.

Hyperkalemia is one of the most serious complications in ARF because it can cause life-threatening cardiac arrhythmias. The various therapies used to treat elevated potassium levels are listed in Table 45-4. Both insulin and sodium bicarbonate temporarily shift potassium into the cells, but it will eventually shift back out. Calcium gluconate raises the threshold at which arrhythmias will occur. Only sodium polystyrene sulfonate (Kayexalate) and dialysis actually remove potassium from the body. Sodium polystyrene sulfonate should never be given to a patient with a paralytic ileus because bowel necrosis can occur.

TABLE 45-3   Collaborative Care
Acute Renal Failure

Diagnostic
History and physical examination
Identification of precipitating cause
Serum creatinine and BUN levels
Serum electrolytes
Urinalysis
Renal ultrasound
Renal scan (as indicated)
CT scan or MRI (as indicated)
Retrograde pyelogram (as indicated)

Collaborative Therapy
Treatment of precipitating cause
Fluid restriction (600 ml plus previous 24-hour fluid loss)
Nutritional therapy
- Adequate protein intake (0.6 to 2 g/kg per day) depending on degree of catabolism
- Potassium restriction
- Phosphate restriction
- Sodium restriction
Measures to lower potassium (if elevated)*
Calcium supplements or phosphate-binding agents
Total parenteral nutrition (if indicated)†
Enteral nutrition (if indicated)†
Initiation of dialysis (if necessary)
Continuous renal replacement therapy (if necessary)

BUN, Blood urea nitrogen; *CT*, computed tomography; *MRI*, magnetic resonance imaging.
*See Table 45-4.
†Renal formulations of these two forms of nutrition are available.

TABLE 45-4   Therapies to Treat Elevated Potassium Levels

1. **Regular Insulin Administration IV**
   Potassium moves into cells when insulin is given. Glucose is given concurrently to prevent hypoglycemia. When effects of insulin diminish, potassium shifts back out of cells.

2. **Sodium Bicarbonate**
   Therapy can correct acidosis and causes shift of potassium into cells.

3. **Calcium Gluconate IV**
   Therapy is given IV and generally used in advanced cardiac toxicity. Calcium raises the threshold for excitation, resulting in arrhythmias.

4. **Dialysis**
   Hemodialysis can bring potassium levels to normal within 30 min to 2 hr.

5. **Sodium Polystyrene Sulfonate (Kayexalate)**
   Cation-exchange resin is administered by mouth or retention enema. When resin is in the bowel, potassium is exchanged for sodium. Therapy removes 1 mEq of potassium per gram of drug. It is mixed in water with sorbitol to produce osmotic diarrhea, allowing for evacuation of potassium-rich stool from body.

6. **Dietary Restriction**
   Daily potassium intake is limited to 40 mEq.

IV, Intravenous.

The most common indications for dialysis in ARF include (1) volume overload, resulting in compromised cardiac and/or pulmonary status; (2) elevated potassium level with ECG changes; (3) metabolic acidosis (serum bicarbonate level less than 15 mEq/L [15 mmol/L]); (4) BUN level greater than 120 mg/dl (43 mmol/L); (5) significant change in mental status; and (6) pericarditis, pericardial effusion, or cardiac tamponade. Laboratory values are only rough parameters, and clinical assessment is the most important guide in determining the need for dialysis.

If dialysis is required, two options are available: hemodialysis (HD) and peritoneal dialysis (PD). HD is the method of choice when rapid changes are required in a short time. It is technically more complicated because specialized staff and equipment and vascular access are required. Anticoagulation therapy may be necessary to prevent blood clotting when blood contacts the foreign membrane material in the dialysis blood circuit. Rapid fluid shifts during HD may cause hypotension. HD is preferred for the hypercatabolic patient and for the individual who has had abdominal or thoracic trauma or surgery. PD is much simpler than HD, but it carries the risk of peritonitis, is less efficient in the catabolic patient, and requires longer treatment times. PD may be preferred for the individual with intracranial bleeding or cardiovascular instability. (HD and PD are discussed later in this chapter.)

Continuous renal replacement therapy (CRRT) may also be used in the treatment of ARF. (CRRT is discussed later in this chapter.) In the hemodynamically unstable patient, CRRT provides gradual removal of excess fluid and solutes. It is technically similar to HD and requires extracorporeal blood circulation via cannulation of two veins or an artery and vein. Blood removed from the artery or vein passes through a hemofilter where solutes and water are removed, and then the blood is returned to the patient. CRRT runs continuously and requires at least 12 to 24 hours to accomplish what can be done with 3 to 4 hours of HD. Larger amounts of fluid may be removed than with intermittent HD. It is the preferred treatment in the hemodynamically unstable patient with mild to moderate ARF with fluid overload.

Nutritional Therapy. The challenge of nutritional management in renal failure is to provide adequate calories to prevent catabolism despite the restrictions required to prevent electrolyte and fluid disorders and azotemia. If the patient does not receive adequate nutrition, catabolism of body protein will occur.[4] This process causes increased urea, phosphate, and potassium levels. Adequate energy should be provided from carbohydrate and fat sources to prevent ketosis from endogenous fat breakdown and gluconeogenesis from muscle protein breakdown.[5] The daily caloric intake should be about 30 to 35 kcal/kg of body weight. Protein intake is generally 1.2 to 1.3 g/kg but can be as high as 2 g/kg if the patient is catabolic.[6] Essential amino acid supplements (e.g., Amin-Aid) can be given for amino acid and caloric supplementation.

Potassium and sodium are regulated in accordance with plasma levels. Sodium is restricted as needed to prevent edema, hypertension, and CHF. Dietary fat intake is increased so that the patient receives at least 30% to 40% of total calories from fat. Fat emulsion IV infusions can also be given as a nutritional supplement and provide a good source of nonprotein calories (see Chapter 39). If a patient cannot maintain adequate oral intake, enteral nutrition is the preferred route for nutritional support (see Chapter 39). When the GI tract is not functional, total parenteral nutrition (TPN) is necessary for the provision of adequate nutrition. The patient treated with TPN may need daily HD or CRRT to remove the excess fluid. Concentrated TPN formulas are available to minimize fluid volume.[7]

NURSING MANAGEMENT
ACUTE RENAL FAILURE

■ Nursing Assessment

An assessment of the patient in ARF includes the specific areas presented in Table 45-2. It is important to monitor the vital signs and intake and output. The urine should be examined for color, specific gravity, glucose, protein, blood, or sediment. The patient's general appearance should be assessed, including skin color, peripheral edema, neck vein distention, and bruises.

If the patient is receiving dialysis, the access site should be observed for signs of inflammation. The patient's mental status and level of consciousness should also be evaluated. The oral mucosa should be examined for dryness and inflammation. The lungs should be auscultated for crackles and rhonchi or diminished breath sounds. The heart should be monitored for the presence of an S_3, other murmurs, or a pericardial friction rub. ECG readings should be assessed for the presence of arrhythmias. Laboratory values and diagnostic test results should be reviewed. All of the previous data are essential for developing a collaborative plan of care.

■ Nursing Diagnoses

Nursing diagnoses and potential complications for the patient with ARF include, but are not limited to, the following:
- Excess fluid volume *related to* renal failure and fluid retention
- Risk for infection *related to* invasive lines, uremic toxins, and altered immune responses secondary to kidney failure
- Imbalanced nutrition: less than body requirements *related to* altered metabolic state and dietary restrictions
- Disturbed thought processes *related to* effects of uremic toxins on central nervous system (CNS)
- Fatigue *related to* anemia, metabolic acidosis, and uremic toxins
- Anxiety *related to* disease process, therapeutic interventions, and uncertainty of prognosis
- Potential complication: arrhythmias *related to* electrolyte imbalances
- Potential complication: metabolic acidosis *related to* inability to excrete H^+, impaired HCO_3^- reabsorption, and decreased synthesis of ammonia

■ Planning

The overall goals are that the patient with ARF will (1) completely recover without any loss of kidney function, (2) be maintained in normal fluid and electrolyte balance, (3) have decreased anxiety, and (4) comply with and understand the need for careful follow-up care.

■ Nursing Implementation

Health Promotion. Prevention of ARF is essential because of the high mortality rate and is primarily directed toward identifying and monitoring high-risk populations, controlling nephrotoxic drugs and industrial chemicals, and preventing prolonged episodes of hypotension and hypovolemia. In the hospital, the factors that increase the risk for developing ARF are advanced age, massive trauma, major surgical procedures, extensive burns, cardiac failure, sepsis, obstetric complications, or baseline renal insufficiency caused by hypertension or diabetes mellitus. Careful monitoring of intake and output and fluid and electrolyte balance is essential. Extrarenal losses of fluid from vomiting, diarrhea, and hemorrhage and increased insensible losses must be assessed and recorded. Prompt replacement of significant fluid losses will help prevent ischemic tubular damage associated with trauma, burns, and extensive surgery. Intake and output records and the patient's weight provide valuable indicators of fluid volume status. Aggressive diuretic therapy for the patient with fluid overload resulting from any cause can lead to inadequate renal vascular perfusion.

Streptococcal infections must be identified and treated with antibiotics. Compliance with the antibiotic regimen is critical to eliminate the source of infection and prevent complications such as acute poststreptococcal glomerulonephritis and rheumatic heart disease.

For the older adult or diabetic patient who is undergoing diagnostic studies requiring intravenous (IV) contrast media, special attention must be given to prevent a nephrotoxic injury secondary to the dye. Adequate hydration before and after the test is critical. Patients with urinary tract infections need prompt treatment and careful follow-up care. Chemotherapeutic drugs that cause hyperuricemia also can put a patient at risk for renal injury.

The individual who is taking drugs that are potentially nephrotoxic (see Table 43-3) must have renal function monitored. Nephrotoxic drugs should be used sparingly in the high-risk patient. When these drugs must be used, they should be given in the smallest effective doses for the shortest possible periods. The patient should be cautioned about the abuse of over-the-counter analgesics (especially nonsteroidal antiinflammatory drugs [NSAIDs]) because some of these may worsen renal function in the patient with borderline renal insufficiency by decreasing glomerular pressure. Angiotensin-converting enzyme (ACE) inhibitors can also decrease perfusion pressure and cause hyperkalemia and are contraindicated in renal insufficiency. Industrial and agricultural chemicals and products (organic solvents, insecticides, cleaning agents) must be monitored regularly to assess their safety for employees and the general population.

Acute Intervention. The patient with ARF is critically ill and suffers not only from the effects of renal disease but also from the effects of comorbid diseases or conditions (e.g., diabetes, cardiovascular disease) that also affect renal function. The nurse must focus on the patient as a total person with many physical and emotional needs. Usually the changes caused by ARF come on suddenly. Both the patient and the family need assistance in understanding that the functioning of the whole body can be disrupted by renal failure but that these changes are generally reversible with time.

The nurse has an important role in managing fluid and electrolyte balance during the oliguric and diuretic phases. Observing and recording accurate intake and output are essential. Daily weights measured with the same scale at the same time each day allow for the evaluation and detection of excessive gains or losses of body fluid (1 kg is equivalent to 1000 ml of fluid). The nurse must be knowledgeable about the common signs and symptoms of hypervolemia (in the oliguric phase) or hypovolemia (in the diuretic phase), potassium and sodium disturbances, and other electrolyte imbalances that may occur in ARF (see Chapter 16). Hyperkalemia is a leading cause of death in the oliguric phase of

ARF. Most typically, hyperkalemia is manifested by arrhythmias and impairment of neuromuscular function including muscle weakness, abdominal cramps, flaccid paralysis, and absence of deep tendon reflexes. Cardiac conduction abnormalities to watch for include a prolonged PR interval, prolonged QRS interval, peaked T wave, and depressed ST segment.

Because infection is the leading cause of death overall in ARF, meticulous aseptic technique is critical. The patient should be protected from other individuals with infectious diseases. The nurse should be alert for local manifestations of infection (e.g., swelling, redness, pain) and systemic manifestations (e.g., malaise, leukocytosis) because an elevated temperature may not be present. Patients with renal failure have a blunted febrile response to an infection (e.g., pneumonia). If antibiotics are used to treat an infection, the type, frequency, and dosage must be carefully considered because the kidneys are the primary route of excretion for many antibiotics. Nephrotoxic drugs (see Table 43-3) should not be used unless there is no other alternative.

Respiratory complications, especially pneumonitis, can be prevented. Humidified oxygen, incentive spirometry; coughing, turning, and deep breathing; and ambulation are measures the nurse can use to help maintain adequate respiratory ventilation.

Skin care and measures to prevent pressure ulcers should be performed because the patient usually develops edema, as well as decreased muscle tone. Mouth care is important to prevent stomatitis, which develops when ammonia (produced by bacterial breakdown of urea) in saliva irritates the mucous membranes.

Ambulatory and Home Care. Recovery from ARF is highly variable and depends on the underlying illness, the general condition and age of the patient, the length of the oliguric phase, and the severity of nephron damage. Good nutrition, rest, and activity are necessary. The diet should be high in calories. Protein and potassium intake should be regulated in accordance with renal function. Follow-up care and regular evaluation of renal function are necessary. The patient should be taught the signs and symptoms of recurrent kidney disease. Measures to prevent the recurrence of ARF must be emphasized.

The long-term convalescence of 3 to 12 months may cause psychosocial and financial hardships for the family, and appropriate counseling and social work and psychiatry referrals should be made as indicated. If the kidneys do not recover, the patient will eventually need dialysis and transplantation.

■ Evaluation

The expected outcomes are that the patient with ARF will
- regain and maintain normal fluid and electrolyte balance
- comply with treatment regimen
- experience no infectious complications
- have complete recovery

■ Gerontologic Considerations: Acute Renal Failure

The older adult is more susceptible than the younger adult to ARF as the number of functioning nephrons decrease with age. Impaired function of other organ systems (e.g., cardiovascular disease, impaired pancreas function) can increase the risk of developing ARF. The aging kidney is less able to compensate for changes in fluid volume, solute load, and cardiac output. Common causes of ARF in the older adult include dehydration, hypotension, diuretic therapy, aminoglycoside therapy, obstructive disorders (e.g., prostatic hyperplasia), surgery, infection, and radiocontrast agents. The prognosis after an episode of ARF is generally worse in the older adult than in the younger person. The mortality rate of ARF is 5% to 25% higher in the older adult than in the younger adult, and death is usually caused by infection, GI hemorrhage, or myocardial infarction.[2] ■

CHRONIC KIDNEY DISEASE

Chronic kidney disease (CKD) involves progressive, irreversible destruction of the nephrons in both kidneys. Among individuals with CKD, the stages are defined based on the level of kidney function (Table 45-5). The last stage of kidney failure **(end-stage renal disease** [ESRD]) occurs when the GFR is less than 15 ml per minute. At this point, renal replacement (dialysis or transplantation) is required. Although there are many different causes of chronic kidney disease (Fig. 45-2), the end result is a systemic disease involving every body organ. (The specific disease processes are discussed in Chapter 44.)

The kidneys have remarkable functional reserve. Up to 80% of the GFR (reflected in creatinine clearance measurements) may be lost with few overt changes in the functioning of the body. A person is born with about 2 million nephrons and can survive without dialysis until almost 90% of the nephrons are lost. In the majority of cases the individual passes through the early stages of CKD without recognizing the disease state because the remaining nephrons hypertrophy to compensate. The prognosis and course of CKD are highly variable depending on the etiology, patient's condition and age, and adequacy of medical follow-up. Some individuals live normal, active lives with compensated renal failure, whereas others may rapidly progress to end-stage renal failure. When the creatinine clearance falls below 15 ml per minute (from the normal range of 85 to 135 ml per minute for the average adult), some form of dialysis or transplantation is required for survival.

In the United States at the end of 2002, over 345,000 individuals with ESRD were being treated for CKD. Of these, more than 245,000 were dialysis patients. and more than 100,000 had a functioning kidney transplant. Over the past 5 years, the number of new patients with kidney failure has averaged about 80,000 annually.

This number of patients with ESRD is expected to reach 660,000 by 2010. Each year about 70,000 people die from causes related to renal failure. At least 40 million Americans are at risk for CKD. In the United States the leading causes of ESRD are diabetes mellitus and hypertension[8] (see Fig. 45-2). In Canada, the primary causes are diabetes mellitus and glomerulonephritis.

In 1973, dramatic legislative changes related to chronic kidney disease occurred when the federal government enacted a law providing financial assistance through Medicare to all eligible persons who had ESRD and required treatment. Under this law, Medicare pays 80% of the cost of health care for ESRD patients who have worked long enough to qualify for benefits.

Since 1973 many deaths have been prevented through the use of maintenance dialysis and renal transplantation. Most patients are treated with dialysis because (1) there is a lack of donated organs, (2) some patients are physically or mentally unsuitable for transplantation, or (3) some patients do not want transplants. With the advancement of medical science, an increasing number of individuals are receiving maintenance dialysis, including the elderly and those with complex medical problems. Every patient with ESRD, regardless of age, should be offered dialysis unless

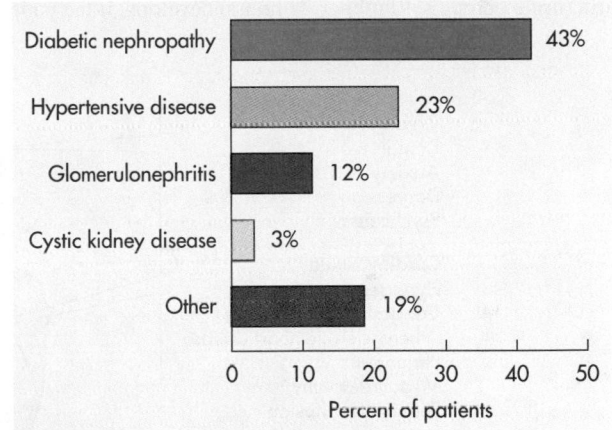

FIG. 45-2 Incidence of primary renal disease leading to end-stage renal disease (United States Renal Data Systems).

TABLE 45-5	**Stages and Descriptions of Chronic Kidney Disease***		
	DESCRIPTION	**GFR (ml/min/1.73 m²)**	**ACTION†**
	At increased risk for CKD	≥90 (with CKD risk factors)	Screening CKD risk reduction
Stage 1	Kidney damage with normal or ↑ GFR	≥90	Diagnosis and treatment Treatment of comorbid conditions CVD risk reduction
Stage 2	Kidney damage with mild ↓ GFR	60-89	Estimation of progression
Stage 3	Moderate ↓ GFR	30-59	Evaluation and treatment of complications
Stage 4	Severe ↓ GFR	15-29	Preparation for renal replacement therapy
Stage 5	Kidney failure	<15 (or dialysis)	Renal replacement (if uremia present)

Source: Kidney/Disease Outcomes Quality Initiative clinical practice guidelines for chronic kidney disease: evaluation, classification, and stratification, National Kidney Foundation.
Stages 1 to 5 identify patients who have chronic kidney disease.
*Chronic kidney disease is defined as either kidney damage or GFR <60 ml/min/1.73 m² for ≥3 months. Kidney damage is defined as pathologic abnormalities or markers of damage, including abnormalities in blood or urine tests or imaging studies.
†Includes actions from preceding stages.
GFR, Glomerular filtration rate; *CKD,* chronic kidney disease; *CVD,* cardiovascular disease.

it is medically contraindicated or the patient refuses treatment. If a patient is not covered by Medicare, a variety of state and private programs are available to provide financial assistance.

Clinical Manifestations

As renal function progressively deteriorates, every body system becomes affected. The clinical manifestations are a result of retained substances, including urea, creatinine, phenols, hormones, electrolytes, water, and many other substances. **Uremia** is a syndrome that incorporates all the signs and symptoms seen in the various systems throughout the body in chronic kidney disease (Fig. 45-3). It is important to recognize that the manifestations of uremia vary among patients, according to the cause of the kidney disease, comorbid conditions, age, and degree of compliance with the prescribed medical regimen. Many patients are very tolerant of the changes that occur because they develop gradually.

Urinary System. In the early stage of renal insufficiency, polyuria results from the inability of the kidneys to concentrate urine. This happens most often at night, and the patient must arise several times to urinate (nocturia). Because of the decrease in renal concentrating ability, the specific gravity of urine gradually becomes fixed at around 1.010 (the osmolar concentration of plasma). As CKD worsens, oliguria develops and eventually anuria (urine output <40 ml per 24 hours) develops. If the patient is still producing urine, proteinuria, casts, pyuria, and hematuria could be present depending on the cause of the kidney disease.

Metabolic Disturbances

Waste product accumulation. As the GFR decreases, the BUN and serum creatinine levels increase. The BUN is increased not only by the kidney failure but also by protein intake, fever, corticosteroids, and catabolism. For this reason, serum creatinine and creatinine clearance determinations are considered more accurate indicators of kidney function than BUN. As the BUN increases, nausea, vomiting, lethargy, fatigue, impaired thought processes, and headaches become common as a result of the presence of waste products in the CNS and GI tissues.

The serum creatinine level in an older adult patient with ESRD will be lower than in a younger person with the same degree of renal dysfunction. Decreased muscle mass and decreased muscle activity from aging account for this finding because creatinine is an end product of muscle metabolism.

Altered carbohydrate metabolism. Defective carbohydrate metabolism is caused by impaired glucose use resulting from cellular insensitivity to the normal action of insulin. The exact nature of this insulin resistance is unclear, but it may be related to circulating insulin antagonists, alterations in hormone receptors, or abnormalities of transport mechanisms. Moderate hyperglycemia, hyperinsulinemia, and abnormal glucose tolerance

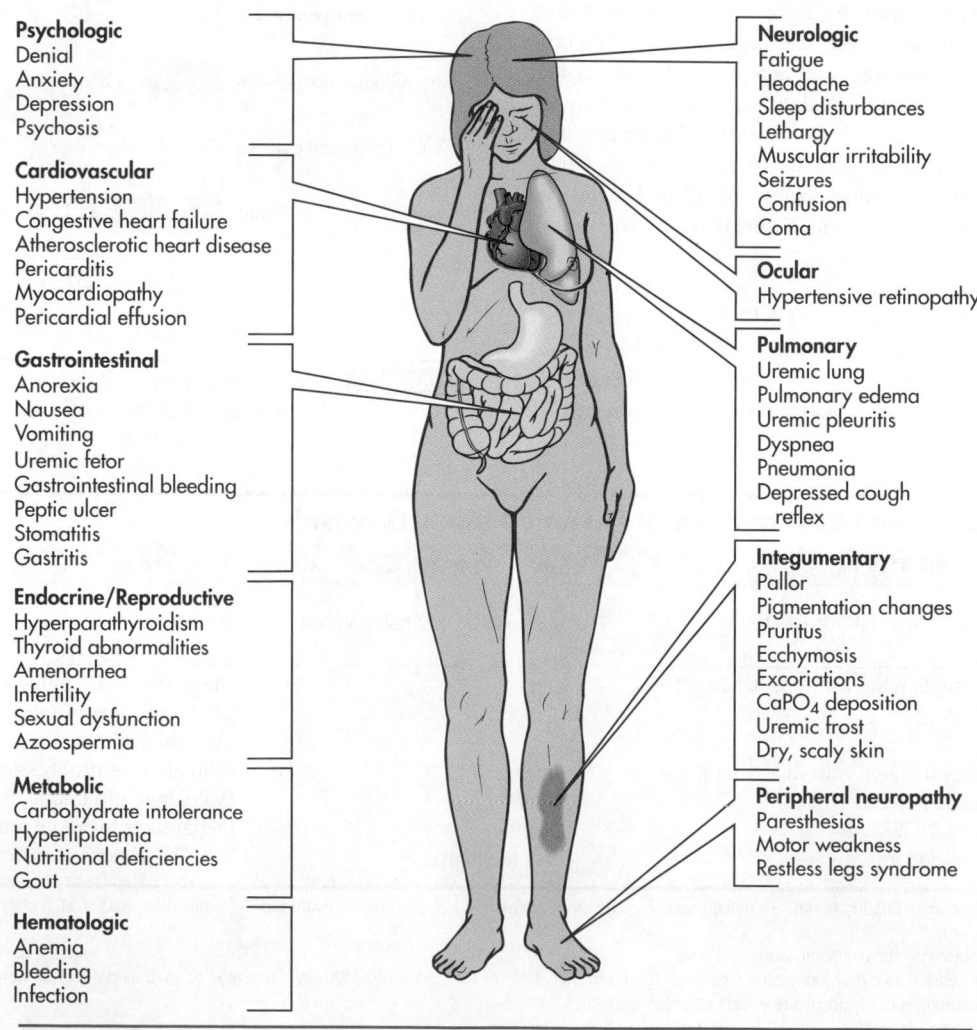

Psychologic
Denial
Anxiety
Depression
Psychosis

Cardiovascular
Hypertension
Congestive heart failure
Atherosclerotic heart disease
Pericarditis
Myocardiopathy
Pericardial effusion

Gastrointestinal
Anorexia
Nausea
Vomiting
Uremic fetor
Gastrointestinal bleeding
Peptic ulcer
Stomatitis
Gastritis

Endocrine/Reproductive
Hyperparathyroidism
Thyroid abnormalities
Amenorrhea
Infertility
Sexual dysfunction
Azoospermia

Metabolic
Carbohydrate intolerance
Hyperlipidemia
Nutritional deficiencies
Gout

Hematologic
Anemia
Bleeding
Infection

Neurologic
Fatigue
Headache
Sleep disturbances
Lethargy
Muscular irritability
Seizures
Confusion
Coma

Ocular
Hypertensive retinopathy

Pulmonary
Uremic lung
Pulmonary edema
Uremic pleuritis
Dyspnea
Pneumonia
Depressed cough
  reflex

Integumentary
Pallor
Pigmentation changes
Pruritus
Ecchymosis
Excoriations
$CaPO_4$ deposition
Uremic frost
Dry, scaly skin

Peripheral neuropathy
Paresthesias
Motor weakness
Restless legs syndrome

FIG. 45-3 Clinical manifestations of chronic uremia.

tests may be seen. Insulin and glucose metabolism may improve (but not to normal values) after the initiation of dialysis.

Diabetics who become uremic may require less insulin than before the onset of chronic kidney disease. This is because insulin, which is dependent on the kidneys for excretion, remains in circulation longer. The insulin dosing must be individualized and glucose levels monitored carefully.

Elevated triglycerides. Hyperinsulinemia stimulates hepatic production of triglycerides. Almost all patients with uremia develop hyperlipidemia, with elevated very-low-density lipoproteins (VLDLs), normal or decreased low-density lipoproteins (LDLs), and lowered high-density lipoproteins (HDLs). The reason for the altered lipid metabolism is related to decreased levels of the enzyme lipoprotein lipase that is important in the breakdown of lipoproteins. Hyperlipidemia is a definite risk factor for accelerated atherosclerosis (see Chapter 33). This can worsen atherosclerotic changes in diabetics with ESRD.

The serum level of triglycerides does not usually decrease after dialysis is started. For patients receiving chronic PD, the level frequently becomes higher as a result of the increased amounts of glucose absorbed from the peritoneal dialysate fluid. Elevated glucose levels lead to increased insulin levels. Insulin stimulates the liver to produce triglycerides.

Electrolyte and Acid-Base Imbalances

Potassium. Hyperkalemia is the most serious electrolyte disorder associated with kidney disease. Fatal arrhythmias can occur when the serum potassium level reaches 7 to 8 mEq/L (7 to 8 mmol/L). Hyperkalemia results from the decreased excretion by the kidneys, the breakdown of cellular protein, bleeding, and metabolic acidosis. Potassium may also come from the food consumed, dietary supplements, drugs, and IV infusions.

Sodium. Sodium may be normal or low in renal failure. Because of impaired sodium excretion, sodium along with water is retained. If large quantities of body water are retained, dilutional hyponatremia occurs. Sodium retention can contribute to edema, hypertension, and congestive heart failure. Sodium intake must be individually determined but is generally restricted to 2 g per 24 hours.

Calcium and phosphate. Calcium and phosphate alterations are discussed in the section on ARF (p. 1213) and in the section on the musculoskeletal system (p. 1220).

Magnesium. Magnesium is primarily excreted by the kidneys. Hypermagnesemia is generally not a problem unless the patient is ingesting magnesium (e.g., milk of magnesia, magnesium citrate, antacids containing magnesium). Clinical manifestations of hypermagnesemia can include absence of reflexes, decreased mental status, cardiac arrhythmias, hypotension, and respiratory failure.

Metabolic acidosis. Metabolic acidosis results from the impaired ability of the kidneys to excrete the acid load (primarily ammonia) and from defective reabsorption and regeneration of bicarbonate. The average adult produces 80 to 90 mEq of acid per day. In renal failure, plasma bicarbonate, which is an indirect measure of acidosis, usually falls to a new steady state at around 16 to 20 mEq/L (16 to 20 mmol/L). It generally does not progress below this level because hydrogen ion production is usually balanced by buffering from demineralization of the bone (the phosphate buffering system). Although Kussmaul respiration is uncommon in CRF, this breathing pattern reduces the severity of acidosis by increasing carbon dioxide excretion.

Hematologic System

Anemia. The anemia associated with CKD is classified as normocytic, normochromic. It is due to decreased production of the hormone erythropoietin by the kidneys, resulting in decreased erythropoiesis by the bone marrow.[9] Erythropoietin stimulates precursor cells in the bone marrow to produce RBCs. Other factors contributing to anemia are nutritional deficiencies, decreased RBC life span, increased hemolysis of RBCs, frequent blood samplings, and bleeding from the GI tract. For patients receiving maintenance HD, blood loss in the dialyzer may also contribute to the anemic state. Elevated levels of PTH (produced to compensate for low serum calcium levels) can inhibit erythropoiesis, shorten survival of RBCs, and cause bone marrow fibrosis, which can result in decreased numbers of hematopoietic cells.

Sufficient iron stores are needed for erythropoiesis. Many patients with renal failure are iron deficient and require iron replacement. Folic acid, which is essential for RBC maturation, is dialyzable. If it is not adequately replaced in the diet or by drugs, megaloblastic anemia may develop in a patient receiving chronic HD.

Bleeding tendencies. The most common cause of bleeding in uremia is a qualitative defect in platelet function. This dysfunction is caused by impaired platelet aggregation and impaired release of platelet factor 3. In addition, alterations in the coagulation system with increased concentrations of both factor VIII and fibrinogen are found in the serum of these patients. The altered platelet function, hemorrhagic tendencies, and GI bleeding can usually be corrected with regular HD or PD.

Infection. Infectious complications are caused by changes in leukocyte function and altered immune response and function. There is a diminished inflammatory response because of an altered chemotactic response by both neutrophils and monocytes. This impairment significantly decreases the accumulation of WBCs at the site of injury or infection. Both cellular and humoral immune responses are suppressed. Characteristic clinical findings include lymphopenia, lymphoid tissue atrophy (especially of the thymus), decreased antibody production, and suppression of the delayed hypersensitivity response. Other factors contributing to the increased risk of infection include malnutrition, hyperglycemia, and external trauma (e.g., catheters, needle insertions into vascular access sites).

Increased incidence of cancer. There is a significant increase in the incidence of neoplasms in the patient with renal failure who has not had a transplant compared with the general population. Lung, breast, uterus, colon, prostate, and skin malignancies are most commonly found.

Cardiovascular System. The most common cardiovascular abnormality is hypertension, which usually exists pre-ESRD and is worsened by sodium retention and increased extracellular fluid volume. In some individuals, increased renin production contributes to the problem (see Fig. 43-4). Hypertension accelerates atherosclerotic vascular disease, produces intrarenal arterial spasm, and eventually leads to left ventricular hypertrophy and congestive heart failure.[10] Hypertension also causes retinopathy, encephalopathy, and nephropathy.

The vascular changes from long-standing hypertension and the accelerated atherosclerosis from elevated triglyceride levels are responsible for many cardiovascular complications (e.g., myocardial infarction, stroke). These are leading causes of death for patients receiving chronic dialysis. Diabetes mellitus is a major risk factor for the development of vascular problems.

CHF from left ventricular hypertrophy can lead to pulmonary edema. Peripheral edema is often present. Cardiac arrhythmias may result from hyperkalemia, hypocalcemia, and decreased coronary artery perfusion.

Uremic pericarditis can develop and occasionally progresses to pericardial effusion and cardiac tamponade. Pericarditis is manifested by a friction rub, chest pain, and low-grade fever.

Respiratory System. Respiratory changes include Kussmaul respiration, dyspnea from fluid overload, pulmonary edema, uremic pleuritis (pleurisy), pleural effusion, and a predisposition to respiratory infections, which may be related to decreased pulmonary macrophage activity. The sputum is thick and tenacious. The cough reflex is depressed. "Uremic lung," or uremic pneumonitis, is typically found in CKD and shows up as interstitial edema on chest x-ray. This condition usually responds to vigorous fluid removal during dialysis treatments.

Gastrointestinal System. Every part of the GI system is affected as a result of inflammation of the mucosa caused by excessive urea. Mucosal ulcerations, found throughout the GI tract, are caused by the increased ammonia produced by bacterial breakdown of urea. Stomatitis with exudates and ulcerations, a metallic taste in the mouth, and *uremic fetor* (a urinous odor of the breath) are commonly found. Anorexia, nausea, and vomiting caused by irritation of the GI tract by waste products contribute to weight loss and malnutrition. Diabetic gastroparesis can compound these problems for patients with diabetes. GI bleeding is also a risk because of irritation of the mucosa by waste products coupled with the platelet defect. Diarrhea may occur because of hyperkalemia and altered calcium metabolism. Constipation may be due to the ingestion of iron salts and/or calcium-containing phosphate binders. Constipation can be made worse by the limited fluid intake and inactivity.

Neurologic System. Neurologic changes are expected as renal failure progresses. They are attributed to increased nitrogenous waste products, electrolyte imbalances, metabolic acidosis, and axonal atrophy and demyelination of nerve fibers.[11] High levels of uremic toxins have been implicated in axonal damage.

In renal failure a general depression of the CNS results in lethargy, apathy, decreased ability to concentrate, fatigue, irritability, and altered mental ability. Seizures and coma may result from a rapidly increasing BUN and hypertensive encephalopathy. Dialysis encephalopathy (dialysis dementia), a progressive neurologic impairment associated with aluminum toxicity, is characterized by speech disturbances, dementia, lack of muscle coordination, and myoclonic seizures. Aluminum toxicity is now uncommon as aluminum-based drugs have been replaced.

Peripheral neuropathy is initially manifested by a slowing of nerve conduction to the extremities. The patient complains of restless legs syndrome and may describe it as "bugs crawling inside the leg." Paresthesias are most often in the feet and legs and may be described by the patient as a burning sensation. Eventually, motor involvement may lead to bilateral foot drop, muscular weakness and atrophy, and loss of deep tendon reflexes. Muscle twitching, jerking, *asterixis* (hand-flapping tremor), and nocturnal leg cramps also occur. In patients with diabetes, uremic neuropathy is compounded by the neuropathy associated with diabetes mellitus.

The treatment for neurologic problems is dialysis or transplantation. Altered mental status is often the signal that dialysis must be initiated. Dialysis should improve the general CNS symptoms and may slow or halt the progression of neuropathies. However, motor neuropathy may not be reversible.

Musculoskeletal System. **Renal osteodystrophy** is a syndrome of skeletal changes found in chronic kidney disease.[12] This syndrome is a result of alterations in calcium and phosphate metabolism (Fig. 45-4). Normally the calcium/phosphate ratio maintains the electrolytes in a soluble state. As the GFR decreases, urinary phosphate excretion is impaired, and the serum phosphate increases.

The kidneys metabolize vitamin D (formed in the skin or ingested) to its active form. The active form of vitamin D is needed for calcium absorption from the GI tract. In renal failure the kidneys fail to activate vitamin D, calcium absorption is impaired, and serum calcium decreases. Low serum calcium stimulates the release of PTH, which causes resorption of calcium and phosphate from the bone. This release increases serum calcium, as well as serum phosphate. The excess phosphate will bind with calcium, leading to the formation of insoluble metastatic calcifications that are deposited throughout the body. Common sites are the blood vessels, joints, lungs, muscles, myocardium, and eyes.[13] "Uremic red eye" is caused by the irritation from deposits in the eye. Metastatic calcifications in the arteries of the fingers and toes may cause gangrene. Intracardiac calcifications can disrupt the conduction system and cause cardiac arrest.

Two types of renal osteodystrophy are associated with ESRD:

1. *Osteomalacia.* This condition results from lack of mineralization of newly formed bone. It can be a result of hypocalcemia. It can also be caused by aluminum accumulation because the primary route for aluminum excretion is through the kidneys. The primary source of aluminum is aluminum-based phosphate binders. Over the past decade, there has been a decreased use of aluminum-based phosphate binders and a concomitant decrease in the incidence of osteomalacia.

2. *Osteitis fibrosa.* This condition results from calcium resorption from the bone and replacement with fibrous tissue. Osteitis fibrosa is primarily a result of markedly elevated levels of PTH that cause bone resorption.

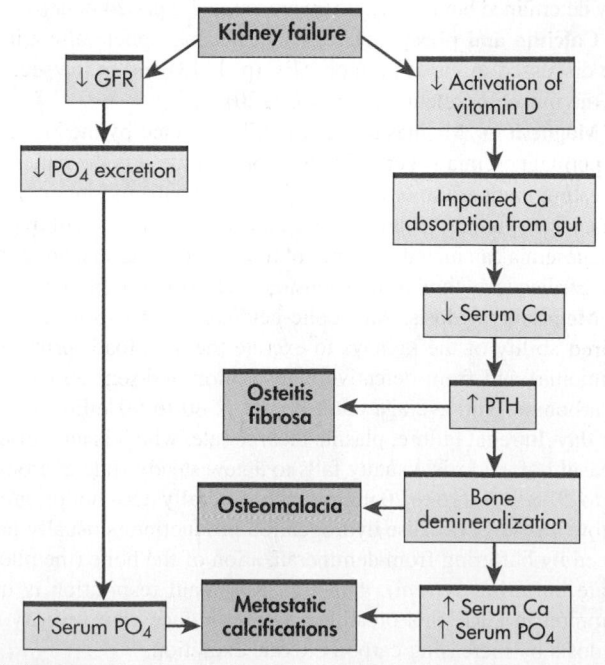

FIG. 45-4 Mechanisms of renal osteodystrophy. *GFR*, Glomerular filtration rate.

Integumentary System. The most noticeable change in the integumentary system is a yellow-gray discoloration of the skin. This change is a result of the absorption and retention of urinary pigments that normally give the characteristic color to urine. The skin also appears pale as a result of anemia and is dry and scaly because of a decrease in oil and sweat gland activity. Decreased perspiration results from a decrease in the size of the sweat glands.

Pruritus most commonly results from a combination of the dry skin, calcium-phosphate deposition in the skin, and sensory neuropathy. The itching may be so intense that it can lead to bleeding or infection secondary to scratching. Uremic frost is a rare condition in which urea crystallizes on the skin and is usually seen only when BUN levels are extremely high. It occurs when a patient refuses dialysis or is withdrawn from dialysis.

The hair is dry and brittle and may fall out. The nails are thin, brittle, and ridged. Petechiae and ecchymoses may be present and are due to platelet abnormalities.

Reproductive System. Both sexes characteristically experience infertility and a decreased libido. Women usually have decreased levels of estrogen, progesterone, and luteinizing hormone, causing anovulation and menstrual changes (usually amenorrhea). Menses and ovulation may return after dialysis is started. Men experience loss of testicular consistency, decreased testosterone levels, and low sperm counts. Sexual dysfunction in both sexes may also be caused by anemia, which causes fatigue and decreased libido. In addition, peripheral neuropathy can cause impotence in men and anorgasmy in women. Additional factors that may cause changes in sexual function are psychologic problems (e.g., anxiety, depression), physical stress, and side effects of drugs.

Sexual function may improve with maintenance dialysis and may become normal with successful transplantation. Pregnant dialysis patients have been able to carry a fetus to term, but there is significant risk to the mother and infant. Pregnancy in transplant patients is more common, but there is also a risk to both the mother and fetus.

Endocrine System. Many patients with chronic kidney disease exhibit some clinical manifestations of hypothyroidism. Tests of thyroid function may yield low to low-normal levels for serum triiodothyronine (T_3) and thyroxine (T_4) levels. Neither the clinical significance nor the exact cause of these findings is known.

Psychologic Changes. Personality and behavioral changes, emotional lability, withdrawal, and depression are commonly observed. Fatigue and lethargy contribute to the feeling of illness. The changes in body image caused by edema, integumentary disturbances, and access devices (e.g., fistulas, catheters) lead to further anxiety and depression. Decreased ability to concentrate and slowed mental activity can give the appearance of dullness and disinterest in the environment. There are also significant changes in lifestyle, occupation, family responsibilities, and financial status that must be dealt with by the patient. Long-term survival depends on drugs, dietary restrictions, dialysis, and possibly transplantation. The patient will also grieve the loss of renal function. This can be a prolonged process for some individuals.

Diagnostic Studies

Adverse outcomes of CKD can often be prevented or delayed through early detection and treatment. Early stages of CKD can be detected through routine laboratory measurements (Table 45-6).

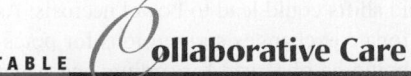

TABLE 45-6 Collaborative Care
Conservative Therapy of Chronic Kidney Disease

Diagnostic
History and physical examination
Identification of reversible renal disease
  Renal ultrasound
  Renal scan
  CT scan
  Renal biopsy
BUN, serum creatinine, and creatinine clearance levels
Serum electrolytes
Protein-to-creatinine ratio in first morning voided specimen
Urinalysis and urine culture
Hematocrit and hemoglobin levels

Collaborative Therapy
Correction of extracellular fluid volume overload or deficit
Nutritional therapy*
Erythropoietin therapy
Calcium supplementation, phosphate binders, or both
Antihypertensive therapy
Measures to lower potassium†
Adjustment of drug dosages to degree of renal function

BUN, Blood urea nitrogen; CT, computed tomography.
*See Tables 45-7 and 45-8.
†See Table 45-4.

Serum creatinine is used to estimate GFR. A protein-to-creatinine ratio or albumin-to-creatinine ratio in a first morning or random urine specimen can be done. A urinalysis can be done to detect RBCs, WBCs, protein, and glucose. Imaging of the kidneys is usually done by ultrasound.

Collaborative Care: Conservative Therapy of Chronic Kidney Disease

When a patient is diagnosed as having CKD, conservative therapy is attempted before maintenance dialysis begins (see Table 45-6). Every effort is made to detect and treat potentially reversible causes of renal failure (e.g., cardiac failure, dehydration, infections, nephrotoxins, urinary tract obstruction, renal artery stenosis). A renal biopsy may be necessary to provide a definitive diagnosis. The goals of conservative therapy are to preserve existing renal function, treat the clinical manifestations, prevent complications, and provide for the patient's comfort. Drug and nutritional therapy and supportive care are essential components of the conservative treatment plan.

Drug Therapy

Hyperkalemia. There are multiple strategies for managing hyperkalemia (see Table 45-4). Every effort is made to control hyperkalemia with the restriction of high-potassium foods and drugs. Acute hyperkalemia may require treatment with IV glucose and insulin or IV 10% calcium gluconate. Sodium polystyrene sulfonate (Kayexalate), a cation-exchange resin, is commonly used to lower potassium levels and can be administered on an outpatient basis. The patient should be told to expect some diarrhea because this preparation contains sorbitol, a bulk laxative that ensures evacuation of the potassium from the bowel. It should never be given to a patient with a hypoactive bowel (paralytic ileus) because fluid shifts could lead to bowel necrosis. As sodium polystyrene sulfonate exchanges sodium ions for potassium ions, the patient should be observed for sodium and water retention. If life-threatening arrhythmias are present, dialysis may be required.

Hypertension. The progression of chronic kidney disease can be delayed by controlling hypertension.[14] Treatment of hypertension initially consists of sodium and fluid restriction and the administration of antihypertensive drugs. The antihypertensive drugs most commonly used are diuretics (e.g., furosemide [Lasix]), β-adrenergic blockers (e.g., metoprolol [Lopressor]), calcium channel blockers (e.g., nifedipine [Procardia], and ACE inhibitors (e.g., captopril [Capoten], enalapril [Vasotec]) (see Chapter 32). Diuretics and β-adrenergic blockers are the recommended initial therapy. β-Adrenergic blockers also decrease the incidence of cardiovascular events and mortality from myocardial infarction.[15] ACE inhibitors decrease proteinuria and delay the progression of renal failure. They must be used cautiously when ESRD occurs because they can further decrease the GFR and increase serum potassium levels.

The BP should periodically be measured in supine, sitting, and standing positions to effectively monitor the effect of antihypertensive drugs. The patient should be taught how to monitor the blood pressure (BP) at home and what BP readings require immediate intervention. BP control is essential to slow atherosclerotic changes that could further impair renal function.

Renal osteodystrophy. Phosphate intake is generally restricted to less than 1000 mg per day, but usually dietary control is not adequate. Calcium-based phosphate binders such as calcium carbonate (e.g., Tums) and calcium acetate (e.g., PhosLo) are used to bind the phosphate, which is then excreted in the stool. Giving a calcium-based binder when the phosphate levels are still high (6 mg/dl [1.98 mmol/L]) may cause the formation of calcium-phosphate deposits. Sevelamer (Renagel) is a new phosphate binder that does not contain either calcium or aluminum. It has the added benefits of lowering cholesterol and LDLs.[16]

Because dementia and bone disease (osteomalacia) are associated with excessive absorption of aluminum, aluminum hydroxide gels or antacids (e.g., Alu-Caps, Amphojel, Basaljel, Alternagel) should not be used to bind phosphate. Magnesium-containing antacids (Maalox, Mylanta) should not be given because magnesium is dependent on the kidneys for excretion. Phosphate binders should be administered with each meal to be effective because most phosphate is absorbed within 1 hour after eating. Hypercalcemia may occur with calcium supplementation and is associated with increased cardiac calcifications and mortality in ESRD patients. Constipation is a frequent side effect of phosphate binders and may necessitate the use of stool softeners.

Hypocalcemia is often a problem because of the inability of the GI tract to absorb calcium in the absence of vitamin D. If hypocalcemia persists in the setting of controlled serum phosphate levels and supplemental calcium, the active form of vitamin D should be given. It is commercially available in oral preparations such as calcitriol (Rocaltrol) and in IV form as calcitriol (Calcijex). Paricalcitol (Zemplar) and doxercalciferol (Hectorol) are new synthetic vitamin D_2 analogs that are designed to reduce PTH levels. They cause less hypercalcemia and hyperphosphatemia than the older analogs.[16] It is important to lower the phosphate level before administering calcium or vitamin D because these drugs may contribute to soft tissue calcification if both calcium and phosphate levels are elevated.

If renal osteodystrophy remains severe despite conservative therapy, a subtotal parathyroidectomy may be performed to decrease the synthesis and secretion of PTH. In some situations a total parathyroidectomy is performed, and some parathyroid tissue is transplanted into the forearm. The transplanted cells produce PTH as needed. If production of PTH becomes excessive, some of the cells can be removed from the forearm using local anesthesia.

The most common methods for evaluating the status of the bone disease are skeletal x-rays, bone scans, bone biopsy, and bone densitometry. PTH and alkaline phosphatase levels should also be measured. Alkaline phosphatase is elevated when there is demineralization of the bone but can also be increased by liver disease.

Anemia. The most important cause of anemia is a decreased production of erythropoietin. With the use of recombinant deoxyribonucleic acid (DNA) technology (see Fig. 13-15), erythropoietin (Epogen, Procrit) is made in large amounts and is available for the treatment of anemia.[9] It can be administered intravenously or subcutaneously. It has been very effective in treating anemia. A significant increase in hematocrit is usually not seen for 2 to 3 weeks. The patient who is receiving erythropoietin has improved cardiac performance and exercise tolerance and an enhanced quality of life. Darbepoetin (Aranesp) is a long-acting form of erythropoietin that is now available.

A common adverse effect of exogenous erythropoietin is the development or acceleration of hypertension. The underlying mechanism is related to the hemodynamic changes (e.g., increased whole blood viscosity) that occur as the anemia is corrected. Another side effect of erythropoietin therapy is the development of functional iron deficiency resulting from the increased demand for iron to support erythropoiesis. Most patients receive oral iron supplements. The GI side effects of iron, including gastric irritation and constipation, may lead to noncompliance. Orally administered iron should not be taken at the same time as phosphate binders because calcium binds the iron. The patient should be advised that iron may make the stool dark in color. Parenteral iron (Venofer, Ferrlecit) is used if iron deficiencies persist in spite of oral iron intake. Supplemental folic acid (1 mg daily) is usually given because it is needed for RBC formation and is removed by dialysis.

Blood transfusions should be avoided in treating anemia unless the patient experiences an acute blood loss or has symptomatic anemia (i.e., dyspnea, excess fatigue, tachycardia, palpitations, chest pain). Undesirable effects of transfusions are the suppression of erythropoiesis as a result of a decrease in the hypoxic stimulus, the possible transmission of hepatitis B or C or human immunodeficiency virus (HIV), and the possibility of iron overload because each unit of blood contains about 250 mg of iron.

Complications of drug therapy. Many drugs are partially or totally excreted by the kidneys. Drug toxicity is a serious problem in the patient with uremia. Delayed and decreased elimination lead to an accumulation of drugs in the body. Drug doses and frequency of administration must be adjusted based on the severity of the kidney disease. Increased sensitivity may result as drug levels increase in the blood and tissues. Drugs of particular concern include digitalis preparations, antibiotics, and pain medication.

Digitalis preparations are excreted largely by the kidneys. Loading doses may not have to be changed, but maintenance doses and frequency may have to be adjusted. Many patients require only 0.125 mg every other day. Dialysis does not affect body levels of digoxin, but it does affect potassium levels. Hypokalemia can potentiate the action of digitalis.

Aminoglycosides (gentamicin, amikacin), penicillin in high doses, and tetracyclines are potentially nephrotoxic and require dose and frequency adjustments. The frequency and dose of vancomycin and gentamicin must be decreased because they are dependent on the kidney for excretion. These drugs can accumulate to toxic levels if appropriate adjustments are not made.

Meperidine (Demerol) should never be administered to a patient with CKD because the liver metabolizes it to normeperidine, which is dependent on the kidneys for excretion. If normeperidine accumulates, seizures can result. Other pain medications may be given, but less frequently and in smaller doses (e.g., oxycodone with acetaminophen, morphine sulfate).

Patients should be advised to avoid NSAIDs. These drugs block the synthesis of the renal prostaglandins that promote vasodilation. This can worsen renal hypoperfusion. Many NSAIDs are available over the counter, so it is essential that the patient be cautioned. Acetaminophen can be substituted.

Nutritional Therapy

Protein restriction. The current diet is designed to be as normal as possible to maintain good nutrition (Table 45-7). Protein is restricted because BUN is an end product of protein metabolism. For the patient who is not undergoing dialysis, one guide is to restrict protein intake to 0.6 to 0.75 g/kg of ideal body weight (IBW) per day when the creatinine clearance is less than 25 ml per minute.[17] Some treatment centers use a routine 40-g protein diet. Because this diet is deficient in vitamins and water-soluble vitamins are lost through dialysis, multivitamins are prescribed.

Protein restriction may reduce the decline of renal function in the patient with chronic renal insufficiency. A low-protein (0.6 to 0.8 g/kg body weight per day), low-phosphorus diet supplemented with amino acids and their ketoanalogues can slow the progression of renal failure.[18] Keto acids of essential amino acids are a dietary supplement. The rationale for using this treatment is that in the body, nonessential amino acids transfer amine groups to the essential keto acids synthesizing essential amino acids. The nitrogen present in nonessential amino acids is used, and the total nitrogen intake is kept to an absolute minimum. Keto acid supplements are available in liquid preparations. Modest protein restriction (0.6 to 0.8 g/kg per day) appears to be a relatively safe therapeutic option for patients with moderate renal insufficiency. For patients with more severe renal insufficiency, low-protein diets should be used with caution because these patients are at risk for developing malnutrition.

Once the patient starts dialysis, protein intake can be increased to 1.2 to 1.3 g/kg of IBW per day. Dietary protein guidelines for PD differ from those for HD because excessive amounts of protein are lost in the dialysate. The protein intake must be high enough to compensate for the losses so that the nitrogen balance is maintained. The recommended protein intake is at least 1.2 g/kg of IBW per day and can be increased depending on the individual needs of the patient. At least 50% of protein intake should have high biologic value containing all of the essential amino acids (e.g., eggs, milk, meat, poultry).

Sufficient calories from carbohydrates and fat are needed to minimize catabolism of body protein and to maintain body weight. Therefore 100 g of carbohydrates and an appropriate amount of fat are prescribed to maintain an intake of 30 to 35 kcal/kg body weight per day. See Table 45-7 for specific guidelines.

For patients with malnutrition or inadequate caloric intake, commercially prepared products that are high in calories and low in protein, sodium, and potassium are available. Liquid and powder preparations include Nepro, Microlipid, SumaCal, Suplena, and Polycose. Products containing only the essential amino acids (Amin-Aid) can also be used as dietary supplements.

Water restriction. Water intake depends on the daily urine output. Generally, 600 ml (from insensible loss) plus an amount equal to the previous day's urine output is allowed for a patient with chronic kidney disease who is not receiving dialysis. Foods that are liquid at room temperature (e.g., gelatin, ice cream) should be counted as fluid intake. The fluid allotment should be

TABLE 45-7   **Nutritional Therapy**

Daily Requirements for the Patient with Chronic Kidney Disease

	CONSERVATIVE MANAGEMENT	HEMODIALYSIS	PERITONEAL DIALYSIS
Fluid allowance	Urine output plus 600 ml	Urine output plus 600 ml	Often no restriction
Protein*	0.6-0.75 g/kg body weight	1.2-1.3 g/kg IBW	≥1.2-1.3 g/kg IBW
Calories	30-35 kcal/kg EDW	30-35 kcal/kg EDW†	30-35 kcal/kg IBW†
Fat	Determined by caloric requirement	Determined by caloric requirement	Determined by caloric requirement
Carbohydrate	Unlimited intake of sugars, starches; bread and cereal products limited due to protein restriction	Same as for conservative management	Dependent on individual patient needs
Iron	Variable	Variable	Variable
Potassium	2-3 g	2-3 g	3-4 g, no restrictions
Sodium	2-3 g	2-3 g	2-4 g
Phosphorus	800-1000 mg	1000 mg	1000 mg
Calcium	Variable	1000-1500 mg	1000-1500 mg
Folic acid	1 mg supplement	1 mg supplement	1 mg supplement

EDW, Estimated dry weight; *IBW,* ideal body weight.
*At least 50% of protein intake should be of high biologic value (e.g., coming from eggs, milk, meat).
†Includes dialysate calories.

TABLE 45-8	Nutritional Therapy	
High-Potassium Foods		
Fruits/Fruit Juices	**Vegetables**	**Cereal**
Apple juice	Beans, white and pinto*	All-bran*
Grapefruit juice	Broccoli	Raisin bran*
Orange juice*	Carrots	**Meat and Poultry**
Prune juice*	Lima beans, cooked*	Beef*, pork, cooked
Tomato juice*	Mushrooms, fresh*	Chicken
Oranges	Potato, baked*	Turkey
Tomatoes	Squash, baked*	**Miscellaneous**
Honeydew melons*	Spinach, cooked*	Chocolate
Raisins*	**Dairy**	Molasses
Avocados*	Milk*	Sunflower seeds*
Bananas*	Yogurt*	
Prunes*		

*Greater than 10 mEq of potassium per serving.

spaced throughout the day so that the patient does not become thirsty. For the chronic HD patient, fluid intake is adjusted so that weight gains are no more than 1 to 3 kg between dialyses.

Sodium and potassium restriction. The sodium and potassium restriction depends on the ability of the kidneys to excrete these electrolytes. Sodium-restricted diets may vary from 2 to 4 g depending on the degree of edema and hypertension. Sodium and salt should not be equated because the sodium content in 1 g of sodium chloride is equivalent to 400 mg of sodium. The patient should be instructed to avoid high-sodium foods such as cured meats, pickled foods, canned soups and stews, frankfurters, cold cuts, soy sauce, and salad dressings (see Tables 34-9 through 34-11). Most salt substitutes should not be used because they contain potassium chloride.

Dietary restrictions for potassium range from about 2 to 4 g (39 mg = 1 mEq). Some PD patients do not need potassium restrictions. Some foods with high potassium content that should be avoided are oranges, bananas, melons, tomatoes, prunes, raisins, deep green and yellow vegetables, beans, and legumes (Table 45-8).

Phosphate restriction. Phosphate should be limited to approximately 1000 mg a day. Foods that are high in phosphate include dairy products (e.g., milk, ice cream, cheese, yogurt) or foods containing dairy products (pudding). Most foods that are high in phosphate are also high in calcium. Restricting phosphate will restrict calcium intake.

NURSING MANAGEMENT
CONSERVATIVE THERAPY OF CHRONIC KIDNEY DISEASE

■ Nursing Assessment

The nurse should obtain a complete history of any existing renal disease or family history of renal disease because some renal disorders have a hereditary basis. Information on long-term health problems such as hypertension, diabetes, recurrent urinary tract infections, and systemic lupus erythematosus should be ob-

tained. Because many drugs are potentially nephrotoxic, both current and past use of prescription and over-the-counter drugs must be reviewed.

The nurse should assess the patient's dietary habits and discuss any problems. The height and weight should be measured, and any recent weight changes must be evaluated.

Clinical manifestations of CKD are apparent in multiple body systems (see Fig. 45-3). Fatigue, lethargy, and pruritus are often the early symptoms of CKD. Hypertension and changes in urine characteristics are often the first signs.

Support systems should be assessed. The chronicity of renal disease and the long-term nature of treatment modalities affect every area of a person's life, including family relationships, social and work activities, and self-image. The choice of treatment modality may be related to support systems available to the patient. Recognition that CKD is a lifelong illness will facilitate the care.

■ Nursing Diagnoses

Nursing diagnoses for CKD may include, but are not limited to, those presented in NCP 45-1.

■ Planning

The overall goals are that a patient with CKD will (1) demonstrate knowledge and ability to comply with the therapeutic regimen, (2) participate in decision making for the plan of care and future treatment modality, (3) demonstrate effective coping strategies, and (4) continue with activities of daily living within physiologic limitations.

■ Nursing Implementation

Health Promotion. Individuals at risk for CKD must be identified. These include people with a history (or a family history) of renal disease, hypertension, diabetes mellitus, and repeated urinary tract infection. These individuals should have regular checkups including serum creatinine, BUN, and urinalysis. They should be advised that any changes in urine appearance (color, odor), frequency, or volume must be reported to the health care provider. If a patient must be prescribed a potentially nephrotoxic drug, it is important to monitor renal function with serum creatinine and BUN.

Individuals identified as at risk need to take measures to prevent or delay the progression of CKD. These include glycemic control for patients with diabetes (see Chapter 47), BP control, and early and definitive treatment of urinary tract infections.

Acute Intervention. The specific nursing management of the patient with CKD is detailed in NCP 45-1. It is important to teach the patient and family because diet, drugs, and follow-up medical care are the responsibilities of the patient (Table 45-9). The patient should check a daily weight; learn to take daily BPs; and be able to identify signs and symptoms of fluid overload, hyperkalemia, and other electrolyte imbalances. The patient and family must understand the importance of strict dietary adherence. The dietitian should meet with the patient and family on a regular basis for diet planning. A diet history and consideration of cultural variations will facilitate diet planning and adherence.

The patient needs a complete understanding of the drugs, the dosages, and the common side effects. It may be helpful to make

NURSING CARE PLAN 45-1

Patient with Chronic Kidney Disease

EXPECTED PATIENT OUTCOMES	NURSING INTERVENTIONS and *RATIONALES*
NURSING DIAGNOSIS	**Excess fluid volume** *related to* inability of kidneys to excrete fluid, inadequate dialysis, and excessive fluid intake *as manifested by* edema, hypertension, bounding pulse, weight gain, shortness of breath, pulmonary edema.
• No edema • No evidence of dyspnea • Dry weight remaining within 4 lb (2 kg) of patient's dry weight • BP and pulse within limits for patient	• Monitor for increase in BP, periorbital sacral and peripheral edema, dyspnea, and pericardial friction rub, *which are indicators of fluid excess.* • Teach patient how to maintain a low-sodium diet *to help control edema and hypertension.* • Teach patient fluid control measures and importance of daily weights *to help monitor and control fluid overload and related hypertension.*
NURSING DIAGNOSIS	**Impaired skin integrity** *related to* decrease in oil and sweat gland activity, hyperphosphatemia, deposition of calcium-phosphate precipitates, capillary fragility, excess fluid, and neuropathy *as manifested by* itching, bruising, dry skin, edema, excoriation.
• No itching or skin dryness • Intact, clean skin • No calcium-phosphate deposits	• Assess skin for changes in color, texture, turgor, and vascularity *to provide information for appropriate interventions.* • Inspect patient for bruises, purpura, and signs of infection *to detect early signs of problems.* • Provide skin care with tepid water, bath oils, super-fatted soaps, or oatmeal *to relieve itching and moisturize dry skin.* • Apply ointments or creams (lanolin, Aquaphor) following bath or shower *to relieve itching and promote comfort.* • Administer antihistamines and antipruritics as prescribed *to relieve itching.* • Monitor serum calcium and phosphate levels *because elevated blood levels may lead to severe pruritus and calcium-phosphate precipitation in the skin.*
NURSING DIAGNOSIS	**Risk for injury** (fracture) *related to* alterations in the absorption of calcium and excretion of phosphate, altered vitamin D metabolism.
• Slowing of bone disease • Serum calcium levels >8 mg/dl (2 mmol/L) and phosphate levels <5.5 mg/dl (1.8 mmol/L) • No bone fractures	• Assess for hypocalcemia and hyperphosphatemia *to determine degree of bone demineralization and potential risk for injury.* • Provide safe environment *to reduce the risk of injury.* • Administer calcium supplements, vitamin D, and phosphate binders as ordered *to prevent and/or treat the bone demineralization.* • Give calcium supplement or phosphate binder with meals *to increase effectiveness.* • Ensure that patient understands and follows phosphate restrictions and can state the purpose of phosphate binders, calcium supplements, and vitamin D supplements. • Observe for hypercalcemia when using calcium supplements. • Explain to patient the potential for fracture *to reduce the risk of unsafe practices that might result in a traumatic or pathologic fracture.*
NURSING DIAGNOSIS	**Activity intolerance** *related to* anemia and neuropathy *as manifested by* fatigability, shortness of breath, pallor, dyspnea, tachycardia.
• Hematocrit and hemoglobin levels in acceptable range • Transferrin percent saturation and ferritin in acceptable range • Able to perform activities of daily living without undue fatigue	• Monitor hematocrit and hemoglobin levels *as an indicator of the patient's oxygen-carrying capacity.* • Monitor response of hematocrit and hemoglobin to erythropoietin (if ordered). • Monitor transferrin percent saturation and ferritin as indicators of iron available for erythropoiesis. • Administer oral iron between meals and IV iron (as ordered) and erythropoietin (as ordered) *to maintain normal erythropoiesis and stimulate production of RBCs.* • Administer folic acid after hemodialysis *because folic acid is dialyzable and would be lost in the dialysate.* • Provide adequate periods of rest *to enable patient to recuperate from past activities and participate in future activity.* • Teach patient to plan activities *to avoid fatigue.*

Continued

NURSING CARE PLAN 45-1

Patient with Chronic Kidney Disease—cont'd

EXPECTED PATIENT OUTCOMES	NURSING INTERVENTIONS and *RATIONALES*
NURSING DIAGNOSIS	**Imbalanced nutrition: less than body requirements** *related to* restricted intake of nutrients (especially protein), nausea, vomiting, anorexia, and stomatitis *as manifested by* loss of appetite and weight.
• Maintenance of ideal body weight • Prealbumin, transferrin, and albumin within acceptable limits	• Monitor weight, BUN, serum creatinine, prealbumin, total protein, and serum electrolytes *as indicators of effectiveness of dialysis, nutritional status, and response to treatment.* • Provide frequent mouth care *to prevent stomatitis, remove bad taste, and increase patient's comfort.* • Provide small, frequent meals *to reduce nausea and vomiting.* • Administer H_2 histamine blockers (e.g., famotidine [Pepcid]), proton pump inhibitors (e.g., omeprazole [Prilosec]), and GI promotility agents (e.g., metoclopramide [Reglan]) (as ordered) *to minimize GI irritation and facilitate motility.* • Allow patient freedom in choosing food and fluid intake within limitations *to increase the patient's sense of control.* • Provide at least 30-35 kcal/kg body weight/day with a high carbohydrate intake *to minimize catabolism of body protein and maintain body weight.* • Restrict protein and phosphate to prescribed amount *to decrease the metabolic end products of urea, potassium, phosphate, and hydrogen.* • Provide hard candy, gum, and lollipops *to improve taste and increase carbohydrate/calorie intake. If diabetic, sugar-free gum or hard candy may be substituted.*
NURSING DIAGNOSIS	**Anticipatory grieving** *related to* loss of kidney function *as manifested by* expression of feelings of sadness, anger, inadequacy, hopelessness.
• Acceptance of chronic disease	• Listen to the concerns of patient *to convey a caring attitude and foster a relationship to determine how patient is handling the situation.* • Allow patient time to mourn loss of body function *so that patient can deal with feelings and identify ways of coping with losses more effectively.* • Include family members in discussions of patient's concerns *to enable them to assist the patient and foster their support and understanding.*
NURSING DIAGNOSIS	**Risk for infection** *related to* suppressed immune system, access sites, and malnutrition secondary to dialysis and uremia.
• No infections • WBC within normal range	• Assess for local (pain on urination, hematuria, cloudy urine; redness, swelling, or drainage in areas of skin breaks) and systemic (chills, fever, tachycardia) manifestations of infection *to ensure early identification and treatment.* • Instruct patient to avoid exposure to people with infections *to decrease risk of infection.* • Maintain aseptic technique when performing dialysis or other invasive procedures (IV insertion, urinary catheter insertion) *to prevent the introduction of organisms.*

COLLABORATIVE PROBLEMS

NURSING GOALS	NURSING INTERVENTIONS and *RATIONALES*
POTENTIAL COMPLICATION	**Hypertension** *related to* sodium and water retention and alterations of renin-angiotensin system.
• Monitor for hypertension • Report deviations from acceptable parameters • Carry out appropriate medical and nursing interventions	• Assess patient for elevated BP, headache, dizziness, shortness of breath, chest pain, and edema *to identify the presence and effects of hypertension.* • Take vital signs *to provide a database for ongoing analysis of patient's response to treatment.* • Administer antihypertensive drugs (as ordered) after checking BP. • Observe for orthostatic hypotension and other side effects of antihypertensive drugs *because overtreatment may cause problems.* • Instruct patient to change positions slowly *to minimize dizziness caused by orthostatic hypotension.* • Explain the actions and side effects of antihypertensive drugs and risks of uncontrolled hypertension (e.g., stroke) *to foster adherence to drug regimen.*

NURSING CARE PLAN 45-1

Patient with Chronic Kidney Disease—cont'd

COLLABORATIVE PROBLEMS—cont'd

NURSING GOALS	NURSING INTERVENTIONS and *RATIONALES*
POTENTIAL COMPLICATION • Monitor for signs of hyperkalemia • Report deviations from acceptable parameters • Carry out appropriate medical and nursing interventions	**Hyperkalemia** *related to* decreased renal function, increased tissue catabolism, and shift of potassium into extracellular fluid secondary to metabolic acidosis. • Assess for manifestations of hyperkalemia such as serum potassium >5.5 mEq/L (5.5 mmol/L), muscle weakness, arrhythmias (peaked T waves, widened QRS, depressed ST segment on ECG), paresthesias, abdominal cramping, and diarrhea *to ensure early identification and treatment*. • Do not administer IV solutions, drugs (e.g., potassium penicillin IV), or nutritional supplements that contain potassium. • Discuss importance of following prescribed diet and avoiding foods high in potassium and receiving regular dialysis *to prevent complications of hyperkalemia*. • Monitor serum potassium and notify physician of elevated levels and abnormal ECG results *because elevated potassium can cause life-threatening cardiac arrhythmias*. • Be prepared to administer treatment for hyperkalemia *because this is a medical emergency requiring prompt treatment*. (See Table 45-4 for treatments.)
POTENTIAL COMPLICATION • Monitor for peripheral neuropathies • Report deviations from acceptable parameters • Carry out appropriate medical and nursing interventions	**Peripheral neuropathy** *related to* effects of uremia on peripheral nerves. • Assess patient for decreased sensation in feet, numbness and burning of feet, muscle cramps, restlessness of legs, loss of muscle strength, footdrop *to identify the presence of peripheral neuropathy*. • Explain to patient the reason for neuropathy *to increase understanding and decrease anxiety*. • Prevent trauma and excess stimulation to extremities *because areas with diminished sensation are extremely prone to injury*. • Teach patient to examine areas of decreased sensation *to observe for injury*. • In collaboration with physical therapy department, develop exercise regimen *to maintain prescribed level of activity*.

a list of the drugs and the times of administration that can be posted in the home. The patient must be instructed to avoid certain over-the-counter drugs such as NSAIDs and magnesium-based laxatives and antacids. The patient should also be aware that meperidine and ACE inhibitors may be harmful because of renal insufficiency.

Motivation to assume the primary role in the management of their disease is essential. The period of conservative management provides an opportunity to evaluate each patient's ability to manage the disease. This knowledge will be helpful when determining the treatment modality.

Ambulatory and Home Care. The length of time that a patient can receive conservative therapy is highly variable and depends on the progression of renal failure and the presence of other comorbid conditions. When conservative therapy is no longer effective, HD, PD, and transplantation are the available treatment options.

While the patient is receiving conservative therapy, the decision regarding future therapies should be made. This should be done before complications such as mental status changes, bleeding, progressive neuropathies, and fluid overload occur.[19]

The patient and family need a clear explanation of what is involved in dialysis and transplantation. If alternative treatments are presented early in the course of therapy, there will be an opportunity to carefully consider choices. Providing information about the treatment options will allow the patient to be active in

TABLE 45-9

Patient & Family Teaching Guide
Chronic Kidney Disease

1. Explain dietary (protein, sodium, potassium, phosphate) and fluid restrictions.
2. Encourage discussion of difficulties in modifying diet and fluid intake.
3. Explain signs and symptoms of electrolyte imbalance, especially high potassium.
4. Teach alternative ways of reducing thirst, such as sucking on ice cubes, lemon, or hard candy.
5. Explain the rationale for prescribed drugs and common side effects. Examples:
   Phosphate binders should be taken with meals.
   Iron supplements should be taken between meals.
6. Explain the importance of reporting any of the following:
   Weight gain greater than 4 lb (2 kg)
   Increasing BP
   Shortness of breath
   Edema
   Increasing fatigue or weakness
   Confusion or lethargy
7. Encourage patient and family to share concerns about lifestyle changes, living with a chronic illness, and decisions about type of dialysis or transplantation.

NURSING RESEARCH
Uncertainty and Coping in Family Members of Patients with End-Stage Renal Disease

Citation   Pelletier-Hibbert M, Sohi P: Sources of uncertainty and coping strategies used by family members of individuals living with end-stage renal disease, *Nephrology Nursing J* 28:411, 2000.

Purpose   To describe sources of uncertainty and common coping strategies used by family members of patients with end-stage renal disease (ESRD).

Methods   Using a qualitative-descriptive-exploratory design, 41 family members of patients receiving dialysis in eastern Canada were interviewed in focus groups. They were asked to describe the experience of living with a loved one who required dialysis. Open-ended questions were used during the audiotaped sessions. The interviews were analyzed by thematic analysis.

Results and Conclusions   Family members reported that uncertainty was a major source of stress. There were four themes identified as sources of uncertainty: (1) patient's health, (2) dialysis treatment, (3) potential loss, and (4) availability of renal transplant. Coping strategies included "living each day as it comes," finding positive meaning in the illness and treatment, hoping for a transplant, and believing in God. Uncertainty was attributed to the unpredictability of ESRD and its effects on all aspects of life. Uncertainty was felt most intensely by those who live day-to-day with the patient. Family members used coping strategies that included day-to-day rather than long-term planning.

Implications for Nursing Practice   It is essential that the nurses caring for ESRD patients recognize potential sources of uncertainty for both patients and the family members. Teaching and care can be directed at alleviating sources of uncertainty and assisting in the development of effective coping strategies for the patient and the family members.

the decision-making process and give a sense of control over life-altering decisions. The patient should be informed that if dialysis is chosen, the option of transplantation still remains. It should be emphasized that if a transplanted organ fails, the patient can return to dialysis. The patient should also be counseled that retransplantation is also an option.

■ Evaluation

The expected outcomes for the patient with chronic kidney disease are presented in NCP 45-1.

Dialysis

Dialysis is the movement of fluid and molecules across a semipermeable membrane from one compartment to another. Clinically, dialysis is a technique in which substances move from the blood through a semipermeable membrane and into a dialysis solution (dialysate). It is used to correct fluid and electrolyte imbalances and to remove waste products in renal failure. It can also be used to treat drug overdoses. The two methods of dialysis available are **peritoneal dialysis** (PD) and **hemodialysis** (HD) (Table 45-10). In PD the peritoneal membrane acts as the semipermeable membrane. In HD an artificial membrane (usually made of cellulose-based or synthetic materials) is used as the semipermeable membrane and is in contact with the patient's blood.

Dialysis is begun when the patient's uremia can no longer be adequately managed conservatively. Generally dialysis is initiated when the GFR (or creatinine clearance) is less than 15 ml per minute. This criterion can vary widely in different clinical situations and the physician will determine when to start dialysis based on the patient's clinical status. Certain uremic complications, including encephalopathy, neuropathies, uncontrolled hyperkalemia, pericarditis, and accelerated hypertension, indicate a need for immediate dialysis.

TABLE 45-10   Comparison of Peritoneal Dialysis and Hemodialysis

PERITONEAL DIALYSIS		HEMODIALYSIS	
ADVANTAGES	DISADVANTAGES	ADVANTAGES	DISADVANTAGES
Immediate initiation in almost any hospital	Bacterial or chemical peritonitis	Rapid fluid removal	Vascular access problems
Less complicated than hemodialysis	Protein loss into dialysate	Rapid removal of urea and creatinine	Dietary and fluid restrictions
Portable system with CAPD	Exit site and tunnel infections	Effective potassium removal	Heparinization may be necessary
Fewer dietary restrictions	Self-image problems with catheter placement	Less protein loss	Extensive equipment necessary
Relatively short training time	Hyperglycemia	Lowering of serum triglycerides	Hypotension during dialysis
Usable in the patient with vascular access problems	Aggravated hyperlipidemia	Home dialysis possible	Added blood loss that contributes to anemia
Less cardiovascular stress	Surgery for catheter placement	Temporary access can be placed at bedside	Specially trained personnel necessary
Home dialysis possible	Contraindication in the patient with multiple abdominal surgeries, trauma, unrepaired hernia		Surgery for permanent access placement
Preferable for the diabetic patient	Specially trained personnel needed		Self-image problems with permanent access
	Catheter can migrate		

CAPD, Continuous ambulatory peritoneal dialysis.

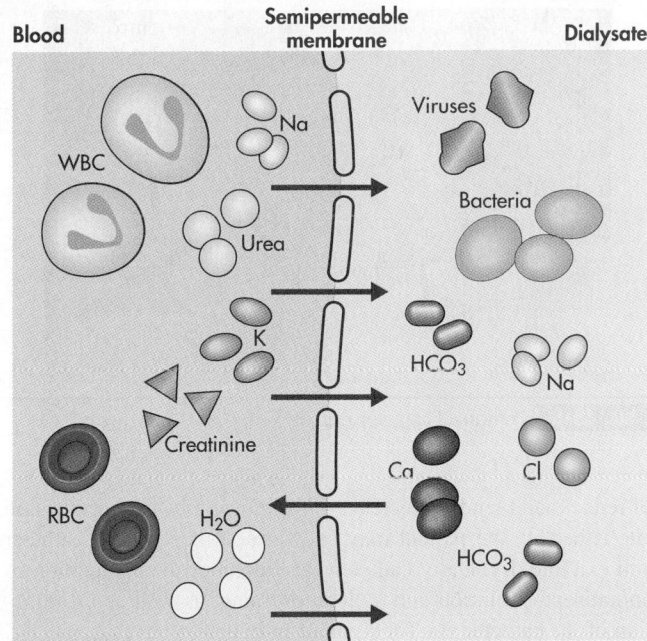

FIG. 45-5 Osmosis and diffusion across a semipermeable membrane.

General Principles of Dialysis

Solutes and water move across the semipermeable membrane from the blood to the dialysate or from the dialysate to the blood in accordance with concentration gradients. The principles of diffusion, osmosis, and ultrafiltration are involved in dialysis (Fig. 45-5). *Diffusion* is the movement of solutes from an area of greater concentration to an area of lesser concentration. In renal failure, urea, creatinine, uric acid, and electrolytes (potassium, phosphate) move from the blood to the dialysate with the net effect of lowering their concentration in the blood. RBCs, WBCs, and plasma proteins are too large to diffuse through the pores of the membrane. Bacteria and viruses that may be present in the dialysate are too large to migrate through the pores into the blood.

Osmosis is the movement of fluid from an area of lesser to an area of greater concentration of solutes. Glucose is added to the dialysate and creates an osmotic gradient across the membrane, pulling excess fluid from the blood.

Ultrafiltration (water and fluid removal) results when there is an osmotic gradient or pressure gradient across the membrane. In PD, excess fluid is removed by increasing the osmolality of the dialysate (osmotic gradient) with the addition of glucose. In HD, the gradient is created by increasing pressure in the blood compartment (positive pressure) or decreasing pressure in the dialysate compartment (negative pressure). Extracellular fluid moves into the dialysate because of the pressure gradient. The excess fluid is removed by creating a pressure differential between the blood and the dialysate solution with a combination of positive pressure in the blood compartment or a negative pressure in the dialysate compartment.

PERITONEAL DIALYSIS

Although PD was first used in 1923, it did not come into widespread use for chronic treatment until the 1970s with the development of soft, pliable peritoneal solution bags and the intro-

duction of the concept of continuous PD. In the United States, approximately 10% of patients receiving dialysis treatments are on PD.[8] In Canada, approximately 36% of patients are receiving PD because of the decreased availability of HD. In recent years the use of PD to treat chronic kidney disease has decreased in the United States.

Catheter Placement

Peritoneal access is obtained by inserting a catheter through the anterior abdominal wall (Fig. 45-6). The prototype of the catheter that is used was developed by Tenckhoff in 1968 and is made of silicone rubber tubing. The catheters are about 60 cm long and have two Dacron cuffs on the subcutaneous and peritoneal portions of the catheter that act as anchors and prevent the migration of microorganisms down the shaft from the skin. Within a few weeks, fibrous tissue grows into the Dacron cuff, holding the catheter in place and preventing bacterial penetration into the peritoneal cavity. The tip of the catheter rests in the peritoneal cavity and has many perforations spaced along the distal end of the tubing to allow fluid to flow in and out of the catheter. Bent or "swan neck" catheters with curled, "pigtail" ends are preferred because they prevent catheter migration and kinking and allow for easier fills and drains. There are numerous variations of the Tenckhoff catheter, including the Toronto-Western, Purdue Column-Disc, and Gore-Tex catheters (Fig. 45-7).

The technique for catheter placement varies. Although it is possible to place a permanent catheter in the peritoneal cavity at the bedside with a trocar, it is usually done via surgery so that its placement can be directly visualized, minimizing potential complications. Preparation of the patient for catheter insertion includes emptying the bladder and bowel, weighing the patient, and obtaining a signed consent form.

In the nonsurgical (bedside) approach, an area approximately 2 cm below the umbilicus is numbed with a local anesthetic, and a small stab wound is made. A stylet is inserted, and the abdomen is distended with dialysis solution. The catheter is then placed

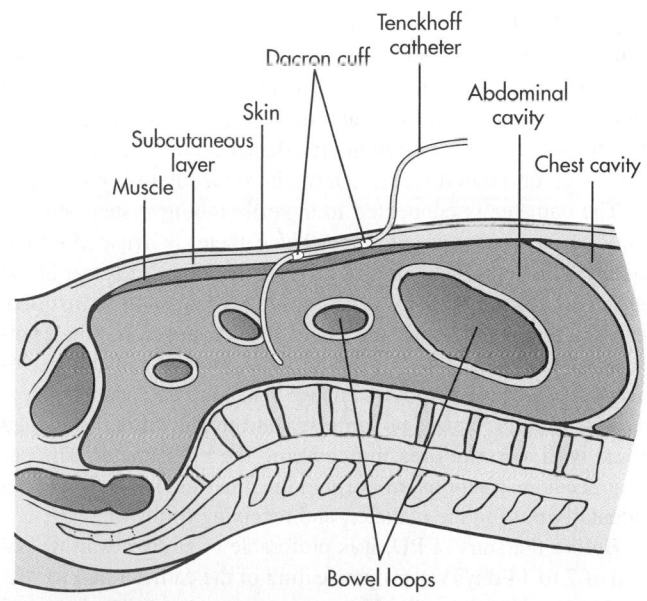

FIG. 45-6 Tenckhoff catheter used in peritoneal dialysis.

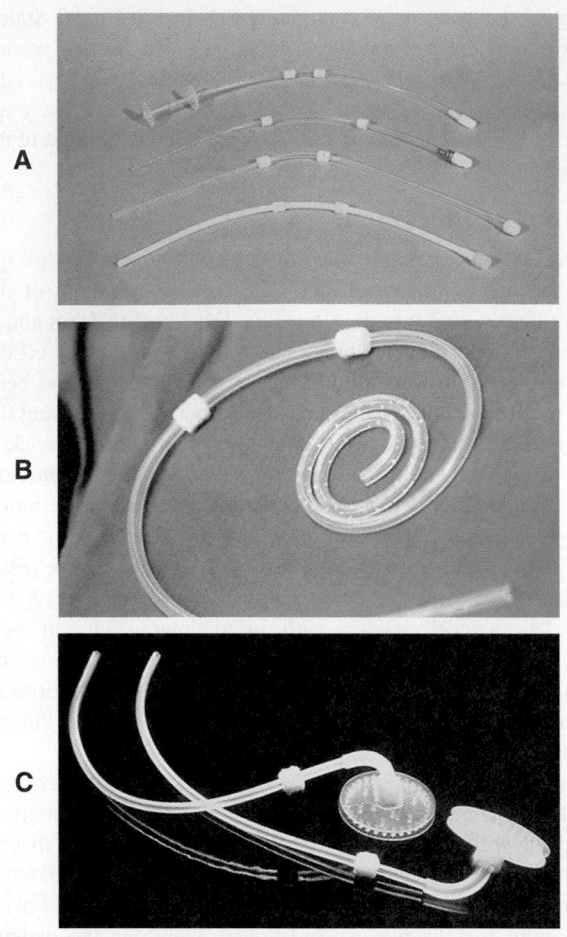

FIG. 45-7 A, Peritoneal catheters used for peritoneal dialysis. B, Bent neck, curl catheters. C, Disc catheters.

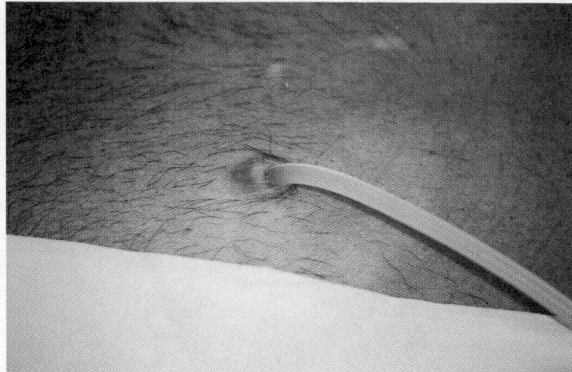

FIG. 45-8 Peritoneal catheter exit site.

into the peritoneal cavity. When the patient feels pressure in the rectal area and has the urge to defecate, the catheter is in place.

In the surgical approach, a midline umbilical incision is made, and a small puncture is made to one side and below this incision. The distal end of the catheter is placed in the peritoneum, and it is tunneled under the skin to the puncture site. The tunnel helps prevent peritonitis. After the catheter is inserted, the skin is cleaned with an antiseptic solution, and a sterile dressing is applied. Complications of catheter insertion include perforation of the bladder, the bowel, or a blood vessel and the introduction of bacteria.

The catheter is connected to a sterile tubing system and secured to the abdomen with tape. The catheter is irrigated immediately with heparinized dialysate (usually 500 ml) to clear blood and fibrin from it. Prophylactic antibiotics may also be instilled. The irrigations may continue for 12 to 24 hours using small volumes of dialysate. This procedure helps prevent catheter occlusion that can lead to poor drainage and inflow. Catheter placement is usually same-day surgery, and the patient is discharged home with a sterile dressing covering the PD catheter. The patient needs instructions on keeping the dressing dry, avoiding accidentally pulling the catheter, and receiving follow-up care.

Before the start of PD, it is preferable to allow a waiting period of 7 to 14 days for proper sealing of the catheter and for tissue to grow into the cuffs. However, some centers start dialysis 5 to 7 days after catheter insertion. About 2 to 4 weeks after catheter implantation, the exit site should be clean, dry, and free

of redness and tenderness (Fig. 45-8). Once the catheter incision site is healed, the patient may shower and then pat the catheter and exit site dry. Daily catheter care includes the application of an antiseptic solution and a clean dressing, as well as examination of the catheter site for signs of infection.

Dialysis Solutions and Cycles

Dialysis solutions are available commercially in 1- or 2-L (and sometimes smaller or larger volume) plastic bags (Dianeal, Inpersol) with glucose concentrations of 1.5%, 2.5%, and 4.25%. The electrolyte composition is similar to that of plasma. The dialysis solution is warmed to body temperature using dry heat to increase peritoneal clearance, prevent hypothermia, and enhance comfort.

Ultrafiltration (fluid removal) during PD depends on osmotic forces, with glucose being the most effective osmotic agent currently available. However, the problems arising from high rates of peritoneal glucose absorption, such as obesity, hypertriglyceridemia, and difficult control of blood glucose in the diabetic patient, have led to a search for alternative osmotic agents, including amino acid solutions. Many of these agents are currently under investigation.

The three phases of the PD cycle are *inflow* (fill), *dwell* (equilibration), and *drain*. The three phases are called an *exchange*. The patient dialyzing at home will receive about four exchanges per day. An acutely ill hospitalized patient may receive 12 to 24 exchanges per day. During inflow, a prescribed amount of solution, usually 2 L, is infused through an established catheter over about 10 minutes. The flow rate may be decreased if the patient has pain. After the solution has been infused, the inflow clamp is closed before air enters the tubing.

The next part of the cycle is the dwell phase, or equilibration, during which diffusion and osmosis occur between the patient's blood and the peritoneal cavity. The duration of the dwell time can last 20 to 30 minutes to 8 or more hours, depending on the method of PD. Drain time takes 15 to 30 minutes and may be facilitated by gently massaging the abdomen or changing position. The cycle starts again with the infusion of another 2 L of solution. For manual PD, a period of about 30 to 50 minutes is required to complete an exchange.

Peritoneal Dialysis Systems

Two types of PD currently being used are **automated peritoneal dialysis** (APD) and **continuous ambulatory peritoneal dialysis** (CAPD).

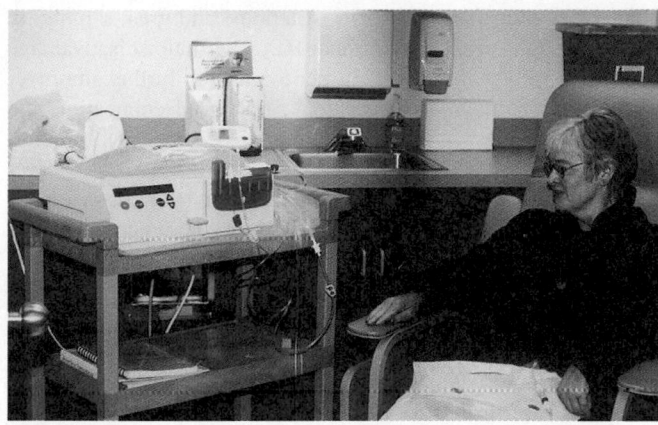

FIG. 45-9 Automated peritoneal dialysis cycler, which can be used while the patient is sleeping at night or for hospitalized patients who require frequent exchanges.

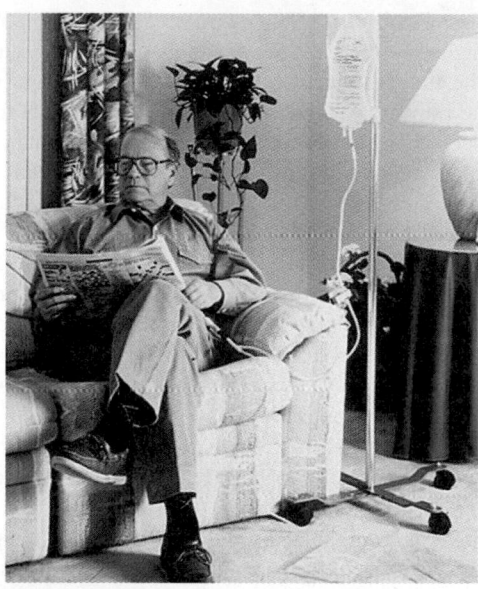

FIG. 45-10 Infusion period for a continuous ambulatory peritoneal dialysis patient.

Automated Peritoneal Dialysis. An automated device called a cycler is used to deliver the dialysate for APD (Fig. 45-9). The automated cycler times and controls the fill, dwell, and drain phases. The machine cycles four or more exchanges per night with 1 to 2 hours per exchange. Alarms and monitors are built into the system to make it safe for the patient to dialyze while sleeping. It may be easier to teach the patient and family to use the PD machine at home compared with the HD machine. The patient disconnects from the machine in the morning and usually leaves fluid in the abdomen during the day. One to two daytime manual exchanges may also be prescribed to ensure adequate dialysis. It is difficult to achieve the required solute and fluid clearance with solely nighttime APD. Older cyclers were quite large. With new technology cyclers are now about the size of a VCR or DVD player and have longer tubing to allow greater mobility.

Continuous Ambulatory Peritoneal Dialysis. CAPD is carried out manually by exchanging 1.5 to 3 L (usually 2 L) of peritoneal dialysate at least four times daily with dwell times of 4 to 10 hours. For example, one schedule starts the exchanges at 7 AM, 12 noon, 5 PM, and 10 PM. In this procedure the person instills 2 L of dialysate from a collapsible plastic bag into the peritoneal cavity through a disposable plastic tube.

Technical advances in CAPD systems allow the bag and line to be disconnected after the instillation of the fluid, decreasing the risk of peritonitis. After the equilibration period, the line is reconnected to the catheter, the dialysate (effluent) is drained from the peritoneal cavity, and a new 2-L bag of dialysate solution is infused (Fig. 45-10). It is critical in PD to maintain aseptic technique to avoid peritonitis. Several tubing connections and devices are commercially available to help maintain an aseptic system.

Contraindications for PD include the following:

1. History of multiple abdominal surgical procedures or severe abdominal pathologic condition (e.g., severe pancreatitis, diverticulitis)
2. Recurrent abdominal wall or inguinal hernias
3. Excessive obesity with large abdominal wall and fat deposits
4. Preexisting vertebral disease (e.g., chronic back problems)
5. Severe obstructive pulmonary disease

Complications of Peritoneal Dialysis

Exit Site Infection. Infection of the peritoneal catheter exit site is most commonly caused by *Staphylococcus aureus* or *S. epidermidis* (from skin flora). Superficial exit site infections caused by these organisms are generally resolved with antibiotic therapy. Clinical manifestations of an exit site infection include redness at site, tenderness, and drainage. If not treated immediately, subcutaneous tunnel infections usually result in abscess formation and may cause peritonitis, necessitating catheter removal.

Peritonitis. Peritonitis results from contamination of the dialysate or tubing or from progression of an exit site or tunnel infection. Less commonly, peritonitis results from bacteria in the intestine crossing over into the peritoneal cavity. Peritonitis is usually caused by *S. aureus* or *S. epidermidis*.[20] The primary clinical manifestation of peritonitis is a cloudy peritoneal effluent that has a WBC count of over 100 cells/μl (particularly neutrophils). GI manifestations may also be present, including diffuse abdominal pain, diarrhea, vomiting, abdominal distention, and hyperactive bowel sounds. Fever may or may not be present. Cultures, Gram stain, and a cell count with WBC differential of the peritoneal effluent are used to confirm the diagnosis of peritonitis. Antibiotics can be given by mouth, IV, or intraperitoneal. The patient is usually treated on an outpatient basis. Repeated infections may require the removal of the peritoneal catheter and termination of PD. The formation of adhesions in the peritoneum can result from repeated infections and interferes with the peritoneal membrane's ability to act as a dialyzing surface.

Abdominal Pain. Although not severe, pain is a common complication caused by the low pH of the dialysate solution, peritonitis, intraperitoneal irritation (which usually subsides in 1 to 2 weeks), and placement of the catheter. Pain can also occur when the tip of the catheter touches the bladder, bowel, or peritoneum. A change in the position of the catheter should correct this problem. Accidental infusion of air or infusing the dialysate too rapidly may cause referred pain in the shoulder. If the infusion rate is decreased, the pain usually subsides.

Outflow Problems. When outflow is less than 80% of inflow immediately after catheter placement, it may be caused by a kink in the tunnel segment of the catheter, omentum wrapped around the catheter, or migration of the catheter out of the pelvic region. Persistent outflow problems may require radiologic or surgical manipulation of the catheter. Outflow problems after the catheter has settled into place are often the result of a full colon. Bowel evacuation frequently relieves the problem.

Hernias. Because of increased intraabdominal pressure secondary to the dialysate infusion, hernias can develop in predisposed individuals such as multiparous women and older men. However, in most situations after hernia repair, PD can be resumed after several days using small dialysate volumes and by keeping the patient supine.

Lower Back Problems. Increased intraabdominal pressure can cause or aggravate lower back pain. The lumbosacral curvature is increased by intraperitoneal infusion of dialysate. Orthopedic binders and a regular exercise program for strengthening the back muscles have been beneficial for some patients.

Bleeding. Effluent drained after the first few exchanges may be pink or slightly bloody because of the trauma of catheter insertion. Bloody effluent over several days or the new appearance of blood in the effluent can indicate active intraperitoneal bleeding. If this occurs, the BP and hematocrit should be checked. Blood may also be present in the effluent of women who are menstruating or ovulating, and this requires no intervention.

Pulmonary Complications. Atelectasis, pneumonia, and bronchitis may occur from repeated upward displacement of the diaphragm, resulting in decreased lung expansion. The longer the dwell time, the greater the likelihood of pulmonary problems. Frequent repositioning and deep-breathing exercises can help. When lying in bed, elevation of the head of the bed may prevent these problems.

Protein Loss. The peritoneal membrane is permeable to plasma proteins, amino acids, and polypeptides. These substances are lost in the dialysate fluid. The amount of loss may be as much as 5 to 15 g per day. This loss may increase up to 40 g per day during episodes of peritonitis as the membrane becomes more permeable. Positive nitrogen balance can be maintained with adequate protein intake.

Carbohydrate and Lipid Abnormalities. Dialysate glucose is absorbed via the peritoneum and may be as much as 100 to 150 g per day. Continuous absorption of glucose results in increased insulin secretion and increased plasma insulin levels. The hyperinsulinemia stimulates hepatic production of triglycerides.

Encapsulating Sclerosing Peritonitis and Loss of Ultrafiltration. *Encapsulating sclerosing peritonitis* is a term applied to the development of a thick fibrous membrane that surrounds and compresses the bowel. Intestinal obstruction and strangulation are common complications. This condition generally necessitates changing the patient to HD because of the loss of ultrafiltration. It can occur for unknown reasons or from accidental infusion of disinfecting agents. Loss of ultrafiltration is associated with rapid glucose absorption.

Effectiveness of and Adaptation to Chronic Peritoneal Dialysis

The technique is associated with a short training program, independence, and ease of traveling. Clinically, the patient receiving PD does as well as the patient receiving HD and sometimes better. There are fewer dietary restrictions, and greater mobility is possible than with conventional HD. The major disadvantage is the possibility of developing peritonitis. As further improvements in techniques are made (e.g., improved connecting and sterilizing devices, in-line filters, improved catheters), the incidence of peritonitis should decrease.

PD is especially indicated for the individual who has vascular access problems or responds poorly to the hemodynamic stresses of HD (e.g., the older adult patient with diabetes and cardiovascular disease). The diabetic patient with ESRD does better with PD than with HD. The advantages of PD for the diabetic patient include better BP control, less hemodynamic instability because fluid shifts are gradual, better control of blood glucose by using intraperitoneal insulin (which can often eliminate the need for subcutaneous insulin), and prevention of retinal hemorrhage because heparin is not required as it is in HD.

HEMODIALYSIS

In 1943 Willem Kolff in the Netherlands performed the first successful dialysis on a human being with the use of a rotating-drum dialyzer. He initiated dialysis treatment in the United States in 1948.[21] Tremendous technologic advances have been made in HD since the 1940s, allowing for safer, shorter treatments using sophisticated equipment.

Vascular Access Sites

Obtaining vascular access is one of the most difficult problems associated with HD. To carry out HD, a very rapid blood flow is required, and access to a large blood vessel is essential. The types of vascular access in current use include arteriovenous fistulas (AVFs) and grafts (AVGs), temporary and semipermanent catheters, subcutaneous ports, and shunts.

Shunts. In the past external shunts were used, but today they are rarely used except with CRRT because of the numerous complications associated with them. The shunt consists of a U-shaped Silastic tube divided at the midpoint, and each of the two ends is placed in an artery and a vein (Fig. 45-11, *A*).

Internal Arteriovenous Fistulas and Grafts. In 1966 the use of the subcutaneous internal arteriovenous native (using the person's own blood vessels) fistula (see Fig. 45-11, *B*) was introduced. An arteriovenous native fistula (AVF) is created most commonly in the forearm with an anastomosis between an artery (usually radial or ulnar) and a vein (usually cephalic). The fistula provides for arterial blood flow through the vein. The arterial blood flow is essential to provide the rapid blood flow required for HD. The increased pressure of the arterial blood flow through the vein makes the vein dilate and become tough, making it amenable to repeated venipuncture. The vein is accessed using two large-gauge needles.

Native fistulas have the best overall patency rates and least number of complications of all vascular accesses. However, they are suitable only for the patient with relatively healthy blood vessels.[22] AVFs may not be possible in patients with a history of severe hypertension, peripheral vascular disease, diabetes, prolonged IV drug use, or previous multiple IV procedures in the forearm.

For these individuals a synthetic graft is usually required. **Arteriovenous grafts** (AVGs), first introduced in 1976, are made of synthetic materials (polytetrafluoroethylene [PTFE], Teflon) and form a "bridge" between the arterial and venous blood supplies.

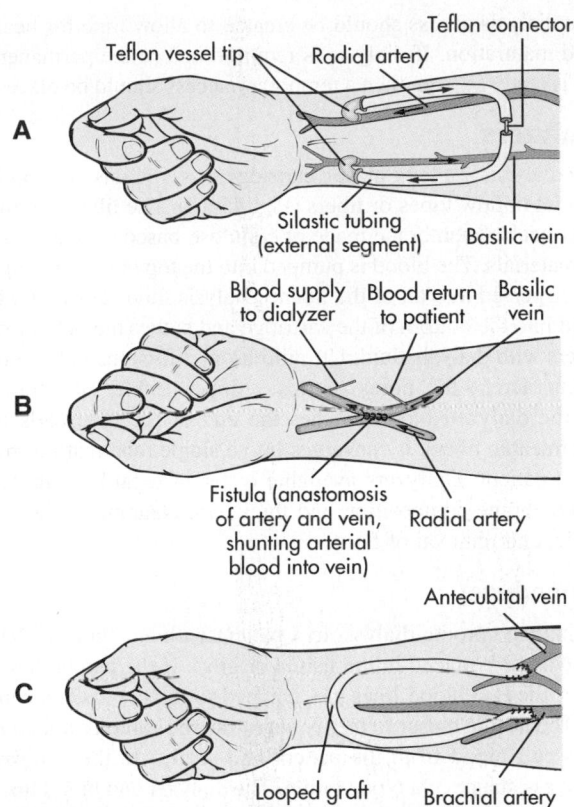

FIG. 45-11 Vascular access for hemodialysis. **A,** External shunt. **B,** Internal arteriovenous fistula. **C,** Internal arteriovenous graft.

Grafts are surgically anastomosed between an artery (usually brachial) and a vein (usually antecubital) (see Fig. 45-11, *C*). The graft, like the fistula, is under the skin and accessed using two large-gauge needles. The graft material is self-healing, meaning it should close over any puncture site after the needle is removed. Because grafts are made of artificial materials, they can become infected easily and are thrombogenic.

The AVF requires 4 to 6 weeks to mature (dilate and toughen) sufficiently for use. When an AVG is placed, an interval of 2 to 4 weeks is usually necessary to allow the graft to heal, but some centers may use it earlier.

Two 14- to 16-gauge needles are inserted into the fistula or graft to obtain vascular access. One needle is placed to pull blood from the circulation to the HD machine, and the other needle is used to return the dialyzed blood to the patient. The needles are attached via tubing to dialysis lines. Normally, a *thrill* can be felt by palpating the area of anastomosis, and a *bruit* can be heard with a stethoscope. The bruit and thrill are created by arterial blood rushing into the vein. BPs, IV insertion, and venipuncture should not be performed on the affected extremity. This prevents infection and clotting of the vascular access. Vascular access can be difficult to obtain for patients with ESRD. Protection of the vascular access site is of paramount importance.

The AVF is much less likely to clot and become infected than a graft. Thrombosis in AVGs is common but can often be corrected with interventional radiology techniques or a surgical procedure. AVGs can cause the development of distal ischemia *(steal syndrome)* because too much of the arterial blood is being shunted or "stolen" from the distal extremity. This is usually seen soon after surgery and may require surgical correction.

Aneurysms can also develop at the fistula site and can rupture if left untreated. AVG infections are not uncommon, and immediate treatment is essential to salvage the graft and prevent bacteremia. Severe AVG infections may necessitate graft removal.

Temporary Vascular Access. In some situations when immediate vascular access is required, percutaneous cannulation of the internal jugular or femoral vein is performed. In the past, the subclavian vein was often cannulated, but the central stenosis that can occur with this approach has made it the option of last resort. A flexible Teflon, silicone rubber, or polyurethane catheter is inserted at the bedside into one of these large veins and provides access to circulation without surgery (Fig. 45-12, *A*). The catheters usually have a double external lumen with an internal septum separating the two internal segments (Fig. 45-12, *B*). One lumen is used for blood removal and the other for blood return. Temporary catheters in the jugular or subclavian veins can be left in place for 1 to 3 weeks. Femoral vein cannulas can remain in place for up to 1 week.

Jugular vein cannulation is associated with a low incidence of thrombosis. That is the primary reason this method is preferred over subclavian cannulation. Short-term jugular vein access with stiff catheters may be uncomfortable and restrict neck movement. Bent catheters can ease this problem (see Fig. 45-12, *A*). In addition to vessel thrombosis and stenosis, subclavian vein cannulation has been associated with pneumothorax, brachial plexus neuropathies, and hemothorax. Both types of catheter placements pose the risk of infection.

Disadvantages of femoral vessel cannulation include the following: (1) the catheter can remain in place only a short time, (2) the location encourages catheter kinking, and (3) the groin is not a clean site. Potential complications of femoral catheterization are femoral vein thrombosis with pulmonary emboli (especially if the treatment is prolonged), infections, immobility, and inad-

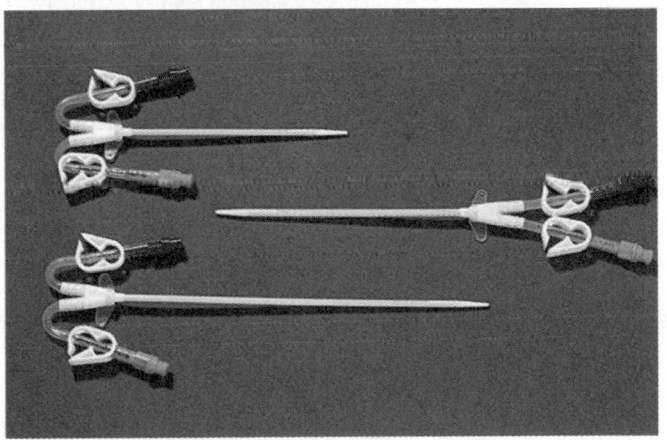

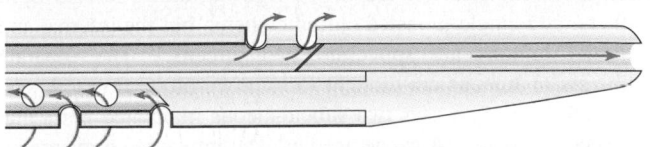

FIG. 45-12 Temporary double-lumen vascular access catheter for acute hemodialysis. **A,** Soft, flexible dual-lumen tube is attached to a Y hub. **B,** Blood is withdrawn continuously through the red lumen (upstream) and returned through the blue lumen (downstream), thus reducing recirculation.

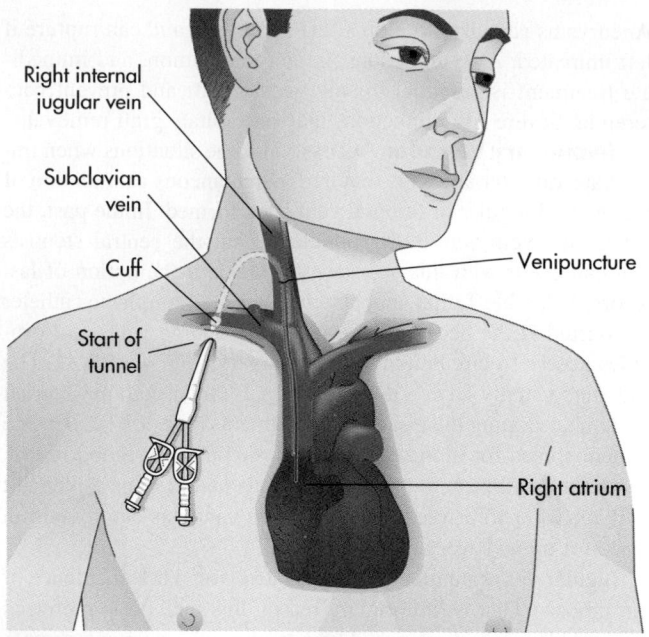

Right internal
jugular vein

Subclavian
vein

Cuff

Start of
tunnel

Venipuncture

Right atrium

FIG. 45-13 Right internal jugular placement for a tunneled, cuffed semipermanent catheter.

vertent blood vessel punctures with hematoma formation. The patient must be on bed rest while the femoral catheter is in place to prevent trauma to the vessel.

For all temporary catheters, no drugs should be administered or blood withdrawn via the catheter by nondialysis staff. This is to minimize the risk of infection, catheter loss, and accidental injection of heparin. Trained dialysis staff will instill heparin into the lumens of the catheter at the end of each treatment to ensure patency and withdraw it before the next treatment.

Semipermanent, soft, flexible Silastic double-lumen catheters (Davol, Bard, Permcath) are being used more often. These catheters can be used as temporary access while awaiting fistula placement and development or as long-term access when other forms of access have failed. This type of catheter exits on the upper chest wall and is tunneled subcutaneously to the internal or external jugular vein (Fig. 45-13). The catheter tip rests in the right atrium. It has one or two subcutaneous Dacron cuffs that prevent infection from tracking along the catheter and anchor the catheter, eliminating the need for sutures.

Several new semipermanent silicone and polyurethane catheters are now available. The aim of all of the new catheters is to increase blood flow rates while decreasing rates of infections and catheter loss from clotting or the development of fibrin sheaths on the catheter exterior. The Tesio catheters involve two tunneled cuffed catheters that are placed through separate tunnels. Both catheter tips are in the right atrium. The Ash Split catheter is a single tunneled cuffed catheter, but the internal and external lumens are split into two lumens.[23] The separate catheters or lumens are thought to improve blood flows. A system called LifeSite uses two subcutaneous implanted ports that are accessed using 14-gauge needles. The implanted ports are attached to internal silicone catheters that are usually tunneled into the internal or external jugular vein.[24]

Advance planning is essential for management of the patient with renal failure who is approaching end-stage disease and dialysis. Several months before the estimated start of dialysis, a per-

manent dialysis access should be created to allow time for healing and maturation. If dialysis is required before the permanent access is ready for use, then a temporary access should be placed.

Dialyzers

The dialyzer is a long plastic cartridge that contains thousands of parallel hollow tubes or fibers (Fig. 45-14). The fibers are the semipermeable membrane made of cellulose-based or other synthetic materials. The blood is pumped into the top of the cartridge and is dispersed into all of the fibers. Dialysis fluid (*dialysate*) is pumped into the bottom of the cartridge and bathes the outside of the fibers with dialysis fluid. Ultrafiltration, diffusion, and osmosis occur across the pores of this semipermeable membrane. When the dialyzed blood reaches the end of the thousands of semipermeable fibers, it converges into a single tube that returns it to the patient. Dialyzers available differ in regard to surface area, membrane composition and thickness, clearance of waste products, and removal of fluid.

Procedure

To initiate chronic dialysis in a patient with an AVG or AVF, two needles are placed in the fistula or graft. If the patient has a catheter, the two blood lines are attached to the two catheter lumens. The needle closer to the fistula or the red catheter lumen is used to pull blood from the patient and send it to the dialyzer with the assistance of a blood pump. The dialyzer and blood lines are usually primed with up to 1000 ml of saline solution to eliminate air from the system. Heparin is added to the blood as it flows into the dialyzer because any time blood contacts a foreign substance it has a tendency to clot. When the blood enters the extracorporeal circuit, it is propelled through the top of the dialyzer by a blood pump at a flow rate of 200 to 500 ml per minute, while the dialysate (warmed to body temperature) circulates in the opposite direction at a rate of 300 to 900 ml per minute. Blood is returned from the dialyzer to the patient through the second needle or blue catheter lumen.

In addition to the dialyzer, there is a dialysate delivery and monitoring system (Fig. 45-15). This system pumps the dialysate through the dialyzer, countercurrent to the blood flow. Adjustments can be made for ultrafiltration by creating a positive pressure on the blood side or a negative pressure on the dialysate side or by a combination of both. The newest dialysis delivery systems have ultrafiltration controllers that equalize negative and positive pressures for the removal of the precise amount of fluid per hour. The dialysis system has alarm systems to warn of blood leaking into the dialysate or air leaking into the blood; alterations in dialysate temperature, concentration, or pressure; and extremes in BP readings.

Dialysis is terminated by flushing the dialyzer with saline solution to return all blood through the access. The needles are then removed from the patient, and firm pressure is applied to the venipuncture sites until the bleeding stops. On occasion the access site can begin to bleed again. If this occurs, pressure should be reapplied, but not so firmly that flow is occluded because this could cause thrombosis. For patients with a catheter, the blood lines are clamped and removed from the catheter lumens.

Before beginning treatment, the nurse must complete an assessment that includes fluid status (weight, BP, peripheral edema, lung and heart sounds), condition of vascular access, temperature, and general skin condition. The difference between the last

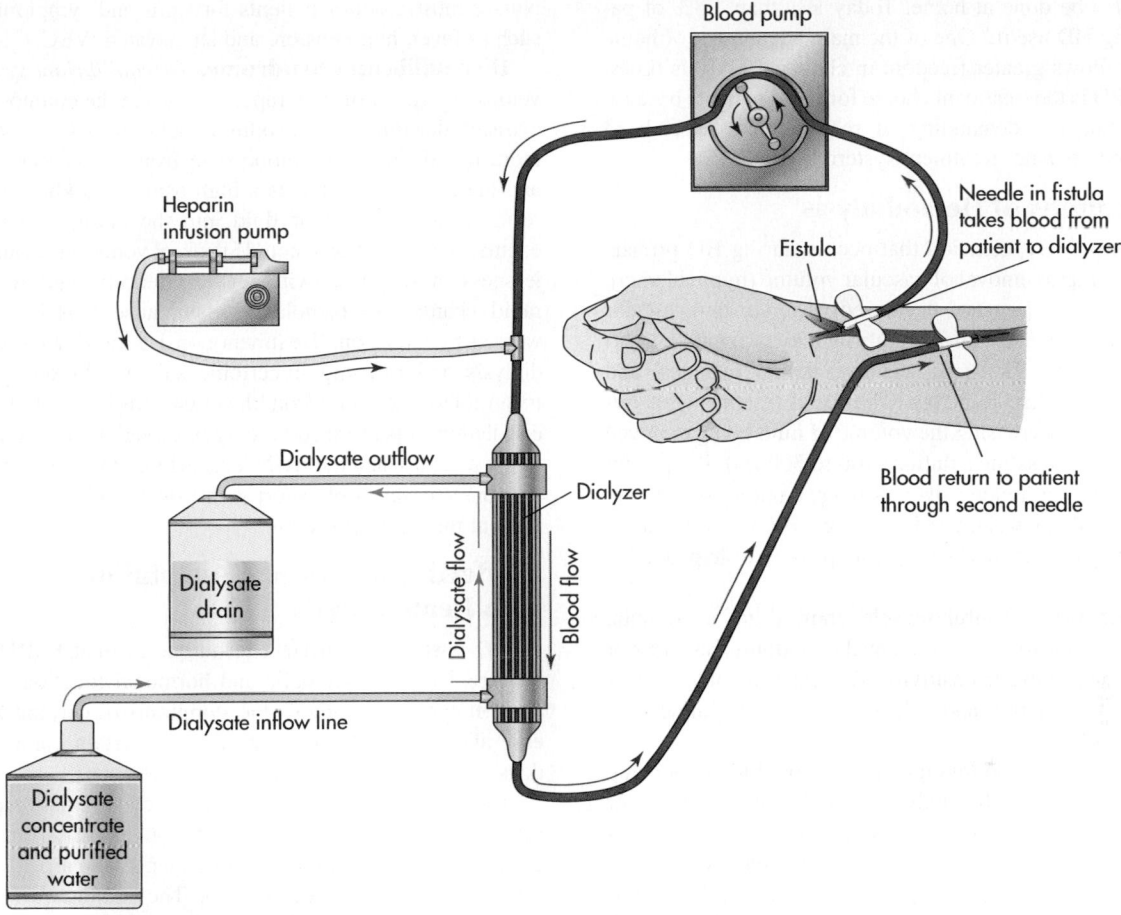

FIG. 45-14 Components of a hemodialysis system. Blood is removed via a needle inserted in a fistula or via catheter lumen. It is propelled to the dialyzer by a blood pump. Heparin is infused to prevent clotting. Dialysate is pumped in and flows in the opposite direction of the blood. The dialyzed blood is returned to the patient through a second needle or catheter lumen. Old dialysate and ultrafiltrate are drained and discarded.

postdialysis weight and the present predialysis weight determines the ultrafiltration or the amount of weight to be removed. Ideally, no more than 1 to 1.5 kg should be gained between treatments to avoid causing hypotension associated with the removal of larger volumes of fluid. Many patients gain 2 to 3 kg between treatments, and this volume usually can be removed if their BP is not labile. While the patient is on dialysis, vital signs should be taken at least every 30 to 60 minutes because rapid changes may occur in the BP.

Most maintenance dialysis units use reclining chairs that allow for elevation of the feet if hypotension develops. Most people sleep, read, talk, or watch television during dialysis. Treatments usually last 3 to 5 hours and are done three times per week to achieve adequate clearance and maintain fluid balance.

Settings for Hemodialysis. HD can be done in an inpatient (hospital) or outpatient (clinic or hospital) setting. Inpatient dialysis is used for treating hospitalized patients. In outpatient dialysis the patient comes to the unit for treatment. The patient may choose to do self-care with backup support from trained personnel if needed. Self-care patients put in the dialysis needles, set up the machine, and monitor the course of the treatment.

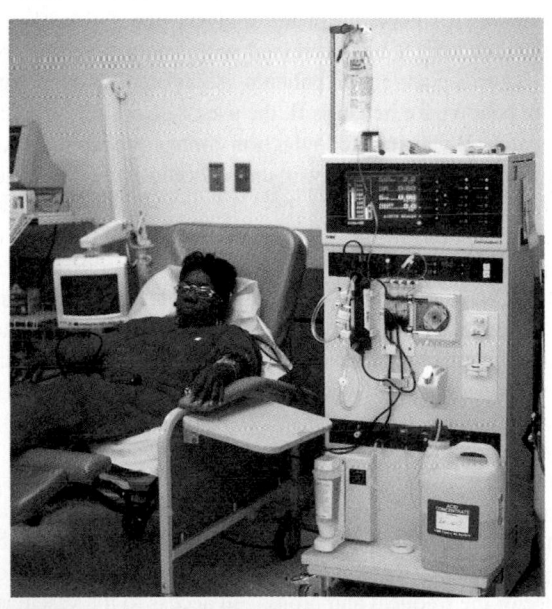

FIG. 45-15 Patient receiving in-center hemodialysis.

HD can also be done at home. Today less than 1.3% of patients receiving HD use it.[8] One of the main advantages of home HD is that it allows greater freedom in choosing dialysis times. Today home PD is the treatment choice for more patients because it is less technically demanding, it requires less specialized equipment, and no water treatment system is needed.

Complications of Hemodialysis

Hypotension. Hypotension that occurs during HD primarily results from rapid removal of vascular volume (hypovolemia), decreased cardiac output, and decreased systemic intravascular resistance. The drop in BP during dialysis may precipitate light-headedness, nausea, vomiting, seizures, vision changes, and chest pain from cardiac ischemia. The usual treatment for hypotension includes decreasing the volume of fluid being removed and infusion of 0.9% saline solution (100 to 300 ml). If a patient experiences recurrent hypotensive episodes, a reassessment may have to be done of dry weight and BP drugs. BP drugs should be held before dialysis if there are frequent episodes of hypotension during dialysis.

Muscle Cramps. Painful muscle cramps are a common problem. They result from rapid removal of sodium and water or from neuromuscular hypersensitivity. Treatment includes reducing the ultrafiltration rate and infusing hypertonic saline or a normal saline bolus.

Loss of Blood. Blood loss may result from blood not being completely rinsed from the dialyzer, accidental separation of blood tubing, dialysis membrane rupture, or bleeding after the removal of needles at the end of dialysis. If a patient has received too much heparin or has clotting problems, there can be significant postdialysis bleeding. It is essential to rinse back all blood, to closely monitor heparinization to avoid excess anticoagulation, and to hold firm but nonocclusive pressure on access sites until the risk of bleeding has passed.

Hepatitis. The causes of hepatitis B and C in dialysis patients include blood transfusions or the lack of adherence to precautions used to prevent the spread of infection. As blood is now screened for hepatitis B and C, blood is an unlikely source of infection. IV drug abuse and unprotected sex can also contribute to the incidence of hepatitis in the dialysis population. The incidence of hepatitis B has decreased with frequent testing for hepatitis B surface antigen in patients, isolation of dialysis patients who are positive for hepatitis B, the use of disposable equipment, the hepatitis B vaccine, and infection control precautions. All patients and personnel in dialysis units should receive hepatitis B vaccine.

Currently, hepatitis C is responsible for the majority of cases of hepatitis in dialysis patients. (Hepatitis is discussed in more detail in Chapter 42.) The Centers for Disease Control and Prevention does not recommend isolation of the HD patient who has hepatitis C. Infection control precautions are mandated in the care of the patient with hepatitis C to protect the patient and staff. (Infection control precautions are discussed in Chapter 12.) Currently, no vaccine is available for hepatitis C.

Sepsis. Sepsis is most often related to infections of vascular access sites. Bacteria can also be introduced during the dialysis treatment as a result of poor technique or interruption of blood tubing or dialyzer membranes. Bacterial endocarditis can occur because of the frequent and prolonged access to the vascular system. Aseptic technique is essential to prevent this problem.

Nurses must monitor patients for signs and symptoms of sepsis such as fever, hypotension, and an elevated WBC.

Disequilibrium Syndrome. *Disequilibrium syndrome* develops as a result of very rapid changes in the composition of the extracellular fluid. Urea, sodium, and other solutes are removed more rapidly from the blood than from the cerebrospinal fluid and the brain. This creates a high osmotic gradient in the brain resulting in the shift of fluid into the brain, causing cerebral edema. Manifestations include nausea, vomiting, confusion, restlessness, headaches, twitching and jerking, and seizures. The rapid changes in osmolality may cause muscle cramps and worsen hypotension. Treatment consists of slowing or stopping dialysis and infusing hypertonic saline solution, albumin, or mannitol to draw fluid from the brain cells back into the systemic circulation. It is more commonly observed in the initial treatment of the patient when the BUN level is high. First dialysis treatment sessions are purposely short with limited total solute removal to prevent this rare syndrome.

Effectiveness of and Adaptation to Hemodialysis

HD is still an imperfect technique to treat ESRD. It cannot fully replace the metabolic and hormonal functions of the kidneys. It can ease many of the symptoms of chronic kidney disease and, if started early, can prevent certain complications. It does not alter the accelerated atherosclerosis.

The yearly death rate of patients receiving maintenance dialysis has increased to 22%.[8] The major reason for this is the increased proportion of older adult patients who are now receiving dialysis as maintenance therapy. The majority of deaths are caused by cardiovascular disease (stroke or myocardial infarction). Infectious complications are the second leading cause of death.

Individual adaptation to maintenance HD varies considerably. Initially many patients feel positive about the dialysis because it makes them feel better and keeps them alive, but there is often great ambivalence about whether it is worthwhile. Dependence on a machine is a reality, and some have dreams about being tied to the machine. In response to their illness, dialysis patients may demonstrate noncompliance, depression, and suicidal tendencies. The primary nursing goals are to help the patient regain or maintain positive self-esteem and control of his or her life and to continue to be productive in society.[25]

CONTINUOUS RENAL REPLACEMENT THERAPY

Continuous renal replacement therapy (CRRT) is an alternative or adjunctive method for treating ARF. CRRT provides a means by which solutes and a large volume of fluid can be removed slowly and continuously from a hemodynamically unstable patient. Continuous renal replacement therapies are contraindicated if a patient has life-threatening manifestations of uremia (hyperkalemia, pericarditis) that require rapid resolution.[26] CRRT can be used in conjunction with HD for continuous fluid removal.

There are several technical variations of CRRT. Both fluid and solute removal can be achieved with continuous therapies. There are two types of CRRT differentiated by whether arterial or venous access is required and if a blood pump is needed (Table 45-11). The continuous arteriovenous therapies (CAVTs) require arterial

TABLE 45-11 **Types of Continuous Renal Replacement Therapies**

ACRONYM	THERAPY	PURPOSE
SCUF (AV)	Slow continuous ultrafiltration	Fluid removal via ultrafiltration
CVVU (VV)	Continuous venovenous ultrafiltration	Solute loss via convection
CAVH (AV)	Continuous arteriovenous hemofiltration	Fluid removal via ultrafiltration
CVVH (VV)	Continuous venovenous hemofiltration	Solute loss via convection; hemodilution using replacement fluid
CAVHD (AV)	Continuous arteriovenous hemodialysis	Fluid removal via ultrafiltration and osmosis
CVVHD (VV)	Continuous venovenous hemodialysis	Solute loss via convection and diffusion

AA, Arteriovenous; *VV,* venovenous.

access because the arterial pressure is needed to pump blood through the circuit that is placed between the arterial and venous catheters (Fig. 45-16). Vascular access is usually achieved by cannulation of the femoral artery and femoral, jugular, or subclavian vein. Rarely, an external shunt may be placed. The CAVTs include slow continuous ultrafiltration (SCUF), continuous arteriovenous

hemofiltration (CAVH), and continuous arteriovenous hemodialysis (CAVHD). There are other more complex mixed modalities.

Continuous venovenous therapies (CVVTs) achieve the same goals as CAVT but use venous dual-lumen catheters for access, necessitating the use of a blood pump to propel the blood through the circuit (Fig. 45-17). The CVVTs include continuous venovenous ultrafiltration (CVVU), continuous venovenous hemofiltration (CVVH), and continuous venovenous hemodialysis (CVVHD). In many clinical situations, CVVT is preferred because it is difficult to obtain and maintain arterial access for long periods.

In CRRT a highly permeable, hollow fiber hemofilter placed between the two catheter lumens removes plasma water and nonprotein solutes, which are collectively termed *ultrafiltrate.* Under the influence of hydrostatic pressure and osmotic pressure, water and nonprotein solutes pass out of the filter into the extracapillary space and drain through the ultrafiltrate port into a collection device (see Fig. 45-16). The remaining fluid continues through the filter and returns to the patient through the second catheter or catheter lumen. While the ultrafiltrate drains out of the hemofilter, fluid and electrolyte replacements can be infused into the venous line infusion port. This fluid is designed to replace volume and solutes such as sodium, chloride, bicarbonate, and glucose. It will also further dilute intravascular fluid, decreasing the concentration of unwanted solutes such as BUN, creatinine, and potassium. The infusion rate of replacement fluid is determined by the degree of fluid and electrolyte imbalance. Replacement fluid may also be infused into the arterial line infusion port. This method allows for greater clearance of urea and can decrease filter clotting.

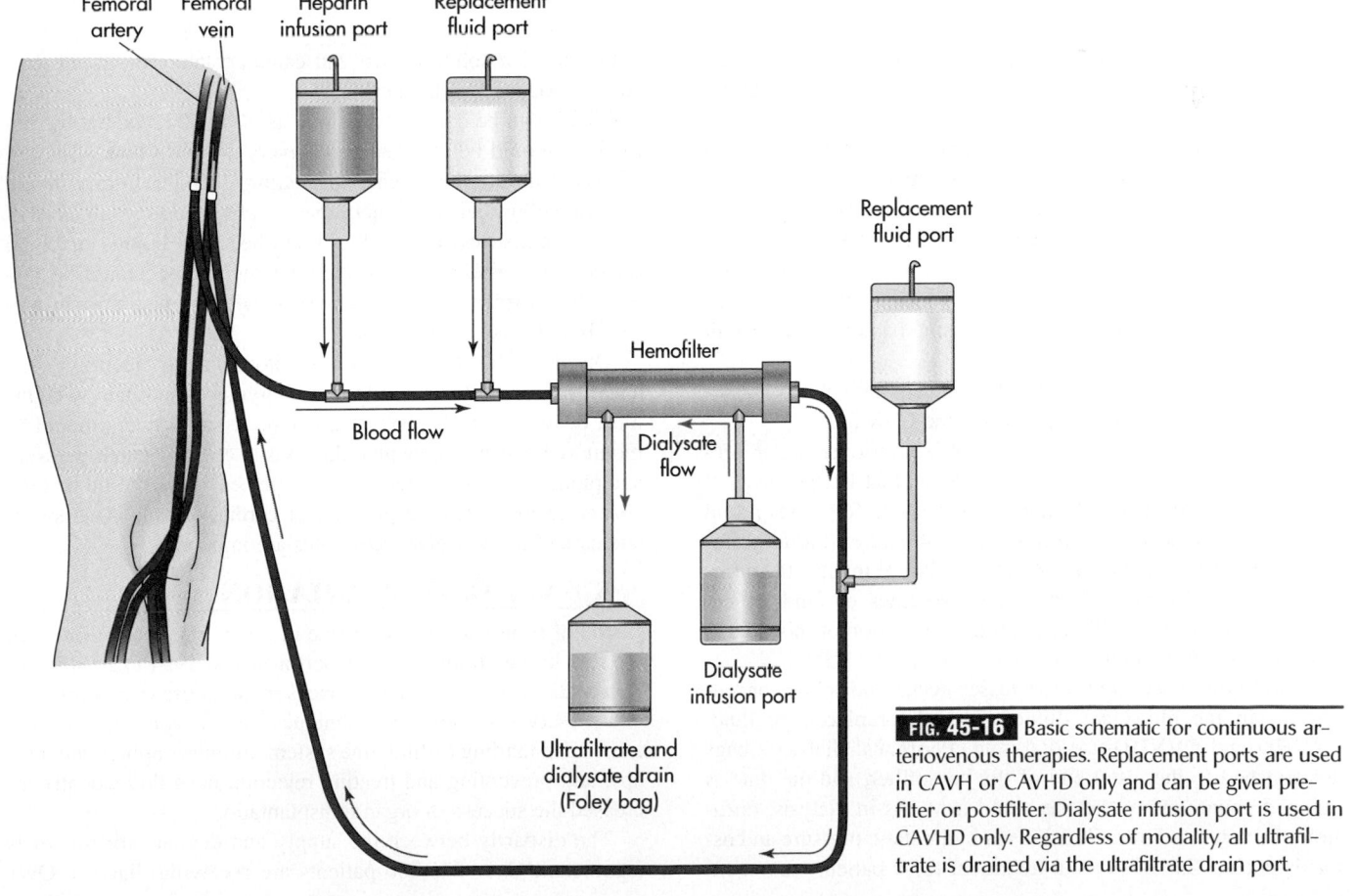

FIG. 45-16 Basic schematic for continuous arteriovenous therapies. Replacement ports are used in CAVH or CAVHD only and can be given prefilter or postfilter. Dialysate infusion port is used in CAVHD only. Regardless of modality, all ultrafiltrate is drained via the ultrafiltrate drain port.

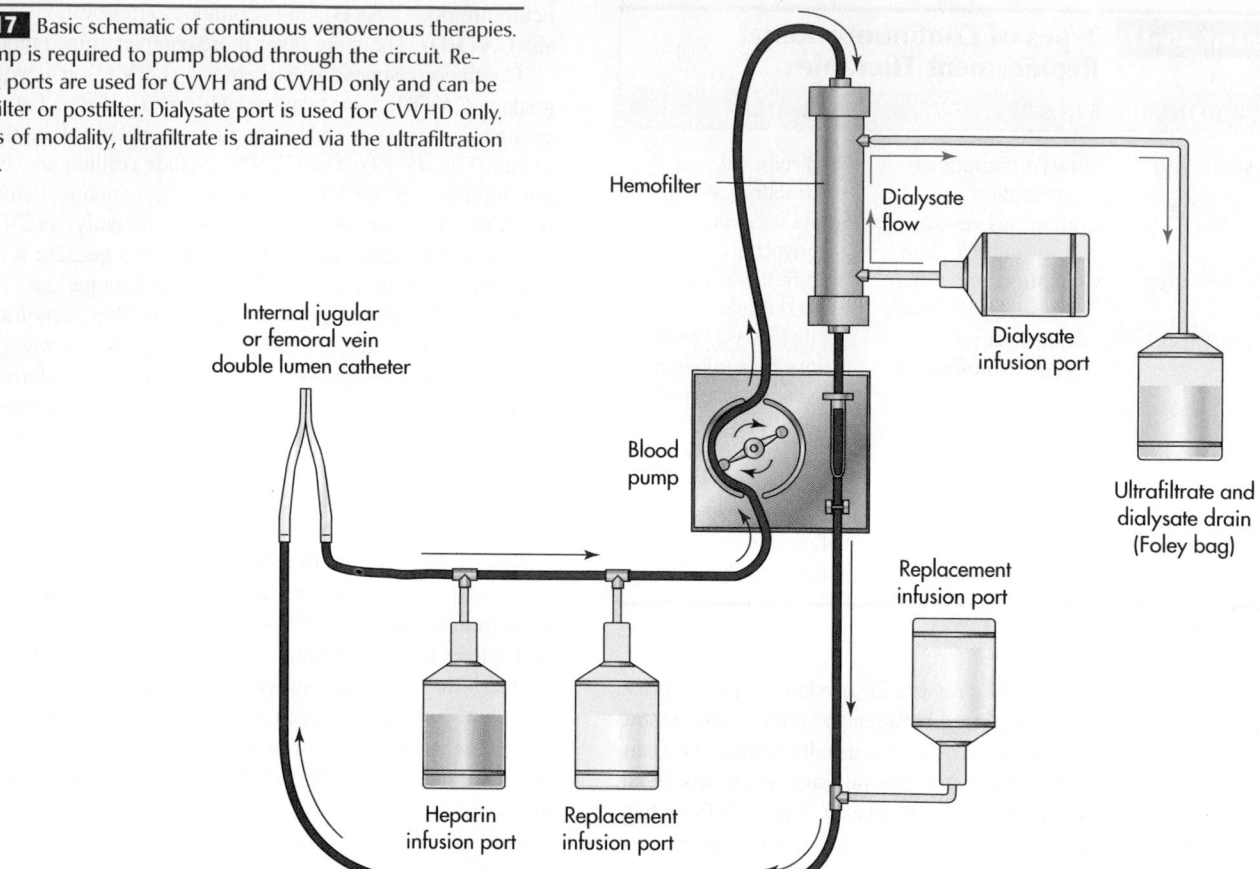

FIG. 45-17 Basic schematic of continuous venovenous therapies. Blood pump is required to pump blood through the circuit. Replacement ports are used for CVVH and CVVHD only and can be given prefilter or postfilter. Dialysate port is used for CVVHD only. Regardless of modality, ultrafiltrate is drained via the ultrafiltration drain port.

Hemofilter

Dialysate flow

Dialysate infusion port

Ultrafiltrate and dialysate drain (Foley bag)

Internal jugular or femoral vein double lumen catheter

Blood pump

Replacement infusion port

Heparin infusion port

Replacement infusion port

Like HD, CRRT provides for the removal of fluid, electrolytes, and solutes. However, several of its features differ from HD, including the following:

1. It is continuous rather than intermittent. Large volumes can be removed over days versus hours.
2. Solute removal can occur by *convection* (no dialysate required) in addition to osmosis and diffusion.
3. It causes less hemodynamic instability (e.g., hypotension).
4. It does not require constant monitoring by a specialized HD nurse but does require a trained intensive care unit (ICU) nurse.
5. It does not require complicated HD equipment, but a modified blood pump is required for the CVVTs.

Regardless of whether the modality is arteriovenous or venovenous, each modality has three therapies that have equivalent outcomes. SCUF and CVVU are strictly for ultrafiltration or fluid removal. There is some convective loss of solutes, but no diffusion or osmosis is involved. CAVH and CVVH involve the introduction of replacement fluids. Large volumes of fluid are removed hourly (600 to 900 ml), and then a portion of this fluid is replaced (500 to 800 ml).

Ultrafiltration and convective losses occur, and solute concentrations in the blood are diluted with the replacement fluid. CAVHD and CVVHD use dialysate. Peritoneal dialysate bags are attached to the distal end of the hemofilter, and the fluid is pumped countercurrent to the blood flow. As in dialysis, diffusion of solutes and ultrafiltration via hydrostatic pressure and osmosis occur. This is an ideal treatment for a patient who needs both fluid and solute control but cannot tolerate the rapid fluid shifts associated with HD.[27]

CRRT can be continued as long as 30 to 40 days, but the hemofilter should be changed about every 24 to 48 hours because of loss of filtration efficiency or clotting. The ultrafiltrate should be clear yellow, and specimens may be obtained for evaluation of serum chemistries. If the ultrafiltrate becomes bloody or blood tinged, a possible rupture in the filter membrane should be suspected, and treatment should be suspended immediately to prevent blood loss and infection.

During CRRT the nurse must monitor fluid and electrolyte balance. Hourly intake and output measurements and daily weights must be recorded. Vital signs and hemodynamic status should be monitored hourly. Although reductions in central venous pressure and pulmonary artery pressure are expected, there should be little change in mean arterial pressure or cardiac output. Assessment and care of the vascular access sites are important.

KIDNEY TRANSPLANTATION

Major progress has been made in organ transplantation since the first kidney transplant was performed in 1954 in Boston between identical twins. The advances made in organ procurement and preservation, surgical techniques, tissue typing and matching, understanding the immune system, immunosuppressant therapy, and preventing and treating rejection have dramatically increased the success of organ transplantation.

The disparity between the supply and demand for organs is significant. Over 245,000 patients are receiving dialysis. Over

54,000 patients are currently awaiting cadaveric kidney transplants, but only about 8000 cadaveric transplants were performed in 2002. Over 5200 living donor kidney transplants were done in 2002. Transplantation from a cadaver donor usually requires a prolonged waiting period, with median waiting times of 18 months to 4 years depending on blood type and other factors. Blood types B and O have the longest waiting times.[28]

Kidney transplantation is extremely successful, with 1-year graft survival rates of about 90% for cadaver transplants and 95% for live donor transplants.[28] An advantage of kidney transplantation when compared with dialysis is that it reverses many of the pathophysiologic changes associated with renal failure when normal kidney function is restored. It also eliminates the dependence on dialysis and the accompanying dietary and lifestyle restrictions. Transplantation is also less expensive than dialysis after the first year.

Recipient Selection

Appropriate recipient selection is important for a successful outcome. Candidacy is determined by a variety of medical and psychosocial factors that vary among transplant centers. A careful evaluation is completed in an attempt to identify and minimize potential complications after transplantation. Certain patients, particularly those with cardiovascular disease and diabetes mellitus, are considered high risk. With careful evaluation and monitoring, high-risk patients can achieve the same success rates as other patients.[29] Some patients who are approaching ESRD can receive a transplant before dialysis is required if they have a living donor. This approach is most advantageous for patients with diabetes, who have a much higher mortality rate on dialysis than nondiabetics.

Contraindications to transplantation include disseminated malignancies, refractory or untreated cardiac disease, chronic respiratory failure, extensive vascular disease, chronic infection, and unresolved psychosocial disorders (e.g., noncompliance with medical regimens, alcoholism, drug addiction). The presence of hepatitis B or C is not a contraindication to transplantation.

Surgical procedures may be required before transplantation based on the results of the recipient evaluation. Coronary artery bypass may be indicated for advanced coronary artery disease. Cholecystectomy may be necessary for patients with a history of gallstones, biliary obstruction, or cholecystitis. On rare occasions, bilateral nephrectomies may be done for patients with refractory hypertension, recurrent urinary tract infections, or grossly enlarged kidneys resulting from polycystic kidney disease.

Histocompatibility Studies

Histocompatibility testing is discussed in Chapter 13 on p. 256.

Donor Sources

Kidneys for transplantation may be obtained from compatible blood type cadaver donors, blood relatives, emotionally related living donors (e.g., spouses, friends), and altruistic living donors who are unknown to the recipient. Expanding the living donor pool is one of the best possibilities for decreasing the size of the cadaveric waiting list and reducing waiting times.

Live Donors. Live donors must undergo an extensive multidisciplinary evaluation to be certain that they are in good health and have no history of disease that would place them at risk for

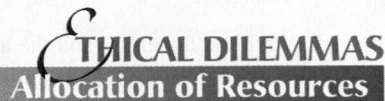

ETHICAL DILEMMAS
Allocation of Resources

Situation

A transplant nurse coordinator is considering her feelings about two patients who are being evaluated for placement on the cadaveric kidney transplant waiting list. One patient is a 40-year-old African American school teacher. She is married and has two children. The other patient is a 22-year-old unemployed white male who is actively using cocaine. He misses 3 to 4 dialysis treatments per month and does not take his phosphate binders or antihypertensive drugs consistently.

Important Points for Consideration

- It is tempting to believe that nurses can be neutral, basing allocation of scarce resources on need rather than worth. However, it is difficult to practice patient-neutral care.
- Psychologic, physiologic, and adherence factors are included in the assessment process for eligibility for organ transplantation.
- In kidney transplantation, the organ is transplanted into the patient who has received the most points based on a scoring system, regardless of the health care provider's opinion of the patient's worth. If a patient is denied transplant candidacy on this basis, he or she must be given a chance to change or improve the problem or condition in a specified period.
- The national organ procurement system is designed to be unbiased about the patient in all respects. Once a patient is placed on the list for transplantation, that patient is deemed of no greater or lesser worth than any other patient.
- Because organ donation is voluntary and altruistic in the United States, any concerns that the system of procurement and transplantation is not fair may negatively affect the pool of available organs.

Critical Thinking Questions

1. What does the 2001 American Nurses Association (ANA) Code of Ethics say about how nurses should view patients?
2. What are your feelings about which of the patients should receive the next available organ?

developing kidney failure or operative complications. Psychosocial and financial evaluations are done as well. Crossmatches are done at the time of the evaluation and about a week before the transplant to ensure that no antibodies to the donor are present or that the antibody titer is below the allowed level. Advantages of a live donor kidney include better patient and graft survival rates regardless of histocompatibility match, immediate organ availability, immediate function because of minimal cold time (kidney out of body and not getting blood supply), and the opportunity to have the recipient in the best possible medical condition because the surgery is elective.

As a result of advances in technology and immunology, living donors do not necessarily need to be ABO compatible with the recipient. Plasmapheresis can be used to remove the antibodies to the incompatible blood group, and potent immunosuppression and immunomodulation with IV immune globulin dampen the response to the antibody. It is also possible to have some antibodies to the donor human leukocyte antigens (HLA) present and still proceed with the transplant. These antibodies can also be removed with plasmapheresis and the antibody level reduced with significant immunosuppression and immunomodulation. ABO incompatibility or the presence of antibody to the donor's HLA complicates the transplant process. However, because the donor shortage is severe, complex measures are necessary to ensure that as many patients as possible are transplanted.

The donor will see a nephrologist for a complete history and physical and laboratory and diagnostic studies. Laboratory studies include a 24-hour urine study for creatinine clearance and total protein, complete blood count, and chemistry and electrolyte profiles. Hepatitis B and C, HIV, and cytomegalovirus (CMV) testing are done to assess for the presence of any transmissible diseases. An ECG and chest x-ray are also done. A renal ultrasound and a renal arteriogram or three-dimensional CT are performed to ensure that the blood vessels supplying each kidney are adequate and that there are no anomalies and to determine which kidney will be removed.

A transplant psychologist or social worker will determine if the individual is emotionally stable and able to deal with the issues related to organ donation. All donors must be informed about the risks and benefits of donation, the potential short-term and long-term complications, and what can be expected during the hospitalization and recovery phases. Although the cost of the evaluation and surgery are covered by the recipient's insurance, there is no compensation available for lost wages during the posthospitalization recovery period. This period can last 6 weeks or longer. The laparoscopic donor nephrectomy procedure shortens the amount of time before a person can return to work or other usual activities.[30]

Cadaver Donors. Cadaver kidney donors are relatively healthy individuals who have suffered an irreversible brain injury. The most common causes of injury are cerebral trauma from motor vehicle accidents or gunshot wounds, intracerebral or subarachnoid hemorrhage, and anoxic brain damage caused by cardiac arrest. The brain-dead donor must have effective cardiovascular function and be supported on a ventilator to preserve the organs. The age range of most suitable kidney donors is from 2 to 70 years. The age of the donor is less important than the quality of kidney function. The donor must be free of active IV drug abuse; severe hypertension; long-standing diabetes mellitus; malignancies; sepsis; and communicable diseases, including HIV, hepatitis B and C, syphilis, and tuberculosis. Permission from the donor's legal next-of-kin is required after brain death is determined even if the donor carried a signed donor card.

The kidneys are removed and preserved. They can be preserved for up to 72 hours, but most transplant surgeons prefer to transplant kidneys before the cold time reaches 24 hours. Experience has shown that prolonged cold time increases the likelihood that the kidney will not function immediately, and the transplant recipient will require dialysis until the ATN from the extended cold time resolves.

Cadaveric kidneys are distributed by the United Network for Organ Sharing using an objective computerized point system. The ABO group, HLA typing, age, antibody level, and length of time waiting are entered into the national computer for each candidate when they are listed. When a donor becomes available, the donor's HLA data, ABO type, and other key information are compared with the data of all patients awaiting transplantation locally and nationwide. Donors rend recipients must have the same blood type. Points are given for how close the HLA match is, how long the patient has been waiting, if the antibody level is unusually high, and if the recipient is less than 19 years old. Extra points are given for high antibody levels because this can severely limit the number of donors with which the patient will not have a positive crossmatch. The kidney is offered to the recipient with the most points in the local area. If there are no patients in the local area who are suitable, the organ is then offered in the region and then to the nation. When a kidney arrives at the recipient's transplant center, a final crossmatch is done. The final crossmatch must be negative for the cadaveric transplant to proceed. (Crossmatching is discussed in Chapter 13.)

The only exception to the previous plan is if a patient needs an emergency transplant or if a donor and recipient do not mismatch on any of the six HLA antigens (zero antigen mismatch). In these situations, the patient meeting either one of these criteria goes to the top of the list. Emergency transplants are given priority because the patient is facing imminent death if not transplanted (for example, a patient who had no vascular access sites left and can no longer dialyze). Zero antigen mismatches are given priority because statistically these grafts have much better survival rates. If a zero antigen mismatch patient is identified nationally, one of the donor kidneys must be sent to that recipient's transplant center regardless of location.

Surgical Procedure

Live Donor. The donor nephrectomy is performed by a urologist or transplant surgeon. The donor's surgery begins an hour or two before the recipient's surgery is started. The recipient is surgically prepared for the kidney transplant in a nearby operating room. For a conventional nephrectomy, the donor is placed in the lateral decubitus position on the operating table so that the flank is presented laterally. An incision is made at the level of the eleventh rib. The rib may have to be removed to provide adequate visualization of the kidney. After removal of the kidney, it is flushed with a chilled, sterile electrolyte solution and prepared for immediate transplant into the recipient. The nephrectomy takes about 3 hours. The short cold time is the primary reason for the success of living donor transplants.

Laparoscopic donor nephrectomy is an alternative to a conventional nephrectomy. (Laparoscopic nephrectomy is discussed in Chapter 44.) This procedure is now being used as the primary method of live kidney procurement. The laparoscopic approach significantly decreases the hospital stay, pain, operative blood loss, debilitation, and length of time off work. For these reasons, the number of people willing to donate a kidney has increased significantly.[31]

Kidney Transplant Recipient

The transplanted kidney is usually placed extraperitoneally in the iliac fossa. The right iliac fossa is preferred to facilitate anastomoses and minimize the occurrence of ileus.

Before any incisions are made, a urinary catheter is placed into the bladder. An antibiotic solution is instilled to distend the bladder and decrease the risk of infection. A crescent-shaped incision is made extending from the iliac crest to the symphysis pubis (Fig. 45-18). The peritoneum is left intact. The iliac and hypogastric vessels are dissected free.

Rapid revascularization is critical to prevent ischemic injury to the kidney. The donor artery is anastomosed to the recipient's internal iliac (hypogastric) or external iliac artery. The donor vein is anastomosed to the recipient's external iliac vein. Kidney transplants with living donors can be technically more difficult because the blood vessel lengths can be shorter than in cadaveric transplants.

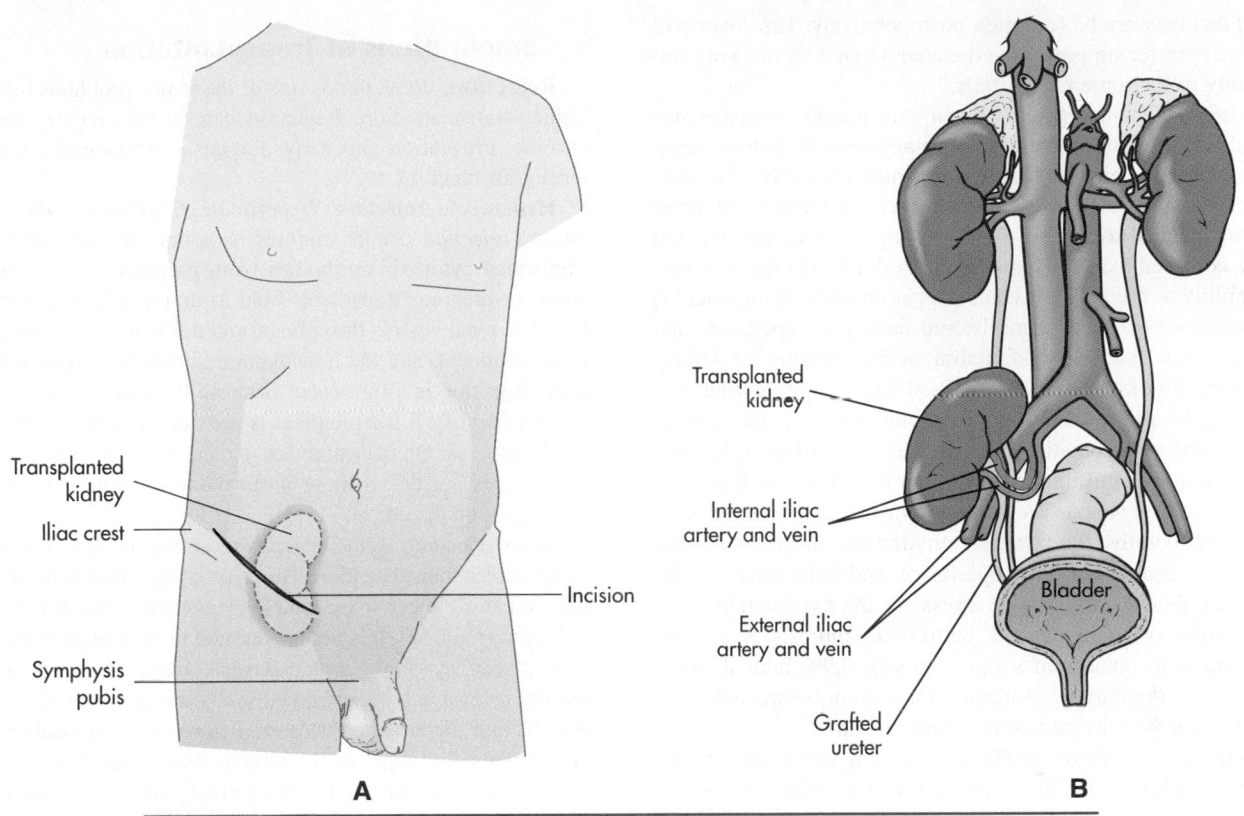

FIG. 45-18 A, Surgical incision for a renal transplant. B, Surgical placement of transplanted kidney.

When the anastomoses are complete, the clamps are released, and blood flow to the kidney is reestablished. The kidney should become firm and pink. Urine may begin to flow from the ureter immediately. Mannitol or furosemide (Lasix) may be administered to promote diuresis.

The donor ureter in most cases is then tunneled through the bladder submucosa before entering the bladder cavity and being sutured in place. This approach is called *ureteroneocystostomy*. This allows the bladder wall to compress the ureter as it contracts for micturition, thereby preventing reflux of urine up the ureter into the transplanted kidney. The transplant surgery takes approximately 3 to 4 hours.

NURSING MANAGEMENT
KIDNEY TRANSPLANT RECIPIENT

The successful recovery and rehabilitation of the recipient are made possible with careful nursing assessment, diagnosis, intervention, and evaluation of all body systems. With a hospital length of stay averaging 4 to 5 days, discharge planning and teaching needs must be identified and addressed early in the hospital course.

■ Preoperative Care

Nursing care of the patient in the preoperative phase includes emotional and physical preparation for surgery. Because the patient and family may have been waiting years for the kidney transplant, a review of the operative procedure and what can be expected in the immediate postoperative recovery period is necessary. It is important to stress that there is a chance the kidney may not function immediately, and dialysis may be required for

days to weeks. The need for immunosuppressive drugs and measures to prevent infection must be reviewed.

To ensure the patient is in optimal physical condition for surgery, an ECG, chest x-ray, and laboratory studies are ordered. Dialysis may be required before surgery for any significant abnormality such as fluid overload or hyperkalemia. A patient on PD must empty the peritoneal cavity of all dialysate solution before going to surgery. Because dialysis may be required after transplant, the patency of the vascular access must be maintained. The vascular access extremity should be labeled "dialysis access, no procedures" to prevent use of the affected extremity for BP measurement, blood drawing, or IV infusions.

■ Postoperative Care

Live Donor. The usual postoperative care for the donor is similar to that following conventional or laparoscopic nephrectomy (see Chapter 44). Close monitoring of renal function to assess for impairment and of the hematocrit to assess for bleeding is essential. The creatinine should be less than 1.4 mg/dl, and the hematocrit should not fall more than 3 to 6 points. The pain that a donor who has had a conventional nephrectomy experiences is greater than that of the donor who had a laparoscopic procedure. Generally, all donors have more pain than their recipients. Conventional donors are ready to be discharged from the hospital in 4 to 7 days and can usually return to work in 6 to 8 weeks. Laparoscopic donors are able to be discharged from the hospital in 2 to 4 days and can return to work in 4 to 6 weeks. The donor is seen by the surgeon 1 to 2 weeks after discharge.

Nurses caring for the living donor need to acknowledge the precious gift that this person has given. The donor has taken physical, emotional, and financial risks to assist the recipient. It is vital that they not be forgotten postoperatively. The donor will need even greater support if the donated organ does not work immediately or for some reason fails.

Recipient. The first priority during this period is maintenance of fluid and electrolyte balance. In many centers, kidney transplant recipients spend the first 12 to 24 hours in the ICU because of the close monitoring required. Very large volumes of urine may be produced soon after the blood supply to the transplanted kidney is reestablished. This diuresis is due to (1) the new kidney's ability to filter BUN, which acts as an osmotic diuretic; (2) the abundance of fluids administered during the operation; and (3) initial renal tubular dysfunction, which inhibits the kidney from concentrating urine normally. Urine output during this phase may be as high as 1 L per hour and gradually decreases as the BUN and serum creatinine levels return toward normal. Urine output is replaced milliliter for milliliter hourly for the first 12 to 24 hours. Central venous pressure readings are essential for monitoring postoperative fluid status. Dehydration must be avoided to prevent subsequent renal hypoperfusion and renal tubular damage. Electrolyte monitoring to assess for the hyponatremia and hypokalemia often associated with rapid diuresis is critical. Treatment with potassium supplements or 0.9% normal saline solution infusion may be indicated. IV sodium bicarbonate may also be required if the patient becomes acidotic.

Acute tubular necrosis (ATN) is becoming more common because of prolonged cold times and the use of marginal donors. The ischemic damage from extended cold times causes ATN. While the patient is in ATN, dialysis is required to maintain fluid and electrolyte balance. Some patients have high-output ATN with the ability to excrete fluid, but not metabolic wastes or electrolytes. Other patients have oliguric or anuric ATN. These patients are at risk for fluid overload in the immediate postoperative period and must be assessed closely for the need for dialysis. The period of ATN can last anywhere from days to weeks, with gradually improving kidney function. Most patients with ATN will be discharged from the hospital on dialysis. This is extremely discouraging for the patient, who will need reassurance that renal function usually improves. Dialysis will be discontinued when urine output increases and serum creatinine and BUN begin to normalize.

A sudden decrease in urine output in the early postoperative period is a cause for concern. It may be due to dehydration, rejection, a urine leak, or obstruction. A common cause of early obstruction is a blood clot in the urinary catheter. Catheter patency must be maintained as the catheter remains in the bladder for 3 to 5 days to allow the bladder anastomosis to heal. If blood clots are suspected, gentle catheter irrigation with an order from the health care provider can reestablish patency.

Postoperative teaching should include the prevention and treatment of rejection, infection, and complications of surgery and the purpose and side effects of immunosuppression. Patients should be aware that rejection is a common occurrence during the first 3 months after transplant. Frequent blood tests and clinic visits help detect rejection early. Patient education to ensure a smooth transition from hospital to home is an integral part of the nursing care.[32]

Immunosuppressive Therapy

The goal of immunosuppression is to adequately suppress the immune response to prevent rejection of the transplanted kidney while maintaining sufficient immunity to prevent overwhelming infection. Immunosuppressive therapy is discussed in Chapter 13 and in Table 13-17.

Complications of Transplantation

Rejection. Rejection is one of the major problems following kidney transplantation. Rejection can be hyperacute, acute, or chronic. Prevention and early diagnosis are essential for long-term graft function.

Hyperacute rejection. *Hyperacute (antibody-mediated, humoral) rejection* occurs minutes to hours after transplantation. Preformed cytotoxic antibodies from pregnancy, blood transfusions, or previous transplants bind to donor antigens in the kidney. The renal vessels thrombose, and the kidney necroses. There is no treatment, and the transplanted kidney is removed. Hyperacute rejection is a rare event because the final crossmatch will usually identify if the recipient is sensitized to any of the donor HLA antigens. On occasion, for unclear reasons, the final crossmatch does not detect these preformed antibodies, and hyperacute rejection occurs.

Acute rejection. *Acute rejection* most commonly occurs days to months after transplantation. This type of rejection is mediated by the recipient's T cytotoxic lymphocytes, which attack the foreign kidney (Fig. 45-19). It is not uncommon to have at least one rejection episode, especially with cadaver kidneys. These episodes are usually reversible with additional immunosuppressive therapy that may include increased corticosteroid doses or polyclonal or monoclonal antibodies. Signs of rejection include elevated creatinine and BUN, fever, weight gain, decreased urine output, increased BP, and tenderness over the transplanted kidney. It is sometimes difficult to distinguish between acute rejection and nephrotoxicity caused by high cyclosporine or tacrolimus (Prograf) levels.

Chronic rejection. *Chronic rejection* is a process that occurs over months or years and is irreversible. The kidney is infiltrated with large numbers of T and B cells characteristic of an ongoing,

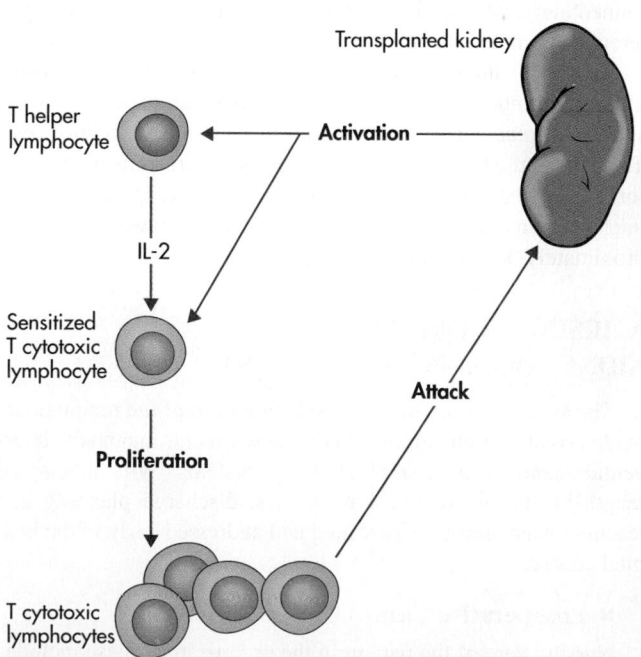

FIG. 45-19 Mechanism of action of T cytotoxic lymphocyte activation and attack of renal transplanted tissue. The transplanted kidney is recognized as foreign and activates the immune system. T helper cells are activated to produce IL-2, and T cytotoxic lymphocytes are sensitized. After these T cytotoxic cells proliferate, they attack the transplanted kidney.

low-grade immune-mediated injury. Chronic rejection is associated with a gradual occlusion of the renal blood vessels. Signs include proteinuria, hypertension, and increasing serum creatinine levels. There is no definitive therapy for this type of rejection. Changing immunosuppressive therapy to include tacrolimus or mycophenolate mofetil (CellCept) has brought some improvement for some patients who were not previously taking these drugs. Treatment is mainly supportive. This type of rejection is difficult to manage and is not associated with the optimistic prognosis of acute rejection. Patients with chronic rejection should be put on the transplant list in the hope that they can be retransplanted before dialysis is required.

Infection. Infection remains a significant cause of morbidity and mortality after transplantation.[33] The transplant recipient is at risk for infection because of suppression of the body's normal defense mechanisms by surgery, immunosuppressive drugs, and the effects of ESRD. Underlying systemic illness such as diabetes mellitus or systemic lupus erythematosus, malnutrition, and older age can further compound the negative effects on the immune response. At times the signs and symptoms of infection can be subtle. Nurses caring for transplant recipients must be astute in their observation and assessment because prompt diagnosis and treatment of infections will improve patient outcomes.

The most common infections observed in the first month after transplantation are similar to those acquired by any postoperative patient, such as pneumonia, wound infections, IV line and drain infections, and urinary tract infections. Fungal and viral infections are not uncommon because of the patient's immunosuppressed state. Fungal infections can include *Candida, Cryptococcus, Aspergillus,* and *Pneumocystis carinii.* Fungal infections are difficult to treat, require prolonged treatment periods, and often involve the administration of nephrotoxic drugs. Transplant recipients usually receive prophylactic antifungal drugs to prevent these infections, such as clotrimazole (Mycelex), fluconazole (Diflucan), and sulfamethoxazole-trimethoprim (Bactrim).

Viral infections including CMV, Epstein-Barr virus, herpes simplex virus (HSV), varicella-zoster virus, and polyomavirus (e.g., BK virus) can be primary or reactivation of existing disease.[34,35] Primary infections occur as new infections after transplantation from an exogenous source such as the donated organ or blood transfusion. Reactivation occurs when a virus exists in a patient and becomes reactivated after transplantation because of immunosuppression.

CMV is one of the most common viral infections. If a recipient has never had CMV and receives an organ from a donor with a history of CMV, antiviral prophylaxis will be administered (ganciclovir IV, valganciclovir [Valcyte]). If a primary active CMV infection is diagnosed or there is symptomatic reactivation of CMV, IV ganciclovir will be given along with an immune globulin that contains CMV antibodies. To prevent HSV infections, oral acyclovir is given for several months after the transplant.

Cardiovascular Disease. Transplant recipients have an increased incidence of atherosclerotic vascular disease. Cardiovascular disease is the leading cause of death after renal transplantation.[8] Hypertension, hyperlipidemia, diabetes mellitus, smoking, rejection, infections, and increased homocysteine levels can all contribute to cardiovascular disease. Immunosuppressants can worsen hypertension and hyperlipidemia. It is important that the patient be taught to control risk factors such as elevated cholesterol, triglycerides, and blood glucose and weight gain. Adherence to the prescribed antihypertensive regimen is essential not only to prevent cardiovascular events but also to prevent damage to the new kidney. (Hypertension is discussed in Chapter 32.)

Malignancies. The overall incidence of malignancies in kidney transplant recipients is about 6%, which is 100 times greater than in the general population. The primary cause of this increased incidence is the immunosuppressive therapy. Not only do immunosuppressants suppress the immune system, but they also suppress the ability to fight infection and the production of abnormal cells such as cancer cells. The malignancies include cancer of the skin, lips, kidney, hepatobiliary system, vulva, and perineum; lymphomas; and Kaposi's sarcoma and other sarcomas. Regular screening for cancer is an important part of the transplant recipient's preventive care. The patient must also be advised to avoid sun exposure by using protective clothing and sunscreens to minimize the incidence of skin cancers.

Recurrence of Original Renal Disease. Recurrence of the original disease that destroyed the native kidneys occurs in some kidney transplant recipients. It is most common with certain types of glomerulonephritis, IgA nephropathy, diabetes mellitus, and focal segmental sclerosis. Disease recurrence can result in the loss of a functioning kidney transplant. Patients must be advised before transplant if they have a disease known to recur.

Corticosteroid-Related Complications. Aseptic necrosis of the hips, knees, and other joints can result from chronic corticosteroid therapy and renal osteodystrophy. Other significant problems related to corticosteroids include peptic ulcer disease, glucose intolerance and diabetes, cataracts, hyperlipidemia, and an increased incidence of infections and malignancies. In the first year after transplant, corticosteroid doses are usually decreased to 5 to 10 mg a day. The use of tacrolimus and cyclosporine has allowed for the corticosteroid doses to be much lower than they were in the past. Some patients have been successfully withdrawn from corticosteroids 1½ to 2 years after transplantation, thus eliminating these problems. Vigilant monitoring for side effects of corticosteroids and early treatment is essential.

■ Gerontologic Considerations: Chronic Kidney Disease

The incidence of ESRD in the United States and Canada is increasing most rapidly in older patients. The mean age of the United States ESRD population has increased. Recent data indicate that of all the patients who have ESRD about 48% are 65 or older.[8] The most common diseases leading to renal failure in the older adult are hypertension and diabetes. Medicare and non-Medicare expenditures can be expected to increase as the ESRD population ages and as a result has a greater number of comorbid conditions.

The care of the geriatric ESRD patient is particularly challenging, not only because of the normal physiologic changes of aging that occur but also because of the number of comorbid conditions that develop.[36] Physiologic changes of clinical importance in the older ESRD patient include diminished cardiopulmonary function, bone loss, immunodeficiency, altered protein synthesis, impaired cognition, and altered drug metabolism. Malnutrition is common in the older ESRD patient for a variety of reasons, including lack of mobility, lack of understanding of basic nutritional requirements, social isolation, physical disability, impaired cognitive function, and malabsorption problems.[37,38]

The older patient needs to consider what is the best treatment modality based on his or her health, personal preferences, and support available. Home PD allows the patient to be more mobile and to enjoy an increased sense of control over the illness. PD causes less hemodynamic instability than HD but does require self-care or assistance from another person. The older adult may not have adequate help in the home to provide assistance. Establishing vascular access for HD may be difficult in an older patient because of atherosclerotic changes. Travel to and from the HD unit may also be problematic if the patient does not drive or have access to reliable public transportation. Although transplantation is an option, elderly patients must be carefully screened to ensure that the benefits outweigh the risks. A living donor is preferable so that there is not a prolonged waiting time.

The most common cause of death in the elderly ESRD patient is cardiovascular disease (MI, stroke) followed by withdrawal from dialysis. If a competent patient decides to withdraw from dialysis, it is essential to support the patient and family. Ethical issues (see the Ethical Dilemmas box) to be considered in this situation include patient competency, benefit versus burden of treatment, and futility of treatment.[36] Withdrawal from treatment is not a failure if the patient is well informed and comfortable with the decision.

The increasing number of elderly, debilitated ESRD patients receiving dialysis has raised a number of ethical concerns about the use of scarce resources in a population with a limited life expectancy. Substantial evidence exists showing success of dialysis (especially PD) in the elderly. Quality of life has also been reported to be good to excellent in many older ESRD patients. There appears to be no justification for excluding the older adult from dialysis programs. Rationing dialysis on the basis of age alone is not supported based on current outcome and quality-of-life data. ■

*E*THICAL DILEMMAS
Withdrawing Treatment

Situation

A 70-year-old patient with diabetes mellitus and chronic renal failure who has been receiving dialysis for 10 years tells the nurse that he wants to discontinue his dialysis. His quality of life has diminished during the past 2 years since his wife died. He is not a prospective transplant patient.

Important Points for Consideration

- Quality of life is an important consideration for patients when weighing whether to begin or discontinue treatment.
- Quality-of-life decisions often weigh the benefit against the burden of treatment. When a treatment becomes too burdensome, the patient (if competent) may request to withdraw the treatment.
- A determination must be made if there is some other treatable problem such as depression that may be clouding the patient's judgment.
- Patient autonomy, or the patient's right to self-determination regarding treatment decisions, applies both to initiating and discontinuing treatment.
- If a decision is made to withdraw treatment, the health care team, patient, and family should develop an appropriate follow-up plan that includes palliative care and hospice support.

Critical Thinking Questions

1. How should the nurse respond to the patient's request?
2. What is the ANA's position on withdrawing or withholding treatment that no longer benefits the patient or causes suffering?

CRITICAL THINKING EXERCISES

Case Study
Chronic Kidney Disease

Patient Profile. Juanita, a 46-year-old Native American school teacher, has been treated for type 2 diabetes mellitus since the age of 25. She has been observed by her nephrologist for the past several years for manifestations of progressive chronic kidney disease. Eight weeks ago she had an arteriovenous fistula created in preparation for starting hemodialysis. Over the past week she has experienced anorexia, nausea, vomiting, problems with concentration, and pruritus.

Subjective Data

- Complains of swelling in her feet and hands
- Has gained 10 lb (4.5 kg) in the past 2 weeks
- Complains of dyspnea and weakness when walking

Objective Data

Laboratory Data

- Creatinine clearance: 8.2 ml/min
- Serum creatinine: 12.8 mg/dl (1132 mmol/L)
- BUN: 125 mg/dl (45 mmol/L)
- Potassium: 6 mEq/L (6 mmol/L)
- Hematocrit: 20%

Chest X-ray

- Pulmonary edema

CRITICAL THINKING QUESTIONS

1. Explain the basic pathophysiologic changes that resulted in the development of her diabetic nephropathy.
2. What are the indications for dialysis in this patient?
3. Identify the abnormal diagnostic study results and why each would occur.
4. Explain why Juanita developed each of her clinical manifestations.
5. What are important nursing interventions for Juanita and her family?
6. Based on the assessment data provided, write one or more nursing diagnoses. Are there any collaborative problems?

Nursing Research Issues

1. What is the psychosocial impact of dialysis on the spouse and family?
2. What nursing strategies promote compliance in the dialysis patient?
3. Are the stressors for older (>65 years) dialysis patients different from those of younger patients?
4. What is the quality of life for a living-related donor following surgery?
5. What are the needs of the family when a patient chooses to withdraw from dialysis treatment?

REVIEW QUESTIONS

The number of the question corresponds to the same-numbered objective at the beginning of the chapter.

1. A patient is admitted to the hospital with chronic kidney disease. The nurse understands that this condition is characterized by
   a. progressive irreversible destruction of the kidneys.
   b. a rapid decrease in urinary output with an elevated BUN.
   c. an increasing creatinine clearance with a decrease in urinary output.
   d. prostration, somnolence, and confusion with coma and imminent death.

2. Prerenal causes of ARF include
   a. prostate cancer and calculi formation.
   b. hypovolemia and myocardial infarction.
   c. acute glomerulonephritis and neoplasms.
   d. septic shock and nephrotoxic injury from drugs.

3. During the oliguric phase of ARF, the nurse monitors the patient for
   a. hypernatremia and CNS depression.
   b. pulmonary edema and ECG changes.
   c. Kussmaul respirations and hypotension.
   d. urine with high specific gravity and low sodium concentration.

4. If a patient is in the diuretic phase of ARF, the nurse must monitor for which serum electrolyte imbalances?
   a. Hyperkalemia and hyponatremia
   b. Hyperkalemia and hypernatremia
   c. Hypokalemia and hyponatremia
   d. Hypokalemia and hypernatremia

5. A systemic effect of chronic kidney disease that is usually reversed by the initiation of dialysis is
   a. anemia.
   b. hyperlipidemia.
   c. psychologic changes.
   d. nausea and vomiting.

6. Measures indicated in the conservative therapy of chronic kidney disease include
   a. decreased fluid intake, carbohydrate intake, and protein intake.
   b. increased fluid intake, decreased carbohydrate intake and protein intake.
   c. decreased fluid intake and protein intake, increased carbohydrate intake.
   d. decreased fluid intake and carbohydrate intake, increased protein intake.

7. One of the major disadvantages of peritoneal dialysis is that
   a. hypotension is a constant problem because of continuous fluid removal.
   b. blood loss can be extensive because of the use of heparin to keep the catheter patent.
   c. solutes are removed more rapidly from the blood than from the CNS, causing disequilibrium syndrome.
   d. high glucose concentrations of the dialysate necessary for ultrafiltration cause carbohydrate and lipid abnormalities.

8. To assess the patency of a newly placed arteriovenous graft for dialysis, the nurse should
   a. irrigate the graft daily with low-dose heparin.
   b. monitor for any increase in BP in the affected arm.
   c. listen with a stethoscope over the graft for the presence of a bruit.
   d. frequently monitor the pulses and neurovascular status distal to the graft.

9. A patient in ESRD receiving hemodialysis is considering asking a relative to donate a kidney for transplant. In assisting the patient to make a decision about treatment, the nurse informs the patient that
   a. successful transplantation usually provides better quality of life than that offered by dialysis.
   b. if rejection of the transplanted kidney occurs, no further treatment for the renal failure is available.
   c. the immunosuppressive therapy that is required following transplantation causes fatal malignancies in many patients.
   d. hemodialysis replaces the normal functions of the kidneys and patients do not have to live with the continual fear of rejection.

10. Following a kidney transplant, the nurse teaches the patient that signs of rejection include
    a. fever, weight loss, increased urinary output, increased BP.
    b. fever, weight gain, increased urinary output, increased BP.
    c. fever, weight loss, increased urinary output, decreased BP.
    d. fever, weight gain, decreased urinary output, increased BP.

11. Most of the long-term problems that occur in the patient with a kidney transplant are a result of
    a. chronic rejection.
    b. immunosuppressive therapy.
    c. recurrence of the original renal disease.
    d. failure of the patient to follow the prescribed regimen.

REFERENCES

1. Brady H et al: Acute renal failure. In Brenner BM, editor: *The kidney*, Philadelphia, 2000, WB Saunders.
2. Agrawal M, Swartz R: Acute renal failure, *Am Fam Physician* 61:2077, 2000.
3. Johnson DC, Anderson RJ: Acute renal failure, part 2: zeroing in on the diagnosis: early remedial efforts can stop disease progression, *J Crit Illn* 17:301, 2002.
4. Bozfakioglu S: Nutrition in patients with acute renal failure, *Nephrol Dial Transplant* 16:S6, 2001.
5. Richard C: Renal disorders. In Lancaster L, editor: *Core curriculum for nephrology nursing*, ed 4, New Jersey, 2001, Anthony Janetti.
6. Druml W: Nutritional management of acute renal failure, *Am J Kidney Dis* 37:S89, 2001.
7. Greene JH, Hoffart N: Nutrition in renal failure, dialysis, and transplant. In Lancaster L, editor: *Core curriculum for nephrology nursing*, ed 4, New Jersey, 2001, Anthony Janetti.
8. US Renal Data System: USRDS 2001 annual data report: Atlas of end-stage renal disease, Bethesda, MD, 2001, National Institutes of Health, National Institute of Diabetes & Digestive and Kidney Diseases.

9. Foret JP: Diagnosing and treating anemia and iron deficiency in hemodialysis patients, *Nephrol Nurs J* 29:292, 2002.

10. Levin A, Stevens L, McCullough P: Cardiovascular disease and the kidney: tracking a killer in chronic kidney disease, *Postgrad Med* 111:53, 2002.

11. Laaksonen S et al: Does dialysis therapy improve autonomic and peripheral nervous system abnormalities in chronic uraemia? *J Intern Med* 248:21, 2000.

12. Lancaster L: Systemic manifestations of renal failure. In Lancaster L, editor: *Core curriculum for nephrology nursing*, ed 4, New Jersey, 2001, Anthony Janetti.

13. Roth C, Culp K: Renal osteodystrophy in older adults with end-stage renal disease, *J Gerontol Nurs* 27:46, 2001.

14. Andrews L, Gibbs M: Antihypertensive medications and renal disease, *Nephrol Nurs J* 29:379, 2002.

15. Chorzempa A, Tabloski P: Post myocardial infarction: treatment in the older adult, *Nurse Pract* 26:36, 2001.

16. Markauskas I: The complexities of renal bone disease, *Nephrol News Issues* 15:41, 2001.

17. Kopple J: National Kidney Foundation K/DOQI clinical practice guidelines for nutrition in chronic renal failure, *Am J Kidney Dis* 37(suppl 2):S66, 2001.

18. Hartley GH: Nutritional status, delaying progression and risks associated with protein restriction, *Edtna-Erca Journal* 27:101, 2001.

19. Compton A, Provenzano R, Johnson C: The nephrology nurse's role in improved care of patients with chronic kidney disease, *Nephrol Nurs J* 29:331, 2002.

20. Finkelstein ES et al: Patterns of infection in patients maintained on long-term peritoneal dialysis therapy with multiple episodes of peritonitis, *Am J Kidney Dis* 39:1278, 2002.

21. Work J: Introduction: advances in hemodialysis access, *Adv Ren Replac Ther* 9:71, 2002.

22. Trerotola S: Hemodialysis catheter placement and management, *Radiology* 215:651, 2000.

23. Richard HM et al: A randomized, prospective evaluation of the Tesio, Ash Split, and Opti-flow hemodialysis catheters, *J Vasc Interv Radiol* 12:431, 2001.

24. Beathard GA, Posen GA: Initial clinical results with Life-site® hemodialysis access system, *Kidney Int* 58:2221, 2000.

25. Morgan L: A decade review: methods to improve adherence to the treatment regimen among hemodialysis patients, *Nephrol Nurs J* 27:299, 2000.

26. Kaplow R, Richard B: Continuous renal replacement therapies: a more gentle blood filtering technique allows for fewer complications, *Am J Nsg* 102:26, 2002.

27. Bellmann R et al: Elimination of levofloxacin in critically ill patients with renal failure: influence of continuous veno-venous hemofiltration, *Int J Clin Pharmacol Ther* 40:142, 2002.

28. United Network for Organ Sharing: 2001 Annual report: the US scientific registry of transplant recipients and the organ procurement and transplantation network, 2001, Department of Health and Human Services.

29. Dabbs A et al: Rejection after organ transplantation: a historical review, *Am J Crit Care* 9:419, 2000.

30. Connerney I et al: Laparoscopic nephrectomy program boosts successful outcomes at university, *Inside Case Management* 6:6, 1999.

31. Ratner LE, Montgomery RA, Kavoussi LR: Laparoscopic live-donor nephrectomy: the four year Johns Hopkins University experience, *Nephrol Dial Transplant* 14:2090, 1999.

32. Manuel P et al: Strategies to improve long-term outcomes after renal transplantation, *N Engl J Med* 346:580, 2002.

33. Andany M, Kasiske B: Care of the kidney transplant recipient: vigilant monitoring creates the best outcome, *Postgrad Med* 112:93, 2002.

34. Pellegrin I et al: New molecular assays to predict occurrence of cytomegalovirus disease in renal transplant recipients, *J Infect Dis* 182:36, 2000.

35. Hopwood P, Crawford DH: The role of EBV in post-transplant malignancies: a review, *J Clin Pathol* 53:248, 2000.

36. Brown WW: The geriatric dialysis patient. In Henrick WL, editor: *Principles and practice of dialysis*, ed 2, Baltimore, 1999, Lippincott Williams & Wilkins.

37. Wolfson M: Nutrition in elderly dialysis patients, *Seminars in Dialysis* 15:113, 2002.

38. Thomas LK et al: Identification of the factors associated with compliance to therapeutic diets in older adults with end stage renal disease, *Journal of Renal Nutrition* 11:80, 2001.

RESOURCES

American Association of Kidney Patients (AAKP)
3505 East Frontage Road, Suite 315
Tampa, FL 33607
800-749-2257
Fax: 813-636-8122
www.aakp.org

American Kidney Fund (AKF)
6110 Executive Boulevard, Suite 1010
Rockville, MD 20852
800-638-8299
www.ukfinc.org

American Nephrology Nurses' Association
ANNA National Office
East Holly Avenue, Box 56
Pitman, NJ 08071-0056
888-600-ANNA (2662) or 856-256-2320
Fax: 856-589-7463
http://anna.inurse.com

American Organ Transplant Association
P.O. Box 441766
Houston, TX 77244
281-493-2047
Fax: 281-493-2099
www.a-o-t-a.org

International Society of Nephrology (ISN)
www.isn-online.org

International Transplant Nurses Society
1739 East Carson Street, Box 351
Pittsburgh, PA 15203
412-343-ITNS
Fax: 412-343-3959
www.itns.org

Kidney Transplant/Dialysis Association, Inc.
P.O. Box 51362 GMF
Boston, MA 02205-1362
781-641-4000
http://users.rcn.com/ktda1

National Association of Transplant Coordinators (NATCO)
P.O. Box 15384
Lenexa, KS 66285-5384
913-492-3600
Fax: 913-599-5340
www.natco1.org

National Institute of Diabetic and Digestive and Kidney Diseases Information (NIDDK)
Office of Communications and Public Liaison
NIH, Building 31, Room 9A04
31 Center Drive MSC 2560
Bethesda, MD 20892-2560
www.niddk.nih.gov/

National Kidney Foundation
30 East 33rd Street, Suite 1100
New York, NY 10016
800-622-9010 or 212-889-2210
Fax: 212-689-9261
www.kidney.org

RENALNET
www.renalnet.org

RenalWEB Patient Education
www.renalweb.com/topics/patiented/patiented.htm

United Network for Organ Sharing
1100 Boulders Parkway, Suite 500
Richmond, VA 23225-8770
888-TX-INFO-1 or 804-330-8541
www.unos.org

For additional Internet resources, see the website for this book at *http://evolve.elsevier.com/Lewis/medsurg/.*

Problems Related to Regulatory Mechanisms

SECTION OUTLINE

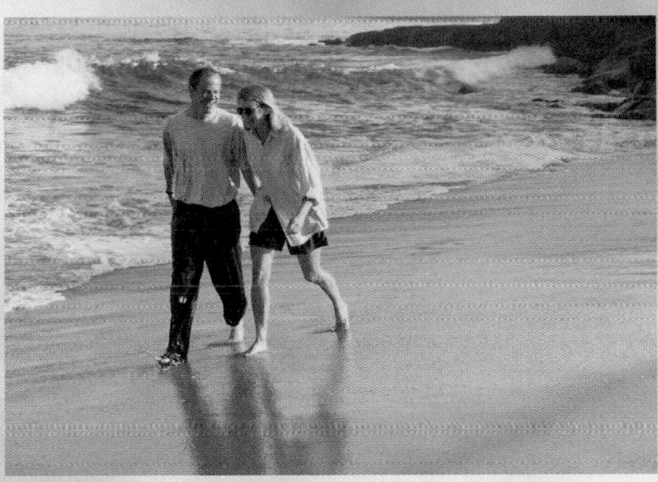

CHAPTER *46*

NURSING ASSESSMENT
Endocrine System

Jean Foret Giddens

LEARNING OBJECTIVES

1. Identify the common characteristics and functions of hormones.
2. Identify the locations of the endocrine glands.
3. Describe the functions of hormones secreted by the pituitary, thyroid, parathyroid, and adrenal glands and the pancreas.
4. Describe the locations and roles of hormone receptors.
5. Identify the significant subjective and objective assessment data related to the endocrine system that should be obtained from a patient.
6. Describe the appropriate technique used in the physical assessment of the thyroid gland.
7. Describe age-related changes in the endocrine system and differences in assessment findings.
8. Differentiate normal from common abnormal findings in the assessment of the endocrine system.
9. Describe the purpose, significance of results, and nursing responsibilities related to diagnostic studies of the endocrine system.

KEY TERMS

aldosterone, p. 1255	insulin, p. 1255
antidiuretic hormone, p. 1253	islets of Langerhans, p. 1255
calcitonin, p. 1254	negative feedback, p. 1249
catecholamines, p. 1254	oxytocin, p. 1254
corticosteroid, p. 1255	parathyroid hormone, p. 1254
cortisol, p. 1255	target tissue, p. 1248
glucagon, p. 1255	thyroxine, p. 1254
growth hormone, p. 1253	triiodothyronine, p. 1254
hormone, p. 1248	tropic hormones, p. 1252

The endocrine system and the nervous system are two of the primary communicating and coordinating systems in the body. The nervous system communicates through nerve impulses; the endocrine system communicates through chemical substances known as hormones, and it plays a role in reproduction, growth and development, and regulation of energy. The endocrine system is composed of glands or glandular tissues that produce, store, and secrete hormones that travel through the blood to specific target cells throughout the body.

The endocrine glands include the hypothalamus, pituitary, thyroid, parathyroids, adrenals, pancreas, ovaries, testes, pineal, and thymus (Fig. 46-1). The thymus gland is important in the function of the immune system and is discussed in Chapter 13. The pineal gland, which secretes melatonin, is not discussed in this chapter, because the significance of this gland in humans is not well understood.[1] In addition to the endocrine glands, other body organs secrete hormones. For example, the kidneys secrete erythropoietin, the heart secretes atrial natriuretic hormone, and the gastrointestinal tract secretes numerous peptide hormones (e.g., gastrin). These hormones are discussed in their respective assessment chapters.

STRUCTURES AND FUNCTIONS OF THE ENDOCRINE SYSTEM

Glands

The organs of the endocrine system are referred to as *glands*. Endocrine glands produce chemical substances called *hormones* and secrete them into blood, where they eventually affect specific target tissues. A **target tissue** is the body tissue or organ that the hormone has its effect on. For example, the thyroid (gland) synthesizes thyroxine (the hormone), which influences all body tissues (target tissue). It is important to note that not all glands in the body belong to the endocrine system. There are two types of glands—*exocrine glands* and *endocrine glands*. Exocrine glands secrete their substances into ducts that then empty into a body cavity or onto a surface (e.g., skin). For example, salivary glands produce saliva, which is secreted through salivary ducts into the mouth. By contrast, endocrine glands do not have ducts. They secrete their substances directly into the blood.

Hormones

Classifications and Functions. A **hormone** is a chemical substance synthesized and secreted by a specific organ or tissue. Most hormones have common characteristics, including (1) secretion in small amounts at variable but predictable rates, (2) circulation through the blood, and (3) binding to specific cellular receptors either in the cell membrane or within the cell.

Hormones are classified by their chemical structure: lipid-soluble hormones and water-soluble (protein-based) hormones. Lipid-soluble hormones include steroid hormones (all hormones produced by the adrenal cortex and sex glands) and thyroid hormones. All other hormones are water soluble.[2] The differences in solubility become important in understanding how the hormone interacts with the target cell.

As mentioned previously, the hormones control a number of physiologic activities. Important hormonal functions are related to reproduction, response to stress and injury, electrolyte balance, energy metabolism, growth, maturation, and aging. Hormones also play a role in nervous system function. Some hormones have a regulatory effect on nervous tissue. For example, catechol-

Reviewed by Rebecca B. Griffin, RN, MS, Instructor, McLennan Community College, Waco, Tex.

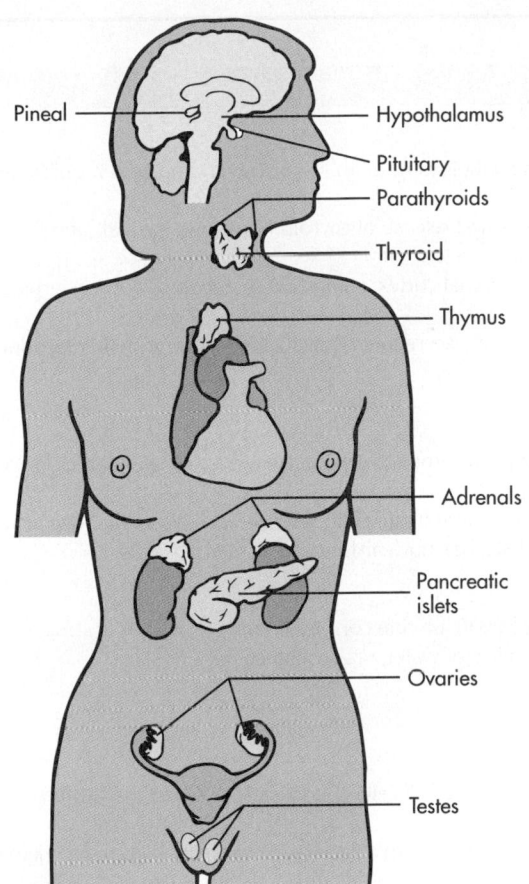

FIG. 46-1   Location of the major endocrine glands. The parathyroid glands actually lie on the posterior surface of the thyroid.

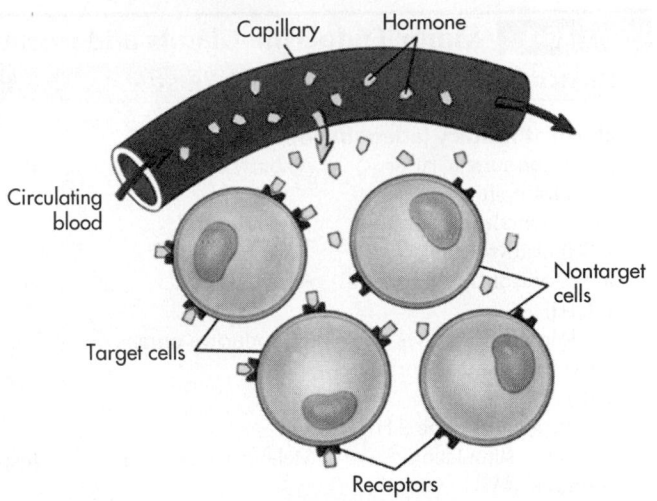

FIG. 46-2   The target cell concept. Hormones act only on cells that have receptors specific to that hormone, because the shape of the receptor determines which hormone can react with it. This is an example of the lock-and-key model of biochemical reactions.

amines are hormones when they are secreted by the adrenal medulla, but act as neurotransmitters when secreted by nerve cells in the brain and peripheral nervous system. When epinephrine travels through the blood, it is a hormone and affects target tissues. When it travels across synaptic junctions, it acts as a neurotransmitter. Hormones can also influence behavior.[3] For example, excess growth hormone, cortisol, and parathyroid hormone can cause mood swings. Depression has been associated with adrenal insufficiency. Table 46-1 summarizes the major hormones, glands or tissues from which they are synthesized, target organs or tissues, and functions.

Hormone Transport. Hormones are carried by the blood to other sites in the body where their actions are exerted. Some hormones (e.g., steroid and thyroid hormones) are not water soluble. Therefore these types of hormones are bound to plasma proteins for transport in the blood. Although hormones are inactive when bound to plasma proteins, they can be released when appropriate and immediately exert their action at the target tissue. Water-soluble hormones (e.g., protein hormones, catecholamines) circulate freely in the blood and are not dependent upon proteins for transport.

Targets and Receptors. As mentioned above, hormones exert their effects on target tissue. The hormone recognizes the target tissue through receptors (the site that interacts with the hormone) on or within cells of the target tissue. The specificity of hormone–target cell interaction is determined by receptors in a "lock-and-key" type of mechanism. Thus a hormone will act only

on cells that have a receptor specific for that hormone (Fig. 46-2). It is important to note there are two types of receptors: those that are within the cell (e.g., steroid and thyroid hormone receptors) and those that are on the cell membrane (e.g., protein-type hormone receptors). The location of the receptor sites affects the mechanism of action for the hormone.

Steroid hormone receptors. Steroid and thyroid hormone receptors are located inside the cell. Because these hormones are lipid soluble, they pass through the target cell membrane by passive diffusion and bind to receptor sites located in the cytoplasm or nucleus of the target cell.[4] Intracellular hormone-receptor complexes, such as those seen in steroid hormone action, bind to specific sites on deoxyribonucleic acid (DNA) to stimulate or inhibit the synthesis of messenger ribonucleic acid (mRNA). When new mRNA is synthesized, it migrates to the cytoplasm, where it stimulates the synthesis of new protein. These new proteins produce specific effects in the target cell (Fig. 46-3).

Protein hormone receptors. Protein hormone action is a two-step process. The receptor is located in the target cell membrane; thus the hormone itself acts as a "first messenger." The hormone-receptor interaction stimulates the production of a "second messenger" such as cyclic adenosine monophosphate (cAMP). cAMP works by activating enzymes to regulate intracellular activity (see Fig. 46-3).

Regulation of Hormonal Secretion. The regulation of endocrine activity is controlled by specific mechanisms of varying levels of complexity. These mechanisms stimulate or inhibit hormone synthesis and secretion and include simple feedback, complex feedback, nervous system control, and physiologic rhythms.

Simple feedback. The regulation of hormone levels in the blood depends on a highly specialized mechanism called *feedback.* Feedback is based on the blood level of a particular substance. This substance may be a hormone or other chemical compound regulated by, or responsive to, a hormone. With **negative feedback,** the most common type of feedback system, the gland responds by increasing or decreasing the secretion of a hormone based on feedback from various factors.[5] Negative

TABLE 46-1	Major Endocrine Glands and Hormones	
HORMONES	**TARGET TISSUE**	**FUNCTIONS**
Anterior Pituitary (adenohypophysis)		
Growth hormone (GH) or somatotropin	All body cells	Promotes protein anabolism (growth, tissue repair) and lipid mobilization and catabolism
Thyroid-stimulating hormone (TSH) or thyrotropin	Thyroid gland	Stimulates synthesis and release of thyroid hormones, growth and function of thyroid gland
Adrenocorticotropic hormone (ACTH)	Adrenal cortex	Fosters growth of adrenal cortex; stimulates secretion of corticosteroids
Gonadotropic hormones • Follicle-stimulating hormone (FSH) • Luteinizing hormone (LH)	Reproductive organs	Stimulates sex hormone secretion, reproductive organ growth, reproductive processes
Melanocyte-stimulating hormone (MSH)	Melanocytes in skin	Increases melanin production in melanocytes to make skin darker in color
Prolactin	Ovary and mammary glands in females	Stimulates milk production in lactating women; increases response of follicles to LH and FSH; has unclear function in men
Posterior Pituitary (neurohypophysis)		
Oxytocin	Uterus; mammary glands	Stimulates milk secretion, uterine contractility
Antidiuretic hormone (ADH) or vasopressin	Renal tubules, vascular smooth muscle	Promotes reabsorption of water, vasoconstriction
Thyroid		
Thyroxine (T_4)	All body tissues	Precursor to T_3
Triiodothyronine (T_3)	All body tissues	Regulates metabolic rate of all cells and processes of cell growth and tissue differentiation
Calcitonin	Bone tissue	Regulates calcium and phosphorus blood levels; decreases serum Ca^{2+} levels
Parathyroids		
Parathyroid hormone (PTH) or parathormone	Bone, intestine, kidneys	Regulates calcium and phosphorus blood levels; promotes bone demineralization and increases intestinal absorption of Ca^{2+}; increases serum Ca^{2+} levels
Adrenal Medulla		
Epinephrine (Adrenaline)	Sympathetic effectors	Response to stress; enhances and prolongs effects of sympathetic nervous system
Norepinephrine	Sympathetic effectors	Response to stress; enhances and prolongs effects of sympathetic nervous system
Adrenal Cortex		
Corticosteroids (e.g., cortisol, hydrocortisone)	All body tissues	Promotes metabolism, response to stress
Androgens (e.g., testosterone, androsterone) and estrogen	Reproductive organs	Promotes masculinization in men, growth and sexual activity in women
Mineralocorticoids (e.g., aldosterone)	Kidney	Regulates sodium and potassium balance and thus water balance
Pancreas		
Islets of Langerhans		
Insulin (from beta cells)	General	Promotes movement of glucose out of blood and into cells
Glucagon (from alpha cells)	General	Promotes movement of glucose from glycogen (glycogenolysis) and into blood
Somatostatin	Pancreas	Inhibits insulin and glucagon secretion
Pancreatic polypeptide	General	Influences regulation of pancreatic exocrine function and metabolism of absorbed nutrients
Gonads		
Women: Ovaries		
Estrogen	Reproductive system, breasts	Stimulates development of secondary sex characteristics, preparation of uterus for fertilization and fetal development; stimulates bone growth
Progesterone	Reproductive system	Maintains lining of uterus necessary for successful pregnancy
Men: Testes		
Testosterone	Reproductive system	Stimulates development of secondary sex characteristics, spermatogenesis

A

B

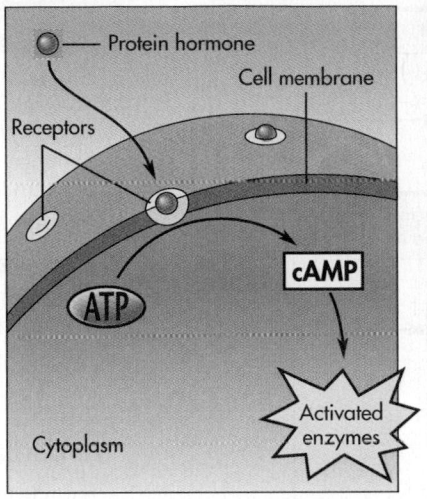

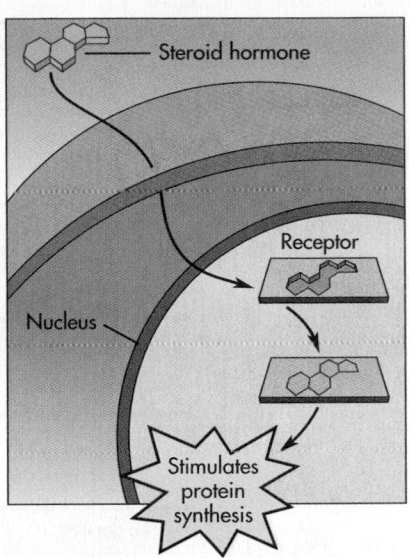

FIG. 46-3 **A,** Protein hormones bind to receptors located on the surface of the cell membrane. The hormone-receptor interaction stimulates the formation of cAMP, thereby activating various cell processes. **B,** Steroid hormones penetrate the cell membrane and interact with intracellular receptors. The hormone-receptor complex activates the cell by stimulating protein synthesis.

feedback is similar to the functioning of a thermostat in which cold air in a room activates the thermostat to release heat, and hot air turns off the thermostat to prevent more warm air from entering the room.

The pattern of insulin secretion is a physiologic example of negative feedback between glucose and insulin. Elevated blood glucose levels stimulate the secretion of insulin from the pancreas. As blood glucose levels decrease, the stimulus for insulin secretion also decreases (Fig. 46-4). The homeostatic mechanism

is considered negative feedback because it reverses the change in blood glucose level. Another example of negative feedback is the relationship between calcium and parathyroid hormone (PTH). Low blood levels of calcium stimulate the parathyroid gland to release PTH, which acts on bone, the intestine, and kidneys to increase blood calcium levels. The increased blood calcium levels then inhibit further PTH release (Fig. 46-5).

Complex feedback. Another level of complexity exists in feedback systems. An example of this is regulation of thyroid hormones (Fig. 46-6). The synthesis and release of thyroid stimulating hormone (TSH) or thyrotropin from the anterior pituitary is stimulated by thyrotropin-releasing hormone (TRH), which is secreted by the hypothalamus. The thyroid hormones, T_3 and T_4, have an inhibitory effect on the secretion of both TRH from the hypothalamus and TSH from the anterior pituitary.

Nervous system control. In addition to chemical regulation, some endocrine glands are directly affected by the activity of the nervous system. Pain, emotion, sexual excitement, and stress can stimulate the nervous system to modulate hormone secretion. Neural involvement is initiated by the central nervous system (CNS) and implemented by the sympathetic nervous system (SNS). For example, stress is sensed by the CNS, and the SNS secretes catecholamines that increase heart rate and blood pressure to deal with stress more effectively. (Effects of stress are discussed in Chapter 8.)

Rhythms. Another regulatory mechanism affecting many hormonal secretions involves the rhythms of secretions. These rhythms originate in brain structures. A common physiologic rhythm is the *circadian rhythm,* in which a hormone level fluctuates predictably during a 24-hour period.[6] These rhythms may be

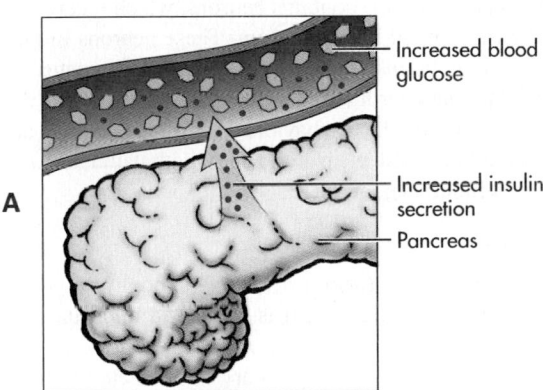

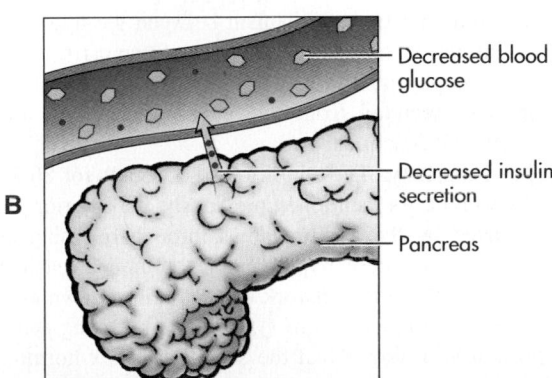

A

Increased blood glucose

Increased insulin secretion

Pancreas

B

Decreased blood glucose

Decreased insulin secretion

Pancreas

FIG. 46-4 Feedback mechanism between blood glucose and insulin. Increased blood glucose stimulates increased insulin secretion from the pancreas. As blood glucose levels decline, insulin secretion decreases.

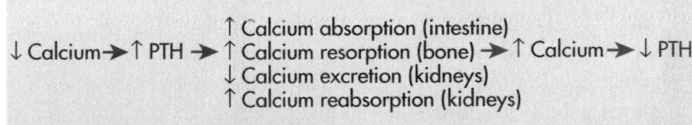

↓ Calcium → ↑ PTH → ↑ Calcium absorption (intestine)
↑ Calcium resorption (bone) → ↑ Calcium → ↓ PTH
↓ Calcium excretion (kidneys)
↑ Calcium reabsorption (kidneys)

FIG. 46-5 Feedback mechanism between parathyroid hormone (PTH) and calcium.

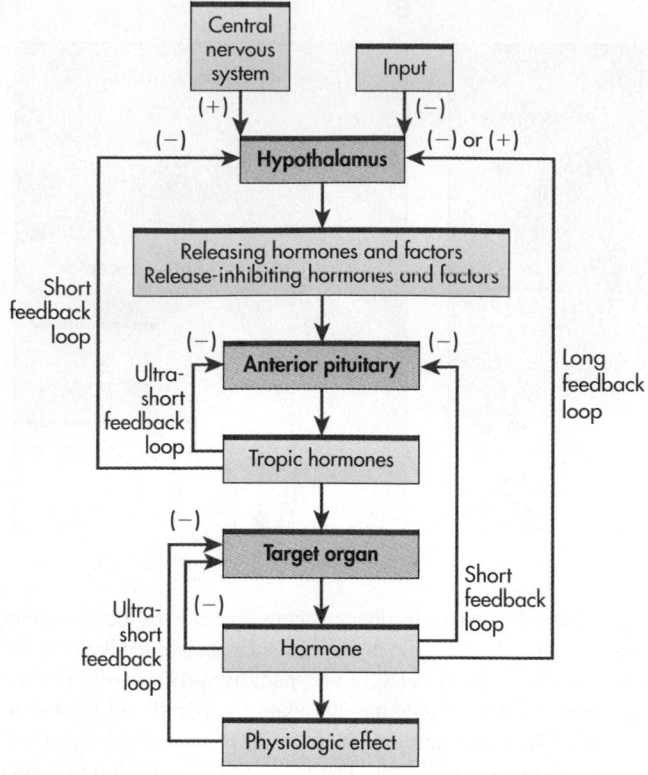

FIG. 46-6 General model for control and negative feedback to hypothalamus-pituitary target organ systems. Negative feedback regulation is possible at three levels: target organ (ultrashort feedback), anterior pituitary (short feedback), and hypothalamus (long feedback).

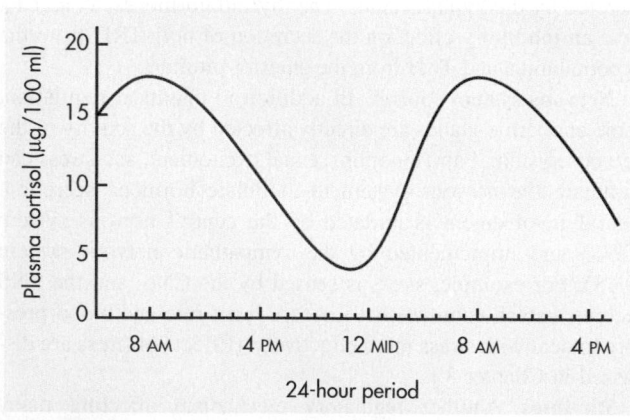

FIG. 46-7 Circadian rhythm of cortisol secretion.

related to sleep-wake or dark-light cycles. For example, cortisol rises early in the day, declines toward evening, and rises again toward the end of sleep to peak by morning (Fig. 46-7). Growth hormone (GH) and prolactin secretion peak during sleep. TSH secretion is also maximal during sleep and ebbs 3 hours after a person awakens in the morning. The menstrual cycle is an example of a body rhythm that is longer than 24 hours (*ultradian*). These rhythms must be considered when interpreting hormone levels on laboratory results. (See diagnostic studies section in this chapter and Chapter 49.)

TABLE 46-2	Hormones of the Hypothalamus

Releasing Hormones
Corticotropin-releasing hormone (CRH)
Thyrotropin-releasing hormone (TRH)
Growth hormone–releasing factor or somatotropin-releasing hormone
Gonadotropin-releasing hormone (GnRH)
Prolactin-releasing hormone

Inhibiting Hormones
Somatostatin (inhibits growth hormone release)
Prolactin-inhibiting hormone

Hypothalamus

The relationship between the hypothalamus and the pituitary gland is one of the most important aspects of the endocrine system. Although the pituitary gland has been referred to as the "master gland," most of its functions rely on an interrelationship with the hypothalamus. The hypothalamus and pituitary gland integrate communication between nervous and endocrine systems.

The hypothalamus is located in the most central part of the diencephalon area of the brain (see Fig. 46-1). Although it is really part of the brain, the hypothalamus secretes many hormones. Two important groups of hormones from the hypothalamus are *releasing* hormones and *inhibiting* hormones. The function of these hormones is to either stimulate (release) or inhibit the secretion of hormones from the anterior pituitary (Table 46-2).

The hypothalamus also contains neurons, which receive input from the brainstem and limbic system. These neurons influence the limbic system, brainstem, and spinal cord. This creates a circuit to facilitate the coordination of the endocrine system, ANS, and expression of complex behavioral responses, such as anger and feelings of fear and pleasure. The hypothalamus may also have a role in libido (sex drive).[7]

Pituitary

The pituitary gland (also called the hypophysis) is very small—about the size of a pea. It is located in the sella turcica under the hypothalamus at the base of the brain above the sphenoid bone (see Fig. 46-1). The pituitary is connected to the hypothalamus by the infundibular (hypophyseal) stalk. This stalk serves as a communication mechanism between the hypothalamus and the pituitary. The pituitary consists of two parts, the *anterior* (adenohypophysis) and the *posterior* (neurohypophysis) lobes. Hormones secreted from each of these pituitary lobes serve very different functions.

Anterior Pituitary. The anterior lobe accounts for 80% of the gland by weight. As mentioned previously, the anterior pituitary is regulated by the hypothalamus through releasing and inhibiting hormones. These hypothalamic hormones reach the anterior pituitary through a network of capillaries known as the *hypothalamus-hypophyseal portal system*. The releasing and inhibiting hormones in turn affect the secretion of six hormones from the anterior pituitary (Fig. 46-8; see Table 46-2).

Tropic hormones. Several hormones secreted by the anterior pituitary are referred to as **tropic hormones.** These are hormones that control the secretion of hormones by other glands.

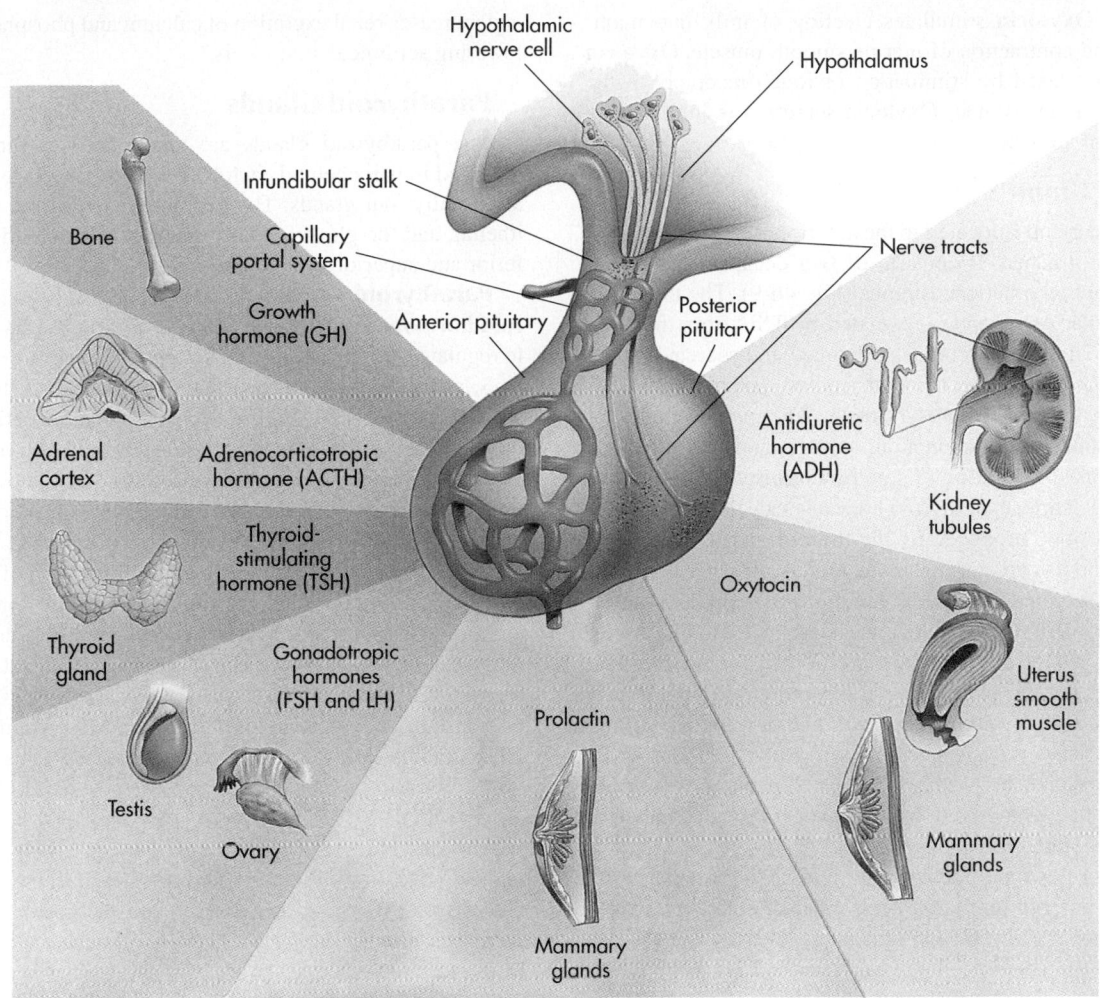

FIG. 46-8 Relationship between the hypothalamus, pituitary, and target organs. The hypothalamus communicates with the anterior pituitary via a capillary system and with the posterior pituitary via nerve tracts. The anterior and posterior pituitary hormones are shown with their target tissues.

Thyroid-stimulating hormone (TSH) stimulates the thyroid gland to secrete thyroid hormones. Adrenocorticotropic hormone (ACTH) stimulates the adrenal cortex to secrete corticosteroids. Follicle-stimulating hormone (FSH) stimulates secretion of estrogen and the development of ova in the female and sperm development in the male. Luteinizing hormone (LH) stimulates ovulation in the female and secretion of sex hormones in both the male and female.

Growth hormone. Growth hormone (GH) has effects on all body tissue. GH, as its name suggests, affects the growth and development of skeletal muscles and long bones, affecting a person's size and height. It also has numerous biologic actions, including a role in protein, fat, and carbohydrate metabolism.[8]

Prolactin. Prolactin is a hormone that stimulates breast development necessary for lactation after childbirth. Prolactin is also referred to as lactogenic hormone.

Posterior Pituitary. The posterior pituitary is composed of nerve tissue and is essentially an extension of the hypothalamus. The communication between the hypothalamus and posterior pituitary occurs through nerve tracts known as the *median eminence*. The hormones secreted by the posterior pituitary, **antidiuretic hormone** (ADH) and oxytocin, are actually produced in the hypo-

thalamus. These hormones travel down the nerve tracts from the hypothalamus to the posterior pituitary and are stored until their release is triggered by the appropriate stimuli (see Fig. 46-8).

Antidiuretic hormone. The major physiologic role of ADH is regulation of fluid volume by stimulating reabsorption of water in the renal tubules. ADH, also called vasopressin, is also a potent vasoconstrictor.

The most important stimulus to ADH secretion is plasma osmolality (a measure of solute concentration of circulating blood). Plasma osmolality will increase when there is a decrease in extracellular fluid or an increase in solute concentration. The increased plasma osmolality activates osmoreceptors, which are extremely sensitive, specialized neurons in the hypothalamus. These activated osmoreceptors stimulate ADH release. ADH secretion is also stimulated by decreased blood volume, orthostatic changes in blood pressure, hypotension, pain, nausea, vomiting, and many drugs (e.g., anesthetic drugs, narcotics).[2] When ADH is released, the renal tubules reabsorb water, creating a more concentrated urine. The release of ADH is inhibited by an increase in fluid volume, β-adrenergic agonists, and alcohol. When ADH release is inhibited, renal tubules do not reabsorb water, thus creating a more dilute urine.

Oxytocin. Oxytocin stimulates ejection of milk into mammary ducts and contraction of uterine smooth muscle. Oxytocin secretion is increased by stimulation of touch receptors in the nipples of lactating women. Oxytocin secretion is inhibited by endorphins and alcohol.

Thyroid Gland

The thyroid gland is located in the anterior portion of the neck in front of the trachea. It consists of two encapsulated lateral lobes connected by a narrow isthmus (Fig. 46-9). The thyroid is a highly vascular organ and is regulated by TSH from the anterior pituitary. The three hormones produced and secreted by the thyroid gland are thyroxine, triiodothyronine, and calcitonin.

Thyroxine and Triiodothyronine. The major function of the thyroid gland is the production, storage, and release of the thyroid hormones, **thyroxine** (T_4) and **triiodothyronine** (T_3). T_4 is by far the most abundant thyroid hormone, accounting for 90% of thyroid hormone produced by the thyroid gland. T_3 is much more potent and has greater metabolic effects. About 10% of circulating T_3 is secreted directly by the thyroid gland, and the remainder is obtained by peripheral conversion of T_4. Iodine is necessary for the synthesis of thyroid hormones. T_4 and T_3 affect metabolic rate, caloric requirements, oxygen consumption, carbohydrate and lipid metabolism, growth and development, brain functions, and nervous system activity. More than 99% of thyroid hormones are bound to plasma proteins, especially thyroxine-binding globulin synthesized by the liver. Only the unbound "free" hormones are biologically active.

Thyroid hormone production and release is stimulated by TSH from the anterior pituitary gland. When circulating levels of thyroid hormone are low, the hypothalamus releases TRH, which in turn causes the anterior pituitary to release TSH. High circulating thyroid hormone levels have an inhibitory effect on the secretion of both TRH from the hypothalamus and TSH from the anterior pituitary.[9]

Calcitonin. Calcitonin is a hormone produced by C cells (parafollicular cells) of the thyroid gland in response to high circulating calcium levels. Calcitonin inhibits calcium *resorption* (loss of substance) from bone, increases calcium storage in bone, and increases renal excretion of calcium and phosphorus, thereby lowering serum calcium levels.[2]

Parathyroid Glands

The parathyroid glands are small, oval structures usually arranged in pairs behind each thyroid lobe (see Fig. 46-9). There are usually four glands. The major cell type of the glands is epithelial, and the gland is richly supplied with blood from the inferior and superior thyroid arteries.

Parathyroid Hormone. The parathyroids secrete **parathyroid hormone** (PTH), also called *parathormone*. Its major role is to regulate the blood level of calcium. PTH acts on bone, the kidneys, and indirectly the gastrointestinal (GI) tract. In bone, PTH stimulates bone resorption and inhibits bone formation, resulting in the release of calcium and phosphate into the blood. In the kidney, PTH increases calcium reabsorption and phosphate excretion. In addition, PTH stimulates the renal conversion of vitamin D to its most active form (1,25-dihydroxyvitamin D_3). This active vitamin D then enhances the intestinal absorption of calcium.

PTH is not under pituitary and hypothalamic control. The secretion of this hormone is directly regulated by a feedback system (see Fig. 46-5). When the serum calcium level is low, PTH secretion increases; when the serum calcium level rises, PTH secretion falls. In addition, high levels of active vitamin D inhibit PTH and low levels of magnesium stimulate PTH secretion.

Adrenal Glands

The adrenal glands are small, paired, highly vascularized glands located on the upper portion of each kidney. Each gland consists of two parts, the medulla and the cortex (Fig. 46-10). Each has distinct functions, and the glands act independently from one another.

Adrenal Medulla. The adrenal medulla constitutes 10% to 20% of the gland and consists of sympathetic postganglionic neurons. The medulla secretes the catecholamines epinephrine (the major hormone [75%]), norepinephrine (25%), and dopamine. **Catecholamines,** usually considered neurotransmitters, are hormones when secreted by the adrenal medulla, because they are released into the circulation and transported to their target organs.

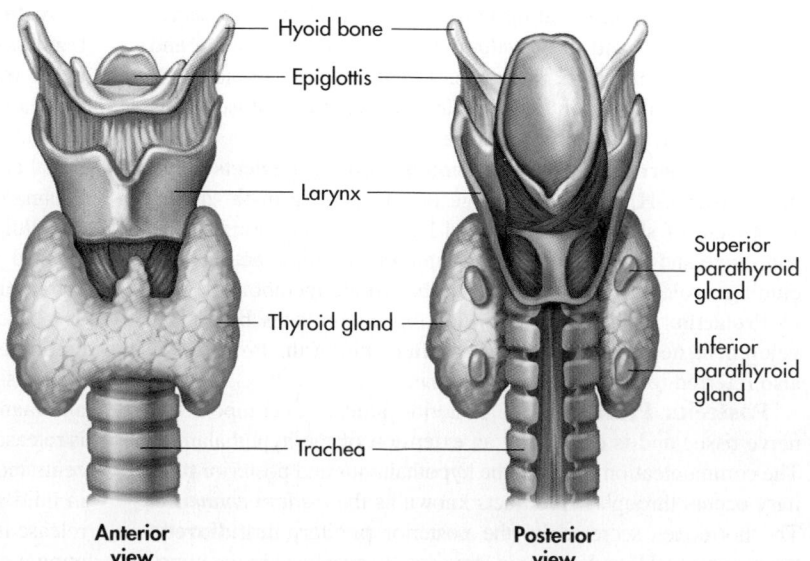

FIG. 46-9 Thyroid and parathyroid glands. Note the surrounding structures.

Anterior view

Posterior view

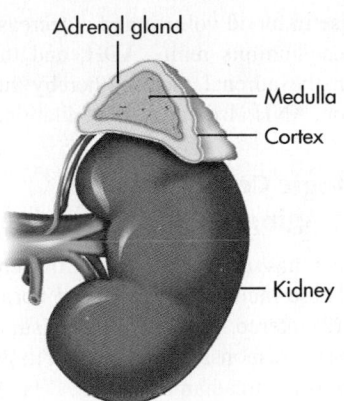

FIG. 46-10 The adrenal gland is composed of the adrenal cortex and the adrenal medulla.

Catecholamines exert their effects after binding to adrenergic receptors on cells, and they have widespread effects on all body systems. Catecholamines are an essential part of the body's response to stress (see Chapter 8).

Adrenal Cortex. The adrenal cortex, the outer part of the adrenal gland, constitutes 80% to 90% of the gland. It secretes more than 50 steroid hormones, which are classified as glucocorticoids, mineralocorticoids, and androgens. Cholesterol is the precursor for steroid hormone synthesis. Glucocorticoids (e.g., cortisol) are named for their effects on glucose metabolism. Mineralocorticoids (e.g., aldosterone) are essential for the maintenance of fluid and electrolyte balance. Adrenal androgens are produced and secreted in small but significant amounts. The term **corticosteroid** refers to any of the hormones synthesized by the adrenal cortex (excluding androgens).

Cortisol. Cortisol, the most abundant and potent glucocorticoid, is necessary to maintain life. One major function of cortisol is the regulation of blood glucose concentration. Cortisol increases blood glucose through facilitation of hepatic gluconeogenesis by promoting conversion of amino acids to glucose and inhibiting protein synthesis.[5] Cortisol also decreases peripheral glucose use in the fasting state. Additionally, glucocorticoids stimulate lipolysis in adipose tissue, thereby mobilizing glycerol and free fatty acids.

Another major effect of glucocorticoids is their antiinflammatory action and supportive actions in response to stress. A marked increase in the rate of cortisol secretion by the adrenal cortex aids the body in coping more effectively with stressful situations (see Chapter 8). Cortisol decreases the inflammatory response by stabilizing the membranes of cellular lysosomes and preventing increased capillary permeability. The lysosomal stabilization reduces the release of proteolytic enzymes and thereby their destructive effects on surrounding tissue. Cortisol can also inhibit production of prostaglandins, thromboxanes, and leukotrienes (see Chapter 12, Fig. 12-7) and alter the cell-mediated immune response.

Cortisol helps maintain vascular integrity and fluid volume. It has a mineralocorticoid effect because it can bind to mineralocorticoid receptor.

Cortisol is secreted in a diurnal pattern (see Fig. 46-7). The major control of cortisol is by means of a negative feedback mechanism that involves the secretion of corticotropin-releasing hormone (CRH) from the hypothalamus. CRH stimulates the secretion of ACTH by the anterior pituitary. Cortisol levels are also increased by surgical stress, burns, infection, fever, psychoses, acute anxiety, and hypoglycemia.

Aldosterone. Aldosterone is a potent mineralocorticoid that maintains extracellular fluid volume. It acts at the renal tubule to promote renal reabsorption of sodium and excretion of potassium and hydrogen ions. Aldosterone synthesis and secretion are stimulated by angiotensin II, hyponatremia, and hyperkalemia and inhibited by atrial natriuretic hormone and hypokalemia.

Adrenal androgens. The third class of steroids synthesized and secreted by the adrenal cortex are the androgens. Normally, the adrenal cortex secretes small amounts of androgens. Adrenal androgens stimulate pubic and axillary hair growth and sex drive in females. In the female, androgens are converted to estrogen in the peripheral tissues. In postmenopausal women the major source of estrogen is from the peripheral conversion of adrenal androgen to estrogen. The effects of adrenal androgen in men are negligible in comparison with testosterone secreted by the testes.

Pancreas

The pancreas is a long, tapered, lobular, soft gland located behind the stomach and anterior to the first and second lumbar vertebrae. The pancreas has both exocrine and endocrine functions (see Chapter 38). The hormone-secreting portion of the pancreas is referred to as the **islets of Langerhans.** The islets account for less than 2% of the gland and consist of four types of hormone-secreting cells: alpha, beta, delta, and F cells. Alpha cells produce and secrete the hormone glucagon. Insulin is produced and secreted by beta cells. Somatostatin is produced and secreted by the delta cells. Pancreatic polypeptide is secreted by the F (or PP) cells.

Glucagon. Glucagon is synthesized and released from pancreatic alpha cells in response to low levels of blood glucose, protein ingestion, and exercise. It increases blood glucose by stimulating glycogenolysis, gluconeogenesis, and ketogenesis. Usually, glucagon and insulin function in a reciprocal manner to maintain normal blood glucose levels. The exception is after ingestion of a high-protein carbohydrate-free diet, in which case both hormones are secreted. In this instance, glucagon counteracts the inhibitory effect of insulin on gluconeogenesis, and normal blood glucose levels are maintained.

Insulin. Insulin is the principal regulator of the metabolism and storage of ingested carbohydrates, fats, and proteins. Insulin facilitates glucose transport across cell membranes in most tissues. However, the brain, nerves, the lens of the eye, hepatocytes, erythrocytes, and cells in the intestinal mucosa and kidney tubules are not dependent on insulin for glucose uptake. An increased blood glucose level is the major stimulus for insulin synthesis and secretion. Other stimuli to insulin secretion are increased amino acid levels and vagal stimulation. Insulin secretion is usually inhibited by low blood glucose levels, glucagon, somatostatin, hypokalemia, and catecholamines (Table 46-3).

A major effect of insulin on glucose metabolism occurs in the liver, where the hormone enhances glucose incorporation into glycogen and triglycerides by altering enzymatic activity and inhibiting gluconeogenesis. Another major effect occurs in peripheral tissues where insulin facilitates glucose transport into cells, transport of amino acids across muscle membranes and their synthesis into protein, and transport of triglycerides into adipose tissue. Thus insulin is a storage, or *anabolic*, hormone.

The endocrine system is concerned with the regulation of body processes and the maintenance of internal homeostasis despite

TABLE 46-3	Factors Influencing Insulin Secretion

Stimulate Secretion	Inhibit Secretion
↑ Glucose levels	↓ Glucose levels
↑ Amino acid levels	↓ Amino acid levels
↑ Gastrointestinal hormone levels	↓ Potassium levels
↑ Vagal stimulation	↑ Corticosteroid hormone levels
↑ Fats	↑ Catecholamine levels
	↑ Somatostatin levels
	↑ Glucagon levels (usually)
	↑ Insulin levels

vastly changing substrates, as is seen in glucose homeostasis after food ingestion. After a meal, insulin is responsible for the storage of nutrients (anabolism). In the fasting state (during which ingested glucose is not readily available), hormones such as catecholamines, cortisol, and glucagon break down stored complex fuels (catabolism) to provide simple glucose as fuel for energy.

Heart

Atrial Natriuretic Hormone. *Natriuretic hormones* are a family of peptides; the most abundant is atrial natriuretic hormone (ANH). ANH is produced from cells in the right atrium in response to an increase in the stretch of the atrial wall caused by an abnormally high blood volume or blood pressure. These receptors in the atrium are also stimulated by high serum sodium levels. ANH acts on the kidneys to increase sodium loss. Increased loss of urinary sodium pulls water into the urine, result-

ing in a decrease in blood volume and a decrease in blood pressure.[10] ANH also inhibits renin, ADH, and the action of angiotensin II on the adrenal glands, thereby suppressing aldosterone secretion. ANH also causes vasodilation.

■ Gerontologic Considerations: Effects of Aging on the Endocrine System

Normal aging has many effects on the endocrine system (Table 46-4). These include (1) decreased hormone production and secretion, (2) altered hormone metabolism and biologic activity, (3) decreased responsiveness of target tissues to hormones, and (4) alterations in circadian rhythms.

Assessment of the effects of aging on the endocrine system is difficult because the subtle changes of aging often mimic manifestations of endocrine disorders. Some endocrine changes associated with aging are obvious; others are subtle. The nurse must be aware that endocrine problems may manifest differently in an older adult than in a younger person. Additionally, symptoms of endocrine dysfunction such as fatigue, constipation, or mental impairment in the older adult are often missed because they are attributed solely to aging.[11] It is important that the nurse consider age-related endocrine changes when assessing the older adult.[12-14] ■

ASSESSMENT OF THE ENDOCRINE SYSTEM

Hormones affect every body tissue and system, causing great diversity in the signs and symptoms of endocrine dysfunction.[3] Therefore assessment of the endocrine system is often difficult and requires keen clinical skills to detect manifestations of disorders. Endocrine dysfunction may result from deficient or ex-

| TABLE 46-4 | **𝒢erontologic Differences in Assessment** Effects of Aging on the Endocrine System |

GLAND	CHANGES	CLINICAL SIGNIFICANCE
Thyroid	Atrophy of thyroid gland. TSH and T_3 secretion is decreased	Increased incidence of hypothyroidism with aging. However, most older adults maintain adequate thyroid function
Parathyroid	Increased basal level of PTH and increased secretion	Increased calcium resorption from bone; hypercalcemia, hypercalciuria
Adrenal cortex	Adrenal cortex becomes more fibrotic and slightly smaller	Unknown. Possibly contributes to a decreased response to sodium restriction and upright posture
	Higher plasma levels of cortisol	
	Decreased plasma levels of adrenal androgens and aldosterone	
Adrenal medulla	Increased secretion and basal level of norepinephrine	Decreased responsiveness to β-adrenergic agonists and receptor blockers
	No change in plasma epinephrine levels with aging	
	Decreased β-adrenergic receptor response to norepinephrine	May partly explain increased incidence of hypertension with aging
Pancreas	Increase in fibrosis and fatty deposits in pancreas	May partly contribute to increased incidence of diabetes mellitus with advanced aging
	Increased glucose intolerance and decreased sensitivity to insulin	
Gonads	*Females:* decline in estrogen secretion	Women experience symptoms associated with menopause and have increased risk for atherosclerosis and osteoporosis
	Males: decline in testosterone secretion	Men may or may not experience symptoms

PTH, Parathyroid hormone; *TSH,* thyroid-stimulating hormone; T_3, triiodothyronine; T_4, thyroxine.

cessive hormone secretion, transport abnormalities, an inability of the target tissue to respond to a hormone, or inappropriate stimulation of the target-tissue receptor.

Endocrine disorders may have specific or nonspecific (vague) clinical manifestations. Specific signs and symptoms such as the classic "polys" (polyuria, polydipsia, and polyphagia) in diabetes mellitus make the assessment easier; nonspecific signs and symptoms such as tachycardia, palpitations, fatigue, or altered

mood are more problematic. Nonspecific changes should alert the health care provider to the possibility of an endocrine disorder. The most common nonspecific symptoms, fatigue and depression, often are accompanied by other manifestations such as changes in energy level, alertness, sleep patterns, mood, affect, weight, skin, hair, personal appearance, and sexual function (Table 46-5).

TABLE 46-5	Health History
	Endocrine System

Health Perception–Health Management
- What is your usual day like?
- Have you noticed any changes in your ability to perform your usual activities compared with last year? 5 years ago?*

Nutritional-Metabolic
- What is your weight and height?
- How much do you want to weigh?
- Have there been any changes in your appetite or weight?*
- Have you noticed any changes in the distribution of the hair anywhere on your body?*
- Have you noticed any changes in the color of your skin, particularly on your face, neck, hands, or body creases?*
- Has the texture of your skin changed? For example, does it seem thicker and drier than it used to?*
- Have you noticed any difficulty swallowing, or are your shirts more difficult to button?*
- Do you feel more nervous than you used to? Do you notice your heart pounding, or that you sweat when you do not think you should be sweating?
- Do you have difficulty holding things because of shakiness of your hands?*
- Do you feel that most rooms are too hot or too cold? Do you frequently have to put on a sweater, or feel as though you need to open windows when others in the room seem comfortable?*

Elimination
- Do you have to get up at night to urinate? If so, how many times? Do you keep water by your bed at night?
- Have you ever had a kidney stone?*
- Describe your usual bowel pattern. Have you noted any bowel changes?*
- Do you use anything, such as laxatives, to help you move your bowels?*

Activity-Exercise
- What is your usual activity pattern during a typical day?
- Do you have a planned exercise program? If yes, what is it and have you had to make any changes in this routine lately? If so, why and what kinds of changes?
- Do you experience fatigue with or without activity?*

Sleep-Rest
- How many hours do you sleep at night? Do you feel rested on awakening?
- Are you ever awakened by sweating during the night?*
- Do you have nighmares?*
- Does anyone in your family complain about your snoring?*

Cognitive-Perceptual
- How is your memory? Have you noticed any changes?
- How long can you concentrate on any one thing? Has this changed lately?
- Have you experienced any blurring or double vision?*
- When was your last eye examination?

Self-Perception–Self Concept
- Have you noticed any changes in your physical appearance or size?*
- Are you concerned about your weight?*
- Do you feel you are able to do what you think you should be capable of doing? If not, why not?
- Does your health problem affect how you feel about yourself?*

Role-Relationship
- Are you married? Do you have any children? Do you think you are able to take care of your family, home? If no, why not?
- Where do you work? What kind of work do you do? Are you able to do what is expected of you and what you expect of yourself?
- If retired, what do you do with your time? What did you do before you retired?
- If unemployed, are you looking for work?
- Is your income adequate for your needs?

Sexuality-Reproductive
Women
- When did you start to menstruate? Was this earlier or later than other women in your family? Do you have scant, heavy, or irregular menstrual flows?
- How many children have you had? How much did they weigh at birth? Were you told you had diabetes during any pregnancy?*
- Were you able to nurse your children if you wanted to?
- Are you attempting to get pregnant but cannot?*
Men
- Have you noticed any changes in your ability to have an erection?*
- Are you trying to have children but cannot?*

Coping-Stress Tolerance
- What kind of stressors do you have?
- How do you deal with stress or problems?
- What is your support system? To whom do you turn when you have a problem?

Value-Belief
- Do you think medicine should still be taken even though you feel OK?
- Do any of your prescribed therapies cause any conflict in your value-belief system?*

*If yes, describe.

TABLE 46-6 Common Assessment Abnormalities
Endocrine System

FINDING	DESCRIPTION	POSSIBLE ETIOLOGY AND SIGNIFICANCE
Head, Neck		
Visual changes	Decreased visual acuity and/or decreased peripheral vision	Enlargement of pituitary gland or pituitary tumor can result in pressure on the optic nerve.
Exophthalmos	Protrusion of the eyeballs from the orbits	Classic finding associated with hyperthyroidism; results from fluid accumulation in the eye and retroorbital tissues.
Moon face	Periorbital edema and facial fullness	Classic finding associated with Cushing syndrome.
Myxedema	Puffiness, periorbital edema, masklike affect	Accumulation of hydrophilic mucopolysaccharides in the dermis; associated with long-standing hypothyroidism.
Goiter	Enlargement of the thyroid gland	Thyroid dysfunction or iodine deficiency; seen in hyperthyroidism and hypothyroidism.
Integument		
Hyperpigmentation	Darkening of the skin, particularly in creases and skinfolds	Addison's disease caused by increased secretion of melanocyte-stimulating hormone.
Striae	Purplish red marks below the skin surface—usually seen on abdomen, breasts, and buttocks	Cushing syndrome.
Changes in skin texture	Thick, cold, dry skin	Hypothyroidism.
	Thick, leathery, oily skin	Growth hormone excess (acromegaly).
	Warm, smooth, moist skin	Hyperthyroidism.
Changes in hair distribution	Hair loss	Hypothyroidism, hyperthyroidism, decreased pituitary secretion.
	Diminished axillary and pubic hair	Cortisol deficiency.
	Hirsutism (excessive facial hair on women)	Cushing syndrome, prolactinoma (a pituitary tumor).
Skin ulceration	Areas of ulcerated skin, most commonly found on the legs and feet	Peripheral neuropathy and peripheral vascular disease are contributory factors in the development of diabetic foot ulcers.
Musculoskeletal		
Changes in muscular strength or muscle mass	Generalized weakness and/or fatigue	Common symptoms associated with many endocrine problems, including pituitary, thyroid, parathyroid, and adrenal dysfunctions; diabetes mellitus; diabetes insipidus.
	Decreased muscle mass	Specifically seen in those with growth hormone deficiency and in Cushing syndrome secondary to protein wasting.
Enlargement of bones and cartilage	Coarsening of facial features; increases in size of hand and feet over a period of several years	Gradual enlargement and thickening of bony tissue occurs with growth hormone excess in adults as seen in acromegaly.
Nutrition		
Changes in weight	Weight loss	Hyperthyroidism due to increases in metabolism.
	Weight gain	Hypothyroidism, Cushing syndrome.
Altered glucose levels	Increased serum glucose	Diabetes mellitus, Cushing syndrome, growth hormone excess.
Neurologic		
Lethargy	State of mental sluggishness or somnolence	Hypothyroidism.
Tetany	Intermittent involuntary muscle spasms usually involving the extremities	Severe calcium deficiency that can occur with hypoparathyroidism.
Seizure	Sudden involuntary contraction of muscles	Consequence of a pituitary tumor; fluid and electrolyte imbalance associated with excessive ADH secretion; complications of diabetes mellitus; severe hypothyroidism.
Gastrointestinal		
Constipation	Passage of infrequent hard stools	Hypothyroidism; hyperparathyroidism due to calcium imbalances.

ADH, Antidiuretic hormone.

TABLE 46-6 Common Assessment Abnormalities
Endocrine System—cont'd

FINDING	DESCRIPTION	POSSIBLE ETIOLOGY AND SIGNIFICANCE
Reproductive		
Changes in reproductive function	Menstrual irregularities, decreased libido, decreased fertility, impotence	Reproductive function is significantly affected by various endocrine abnormalities, including pituitary hypofunction, growth hormone excess, thyroid dysfunction, and adrenocortical dysfunction.
Other		
Polyuria	Excessive urinary output	Diabetes mellitus (secondary to hyperglycemia) or diabetes insipidus (associated with decreased ADH).
Polydipsia	Excessive thirst	Extreme water losses in diabetes mellitus (with severe hyperglycemia) and diabetes insipidus.
Thermoregulation	Cold insensitivity Heat intolerance	Hypothyroidism caused by a slowing of metabolic processes. Hyperthyroidism caused by excessive metabolism.

Subjective Data

The lack of clear-cut manifestations of endocrine problems requires a conscientious and detailed health history. A careful health history will yield data to help sort out possible causes and the effect of the problem on the person's life (Table 46-6).

Important Health Information

Past health history. During an assessment, the patient should be questioned about the general state of health and if there have been any changes. In addition, the patient or significant other should be specifically questioned about previous or current endocrine abnormalities and abnormal patterns of growth and development.

Medications. The patient should be questioned about the use of all medications (both prescription and over-the-counter drugs) and the use of herbs and dietary supplements. The patient should be asked the reason for taking the drug, dose, and the length of time taken. The patient should specifically be asked about the use of hormone replacements. Information that the patient is currently taking hormone replacements such as insulin, thyroid, or corticosteroids (e.g., prednisone) helps direct the nurse regarding possible problems associated with the use of these agents. For example, corticosteroids may cause glucose intolerance in the susceptible patient by increasing glycogenolysis and insulin resistance. The side and adverse effects of many nonhormone medications can contribute to problems affecting endocrine function. For example, many drugs can affect blood glucose levels (see Chapter 47, Table 47-8).

Surgery or other treatments. The nurse should inquire about previous hospitalizations, surgery, chemotherapy, and radiation therapy (especially of the neck). Surgery of the brain or a severe blow to the head could have resulted in pituitary or hypothalamic alterations.

Functional Health Patterns

Health perception–health management pattern. Inquiry should be made about the patient's general health care and health care behaviors. Such an inquiry might result in the identification of vague, nonspecific symptoms that could suggest an endocrine problem.

Heredity can play a major role in the occurrence of endocrine problems. The patient should be questioned about the following conditions in family members: diabetes mellitus or insipidus; hyperthyroidism or hypothyroidism, goiter; hypertension or hypotension; obesity; infertility; growth problems; pheochromocytoma (neoplastic tumor of the adrenal medulla or sympathetic ganglia); autoimmune diseases (e.g., Addison's disease); and adrenal hyperplasia. Further information may be elicited by asking additional questions such as the following: Are there any other members of your family who have, or have had, a similar problem? This frequently uncovers evidence of a familial tendency.

Nutritional-metabolic pattern. Because a major function of the endocrine system is regulating metabolism and maintaining homeostasis, the patient with endocrine dysfunction will often experience alterations in nutritional-metabolic patterns. Reported changes in appetite and weight can indicate endocrine dysfunction. Weight loss with increased appetite may indicate hyperthyroidism or diabetes mellitus, particularly type 1. Weight loss with decreased appetite may indicate hypopituitarism, hypocortisolism, or gastroparesis (decreased gastric motility and emptying) from diabetes mellitus. Weight gain may indicate hypothyroidism and, if the weight gain is concentrated in the truncal area, hypercortisolism. In addition, weight gain in a genetically susceptible patient may increase the risk for type 2 diabetes mellitus.

Difficulty swallowing or a change in neck size may indicate a thyroid disorder or inflammation. Questions related to increased sympathetic nervous system activity (e.g., nervousness, palpitations, sweating, tremors) may assist the nurse in identifying a thyroid disorder or pheochromocytoma. Heat or cold intolerance may indicate hyperthyroidism or hypothyroidism, respectively.

The patient should be questioned about dietary intake. This record should be examined for the presence of foods that contain thyroid-inhibiting substances (goitrogens) (see Chapter 48, Table 48-8).

The patient should also be asked about changes to his or her skin or hair. Hair distribution and skin and hair color and texture can all indicate endocrine dysfunction. Hair loss can indicate hypopituitarism, hypothyroidism, hypoparathyroidism, or increased testosterone and other androgens. Increased body hair may indicate hypercortisolism. Decreased skin pigmentation can occur in hypopituitarism, hypothyroidism, and hypoparathyroidism, whereas increased skin pigmentation, particularly in sun-exposed areas, can indicate hypocortisolism. A patient with hypothyroidism or excess growth hormone may complain of coarse, leathery skin. A patient with hyperthyroidism may comment about fine, silky hair.

Elimination pattern. Because maintenance of fluid balance is a major role of the endocrine system, questions related to elimination patterns may uncover endocrine dysfunction. For example, increased thirst and urination can indicate diabetes mellitus or insipidus. The patient should be asked about the frequency and consistency of bowel movements. Frequent defecation may indicate hyperthyroidism. Large-volume, watery stools or fecal incontinence may indicate autonomic neuropathy of diabetes mellitus. Constipation is also seen in the patients with diabetes mellitus, as well as in hypothyroidism, hypoparathyroidism, and hypopituitarism.

Activity-exercise pattern. The nurse should ask about energy levels, particularly as compared with the patient's past energy level. Fatigue and hyperactivity are two common problems associated with endocrine problems. The major effect of endocrine dysfunction on activity-exercise pattern is an inability to maintain previous activity levels.

Sleep-rest pattern. It is important that the nurse obtain a detailed sleep history. Sleep disturbances are frequently seen in endocrine dysfunction. The patient with diabetes mellitus or insipidus will complain of nocturia, which can severely disrupt normal sleep patterns. The patient with type 1 diabetes mellitus on a tight glucose control regimen who complains of sweating or nightmares may be experiencing hypoglycemia. The hyperthyroid patient may complain of inability to sleep, as may one with hypercortisolism. The patient with hypothyroidism, hypocortisolism, or hypopituitarism may tell the nurse of sleeping all the time, yet still being fatigued.

Cognitive-perceptual pattern. A patient with an endocrine dysfunction will frequently manifest apathy and depression. The nurse can question both the patient and significant other to determine if any cognitive changes are present. Memory deficits and an inability to concentrate are common in endocrine disorders. A patient report of visual changes such as blurring or double vision could be an indication of endocrine problems.

Self-perception–self-concept pattern. Endocrine disorders may affect the patient's self-perception because of associated physical changes affecting appearance. Changes in weight, size, and level of fatigue should be determined. The chronicity of many endocrine disorders and need for continued therapy can affect the patient's self-perception. The patient can be asked to describe the effects of the present illness on self-perception.

Role-relationship pattern. The nurse should ask whether there have been any changes in the patient's ability to maintain roles at home, at work, or in the community. Often the patient with an endocrine disorder will be unable to sustain life's roles. However, in most cases the patient can be advised that, with adequate management, previous roles can be resumed. This can be very reassuring for the patient and family.

Sexuality-reproductive pattern. The development of abnormal secondary sex characteristics (e.g., facial hair in a woman or decreased need for shaving in a man) should be documented. Problems with menstruation and pregnancy in a woman may indicate an endocrine disorder. Consequently, a detailed history of menstruation and pregnancy should be obtained. Menstrual irregularities are seen in disorders of the ovaries, pituitary, thyroid, and adrenal glands. A female patient with a history of large ba-

bies may have had undiagnosed gestational diabetes, which may put her at a higher risk to develop diabetes mellitus. A history of inability to lactate may indicate a pituitary disorder.

Male sexual dysfunction is also frequently seen in endocrine disorders. It usually takes the form of impotence, although retrograde ejaculation can occur. Infertility in either sex warrants a full reproductive and endocrine workup.

Coping–stress tolerance pattern. Stressors of all kinds affect the endocrine system. Areas that can cause a great deal of stress should be investigated. The patient should be asked about place of employment, kind of work, ability to meet job requirements, and the amount of stress involved. The nurse should ask whether the job provides an adequate income in order to identify financial stressors. Usual coping patterns are also discussed. The nurse then determines whether previous coping patterns are still successful. It is often useful to ask family members or a significant other about the patient's coping strategies and reaction to stress.

Value-belief pattern. When dealing with a patient with a chronic condition, identification of the patient's value-belief patterns can assist the health care team to identify appropriate regimens. This is particularly important in a condition such as diabetes mellitus, which may require major lifestyle changes for successful management. Other endocrine disorders, such as hypothyroidism or hypocortisolism, can be easily managed with oral medication taken faithfully. Identification of a patient's ability to make lifestyle changes or take daily medication (and increase this medication as indicated) is an important nursing function.

Objective Data

Most endocrine glands are inaccessible to direct examination. With the exception of the thyroid and male gonads, the glands are deeply encased in the body, protected against injury and trauma. However, assessment can be accomplished using a variety of objective data. It is imperative that the nurse understand the actions of hormones so that the function of a gland can be assessed by monitoring the target tissue.

Physical Examination. It is important to keep in mind that the endocrine system affects every body system. Clinical manifestations of endocrine function vary significantly depending on the gland involved. Specific clinical findings for the various endocrine problems are discussed in Chapters 47 and 48. Regardless of the type of endocrine dysfunction, the following general examination procedure should be followed.

Vital signs. A full set of vital signs is taken at the beginning of the examination. Variations in temperature may be associated with thyroid dysfunction. Cardiovascular changes such as tachycardia, bradycardia, hypotension, or hypertension may be seen with a variety of endocrine-related problems.

Height and weight. Assessment of the endocrine system includes a history of growth and development patterns, weight distribution and changes, and comparisons of these factors with normal findings. Growth pattern abnormalities suggest problems associated with growth hormone. Changes in weight also may be associated with endocrine dysfunction. Thyroid disorders and diabetes mellitus are examples of endocrine disorders that can affect body weight. Body mass index (BMI) is a height-to-weight ratio used to assess nutritional status (see Chapter 39, Fig. 39-6).

It may also be helpful to compare the patient's current body weight to her or his usual body weight in order to assess changes. Weight change (%) is calculated by dividing the current body weight by usual body weight and multiplying by 100. Weight change greater than 5% in 1 month, 7.5% in 3 months, or 10% in 6 months is considered significant.[15]

Mental-emotional status. Throughout the examination the patient's orientation, alertness, memory, affect, personality, anxiety, and appropriateness of dress and speech pattern should be objectively assessed. Endocrine disorders can commonly cause changes in mental and emotional status.

Integument. The nurse should note the color and texture of the skin, hair, and nails. The overall skin color should be noted, as well as pigmentation and possible ecchymosis. Hyperpigmentation of the skin (particularly on the knuckles, elbows, knees, genitalia, and palmar creases) is a classic finding in Addison's disease, but also is seen with ACTH-producing tumors and acromegaly.[3] The skin should be palpated for skin texture and presence of moisture. The hair distribution should be examined not only on the head, but also on the face, trunk, and extremities. The appearance and texture of the hair should be examined. Dull, brittle hair; excessive hair growth; or hair loss may indicate endocrine dysfunction.

Head. The size and contour of the head should be inspected. Facial features should be symmetric. Eyes should be inspected for position, symmetry, shape and eye movement, opacity over the lens, lid lag, and edema. Visual acuity should also be checked because changes may be associated with a pituitary tumor. In the mouth, the nurse should inspect the buccal mucosa and the condition of teeth, malocclusion and mottling, tongue size, and fasciculations (localized, uncoordinated, uncontrollable twitching of a single muscle group).

Neck. When inspecting the thyroid gland, observation should be made first in the normal position (preferably with side lighting), then in slight extension, and then as the patient swallows some water. The trachea should be midline and the neck should appear symmetric. Any unusual bulging over the thyroid area should be noted. If there is no noticeable enlargement of the thyroid gland, palpation can be done. (Because palpation can trigger the release of thyroid hormones, palpation should be deferred in the patient with a visibly enlarged thyroid gland.) When an enlarged thyroid is noted, the lateral lobes should be auscultated with the stethoscope bell to determine the presence of a bruit.

The thyroid gland is difficult to palpate. Thyroid palpation requires considerable practice, as well as validation by a more experienced examiner. Water should always be available for the patient to swallow as part of this examination. There are two acceptable approaches to thyroid palpation: anterior or posterior. For anterior palpation the nurse stands in front of the patient, with the patient's neck flexed. The nurse places the thumb horizontally with the upper edge along the lower border of the cricoid cartilage. The thumb is then moved over the isthmus as the patient swallows water. The fingers are then placed laterally to the anterior border of the sternocleidomastoid muscle, and each lateral lobe is palpated before and while the patient swallows water.

For posterior palpation the examiner stands behind the patient. With the thumbs of both hands resting on the nape of the patient's neck, the nurse uses the index and middle fingers of both hands to feel for the thyroid isthmus and for the anterior surfaces of the lateral lobes. To facilitate the examination of each lobe and to relax the neck muscles, the nurse asks the patient to flex the neck slightly forward and to the right. The thyroid cartilage is displaced to the right by the left hand and fingers. The nurse palpates with the right hand after placing the thumb deep

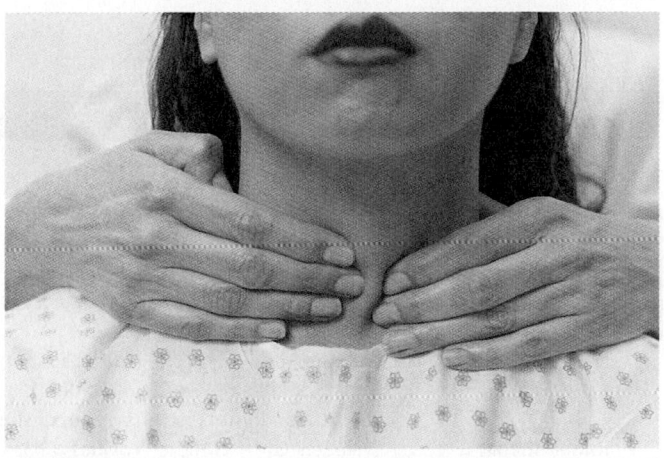

FIG. 46-11 Posterior palpation of the thyroid gland.

and behind the sternocleidomastoid muscle with the index and middle fingers in front of it; the area is palpated with the right hand (Fig. 46-11). While this is done, the patient is asked to swallow water. This procedure is then repeated on the left side. The thyroid is palpated for its size, shape, symmetry, and tenderness and for any nodules.

In a normal person the thyroid is often not palpable. If palpable, it usually feels smooth, with a firm consistency, and is not tender with gentle pressure. Nodules, enlargement, asymmetry, or hardness is abnormal, and the patient should be referred for further evaluation.

Thorax. The thorax should be inspected for shape and characteristics of the skin. The presence of gynecomastia in men should be noted. Lung sounds and heart sounds are auscultated, noting the presence of adventitious lung sounds or extra heart sounds.

Abdomen. There are no specific abdominal examination findings for endocrine dysfunction other than skin characteristics and hyperactive or hypoactive bowel sounds.

Extremities. The size, shape, symmetry, and general proportion of hand and feet size should be assessed. The skin should be inspected for changes in pigmentation and presence of lesions and edema. Muscle strength should be evaluated, as well as deep tendon reflexes. In the upper extremities, the presence of tremors is assessed by placing a piece of paper in the outstretched fingers, palm down.

Genitalia. The hair distribution pattern should be inspected. A diamond pattern in women is an abnormal finding and may indicate endocrine dysfunction. For males, the testes should be palpated; for females, any clitoral enlargement should be noted.

Common assessment abnormalities related to the endocrine system are presented in Table 46-6.

DIAGNOSTIC STUDIES OF THE ENDOCRINE SYSTEM

Accurately performed laboratory tests and radiologic examinations contribute to the diagnosis of an endocrine problem. Laboratory tests usually involve blood and urine testing. Radiologic tests include regular x-ray, computed tomography (CT), and magnetic resonance imaging (MRI). With all diagnostic testing, the nurse is responsible for explaining the procedure to the patient and family. Diagnostic studies common to the endocrine system are presented in Table 46-7.

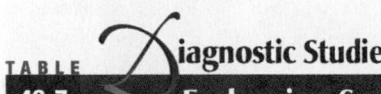

TABLE 46-7

Diagnostic Studies
Endocrine System

STUDY	PURPOSE AND DESCRIPTION	NURSING RESPONSIBILITY
Pituitary Studies **Serum Studies**		
• Growth hormone (GH) (Somatotropin)	Evaluates GH secretion. Used to identify GH deficiency or GH excess. GH levels are affected by time of day, food intake, and stress. GH should be <5 ng/ml (5.0 μg/L) in men and <10 ng/ml (10.0 μg/L) in women. Values >50 ng/ml (50.0/μg/L) suggest acromegaly.	Make sure that patient has been fasting and has not recently been emotionally or physically stressed. Indicate patient fasting status and recent activity level on the laboratory slip. Send blood sample to laboratory immediately.
• Somatomedin C (insulin-like growth factor 1 [IGF-1])	Evaluates GH secretion. Provides a more accurate reflection of mean plasma concentration of GH because it is not subject to circadian rhythm and fluctuations. *Normal values* are 135-250 ng/ml; low levels indicate GH deficiency, all high levels indicate GH excess.	Overnight fasting is preferred but not necessary.
• Growth hormone stimulation test	Needed to adequately diagnose GH deficiency. Measures GH secretion in response to stimulation (insulin, arginine). For insulin, baseline blood levels for GH, glucose, and cortisol are obtained. Insulin is then administered intravenously; blood samples for GH are obtained 30, 60, and 90 minutes after insulin is administered; blood glucose levels are monitored at 15- to 30-minute intervals. Blood glucose should drop to less than 40 mg/dl for effective testing. GH level should rise twofold to threefold over baseline levels. Response is subnormal or absent in GH deficiency.	Ensure patient/family understands this procedure. Patient must be NPO after midnight. Water is permitted on morning of the test. IV access is established for administration of medications and frequent blood sampling. Nurse must continually assess for hypoglycemia and hypotension. 50% dextrose and 5% dextrose IV solution should be kept at the bedside in case severe hypoglycemia occurs.
• Gonadotropin levels Follicle-stimulating hormone (FSH) Luteinizing hormone (LH)	Useful in distinguishing primary gonadal problems from pituitary insufficiency. Normal levels vary according to age and sex. In women, there are marked differences during menstrual cycle and in postmenopausal period. Levels are low in pituitary insufficiency and high in primary gonadal failure. In women, values for FSH are basal rate—2-15 mIU/ml (2-15 IU/L); ovulatory surge—8-40 mIU/ml (8-40 IU/L); and postmenopausal level—greater than 50 mIU/ml (50 IU/L). In women, values for LH are basal rate—2-20 mIUml (2-20 IU/L); ovulatory surge—30-140 mIU/ml (30-140 IU/L); and postmenopausal level—greater than 50 mIU/ml (50 IU/L). In men, values for FSH are 2-15 mIU/ml (2-15 IU/L) and values for LH are 3-25 mIU/ml (3-25 IU/L).	There is no special preparation of the patient. Only one blood tube is needed for both FSH and LH. Note on the laboratory slip time of menstrual cycle or whether she is postmenopausal.
• Water deprivation test	Used to differentiate causes of polyuria, including central diabetes insipidus (DI), nephrogenic DI, syndrome of inappropriate antidiuretic hormone (SIADH), and psychogenic polydipsia. ADH or vasopressin is administered intravenously or subcutaneously. In normal patients and those with psychogenic DI, urine osmolality and plasma osmolality are normal after ADH administration. In patients with central DI, urine osmolality increases after ADH administration. In patients with nephrogenic DI, there is little or no response to ADH.	Have patient discontinue fluids and smoking after midnight. Obtain baseline weight and urine and plasma osmolality. Weigh patient and take three postural BP measurements (lying and standing BP measurements separated by 2 minutes) hourly. Assess urine hourly for volume and specific gravity. Send hourly samples for urine osmolality. Draw sample for plasma osmolality when (1) urine samples are collected and (2) orthostatic hypotension and postural tachycardia appear. Assess weight at 4, 6, 7, and 8 hours. Patients must be very closely supervised during this test.

BP, Blood pressure; *IV,* intravenous; *NPO,* nothing by mouth.

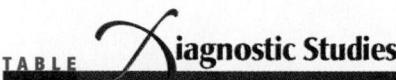

TABLE
46-7

Diagnostic Studies
Endocrine System—cont'd

STUDY	PURPOSE AND DESCRIPTION	NURSING RESPONSIBILITY
Pituitary Studies—cont'd		
Serum Studies—cont'd • Prolactin level	Evaluates prolactin levels. Decreased levels in postpartum women attempting to nurse may be associated with Sheehan syndrome. *Normal values* <20 ng/ml (<20 μg/L) (nonlactating); levels >200 ng/ml (200 μg/L) indicate pituitary tumors.	Draw blood within 3-4 hours after patient awakens. Specimen must be sent to the laboratory immediately. If there is a delay, the specimen is placed on ice.
Radiologic Studies • Magnetic resonance imaging (MRI)	Examination of choice for radiologic evaluation of the pituitary gland and hypothalamus. Useful in identification of tumors involving the hypothalamus or pituitary.	Inform patient of the need to lie as still as possible during the test; explain that tests are painless and noninvasive.
Thyroid Studies		
Serum Studies • Thyroid-stimulating hormone (TSH)	Measures levels for TSH. *Normal values* are 0.3-5.4 μU/ml (0.3-5.4 mU/L). Considered the most sensitive method for evaluating thyroid disease. Generally recommended as first diagnostic test for thyroid dysfunction.	Explain blood draw procedure to the patient. No specific preparations are necessary.
• Thyroxine (T_4)	Measures total serum level of T_4. Useful in evaluating thyroid function and monitoring thyroid therapy. *Normal values* are 5-12 μg/dl (51-142 nmol/L).	See above.
• Triiodothyronine (T_3)	Measures serum levels of T_3. It is helpful in diagnosing hyperthyroidism if T_4 levels are normal. *Normal values* are 65-195 ng/dl (1.0-3.0 nmol/L).	See above.
• Free T_4	Measures active component of total T_4. *Normal values* are 1.0-3.5 ng/dl (12.9-45.0 pmol/L). Because level remains constant, this is considered better indication of thyroid function than T_4.	See above.
• T_3 resin uptake (T_3RU)	Indirectly measures binding capacity of thyroid-binding globulin. *Normal values* are 25%-35%.	See above.
Radiologic Studies • Radioactive iodine uptake (RAIU)	Provides direct measure of thyroid activity. Useful for evaluation of functional activity of solitary thyroid nodules. Patient is given radioactive iodine either orally or intravenously. The uptake by the thyroid gland is measured with a scanner at several time intervals such as 2 to 4 hours and at 24 hours. The values of RAIU are expressed in percentage of uptake. For 2-4 hours *normal values* are 3%-19%; for 24 hours, they are 11%-30%.	Patient should be NPO for 6-8 hours before test, but can resume eating 1 hour after oral iodine dose is taken. Patient should not have supplemental iodine for several weeks before the test. Thyroid medications interfere with test results.
• Thyroid scan	Used to evaluate nodules of the thyroid. Radioactive isotopes are given orally or intravenously. Scanner passes over thyroid and makes graphic record of radiation emitted. Normal thyroid scan reveals homogeneous pattern with symmetric lobes. Benign nodules appear as warm spots because they take up the radionuclide; malignant tumors appear as cold spots because they tend not to take up the radionuclide.	Explain procedure to the patient; be sure patient understands that radioactive iodine taken orally is harmless. No special preparation is required.

Continued

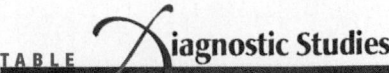

TABLE
46-7
Diagnostic Studies
Endocrine System—cont'd

STUDY	PURPOSE AND DESCRIPTION	NURSING RESPONSIBILITY
Parathyroid Studies **Serum Studies**		
• Parathyroid hormone (PTH)	Measures PTH level in serum. Normal range depends on assay used (check with laboratory). This study must be interpreted in terms of concomitantly drawn serum calcium level.	Fasting specimen preferred. Inform patient that blood sample will be drawn. Sample must be kept on ice. Observe venipuncture site for bleeding or hematoma formation.
• Total serum calcium	Measures total serum calcium to help detect bone and parathyroid disorders. Hypercalcemia can indicate primary hyperparathyroidism, and hypocalcemia can indicate hypoparathyroidism. *Normal values* are 9.0-11.0 mg/dl or 4.5-5.5 mEq/L (2.25-2.74 mmol/L).	Fasting specimen preferred. Inform patient that blood sample will be drawn. Observe venipuncture site for bleeding or hematoma formation. Ensure that prolonged tourniquet application does not cause falsely elevated values.
• Serum phosphate	Measures inorganic phosphorus. Hyperphosphatemia indicates primary hypoparathyroidism or secondary causes (e.g., renal failure); hypophosphatemia indicates hyperparathyroidism. Phosphorus and calcium levels are inversely related. *Normal values* are 2.8-4.5 mg/dl (0.90-1.45 mmol/L).	Need for fasting varies with laboratory. Determine fasting requirement. Inform patient that blood sample will be drawn. Observe venipuncture site for bleeding or hematoma formation.
Adrenal Studies **Serum Studies**		
• Cortisol	Measures amount of total cortisol in serum and evaluates status of adrenal cortex function. *Normal values* are 5-25 μg/dl (0.14-0.69 μmol/L) at 8 AM, 10 mg/dl (0.28 mmol/L) at 8 PM.	Cortisol has diurnal variation—levels are higher in the morning than in evening. Sample should be drawn in morning—evening samples may also be ordered. Mark time of blood draw on laboratory slip. Patient anxiety should be minimized.
• Aldosterone	Aldosterone levels are drawn to evaluate for hyperaldosteronism. *Normal values* are 5-20 ng/dl (140-556 pmol/L) (upright posture) and 8.5 ng/dl (237 pmol/L) (supine position).	Usually morning blood sample is preferred. Indicate patient position (supine, sitting, standing) during venipuncture.
• Adrenocorticotropic hormone (ACTH, corticotropin)	Measures the plasma level of ACTH. Although ACTH is a pituitary hormone, it controls adrenal cortex secretion, thus helps to determine if underproduction or overproduction of cortisol is caused by dysfunction of the adrenal gland or pituitary gland. *Normal values* are morning: <80 pg/ml (18 pmol/L); evening: <50 pg/ml (<11 pmol/L).	Patient should be NPO after midnight before morning blood draw. Minimize stress. Diurnal levels correspond with variation of cortisol levels; that is, levels are higher in morning, lower in evening. ACTH is very unstable; blood tube must be placed on ice and sent to laboratory immediately.
• ACTH stimulation with cosyntropin	Used to evaluate adrenal function. After baseline samples are drawn, 250 mg cosyntropin (synthetic ACTH) is given as IV or IM bolus; samples are drawn 30 and 50 minutes after bolus. Baseline ACTH sample is often drawn in case results are abnormal. Plasma cortisol at 60 minutes should be (1) greater than baseline and (2) greater than 20 μg/dl.	Obtain baseline cortisol level at beginning of cosyntropin infusion. Inject cosyntropin with a plastic syringe and collect blood samples in plastic heparinized tubes. Administer test with continuous-infusion method. Monitor site and rate of IV infusion. Ensure sample collection at appropriate times.
• ACTH suppression (dexamethasone suppression)	Assesses adrenal function and is especially helpful if hyperactivity is suspected. Useful in evaluation of Cushing syndrome. Dexamethasone (Decadron) 2 mg is given at 11 PM to suppress secretion of corticotropin-releasing hormone. Plasma cortisol sample is drawn at 8 AM. Cortisol level <5 μg/dl (138 nmol/L) indicates normal adrenal response (50% decrease in cortisol production).	Ensure that patient has fasted. Inform patient that blood sample will be taken. Observe venipuncture site for bleeding and hematoma formation. Do not test acutely ill patients; those under stress are not tested. ACTH may override suppression. Screen patient for drugs such as estrogen and glucocorticoids, which may give false-positive results. Ensure accurate timing of medication and sample collection.

IM, Intramuscular.

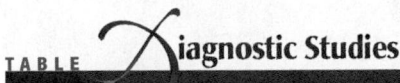

TABLE
46-7   Diagnostic Studies
Endocrine System—cont'd

STUDY	PURPOSE AND DESCRIPTION	NURSING RESPONSIBILITY
Urine Studies		
• 17-Ketosteroids	Measures androgen metabolites in urine and evaluates adrenocortical and gonadal function. *Normal values* are 10-22 mg/day (35-76 μmol/day) for men and 6-16 mg/day (21-55 μmol/day) for women.	Instruct patient regarding 24-hour urine collection. Tell patient that specimen must be kept refrigerated or iced during collection. Determine whether preservative is required for method used.
• Aldosterone	Measures urinary aldosterone level to evaluate adrenal function. Useful in determining therapy for hypertension. *Normal values* are 2-26 μg/24 hours (5.5-72 nmol/day).	Ensure that patient is on unrestricted diet with normal salt intake and no medication for 3 weeks before collection. Instruct patient regarding 24-hour urine collection.
• Free cortisol	Measures free (unbound) cortisol. Preferred test to evaluate hypercortisolism. *Normal values* are <100 μg/24 hours.	Instruct patient about 24-hour urine collection and avoidance of stressful situations and excessive physical exercise. Some drugs (e.g., reserpine, diuretics, phenothiazines, amphetamines) may elevate levels. Ensure that patient is on low-sodium diet.
• Vanillylmandelic acid	Measures urinary excretion of catecholamine metabolite and is helpful in diagnosing pheochromocytoma. *Normal values* are <8 mg/24 hours (40 μmol/day); pheochromocytoma is indicated with values of 10-250 mg/24 hours (51-126 μmol/day).	Keep 24-hour urine collection at pH of less than 3.0 with hydrochloric acid as preservative. Know that newer methods are not affected by dietary intake. Consult with laboratory or physician about patient discontinuing any drugs 3 days before urine collection.
Radiologic Tests		
• Computed tomography (CT)	Abdominal CT is the radiologic examination of choice for the adrenal gland. Used to detect tumor and size of tumor mass or metastatic spread. Oral and/or IV contrast medium may be used.	Inform patient of procedure. Patient must lie still during the procedure. If IV contrast is used, check for iodine allergy.
Pancreatic Studies		
Serum Studies		
• Fasting blood sugar (FBS) level	Measures circulating glucose level. *Normal values* for adults are 70-110 mg/dl (3.9-6.7 mmol/L); for pregnant women they are 60-90 mg/dl (3.3-5 mmol/L).	Patient should fast for at least 4-8 hours—water intake is permitted. If patient has an IV infusion containing dextrose, test is not considered valid.
• Oral glucose tolerance	A. 2-hour test used to diagnose diabetes mellitus if FBS is equivocal. Patient drinks 75 g of glucose; samples for glucose are drawn immediately and at 30, 60, and 120 minutes. *Normal values* are <200 mg/dl (11.1 mmol/L) at 30, 60, and 90 minutes and <140 mg/dl (7.8 mmol/L) at 120 minutes. B. 5-hour test used to evaluate hypoglycemia. Patient drinks 100 g of glucose; samples of glucose are drawn immediately and at 30, 60, 90, 120, 180, 240, and 300 minutes. Baseline cortisol level test is done if patient becomes symptomatic. Patients with reactive hypoglycemia have adrenergic symptoms and glucose <60 mg/dl (3.3 mmol/L) between 30 minutes and 5 hours after glucose ingestion.	Ensure that tests are not done on patients who are malnourished, confined to bed for over 3 days, or severely stressed. Instruct patient to refrain from smoking and caffeine and to fast for 12 hours before test. Ensure that patient's diet 3 days before test included 150-300 g of carbohydrate with intake of at least 1500 calories per day. Screen for estrogens, phenytoin (Dilantin), and corticosteroids, and check for hypokalemia, which may impair glucose tolerance. Simultaneously monitor glucose levels with capillary glucose monitoring.
• Capillary glucose monitoring	Used to give immediate glucose values with glucose oxidase or electrochemical methods. Capillary values (whole blood) are usually 10%-15% less than serum values.	Obtain large drop of blood from clean finger, touch strip to drop of blood (not finger), time accurately, and compare colors in good lighting, if using visual method. Use digital readout if available. Use automatic finger-puncture device if available. Be sure to change section of device that touches patient's fingers between patients.
• Glycosylated hemoglobin (Hb A$_{1c}$ [A1C])	Measures degree of glucose control during previous 3 months (life span of hemoglobin molecule). *Normal values* are 4%-6% (values vary widely; check with laboratory).	Inform patient that fasting is not necessary and that blood sample will be drawn. Observe venipuncture site for bleeding or hematoma formation.

Continued

TABLE 46-7 Diagnostic Studies — Endocrine System—cont'd

STUDY	PURPOSE AND DESCRIPTION	NURSING RESPONSIBILITY
Urine Studies		
• Glucose	Estimate amount of glucose in urine by using an enzymatic method. Dipstick is dipped into the urine and read for color changes after 1 minute. Normal results will show negative glucose in the urine.	Use freshly voided urine specimen collected at appropriate time. Know that many different drugs alter glucose readings and that errors are great if directions for timing are not followed exactly. Follow package directions.
• Ketones	Measures amount of acetone excreted in urine as result of incomplete fat metabolism. Tested with a dipstick as described above. Normal value is negative or trace ketone. Positive result can indicate lack of insulin and diabetic acidosis.	Use freshly voided urine specimen. Test is often done with glucose test. Directions must be followed exactly. Certain drugs can produce false-positive and false-negative results.
Radiologic Tests		
• Computed tomography (CT)	Abdominal CT is the radiologic examination of choice for pancreas. Used to identify tumors or cysts. Oral and/or intravenous contrast medium may be ordered.	Inform patient of procedure. Patient must lie still during the procedure. If IV contrast is used, check for iodine allergy.

Laboratory Studies

Laboratory studies used to diagnose endocrine problems may include direct measurement of the hormone level, or they may involve an indirect indication of gland function by evaluating blood or urine components affected by the hormone (e.g., electrolytes).

Hormones with fairly constant basal levels (e.g., T_4) require only a single measurement. Notation of sample time on the laboratory slip and sample is important for hormones with circadian or sleep-related secretion (e.g., cortisol). Evaluation of other hormones may require multiple blood sampling such as in suppression (e.g., dexamethasone) and stimulation (e.g., glucose tolerance) tests. In these situations, it is often necessary to obtain intravenous access to administer medications and fluids and to draw multiple blood samples.

Nursing interventions common to all patients requiring venipuncture for blood sampling include explaining the procedure to the patient, use of sterile technique, and applying pressure to the venipuncture site to minimize development of a hematoma. Many tests of endocrine function require the patient to fast and require the elimination of as many environmental stimuli as possible.[16] Normal values and collection procedures vary among laboratories. It is therefore important to refer to institutional policy and procedure for collection and handling of the various laboratory specimens, as well as established normal values for test results.

Pituitary Studies. Disorders associated with the pituitary gland can manifest in a wide variety of ways because of the number of hormones produced. There are many diagnostic studies that evaluate these hormones either directly or indirectly. The studies used to assess function of the anterior pituitary hormones relate to growth hormone, prolactin, follicle-stimulating hormone, luteinizing hormone, thyroid-stimulating hormone (TSH), and adrenocorticotropic hormone.

Thyroid Studies. There are a number of tests available to evaluate thyroid function. The most sensitive and accurate laboratory test is measurement of TSH; thus it is often recommended as a first diagnostic test for evaluation of thyroid function.[9] Common additional tests ordered in the presence of abnormal TSH include total serum thyroxine (T_4), free T_4, and total serum triiodothyronine (T_3). Free T_4 is the unbound thyroxine and is a more accurate reflection of thyroid function than total T_4. Less common tests that help in the differentiation of various types of thyroid disease include T_3, free T_3 resin uptake, thyroid autoantibodies, thyroid scanning, ultrasound, and biopsy. These tests are done to help differentiate various types of thyroid disorders.

Parathyroid Studies. The only hormone secreted by the parathyroid glands is parathyroid hormone (PTH). Because the function of PTH is to regulate serum calcium and phosphate levels, abnormalities in PTH secretion are reflected in the calcium and phosphate levels.[16] For this reason, diagnostic tests for the parathyroid gland typically include PTH, serum calcium, and serum phosphate.

Adrenal Studies. Diagnostic tests associated with the adrenal glands focus on the three types of hormones secreted: glucocorticoids, mineralocorticoids, and androgens. These hormone levels can be measured both in blood plasma and in urine. If urine studies are done, these will usually be done as 24-hour urine collection. The major advantage of a 24-hour urine sample is that the short-term fluctuations in hormone levels seen in plasma samples are eliminated.[17]

Pancreatic Studies. The tests found in Table 46-7 are geared toward evaluating the metabolism of glucose. The best way to diagnose diabetes mellitus is the oral glucose tolerance test. However, other tests listed are useful in management of diabetes. (Diagnostic studies for diabetes are discussed in Chapter 47.)

Radiologic Studies

A variety of radiologic studies are done to evaluate the endocrine system. Basic x-ray, CT, MRI, and radiologic isotope tests are examples of procedures commonly done. These studies are helpful in identifying the size of the gland or the presence of lesions or tumor on the gland, and in some cases the function of the gland. Nursing interventions common for patients undergoing radiologic testing include explaining the procedure to the patient. Some procedures may involve injection of a contrast medium; therefore the nurse must check for allergies.

REVIEW QUESTIONS

The number of the question corresponds to the same-numbered objective at the beginning of the chapter.

1. A characteristic common to all hormones is that they
   a. circulate in the blood bound to plasma proteins.
   b. influence cellular activity of specific target tissues.
   c. accelerate the metabolic processes of all body cells.
   d. enter cells to alter the cell's metabolism or gene expression.

2. A patient is receiving radiation therapy for cancer of the kidney. The nurse monitors the patient for signs and symptoms of damage to the
   a. pancreas.
   b. thyroid gland.
   c. adrenal glands.
   d. posterior pituitary gland.

3. A patient has a serum sodium level of 152 mEq/L (152 mmol/L). The normal hormonal response to this situation is
   a. release of ADH.
   b. release of renin.
   c. secretion of aldosterone.
   d. secretion of corticotropin-releasing hormone.

4. All cells in the body are believed to have intracellular receptors for
   a. insulin.
   b. glucagon.
   c. growth hormone.
   d. thyroid hormone.

5. When obtaining subjective data from a patient during assessment of the endocrine system, the nurse asks specifically about
   a. energy level.
   b. intake of vitamin C.
   c. employment history.
   d. frequency of sexual intercourse.

6. An appropriate technique to use during physical assessment of the thyroid gland is
   a. asking the patient to hyperextend the neck during palpation.
   b. percussing the neck for dullness to define the size of the thyroid.
   c. having the patient swallow water during inspection and palpation of the gland.
   d. using deep palpation to determine the extent of a visibly enlarged thyroid gland.

7. Endocrine disorders often go unrecognized in the older adult because
   a. symptoms are often attributed to aging.
   b. older adults rarely have identifiable symptoms.
   c. endocrine disorders are relatively rare in the older adult.
   d. older adults usually have subclinical endocrine disorders that minimize symptoms.

8. An abnormal finding by the nurse during an endocrine assessment would be
   a. blood pressure of 100/70.
   b. soft, formed stool every other day.
   c. excessive facial hair on a woman.
   d. 5 lb weight gain over last 6 months.

9. A patient has a total serum calcium level of 3 mg/dl (1.5 mEq/L). If this finding reflects hypoparathyroidism, the nurse would expect further diagnostic testing to reveal
   a. decreased serum PTH.
   b. increased serum ACTH.
   c. increased serum glucose.
   d. decreased serum cortisol levels.

REFERENCES

1. Molitch M: Neuroendocrinology. In Felig P, Frohman LA, editors: *Endocrinology and metabolism,* ed 4, New York, 2001, McGraw-Hill.
2. McCance KL, Huether SE: *Pathophysiology: the biologic basis for disease in children and adults,* ed 4, St Louis, 2002, Mosby.
3. Frohman LA, Felig P: The clinical manifestations of endocrine disease. In Felig P, Frohman LA, editors: *Endocrinology and metabolism,* ed 4, New York, 2001, McGraw-Hill.
4. Rasenick MM, Jaffe RC: Molecular mechanism of hormone action: biology of signal transduction. In Felig P, Frohman LA, editors: *Endocrinology and metabolism,* ed 4, New York, 2001, McGraw-Hill.
5. Herlihy B, Maebius NK: *The human body in health and illness,* Philadelphia, 2000, WB Saunders.
6. Becker KL, editor: *Principles and practice of endocrinology and metabolism,* ed 3, Philadelphia, 2001, Lippincott Williams & Wilkins.
7. Cooper PE: Physiology and pathophysiology of the endocrine brain and hypothalamus. In Becker KL, editor: *Principles and practice of endocrinology and metabolism,* ed 3, Philadelphia, 2001, Lippincott Williams & Wilkins.
8. Baumann G: Growth hormone and its disorders. In Becker KL, editor: *Principles and practice of endocrinology and metabolism,* ed 3, Philadelphia, 2001, Lippincott Williams & Wilkins.
9. Larson J, Anderson EH, Koslawy M: Thyroid disease: a review for primary care, *J Am Acad Nurse Pract* 12:226, 2000.
10. McCance KL, Huether SE: *Pathophysiology: the biologic basis for disease in children and adults,* ed 4, St Louis, 2002, Mosby.
11. Gruenewald DA: Endocrinology and aging. In Becker KL, editor: *Principles and practice of endocrinology and metabolism,* ed 3, Philadelphia, 2001, Lippincott Williams & Wilkins.
12. Fletcher KR: Physical and laboratory assessment. In Stone JT, Wyman JF, Salisbury SA, editors: *Clinical gerontological nursing,* ed 2, Philadelphia, 1999, WB Saunders.
13. Dellasega C, Yonushonis ME, Johnson AD: The aging endocrine system. In Stanley M, Beare PG: *Gerontological nursing,* ed 2, Philadelphia, 1999, FA Davis.
14. Kessenich CR, Cichon MJ: Hormonal decline in elderly men and male menopause, *Geriatr Nurs* 22:24, 2001.
15. Wilson SF, Giddens JF: *Health assessment for nursing practice,* ed 2, St Louis, 2001, Mosby.
16. Pagana KD, Pagana TJ: *Diagnostic and laboratory test reference,* ed 5, St Louis, 2001, Mosby.
17. Corbett JG: *Laboratory tests and diagnostic procedures with nursing diagnoses,* ed 5, Upper Saddle River, NJ, 2000, Prentice-Hall.

RESOURCES

Resources for this chapter are listed in Chapter 47 on page 1302 and Chapter 48 on page 1338.

CHAPTER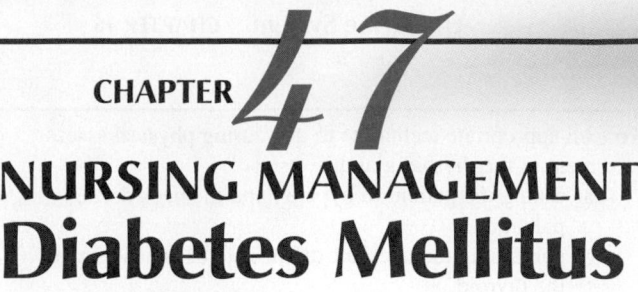

NURSING MANAGEMENT
Diabetes Mellitus

Susan Semb

LEARNING OBJECTIVES

1. Describe the pathophysiology and clinical manifestations of diabetes mellitus.
2. Describe the differences between type 1 and type 2 diabetes mellitus.
3. Describe the collaborative care of the patient with diabetes mellitus.
4. Describe the role of nutrition and exercise in the management of diabetes mellitus.

5. Describe the nursing management of a patient with newly diagnosed diabetes mellitus.
6. Describe the nursing management of the patient with diabetes mellitus in the ambulatory and home care settings.
7. Identify the pathophysiology and clinical manifestations of acute and chronic complications of diabetes mellitus.
8. Explain the collaborative care and nursing management of the patient with acute and chronic complications of diabetes mellitus.

KEY TERMS

angiopathy, p. 1296
diabetes mellitus, p. 1268
diabetic ketoacidosis, p. 1271
diabetic nephropathy, p. 1297
diabetic neuropathy, p. 1298
diabetic retinopathy, p. 1297
hyperosmolar hyperglycemic nonketotic syndrome, p. 1293
hypoglycemic unawareness, p. 1295
impaired fasting glucose, p. 1272
impaired glucose tolerance, p. 1271

insulin pump, p. 1276
insulin resistance, p. 1271
insulin resistance syndrome, p. 1271
intensive insulin therapy, p. 1277
lipodystrophy, p. 1278
prediabetes, p. 1271
self-monitoring of blood glucose, p. 1283
Somogyi effect, p. 1278

Diabetes Mellitus

Diabetes mellitus is a multisystem disease related to abnormal insulin production, impaired insulin utilization, or both. Diabetes mellitus is a serious health problem throughout the world. In the United States an estimated 17 million people, or 6.2% of the population, have diabetes mellitus. More than 2 million Canadians have diabetes. About one third of the people with diabetes mellitus are not diagnosed, and these individuals are unaware that they have the disease. Diabetes mellitus is the fifth leading cause of death in the United States, with 210,000 deaths annually. Nearly 20% of people over age 65 years have diabetes. The incidence of diabetes is expected to increase 165% in the next 50 years.[1]

Diabetes is the leading cause of heart disease, stroke, adult blindness, and nontraumatic lower limb amputations. People with diabetes mellitus have at least a twofold risk for the devel-

opment of coronary artery disease, and more than 65% have hypertension. The staggering annual cost due to medical expenditures attributable to diabetes is estimated at $98 billion. Hospitalization costs account for the greatest proportion of medical costs.[1] These dollar amounts do not reflect the impact that this disease has on the quality of the lives of the affected people and their families.

Etiology and Pathophysiology

Current theories link the causes of diabetes, singly or in combination, to genetic, autoimmune, viral, and environmental factors (e.g., obesity, stress). Regardless of its cause, diabetes is primarily a disorder of glucose metabolism related to absent or insufficient insulin supplies and/or poor utilization of the insulin that is available.

Although the American Diabetes Association (ADA) recognizes 11 different classifications of the disease, most of these types

CULTURAL & ETHNIC CONSIDERATIONS
Diabetes Mellitus

- The highest incidence of diabetes is among Native Americans, 15% of whom are treated for diabetes.
- Pima Indians in Arizona have the highest rate of diabetes in the world, with 50% of adults having diabetes.
- Complications of diabetes are more common in Native Americans and African Americans than in whites.
- Complications from diabetes are the major causes of death in most Native American populations.
- The rate of end-stage renal failure is six times higher among Native Americans than among other people with diabetes.
- Amputation rates among Native Americans are three to four times higher than in other populations with diabetes.
- The incidence of diabetes is higher among African Americans and Hispanics than whites, with 10% of Hispanics and 13% of African Americans having diabetes.
- Type 2 diabetes tends to affect a younger-age population in nonwhites than in whites.

Reviewed by Elizabeth Alden, RNC, BSN, CDE, Clinical Diabetic Educator, Diabetes Disease Management Team, University of New Mexico Hospital, Albuquerque, N.M.; and M. Susan Grinslade, RN, PhD(c), Assistant Professor, School of Nursing, University of Texas Health Science Center, San Antonio, Tex.

TABLE 47-1	Characteristics of Type 1 and Type 2 Diabetes Mellitus	
FACTOR	**TYPE 1 DIABETES MELLITUS**	**TYPE 2 DIABETES MELLITUS**
Age at onset	More common in young person but can occur at any age	Usually age 35 yr or older but can occur at any age Incidence is increasing in children
Type of onset	Signs and symptoms abrupt, but disease process may be present for several years	Insidious
Prevalence	Accounts for 5%-10% of all types of diabetes	Accounts for 90% of all types of diabetes
Environmental factors	Virus, toxins	Obesity, lack of exercise
Islet cell antibodies	Often present at onset	Absent
Endogenous insulin	Minimal or absent	Possibly excessive; adequate but delayed secretion or reduced utilization
Nutritional status	Thin, catabolic state	Obese or possibly normal
Symptoms	Thirst, polyuria, polyphagia, fatigue	Frequently none or mild
Ketosis	Prone at onset or during insulin deficiency	Resistant except during infection or stress
Nutritional therapy	Essential	Essential, possibly sufficient for glycemic control
Insulin	Required for all	Required for some
Oral hypoglycemic agents	Not beneficial	Usually beneficial
Vascular and neurologic complications	Frequent	Frequent

are rarely encountered in routine nursing practice (Table 47-1).[2] The two most common types of diabetes are classified as type 1 or type 2 diabetes mellitus. Gestational diabetes and secondary diabetes are other classifications of diabetes commonly seen in clinical practice (discussed later in this chapter).

Normal Insulin Metabolism. Insulin is a hormone produced by the β cells in the islets of Langerhans of the pancreas. Under normal conditions, insulin is continuously released into the bloodstream in small pulsatile increments (a basal rate), with increased release (bolus) when food is ingested (Fig. 47-1). The activity of released insulin lowers blood glucose and facilitates a stable, normal glucose range of approximately 70 to 120 mg/dl (3.9 to 6.66 mmol/L). The average amount of insulin secreted daily by an adult is approximately 40 to 50 U, or 0.6 U/kg of body weight.

Other hormones (glucagon, epinephrine, growth hormone, and cortisol) work to oppose the effects of insulin and are often referred to as *counterregulatory hormones.* These hormones work to increase blood glucose levels by stimulating glucose production and output by the liver and by decreasing the movement of glucose into the cells. Insulin and these counterregulatory hormones provide a sustained but regulated release of glucose for energy during food intake and periods of fasting and usually maintain blood glucose levels within the normal range. An abnormal production of any or all of these hormones may be present in diabetes.

Insulin is released from the pancreatic β cells as its precursor, proinsulin, and is then routed through the liver. Proinsulin is composed of two polypeptide chains, chain A and chain B, which are linked by the C-peptide chain. Insulin is formed when enzymes cleave C off, leaving the A and B chains. The presence of C peptide in serum and urine is a useful indicator of β cell function.

Insulin promotes glucose transport from the bloodstream across the cell membrane to the cytoplasm of the cell. The rise in plasma insulin after a meal stimulates storage of glucose as glycogen in liver and muscle, inhibits gluconeogenesis, enhances

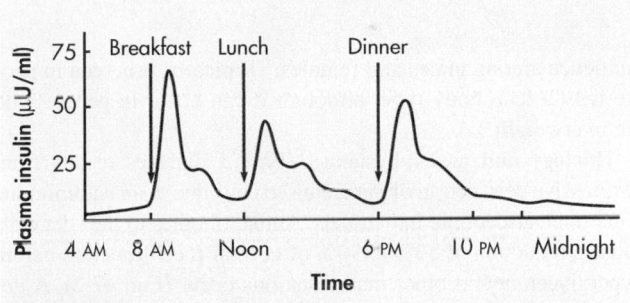

FIG. 47-1 Normal endogenous insulin secretion. In the first hour or two after meals, insulin concentrations rise rapidly in blood and peak at about 1 hour. After meals, insulin concentrations promptly decline toward preprandial values as carbohydrate absorption from the gastrointestinal tract declines. After carbohydrate absorption from the gastrointestinal tract is complete and during the night, insulin concentrations are low and fairly constant, with a slight increase at dawn.

fat deposition in adipose tissue, and increases protein synthesis. The fall in insulin level during normal overnight fasting facilitates the release of stored glucose from the liver, protein from muscle, and fat from adipose tissue. For this reason insulin is known as the *anabolic* or storage hormone.

Skeletal muscle and adipose tissue have specific receptors for insulin and are considered insulin-dependent tissues. Other tissues (e.g., brain, liver, blood cells) do not directly depend on insulin for glucose transport but require an adequate glucose supply for normal function. Although liver cells are not considered insulin-dependent tissue, insulin receptor sites on the liver facilitate the hepatic uptake of glucose and its conversion to glycogen.

Type 1 Diabetes Mellitus. Formerly known as "juvenile onset" or "insulin dependent" diabetes, *type 1 diabetes mellitus* most often occurs in people who are under 30 years of age, with a peak onset between ages 11 and 13. The rate of type 1 diabetes is 1.5 to 2 times higher in whites than nonwhites, with a similar

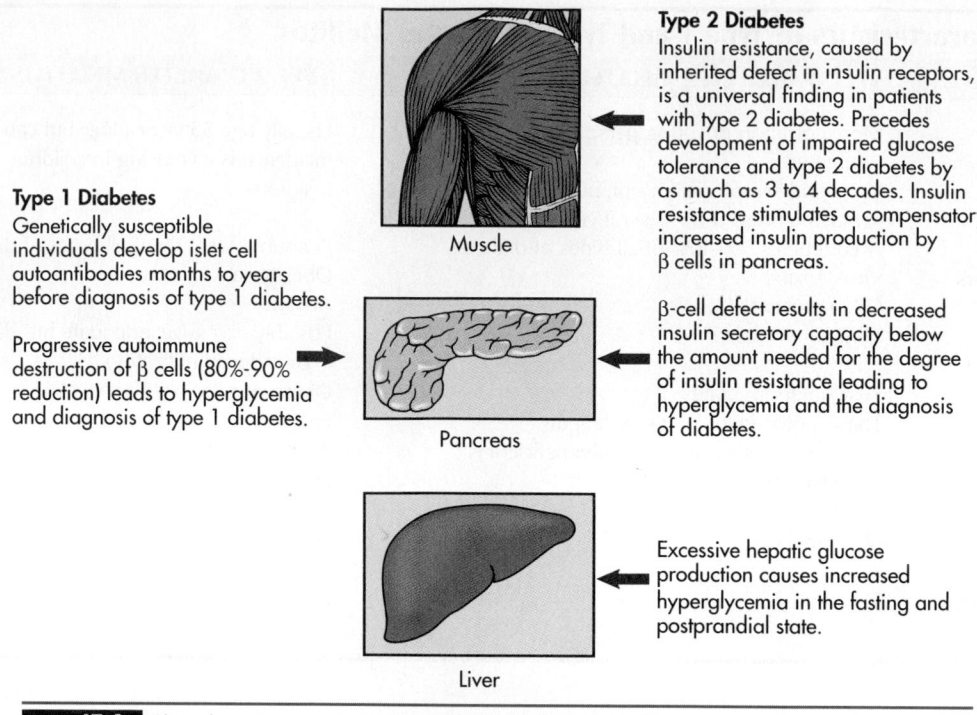

Type 1 Diabetes
Genetically susceptible individuals develop islet cell autoantibodies months to years before diagnosis of type 1 diabetes.

Progressive autoimmune destruction of β cells (80%-90% reduction) leads to hyperglycemia and diagnosis of type 1 diabetes.

Muscle

Pancreas

Liver

Type 2 Diabetes
Insulin resistance, caused by inherited defect in insulin receptors, is a universal finding in patients with type 2 diabetes. Precedes development of impaired glucose tolerance and type 2 diabetes by as much as 3 to 4 decades. Insulin resistance stimulates a compensatory increased insulin production by β cells in pancreas.

β-cell defect results in decreased insulin secretory capacity below the amount needed for the degree of insulin resistance leading to hyperglycemia and the diagnosis of diabetes.

Excessive hepatic glucose production causes increased hyperglycemia in the fasting and postprandial state.

FIG. 47-2 Altered mechanisms in type 1 and type 2 diabetes mellitus.

incidence among males and females.[3] Typically, it is seen in people with a lean body type, although it can occur in people who are overweight.

Etiology and pathophysiology. Type 1 diabetes results from progressive destruction of pancreatic β cells due to an autoimmune process in susceptible individuals. Autoantibodies to the islet cells cause a reduction of 80% to 90% of normal β cell function before hyperglycemia and other manifestations occur (Fig. 47-2). A genetic predisposition and exposure to a virus are factors that may contribute to the pathogenesis of type 1 diabetes.

Predisposition to type 1 diabetes is believed to be related to human leukocyte antigens (HLAs). (See Chapter 13 for a discussion of HLAs and disease associations). Theoretically, when an

individual with certain HLA types is exposed to viral infections, the β cells of the pancreas are destroyed, either directly or through an autoimmune process. The HLA types associated with an increased risk for type 1 diabetes include HLA-DR3 and HLA-DR4 (see Genetics in Clinical Practice box).

Onset of disease. Type 1 diabetes is associated with a long preclinical period. The islet cell autoantibodies responsible for β cell destruction are present for months to years before the onset of symptoms. Manifestations of type 1 diabetes develop when the person's pancreas can no longer produce insulin. Once this occurs, the onset of symptoms is usually rapid, and the patient comes to the emergency department with impending or actual ketoacidosis. The patient usually has a history of recent and sudden

GENETICS in CLINICAL PRACTICE
Types 1 and 2 Diabetes Mellitus

	TYPE 1 DIABETES MELLITUS	TYPE 2 DIABETES MELLITUS
Genetic basis	Associations between specific human leukocyte antigens (HLA-DR3, HLA-DR4)	Polygenic
	Possible mutation in insulin gene on chromosome 11	Major genes have not yet been identified
		Maturity-onset diabetes of the young (MODY)
		MODY1—linked to chromosome 20
		MODY2—linked to chromosome 7
		MODY3—linked to chromosome 12
Incidence	Accounts for about 5%-10% of cases in the United States	Accounts for about 90% of cases in the United States
Risk to offspring	Risk to offspring of diabetic mothers is only 1%-3%	Risk to first-degree relatives is 10%-15%
	Risk to offspring of diabetic fathers is 4%-6%	Identical twin concordance often exceeds 90%
	Identical twin concordance is 30%-50%	
Genetic testing	Currently under investigation	Currently under investigation
Clinical implications	Most individuals with type 1 diabetes do not have a first-degree relative with disorder	Most important risk factors include family history and obesity

weight loss, as well as the classic symptoms of *polydipsia* (excessive thirst), *polyuria* (frequent urination), and *polyphagia* (excessive hunger).

The individual with type 1 diabetes requires a supply of insulin from an outside source *(exogenous insulin),* such as an injection, in order to sustain life. Without insulin, the patient will develop **diabetic ketoacidosis** (DKA), a life-threatening condition resulting in metabolic acidosis. Newly diagnosed patients with type 1 diabetes often experience a remission, or "honeymoon period," soon after treatment is initiated. During this time, the patient requires very little injected insulin because β cell mass remains sufficient for glucose control as the progressive destruction continues to occur. Eventually, as more β cells are destroyed, blood glucose levels increase, more insulin is needed, and the honeymoon period ends. The honeymoon period usually lasts 3 to 12 months, after which the person will require insulin on a permanent basis.

Type 2 Diabetes Mellitus. *Type 2 diabetes mellitus* is, by far, the most prevalent type of diabetes, accounting for over 90% of patients with diabetes. Type 2 diabetes usually occurs in people over 40 years of age, and 80% to 90% of patients are overweight at the time of diagnosis. It has a tendency to run in families and probably has a genetic basis (see Genetics in Clinical Practice box). Prevalence of this type of diabetes is greater in some ethnic populations. The highest rates occur among Native Americans, who are about three times as likely to have type 2 diabetes as non-Hispanic whites of similar age. Hispanics also have higher rates, being about twice as likely to have diabetes as age-matched white counterparts. African Americans are about 1.7 times as likely to have diabetes as non-Hispanic whites of similar age.[1]

Prevalence of type 2 diabetes increases with age, with about half of the people diagnosed being older than 55. In the past, type 2 diabetes was known as "adult onset" diabetes. This term is no longer considered appropriate because the disease is now being seen in a rapidly growing number of children and adolescents.

Etiology and pathophysiology. In type 2 diabetes, the pancreas usually continues to produce some *endogenous* (self-made) insulin. However, the insulin that is produced is either insufficient for the needs of the body and/or is poorly utilized by the tissues. In contrast, there is a virtual absence of endogenous insulin in type 1 diabetes. The presence of endogenous insulin is the major pathophysiologic distinction between type 1 and type 2 diabetes.

Genetic mutations that lead to insulin resistance and a higher risk for obesity have been found in many people with type 2 diabetes. It is likely that multiple genes are involved in this complex, multifactorial disorder (see Genetics in Clinical Practice box).

Three major metabolic abnormalities have a role in the development of type 2 diabetes. The first factor is **insulin resistance,** which is a condition in which body tissues do not respond to the action of insulin. This is due to insulin receptors that are either unresponsive to the action of insulin and/or insufficient in number. Most insulin receptors are located on skeletal muscle, fat, and liver cells. When insulin is not properly used, the entry of glucose into the cell is impeded, resulting in hyperglycemia. In the early stages of insulin resistance, the pancreas responds to high blood glucose by producing greater amounts of insulin (if β cell function is normal). This creates a temporary state of hyperinsulinemia that coexists with the hyperglycemia.

A second factor in the development of type 2 diabetes is a marked decrease in the ability of the pancreas to produce insulin, as the β cells become fatigued from the compensatory overproduction of insulin. **Impaired glucose tolerance** (IGT), often called **prediabetes,** usually occurs when the alteration in β cell function is mild. IGT is a condition in which blood glucose levels are higher than normal but not high enough for a diagnosis of diabetes. Most people with IGT are at increased risk for developing type 2 diabetes and will develop it within 10 years. It is estimated that about 16 million Americans have IGT.

A third factor is inappropriate glucose production by the liver. Instead of properly regulating the release of glucose in response to blood levels, the liver does so in a haphazard way that does not correspond to the body's needs at the time. However, this is not considered a primary factor in the development of type 2 diabetes. Figure 47-2 depicts the altered mechanisms in type 1 and type 2 diabetes.

Insulin resistance syndrome (also known as *syndrome X,* metabolic syndrome, and cardiovascular dysmetabolic syndrome) is a cluster of abnormalities that act synergistically to greatly increase the risk for cardiovascular disease. Insulin resistance syndrome is characterized by elevated insulin levels, high levels of triglycerides, decreased levels of high-density lipoproteins (HDLs), increased levels of low-density lipoproteins (LDLs), and hypertension. Risk factors for insulin resistance syndrome include central obesity, sedentary lifestyle, polycystic ovary syndrome, urbanization/Westernization, ethnicity (Native Americans, Hispanics, and African Americans), family history, gestational diabetes, and increased age. Overweight people with IGT can prevent or delay the onset of diabetes through a program of weight loss and regular physical activity.[4]

Onset of disease. Disease onset in type 2 diabetes is usually gradual. The person may go for many years with undetected hyperglycemia that might produce few, if any, symptoms. If the patient with type 2 diabetes has marked hyperglycemia (e.g., 500 to 1000 mg/dl [27.6 to 55.1 mmol/L]), a sufficient endogenous insulin supply may prevent DKA from occurring. However, osmotic fluid and electrolyte loss related to hyperglycemia may become severe and lead to hyperosmolar coma. (Complications of diabetes are discussed later in this chapter.)

Gestational Diabetes. *Gestational diabetes* develops during pregnancy and occurs in about 4% of pregnancies in the United States. It is detected at 24 to 28 weeks of gestation, usually following an oral glucose tolerance test (OGTT). Women with gestational diabetes have a higher risk for cesarean delivery, perinatal death, and neonatal complications. Although most women with gestational diabetes will have normal glucose levels within 6 weeks postpartum, their risk for developing type 2 diabetes in 5 to 10 years is increased. Nutritional therapy is considered to be the first-line therapy. If nutritional therapy alone does not achieve desirable fasting blood glucose levels, insulin therapy is usually indicated. Gestational diabetes and management of the pregnant patient with diabetes is a specialized area not covered in detail in this chapter. The reader is advised to consult an obstetric text for information about this area.

Secondary Diabetes. Diabetes occurs in some people because of another medical condition or due to the treatment of a medical condition that causes abnormal blood glucose levels. Conditions that may cause secondary diabetes include Cushing syndrome, hyperthyroidism, and the use of parenteral nutrition.

Commonly used medications that can induce diabetes in some people include corticosteroids (prednisone), phenytoin (Dilantin), and atypical antipsychotics (e.g., clozapine [clozapril]). Secondary diabetes usually resolves when the underlying condition is treated. (Drugs that can alter blood glucose levels are listed in Table 47-8 later in this chapter.)

Clinical Manifestations

Type 1 Diabetes Mellitus. Because the onset of type 1 diabetes is rapid, the initial manifestations are usually acute. The classic symptoms are *polyuria* (frequent urination), *polydipsia* (excessive thirst), and *polyphagia* (excessive hunger). The osmotic effect of glucose produces the manifestations of polydipsia and polyuria. Polyphagia is a consequence of cellular malnourishment when insulin deficiency prevents utilization of glucose for energy. Weight loss may occur as the body cannot get glucose and turns to other energy sources, such as fat and protein. Weakness and fatigue may also be experienced, as body cells lack needed energy from glucose. Ketoacidosis, a complication associated with untreated type 1 diabetes, is associated with additional clinical manifestations that are discussed later in this chapter.

Type 2 Diabetes Mellitus. The clinical manifestations of type 2 diabetes are often nonspecific, although it is possible that an individual with type 2 diabetes will experience some of the classic symptoms associated with type 1. Some of the more common manifestations associated with type 2 diabetes include fatigue, recurrent infections, prolonged wound healing, and visual changes. Unfortunately the clinical manifestations appear so gradually that before the person knows it, he or she may have complications.

Complications

Complications of diabetes are discussed in detail later in this chapter.

Diagnostic Studies

Regardless of the type, the diagnosis of diabetes mellitus can be made through one of three methods. Whichever method is used, diagnosis of diabetes must be confirmed on a subsequent day by any of the three methods.[2] These methods and their criteria for diagnosis are as follows:

- Fasting plasma glucose level exceeding 126 mg/dl (7.0 mmol/L).
- Random, or casual, plasma glucose measurement exceeding 200 mg/dl (11.1 mmol/L), plus manifestations of diabetes, such as polyuria, polydipsia, and unexplained weight loss. *Casual* is defined as any time of day without regard to the time of the last meal.
- Two-hour OGTT level exceeding 200 mg/dl (11.1 mmol/L), using a glucose load of 75 g.

The fasting plasma glucose (FPG) test, confirmed by repeat testing on another day, is the preferred method of diagnosis. When overt symptoms of hyperglycemia (polyuria, polydipsia, and polyphagia) coexist with fasting plasma glucose levels of 126 mg/dl (7.0 mmol/L) or greater, further testing using the oral glucose tolerance test (OGTT) may not be necessary to make a diagnosis.[2]

When OGTT is used, the accuracy of test results depends on adequate patient preparation and attention to the many factors that may influence the outcome of such tests. For example, factors that can cause falsely elevated values include recent severe restrictions of dietary carbohydrate, acute illness, medications (e.g., contraceptives, glucocorticosteroids), and restricted activity such as bed rest. A patient with impaired gastrointestinal absorption may also have false-negative test results.

Impaired glucose tolerance (IGT) and impaired fasting glucose (IFG) each represent an intermediate stage between normal glucose homeostasis and diabetes. When the fasting blood glucose level is greater than 110 mg/dl (6.1 mmol/L) but less than 126 mg/dl (7.0 mmol/L), the individual is considered to have **impaired fasting glucose.** *Impaired glucose tolerance* is classified as a 2-hour plasma glucose level higher than normal but lower than that considered diagnostic for diabetes mellitus (between 140 mg/dl [7.8 mmol/L] and 200 mg/dl [11.1 mmol/L]).[2] IGT and IFG are risk factors for diabetes, as well as cardiovascular disease.

Measurement of glycosylated hemoglobin, also known as the *hemoglobin A$_{1c}$* (A1C) test, is useful in determining glycemic levels over time. The test works by showing the amount of glucose that has been attached to hemoglobin molecules over their life span. When blood glucose is elevated over time, the amount of glucose attached to the hemoglobin molecule increases and remains attached to the red blood cell (RBC) for the life of the cell (approximately 120 days). Therefore a glycosylated hemoglobin test indicates the overall glucose control for the previous 90 to 120 days. All patients with diabetes should have regular assessments of A1C done. Major studies have demonstrated that people with diabetes who can maintain near-normal A1C levels over time have a greatly reduced risk for the development of retinopathy, nephropathy, and neuropathy. For people with diabetes, the ideal A1C goal is 7.0% or less. Diseases affecting RBCs (e.g., sickle cell anemia) can affect the A1C results and should be taken into consideration in the interpretation of this test result.

Collaborative Care

The goals of diabetes management are to reduce symptoms, promote well-being, prevent acute complications of hyperglycemia, and delay the onset and progression of long-term complications. These goals are most likely to be met when the patient is able to maintain blood glucose levels as near to normal as possible. Patient teaching, which enables the patient to become the most active participant in his or her own care, is essential for a successful treatment plan. Nutritional therapy, drug therapy, exercise, and self-monitoring of blood glucose are the tools used in the management of diabetes (Table 47-2). The two types of glucose-lowering agents (GLAs) used in the treatment of diabetes are insulin and oral agents (OAs). All individuals with type 1 diabetes require insulin. For some people with type 2 diabetes, a regimen of proper nutrition, regular physical activity, and maintenance of desirable body weight will be sufficient to attain an optimal level of blood glucose control. For the majority, however, drug therapy will be necessary.

Drug Therapy: Insulin

Exogenous (injected) insulin is needed when a patient has inadequate insulin to meet specific metabolic needs and the combination of nutritional therapy, exercise, and OAs cannot maintain a satisfactory blood glucose level. Exogenous insulin is required for the management of type 1 diabetes. Exogenous insulin may be prescribed for the patient with type 2 diabetes who

TABLE 47-2 Collaborative Care — Diabetes Mellitus

Diagnostic
History and physical examination
Blood tests, including fasting blood glucose, postprandial blood glucose, glycosylated hemoglobin (A1C), lipid profile, blood urea nitrogen and serum creatinine, electrolytes
Urine for complete urinalysis, microalbuminuria, glucose and acetone (if indicated)
Funduscopic examination–dilated eye examination
Neurologic examination, including monofilament test for sensation to lower extremities
ECG
Blood pressure
Monitoring of weight
Doppler scan (if indicated)
Dental examination
Foot (podiatric) examination

Collaborative Therapy
Nutritional therapy (see Table 47-9)
Exercise therapy (see Tables 47-10 and 47-11)
Drug therapy
▪ Insulin (see Fig. 47-3 and Tables 47-3 and 47-4)
▪ Oral agents (see Table 47-7)
▪ Enteric-coated aspirin (325 mg)
▪ Angiotension-converting enzyme (ACE) inhibitors (see Table 32-8)
▪ Antilipidemic drugs (if indicated) (see Chapter 33, Table 33-6)
Self-monitoring of blood glucose (SMBG)
Patient and family teaching and follow-up programs

ECG, Electrocardiogram.

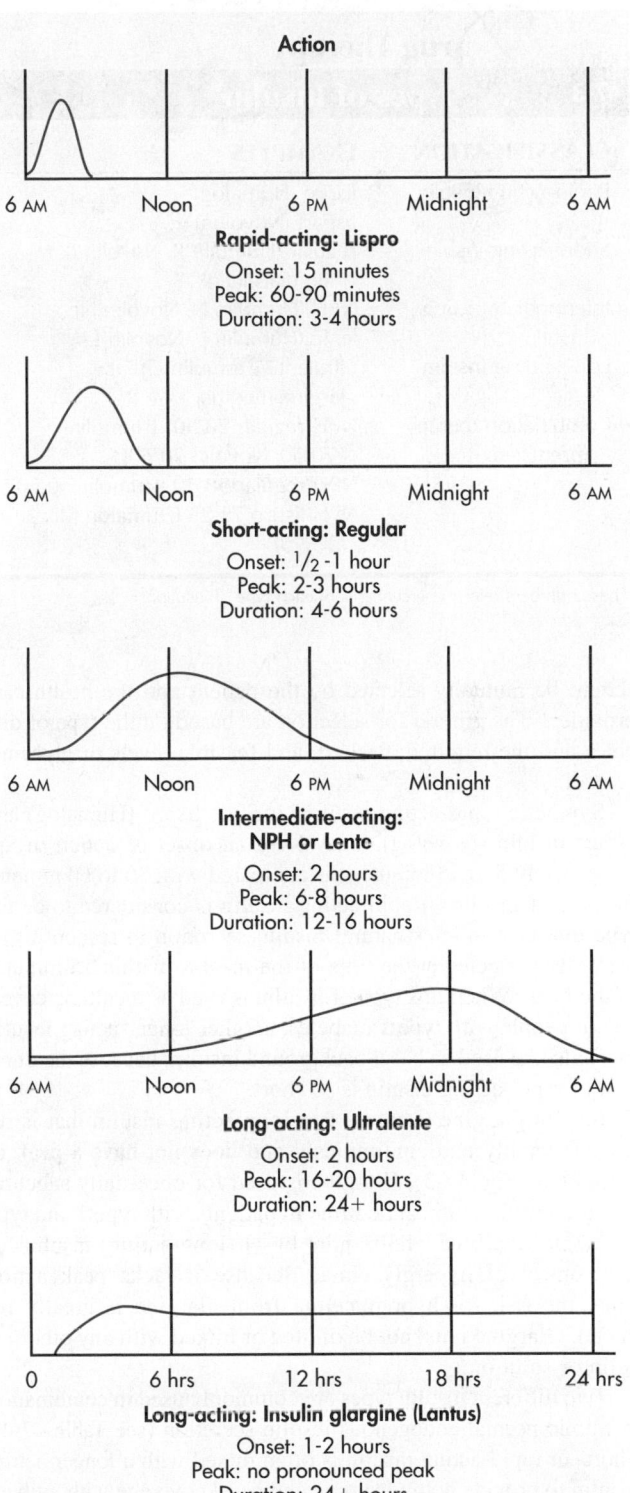

FIG. 47-3 Commercially available insulin preparations showing onset, peak, and duration of action.

cannot control blood glucose by other means, especially during periods of severe stress, such as illness or surgery.[5]

Types of Insulin. In the past, purified preparations of insulin made from beef and pork pancreas were used. However, human insulin is now the most widely used type of insulin. Human insulin is not directly harvested from human organs, but is derived from common bacteria (e.g., *Escherichia coli*) or yeast cells using recombinant DNA technology (see Chapter 13, Fig. 13-15). Although some patients who have had diabetes for many years may still be using animal insulin, newly diagnosed patients using insulin use the synthetically derived human insulin. The major advantage of human insulin is cost-effectiveness and decreased likelihood of causing an allergic reaction to animal insulin or additives to regular insulin.

Insulins differ in regard to onset, peak action, and duration (Fig. 47-3). The specific properties of each type of insulin are matched with the patient's diet and activity. Different combinations of these insulins can be used to tailor treatment to the patient's specific pattern of blood glucose levels, lifestyle, eating, and activity patterns. Different types of insulin are listed in Table 47-3. All insulin preparations start with regular insulin as a base. By adding zinc, acetate buffers, and protamine to insulin in various ways, the onset of activity, peak, and duration times can be manipulated. Zinc is added to make lente insulin, and zinc and protamine are added to make NPH. These additives can cause an allergic reaction at the injection site.

The timing of insulin administration in relation to meals is important. Regular insulin should be taken 30 to 45 minutes before meals to ensure the onset of action in conjunction with meal absorption. Examples of insulin combination regimens, onset, peak, and descriptions of the advantages and disadvantages of each regimen are presented in Table 47-4. Ideally, regimens

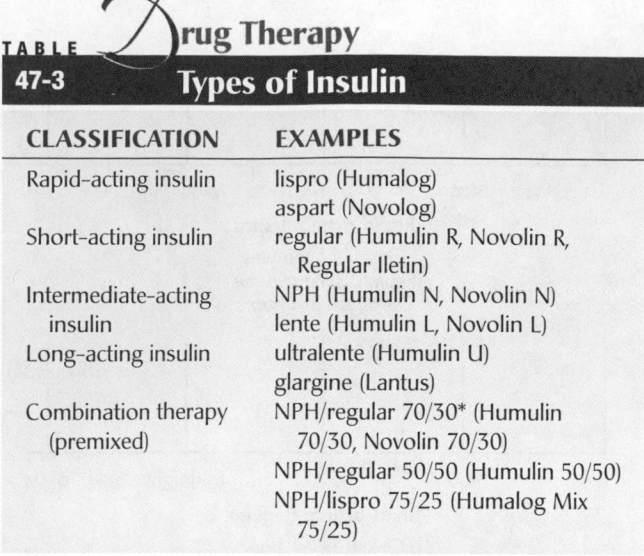

TABLE 47-3 Drug Therapy: Types of Insulin

CLASSIFICATION	EXAMPLES
Rapid-acting insulin	lispro (Humalog)
	aspart (Novolog)
Short-acting insulin	regular (Humulin R, Novolin R, Regular Iletin)
Intermediate-acting insulin	NPH (Humulin N, Novolin N)
	lente (Humulin L, Novolin L)
Long-acting insulin	ultralente (Humulin U)
	glargine (Lantus)
Combination therapy (premixed)	NPH/regular 70/30* (Humulin 70/30, Novolin 70/30)
	NPH/regular 50/50 (Humulin 50/50)
	NPH/lispro 75/25 (Humalog Mix 75/25)

*These numbers refer to percentages of each type of insulin.

should be mutually selected by the patient and the health care provider.[6] The criteria for selection are based on the type of diabetes and the required, desired, and feasible levels of glycemic control.

Synthetic rapid-acting insulins include lispro (Humalog) and aspart insulin (Novolog). They have an onset of action of approximately 5 to 15 minutes (as compared with 30 to 60 minutes for regular insulin). Rapid-acting insulin is considered to be the type that best mimics natural insulin secretion in response to a meal. It is injected at the time of the meal to within 15 minutes of the meal. When this type of insulin is used as mealtime coverage in people with type 1 diabetes, another longer-acting insulin must also be used as basal background insulin, because the duration of rapid-acting insulin is so short.

Insulin glargine (Lantus) is a long-acting insulin that is released steadily and continuously and does not have a peak of action (see Fig. 47-3). Glargine is used for once-daily subcutaneous administration at bedtime in patients with type 1 and type 2 diabetes mellitus who require basal (long-acting) insulin for the control of hyperglycemia. Because it lacks peak action time, the risk for hypoglycemia from glargine is greatly reduced. Glargine must not be diluted or mixed with any other insulin or solution.[7]

Two different insulin types are commonly used in combination to mimic normal endogenous insulin secretion (see Table 47-4). Short- or rapid-acting insulin is often mixed with a longer-acting insulin to provide both mealtime and basal coverage without having to administer two separate injections. Patients may mix the two types of insulin themselves or may use a commercially premixed formula (see Table 47-3). These offer convenience to patients and are especially helpful to those who lack the visual, manual, or cognitive skills to mix insulin themselves. However, the convenience of these formulas sacrifices the potential for optimal blood glucose control, because there is less opportunity for flexible dosing based on need.

As a protein, insulin requires special storage considerations. Heat and freezing alter the insulin molecule. Insulin vials that the patient is currently using may be left at room temperature for up to 4 weeks unless the room temperature is higher than 86° F (30° C) or below freezing (less than 37° F [2° C]). Prolonged exposure to direct sunlight should be avoided. Extra insulin may be stored in the refrigerator. The same principles apply for a patient who is traveling. Insulin can be stored in a thermos or cooler to keep it cool (not frozen) if the patient is traveling in hot climates.

Prefilled syringes are stable for up to 30 days when stored in the refrigerator. This may be beneficial to patients who are sight impaired or who lack the manual dexterity to fill their own syringes at home. In these cases family members, friends, and caregivers may prefill syringes on a periodic basis. Syringes prefilled with a cloudy solution should be stored in a vertical position with the needle pointed up to avoid clumping of suspended insulin binders in the needle.[8] When stored properly, prefilled syringes with mixed insulins should maintain potency for 30 days. Likewise, commercially prepared mixtures may be prefilled and stored for later use. Some insulin combinations are not appropriate for prefilling and storage because the mixture can alter the onset, action, and/or peak times of either of the types. Pharmacy references should be consulted as needed when mixing and prefilling different types of insulin. Prefilled syringes should be gently rolled between the palms before injection to warm the refrigerated insulin and to resuspend the particles.

Administration of Insulin. Because insulin is inactivated by gastric juices, it cannot be taken orally. Injection is the only route of administration currently approved for self-administration. Routine administration of insulin is most commonly done by means of subcutaneous (SQ) injection, although intravenous (IV) administration of regular insulin can be done when immediate onset of action is desired.

Injection. The steps in administering an SQ insulin injection are outlined in Table 47-5. The technique should be taught to new insulin users and reviewed periodically with long-term users. It should never be assumed that because insulin is being used, the patient knows and practices the correct insulin injection technique. Inaccurate preparation is often caused by poor eyesight. Air bubbles in the syringe may not be seen, or the scale on the syringe may be read improperly.

The patient receiving mixed insulins (e.g., regular and an intermediate-acting insulin) needs to learn the proper technique for combining both in the same syringe if commercially prepared premixed insulins are not used (Fig. 47-4). Insulins should not be mixed if they differ in purity or species origin.

The speed with which peak serum concentrations are reached varies with the anatomic site for injection. The fastest absorption is from the abdomen, followed by the arm, thigh, and buttock. Appropriate sites for insulin injection are noted in Fig. 47-5, although the abdomen is the preferred site. The patient should be cautioned about injecting into a site that is to be exercised. For example, the patient should not inject insulin into the thigh and then go jogging. Exercise of the area containing the injection site together with the increased body heat generated by the exercise may increase the rate of absorption and speed the onset of insulin action.

Before purified human insulins were widely used, patients were advised to rotate anatomic injection sites to prevent *lipodystrophy*, a condition that produces lumps and dents in the skin from repeated injection in the same spot. The use of

Drug Therapy

TABLE 47-4   Insulin Regimens

REGIMEN	TYPE OF INSULIN USED	TIME ADMINISTERED AND EXPECTED TIME-ACTION CURVE*	ADVANTAGES	DISADVANTAGES
Single dose	Intermediate insulin (I)		One injection should cover noon and PM meal. Hypoglycemia during sleep is not a problem.	No fasting, breakfast, or nighttime coverage of hyperglycemia is available.
Split-mixed dose (70/30 premix)	Intermediate and regular or Humalog insulin (I + R or I + H)		Two injections provide coverage for 24 hr.	Two injections are required. Patient must adhere to a set meal pattern.
Split-mixed dose	Intermediate and regular or Humalog insulin (I + R or I + H)		Three injections provide coverage for 24 hr, particularly during early AM hours. Potential is reduced for 2-3 AM hypoglycemia.	Three injections are required.
Multiple dose	Intermediate and regular or Humalog insulin (I + R or I + H)		More flexibility is allowed at mealtimes and for amount of food intake.	Four injections are required. Premeal blood glucose checks, establishing and following individualized algorithm are necessary. Patients with type 1 will require basal insulin (I or LA) during the day.
Multiple dose† (split dose long-acting insulin [ultralente])	Regular or Humalog and long-acting insulin (R + LA or H + LA)		Insulin delivery pattern more closely simulates normal endogenous insulin pattern. Some flexibility is allowed in food intake pattern. Regimen gives a basal insulin coverage and regular or Humalog insulin covers meal blood glucose excursions.	Required three or four injections and blood glucose check premeal and on retiring. Establishing and following individualized algorithm are necessary.

H, lispro (Humalog) or rapid-acting insulin (R) = ———; I, intermediate insulin = ———; LA, long-acting insulin = —·—·—; R, regular insulin = ———.
*Insulin delivery through a pump is similar to this regimen.

TABLE 47-5 Patient & Family Teaching Guide
Insulin Therapy

1. Wash hands thoroughly.
2. Roll intermediate or long-acting insulin bottle between palms of hands to mix insulin. *Note:* Always inspect insulin bottle before using it. Make sure that it is of proper type and concentration, expiration date has not passed, and top of bottle is in perfect condition.
3. Prepare insulin injection in same manner as for any injection.
4. Select proper injection site and inject following procedure for any SQ injection (see Fig. 47-5). In sites where SQ tissue is adequate, inject commercial insulin needles at 90-degree angle. For sites with minimal SQ tissue, pinch up skin and insert needle at 45-degree angle.
5. If blood appears in syringe after needle is inserted, select new site for injection. Aspiration of syringe is not necessary.
6. After injecting insulin, apply some pressure with dry cotton ball (or 2 × 2 gauze pad) at site when withdrawing needle.
7. Hold ball in place for a few seconds but do not massage.
8. Destroy and dispose of single-use syringe safely. *Note:* When instructing patient to self-inject insulin, use the following guidelines (if appropriate):
   - Aspiration does not need to be done before injection.
   - The injection site does not need to be cleansed with alcohol.

SQ, Subcutaneous.

1 Wash hands.
2 Gently rotate NPH insulin bottle.
3 Wipe off tops of insulin vials with alcohol sponge.
4 Draw back amount of air into the syringe that equals total dose.

5 Inject air equal to NPH dose into NPH vial. Remove syringe from vial.

6 Inject air equal to regular dose into regular vial.

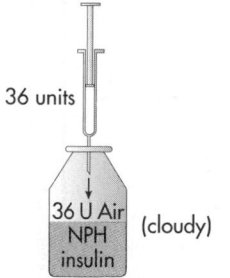

36 units

36 U Air NPH insulin (cloudy)

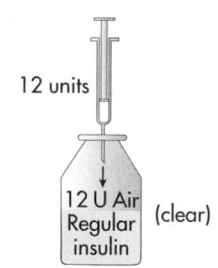

12 units

12 U Air Regular insulin (clear)

7 Invert regular insulin bottle and withdraw regular insulin dose.

8 Without adding more air to NPH vial, carefully withdraw NPH dose.

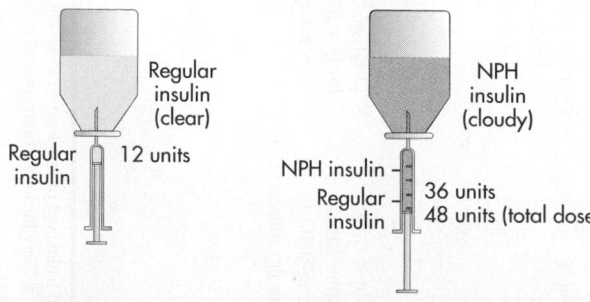

Regular insulin (clear)

Regular insulin   12 units

NPH insulin (cloudy)

NPH insulin –
Regular insulin   36 units
48 units (total dose)

FIG. 47-4 Mixing insulins. This step-order process avoids the problem of contaminating regular insulin with intermediate–acting insulin.

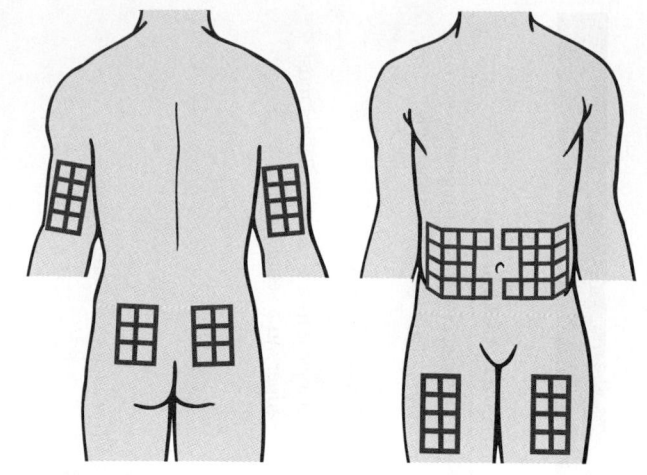

FIG. 47-5 Injection sites for insulin.

human insulin reduces the risk for lipodystrophy. Because of this, and because rotating sites causes variability in insulin absorption, rotation of injection sites to different anatomic sites is no longer the recommended practice. Instead, patients are advised to rotate the injection within one particular site, such as the abdomen. Sometimes it is helpful to think of the entire abdomen as a checkerboard, with each square representing an injection site as the patient rotates sites systematically across the board.

Most commercial insulin is available as U100, indicating that 1 ml contains 100 U of insulin. U100 insulin must be used with a U100-marked syringe. Disposable plastic insulin syringes are available in a variety of sizes, including 1, 0.5, and 0.3 ml. The 0.5 ml size may be used for doses of 50 U or less, and the 0.3 ml syringe can be used for doses of 30 U or less. Smaller syringes offer a number of advantages. The major benefit is increased accuracy and reliability when delivering smaller doses because wider line markings are easier to see. Patients should be cautioned to check dosage lines carefully when changing syringe types because some use a scale of 1 U increments and others use a 2 U increment.

Recapping should *only* be done by the person using the syringe. The nurse must never recap a needle that has been used by a patient. The use of an alcohol swab on the site before self-injection is no longer recommended. Routine hygiene such as washing with soap and rinsing with water is adequate. This applies primarily to patient self-injection technique. When injection occurs in a health care facility, policy may dictate site preparation with alcohol to prevent nosocomial infection.

An insulin pen is a compact portable device that serves the same function as a needle and syringe but is handier to use (Fig. 47-6, *A*). The pen usually comes preloaded with insulin. One of the advantages of insulin pens is that they are less "medical" looking. A new type of pen is the InDuo, which combines an insulin pen and a blood glucose monitor (Fig. 47-6, *B*).

Alternate delivery methods. Continuous subcutaneous insulin infusion can be administered using an **insulin pump,** a small battery-operated device that resembles a standard paging device in size and appearance (Fig. 47-7). Usually worn on the belt, the pump is connected via a small plastic tube to a catheter inserted into the subcutaneous tissue in the abdominal wall.

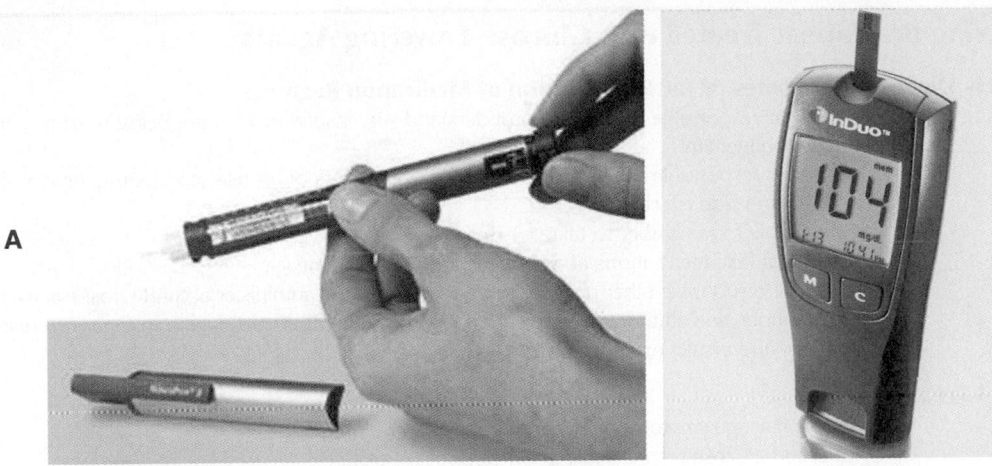

FIG. 47-6 **A**, NovoPen insulin pen. **B**, Blood glucose monitor by InDuo is used to measure blood glucose levels.

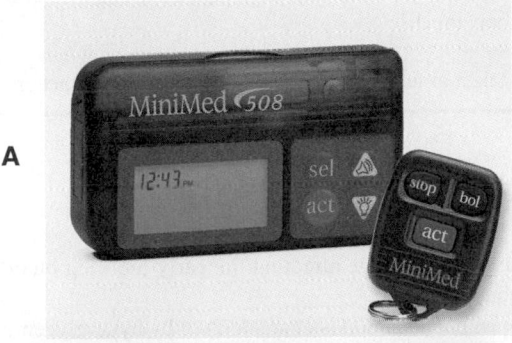

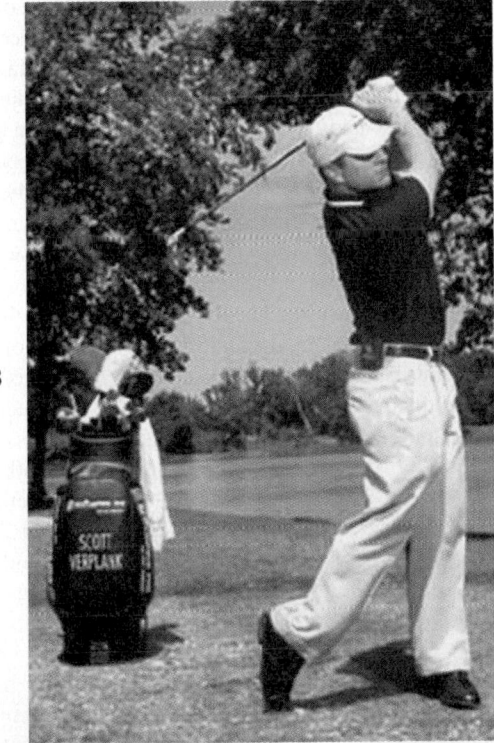

FIG. 47-7 **A**, MiniMed insulin pump. **B**, Professional golfer Scott Verplank wearing his MiniMed pump at the Ryder Cup 2002.

Every 2 to 3 days the insertion site is changed and the pump is refilled with insulin and reprogrammed. The device is programmed to deliver a continuous infusion of short-acting insulin 24 hours a day, known as the "basal rate." At mealtime, the user programs the pump to deliver a bolus infusion of insulin appropriate to the amount of carbohydrate ingested and to bring down high premeal blood glucose, if necessary. A major advantage of the insulin pump is the potential for tight glucose control.[9] This is possible because insulin delivery becomes very similar to the normal physiologic pattern. Pumps also offer the benefit of a more normal lifestyle, allowing users more flexibility with meal and activity patterns. The insertion site should be checked daily for redness and swelling.[10]

An alternative to the insulin pump is **intensive insulin therapy,** which consists of multiple daily insulin (MDI) injections together with frequent self-monitoring of blood glucose. The goal is to achieve a near-normal glucose level of 80 to 120 mg/dl (4.45 to 6.7 mmol/L) before meals. The Diabetes Control and Complications Trial (DCCT) demonstrated that people with type 1 diabetes who have tight glucose control through intensive management develop fewer and less severe complications.[11] Studies have shown comparable control outcomes in patients receiving intensive therapy and patients with an insulin pump. The disadvantages of MDI are that three or more injections are needed daily. In addition, intermediate- and long-acting insulins (NPH, lente, ultralente, glargine) must be used as the basal component.

Problems with Insulin Therapy. Hypoglycemia, allergic reactions, lipodystrophy, and Somogyi effect are the problems associated with insulin therapy. Hypoglycemia is discussed in detail later in this chapter. (Guidelines for assessing patients treated with insulin are presented in Table 47-6.)

Allergic reactions. Local inflammatory reactions to insulin may occur, such as itching, erythema, and burning around the injection site. Local reactions may be self-limiting within 1 to 3 months or may improve with a low dose of antihistamine. A true insulin allergy is a systemic response with urticaria and possibly anaphylactic shock generally resulting from the use of animal

TABLE 47-6   Assessing the Patient Treated with Glucose-Lowering Agents

For Patient with Newly Diagnosed Diabetes or for Reevaluation of Medication Regimen

Cognitive	Is patient or responsible other able to understand why insulin or OAs are being used as part of diabetes management?
	Is patient or responsible other able to understand concepts of asepsis, combining insulins, insulin-OA actions, and side effects?
	Is patient able to remember to take >1 dose/day?
	Does patient take medications at right times in relation to meals?
Psychomotor	Is patient or responsible other physically able to prepare and administer accurate doses of the medication?
Affective	What emotions and attitudes are patient and responsible others displaying in regard to diagnosis of diabetes and insulin or OA treatment?

For Follow-up of GLA-treated Patient

Effectiveness of therapy	Is patient having symptoms of hyperglycemia?
	Does blood glucose record show good or poor control?
	Is glycosylated hemoglobin consistent with glucose records?
Side effects of therapy	Is atrophy or hypertrophy present at injection sites?
	Has patient had hypoglycemic episodes? If so, how often? What time of day?
	Are there complaints of nightmares, night sweats, or early morning headaches?
	Has patient had skin rash or GI upset since taking OA?
Self-management behaviors	If patient is having hypoglycemic episodes, how are those episodes managed?
	How much insulin or OA is the patient taking and at what time of day? Is patient adjusting insulin or OA dose? Under what circumstances and by how much?
	Has exercise pattern changed?
	Is patient adhering to the meal plan? Are meals taken at times corresponding to peak insulin action?

GI, Gastrointestinal; *GLA,* glucose-lowering agent; *OAs,* oral agents.

insulins. Fortunately, this type of allergy is rare, particularly since human insulin has become available.

Lipodystrophy. **Lipodystrophy** (hypertrophy or atrophy of SQ tissue) may occur if the same injection sites are used frequently. Hypertrophy, a thickening of the SQ tissue, eventually regresses if the patient does not use the site for at least 6 months. The use of hypertrophied sites may result in erratic insulin absorption. Lipodystrophies have been most commonly associated with beef or beef and pork insulin and rarely with human insulin. Site rotation on a daily or weekly basis is not necessary with human insulin.

Somogyi effect and dawn phenomenon. Wide differences in early morning (low) and fasting (high) glucose levels characterize the **Somogyi effect** (Fig. 47-8). Usually occurring during the hours of sleep, the Somogyi effect produces a decline in blood glucose level in response to too much insulin. Counterregulatory hormones are released, stimulating lipolysis, gluconeogenesis, and glycogenolysis, which in turn produce rebound hyperglycemia and ketosis. The danger of this effect is that when blood glucose levels are measured in the morning, hyperglycemia is apparent and the patient (or the health care professional) may increase the insulin dose. The Somogyi effect is associated with the occurrence of undetected hypoglycemia during sleep, although it can happen at any time.

The patient may report headaches on awakening and may recall night sweats or nightmares. If the Somogyi effect is suspected as a cause for early morning high blood glucose, the patient may be advised to check blood glucose levels between 2:00 and 4:00 AM to determine if hypoglycemia is present at that time.

If it is, the insulin dosage affecting the early morning blood glucose is reduced.

The *dawn phenomenon* is characterized by hyperglycemia that is present on awakening in the morning due to the release of counterregulatory hormones in the predawn hours. It has been suggested that growth hormone and/or cortisol are possible factors in this occurrence. The dawn phenomenon affects the majority of people with diabetes and tends to be most severe when growth hormone is at its peak in adolescence and young adulthood.

Careful assessment is required to document each phenomenon because the treatment for each differs. The treatment for Somogyi effect is less insulin. The treatment for dawn phenomenon is an adjustment in the timing of insulin administration or an increase in insulin. The assessment must include insulin dose, injection sites, and variability in the time of meals or insulin administration. In addition, the patient is asked to measure and document bedtime, nighttime (between 2:00 and 4:00 AM), and morning fasting blood glucose levels on several occasions. If the predawn levels are below 60 mg/dl (3.3 mmol/L) and signs and symptoms of hypoglycemia are present, the insulin dosage should be reduced. If the 2:00 to 4:00 AM blood glucose is high, the insulin dosage should be increased. In addition, the patient should be counseled on appropriate bedtime snacks.

Drug Therapy: Oral Agents

Oral agents (OAs) are not insulin, but they work to improve the mechanisms by which insulin and glucose are produced and used by the body. For any of the OAs to be effective, the patient

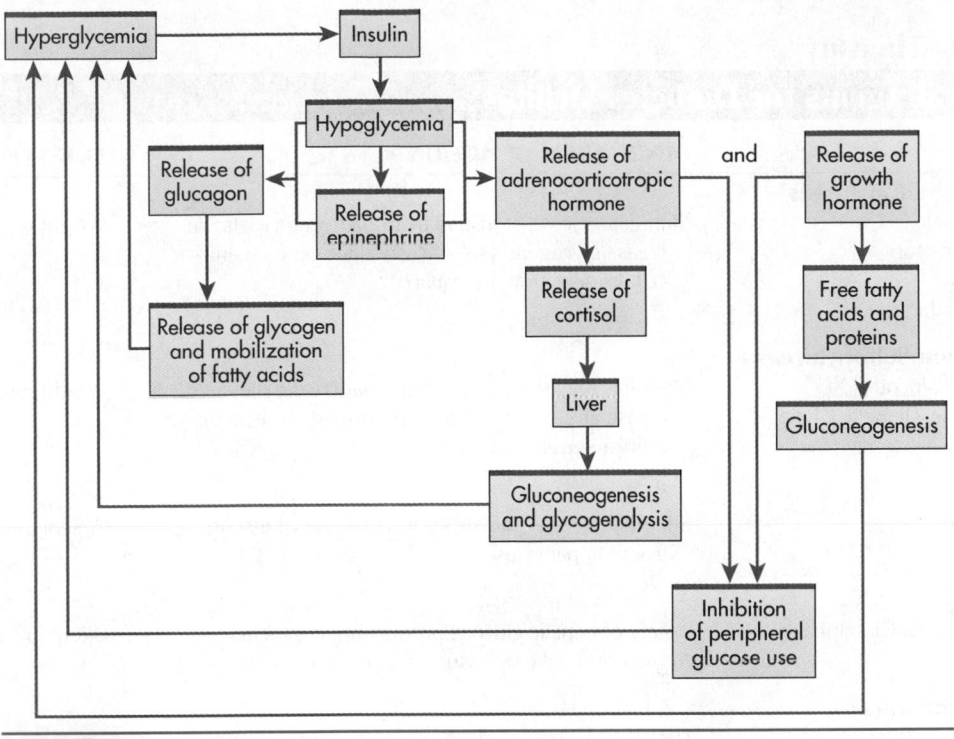

FIG. 47-8 The Somogyi effect.

must have some circulating endogenous insulin. There are currently no OAs for the treatment of type 1 diabetes. OAs may be used in combination with agents from other classes or with insulin to achieve blood glucose targets. Guidelines for assessing patients receiving OAs are shown in Table 47-6.

Currently, five classes of oral medications are available to improve diabetes control for patients with type 2 diabetes.[12] These agents are listed in Table 47-7.

Sulfonylureas. Sulfonylureas have been widely used to treat type 2 diabetes since the 1950s. They are called *first generation* or *second generation* depending on when they were introduced into clinical use in the United States. The first generation of these drugs used in the treatment of diabetes mellitus includes tolbutamide (Orinase), acetohexamide (Dymelor), tolazamide (Tolinase), and chlorpropamide (Diabinese). The second generation of sulfonylureas includes glipizide (Glucotrol, Glucotrol XL), glyburide (Micronase, DiaBeta, Glynase), and glimepiride (Amaryl). Second-generation drugs have fewer adverse effects and are more potent by weight, but they are more expensive.

The primary action of the sulfonylureas is to increase insulin production from the pancreas. Therapy with sulfonylureas is generally more effective early in the course of type 2 diabetes. About 10% of patients will experience decreased effectiveness of these medications after prolonged use.[13]

Meglitinides. Like the sulfonylureas, repaglinide (Prandin) and nateglinide (Starlix) increase insulin production from the pancreas. But because they are more rapidly absorbed and eliminated, they offer a reduced potential for hypoglycemia. When taken just before meals, pancreatic insulin production increases during and after the meal, mimicking the normal blood glucose response to eating. Patients should be instructed to take meglitinides anytime from 30 minutes before each meal right up to the time of the meal.

Biguanides. Metformin (Glucophage) is a biguanide glucose-lowering agent. It can be used alone or with sulfonylureas, other OAs, or insulin to treat type 2 diabetes. The primary action of metformin is to reduce glucose production by the liver. It also enhances insulin sensitivity at the tissue level and improves glucose transport into the cells. Besides being an effective blood glucose–lowering agent, metformin has other advantages. Unlike sulfonylureas and insulin, metformin does not promote weight gain. It also has beneficial effects on plasma lipids. Metformin is also used to treat prediabetes, especially in individuals who are obese and have diabetes.

Combination therapy that combines metformin with another drug is available as one tablet. These combinations include metformin with glyburide (Glucovance), with rosiglitazone (Avandia), and with glipizide (Metaglip).[6]

***α*-Glucosidase inhibitors.** Also known as "starch blockers," these drugs work by slowing down the absorption of carbohydrate in the small intestine. Acarbose (Precose) and miglitol (Glyset) are the available drugs in this class. Taken with the first bite of each main meal, they are most effective in lowering postprandial blood glucose. Effectiveness of these medications is measured by checking 2-hour postprandial glucose levels. Medications from this class are not effective against fasting hyperglycemia.[13]

Thiazolidinediones. Sometimes referred to as "insulin sensitizers," these agents include pioglitazone (Actos) and rosiglitazone (Avandia). They are most effective for people who have insulin resistance. They improve insulin sensitivity, transport, and

Drug Therapy

TABLE 47-7   Oral Agents for Diabetes Mellitus

TYPE	MECHANISM OF ACTION	SIDE EFFECTS
First-Generation Sulfonylureas* tolbutamide (Orinase) acetohexamide (Dymelor) tolazamide (Tolinase) chlorpropamide (Diabinese)	Stimulate release of insulin from pancreatic islets; decrease glycogenolysis and gluconeogenesis; enhance cellular sensitivity to insulin	Weight gain, hypoglycemia
Second-Generation Sulfonylureas glipizide (Glucotrol, Glucotrol XL) glyburide (Micronase, DiaBeta, Glynase) glimepiride (Amaryl)	Stimulate release of insulin from pancreatic islets; decrease glycogenolysis and gluconeogenesis; enhance cellular sensitivity to insulin	Weight gain, hypoglycemia
Meglitinides repaglinide (Prandin) nateglinide (Starlix)	Stimulate a rapid and short-lived release of insulin from the pancreas	Weight gain, hypoglycemia
Biguanide metformin (Glucophage, Glucophage XR)	↓ Rate of hepatic glucose production; augments glucose uptake by tissues, especially muscles	Diarrhea, lactic acidosis
α-Glucosidase Inhibitors acarbose (Precose) miglitol (Glyset)	Delay absorption of glucose from GI tract	Gas, abdominal pain, diarrhea
Thiazolidinediones pioglitazone (Actos) rosiglitazone (Avandia)	↑ Glucose uptake in muscle; ↓ endogenous glucose production	Weight gain, edema
Combination Therapy Glucovance Avandamet Metaglip	Combination of metformin and glyburide Combination of rosiglitazone and metformin Combination of metformin and glipizide	Nausea, diarrhea, abdominal pain, lactic acidosis, weight gain, hypoglycemia

*These drugs are not commonly used because they have been replaced by the second-generation sulfonylureas.

utilization at target tissues. Because they do not increase insulin production, thiazolidinediones will not cause hypoglycemia when used alone, but the risk is still present when a thiazolidinedione is used in combination with a sulfonylurea or insulin. Patients taking these medications may experience a secondary benefit of improved lipid profiles and blood pressure levels.[13,14]

Other Drugs Affecting Blood Glucose Levels. Both the patient and the health care provider must be aware of drug interactions that can potentiate hypoglycemic and hyperglycemic effects. For example, β-adrenergic blockers can mask symptoms of hypoglycemia and prolong the hypoglycemic effects of insulin. Thiazide and loop diuretics can potentiate hyperglycemia by inducing potassium loss, although low-dose therapy with a thiazide is usually considered safe. A list of medications that may influence glycemic control is presented in Table 47-8.

Nutritional Therapy

Although nutritional therapy is the cornerstone of care for the person with diabetes, it is also the most challenging for many people. Achieving nutritional goals requires a coordinated team effort that takes into account the behavioral, cognitive, socioeco-

nomic, cultural, and religious aspects of the person. Because of these complexities it is recommended that a diabetes nurse educator and a registered dietitian, with expertise in diabetes management, be members of the team.

Many people, both lay and professional, are misinformed about the nutritional management of diabetes. Although it is still used in many settings, the term "ADA diet" is no longer recommended because the American Diabetes Association (ADA) no longer endorses a single meal plan. Instead, nutritional therapy for the management of diabetes is based on a plan of healthy eating that is appropriate and beneficial to most people, whether they have diabetes or not. In an institutional setting, the prescribed diet is often labeled "ADA," indicating that the meal plan follows the ADA's current nutritional recommendations.

Recently issued guidelines from the ADA indicate that within the context of an overall healthy eating plan, a person with diabetes can eat the same foods as a person who does not have diabetes. This means that the same principles of good nutrition that apply to the general population also apply to the person with diabetes. The Food Guide Pyramid (see Chapter 39, Fig. 39-1) summarizes and illustrates nutritional guidelines and nutrient needs. These are also appropriate in guiding the food choices of

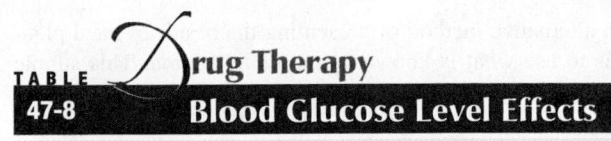

TABLE 47-8   Drug Therapy
Blood Glucose Level Effects

Glucose-Lowering Effect

acetaminophen (Tylenol)	Monoamine oxidase inhibitors
allopurinol (Zyloprim)	phenylbutazone
α-Glucosidase inhibitors	Potassium salts
Anabolic steroids	probenecid
β-Adrenergic blockers	Salicylates in large doses
Biguanides	Sulfonylureas
chloramphenicol	Thiazolidinediones
clofibrate (Atromid)	Tricyclic antidepressants
Insulin	Urinary acidifiers

Glucose-Raising Effect

acetazolamide (Diamox)	Glucagon
Alcohol	Glucose
asparaginase (Elspar)	Glycerin
Caffeine in large doses	Glycerol
Arginine	levodopa
Barbiturates	lithium
Birth control pills	Niacin
calcitonin	Marijuana
Calcium channel blockers	Nicotine
cholestyramine (Questran)	nifedipine (Procardia)
clonidine (Catapres)	phenobarbital
Corticosteroids	Phenothiazines
cyclosporine	phenytoin (Dilantin)
ethacrynic acid (Edecrin)	rifampin
morphine	tacrolimus (Prograf)
epinephrine	Thiazide diuretics
furosemide (Lasix)	Urinary alkalizing agents

people with diabetes. Tools used to measure the effectiveness of nutritional therapy include blood glucose, A1C and lipid values, tests of renal status, and clinical measurements such as body weight and blood pressure.[15] Table 47-9 describes nutritional therapy for type 1 and type 2 diabetes.

According to the ADA, the overall goal of nutritional therapy is to assist people with diabetes in making changes in nutrition and exercise habits that will lead to improved metabolic control. Additional specific goals include the following:[16]

1. Maintain blood glucose levels to as near normal as safely possible to prevent or reduce the risk for complications of diabetes.
2. Achieve lipid profiles and blood pressure levels that reduce the risk for cardiovascular disease.
3. Modify lifestyle as appropriate for the prevention and treatment of obesity, dyslipidemia, cardiovascular disease, and nephropathy.
4. Improve health through healthy food choices and physical activity.
5. Address individual nutritional needs while taking into account personal and cultural preferences and respecting the individual's willingness to change.

Type 1 Diabetes Mellitus. Meal planning should be based on the individual's usual food intake and balanced with insulin and exercise patterns. The insulin regimen should be developed with the patient's eating habits and activity pattern in mind. Patients using rapid-acting insulin can make adjustments in dosage before the meal based on the current blood glucose level and the carbohydrate content of the meal. Intensified insulin therapy, such as multiple daily injections or the use of an insulin pump, allows considerable flexibility in food selection and can be adjusted for deviations from usual eating and exercise habits.

Type 2 Diabetes Mellitus. The emphasis for nutritional therapy in type 2 diabetes should be placed on achieving glucose, lipid, and blood pressure goals. Because 80% to 90% of people with type 2 diabetes are overweight, calorie reduction is a goal.[17]

There is no one proven strategy or method that can be uniformly recommended. A nutritionally adequate meal plan with a reduction of total fat, especially saturated fats, and simple sugars can bring about decreased calorie and carbohydrate consumption. Spacing meals is another strategy that can be adopted to spread nutrient intake throughout the day. A weight loss of 5% to 7% of body weight often improves glycemic control, even if desirable body weight is not achieved. Weight loss is best attempted by a moderate decrease in calories and an increase in caloric expenditure. Regular exercise and learning new behaviors and attitudes can help facilitate long-term lifestyle changes. Monitoring of blood glucose levels, A1C, lipids, and blood pressure provide

TABLE 47-9   Nutritional Therapy
Diabetes Mellitus

FACTOR	TYPE 1 DIABETES MELLITUS	TYPE 2 DIABETES MELLITUS
Total calories	Increase in caloric intake possibly necessary to achieve desirable body weight and restore body tissues	Reduction in caloric intake desirable for overweight or obese patient
Effect of diet	Diet and insulin necessary for glucose control	Diet alone possibly sufficient for glucose control
Distribution of calories	Equal distribution of carbohydrates through meals or adjustment of carbohydrates for insulin activity	Equal distribution recommended; low-fat diet desirable; consistency of carbohydrate at meals desirable
Consistency in daily intake	Necessary for glucose control	Desirable for weight reduction and moderation of blood glucose levels
Uniform timing of meals	Crucial for NPH/lente insulin programs; flexibility with multidose rapid-acting insulin	Desirable but not essential
Intermeal and bedtime snacks	Frequently necessary	Not usually recommended
Nutritional supplement for exercise programs	Carbohydrates 20 g/hr for moderate physical activities	May be necessary if patient controlled on sulfonylurea or insulin

feedback on how well the goals of nutritional therapy are being met.

Food Composition. The meal plan for people with diabetes does not prohibit the consumption of any one type of food. All food groups should be represented in a daily meal plan that is nutritionally balanced. Although an individualized meal plan should be developed with a dietitian, general guidelines and recommendations for people with diabetes include the following:[15]

- *Protein*—15% to 20% of total daily calories. Those with nephropathy should limit protein intake to 10%.
- *Fat*—less than 10% of daily calories from saturated fat. Cholesterol intake should be less than 300 mg/day.
- *Carbohydrate*—should constitute the remaining percentage of calories after determining protein and fat needs. Carbohydrates should include whole grains, fresh vegetables, and fresh fruits. Although overall intake of simple sugar should be limited as much as possible, its consumption is acceptable in moderate amounts when counted as part of total carbohydrate intake.
- *Sodium*—intake should be less than 2400 mg/day.
- *Fiber*—approximately 25 to 30 g/day from a variety of food sources.

Alcohol. Alcohol is high in calories, has no nutritive value, and promotes hypertriglyceridemia. In addition, it has detrimental effects on the liver (see Chapter 42). The inhibitory effect of alcohol on glucose production by the liver can cause severe hypoglycemia in patients on insulin or oral hypoglycemic medications that increase insulin secretion. Patients should be cautioned to honestly discuss the use of alcohol with their health care providers because its use can make blood glucose more difficult to control.

Alcohol can also cause other serious adverse effects when used in conjunction with certain oral medications used to treat diabetes. For example, it may produce a disulfiram (Antabuse) effect (nausea and vomiting, flushing, respiratory distress, chest pain) when ingested with some sulfonylurea medications, such as chlorpropamide (Diabinese). It can also increase the risk of lactic acidosis in patients who use metformin (Glucophage).

Moderate alcohol consumption can sometimes be safely incorporated into the meal plan if blood glucose levels are well controlled and if the patient is not on medications that will cause adverse effects. A patient can reduce the risk for alcohol-induced hypoglycemia by eating carbohydrates when drinking alcohol. One drink has approximately 135 calories. The patient with diabetes should drink alcohol with food, use sugar-free mixes, and drink dry, light wines.

Diet Teaching. Most often, the dietitian initially teaches the principles of the nutrition therapy prescription. Whenever possible, nurses should be prepared to work with dietitians as part of an interdisciplinary diabetes care team. In some instances, access to a dietitian is not possible for patients with limited insurance coverage or who live in remote areas. In these cases, nurses often assume responsibility for teaching basic dietary management to patients with diabetes.

The Food Guide Pyramid is an appropriate teaching tool for people with diabetes (see Chapter 39, Fig. 39-1). The pyramid helps the patient visualize the recommended amounts of foods that should be eaten from each group on a daily basis. For many people, the graphic representation of the pyramid makes this method of meal planning more approachable and easier to understand than exchange lists.

An alternative method of presenting the basics of meal planning is to use what is known as the *plate method*. This simple method helps the patient visualize the amount of vegetables, starch, and meat that should fill a 9-inch plate. For lunch and dinner one half of the plate is filled with nonstarchy vegetables, one fourth is filled with a starch, and one fourth is filled with 2 to 3 oz of lean meat. A glass of low-fat milk and a small piece of fresh fruit complete the meal. The breakfast plate is filled halfway with starch, and one fourth of the plate contains an optional protein. Low-fat milk and fresh fruit complete the breakfast. Assuming low-fat and nonfat foods are selected, following the plate method will provide 1200 to 1400 calories per day and a properly balanced meal plan.[18]

Diet teaching should include the patient's family and significant others whenever possible. It is most effective to direct teaching efforts to the person who will be cooking. It is important, however, that the responsibility for maintaining a diabetic diet not fall to someone other than the patient with diabetes. Reliance on another person to make health decisions fosters dependence and should be avoided except in special situations.

Exercise

Regular, consistent exercise is considered an essential part of diabetes management. Exercise increases insulin sensitivity and can have a direct effect on lowering the blood glucose levels. It also contributes to weight loss, which also decreases insulin resistance. The therapeutic benefits of regular physical activity may result in a decreased need for diabetes medicines in order to reach target blood glucose goals. Regular exercise may also help reduce triglyceride and LDL cholesterol levels, reduce blood pressure, and improve circulation.[19]

Patients who use insulin, sulfonylureas, or meglitinides are at increased risk for hypoglycemia when there is an increase in physical activity, especially if the patient exercises at the time of peak drug action or if food intake has not been sufficient to maintain adequate blood glucose levels. This can also occur if a normally sedentary patient with diabetes has an unusually active day. The glucose-lowering effects of exercise can last up to 48 hours after the activity, so it is possible for hypoglycemia to occur for that long after the activity. It is recommended that patients who use medications that can cause hypoglycemia schedule exercise about 1 hour after a meal, or that they have a 10 to 15 g carbohydrate snack before exercising. Several small carbohydrate snacks can be taken every 30 minutes during exercise to prevent hypoglycemia.[15] Patients using medications that place them at risk for hypoglycemia should always carry a fast-acting source of carbohydrate, such as glucose tablets or hard candies, when exercising. Table 47-10 gives guidelines on the number of calories burned per hour for different activities.

Although exercise is generally beneficial to blood glucose levels, strenuous activity can be perceived by the body as a stress, causing a release of counterregulatory hormones that results in a temporary elevation of blood glucose. As a result, hyperglycemia may occur in cases of poorly controlled type 2 diabetes or in patients with type 1 diabetes who exercise at a time of day when insulin action is waning. Some patients may have to inject a small bolus of rapid-acting or regular insulin if the blood glucose level is elevated before exercising to prevent progressive hyperglycemia. Furthermore, patients should exercise with caution if the blood glucose is greater than 300 mg/dl and there are no ketones, or if the blood glucose is greater than 250 mg/dl and ketones are present in the urine.[20] Additional information about exercise and diabetes that is important for both the patient and the health care provider is provided in the patient and family teaching guide (Table 47-11).

Monitoring Blood Glucose

Self-monitoring of blood glucose (SMBG) is a cornerstone of diabetes management. By providing a current blood glucose reading, SMBG enables the patient to make self-management decisions regarding diet, exercise, and medication. SMBG is also important for detecting episodic hyperglycemia and hypoglycemia. In the past, monitoring was accomplished by checking for the presence and degree of glucose in the urine. This is rarely used anymore because urine testing does not provide current blood glucose levels, making it much less useful for self-management decisions and the early detection and treatment of hypoglycemia.

Portable blood glucose meters are used at the hospital bedside and by patients who perform SMBG. A wide variety of blood glucose meters are available. Disposable lancets are usually used to obtain a small drop of capillary blood (usually from a finger stick) that is placed onto a reagent strip. After a specified time, the meter displays a digital reading of the blood glucose. The technology of SMBG is a rapidly changing field with newer and more convenient systems being introduced every year. Newer systems allow the user to collect blood from alternative sites such as the forearm. Noninvasive approaches to blood glucose monitoring have also been developed. The G2 Biographer from GlucoWatch is a device worn on the wrist. It pulls glucose through the skin using low electric current. It then measures glucose levels for 13 hours and sends an alarm if the reading is abnormal. Another device already in use in Europe measures glucose using infrared rays directed at the skin.

The blood glucose level reported by a laboratory is sometimes higher than the patient's home glucose monitor or the hospital's portable meter. This is because some meters give capillary blood glucose values from whole blood (via finger stick), whereas venous samples taken in the laboratory provide plasma readings. Plasma samples, or venous samples, are approximately 10% to 12% higher. Some meters are automatically calibrated to give a "plasma" test result (although whole blood was used for the sample) so that the home readings can be more readily compared with laboratory values. The literature accompanying a meter will identify if that particular meter is calibrated to give plasma or whole blood readings.

Instructions for using a blood glucose meter also accompany each product. Because errors in monitoring technique can cause errors in management strategies, thorough patient training is crucial. Initial training should be followed up at regular intervals with reassessment. In addition, patients must be taught to use and interpret calibration and control solutions that are a part of each blood glucose monitoring kit.[20] Table 47-12 lists the steps that should be taught to the patient learning to perform SMBG.

TABLE 47-10	Activities That Affect Caloric Expenditure	
LIGHT ACTIVITY (100-200 kcal/hr)	**MODERATE ACTIVITY (200-350 kcal/hr)**	**VIGOROUS ACTIVITY (400-900 kcal/hr)**
Driving a car	Active housework	Aerobic exercise
Fishing	Bicycling (light)	Bicycling (vigorous)
Light housework	Bowling	Hard labor
Secretarial work	Dancing	Ice skating
Teaching	Gardening	Outdoor sports
Walking casually	Golf	Running
	Roller skating	Soccer
	Walking briskly	Tennis
		Wood chopping

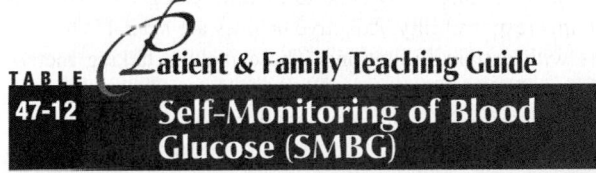

TABLE 47-11 Patient & Family Teaching Guide
Exercise for Patients with Diabetes Mellitus

1. Exercise does not have to be vigorous to be effective. The blood glucose–reducing effects of exercise can be attained with exercise such as brisk walking. The exercises selected should be enjoyable to foster regularity.
2. Exercise is best done after meals, when the blood glucose level is rising.
3. Exercise plans should be individualized for each patient and monitored by the health care provider.
4. It is important to self-monitor blood glucose levels before, during, and after exercise to determine the effect exercise has on blood glucose level at particular times of the day.
5. Be alert to the possibility of delayed exercise-induced hypoglycemia, which may occur several hours after the completion of exercise.
6. Taking a glucose-lowering medication does not mean that planned or spontaneous exercise cannot occur.
7. It is important to compensate for extensive planned and spontaneous activity by monitoring blood glucose level to make adjustments in the insulin dose (if taken) and food intake.

TABLE 47-12 Patient & Family Teaching Guide
Self-Monitoring of Blood Glucose (SMBG)

1. Wash hands in warm water. It is not necessary to clean the site with alcohol, and it may interfere with test results.
2. If it is difficult to obtain an adequate drop of blood for testing, warm the hands in warm water or let the arms hang dependently for a few minutes before the finger puncture is made.
3. If the puncture is made on the finger, use the side of the finger pad rather than near the center. Fewer nerve endings are along the side of the finger pad. If an alternative site is used (e.g., forearm), special equipment may be needed. Refer to manufacturer's instructions for alternative site use.
4. The puncture should be only deep enough to obtain a sufficiently large drop of blood. Unnecessarily deep punctures may cause pain and bruising.

The chief advantage of SMBG is that it supplies immediate information about blood glucose levels that can be used to make adjustments in food intake, activity patterns, and medication dosages. It also produces accurate records of daily glucose fluctuations and trends, as well as alerting the patient to acute episodes of hyperglycemia and hypoglycemia. Furthermore, it provides patients with a tool for achieving and maintaining specific glycemic goals. SMBG is recommended for all insulin-treated patients with diabetes. Other patients with diabetes frequently use SMBG to help achieve and maintain glycemic goals, as well as monitor for acute fluctuations in blood glucose.

The frequency of monitoring depends on several factors, including the patient's glycemic goals, the type of diabetes that the patient has, the patient's ability to perform the test independently, and the patient's willingness to test. Patients with type 1 diabetes typically test four times per day (before meals and at bedtime). Those using an insulin pump may test more frequently. Patients with type 2 diabetes will have more variable and individualized testing regimens.

Testing is most often done before meals, but certain situations warrant more frequent monitoring. For example, the patient should be instructed to test blood glucose before and after exercise to determine its effects on metabolic control. This is especially important in the patient with type 1 diabetes. Blood glucose testing should also be performed whenever hypoglycemia is suspected so that immediate action can be taken if necessary. When the person with diabetes is ill, the blood glucose should be tested at 4-hour intervals to determine the effects of this stressor on the blood glucose level.[20]

SMBG is an empowering tool that allows the patient to be an active partner in the treatment of diabetes. Achieving the desired level of patient participation does require time and effort from the health care professional. The nurse involved in this aspect of management should anticipate a close working relationship with patients as they refine their techniques and learn appropriate decision making about managing their diabetes. A patient who is visually impaired, cognitively impaired, or limited in manual dexterity needs careful evaluation of the degree to which SMBG can be performed independently. Nurses working in home health and outpatient settings may need to identify caregivers who can assume this responsibility. Adaptive devices are available to help patients with certain limitations. These include talking meters and other equipment for the visually impaired, as well as devices to stabilize insulin vials and syringes for those with limitations affecting dexterity.

Pancreas Transplantation. Pancreas transplantation is used as a treatment option for patients with type 1 diabetes mellitus who have end-stage renal disease and who have had or plan to have a kidney transplant. Kidney and pancreas transplants are often done together. If renal failure is not present, the ADA recommends that pancreas transplantation should only be considered for patients who exhibit the following three criteria: (1) a history of frequent, acute, and severe metabolic complications (e.g., hypoglycemia, hyperglycemia, ketoacidosis) requiring medical attention; (2) clinical and emotional problems with exogenous insulin therapy that are so severe as to be incapacitating; and (3) consistent failure of insulin-based management to prevent acute complications.

Successful pancreas transplantation can improve the quality of life of people with diabetes, primarily by eliminating the need for exogenous insulin, frequent daily blood glucose measurements, and many of the dietary restrictions imposed by the disorder. Transplantation can also eliminate the acute complications commonly experienced by patients with type 1 diabetes (e.g., hypoglycemia, hyperglycemia). However, pancreas transplantation is only partially successful in reversing the long-term renal and neurologic complications of diabetes.

Patients who undergo pancreas transplantation require immunosuppression to prevent rejection of the graft and potential recurrence of the autoimmune process that might again destroy pancreatic islet cells. (Immunosuppressive therapy is discussed in Chapter 13.)

Pancreatic islet cell transplantation is another potential treatment measure. However, at this time, islet cell transplantation is an experimental procedure.

New Developments in Diabetic Therapy

Many new insulin delivery systems are being researched. However, these products are still not approved by the Food and Drug Administration. These include the following: (1) *inhaled insulin,* which delivers a dose of liquid or dry powder insulin through the mouth and directly into the lungs, where it enters the blood as rapid-acting insulin; (2) a *skin patch* containing a reservoir of insulin, which can be changed after 12 to 24 hours of wear; (3) an *oral spray,* which is a liquid aerosol version of insulin that is absorbed by mucous membranes in cheeks, tongue, and throat; and (4) *insulin pills* with a special delivery system that prevents enzymatic breakdown as they go through the digestive system. The insulin in the pills is then absorbed in the small intestine, enters the circulation, and is available for use.

■ Culturally Competent Care: Diabetes Mellitus

Because culture can have a strong influence on dietary preferences and meal preparation practices, culturally competent care has special relevance for the care of the patient with diabetes. This is especially pertinent when considering the prevalence of diabetes in such diverse cultural groups as Hispanics, Native Americans, and African Americans. The influences of culture on food choices and meal planning should be explored with the patient as part of the health history. When giving diet instructions, efforts should be made to consider the food preferences of the cultural group. Nutritional resources specifically designed for members of different cultural groups are available from the American Diabetes Association and the American Dietetic Association. ■

NURSING MANAGEMENT
DIABETES MELLITUS

■ Nursing Assessment

Table 47-13 provides initial subjective and objective data that might be obtained from a person with diabetes mellitus. After the initial assessment, periodic patient assessments should be done on a regular basis.

■ Nursing Diagnoses

Nursing diagnoses related to diabetes mellitus may include, but are not limited to, those found in NCP 47-1.

TABLE 47-13	Nursing Assessment
Diabetes Mellitus	

Subjective Data	**Objective Data**
Important Health Information	**Eyes**
Past health history: Mumps, rubella, coxsackievirus or other viral infections; recent trauma, infection, or stress; pregnancy, gave birth to infant >9 lb; chronic pancreatitis; Cushing syndrome, acromegaly; family history of type 1 or type 2 diabetes mellitus	Soft, sunken eyeballs; vitreal hemorrhages, cataracts
	Integumentary
	Dry, warm, inelastic skin; pigmented lesions (on legs); ulcers (especially on feet), loss of hair on toes
Medications: Use of and compliance with insulin or OAs; use of corticosteroids, diuretics, phenytoin (Dilantin)	**Respiratory**
Surgery or other treatments: Any recent surgery	Rapid, deep respirations (Kussmaul respirations)
Functional Health Patterns	**Cardiovascular**
Health perception–health management: Positive family history; malaise; date of last eye and dental examination	Hypotension; weak, rapid pulse
	Gastrointestinal
Nutritional-metabolic: Obesity; weight loss (type 1), weight gain (type 2): thirst, hunger; nausea and vomiting; poor healing especially involving the feet, compliance with diet in patients with previously diagnosed diabetes	Dry mouth, vomiting, fruity breath
	Neurologic
	Altered reflexes, restlessness, confusion, stupor, coma
	Musculoskeletal
Elimination: Constipation or diarrhea; frequent urination, nocturia, urinary incontinence; skin infections	Muscle wasting
	Possible Findings
Activity-exercise: Muscle weakness, fatigue	Serum electrolyte abnormalities; fasting blood glucose level >126 mg/dl (7.0 mmol/L); glucose tolerance test ≥200 mg/dl (11.1 mmol/L); leukocytosis; ↑ blood urea nitrogen, creatinine, triglycerides, cholesterol, LDL, VLDL; ↓ HDL; glycosylated hemoglobin ≥6%; glycosuria; ketonuria; albuminuria; acidosis
Cognitive-perceptual: Abdominal pain, headache; blurred vision; numbness or tingling of extremities; pruritus	
Sexuality-reproductive: Impotence; frequent vaginal infections; decreased libido	
Coping–stress tolerance: Depression, irritability, apathy	
Value-belief: Commitment to lifestyle changes involving diet, medication, and activity patterns	

HDL, High–density lipoprotein; *LDL,* low-density lipoprotein; *OA,* oral agents; *VLDL,* very-low-density lipoprotein.

■ Planning

The overall goals for the patient with diabetes mellitus include the following: (1) to be an active participant in the management of the diabetes regimen; (2) to experience few or no episodes of acute hyperglycemic emergencies or hypoglycemia; (3) to maintain blood glucose levels at normal or near-normal levels; (4) to prevent, minimize, or delay the occurrence of chronic complications of diabetes; and (5) to adjust lifestyle to accommodate diabetes regimen with a minimum of stress.

■ Nursing Implementation

Health Promotion. The role of the nurse in health promotion and maintenance relates to the identification, monitoring, and education of the patient at risk for the development of diabetes mellitus. Obesity is the number one predictor of type 2 diabetes mellitus. The Diabetes Prevention Program found that a modest weight loss of 5% to 7% of body weight and regular exercise of 30 minutes five times a week lowered the risk of developing type 2 diabetes up to 58%.[1]

The ADA recommends routine screening for diabetes for all overweight adults over age 45. If normal, it should be repeated at 3-year intervals. The FPG is the preferred method for screening in clinical settings, although the OGTT is also suitable. Testing should be considered at a younger age or be carried out more frequently in individuals who meet the criteria listed in Table 47-14.[2] It is important to know where an individual is on the glucose continuum (Fig. 47-9).

Acute Intervention. Acute situations involving the patient with diabetes include hypoglycemia, diabetic ketoacidosis (DKA), and hyperosmolar hyperglycemic nonketotic syndrome (HHNS). Nursing management for these situations is discussed in more detail later in this chapter. Other areas of acute intervention relate to management during stress, such as during acute illness and surgery.

Stress of acute illness and surgery. Both emotional and physical stress can increase the blood glucose level and result in hyperglycemia. Because it is impossible to avoid stress totally in life, certain situations may require more intense management, such as extra insulin, to maintain glycemic goals and avoid hyperglycemia.

Acute illness, injury, and surgery are situations that may evoke a counterregulatory hormone response resulting in hyperglycemia. Even minor illnesses such as a viral upper respiratory infection or the flu can cause this. When patients with diabetes are ill, they should continue with the regular meal plan while increasing the intake of noncaloric fluids, such as broth, water, and other decaffeinated beverages. They should also continue taking oral agents and insulin as prescribed and check blood glucose at least every 4 hours. If the glucose is greater than 240 mg/dl (13.3 mmol/l), urine should be tested for ketones every 3 to 4 hours. Patients should report moderate to large ketone levels to the health care provider.

When the illness causes the patient to eat less than normal, she or he should continue to take oral hypoglycemic medications and/or insulin as prescribed while supplementing food

NURSING CARE PLAN 47-1

Patients with Diabetes Mellitus

NURSING DIAGNOSIS **Ineffective therapeutic regimen management** *related to* inadequate knowledge *as manifested by* continued hyperglycemia, inaccurate statements regarding diabetes and its management, and self-professed confusion regarding the pathophysiology of diabetes and its treatment.

OUTCOMES—NOC	INTERVENTIONS—NIC and *RATIONALES*
Knowledge: Diabetes Management (1820)	**Teaching: Disease Process (5602)**
▪ Description of insulin function _____	▪ Assess the patient's current level of knowledge related to specific disease process *to determine the scope and extent of required teaching.*
▪ Description of role of nutrition in controlling blood glucose level _____	▪ Describe the disease process and treatment recommendations *to enable patient to better understand rationale behind treatment regimen and lifestyle changes.*
▪ Description of hyperglycemia and related symptoms _____	▪ Discuss lifestyle changes that may be required to control the disease process *to encourage patient to actively participate in determining changes that will be acceptable.*
▪ Description of target blood glucose range _____	
▪ Identification of actions to be taken in relation to blood glucose levels _____	▪ Describe possible chronic complications *to increase awareness of the long-term effects of inadequate control of disease process.*
▪ Demonstration of proper technique to draw up and administer insulin _____	▪ Plan individualized exercise program with patient *because exercise is an integral part of diabetes management.*
	▪ Review steps to prevent hyperglycemia and hypoglycemia *because activity changes can cause changes in insulin needs.*
Outcome Scale	▪ Review insulin administration (if used); have patient give return demonstration of insulin injection *to ensure proper technique.*
1 = None	
2 = Limited	
3 = Moderate	
4 = Substantial	
5 = Extensive	

NURSING DIAGNOSIS **Fatigue** *related to* nutritional deficits secondary to mismanaged diabetes *as manifested by* inability to perform ADLs secondary to malaise, desire for frequent naps during the daytime, and lethargy that is unrelieved by sleep.

OUTCOMES—NOC	INTERVENTIONS—NIC and *RATIONALES*
Endurance (0001)	**Energy Management (0180)**
▪ Performance of usual routine _____	▪ Assist the patient in assigning priority to activities to accommodate energy levels *so that the most energy costly activities are performed during periods of peak energy.*
▪ Lethargy not present _____	▪ Assist the patient to identify tasks that family and friends can perform in the home *to prevent fatigue and to relieve patient stress regarding activities of daily living.*
▪ Concentration _____	
▪ Rested appearance _____	**Hyperglycemia Management (2120)**
▪ Energy restored after rest _____	▪ Monitor for signs and symptoms of hyperglycemia: polyuria, polydipsia, polyphagia, weakness, lethargy, malaise, blurring of vision, or headache *to alert patient to glucose/insulin imbalance and need for treatment.*
	▪ Anticipate situations in which insulin requirements will increase (e.g., times of stress and illness) *to allow patient to adjust insulin dosage appropriately and avoid undue fatigue.*
Outcome Scale	▪ Facilitate diet and exercise regimen *to promote and preserve energy balance.*
1 = Extremely compromised	▪ Restrict exercise when blood glucose levels are >250 mg/dl *to decrease the body's requirement for already unavailable glucose.*
2 = Substantially compromised	
3 = Moderately compromised	
4 = Mildly compromised	
5 = Not compromised	

ADLs, Activities of daily living.

intake with carbohydrate-containing fluids. Examples include soups, juices, and regular decaffeinated soft drinks.[20] The health care provider should be notified promptly if the patient is unable to keep anything down. The patient should understand that medication for diabetes, including insulin, should not be withheld during times of illness because counterregulatory mechanisms often increase the blood glucose level dramatically. Food intake is also important during this time because the body requires extra energy to deal with the stress of the illness. Extra insulin may be necessary to meet this demand and to prevent the onset of DKA in the patient with type 1 diabetes.[21]

During the intraoperative period adjustments in the diabetes regimen can be planned to ensure glycemic control. The patient

NURSING CARE PLAN 47-1

Patients with Diabetes Mellitus—cont'd

NURSING DIAGNOSIS   **Risk for infection** *related to* compromised immune system secondary to diabetes and decreased sensory percpetion secondary to diminished peripheral vascular circulation.

OUTCOMES—NOC	INTERVENTIONS—NIC and *RATIONALES*
Immune Status (0702) ▪ Skin integrity _____ ▪ Recurrent infections not present _____ ▪ Chronic fatigue not present _____	**Skin Surveillance (3590)** ▪ Observe extremities for color, warmth, swelling, pulses, texture, edema, and ulcerations *to detect early signs and symptoms of infection and decreased circulation.* ▪ Monitor skin for excessive dryness and moistness *to prevent conditions that favor skin breakdown.* **Infection Protection (6550)** ▪ Promote sufficient nutritional intake *to prevent illness and encourage wound healing.* ▪ Encourage fluid intake *to maintain adequate hydration and blood viscosity.* ▪ Encourage rest periods *to allow the body to rejuvenate itself and decrease stress.*
Outcome Scale 1 = Extremely compromised 2 = Substantially compromised 3 = Moderately compromised 4 = Mildly compromised 5 = Not compromised	▪ Encourage increased mobility and exercise *to promote and increase circulation to prevent the formation of pressure ulcers and to improve the efficiency of the body's use of insulin.* ▪ Teach patient and family about signs and symptoms of infection (and ask for return demonstration) and when to report them to health care provider *to promote early detection.*

NURSING DIAGNOSIS   **Powerlessness** *related to* sudden change in lifestyle and restrictions placed on normal eating habits secondary to diagnosis of diabetes *as manifested by* anger and statements alluding to lack of control over the situation.

OUTCOMES—NOC	INTERVENTIONS—NIC and *RATIONALES*
Health Beliefs (1700) ▪ Perceived importance of taking action _____ ▪ Perceived threat from inaction _____ ▪ Perceived ability to perform action _____ ▪ Perceived absence of barriers to action _____	**Self-Responsibility Facilitation (4480)** ▪ Hold patient responsible for own behavior *to encourage patient to view self as responsible for health outcomes.* ▪ Encourage verbalization of feelings, perceptions, and fears about assuming responsibility *to identify barriers to patient assuming responsibility for health care.* ▪ Monitor level of responsibility that patient assumes *to determine whether changes need to be made.*
Outcome Scale 1 = Very weak 2 = Weak 3 = Moderate 4 = Strong 5 = Very strong	▪ Discuss consequences of not dealing with own responsibilities *so that patient will have realistic knowledge of the health implications of inaction.* ▪ Provide positive feedback for accepting additional responsibility *to reinforce positive behavior.*

is given IV fluids and insulin immediately before, during, and after surgery when there is no oral intake. The type 2 diabetic patient who uses OAs is usually instructed to discontinue them 48 hours before surgery and is treated with insulin during the surgical period. The patient should understand that this is a temporary measure and is not to be interpreted as a worsening of diabetes.

The nurse caring for an unconscious surgical patient receiving insulin must be alert for hypoglycemic signs such as sweating, tachycardia, and tremors. Frequent monitoring of blood glucose will prevent episodes of severe hypoglycemia in this patient.

Ambulatory and Home Care. Successful management of diabetes requires ongoing interaction among the patient, the family,

and the health care team. It is important that a diabetes nurse educator be involved in the care of the patient and the family. This person provides expertise in many areas of specialized care needs.

Because diabetes is a complex, chronic condition, a great deal of patient contact takes place in outpatient and home settings. The major goal of patient care in these settings is to enable the patient or caregiver to reach an optimal level of independence in self-care activities. Unfortunately, many patients with diabetes face challenges in reaching these goals. Diabetes increases the risk for other chronic conditions that can affect self-care activities. These include visual impairment, lower extremity problems that affect mobility, and other functional limitations related to cerebrovascular disease. Therefore important nursing

TABLE 47-14 Criteria for Testing in Asymptomatic, Undiagnosed Individuals

Type 1 Diabetes Mellitus

Testing presumably healthy individuals for the presence of any immune markers (e.g., HLA), outside of a clinical trials setting, is not recommended.

Type 2 Diabetes Mellitus

In asymptomatic, undiagnosed individuals, testing for diabetes should be considered in all individuals at age 45 years and above and, if normal, it should be repeated at 3-year intervals. Testing* should be considered at a younger age, or be carried out more frequently, in individuals who

- are overweight (body mass index [BMI] ≥25 kg/m²).
- have a first-degree relative with diabetes.
- are members of a high-risk ethnic population (African American, Hispanic, Native American, Asian American, Pacific Islander).
- have delivered a baby weighing >9 lb or were diagnosed with gestational diabetes mellitus.
- are hypertensive (≥140/90 mm Hg).
- have an HDL cholesterol level ≤35 mg/dl (0.90 mmol/L) and/or a triglyceride level ≥250 mg/dl (2.82 mmol/L).
- on previous testing, had impaired glucose tolerance or increased fasting glucose.

Adapted from American Diabetes Association Clinical Practice Recommendations.
*Testing may include fasting plasma glucose (FPG) or oral glucose tolerance test (OGTT). The FPG is the recommended diagnostic test because of its ease of administration, convenience, acceptability to patients, and lower cost.
HDL, High-density lipoprotein.

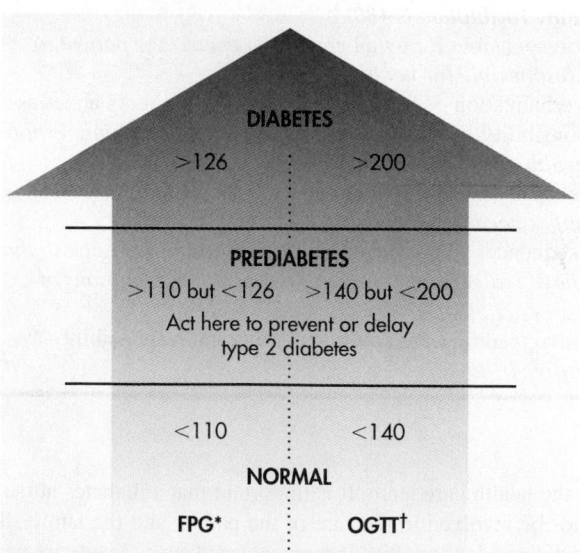

* The fasting plasma glucose (FPG) test: After an overnight fast, blood glucose is measured in the morning.

† The 2-hour oral glucose tolerance test (OGTT): Includes a fasting blood glucose test and glucose measurements 2 hours after drinking a glucose-containing solution.

Note: The American Diabetes Association and the National Institute of Diabetes and Digestive and Kidney Diseases believe either test is appropriate to measure prediabetes and diabetes.

FIG. 47-9 The glucose continuum. Numbers represent blood glucose levels in mg/dl.

functions are to assess the ability of patients and caregivers in such activities as SMBG and insulin injection techniques. Assistive devices for self-administration of insulin include syringe magnifiers, vial stabilizers, and dosing aids for the visually impaired. In some cases, the nurse will make referrals to others who can help the patient achieve the self-care goal. These may include an occupational therapist, a social worker, a home health aid, or a dietitian.

A diagnosis of diabetes affects the patient in many profound ways. Patients with diabetes must continually contend with lifestyle choices that affect the food they eat, the activity they engage in, and demands on their time and energy. In addition, they face the potential of becoming victim to the devastating complications of this disease. Careful assessment of what it means to the patient to have diabetes should be the starting point of patient teaching. The nurse can help patients make adjustments by displaying an attitude that is supportive and nonjudgmental. The goals of teaching should be mutually determined by the patient and the nurse based on individual needs, as well as therapeutic requirements.

The patient's support system must be identified. If this is the family, they need to be involved in teaching so they can care for the patient when self-care is no longer possible. The family and significant others need to be encouraged to provide emotional support and encouragement as the patient deals with the reality of living with a chronic disease.

Insulin therapy. Nursing responsibilities for the patient receiving insulin include proper administration, assessment of the

ℰVIDENCE-BASED PRACTICE
Self-Management Education of Type 2 Diabetes Mellitus

Clinical Problem

What is the effectiveness of diabetes self-management education in patients with type 2 diabetes mellitus?

Best Clinical Practice

- Self-management education in patients with type 2 diabetes mellitus is effective.
- Interventions involving active participation have been effective in improving diabetes knowledge, self-monitoring of blood glucose levels, self-reported dietary habits, and glycemic control.
- Interventions involving active patient participation are more effective than didactic interventions.

Implications for Nursing Practice

- The nurse needs to realize that patients need to be in control of their own health and encourage patients to assume this role.
- Knowledge can empower a person to take a central role in his or her own health care.
- Teaching should involve getting the patient actively involved in the learning process (see Chapter 4).

References for Evidence

Norris SL, Engelgau MM, Venkat Narayan KM: Effectiveness of self-management training in type 2 diabetes. A systematic review of randomized controlled trials, *Diabetes Care* 24:561, 2001.
Review: self-management training in type 2 diabetes mellitus is effective in the short term, *ACP Journal* 135:45, 2001.

patient's response to insulin therapy, and education of the patient regarding administration, adjustment to, and side effects of insulin (see Table 47-5). Table 47-6 lists guidelines for the nurse assessing a patient using glucose-lowering agents, including insulin and OAs.

Assessment of the patient who is new to insulin must include an evaluation of his or her ability to manage this therapy safely. This includes the ability to understand the interaction of insulin, diet, and activity and to be able to recognize and treat the symptoms of hypoglycemia appropriately. If the patient does not have the cognitive skills to do these things, another responsible person must be identified and trained. The patient or caregiver must also have the cognitive and manual skills needed to prepare and inject the insulin. If the patient or family lacks these, additional resources will be needed to assist the patient.

Many patients are fearful when they first begin using insulin. Some patients find it difficult to self-inject because they are afraid of needles or the pain associated with an injection. Some are afraid they will hurt themselves by giving too much or too little insulin. And in some cases, the patient believes that using insulin is a "last ditch" effort and that he or she is now in the final stages of the disease process. Therefore it is important to explore the patient's underlying fears before beginning the teaching.

Follow-up assessment of the patient who has been using insulin therapy includes an inspection of injection sites for signs of lipodystrophy and other reactions, review of insulin preparation and injection technique, a history pertaining to the occurrence of hypoglycemic episodes, and the patient's method for handling hypoglycemic episodes. A review of the patient's recorded blood glucose tests is also important in assessing overall glycemic control.

Oral agents. Nursing responsibilities for the patient taking OAs are similar to those for the patient taking insulin. Proper administration, assessment of the patient's use of and response to the OA, and education of the patient and the family about OAs are all part of the nurse's function.

The nurse's assessment can be extremely valuable in determining the most appropriate OA for a patient. Factors such as the patient's mental status, eating habits, home environment, attitude toward diabetes, and medication history all play a significant role in determining the most appropriate OA for the individual patient. For example, frail older adults who live alone are at high risk for severe hypoglycemia because low blood glucose is frequently undetected and/or untreated in this population. This is especially true if the patient has a short-term memory deficit. In these cases, an OA that does not cause hypoglycemia, or a shorter-acting OA, would be most appropriate.

Patient teaching is an essential nursing function when caring for the patient who uses OAs for blood glucose control. Some patients may assume that their diabetes is not a serious condition if they are taking only a pill for glycemic control. Therefore the patient should be instructed that these agents will help keep blood glucose controlled and will help prevent serious long- and short-term complications of diabetes. Patients should be instructed that OAs are used in addition to diet and activity as therapy for diabetes and that they should continue with their meal and activity plans. Patients should not take extra pills if overeating has occurred, unless specifically instructed to do so by their health care

provider. If the patient uses sulfonylureas, instructions should be given with regard to prevention, symptom recognition, and management of hypoglycemia.

The patient should also be instructed to contact a health care provider if periods of illness or extreme stress occur. During such a period, insulin therapy may be required to prevent or treat hyperglycemic symptoms and avoid an acute hyperglycemia emergency.

Personal hygiene. The potential for microvascular complications and infections requires diligent skin and dental hygiene practices on the part of the patient. Because of the susceptibility to periodontal disease, daily brushing and flossing should be encouraged in addition to regular visits to the dentist. When dental work must be done, the dentist should be informed that the patient has diabetes.

Routine care should include regular bathing, with particular emphasis given to foot care. Problems associated with the feet and lower extremities are presented later in this chapter. If cuts, scrapes, or burns occur, they should be treated promptly and monitored carefully. The area should be washed, and a nonabrasive or nonirritating antiseptic ointment may be applied. The area should be covered with a dry, sterile pad. If the injury does not begin to heal within 24 hours or if signs of infection develop, the health care provider should be notified immediately.

Medical identification and travel. The patient should be instructed to carry medical identification at all times indicating that he or she has diabetes. Police, paramedics, and many private citizens are aware of the need to look for this identification when working with sick or unconscious persons. Every person with diabetes should wear a medical alert bracelet or necklace. An identification card (Fig. 47-10) can supply valuable information, such as the name of the health care provider and the type and dose of insulin or OA.

Travel for a patient with diabetes requires advance planning. The patient should have a full set of diabetes care supplies in the carry-on luggage when traveling by plane, train, or bus. This includes blood glucose monitoring equipment, insulin, and syringes. When syringes and lancing devices are carried onto a

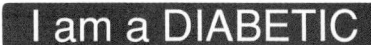

I am a DIABETIC

If unconscious or behaving abnormally, I may be having a reaction associated with diabetes or its treatment.

If I can swallow, give me a sweet drink, orange juice, Lifesavers, or lowfat milk.

If I do not recover promptly, call a physician or send me to the hospital.

If I am unconscious or cannot swallow, do not attempt to give me anything by mouth, but call a physician or send me to the hospital immediately.

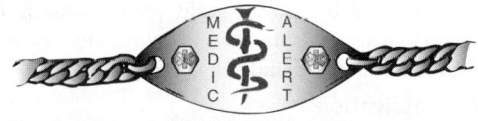

FIG. 47-10 Medical alerts. A patient with diabetes should carry a card and wear a bracelet or necklace that indicates diabetes. If the patient with diabetes is unconscious, these measures will ensure prompt and appropriate attention.

commercial airliner, a letter from the prescribing health care provider indicating medical necessity may prevent delays at security checkpoints. For patients who use insulin or an OA that can cause hypoglycemia, snack items and a quick-acting carbohydrate source for treating hypoglycemia should be included in the carry-on luggage. Extra insulin should be available in case a bottle breaks or gets lost. In addition, the patient should carry a full day's supply of food in the event of cancelled flights, delayed meals, or closed restaurants. If the patient is planning a trip out of the country, it is wise to have a letter from the health care provider explaining that the patient has diabetes and requires all the materials, particularly syringes, for ongoing health care.

Some travel involves time changes such as traveling coast to coast or across the International Date Line. The patient should contact the health care provider to plan an appropriate insulin schedule. Many patients find it easier and more predictable to take only regular insulin every 4 to 6 hours to cover insulin needs while on long airplane trips instead of trying to anticipate the peak of intermediate insulin and the availability of meals. During travel, most patients find it helpful to keep watches set to the time of the city of origin until they reach their destination. The key to travel when taking insulin is to know the type of insulin being taken, its onset of action, the anticipated peak time, and meal times.

Patient and family teaching. The goals of diabetes self-management education are to enable the patient to become the most active participant in his or her care, while matching level of self-management to the ability of the individual patient. Patients who actively manage their diabetes care have better outcomes than those who do not. For this reason, an educational approach that facilitates informed decision making on the part of the patient is widely advocated. Sometimes this is referred to as the *empowerment approach* to education.

Unfortunately, patients can encounter a variety of physical, psychologic, and emotional barriers when it comes to effectively managing their diabetes. These barriers may include feelings of inadequacy about one's own abilities, unwillingness to make the necessary behavioral changes, ineffective coping strategies, and cognitive deficits. If the patient is not able to manage the disease, a family member may be able to assume part of this role. If the patient or the family cannot

make decisions related to diabetes management, the nurse may refer the patient to a social worker or other resources within the community. These resources can assist the patient and the family in outlining a feasible treatment program that meets their capabilities. Patient and health care provider resources are listed at the end of this chapter.

An assessment of the patient's knowledge of diabetes and lifestyle preferences is useful in planning a teaching program. Table 47-15 presents guidelines to use for patient teaching. The nurse should assess the patient's knowledge base frequently so that gaps in knowledge or incorrect or inaccurate ideas can be quickly corrected.

The ADA and the American Association of Diabetes Educators offer pamphlets, booklets, and a bimonthly magazine called *Diabetes Forecast.* Affiliates of the ADA are located in all states and most can be reached by dialing 1-800-DIABETES. The ADA also publishes materials and sponsors conferences for health care professionals concerned with diabetes education, research, and management of patients. This organization also gives recognition to education programs that meet the national standards of diabetes education and can provide a list of these programs. Drug companies manufacturing diabetes-related products also have free educational materials for patients and health care providers.

■ Evaluation

The expected outcomes for the patient with diabetes mellitus are addressed in NCP 47-1.

Acute Complications of Diabetes Mellitus

The acute complications of diabetes mellitus arise from events associated with hyperglycemia and insufficient insulin. A problem that may arise from too much insulin or an excessive dose of an OA is *hypoglycemia* (also referred to as *insulin reaction* or *low blood glucose*). It is important for the health care provider to be able to distinguish between hyperglycemia and hypoglycemia because hypoglycemia worsens rapidly and constitutes a serious threat if action is not immediately taken. Table 47-16 compares the manifestations, causes, management, and prevention of hyperglycemia and hypoglycemia.

DIABETIC KETOACIDOIS

Etiology and Pathophysiology

Diabetic ketoacidosis (DKA), also referred to as *diabetic acidosis* and *diabetic coma,* is caused by a profound deficiency of insulin and is characterized by hyperglycemia, ketosis, acidosis, and dehydration. It is most likely to occur in people with type 1 diabetes but may be seen in type 2 in conditions of severe illness or stress when the pancreas cannot meet the extra demand for insulin. Precipitating factors include illness and infection, inadequate insulin dosage, undiagnosed type 1 diabetes, poor self-management, and neglect.

When the circulating supply of insulin is insufficient, glucose cannot be properly used for energy so that the body breaks down fat stores as a secondary source of fuel (Fig. 47-11). Ketones are acidic by-products of fat metabolism that can cause serious prob-

---

COMPLEMENTARY & ALTERNATIVE THERAPIES
Herbs That Affect Glucose Levels

Effects
Herbs can affect glycemic control. Herbs that can increase the antidiabetic effect of medications (i.e., lower blood glucose) include bay, basil, bee pollen, garlic, ginger, ginseng, milk thistle, and sage. Herbs that can decrease the antidiabetic effect of medications include St. John's wort.

Nursing Implications
It is very important that patients with diabetes consult with their health care provider before using herbs or nutritional supplements. Patients who use herbs should monitor their blood glucose levels carefully and regularly.

TABLE 47-15   Patient & Family Teaching Guide
General Guidelines for Management of Diabetes Mellitus

	DO	DON'T
Blood glucose	• Monitor your blood glucose at home and record results in a log. • Take your insulin or OA as prescribed. • Obtain a hemoglobin A1C blood test every 3-6 mo as an indicator of your long-term blood glucose control. • Carry some form of glucose at all times so you can treat hypoglycemia quickly. • Instruct family members in the use of glucagon administration in the case of emergencies due to hypoglycemia.	• Skip doses of your insulin, especially when you are sick. • Run out of insulin. • Enroll in a fad diet. • Rub the area where insulin was administered.
Exercise	• Learn how exercise and food affect your blood glucose levels. • Begin a medically supervised exercise program.	• Forget that exercise will lower your blood glucose level. • Exercise if your blood glucose levels are very elevated. This may lead to a temporary worsening of your blood glucose levels.
Diet	• Follow your diet, eating regular meals at regular times. • Eat slowly and chew food thoroughly. • Choose foods low in saturated fats. • Limit the amount of alcohol you drink. • Learn your cholesterol level.	• Drink excessive amounts of alcohol because this may lead to unpredictable low blood glucose reactions. • Eat fried foods.
Other guidelines	• Obtain an annual eye examination by an ophthalmologist. • Obtain annual urine testing for protein. • Examine your feet at home. • Wear comfortable, well-fitting shoes to help prevent foot injury. Break in new shoes gradually. • Always carry identification that says you have diabetes. • Have other medical problems treated, especially high blood pressure. • Know the symptoms of hypoglycemia and hyperglycemia. • Quit smoking.	• Smoke. • Apply hot or cold directly to your feet. • Go barefoot. • Ignore the symptoms of hypoglycemia and hyperglycemia. • Put baby oil or lotion between your toes.

OA, Oral agent.

lems when they become excessive in the blood. Ketosis alters the pH balance, causing metabolic acidosis to develop. Ketonuria is a process that begins when ketone bodies are excreted in the urine. During this process, electrolytes become depleted as cations are eliminated along with the anionic ketones in an attempt to maintain electrical neutrality.

Insulin deficiency impairs protein synthesis and causes excessive protein degradation. This results in nitrogen losses from the tissues. Insulin deficiency also stimulates the production of glucose from amino acids (from proteins) in the liver and leads to further hyperglycemia. But because there is a deficiency of insulin, the additional glucose cannot be used and the blood glucose level rises further, adding to the osmotic diuresis. Untreated, this leads to severe depletion of sodium, potassium, chloride, magnesium, and phosphate. Vomiting caused by the acidosis results in more fluid and electrolyte losses. Eventually, hypovolemia followed by shock will ensue.

Renal failure may eventually occur from hypovolemic shock. This causes the retention of ketones and glucose, and the acidosis progresses. Untreated, the patient becomes comatose as a result of dehydration, electrolyte imbalance, and acidosis. If the condition is not treated, death is inevitable.

Clinical Manifestations

Signs and symptoms of DKA include manifestations of dehydration such as poor skin turgor, dry mucous membranes, tachycardia, and orthostatic hypotension. Early symptoms may include lethargy and weakness. As the patient becomes severely dehydrated, the skin becomes dry and loose, and the eyeballs become soft and sunken. Abdominal pain is another symptom of DKA that may be accompanied by anorexia and vomiting. Finally, Kussmaul respirations (rapid, deep breathing associated with dyspnea) are the body's attempt to reverse metabolic acidosis through the exhalation of excess carbon dioxide. Acetone is noted on the breath as a sweet, fruity odor. (See Chapter 16 for a discussion of respiratory compensation of metabolic acidosis.) Laboratory findings include a blood glucose level above 250 mg/dl, arterial blood pH below 7.35, serum bicarbonate level less than 15 mEq/L, and ketones in the blood and urine.[21]

Collaborative Care

Before the advent of self-monitoring of blood glucose, patients with DKA required hospitalization for treatment. Today, hospitalization may not be required. In instances where fluid and

TABLE 47-16 Comparison of Hyperglycemia and Hypoglycemia

HYPERGLYCEMIA	HYPOGLYCEMIA	HYPERGLYCEMIA	HYPOGLYCEMIA
Manifestations*		**Treatment**	
Elevated blood glucose†	Blood glucose <50 mg/dl (2.8 mmol/L)	Physician's attention	Immediate ingestion of 5-20 g of simple carbohydrates
Increase in urination	Cold, clammy skin	Continuance of diabetes medication as ordered	Ingestion of another 5-20 g of simple carbohydrates in 15 min if no relief obtained
Increase in appetite followed by lack of appetite	Numbness of fingers, toes, mouth	Frequent checking of blood and urine specimens and recording of results	Contacting of physician if no relief obtained
Weakness, fatigue	Rapid heartbeat	Hourly drinking of fluids	Discussion with physician about medication dosage
Blurred vision	Emotional changes		
Headache	Headache		
Glycosuria	Nervousness, tremors	**Preventive Measures**	
Nausea and vomiting	Faintness, dizziness	Taking prescribed dose of medication at proper time	Taking prescribed dose of medication at proper time
Abdominal cramps	Unsteady gait, slurred speech	Accurate administration of insulin/OA	Accurate administration of insulin/OA
Progression to DKA or HHNS	Hunger	Maintenance of diet	Ingestion of all ordered diet foods at proper time
	Changes in vision	Maintenance of good personal hygiene	Provision of compensation for exercise
	Seizures, coma	Adherence to sick-day rules when ill	Ability to recognize and know symptoms and treat them immediately
Causes		Checking of blood for glucose as ordered	Carrying of simple carbohydrates
Too much food	Alcohol intake with food	Contacting of physician regarding ketonuria	Education of friends, family, fellow employees about symptoms and treatment
Too little or no diabetes medication	Too little food—delayed, omitted, inadequate intake	Wearing of diabetic identification	Checking blood glucose as ordered
Inactivity	Too much diabetic medication		Wearing medical alert (diabetic) identification
Emotional, physical stress	Too much exercise without compensation		
Poor absorption of insulin	Diabetes medication or food taken at wrong time		
	Loss of weight with change in medication		
	Use of β-adrenergic blockers interfering with recognition of symptoms		

*There is usually a gradual onset of symptoms in hyperglycemia and a rapid onset in hypoglycemia.
†Specific clinical manifestations related to elevated levels of blood glucose vary according to the patient.
DKA, Diabetic ketoacidosis; *HHNS,* hyperosmolar hyperglycemic nonketotic syndrome; *OA,* oral agent.

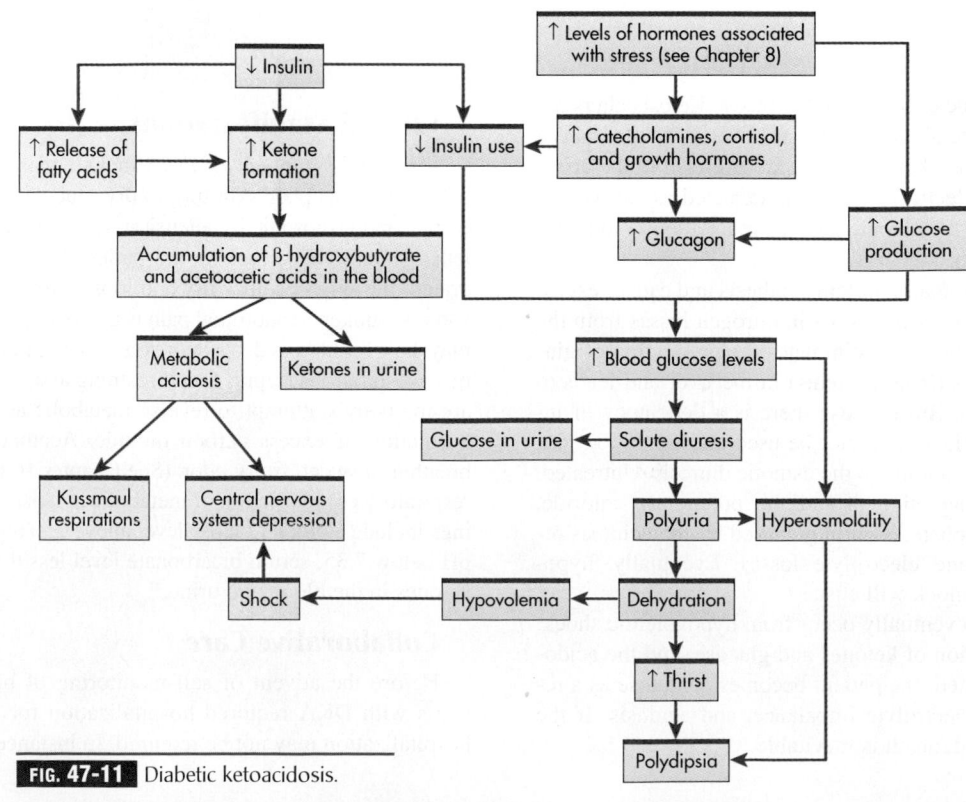

FIG. 47-11 Diabetic ketoacidosis.

electrolyte imbalances are not severe and blood glucose levels can be safely monitored at home, less severe forms of DKA may be managed on an outpatient basis (Table 47-17). However, other factors must be considered as to the location of where the patient is managed. These include the presence of fever, nausea, vomiting, and diarrhea; altered mental status; nature of the cause of the ketoacidosis; and availability of frequent communication with the health care provider (every few hours).

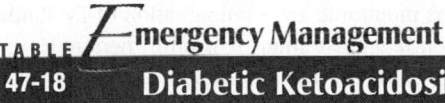

TABLE 47-17	Collaborative Care

Diabetic Ketoacidosis (DKA) and Hyperosmolar Hyperglycemic Nonketotic Syndrome (HHNS)

Diagnostic
History and physical examination
Blood studies, including immediate blood glucose, complete blood count, ketones, pH, electrolytes, blood urea nitrogen, arterial blood gases
Urinalysis, including specific gravity, pH, glucose, acetone

Collaborative Therapy
Intravenous administration of rapid-acting insulin
Administration of intravenous fluids
Electrolyte replacement
Assessment of mental status
Recording of intake and output
Central venous pressure monitoring (if indicated)
Assessment of blood glucose levels
Assessment of blood and urine for ketones
ECG monitoring
Assessment of cardiovascular and respiratory status

ECG, Electrocardiogram.

Regardless of the setting in which it occurs, DKA is a serious condition that proceeds rapidly and must be treated promptly. (See Table 47-18 for the emergency management of a patient with DKA.) Because fluid imbalance is potentially life threatening, the initial goal of therapy is to establish intravenous access and begin fluid and electrolyte replacement. Typically, an infusion of 0.45% or 0.9% NaCl at a rate to restore urine output to 30 to 60 ml/hr and to raise blood pressure constitutes the initial fluid therapy regimen. When blood glucose levels approach 250 mg/dl (13.9 mmol/L), 5% dextrose is added to the fluid regimen to prevent hypoglycemia.[22]

The aim of fluid and electrolyte therapy is to replace extracellular and intracellular water and to correct deficits of sodium, chloride, bicarbonate, potassium, phosphate, magnesium, and nitrogen. Early potassium replacement is essential because hypokalemia is a significant cause of unnecessary and avoidable death during treatment of DKA. Although initial serum potassium may be normal or high, levels can rapidly decrease once therapy starts as insulin drives potassium into the cells, leading to life-threatening hypokalemia.

IV insulin administration is therapy directed toward correcting hyperglycemia and hyperketonemia. Insulin therapy is withheld until fluid resuscitation is underway, because insulin allows water to enter the cell along with glucose and can lead to a depletion of vascular volume. Initially a bolus of insulin is delivered, followed by a continuous infusion.

HYPEROSMOLAR HYPERGLYCEMIC NONKETOTIC SYNDROME

Hyperosmolar hyperglycemic nonketotic syndrome (HHNS) is a life-threatening syndrome than can occur in the patient with diabetes who is able to produce enough insulin to prevent DKA but not enough to prevent severe hyperglycemia, osmotic diuresis, and extracellular fluid depletion (Fig. 47-12). The main difference be-

TABLE 47-18	Emergency Management

Diabetic Ketoacidosis

ETIOLOGY	ASSESSMENT FINDINGS	INTERVENTIONS
• Undiagnosed diabetes mellitus • Inadequate treatment of existing diabetes mellitus • Insulin not taken as presribed • Infection • Change in diet, insulin, or exercise regimen	• Dry mouth • Thirst • Abdominal pain • Nausea and vomiting • Gradually increasing restlessness, confusion, lethargy • Flushed, dry skin • Eyes appear sunken • Breath odor of ketones • Rapid, weak pulse • Labored breathing (Kussmaul respirations) • Fever • Urinary frequency • Serum glucose >300 mg/dl (16.7 mmol/L) • Glucosuria and ketonuria	**Initial** • Ensure patent airway. • Administer oxygen via nasal cannula or non-rebreather mask. • Establish IV access with large-bore catheter. • Begin fluid resuscitation with 0.9% NaCl solution 1 L/hr until BP stabilized and urine output 30-60 ml/hr. • Begin continuous regular insulin drip 0.1 U/kg/hr. • Identify history of diabetes, time of last food, and time/amount of last insulin injection. **Ongoing Monitoring** • Monitor vital signs, level of consciousness, cardiac rhythm, oxygen saturation, and urine output. • Assess breath sounds for fluid overload. • Monitor serum glucose and serum potassium. • Administer potassium to correct hypokalemia. • Administer sodium bicarbonate if severe acidosis (pH <7.0).

BP, Blood pressure; IV, intravenous.

tween HHNS and DKA is that the patient with HHNS usually has enough circulating insulin so that ketoacidosis does not occur. Because HHNS produces fewer symptoms in the earlier stages, blood glucose levels can climb quite high before the problem is recognized. The higher blood glucose levels increase serum osmolality and produce more severe neurologic manifestations, such as somnolence, coma, seizures, hemiparesis, and aphasia. HHNS often occurs in the older adult patient with type 2 diabetes and is often related to impaired thirst sensation and/or a functional inability to replace fluids. There is usually a history of inadequate fluid intake, increasing mental depression, and polyuria. Laboratory values in HHNS include blood glucose greater than 400 mg/dl and a marked increase in serum osmolality. Ketone bodies are absent or minimal in both blood and urine.

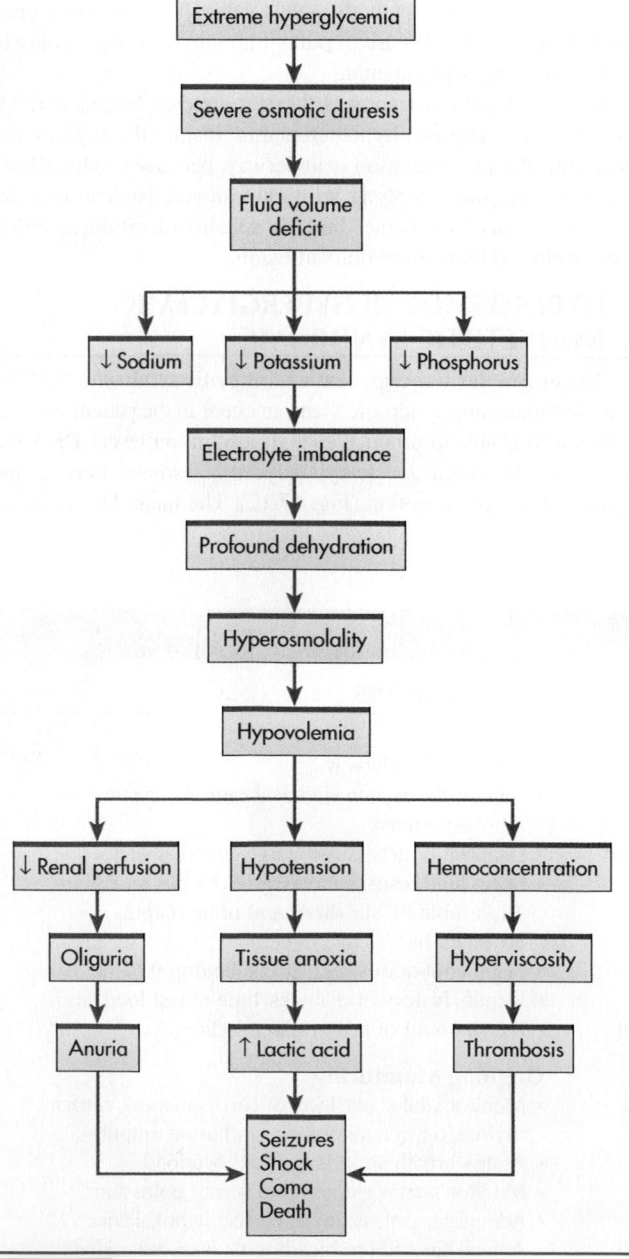

FIG. 47-12 Pathophysiology of hyperosmolar hyperglycemic nonketotic syndrome (HHNS).

Collaborative Care

HHNS constitutes a medical emergency and has a high mortality rate. Therapy is similar to that for the treatment of DKA and includes immediate IV administration of either 0.9% or 0.45% NaCl at a rate that is dependent on cardiac status and the degree of fluid volume deficit. Regular insulin is given by IV bolus, followed by an infusion after fluid replacement therapy is instituted to aid in reducing the hyperglycemia. When blood glucose levels fall to approximately 250 mg/dl (13.9 mmol/L), IV fluids containing glucose are administered to prevent hypoglycemia. Electrolytes are monitored and replaced as needed. Hypokalemia is not as significant in HHNS as it is in DKA, although fluid losses may result in milder potassium deficits that require replacement. Vital signs, intake and output, tissue turgor, laboratory values, and cardiac monitoring are assessed to monitor the efficacy of fluid and electrolyte replacement. Patients with renal or cardiac compromise require special monitoring to avoid fluid overload during fluid replacement. This includes monitoring of serum osmolality and frequent assessment of cardiac, renal, and mental status.

The management for both DKA and HHNS is similar, except that HHNS requires greater fluid replacement (see Table 47-17). Once the patient is stabilized, attempts to detect and correct the underlying precipitating cause should be initiated.

NURSING MANAGEMENT
DIABETIC KETOACIDOSIS AND HYPEROSMOLAR HYPERGLYCEMIC NONKETOTIC SYNDROME

When hospitalized, the patient is closely monitored with appropriate blood and urine tests. The nurse is responsible for monitoring blood glucose and urine for output and ketones, as well as using laboratory data to direct care.

Areas that must be monitored are administration of IV fluids to correct dehydration, administration of insulin therapy to reduce blood glucose and serum acetone, administration of electrolytes to correct electrolyte imbalance, assessment of renal status, assessment of the cardiopulmonary status related to hydration and electrolyte levels, and monitoring of the level of consciousness.

The nurse must also monitor the signs of potassium imbalance resulting from hypoinsulinemia and osmotic diuresis (see Chapter 16). When treatment for hyperglycemia is begun with insulin, serum potassium levels may decrease rapidly as potassium moves into the cells once insulin becomes available. This movement of potassium into and out of extracellular fluid influences cardiac functioning. Cardiac monitoring is a useful aid in detecting hyperkalemia and hypokalemia because characteristic changes indicating potassium excess or deficit are observable on ECG tracings (see Chapter 16, Fig. 16-14). Vital signs should be assessed often to determine the presence of fever, hypovolemic shock, tachycardia, and Kussmaul breathing.

HYPOGLYCEMIA

Hypoglycemia, or low blood glucose, occurs when there is too much insulin in proportion to available glucose in the blood. This causes the blood glucose level to drop to less than 70 mg/dl (3.9 mmol/L). Because the brain requires a constant supply of glucose in sufficient quantities to function properly, hypoglycemia can affect mental functioning. Common manifestations of hypoglycemia include confusion, irritability, diaphoresis, tremors, hunger, weakness, and visual disturbances. Manifestations of hypoglycemia can mimic alcohol intoxication. Untreated hypoglycemia can progress to loss of consciousness, seizures, coma, and death.

Hypoglycemic unawareness is a condition in which a person does not experience the warning signs and symptoms of hypoglycemia, increasing his or her risk for dangerously low blood glucose levels. This is often related to autonomic neuropathy of diabetes that interferes with the secretion of counterregulatory hormones that produce these symptoms. Elderly patients and patients who use β-adrenergic blockers are also at risk for hypoglycemic unawareness. It is usually not safe for patients with risk factors for hypoglycemic unawareness to aim for tight blood glucose control, because a major drawback of intensive treatment is hypoglycemia. These patients are usually managed with blood glucose goals that are somewhat higher than patients who are able to detect and manage the onset of hypoglycemia.

Hypoglycemic symptoms may occur when a very high blood glucose level falls too rapidly (e.g., a blood glucose level of 300 mg/dl [16.7 mmol/L] falling quickly to 180 mg/dl [10 mmol/L]). Although the blood glucose level is above normal by definition and measurement, the sudden metabolic shift can evoke hypoglycemic symptoms. Too vigorous management of hyperglycemia with insulin can induce this type of situation.

Causes of hypoglycemia are often related to a mismatch in the timing of food intake and the peak action of insulin or oral hypoglycemic agents that increase endogenous insulin secretion. The balance between blood glucose and insulin can be disrupted by the administration of too much insulin or medication, the ingestion of too little food, delaying the time of eating, and performing unusual amounts of exercise. Insulin reactions can occur at any time, but most reactions occur when the OA or insulin is at its peak of action or when the patient's daily routine is disrupted without adequate adjustments in diet, medications, and activity. Although hypoglycemia is more common with insulin therapy, it can occur with OAs and may be severe and persist for an extended time because of the longer duration of action.

NURSING *and* COLLABORATIVE MANAGEMENT HYPOGLYCEMIA

With effective treatment, hypoglycemia can usually be quickly reversed. At the first sign of hypoglycemia, the blood glucose should be checked if possible (Table 47-19). If it is below 70 mg/dl (3.9 mmol/L), the patient should immediately begin treatment for hypoglycemia. If the blood glucose is above 70 mg/dl (3.9 mmol/L), other causes of the signs and symptoms should be investigated. If the patient has manifestations of hypoglycemia and monitoring equipment is not available, hypoglycemia should be assumed and treatment should be initiated.

Hypoglycemia is treated by ingesting 10 to 15 g of a simple (fast-acting) carbohydrate, such as 4 to 8 oz of fruit juice or regular (non-diet) soft drink or 8 oz of low-fat milk. Commercial products such as gels or tablets containing specific amounts of glucose are convenient for carrying in a purse or pocket to be used in such situations.

TABLE 47-19	Collaborative Care — Hypoglycemia

Diagnostic
Stat blood glucose
History (if possible) and physical examination

Collaborative Therapy
Determination of cause of hypoglycemia (after correction of condition)

Conscious Patient
Administration of 15-20 g of quick-acting carbohydrate (e.g., 6–8 oz of regular soda, 8–10 LifeSavers, 1 tb syrup or honey, 4 tsp jelly, 4–6 oz orange juice, 8 oz low-fat milk, commercial dextrose products [per label instructions])
Repetition of treatment in 15 min (if no improvement)
Administration of additional food of longer-acting carbohydrate (e.g., slice of bread, crackers) after symptoms subside
Immediate notification of health care provider or emergency service (if patient outside hospital) if symptoms do not subside after two to three administrations of quick-acting carbohydrate

Worsening Symptoms or Unconscious Patient
Subcutaneous or intramuscular injection of 1 mg glucagon
Intravenous administration of 50 ml 50% glucose

Treatment with sweet foods that also contain fat, such as candy bars, cookies, and ice cream, should be avoided because the fat in them will slow down the absorption of the sugar and delay the response to treatment. Overtreatment with large quantities of quick-acting carbohydrates should also be avoided so that a rapid fluctuation to hyperglycemia does not occur. A prompt but moderate approach is best. Blood glucose should be checked about 15 minutes following the initial treatment for hypoglycemia, and treatment should be repeated if the blood glucose remains below 70 mg/dl (3.9 mmol/L). Once the blood glucose is greater than 70 mg/dl (3.9 mmol/L), the patient should eat the regularly scheduled meal or a snack to prevent hypoglycemia from recurring. Good snacks include peanut butter and cheese and crackers. Blood glucose should also be checked again about 45 minutes after treatment to ensure that hypoglycemia is not recurring.

If there is no significant improvement in the patient's condition after two to three doses of 10 to 15 g of simple carbohydrate, or if the patient is not alert enough to swallow, 1 mg of glucagon may be administered by intramuscular (IM) or SQ injection. An IM injection in a site such as the deltoid muscle will result in a quicker response. Glucagon stimulates a strong hepatic response to convert glycogen to glucose and therefore makes glucose rapidly available. Rebound hypoglycemia is a potential adverse effect of glucagon. Having the patient ingest a complex carbohydrate after recovery may prevent this from happening.

Once the acute hypoglycemia has been reversed, the nurse should explore with the patient the reasons why the situation developed. This assessment may indicate the need for additional education of the patient and the family to avoid future episodes of hypoglycemia. The danger of hypoglycemic reactions must be stressed because memory and learning impairment can result from repeated episodes of severe hypoglycemia.

Chronic Complications of Diabetes Mellitus

Chronic complications of diabetes are primarily those of end-organ disease that result from damage to the large and small blood vessels from chronic hyperglycemia. Several theories exist as to how and why chronic hyperglycemia damages cells and tissues. Possible causes include (1) the accumulation of damaging by-products of glucose metabolism, such as sorbitol, which is associated with damage to nerve cells; (2) the formation of abnormal glucose molecules in the basement membrane of small blood vessels such as those that circulate to the eye and kidney; and (3) a derangement in red blood cell function that leads to a decrease in oxygenation to the tissues.

The Diabetes Control and Complication Trial (DCCT) was a landmark study that has greatly influenced diabetes management since its results were announced in 1993.[23] This study demonstrated that in patients with type 1 diabetes the risk for microvascular complications could be significantly reduced by keeping blood glucose levels as near to normal as possible for as much of the time as possible (tight glucose control). In this study, patients were randomly assigned to one of two groups: intensive or standard treatment. The intensive treatment group took three or more insulin injections a day or used an insulin pump. The patients in the standard treatment group took one to two injections a day and tested their blood glucose once or twice a day. The average A1C in the intensive treatment group was 7.2% and in the standard treatment group was 9%. (The normal range for A1C in a person without diabetes is 4.0% to 6.05%.)

In addition, the results found that the subjects in the intensive therapy group reduced their risk for the development of retinopathy and nephropathy. The main adverse effect associated with intensive therapy was an increase in cases of severe hypoglycemia.

Based on the findings of the DCCT, the ADA issued recommendations for the management of diabetes that included treatment goals to maintain blood glucose levels as near to normal as possible. Specific targets for individual patients must take into account the risk for severe or undetected hypoglycemia as a side effect of tight glucose control.

More recently, the United Kingdom Prospective Diabetes Study (UKPDS) demonstrated that intensive treatment of type 2 diabetes can also significantly lower the risk for developing diabetes-related eye, kidney, and neurologic problems. The findings from this study included a 25% reduction of microvascular disease in subjects who maintained long-term glycemic control.[24]

Because of the devastating effects of long-term complications, patients with diabetes require scheduled and ongoing monitoring for the detection and prevention of chronic complications.[25] The ADA recommendations for ongoing evaluation are listed in Table 47-20. It is imperative that patients understand the importance of participating in regular follow-up examinations.

ANGIOPATHY

Angiopathy, or blood vessel disease, is estimated to account for the majority of deaths among patients with diabetes. These chronic blood vessel dysfunctions are divided into two categories: macrovascular complications and microvascular complications.

Macrovascular Complications

Macrovascular complications are diseases of the large and medium-sized blood vessels that occur with greater frequency and with an earlier onset in people with diabetes. Although atherosclerotic plaque formation is believed to have a genetic origin, its development seems to be promoted by the altered lipid metabolism common to diabetes. Tight glucose control may help delay the atherosclerotic process.[23] Macrovascular diseases include cerebrovascular, cardiovascular, and peripheral vascular disease. Although genetic makeup cannot be altered, a patient with diabetes can diminish other risk factors associated with macroangiopathy, such as obesity, smoking, hypertension, high fat intake, and sedentary lifestyle. Smoking, which is detrimental to health in general, is especially injurious to people with diabetes. Smoking significantly increases the risk for blood vessel disease in people with diabetes and increases the risk for cardiovascular disease, stroke, and lower extremity amputation.

Insulin resistance seems to play an important role in the development of cardiovascular disease and is implicated in the pathogenesis of essential hypertension and dyslipidemia. The term *insulin resistance syndrome* is applied to the clinical associ-

TABLE 47-20 Prevention, Detection, and Monitoring of Long-Term Complications of Diabetes Mellitus*

COMPLICATION	TYPE OF EXAMINATION	FREQUENCY
Retinopathy	• Funduscopic–dilated eye examination	• Annually
Nephropathy	• Urinalysis for microalbuminuria	• Annually
Neuropathy (foot and lower extremities)	• Visual examination of foot	• Daily by patient; every visit by health care provider

	• Comprehensive foot examination:
	  –Visual examination
	  –Sensory examination with monofilament and tuning fork
	  –Palpation (pulses, temperature, callus formation)
		• Annually

Cardiovascular disease	• Blood pressure • Lipid panel • Exercise stress testing (may include stress ECG, stress echocardio-gram, perfusion imaging)	• Every visit • Annually • As needed based on risk factors

ECG, Electrocardiogram.
*Based on the recommendations of the American Diabetes Association.

ation of insulin resistance, hypertension, and increased very-low-density lipoprotein (VLDL) and decreased high-density lipoprotein (HDL) cholesterol concentrations. The role of insulin resistance in the pathogenesis of cardiovascular disease is not well understood, but it seems to combine with dyslipidemia in contributing to greater risk of cardiovascular disease in patients with diabetes mellitus.[22] All patients with diabetes should be screened for dyslipidemia at the time diabetes is diagnosed. These abnormalities typically include an elevated triglyceride level and reduced HDL cholesterol.

Microvascular Complications

Microvascular complications result from thickening of the vessel membranes in the capillaries and arterioles in response to conditions of chronic hyperglycemia. They differ from the macrovascular complications in that they are specific to diabetes. Although microangiopathy can be found throughout the body, the areas most noticeably affected are the eyes (retinopathy), the kidneys (nephropathy), and the skin (dermopathy). Thickening of the basement membrane has been found in some persons with diabetes before or at the time of diagnosis or before the onset of symptoms of diabetes mellitus. However, clinical manifestations usually do not appear until 10 to 20 years after the onset of diabetes.

DIABETIC RETINOPATHY

Etiology and Pathophysiology

Diabetic retinopathy refers to the process of microvascular damage to the retina as a result of chronic hyperglycemia in patients with diabetes. After 15 years with diabetes mellitus, nearly all patients with type 1 diabetes and 80% with type 2 diabetes will have some degree of retinal disease. Diabetic retinopathy is estimated to be the most common cause of new cases of blindness in people ages 20 to 74 years.[26]

Retinopathy can be classified as nonproliferative or proliferative. In *nonproliferative retinopathy*, the most common form, partial occlusion of the small blood vessels in the retina causes the development of microaneurysms in the capillary walls. The walls of these microaneurysms are so weak that capillary fluid leaks out, causing retinal edema and eventually hard exudates or intraretinal hemorrhages. Vision may be affected if the macula is involved.

Proliferative retinopathy, the most severe form, involves the retina and the vitreous. When retinal capillaries become occluded, the body compensates by forming new blood vessels to supply the retina with blood, a pathologic process known as *neovascularization*. These new vessels are extremely fragile and hemorrhage easily, producing vitreous contraction. Eventually light is prevented from reaching the retina as the vessels become torn and bleed into the vitreous cavity. The patient sees black or red spots or lines. If these new blood vessels pull the retina while the vitreous contracts, causing a tear, partial or complete retinal detachment will occur. If the macula is involved, vision is lost. Without treatment, more than half of patients with proliferative diabetic retinopathy will be blind.

Collaborative Care

The earliest and most treatable stages of diabetic retinopathy often produce no changes in the vision. Because of this, the patient with diabetes must have regular dilated eye examinations by an ophthalmologist or a specially trained optometrist for early detection and treatment.

The most common forms of treatment for diabetic retinopathy are early photocoagulation of the retina, cryotherapy (cryoprexy), and vitrectomy. Photocoagulation by laser destroys the ischemic areas of the retina that produce growth factors that encourage neovascularization.[27] (Photocoagulation is discussed in Chapter 21.)

Cryotherapy (cryoprexy) is sometimes used to treat peripheral areas of the retina that cannot be reached with lasers or when retinal hemorrhage prevents complete photocoagulation. In this procedure, topical anesthesia is used so that a cryoprobe can be placed directly on the surface of the eye. When the probe is properly located, its tip creates a frozen area that extends through the external tissue through the eyeball until it reaches a specific point on the retina. Multiple points on the retina can be treated in this way. (Cryotherapy is discussed in Chapter 21.)

Vitrectomy is the aspiration of blood, membrane, and fibers from the inside of the eye through a small incision just behind the cornea. Vitrectomy is indicated when there is vitreal hemorrhage that does not clear in 6 months or when there is threatened or actual retinal detachment. (Vitrectomy is discussed in Chapter 21.)

Persons with diabetes are also prone to other visual problems. Glaucoma occurs as a result of the occlusion of the outflow channels secondary to neovascularization. This type of glaucoma is difficult to treat and often results in blindness. Cataracts develop at an earlier age and progress more rapidly in people with diabetes.

NEPHROPATHY

Diabetic nephropathy is a microvascular complication associated with damage to the small blood vessels that supply the glomeruli of the kidney. It is the leading cause of end-stage renal disease (ESRD) in the United States. The risk of nephropathy is about the same in patients with either type 1 or type 2 diabetes. Risk factors for the development of diabetic nephropathy include hypertension, genetic predisposition, smoking, and chronic hyperglycemia. Results of the DCCT and UKPDS studies have demonstrated that kidney disease can be significantly reduced when near-normal blood glucose control is achieved and maintained.[11,24]

Hypertension significantly accelerates the progression of diabetic nephropathy. Therefore aggressive blood pressure management is indicated for all patients with diabetes. Angiotensin-converting enzyme (ACE) inhibitor drugs (e.g., lisinopril [Prinivil, Zestril]) are commonly prescribed to patients with diabetes because they are effective blood pressure–lowering agents with few side effects. In addition, ACE inhibitors are often prescribed to patients with diabetes even when they are not hypertensive. This is because drugs in this class have a protective effect on the kidney that prevents the progression of diabetic nephropathy independent of hypertension control.[28] Angiotensin II receptor antagonists (e.g., losartan [Cozaar]) may also be used for their kidney-protective benefits. (See Chapter 32 for a discussion of hypertension and Chapter 45 for a discussion of renal failure.)

Standards for the prevention and detection of nephropathy in patients with diabetes include yearly screening for the presence of microalbuminuria (MAU) in the urine. This test detects kidney damage at an earlier stage than the standard dipstick test for urine protein. The presence of protein in the urine as detected by MAU urinalysis should be followed with an albumin/creatinine ratio or 24-hour urine collection for determination of creatinine clearance and serum creatinine.

NEUROPATHY

Diabetic neuropathy is nerve damage that occurs because of the metabolic derangements associated with diabetes mellitus. About 60% to 70% of patients with diabetes have some degree of neuropathy, with neurologic complications occurring equally in type 1 and type 2 diabetes.[1,29] The most common type of neuropathy affecting persons with diabetes is sensory neuropathy. This can lead to the loss of protective sensation in the lower extremities, and, coupled with other factors, this significantly increases the risk for complications that result in a lower limb amputation.

Etiology and Pathophysiology

The pathophysiologic processes of diabetic neuropathy are not well understood. Several theories exist, including metabolic, vascular, and autoimmune elements. The prevailing theory suggests that persistent hyperglycemia leads to an accumulation of sorbitol and fructose in the nerves that causes damage by an unknown mechanism. The result is reduced nerve conduction and demyelinization. Ischemia in blood vessels damaged by chronic hyperglycemia that supply the peripheral nerves is also implicated in the development of diabetic neuropathy. Neuropathy can precede, accompany, or follow the diagnosis of diabetes.

Classification

The two major categories of diabetic neuropathy are *sensory neuropathy,* which affects the peripheral nervous system, and *autonomic neuropathy.* Each of these types can take on several forms.

Sensory Neuropathy. The most common form of sensory neuropathy is distal symmetric neuropathy, which affects the hands and/or feet bilaterally. This is sometimes referred to as "stocking-glove neuropathy." Characteristics of distal symmetric neuropathy include loss of sensation, abnormal sensations, pain, and paresthesias. The pain, which is often described as burning, cramping, crushing, or tearing, is usually worse at night and may occur only at that time. The paresthesias may be associated with tingling, burning, and itching sensations. The patient may report a feeling of walking on pillows or numb feet. At times the skin becomes so sensitive (hyperesthesia) that even light pressure from bedsheets cannot be tolerated. Complete or partial loss of sensitivity to touch and temperature is common. Foot injury and ulcerations can occur without the patient ever having pain (Fig. 47-13). Neuropathy can also cause atrophy of the small muscles of the hands and feet, causing deformity and limiting fine movement.

Control of blood glucose is the only treatment for diabetic neuropathy. It is effective in many, but not all, cases. Drug therapy may be used to treat neuropathic symptoms, particularly pain. Medications commonly used include topical creams (e.g., capsaicin [Zostrix]), tricyclic antidepressants (e.g., amitriptyline [Elavil]), and antiseizure medications (e.g., gabapentin [Neurontin]). Capsaicin is a moderately effective topical cream made from chili peppers. It depletes the accumulation of pain-mediating chemicals in the peripheral sensory neurons. The cream is applied three to four times a day. There is usually an increase in symptoms at the start of therapy, which is followed by relief of pain in 2 to 3 weeks.[29] Tricyclic antidepressants are also moderately effective in treating the symptoms of diabetic neuropathy. They work by inhibiting the reuptake of norepinephrine and serotonin, which are

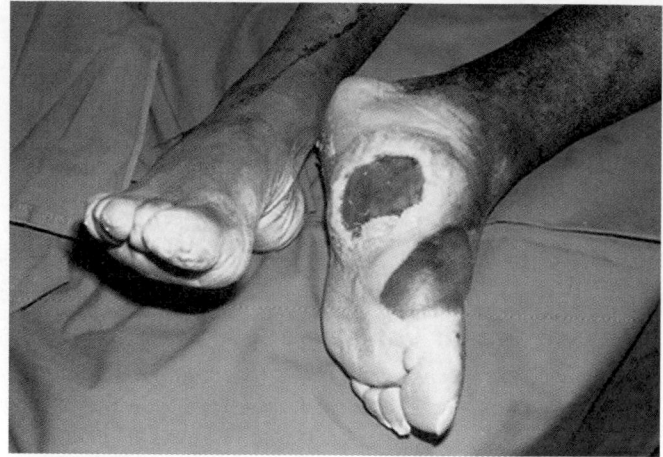

FIG. 47-13 Neuropathy: neurotrophic ulceration.

neurotransmitters that are believed to play a role in the transmission of pain through the spinal cord.[29] Although gabapentin has been found to be effective in treating the pain of diabetic neuropathy, its mechanism of action is not well understood.

Autonomic Neuropathy. Autonomic neuropathy can affect nearly all body systems and lead to hypoglycemic unawareness, bowel incontinence and diarrhea, and urinary retention. Delayed gastric emptying (gastroparesis) is a complication of autonomic neuropathy that can produce anorexia, nausea, vomiting, gastroesophageal reflux, and persistent feelings of fullness. Gastroparesis can trigger hypoglycemia by delaying food absorption. Cardiovascular abnormalities associated with autonomic neuropathy are postural hypotension, resting tachycardia, and painless myocardial infarction. A patient with postural hypotension should be instructed to change from a lying or sitting position slowly.

Diabetes can affect sexual function in men and women. Erectile dysfunction associated with diabetes mellitus is believed to result from damage to the sacral parasympathetic nerves. Determining whether this problem is of organic or psychologic origin is an important part of the assessment. Decreased libido is a problem with some women with diabetes. Monilial and nonspecific vaginitis are also common. Organic impotence or sexual dysfunctioning in either the male or the female patient requires sensitive therapeutic counseling for both the patient and the patient's partner. (See Chapter 53 for a further discussion of impotence.)

A neurogenic bladder may develop as sensation in the inner bladder wall decreases, causing urinary retention. A patient with retention has infrequent voiding, difficulty in voiding, and a weak stream of urine. Emptying the bladder every 3 hours in a sitting position helps prevent stasis and subsequent infection. Tightening the abdominal muscles during voiding and using the Credé maneuver (mild massage downward over the lower abdomen and bladder) may also help with complete bladder emptying. Cholinergic agonist drugs such as bethanechol (Urecholine) may be used. The patient may also have to learn self-catheterization (see Chapter 44).

COMPLICATIONS OF THE FOOT AND LOWER EXTREMITY

Foot complications are the most common cause of hospitalization in the person with diabetes.[30] The development of diabetic foot complications is a multifactorial process. They result from a combination of microvascular and macrovascular diseases that place the patient at risk for injury and serious infection that may lead to amputation. Sensory neuropathy and peripheral vascular disease (PVD) are risk factors, and clotting abnormalities, impaired immune function, and autonomic neuropathy also play important roles. Smoking is deleterious to the health of lower extremity blood vessels and increases the risk for amputation.

PVD increases the risk for amputation by causing a reduction in blood flow to the lower extremities. When blood flow is decreased, oxygen, white blood cells, and vital nutrients are not available to the tissues. Therefore wounds take longer to heal and the risk for infection increases. Signs of PVD include intermittent claudication, pain at rest, cold feet, loss of hair, delayed capillary filling, and dependent rubor (redness of the skin that occurs when the extremity is in a dependent position). The disease is diagnosed by history, Doppler findings, and angiography. Management includes control or reduction of risk factors, particularly smoking, high cholesterol intake, and hypertension. Bypass or graft surgery is indicated in some patients. Proper care of the feet is essential for the patient with PVD. Guidelines for patient teaching are listed in Table 47-21.

Sensory neuropathy is a major risk factor for lower extremity amputation in the person with diabetes. Loss of protective sensation (LOPS) often prevents the patient from becoming aware that a foot injury has occurred. Improper footwear and injury from stepping on foreign objects while barefoot are common causes of undetected foot injury in the person with LOPS. Because the primary risk factor for lower extremity amputation is LOPS, annual screening using a *monofilament* is an extremely important preventive measure. This is done by applying a thin, flexible filament to several spots on the plantar surface of the foot and asking the patient to report if it is felt. Insensitivity to a 10 g Semmes-Weinstein monofilament has been shown to greatly increase the risk for diabetic foot ulcers that can lead to amputation. If the patient has LOPS, aggressive measures must be taken to teach the patient how to prevent foot ulceration. These measures include the selection of proper footwear, including prescription shoes. Other measures are to carefully avoid injury to the foot, to practice diligent skin and nail care, to inspect the foot thoroughly each day, and to treat small problems promptly.

The Doppler instrument is used to diagnose the presence or degree of PVD. Similar to an electronic stethoscope, this device amplifies sound. The procedure is noninvasive and can measure blood pressure in the lower extremities and blood flow velocity. It can indicate areas of stenosis or occlusion and is useful as an indicator of the need for additional vascular tests.

Neuropathic arthropathy, or *Charcot foot*, results in ankle and foot changes that ultimately lead to joint dysfunction and footdrop. These changes occur gradually and promote an abnormal distribution of weight over the foot, further increasing the chances of developing a foot ulcer as new pressure points emerge. Neuropathic ulcers resemble a "BB shot" or "punched out" wound and are usually painless. Infection is a danger and necessitates the long-term use of antibiotics and weeks of avoidance of weight bearing on the affected limb.

INTEGUMENTARY COMPLICATIONS

Skin disorders such as diabetic dermopathy and necrobiosis lipoidica diabeticorum are attributed to microangiopathy. Shin spots are brown spots located on the anterior surfaces of the lower extremities. They are harmless and painless and initially measure less than 1 cm in diameter. *Necrobiosis lipoidica dia-*

TABLE 47-21   Patient & Family Teaching Guide — Foot Care

1. Wash feet daily with a mild soap and *warm* water. Test water temperature with hands first.
2. Pat feet dry gently, especially between toes.
3. Examine feet daily for cuts, blisters, swelling, and red, tender areas. Do not depend on feeling sores. If eyesight is poor, have others inspect feet.
4. Use lanolin on feet to prevent skin from drying and cracking. Do not apply between toes.
5. Use mild foot powder on sweaty feet.
6. Do not use commercial remedies to remove calluses or corns.
7. Cleanse cuts with *warm* water and mild soap, covering with clean dressing. Do not use iodine, rubbing alcohol, or strong adhesives.
8. Report skin infections or nonhealing sores to health care provider immediately.
9. Cut toenails even with rounded contour of toes. Do not cut down corners. The best time to trim nails is after a shower or bath.
10. Separate overlapping toes with cotton or lamb's wool.
11. Avoid open-toe, open-heel, and high-heel shoes. Leather shoes are preferred to plastic ones. Wear slippers with soles. Do not go barefoot. Shake out shoes before putting on.
12. Wear clean, absorbent (cotton or wool) socks or stockings that have not been mended. Colored socks must be colorfast.
13. Do not wear clothing that leaves impressions, hindering circulation.
14. Do not use hot water bottles or heating pads to warm feet. Wear socks for warmth.
15. Guard against frostbite.
16. Exercise feet daily either by walking or by flexing and extending feet in suspended position. Avoid prolonged sitting, standing, and crossing of legs.

beticorum is believed to be the result of the breakdown of collagen in the skin. It usually appears as red-yellow lesions, with atrophic skin that becomes shiny and transparent revealing tiny blood vessels under the surface. Because the thin skin is prone to injury, special care must be taken to protect affected areas from injury and ulceration. This condition is not common, but it may appear before other clinical signs or symptoms of diabetes. It is more frequently seen in young women.

INFECTION

A patient with diabetes is more susceptible to infections than other patients. The mechanisms for this phenomenon include a defect in the mobilization of inflammatory cells and an impairment of phagocytosis by neutrophils and monocytes. Recurring or persistent infections such as *Candida albicans,* as well as boils and furuncles, in the undiagnosed patient often lead the health care provider to suspect diabetes. Loss of sensation (neuropathy) may delay the detection of an infection.

Persistent glycosuria may predispose to bladder infections, especially in patients with a neurogenic bladder. Decreased circulation resulting from angiopathy can prevent or delay the immune response. Antibiotic therapy has prevented infection from being a major cause of death in diabetic patients. The treatment of infections must be prompt and vigorous.

Gerontologic Considerations: Diabetes Mellitus

Diabetes is more prevalent in older populations. A major reason for this is that the process of aging involves insulin resistance and glucose intolerance, which are believed to be precursors to type 2 diabetes.[31] Aging is also associated with a number of conditions that are more likely to be treated with medications that impair insulin action (e.g., corticosteroids, antihypertensives, phenothiazines). Undiagnosed and untreated diabetes is more common in the elderly, partly because many of the normal physiologic changes of aging resemble those of diabetes, such as visual changes and decreased glomerular filtration.

Although good glycemic control is important to people of all ages with diabetes, several factors are taken into account when determining glycemic goals for an older adult. One is that hypoglycemic unawareness is more common in this age-group, making these patients more likely to suffer adverse consequences from blood glucose–lowering therapy. They may also have delayed psychomotor function that could interfere with the ability to treat hypoglycemia. Other factors to consider in establishing glycemic goals for the older patient include the patient's own desire for treatment and other coexisting medical problems such as cognitive impairment. Although it is generally agreed that treatment is indicated for older adults with diabetes to prevent acute complications and avoid unpleasant symptoms, strict glycemic control may be difficult to achieve.[32,33]

As with any group, diet and exercise are recommended as therapy for older adult patients with diabetes. This should take into account functional limitations that may interfere with physical activity and the ability to prepare meals. Because of the physiologic changes that occur with aging, the therapeutic outcome for the older adult with diabetes who receives OAs may be altered. First-generation sulfonylureas, such as tolazamide (Tolinase), are generally avoided in this age-group because the long half-life of these drugs increases the risk for hypoglycemia. The second-generation sulfonylurea drugs (e.g., glyburide [Micronase]) are usually well tolerated and have increased potency but appear to have fewer side effects and fewer drug interaction problems when compared with the first-generation agents. Other OAs described earlier in this chapter may also be used in older patients with diabetes. Insulin therapy may be instituted if OAs fail. However, it is important to recognize that elderly patients are more likely to have limitations in manual dexterity and visual acuity, both of which are necessary for accurate insulin administration.

Patient teaching should be based on the individual's needs, using a slower pace with simple printed or audio materials. It is important to include family or a support person in the teaching. The patient education issues for the older patient include those related to vision, mobility, mental status, functional ability, financial and social situation, the effect of multiple medications, eating habits, the potential for undetected hypoglycemia, and quality-of-life issues.[34] ■

CRITICAL THINKING EXERCISES

Case Study
Diabetic Ketoacidosis
Patient Profile. John, a 34-year-old Native American man, was admitted to the emergency department after he was found comatose in his apartment by his wife.

Subjective Data (provided by wife)
- Was diagnosed with diabetes mellitus 12 months ago
- Was taking 48 U of insulin daily: 12 U of regular insulin plus 20 U of NPH before breakfast, 8 U of regular insulin before dinner, and 8 U of NPH at bedtime
- Has history of flu for 1 week with vomiting and anorexia
- Stopped taking insulin 2 days ago when he was unable to eat

Objective Data
Physical Examination
- Breathing is deep and rapid
- Acetone smell on breath
- Skin flushed and dry

Diagnostic Studies
- Blood glucose level of 730 mg/dl (40.5 mmol/L)
- Blood pH of 7.26

CRITICAL THINKING QUESTIONS
1. Briefly explain the pathophysiology of the development of diabetic ketoacidosis (DKA) in this patient.
2. What clinical manifestations of DKA does this patient exhibit?
3. What factors precipitated this patient's DKA?
4. What distinguishes this case history from one of hyperosmolar hyperglycemic nonketotic syndrome (HHNS) or hypoglycemia?
5. What teaching should be done with this patient and his family?
6. What role should John's wife have in the management of his diabetes?
7. Based on the assessment data presented, write one or more appropriate nursing diagnoses. Are there any collaborative problems?

Nursing Research Issues
1. What degree of pain does the patient associate with capillary blood glucose monitoring?
2. How often does the patient make phone contact with a diabetes nurse educator when this service is available free as compared with when there is a charge?
3. What factors contribute to a patient's willingness to maintain tight glycemic control in the present to prevent chronic complications from diabetes in the future?
4. Does the frequency of review of major diabetes education issues affect the frequency of occurrence of acute complications of diabetes?

REVIEW QUESTIONS

The number of the question corresponds to the same-numbered objective at the beginning of the chapter.

1. The polydipsia and polyuria related to diabetes mellitus are primarily caused by
   a. the release of ketones from cells during fat metabolism.
   b. fluid shifts resulting from the osmotic effect of hyperglycemia.
   c. damage to the kidneys from exposure to high levels of glucose.
   d. changes in RBCs resulting from attachment of excessive glucose to hemoglobin.

2. When a patient with type 2 diabetes mellitus is admitted to the hospital with pneumonia, the nurse recognizes that the patient
   a. must receive insulin therapy to prevent the development of ketoacidosis.
   b. has islet cell antibodies that have destroyed the ability of the pancreas to produce insulin.
   c. has minimal or absent endogenous insulin secretion and requires daily insulin injections.
   d. may have sufficient endogenous insulin to prevent ketosis but is at risk for development of hyperosmolar hyperglycemic nonketotic syndrome.

3. Effective collaborative management of diabetes includes
   a. using insulin with all patients to achieve glycemic goals.
   b. relying on the health care provider as the central figure in the program for good control.
   c. relying solely on nutritional therapy as the initial treatment modality for all patients with diabetes.
   d. aiming for a balance of diet, activity, and medications together with appropriate monitoring and patient and family teaching.

4. The nurse assists the patient with nutritional therapy of diabetes with the knowledge that a "diabetic diet" is designed
   a. to be used only for type 1 diabetes.
   b. for use during periods of high stress.
   c. to normalize blood glucose by elimination of sugar.
   d. to help normalize blood glucose through a balanced diet.

5. In teaching a newly diagnosed type 1 diabetic "survival skills," the nurse includes information about
   a. weight loss measures.
   b. elimination of sugar from diet.
   c. need to reduce physical activity.
   d. self-monitoring of blood glucose.

6. An appropriate teaching measure for the patient with diabetes mellitus related to care of the feet is to
   a. use heat to increase blood supply.
   b. avoid softening lotions and creams.
   c. inspect all surfaces of the feet daily.
   d. use iodine to disinfect cuts and abrasions.

7. A diabetic patient has a serum glucose level of 824 mg/dl (45.7 mmol/L) and is unresponsive. Following assessment of the patient, the nurse suspects diabetic ketoacidosis rather than hyperosmolar hyperglycemic nonketotic syndrome based on the finding of
   a. polyuria.
   b. severe dehydration.
   c. rapid, deep respirations.
   d. decreased serum potassium.

8. Which of the following is not an appropriate therapy for patients with diabetes mellitus?
   a. Use of diuretics to treat renal problems
   b. Use of ACE inhibitors to treat renal problems
   c. Use of laser photocoagulation to treat retinopathy
   d. Use of regular insulin for a patient with type 2 diabetes during the intraoperative period

REFERENCES

1. American Diabetes Association: Available at *www.ada.org* (accessed Nov 1, 2002).
2. Report of the expert committee on the diagnosis and classification of diabetes mellitus, *Diabetes Care* 25(suppl 1):5, 2002.
3. Edelman SV, Henry RR. *Diagnosis and management of type 2 diabetes,* ed 3, Caddo, Okla, 1999, Professional Communications.
4. National Institute of Diabetes and Digestive and Kidney Disease: Diet and exercise dramatically delay type 2 diabetes: diabetes medication metformin also effective. Available at *www.niddk.nih.gov* (accessed Nov 1, 2002).
5. Stoller WA: Individualizing insulin management: three practical cases, rules for regimen adjustment, *Postgrad Med* 111:51, 2002.
6. Mayerson AB, Inzucchi SE: Type 2 diabetes therapy: a pathophysiologically based approach, *Postgrad Med* 111:83, 2002.
7. Aventis Pharmaceuticals: Lantus prescribing information. Available at *www.aventispharma-us.com* (accessed Nov 1, 2002).
8. American Diabetes Association: Position statement: insulin administration, *Diabetes Care* 25(suppl 1):112, 2002.
9. Bode BW, Tamborlane WV, Davidson PC: Insulin pump therapy in the 21st century: strategies for successful use in adults, adolescents, and children with diabetes, *Postgrad Med* 111:69, 2002.
10. Fain JA: Delivering insulin 'round the clock, *Nursing* 32:54, 2002.
11. American Diabetes Association: Position statement: implications of the Diabetes Control and Complication Trial, *Diabetes Care* 25(suppl 1):25, 2002.
12. Ahmann AJ, Riddle MC: Current oral agents for type 2 diabetes: many options, but which to choose when? *Postgrad Med* 111:32, 2002.
13. Funnell MM, Barlage DL: Saying a mouthful about oral diabetes drugs, *Nursing* 30:34, 2000.
14. Takeda Pharmaceuticals America, Eli Lilly and Company: Actos product insert, no date.
15. American Diabetes Association: Position statement: nutritional recommendations and principles for people with diabetes mellitus, *Diabetes Care* 25(suppl 1):61, 2002.
16. American Diabetes Association: Position statement: evidence-based nutrition principles and recommendations for the treatment and prevention of diabetes and related complications, *Diabetes Care* 25:50, 2002.
17. American Diabetes Association: *Medical management of type 2 diabetes,* ed 4, Alexandria, Va., 1998, American Diabetes Association.
18. Funnell MM et al: *Life with diabetes,* ed 2, Alexandria, Va., 2000, American Diabetes Association.
19. Flood L, Constance A: Diabetes and exercise safety, *Am J Nurs* 102:47, 2002.

20. American Diabetes Association: *The diabetes ready-reference guide for health care professionals,* Alexandria, Va., 2000, American Diabetes Association.

21. Konick-McMahan J: Riding out a diabetic emergency, *Nursing* 29:9, 1999.

22. American Diabetes Association: Position statement: insulin administration, *Diabetes Care* 25(suppl 1):112, 2002.

23. Diabetes Control and Complications Trial Research Group: The effect of intensive treatment of diabetes on the development and progression of long-term complications in insulin-dependent diabetes mellitus, *N Engl J Med* 329:977, 1993.

24. American Diabetes Association: Position statement: implications of the United Kingdom Prospective Diabetes Study, *Diabetes Care* 25(suppl 1):28, 2002.

25. American Diabetes Association: Position statement: standards of medical care for patients with diabetes mellitus, *Diabetes Care* 25(suppl 1):33, 2002.

26. American Diabetes Association: Position statement: diabetic retinopathy, *Diabetes Care* 25(suppl 1):90, 2002.

27. Grand MG et al: Eye disease. In Levin ME, Pfeifer MA, editors: *The uncomplicated guide to diabetes complications,* Alexandria, Va., 1998, American Diabetes Association.

28. American Diabetes Association: Position statement: diabetic nephropathy, *Diabetes Care* 25(suppl 1):85, 2002.

29. Vinik AI: Diagnosis and management of diabetic neuropathy, *Advances in the Care of Older People with Diabetes* 15:293, 1999.

30. Mulder GD: Evaluating and managing the diabetic foot, *Adv Skin Wound Care* 13:33, 2000

31. Barzilai N et al: Advances in diabetes management: application to the geriatric patient, *Ann Long Term Care* 8:58, 2000.

32. Chau D, Edelman SV: Clinical management of diabetes in the elderly, *Clinical Diabetes* 19:172, 2001.

33. Gabriely I, Barzilai N: Management of insulin resistance in the elderly patient with diabetes, *Clin Geriatr* 10:38, 2002.

34. Strachan M: Cognitive decline and the older patient with diabetes, *Clin Geriatr* 10:29, 2002.

RESOURCES

American Association of Diabetes Educators
100 West Monroe Street, Suite 400
Chicago, IL 60603
800-338-3633
Fax: 312-424-2427
www.aadenet.org/

American Diabetes Association
1701 North Beauregard Street
Alexandria, VA 22311
800-DIABETES (342-2383)
Fax: 703-549-6995
www.diabetes.org/

American Dietetic Association
216 West Jackson Boulevard
Chicago, IL 60606-6995
800-877-1600 or 312-899-0040
www.eatright.org/

Juvenile Diabetes Research Foundation International
120 Wall Street
New York, NY 10005-4001
800-533-CURE (2873) or 212-785-9500
Fax: 212-785-9595
www.jdrf.org/index.php

National Diabetes Information Clearinghouse
1 Information Way
Bethesda, MD 20892-3560
301-654-3327
Fax: 301-907-8906
www.niddk.nih.gov/

For additional Internet resources, see the website for this book at *http://evolve.elsevier.com/Lewis/medsurg/.*

CHAPTER 48

NURSING MANAGEMENT
Endocrine Problems

Jean Foret Giddens

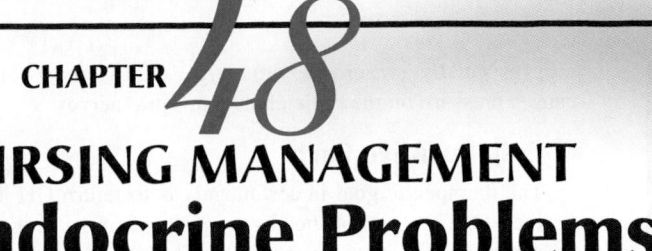

LEARNING OBJECTIVES

1. Describe the pathophysiology, clinical manifestations, collaborative care, and nursing management of the patient with an imbalance of hormones produced by the anterior pituitary gland.
2. Describe the pathophysiology, clinical manifestations, collaborative care, and nursing management of the patient with an imbalance of antidiuretic hormone secretion.
3. Describe the pathophysiology, clinical manifestations, collaborative care, and nursing management of the patient with thyroid dysfunction.
4. Describe the pathophysiology, clinical manifestations, collaborative care, and nursing management of the patient with an imbalance of the hormone produced by the parathyroid glands.
5. Describe the pathophysiology, clinical manifestations, collaborative care, and nursing management of the patient with an imbalance of hormones produced by the adrenal cortex.
6. Describe the pathophysiology, clinical manifestations, collaborative care, and nursing management of the patient with an excess of hormones produced by the adrenal medulla.
7. Describe the side effects of corticosteroid therapy.
8. List common nursing assessments, interventions, rationales, and expected outcomes related to patient teaching for management of chronic endocrine problems.

KEY TERMS

acromegaly, p. 1303
Addison's disease, p. 1331
cretinism, p. 1319
Cushing syndrome, p. 1326
diabetes insipidus, p. 1309
exophthalmos, p. 1312
goiter, p. 1311
goitrogens, p. 1317
Graves' disease, p. 1311
hyperaldosteronism, p. 1334
hyperparathyroidism, p. 1323
hyperthyroidism, p. 1311

hypoparathyroidism, p. 1325
hypopituitarism, p. 1306
hypothyroidism, p. 1319
myxedema, p. 1320
pheochromocytoma, p. 1335
syndrome of inappropriate anti-diuretic hormone, p. 1307
tetany, p. 1324
thyroiditis, p. 1318
thyrotoxic crisis, p. 1312
thyrotoxicosis, p. 1311

Disorders of the Anterior Pituitary Gland

GROWTH HORMONE EXCESS

Etiology and Pathophysiology

Growth hormone (GH), an anabolic hormone, promotes protein synthesis and mobilizes glucose and free fatty acids. GH is produced by the anterior pituitary and stimulates the liver to produce insulin-like growth factor–1 (IGF-1), also known as somatomedin C. IGF-1 stimulates growth of bones and soft tissues. Normally IGF-1 also signals the anterior pituitary to reduce GH production. Overproduction of GH is almost always caused by a benign pituitary adenoma (tumor). The pituitary tumor secretes GH despite elevated IGF-1 levels, leading to unwanted growth of bones and other soft tissue. Overproduction of GH also causes elevation of blood glucose through insulin antagonism. Prolonged elevated glucose levels associated with elevation in GH leads to glucose intolerance.

In children, excessive secretion of GH results in *gigantism*. When the onset of GH excess occurs before closure of the epiphyses, the long bones are still capable of longitudinal growth. The excessive growth is usually proportional. These children may grow as tall as 8 feet (240 cm) and weigh more than 300 lb (136 kg).

In adults, excessive secretion of GH results in acromegaly. **Acromegaly** is characterized by an overgrowth of the bones and soft tissues. Because the problem develops after epiphyseal closure in adults, the bones are unable to grow longer. Instead, the bones increase in thickness and width. Acromegaly is relatively rare. Only three out of every 1 million adults in the United States is diagnosed with this disease each year, with a prevalence of 40 to 60 out of every 1 million individuals.[1] Both genders are affected equally.

Untreated, acromegaly leads to a number of changes in the body. Effects on the cardiovascular system include cardiomegaly, left ventricular hypertrophy, and hypertension. For this reason, disease of the cardiovascular system is associated with increased mortality rates in these individuals. Other systems that undergo changes include the gastrointestinal, genitourinary, musculoskeletal, and nervous systems.

Clinical Manifestations

Manifestations of acromegaly begin gradually, usually in the third and fourth decades of life. Typically there is an average of 7 to 9 years between the initial onset of symptoms and final diagnosis. Individuals experience enlargement of the hands and

Reviewed by Karla Jones, RN, MS, Nursing Faculty, Treasure Valley Community College, Ontario, Ore.; JoAnne Konick-McMahan, RN, MSN, CCRN, Advance Practice Nurse, School of Nursing, University of Pennsylvania, Philadelphia, Pa.; Debra A. Morgan, RN, EdD, Assistant Professor, College of Health Sciences and Human Services, Midwestern State University, Wichita Falls, Tex.

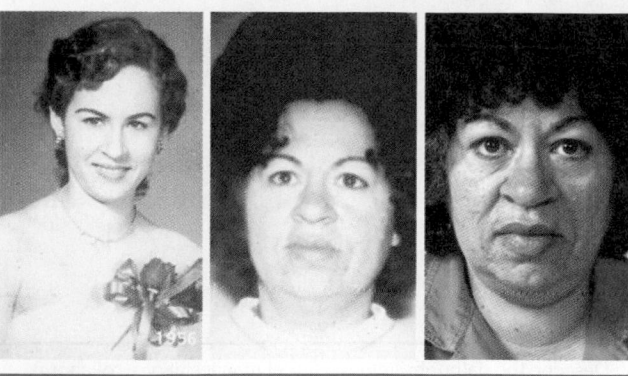

FIG. 48-1 Progressive development of facial features of acromegaly.

feet. The fingertips develop a tufted or clubbed-like appearance. The enlargement of the bones and cartilage may cause symptoms that range from mild joint pain to deforming, crippling arthritis. Changes in physical appearance occur with thickening and enlargement of bony and soft tissue on the face and head (Fig. 48-1). Enlargement of the mandible causes the jaw to jut forward. The paranasal and frontal sinuses enlarge, as does the bony tissue of the forehead. Enlargement of soft tissue around the eyes, nose, and mouth results in a coarsening of facial features. Enlargement of the tongue results in speech difficulties, and the voice deepens as a result of hypertrophy of the vocal cords.

Sleep apnea may also occur and is thought to be related to upper airway narrowing resulting from changes in pharyngeal soft tissues.[2] The skin becomes thick, leathery, and oily. Persons with acromegaly may also experience peripheral neuropathy and proximal muscle weakness. Women may develop menstrual disturbances. The patient may also exhibit manifestations of diabetes mellitus such as polydipsia and polyuria. Cardiovascular disease may manifest as hypertension, angina pectoris, and congestive heart failure.

The enlarged pituitary tumor gland can exert pressure on surrounding structures within the brain, leading to visual disturbances and headaches. Because GH mobilizes stored fat for energy, it increases free fatty acid levels in the blood and predisposes the patient to atherosclerosis. The hormone also antagonizes the action of insulin and causes hyperglycemia. Prolonged secretion of GH leads to glucose intolerance.

Diagnostic Studies

In addition to the history and physical examination, diagnosis of GH excess requires evaluation of plasma GH, plasma IGF-1 levels, IGF binding protein–3 (IGFBP-3) levels, and GH response to an oral glucose challenge. A single measurement of serum GH is of limited value in the diagnosis of acromegaly because GH levels normally fluctuate. IGF-1 levels are more constant and thus provide a more reliable measure than GH levels. The definitive test for acromegaly is the oral glucose challenge test. Normally GH concentration falls during an oral glucose tolerance test. In acromegaly, these levels do not fall.[3]

Magnetic resonance imaging (MRI) is indicated for the identification, localization, and determination of the extension of the pituitary tumor into surrounding tissue. High-resolution computed tomography (CT) scanning with contrast media may also be used to localize the tumor. A complete ophthalmologic examination, including visual fields, is typically done because the tu-

mor (especially a macroadenoma larger than 10 mm) potentially causes pressure on the optic chiasm or optic nerves.

Collaborative Care

The therapeutic goal in acromegaly is to return GH levels to normal. This is accomplished by surgery, radiation, drug therapy, or a combination of these therapies. The prognosis depends on age at onset, age when treatment is initiated, and tumor size. Usually bone growth can be arrested and soft tissue hypertrophy can be reversed. However, sleep apnea and diabetic and cardiac complications may persist in spite of treatment.

Surgical Therapy. Surgery (hypophysectomy) is the treatment of choice and offers the best hope for a cure, especially for smaller tumors (microadenomas smaller than 10 mm). More than 97% of surgeries done to remove pituitary tumors associated with acromegaly are accomplished with the *transsphenoidal* approach.[4] With this procedure, an incision is made in the inner aspect of the upper lip and gingiva. The sella turcica is entered through the floor of the nose and sphenoid sinuses (Fig. 48-2).

The goal of transsphenoidal surgery is to remove only the tumor that is causing GH secretion. This procedure produces an immediate reduction in GH levels followed by a drop in IGF-1 levels within a few weeks. Although 94% of these procedures are effective, some patients (especially those with larger tumors or those with GH levels greater than 50 ng/ml) do not obtain a cure with the surgery and require adjunctive radiation or drug therapy to control GH hypersecretion.[4] In some cases, the entire pituitary gland is removed during surgery *(hypophysectomy),* resulting in a permanent absence of pituitary hormones. Rather than replacing the pituitary (tropic) hormones, which requires parenteral administration, the essential hormones produced by target organs (glucocorticoids, thyroid hormone, and sex hormones) can be given orally. Hormone replacement must be continued throughout life.

Radiation Therapy. Irradiation of the tumor is considered a secondary treatment option. It is indicated when surgery has failed to produce complete remission. External radiation can successfully reduce GH levels in 30% to 70% of patients, but the primary disadvantage is the long delay (months to years) for GH levels to normalize.[4] Because of the length of time it takes to achieve GH reduction, radiation therapy is usually offered in combination

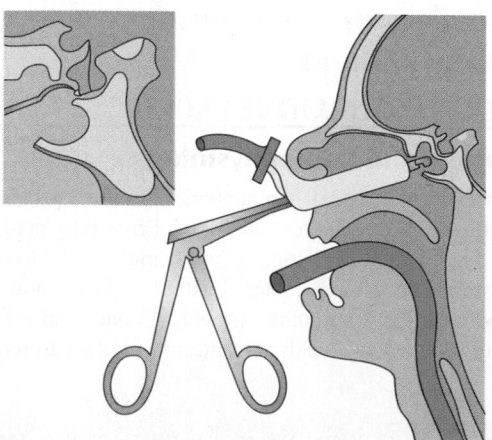

FIG. 48-2 Surgery on the pituitary gland is most commonly performed with the transsphenoidal approach. An incision is made in the inner aspect of the upper lip and gingiva. The sella turcica is entered through the floor of the nose and sphenoid sinuses.

with drugs that reduce GH levels. If a tumor is large or has extensive spread, surgery may be followed by radiation. Radiation has also been used to reduce the size of a tumor before surgery. Depending on the amount of radiation and the patient's susceptibility, the patient may experience local skin changes, alopecia, or oral complications. Hypopituitarism commonly results from radiation therapy and requires hormone replacement therapy.

Stereotactic radiosurgery (gamma surgery) may be used for small, surgically inaccessible pituitary tumors (see Chapter 55). This procedure consists of radiation delivered to a single site from multiple angles and can be used to occlude blood vessels feeding the tumor, thereby starving it.[5,6]

Drug Therapy. Three groups of agents are used in the treatment of acromegaly: somatostatin analogs, dopamine agonists, and GH receptor antagonists. These drugs reduce GH levels and are often used as initial treatment or as adjunct therapy to surgery or radiation. The use of drug therapy as primary treatment has been considered, but the safety and cost of long-term drug treatment have yet to be established.[5]

The most common drug used for acromegaly is octreotide (Sandostatin), a somatostatin analog that reduces GH levels to within the normal range in many patients. Octreotide is given by subcutaneus injection three times a week. Two newer long-acting analogs, octreotide (Depot, Sandostatin LAR) and lanreotide SR (Ipstyl), are now available that are administered as intramuscular (IM) injections every 2 to 4 weeks. Another group of agents, dopamine agonists, are useful in the treatment of acromegaly because these agents suppress GH secretion. Cabergoline (Dostincx) has essentially replaced bromocriptine (Parlodel) because it is more effective and is associated with fewer side effects.

A GH receptor antagonist, pegvisomant (Somavert), has recently been developed for use in the treatment of acromegaly and is considered an alternative to dopamine agonists or somatostatin analogs. This agent is best used to control disease for patients who have received radiation therapy, but still have hypersecretion of GH.[7] It is not considered appropriate for primary treatment because this agent only blocks hormone action rather than acting on the tumor.

NURSING MANAGEMENT
GROWTH HORMONE EXCESS

■ Nursing Assessment

The nurse needs to assess for signs and symptoms of abnormal tissue growth and evaluate changes in the physical size of each patient. The adult should be questioned about increases in hat, ring, glove, and shoe sizes. The patient can be questioned about changes in appearance. Photographs are helpful to evaluate any changes. Because physical changes occur slowly and over a long period of time, it is possible that the individual is not even aware of such changes. The patient needs unconditional acceptance by health care workers and considerable emotional support during the periods of diagnosis and treatment.

■ Nursing Diagnoses

Nursing diagnoses for the patient with GH excess include, but are not limited to, the following:

- Disturbed body image *related to* enlargement of the hands, feet, jaw, and soft body tissue
- Deficient fluid volume *related to* polyuria

- Disturbed sleep pattern *related to* soft tissue swelling
- Disturbed sensory perception (visual) *related to* enlarged pituitary gland

■ Planning

The overall goals are that the patient with GH excess will (1) accept and cope effectively with altered body image, (2) maintain adequate fluid volume, (3) experience restful sleep patterns, (4) develop no complications, and (5) obtain long-term follow-up care.

■ Nursing Implementation

Acute Intervention. Patients typically have many questions and concerns regarding surgery. It is important for the nurse to offer reassurance and to provide accurate information regarding this process. An explanation regarding hormonal replacement, should it be necessary, is also important.

The individual treated surgically needs skilled neurosurgical nursing care and must be prepared before surgery for postoperative care. Nursing interventions include preoperative installation of antibiotic nose drops, discussion of mouth breathing, mouth care, ambulation, pain control, activity, and hormone replacement. The patient should be instructed to avoid vigorous coughing, sneezing, and straining at stool (Valsalva maneuver) to prevent cerebrospinal fluid leakage from the point at which the sella turcica was entered.

After surgery in which a transsphenoidal approach has been used, the head of the patient's bed should be elevated at a 30-degree angle at all times. This elevation avoids pressure on the sella turcica and decreases headaches, a frequent postoperative problem. Monitoring neurologic status, including pupillary response, should be done in order to detect neurologic complications.

Any clear nasal drainage should be sent to the laboratory to be tested for glucose. A glucose level greater than 30 mg/dl (1.67 mmol/L) indicates cerebrospinal fluid leakage from an open connection to the brain. If this happens, the patient is at an increased risk for meningitis. Complaints of persistent and severe generalized or supraorbital headache may indicate cerebrospinal fluid leakage into the sinuses. A cerebrospinal fluid leak usually resolves within 72 hours when treated with head elevation and bed rest. If the leak persists, daily spinal taps may be done to reduce pressure to below normal levels and allow the fossa to heal. Intravenous (IV) antibiotics are usually administered when there is a cerebrospinal fluid leak to prevent meningitis. If the leak does not respond to treatment in 72 hours, surgical intervention may be required.

Mild analgesia is given for headaches. The nurse should perform mouth care every 4 hours to keep the surgical area clean and free of debris and to promote patient comfort. Toothbrushing should be avoided for at least 10 days to prevent disrupting the suture line and to avoid discomfort.

If stereotactic radiosurgery is used, the patient is usually moved from the specialized radiation center to the neurosurgical nursing unit for overnight observation. The patient will be in a stereotactic head frame. Vital signs, neurologic status, and fluid volume status must be carefully monitored. Possible complications include increased headaches, seizures, nausea, and vomiting. The patient with a history of seizures is at increased risk for seizures for at least 24 hours after the procedure. All staff should know how to remove a stereotactic frame in case of an emergency. The patient may experience discomfort at the pin sites. Pin-site care should be done according to institutional policy. Family members can be instructed in pin-site care if the patient is discharged the day after the procedure.

A possible postoperative complication is transient diabetes insipidus (DI). This may occur because of the loss of antidiuretic hormone (ADH), which is stored in the posterior lobe of the pituitary gland, or cerebral edema related to manipulation of the pituitary during surgery. To assess for DI, urine output and serum and urine osmolarity must be closely monitored. Clinical manifestations and treatment of DI are discussed in more detail later in this chapter.

Ambulatory and Home Care. If a hypophysectomy is performed or the pituitary is damaged, hormone replacement will be necessary. ADH, cortisol, and thyroid hormone replacement will be needed. Because these medications need to be taken for life, careful patient teaching is essential when replacement of these hormones is necessary.

Because surgery may result in permanent hormone deficiencies and possible decreased fertility, the patient needs assistance in working through the grieving process associated with these losses. The need for continued drug therapy reduces the patient's perception of independence and requires considerable emotional adjustment. The nurse must consider the emotional impact of a hypophysectomy when counseling the patient and planning the educational program related to hormone replacement.

▪ Evaluation

The expected outcomes are that the patient with GH excess will
- experience no complications postoperatively
- know how and when to take hormone replacements (if indicated)
- state symptoms requiring immediate attention and appropriate actions
- state the importance of long-term follow-up
- have a follow-up medical appointment

EXCESSES OF OTHER TROPIC HORMONES

Excesses of tropic hormones and overproduction of a single anterior pituitary hormone usually produce syndromes related to hormone excess from the target organ. If adrenocorticotropic hormone (ACTH) is increased, Cushing's disease results; if thyroid-stimulating hormone (TSH) levels are excessive, hyperthyroidism develops.

Prolactinomas (prolactin-secreting adenomas) are the most frequently occurring pituitary tumor, accounting for 40% to 60% of all hyperfunctioning pituitary tumors.[8] Common manifestations experienced by women with prolactinomas include galactorrhea, ovulatory dysfunction (anovulation, infertility), menstrual dysfunction (oligomenorrhea or amenorrhea), decreased libido, and hirsutism. In men, impotence and decreased libido and sperm density may result. The affected patient may also experience headaches and visual problems. The visual problems are secondary to pressure on the optic chiasm. Because prolactinomas do not typically progress in size, drug therapy is usually the first-line treatment.[8] Dopamine agonists such as bromocriptine (Parlodel), cabergoline (Dostinex), and pergolide (Permax) have successfully been used to treat this disorder. Surgery using the transsphenoidal approach (discussed previously) may be considered depending on the size and extent of the tumor. Use of radiation for treatment of prolactinomas has been somewhat limited, but is mainly used in those patients who have failed to respond to medical or surgical therapy.

HYPOFUNCTION OF THE PITUITARY GLAND

Hypopituitarism is a rare disorder that involves a decrease in one or more of the pituitary hormones. The anterior pituitary gland secretes ACTH, TSH, follicle-stimulating hormone (FSH), luteinizing hormone (LH), GH, and prolactin; the posterior pituitary gland secretes ADH and oxytocin. A deficiency of only one pituitary hormone is referred to as *selective hypopituitarism*. Total failure of the pituitary gland results in deficiency of all pituitary hormones—a condition referred to as *panhypopituitarism*. The most common hormone deficiencies associated with hypopituitarism involve GH and gonadotropins. TSH, ACTH, and ADH are less frequently involved.[9]

Etiology and Pathophysiology

The most common cause of pituitary hypofunction is a pituitary tumor. Autoimmune disorders, infections, pituitary infarction (Sheehan syndrome), or destruction of the pituitary gland (as a result of trauma, radiation, and surgical procedures) also can cause hypopituitarism. *Sheehan syndrome* is a postpartum condition of pituitary necrosis and hypopituitarism after circulatory collapse resulting from uterine hemorrhaging.

Hormone deficiencies involving anterior pituitary hormones lead to end-organ failure; thus the effects of hypopituitarism depend on the specific pituitary hormone or hormones that are lacking. For example, infertility may be the first indication of pituitary hypofunction associated with a pituitary tumor. Deficiencies of TSH and ACTH are life threatening. ACTH deficiency causes a tendency toward shock and may result in an episode of acute adrenal insufficiency (refractory and life-threatening shock from sodium and water depletion). (Adrenal shock is discussed later in this chapter.)

Clinical Manifestations

The signs and symptoms associated with pituitary hypofunction vary with the degree and speed of onset of pituitary dysfunction and are related to hyposecretion of the target glands and/or a growing pituitary tumor. Common symptoms associated with a space-occupying lesion include headaches, visual changes (decreased peripheral vision or decreased visual acuity), *anosmia* (loss of the sense of smell), and seizures.

Adults with GH deficiency often have subtle nonspecific clinical findings. They have truncal obesity and decreased muscle mass causing reduced strength, decreased energy, and reduced exercise capability. Decreased bone density and pathologic fractures may occur.[10] They may have a flat affect or appear depressed. Impaired psychologic well-being is a common finding associated with GH deficiency in adults.

FSH and LH deficiencies in the adult woman are first manifested as menstrual irregularities, diminished libido, and changes in secondary sex characteristics (e.g., decreased breast size). Men with FSH and LH deficiencies experience testicular atrophy, diminished spermatogenesis, loss of libido, impotence, and decreased facial hair and muscle mass.

Deficiency of ACTH and cortisol often produce a nonspecific clinical picture. Signs and symptoms may include weakness, fatigue, headache, dry and pale skin, and diminished axillary and pubic hair. Individuals may have postural hypotension, fasting hypoglycemia, diminished tolerance for stress, and poor resistance to infection.

The clinical presentations of individuals with thyroid hormone deficiency associated with hypopituitarism are similar (although usually milder) to those seen with primary hypothyroidism. Common symptoms include cold intolerance, constipation, fatigue, lethargy, and weight gain. (Hypothyroidism is discussed in greater detail later in this chapter.)

Diagnostic Studies

In addition to conducting a history and physical examination, diagnostic studies are useful in the diagnosis and treatment of hypopituitarism. Radiologic tests such as MRI and CT are indicated to determine the presence of a pituitary tumor. The laboratory tests indicated for hypopituitarism vary widely, but generally involve the direct measurement of pituitary hormones or an indirect determination of the hormone level. Diagnostic tests are also used to evaluate the effectiveness of therapy. See Chapter 46 for more information regarding diagnostic studies.

Collaborative Care

Treatment of hypopituitarism consists of surgery or radiation for tumor removal, followed by permanent hormone replacement. Surgery and radiation of pituitary tumors are discussed earlier in this chapter. Hormone replacement therapy is carried out with the appropriate hormone needed (e.g., GH, corticosteroids, thyroid hormone, and sex hormones). Hormone replacement therapies for thyroid hormone and corticosteroids are discussed later in this chapter.

Somatropin (Genotropin, Humatrope) is used for GH replacement therapy. Adults with GH deficiency respond well to GH replacement and experience increased energy, increased lean body mass, a feeling of well-being, and improved body image. The side effects most commonly reported by adults include swelling in the feet and hands, pain in the joints, and headache. Somatropin is given as a subcutaneous injection. The dosing is variable because it is adjusted based on relief of symptoms, IGF-1 levels, and the development of adverse effects.

Although gonadal deficiency is not life threatening, replacement therapy is offered to improve sexual function and general well-being. This therapy, however, is contraindicated in individuals with certain medical conditions, such as breast cancer, phlebitis, and pulmonary embolism in women and prostate cancer in men. Testosterone is used to treat men with gonadotropin deficiency. The benefits achieved with testosterone therapy include a return of male secondary sex characteristics, improvement in libido, and increase in muscle mass, bone mass, and bone density. Testosterone can be administered via a transdermal patch, topical gel, self-administered IM injection, or orally. Because oral preparations are often ineffective and have more side effects, their use is limited.[9] Dosing is adjusted to keep serum testosterone levels within a normal range.

Estrogen and progesterone replacement therapy may be indicated for hypogonadal women to treat hot flashes, vaginal dryness, and decreased libido. Hormone replacement for women is discussed in greater detail in Chapter 52.

NURSING MANAGEMENT
HYPOFUNCTION OF THE PITUITARY GLAND

A primary nursing role in anterior pituitary insufficiency is assessment and recognition of signs and symptoms associated with hypopituitarism. Nursing management is directed at pro-

viding interventions associated with problems that result from hormone deficiency. The nurse also plays a pivotal role in teaching the patient about diagnostic procedures, the disease process, and collaborative care options. Because of the need for lifelong hormonal therapy, patient teaching is important regarding hormonal administration, side effects, and follow-up therapy. Because individuals with hypopituitarism incur a number of health-related costs and are more likely to take sick days compared with the general population, the nurse should also explore concerns associated with finances and role performance at both home and work.[11]

Disorders Associated with Antidiuretic Hormone Secretion

The two primary conditions associated with antidiuretic hormone (ADH) secretion are a result of either overproduction or underproduction of ADH. Overproduction or oversecretion of ADH results in a condition known as *syndrome of inappropriate antidiuretic hormone* (SIADH). Underproduction or undersecretion of ADH results in a condition referred to as *diabetes insipidus* (DI).

ADH, also referred to as *arginine vasopressin* (AVP), is synthesized in the hypothalamus and then transported and stored in the posterior pituitary gland. It plays a major role in the regulation of water balance and osmolarity (see Chapter 46).

SYNDROME OF INAPPROPRIATE ANTIDIURETIC HORMONE

Etiology and Pathophysiology

Syndrome of inappropriate antidiuretic hormone (SIADH) occurs when ADH is released despite normal or low plasma osmolarity (Fig. 48-3). SIADH results from an abnormal production or sustained secretion of ADH and is characterized by fluid retention, serum hypoosmolality, dilutional hyponatremia, hypochloremia, concentrated urine in the presence of normal or increased intravascular volume, and normal renal function. This syndrome occurs more commonly in older adults. SIADH is thought to be the most common cause of hyponatremia in older adults.[12]

SIADH has various causes (Table 48-1). The most common cause is malignancy, especially small cell lung cancer. These cancerous cells are capable of producing, storing, and releasing ADH.[13]

SIADH tends to be self-limiting when caused by head trauma or drugs but is chronic in nature when associated with tumors or metabolic diseases. Treatment of the underlying cause or discontinuing the causal medication is indicated to improve the clinical course.

Clinical Manifestations

The excess ADH increases distal tubule and collecting duct permeability and reabsorption of water into the circulation. Consequently, extracellular fluid volume expands, plasma osmolality declines, the glomerular filtration rate increases, and sodium levels decline (dilutional hyponatremia). Hyponatremia causes muscle cramps and weakness. The patient with SIADH will experience low urinary output and increased body weight.[14] As the serum sodium level falls (usually less than 120 mEq/L [120 mmol/L]),

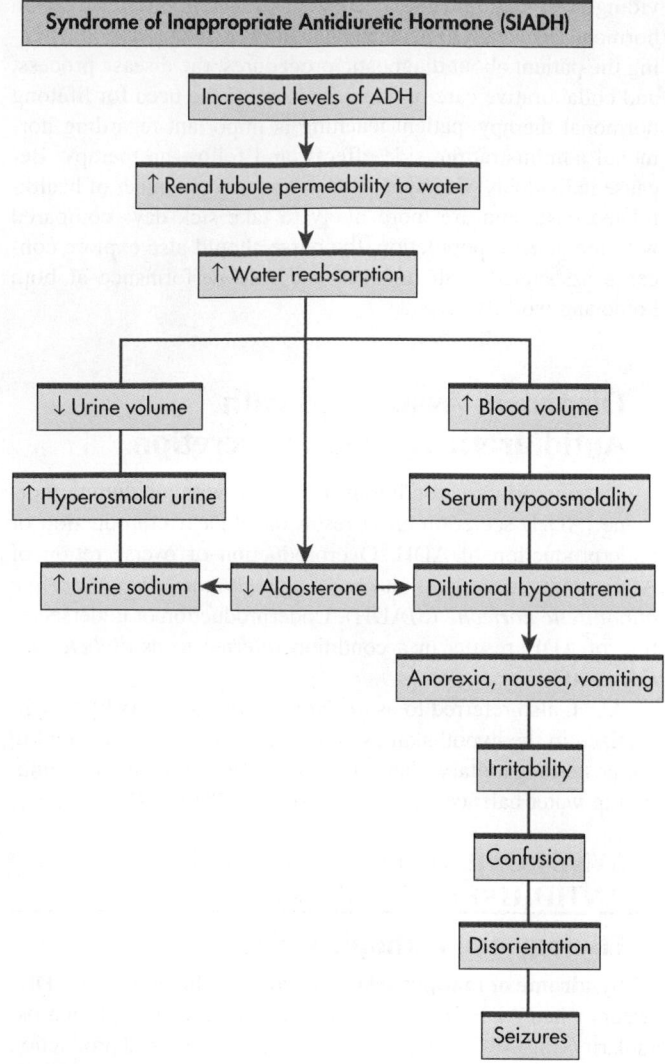

Syndrome of Inappropriate Antidiuretic Hormone (SIADH)

Increased levels of ADH

↓

↑ Renal tubule permeability to water

↓

↑ Water reabsorption

↓ Urine volume   ↑ Blood volume

↑ Hyperosmolar urine   ↑ Serum hypoosmolality

↑ Urine sodium ← ↓ Aldosterone → Dilutional hyponatremia

↓

Anorexia, nausea, vomiting

↓

Irritability

↓

Confusion

↓

Disorientation

↓

Seizures

FIG. 48-3 Pathophysiology of syndrome of inappropriate antidiuretic hormone (SIADH).

TABLE 48-1	Causes of Syndrome of Inappropriate Antidiuretic Hormone

Malignant Tumors
Small cell carcinoma of the lung
Pancreatic cancer
Lymphoid cancers (Hodgkin's disease, non-Hodgkin's lymphoma, lymphocytic leukemia)
Thymus cancer
Prostate cancer
Colorectal cancer

Central Nervous System Disorders
Head injury (skull fracture, subdural hematoma, subarachnoid hemorrhage)
Cerebrovascular injury
Brain tumors
Infection (encephalitis, meningitis)
Cerebral atrophy
Guillain-Barré syndrome
Systemic lupus erythematosus

Drug Therapy
carbamazepine (Tegretol)
chlorpropamide (Diabinese)
General anesthesia agents
Opioids
Oxytocin
Thiazide diuretics
Tricyclic antidepressants
Antineoplastic agents (vincristine [Oncovin], vinblastine [Velban], cyclophosphamide [Cytoxan])

Miscellaneous Conditions
Hypothyroidism
Lung infection (pneumonia, tuberculosis, lung abscess)
Chronic obstructive pulmonary disease
Positive pressure mechanical ventilation

manifestations become more severe and include vomiting, abdominal cramps, muscle twitching, and seizures. As plasma osmolality and serum sodium levels continue to decline, cerebral edema may occur, leading to lethargy, anorexia, confusion, headache, seizures, and coma.

Diagnostic Studies

The diagnosis of SIADH is made by simultaneous measurements of urine and serum osmolality. The dilutional hyponatremia is indicated by a serum sodium less than 134 mEq/L, serum osmolality less than 280 mOsm/kg (280 mmol/kg), and a urine specific gravity greater than 1.005. A serum osmolality much lower than the urine osmolality indicates the inappropriate excretion of concentrated urine in the presence of dilute serum. Initially, thirst, dyspnea on exertion, fatigue, and dulled sensorium may be evident. Other laboratory findings are decreased blood urea nitrogen, creatinine clearance, hemoglobin, and hematocrit.

Collaborative Care

Once SIADH is identified, treatment is directed at the underlying cause of the disorder. Medications that stimulate the release of ADH should be avoided or discontinued. The immediate treatment goal is to restore normal fluid volume and osmolality. If symptoms are mild and serum sodium is greater than 125 mEq/L (125 mmol/L), the only treatment may be restriction of fluids to 800 to 1000 ml per day. This restriction should result in gradual, daily reductions in weight, a progressive rise in serum sodium concentration and osmolality, and symptomatic improvement. In cases of severe hyponatremia (less than 120 mEq/L), especially in the presence of neurologic symptoms such as seizures, intravenous hypertonic saline solution (3% to 5%) may be administered. Hypertonic saline requires a very slow infusion rate on an infusion pump to avoid too rapid a rise in sodium. A diuretic such as furosemide (Lasix) may be used to promote diuresis, but only if the serum sodium is at least 125 mEq/L (125 mmol/L), because it may promote further loss of sodium. Because furosemide increases potassium excretion, potassium supplements may be needed. A fluid restriction of 500 ml per day is also indicated for those with severe hyponatremia.

In chronic SIADH, water restriction of 800 to 1000 ml per day is recommended. Because this degree of restriction may not be tolerated, demeclocycline (Declomycin) and lithium may be administered. These agents block the effect of ADH on the renal tubules, thereby allowing a more dilute urine.

NURSING MANAGEMENT
SYNDROME OF INAPPROPRIATE ANTIDIURETIC HORMONE

The nurse can be instrumental in the early detection and treatment of SIADH. An appropriate nursing assessment (Table 48-2) should be conducted for those at risk and those who have confirmed SIADH. Specifically, the nurse should be alert for low urinary output with a high specific gravity, a sudden weight gain, or a serum sodium decline. Nursing management of acute onset of SIADH is presented in Table 48-2.

When SIADH is chronic, the patient must learn to self-manage treatment regimens. Fluids are restricted to 800 to 1000 ml per day. Sucking on hard candy or ice chips can help decrease thirst.[14] If drinking liquids is an aspect of socialization, the patient should be assisted in planning fluid intake so liquid allowances are saved for social occasions. The patient may be treated with a diuretic to remove excess fluid volume. The diet should be supplemented

---

TABLE 48-2 Nursing Assessment and Management: Syndrome of Inappropriate Antidiuretic Hormone

Assessment
- Hourly vital signs
- Hourly intake (oral and parenteral) and output
- Hourly measurement of urine specific gravity
- Daily weights
- Level of consciousness
- Observe for signs of hyponatremia (e.g., decreased neurologic function, seizures, nausea and vomiting, muscle cramping)
- Monitor heart and lung sounds

Management
- Restrict total fluid intake to no more than 1000 ml/day (including that taken with medications)
- Position head of bed flat or with no more than 10 degrees of elevation to enhance venous return to heart and increase left atrial filling pressure, reducing ADH release
- Protect from injury (i.e., assist with ambulation, side rails up on bed) because of potential alterations in mental status
- Seizure precautions
- Frequent turning, positioning, and range-of-motion exercise (if patient is bedridden)
- Frequent oral hygiene
- Provide distractions to decrease the discomfort of thirst related to fluid restrictions

ADH, Antidiuretic hormone.

---

with sodium and potassium, especially if diuretics are prescribed. Solutions of these electrolytes must be well diluted to prevent gastrointestinal (GI) irritation or damage. They are best taken at mealtime to allow mixing with and dilution by food. The patient should be taught the symptoms of fluid and electrolyte imbalances, especially those involving sodium and potassium, so that responses to treatment can be monitored (see Chapter 16). If a patient is to be treated with demeclocycline (Declomycin), the need for close follow-up care should be stressed because of the nephrotoxic side effects and the potential for fungal infections associated with this drug.

DIABETES INSIPIDUS

Etiology and Pathophysiology

Diabetes insipidus (DI) is a group of conditions associated with a deficiency of production or secretion of ADH or a decreased renal response to ADH. The decrease in ADH results in fluid and electrolyte imbalances caused by increased urinary output and increased plasma osmolality (Fig. 48-4). Depending on the cause, DI may be transient or a chronic lifelong condition.

There are several classifications of DI (Table 48-3). *Central DI* (also known as *neurogenic DI*) occurs when any organic lesion of the hypothalamus, infundibular stem, or posterior pituitary interferes with ADH synthesis, transport, or release.

Nephrogenic DI (NDI) describes conditions in which there is adequate ADH, but there is a decreased response to ADH in the kidney. Lithium is one of the most common causes of drug-induced NDI.[15,16]

Dispogenic DI, a less common condition, is associated with excessive water intake. This can be caused by a structural lesion in the thirst center or may be caused by a psychologic disorder most commonly associated with schizophrenia.[17]

Clinical Manifestations

DI is characterized by increased thirst (polydipsia) and increased urination (polyuria) (see Fig. 48-4). The primary characteristic of DI is the excretion of large quantities of urine (5 to 20 L per day) with a very low specific gravity (less than 1.005) and urine osmolality of <100 mOsm/kg (<100 mmol/kg). Serum osmolality is elevated (usually greater than 295 mOsm/kg [295 mmol/kg]) as a result of hypernatremia due to pure water loss in the kidney. In partial central DI, urinary output may be lower (2 to 4 L per day). Most patients compensate for fluid loss by drinking great amounts of water so that serum osmolality is normal or only moderately elevated. The patient with central DI particularly favors cold or iced drinks. The patient may be fatigued from nocturia and may experience generalized weakness.

Central DI usually occurs suddenly with excessive fluid loss. After intracranial surgery, DI usually has a triphasic pattern: the acute phase with abrupt onset of polyuria; an interphase, where urine volume apparently normalizes; and a third phase, where central DI is permanent. The third phase is usually apparent within 10 to 14 days postoperatively. Central DI that results from head trauma is usually self-limiting and improves with treatment of the underlying problem. DI following cranial surgery is more likely to be permanent. Although the clinical manifestations of NDI are similar, the onset and amount of fluid losses are less dramatic.

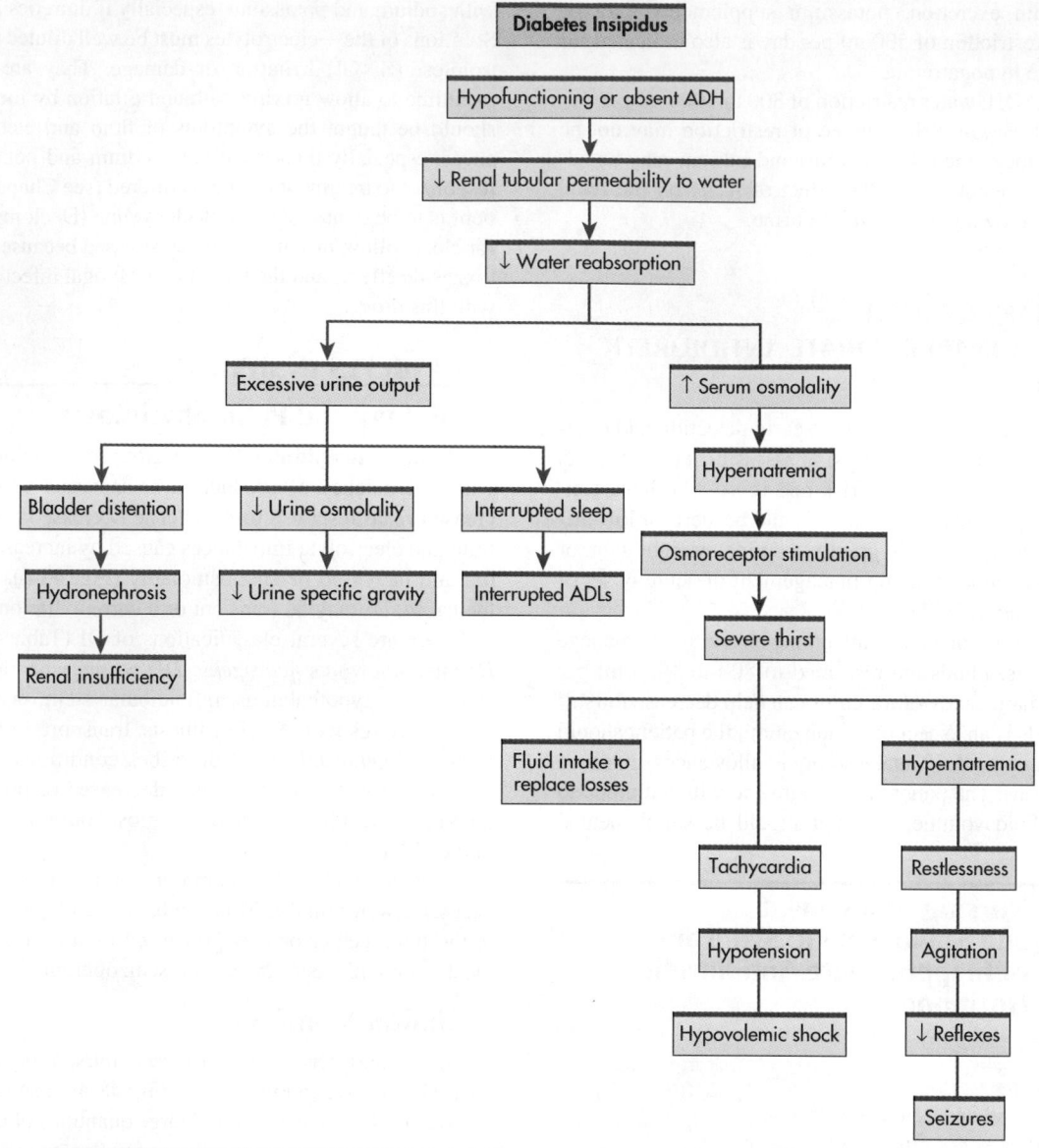

FIG. 48-4 Pathophysiology of diabetes insipidus (DI). *ADH,* Antidiuretic hormone; *ADLs,* activities of daily living.

TABLE 48-3	Types and Causes of Diabetes Insipidus (DI)	
TYPES	**CAUSES**
Central DI	Problem stems from an interference with ADH synthesis or release. Multiple causes include brain tumor, head injury, brain surgery, CNS infections.
Nephrogenic DI	Problem stems from inadequate renal response to ADH despite presence of adequate ADH. Caused by drug therapy (especially lithium), renal damage, or hereditary renal disease.
Dispogenic DI	Problem stems from excessive water intake. Caused by structural lesion in thirst center or psychologic disorder.

ADH, Antidiuretic hormone; *CNS,* central nervous system.

If oral fluid intake cannot keep up with urinary losses, severe fluid volume deficit results. This deficit is manifested by weight loss, constipation, poor tissue turgor, hypotension, tachycardia, and shock. In addition, the patient shows central nervous system (CNS) manifestations, ranging from irritability and mental dullness to coma. These manifestations are related to increasing serum osmolality and hypernatremia. Because of the polyuria, severe dehydration and hypovolemic shock may occur.

Diagnostic Studies

Because DI may be central, nephrogenic, or dispogenic in origin, identification of the cause is the initial step. A complete history and physical is done. Dispogenic DI is associated with overhydration and hypervolemia rather than with dehydration and hypovolemia seen in other forms of DI. A water deprivation test is usually done to confirm the diagnosis of central DI. Before a water deprivation test is done, the patient's baseline weight, pulse, urine and plasma osmolalities, specific gravity of urine, and blood pressure are obtained. All fluids are withheld for 8 to 16 hours. The patient may be anxious and should be reassured that the test will be stopped if fluid volume deficit becomes severe. The patient should be observed throughout the test because of the craving to drink. During the test, the patient's blood pressure, weight, and urine osmolality are assessed hourly. The test continues until urine osmolalities stabilize (hourly increase less than 30 mOsm/kg [30 mmol/kg] in 2 consecutive hours) or body weight declines by 5%, or orthostatic hypotension develops. ADH is then given, and urine osmolality is measured 1 hour later. In central DI, the rise in urinary osmolality after vasopressin exceeds 9%.

Collaborative Care

Determining and treating the primary cause is central to the collaborative management of DI. The therapeutic goal is maintenance of fluid and electrolyte balance.

For central DI, fluid and hormonal replacement is the cornerstone of treatment. In acute DI, hypotonic saline is administered intravenously, titrated to replace urinary output.[17] Hormone replacement is necessary because of the lack of ADH production or secretion. Desmopressin acetate (DDAVP), an analog of ADH, is the hormone replacement of choice for central DI. DDAVP can be administered orally, intravenously, or as a nasal spray. Several other drugs are available for ADH replacement, including aqueous vasopressin (Pitressin), vasopressin tannate, and lysine vasopressin (Diapid). Several drugs can be used for the treatment of partial central DI, including chlorpropamide (Diabinese), clofibrate (Atromid), and carbamazepine (Tegretol). Chlorpropamide, thought to potentiate the action of ADH and stimulate endogenous release, is considered the most consistently effective and safest of these agents.

Hormone replacement and chlorpropamide have little effect in the treatment of NDI because the kidney is unable to respond to ADH. Instead, the treatment for NDI revolves around dietary measures (low-sodium diet) and thiazide diuretics. Limiting sodium intake to no more than 3 g per day is thought to help decrease urine output.[17] Interestingly, thiazide diuretics are used in the treatment of NDI. Although it seems paradoxic to treat a condition associated with polyuria with a diuretic, thiazides produce a net decrease in urine output. The thiazides are able to slow the glomerular filtration rate, allowing the kidney to reabsorb more water in the loop of Henle and distal tubles.[18] Thiazide diuretics most commonly used are hydrochlorothiazide (HydroDiuril) and chlorothiazide (Diuril). When low-sodium diet and thiazides are not effective, indomethacin (Indocin) may be prescribed. Indomethacin, a nonsteroidal antiinflammatory agent, helps increase renal responsiveness to ADH.

NURSING MANAGEMENT
DIABETES INSIPIDUS

Nursing management of the patient with DI revolves around early detection, maintenance of adequate hydration, and patient teaching for long-term management.

During acute DI, the nurse administers fluids and hormone replacement. Fluids are replaced orally or intravenously, depending on the patient's condition and ability to drink copious amounts of fluids. Adequate fluids should be kept at the bedside. If IV glucose solutions are used, urine should be assessed for glucose. If urine is positive for glucose, the health care provider should be notified, because glucosuria causes an osmotic diuresis, which increases the fluid volume deficit. Accurate records of intake and output, urine specific gravity, and daily weights are mandatory in the assessment of fluid volume status.

Nursing interventions also include the administration of DDAVP. The patient should be assessed for weight gain, headache, restlessness, and chest pain. The adequacy of treatment is assessed by monitoring fluid intake and output and by urine specific gravity. Increased urine volume with low specific gravity is related to an inadequate pharmacologic effect, and the health care provider should be notified immediately.

The patient with chronic DI requiring long-term ADH replacement needs instruction in self-management. DDAVP can be taken orally or intranasally. Nasal irritation, headache, and nausea may indicate overdosage, whereas failure to improve may indicate underdosage. The patient should be instructed to report any of these symptoms. Patients taking DDAVP should be instructed to monitor their weight daily. Increases in weight may indicate fluid retention. The need for close follow-up should be stressed.

Disorders of the Thyroid Gland

Thyroid hormones, thyroxine (T_4) and triiodothyronine (T_3), regulate energy metabolism and growth and development. Thyroid disorders include hyperfunction, hypofunction, inflammation, and enlargement of the thyroid. Thyroid enlargement is referred to as **goiter.** A goiter may interfere with surrounding structures and can be associated with increased, normal, or decreased hormone production.

HYPERTHYROIDISM

Hyperthyroidism is a clinical syndrome in which there is a sustained increase in synthesis and release of thyroid hormones by the thyroid gland. The term **thyrotoxicosis** refers to the physiologic effects of hypermetabolism that result from excess circulating levels of T_4, T_3, or both. Hyperthyroidism and thyrotoxicosis usually occur together as in Graves' disease. However, in some forms of thyroiditis, thyrotoxicosis may occur without hyperthyroidism.[19]

Hyperthyroidism occurs in approximately 2% of women and only 0.2% men; the highest frequency is in the 30- to 50-year-old age group. The most common form of hyperthyroidism is Graves' disease. Other causes include toxic nodular goiter, thyroiditis, exogenous iodine excess, pituitary tumors, and thyroid cancer.[19]

Etiology and Pathophysiology

Graves' Disease. Graves' disease is an autoimmune disease of unknown etiology marked by diffuse thyroid enlargement and excessive thyroid hormone secretion. Precipitating factors such as insufficient iodine supply, infections, and stressful life events may interact with genetic factors that control the immune response and metabolic abnormalities to cause Graves' disease. A concordance rate of 50% in identical twins indicates genetic and environmental components in the expression of the disease.

Graves' disease accounts for 75% of the cases of hyperthyroidism. The patient develops antibodies to the TSH receptor. These antibodies attach to the receptors and stimulate the thyroid

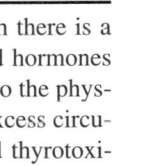

gland to release T_3, T_4, or both. The excessive release of thyroid hormones leads to the clinical manifestations associated with thyrotoxicosis.

The disease is characterized by remissions and exacerbations, with or without treatment. It may progress to destruction of thyroid tissue, causing hypothyroidism.

Toxic Nodular Goiters. Nodular goiters are characterized by thyroid hormone–secreting nodules that are independent of TSH stimulation. If associated with signs of hyperthyroidism, a nodule is termed *toxic.* There may be multiple nodules (multinodular goiter) or a single nodule (solitary autonomous nodule). The nodules are usually benign follicular adenomas. Toxic nodular goiters occur equally in men and women. Although they can appear at any age, the frequency of toxic multinodular goiter is greatest in people over 40 years of age. Small solitary autonomous nodules do not usually secrete enough thyroid hormone to cause clinical thyrotoxicosis. However, larger nodules (greater than 3 cm) may result in clinical disease.

Clinical Manifestations

The clinical manifestations of hyperthyroidism are related to the effects of excess thyroid hormones in two ways. The first is the direct effect of hormones on increasing metabolism. The second is increased tissue sensitivity to stimulation by the sympathetic nervous system. Thyroid hormones increase the number of β-adrenergic receptors, thereby increasing sensitivity to the action of catecholamines (epinephrine and norepinephrine). However, the absolute levels of these hormones are not elevated.

Palpation of the thyroid gland may reveal a goiter. When the thyroid gland is excessively large, a goiter may be noted on inspection. Auscultation of the thyroid gland may reveal bruits. Another common finding associated with hyperthyroidism is *ophthalmopathy,* a term used to describe abnormal eye appearance or function. A classic finding in Graves' disease is **exophthalmos,** a protrusion of the eyeballs from the orbits (Fig. 48-5). Exophthalmos is a type of infiltrative ophthalmopathy that is due to impaired venous drainage from the orbit, which causes increased fat

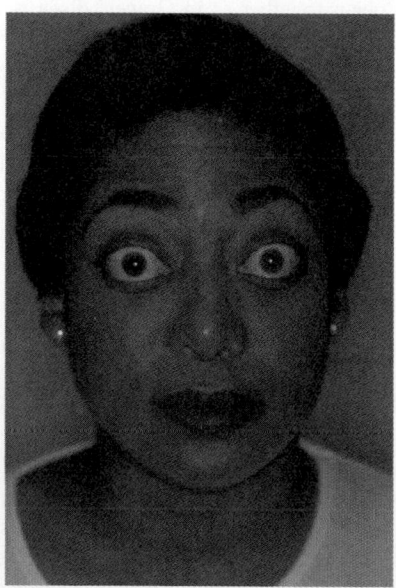

FIG. 48-5 Graves' disease. This woman has a diffuse goiter and exophthalmos.

deposits and fluid (edema) in the retroorbital tissues. Because of increased pressure, the eyeballs are forced outward and protrude. This sign is seen in 20% to 40% of patients with Graves' disease. It is usually bilateral but can be unilateral or asymmetric. In noninfiltrative ophthalmopathy, the upper lids are usually retracted and elevated, with the sclera visible above the iris. When the eyelids do not close completely, the exposed corneal surfaces become dry and irritated. Serious consequences, such as corneal ulcers and eventual loss of vision, can occur.

Other common manifestations of thyroid hyperfunction are summarized in Table 48-4. A patient with advanced disease may exhibit many of the manifestations, whereas a patient in the early stages of hyperthyroidism may exhibit only weight loss and increased nervousness. Symptoms in the elderly patient with this disorder may be very different (referred to as *apathetic hyperthyroidism*) and may include anorexia, apathy, lassitude, depression, and confusion.[20] Table 48-5 compares features of hyperthyroidism in younger and older adult patients.

Complications

Thyrotoxic crisis (also called *thyroid storm*) is an acute, rare condition in which all hyperthyroid manifestations are heightened. Although it is considered a life-threatening emergency, death is rare when treatment is vigorous and initiated early. The cause is presumed to be stressors (e.g., infection, trauma, surgery) in a patient with preexisting hyperthyroidism, either diagnosed or undiagnosed. The physiologic factor or factors that initiate thyrotoxic crisis are unknown.[19]

Manifestations include severe tachycardia, heart failure, shock, hyperthermia (up to 105.3° F [40.7° C]), restlessness, agitation, seizures, abdominal pain, nausea, vomiting, diarrhea, delirium, and coma. Aggressive measures must be taken to prevent death. Treatment is aimed at reducing circulating thyroid hormone levels and the clinical manifestations of this disorder by appropriate drug therapy. Therapy is directed at fever reduction, fluid replacement, and elimination or management of the initiating stressor(s).

Diagnostic Studies

The two primary laboratory findings used to confirm the diagnosis of hyperthyroidism are decreased TSH levels and elevated free thyroxine (FT_4) levels.[21] Total T_3 and T_4 may also be assessed, but these are not as useful. Measurements of total T_3 and T_4 measure both free and bound (to protein) hormone levels. In the body, the free hormone is the only form of the hormone that is biologically active.

The radioactive iodine uptake (RAIU) test is indicated to differentiate Graves' disease from other forms of thyroiditis. The patient with Graves' disease will show a diffuse, homogeneous uptake of 35% to 95%, whereas the patient with thyroiditis will show an uptake of less than 2%. The person with nodular goiter will show an uptake in the high-normal range (Table 48-6).

Collaborative Care

The overall goal in the treatment of hyperthyroidism is to block the adverse effects of thyroid hormones and stop their oversecretion. The three primary treatment options for the patient with hyperthyroidism are antithyroid medications, radioactive iodine therapy, and subtotal thyroidectomy (see Table 48-6). In general, the treatment of choice in nonpregnant adults is radioac-

TABLE 48-4   Clinical Manifestations: Thyroid Hormone Dysfunction

HYPOFUNCTION	HYPERFUNCTION	HYPOFUNCTION	HYPERFUNCTION
Cardiovascular System		**Musculoskeletal System**	
Increased capillary fragility	Systolic hypertension	Fatigue	Fatigue
Decreased rate and force of contraction	Increased rate and force of cardiac contractions	Weakness	Muscle weakness
Varied changes in blood pressure	Bounding, rapid pulse	Muscular aches and pains	Proximal muscle wasting
Cardiac hypertrophy	Increased cardiac output	Slow movements	Pretibial myxedema
Distant heart sounds	Cardiac hypertrophy	Arthralgia	Dependent edema
Anemia	Systolic murmurs		Osteoporosis
Tendency to develop congestive heart failure, angina, myocardial infarction	Arrhythmias	**Nervous System**	
	Palpitations	Apathy	Difficulty in focusing eyes
	Atrial fibrillation (more common in the older adult)	Lethargy	Nervousness
	Angina	Fatigue	Fine tremor (of fingers and tongue)
Respiratory System		Forgetfulness	Insomnia
Dyspnea	Increased respiratory rate	Slowed mental processes	Lability of mood, delirium
Decreased breathing capacity	Dyspnea on mild exertion	Hoarseness	Restlessness
		Slow, slurred speech	Personality changes of irritability, agitation
Gastrointestinal System		Prolonged relaxation of deep tendon muscles	Exhaustion
Decreased appetite	Increased appetite, thirst	Stupor, coma	Hyperreflexia of tendon reflexes
Nausea and vomiting	Weight loss	Paresthesias	Depression, fatigue, apathy (in the older adult)
Weight gain	Increased peristalsis	Anxiety, depression	Lack of ability to concentrate
Constipation	Diarrhea, frequent defecation	Polyneuropathy	Stupor, coma
Distended abdomen	Increased bowel sounds		
Enlarged, scaly tongue	Splenomegaly	**Reproductive System**	
	Hepatomegaly	Prolonged menstrual periods or amenorrhea	Menstrual irregularities
		Decreased libido	Amenorrhea
Integumentary System		Infertility	Decreased libido
Dry, thick, inelastic, cold skin	Warm, smooth, moist skin		Impotence in men
Thick, brittle nails	Thin, brittle nails detached from nailbed (onycholysis)		Gynecomastia in men
Dry, sparse, coarse hair	Hair loss (may be patchy)	**Other**	Decreased fertility
Poor turgor of mucosa	Clubbing of fingers	Increased susceptibility to infection	Intolerance to heat
Generalized interstitial edema	Palmar erythema	Increased sensitivity to narcotics, barbiturates, anesthesia	Increased sensitivity to stimulant drugs
Puffy face	Fine silky hair	Intolerance to cold	Elevated basal temperature
Decreased sweating	Premature graying (in men)	Decreased hearing	Lid lag, stare
Pallor	Diaphoresis	Sleepiness	Eyelid retraction
	Vitiligo	Goiter	Exophthalmos
			Goiter
			Rapid speech

TABLE 48-5   Comparison of Hyperthyroidism in Younger and Older Adults

	YOUNGER ADULT	OLDER ADULT
Common causes	Graves' disease in >90% of cases	Graves' disease or toxic nodular goiter
Common symptoms	Nervousness, irritability, weight loss, heat intolerance, warm, moist skin	Anorexia, weight loss, apathy, lassitude, depression, confusion
Goiter	Present in >90% of cases	Present in about 50% of cases
Ophthalmopathy	Exophthalmos present in 20%-40% of cases	Exophthalmos less common
Cardiac features	Tachycardia and palpitations common, but without heart failure	Angina, arrhythmia, congestive heart failure may occur

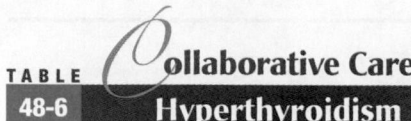

TABLE 48-6	Collaborative Care Hyperthyroidism

Diagnostic
History and physical examination
Ophthalmologic examination
ECG
Laboratory tests
• Serum free T_4, TSH levels
• TRH stimulation test
Radioactive iodine uptake (RAIU)

Collaborative Therapy
Drug Therapy
Antithyroid drugs
• propylthiouracil (PTU)
• methimazole (Tapazole)
Iodine
β-Adrenergic blockers (e.g., propranolol [Inderal]
Radiation Therapy
Radioactive iodine
Surgical Therapy
Subtotal thyroidectomy
Nutritional Therapy
High-calorie diet
High-protein diet
Frequent meals

ECG, Electrocardiogram; *TRH*, thyrotropin-releasing hormone; *TSH*, thyroid-stimulating hormone.

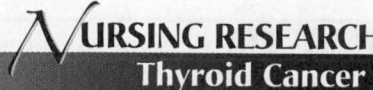

NURSING RESEARCH
Thyroid Cancer

Citation
Stajduhar KI et al: Thyroid cancer: patients' experiences of receiving I[131] therapy, *Oncol Nurs Forum* 27:1213, 2000.

Purpose
To enhance the understanding of experiences and needs of patients with thyroid cancer receiving iodine-131 therapy.

Methods
Data for this qualitative study were collected through focus groups, telephone interviews, and field notes. Tape recordings were made of the interviews. Data were subjected to thematic analysis.

Results and Conclusions
Four major themes emerged from data analysis: recognizing the totality of the cancer experience, isolation, recognizing the totality of the treatment experience, and understanding barriers to treatment. Based on the data, it was concluded that health care workers involved with patients with thyroid cancer lack an understanding of thyroid disease and the effects of therapy. Educational programs are needed to adequately prepare both nurses and patients.

Implications for Nursing Practice
An improvement in the care and education provided to patients receiving I[131] therapy is needed. Nurse education, as well as patient education, is needed. In order for nurses to provide comprehensive cancer care, psychosocial and physical needs must be addressed, requiring a collaborative approach among patient, nurses, and other health care professionals.

tive iodine therapy. However, the choice of treatment is influenced by the patient's age, severity of the disorder, complicating features (including pregnancy), and patient's preferences. If surgery is to be performed, the patient is usually given antithyroid drugs and iodine to produce a euthyroid state and possibly β-adrenergic blockers to relieve symptoms preoperatively.

Drug Therapy. Drugs used in the treatment of hyperthyroidism include antithyroid drugs, iodine, and β-adrenergic blockers. It is important to note that although these drugs are useful in the treatment of thyrotoxic states, they are not considered curative. Radiation therapy or surgery may ultimately be required.

Antithyroid drugs. The first-line antithyroid drugs used in the treatment of hyperthyroidism are propylthiouracil (PTU) and methimazole (Tapazole). These drugs inhibit the synthesis of thyroid hormones. PTU also blocks peripheral conversion of T_4 to T_3. Although there is considerable individual variation, improvement usually begins 1 to 2 weeks after the initiation of therapy, and good results are seen within 4 to 8 weeks. Therapy is usually continued for 6 months to 2 years to allow for spontaneous remission. These drugs are not curative. The major disadvantages of these drugs are patient noncompliance and a high rate of recurrence of hyperthyroidism when the drugs are discontinued. In addition, agranulocytosis may occur in rare situations. Indications for use of antithyroid drugs include Graves' disease in the young patient, hyperthyroidism during pregnancy, and the need to attain a euthyroid state before surgery or radiation therapy.

Iodine. Iodine is useful in conjunction with other antithyroid drugs in the preparation of a patient for thyroidectomy or for treatment of thyrotoxic crisis. The administration of iodine in

large doses rapidly inhibits synthesis of T_3 and T_4 and blocks the release of these hormones into circulation. It also decreases the vascularity of the thyroid gland, making surgery safer and easier. The maximal effect of iodine is usually seen within 1 to 2 weeks. After that time, a reduction in the therapeutic effect may be seen. For this reason, long-term iodine therapy is not effective in controlling hyperthyroidism. Iodine is available in the form of saturated solution of potassium (SSKI) and Lugol's solution.

β-Adrenergic blockers. β-Adrenergic blockers are used for symptomatic relief of thyrotoxicosis that results from increased β-adrenergic receptor stimulation caused by excess thyroid hormones. Propranolol (Inderal), the most frequently used β-adrenergic blocker, is usually administered with other antithyroid agents and rapidly provides symptomatic relief. Atenolol (Tenormin) is the preferred β-adrenergic blocker for use in the hyperthyroid patient with asthma or heart disease.

Radioactive Iodine Therapy. As mentioned previously, radioactive iodine therapy (RAI) is the treatment of choice for most nonpregnant adults. (A pregnancy test is done on all women who experience menstrual cycles before initiation of therapy.) RAI damages or destroys thyroid tissue, thus limiting thyroid hormone secretion. Radioactive iodine has a delayed response, and maximum effects may not be seen for 2 to 3 months. For this reason, the patient is usually treated with antithyroid drugs and propranolol before and during the first 3 months after the initiation of RAI until the effects of irradiation become apparent. Although this method of treatment is usually effective, the biggest disadvantage is the high incidence of posttreatment hypothyroidism, resulting in the need for lifelong thyroid hormone replacement.[21]

Surgical Therapy. Another effective treatment option for the individual with hyperthyroidism is a thyroidectomy. A *subtotal thyroidectomy* is the preferred surgical procedures and involves the removal of a significant portion of the thyroid gland. For subtotal thyroidectomy to be effective, approximately 90% of thyroid tissue must be removed. If too much tissue is taken, the gland will not regenerate after surgery and hypothyroidism will result. Thyroidectomy is indicated for individuals who have been unresponsive to antithyroid therapy, for individuals with very large goiters causing tracheal compression, and for individuals with a possible malignancy. Additionally, this surgery may be done when an individual is not a good candidate for RAI or does not want to take RAI.[22,23] One advantage thyroidectomy has over RAI is a more rapid reduction in T_3 and T_4 levels.

Endoscopic thyroidectomy is a minimally invasive procedure. It is an appropriate procedure for patients with small nodules (less than 3 cm) where there is no evidence of malignancy. An advantage of endoscopic thyroidectomy over the traditional approach is less scarring, less pain, and a faster return to normal activity.

Before surgery, antithyroid drugs, iodine, and β-adrenergic blockers may be administered to achieve a euthyroid state and to control symptoms. Iodine reduces vascularization of the gland, reducing the risk of hemorrhage. Other associated disorders such as cardiac disease or diabetes mellitus must also be controlled. Postoperative complications include hypothyroidism, damage to or inadvertent removal of parathyroid glands causing hypoparathyroidism and hypocalcemia, hemorrhage, injury to the recurrent or superior laryngeal nerve, thyrotoxic crisis, and infection.

Nutritional Therapy. The potential for nutritional deficits is high when an increased metabolic rate is present. A high-calorie diet (4000 to 5000 kcal/day) may be ordered to satisfy hunger and prevent tissue breakdown. This is accomplished with six full meals a day and snacks high in protein, carbohydrates, minerals, and vitamins, particularly vitamin A, thiamine, vitamin B_6, and vitamin C. The protein allowance should be 1 to 2 g/kg of ideal body weight. Increased carbohydrates should compensate for disturbed metabolism, provide energy, and spare body protein stores. Highly seasoned and high-fiber foods should be avoided because they stimulate the already hyperactive gastrointestinal tract. Substitutes should be provided for caffeine-containing liquids such as coffee, tea, and cola because the stimulating effects of these fluids increase restlessness and sleep disturbances. Milk is an excellent food source that provides calcium and protein. A dietitian should be consulted for guidance in meeting the nutritional needs of a patient with hyperthyroidism.

NURSING MANAGEMENT
HYPERTHYROIDISM

■ Nursing Assessment

Subjective and objective data that should be obtained from an individual with hyperthyroidism are presented in Table 48-7.

■ Nursing Diagnoses

Nursing diagnoses for the patient with hyperthyroidism include, but are not limited to, those presented in NCP 48-1.

■ Planning

The overall goals are that the patient with hyperthyroidism will (1) experience relief of symptoms, (2) have no serious complications related to the disease or treatment, and (3) cooperate with the therapeutic plan.

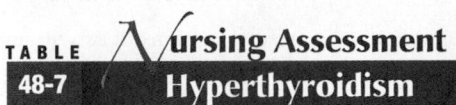

TABLE 48-7	Nursing Assessment Hyperthyroidism

Subjective Data

Important Health Information

Past health history: Preexisting goiter; recent infection or trauma, immigration from iodine-deficient area, autoimmune disease

Medications: Use of thyroid hormones

Functional Health Patterns

Health perception–health management: Positive family history of thyroid or autoimmune disorders

Nutritional-metabolic: Insufficient iodine intake; weight loss; increased appetite, thirst; nausea

Elimination: Diarrhea; polyuria; sweating

Activity-exercise: Dyspnea on exertion; palpitations; muscle weakness, fatigue

Sleep-rest: Insomnia

Cognitive-perceptual: Chest pain; nervousness; heat intolerance; pruritus

Sexuality-reproductive: Decreased libido; impotence; gynecomastia (in men); amenorrhea (in women)

Coping–stress tolerance: Emotional lability, irritability, restlessness, personality changes, delirium

Objective Data

General Observation

Agitation, rapid speech and body movements; hyperthermia, enlarged or nodular thyroid gland

Eyes

Exophthalmos, eyelid retraction; infrequent blinking

Integumentary

Warm, diaphoretic, velvety skin; thin, loose nails; fine, silky hair and hair loss; palmar erythema; clubbing; white pigmentation of skin (vitiligo), diffuse edema of legs and feet

Respiratory

Tachypnea

Cardiovascular

Tachycardia, bounding pulse, systolic murmurs, arrhythmias, hypertension

Gastrointestinal

Increased bowel sounds; hepatosplenomegaly

Neurologic

Hyperreflexia; diplopia; fine tremors of hands, tongue, eyelids; stupor; coma

Musculoskeletal

Muscle wasting

Reproductive

Menstrual irregularities, infertility; impotence, gynecomastia in men

Possible Findings

↑ T_3, ↑ T_4; ↑ T_3 resin uptake; ↓ serum thyroid-stimulating hormone (TSH); chest x-ray showing enlarged heart

NURSING CARE PLAN 48-1

Patient with Hyperthyroidism

EXPECTED PATIENT OUTCOMES	NURSING INTERVENTIONS and *RATIONALES*
NURSING DIAGNOSIS	**Activity intolerance** *related to* fatigue, exhaustion, and heat intolerance secondary to hypermetabolism *as manifested by* complaints of weakness, hyperactivity, short attention span, memory lapses, dyspnea, tachycardia, irritability.
• Decreased perception of weakness and fatigue	• Assess for signs of activity intolerance *because hyperthyroidism results in protein catabolism, overactivity, and increased metabolism leading to exhaustion.* • Monitor vital signs q4hr and before and after activities *because tachycardia and BP elevations can indicate excessive thyroid hormone activity.* • Assist patient with self-care as needed *to make certain patient's daily needs are met.* • Schedule activities of daily living and treatments *to promote adequate rest periods.*
NURSING DIAGNOSIS	**Risk for injury** (corneal ulceration) *related to* decreased blinking or inability to close eyelids secondary to exophthalmos.
• No evidence of corneal damage	• Assess patient for complaints of eye pain, feeling of grittiness or "sand" in eyes, inability to close eyelids completely, lid lag, lid retraction, visible sclera above iris, and "stare" *to determine if risk factors are present for corneal ulcers and initiate appropriate interventions.* • Teach patient to exercise extraocular muscles daily *to maintain flexibility.* • Cover patient's eyes with mask or tape shut if eyes will not close *to prevent corneal drying and, at night, to promote sleep.* • Apply methylcellulose eyedrops (artificial tears) *to soothe and moisten conjunctival membranes.*
NURSING DIAGNOSIS	**Imbalanced nutrition: less than body requirements** *related to* hypermetabolism and inadequate diet *as manifested by* complaints of weight loss; less than optimal body weight.
• Maintenance of weight (or gain weight) • Alleviation (or prevention) of nutritional deficiency	• Assess patient's eating habits and weight pattern *to determine extent of the problem and plan appropriate interventions.* • Teach and provide high-calorie, high-vitamin, high-mineral diet that includes between-meal and bedtime snacks *because hyperthyroidism increases metabolic rate.* • Weigh patient daily *to evaluate effectiveness of nutritional plan.* • Arrange dietary consultation if indicated.
NURSING DIAGNOSIS	**Anxiety** *related to* lack of knowledge about management and course of disease and hypermetabolism *as manifested by* verbalization of inability to cope with stress.
• Verbalization of knowledge of management and course of disease • Verbalization of decrease in anxiety	• Teach patient about disease management, including medication regimen, potential for hypertension, chronic nature of disease, and dietary implications, *because knowledge decreases anxiety and increases a sense of control.* • Promote rest and relaxation *because anxiety often causes difficulty with rest and sleep.* • Teach patient strategies for coping with stress *to prevent increasing anxiety.* • Administer medications as ordered *because decrease in clinical manifestations will decrease anxiety.*

■ Nursing Implementation

Acute Intervention. Individuals who have hyperthyroidism are usually treated in an outpatient setting. However, patients who develop acute thyrotoxicosis or those who undergo thyroidectomy require hospitalization and acute care.

Acute thyrotoxicosis. Acute thyrotoxicosis is a systemic syndrome that requires aggressive treatment, often in an intensive care unit. The nurse needs to administer medications (previously discussed) that block thyroid hormone production. Nursing management also includes provisions for supportive therapy. Having an understanding of the major organ response to the hypermetabolic state is a critical aspect of nursing management. Supportive therapy includes monitoring for cardiac arrhythmias and decompensation, ensuring adequate oxygenation, and administration of intravenous fluids to replace fluid and electrolyte losses. This is especially important in the patient who develops vomiting and diarrhea.[24,25]

A calm, quiet room should be provided because increased metabolism causes sleep disturbances. Provision of adequate rest may be a challenge because of the patient's irritability and restlessness. Specific interventions may include (1) placing the patient in a cool room, away from very ill patients and noisy, high-traffic areas; (2) using light bed coverings and changing the linen frequently if the patient is diaphoretic; (3) encouraging and assisting with exercise involving large muscle groups (tremors can interfere with small-muscle coordination) to allow the release of nervous tension and restlessness; (4) restricting visitors who upset the patient; and (5) establishing a supportive, trusting relationship to help the patient cope with aggravating events and lessen anxiety.

If exophthalmos is present, there is a potential for corneal injury related to irritation and dryness. The patient may also have orbital pain. Nursing interventions to relieve eye discomfort and prevent corneal ulceration include applying artificial tears to soothe and moisten conjunctival membranes. Salt restriction may help reduce periorbital edema. Elevation of the patient's head promotes fluid drainage from the periorbital area; the patient should sit upright as much as possible. Dark glasses reduce glare and prevent irritation from smoke, air currents, dust, and dirt. If the eyelids cannot be closed, they should be lightly taped shut for sleep. To maintain flexibility, the patient should be taught to exercise the intraocular muscles several times a day by turning the eyes in the complete range of motion. Good grooming can be helpful in reducing the loss of self-esteem that can result from an altered body image. If the exophthalmos is severe, treatment may involve suturing the eyelids together, administering corticosteroids, radiation of retroorbital tissues, orbital decompression, or corrective lid or muscle surgery.

Thyroid surgery. When subtotal thyroidectomy is the treatment of choice, the patient must be adequately prepared to avoid postoperative complications. The signs and symptoms of thyrotoxicosis must be alleviated as much as possible, and cardiac problems must be controlled before surgery. If iodine is used to relieve hyperthyroid symptoms, it should be mixed with water or juice, sipped through a straw, and administered after meals. The patient must be assessed for signs of iodine toxicity such as swelling of buccal mucosa and other mucous membranes, excessive salivation, nausea and vomiting, and skin reactions. If toxicity occurs, iodine administration should be discontinued and the physician notified.

Preoperative teaching should include comfort and safety measures in which the patient can participate. Coughing, deep breathing, and leg exercises should be practiced and their importance explained. The patient should be taught how to support the head manually while turning in bed, because this maneuver minimizes stress on the suture line after surgery. Range-of-motion exercises of the neck should be practiced. The nurse should explain routine postoperative care such as IV infusions. The patient should be told that talking is likely to be difficult for a short time after surgery.

The hospital room must be prepared before the patient's return from surgery. Oxygen, suction equipment, and a tracheostomy tray should be readily available. A tracheostomy tray is required in case airway obstruction occurs. Although this rarely occurs, it is an emergency situation the nurse must be prepared for. Recurrent laryngeal nerve damage leads to vocal cord paralysis. If there is paralysis of both cords, spastic airway obstruction will occur, requiring an immediate tracheostomy.

Respiration may also become difficult because of excess swelling of the neck tissues, hemorrhage, hematoma formation, and laryngeal stridor. *Laryngeal stridor* (harsh, vibratory sound) may occur during inspiration and expiration as a result of tetany, which occurs if the parathyroid glands are removed or damaged during surgery. To treat tetany, calcium salts such as calcium gluconate and calcium chloride should be readily available for IV administration.

After a thyroidectomy the nurse should do the following:

1. Assess the patient every 2 hours for 24 hours for signs of hemorrhage or tracheal compression such as irregular breathing, neck swelling, frequent swallowing, sensations of fullness at the incision site, choking, and blood on the anterior or posterior dressings.
2. Place the patient in a semi-Fowler position and support the patient's head with pillows, avoiding flexion of the neck and any tension on the suture lines.
3. Monitor vital signs. Complete the initial assessment by checking for signs of tetany secondary to hypoparathyroidism (e.g., tingling in toes, fingers, or around the mouth; muscular twitching; apprehension) and by evaluating difficulty in speaking and hoarseness. Trousseau's sign and Chvostek's sign should be monitored for 72 hours (see Chapter 16, Fig. 16-15). Some hoarseness is to be expected for 3 to 4 days after surgery because of edema.
4. Control postoperative pain by giving medication.

If postoperative recovery is uneventful, the patient is ambulated within hours after surgery, is permitted to take fluid as soon as tolerated, and eats a soft diet the day after surgery.

The appearance of the incision may be highly distressing to the patient. The patient can be reassured that the scar will fade in color and eventually look like a normal neck wrinkle. A scarf, jewelry, high collar, or other covering can effectively camouflage a fresh scar.

Ambulatory and Home Care

Postoperative care. Discharge teaching for the patient following surgery is an important aspect of nursing care. The patient and family need to be aware that thyroid hormone balance should be monitored periodically to ensure that normal function has returned. Most patients experience a period of relative hypothyroidism soon after surgery because of the substantial reduction in the size of the thyroid. However, the remaining tissue usually hypertrophies, recovering the capacity to produce the hormone needed by the body, but this takes time. The administration of thyroid hormone is avoided because exogenous hormone inhibits pituitary production of TSH and delays or prevents the restoration of normal gland function and thyroid tissue regeneration.

The patient can do a great deal to prevent complications and promote a return to normal function during the hypothyroid period after surgery. Caloric intake must be reduced substantially below the amount that was required before surgery to prevent weight gain. The patient may be advised to avoid **goitrogens** (foods that contain thyroid-inhibiting substances) (Table 48-8). Adequate iodine is necessary to promote thyroid function, but excesses inhibit the thyroid. Seafood once or twice a week or normal use of iodized salt should provide sufficient intake.

Regular exercise helps stimulate the thyroid gland and should be encouraged. High environmental temperature should be avoided because it inhibits thyroid regeneration.

Regular follow-up care is necessary. The patient should be seen biweekly for a month and then at least semiannually to assess for the development of hypothyroidism. If a complete thyroidectomy has been performed, the patient needs instruction in lifelong thyroid replacement. Failure of thyroid function is considered the normal end stage of Graves' disease. The patient should be taught the signs and symptoms of progressive thyroid failure and instructed to seek medical care if these develop.

TABLE 48-8   Common Exogenous Goitrogens

Foods	Drugs
Potent Goitrogens	**Thyroid Inhibitors**
Turnips	propylthiouracil (PTU)
Rutabagas	methimazole (Tapazole)
Soybeans	Iodine in large doses
Skins of peanuts	**Others**
Milk from kale-fed cattle	Sulfonamides
Less Potent Goitrogens	Salicylates
Seafood	p-Aminosalicylic acid
Green leafy vegetables	phenylbutazone (Butazolidin)
Peanuts	lithium
Peaches	amiodarone (Cardarone)
Peas	
Strawberries	
Carrots	
Cabbage	
Mustard seed	
Radishes	

Hypothyroidism is relatively easy to manage with oral administration of thyroid replacement.

Radioactive iodine therapy. Radioactive iodine therapy is administered on an outpatient basis and is the therapy of choice for the nonpregnant adult. Because the therapeutic dose of radioactive iodine is low, no radiation safety precautions are necessary. The patient should be instructed that radiation thyroiditis and parotiditis are possible and may cause dryness and irritation of the mouth and throat. Relief may be obtained with frequent sips of water, ice chips, or the use of a salt and soda gargle three or four times per day. This gargle is made by dissolving 1 teaspoon of salt and 1 teaspoon of baking soda in 2 cups of warm water. The discomfort should subside in 3 to 4 days. If dryness and irritation persist, the patient should contact his or her health care provider. Because of the high frequency of hypothyroidism after radioactive iodine therapy, the patient and significant others should be taught the symptoms of hypothyroidism and instructed to seek medical help if these symptoms occur.

▪ Evaluation

The expected outcomes are that the patient with hyperthyroidism will
- experience relief of symptoms
- have no serious complications related to the disease or treatment
- cooperate with the therapeutic plan

THYROID ENLARGEMENT

Goiter is hypertrophy of the thyroid gland caused by excess TSH stimulation, which in turn can be caused by inadequate circulating thyroid hormones. Goiter may also be caused by growth-stimulating immunoglobulins and other growth factors. Goitrogens (see Table 48-8), which inhibit synthesis of thyroid hormone, can cause goiter but usually only in the individual who lives in an iodine-deficient area (endemic goiter). A goiter is also commonly found in patients with Graves' disease.

TSH and T_4 levels are measured to determine whether a goiter is associated with hyperthyroidism, hypothyroidism, or nor-

mal thyroid function. Thyroid antibodies are measured to assess for thyroiditis. Treatment with thyroid hormone may prevent further thyroid enlargement. Surgery to remove large goiters may be necessary.

THYROID NODULES

A thyroid nodule, a palpable deformity of the thyroid gland, may be benign or malignant. Benign nodules are usually not dangerous, but they can cause tracheal compression if they become too large. Malignant tumors of the thyroid gland are not common. The American Cancer Society estimated 20,700 new cases of thyroid cancer were diagnosed in 2002.[26] The four major types of thyroid cancer are papillary, follicular, medullary, and anaplastic. The major sign of thyroid cancer is the presence of a hard, painless nodule or nodules on an enlarged thyroid gland.

Nodular enlargement of the thyroid gland or palpation of a mass usually requires radiologic evaluation. Ultrasound is often the first radiologic test used in the diagnostic workup of a thyroid nodule. Computed tomography (CT), magnetic resonance imaging (MRI), and ultrasound-guided fine-needle aspiration (FNA) are other diagnostic options. FNA is indicated when a tissue sample for pathologic examination is necessary. FNA is considered one of the most effective methods to identify malignancy.[27] A thyroid scan may also be done to evaluate for possible malignancy. The scan shows whether nodules on the thyroid are "hot" or "cold." Thyroid tumors may or may not take up radioactive iodine. Tumors that take up the radioactive iodine are called "hot" nodules and are nearly always benign. If the nodule does not take up the radioactive iodine, it appears as "cold" and has a higher risk of being malignant. Measurement of serum calcitonin is also helpful in diagnosis, because increased levels are associated with medullary thyroid carcinoma.

Surgical removal of the tumor is usually indicated in the treatment of thyroid cancer. Surgical procedures may range from unilateral total lobectomy with removal of the isthmus to total thyroidectomy with bilateral lobectomy. Many thyroid cancers are TSH dependent, and thyroid hormone in hyperphysiologic doses is often prescribed to inhibit pituitary secretion of TSH. Radiation therapy may also be indicated to prolong survival.

Nursing care for the patient with thyroid tumors is similar to care for the patient who has undergone thyroidectomy and also includes general nursing measures for the patient with cancer (see Chapter 15).

THYROIDITIS

Thyroiditis is an inflammatory process in the thyroid and can have several causes. *Subacute granulomatous thyroiditis* (de Quervain's thyroiditis), which causes thyrotoxicosis, is thought to be caused by a viral infection. *Acute thyroiditis* is due to bacterial or fungal infection. Subacute and acute forms of thyroiditis have abrupt onsets and the thyroid gland is painful. *Chronic autoimmune thyroiditis* (Hashimoto's thyroiditis), leading to hypothyroidism, is insidious in onset. Hashimoto's thyroiditis is a chronic autoimmune disease in which thyroid tissue is replaced by lymphocytes and fibrous tissue. It is the most common cause of goiterous hypothyroidism in the United States. *Silent thyroiditis,* a form of lymphocytic thyroiditis, has a variable onset. In women, this condition may occur in the postpartal period. It is believed to be an autoimmune disease and may be early Hashimoto's thyroiditis.

T_4 and T_3 are initially elevated in subacute, acute, and silent thyroiditis but may become depressed with time. TSH levels are low and then elevated. Thyroid hormone levels are usually low in chronic Hashimoto's thyroiditis, and TSH is high. Suppression of RAIU is seen in subacute and silent thyroiditis. Antithyroid antibodies are present in Hashimoto's thyroiditis.

Recovery from thyroiditis may be complete in weeks or months without treatment. If the condition is bacterial in origin, treatment may include specific antibiotics or surgical drainage. In subacute and acute forms, salicylates and nonsteroidal antiinflammatory drugs are used. If there is no response to these drugs in 48 hours, corticosteroids are given. Propranolol (Inderal) or atenolol (Tenormin) may be used for the cardiovascular symptoms of a hyperthyroid condition. Thyroid hormone replacement is indicated if the patient is hypothyroid.

Nursing care of the patient with thyroiditis depends, in part, on the therapeutic management. Education regarding treatment and encouraging compliance are important for all types of thyroiditis. The patient should be instructed to remain under close health care supervision so that progress can be monitored and to report any change in symptoms to the health care provider.

The patient with thyroiditis of autoimmune origin may be susceptible to other autoimmune diseases such as Addison's disease, pernicious anemia, premature gonadal failure, or Graves' disease. The patient should be taught the signs and symptoms of these disorders, particularly Addison's disease. The patient should also be given a list of common goitrogens (see Table 48-8) and encouraged to avoid them as much as possible. A patient receiving thyroid hormone replacement must be taught the expected side effects of these drugs and measures to manage them. This information is covered in greater detail in the following section. The patient treated surgically needs care similar to that given to the person undergoing thyroidectomy.

HYPOTHYROIDISM

Etiology and Pathophysiology

Hypothyroidism is one of the most common medical disorders in the United States, affecting 8% of women and 2% of men over 50 years of age.[28] Hypothyroidism results from insufficient circulating thyroid hormone as a result of a variety of abnormalities. Hypothyroidism can be primary (related to destruction of thyroid tissue or defective hormone synthesis) or secondary (related to pituitary disease with decreased TSH secretion or hypothalamic dysfunction with decreased thyrotropin-releasing hormone [TRH] secretion). It may also be transient, related to thyroiditis or discontinuance of thyroid hormone therapy.[19]

Iodine deficiency is the most common cause of hypothyroidism worldwide and is most prevalent in iodine-deficient areas of the world. In areas where iodine intake is adequate, such as the United States, the most common cause of primary hypothyroidism in the adult is atrophy of the thyroid gland. This atrophy is the end result of Hashimoto's thyroiditis and Graves' disease. These autoimmune diseases destroy the thyroid gland. Hypothyroidism also may develop as a consequence of treatment for hyperthyroidism, specifically the surgical removal of the thyroid glands, or radioactive iodine therapy. Occasionally, hypothyroidism develops as a result of the ingestion of excessive amounts of goitrogens (see Table 48-7).

Although the typical patient with hypothyroidism is a woman over 50 years of age, the disease can occur at any age and in either sex. Hypothyroidism that develops in infancy (termed **cretinism**) is caused by thyroid hormone deficiencies during fetal or early neonatal life.

Clinical Manifestations

All hypothyroid states have certain features in common, regardless of the cause. Manifestations vary depending on the severity and the duration of thyroid deficiency, as well as the patient's age at onset of the deficiency.[29]

Hypothyroidism has systemic effects characterized by an insidious and nonspecific slowing of body processes. The clinical presentation can range from a patient with no symptoms to a patient with classic symptoms and physical changes easily detected on examination (Fig. 48-6). Unless hypothyroidism occurs after thyroidectomy or thyroid ablation, or during treatment with antithyroid drugs, the onset of symptoms may occur over months to years. The development of symptoms is so slow and subtle that medical attention is seldom sought. The patient's family and friends are often unaware of the changes. The severity of symptoms experienced depends on the degree of thyroid hormone deficiency and the long-term physiologic effects of thyroid hormone deficiency. Long-term effects may involve any body system but are more pronounced in the neurologic, cardiovascular, GI, reproductive, and hematologic systems.

The adult with hypothyroidism often is fatigued, lethargic, and experiences personality and mental changes.[29] The mental changes seen in hypothyroidism include impaired memory, slowed speech, decreased initiative, and somnolence. Many individuals with hypothyroidism appear depressed. Although the patient with hypothyroidism sleeps long periods of time, the stages of sleep are altered.

Although hypothyroidism affects cardiac function, it is usually significant only in the presence of coexisting cardiac disease. Hypothyroidism is associated with decreased cardiac output and decreased cardiac contractility. Thus the patient may experience

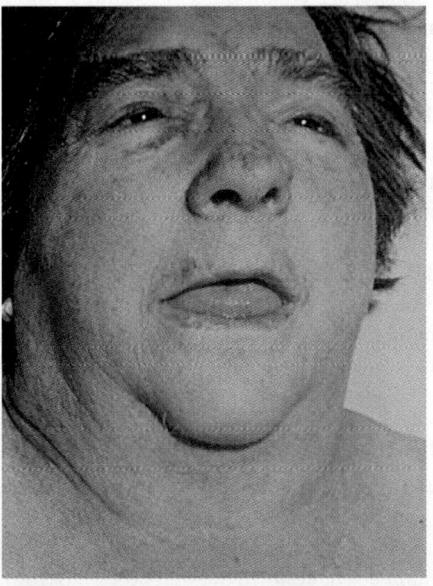

FIG. 48-6 Myxedema facies with dull, puffy skin; coarse, sparse hair; periorbital edema; and prominent tongue.

low exercise tolerance and shortness of breath on exertion. In the patient with a preexisting cardiovascular condition, hypothyroidism may cause significant hemodynamic compromise. Anemia is a common feature of hypothyroidism. Erythropoietin levels may be low or normal. Oxygen demand is decreased, and there is a hypocellular bone marrow. The result is a low hematocrit. Other hematologic problems are related to cobalamin, iron, and folate deficiencies. The patient may bruise easily. Increased serum cholesterol and triglyceride levels and the accumulation of mucopolysaccharides in the intima of small blood vessels can result in coronary atherosclerosis. This accumulation is seldom symptomatic (i.e., characterized by angina) because of the decreased myocardial oxygen consumption that has been observed in hypothyroidism.

GI motility is decreased in hypothyroidism, and achlorhydria (absence or decrease of hydrochloric acid) is common. Constipation, which is a common complaint, may progress to obstipation and, rarely, to intestinal obstruction. The underlying metabolic disease makes the individual a high risk candidate for intestinal surgery.

Other physical changes include cold intolerance, hair loss, dry and coarse skin, brittle nails, hoarseness, muscle weakness and swelling, and weight gain.[29] Weight gain is most likely a result of decreased metabolic rate. Those with severe long-standing hypothyroidism may display **myxedema,** the accumulation of hydrophilic mucopolysaccharides in the dermis and other tissues (see Fig. 48-6). This mucinous edema causes the characteristic facies of hypothyroidism (i.e., puffiness, periorbital edema, and masklike affect). Individuals with hypothyroidism may describe an impaired self-image in regard to their disabilities and altered appearance. Women with hypothyroidism frequently complain of menorrhagia. Some affected individuals have been treated for menorrhagia for years and may have undergone hysterectomy before the hypothyroidism was diagnosed. In addition, anovulatory cycles with subsequent infertility may occur.

In the older adult, the typical manifestations of hypothyroidism (including fatigue, cold and dry skin, hoarseness, hair loss, constipation, and cold intolerance) may be attributed to normal aging. For this reason, these symptoms may not raise suspicion of an underlying condition. Older adults who have confusion, lethargy, and depression should be evaluated for thyroid disease.

Complications

The mental sluggishness, drowsiness, and lethargy of hypothyroidism may progress gradually or suddenly to a notable impairment of consciousness or coma. This situation, termed *myxedema coma,* constitutes a medical emergency. Myxedema coma can be precipitated by infection, drugs (especially narcotics, tranquilizers, and barbiturates), exposure to cold, and trauma. It is characterized by subnormal temperature, hypotension, and hypoventilation. For the patient to live, vital functions must be supported and IV thyroid hormone replacement must be administered.

Diagnostic Studies

The most common and reliable laboratory tests used to evaluate thyroid function are those that measure TSH and FT$_4$. These values, correlated with symptoms gathered from the history and physical examination, confirm the diagnosis.[29] Serum TSH levels help determine the cause of hypothyroidism. Serum TSH is high when the defect is in the thyroid and low when it is in the pitu-

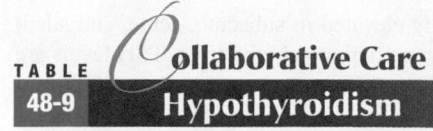

TABLE 48-9	Collaborative Care Hypothyroidism

Diagnostic
History and physical examination
Serum TSH and free T$_4$
Serum T$_3$ and T$_4$
TRH stimulation test

Collaborative Therapy
Thyroid hormone replacement (e.g., levothyroxine)
Monitor thyroid hormone levels and adjust dosage (if needed)
Nutritional therapy to promote weight loss
Patient and family teaching (see Table 48-10)

TRH, Thyrotropin-releasing hormone; *TSH,* thyroid-stimulating hormone.

itary or hypothalamus. An increase in TSH after TRH injection suggests hypothalamic dysfunction, whereas no change suggests anterior pituitary dysfunction (Table 48-9). Other abnormal laboratory findings are elevated cholesterol and triglycerides, anemia, and increased creatine kinase.

Collaborative Care

The overall goal for treatment in a patient with hypothyroidism is restoration of a euthyroid state as safely and rapidly as possible with hormone replacement therapy. A low-calorie diet is indicated to promote weight loss.

Levothyroxine (Synthroid, Levothroid) is the drug of choice to treat hypothyroidism.[19] In the young and otherwise healthy patient, the maintenance replacement dose can be started at once. The typical initial adult dose usually starts at 0.05 mg taken orally daily. The maintenance dose is adjusted according to the patient's response and laboratory findings. In the older adult patient and the person with compromised cardiac status, a smaller initial dose (0.0125 to 0.025 mg/day) is recommended because the usual dose may increase myocardial oxygen demand. The increased oxygen demand may cause angina and cardiac arrhythmias. Any chest pain experienced by a patient starting thyroid replacement should be reported immediately, and electrocardiogram (ECG) and serum cardiac enzyme tests must be performed. In the patient without side effects the dose is increased at 1- to 4-week intervals. It is important that the patient take replacement medication regularly. Lifelong thyroid replacement therapy is usually required.

NURSING MANAGEMENT HYPOTHYROIDISM

■ Nursing Assessment

The nurse plays an important role in the detection of hypothyroidism. Careful assessment may reveal the early and subtle changes that indicate dysfunction, particularly when caring for the patient with a condition that may predispose him or her to endocrine dysfunction. Assessment of the patient who is suspected of having hypothyroidism should include questions about weight gain, mental changes, fatigue, slowed and slurred speech, cold intolerance, skin changes such as increased dryness or thickening, constipation, and dyspnea. In addition, the nurse should assess for recent introduction of iodine-containing medications or ingestion of large amounts of goitrogens (see Table 48-8). The patient should be assessed for bradycardia; distended abdomen; dry, thick, cold skin; thick, brittle nails; paresthesias; and muscular aches and pains.

■ Nursing Diagnoses

Nursing diagnoses for the patient with hypothyroidism may include, but are not limited to, those presented in NCP 48-2.

■ Planning

The overall goals are that the patient with hypothyroidism will (1) experience relief of symptoms, (2) maintain a euthyroid state, (3) maintain a positive self-image, and (4) comply with lifelong thyroid replacement therapy.

■ Nursing Implementation

Health Promotion. There is currently no consensus regarding thyroid function screening. Although hypothyroidism is relatively common, particularly among women over age 50, there does not appear to be strong justification to screen the general population. However, some research indicates that it might be reasonable to screen certain adult populations such as individuals with family history of thyroid disease, those with history of neck radiation, women over 50, and all persons over 60.[30,31]

Acute Intervention. Most individuals with hypothyroidism do not require acute nursing care, because most are managed on an outpatient basis. However, the patient who develops

NURSING CARE PLAN 48-2

Patient with Hypothyroidism

EXPECTED PATIENT OUTCOMES	NURSING INTERVENTIONS and *RATIONALES*
NURSING DIAGNOSIS	**Hypothermia** *related to* cold intolerance *as manifested by* complaints of feeling cold, shivering.
• Satisfaction with temperature of environment • Personal comfort	• Provide extra clothing, blankets, warm environment *to increase patient's comfort.* • Explain to patient and significant others that decreased heat production causes discomfort *to increase patient's understanding of disease.*
NURSING DIAGNOSIS	**Imbalanced nutrition: more than body requirements** *related to* hypometabolism *as manifested by* weight gain.
• Maintenance of weight in usual range	• Provide low-calorie, high-protein diet; include foods high in cobalamin (vitamin B_{12}), folic acid, iron, and vitamin C *to reduce tendency for weight gain while preventing muscle wasting and anemia.* • Explain the need for fewer calories *so patient will be more agreeable to dietary restrictions.* • Assist patient to develop method of monitoring weight and caloric intake *so excess weight gain can be avoided.* • Encourage small, frequent meals *because eating frequently will prevent feelings of hunger and overeating.*
NURSING DIAGNOSIS	**Constipation** *related to* gastrointestinal hypomotility *as manifested by* irregular, hard stools.
• Regular soft, formed stool	• Assess bowel pattern and characteristics *to plan appropriate interventions.* • Provide 2-3 L of fluids per day *to maintain soft stool.* • Offer foods high in bulk and roughage *to increase fecal mass.* • Encourage activity *to stimulate peristalsis.* • Administer laxatives or stool softeners if necessary *to stimulate GI motility.*
NURSING DIAGNOSIS	**Activity intolerance** *related to* decreased metabolic rate and mucin deposits in joints and interstitial spaces *as manifested by* generalized weakness and muscle and joint stiffness.
• Able to participate in self-care activities with minimal discomfort and fatigue	• Assess ability to participate in self-care activities *to determine extent of problem and plan appropriate interventions.* • Monitor vital signs and comfort level *to determine effect of activities and plan activity increases.* • Administer thyroid hormone replacement as ordered *to correct hypometabolic state.* • Plan frequent rest periods *to improve patient's tolerance and comfort level.* • Pace activities to match patient's abilities *to allow maximum participation.*
NURSING DIAGNOSIS	**Disturbed thought processes** *related to* diminished cerebral blood flow secondary to decreased cardic output *as manifested by* forgetfulness, memory loss, and personality changes.
• Maintenance of orientation to reality to highest level possible	• Assess thinking processes such as memory, attention span, orientation *to enable appropriate planning.* • Repeat information to patient *because he or she requires more time to comprehend.* • Explain cause of problems to patient and family *to reduce anxiety and frustration.* • Provide clock and calendar *to maintain orientation to time and day.* • Provide written handouts with all instructions *to help patient adhere to regimen.*

myxedema coma requires acute nursing care, often in an intensive care setting. Mechanical respiratory support is frequently necessary, and the patient will require cardiac monitoring. The nurse will administer thyroid hormone replacement therapy and all other medications intravenously because the paralytic ileus associated with myxedema coma causes unreliable absorption of oral medications. If the patient is hyponatremic, hypertonic saline may be administered until the serum sodium reaches at least 130 mEq/L (130 mmol/L). The nurse should monitor core temperature because the patient with myxedema coma is often hypothermic.[25]

For assessment of the patient's progress, vital signs, body weight, fluid intake and output, and visible edema should be monitored. Cardiac assessment is especially important because the cardiovascular response to the hormone determines the medication regimen. Energy level and mental alertness should be noted. These should increase within 2 to 14 days and continue to rise steadily to normal levels.

Ambulatory and Home Care. Patient teaching is imperative for the patient with hypothyroidism. A patient and family teaching guide is provided in Table 48-10. Initially the hypothyroid patient needs more time than usual to comprehend all of the necessary information. It is important to provide written instructions, repeat the information often, and assess the patient's comprehension level regularly.

The need for lifelong drug therapy must be stressed. The patient should be instructed in expected and unexpected side effects. Specifically, the signs and symptoms of hypothyroidism or hyperthyroidism that indicate hormone imbalance should be included in the teaching plan. Toxic symptoms should be clearly defined. Table 48-4 lists signs of hyperthyroidism that are the same as toxic symptoms of thyroid hormone replacement.

TABLE 48-10 Patient & Family Teaching Guide — Hypothyroidism

1. Explain the nature of thyroid hormone deficiency and self-care practices necessary to prevent complications. Patient and family must understand thyroid replacement therapy. It is especially important to emphasize the need for lifelong replacement, the need to continually take the medication, and the need for regular follow-up care.
2. Emphasize the need for a comfortable, warm environment because of intolerance to cold.
3. Teach measures to prevent skin breakdown. Soap should be used sparingly and lotion applied to skin.
4. Caution the patient to avoid sedatives. If they must be used, suggest that the lowest dose be used. Family members should closely monitor mental status, level of consciousness, and respirations.
5. Discuss with the patient measures to minimize constipation. Suggestions should include a gradual increase in activity and exercise, increased fiber in diet, use of stool softeners, and maintenance of a regular bowel elimination time. Use of enemas should be avoided because they produce vagal stimulation, which can be hazardous if cardiac disease is present.

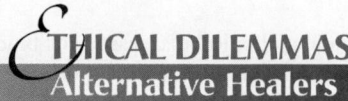
ETHICAL DILEMMAS — Alternative Healers

Situation
The nurse is caring for a Hispanic woman with thyroid disease. Thyroid replacement therapy is the planned treatment. The patient's cultural healer tells her not to take the medication and suggests that she should begin an herbal regimen instead. Should the nurse intervene?

Important Points for Consideration
- Culturally competent nursing care should incorporate the patient's cultural and religious values and beliefs.
- Patient autonomy, the patient's right to choose a treatment plan, should be respected.
- Having adequate, understandable information about available treatment options and their possible consequences facilitates an informed choice.

Critical Thinking Questions
1. What information should the nurse obtain from the patient? What information should the nurse provide for the patient?
2. How should the nurse proceed? Should the nurse try to incorporate the healer's herbal regimen into the plan of care while attempting to persuade the woman of the need for the thyroid replacement therapy?

The patient must be taught to contact a health care provider immediately if signs of overdose such as orthopnea, dyspnea, rapid pulse, palpitations, nervousness, or insomnia appear. The patient with diabetes mellitus should test his or her capillary blood glucose at least daily because return to the euthyroid state frequently increases insulin requirements. In addition, thyroid preparations potentiate the effects of other common drug groups, such as anticoagulants, antidepressants, and digitalis compounds. Thus the patient should be taught the toxic signs and symptoms of these medications and should remain under close medical observation until stable.

It is sometimes difficult for the patient to recognize signs of overdosage or underdosage of drug therapy; therefore a family member or friend should be included in the instruction process. Handouts for the patient should be written in understandable language and should accompany verbal instruction. The handouts should be reviewed with the patient and family to assess understanding, and information should be clarified when necessary.

With treatment, striking transformations occur in both appearance and mental function. Most adults return to a normal state. Cardiovascular conditions and (occasionally) psychosis may persist despite corrections of the hormonal imbalance. Relapses occur if treatment is interrupted.

■ Evaluation

The expected outcomes are that the patient with hypothyroidism will
- have relief from symptoms
- maintain a euthyroid state as evidenced by normal thyroid hormone and TSH levels
- state the need for and a plan to adhere to lifelong therapy

Disorders of the Parathyroid Glands

HYPERPARATHYROIDISM

Etiology and Pathophysiology

Hyperparathyroidism is a condition involving increased secretion of parathyroid hormone (PTH). PTH helps regulate calcium and phosphate levels by stimulating bone resorption of calcium, renal tubular reabsorption of calcium, and activation of vitamin D. Thus oversecretion of PTH is associated with increased serum calcium levels. Hyperparathyroidism affects approximately 0.1% of the general population.[32]

Hyperparathyroidism is classified as primary, secondary, or tertiary. *Primary hyperparathyroidism* is due to an increased secretion of PTH leading to disorders of calcium, phosphate, and bone metabolism. The most common cause is a benign neoplasm or a single adenoma (80% of cases) in the parathyroid gland. Primary hyperparathyroidism is more common in women and usually occurs between 30 and 70 years of age.[32] The peak incidence is in the fifth and sixth decades of life. Patients who have previously undergone head and neck radiation may have an increased predisposition to the development of parathyroid adenoma.

Secondary hyperparathyroidism appears to be a compensatory response to states that induce or cause hypocalcemia, the main stimulus of PTH secretion. Disease conditions associated with secondary hyperparathyroidism include vitamin D deficiencies, malabsorption, chronic renal failure, and hyperphosphatemia. *Tertiary hyperparathyroidism* occurs when there is hyperplasia of the parathyroid glands and a loss of negative feedback from circulating calcium levels. Thus there is autonomous secretion of PTH, even with normal calcium levels. It is observed in the patient who has had a kidney transplant after a long period of dialysis treatment for chronic renal failure (see Chapter 45).

The excessive levels of circulating PTH usually lead to hypercalcemia and hypophosphatemia, creating a multisystem effect (Table 48-11). In the bones, subperiosteal bone resorption, decreased bone density, cyst formation, and general weakness can occur as a result of the effect of PTH on osteoclastic (bone resorption) and osteoblastic (bone formation) activity. In the kidneys, the excess calcium cannot be reabsorbed, leading to increased levels of calcium in the urine (hypercalciuria). This urinary calcium, along with a large amount of urinary phosphate, can lead to calculi formation. In addition, PTH stimulates the synthesis of a biologically active form of vitamin D, a potent stimulator of calcium transport in the intestine. In this way, PTH indirectly increases GI absorption of calcium, contributing further to the high serum calcium levels.

Clinical Manifestations and Complications

Clinical manifestations of hyperparathyroidism range from the asymptomatic individual (who is diagnosed through testing for unrelated problems) to the patient with overt symptoms. Most clinical manifestations are associated with hypercalcemia and are summarized in Table 48-11. The major manifestations include weakness, loss of appetite, constipation, increased need for sleep, emotional disorders, and shortened attention span. Major signs include loss of calcium from bones (osteoporosis), fractures, and kidney stones (nephrolithiasis). Neuromuscular abnormalities are characterized by muscle weakness, particularly in the proximal muscles of the lower extremities. Asymptomatic cases are being identified with increasing frequency with routine calcium screening. Serious complications of hyperparathyroidism are renal failure; pancreatitis; cardiac changes; and long bone, rib, and vertebral fractures.

Diagnostic Studies

PTH, as measured by radioimmunoassay, is elevated with hyperparathyroidism. Serum calcium levels usually exceed 10 mg/dl (2.50 mmol/L). Because of its inverse relation with calcium, the serum phosphorus level is usually below 3 mg/dl (0.1 mmol/L). Elevations in other laboratory tests include urine calcium, serum chloride, uric acid, creatinine, amylase (if pancreatitis is present), and alkaline phosphatase (in the presence of bone disease). Bone density measurements may also be used to detect bone loss. Imaging, such as MRI, CT scanning, and ultrasound, may be used for localization of the adenoma.

Collaborative Care

The treatment objectives are to relieve the manifestations and prevent complications caused by excess PTH. The choice of therapy depends on the urgency of the clinical situation, the degree of hypercalcemia, the underlying disorder, renal and hepatic function, the clinical presentation of the patient, and the particular advantages and disadvantages of the different therapeutic modalities.

Surgical Therapy. The most effective treatment of primary and secondary hyperparathyroidism is surgical intervention.[19] Parathyroidectomy leads to rapid reduction of chronically high calcium levels. Criteria for surgery include serum calcium levels greater than 12 mg/dl (3.0 mmol/L), hypercalciuria (greater than 400 mg/day), markedly reduced bone mineral density, overt symptoms (i.e., neuromuscular effects, nephrolithiasis), or those under age 50.[33] The surgical procedure involves partial or complete removal of the parathyroid glands. In the past, this surgery always involved an open surgical approach. However, this procedure is now being done using an endoscope on an outpatient basis in many health care facilities. Autotransplantation of normal parathyroid tissue in the forearm or near the sternocleidomastoid muscle may be done, allowing PTH secretion to continue with normalization of calcium levels. If autotransplantation is not possible, or if it fails, the patient will need to take calcium supplements for life.

Nonsurgical Therapy. If the patient does not meet the criteria for surgical intervention, or if the patient is elderly or at increased surgical risk from other health problems, a conservative management approach is used. This includes an annual examination with tests for serum PTH, calcium, phosphorus, and alkaline phosphatase levels; renal function; x-rays to assess for metabolic bone disease; and measurement of urinary calcium excretion. Continued ambulation and the avoidance of immobility are critical aspects of management. Dietary measures also include maintenance of a high fluid intake and a moderate calcium intake. The diet should contain 8 to 10 g of sodium per day to replace losses from increased urine output.

Phosphorus is usually supplemented unless contraindicated by an increased risk for urinary calculi formation. Several drugs currently used in the treatment of hyperparathyroidism are helpful in

TABLE 48-11	Clinical Manifestations: Parathyroid Dysfunction	
SYSTEM	**HYPOFUNCTION**	**HYPERFUNCTION**
Cardiovascular	Decreased contractility of heart muscle Decreased cardiac output Prolongation of QT and ST intervals on ECG Arrhythmias	Arrhythmias Shortened QT interval on ECG Hypertension
Gastrointestinal	Abdominal cramps Fecal incontinence (in older adult)	Vague abdominal pain Anorexia Nausea and vomiting Constipation Pancreatitis Peptic ulcer disease Cholelithiasis Weight loss
Integumentary	Dry, scaly skin Hair loss on scalp and body Brittle nails, transverse ridging Changes in developing teeth, lack of tooth enamel	Skin necrosis Moist skin
Musculoskeletal	Fatigue Weakness Painful muscle cramps Skeletal x-ray changes, osteosclerosis Soft tissue calcification Difficulty in walking	Skeletal pain Backache Weakness, fatigue Pain on weight bearing Osteoporosis Pathologic fractures of long bones Compression fractures of spine Decreased muscle tone
Neurologic	Personality changes Psychiatric manifestations of depression, anxiety Irritability Memory impairment Headache Seizures Positive Chvostek's sign or Trousseau's phenomenon Tremor Paresthesias of perioral area, hands, feet Hyperactive deep-tendon reflexes Disorientation, confusion (in older adult)	Personality disturbances Emotional irritability Memory impairment Psychosis Delirium, confusion, coma Incoordination Hyperactive deep-tendon reflexes Abnormalities of gait Psychomotor retardation Headache
Renal	Urinary frequency Urinary incontinence	Hypercalciuria Kidney stones (nephrolithiasis) Urinary tract infections Polyuria
Other	Eye changes, including lenticular opacities, cataracts, papilledema	Corneal calcification on slit-lamp examination

ECG, Electrocardiogram.

lowering calcium levels, but do not, in themselves, treat the underlying problem. Bisphosphonates (e.g., alendronate [Fosamax]) inhibit osteoclastic bone resorption and rapidly normalize serum calcium levels. Estrogen or progestin therapy can reduce serum and urinary calcium levels in the postmenopausal woman and may retard demineralization of the skeleton. Oral phosphate may be used to inhibit the calcium-absorbing effects of vitamin D in the intestine. Phosphates should only be used if the patient has normal renal function and low serum phosphate levels. Diuretics may be given to increase the urinary excretion of calcium.

Calcimimetic agents (such as R-586) are a new class of drugs that increase the sensitivity of the calcium receptor on the parathyroid gland, resulting in decreased PTH secretion and calcium

blood levels, thus sparing calcium stores in the bone. Although these agents are still under clinical investigation, initial studies have been encouraging.[34,35]

NURSING MANAGEMENT
HYPERPARATHYROIDISM

Nursing management of the patient with hyperparathyroidism is somewhat dependent on the collaborative treatment strategy. Nursing care for the patient following a parathyroidectomy is similar to that for a patient after thyroidectomy. The major postoperative complications are associated with hemorrhage and fluid and electrolyte disturbances. **Tetany,** a condition of neuromuscular hyperexcitability associated with sudden decrease in calcium levels, is another concern. It is usually apparent early in the postoperative period but may develop over several days. Mild tetany, characterized by unpleasant tingling of the hands and around the mouth, may be present but should abate without problems. If tetany becomes more severe (e.g., muscular spasms or laryngospasms develop), IV calcium may be given. IV calcium gluconate should be readily available for patients following parathyroidectomy in the event that acute tetany occurs.

Strict monitoring of intake and output is necessary to evaluate fluid status. Calcium, potassium, phosphate, and magnesium levels are assessed frequently, as well as Chvostek's and Trousseau's signs (see Chapter 16, Fig. 16-15). Mobility is encouraged to promote bone calcification.

If surgery is not performed, treatment to relieve symptoms and prevent complications is initiated. The nurse can assist the patient with hyperparathyroidism to adapt the meal plan to his or her lifestyle. A referral to a dietitian may be useful. Because immobility can aggravate the bone loss, the nurse can assist the patient to implement an exercise program and identify resources, such as shopping malls and YMCAs as places to exercise safely. The patient should be encouraged to keep the regular appointments, and the tests being performed should be explained. The patient should also be instructed in the symptoms of hypocalcemia or hypercalcemia and to report these should they occur. Hypocalcemia and hypercalcemia are discussed in Chapter 16.

HYPOPARATHYROIDISM

Etiology and Pathophysiology

Hypoparathyroidism, a condition associated with inadequate circulating PTH, is uncommon. It is characterized by hypocalcemia resulting from a lack of PTH to maintain serum calcium levels. PTH resistance at the cellular level may also occur (pseudohypoparathyroidism). This is caused by a genetic defect resulting in hypocalcemia in spite of normal or high PTH levels and is often associated with hypothyroidism and hypogonadism.

The most common cause of hypoparathyroidism is iatrogenic. This may include accidental removal of the parathyroids or damage to the vascular supply of the glands during neck surgery (e.g., thyroidectomy, radical neck surgery). Idiopathic hypoparathyroidism resulting from the absence, fatty replacement, or atrophy of the glands is a rare disease that usually occurs early in life and may be associated with other endocrine disorders. Affected patients may have antiparathyroid antibodies. Severe hypomagnesemia also leads to a suppression of PTH secretion.[36]

Clinical Manifestations

The clinical features of acute hypoparathyroidism are due to a low serum calcium level (see Table 48-11). Sudden decreases in calcium concentration cause tetany. This state is characterized by tingling of the lips, fingertips, and occasionally feet and increased muscle tension leading to paresthesias and stiffness. Painful tonic spasms of smooth and skeletal muscles (particularly of the extremities and face), dysphagia, a constricted feeling in the throat, and laryngospasms are also present. Chvostek's sign and Trousseau's sign are usually positive. Respiratory function may be severely compromised by accessory muscle spasm and laryngospasm-induced airway obstruction. Patients are usually anxious and apprehensive. Abnormal laboratory findings include de-

creased serum calcium and PTH levels and increased serum phosphate levels. Other causes of chronic hypocalcemia include chronic renal failure, vitamin D deficiency, and hypomagnesemia.

NURSING *and* COLLABORATIVE MANAGEMENT HYPOPARATHYROIDISM

The primary management objectives for a patient with hypoparathyroidism are to treat acute complications such as tetany, maintain normal serum calcium levels, and prevent long-term complications. Emergency treatment of tetany requires the administration of IV calcium. Generally, in adults, 10 to 20 ml of a 10% solution of calcium gluconate is infused over 10 minutes.[37] Calcium must be infused slowly because high blood levels can cause hypotension, serious cardiac arrhythmias, or cardiac arrest. Thus ECG monitoring is indicated when calcium is administered. The patient who takes digoxin is particularly vulnerable. In addition, IV calcium can cause venous irritation and inflammation. Extravasation may cause cellulitis, necrosis, and tissue sloughing. IV patency should be assessed before administration.

Rebreathing may partially alleviate acute neuromuscular symptoms associated with hypocalcemia such as generalized muscle cramps or mild tetany. The patient who can cooperate should be instructed to breathe in and out of a paper bag or breathing mask. This reduces carbon dioxide excretion from the lungs, increases carbonic acid levels in the blood, and lowers the pH.

Calcium is present in serum as free calcium (ionized), bound to protein, or complexed with phosphate, citrate, or carbonate. The free (ionized form) of calcium is the biologically active form. Because an acidic environment enhances the degree of ionization of calcium, the proportion of total body calcium available in the active form is increased, temporarily relieving the manifestations of hypocalcemia.

The patient with hypoparathyroidism needs instruction in the management of long-term drug therapy and nutrition. Oral calcium supplements of at least 1 g per day in divided doses for the patient under 40 years of age and 2 g per day in divided doses for the patient more than 40 years of age are usually prescribed. Specific hormone replacement of PTH is not used to treat hypoparathyroidism because of expense and the need for parenteral administration. Vitamin D is used in chronic and resistant hypocalcemia to enhance intestinal calcium absorption and bone resorption. The preferred preparations are dihydrotachysterol (Hytakerol) and 1,25-dihydroxycholecalciferol (calcitriol [Rocaltrol]). These drugs raise calcium levels rapidly and are quickly metabolized. Rapid metabolism is desired because vitamin D is a fat-soluble vitamin and toxicity can cause irreversible renal impairment. Ergocalciferol (Calciferol) may also be prescribed.

A high-calcium meal plan includes foods such as dark green vegetables, soybeans, and tofu. The patient should be told that foods containing oxalic acid (e.g., spinach, rhubarb), phytic acid (e.g., bran, whole grains), and phosphorus reduce calcium absorption.

The patient should be instructed about the need for lifelong treatment and follow-up care. The patient's calcium levels should be monitored three to four times a year. Treatment modification is often necessary because hypercalcemia can develop without apparent cause. The patient must also be taught to recognize signs and symptoms of hypocalcemia and hypercalcemia, and to contact the health care provider if they occur.

Disorders of the Adrenal Cortex

There are three main classifications of adrenal steroid hormones. Glucocorticoids regulate metabolism, increase blood glucose levels, and are critical in the physiologic stress response. In humans the primary glucocorticoid is cortisol. Mineralocorticoids regulate sodium and potassium balance. The primary mineralocorticoid is aldosterone. Androgens contribute to growth and development in both genders and to sexual activity in adult women. The term *corticosteroid* refers to any one of these three types of hormones produced by the adrenal cortex.

CUSHING SYNDROME

Etiology and Pathophysiology

Cushing syndrome is a spectrum of clinical abnormalities caused by excess corticosteroids, particularly glucocorticoids. Several conditions can cause Cushing syndrome (Table 48-12). The most common cause is iatrogenic administration of exogenous corticosteroids (e.g., prednisone). Approximately 85% of endogenous Cushing syndrome is due to an ACTH-secreting pituitary tumor (Cushing's disease). Other causes of Cushing syndrome include adrenal tumors and ectopic ACTH production by tumors outside the hypothalamic-pituitary-adrenal axis (usually of the lung or pancreas). Cushing's disease and primary adrenal tumors are more common in women in the 20- to 40-year age-group; ectopic ACTH production is more common in men.

Clinical Manifestations

The clinical manifestations of Cushing syndrome can be seen in most body systems and are related to excess levels of corticosteroids (Table 48-13). Although manifestations of glucocorticoid excess usually predominate, symptoms of mineralocorticoid and androgen excess may also be seen.

Corticosteroid excess causes pronounced changes in physical appearance (Fig. 48-7). Weight gain, the most common feature, results from the accumulation of adipose tissue in the trunk, face, and cervical area (Fig. 48-8). Transient weight gain from sodium and water retention may be present because of the mineralocorticoid effects of cortisol. Hyperglycemia occurs because of glucose intolerance (associated with cortisol-induced insulin resistance) and increased gluconeogenesis by the liver.

Protein wasting is caused by the catabolic effects of cortisol on peripheral tissue. Muscle wasting leads to muscle weakness, especially in the extremities. Loss of protein matrix in bone leads to osteoporosis with subsequent pathologic fractures (e.g., vertebral compression fractures) and bone and back pain. Loss of collagen makes the skin weaker and thinner. Therefore the skin bruises easier. Catabolic processes predominate, and wound healing is delayed. Mood disturbances (irritability, anxiety, euphoria), insomnia, irrationality, and occasionally psychosis may occur.

TABLE 48-12   Causes of Cushing Syndrome

- Prolonged administration of high doses of corticosteroids
- ACTH-secreting pituitary tumor (Cushing's disease)
- Cortisol-secreting neoplasm within the adrenal cortex that can be either carcinoma or adenoma
- Excess secretion of ACTH from carcinoma of the lung or other malignant growth outside the pituitary or adrenal glands

ACTH, Adrenocorticotropic hormone.

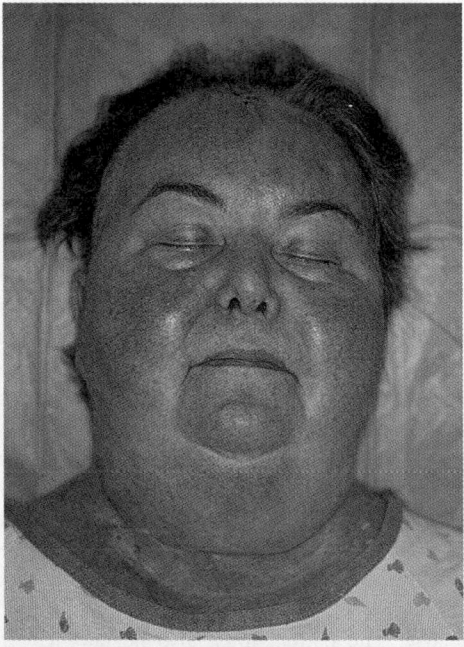

FIG. 48-7 Cushing syndrome. Facies include a rounded face ("moon face") with thin, reddened skin. Hirsutism may also be present.

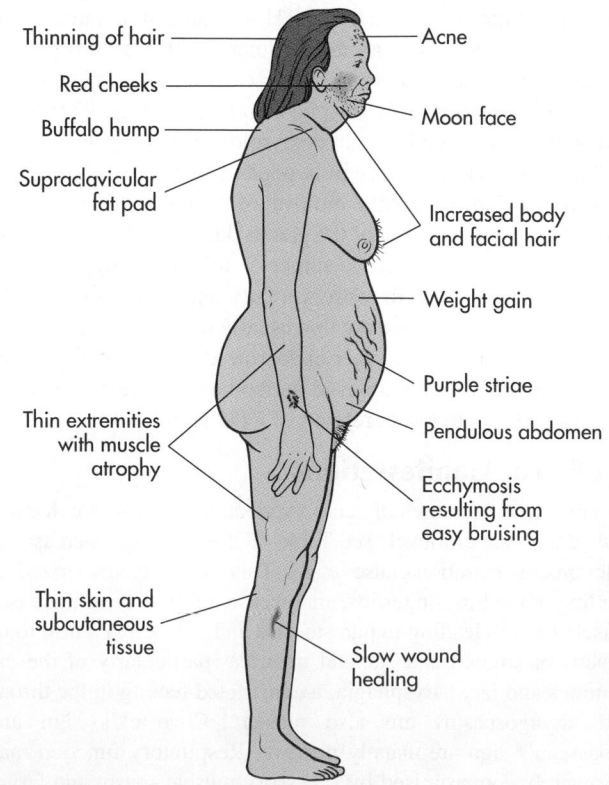

FIG. 48-8 Common characteristics of Cushing syndrome.

Thinning of hair
Red cheeks
Buffalo hump
Supraclavicular fat pad
Thin extremities with muscle atrophy
Thin skin and subcutaneous tissue
Acne
Moon face
Increased body and facial hair
Weight gain
Purple striae
Pendulous abdomen
Ecchymosis resulting from easy bruising
Slow wound healing

TABLE 48-13 **Clinical Manifestations: Adrenocortical Hormone Dysfunction**

SYSTEM	HYPOFUNCTION (ADDISON'S DISEASE)	HYPERFUNCTION (CUSHING SYNDROME)
Glucocorticoids		
General appearance	Weight loss	Truncal (centripedal) obesity, thin extremities, rounding of face (moon face), fat deposits on back of neck and on shoulders ("buffalo hump")
Integumentary	Bronzed or smoky hyperpigmentation of face, neck, hands (especially creases), buccal membranes, nipples, genitalia, and scars (if pituitary function normal); vitiligo, alopecia	Thin, fragile skin; purplish red striae; petechial hemorrhages; bruises; florid cheeks (plethora); acne; poor wound healing
Cardiovascular	Hypotension, tendency to develop refractory shock, vasodilation	Hypervolemia, hypertension, edema of lower extremities
Gastrointestinal	Anorexia, nausea and vomiting, cramping abdominal pain, diarrhea	Increase in secretion of pepsin and hydrochloric acid, anorexia
Urinary		Glycosuria, hypercalciuria, kidney stones
Musculoskeletal	Fatigability	Muscle wasting in extremities, proximal muscle weakness, fatigue, osteoporosis, awkward gait, back and joint pain, weakness
Immune	Propensity toward co-existing autoimmune diseases	Inhibition of immune response, suppression of allergic response, inhibition of inflammation
Hematologic	Anemia, lymphocytosis	Leukocytosis, lymphopenia, polycythemia, increased coagulability
Fluids and electrolytes	Hyponatremia, hypovolemia, dehydration, hyperkalemia	Sodium and water retention, edema, hypokalemia
Metabolic	Hypoglycemia, insulin sensitivity, fever	Hyperglycemia, negative nitrogen balance, dyslipidemia
Emotional	Neurasthenia, depression, exhaustion or irritability, confusion, delusions	Psychic stimulation, euphoria, irritability, hypomania to depression, emotional lability
Mineralocorticoids		
Fluid and electrolytes	Sodium loss, decreased volume of extracellular fluid, hyperkalemia, salt craving	Marked sodium and water retention, tendency toward edema, marked hypokalemia
Cardiovascular	Hypovolemia, tendency toward shock, decreased cardiac output, decreased heart size	Hypertension, hypervolemia
Androgens		
Integumentary	Decreased axillary and pubic hair (in women)	Hirsutism, acne
Reproductive	No effect in men, decreased libido in women	Menstrual irregularities and enlargement of clitoris (in females); gynecomastia and testicular atrophy (in males)
Musculoskeletal	Decrease in muscle size and tone	Muscle wasting and weakness

Mineralocorticoid excess may cause hypertension (secondary to fluid retention), whereas adrenal androgen excess may cause pronounced acne, virilization in women, and feminization in men. Menstrual disorders and hirsutism in women and gynecomastia and impotence in men are seen more commonly in adrenal carcinomas.

The clinical presentation, as revealed by the history and physical examination, is the first indication of Cushing syndrome. Of particular importance are (1) centripedal (truncal) obesity or generalized obesity; (2) "moon facies" (fullness of the face) with facial plethora; (3) purplish red striae, which are usually depressed below the skin surface, on the abdomen, breast, or buttocks; (4) hirsutism in women; (5) menstrual disorders in women; (6) hypertension; and (7) unexplained hypokalemia.

Diagnostic Studies

When Cushing syndrome is suspected, a 24-hour urine collection for free cortisol and a low-dose dexamethasone suppression test are done (see Chapter 46). If these results are borderline, a high-dose dexamethasone suppression test is done. False-positive results can occur in patients with depression, those under acute stress, and those who are active alcoholics. Plasma cortisol (the primary glucocorticoid) levels may be elevated, with loss of diurnal variation. CT scanning and MRI may be used for tumor localization.

Other findings on diagnostic tests associated with, but not diagnostic of, Cushing syndrome include granulocytosis, lymphopenia, eosinopenia, hyperglycemia, glycosuria, hypercalciuria, and osteoporosis. Hypokalemia and alkalosis are seen in ectopic

ACTH syndrome and adrenal carcinoma. Plasma ACTH levels may be low, normal, or elevated depending on the underlying problem. High or normal levels indicate ACTH-dependent Cushing's disease, whereas low or undetectable levels indicate an adrenal or exogenous etiology.

Collaborative Care

The primary goal of treatment for Cushing's disease is to normalize hormone secretion. The specific treatment is dependent on the underlying cause (Table 48-14). If the underlying cause is a pituitary adenoma, the standard treatment is surgical removal of the pituitary tumor using the transsphenoidal approach.[38] (Transsphenoidal approach is discussed earlier in this chapter.) Radiation to the pituitary adenoma may be necessary if surgical outcomes are not optimal or if the patient is not a good surgical candidate. Adrenalectomy is indicated for Cushing syndrome caused by adrenal tumors or hyperplasia. Occasionally, bilateral adrenalectomy is necessary. Laparoscopic adrenalectomy is considered an appropriate surgical approach except for patients with known or suspected malignant adrenal tumors. An open surgical adrenalectomy is the treatment of choice for adrenal cancer.[39] Patients with ectopic ACTH-secreting tumors are managed by treating the primary neoplasm.

Drug therapy as a treatment measure for Cushing syndrome is usually indicated when surgery is contraindicated. The goal of drug therapy is the inhibition of adrenal function. Mitotane (Lysodren) suppresses cortisol production, alters peripheral metabolism of cortisol, and decreases plasma and urine corticosteroid levels. This drug essentially results in a "medical adrenalectomy." Metyrapone, ketoconazole (Nizoral), and aminoglutethimide (Cytaden) are used to inhibit cortisol synthesis. The relatively common side effects of these agents include anorexia, nausea and vomiting, GI bleeding, depression, vertigo, skin rashes, and diplopia. The GI side effects may be minimized by administering mitotane (Lysodren) with meals and with a bedtime snack.

If Cushing syndrome has developed during the course of prolonged administration of corticosteroids (e.g., prednisone), one or more of the following alternatives may be tried: (1) gradual discontinuance of corticosteroid therapy, (2) reduction of the corticosteroid dose, and (3) conversion to an alternate-day regimen. Gradual tapering of the corticosteroids is necessary to avoid potentially life-threatening adrenal insufficiency. An alternate-day regimen is one in which twice the daily dosage of a shorter-acting corticosteroid is given every other morning to minimize hypothalamic-pituitary-adrenal suppression, growth suppression, and altered appearance. This regimen is not used when the corticosteroids are given as endocrine replacement therapy.

TABLE 48-14	**Collaborative Care** **Cushing Syndrome**

Diagnostic
History and physical examination
Mental status examination
Plasma cortisol levels for diurnal variations
Plasma ACTH level
Complete blood count
Blood chemistries for sodium, potassium, glucose
Dexamethasone suppression test
24-hour urine for free cortisol
Examination of visual field
CT scan, MRI

Collaborative Therapy*
Adrenocortical Adenoma, Carcinoma, or Hyperplasia
Adrenalectomy (open or laparoscopic)
Drug therapy
- mitotane (Lysodren)
- metyrapone
- ketoconazole (Nizoral)
- aminoglutethimide (Cytaden)

Pituitary Adenoma
Transsphenoidal resection
Radiation therapy

Ectopic ACTH-secreting Tumor
Treatment of the tumor responsible (surgical removal or radiation)

Exogenous Corticosteroid Therapy
Discontinuance of or alteration in administration of exogenous corticosteroids

*Treatment is based on underlying cause.
ACTH, Adrenocorticotropic hormone; *CT*, computed tomography; *MRI*, magnetic resonance imaging.

NURSING MANAGEMENT
CUSHING SYNDROME

■ **Nursing Assessment**

Subjective and objective data that should be obtained from a patient with Cushing syndrome are presented in Table 48-15.

■ **Nursing Diagnoses**

Nursing diagnoses for the patient with Cushing syndrome may include, but are not limited to, those presented in the NCP 48-3.

■ **Planning**

The overall goals are that the patient with Cushing syndrome will
- experience relief of symptoms
- have no serious complications
- maintain a positive self-image
- actively participate in the therapeutic plan

■ **Nursing Implementation**

Health Promotion. Health promotion is focused on identifying patients at risk for Cushing syndrome. Patients receiving long-term, exogenous cortisol for a variety of diseases are at risk. Patient teaching related to the medication use and monitoring of side effects are important preventive measures.

Acute Intervention. The patient with Cushing syndrome is seriously ill. Because the therapeutic interventions have many side effects, the focus of daily assessment is on signs and symptoms of hormone and drug toxicity and complicating conditions such as cardiovascular disease, diabetes mellitus, infection, nephrolithiasis, and pathologic fractures. Nursing assessment should include monitoring of vital signs, daily weight, glucose, possible infection (especially pain, loss of function, and purulent drainage, because other signs and symptoms of inflammation such as fever and redness may be minimal or absent), and signs

TABLE 48-15	Nursing Assessment	
	Cushing Syndrome	

Subjective Data

Important Health Information

Past health history: Pituitary tumor (Cushing's disease); adrenal, pancreatic or pulmonary neoplasms; GI bleeding; frequent infections

Medications: Use of corticosteroids

Functional Health Patterns

Health perception–health management: Malaise

Nutritional-metabolic: Weight gain, anorexia

Elimination: Polyuria; prolonged wound healing, easy bruising

Activity-exercise: Weakness, fatigue

Sleep: Insomnia, poor sleep quality

Cognitive-perceptual: Headache; back, joint, bone, and rib pain; poor concentration and memory

Self-perception–self concept: Negative feelings regarding changes in personal appearance

Sexuality-reproductive: Amenorrhea, impotence, decreased libido

Coping–stress tolerance: Anxiety, mood disturbances, emotional lability, psychosis

Objective Data

General

Truncal obesity, supraclavicular fat pads, buffalo hump, moon facies

Integumentary

Plethora; hirsutism of body and face, thinning of head hair; thin, friable skin; acne; petechiae; purpura; hyperpigmentation; purplish red striae on breasts, buttocks, and abdomen; edema of lower extremities

Cardiovascular

Hypertension

Musculoskeletal

Muscle wasting, thin extremities, awkward gait

Reproductive

Gynecomastia, testicular atrophy (in men), enlarged clitoris (in women)

Possible Findings

Hypokalemia, hyperglycemia, dyslipidemia; polycythemia, granulocytosis, lymphocytopenia, eosinopenia; ↑ plasma cortisol; high, low, or normal ACTH levels; abnormal dexamethasone suppression test; ↑ urine free cortisol, 17-ketosteroids; glycosuria, hypercalciuria; osteoporosis on x-ray

ACTH, Adrenocorticotropic hormone; *GI,* gastrointestinal.

---

and symptoms of abnormal thromboembolic phenomena, such as sudden chest pain, dyspnea, or tachypnea.

Another important focus of nursing care is emotional support. Changes in appearance such as centripedal obesity, multiple bruises, hirsutism in women, and gynecomastia in men can be distressing. The patient may feel unattractive, repulsive, or unwanted.[40] The nurse can help by remaining sensitive to the patient's feelings and offering respect and unconditional acceptance. The patient can be reassured that the physical changes and much of the emotional lability will resolve when hormone levels return to normal.

If treatment involves surgical removal of a pituitary adenoma, an adrenal tumor, or one or both adrenal glands, nursing care will have an additional focus on preoperative and postoperative care.

Preoperative care. Before surgery the patient should be brought to optimal physical condition. Hypertension and hyperglycemia must be controlled, and hypokalemia is corrected with diet and potassium supplements. A high-protein meal plan helps correct the protein depletion. Preoperative teaching will depend on the type of surgical approach planned (hypophysectomy or adrenalectomy), but should include information regarding the postoperative care the patient should anticipate. In the postoperative period (for both open and laparoscopic adrenalectomy), patients will probably have a nasogastric tube, urinary catheter, intravenous therapy, central venous pressure monitoring, and leg sequential compression devices to prevent emboli.[38]

Postoperative care. Surgery on glands poses risks beyond those of other types of operations. Because glands are highly vascular, the risk of hemorrhage is increased. Manipulation of glandular tissue during surgery may release large amounts of hormone into the circulation, producing marked fluctuations in the metabolic processes affected by these hormones. Postopera-

tively, blood pressure, fluid balance, and electrolyte levels tend to be unstable because of these hormone fluctuations. High doses of corticosteroids (e.g., hydrocortisone [Solu-Cortef]) are administered intravenously during surgery and for several days afterward to ensure adequate responses to the stress of the procedure. If large amounts of endogenous hormone have been released into the systemic circulation during surgery, the patient is likely to develop hypertension, increasing the risk of hemorrhage. High levels of corticosteroids also increase susceptibility to infection and delay wound healing.

Any rapid or significant changes in blood pressure, respirations, or heart rate should be reported. Fluid intake and output should be monitored carefully and assessed for potential imbalances. The critical period for circulatory instability ranges from 24 to 48 hours after surgery. IV corticosteroids are given, and the dose and rate of flow are adjusted to the patient's clinical manifestations and fluid and electrolyte balance. Oral doses are given as tolerated. The IV line may be kept in place after IV corticosteroids are withdrawn to keep a line open for quick administration of corticosteroids or vasopressors. Morning urine levels of cortisol (obtained at the same time each morning) are measured to evaluate the effectiveness of the surgery.

If corticosteroid dosage is tapered too rapidly after surgery, acute adrenal insufficiency may develop. Vomiting, increased weakness, dehydration, and hypotension may indicate hypocortisolism. In addition, the patient may complain of painful joints, pruritus, or peeling skin and may experience severe emotional disturbances. These signs and symptoms should be reported so that drug doses can be adjusted. The nurse must constantly be alert for signs of corticosteroid imbalance. After surgery the patient is usually maintained on bed rest until the blood pressure stabilizes. The nurse must be alert for subtle signs of postopera-

NURSING CARE PLAN 48-3

Patient with Cushing Syndrome

EXPECTED PATIENT OUTCOMES	NURSING INTERVENTIONS and *RATIONALES*
NURSING DIAGNOSIS	**Risk for infection** *related to* lowered resistance to stress and suppression of immune system.
• No infection • Early detection and treatment of any infectious process	• Assess for inadequate protein stores, proteinuria, muscle wasting, poor wound healing *as indicators of risk for infection.* • Assess potential infection sites such as urinary and respiratory tracts, skin, and IV lines *so infection can be detected early and treatment initiated promptly.* • Note pain, loss of function, and purulent drainage and teach patient and family to be aware of these signs *because other signs and symptoms of infecton may be minimal or absent.* • Provide private room, if possible; maintain meticulous asepsis and prevent contact with contagious individuals *to reduce the risk of cross-contamination.* • Instruct patient in self-care practices *to avoid infection (e.g., hand washing).* • Refer patient to dietitian for high-protein diet instruction *to help correct the protein depletion caused by excess corticosteroids.*
NURSING DIAGNOSIS	**Imbalanced nutrition: more than body requirements** *related to* increased appetite, high caloric content of foods, and inactivity *as manifested by* statement of increased appetite; weight 10% or more than optimum for height.
• Maintenance of body weight if appropriate or no more than 1 to 2 lb loss per week	• Obtain dietary consult for instruction in low-calorie, high-nutrition diet (including protein and calcium) *because excess corticosteroids produce weight gain and calcium and protein loss.* • Assist with appropriate menu choices *to reinforce dietary instructions.* • Provide low-calorie, high-vitamin snacks.
NURSING DIAGNOSIS	**Disturbed self-esteem** *related to* altered body image, emotional lability, and diminished physical capabilities *as manifested by* verbalization of negative feelings regarding personal appearance and inability to perform usual activities.
• Verbalization of acceptance of appearance by patient and family • Self-care methods to improve appearance	• Explain to patient and family that physical and emotional changes are related to hormone imbalance and that most will disappear when hormone imbalance is corrected *to increase their understanding and assist with coping.* • Accept and respect patient as a person *to maintain patient's self-worth.* • Encourage good grooming and use of attractive attire *to improve patient's appearance and self-esteem.* • Compliment patient when appropriate *to boost morale by providing positive feedback.*
NURSING DIAGNOSIS	**Impaired skin integrity** *related to* excess corticosteroids, immobility, and altered skin fragility *as manifested by* edema; thin, fragile skin; impaired healing.
• Intact skin	• Assess skin *for early detection of trauma.* • Protect patient from bumping and bruising *to prevent injury to easily traumatized tissue.* • Change patient's position frequently *to minimize pressure over bony prominences and improve circulation in edematous tissue.* • Provide good skin care, particularly to edematous areas and areas over bony prominences *because these areas have decreased circulation.*

tive infections because the usual inflammatory responses are suppressed. Meticulous care must be used when changing the dressing and during any other procedures that necessitate access to body cavities, circulation, or areas under the skin so that infection is prevented.

Ambulatory and Home Care. Discharge instructions are based on the patient's lack of endogenous corticosteroids and resulting inability to react to stressors physiologically. Patients should wear Medic Alert bracelets at all times and carry medical identification and instructions in a wallet or purse. Exposure to extremes of temperature, infections, and emotional disturbances should be avoided as much as possible. Stress may produce or precipitate acute

adrenal insufficiency because the remaining adrenal tissue cannot meet an increased hormonal demand. Many patients can be taught to adjust their corticosteroid replacement therapy in accordance with their stress levels. The nurse should consult with each patient's health care provider to determine the parameters for dosage changes if this plan is feasible. If the patient cannot adjust his or her own medication or if weakness, fainting, fever, or nausea and vomiting occur, the patient should contact the health care provider for a possible adjustment in corticosteroid dosage. Lifetime replacement therapy is required by many patients. However, it may take several months to adjust the hormone dose satisfactorily, and patients should be prepared for this.

■ Evaluation

Expected outcomes for the patient with Cushing's syndrome are addressed in NCP 48-3.

ADRENOCORTICAL INSUFFICIENCY

Etiology and Pathophysiology

Adrenocortical insufficiency (hypofunction of the adrenal cortex) may be from a primary cause (known as **Addison's disease**) or a secondary cause (lack of pituitary ACTH secretion). In Addison's disease, all three classes of adrenal corticosteroids (glucocorticoids, mineralocorticoids, and androgens) are reduced. In secondary adrenocortical insufficiency, corticosteroids and androgens are deficient but mineralocorticoids rarely are. ACTH deficiency may be caused by pituitary disease or suppression of the hypothalamic-pituitary axis as a result of the administration of exogenous corticosteroids.

The most common cause of Addison's disease is an autoimmune response. Adrenal tissue is destroyed by antibodies against the patient's own adrenal cortex. Often, other endocrine conditions are present and Addison's disease is considered a component of *polyendocrine deficiency syndrome.* Tuberculosis can cause Addison's disease, but this is now rare. Other causes include infarction, fungal infections (e.g., histoplasmosis), acquired immunodeficiency syndrome (AIDS), and metastatic cancer. Iatrogenic Addison's disease may be due to adrenal hemorrhage, often related to anticoagulant therapy, antineoplastic chemotherapy, ketoconazole (Nizoral) therapy for AIDS, or bilateral adrenalectomy. Although adrenal insufficiency most often occurs in adults between 30 and 60 years of age and affects both genders equally, Addison's disease caused by an autoimmune response is most common in white females.[41]

Clinical Manifestations

Because manifestations do not tend to become evident until 90% of the adrenal cortex is destroyed, the disease is often advanced before it is diagnosed. The manifestations have a very slow (insidious) onset and include progressive weakness, fatigue, weight loss, and anorexia as primary features. Skin hyperpigmentation, a striking feature, is seen primarily in sun-exposed areas of the body, at pressure points, over joints, and in creases, especially palmar creases. It is most likely due to increased secretion of β-lipotropin (which contains melanocyte-stimulating hormone [MSH]) or ACTH. These tropic hormones are increased because of decreased negative feedback and subsequent low corticosteroid levels. Other frequent manifestations are hypotension, hyponatremia, hyperkalemia, nausea and vomiting, and diarrhea.

Patients with secondary adrenocortical hypofunction may have many signs and symptoms in common with patients with Addison's disease but are characteristically not hyperpigmented because ACTH and related peptide levels are low. When severe dehydration, hyponatremia, and hyperkalemia are present, a diagnosis of primary adrenocortical insufficiency is favored because of the mineralocorticoid insufficiency associated with this disorder.

Complications

Patients with adrenocortical insufficiency are at risk for an acute adrenal insufficiency (addisonian crisis), a life-threatening emergency caused by insufficient adrenocortical hormones or a sudden sharp decrease in these hormones. Addisonian crisis is triggered by stress (e.g., from infection, surgery, trauma, hemorrhage, or psychologic distress); following sudden withdrawal of corticosteroid hormone replacement therapy (which is often done by a patient who lacks knowledge of the importance of replacement therapy); after adrenal surgery; or following sudden pituitary gland destruction.

During acute adrenal insufficiency, severe manifestations of glucocorticoid and mineralocorticoid deficiencies are exhibited, including hypotension (particularly postural), tachycardia, dehydration, hyponatremia, hyperkalemia, hypoglycemia, fever, weakness, and confusion. Hypotension may lead to shock. Circulatory collapse associated with adrenal insufficiency is often unresponsive to the usual treatment (vasopressors and fluid replacement). GI manifestations include nausea, vomiting, diarrhea, and vague abdominal pain.

Diagnostic Studies

In addition to clinical features, a diagnosis of Addison's disease can be made when cortisol levels are subnormal or fail to rise over basal levels with an ACTH stimulation test. A failure of cortisol levels to rise in response to ACTH stimulation indicates primary adrenal disease. A positive response to ACTH stimulation indicates a functioning adrenal gland and points to a probable pituitary disease (see Chapter 46). Other abnormal laboratory findings include hyperkalemia, hypochloremia, hyponatremia, hypoglycemia, anemia, and increased blood urea nitrogen levels. Urine levels of free cortisol are low. An ECG may show low voltage and a vertical QRS axis. In addition, peaked T waves caused by hyperkalemia may be evident. CT scans and MRI are used to localize tumors or identify adrenal calcifications or enlargement (Table 48-16).

Collaborative Care

Treatment of adrenocortical insufficiency is focused on management of the underlying cause when possible. The mainstay of treatment for adrenocortical insufficiency is replacement therapy (see Table 48-16). Hydrocortisone, the most commonly used form of replacement therapy, has both glucocorticoid and mineralocorticoid properties. During situations associated with physi-

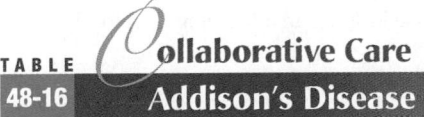

TABLE 48-16   *Collaborative Care*   **Addison's Disease**

Diagnostic
History and physical examination
Plasma cortisol levels
Serum electrolytes
ACTH-stimulation test
CT scan, MRI

Collaborative Therapy
Daily glucocorticoid replacement (two thirds on awakening in morning, one third in late afternoon)*
Daily mineralocorticoid in morning*
Salt additives for excess heat or humidity

*For conditions of normal daily stress in individuals with usual daytime activity.
ACTH, Adrenocorticotropic hormone; *CT,* computed tomography; *MRI,* magnetic resonance imaging.

ologic stress, glucocorticoid dosage must be increased to prevent addisonian crisis.[42]

Addisonian crisis is a life-threatening emergency requiring aggressive management. Treatment must be directed toward shock management and high-dose hydrocortisone replacement. Large volumes of 0.9% saline solution and 5% dextrose are administered to reverse hypotension and electrolyte imbalances until blood pressure returns to normal.[41]

NURSING MANAGEMENT
ADDISON'S DISEASE

■ Nursing Implementation

Acute Intervention. When the patient with Addison's disease is hospitalized, whether for diagnosis, an acute crisis, or some other health problem, frequent nursing assessment is necessary. Vital signs and signs of fluid volume deficit and electrolyte imbalance should be assessed every 30 minutes to 4 hours for the first 24 hours depending on the patient's instability. In addition, daily weights, diligent corticosteroid administration, protection against exposure to infection, and complete assistance with daily hygiene should be practiced. The patient should be protected from noise, light, and environmental temperature extremes. The patient cannot cope with these stresses because he or she cannot produce corticosteroids.

If the hospitalization was due to adrenal crisis, the patient usually responds by the second day and can start oral corticosteroid replacement. Because discharge frequently occurs before the usual maintenance dose of corticosteroids is reached, the patient should be instructed on the importance of keeping scheduled follow-up appointments.

Ambulatory and Home Care. The nurse has an important role in the long-term management of Addison's disease. The serious nature of the disease and the need for lifelong replacement therapy necessitate a well-organized and carefully presented

TABLE 48-17 *Patient & Family Teaching Guide*
Addison's Disease

The following should be included in a teaching plan for the patient and family.
1. Names and dosages of drugs
2. Actions of drugs
3. Symptoms of overdosage and underdosage
4. Conditions requiring increased medication (e.g., trauma, infection, surgery, emotional crisis)
5. Course of action to take relative to changes in medication
   a. Increase in dose of corticosteroid
   b. Administration of large dose of corticosteroid intramuscularly, including demonstration and return demonstration
   c. Consultation with health care provider
6. Prevention of infection and need for prompt and vigorous treatment of existing infections
7. Need for lifelong replacement therapy
8. Need for lifelong medical supervision
9. Need for medical identification device

teaching plan. Table 48-17 outlines the major areas that must be included in the teaching plan.

Glucocorticoids are usually given in divided doses, two thirds in the morning and one third in the afternoon. Mineralocorticoids are given once daily, preferably in the morning. This dosage schedule reflects normal circadian rhythm in endogenous hormone secretion and decreases the side effects associated with corticosteroid replacement therapy. A hormone-deficit patient receiving glucocorticoid replacement is less apt to exhibit harmful symptoms from the medication than a patient receiving pharmacologic doses of these drugs. Because the aim of replacement therapy is to return to normal hormone levels, nursing care is designed to help the patient maintain hormone balance and manage the medication regimen.

Because the patient with Addison's disease is unable to tolerate physical or emotional stress without additional exogenous corticosteroids, long-term care revolves around recognizing the need for extra medication and techniques for stress management. The need for corticosteroid hormone is proportional to stress levels. A patient who cannot produce endogenous hormone must adjust the dose of exogenous hormone to the stress level. Examples of situations requiring corticosteroid adjustment are fever, influenza, extraction of teeth, and rigorous physical activity, such as playing tennis on a hot day or running a marathon. Doses are usually doubled when minor stress occurs (e.g., a respiratory infection, dental work) and tripled when major stress occurs. When in doubt, it is better to err on the side of overreplacement. If vomiting or diarrhea occurs, as may happen with influenza, the health care provider must be notified immediately because electrolyte replacement may be necessary. In addition, these manifestations may be early indicators of crisis. Overall, patients who take their medications consistently can anticipate a normal life expectancy.

Patients must be taught the signs and symptoms of corticosteroid deficiency and excess and to report to their clinicians so that the dose can be adjusted to each patient's need. It is critical that the patient wear an identification bracelet (Medic Alert) and carry a wallet card stating that the patient has Addison's disease so that appropriate therapy can be initiated in case of an unexpected trauma, accident, or crisis. The patient should be instructed and given handouts related to other medications that cause a need to increase glucocorticoid dosage (e.g., phenytoin [Dilantin], barbiturates, rifampin [Rifadin], and antacids). Estrogen inhibits steroid metabolism. Patients using mineralocorticoid therapy should be instructed how to take their blood pressure and given parameters to report to their health care providers, because untoward changes may indicate a need for dosage adjustment.

The patient should carry an emergency kit at all times. The kit should consist of 100 mg of IM hydrocortisone, syringes, and instructions for use. The patient and significant others should be instructed in how to give an IM injection in case the replacement therapy cannot be taken orally. The patient should verbalize instructions, practice IM injections with saline, and have written instructions as to when to alter the dose.

CORTICOSTEROID THERAPY

Cortisol and related glucocorticoids are used to relieve the signs and symptoms associated with many diseases (Table 48-18). The long-term administration of corticosteroids in therapeutic doses of-

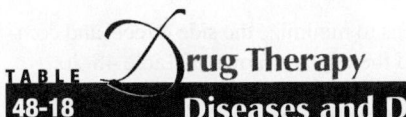

TABLE 48-18 Drug Therapy: Diseases and Disorders Treated with Corticosteroids

Hormone Replacement
Adrenal insufficiency
Congenital adrenal hyperplasia

Therapeutic Effect
Allergic reactions
- Anaphylaxis
- Bee stings
- Contact dermatitis
- Drug reactions
- Serum sickness
- Urticaria

Collagen diseases
- Giant cell arteritis
- Mixed connective tissue disorders
- Polymyositis
- Polyarteritis nodosa
- Rheumatoid arthritis
- Systemic lupus erythematosus

Inflammation
Gastrointestinal diseases
- Inflammatory bowel disease
- Nontropical sprue

Endocrine diseases
- Hypercalcemia
- Hashimoto's thyroiditis
- Thyroid storm

Immunosuppression (after organ transplantation)

Liver diseases
- Alcoholic hepatitis
- Autoimmune hepatitis

Nephrotic syndrome

Neurologic disease
- Prevention of cerebral edema and increased intracranial pressure
- Head trauma

Pulmonary diseases
- Aspiration pneumonia
- Asthma
- Chronic obstructive pulmonary disease

Skin diseases

Malignancies, leukemia, lymphoma

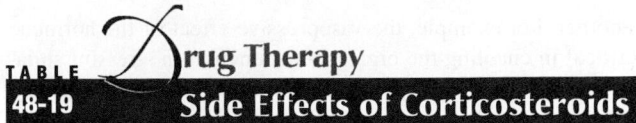

TABLE 48-19 Drug Therapy: Side Effects of Corticosteroids

- Hypokalemia may develop.
- Predisposition to peptic ulcer disease.
- Skeletal muscle atrophy and weakness occurs.
- Mood and behavior changes may be observed.
- Glucose intolerance predisposes to diabetes mellitus.
- Fat from extremities is redistributed to trunk and face.
- Hypocalcemia related to anti–vitamin D effect may occur.
- Healing is delayed. At increased risk for wound dehiscence.
- Susceptibility to infection is increased. Infection develops more rapidly and spreads more widely.
- Suppression of pituitary ACTH synthesis occurs. Corticosteroid deficiency is likely if hormones are withdrawn abruptly.
- Increased blood pressure occurs because of excess blood volume and potentiation of vasoconstrictor effects. Hypertension predisposes to heart failure.
- Protein depletion decreases bone formation, density, and strength. Predisposes to pathologic fractures, especially compression fractures of the vertebrae (osteoporosis).

ACTH, Adrenocorticotropic hormone.

ten leads to serious complications and side effects (Table 48-19). For this reason, corticosteroid therapy is not recommended for minor chronic conditions. Therapy should be reserved for diseases in which there is a risk of death or permanent loss of function and conditions in which short-term therapy is likely to produce remission or recovery. The potential benefits of treatment must always be weighed against the risks.

Effects of Corticosteroid Therapy

There are multiple effects of corticosteroid therapy. Although these actions can prove to be beneficial and therapeutic in some situations, they can also contribute to adverse effects as well. The expected effects of corticosteroid therapy include the following:

1. *Antiinflammatory action.* Corticosteroids decrease the number of circulating lymphocytes, monocytes, and eosinophils. They enhance the release of polymorphonuclear leukocytes from bone marrow, inhibit the accumulation of leukocytes at the site of inflammation, and inhibit the release of substances involved in the inflammatory response (e.g., kinins, prostaglandins, histamine) from the leukocytes. Therefore manifestations of inflammation, including redness, tenderness, heat, swelling, and local edema, are suppressed.

2. *Immunosuppression.* Corticosteroids cause atrophy of lymphoid tissue, suppress the cell-mediated immune responses, and decrease the production of antibodies.

3. *Maintenance of normal blood pressure.* Corticosteroids potentiate the vasoconstrictor effect of norepinephrine and act on the renal tubules to increase sodium reabsorption and enhance potassium and hydrogen excretion. Retention of sodium (and subsequently water) increases blood volume and helps maintain blood pressure. Mineralocorticoids have a direct effect on sodium reabsorption in the distal tubule of the kidney and as a result increase sodium and water retention.

4. *Carbohydrate and protein metabolism.* Corticosteroids antagonize the effects of insulin and can induce glucose intolerance by increasing hepatic glycogenolysis and insulin resistance. They also stimulate the breakdown of protein for gluconeogenesis, which can lead to skeletal muscle wasting. Although corticosteroids mobilize free fatty acids and redistribute fat in cushingoid patterns, the mechanism for this process is unknown.

Complications Associated with Corticosteroid Therapy

As mentioned previously, the effects of corticosteroids can prove to be beneficial or harmful based on the physiologic actions. A beneficial effect in one situation may be a harmful one in another. For example, the vasopressive effect of the hormone is critical in enabling the organism to function in stressful situations but can produce hypertension when used for drug therapy. Suppression of inflammation and the immune response may help save the lives of the victim of anaphylaxis and the transplant recipient, but it causes reactivation of latent tuberculosis and greatly reduces resistance to other infections. In addition, corticosteroids inhibit the antibody response to vaccines. Specific side effects related to corticosteroid therapy are listed in Table 48-19.

NURSING *and* COLLABORATIVE MANAGEMENT
CORTICOSTEROID THERAPY

Many patients receive corticosteroid therapy, in particular glucocorticoid therapy, for nonendocrine reasons (see Table 48-18). Thorough instruction is necessary to ensure patient compliance. When corticosteroids are used as nonreplacement therapies, they are taken once daily or once every other day. They should be taken early in the morning with food to decrease gastric irritation. Because exogenous corticosteroid administration may suppress endogenous ACTH and therefore endogenous cortisol (suppression is time and dose dependent), the danger of abrupt cessation of corticosteroid therapy must be emphasized to patients and significant others.

Because patients often receive corticosteroid treatment for prolonged periods of time (greater than 3 months), corticosteroid-induced osteoporosis is an important concern. Therapies to reduce the resorption of bone may include increased calcium intake, vitamin D supplementation, bisphosphonates (e.g., alendronate [Fosamax]), and institution of a low-impact exercise program. Further instruction and interventions to minimize the side effects and complications of corticosteroid therapy are shown in Table 48-20.

HYPERALDOSTERONISM
Etiology and Pathophysiology

Hyperaldosteronism is characterized by excessive aldosterone secretion. The main effects of aldosterone are sodium retention and potassium and hydrogen ion excretion. Thus the hallmark of this disease is hypertension with hypokalemic alkalosis. *Primary hyperaldosteronism* (PA) is most commonly caused by a small solitary aldosterone-producing adenoma of the adrenal zona glomerulosa. Occasionally multiple lesions are involved and are associated with adrenal hyperplasia. PA affects both genders equally and occurs most frequently between 30 and 50 years of age.[43] It is estimated that approximately 1 of every 200 cases of hypertension is caused by PA.[44] *Secondary hyperaldosteronism* occurs in response to a nonadrenal cause of elevated aldosterone levels such as renal artery stenosis, renin-secreting tumors, and chronic renal disease.

Clinical Manifestations

Elevated levels of aldosterone are associated with sodium retention and elimination of potassium. Sodium retention leads to hypernatremia, hypertension, and headache. Edema does not usually occur because the rate of sodium excretion increases, which prevents more severe sodium retention. The potassium wasting leads to hypokalemia, which causes generalized muscle weakness, fatigue, cardiac arrhythmias, glucose intolerance, and metabolic alkalosis that may lead to tetany.[43]

Diagnostic Studies

The diagnosis of hyperaldosteronism should be suspected in all hypertensive patients with hypokalemia who are not being treated with diuretics. PA is associated with elevated plasma aldosterone levels, elevated sodium levels, decreased serum potassium levels, and decreased plasma renin activity.[44] An IV saline infusion test is often performed. In this test, 2 L of normal saline is infused over 4 hours, with plasma aldosterone levels measured at the beginning and end of the infusion. If aldosterone levels fail to decrease (i.e., levels are >10 ng/dl [277 pmol/L]), the patient probably has hyperaldosteronism. Adenomas are localized by means of a CT scan. If a tumor is not found, plasma 18-hydroxycorticosterone is measured after overnight bed rest. A level >50 ng/dl (1387 pmol/L) indicates an adenoma.

NURSING *and* COLLABORATIVE MANAGEMENT
PRIMARY HYPERALDOSTERONISM

The preferred treatment for PA is surgical removal of the adrenal gland that has the adenoma (adrenalectomy). Although this surgery can be done as an open procedure, laparoscopic adrenalectomy is increasingly performed because of the benefits this minimally invasive surgery offers.[44] Before surgery, patients should be treated with a low-sodium diet, potassium-sparing diuretics (spironolactone [Aldactone], eplerenone [Inspra]), and antihypertensive agents to normalize serum potassium levels and blood pressure. Spironolactone and eplerenone block the binding of aldosterone to the mineralocorticoid receptor in the terminal distal tubules and collecting ducts of the kidney, thus increasing the excretion of sodium and water and retention of potassium.

TABLE 48-20

*P*atient & Family Teaching Guide
Corticosteroid Therapy

The nurse needs to teach the patient and family the following:
1. Plan a diet high in protein, calcium (at least 1500 mg per day), and potassium but low in fat and concentrated simple carbohydrates such as sugar, honey, syrups, and candy.
2. Identify measures to ensure adequate rest and sleep, such as daily naps and avoidance of caffeine late in the day.
3. Develop and maintain an exercise program to help maintain bone integrity.
4. Recognize edema and ways to restrict sodium intake to less than 2000 mg per day if edema occurs.
5. Monitor glucose levels and recognize symptoms and signs of hyperglycemia (e.g., polydipsia, polyuria, blurred vision) and glycosuria (glucose in the urine). The patient should be instructed to report hyperglycemic symptoms or capillary glucose levels greater than 180 mg/dl (10 mmol/L) or urine positive for glucose.
6. Notify health care provider if experiencing postprandial heartburn or epigastric pain that is not relieved by antacids.
7. See an eye specialist yearly to assess development of possible cataracts.
8. Use safety measures such as getting up slowly from bed or a chair and use good lighting to avoid accidental injury.
9. Maintain good hygiene practices and avoid contact with persons with colds or other contagious illnesses to avoid infection.

Oral potassium supplements and sodium restrictions are also necessary. Potassium supplementation and a potassium-sparing diuretic should not be started simultaneously because of the danger of hyperkalemia.

Patients with bilateral adrenal hyperplasia are treated with spironolactone; amiloride (Midamor), which is another potassium-sparing diuretic; or aminoglutethimide (Cytadren), which blocks aldosterone synthesis. Calcium channel blockers may also be used to control blood pressure. A new drug that is available for the treatment of hyperaldosteronism is eplerenone (Inspra). Eplerenone is the first agent of a new class of drugs known as selective aldosterone receptor antagonists.[45]

Nursing care includes careful assessment for signs of fluid and electrolyte balance (especially potassium) and cardiovascular status. Blood pressure should be monitored frequently before and after surgery because unilateral adrenalectomy is successful in controlling hypertension in only 50% of patients with adenoma. Patients receiving maintenance therapy with spironolactone or amiloride need instruction about the possible side effects of gynecomastia, impotence, and menstrual disorders, as well as knowledge about the signs and symptoms of hypokalemia and hyperkalemia. Patients should be taught how to monitor their own blood pressure and the need for frequent monitoring. The need for continued health supervision should be stressed.

Disorders of the Adrenal Medulla

PHEOCHROMOCYTOMA

Etiology and Pathophysiology

Pheochromocytoma is a rare condition characterized by a tumor of the adrenal medulla that produces excessive catecholamines (epinephrine, norepinephrine). Pheochromocytoma can occur at any age and in either gender, but it is found most commonly in young to middle-aged adults. In most cases affecting adults, the tumor is benign, encapsulated, unilateral, and solitary.[46] Occasionally bilateral tumors are found. The secretion of excessive catecholamines results in severe hypertension. If undiagnosed and untreated, pheochromocytoma may be fatal.

Clinical Manifestations

The most striking clinical features of pheochromocytoma include severe, episodic hypertension accompanied by the classic triad of severe, pounding headache, tachycardia, and profuse sweating. Attacks of episodic hypertension are due to sympathetic nervous system stimulation and are often accompanied by anxiety and palpitations. Attacks may be provoked by many medications, including antihypertensives, opioids, radiologic contrast media, and tricyclic antidepressants. The duration of the attacks may vary from a few minutes to several hours. Untreated, pheochromocytoma may lead to diabetes mellitus, cardiomyopathy, manifestations of uncontrolled hypertension, and death.

Diagnostic Studies

Although pheochromocytoma is associated with a number of symptoms, correct diagnosis is often missed. Pheochromocytoma is an uncommon cause of hypertension, accounting for only 0.1% of all cases of hypertension.[47] This condition should be considered in patients who do not respond to traditional hypertensive treatments.

The measurement of urinary metanephrines (catecholamine metabolites), usually done as a 24-hour urine collection, is the simplest and most reliable test. Values are elevated in at least 90% of persons with pheochromocytoma. Vanillylmandelic acid (VMA) may also be measured in a 24-hour urine sample. However, this test has more false negatives than urine metanephrines. Plasma catecholamines are also elevated. It is preferable to measure serum catecholamines during an "attack." CT scans and MRI are used for tumor localization.

NURSING *and* COLLABORATIVE MANAGEMENT
PHEOCHROMOCYTOMA

The primary treatment consists of surgical removal of the tumor. Before surgery the patient is hospitalized for treatment to correct cardiovascular complications to decrease the risk of surgery. Preoperatively, sympathetic blocking agents (e.g., phenoxybenzamine [Dibenzyline], prazosin [Minipress], terazosin [Hytrin], or doxazosin [Cardura]) are administered to reduce the blood pressure and alleviate other symptoms of catecholamine excess. Because this management may result in orthostatic hypotension, the patient must be advised to make postural changes cautiously. Calcium channel blockers may be used to treat the hypertension and to avoid problems with orthostatic hypotension in patients with preexisting cardiovascular disease.

Surgery is done via laparoscopic adrenalectomy or by open abdominal incision. Complete removal of the adrenal tumor cures the hypertension in the majority of individuals, but hypertension persists in approximately 10% to 30% of patients.[47] For these individuals, blood pressure management involves standard antihypertensive drug therapy. If surgery is not an option, metyrosine is used to diminish catecholamine production by the tumor and simplify chronic management.

Case finding is an important nursing function. Any patient with hypertension accompanied by symptoms of sympathoadrenal discharge should be referred to a health care provider for definitive diagnosis. An important part of the nursing assessment is observation of the patient for the classic triad of symptoms of pheochromocytoma (severe pounding headache, tachycardia, and profuse sweating). Blood pressure should be monitored immediately if the patient is experiencing an "attack." The nurse should be prepared to check blood pressure when any of the drugs that might precipitate an attack are given.

The nurse should attempt to make the patient with pheochromocytoma as comfortable as possible. All diagnostic samples should be collected appropriately. Capillary blood glucose levels should be monitored to assess for diabetes mellitus. Patients should be monitored closely if any medications are used that may precipitate an "attack." Patients need rest, nourishing food, and emotional support during this period. Preoperative and postoperative care is similar to that for any patient undergoing adrenalectomy except that blood pressure fluctuations from catecholamine excesses tend to be severe and must be carefully monitored. Because hypertension may persist even when the tumor is removed, the nurse should stress the importance of follow-up care and routine blood pressure monitoring. If metyrosine is being used, the patient should be instructed to rise slowly and hold onto a secure object, because this medication can cause orthostatic hypotension.

CRITICAL THINKING EXERCISES

Case Study
Graves' Disease

Patient Profile. Sally C., a 43-year-old white woman, was admitted to the hospital with a high fever. Following an endocrine workup, she was diagnosed as having Graves' disease.

Subjective Data
- Reports recent job loss because of inability to cope with job stress
- Reports symptoms including fatigue, unintentional weight loss, insomnia, palpitations, and heat intolerance

Objective Data
Physical Examination
- Has a fever of 104° F (40° C)
- Has blood pressure of 150/78, pulse of 118, and respiratory rate of 24
- Has hot, moist skin
- Has fine tremors of the hands
- Has 4+ deep tendon reflexes and muscle strength of 1 to 2

Collaborative Care
- Subtotal thyroidectomy planned for 2 months later
- Started on propylthiouracil (PTU) and propranolol (Inderal)

CRITICAL THINKING QUESTIONS
1. What is the etiology of the patient's symptoms?
2. What diagnostic studies were probably ordered? What would the results have been to establish the diagnosis of Graves' disease?
3. Why was surgery delayed?
4. What was the purpose of the drug therapy?
5. What are the patient's immediate learning needs and her learning needs preoperatively and postoperatively?
6. What are the nursing interventions for successful long-term management of this patient after the subtotal thyroidectomy?
7. Based on the assessment data presented, write one or more appropriate nursing diagnoses pertinent to this patient while hospitalized. Are there any collaborative problems?

Nursing Research Issues
1. Is sucking on hard candy or ice chips more effective in decreasing the subjective sensation of thirst in patients with SIADH?
2. What is the difference in the mental status of hypothyroid patients before and after thyroid replacement therapy?
3. What are the symptoms of infection in patients with Cushing syndrome?
4. Is a nurse-directed dosage adjustment more effective than a patient-directed dosage adjustment in preventing symptoms in the patient lacking endogenous cortisol who is exposed to stress?
5. Does regular exercise prevent bone loss in patients receiving glucocorticoid therapy?

REVIEW QUESTIONS

The number of the question corresponds to the same-numbered objective at the beginning of the chapter.

1. Following a hypophysectomy for treatment of acromegaly, a patient develops hypopituitarism. The nurse teaches the patient that
   a. hormone replacement with ACTH, TSH, FSH, and LH will be necessary.
   b. permanent ADH replacement will be needed if the postoperative diabetes insipidus does not reverse.
   c. frequent monitoring of blood and urine glucose is needed to identify the development of diabetes mellitus.
   d. the elimination of the source of excess growth hormone will reverse the physiologic effects of acromegaly.
2. A patient with a head injury develops SIADH. Symptoms the nurse would expect to find include
   a. edema.
   b. weight gain.
   c. urine specific gravity of 1.004.
   d. serum sodium of 140 mEq/L (140 mmol/L).
3. The health care provider prescribes levothyroxine for a patient with myxedema. Following teaching regarding this therapy, the nurse determines that further instruction is needed when the patient says,
   a. "I can expect to return to normal function with the use of this drug."
   b. "I can expect the medication dose to be increased every several weeks."
   c. "I will only need to take this medication until my symptoms are improved."
   d. "I will report any chest pain or difficulty breathing to the doctor right away."
4. Following thyroid surgery, the nurse suspects damage or removal of the parathyroid glands when the patient develops
   a. laryngeal stridor.
   b. muscle weakness.
   c. hoarseness and difficulty swallowing.
   d. hyperthermia and severe tachycardia.

Continued

REVIEW QUESTIONS—cont'd

5. An important nursing intervention when caring for a patient with Cushing syndrome is to
   a. restrict protein intake.
   b. observe for signs of hypotension.
   c. administer medication in equal doses.
   d. protect the patient from exposure to infection.

6. After an adrenalectomy for pheochromocytoma, the patient is most likely to experience
   a. hypokalemia.
   b. hyperglycemia.
   c. marked sodium and water retention.
   d. marked fluctuations in blood pressure.

7. To control the side effects of pharmacologic corticosteroid therapy, the nurse teaches the patient to
   a. increase calcium intake to 1500 mg per day.
   b. perform glucose monitoring for hypoglycemia.
   c. carry an emergency kit of hydrocortisone in case of severe stress.
   d. avoid abrupt position changes because of orthostatic hypotension.

8. The nurse teaches the patient that the best time to take corticosteroids for replacement purposes is
   a. once a day at bedtime.
   b. every other day on awakening.
   c. on arising and in the late afternoon.
   d. at consistent intervals every 6 to 8 hours.

REFERENCES

1. Sachse D: Acromegaly: early recognition of this rare multisystem disorder results in considerable benefit to patients, *Am J Nurs* 101:69, 2001.
2. Dostalova S et al: Craniofacial abnormalities and their relevance for sleep apnea syndrome aetiopathogenesis in acromegaly, *Eur J Endocrinol* 144:491, 2001.
3. Quabbe HJ, Plockinger U: Somatotroph adenomas. In Thapar K et al, editors: *Diagnosis and management of pituitary tumors,* Totowa, NJ, 2001, Humana Press.
4. Laws ER, Vance ML, Thapar K: Pituitary surgery for the management of acromegaly, *Horm Res* 53(suppl 3):71, 2000.
5. Darzy DH, Shalet SM: Evolving therapeutic strategies for acromegaly, *J Endocrinol Invest* 24:468, 2001.
6. Zhang N et al: Radiosurgery for growth hormone-producing pituitary adenomas, *J Neurosurg* 93(suppl 3):6, 2000.
7. van der Lely AJ et al: Long-term treatment of acromegaly with pegvisomant, a growth hormone receptor antagonist, *Lancet* 358:1754, 2001.
8. Abbound CF, Ebersold MJ: Prolactinomas. In Thaper K et al: *Diagnosis and management of pituitary tumors,* Totowa, NJ, 2001, Humana Press.
9. Pinzone JJ: Hypopituitarism. In Becker KL, editor: *Principles and practice of endocrinology and metabolism,* ed 3, Philadelphia, 2001, Lippincott Williams & Wilkins.
10. Wuster C: Fracture rates in patients with growth hormone deficiency, *Horm Res* 54(suppl 1):31, 2000.
11. Ehrnborg C et al: Cost of illness in adult patients with hypopituitarism, *Pharmacoeconomics* 17:621, 2000.
12. Anpalahan M: Chronic idopathic hyponatremia in older people due to syndrome of inappropriate antidiuretic hormone secretion (SIADH) possibly related to aging, *J Am Geriatr Soc* 49:788, 2001.
13. Abrams C: ADH-associated pathologies, *Medical Laboratory Observer* 32:24, 2000.
14. Terpstra TL, Terpstra TL: Syndrome of inappropriate antidiuretic hormone secretion: recognition and management, *Medsurg Nurs* 9:61, 2000.
15. Bendz H, Aurell M: Drug-induced diabetes insipidus: incidence, prevention and management, *Drug Safety* 21:449, 1999.
16. Bichet DG: Nephrogenic diabetes insipidus, *Am J Med* 105:431, 1998.
17. Nickolaus MJ: Diabetes insipidus: a current perspective, *Crit Care Nurse* 19:18, 1999.
18. Magaldi AJ: New insights into the paradoxical effects of thiazides in diabetes insipidus therapy, *Nephrol Dial Transplant* 15:1903, 2000.
19. Trotto NE: Hypothyroidsm, hyperthyroidism, hyperparathyroidism, *Patient Care* 33:186, 1999.
20. Bailes BK: Hyperthyroidism in elderly patients, *AORN J* 69:254, 1999.
21. Larson J, Anderson EH, Koslawy M: Thyroid disease: a review for primary care, *J Am Acad Nurse Pract* 12:226, 2000.
22. Clement B: Thyrotoxicosis, *Semin Periop Nurs* 7:152, 1998.
23. Burman KD: Hyperthyroidism. In Becker KL, editor: *Principles and practice of endocrinology and metabolism,* ed 3, Philadelphia, 2001, Lippincott Williams & Wilkins.
24. Dahlen R: Managing patients with acute thyrotoxicosis, *Crit Care Nurse* 22:62, 2002.
25. Rignel MD: Management of hypothyroidism and hyperthyroidism in the intensive care unit, *Crit Care Clin* 17:59, 2001.
26. American Cancer Society: CA facts and figures 2002. Available at *www.cancer.org* (accessed Feb 26 2003)
27. Weber AL, Randolph G, Askoy FG: The thyroid and parathyroid glands: CT and MR imaging and correlation with pathology and clinical findings, *Radiol Clin North Am* 38:1005, 2000.
28. Canaris GJ et al: The Colorado thyroid disease prevalence study, *Arch Intern Med* 160:526, 2000.
29. Elliott B: Diagnosing and treating hypothyroidism, *Nurse Pract* 25:92, 2000.
30. American College of Physicians: Screening for thyroid disease: clinical guide part 1, *Ann Intern Med* 129:141, 1998.
31. Helfand M, Redfern CC: Screening for thyroid disease: clinical guide part 2, *Ann Intern Med* 129:144, 1998.
32. Silverberg SJ: Natural history of primary hyperparathyroidism, *Endocrinol Metab Clin North Am* 29:451, 2000.
33. National Institutes of Health consensus development conference statement on primary hyperparathyroidism, *J Bone Miner Res* 6(suppl 2):S9, 1991.
34. Strewler GJ: Medical approaches to primary hyperparathyroidism, *Endocrinol Metab Clin North Am* 29:523, 2000.
35. Weigel RJ: Nonoperative management of hyperparathyroidism: present and future, *Curr Opin Oncol* 13:33, 2001.
36. Dacey MJ: Hypomagnesemic disorders, *Crit Care Clin* 17:155, 2001.
37. DeBeur SM, Streeten EA, Levine MA: Hypoparathyroidism and other causes of hypocalcemia. In Becker KL, editor: *Principles and practice of endocrinology and metabolism,* ed 3, Philadelphia, 2001, Lippincott Williams & Wilkins.

38. Williams M: Disorders of the adrenal gland, *Semin Periop Nurs* 7:179, 1998.
39. Gill IS: The case for laparoscopic adrenalectomy, *J Urol* 166:429, 2001.
40. Gotch P: Cushing's syndrome from the patient's perspective, *Endocrinol Metab Clin North Am* 23:607, 1994.
41. Leuken K: Clinical manifestations and management of Addison's disease, *J Am Acad Nurse Pract* 11:151, 1999.
42. Oelkers W, Diederich S, Bahr V: Therapeutic strategies in adrenal insufficiency, *Ann Endocrinol* 62:212, 2001.
43. Gill JR: Hyperaldosteronism. In Becker KL, editor: *Principles and practice of endocrinology and metabolism,* ed 3, Philadelphia, 2001, Lippincott Williams & Wilkins.
44. Rossi H, Kim A, Prinz R: Primary hyperaldosteronism in the era of laparoscopic adrenalectomy, *Am Surg* 68:253, 2002.
45. Pitt OL, Young WF, MacDonald TM: A review of the medical treatment of primary aldosteronism, *J Hypertens* 19:353, 2001.
46. Landsberg L, Young JB: Pheochromocytoma. In *Harrison's online,* 2002, McGraw-Hill. Available at *www.harrisonsonline.com* (accessed Feb 26, 2003)
47. Lo CY et al: Adrenal pheochromocytoma remains a frequently overlooked diagnosis, *Am J Surg* 179:212, 2000.

RESOURCES

American Association of Clinical Endocrinologists (AACE)
1000 Riverside Avenue, Suite 205
Jacksonville, FL 32204
904-353-7878
Fax: 904-353-8185
www.aace.com

American Society for Bone and Mineral Research
2025 M Street, NW, Suite 800
Washington, DC 20036-3309
202-367-1161
Fax: 202-367-2161
www.asbmr.org

American Thyroid Association
6066 Leesburg Pike, Suite 650
Falls Church, VA 22041
703-998-8890
Fax: 703-998-8893
www.thyroid.org

Endocrine Nurses Society (ENS)
4350 East West Highway, Suite 500
Bethesda, MD 20814-4410
301-941-0249
Fax: 301-941-0259
www.endo-nurses.org

Endocrine Society
4350 East West Highway, Suite 500
Bethesda, MD 20814-4426
301-941-0200
Fax: 301-941-0259
www.endo-society.org

National Institute of Diabetes and Digestive and Kidney Diseases (Addison's Disease)
2 Information Way
Bethesda, MD 20892-3570
www.niddk.nih.gov

Pituitary Tumor Network Association
P.O. Box 1958
Thousand Oaks, CA 91358
805-499-9973
Fax: 805-480-0633
www.pituitary.com

Thyroid Federation International
96 Mack Street
Kingston, ON
K7L 1N9 Canada
613-544-8364
Fax: 613-544-9731
www.thyroid-fed.org

For additional Internet resources, see the website for this book at *http://evolve.elsevier.com/Lewis/medsurg/.*

CHAPTER *49*

NURSING ASSESSMENT
Reproductive System

Jean Foret Giddens

LEARNING OBJECTIVES

1. Describe the structures and functions of the male and female reproductive systems.
2. Explain the functions of the major hormones essential for the structure and function of the reproductive systems.
3. Describe the physiologic and psychologic changes of a man and of a woman during the stages of sexual response.
4. Describe age-related changes in the reproductive systems and differences in assessment findings.
5. Identify significant subjective and objective data related to the reproductive systems and information about sexual function that should be obtained from a patient.
6. Describe noninvasive techniques used in the physical assessment of the reproductive systems.
7. Differentiate normal from abnormal findings obtained from a physical assessment of the reproductive systems.
8. Describe the purpose, significance of results, and nursing responsibilities related to diagnostic studies of the reproductive systems.

KEY TERMS

amenorrhea, p. 1345
clitoris, p. 1343
ductus deferens, p. 1339
dyspareunia, p. 1350
epididymis, p. 1339
gonads, p. 1339

menarche, p. 1344
menopause, p. 1345
menstrual cycle, p. 1345
mons pubis, p. 1342
nulliparous, p. 1341
spermatogenesis, p. 1339

STRUCTURES AND FUNCTIONS OF THE MALE AND FEMALE REPRODUCTIVE SYSTEMS

The reproductive system of both males and females consists of primary (or essential) organs and secondary (or accessory) organs. The primary reproductive organs are referred to as **gonads.** The female gonads are the ovaries; the male gonads are the testes. The primary responsibility of the gonads is secretion of hormones and production of gametes (ova and sperm). Secondary or accessory organs are responsible for transporting and nourishing the ova and sperm, as well as preserving and protecting the fertilized eggs.

Male Reproductive System

The three primary roles of the male reproductive system are (1) production and transportation of sperm, (2) deposit of sperm in the female reproductive tract, and (3) secretion of hormones. The primary reproductive organs in the male are the testes. Secondary reproductive organs include ducts (epididymis, ductus deferens, ejaculatory duct, and urethra), sex glands (prostate gland, Cowper's glands, and seminal vesicles), and the external genitalia (scrotum and penis)[1] (Fig. 49-1).

Reviewed by Susan K. Goebel, RNC, MS, WHNP, SANE, Assistant Professor of Nursing, Mesa State College, Grand Junction, Colo.; Nurse Practitioner, Mesa County Health Department.

Testes. The paired testes are ovoid, smooth, firm organs measuring 3.5 to 5.5 cm long and 2 to 3 cm wide. They are within the scrotum—a pouchlike structure composed of a thin, loose outer layer of skin over a tough connective tissue layer. Within the testes coiled structures known as seminiferous tubules form *spermatozoa* (immature sperm). The process of sperm production is called **spermatogenesis.** Interstitial cells of the testes lie between the seminiferous tubules and produce the male sex hormone testosterone.

Ducts. Sperm formed in the seminiferous tubules move through a series of ducts. These ducts transport the sperm from the testes to the outside of the body. As sperm exit the testes they enter and pass through the epididymis, ductus deferens, ejaculatory duct, and urethra.

The **epididymis** is a comma-shaped structure located on the top and behind each testis inside the scrotum (Figs. 49-1 and 49-2). It is a very long, tightly coiled structure that measures about 20 feet in length.[1] The epididymis transports the sperm as they mature. Sperm exit the epididymis through a long, thick tube known as the ductus deferens.

The **ductus deferens** (also known as the *vas deferens*) is continuous with the epididymis within the scrotal sac. It travels upward through the scrotum and continues through the inguinal ring into the abdominal cavity. The spermatic cord is a connective tissue sheath that encloses the ductus deferens, arteries, veins, nerves, and lymph vessels as it ascends up through the inguinal canal (see Fig. 49-2). In the abdominal cavity, the ductus deferens travels up, over, and behind the bladder. Behind the bladder the ductus deferens joins the seminal vesicle to form the ejaculatory duct (see Fig. 49-1).

The ejaculatory duct passes downward through the prostate gland, connecting with the urethra. The urethra extends from the bladder, through the prostate, and ends in a slitlike opening (the meatus) on the ventral side of the *glans,* the tip of the penis. During the process of ejaculation, sperm travels through the urethra and out of the body.

Glands. The seminal vesicles, prostate gland, and Cowper's (bulbourethral) glands are the accessory glands of the male repro-

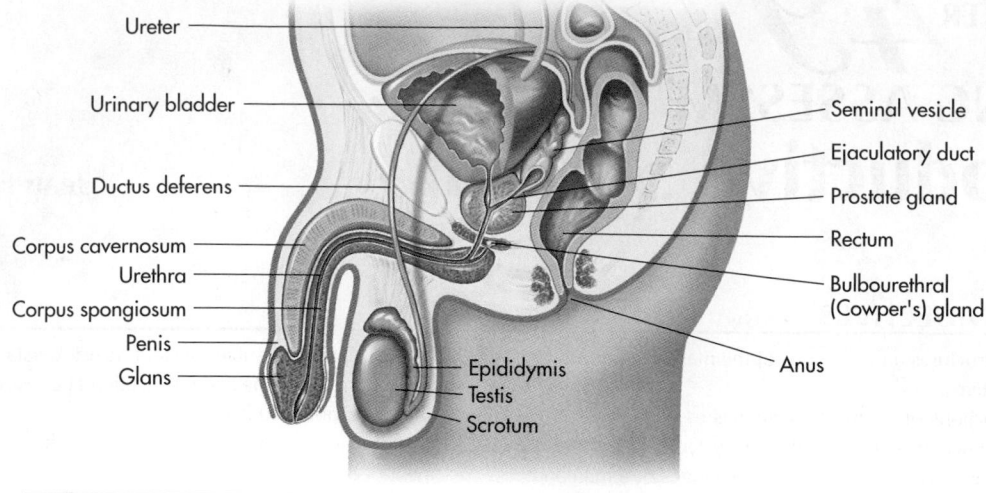

FIG. 49-1 External and internal male sex organs.

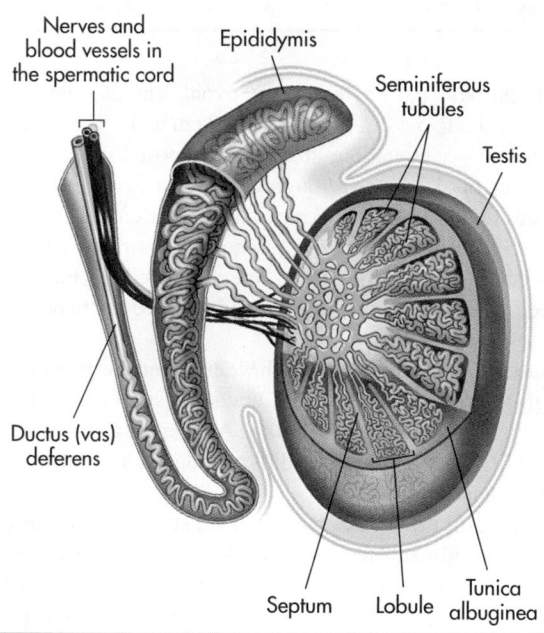

FIG. 49-2 Seminiferous tubules, testis, epididymis, and ductus (vas) deferens.

ductive system. These glands produce and secrete seminal fluid (semen), which surrounds the sperm and forms the *ejaculate*.

The seminal vesicles lie just behind the bladder and between the rectum and the bladder. The ducts of the seminal vesicles fuse with the ductus deferens to form the ejaculatory ducts that enter the prostate gland. The prostate gland lies underneath the bladder. Its posterior surface approximates the rectal wall. The prostate normally measures 2 cm wide and 3 cm long and is divided into the right and left lateral lobes and an anteroposterior median lobe. Cowper's glands lie on each side of the urethra and slightly posterior to it, just below the prostate. The ducts of these glands enter directly into the urethra.

The secretion from the seminal vesicles and prostate makes up most of the fluid in the ejaculate. By comparison, the seminal vesicles and Cowper's glands contribute a minimum amount of fluid to the ejaculate. These various secretions serve as a medium

for the transport of sperm and create an alkaline, nutritious environment that promotes sperm motility and survival.

External Genitalia. The external genitalia consist of the penis and the scrotum. The penis consists of a shaft, and the tip is known as the glans. The glans is covered by a fold of skin, the prepuce (or foreskin), that forms at the junction of the glans and the shaft of the penis. In circumcised men the prepuce has been removed. The broadened segment of the glans at the junction is the corona. The shaft of the penis consists of erectile tissue composed of the corpus cavernosum, the corpus spongiosum, the fibrous sheath that encases the erectile tissue, and the urethra. The skin covering the penis is thin, loose, and essentially hairless.

Female Reproductive System

The three primary roles of the female reproductive system are (1) production of ova (eggs), (2) secretion of hormones, and (3) protection and facilitation of the development of the fetus in a pregnant female. Like the male, the female has primary and secondary reproductive organs. The primary reproductive organs in the female are the paired ovaries. Secondary reproductive organs include ducts (fallopian tubes), the uterus, the vagina, sex glands (Bartholin's glands and breasts), and the external genitalia (vulva).

Pelvic Organs

Ovaries. The ovaries are usually located on either side of the uterus, just behind and below the fallopian (uterine) tubes (Figs. 49-3 and 49-4). The ovaries are firm and solid, approximately 1.5 cm wide, and 3 cm long. Their functions include *ovulation,* as well as secretion of the two major reproductive hormones, estrogen and progesterone. The outer zone of the ovary contains follicles with germ cells, or *oocytes.* Each follicle contains a primordial (immature) oocyte surrounded by granulosa and theca cells. These two layers protect and nourish the oocyte until the follicle reaches maturity and ovulation occurs. However, not all follicles reach maturity. In a process termed *atresia,* most of the primordial follicles become smaller and are reabsorbed by the body; thus the number of follicles declines from 2 million to 4 million at birth to approximately 300,000 to 400,000 at menarche. This number continues to de-

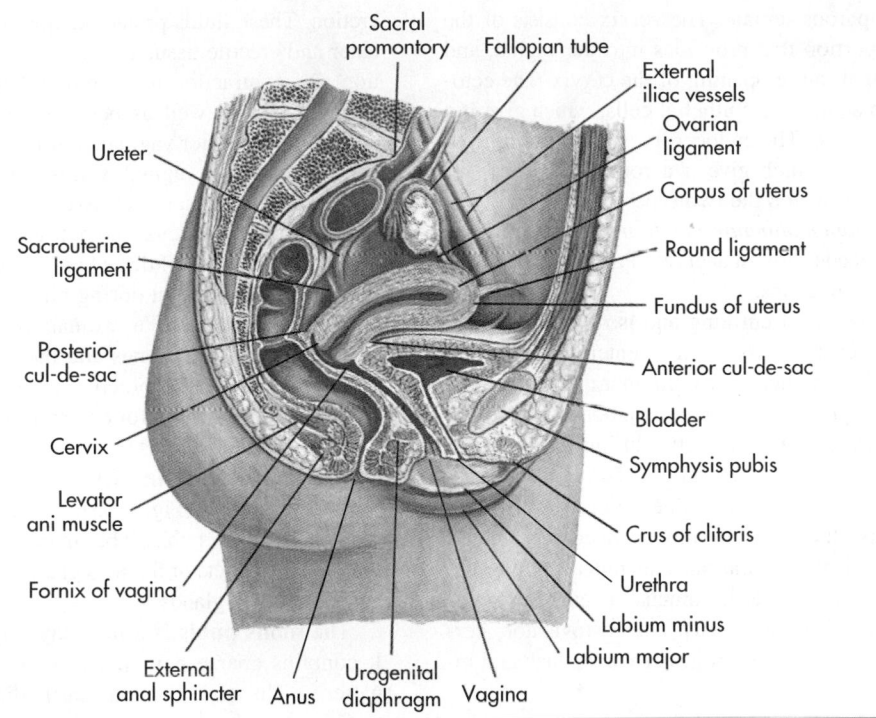

FIG. 49-3 Female reproductive tract and related organs.

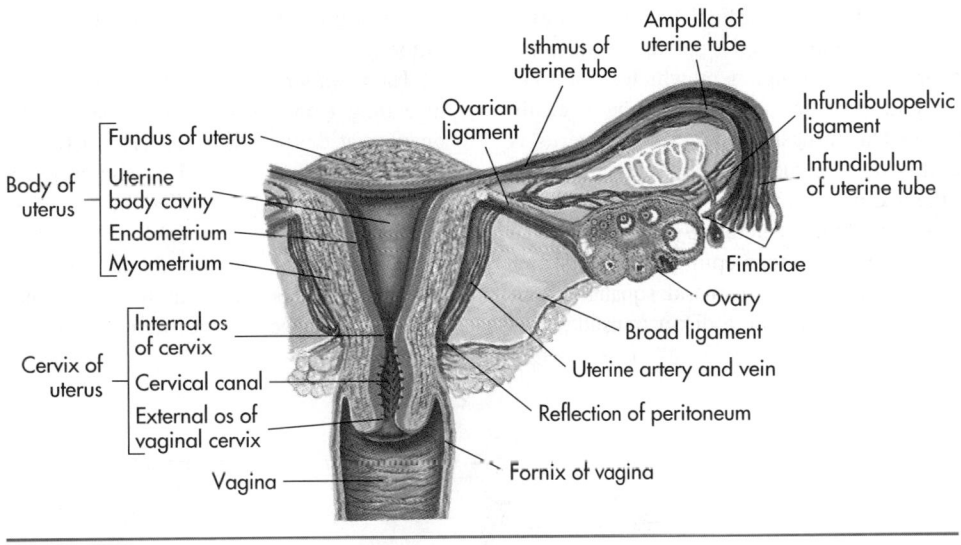

FIG. 49-4 Female reproductive tract: anterior view.

crease throughout a woman's reproductive years. Fewer than 500 oocytes are actually released by ovulation during the reproductive years of the normal healthy woman.

Fallopian tubes. Normally, each month during a woman's reproductive years, one ovarian follicle reaches maturity, and the ovum is ovulated, or expelled, from the ovary through the stimulus of the gonadotropic hormones, follicle-stimulating hormone (FSH) and luteinizing hormone (LH). The ovum then travels up a fallopian tube where fertilization by sperm may occur, if they are present. An ovum can be fertilized up to 72 hours after its release.

The distal ends of the fallopian tubes consist of fingerlike projections called *fimbriae* that "massage" the ovaries at ovulation to help extract the mature ovum. The tubes, which average 4.8 inches (12 cm) in length, extend from the fimbriae to the superior lateral borders of the uterus. Fertilization usually takes place within the outer one third of the fallopian tubes.

Uterus. The uterus is a pear-shaped, hollow, muscular organ (see Figs. 49-3 and 49-4). It is located between the bladder and the rectum. In the mature **nulliparous** (never pregnant) female, the uterus is approximately 6 cm long and 4 cm wide. The uterine walls consist of an outer serosal layer, the perimetrium; a middle muscular layer, the myometrium; and an inner mucosal layer, the endometrium.

The uterus consists of the fundus, body (or corpus), and cervix (see Fig. 49-4). The body makes up about 80% of the uterus and connects with the cervix at the isthmus, or neck. The cervix is the lower portion of the uterus that projects into the anterior wall of the vaginal canal. It makes up about 15% to 20% of the uterus in the nulliparous female. The cervix consists of the *ectocervix,* the outer portion that protrudes into the vagina, and the *endocervix,* the canal in the opening of the cervix. The ectocervix is covered with squamous epithelial cells, which give it a smooth, pinkish appearance. The endocervix contains a lining of columnar epithelial cells, which give it a rough, reddened appearance. The junction at which the two types of epithelial cells meet is termed the *squamocolumnar junction* and contains the optimal types of cells needed for an accurate Papanicolaou (Pap) smear to screen for malignancies.

The cervical canal is 2 to 4 cm long and is relatively tightly closed. The cervix, however, allows sperm to enter the uterus and also allows menses to be expelled. The columnar epithelium, under hormonal influence, provides elasticity at labor for the cervix to stretch to allow for the passage of a fetus during the birth process. The entrance of sperm into the uterus is facilitated by mucus produced by the cervix under the influence of estrogen. Under normal conditions, the cervical mucus becomes watery, stretchy, and more abundant at ovulation. This mucus, referred to as *spinnbarkeit,* is considered "fertile mucus" because it facilitates the passage of sperm into the uterus. The postovulatory cervical mucus, under the influence of progesterone, is thick and inhibits sperm passage.

The anterior and posterior peritoneal covering of the uterus is called the *broad ligament.* It separates the uterus from the bladder and the rectum but does not provide support for the uterus or the *adnexa* (ovaries and tubes). The cardinal ligaments, which extend from the isthmus of the uterus to the pelvic wall, also offer only minimal support. The round ligament, which extends anteriorly to the labia majora, provides some support but is easily weakened by pregnancy. The firmest support for the uterus is provided by the uterine sacral ligaments, which pull the uterus back and away from the vaginal orifice.

Vagina. The vagina is a tubular structure 3 to 4 inches (8 to 10 cm) long that is lined with squamous epithelium. The secretions of the vagina consist of cervical mucus, desquamated epithelium, and, during sexual stimulation, a direct transudate secretion. These fluids protect against vaginal infection. The muscular and erectile tissue of the vaginal walls allows enough dilation and contraction to accommodate the passage of the fetus during labor, as well as penetration of the penis during intercourse. The anterior vaginal wall lies along the urethra and bladder. The posterior vaginal wall is adjacent to the rectum.

Pelvis. The female pelvis consists of four bones (two hipbones, sacrum, coccyx) held together by several strong ligaments. The sections of these bones that lie below the iliopectineal line are very important during birth and are often a factor determining the ability of a woman to deliver a child vaginally. Knowledge of these bones and the landmarks that they form in the pelvis allows the practitioner to estimate pelvic measurements and the potential for a woman's pelvis to accommodate the birth of a full-term fetus.

External Genitalia. The external portion of the female reproductive system (Fig. 49-5), commonly called the *vulva,* consists of the mons pubis, labia majora, labia minora, clitoris, urethral meatus, ducts of Skene's glands, vaginal introitus (opening), and Bartholin's glands.

The **mons pubis** is a fatty layer lying over the pubic bone. It contains coarse hair that lies in an upside-down triangular pattern. (The male hair pattern is diamond shaped.) The labia majora are folds of adipose tissue that form the outer borders of the vulva. These hair-covered folds contain sweat glands and sebaceous glands. The hairless labia minora form the borders of the vaginal orifice and extend anteriorly to enclose the clitoris.[2]

The *vestibule* is a boat-shaped fossa between the labia minora, extending from the clitoris at the anterior end to the vaginal opening at the posterior end. The perineum is the area between the vagina and the anus. The vaginal introitus is surrounded by thin membranous tissue called the *hymen.* In the adult female, the hymen usually appears as folds or hymenal tags and separates the external genitalia from the vagina. Although all females have this structure, there is wide anatomic variation in its morphology. At the posterior aspect of the vagina, a tense band of mucous mem-

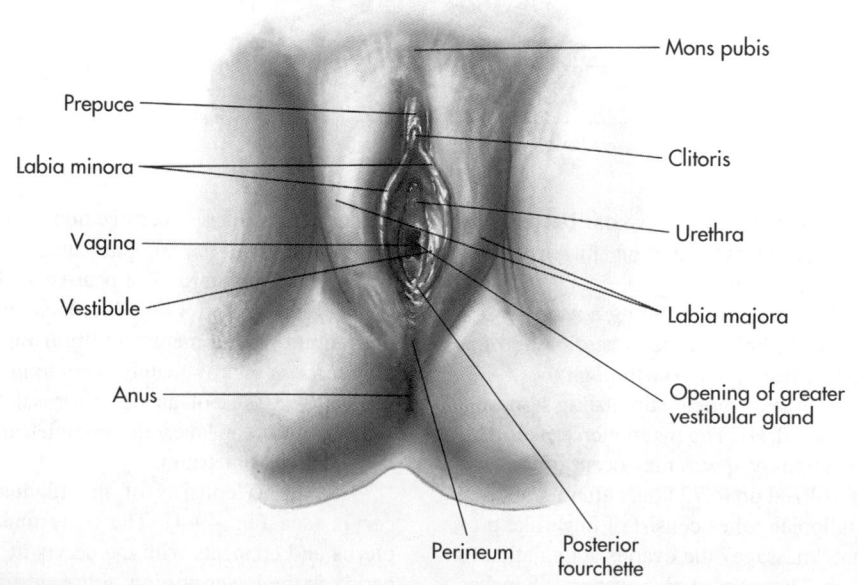

Prepuce

Labia minora

Vagina

Vestibule

Anus

Mons pubis

Clitoris

Urethra

Labia majora

Opening of greater vestibular gland

Perineum   Posterior fourchette

FIG. 49-5 External female genitalia.

brane connecting the posterior ends of the labia minora is referred to as the *posterior fourchette.*

The **clitoris** is erectile tissue that becomes engorged during sexual excitation. It lies anterior to the urethral meatus and the vaginal orifice and is usually covered by the prepuce, or hood.[2] Clitoral stimulation is an important part of sexual activity for many women.

Ducts of the Skene's glands lie alongside the urinary meatus and are thought to help lubricate the urinary meatus.[3] The Bartholin's glands, located at the posterior and lateral aspects of the vaginal orifice, secrete a thin, mucoid material believed to contribute slightly to lubrication during sexual intercourse. These glands are not usually palpable unless sebaceous-like cysts form or in the presence of an infection, such as a sexually transmitted disease.

Breasts. The breasts are a secondary sex characteristic that develops during puberty in response to estrogen and progesterone. Cyclic hormonal changes lead to regular changes in breast tissue to prepare it for lactation when fertilization and pregnancy occur. The breasts are also considered a major organ of sexual stimulation and response in some cultures.

The breasts extend from the second to the sixth ribs, with the tail reaching the axilla (Fig. 49-6). The fully mature breast is dome shaped and contains a pigmented center termed the *areola.* The areolar region contains Montgomery's tubercles, which are similar to sebaceous glands and assist in lubricating the nipple. During lactation, the alveoli, or acini, secrete milk. The milk then flows into a ductal system and is transported to the lactiferous sinuses. The nipple contains 15 to 20 tiny openings through which the milk flows during breastfeeding. The fibrous and fatty tissue that supports and separates the channels of the mammary duct system is primarily responsible for the varying sizes and shapes of the breasts in different individuals.

The breast's rich lymphatic network drains primarily into the axillary, infraclavicular, and supraclavicular channels (Fig. 49-7). Superficial lymph nodes are located in the axilla and are accessible to

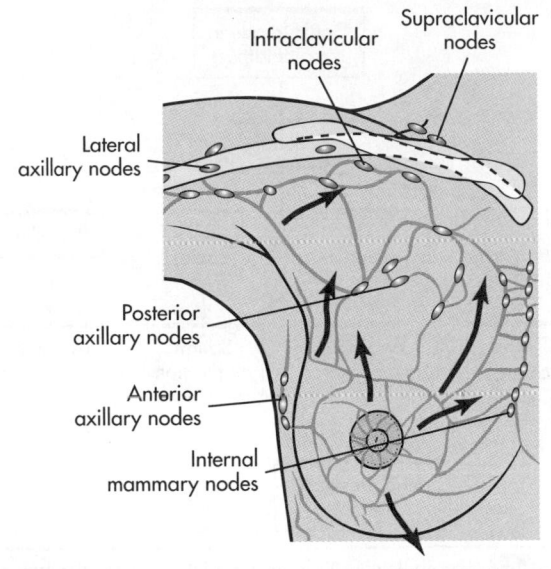

FIG. 49-7 Lymphatic drainage of the breast. *Arrows* indicate direction of drainage.

examination. This system is often responsible for the metastasis of a malignant tumor from the breast to other parts of the body.

Neuroendocrine Regulation of the Reproductive System

The hypothalamus, the pituitary gland, and the gonads secrete numerous hormones (Fig. 49-8). (Endocrine hormones are discussed in Chapter 46.) These hormones regulate the processes of ovulation, spermatogenesis (formation of sperm), and fertilization and the formation and function of the secondary sex characteristics. The amounts of hormones secreted by the anterior pituitary gland cause cyclic changes in the ovaries. The hypothalamus

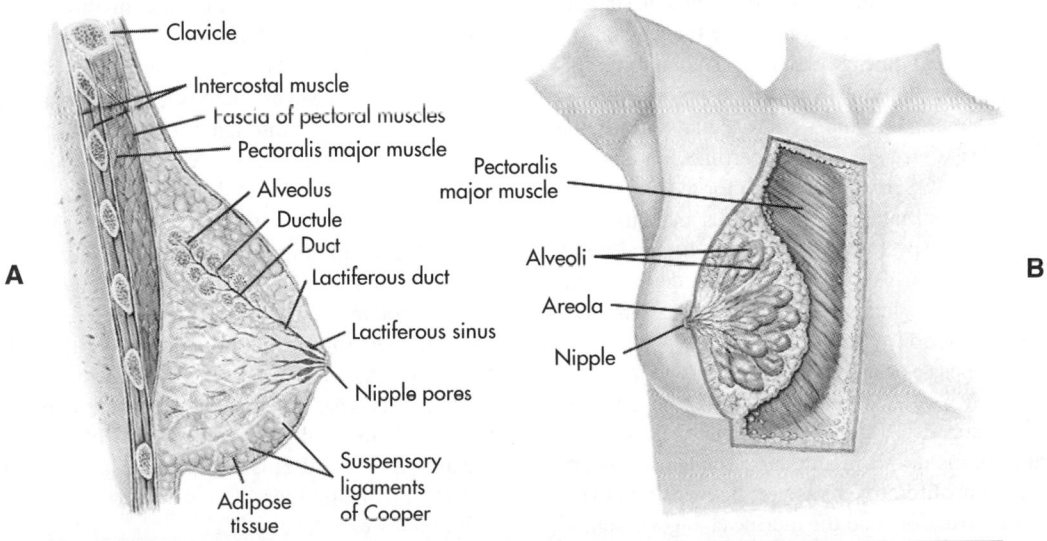

FIG. 49-6 The female breast. **A,** Sagittal section of a lactating breast. Notice how the glandular structures are anchored to the overlying skin and to the pectoral muscle by suspensory ligaments of Cooper. Each lobule of glandular tissues is drained by a lactiferous duct that eventually opens through the nipple. **B,** Anterior view of a lactating breast. In nonlactating breasts, the glandular tissue is much less prominent with adipose tissue making up most of each breast.

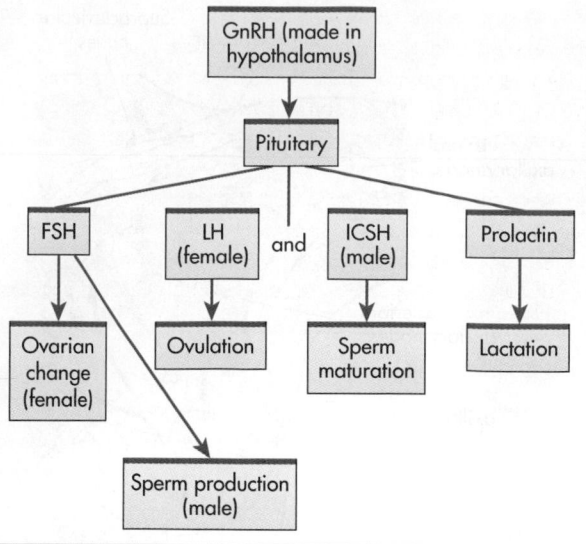

FIG. 49-8 Hypothalamic-pituitary-gonadal axis. Only the major pituitary hormone actions are depicted. *FSH,* Follicle-stimulating hormone; *GnRH,* gonadotropin-releasing hormone; *ICSH,* interstitial cell–stimulating hormone; *LH,* luteinizing hormone.

TABLE 49-1	**Gonadal Feedback Mechanisms**

Negative Feedback

↓ Estrogen → ↑ GnRH → ↑ FSH → ↑ Estrogen
(hypothalamus)   (pituitary)   (ovaries)

Positive Feedback

↑ Estrogen → ↑ GnRH → ↑ LH
(hypothalamus)   (pituitary)

Testes (Negative Feedback)

↓ Testosterone → ↑ GnRH → ↑ FSH → ↑ Testosterone
(hypothalamus)   and   (testes)
ICSH
(pituitary)

FSH, Follicle-stimulating hormone; *GnRH,* gonadotropin-releasing hormone; *ICSH,* interstitial cell–stimulating hormone; *LH,* luteinizing hormone.

secretes gonadotropin-releasing hormone (GnRH), which stimulates the pituitary gland to secrete its hormones, including FSH and LH. LH in males is sometimes called interstitial cell–stimulating hormone (ICSH). The gonadal hormones are estrogen, progesterone, and testosterone.

In women, FSH production by the anterior pituitary stimulates the growth and maturity of the ovarian follicles necessary for ovulation. The mature follicle produces estrogen, which in turn suppresses the release of FSH. Another hormone, inhibin, is also secreted by the ovarian follicle and inhibits both GnRH and FSH secretion. In men, FSH stimulates the seminiferous tubules to produce sperm.

LH contributes to the ovulatory process because it causes follicles to complete maturation and undergo ovulation. It also causes the development of a ruptured follicle, or the area on the ovum where the ovum exited during ovulation. The ruptured follicle develops into a corpus luteum from which progesterone is secreted. Progesterone maintains the rich vascular state of the uterus (secretory phase) in preparation for fertilization and implantation. In men, LH or ICSH is responsible for the production of testosterone by the interstitial cells of the testes and thus is essential for the full maturation of sperm. Prolactin has no known function in men. In women, prolactin stimulates the development and growth of the mammary glands. During lactation, it initiates and maintains milk production.

The gonadal hormones, estrogen and progesterone, are produced by the ovaries in women. Small amounts of an estrogen precursor are also produced in the adrenal cortices. Estrogen is essential to the development and maintenance of the secondary sex characteristics, the proliferative phase of the menstrual cycle immediately after menstruation, and the uterine changes essential to pregnancy. The role and importance of estrogen in men are not well understood. In men, estrogen is produced predominantly in the adrenal cortex.

Progesterone plays a major role in the menstrual cycle but most specifically in the secretory phase. Like estrogen, progesterone is involved in the bodily changes associated with pregnancy. Adequate progesterone is necessary to maintain an implanted egg.

The major gonadal hormone of men, testosterone, is produced by the testes. Testosterone is responsible for the development and maintenance of secondary sex characteristics, as well as for adequate spermatogenesis. Androgens are produced in females by the adrenal glands and ovaries in small amounts.

The circulating levels of gonadal hormones are controlled primarily by a negative feedback process. Receptors within the hypothalamus and pituitary are sensitive to the circulating blood levels of the hormones (Table 49-1). Increased levels of hormones stimulate a hypothalamic response to decrease the high circulating levels. Likewise, low circulating levels provoke a hypothalamic response that increases the low circulating levels. For example, if the circulating level of testosterone in men is low, the hypothalamus is stimulated to secrete GnRH. This stimulates the anterior pituitary to secrete greater amounts of FSH and ICSH, which in turn causes an increase in the production of testosterone. The high levels of testosterone then stimulate a decrease in the production of GnRH and thus of FSH and ICSH.

In women, however, there is a slight variation. The circulating levels are controlled through a combination of both a negative and a positive feedback system. A negative feedback control mechanism exists similar to that described previously. When circulating estrogen levels are low, the hypothalamus is stimulated to increase its production of GnRH. GnRH stimulates the pituitary to secrete greater amounts of FSH and LH, resulting in higher levels of estrogen production by the ovaries. Reciprocally higher levels of circulating estrogen result in a decreasing secretion of GnRH and thus a decrease in the secretion of FSH by the pituitary.

There is also a positive feedback control mechanism in women. Thus, with increasing levels of circulating estrogen, a greater level of GnRH is produced, resulting in an increased level of LH from the pituitary. Likewise, lowered levels of estrogen result in a lowered level of LH.

Menarche

Menarche is the first episode of menstrual bleeding, indicating that a female has reached puberty. This usually occurs at approximately 12 to 13 years of age, although normal onset can be as early as 10 years of age in some individuals.[4] As puberty approaches, there are changes associated with the elevated rate of estrogen and progesterone secretion by the ovaries. These changes include the development of breast buds and pubic hair, and later the development of axillary hair. During this time, there is a decrease in the sensitivity of the hypothalamic-pituitary axis that allows for increased secretion of FSH and LH and a resultant increase in estrogen. It is during this time that the adult pattern of gonadotropin secretion occurs, resulting in the menstrual cycle. Menstrual cycles are often irregular for the first 1 to 2 years following menarche because of *anovulatory cycles* (cycles without ovulation).[4]

Menstrual Cycle

The major functions of the ovaries are ovulation and the secretion of hormones. These functions are accomplished during the normal **menstrual cycle,** a monthly process mediated by the hormonal activity of the hypothalamus, pituitary gland, and ovaries. Menstruation occurs during each month in which an egg is not fertilized (Fig. 49-9). The endometrial cycle is divided into three phases labeled in relation to uterine and ovarian changes: (1) the *proliferative* or *follicular phase,* (2) the *secretory* or *luteal phase,* and (3) the *menstrual* or *ischemic phase.* The length of the menstrual cycle ranges from 20 to 40 days, the average being 28 days.

The menstrual cycle begins on the first day of menstruation, which usually lasts 3 to 7 days. Table 49-2 includes characteristics of the menstrual cycle and related patient teaching. During this time, estrogen and progesterone levels are low, but FSH levels begin to increase. During the follicular phase, a single follicle matures fully under the stimulation of FSH. (The mechanism that ensures that usually only one follicle reaches maturity is not known.) The mature follicle stimulates estrogen production, causing a negative feedback with resulting decreased FSH secretion.

Although the initial stage of follicular maturation is stimulated by FSH, complete maturation and ovulation occur only with the presence of LH. When estrogen levels peak on about the twelfth day of the cycle, there is a surge of LH, which triggers ovulation a day or two later. After ovulation (maturation and release of an ovum), LH promotes the development of the corpus luteum.

The fully developed corpus luteum continues to secrete estrogen and initiates progesterone secretion. If fertilization occurs, high levels of estrogen and progesterone continue to be secreted as a result of the continued activity of the corpus luteum from stimulation by human chorionic gonadotropin (hCG). If fertilization does not take place, menstruation occurs because of a decrease in estrogen production and progesterone withdrawal.

During the follicular phase, the endometrial lining of the uterus also undergoes change. As larger amounts of estrogen are produced, the endometrial lining undergoes proliferative changes, and there is an increase in cellular growth, including an increase in the length of blood vessels and glandular tissue.

With ovulation and the resulting increased levels of progesterone, the luteal (or secretory) phase begins. In this phase, the blood vessels begin to coil, increasing the surface area of the vascular supply. The glandular tissues mature and secrete a glycogen-rich substance, and the glandular ducts dilate. If the corpus luteum regresses (when fertilization does not occur) and estrogen and progesterone levels fall, the endometrial lining can no longer be supported. As a result, the blood vessels contract, and tissue begins to slough (fall away). This sloughing results in the menses and the start of the menstrual phase.

Menopause

Menopause is the physiologic cessation of menses associated with declining ovarian function. It is usually considered complete after 1 year of **amenorrhea** (absence of menstruation).[5] (Menopause is discussed in Chapter 52.)

Phases of the Sexual Response

The sexual response is a complex interplay of psychologic and physiologic phenomena and is influenced by a number of variables, including daily stress, illness, and crisis. The changes that occur during sexual excitement are similar for men and women. Masters and Johnson described the sexual response in terms of the excitement, plateau, orgasmic, and resolution phases.[6]

Male Sexual Response. The penis and the urethra are essential to the transport of sperm into the vagina and the cervix during intercourse. This transport is facilitated by penile erection in response to sexual stimulation during the excitement phase. Erection results from the filling of the large venous sinuses within the erectile tissue of the penis. In the flaccid state the sinuses hold only a small amount of blood, but during the erection stage they are congested with blood. Because the penis is richly endowed with sympathetic, parasympathetic, and pudendal nerve endings, it is readily stimulated to erection. The loose skin of the

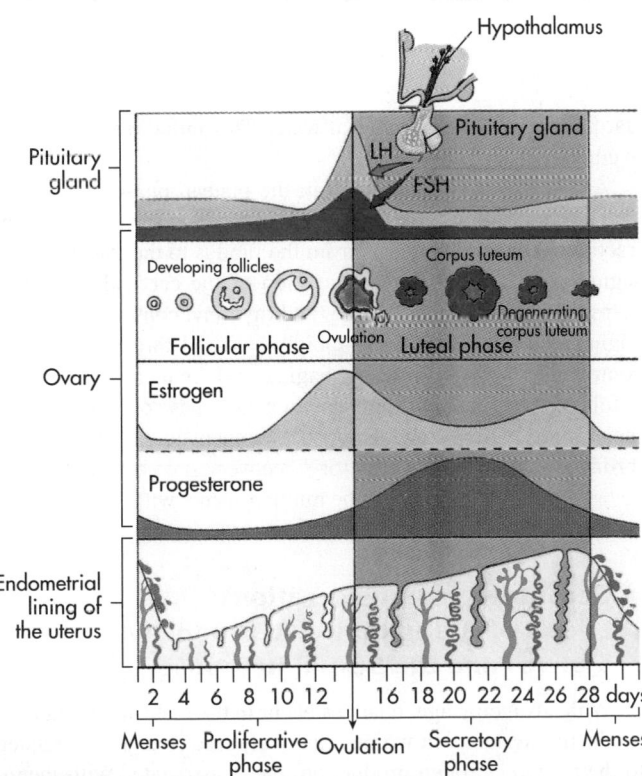

FIG. 49-9   Events of the menstrual cycle. The various lines depict the changes in blood hormone levels, the development of the follicles, and the changes in the endometrium during the cycle. *FSH,* Follicle-stimulating hormone; *LH,* luteinizing hormone.

TABLE 49-2   Patient & Family Teaching Guide

Characteristics of Menstruation

CHARACTERISTIC	PATIENT TEACHING
Menarche Occurs between ages 9 and 16 yr; average age at onset is 12 or 13 yr.	See health care provider regarding possible endocrine or developmental abnormality when delayed.
Interval Usually is 21-35 days, but regular cycles as short as 17 or as long as 45 days are considered normal if pattern is consistent for individual.	Keep written record to identify own pattern of menstrual cycle. Expect some irregularity in premenopausal period. Be aware that drugs (phenothiazines, narcotics, contraceptives) and stressful life events can result in missed periods.
Duration Menstrual flow generally lasts 2-8 days.	Realize that pattern is fairly constant but that wide variations do exist.
Amount Menstrual flow varies from 20-80 ml per menses; average is 30 ml; amount varies among women and in the same woman at different times; it is usually heaviest first 2 days.	Count pads or tampons used per day. The average tampon or pad, when completely saturated, absorbs 20-30 ml. Very heavy flow is indicated by complete soaking of two pads in 1-2 hr. Flow increases and then gradually decreases in premenopausal period. IUD or drugs such as anticoagulants and thiazides can produce heavy menses.
Composition Menstrual discharge is mixture of endometrium, blood, mucus, and vaginal cells; it is dark red and less viscous than blood and usually does not clot.	Clots indicate heavy flow or vaginal pooling.

IUD, Intrauterine device.

penis becomes taut as a result of the intense venous congestion. This erectile tautness allows for easy insertion into the vagina.

As the man reaches the plateau phase, the erection is maintained, and a small increase in diameter occurs as a result of a slight increase in vasocongestion. There is also an increase in testicle size. Sometimes a change in color occurs in the glans penis, which becomes more reddish-purple.

The subsequent contraction of the penile and urethral musculature during the orgasmic phase propels the sperm outward through the meatus. In this process, termed *ejaculation,* sperm are released into the ductus deferens during contractions. Sperm advance through the urethra, where fluids from the prostate and seminal vesicles are added to the ejaculate. The sperm continue their path through the urethra, receiving a small amount of fluid from the Cowper's glands, and are finally ejaculated through the urinary meatus. Orgasm is characterized by the rapid release of the vasocongestion and muscular tension (myotonia) that have developed. The rapid release of muscular tension (through rhythmic contractions) occurs primarily in the penis, prostate gland, and seminal vesicles. After ejaculation, a man enters the resolution phase. During this phase the penis undergoes involution, gradually returning to its unstimulated, flaccid state.

Female Sexual Response. The changes that occur in a woman during sexual excitation are similar to those in a man. In response to stimulation the clitoris becomes congested and vaginal lubrication increases from secretions from the cervix,

Bartholin's glands, and vaginal walls. This initial response is the excitation phase.

As excitation is maintained in the plateau phase, the vagina expands and the uterus is elevated. In the orgasmic phase, contractions occur in the uterus from the fundus to the lower uterine segment. There is a slight relaxation of the cervical os, which helps the entrance of the sperm, and rhythmic contractions of the vagina. Muscular tension is rapidly released through rhythmic contractions in the clitoris, the vagina, and the uterus. This phase is followed by a resolution phase in which these organs return to their preexcitation state. However, women do not have to go through the resolution (refractory) recovery state before they can be orgasmic again. They can be multiorgasmic without resolution between orgasms.

■ Gerontologic Considerations: Effects of Aging on the Reproductive Systems and the Sexual Response

With advancing age, changes occur in the male and female reproductive systems. In women many of these changes are related to the altered estrogen production that is associated with menopause. A reduction in circulating estrogen along with an increase in androgens in postmenopausal women is associated with breast and genital atrophy, reduction in bone mass, and increased rate of atherosclerosis.[7] The decrease in estrogen also contributes to dry,

TABLE 49-3 — Gerontologic Differences in Assessment: Reproductive Systems

CHANGES	DIFFERENCES IN ASSESSMENT FINDINGS
Male	
Penis	
Decreased subcutaneous fat, decreased skin turgor	Easily retractable foreskin (if uncircumcised); decrease in size; fewer sustained erections
Testes	
Decreased testosterone production	Decrease in size; change in position (lower); increase in firmness
Prostate	
Benign hyperplasia	Enlargement
Breasts	
Enlargement	Gynecomastia (abnormal enlargement)
Female	
Breasts	
Decreased subcutaneous fat, increased fibrous tissue, decreased skin turgor	Less resilient, looser, more pendulous tissue; decreased size; duct around nipple may feel like stringy strand
Vulva	
Decreased skin turgor	Atrophy; decreased amount of pubic hair; decreased size of clitoris and labia
Vagina	
Atrophy of tissue, decreased muscle tone	Pale and dry mucosa; relaxation of outlets; mucosa thins; vagina narrower and shorter
Urethra	
Decreased muscle tone	Cystocele (protrusion of bladder through vaginal wall)
Uterus	
Decreased thickness of myometrium	Decrease in size; uterine prolapse
Ovaries	
Decreased ovarian function	Nonpalpable ovaries; decreased size

TABLE 49-4 — Gerontologic Differences in Assessment: Sexual Function

Male
Increased stimulation necessary for erection
Decreased ability to attain erection
Possible decreased response to sexual stimuli

Female
Decreased vaginal lubrication
Possible decreased response to sexual stimuli

effects of these changes, as well as the negative social attitude toward sexuality in older adults, can affect the sexual practices of people in this age-group. Nurses have an important role in providing accurate and unbiased information about sexuality and age. Nurses should emphasize the normalcy of sexual activity in older adults. Counseling may be necessary to help older patients accommodate to these normal physiologic changes. ∎

ASSESSMENT OF THE MALE AND FEMALE REPRODUCTIVE SYSTEMS

Subjective Data

Important Health Information. In addition to general health information, the nurse needs to elicit information specifically relating to the reproductive system. Reproduction and sexual issues are often considered extremely personal and private. The nurse must develop trust to elicit such information. A professional demeanor is important when taking a reproductive or sexual history. The nurse needs to be sensitive, ask gender-neutral questions, and maintain an awareness of a patient's culture and beliefs.[10] It is helpful if the nurse begins with the least sensitive information (e.g., menstrual history) before asking questions about more sensitive issues such as sexual practices or sexually transmitted diseases.

Past health history. The past health history should include information about major illnesses, hospitalizations, and surgeries for both men and women.[2] The nurse should also inquire about any infections involving the reproductive system, including sexually transmitted diseases. Women should also have a complete obstetric and gynecologic history taken.

Common pediatric illnesses that affect reproductive function are mumps and rubella. The occurrence of mumps in young men has been associated with an increase in sterility. Bilateral testicular atrophy can occur secondary to mumps-related orchitis. In the health history the nurse should ask if male patients have had mumps, have been immunized with mumps vaccine, or have any indications of sterility.

Rubella is of primary concern to women of childbearing age. If rubella occurs during the first 3 months of pregnancy, the possibility of congenital anomalies is increased. For this reason, nurses should encourage immunization for all women of childbearing age who have not been immunized for rubella or have not already had the disease. However, women should not be immunized if they are already pregnant. Women are also advised not to conceive for at least 3 months after immunization.

The nurse should also question the patient regarding the patient's current health status and the presence of any acute or

friable vaginal mucosa, causing many women to experience dyspareunia.[8] A gradual hormonal decline in elderly men also occurs and is sometimes referred to as male menopause. Manifestations of hormonal decline in men can be physical, psychologic, or sexual. Some of the changes include an increase in prostate size, decreased testosterone level, decreased sperm production, decreased muscle tone of the scrotum, and a decrease in the size and firmness of the testicles. Impotence and sexual dysfunction occur in some men as a result of these changes.[9] Age-related changes in the reproductive systems and differences in assessment findings are presented in Table 49-3.

Gradual changes resulting from advancing age occur in the sexual responses of men and women (Table 49-4). These changes occur at different rates and to varying degrees. The cumulative

chronic health problems. Problems in other body systems are often related to problems with the reproductive system. Questions relating to possible endocrine disorders, particularly diabetes mellitus (DM), hypothyroidism, and hyperthyroidism, must be asked, because these disorders directly interfere with women's menstrual cycles and with sexual performance. Men who have DM may experience impotence and retrograde ejaculation. In women with uncontrolled DM, pregnancy and the use of oral contraceptives may constitute significant risks to health. Many other chronic illnesses such as cardiovascular disease, respiratory disorders, anemia, cancer, and kidney and urinary tract disorders may affect the reproductive system and sexual functioning.

A history of a stroke should be determined. In men, strokes may cause physiologic or psychologic impotence. Men who have suffered a myocardial infarction (MI) may experience impotence because of the fear of precipitating another heart attack resulting from sexual activity. This same concern is shared by the woman both as a partner of someone who has had an MI and as the person recovering from an MI. Although most patients have concerns about sexual activity following an MI, many are not comfortable expressing these concerns to the nurse.[11] The nurse must be sensitive to this concern. In women, a history of cardiovascular disease (e.g., hypertension, thrombophlebitis, angina) causes a higher incidence of morbidity and mortality with pregnancy or oral contraceptive use.

Medications. A list of all prescription and over-the-counter medications that the patient is taking should be documented, including reason for the medication, the dosage, and the length of time that the medication has been taken. All drugs taken by female patients should be evaluated for possible teratogenic effects in women of childbearing age. The patient should be asked about the use of herbal products and dietary supplements.

Particularly relevant in the assessment of the reproductive system is the use of diuretics (sometimes prescribed for premenstrual edema), psychotropic agents (which may interfere with sexual performance), and antihypertensives (some of which may cause impotence). Thus patients who use drugs such as methyldopa (Aldomet), clonidine (Catapres), guanethidine (Ismelin), and hydralazine (Apresoline) must be closely assessed for these problems. The nurse must also note the use of drugs such as alcohol, marijuana, barbiturates, amphetamines, or phencyclidine hydrochloride (PCP; also called "angel dust"), which can have serious behavioral or physiologic effects on the functioning of the reproductive system.

In women, the use of oral contraceptives or other hormones should be noted. The use of hormone replacement therapy (HRT) is relevant for women because of its potential benefit in preventing osteoporosis. Estrogen may also have beneficial effects on memory and cognitive function in older women. In women with a uterus, the concurrent use of progesterone should be documented. The use of estrogen alone in women who have a uterus has been shown to increase the incidence of endometrial cancer.[5]

Oral contraceptive use can aggravate the symptoms of certain neurologic disorders, such as seizures or migraine headaches. However, the use of lower doses of estrogen in current contraceptives makes these side effects less problematic and may actually be therapeutic. A history of cholecystitis and hepatitis is important information because these conditions may be contraindications for oral contraceptives; cholecystitis is often aggravated by oral contraceptives, and chronic active inflammation of the liver generally precludes the use of estrogen products because they are metabolized by the liver. Chronic obstructive pulmonary disease may be a contraindication to oral contraceptive use because progesterone thickens respiratory secretions.

Surgery or other treatments. Any surgical procedures should be noted in the health history. Surgical procedures involving the reproductive system are listed in Table 49-5. Therapeutic or spontaneous abortions should also be documented.

TABLE 49-5   Surgeries of the Reproductive Systems

SURGERY	DESCRIPTION
Male	
Herniorrhaphy	Repair of hernia
Orchiectomy	Removal of one or both testes
Prostatectomy	Removal of prostate gland
Repair of testicular torsion	Correction of axial rotation of spermatic cord, which cuts off blood supply to the testicle, epididymis, and other structures
Varicocelectomy	Repair of varicose vein of scrotum
Vasectomy	Removal of part of ductus (vas) deferens; can be an elective procedure for sterilization or contraception
Female	
Cryosurgery	Use of subfreezing temperature to destroy tissue, especially in treatment of abnormal cells
Dilation and curettage	Dilation of uterus and scraping of endometrium, performed to diagnose disease of uterus, correct heavy or prolonged vaginal bleeding, or empty uterus of products of conception; also used in the treatment of infertility to correlate state of endometrium and time of cycle
Hysterectomy	Removal of uterus
Mastectomy	Removal of one or both breasts
Oophorectomy	Removal of one or both ovaries
Repair of cystocele	Correction of protrusion of urinary bladder through vaginal wall
Repair of rectocele	Correction of protrusion of rectum into vagina
Salpingectomy	Removal of one or both fallopian tubes
Tubal sterilization	Ligation of fallopian tubes

Functional Health Patterns. The key questions to ask a patient with a reproductive problem are presented in Table 49-6.

Health perception–health management pattern. Two of the primary focuses of this health pattern are the patient's perception of his or her own health and measures that the patient takes to maintain health. Specifically, it is important to ask about self-examination practices and screenings. Monthly breast self-examination (BSE), mammography according to age-specific guidelines (see Chapter 50), and routine Pap smears are integral to a woman's health. Testicular self-examination (TSE) should be practiced by all men, starting in adolescence. Regular prostate examination should be encouraged as well. The American Cancer Society recommends that men over age 50 have digital rectal examination (DRE) yearly.[12]

Family history is also a component of this health pattern. The nurse should inquire about a history of cancer, particularly cancer of the reproductive organs. First-degree relatives who have cancer of the breast, ovaries, uterus, or prostate significantly increases the risk of cancer for the patient. Determination of a familial tendency for diabetes mellitus, hypothyroidism, hyperthyroidism, hypertension, stroke, angina, myocardial infarction, endocrine disorders, or anemia is also important.

Assessment of the reproductive system is incomplete without a knowledge of the patient's lifestyle choices. The nurse should know whether a woman uses cigarettes, alcohol, caffeine, or other drugs because these substances can be detrimental to both mother and fetus. Cigarette smoking may delay conception. Cigarette smoking also can increase the risk of morbidity in women using oral contraceptives and is associated with early menopause. These substances may also adversely affect the sperm count in men and cause impotence or decreased libido.

TABLE 49-6 Health History — Reproductive System

Health Perception–Health Management
- How would you describe your overall health?
- *Women:* Explain how you examine your breasts. When was your last Pap smear? Mammogram? What were the results?
- *Men:* Explain how you examine your testes. When was your last prostate examination?
- Describe the health of your family members. Any history of breast, uterine, ovarian, or prostate cancer?
- Do you use tobacco products, alcohol, or drugs?*

Nutritional-Metabolic
- Describe what you usually eat and drink.
- Have you experienced any changes in weight?*
- How do you feel about your current weight?
- Do you take any nutritional supplements such as calcium or vitamins?*
- Do you have any dietary restrictions?*

Elimination
- Do you experience problems with urination (e.g., pain, burning, dribbling, incontinence, frequency)?*
- Have you had bladder infections? If so, when? How often?
- Do you experience problems with bowel movements?* Do you use laxatives?*

Activity-Exercise
- What activities do you typically do each day?
- Do you have enough energy for your desired activities?
- Can you dress yourself? Feed yourself? Walk without help?

Sleep-Rest
- How many hours do you typically sleep each night?
- Do you feel rested after sleep?
- Do you experience any problems associated with sleeping?*

Cognitive-Perceptual
- Are you able to read and write?
- Do you experience problems with dizziness?*
- Do you experience pain? If yes, where?
- Do you experience pain during sexual activity or intercourse?*

Self-Perception–Self-Concept
- How would you describe yourself?
- Have there been any changes recently that have made you feel differently about yourself?*
- Are you experiencing any problems that are affecting your sexuality?*

Role-Relationship
- Describe your living arrangements. Who do you live with?
- Do you have a significant other? If yes, is this relationship satisfying?
- Are you experiencing any role-related problems in your family?* At work?*
- What are the relationships among your family members?

Sexuality-Reproductive
- Are you sexually active? If so, how many partners do you have?
- What kind of sex do you engage in (e.g., oral, vaginal, rectal)?
- How do you protect yourself against sexually transmitted disease and unwanted pregnancy?
- Are you satisfied with your present means of sexual expression? If no, explain.
- Have you experienced any recent changes in your sexual practices?*
- *Women:* date of last menstruation, description of menstrual flow, problems with menstruation, age of menarche, age of menopause.
- *Women:* pregnancy history—number of times pregnant, number of living children, number of miscarriages/abortions.

Coping-Stress Tolerance
- Have there been any major changes in your life within the last couple of years?*
- What is stressful in your life right now?
- How do you handle health problems when they occur?

Value-Belief
- What beliefs do you have about your health and illnesses?
- Do you use home remedies?*
- Is religion an important part of your life?*
- Do you feel that any of your personal beliefs or values may be compromised because of your treatment?*

*If yes, describe.

The nurse must determine if the patient is allergic to sulfonamides, penicillin, rubber, or latex. Sulfonamides and penicillin are used frequently in the treatment of reproductive and genitourinary problems such as vaginitis and gonorrhea. Rubber and latex are commonly used in diaphragms and condoms. An allergy to these substances precludes their use as contraceptive methods.

Nutritional-metabolic pattern. Anemia is a common problem in women in their reproductive years, particularly during pregnancy and the postpartum period. The adequacy of the diet should be evaluated with this condition in mind.

A thorough nutritional and psychologic history should be taken to assess for the presence of an eating disorder. Anorexia can cause amenorrhea and the subsequent problems, such as osteoporosis, that are related to estrogen cessation. The nurse has the opportunity to help prevent the debilitating condition of osteoporosis. From early adolescence, women can be counseled regarding adequate calcium intake and the role of calcium in the prevention of osteoporosis. The patient's daily calcium intake should be estimated to determine whether there is a need for supplementation. Folic acid intake for women in their reproductive years should be evaluated because a deficiency can result in spina bifida and other neural tube defects in the fetus.[13]

Elimination pattern. Many gynecologic problems can result in genitourinary problems. Stress and urge incontinence are common in older women because of relaxation of the pelvic musculature caused by multiple births or advancing age. Vaginal infections predispose patients to chronic or recurrent urinary tract infections. The proximity of the reproductive organs and the genitourinary tract makes metastasis of malignant tumors to this site a possibility to be considered. Benign prostatic hyperplasia is a common problem of older men. It can alter normal urination, causing retention and difficulty in initiating the urinary stream.

Activity-exercise pattern. The amount, type, and intensity of activity and exercise should be documented. Lack of stress on bones secondary to lack of exercise is an important factor in the development of osteoporosis. Weight-bearing exercise decreases the risk of osteoporosis in women. Women who engage in excessive exercise may experience amenorrhea. This may result from decreased estrogen related to a low percentage of body fat because estrogen is stored in fat cells. Anemia can result in fatigue and activity intolerance and can interfere with satisfactory performance of the activities of daily living.

Sleep-rest pattern. Sleep patterns may be affected during the postpartum period and also while raising young children. The hot flashes and sweating often present during the perimenopause can cause serious sleep interruption when the woman is awakened in a drenching sweat. The need to change her nightgown and bedding further disrupts her sleep. Insomnia is also a common complaint of perimenopausal women. Daytime fatigue often results from such nighttime awakenings. In men, sleep disturbances may be caused by frequent urination at night associated with prostate enlargement.

Cognitive-perceptual pattern. Pelvic pain is associated with various gynecologic disorders such as pelvic inflammatory disease, ovarian cysts, and endometriosis. **Dyspareunia** (painful intercourse) can be particularly problematic for a woman. The pain associated with intercourse can make her reluctant to participate in sexual activity and strain her relationship with her sexual partner. The woman should be referred to her health care provider if dyspareunia is present.

Self-perception–self-concept pattern. The reproductive changes of aging such as pendulous breasts and vaginal dryness in women and decreased size of the penis in men may lead to emotional distress. The subtle changes associated with sexuality and advancing age may alter the self-concept of many persons.

Role-relationship pattern. The nurse needs to obtain information regarding the family structure and occupation. Questions regarding recent changes in work-related relationships or family conflicts should be asked. It is important to ascertain the patient's role in the family as a starting point in determining family dynamics.

Roles and relationships are affected by changes within the family. The addition of a new baby into the family may change family dynamics. Role-relationship patterns change as children begin their careers and move away from home. Another change occurs when people retire.

Sexuality-reproductive pattern. The extent and depth of the interview about a patient's sexuality depend primarily on the expertise of the interviewer and on the needs and the willingness of the patient. Before taking a sexual history, interviewers should assess their own comfort with their sexuality, because any discomfort in questioning becomes obvious to the patient. Interviews must be carried out in an environment that provides reassurance, confidentiality, and a nonjudgmental attitude. It is best to begin with the least sensitive areas and then move to more sensitive areas.

For women, it is important to obtain a menstrual and an obstetric history. The menstrual history includes the date of the last menstrual period, description of menstrual flow, age of menarche, and, if applicable, age at menopause. Menstrual history data are used in the detection of pregnancy, infertility, and numerous other gynecologic concerns. Changes in the usual menstrual pattern must be explicitly described to determine whether the change is transient and unimportant or connected with a more serious gynecologic problem. *Metrorrhagia* (spotting or bleeding between menstruations), *menorrhagia* (excessive menstrual bleeding), *amenorrhea* (lack of menstruation), and *postcoital bleeding* are examples of such problems. Changes in menstrual patterns associated with the use of contraceptive pills, intrauterine devices (IUDs), subdermal estrogen-only implant (Norplant), or medroxyprogesterone (Depo-Provera) injections must be identified. Contraceptive pills usually decrease the amount and duration of flow, whereas some IUDs may cause an increase in the amount and duration. Some IUDs also increase the severity of dysmenorrhea. However, newer IUDs contain progestin and may be therapeutic. The obstetric history includes the number of pregnancies, full-term births, preterm births, and live births. Other obstetric information should include information about any ectopic pregnancies or abortions, either spontaneous or therapeutic. Any problems that occurred with pregnancy should be documented.

A sexual history should include information regarding sexual activity, beliefs, and practices. Sexual preference (heterosexual, homosexual, bisexual), the frequency and type of sexual activity (penile-vaginal, penile-rectal, recipient rectal, oral), and the number of partners and protective measures against sexually transmitted disease and pregnancy should be explored. The patient's knowledge of safe sexual practices should be determined. A history of multiple sex partners and unprotected sex increases the risk of contracting a sexually transmitted disease. For a woman, this can increase the risk of pelvic inflammatory disease, which can compromise her ability to become pregnant.

TABLE 49-7	Sexual History Format

- How long have you been sexually active?
- Are you currently in a relationship that involves sexual intercourse? If yes, do you have one or multiple partners?
- How frequently do you engage in sexual activities? Are you and your partner(s) satisfied with the sexual relationship?
- How many sexual partners have you had in the past 6 months?
- Do you prefer relationships with men, women, or both? (If the patient is gay or lesbian, inquire if he or she is in a significant relationship and has a partner.)
- Has your sex life changed during the past year? If yes, how?
- Have you ever had a sexually transmitted disease? If yes, what?
- What are you doing to protect yourself from sexually transmitted diseases? If protection is used, what type? Do you use protection every time you have intercourse?
- Are you currently using any birth control measures? If yes, what type? How long have you been using this product? How effective do you feel this has been?
- Have you ever been in a relationship with anyone who hurt you? Have you ever been forced into sexual acts as a child or an adult?
- How often have you experienced impotence (male) or difficulty with vaginal lubrication (female) or pain with intercourse?

Adapted from Wilson SF, Giddens JF: *Health assessment for nursing practice*, ed 2, St Louis, 2001, Mosby.

Table 49-7 outlines specific questions for a sexual history. It should be noted that only a skilled interviewer should approach some of the questions presented in Table 49-7, and then only with discretion.

Both men and women should be asked about their general satisfaction with sexuality. The patient's satisfaction with the opportunities for sexual gratification is important information that should be elicited. The patient should be questioned about sexual beliefs and practices and whether orgasm is achieved. Any unexplained change in sexual practices or performance should be explored. Problems of the reproductive system can cause physiologic or psychologic problems that can lead to painful intercourse, impotence, sexual dysfunction, or infertility. Both the cause and the effect of such problems should be determined.

Coping–stress tolerance pattern. The stress related to situations such as pregnancy or menopause may cause an increased dependence on support systems. It is essential for the nurse to ascertain who the support people are in the patient's life. The diagnosis of a sexually transmitted disease can cause stress to the patient and the partner. Means to manage such stress should be explored.

Value-belief pattern. Sexual and reproductive functioning is closely related to cultural, religious, moral, and ethical values. The nurse should be aware of his or her own beliefs in these areas and should recognize and sensitively react to the patient's personal beliefs associated with reproductive and sexuality issues.

Objective Data

Physical Examination: Male. The examination of the male external genitalia includes inspection and palpation. An examination may be performed with the patient lying or standing. The standing position is generally preferred. The examiner should be seated in front of the standing patient. Gloves should be used during examination of the male genitalia.

Pubis. The nurse observes the distribution and general characteristics of the pubic hair and the skin. Normally, the hair is in a diamond-shaped pattern. The hair is usually coarser than scalp hair. The absence of hair is not a normal finding. The skin is also evaluated.

Penis. The nurse notes the size and skin texture of the penis and any lesions, scars, or swelling. The location of the urethral meatus, as well as the presence or absence of a foreskin, should be noted. If present, the foreskin should be retracted to note cleanliness and replaced over the glans after observation. The glans is compressed to note any discharge and its amount, color, and odor if present. The nurse also palpates the penile shaft for tenderness or masses and observes the ventral and dorsal aspects.

Scrotum and testes. The nurse performs a complete skin examination by lifting each testis to inspect all sides of the scrotal sac. Palpation of the scrotum is done to note changes in consistency or the presence of masses. It is important to note if the testes are descended. The left testis usually hangs lower than the right. Undescended testis is a major risk factor for testicular cancer, as well as a potential cause of male infertility.

Inguinal region and spermatic cord. The examiner inspects the skin overlying the inguinal regions for rashes or lesions. The patient should be asked to bear down or cough. While he is straining, the inguinal area should be inspected for the presence of a bulge. No bulging should be seen.

Examination of the inguinal area continues with palpation. The right and left inguinal rings should be palpated using the index finger or middle finger. The finger should be inserted into the lower aspect of the scrotum and should follow the spermatic cord upward through the triangular, slitlike opening of the inguinal ring. At this point, the patient should be asked to bear down and cough. The nurse determines whether the strain produces a bulging of the intestines through the ring, indicating the presence of a hernia, a condition that requires follow-up. The inguinal lymph nodes should also be palpated. Enlargement of the lymph nodes (termed *lymphadenopathy*) could suggest a pelvic organ infection or malignancy.

Anus and prostate. The anal sphincter and perineal regions are inspected for lesions, masses, and hemorrhoids. A DRE is required for all men who have symptoms of prostate trouble, such as difficulty in initiating the flow and the urge to void frequently. This examination should be performed annually for all men over 50 years of age.

Physical Examination: Female. Physical examination of women often begins with inspection and palpation of the breasts and then proceeds to the abdomen and genitalia. Examination of the abdomen provides an opportunity to detect pain or any masses that may involve the genitourinary system. Abdominal examination is discussed in Chapter 38.

Breasts. Breasts are examined first by visual inspection. The nurse, with the patient seated, observes the breasts for symmetry, size, shape, skin color and texture, vascular patterns, dimpling, and the presence of unusual lesions. The patient is asked to put her arms at her sides, arms overhead, lean forward, and press hands on hips. The nurse observes for any abnormalities during these maneuvers. The axillae and the clavicular areas are then palpated for enlarged lymph nodes.

TABLE 49-8	Normal Physical Assessment of the Reproductive System

MALE	FEMALE
External Genitalia Diamond-shaped hair distribution. Penis circumcised, no lesions or discharge noted. Scrotum symmetric, no masses, descended testes. No inguinal hernia.	**Breasts** Symmetric without dimpling. Nipples soft; no drainage, retraction, or lesions noted. No masses or tenderness; no lymphadenopathy.
Anus No hemorrhoids, fissures, or lesions noted.	**External Genitalia** Triangular hair distribution. Genitalia dark pink, no lesions, redness, swelling, or inflammation in perineal region. No vaginal discharge noted. No tenderness with palpation of Skene's ducts and Bartholin's glands.
	Anus No hemorrhoids, fissures, or lesions noted.

TABLE 49-9	Common Assessment Abnormalities
	Breast

FINDING	DESCRIPTION	POSSIBLE ETIOLOGY AND SIGNIFICANCE
Nipple inversion or retraction	Recent onset, erythematous, pain, unilateral	Abscess, inflammation, cancer
	Recent onset (usually within past year), unilateral presentation, lack of tenderness	Neoplasm
Nipple secretions		
• Galactorrhea (female)	Milky, no relationship to lactation, unilateral or bilateral or intermittent or consistent presentation	Drug therapy, particularly phenothiazines, tricyclic antidepressants, methyldopa; hypofunction or hyperfunction of thyroid or adrenal glands; tumors of hypothalamus or pituitary gland; excessive estrogen; prolonged suckling or breast foreplay
• Galactorrhea (male)	Milky, bilateral presentation	Chorioepithelioma of testes, manifestation of pituitary tumor
• Purulent	Gray-green or yellow color; frequent unilateral presentation; association with pain, erythema, induration, nipple inversion	Puerperal (after birth) mastitis (inflammatory condition of breast) or abscess
	Same as above but usually without nipple inversion	Infected sebaceous cyst
• Serous discharge	Clear appearance, unilateral or bilateral or intermittent or consistent presentation	Intraductal papilloma
• Dark green or multicolored discharge	Thick, sticky, and frequently bilateral	Ductal ectasia (dilation of mammary ducts)
• Serosanguineous or bloody drainage	Unilateral presentation	Papillomatosis (widespread development of nipplelike growths), intraductal papilloma, carcinoma (male and female)
Scaling or irritation of nipple	Unilateral or bilateral presentation, crusting, possible ulceration	Paget's disease, eczema, infection
Nodules, lumps, or masses	Multiple, bilateral, well-delineated, soft or firm, mobile cysts; pain; premenstrual occurrence	Fibrocystic changes
	Rubbery consistency, fluid-filled interior, pain	Ductal ectasia
	Soft, mobile, well-delineated cyst, absence of pain	Lipoma, fibroadenoma
	Erythema, tenderness, induration	Infected sebaceous cysts, abscesses
	Usually singular, hard irregularly shaped, poorly delineated, nonmobile	Neoplasm
Dimpling of breast	Unilateral, recent onset, no pain	Neoplasm

After the patient assumes a supine position, a pillow is placed under the back on the side to be examined. The patient is asked to put her arm above and behind her head. These maneuvers flatten breast tissue and make palpation easier. The breast is then palpated in a systematic fashion using a vertical line, a clockwise, or a spoke approach. The nurse should use the distal finger pads for palpation. The tail of Spence should be included in the examination because this area and the upper outer quadrant are the areas where most breast malignancies develop. Finally, the nurse should palpate the area around the areolae for masses. The nipple should be compressed to determine the presence of discharge or any masses. The color, consistency, and odor of any discharge should be documented.

External genitalia. The nurse uses gloves for examination of the external genitalia. The mons pubis, labia majora, labia minora, posterior fourchette, perineum, and anal region are inspected for characteristics of skin, hair distribution, and contour. Lesions, inflammation, swelling, and discharge are noted. The nurse must separate the labia to fully inspect the clitoris, urethral meatus, and vaginal orifice.

Internal pelvic examination. During the speculum examination, the nurse observes the walls of the vagina and the cervix for inflammation, discharge, polyps, and suspicious growths. During this examination, it is possible to take a Pap smear and collect secretions for culture and microscopic examination. After the speculum examination, a bimanual examination is performed to allow assessment of the size, shape, and consistency of the uterus, ovaries, and tubes. The tubes are not normally palpable.

Pelvic and bimanual examinations are considered advanced skills and are not usually within the scope of the nurse general-ist.[14] For this reason, these parts of the examination are not included in this text. Pelvic and bimanual examinations are described in physical assessment textbooks.

Table 49-8 provides an example of a recording format for the physical assessment findings for the male and female reproductive systems. Tables 49-9 through 49-11 summarize common assessment abnormalities of the breasts, female reproductive system, and male reproductive system, respectively.

DIAGNOSTIC STUDIES OF THE REPRODUCTIVE SYSTEMS

Table 49-12 summarizes the most commonly used diagnostic studies in the assessment of the reproductive systems and the nurse's responsibility regarding these diagnostic tests.

Urine Studies

Pregnancy Testing. Occurrence of pregnancy is generally validated by measuring human chorionic gonadotropin (hCG) in the urine. A solution containing monoclonal antibodies specific for hCG is mixed with a small amount of urine. The presence of hCG causes a change in color of the tested urine.

Home pregnancy test kits use the same assay principle described in the preceding paragraph. Positive results are based on the presence of hCG in urine. Some tests can detect pregnancy as early as the first day following a missed menstrual period. These tests are 98% accurate if the test is performed exactly per instructions. A second test is recommended within a week if the first test is negative (assuming menses has not yet occurred).[15]

Hormone Studies. Although estrogen studies are performed on urine, the results are frequently inaccurate because of

---

TABLE 49-10	**Common Assessment Abnormalities** **Female Reproductive System**	
FINDING	**DESCRIPTION**	**POSSIBLE ETIOLOGY AND SIGNIFICANCE**
• Vulvar discharge	Plaque-like consistency, frequent itching and inflammation, lack of odor or yeast-like smell	Candidiasis (*Candida* or yeast infection), vaginitis
	Grayish color, copious flow, frothy appearance, vulvar irritation	Bacterial vaginosis infection
	Grayish green or yellow color; malodorous or "fishy" odor	*Trichomonas vaginalis*
	Bloody color	*Chlamydia trachomatis* or *Neisseria gonorrhoeae* infection, menstruation, trauma, cancer
• Vulvar erythema	Bright or beefy red color, itching	*Candida albicans*, allergy, chemical vaginitis
	Reddened base, painful vesicles or ulcerations	Genital herpes
	Macules or papules, itching	Chancroid (STD), contact dermatitis, scabies, pediculosis
• Vulvar growths	Soft, fleshy growth; nontender	Condyloma acuminatum
	Flat and warty appearance, nontender	Condyloma latum
	Same as either of above, possible pain	Neoplasm
	Reddened base, vesicles, and small erosions; pain	Lymphogranuloma venereum, genital herpes, chancroid
	Indurated, firm ulcers; lack of pain	Chancre (syphilis), granuloma inguinale
• Abdominal pain or tenderness	Intermittent or consistent tenderness in right or left lower quadrant	Salpingitis (infection of fallopian tube), ectopic pregnancy, ruptured ovarian cyst, PID, tubal or ovarian abscess
	Periumbilical location, consistent occurrence	Cystitis, endometritis (inflammation of endometrium), ectopic pregnancy

PID, Pelvic inflammatory disease; *STD,* sexually transmitted disease.

TABLE 49-11 Common Assessment Abnormalities

Male Reproductive System

FINDING	DESCRIPTION	POSSIBLE ETIOLOGY AND SIGNIFICANCE
• Penile growths or masses	Indurated, smooth, disklike appearance; absence of pain; singular presentation	Chancre
	Papular to irregularly shaped ulceration with pus, lack of induration	Chancroid
	Ulceration with induration and nodularity	Cancer
	Flat, wartlike nodule	Condyloma latum
	Elevated, fleshy, moist, elongated projections with single or multiple projections	Condyloma acuminatum
	Localized swelling with retracted, tight foreskin	Paraphimosis (inability to replace foreskin to its normal position after retraction), trauma
• Vesicles, erosions, or ulcers	Painful, erythematous base; vesicular or small erosions	Genital herpes, balanitis (inflammation of glans penis), chancroid
	Painless, singular, small erosion with eventual lymphadenopathy	Lymphogranuloma venereum, cancer
• Scrotal masses	Localized swelling with tenderness, unilateral or bilateral presentation	Epididymitis (inflammation of epididymis), testicular torsion, orchitis (mumps)
	Swelling, tenderness	Incarcerated hernia
	Unilateral or bilateral presentation; swelling without pain; translucent, cordlike or wormlike appearance	Hydrocele (accumulation of fluid in outer covering of testes), spermatocele (firm, sperm-containing cyst of epididymis), varicocele (dilation of veins that drain testes), hematocele (accumulation of blood within scrotum)
	Firm, nodular testes or epididymis; frequent unilateral presentation	Tuberculosis, cancer
• Penile discharge	Clear to purulent color, minimal to copious flow	Urethritis or gonorrhea, *Chlamydia trachomatis* infection, trauma
• Penile or scrotal erythema	Macules and papules	Scabies, pediculosis
• Inguinal masses	Bulging, unilateral presentation during straining	Inguinal hernia
	Shotty, 1-3 cm nodules	Lymphadenopathy

variable estrogen levels during the normal cycle and the difficulty in estimating the day of the cycle in women with irregular menses. Adrenal androgens are precursors of estrogens and can be measured in the urine of both men and women. FSH can be measured in a 24-hour urine specimen. Increased and decreased FSH levels can indicate gonadal failure resulting from pituitary dysfunction. For more information regarding hormone studies, see Chapter 46.

Blood Studies

Hormone Studies. A common serum hormone test, hCG, is used to identify pregnancy. Serum assays for hCG can detect pregnancy before a woman misses her menstrual period.[16] The prolactin assay is used primarily in the workup of a patient with amenorrhea. High levels of prolactin are normally associated with low levels of estrogen, such as those that occur during lactation. However, the same finding can occur with pituitary adenomas, especially with otherwise unexplained *galactorrhea* (excessive secretion of breast milk). Serum progesterone and estradiol are sometimes measured in ovarian

function assessment, particularly for amenorrhea. In addition, hormonal blood studies are essential components of a thorough fertility workup.

Tumor Markers. Biologic tumor markers are substances associated with malignant disease. Measurement of these markers is useful in monitoring therapy (marker levels rise as disease progresses and fall with disease regression) because marker levels may rise months before new disease or metastasis is evident. α-Fetoprotein (AFP) and hCG are sometimes used as tumor markers for testicular malignancy. A specific tumor antigen such as prostate-specific antigen (PSA) is another type of tumor marker frequently used.[15]

Serology Tests for Syphilis. The Venereal Disease Research Laboratory (VDRL) test and the rapid plasma reagin (RPR) detect the presence of antibodies in the serum of patients infected with syphilis. These tests are inexpensive and reliable but have high levels of false-positive results. The fluorescent treponemal antibody absorption (FTA-ABS) test is highly reliable and should be used after a positive VDRL or RPR, even if it is weakly positive or questionable.[15]

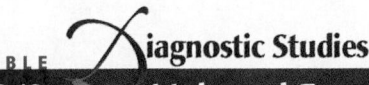

TABLE 49-12 **Diagnostic Studies**

Male and Female Reproductive Systems

STUDY	DESCRIPTION AND PURPOSE	NURSING RESPONSIBILITY
Urine Studies		
• hCG	hCG is detected in urine to ascertain whether a woman is pregnant. Hydatidiform mole and chorioepithelioma (in men and women) may also be detected using hCG.	Obtain thorough menstrual history from patient, including birth control methods. Determine presence or absence of presumptive signs of pregnancy (e.g., breast changes, increased whitish vaginal discharge).
• Testosterone levels	Tumors and developmental anomalies of the testes can be detected.	Instruct patient to collect 24 hr urine specimen. Keep it refrigerated.
• Follicle-stimulating hormone (FSH) assay	Indicates gonadal failure because of pituitary dysfunction. *Female:* Follicular phase: 2-5 IU/24 hr Midcycle: 8-40 IU/24 hr Luteal phase: 2-10 IU/24 hr Postmenopause: 35-100 IU/24 hr *Male:* 2-15 IU/24 hr	Instruct patient to collect 24 hr urine specimen. Indicate phase of menstrual cycle, if menopausal, and if on oral contraceptives or hormones.
Blood Studies		
• Prolactin assay	Detects pituitary dysfunction that can cause amenorrhea.	Observe venipuncture site for bleeding or hematoma formation.
• Prostate specific antigen (PSA)	Used to detect prostate cancer. Also a sensitive test for monitoring response to therapy. Normal finding is <4 ng/ml (<4 μg/L).	No food or fluid restrictions. Collect 5 ml blood. Observe venipuncture site for bleeding.
• Serum hCG assay	hCG is detected in serum to ascertain whether a woman is pregnant; can also be used as a tumor marker for testicular malignancy.	Instruct patient to have blood drawn in laboratory. Elicit where she is in her menstrual cycle, whether she has missed menses, and if so, how late she is.
• Serum androstenedione and testosterone levels	Ascertain whether elevated androgens are due to adrenal or ovarian dysfunction. Serum testosterone is also drawn to assess cause of amenorrhea.	Collect health history to eliminate potential sources of interference with accuracy of results (e.g., use of corticosteroids or barbiturates, presence of hypothyroidism or hyperthyroidism).
• Serum progesterone	Frequently used to detect functioning corpus luteum cyst.	Observe venipuncture site for bleeding or hematoma formation. Include last menstrual period and trimester of pregnancy because progesterone levels vary with gestation.
• Serum estradiol	Measures ovarian function. Particularly useful in assessing estrogen-secreting tumors and states of precocious female puberty. Normal values depend on laboratory that performs test and should be obtained from that laboratory. May be used to confirm perimenopausal status. Increased serum estradiol levels in men may be indicative of testicular tumors.	Observe venipuncture site for bleeding or hematoma formation.
• Serum FSH	Indicates gonadal failure due to pituitary dysfunction; used to validate menopausal status. *Female:* Follicular phase: 2-15 mIU/ml Midcycle: 8-40 mIU/ml Luteal phase: 2-15 mIU/ml Postmenopause: 50-250 mIU/ml *Male:* 2-15 mIU/ml	No food or fluid restrictions required. State phase of menstrual cycle, if menopausal, or if on oral contraceptive or hormones.
• Venereal Disease Research Laboratory (VDRL) (flocculation)	Nonspecific antibody tests used to screen for syphilis. Positive readings can be made within 1-2 wk after appearance of primary lesion (chancre) or 4-15 wk after initial infection.	Observe venipuncture site for bleeding or hematoma formation.
• Rapid plasma reagin (RPR) (agglutination)		Obtain data to determine presence or absence of problems such as hepatitis, pregnancy, and autoimmune diseases that may interfere with the accuracy of results.

hCG, Human chorionic gonadotropin.   *Continued*

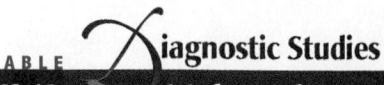

TABLE 49-12	Diagnostic Studies Male and Female Reproductive Systems—cont'd	
STUDY	**DESCRIPTION AND PURPOSE**	**NURSING RESPONSIBILITY**
Blood Studies—cont'd		
• Fluorescent treponemal antibody absorption (FTA-ABS)	Detects syphilis antibodies. Also detects early syphilis with great accuracy. Usually performed if results of above nonspecific tests are questionable.	Inform patient that blood sample will be drawn. Observe venipuncture site for bleeding or hematoma formation.
Cultures and Smears		
• Dark-field microscopy	Direct examination of specimen obtained from potential syphilitic lesion (chancre) is performed to detect *Treponema pallidum*.	Avoid direct skin contact with open lesion.
• Wet mounts	Direct microscopic examination of specimen of vaginal discharge is performed immediately after collection. Determines presence or absence and number of *Trichomonas* organisms, bacteria, white and red blood cells, and candidal buds or hyphae. Other clues or causes of inflammation or infection may be determined.	Explain procedure and purpose to patient. Instruct patient not to douche before examination. Prepare for collection of specimens (glass slide, 10%-20% potassium hydroxide [KOH] solution, sodium chloride [NaCl] solution, and cotton-tipped applicators).
• Cultures	Specimens of vaginal, urethral, or cervical discharge are cultured and used to assess presence of gonorrhea or chlamydia. Rectal and throat cultures may also be taken, depending on data obtained from sexual history.	Obtain specific contact and sexual history inclusive of oral and rectal intercourse. Instruct against douching before examination. Obtain urethral specimen from men before they void. Instruct women who are sexually active with multiple partners to have at least a yearly culture for gonorrhea and chlamydia. Instruct sexually active men to have any discharge evaluated immediately to rule out gonorrhea strains that do not cause classic symptoms of dysuria.
• Gram stain	Used for rapid detection of gonorrhea. Presence of gram-negative intracellular diplococci generally warrants initiation of treatment. Not highly accurate for women. Has also been shown as accurate alternative for *Chlamydia* testing.	Same as above.
Cytologic Studies		
• Pap smear	Microscopic study of exfoliated cells via special staining and fixation technique detects abnormal cells. Cells most commonly studied are those obtained directly from endocervix, cervix, vaginal pool, and endometrial lining of uterine cavity.	Instruct women who are sexually active and who are over age 18 to have Pap smears according to American Cancer Society guidelines. Arrange for smear at midcycle time. Instruct patients not to douche for at least 24 hr before examination. Collect careful menstrual and gynecologic history.
• Nipple discharge test	Cytologic study of nipple discharge is performed.	Indicate whether hormonal preparations or other drugs are being taken, breastfeeding, or history of amenorrhea. Instruct patient during demonstration of breast self-examination or examination of breasts that nipple discharge should always be evaluated.
Radiologic Studies		
• Mammography	Low-dose x-ray image of breast tissue on radiographic film is used to assess breast tissue.	Instruct patient about advantages of the examination. Instruct regarding American Cancer Society recommendations for screening (see Chapter 50).
• Ultrasound	Measures and records high-frequency sound waves as they pass through tissues of variable density. It is very useful in detecting masses greater than 3 cm, such as ectopic pregnancies, IUDs, ovarian cysts, and hydatidiform moles. In men, is used to detect testicular torsion or masses.	Instruct patient that a full bladder may be required depending on the reason for the study.

IUDs, Intrauterine devices.

TABLE 49-12 Diagnostic Studies

Male and Female Reproductive Systems—cont'd

STUDY	DESCRIPTION AND PURPOSE	NURSING RESPONSIBILITY
Radiologic Studies—cont'd		
• Computed tomography (CT) of pelvis	Pelvic CT is used to detect tumor within the pelvis.	Inform patient of procedure. Patient must lie still during the procedure. If intravenous contrast is used, check for iodine allergy.
Invasive Procedures		
• Breast biopsy	Histologic examination of excised breast tissue is performed, either by needle-aspiration or excisional biopsy.	Before surgery, instruct patient about operative procedures and sedation. After surgery, perform wound care and instruct patient about breast self-examination.
• Hysterosalpingogram	Involves instillation of contrast media through cervix into uterine cavity and subsequently through and out fallopian tubes. Spot x-ray images are taken to detect abnormalities of uterus and its adnexa (ovaries and tubes) as contrast progresses through them. Test may be most useful in diagnostic assessment of fertility (e.g., to detect adhesions near ovary, an abnormal uterine shape, blockage of tubal pathways).	Inform patient about procedure and that it may be fairly uncomfortable. Determine possibility of iodine allergy.
• Colposcopy	Direct visualization of cervix with binocular microscope that allows magnification and study of cellular dysplasia and vascular and tissue abnormalities of cervix. This test is used as a follow-up study for abnormal Pap smears and for examination of women exposed to DES in utero. Biopsy of cervix may be taken during colposcopic examination. This test is valuable in decreasing number of false-negative cervical biopsies.	Instruct patient about this outpatient procedure. Inform patient that this examination is similar to speculum examination. Explain purpose of procedure and prepare patient for it.
• Conization	Cone-shaped sample of squamocolumnar tissue of cervix is removed for direct study.	Explain purpose and method of procedure and that it requires use of surgical facilities and anesthesia. Instruct patient to rest for at least 3 days after procedure. Also discuss necessity for 3 wk follow-up check.
• Loop electrosurgical excision of transformation zone (LEETZ)	Excision of cervical tissue via an electrosurgical instrument.	Explain purpose and method of procedure and that it may be done in the physician's office for further diagnostic testing.
• Loop electrosurgical excision procedure (LEEP)	Same as above.	Same as above.
• Culdotomy, culdoscopy, and culdocentesis	Culdotomy is an incision made through posterior fornix of cul-de-sac and allows visualization of peritoneal cavity (i.e., uterus, tubes, and ovaries). Culdoscope can then be used to study these structures closely. This technique is valuable in fertility evaluations. Withdrawal of fluid (culdocentesis) allows examination of fluid characteristics.	Explain purpose and method of procedure. Prepare patient for vaginal operation with preoperative instruction and sedation. Perform assessment of bleeding and discomfort after surgery.
• Laparoscopy (peritoneoscopy)	Allows visualization of pelvic structures via fiberoptic scopes inserted through small abdominal incisions. Instillation of carbon dioxide into cavity improves visualization. This technique is used in diagnostic assessment of uterus, tubes, and ovaries. Can be used in conjunction with tubal sterilization.	Explain purpose and method of procedure. Before surgery, instruct patient about procedure, prepare abdomen, and reassure patient about sedation. Tell patient to rest for 1-3 days after surgery. Inform patient of probability of shoulder pain because of air in the abdomen.
• Dilation and curettage	The operative procedure dilates cervix and allows curetting of endometrial lining. This test is used in assessment of abnormal bleeding patterns and cytologic evaluation of lining.	Before surgery, instruct patient about procedure and sedation. Perform postoperative assessment of degree of bleeding (frequent pad check during first 24 hr).

DES, Diethylstilbestrol.

Continued

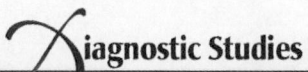

TABLE
49-12
Diagnostic Studies
Male and Female Reproductive Systems—cont'd

STUDY	DESCRIPTION AND PURPOSE	NURSING RESPONSIBILITY
Fertility Studies		
• Semen analysis	Semen is assessed for volume (2-5 ml), viscosity, sperm count (>20 million/ml), sperm motility (60% motile), and percent of abnormal sperm (60% with normal structure).	Instruct patient to bring in fresh specimen within 2 hr after ejaculation.
• Basal body temperature assessment	This measurement indicates indirectly whether ovulation has occurred. (Temperature rises at ovulation and remains elevated during secretory phase of normal menstrual cycle.)	Instruct woman to take her temperature using special basal temperature thermometer (calibrated in tenths of degrees) every morning before getting out of bed. Tell woman to record temperature on graph.
• Huhner test or Sims-Huhner	Mucus sample of cervix is examined within 2-8 hr after intercourse. Total number of sperm is assessed in relation to number of live sperm. This test is performed to determine whether cervical mucus is "hostile" to passage of sperm from vagina into uterus.	Instruct couples to have intercourse at estimated time of ovulation and be present for test within 2-8 hr after intercourse.
• Endometrial biopsy	Small curette is used to obtain piece of endometrial lining to assess endometrial changes common to progesterone secretion after ovulation.	Tell patient that test must be performed postovulation. Explain that procedure should cause only short period of uterine cramping.
• Hysterosalpingogram	Same as operative procedures.	Same as operative procedures.
• Serum progesterone	Same as blood studies.	Same as blood studies.

Cultures and Smears

Cultures and smears are most frequently employed in the diagnosis of sexually transmitted disease. Specimens for cultures and smears are most commonly taken from the vagina, endocervix, and rectum for females and the urethra and rectum for males. For a culture, the specimen is placed on a special culture medium; a smear involves rubbing the specimen on a slide for direct examination. Gram stain smears have been shown to be effective in the diagnosis of chlamydia infection.[17] Dark-field microscopy involves the direct examination of a specimen obtained from a syphilitic chancre for the diagnosis of syphilis.

Cytologic Studies

Cytology involves the study of cells under microscopic examination. The Pap smear is a screening test to detect abnormal cells obtained from the cervix or vagina. It is performed by obtaining cells from the cervical canal, preferably the endocervix, as well as from the vagina, and placing these cells in a fixative for examination by a cytologist for cellular abnormalities. Pap smears are more accurate if performed at midcycle or during the secretory phase of the menstrual cycle because there is a greater likelihood that abnormal cells will be detected during these times. A Pap smear should be performed annually or more frequently in women with a history of dysplasia. Pap smears are necessary in women who have had a hysterectomy because abnormal vaginal cells (if present) can sometimes be detected. Although a Pap smear is highly accurate in detecting cervical cancer, a negative Pap test does not rule out endometrial cancer.

Cytologic study is also indicated for nipple discharge. Cytologic examination discharge can detect the presence of malignant cells as opposed to a discharge associated with infection.

Radiologic Studies

Mammography. Mammography has become one of the most frequently used diagnostic tools in reproductive system assessment. It is used to detect breast masses. Mammography can detect breast masses before they are palpable. Mammography and screening guidelines for mammography are discussed in Chapter 50.

Ultrasound. Ultrasound has many applications for diagnostic study. Pelvic ultrasound is used to obtain images of the pelvic organs. It is used to detect pregnancy in the uterus, ectopic pregnancy, ovarian cysts, and other pelvic masses. Breast ultrasound is useful in the detection of fluid-filled masses. In men, ultrasound is used to detect testicular masses and testicular torsion. Transrectal ultrasound is useful in locating prostate tumors.

Pelvic Computed Tomography (CT) and Magnetic Resonance Imaging (MRI). Pelvic CT or MRI is used to detect primary or metastatic tumors of the reproductive organs. Contrast medium may be used in conjunction with the CT procedure.

REVIEW QUESTIONS

The number of the question corresponds to the same-numbered objective at the beginning of the chapter.

1. A normal reproductive function that may be altered in a patient who undergoes a prostatectomy is
   a. sperm production.
   b. production of testosterone.
   c. production of seminal fluid.
   d. release of sperm from the epididymis.

2. Estrogen production by the mature ovarian follicle causes
   a. decreased secretion of FSH and LH.
   b. increased production of GnRH and FSH.
   c. release of GnRH and increased secretion of LH.
   d. decreased release of FSH and decreased progesterone production.

3. Male orgasm is the result of
   a. clitoral swelling and increased vaginal lubrication.
   b. vaginal enlargement and secretion with penile insertion.
   c. clitoral swelling, vaginal lubrication, and uterine elevation.
   d. rapid release of vasocongestion and muscular tension in the reproductive structures.

4. An age-related finding noted by the nurse during assessment of the older woman's reproductive system is
   a. gynecomastia.
   b. increased vaginal discharge.
   c. decreased amount of pubic hair.
   d. soft, nontender, fleshy vulvar lesions.

5. Significant information about a patient's past medical history related to the reproductive system should include
   a. extent of sexual activity.
   b. general satisfaction with sexuality.
   c. previous sexually transmitted diseases.
   d. self-image and relationships with others.

6. The examination technique used to evaluate the prostate involves
   a. palpation.
   b. percussion.
   c. inspection.
   d. auscultation.

7. An abnormal finding noted during physical assessment of the male reproductive system is
   a. slight clear urethral discharge.
   b. the glans covered with prepuce.
   c. rubbery feeling of the testes on palpation.
   d. urethral meatus on the ventral side of the glans.

8. The screening criteria for assessing prostate cancer include a
   a. baseline ultrasound of the prostate at age 40.
   b. baseline ultrasound of the prostate at age 50.
   c. yearly digital rectal examination for men over age 30.
   d. yearly digital rectal examination for men over age 50.

REFERENCES

1. Thibodeau GA, Patton KT: *The human body in health and disease,* ed 3, St Louis, 2002, Mosby.
2. Di Saia PJ: Clinical anatomy of the female. In Scott JR et al, editors: *Danforth's obstetrics and gynecology,* ed 8, Philadelphia, 1999, Lippincott Williams & Wilkins.
3. McCance KL, Huether SE: *Pathophysiology: the biologic basis for disease in adults and children,* cd 4, St Louis, 2002, Mosby.
4. Arvidson CR: The adolescent gynecologic exam, *Pediatr Nurs* 25:71, 1999.
5. Hammond CB: Climacteric. In Scott JR et al, editors: *Danforth's obstetrics and gynecology,* ed 8, Philadelphia, 1999, Lippincott Williams & Wilkins.
6. Masters WH, Johnson E: *Human sexual response,* Boston, 1966, Little, Brown.
7. Dougherty JD, Knutesen P: The aging female reproductive system. In Stanley M, Beare PG, editors: *Gerontological nursing,* ed 2, Philadelphia, 1999, FA Davis.
8. Stone JT, Wyman JF, Salisbury SA: *Clinical gerontologic nursing: guide to advanced practice,* ed 2, Philadelphia, 1999, WB Saunders.
9. Kessenich CR, Cichon MJ: Hormonal decline in elderly men and male menopause, *Geriatr Nurs* 22:24, 2001.
10. Warner PH, Rowe T, Whipple B: Shedding light on the sexual history, *Am J Nurs* 99:34, 1999.
11. Steinke EE: Sexual counseling after myocardial infarction, *Am J Nurs* 100:38, 2000.
12. American Cancer Society: Prostate cancer reference information. Available at *www.cancer.org* (accessed Feb 20, 2003).
13. Grodner M, Anderson SL, DeYoung S: *Foundations and clinical applications of nutrition: a nursing approach,* ed 2, St Louis, 2000, Mosby.
14. Wilson S, Giddens JF: *Health assessment for nursing practice,* ed 2, St Louis, 2001, Mosby.
15. Corbett JV: *Laboratory tests and diagnostic procedures with nursing diagnosis,* ed 5, Upper Saddle River, NJ, 2000, Prentice Hall.
16. Pagana KD, Pagana TJ: *Mosby's diagnostic and laboratory test reference,* ed 5, St Louis, 2001, Mosby.
17. Mysiuk L, Romanowski B, Brown M: Endocervical Gram stain smears and their usefulness in the diagnosis of *Chlamydia trachomatis, Sexually Transmitted Infections* 77:103, 2001.

RESOURCES

Resources for this chapter are listed in Chapter 52 on p. 1434 and Chapter 53 on p. 1462.

CHAPTER **50**

NURSING MANAGEMENT
Breast Disorders

Shannon Ruff Dirksen

LEARNING OBJECTIVES

1. Assess breast tissue by inspection and palpation using appropriate examination techniques.
2. Teach breast health awareness and breast self-examination, including rationale, technique, and reasons for referral.
3. Describe the types, causes, clinical manifestations, collaborative care, and nursing management of common benign breast disorders.
4. Identify the known risk factors for breast cancer.
5. Describe the pathophysiology, clinical manifestations, and collaborative care of breast cancer.
6. Identify the types of, indications for, and complications of surgical interventions for breast cancer.
7. Explain the physical and psychologic preoperative and postoperative aspects of nursing management for the patient undergoing a mastectomy.
8. Describe the indications for reconstructive breast surgery; types, potential risks, and complications of reconstructive breast surgery; and nursing management after reconstructive breast surgery.

KEY TERMS

ductal ectasia, p. 1365	lymphedema, p. 1370
fibroadenoma, p. 1364	mammoplasty, p. 1378
fibrocystic changes, p. 1364	mastalgia, p. 1363
galactorrhea, p. 1365	mastectomy, p. 1369
gynecomastia, p. 1365	mastitis, p. 1363
intraductal papilloma, p. 1365	Paget's disease, p. 1367
lumpectomy, p. 1370	

Breast disorders are a significant health concern for women. Although most breast pain is of a benign nature, in a woman's lifetime there is a one in eight chance that she will be diagnosed with breast cancer.[1] Whether benign or malignant, intense feelings of shock, fear, and denial often accompany the initial discovery of a lump or change in the breast. These feelings can be associated both with the fear of death and with the possible loss of a breast. Throughout history, the female breast has been regarded as a symbol of beauty, femininity, sexuality, and motherhood. The potential loss of a breast, or part of a breast, may be devastating for many women because of the significant psychologic, social, sexual, and body image implications associated with it. The most frequently encountered breast disorders in women are fibrocystic changes, breast cancer, fibroadenoma, intraductal papilloma, and ductal ectasia. In men, gynecomastia is the most common breast disorder.

ASSESSMENT OF BREAST DISORDERS

It is critical that breast disorders be detected early, diagnosed accurately, and treated promptly.[2] The essential factors in the early detection of breast cancer and other breast-related problems are the regular performance of routine mammography, regular

clinical breast examination (CBE), and breast self-examination (BSE). The frequency of these examinations is determined by the woman's age, the presence of significant risk factors, and her past medical history (Table 50-1). Guidelines established in the United States by the American Cancer Society (ACS) and the National Cancer Institute (NCI) regarding breast surveillance practices include the following:[3]

1. Monthly BSE over age 20
2. Physical examination of the breasts by a trained health professional (CBE) every 3 years between ages 20 and 39 and annually thereafter
3. Annual screening mammography beginning at age 40

The NCI is currently reviewing guidelines on mammography screening for healthy women to determine the best schedule for screening.[4] The benefits of early detection of breast cancer are well established. The use of screening mammography has significantly improved early and accurate detection of breast malignancies. Mammography can identify breast abnormalities that may be cancer before physical symptoms appear. Women at high risk for disease, such as those with a family history of breast cancer, should consult their physician about having mammograms earlier and more frequently.

Breast Self-Examination

Providing education and encouraging women to perform BSE are recommended to decrease mortality rates from breast cancer. In recent years there has been some controversy regarding the value of BSE and its role in reducing mortality rates from breast cancer in women.[5] Until the issue is resolved, women should continue doing BSE with regular screening by mammography and CBE.

Although the reasons that women report for failing to practice regular BSE have changed somewhat over the years, many women still do not regularly examine their breasts. Some reasons cited by women for not practicing BSE are embarrassment, fear of finding a lump, lack of confidence in ability to do BSE, inadequate knowledge of the procedure, and not remembering to do BSE. Factors that increase BSE compliance include positive be-

Reviewed by Rebecca Crane-Okada, RN, PhD, AOCN, Clinical Researcher and Oncology Clinical Nurse Specialist, Joyce Eisenberg Keefer Breast Center, John Wayne Cancer Institute, Saint John's Health Center, Santa Monica, Calif.

TABLE 50-1 Risk Factors for Breast Cancer	
INCREASED RISK	**COMMENTS**
Female	Women account for 99% of breast cancer cases.
Age 50 or over	Majority of breast cancers are found in postmenopausal women.
Family history	Breast cancer in a first-degree relative, particularly when premenopausal or bilateral, increases risk. Gene mutations (BRCA-1 or BRCA-2) play a role in 5%–10% of breast cancer cases.
Personal history of breast cancer, colon cancer, endometrial cancer, ovarian cancer	Personal history significantly increases risk of breast cancer, risk of cancer in other breast, and recurrence.
Early menarche (< age 12); late menopause (> age 55)	A long menstrual history increases the risk of breast cancer.
First full-term pregnancy after age 30; nulliparity	Prolonged exposure to unopposed estrogen increases risk for breast cancer.
Benign breast disease with atypical epithelial hyperplasia	Atypical changes in breast biopsy increase the risk of breast cancer.
Obesity after menopause	Fat cells store estrogen.
Exposure to ionizing radiation	Radiation damages DNA (e.g., prior treatment for Hodgkin's disease).

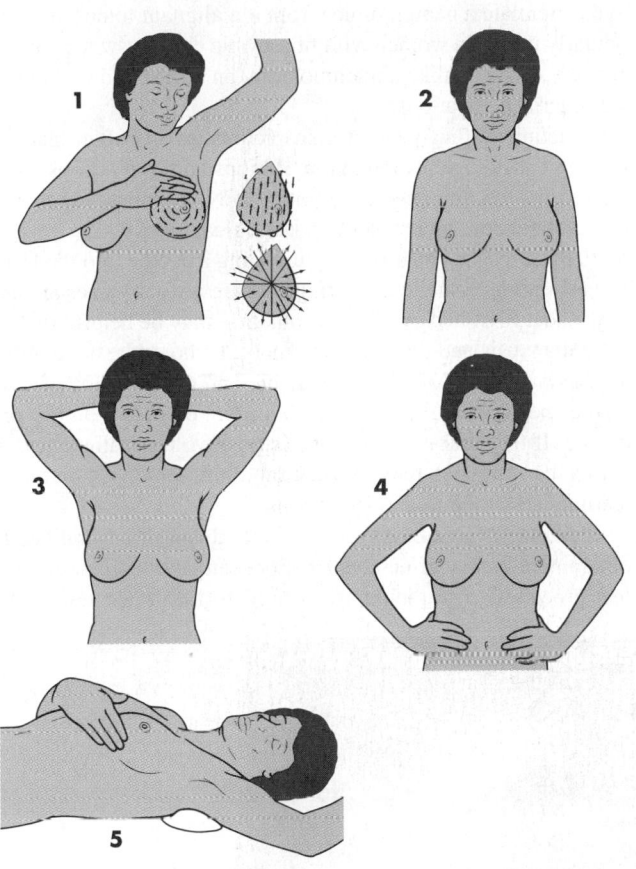

FIG. 50-1 Breast self-examination and patient instruction. *1,* While in the shower or bath, when the skin is slippery with soap and water, examine your breasts. Use the pads of your second, third, and fourth fingers to firmly press every part of the breast. While examining your left breast, use your right hand, and use your left hand to examine your right breast. Using the pads of the fingers on your left hand, examine the entire breast using small circular motions in a spiral or in an up-and-down motion so that the entire breast area is examined. Repeat the procedure using your right hand to examine your left breast. Repeat pattern of palpation under the arm. Check for any lump, hard knot, or thickening of the tissue. *2,* Look at your breasts in a mirror. Stand with your arms at your side. *3,* Raise your arms overhead and check for any changes in the shape of your breasts, dimpling of the skin, or any changes in the nipple. *4,* Next, place your hands on your hips and press down firmly, tightening the pectoral muscles. Observe for asymmetry or changes, keeping in mind that your breasts probably do not exactly match. *5,* While lying down, feel your breasts as described in step 1. When examining your right breast, place a folded towel under your right shoulder and put your right hand behind your head. Repeat the procedure while examining your left breast. Mark your calendar that you have completed your BSE; note any changes or unique characteristics you want to check with your health care provider.

liefs about screening, lower perceived risk, history of breast biopsies, family history of breast cancer, and BSE demonstration.[6]

The nurse who is teaching BSE should emphasize that early detection and treatment enhance survival rates. Efforts must be directed toward teaching women the importance of BSE, how to perform it, and what to do if a problem is detected. BSE teaching techniques should include allowing time for the woman to ask questions about the procedure and to perform a return demonstration. The technique for BSE has been established by the ACS (available on the Internet at *www.cancer.org*) and the NCI (Fig. 50-1). BSE should be done monthly at a regular time when

the breasts are not tender. In premenopausal women, the best time is 7 days after the start of menstruation. At this time, hormonal stimulation of the breasts is at its lowest point. In most women, nodularity and tenderness will be minimal. For women taking oral contraceptives (about 20% to 25% of women ages 15 to 45) the first day of a new package may be a helpful reminder. Postmenopausal women and women who have had hysterectomies should set a regular date for monthly BSE. Many women use the monthly date of a birthday or the first day of the month.

BSE should be done in good light and should include inspection before a mirror and careful, systematic palpation. The entire breast, axilla, and clavicle should be examined. The woman should be taught the BSE procedure by a health care provider using the woman's own hand on her breast. A gentle circular motion over wet, soapy skin is particularly useful if she is in the shower. The woman should be told what to look for, such as a lump, nipple discharge, nipple retraction, redness, pain or tenderness, dimpling of the skin, or edema. Some teaching techniques involve using silicone breast models that simulate normal and abnormal breast tissue to help women learn to identify problems. The woman should be shown the normal variations in her own breasts so that she will be able to detect changes. Finally, she should be reminded that most breast problems are not related to malignancy. At every annual physical examination the health care provider should ask the woman to demonstrate how she performs BSE.

If a problem is suspected such as nipple discharge or finding a lump, the woman should see her primary care provider or contact a comprehensive breast center as soon as possible so that additional diagnostic studies can be promptly initiated. If the problem is not serious, the woman's anxiety can be quickly relieved. If a serious problem is suspected or diagnosed, definitive treatment should not be delayed.

Even when a woman faithfully practices BSE, she should have an annual breast examination by a qualified health care provider and a mammogram if age appropriate. The care and attention to detail shown by the clinician in performing CBE reinforce the practice of BSE by the patient.

Diagnostic Studies

Several techniques can be used to screen for breast disease or provide a diagnosis of a suspicious physical finding. *Mammography* is a method used to visualize the internal structure of the breast using low-dose x-rays (Fig. 50-2). This simple, safe procedure can detect tumors and cysts that cannot be felt by palpation. Improved imaging techniques have reduced the radiation that accompanies mammography to insignificant levels.

Digital mammography has been recently approved by the Food and Drug Administration. In this procedure x-ray images are digitally coded into a computer. This allows for a clearer and more accurate image than conventional mammography x-ray film.

The minimum size of a tumor detectable by physical examination is 1 cm. It may take 10 years or longer for a tumor to grow to this size. Mammography can detect masses of 0.5 cm.

Calcifications are the most easily recognized mammogram abnormality. These deposits of calcium crystals form in the breast for many reasons, such as inflammation, trauma, and aging. Although most calcifications are benign, they also may be associated with preinvasive cancer.[7]

A comparison of current and prior mammograms may show early cancer tissue changes. Because some tumors metastasize late in the preclinical course, early detection by mammography allows for early treatment and the prevention of metastasis of these smaller lesions. In younger women mammography is less sensitive because of the greater density of breast tissue, resulting in more false-negative results.[8] From 10% to 15% of breast cancers cannot be seen on mammography and are detected only by palpation. Suspicious masses should be biopsied even if mammogram findings are unremarkable.

Ultrasound is another diagnostic procedure that can be used to differentiate a benign tumor from a malignant tumor. It is particularly useful in women with fibrocystic changes whose breasts are very dense. Unlike a mammogram, an ultrasound will not detect microcalcifications.

A definitive diagnosis of a suspicious area is often made by means of histologic examination of biopsied tissue. Biopsy techniques include fine-needle aspiration (FNA) biopsy, stereotactic or handheld core biopsy, and open surgical biopsy.

FNA biopsy is performed by inserting a needle into the lesion and aspirating tissue into a syringe. Three or four passes are usually made. FNA and cytologic evaluation may be helpful in making a diagnosis and planning treatment. It should be done only if an experienced cytologist is available and all suspicious lesions read as negative are followed with a more definitive biopsy procedure. If the aspirated specimen is positive for malignancy, the patient can be given this information at the same visit and begin learning about the treatment options.

Stereotactic core biopsy is a reliable diagnostic technique for obtaining a biopsy of an abnormality seen on a mammogram. In this procedure mammography is used to locate the lesion. The

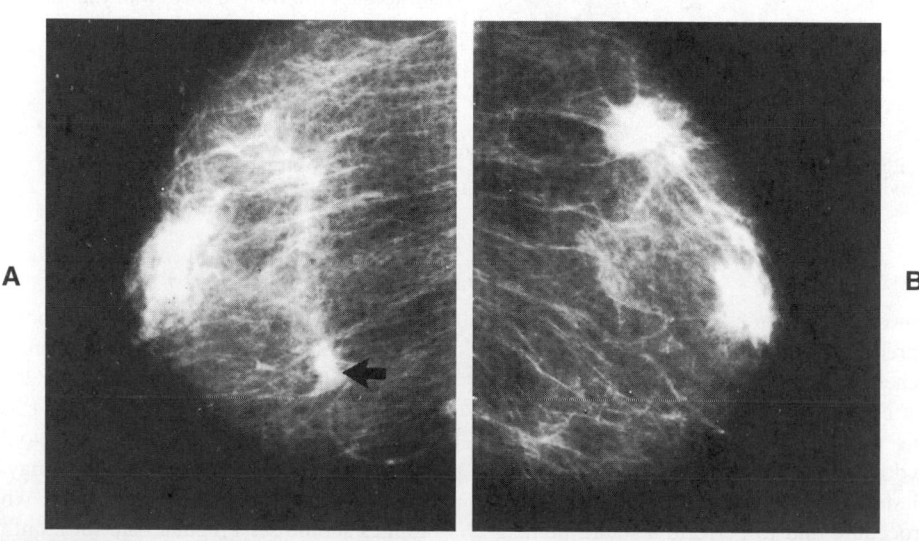

FIG. 50-2   Mammogram showing bilateral invasive ductal carcinoma. **A,** Left breast. The larger left mass was palpable. The smaller right mass was not palpable *(arrow).* **B,** Right breast. Multiple masses are shown.

skin is anesthetized, and a small skin incision is made to allow the entrance of a biopsy gun device. The gun is fired and removes a core sample of the lesion. This is repeated several times, and the core samples are sent for pathologic analysis. This technique has several advantages over an open surgical biopsy, including minimal scarring, the use of local anesthesia, outpatient procedure, reduced cost, and shorter recovery time.[9]

Benign Breast Disorders

MASTALGIA

Mastalgia (breast pain) is the most common breast-related complaint in women. It affects up to 70% of all women.[10] The most common form is *cyclic mastalgia,* which coincides with the menstrual cycle. It is described as diffuse breast tenderness or heaviness. Breast pain may last 2 to 3 days or most of the month. The pain is related to hormonal sensitivity. The symptoms often decrease with menopause. *Noncyclic mastalgia* has no relationship to the menstrual cycle and can continue into menopause.[11] It may be constant or intermittent throughout the month and last for several years. Symptoms include a burning, aching, or soreness in the breast. The etiology of the pain may be due to trauma, fat necrosis, or duct ectasia.

Mammography is frequently done to exclude cancer and provide information on the etiology of mastalgia. Some relief may occur with caffeine and dietary fat reduction; taking vitamins E, A, and B complex and gamma-linolenic acid (evening primrose oil); and the continual wearing of a support bra. Hormonal therapy may be recommended, including oral contraceptives and danazol (Danocrine).

BREAST INFECTIONS

Mastitis

Mastitis is an inflammatory condition of the breast that occurs most frequently in lactating women (Table 50-2). *Lactational mastitis* manifests as a localized area that is erythematous, painful, and tender to palpation. Fever is usually present. The infection develops when organisms, usually staphylococci, gain access to the breast through a cracked nipple. In its early stages, mastitis can be cured with antibiotics. Breastfeeding should continue unless an abscess is forming or a purulent drainage is noted. The mother may wish to use a nipple shield or to hand-express milk from the involved breast until the pain subsides. The woman should see her health care provider promptly to begin a course of antibiotic therapy. Any breast that remains red, tender, and not responsive to antibiotics requires follow-up care and evaluation for inflammatory breast cancer.

Lactational Breast Abscess

If lactational mastitis persists after several days of antibiotic therapy, a lactational breast abscess may have developed. In this condition the skin may become red and edematous over the involved breast, often with a corresponding palpable mass, and the patient may have an elevated temperature. Antibiotics alone constitute insufficient treatment for a breast abscess. Surgical incision and drainage are necessary. The drainage is cultured, sensi-

TABLE 50-2	Differential Diagnosis of Selected Benign Breast Disorders	
DISORDER	**RISK FACTORS**	**CLINICAL MANIFESTATIONS**
Lactation mastitis	Lactating woman	Warm to touch
	Occurs spontaneously in approximately 2% of all postpartum lactating mothers (both primipara and multipara), usually 2-4 wk after birth	Indurated
		Usually unilateral
		Most common etiology is *Staphylococcus aureus*
Nonlactation mastitis	Rare condition	Palpable mass
	Usually women in late adolescence or middle age	Usually an obscure organism
		Should rule out syphilis or tuberculosis
Fibrocystic breast changes	Most common between ages 35 and 50	Not usually discrete masses, nodularity instead; usually accompanied by cyclic pain and tenderness; mass(es) usually cyclic in occurrence (movable, soft)
Cysts	Most common between ages 30 and 50	Palpable mass (movable, soft); may have multiple microcysts
Fibroadenoma	Peak age range between ages 15 and 25	Often bilateral
	Most occur before age 30	Palpable mass (movable, firm)
	Most common among African American women	Most common size at diagnosis is 2-3 cm
		Rapid growth
		Accounts for 2%-3% of all breast masses
Fat necrosis	50% report previous history of trauma to breast	Usually a hard, tender, mobile, indurated mass with irregular borders
Intraductal papilloma	Affects women ages 40-60	Usually associated with serous, serosanguineous, or bloody nipple discharge on affected side
Ductal ectasia	Perimenopausal woman—most common in women in their fifties	Fixation of nipple
	Previous lactation	Usually accompanied by nipple discharge of thick gray material
	Inverted nipples	Often associated with breast pain

tivities are obtained, and therapy with an appropriate antibiotic is begun. Often the woman will find it necessary to express and discard milk from the affected breast until the abscess is resolved.

FIBROCYSTIC CHANGES

Fibrocystic changes in the breast constitute a benign condition characterized by changes in breast tissue (see Table 50-2). The changes include the development of excess fibrous tissue, hyperplasia of the epithelial lining of the mammary ducts, proliferation of mammary ducts, and cyst formation. These changes produce pain by nerve irritation from edema in connective tissue and by fibrosis from nerve pinching. The use of the term *fibrocystic disease* is incorrect because the cluster of problems is actually an exaggerated response to hormonal influence. It has been suggested that the term *fibrocystic condition* or *fibrocystic complex* be used. Fibrocystic changes do not increase the risk of breast cancer for the majority of patients. Masses or nodularities can appear in both breasts and are often found in the upper, outer quadrants and usually occur bilaterally. It is the most frequently occurring breast disorder.

Fibrocystic changes occur most frequently in women between 35 and 50 years of age but often begin in women as young as 20 years of age. Pain and nodularity often increase over time but tend to subside after menopause unless high doses of estrogen replacement are used. The cause of these fibrocystic changes is thought to be heightened responsiveness of breast parenchyma and stroma to circulating estrogen and progesterone. Fibrocystic changes most commonly occur in women with premenstrual abnormalities, nulliparous women, women with a history of spontaneous abortion, nonusers of oral contraceptives, and women with early menarche and late menopause. Symptoms related to fibrocystic changes often worsen in the premenstrual phase and subside after menstruation.

Manifestations of fibrocystic breast changes include one or more palpable lumps that are usually round, well delineated, and freely movable within the breast. Some lumps are fibrous and do not contain cysts. There may be accompanying discomfort ranging from tenderness to pain. The lump is usually observed to increase in size and perhaps in tenderness before menstruation. Cysts may enlarge or shrink rapidly. Nipple discharge associated with fibrocystic breasts is often milky, watery-milky, yellow, or green.

Mammography may be helpful in distinguishing fibrocystic changes from breast cancer. However, in some women the breast tissue is so dense that it is difficult to obtain a worthwhile mammogram study. In these situations, ultrasound may be more useful in differentiating a cystic mass from a solid mass.

NURSING *and* COLLABORATIVE MANAGEMENT
FIBROCYSTIC CHANGES

With the initial discovery of a discrete mass in the breast by a woman or her health care provider, aspiration or surgical biopsy may be indicated. A wait of 7 to 10 days may be planned if the nodularity is recurrent to note changes as the menstrual cycle changes. With large or frequent cysts, surgical removal may be favored over repeated aspiration. An excisional biopsy should be done if no fluid is found on aspiration, if the fluid that is found is hemorrhagic, or if a residual mass remains. This surgery is performed in an office or day surgery unit with the patient under local anesthesia.

Biopsies in women with fibrocystic disease may be indicated for women with an increased risk for breast cancer (see Table 50-1).

Hyperplastic changes approximating the histologic appearance of carcinoma in situ (atypical hyperplasia) and a family history of breast cancer increase the probability of developing breast cancer.

The woman with cystic changes should be encouraged to return regularly for follow-up examinations throughout her life. She should also be taught BSE to self-monitor the problem. Severe fibrocystic changes may make palpation of the breast more difficult. Any new lumps or changes in the breasts should be evaluated, and changes in symptoms should be reported and investigated.

Many types of treatment have been suggested for a fibrocystic condition. These include the use of a good support bra, dietary therapy (low-salt diet, restriction of methylxanthines such as coffee and chocolate), vitamin E therapy, analgesics, danazol (Danocrine), diuretics, hormone therapy, and antiestrogen therapy.[12] Because stress can be a contributing factor in breast discomfort, efforts should also be directed toward the reduction of stress. Although many of these treatments have not been scientifically proven to be beneficial, many women report less discomfort with these nonsurgical measures. Danazol has been used for patients with severe pain. It decreases follicle-stimulating hormone (FSH) and luteinizing hormone (LH), resulting in reduced estrogen production and subsequent decreased pain and nodularity. The androgenic side effects of danazol (acne, edema, hirsutism) often make this therapy intolerable for many women.

The role of the nurse in the care of the patient with fibrocystic breast changes is primarily one of teaching. A woman with fibrocystic breasts should be told that she may expect recurrence of the cysts in one or both breasts until menopause and that cysts may enlarge or become painful just before menstruation. Additionally, she should be reassured that cysts do not "turn into" cancer. Any new lump that does not respond in a cyclic manner over 1 to 2 weeks should be examined by a health care provider promptly. The woman should be carefully instructed in BSE, using her own breasts. The use of silicone breast models can also aid instruction.

FIBROADENOMA

Fibroadenoma is a common cause of discrete benign breast lumps in young women. It generally occurs in women between 15 and 25 years of age and is the most frequent cause of breast masses in women under 25 years of age. Fibroadenomas tend to develop more frequently and at a younger age in African American women.[13] The possible cause of fibroadenoma may be increased estrogen sensitivity in a localized area of the breast. Fibroadenomas are usually small (but can be large, 2 to 3 cm), painless, round, well delineated, and very mobile. They may be soft but are usually solid, firm, and rubbery in consistency. There is no accompanying retraction or nipple discharge. The lump is often painless. The fibroadenoma may appear as a single unilateral mass, although multiple bilateral fibroadenomas have been reported. Growth is slow and often ceases when size reaches 2 to 3 cm. Size is not affected by menstruation. However, pregnancy can stimulate dramatic growth. Fibroadenomas are rarely associated with cancer.

NURSING *and* COLLABORATIVE MANAGEMENT
FIBROADENOMA

Fibroadenomas are easily detected by physical examination and are often visible on mammography. Definitive diagnosis, however, requires biopsy and tissue examination by a pathologist. Treatment of fibroadenomas can include surgical excision, which is not urgent in women under 25 years of age. In women over 35 years of age all new lesions should be examined using an excisional biopsy. Fibroadenomas are not reduced by radiation and are not affected by hormone therapy.

As an alternative to surgery, tumor removal can be accomplished using *cryoablation*. In this procedure a cryoprobe is inserted into the tumor using ultrasound guidance. Extremely cold gas is piped into the tumor. The frozen tumor dies and gradually shrinks.

The nurse frequently has the opportunity to counsel a young woman with fibroadenomas. During this contact the benign nature of the lesion should be stressed and follow-up examinations and BSE should be encouraged.

NIPPLE DISCHARGE

Nipple discharge may occur spontaneously or as a result of nipple manipulation. A milky secretion is due to inappropriate lactation (termed **galactorrhea**) as a result of such problems as drug therapy, endocrine problems, and neurologic disorders. Nipple discharge may also be idiopathic.

Secretions can also be serous, grossly bloody, or brown to green. These may be caused by either benign or malignant disease. A slide can be made of the secretion to detect specific disease. Diseases associated with nipple discharge include malignancies, cystic disease, intraductal papilloma, and ductal ectasia. Treatment depends on identification of the cause. In most cases, nipple discharge is not related to malignancy. If galactorrhea is accompanied by amenorrhea, various gynecologic endocrinopathies should be explored.

Intraductal Papilloma

An **intraductal papilloma** is a benign, wartlike growth found in the mammary ducts, usually near the nipple. Typically, there is an associated bloody nipple discharge, a mass, or both. Intraductal papillomas usually affect women 40 to 60 years of age. A single duct or several ducts may be involved. Treatment includes excision of the papilloma and the involved duct or duct system.

Ductal Ectasia

Ductal ectasia is a benign breast disease of perimenopausal and postmenopausal women involving the ducts in the subareolar area. It usually involves several bilateral ducts. Nipple discharge is the primary symptom. This discharge is multicolored and sticky. Ductal ectasia is initially painless but may progress to burning, itching, and pain around the nipple, as well as swelling in the areolar area. Inflammatory signs are often present, the nipple may retract, and the discharge may become bloody in more advanced disease. Ductal ectasia is not associated with malignancy. If an abscess develops, warm compresses and antibiotics are usually effective treatments. Therapy consists of close follow-up examinations or surgical excision of the involved ducts.

GYNECOMASTIA IN MEN

Gynecomastia, a transient, noninflammatory enlargement of one or both breasts, is the most common breast problem in men (Fig. 50-3). The condition is usually temporary and benign. Gynecomastia in itself is not an established risk factor for breast cancer. The most common cause of gynecomastia is a disturbance of the normal ratio of active androgen to estrogen in plasma or within the breast itself.

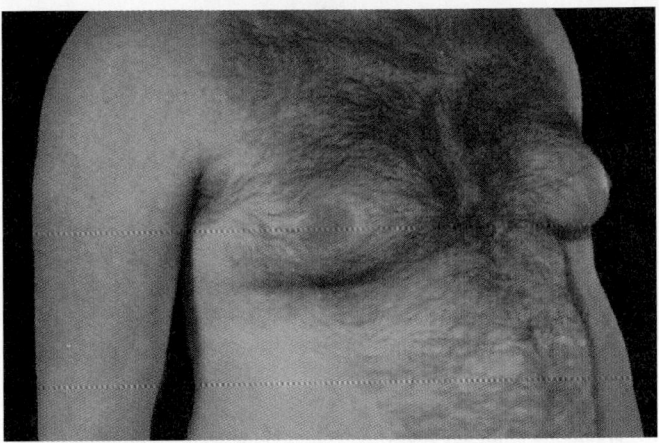

FIG. 50-3   Gynecomastia.

Gynecomastia may also be a symptom of other problems. It is seen accompanying developmental abnormalities of the male reproductive organs. It may also accompany organic diseases, including testicular tumors, cancer of the adrenal cortex, pituitary adenomas, hyperthyroidism, and liver disease.[14] Gynecomastia may occur as a side effect of drug therapy, particularly with administration of estrogens and androgens, digitalis, isoniazid (INH), ranitidine (Zantac), and spironolactone (Aldactone). Use of heroin and marijuana can also cause gynecomastia.

Pubertal Gynecomastia

Pubertal gynecomastia caused by increased estrogen production is seen most often in boys between ages 13 and 17. It is usually limited, although occasionally the localized hyperplasia may measure 2 to 3 cm in size. Pubertal gynecomastia is almost always self-limiting, and disappears within 4 to 6 months of onset. Parents and the affected boy should be reassured that in almost all cases this is a normal physiologic phenomenon that will disappear spontaneously and will require no treatment. Rarely, unilateral gynecomastia in the young male may be marked and fail to regress. This is the only indication for surgical intervention.

Senescent Gynecomastia

Senescent gynecomastia occurs in 40% of older men. A probable cause is the elevation in plasma estrogen in older adult men as the result of increased conversion of androgens to estrogens in peripheral circulation. Although initially unilateral, the tender, firm, centrally located enlargement may become bilateral. When gynecomastia is characterized by a discrete, circumscribed mass, it must be diagnosed to differentiate it from the rarer breast cancer in males. Senescent hyperplasia requires no treatment and generally regresses within 6 to 12 months.

■ Gerontologic Considerations: Age-Related Breast Changes

Loss of subcutaneous fat and structural support and atrophy of mammary glands often result in pendulous breasts in the postmenopausal woman. The nurse should encourage older women to wear a well-fitting bra. Adequate support can improve physical appearance and reduce pain in the back, shoulders, and neck. It can also prevent *intertrigo* (dermatitis caused by friction between opposing surfaces of skin). Surgical lifting of sagging breasts is possible and may be desirable when reconstruction after a mastectomy is performed.

The decrease in glandular tissue in older women makes a breast mass easier to palpate. This decreased density is probably age related and occurs even with women on hormone replacement therapy. Rib margins may be palpable in the older adult woman and can be confused with a mass. As a woman becomes more familiar with her own breasts and is reassured about her findings, the anxiety about this finding should decrease. The nurse should encourage the older woman to continue BSE and to have annual mammograms and clinical examinations because the incidence of breast cancer increases with age. ■

BREAST CANCER

Breast cancer is the most common malignancy in American women except for skin cancer. It is second only to lung cancer as the leading cause of death from cancer in women. An estimated 203,500 new cases of breast cancer were diagnosed in women in the United States in 2002. About 1500 new cases were diagnosed in men.[1] Each year in the United States, approximately 40,000 deaths (39,600 women and 400 men) occur related to breast cancer. The number of deaths of women from breast cancer appears to be leveling off. The largest decreases have been noted in younger women, both African American and white.

Research indicates that 96% of patients diagnosed with localized breast cancer with little or no axillary node involvement will be alive in 5 years. Conversely, only 21% of patients diagnosed with advanced-stage breast cancer with metastases to distant sites will survive 5 years.[2]

Etiology and Risk Factors

Although the etiology is not completely understood, a number of factors are thought to relate to the cause of breast cancer. Heredity or genetically related susceptibility is considered to play a role. Hormonal regulation of the breast is related to the development of breast cancer, but the mechanisms are poorly understood. Sex hormones may act as tumor promoters

CULTURAL & ETHNIC CONSIDERATIONS
Breast Cancer

- African American women have lower survival rates from breast cancer than white women, even when diagnosed at an early stage.
- African American women are diagnosed at a later stage of breast cancer than white women, but this fact alone does not account for the higher mortality rate.
- White women have a higher incidence of breast cancer than nonwhites.
- Breast cancer is the most commonly diagnosed cancer among Hispanic women.
- Hispanic women, especially Mexican Americans, have the lowest rate of cancer screening of any ethnic group.
- Hispanic women tend to have larger, more advanced tumors, which may relate to their higher mortality rate compared with white women.
- Hispanic women are more likely to be diagnosed at a later stage of breast cancer than white women.

if initiating agents have induced malignant changes. Additional factors under study include physical inactivity, dietary fat intake, obesity, and alcohol intake.[2] Environmental factors such as chemical, pesticide, and radiation exposure may also play a role.

Some factors that place a woman at higher risk for breast cancer have been identified (see Table 50-1). Women are at far greater risk than men because 99% of breast cancers occur in women. Increasing age also increases the risk of developing breast cancer. The incidence of breast cancer in women under 25 years of age is very low and increases gradually until age 60. After age 60 the incidence increases dramatically. Positive family history is an important risk factor, especially if the involved member with breast cancer was premenopausal, had bilateral disease, and is a first-degree relative (i.e., mother, sister, daughter). Having any first-degree relative with breast cancer increases a woman's risk of breast cancer 1.5 to 3 times, depending on age. Controversy exists as to whether hormone replacement therapy (HRT), primarily estrogen, in postmenopausal women increases breast cancer risk. Some studies suggest that risk increases only with prolonged HRT use.[15] Limited long-term data suggest that adding progesterone to the estrogen may cause an even higher risk than estrogen therapy alone.[16] The Nurses' Health Study has linked long-term oral contraceptive use to an increased risk of breast cancer.[17]

Risk factors appear to be cumulative and interacting. Therefore the presence of other risk factors may greatly increase the overall risk, especially for those with a positive family history. Identification of risk factors indicates an increased need for careful clinical surveillance of the patient and participation in cancer screening measures. Most women who develop breast cancer have none of the identifiable risk factors.

As many as 5% to 10% of all breast cancer patients may have inherited a specific genetic abnormality contributing to the development of their breast cancer. The first genetic alteration to be identified was in the tumor suppressor gene, p53. The BRCA-1 gene, located on chromosome 17, is a tumor suppressor gene that inhibits tumor development when functioning normally. Women who have BRCA-1 mutations have a 50% to 85% lifetime chance of developing breast cancer.[18] The BRCA-2 gene, located on chromosome 11, is another tumor suppressor gene, and women with a mutation of this gene have a similar risk of breast cancer. Mutations in BRCA genes may cause as many as 10% to 40% of all inherited breast cancers. As many as 1 in 200 to 400 women in the United States may be carriers. These women are also at high risk for developing ovarian cancer.[19] Routine screening for genetic abnormalities in women without evidence of a strong family history of breast cancer is not warranted. Genetic screening is expensive, time consuming, and often not covered by health care insurance.

In women with BRCA-1 or BRCA-2 mutations, prophylactic bilateral oophorectomy can decrease the risk of breast cancer and ovarian cancer.[20,21] In deciding whether to undergo this surgical procedure, women should take into account how long they wish to maintain fertility. In addition, they should receive counseling about the risks and benefits of prophylactic oophorectomy.

A woman who has a high risk of developing breast cancer, related to factors such as family history and prior tissue biopsies, may choose (in consultation with her physician) to undergo pro-

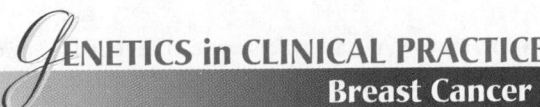

GENETICS in CLINICAL PRACTICE
Breast Cancer

Genetic Basis
- Mutations in genes BRCA-1 and BRCA-2
- Autosomal dominant transmission

Incidence
- Approximately 5% to 10% of breast cancers are related to BRCA-1 and BRCA-2 gene mutations.
- Women with BRCA-1 and BRCA-2 gene mutations have a 50% to 85% lifetime risk of developing breast cancer.
- BRCA-1 and BRCA-2 gene mutations are associated with early-onset breast cancer.
- Family history of both breast and ovarian cancer increases the risk of having a BRCA mutation.

Genetic Testing
- DNA testing is available for BRCA-1 and BRCA-2.

Clinical Implications
- Bilateral oophorectomy reduces the risk of breast cancer in women with BRCA-1 and BRCA-2 mutations.
- Genetic counseling and testing for BRCA mutations should be considered for women whose personal or family history puts them at high risk for a genetic predisposition to breast cancer.

phylactic bilateral mastectomy. This surgery may reduce a women's breast cancer risk by 90%.[22]

Predisposing risk factors in men include states of hyperestrogenism, a family history of breast cancer, and radiation exposure. A thorough examination of the male breast should be a routine part of a physical examination.

Pathophysiology

Various types of breast cancer have been identified based on their histologic characteristics and growth patterns (Table 50-3). The main components of the breast are lobules (milk-producing glands) and ducts (milk passages that connect the lobules and the nipple). In general breast cancer arises from the epithelial lining of the ducts (ductal carcinoma) or from the epithelium of the lobules (lobular carcinoma). Breast cancers may be invasive or in situ. Most breast cancers arise from the ducts and are invasive.

TABLE 50-3 Types of Breast Cancer	
TYPE	**FREQUENCY OF OCCURRENCE**
Infiltrating ductal carcinoma	70%–80%
• Colloid (mucinous)	
• Inflammatory	
• Paget's disease	
• Medullary	
• Papillary	
• Tubular	
Infiltrating lobular carcinoma	10%–15%
Noninvasive	4%–6%
• Ductal carcinoma in situ	

The natural history of breast cancer varies considerably from patient to patient. Cancer growth rate can range from slow to rapid. Factors that affect cancer prognosis are size, axillary node involvement (the more nodes involved, the worse the prognosis), tumor differentiation, DNA content (characteristics of malignant cells), and estrogen and progesterone receptor status. The histologic type of breast cancer seems to have little prognostic significance once the cancer has metastasized.

Noninvasive Breast Cancer. The increased use of screening mammography has led to more women being diagnosed with noninvasive breast cancer. These intraductal cancers include *ductal carcinoma in situ* (DCIS) and *lobular carcinoma in situ* (LCIS). DCIS tends to be unilateral and most likely would progress to invasive breast cancer (usually infiltrating ductal cell carcinoma) if left untreated. LCIS appears to be more of a premalignant breast cancer, and women with this condition have a higher risk of later developing an invasive breast cancer in the same or opposite breast.

Although the management of these two disorders can be controversial, patients with DCIS and LCIS should discuss all treatment options with their physician, including local excision, mastectomy with breast reconstruction, breast-conserving treatment (lumpectomy), radiation therapy, and/or tamoxifen (Nolvadex).

Paget's Disease. Paget's disease is a breast malignancy characterized by a persistent lesion of the nipple and areola with or without a palpable mass. Itching, burning, bloody nipple discharge with superficial erosion, and ulceration may be present. Diagnosis of Paget's disease is confirmed by pathologic examination of the erosion. Nipple changes are often diagnosed as an infection or dermatitis, which can lead to treatment delays. (This is different from Paget's disease of the bone, which is discussed in Chapter 62.) The treatment of Paget's disease is a simple or modified radical mastectomy. Prognosis is good when the cancer remains in the nipple only. The nursing care for the patient with Paget's disease is the same as the care for a patient with breast cancer.

Inflammatory Breast Cancer. Inflammatory breast cancer, the most malignant form of all breast cancers, is rare. It is an aggressive and fast-growing cancer. The skin of the breast looks red, feels warm, and has a thickened appearance that is often described as resembling an orange peel (peau d'orange). Sometimes the breast develops ridges and small bumps that look like hives. The inflammatory changes, often mistaken for an infection, are caused by cancer cells blocking lymph channels. Metastases occur early and widely. Radiation, chemotherapy, and hormone therapy are more likely to be used for treatment than surgery.

Clinical Manifestations

Breast cancer is detected as a single lump or mammographic abnormality in the breast. It occurs most often in the upper, outer quadrant of the breast because it is the location of most of the glandular tissue (Fig. 50-4). The rate at which the lesion grows varies considerably. Slow-growing lesions are often associated with a lower mortality rate. If palpable, breast cancer is characteristically hard, irregularly shaped, poorly delineated, nonmobile, and nontender.

A small percentage of breast cancers cause nipple discharge. The discharge is usually unilateral and may be clear or bloody.

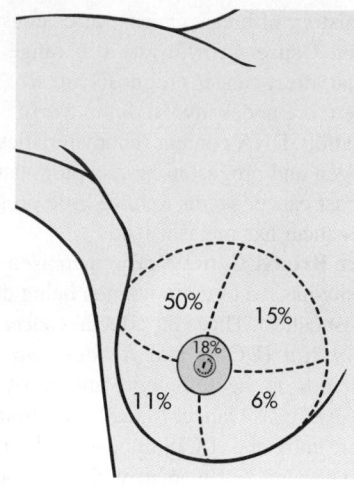

FIG. 50-4 Distribution of where breast cancer occurs.

Nipple retraction may occur. Peau d'orange may occur due to the plugging of the dermal lymphatics. In large cancers, infiltration, induration, and dimpling (pulling in) of the overlying skin may also be noted.

Complications

The main complication of breast cancer is recurrence (Table 50-4). Recurrence may be local or regional (skin or soft tissue near the mastectomy site, axillary or internal mammary lymph nodes) or distant (most commonly involving the bone, lung, brain, and liver). However, metastatic disease can be found in any distant site.

Widely disseminated or metastatic disease involves the growth of colonies of cancerous breast cells in parts of the body distant from the breast. Metastases primarily occur through the lymphatic chains, principally those of the axilla (see Chapter 49, Fig. 49-7). However, the cancer can spread to other parts of the body without invading the axillary nodes even when the primary breast tumor is small. Even in node-negative breast cancer, there is a possibility of distant metastasis.

Diagnostic Studies

In addition to studies used to diagnose breast cancer (see earlier in chapter), other tests are useful in predicting the risk of recurrence or metastatic breast disease. These tests include axillary lymph node status, tumor size, estrogen and progesterone receptor status, DNA content analysis (ploidy status), and cell proliferative indices. Many of these diagnostic studies are useful prognostic indicators of the disease.

Axillary lymph node involvement is one of the most important prognostic factors in early-stage breast cancer.[23] The presence of metastasis in axillary nodes can be determined by pathologic examination of as few as 6 to 10 nodes. The more nodes involved, the greater the risk of recurrence. Patients with four or more positive nodes have the greatest risk of recurrence.

Studies are examining improved methods to assess tumor growth in the regional lymph nodes. This information is important when considering possible adjuvant systemic therapy. A newer surgical technique called *lymphatic mapping* and *sentinel lymph node dissection* (SLND) helps the surgeon identify the lymph

TABLE 50-4	**Common Sites of Breast Cancer Recurrence and Metastasis**
SITE	**CLINICAL PRESENTATION**
Local Recurrence	
Skin	Firm, discrete nodules; occasionally pruritic, usually painless
Regional Recurrence	
Lymph nodes	Enlarged nodes in axilla or supraclavicular area, usually nontender, superior vena caval obstruction from enlarged supraclavicular nodes (oncologic emergency), pain in shoulder and arm of affected side
Distant Metastases	
Skeletal metastasis	Localized pain of gradually increasing intensity, percussion tenderness at involved sites, pathologic fracture caused by involvement of bone cortex, hypercalcemia from skeletal metastasis or endocrine therapy
Spinal cord metastasis	Progressive back pain, localized and radicular; muscular weakness, usually in lower extremities; paresthesias in one or more extremities; bowel or bladder sphincter dysfunction; paralysis from epidural spinal cord compression
Brain metastasis	Headache, unilateral sensory loss, focal muscular weakness, hemiparesis, incoordination (ataxia), visual defects, speech disorder (dysphasia), impaired cognition, behavioral or mental changes, loss of sphincter control, papilledema, persistent nausea and vomiting, seizure activity, progressive decrease in level of consciousness
Pulmonary metastasis (including lung nodules and pleural effusions)	Dependent on sites and extent of pulmonary metastases; chest pain, dyspnea on exertion, shortness of breath, tachypnea, nonproductive cough (not present in all patients); adventitious breath sounds, dullness to percussion, restricted chest-wall expansion on affected side with pleural effusion
Liver metastasis	Abdominal distention; right lower quadrant abdominal pain sometimes with radiation to scapular area; nausea and vomiting, anorexia, weight loss; weakness and fatigue; hepatomegaly, ascites, jaundice; peripheral edema; elevated liver enzymes
Bone marrow metastasis	Anemia; infection; increased bleeding, bruising, petechiae; weakness and fatigue; mild confusion, light-headedness; dyspnea

node(s) that drain first from the tumor site (sentinel node).[24] A radioisotope and/or blue dye is injected into the tumor site, and intraoperatively, it is determined in which node(s) the radioisotope and/or blue dye is located. A local incision is made, and the surgeon dissects the blue-stained sentinel node and/or the radioactive lymph node. The node is then subsequently analyzed by pathologic studies. Assessment of this node can be used to determine if tumor spread has occurred related to the entire axillary area. SLND has been associated with lower morbidity rates and greater accuracy as compared with complete axillary node dissection.[24] National clinical research trials are evaluating whether standard lymph node dissection can be avoided if SLND is performed.

Tumor size is a valuable prognostic variable: the larger the tumor, the poorer the prognosis. The wide variety of histologic types of breast cancer explains the heterogeneity of the disease. In general, the more well differentiated the tumor, the less aggressive it is. Poorly differentiated tumors appear morphologically disorganized and are more aggressive.

Another diagnostic test useful both for treatment decisions and prediction of prognosis is estrogen and progesterone receptor status. Receptor-positive tumors commonly (1) show histologic evidence of being well differentiated, (2) frequently have a *diploid* (more normal) DNA content and low proliferative indices, (3) have a lower chance for recurrence, and (4) are frequently hormone dependent and responsive to hormonal therapy. Receptor-negative tumors (1) are often poorly differentiated histologically, (2) have a high incidence of *aneuploidy* (abnormally high or low DNA content) and higher proliferative indices, (3) frequently recur, and (4) are usually unresponsive to hormonal therapy.

Ploidy status correlates with tumor aggressiveness. Diploid tumors have been shown to have a significantly lower risk of recurrence than aneuploid tumors.

Cell-proliferative indices indirectly measure the rate of tumor cell proliferation. The percent of tumor cells in the S phase of the cell cycle (see Chapter 15, Fig. 15-1) is another important prognostic indicator. Patients with cells that have high S-phase fractions have a higher risk for recurrence and earlier cancer death.

Another prognostic indicator is the genetic marker HER-2/neu (also called c-erb-B2 or neu). Amplification and overexpression of this gene have been associated with a greater risk for recurrence and a poorer prognosis in breast cancer.[25] The presence of this gene assists in the selection and sequence of chemotherapy and predicting patient response to treatment.

Collaborative Care

Historically, a radical **mastectomy** (removal of breast, pectoral muscles, axillary lymph nodes, and all fat and adjacent tissue) was the standard of care. Presently a wide range of treatment options is available to both the patient and the care providers attempting to make critical decisions about what treatment to select (Table 50-5). Prognostic factors are considered when treatment decisions are made about a specific breast cancer. Some of these factors also enter into the staging of breast cancer. The most widely accepted staging method for breast cancer is the American Joint Committee on Cancer's TNM system (Table 50-7).[26] This system uses tumor size (T), nodal involvement (N), and presence of metastasis (M) to determine the stage of disease. The stages range from I to IV, with stage I being very small tumors (less than 2 cm) with no lymph node involvement and no metastasis.

Further classification within these stages depends on the size of the tumor and the number of lymph nodes involved. Stage IV indicates the presence of metastatic spread, regardless of tumor size or lymph node involvement. The therapeutic regimen is often dictated by the clinical stage classification of the cancer.

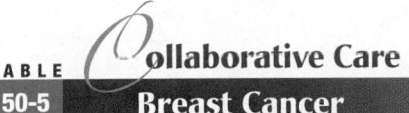

TABLE 50-5	Collaborative Care Breast Cancer

Diagnostic
History including risk factors
Physical examination including breast and lymphatics
Mammography
Ultrasound
Biopsy
MRI (if indicated)

Staging Workup
Complete blood count, platelet count
Calcium and phosphate levels
Liver function tests
Sentinel lymph node dissection
Chest x-ray
Bone scan
CT scan of chest, abdomen, pelvis
MRI (if indicated)

Collaborative Therapy
Surgery
  Breast-conserving (lumpectomy) with sentinel lymph node biopsy/dissection and/or axillary lymph node dissection
  Modified radical mastectomy (may include reconstruction)
Radiation therapy
  Primary radiotherapy
  Adjuvant radiotherapy
  High-dose brachytherapy
  Palliative radiotherapy
Chemotherapy
  Adjuvant chemotherapy
  Chemotherapy for recurrent disease
Hormonal therapy (Table 50-6)
Biologic therapy

CT, Computed tomography; *MRI*, magnetic resonance imaging.

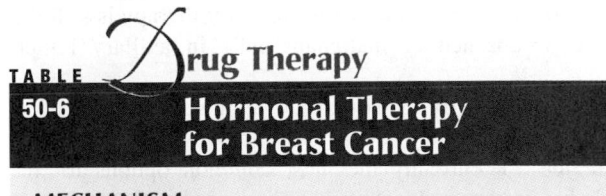

TABLE 50-6	Drug Therapy Hormonal Therapy for Breast Cancer

MECHANISM OF ACTION	EXAMPLES
Blocks estrogen receptors	tamoxifen (Nolvadex)
	toremifene (Fareston)
Destroys estrogen receptors	fulvestrant (Faslodex)
Prevents production of estrogen by inhibiting aromatase	anastrozole (Arimedex)
	letrozole (Femara)
	exemestane (Aromasin)
	vorozole (Rizivor)
	aminoglutethimide (Cytadren)

TABLE 50-7   TNM Classification of Breast Cancer

Primary Tumor (T)

T_0	No evidence of primary tumor
T_{is}	Carcinoma in situ
T_1	Tumor <2 cm
T_2	Tumor 2–5 cm
T_3	Tumor >5 cm
T_4	Extension to chest wall, inflammation

Regional Lymph Nodes (N)

N_0	No tumor in regional lymph nodes
N_1	Metastasis to movable ipsilateral nodes
N_2	Metastasis to matted or fixed ipsilateral nodes
N_3	Metastasis to ipsilateral internal mammary nodes

Distant Metastasis (M)

M_0	No distant metastasis
M_1	Distant metastasis (includes spread to ipsilateral supraclavicular nodes)

Stage Grouping

Stage 0	T_{is}	N_0	M_0
Stage I	T_1	N_0	M_0
Stage IIA	T_0	N_1	M_0
	T_1	N_1	M_0
	T_2	N_0	M_0
Stage IIB	T_2	N_1	M_0
	T_3	N_0	M_0
Stage IIIA	T_0	N_2	M_0
	T_1	N_2	M_0
	T_2	N_2	M_0
	T_3	N_1, N_2	M_0
Stage IIIB	T_4	Any N	M_0
	Any T	N_3	M_0
Stage IV	Any T	Any N	M_1

(Side effects and appropriate nursing management of general treatment modalities for cancer are discussed in Chapter 15.)

In spite of the advent of new prognostic indicators such as determination of DNA content and analysis of cell-cycle phases, the single most powerful prognostic factor related to local recurrence or metastasis after primary therapy is still the presence or absence of malignant cells in axillary lymph nodes.

Surgical Therapy. Breast conservation surgery with radiation therapy and modified radical mastectomy with or without reconstruction are currently the most common options for resectable breast cancer. Most women diagnosed with early-stage breast cancer (tumors smaller than 4 to 5 cm) are candidates for either treatment choice. The overall survival rate with lumpectomy and radiation is about the same as that with modified radical mastectomy.[18]

Axillary node dissection. Axillary lymph node dissection is often performed regardless of the treatment option selected. Examination of nodes provides the most powerful prognostic data currently available and helps determine further treatment (chemotherapy, hormone therapy, or both). For all cases of invasive breast cancer, a typical lymph node dissection has always involved the removal of 10 to 15 lymph nodes. However, this technique may not be necessary or appropriate for some women with very small invasive breast cancers or with noninvasive (in situ) cancers. Sentinel lymph node dissection shows promise for reducing unnecessary lymph node dissection. If the sentinel node does not show any signs of cancer, further lymph nodes may not be removed, depending on the health care setting.

Lymphedema (accumulation of lymph in soft tissue) can occur as a result of the excision or radiation of lymph nodes.[27] When the axillary nodes cannot return lymph fluid to the central circulation, the fluid accumulates in the arm, causing obstructive pressure on the veins and venous return. The patient may experience heaviness, pain, impaired motor function in the arm, and numbness and paresthesia of the fingers as a result of lymphedema. Cellulitis and progressive fibrosis can result from lymphedema.

Although lymphedema is not always preventable, it can be controlled somewhat after surgery or radiation. Frequent and sustained elevation of the arm, performing hand and arm exercises daily, and avoidance of clothing that constricts the arm are all helpful in preventing and reducing lymphedema.[28]

Breast conservation surgery. Breast conservation surgery (termed **lumpectomy**) involves the removal of the entire tumor along with a margin of normal tissue. Following surgery, radiation therapy is delivered to the entire breast, ending with a boost to the tumor bed. If there is evidence of systemic disease, chemotherapy may be given before radiation therapy. Contraindications to breast conservation surgery include breast size too small to yield an acceptable cosmetic result, masses and calcifications that are multifocal (within the same breast quadrant), masses that are multicentric (in more than one quadrant), or diffuse calcifications in more than one quadrant.

One of the main advantages of breast conservation surgery and radiation is that it preserves the breast, including the nipple. The goal of the combined surgery and radiation is to maximize the benefits of both cancer treatment and cosmetic outcome while minimizing risks. Disadvantages of this surgery include the increased cost of the surgery plus radiation over surgery alone and the possible side effects of radiation. Table 50-8 describes treatment options, side effects, complications, and patient issues related to the most common surgical procedures currently used to treat breast cancer.

Modified radical mastectomy. A modified radical mastectomy includes removal of the breast and axillary lymph nodes, but it preserves the pectoralis major muscle. This surgery would be selected over breast conservation therapy if the tumor is too large to excise with good margins and attain a reasonable cosmetic result. Some patients may select this surgical procedure over lumpectomy when presented with the choice of either procedure.

When a modified radical mastectomy is performed, the patient has the option of breast reconstruction. If the patient chooses to have reconstructive surgery, it can be performed immediately following the mastectomy or it can be delayed until postoperative recovery is complete (about 6 months).

Follow-up care. After surgery, the woman must be followed up for the rest of her life at regular intervals. Most women have professional examinations every 6 months for 2 years and then annually thereafter. In addition, the woman must continue to practice monthly BSE on both breasts or the remaining breast and the mastectomy site. The most common site of recurrence of

TABLE 50-8   **Breast Cancer: Surgical Procedures, Side Effects, Complications, and Patient Issues**

PROCEDURES	DESCRIPTION	SIDE EFFECTS	POTENTIAL COMPLICATIONS	PATIENT ISSUES
Modified radical mastectomy	Removal of breast, preservation of pectoralis muscle, axillary node dissection	Chest wall tightens Phantom breast sensations Arm swelling Sensory changes	Short term: skin flap necrosis, seroma, hematoma, infection Long term: sensory loss, muscle weakness, lymphedema	Loss of breast Incision Body image Need for prosthesis Impaired arm mobility
Breast conservation surgery (lumpectomy) with radiation therapy	Wide excision of tumor, sentinel lymph node dissection (SLND) and/or axillary lymph node dissection (ALND), radiation therapy	Breast soreness Breast edema Skin reactions Arm swelling Sensory changes in breast and arm Fatigue	Short term: moist desquamation,* hematoma, seroma, infection Long term: fibrosis, lymphedema,† myositis, pneumonitis,* rib fractures*	Prolonged treatment* Impaired arm mobility† Change in texture and sensitivity of breast
Tissue expansion and breast implants	Expander used to slowly stretch tissue; saline gradually injected into reservoir over weeks to months Insertion of implant under musculofascial layer of chest wall	Discomfort Chest wall tightness	Short term: skin flap necrosis, wound separation, seroma, hematoma, infection Long term: capsular contractions, displacement of implant	Body image Prolonged physician visits to expand implants Additional surgeries for nipple construction, symmetry
Musculocutaneous flap procedures	A musculocutaneous flap (muscle, skin, blood supply) is transposed from latissimus dorsi to transverse rectus abdominis to chest wall‡	Pain related to two surgical sites and extensive surgery	Short term: delayed wound healing, infection, skin flap necrosis, abdominal hernia, hematoma	Prolonged postoperative recovery

*Specific to radiation therapy.
†If ALND (less likely with SLND).
‡Concurrent with mastectomy.

breast cancer is at the surgical site. The woman should also have yearly mammography of the remaining breast or breast tissue.

Postmastectomy pain syndrome. *Postmastectomy pain syndrome* can occur in patients following a mastectomy or axillary node dissection. Common symptoms include chest and upper arm pain, tingling down the arm, numbness, shooting or pricking pain, and unbearable itching that persist beyond the normal 3-month healing time. The pain syndrome is caused by a number of factors including injury to nerves and tissue as a result of surgery, radiation therapy, chemotherapy, or secondary neuroma development. The most common theory for its onset is the injury to intercostobrachial nerves, which are sensory nerves that exit chest wall muscles and provide sensation to the shoulder and upper arm.

Treatments include nonsteroidal antiinflammatory drugs, antidepressants, topical lidocaine patches, EMLA (eutectic mixture of local anesthetics: lidocaine and prilocaine), and antiseizure drugs (e.g., gabapentin [Neurontin]). Other possible treatment modalities include guided imagery training, biofeedback, physical therapy to prevent "frozen shoulder" syndrome as a result of inadequate movement, and psychologic counseling with a person trained in the management of chronic pain syndromes.

Adjuvant Therapy. The decision to recommend adjuvant (additional) therapy after surgery depends on the stage of the disease (number of involved nodes and tumor size), menstrual status and age, cell characteristics, presence or absence of estrogen receptors, and other preexisting health problems that can complicate treatment. Adjuvant therapies include radiation therapy after breast conservation surgery and systemic therapies such as chemotherapy and hormonal therapy.[29]

Radiation therapy. The three situations in which radiation therapy may be used for breast cancer are (1) as the primary treatment to destroy the tumor or as a companion to surgery to prevent local recurrence, (2) to shrink a large tumor to operable size, and (3) as the palliative treatment for pain caused by local recurrence and metastases. Lumpectomy is almost always followed by radiation.

Primary radiation therapy. When radiation therapy is the primary treatment, it is usually performed after local excision of the breast mass. The breast (and the regional lymph nodes in some cases) is radiated daily over the course of approximately 5 to 6 weeks. An external beam of radiation is used to deliver an approximate total dose of 4500 to 5000 cGy (4500 to 5000 rads; 1 rad = 1 cGy). A "boost" treatment to the full breast may also be given, either before or after therapy has been completed. The boost is a dose of radiation delivered to the area in which the original tumor was located. It can be given by external beam and usually adds 10 treatments to the total number given. Fatigue, skin changes, and breast edema may be temporary side effects of external beam radiation therapy. Radiation of the axilla is also effective in decreasing the incidence of axillary recurrence. Chemotherapy may be used systemically to enhance the local effects of radiation. (Nursing management of the patient receiving radiation therapy is discussed in Chapter 15.)

Radiation therapy as adjunct to surgery. Although an uncommon treatment mode, preoperative radiation therapy can be used to reduce the size of a large tumor mass to operable proportions by destroying the cancer cells. Additionally, because the malignant cells are partially or completely destroyed, the rate of local recurrence decreases.

The decision to use radiation therapy after mastectomy is based on the probability of the presence of local residual cancer cells (related to size of cancer and number of involved lymph nodes). Radiating the area will not prevent the appearance of distant metastasis at a later date. The site of radiation therapy (lymph nodes, chest wall, or both) depends on the degree of possible spread of the cancer.

High-dose brachytherapy. High-dose brachytherapy is a new procedure that is an alternative to traditional radiation treatment for early-stage breast cancer. The technique uses a balloon catheter to insert radioactive seeds into the breast after the tumor is removed (Fig. 50-5). The seeds deliver a concentrated dose of radiation directly to the site where the cancer is most likely to occur. Traditional radiation treatments can take 5 to 6 weeks. In contrast, high-dose brachytherapy may require only 5 days.

Palliative radiation therapy. In addition to reducing the primary tumor mass with a resultant decrease in pain, radiation therapy is also used to stabilize symptomatic metastatic lesions in such sites as bone, soft tissue organs, brain, and chest. Radiation therapy relieves pain and is often successful in controlling recurrent or metastatic disease for long periods.

Systemic therapy. The goal of systemic therapy is to destroy tumor cells that may have spread undetected to distant sites. Systemic therapy as an adjuvant to primary local treatment, in the absence of demonstrable metastases, can decrease the rate of recurrence and increase the length of survival.[18] Because of the high risk for recurrent disease, nearly all women with evidence of node involvement, particularly those who are hormone-receptor negative, will have some type of systemic therapy. Certain women, particularly those who are premenopausal, are known to be at higher risk for recurrent or metastatic disease. These women are often recommended for systemic therapy even when no evidence of node involvement is found. Weighing the different risk factors to determine the need for adjuvant therapy in a node-negative patient is a complex process.

Chemotherapy. Chemotherapy refers to the use of cytotoxic drugs to destroy cancer cells. The greatest benefits from chemotherapy have been achieved among premenopausal women with node findings that are positive for malignancy.

In some instances chemotherapy is used preoperatively. Preoperative chemotherapy may be more convenient than postoperative administration and can decrease the size of the primary tumor, possibly permitting less extensive surgery. Also, it has been shown that preoperative chemotherapy suppresses tumor growth and prolongs survival.

Breast cancer is one of the solid tumors that is the most responsive to chemotherapy. The use of combinations of drugs is clearly superior to the use of a single drug. The benefit of combination treatment results from the use of drugs that have different actions on cell growth and division. The more common combination-therapy protocols are cyclophosphamide (Cytoxan), methotrexate, and 5-fluorouracil (5-FU), referred to as

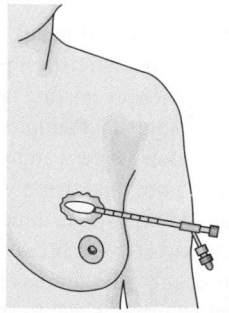 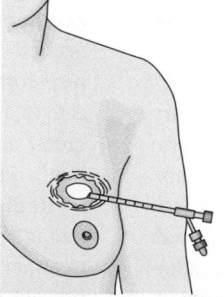 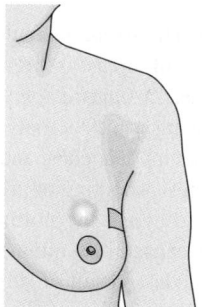

Step 1: During the lumpectomy or shortly thereafter, a deflated balloon is placed inside the cavity created by removal of the tumor.

Step 2: Patient returns to clinic for 1 to 5 days of outpatient treatment, where a radioactive seed is inserted through a catheter into the balloon twice a day for 10 minutes each time. The seed targets radiation to the area where tumors are more likely to recur, while minimizing exposure to healthy tissue.

Step 3: The balloon is deflated and the catheter is removed. No source of radiation remains in the patient's body between treatments or after the final procedure.

FIG. 50-5 High-dose brachytherapy for breast cancer.

CMF; and cyclophosphamide and doxorubicin (Adriamycin), referred to as AC, with or without the addition of a taxane such as paclitaxel (Taxol) or docetaxel (Taxotere); or cyclophosphamide, 5-FU, and epirubicin (Ellence) or doxorubicin, referred to as CEF or CAF, respectively. Paclitaxel, docetaxel, and capecitabine (Xeloda) are used in women whose metastatic breast cancer has not responded to standard chemotherapy.[29] Vinorelbine (Navelbine), a relatively new chemotherapeutic drug for treating metastatic breast cancer, is well tolerated with fewer and milder side effects than other chemotherapy drugs.

Because healthy cells are also affected by chemotherapy, a variety of side effects accompany this treatment modality. The incidence and severity of predictable and commonly observed side effects will be influenced by the specific drug combination, drug schedule, and dose intensity of the drug or drugs. Usually body organs with rapidly growing cells are the most strongly affected. The most common side effects involve the gastrointestinal tract, bone marrow, and hair follicles, resulting in nausea, anorexia, weight loss, bone marrow suppression and subsequent fatigue, and alopecia (hair loss).

Hormonal therapy. Estrogen can promote the growth of breast cancer cells if the cells are estrogen-receptor positive. Hormonal therapy removes or blocks the source of estrogen, thus promoting tumor regression.

Two advances have increased the use of hormone therapy in breast cancer. First, hormone receptor assays, which are reliable diagnostic tests, have been developed to identify women who are likely to respond to hormone therapy. Both estrogen and progesterone receptor status of the tumor can be determined. The importance of these assays is their ability to predict whether hormonal therapy is a treatment option for women with breast cancer, either at the time of initial therapy or if the cancer recurs. Second, drugs have been developed that can inactivate the hormone-secreting glands as effectively as surgery or radiation. Premenopausal and perimenopausal women are more likely to have tumors that are not hormone dependent, whereas women who are postmenopausal are more likely to have hormone-dependent tumors. Chances of tumor regression are significantly greater in women whose tumors contain estrogen and progesterone receptors.

Estrogen deprivation can occur by destroying the ovaries by surgery or radiation therapy or drug therapy (see Table 50-6). Hormonal therapy can (1) block or destroy the estrogen receptors or (2) suppress estrogen synthesis through inhibiting aromatase, an enzyme needed for endogenous estrogen synthesis.[30] Hormonal therapy is widely used to treat recurrent or metastatic cancer but may also be used as an adjuvant to primary treatment.

Tamoxifen (Nolvadex) is the hormonal agent of choice in postmenopausal, estrogen receptor–positive women with or without lymph node involvement. Tamoxifen, an antiestrogen drug, blocks the estrogen receptor sites of malignant cells and thus inhibits the growth-stimulating effects of estrogen. It is commonly used in advanced and early-stage breast cancer to prevent or treat recurrent disease. Tamoxifen may also be used to prevent breast cancer in high risk individuals.[31] Side effects of tamoxifen are minimal but include hot flashes, nausea, vomiting, vaginal discharge, and other effects commonly associated with decreased estrogen. It also increases the risk of blood clots, cataracts, and endometrial cancer in postmenopausal women.[32]

Toremifene (Fareston), an antiestrogen agent similar to tamoxifen, is indicated as first-line treatment for metastatic breast cancer in postmenopausal women with estrogen receptor–positive or estrogen receptor–unknown tumors.

Fulvestrant (Faslodex) may be given to women with advanced breast cancer who no longer respond to tamoxifen. This drug slows cancer progression by destroying estrogen receptors in the breast cancer cells. Fulvestrant is given intramuscularly on a monthly basis.

Aromatase inhibitor drugs, which interfere with the enzyme that synthesizes endogenous estrogen, are used in the treatment of advanced breast cancer in postmenopausal women with disease progression. These drugs include anastrozole (Arimidex), letrozole (Femara), vorozole (Rizivor), exemestane (Aromasin), and aminoglutethimide (Cytadren).

Raloxifene (Evista), a drug used to prevent bone loss, may also reduce the risk of breast cancer without stimulating endometrial growth. Raloxifene acts as an estrogen antagonist at the hormone-sensitive tissues of breast cancer and bone. (Raloxifene is discussed in the section on osteoporosis in Chapter 62.)

Additional drugs that may be used to suppress hormone-dependent breast tumors include megestrol acetate (Megace), diethylstilbestrol (DES), and fluoxymesterone (Halotestin). Less common hormone-deprivation strategies include bilateral oophorectomy, adrenalectomy, and hypophysectomy.

Biologic Therapy. The use of biologic therapy represents an attempt to stimulate the body's natural defenses to recognize and attack cancer cells. Trastuzumab (Herceptin) is an antibody to HER-2/neu, an antigen that often appears on the surface of breast cancer cells. After the antibody attaches to the antigen, it is taken into the cells and eventually kills them. It can be used alone or in combination with other chemotherapy to treat patients with metastatic breast cancer whose tumors overexpress the HER-2 gene. Current research is examining the effectiveness of trastuzumab on early-stage breast cancer.[25] (The use of biologic therapies is discussed in Chapter 15.)

Bone Marrow and Stem Cell Transplantation. Autologous bone marrow or peripheral stem cell transplantation combined with high-dose chemotherapy has been used to treat patients with advanced metastatic breast cancer. In this technique patients donate their own bone marrow or peripheral blood from which stem cells are harvested. Then they receive high doses of chemotherapy, which causes bone marrow suppression. The patient subsequently undergoes autologous bone marrow or stem cell transplantation. These treatments remain under investigation. (Bone marrow and stem cell transplantation are discussed in Chapter 15.)

NURSING MANAGEMENT
BREAST CANCER

■ Nursing Assessment

Many factors need to be considered when a nurse is assessing a patient with a breast problem. The history of the breast disorder assists in establishing the diagnosis. The presence of nipple discharge, pain, rate of growth of the lump, breast asymmetry, and correlation with the menstrual cycle should all be investigated.

The size and location of the lump or lumps should be carefully documented, and the physical characteristics of the lesion, such as consistency, mobility, and shape, should be assessed. If nipple discharge is present, the color and consistency should be noted, as well as whether it occurs from one or both breasts.

Subjective and objective data that should be obtained from an individual suspected of having or diagnosed as having breast cancer are presented in Table 50-9.

TABLE 50-9	Nursing Assessment Breast Cancer

Subjective Data
Important Health Information
Past health history: Benign breast disease with atypical changes; previous unilateral breast cancer; menstrual history (early menarche with late menopause); pregnancy history (nulliparity or first full-term pregnancy after age 30); previous endometrial, ovarian, or colon cancer; hyperestrogenism and testicular atrophy (in men)
Medications: Use of hormones, especially as postmenopausal hormone replacement therapy and in oral contraceptives, infertility treatments
Surgery or other treatments: Exposure to excessive radiation (e.g., thyroid radiation)
Functional Health Patterns
Health perception–health management: Family history (especially mother or sister); mammography history; palpable change found on BSE; alcohol use
Nutritional-metabolic: Obesity; anorexia (possible indicator of metastasis); dietary habits
Cognitive-perceptual: Headache, back, arm, or bone pain (possible indicators of metastasis)
Sexuality-reproductive: Unilateral nipple discharge (clear, milky, or bloody); change in breast contour, size, or symmetry
Coping–stress tolerance: Chronic psychologic stress
Self-perception–self-concept: Anxiety regarding threat to self-esteem

Objective Data
General
Axillary and supraclavicular lymphadenopathy
Integumentary
Firm, discrete nodules at mastectomy site (possible indicator of local recurrence); peripheral edema (possible indicator of metastasis)
Respiratory
Pleural effusions (possible indicator of metastasis)
Gastrointestinal
Hepatomegaly, jaundice; ascites (possible indicators of liver metastasis)
Reproductive
Hard, irregular, nonmobile breast lump most often in upper, outer sector, possibly fixated to fascia or chest wall; nipple inversion or retraction, erosion; edema ("orange peel"), erythema, induration, infiltration, or dimpling (in later stages)
Possible Findings
Finding of mass or change in tissue on breast examination; positive results of mammography or ultrasonography; positive results of FNA or surgical biopsy or similar results with a needle biopsy

BSE, Breast self-examination; *FNA,* fine–needle aspiration.

■ Nursing Diagnoses

Nursing diagnoses related to the care of a patient diagnosed with breast cancer vary. Following diagnosis and before a treatment plan has been selected, the following diagnoses would apply:
- Decisional conflict *related to* lack of knowledge about treatment options and their effects
- Fear *related to* diagnosis of breast cancer
- Disturbed body image *related to* anticipated physical and emotional effects of treatment modalities

If a mastectomy is planned, the nursing diagnoses may include, but are not limited to, those presented in NCP 50-1.

■ Planning

The overall goals are that the patient with breast cancer will (1) actively participate in the decision-making process related to treatment options, (2) fully comply with the therapeutic plan, (3) manage the side effects of adjuvant therapy, and (4) be satisfied with the support provided by significant others and health care providers.

■ Nursing Implementation

Acute Intervention. The time between the diagnosis of breast cancer and the selection of a treatment plan is a difficult period for the woman and her family. Although the primary care provider has discussed treatment options, the woman often relies on the nurse to clarify and expand on these options. During this time, the woman may be very self-focused, verbalizing her conflict and indecision frequently. Appropriate nursing interventions during this period include exploring the woman's usual decision-making patterns, helping the woman accurately evaluate the advantages and disadvantages of the options, providing information relevant to the decision, and supporting the patient once the decision is made.

During this period the woman may exhibit signs of distress or tension, such as tachycardia, increased muscle tension, sleep disturbances, and restlessness, whenever she focuses on the decision to be made. The nurse should assess the woman's body language, motor activity, and affect during periods of high stress and indecision so that appropriate interventions can be carried out.

Regardless of the surgery planned, the patient must be provided with sufficient information to ensure informed consent. Some patients seek extensive, detailed information, whereas others avoid information.[33] Sensitivity to an individual's need for information is essential. Teaching in the preoperative phase includes instruction in turning, coughing, and deep breathing; a review of postoperative exercises; a pain management plan; and an explanation of the recovery period from the time of surgery until discharge.

The woman who has breast conservation surgery usually has an uneventful postoperative course with only a moderate amount of pain. If an axillary lymph node dissection (ALND) has been done or if a woman has had a modified radical mastectomy, specific interventions will be needed.

Restoring arm function on the affected side after mastectomy and axillary lymph node dissection is one of the most important goals of nursing activities. The woman should be placed in a semi-Fowler position with the arm on the affected side elevated on a pillow. Flexing and extending the fingers should begin in the recovery room with progressive increases in activity encouraged. (Information pertaining to arm exercises and care applies to women who have had an axillary node dissection after lumpectomy or total mastectomy.) Postoperative arm and shoulder exercises are instituted gradually at the surgeon's direction (Fig. 50-6). These exercises are designed to prevent contractures and muscle shortening, maintain muscle tone, and improve lymph and blood circulation. The difficulty and pain encountered by the woman in performing the previously simple tasks included in the exercise program may cause frustration and depression. The goal of all exercise is a gradual return to full range of motion within 4 to 6 weeks.

NURSING CARE PLAN 50-1

Patient after a Modified Radical Mastectomy*

EXPECTED PATIENT OUTCOMES	NURSING INTERVENTIONS and *RATIONALES*
NURSING DIAGNOSIS	**Acute pain** *related to* surgical procedure *as manifested by* verbalization regarding presence and degree of pain at operative area.
▪ Absence of or tolerable level of pain ▪ Satisfaction with pain control	▪ Administer analgesics as prescribed *to relieve pain.* Position arm *to prevent tension on suture line and provide support.* ▪ Encourage use of noninvasive pain management strategies such as distraction, imagery, and relaxation *to complement analgesics and decrease need for analgesia.*
NURSING DIAGNOSIS	**Fear** *related to* diagnosis of cancer *as manifested by* insomnia, crying, and questioning of prognosis.
▪ Verbalization of fear ▪ Support of significant others ▪ Confidence in ability to cope ▪ Early recognition of recurrent or metastatic disease	▪ Encourage woman to talk about feelings and diagnosis of cancer *to promote successful resolution of fear and establish effective coping mechanisms.* ▪ Provide opportunity for significant others to discuss situation and learn about support groups *because their fear about the diagnosis and outcome can decrease their effectiveness as a support system.* ▪ Reinforce importance of annual mammogram *because it is a recommended screening technique for identification of local recurrence after mastectomy and for assessing other breast.* ▪ Provide information about signs and symptoms to report to health care provider (i.e., new and persistent problems such as skin changes at surgical site, new changes in breast or chest wall).
NURSING DIAGNOSIS	**Disturbed body image** *related to* loss of body part *as manifested by* verbalization of concern about appearance and feelings of loss of femininity, and refusal to view incision.
▪ Verbalization of feelings about surgery and change in body image ▪ Indication of beginning of resolution of negative feelings toward self ▪ Acceptance of altered body image	▪ Assess degree of self-esteem disturbance *so appropriate interventions can be initiated.* ▪ Arrange for Reach to Recovery visitor or similar community resource *to serve as a role model and provide hope for recovery and a normal future.* ▪ Provide information regarding prosthesis fitting and breast reconstruction (if patient is interested) *so patient can make informed decisions regarding options.* ▪ Assist patient to verbalize feelings and encourage open communication with significant others *to promote grief work and maintain support from family and friends.*
NURSING DIAGNOSIS	**Ineffective therapeutic regimen management** *related to* lack of knowledge regarding postoperative care and breast self-examination (BSE).
▪ Able to change dressings with minimal assistance ▪ Practice of monthly BSE	▪ Demonstrate to patient and significant other how to take care of incision and apply new dressing as appropriate. Have patient return demonstration. ▪ Teach or evaluate BSE performance *to ensure that patient is performing correctly.*
NURSING DIAGNOSIS	**Impaired physical mobility** *related to* pain *as manifested by* limitation in movement or upper extremity on surgical side.
▪ Return to usual arm and shoulder function	▪ Assess degree of mobility impairment *to provide baseline data and to plan appropriate interventions.* ▪ Treat pain *to promote participation in exercise plan.* ▪ Carry out exercises *to prevent contractures and muscle shortening, maintain muscle tone, and improve lymph and blood circulation.* ▪ Assist woman to resume activities of daily living as tolerated or as directed by physician *to reduce dependent behaviors, raise self-esteem, and maintain mobility of affected arm.* ▪ Emphasize bilateral activity of upper extremities *to prevent guarding of operative side and loss of function.*

*These nursing diagnoses may also be applicable to the patient who has had a lumpectomy with an axillary lymph node dissection.

NURSING CARE PLAN 50-1

Patient after a Modified Radical Mastectomy—cont'd

COLLABORATIVE PROBLEM

NURSING GOALS	NURSING INTERVENTIONS and *RATIONALES*
POTENTIAL COMPLICATION • Monitor for signs of lymphedema • Report deviations from acceptable parameters • Carry out appropriate medical and nursing interventions	**Lymphedema** *related to* impaired lymphatic drainage and lack of knowledge of preventive measures. • Assess woman for signs of lymphedema such as edema in hand and/or arm on operative side, heaviness, and/or localized pain *to enable early diagnosis and intervention to prevent and treat the complication.* • Instruct patient about self-care strategies and precautions to reduce risk of lymphedema *so patient will be an active, informed participant in self-care.* • Do not perform venipunctures or take blood pressure measurements on affected arm *to reduce risk of constriction, infection, and lymphedema in affected arm.* • Avoid dependent arm position *to allow proper wound healing and decrease stress to incision site.* • Use elastic sleeve if ordered *to apply mechanical pressure to reduce fluid collection in affected arm and promote venous return.*

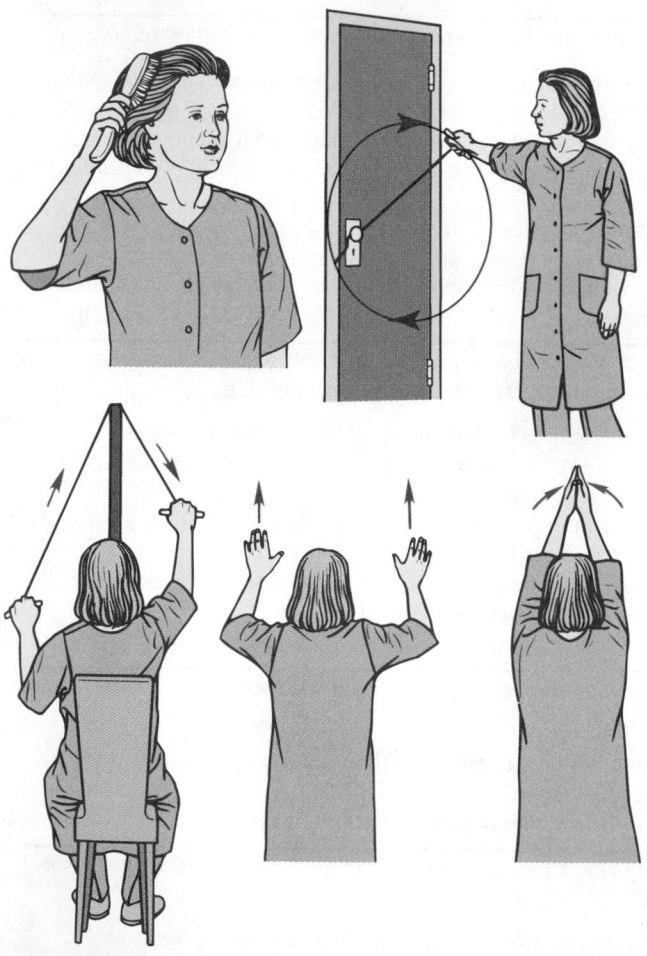

FIG. 50-6 Postoperative exercises for patient with a mastectomy or lumpectomy with axillary lymph node dissection.

Postoperative discomfort can be minimized by administering analgesics about 30 minutes before initiating exercises. When showering is appropriate, the flow of warm water over the involved shoulder often has a soothing effect and reduces joint stiffness. Whenever possible, the same nurse should work with

the woman so that progress can be monitored and problems can be identified.

Measures to prevent or reduce lymphedema after ALND must be used by the nurse and taught to the woman. The affected arm should never be dependent, even while the person is sleeping. Blood pressure readings, venipunctures, and injections should not be done on the affected arm. Elastic bandages should not be used in the early postoperative period because they inhibit collateral lymph drainage. The woman must be instructed to protect the arm on the operative side from even minor trauma such as a pinprick or sunburn. If trauma to the arm occurs, the area should be washed thoroughly with soap and water. A topical antibiotic ointment and a bandage or other sterile dressing should be applied. The surgeon must be advised of the trauma, and the site of injury must be observed closely for evidence of inflammation. The patient must know and understand that she is at risk of developing lymphedema for the rest of her life.[27]

When lymphedema is acute, an intermittent pneumatic compression sleeve may be prescribed. This device applies mechanical massage to the arm. Manual massage is also effective in mobilizing subcutaneous accumulations of fluid. Elevation of the arm so that it is level with the heart, diuretics, and isometric exercises may be recommended to reduce the fluid volume in the arm. The patient may need to wear a fitted elastic pressure-gradient sleeve during waking hours, to maintain maximum volume reduction, and preventively, during air travel.

Psychologic care. Throughout interactions with a woman with breast cancer, the nurse must keep in mind the extensive psychologic impact of the disease. All aspects of care must include sensitivity to the woman's efforts to cope with a life-threatening disease. An open relationship in which the woman can express her fears and feelings is essential. The nurse can help meet the woman's psychologic needs by doing the following:

1. Assisting her to develop a positive but realistic attitude
2. Helping her identify sources of support and strength to her, such as her partner, family, and spiritual practices
3. Encouraging her to verbalize her anger and fears about her diagnosis and the impact it will have on her life

COMPLEMENTARY & ALTERNATIVE THERAPIES
Imagery

Imagery, or visualization, is the process of using mental images to create a desired state.

Clinical Uses
Imagery has many uses, including managing pain, stress, anxiety, asthma, menstrual disorders, gastrointestinal disorders, arthritis, hypertension, and headaches.

Effects
Imagery can promote relaxation, decrease stress, lower blood pressure, relieve pain, reduce side effects of chemotherapy, improve immune function, enhance performance, and enhance wound healing. This behavioral intervention has few side effects.

Nursing Implications
Imagery should be individualized. Images should be avoided that are distressing. People can invent their own imagery or use those that have been created by others. Imagery is well suited as a self-care technique because almost anyone can use it.

4. Promoting open communication of thoughts and feelings between the patient and her family
5. Providing accurate and complete answers to questions about her disease, treatment options, and reproductive or lactation issues (if appropriate)
6. Offering information about community resources, such as Reach to Recovery, Y-Me, CanSurmount, Encore, and local support organizations and groups

The nurse can promote the woman's recovery by arranging a visit from a woman who had similar treatment, such as a Reach to Recovery volunteer, if the service is available. The Reach to Recovery program of the American Cancer Society is a rehabilitation program for women who have had breast surgery. It is designed to help them meet their psychologic, physical, and cosmetic needs. The volunteers, who are all women who have had breast cancer, can answer questions about what to expect at home, how to tell people about the surgery, and what prosthetic devices are available. If a Reach to Recovery volunteer is not available, it is the nurse's responsibility to be knowledgeable about the needs of the woman after breast surgery. The American Cancer Society and the National Cancer Institute can provide excellent materials to assist the nurse in meeting the special needs of women with breast cancer.

The professional staff must never underestimate the tremendous psychologic impact that a diagnosis of cancer and subsequent breast surgery can have on a woman. Emotional complications are common. The nurse's accepting, concerned attitude can do a great deal to relieve the feelings of anger and depression experienced by many patients.

Ambulatory and Home Care. The nurse should explain the follow-up routine to the patient and emphasize the importance of beginning and continuing BSE and annual mammography. Referral to a mental health provider to address individual and family support in addition to coping needs may be indicated. Immediately after surgery, symptoms that should be reported to the clinician include fever, inflammation at the surgical site, erythema, postoperative constipation, and unusual swelling. Other changes to report in the future are new back pain, weakness, shortness of breath, and confusion. If adjuvant therapy is to be used, the woman should have specific instructions about appointment times and treatment locations and management of side effects.

For women who have had a mastectomy, the nurse should stress the importance of wearing a well-fitting prosthesis. A variety of products are available to meet the specific needs of the individual woman. After surgery a temporary camisole prosthesis may be used. A well-trained salesperson can help the woman select a suitable, more permanent weighted prosthesis and bra, generally at 6 weeks postoperatively. There are both physical and psychologic advantages to the use of a prosthesis. The return of a normal external appearance is especially important to most women.

The implications of the loss of a breast on the sexual identity and relationships of the woman vary. A preoperative sexual assessment provides helpful baseline data that the nurse can use to plan postoperative interventions. Often the husband, sexual partner, or family members may need assistance in dealing with their emotional reactions to the diagnosis and surgery for them to act as effective means of support for the patient.[34] There are no physical reasons for a mastectomy to prevent sexual satisfaction. The woman taking tamoxifen may have a decreased sexual drive or vaginal dryness. She may need to use lubrication to prevent discomfort during intercourse. If difficulty in adjustment or other problems develop, counseling may be necessary to deal with the emotional component of a mastectomy and the diagnosis of cancer.

Depression and anxiety may occur with the continued stress and uncertainty of a cancer diagnosis. A woman's self-esteem and identity may also be threatened. Special nursing interventions are necessary, in terms of both psychologic support and self-care teaching, if a recurrence of cancer is found. The support of family and friends and participation in a cancer support group are important aspects of care that are helpful in improving quality of life and have been found to have a clinically significant impact on survival.[35]

■ Evaluation

The expected outcomes for the patient after a modified radical mastectomy are presented in NCP 50-1.

■ Culturally Competent Care: Breast Cancer

Breast cancer does not respect the boundaries of ethnicity or culture. However, there are differences in various ethnic groups related to breast cancer (see Cultural and Ethnic Considerations box on p. 1366 and Nursing Research box on p. 1378). The differences may be due to dietary factors and insufficient use of early detection procedures such as BSE and mammograms.

Cultural values will strongly influence how women will respond to and cope with breast cancer and treatment. It is important for the nurse to be aware of the cultural value of breasts. In addition, the nurse needs to explore cultural factors that relate to the disease of breast cancer. A possible reason that some women may delay treatment after they have discovered a large breast lump is their belief in fatalism—an acceptance of disease as inevitable fate or "God's will." ■

NURSING RESEARCH
Issues of African American Breast Cancer Survivors

Citation

Wilmoth M, Sanders LD: Accept me for myself: African American women's issues after breast cancer, *Oncol Nurs Forum* 28:875, 2001.

Purpose

To identify personal issues and concerns of African American women who are breast cancer survivors.

Methods

Women (*n* = 24) were recruited to participate in two focus group sessions, which were held in a community library. The specific aim of the sessions was to learn the women's perception of the impact that breast cancer had on their personal lives. All sessions were audiotaped and transcribed.

Results and Conclusions

Five themes were identified through content analysis: (1) body appearance (keloid formation and unable to find appropriate color of prosthesis); (2) social support (viewed as both positive and negative); (3) health activism (a need to inform other women of color about the risk); (4) menopause (health care providers had not provided enough information); and (5) learning to live with chronic illness (a sense of survival with a change in priorities).

Implications for Nursing Practice

Nurses play an important role in helping African American women develop awareness of the availability of prostheses and wigs to match their skin tones and hair. Breast cancer survivors should be supported in their own outreach efforts to inform other women in the African American community about breast cancer risk and screening. Providing information to women about the potential for menopausal symptoms should be clearly addressed by health care providers at the same time that other chemotherapy side effects are discussed.

MAMMOPLASTY

Mammoplasty is the surgical change in the size or shape of the breast. It may be done electively for cosmetic purposes to either enlarge or reduce the size of the breasts. It may also be done to reconstruct the breast after a mastectomy.

Health care providers should remain nonjudgmental toward women who desire mammoplasty. The desire to alter the appearance of the breasts has special significance for each woman as she attempts to alter or re-create her body image. It is important for the nurse to be aware of the cultural value placed on the breast by the woman. It is important that the woman have a realistic idea about what mammoplasty can accomplish and about possible complications, such as hematoma formation, hemorrhage, and infection. If an implant is involved, capsular contracture and loss of the implant are possible.

Breast Augmentation

In augmentation mammoplasty (the procedure to enlarge the breasts), an implant is placed in a surgically created pocket between the capsule of the breast and the pectoral fascia, or ideally under the pectoral muscle. Most implants are silicone envelopes filled with a fluid such as dextran, saline, or silicone. Because of their resemblance to the human breast, implants filled with silicone were the most widely used. In 1992 the Food and Drug Administration suspended the routine use of silicone implants in response to potential hazards related to silicone leakage. Allegations of associated immune-related diseases caused or exacerbated by the presence of silicone gel implants have caused considerable controversy and litigation. Currently the use of silicone implants is approved only when medically prescribed in clinical trials.

In the United States saline-filled implants are usually used. Saline-filled implants are silicone shells filled with normal saline. Soybean oil implants are an alternative form of implant. This implant has an outer shell of silicone that is filled with highly refined soybean oil. A major advantage of soybean implants is that it is easier for x-rays to penetrate the implant, so better visualization of the underlying breast tissue is possible with mammography.

Breast Reduction

For some women, large breasts can be a source of pain and embarrassment. They can interfere with normal daily activities such as walking, typing, and driving a car. Overly large breasts can interfere with self-esteem and self-image and can lead to back, shoulder, and neck problems, including degenerative nerve changes. They may make stylish dressing more difficult. Reduction in the size of the breasts can have positive effects on both the psychologic and the physical health of the patient. Reduction mammoplasty is performed by resecting wedges of tissue from the upper and lower quadrants of the breast. The excess skin is removed, and the areola and nipple are relocated on the breast. Lactation can usually be accomplished if massive amounts of tissue are not removed and the nipples are left connected during surgery.

NURSING MANAGEMENT
BREAST AUGMENTATION AND REDUCTION

Breast augmentation and breast reduction may be done in the outpatient surgical area, or it may involve overnight hospitalization. General anesthesia is used. Drains are generally placed in the surgical site to prevent hematoma formation and then removed 2 to 3 days after surgery or when drainage is under 20 ml per day. The drainage must be examined for color and odor to detect postoperative infection or hemorrhage. The woman's temperature should also be monitored. Dressings should be changed as necessary and prescribed using sterile technique. After surgery the woman should be assured that the appearance of the breast will improve when healing is completed. Depending on physician instructions, the patient may be instructed to wear a bra that provides good support continuously for 2 to 3 days after breast reduction or augmentation. Depending on the extent of the operation, most women can resume normal activities within 2 to 3 weeks. Strenuous exercise may not be appropriate until several weeks later.

Breast Reconstruction

Breast reconstructive surgery may be done simultaneously with a mastectomy or some time afterward to achieve symmetry and to restore or preserve body image.[36] The timing of reconstruction surgery should be individualized, based on the psychologic needs of the patient. Immediate breast reconstruction after mastectomy is commonly being performed. The advantages to immediate reconstruction are only one surgical procedure, one anesthesia induction, and one recovery period. Also, surgery takes place before the development of scar tissue or adhesions. Early reconstruction does not delay or influence further treatment or adversely affect predicted survival.

Indications. The main indication for breast reconstruction is to improve the woman's self-image and regain a sense of normality.[37] Present techniques cannot restore lactation, nipple sensation, or erectility. Therefore the erotic functions of the breast are not present. Although the breast will not fully resemble its premastectomy appearance, the reconstructed appearance usually represents an improvement over the mastectomy scar (Fig. 50-7). The contour of the breast is restored without the use of an external prosthesis.

Types of Reconstruction

Breast implants and tissue expansion. Breast implants are placed in a pocket under the pectoralis muscle, which protects the implant and provides soft tissue coverage over the implant. Implants can be placed either at the time of mastectomy or later. Because many mastectomy patients have insufficient tissue, simple placement of an implant may lead to small breast reconstruction that is tight or firm. Autologous tissue reconstruction may then be recommended.

A tissue expander can be used to stretch the skin and muscle at the mastectomy site before inserting implants (Fig. 50-8). The use of tissue expanders and breast implants is the most common breast reconstruction technique currently used.[28] Placement of the expander can be performed at the time of mastectomy or at a later date. The tissue expander, which is minimally inflated at the time of surgery, is gradually filled by weekly injections of sterile water or saline solution, which stretch the skin and muscle. Once the tissue is adequately stretched and the anticipated breast size is reached, the expander is surgically removed and a permanent implant is inserted. Some expanders are designed to remain in place and become the implant, eliminating the need for a second surgical procedure. Tissue expansion does not work well in individuals with extensive scar tissue from surgery or radiation therapy.

The body's natural response to the presence of a foreign substance is the formation of a fibrous capsule around the implant. If excessive capsular formation occurs as a result of infection, hematoma, trauma, or reaction to a foreign body, a contracture can develop, resulting in a deformed breast. Surgeons differ in their approaches to the prevention of contracture formation, although gentle manual massage around the implant is routine. Prevention of the problems that cause excessive capsule formation is critical. Other postoperative complications include skin ulceration, hypertrophic scar formation, intercostal neuralgia, and wound infection.

Musculocutaneous flap procedure. If insufficient muscle is left after mastectomy or if the chest wall has been radiated, the person's own tissue may be used to repair the soft tissue defects. Musculocutaneous flaps are most often taken from the back (latissimus dorsi muscle) or the abdomen (transverse rectus abdominis muscle). In the latissimus dorsi musculocutaneous flap, a block of skin and muscle from the patient's back is used to replace tissue removed during mastectomy.[38] A small implant may

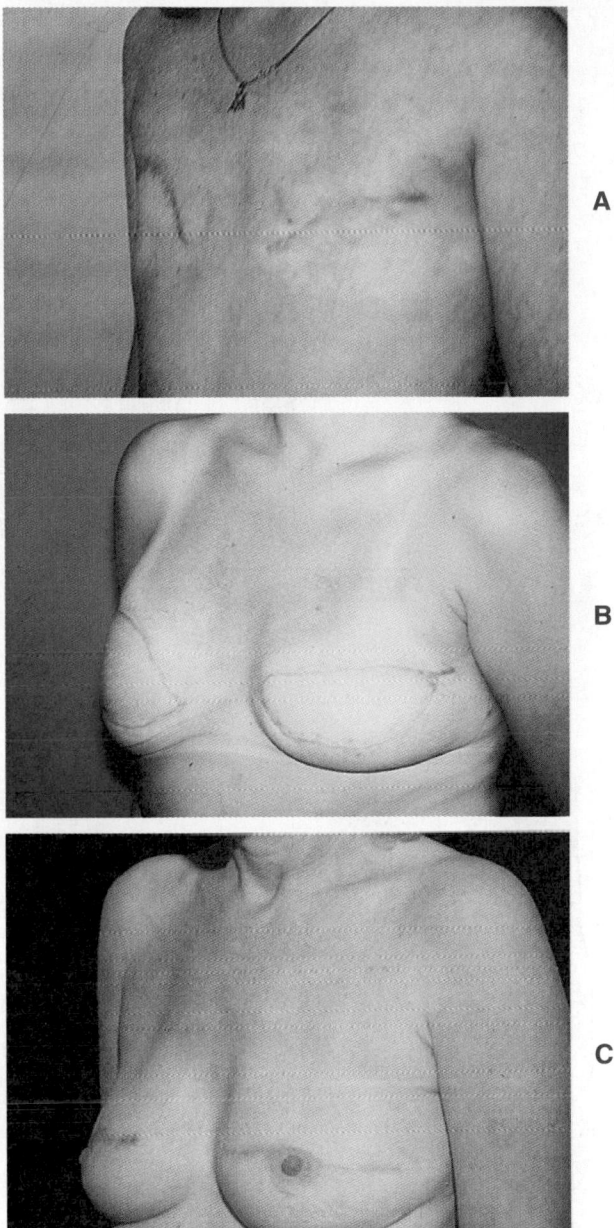

FIG. 50-7 A, Appearance of chest following bilateral mastectomy. B, Postoperative breast reconstruction before nipple-areolar reconstruction. C, Postoperative breast reconstruction after nipple-areolar reconstruction.

be needed beneath the flap to gain reasonable breast shape and size. A disadvantage of this technique is an additional scar on the back.

The *transverse rectus abdominis musculocutaneous* (TRAM) flap is the most frequently used flap operation. The rectus abdominis muscles are paired flat muscles running from the rib cage down to the pubic bone. Arteries running inside the muscle provide branches at many levels, and these branches supply the fat and skin across a large expanse of the abdomen. With this technique the surgeon elevates a large block of tissue from the lower abdominal area, but leaves it attached to the rectus muscle (Fig. 50-9). This tissue is then tunneled or placed as "free flaps"

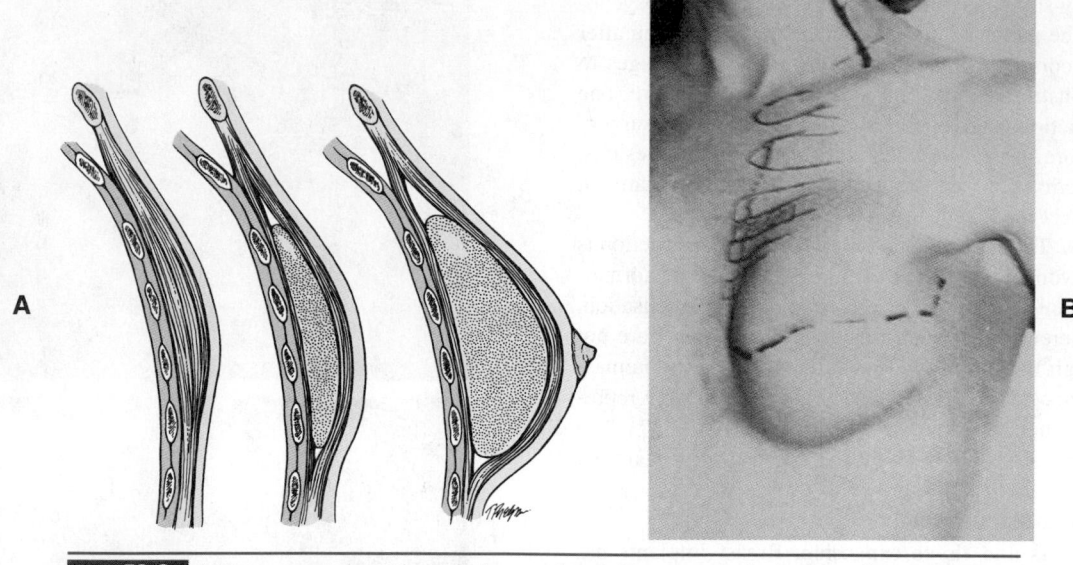

FIG. 50-8 A, Tissue expander with gradual expansion. B, Tissue expander in place after mastectomy.

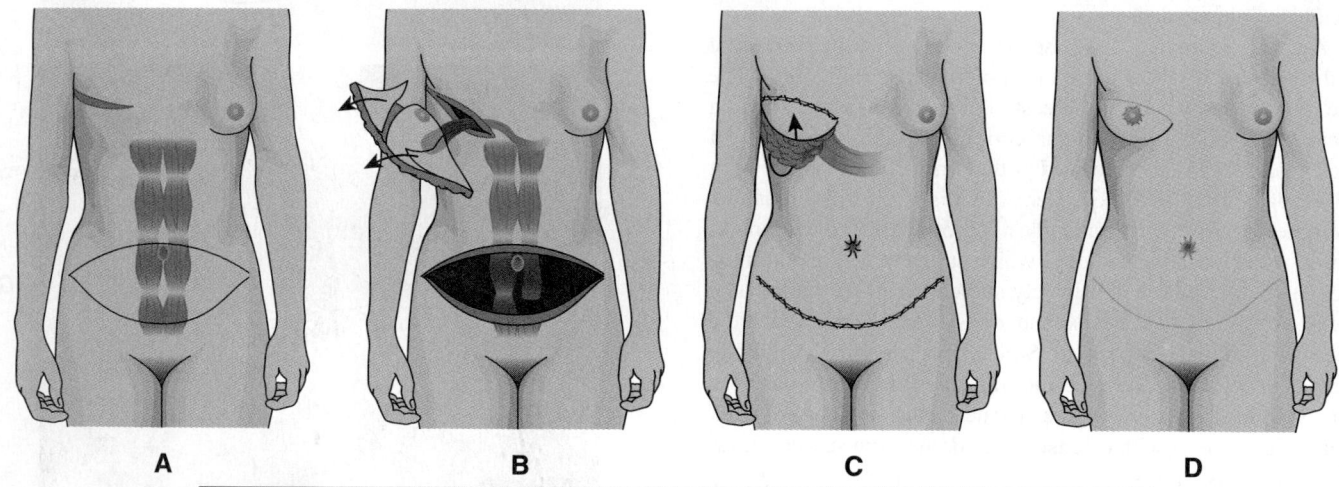

FIG. 50-9 TRAM flap. A, TRAM flap is planned. B, The abdominal tissue, while attached to the rectus muscle, nerve, and blood supply, is tunneled through the abdomen to the chest. C, The flap is trimmed to shape the breast. The lower abdominal incision is closed. D, Nipple and areola are reconstructed after the breast is healed.

under the skin up to the area where the breast will be reconstructed. Then it is molded and fashioned to form a breast. The abdominal incision is closed, giving the patient a result that is similar to having an abdominoplasty. This surgical procedure can last 2 to 8 hours, with recovery taking 4 to 6 weeks. Complications include bleeding, hernia, and infection. An implant may be used in addition to the flap if the flap does not provide the desired cosmetic result alone.

Nipple-areolar reconstruction. The majority of patients who have breast reconstruction also have nipple-areolar reconstruc-

tion. Nipple reconstruction gives the reconstructed breast a much more natural appearance. Nipple-areolar reconstruction is usually done a few months after breast reconstruction. Tissue to construct a nipple may be taken from the opposite breast or from a small flap of tissue on the reconstructed breast mound. The areola may be grafted from the labia, skin in area of the groin, or lower abdominal skin, or it may be tattooed with a permanent pigmented dye. In some patients a small implant may be placed under the completed nipple areolar reconstruction to add additional projection.

CRITICAL THINKING EXERCISES

Case Study
Breast Cancer
Patient Profile. Susan Paulson, a 52-year-old white woman, found a large lump in the upper outer quadrant of her left breast while showering.

Subjective Data
- Has family history of breast cancer—mother diagnosed at age 48 and sister diagnosed at age 45
- Had onset of menarche at age 11
- Has two daughters
- Has no prior history of breast cancer
- States she is afraid she has cancer

Objective Data
- Palpable 1.5 cm mass in upper outer quadrant of left breast
- Left breast mass confirmed by mammogram
- Otherwise normal physical examination
- Fine-needle aspiration biopsy of mass indicates diagnosis of breast cancer

Collaborative Care
- Scheduled for lumpectomy and sentinel lymph node dissection

CRITICAL THINKING QUESTIONS
1. What characteristics of malignancy could be determined by palpation of Susan's breast mass?
2. What in Susan's breast cancer experience with her family members might influence her coping response?
3. What information would the nurse provide to Susan about her planned therapy?
4. What are the possible complications the patient may face after a lumpectomy?
5. What are common postoperative exercises that Susan will need to practice if she has an axillary lymph node dissection?
6. What community resources are available to help Susan and her family adjust to the change in her body and to cope with the diagnosis of cancer? How can the nurse access these resources?
7. What information about breast cancer risks is important to provide to Susan and her daughters? What early detection measures are important for them to know?
8. Based on the assessment data presented, write one or more appropriate nursing diagnoses. Are there any collaborative problems?

Nursing Research Issues
1. What are the major concerns of women who are long-term survivors of breast cancer?
2. Do elderly women experience more or fewer sensory changes after breast surgery than young women?
3. Does perceived susceptibility to breast cancer increase a woman's motivation to participate in breast cancer screening?
4. What effect does dietary intake of caffeine have on a woman's perception of the severity of fibrocystic changes in the breast?
5. What influence does immediate versus delayed reconstruction have on the psychosocial adjustment of a woman after a mastectomy?
6. What is the influence of individualized teaching by a health professional on the frequency of breast self-examination practice in women?

REVIEW QUESTIONS

The number of the question corresponds to the same-numbered objective at the beginning of the chapter.

1. The nurse teaches a patient that BSE involves both the palpation of the breast tissue and
   a. palpation of cervical lymph nodes.
   b. hard squeezing of the breast tissue.
   c. a mammogram to evaluate breast tissue.
   d. inspection of the breasts for any changes.
2. An occupational health nurse is planning a program on BSE for women in the company. To best promote learning and compliance of the participants, the nurse includes
   a. a movie that demonstrates the procedure of BSE.
   b. distribution of detailed written instructions for use at home.
   c. explanations emphasizing the value of early detection of breast cancer.
   d. an opportunity to practice BSE on themselves with individual guidance from the nurse.
3. In teaching a patient with painful fibrocystic breast changes about the condition, the nurse explains that
   a. all discrete breast lumps must be biopsied to rule out malignant changes.
   b. the symptoms will probably subside following menopause unless hormone replacement is used.
   c. the lumps will become progressively larger and more painful, eventually necessitating surgical removal.
   d. restrictions of coffee and chocolate and supplements of vitamin E may relieve the discomfort for many patients.
4. While discussing risk factors for breast cancer with a group of women, the nurse stresses that the greatest known risk factor for breast cancer is
   a. being a woman over age 60.
   b. experiencing menstruation for 40 years or more.
   c. using estrogen replacement therapy during menopause.
   d. having a paternal grandmother with postmenopausal breast cancer.

Continued

REVIEW QUESTIONS—cont'd

5. A patient has an excisional biopsy of a breast nodule that is positive for cancer. The nurse explains that of the other tests done to determine the risk for cancer recurrence or spread, the result that supports the most favorable prognosis is
   a. cells with low S-phase fractions.
   b. absence of an HER-2/neu genetic marker.
   c. absence of axillary lymph node involvement.
   d. estrogen and progesterone receptor–positive tumors.

6. A patient diagnosed with breast cancer has been offered the treatment choice of breast conservation surgery with radiation or a modified radical mastectomy. When questioned by the patient about these options, the nurse informs the patient that the lumpectomy with radiation
   a. preserves the normal appearance and sensitivity of the breast.
   b. provides a shorter treatment period with fewer long-term complications.
   c. has about the same 10-year survival rate as the modified radical mastectomy.
   d. reduces the fear and anxiety that accompany the diagnosis and treatment of cancer.

7. Postoperatively the nurse teaches the patient with a modified radical mastectomy to prevent lymphedema by
   a. using a sling to keep the arm flexed at the side.
   b. exposing the arm to sunlight to increase circulation.
   c. wrapping the arm with elastic bandages during the night.
   d. avoiding unnecessary trauma (e.g., venipuncture, blood pressure measurement) to the arm on the operative side.

8. To prevent capsular formation following breast reconstruction with implants, the nurse teaches the patient to
   a. gently massage the area around the implant.
   b. bind the breasts tightly with elastic bandages.
   c. exercise the arm on the affected side to promote drainage.
   d. avoid strenuous exercise until implant healing has occurred.

REFERENCES

1. Jemal A et al: Cancer statistics 2002, *CA Cancer J Clin* 52:23, 2002.
2. American Cancer Society: *Cancer facts and figures 2002,* Atlanta, 2002, American Cancer Society.
3. Smith R et al: American Cancer Society guidelines for the early detection of cancer, *CA Cancer J Clin* 52:8, 2002.
4. National Cancer Institute: PDQ: detection and prevention. Available at *www.icic.nci.nih.gov/clinpdg/screening/breastcancer-physician.html#1* (accessed Feb 15, 2002).
*5. Kuyl M: The value of breast self-examination: meta analysis of the literature, *Oncol Nurs Forum* 28:815, 2001.
*6. Lauver D et al: Engagement in breast cancer screening behaviors, *Oncol Nurs Forum* 26:545, 1999.
7. Harvard Women's Health Watch: *Benign breast conditions 5:4,* Boston, 1998, Harvard Women's Health.
8. National Cancer Institute: Cancer facts: questions and answers about screening. Available at *http://cis.nci.nin.gov/fact* (accessed Feb. 15, 2002).
9. Cleveland Clinic: Minimally invasive breast biopsy–stereotactic breast biopsy. Available at *www.clevelandclinic.org/breastcenter/services* (accessed Aug 12, 2002).
10. Padden D: Mastalgia: evaluation and treatment, *Nurse Pract Forum* 11:213, 2000.
11. Arona A: Mastalgia. In Hindle W: *Breast care: a clinical guidebook for women's primary health care providers,* New York, 1999, Springer.
12. Cady B et al: Evaluation of common breast problems: guidance for primary care providers, *CA Cancer J Clin* 48:49, 1998.
13. McCance KL, Huether SE, editors: *Pathophysiology: biologic basis for disease in adults and children,* ed 4, St Louis, 2002, Mosby.
14. Jarvis C: *Physical examination and health assessment,* ed 4, St Louis, 2004, WB Saunders.
15. American Cancer Society: *Breast cancer facts and figures 2001-2002,* Atlanta, 2001, American Cancer Society.
16. Schairer C et al: Menopausal estrogen and estrogen-progestin replacement therapy and breast cancer risk, *JAMA* 283:485, 2000.
17. Nurses' Health Study: Risks and benefits of oral contraceptives and postmenopausal hormones, *Nurses' Health Study Newsletter* 5:6, 1998.
18. Giuliano A: Breast. In Tierney L, McPhee S, Papadakis M, editors: *Current medical diagnosis and treatment 2001,* ed 40, New York, 2001, Lange.
19. Vogel V: Breast cancer prevention: a review of current evidence, *CA Cancer J Clin* 50:156, 2000.
20. Kauff ND et al: Risk-reducing salpingo-oophorectomy in women with a BRCA-1 or BRCA-2 mutation, *N Engl J Med* 346:1609, 2002.
21. Rebbeck TR et al: Prohylactic oophorectomy in carriers of BRCA-1 or BRCA-2 mutation, *N Engl J Med* 346:1609, 2002.
22. Hartmann LC, Schaid DJ, Woods JE: Efficiency of bilateral prophylactic mastectomy in women with a family history of breast cancer, *N Engl J Med* 340:77, 1999.
23. Westendorp J: Sentinel lymph node dissection in breast cancer, *Innovations in Breast Cancer Care* 5:94, 2001.
24. Hsueh E, Hansen N, Giuliano A: Intraoperative lymphatic mapping and sentinel lymph node dissection in breast cancer, *CA Cancer J Clin* 50:279, 2000.
25. Hubbard S, Goodman M, Knobf MT: HER-2, herceptin, and breast cancer, *Oncology Nursing Updates* 7:1, 2000.
26. American Joint Committee on Cancer: *Manual for staging of cancer,* ed 4, Philadelphia, 1992, Lippincott.
27. Petrek J, Pressman P, Smith R: Lymphedema: current issues in research and management, *CA Cancer J Clin* 50:292, 2000.
28. Hamolsky D, Facione N: Infiltrating breast cancer. In Miaskowski C, Buchsel P: *Oncology nursing: assessment and clinical care,* St Louis, 1999, Mosby.
29. Aikin J: Adjuvant therapy for breast cancer: choices and challenges, *Innovations in Breast Cancer Care* 5:3, 2000.
30. National Institutes of Health: Adjuvant therapy for breast cancer, *NIH Consensus Statement 2000* 17:1, Nov 2000. Available at *http://consensus.nih.gov* (accessed Dec 28, 2002).
31. Dunn B, Ford L: Breast cancer prevention: results of the National Surgical Adjuvant Breast and Bowel Project (NSABP) breast cancer prevention trial, *Eur J Cancer* 36(suppl 4):S49, 2000.
32. Machia J: Breast cancer: risk, prevention and tamoxifen, *Am J Nurs* 101:26, 2001.
33. Rees C, Bath P: Information-seeking behaviors of women with breast cancer, *Oncol Nurs Forum* 28:899, 2001.
34. Hosleins C, Haber J: Adjusting to breast cancer, *Am J Nurs* 100:26, 2000.
35. Ferrell B et al: Quality of life in breast cancer survivors: implications for developing support services, *Oncol Nurs Forum* 25:887, 1998.

*Nursing research–based reference.

36. Fortunato N, McCullough SM: *Plastic and reconstructive surgery,* St Louis, 1998, Mosby.
*37. Neil K, Armstrong N, Burnett C: Choosing reconstruction after mastectomy: a qualitative analysis, *Oncol Nurs Forum* 25:743, 1998.
38. Thomas S, Greifzu S: Breast reconstruction, *RN* 63:45, 2000.

RESOURCES

American Cancer Society—Reach to Recovery
1599 Clifton Road NE
Atlanta, GA 30329
800-ACS-2345
www.cancer.org

American Society of Plastic Surgeons
Plastic Surgery Education Foundation
444 East Algonquin Road
Arlington Heights, IL
888-475-2784
www.plasticsurgery.org

Breast Cancer Information Center
www.feminist.org/other/bc/bchome.html

Living Beyond Breast Cancer
Survivors' helpline: 888-753-5222
610-645-4567
www.lbbc.org

National Alliance of Breast Cancer Organizations
9 East 37th Street, 10th Floor
New York, NY 10016
888-80-NABCO
212-889-0606
Fax: 212-689-1213
www.nabco.org

National Breast Cancer Coalition
1707 L Street, NW, Suite 1060
Washington, DC 20036
202-296-7477
Fax: 202-265-6854
www.natlbcc.org/

National Cancer Institute
Suite 3036A
6116 Executive Boulevard, MSC8322
Bethesda, MD 20892-8322
800-4-CANCER
www.nci.nih.gov

National Coalition for Cancer Survivorship (NCCS)
1010 Wayne Avenue, Suite 770
Silver Spring, MD 20910
877-622-7936
301-650-9127
Fax: 301-565-9670
www.cansearch.org/

National Lymphedema Network (NLN)
Latham Square
1611 Telegraph Avenue, Suite 1111
Oakland, CA 94612-2138
Hotline: 800-541-3259 or 510-208-3200
Fax: 510-208-3110
www.lymphnet.org/

OncoLink (cancer information site)
University of Pennsylvania Cancer Center
www.oncolink.upenn.edu

Oncology Nursing Society
501 Holiday Drive
Pittsburgh, PA 15220
412-921-7373
Fax: 412-921-6565
www.ons.org

Sisters Network (a national support group for African American breast cancer patients)
8787 Woodway Drive, Suite 4206
Houston, TX 77063
713-781-0255
Fax: 713-780-8998
www.sistersnetworkinc.org

Susan G. Komen Breast Cancer Foundation
800-462-9273
www.komen.org

Y-me National Breast Cancer Organization
212 West Van Buren, Suite 500
Chicago, IL 60607
800-221-2141
312-986-8338
Fax: 312-294-8597
www.Y-me.org

For additional Internet resources, see the website for this book at *http://evolve.elsevier.com/Lewis/medsurg/.*

CHAPTER *51*

NURSING MANAGEMENT
Sexually Transmitted Diseases

Shannon Ruff Dirksen

LEARNING OBJECTIVES

1. Identify the factors contributing to the high incidence of sexually transmitted diseases.
2. Explain the etiology, clinical manifestations, complications, and diagnostic abnormalities of gonorrhea, syphilis, chlamydial infections, genital herpes, and genital warts.
3. Compare primary genital herpes with recurrent genital herpes.
4. Explain the collaborative care and drug therapy of gonorrhea, syphilis, chlamydial infections, genital herpes, and genital warts.

5. Identify the nursing assessment and nursing diagnoses for patients who have a sexually transmitted disease.
6. Describe the nursing role in the prevention and control of sexually transmitted diseases.
7. Describe the nursing management of patients with sexually transmitted diseases.

KEY TERMS

chancres, p. 1387
chlamydial infections, p. 1390
genital herpes, p. 1392
gonorrhea, p. 1385
gummas, p. 1388
lymphogranuloma venereum, p. 1391

sexually transmitted diseases, p. 1384
syphilis, p. 1387
tabes dorsalis, p. 1389
venereal diseases, p. 1384

Sexually Transmitted Diseases

Sexually transmitted diseases (STDs) are infectious diseases transmitted most commonly through sexual contact (Table 51-1). Historically they have been referred to as **venereal diseases.** Many of the agents causing STDs are easily inactivated by drying, heating, and washing. These infections can be bacterial (gonorrhea, chlamydia, syphilis) and/or viral (genital herpes, genital warts). Most infections start as lesions on the genitalia and other sexually exposed mucous membranes. Wide dissemination to other areas of the body can then occur. A latent or subclinical phase is present with all STDs. This can lead to a long-term persistent infection and the transmission of disease from an asymptomatic (but infected) person to another contact. Different STDs can coexist within one person. For example, if a person has gonorrhea, chlamydial infection may also be present.

In the United States all cases of gonorrhea and syphilis, and in most states chlamydial infection, must be reported to the state or local public health authorities. In spite of this requirement, there are many unreported cases of these infections. An estimated 65 million Americans are currently infected with one or more STDs.[1] Every year an additional 15 million Americans are newly infected with an STD.[2] Diseases that are associated with sexual

transmission can also be contracted by other routes such as through blood, blood products, and autoinoculation.

The more commonly diagnosed STDs are discussed in this chapter. Human immunodeficiency virus (HIV) infection and related problems are discussed in Chapter 14. Hepatitis B infection and related problems are discussed in Chapter 42.

Factors Affecting Incidence of Sexually Transmitted Diseases

Many contributing factors are related to the current STD rates. Earlier reproductive maturity and increased longevity have resulted in a longer sexual life span. The increase in the total population has resulted in an increase in the number of susceptible hosts. Other factors include greater sexual freedom, changing roles of women, decreased social control by religious institu-

TABLE 51-1 Microorganisms Responsible for Diseases Transmitted by Sexual Activity

ORGANISM	DISEASE
Chlamydia trachomatis	Nongonococcal urethritis (NGU); cervicitis; lymphogranuloma venereum
Cytomegalovirus (CMV)	Multiple diseases
Hepatitis B virus	Hepatitis B
Herpes simplex virus (HSV)	Genital herpes
Human immunodeficiency virus (HIV)	HIV infection, acquired immunodeficiency syndrome (AIDS)
Human papillomavirus	Genital warts
Poxvirus	Molluscum contagiosum
Neisseria gonorrhoeae	Gonorrhea
Treponema pallidum	Syphilis

Reviewed by Dana Rosdahl, RN-C, PhD(c), FNP, Instructor, Arizona State University, Tempe, Ariz.

tions, and an increased emphasis in the media on sexuality. In addition, increased leisure time, inexpensive travel, and urbanization have brought together people with varying social behaviors and value systems.

Changes in the methods of contraception are also reflected in the incidence of STDs. The condom is considered to be the only contraceptive device that is prophylactic in regard to STDs. Although condom use is increasing in selected populations, it is not used frequently in the general population. Commonly used oral contraceptives cause the secretions of the cervix and the vagina to become more alkaline. This change produces a more favorable environment for the growth of organisms that cause STDs at these sites. Women who take oral contraceptives have a lower risk of pelvic inflammatory disease (PID) as a result of the ability of the cervical mucus to act as a barrier against bacteria. However, the proliferation of chlamydia, the leading cause of non-gonococcal PID, may be enhanced by oral contraceptive use. Whether or not intrauterine device (IUD) users are at increased risk of PID is controversial, but it is clear that IUDs confer no protection against STDs.[3] Long-acting contraceptives such as levonorgestrel (Norplant) and medroxyprogesterone (Depo-Provera) have been shown to lower the concurrent use of condoms, even among women with risk factors for STDs.[4] Both Norplant and Depo-Provera confer no protection against STDs. Lack of awareness of this fact may be a factor leading to STDs in people using these products.

Bacterial Infections

GONORRHEA

Gonorrhea is the second most frequently occurring STD. Following a 73.9% decline in the reported rate of gonorrhea from 1975 to 1997, the gonorrhea rate increased in 1998.[5] The overall rate of gonorrhea in the United States since 1998 has remained essentially unchanged even though true increases may have occurred in some populations and geographic areas. In 2000, 358,995 cases of gonorrhea were reported in the United States. The incidence of gonorrhea is highest among people under 24 years old living in high-density urban areas who have multiple sex partners and unprotected sexual intercourse. Increases have also been noted among men who have sex with men. Most states have enacted laws that permit examination and treatment of minors without parental consent.

Etiology and Pathophysiology

Gonorrhea is caused by *Neisseria gonorrhoeae,* a gram-negative diplococcus. The disease is spread by direct physical contact with an infected host, usually during sexual activity (vaginal, oral, or anal). Mucosa with columnar epithelium is susceptible to gonococcal infection. This tissue is present in the genitalia (urethra in men, cervix in women), the rectum, and the oropharynx. Neonates can develop a gonococcal infection during delivery from an infected mother. The delicate gonococcus is easily killed by drying, heating, or washing with an antiseptic solution. Consequently, indirect transmission by instruments or linens is rare. The incubation period is 3 to 4 days. The disease confers no immunity to subsequent reinfection. Gonococcal infection elicits an inflammatory response, which, if left untreated, leads to the formation of fibrous tissue and adhesions. This fi-

brous scarring is subsequently responsible for many complications in women such as strictures and tubal abnormalities, which can lead to tubal pregnancy, chronic pelvic pain, and infertility.

Clinical Manifestations

Men. The initial site of infection in heterosexual men is usually the urethra. Symptoms of urethritis consist of dysuria and profuse, purulent urethral discharge developing 2 to 5 days after infection (Fig. 51-1). Painful or swollen testicles may also occur. Men generally seek medical evaluation early in the disease because their symptoms are usually obvious and distressing. It is unusual for men with gonorrhea to be asymptomatic.

Women. Most women who contract gonorrhea are asymptomatic or have minor symptoms that are often overlooked, making it possible for them to remain a source of infection. A few women may complain of vaginal discharge, dysuria, or frequency of urination. Changes in menstruation may be a symptom, but these changes are often disregarded by the woman. After the incubation period, redness and swelling occur at the site of contact, which is usually the cervix or urethra (Fig. 51-2). A purulent exudate often develops with a potential for abscess formation. The disease may remain local or can spread by direct tissue extension to the uterus, fallopian tubes, and ovaries. Although the vulva and vagina are uncommon sites for a gonorrheal infection, they may become involved when little or no estrogen is present, as is the case in prepubertal girls and postmenopausal women. Because the vagina acts as a natural reservoir for infectious secretions,

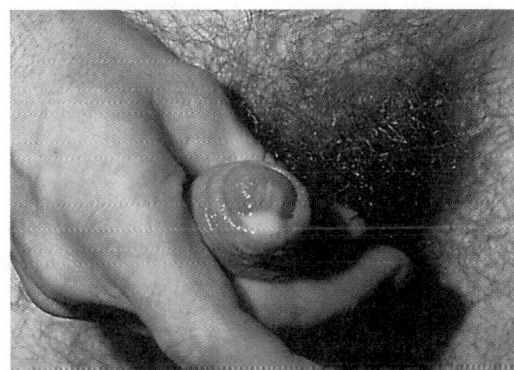

FIG. 51-1 Gonococcal urethritis. Profuse, purulent drainage.

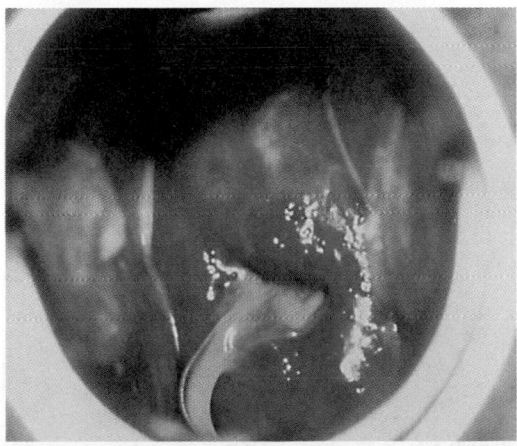

FIG. 51-2 Endocervical gonorrhea. Cervical redness and edema with discharge.

transmission is often more efficient from men to women than it is from women to men.

General. Anorectal gonorrhea may be present and is usually caused by anal intercourse. Symptoms may include soreness, itching, and discharge. Most patients with rectal infections and infections in the throat have few symptoms. A small percentage of individuals develop gonococcal pharyngitis resulting from orogenital sexual contact. When the gonococcus can be demonstrated by a laboratory culture, individuals of either gender are infectious to their sexual partners.

Complications

Because men often seek treatment early in the course of the disease, they are less likely to develop complications. The complications that do occur in men are prostatitis, urethral strictures, and sterility from orchitis or epididymitis. Because women who are asymptomatic seldom seek treatment, complications are more common and usually constitute the reason for seeking medical attention. Pelvic inflammatory disease (PID), Bartholin's abscess, ectopic pregnancy, and infertility are the main complications of gonorrhea in women. A small percentage of infected persons, mainly women, may develop a disseminated gonococcal infection (DGI). In DGI the appearance of skin lesions, fever, arthralgia, or arthritis usually causes the patient to seek medical help (Fig. 51-3).

Eye Infections in Newborns. Almost all states have a health department regulation or law requiring the instillation of a prophylactic drug such as erythromycin (0.5%) ophthalmic ointment or silver nitrate (0.1%) aqueous solution into the eyes of all newborns in a single application. The incidence of gonorrheal eye infections in newborns *(ophthalmia neonatorum)* is therefore relatively rare today. Untreated infected infants develop permanent blindness.

Diagnostic Studies

The immediate identification of *N. gonorrhoeae* is usually made with a Gram stain of smears made from the exudate. The slides should be interpreted by an experienced technician so that a correct diagnosis is made initially, because some patients fail to return for follow-up care. A reliable way to confirm gonococcal infection is to isolate the organism in culture. Cultures of the discharge or secretion can provide a definitive diagnosis after

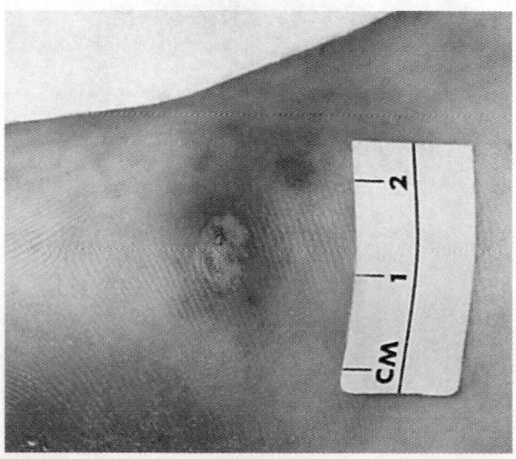

incubation for 24 to 48 hours. Whenever practical, the swab from any mucosal site should be inoculated immediately onto a special growth medium (Thayer-Martin medium) at room temperature, and then placed promptly in an enriched CO_2 environment and incubated. However, various nonnutrient transport media are adequate if the specimen can be transported to the laboratory without refrigeration and inoculated onto the growth medium within 6 hours.

For men, a presumptive diagnosis of gonorrhea is made if there is a history of sexual contact with a new or infected partner followed within a few days by a urethral discharge. Typical clinical manifestations, combined with a positive finding in a Gram-stained smear of the purulent discharge from the penis, gives an almost certain diagnosis. A culture of the discharge is indicated for men whose smears are negative in the presence of strong clinical evidence.

Making a diagnosis of gonorrhea in women on the basis of symptoms is difficult because most women are symptom free or have complaints that may be confused with other conditions. Smears and purulent discharge do not establish a diagnosis of gonorrhea because the female genitourinary tract normally harbors a large number of organisms that resemble *N. gonorrhoeae.* A culture must be performed to confirm the diagnosis. Although the cervix is the most common site of sampling, specimens for culture may also be taken from the urethra, anus, or oropharynx to confirm the diagnosis. The Centers for Disease Control and Prevention (CDC) recommends that all women treated for gonorrhea have a rectal culture done.

A new technique, DNA amplification using polymerase chain reaction (PCR) or ligase chain reaction (LCR), is being used to diagnose gonorrhea. (PCR is discussed in Chapter 13.) This testing technique does not involve culture and is a quicker approach to detecting infection. DNA amplification has a high rate of sensitivity and specificity. The test can be performed on urine, vaginal fluid or discharge, or urethral secretions. This eliminates the need for a urethral swab in male patients and potentially the necessity for pelvic examination in female patients.

Collaborative Care

Drug Therapy. Because of a short incubation period and high infectivity, treatment is generally instituted without awaiting culture results, even in the absence of any signs or symptoms. The treatment of gonorrhea in the early stage is curative. Traditionally, the drug of choice for gonorrheal therapy had been penicillin, but changes have been made because of resistant strains of *N. gonorrhoeae.* As a result of penicillin-resistant strains, ceftriaxone (Rocephin), a penicillinase-resistant cephalosporin, or cefixime (Suprax), ciprofloxacin (Cipro), ofloxacin (Floxin), or levofloxacin (Levaquin) has become part of the treatment plan (Table 51-2). The recommended drug regimen has resulted in a success rate of at least 95% in eliminating uncomplicated urogenital and anorectal gonococcal infections.[6] Resistance to the fluoroquinolones, such as ciprofloxacin (Cipro), has been reported, and although still somewhat rare, is a cause for concern. The high frequency (up to 20% in men and 40% in women) of coexisting chlamydial and gonococcal infections has led to the addition of azithromycin (Zithromax) or doxycycline (Vibramycin) to the treatment regimen. Patients with coexisting syphilis are likely to be cured by the same drugs used for gonorrhea.

All sexual contacts of patients with gonorrhea must be evaluated and treated to prevent reinfection after resumption of sexual

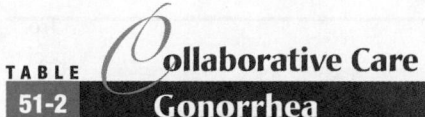

TABLE 51-2	Collaborative Care — Gonorrhea

Diagnostic

History and physical examination
Gram–stained smears of urethral or endocervical exudate
Cultures for *N. gonorrhoeae*
DNA amplification to detect *N. gonorrhoeae*
Testing for other STDs (syphilis, HIV, chlamydia)

Collaborative Therapy

Uncomplicated gonorrhea: cefixime (Suprax) 400 mg orally in a single dose or ceftriaxone (Rocephin) 125 mg IM in a single dose or ciprofloxacin (Cipro) 500 mg orally in a single dose or ofloxacin (Floxin) 400 mg orally in a single dose or levofloxacin (Levaquin) 250 mg orally in a single dose
If chlamydial infection is not ruled out: azithromycin (Zithromax) 1 g orally in a single dose or doxycycline (Vibramycin) 100 mg orally twice a day for 7 days
Patients who are allergic to cephalosporins or quinolones should be treated with spectinomycin
Patients who have uncomplicated gonorrhea and who are treated with any of the above therapies may not need to return to confirm that they are cured
Case finding
Treatment of sexual contacts
Instruction on abstinence from sexual intercourse and alcohol
Reexamination if symptoms persist or recur after completion of treatment

Modified from Centers for Disease Control and Prevention: STD treatment guidelines, *MMWR* 51(RR-6):1, 2002.
HIV, Human immunodeficiency virus; *IM,* intramuscular; *STD,* sexually transmitted disease.

relations. The "ping-pong" effect of reexposure, treatment, and reinfection can cease only when infected partners are treated simultaneously. Additionally, the patient should be counseled to abstain from sexual intercourse and alcohol during treatment. Sexual intercourse allows the infection to spread and can delay complete healing. Alcohol has an irritant effect on the healing urethral walls. Men should be cautioned against squeezing the penis to look for further discharge. Follow-up examination and reculture may be done at least once after treatment, usually in 4 to 7 days. Reinfection, rather than treatment failure, is the main cause for infections identified after treatment has ended.

SYPHILIS

The incidence of **syphilis** reported in the United States in 2000 is at its lowest rate since reporting started in 1941.[7] In 2000 only 5979 cases of syphilis were reported in the United States. The credit for this decline is a national effort that began in 1999 that focuses on community-based prevention programs, faster response to outbreaks, and better access to clinics.[8] However, syphilis remains an important health problem.

Etiology and Pathophysiology

The causative organism of syphilis is *Treponema pallidum,* a spirochete. This bacterium is thought to enter the body through very small breaks in the skin or mucous membranes. Its entry is facilitated by the minor abrasions that often occur during sexual intercourse. Syphilis is a complex disease in which many organs and tissues of the body can become infected by *T. pallidum.* The infection causes the production of antibodies that also react with normal tissues. After a short period of protection, the antibody levels decrease, and a person is susceptible to reinfection.[9] Not all people who are exposed to syphilis acquire the disease; about one third become infected after intercourse with an infected person. In addition to sexual contact, syphilis may be spread through contact with infectious lesions and sharing of needles among intravenous (IV) drug users. *T. pallidum* is extremely fragile and easily destroyed by drying, heating, or washing. The incubation period for syphilis ranges from 10 to 90 days (average 21 days). Congenital syphilis is transmitted from an infected mother to the fetus in utero after the tenth week of pregnancy. The rate of infant death is up to 40% of women untreated for syphilis.[10]

More so than for gonorrhea, those with untreated syphilis tend to be young persons of a low educational and socioeconomic level who have limited access to health care. Racial disparities also exist, with African Americans having syphilis at a rate 30 times greater than the rate of whites.[1]

There is an association between syphilis and HIV infection. Persons at high risk for acquiring syphilis are also at an increased risk for acquiring HIV. Often, both infections may be present in the same person. The presence of syphilitic lesions on the genitals enhances HIV transmission. HIV-infected patients with syphilis appear to be at greatest risk for clinically significant central nervous system (CNS) involvement and may require more intensive treatment with penicillin than do other patients with syphilis. Therefore the evaluation of all patients with syphilis should also include testing for HIV with the patient's consent.

Clinical Manifestations

Syphilis has a variety of signs and symptoms that can mimic a number of other diseases. Consequently, compared with other STDs, it is more difficult to recognize syphilis. If it is not treated, specific clinical stages are characteristic of the progression of the disease (Table 51-3). In the *primary stage* of the bacterial invasion (Fig. 51-4), **chancres** appear. These are painless indurated lesions on the penis, vulva, lips, mouth, vagina, and rectum. They frequently occur 10 to 90 days after inoculation. The chancre lasts 3 to 6 weeks, eventually healing on its own. During this time the draining of the microorganisms into the lymph nodes causes regional lymphadenopathy. Genital ulcers may also be present. Without treatment the infection progresses to the secondary stage.

The *secondary stage* of syphilis is systemic. The stage begins a few weeks after the chancres are first seen. During this stage blood-borne bacteria spread to all major organ systems. Manifestations characteristic of the secondary stage can include cutaneous eruptions, fever, alopecia (hair loss), sore throat, headaches, weight loss, tiredness, and generalized adenopathy. The cutaneous eruptions (Fig. 51-5) include a bilateral, symmetric rash usually involving the palms and soles; mucous patches in the mouth, tongue, or cervix; and condylomata lata (moist, weeping papules) in the anal and genital area.

The *latent* or *hidden stage* of syphilis follows the secondary stage and is a period during which the immune system is able to suppress the infection. The latent stage can be further divided into an early stage, in which the infection has been acquired in the preceding year, and a late stage, in which the infection has been present for greater than 1 year. There are no signs or symptoms of syphilis during this time. During the latent stage, the di-

TABLE 51-3 Stages of Syphilis			
CLINICAL STAGE	CHARACTERISTIC FINDINGS	COMMUNICABILITY	DURATION OF STAGE
Primary	Chancre	Exudate from chancre highly infectious; blood is infectious	3-8 wk
Secondary	Cutaneous eruptions, alopecia, systemic symptoms (malaise, arthralgia, headache, occasionally liver and kidney dysfunction), regional adenopathy 6-12 wk after chancre	Exudate from skin and mucous membrane lesions highly infectious	1-2 yr
Latent	Absence of signs or symptoms	Noninfectious after 4 yr, possible placental transmission	Throughout life or progression to late stage
Late*	Appearance 3-20 yr after initial infection	Noninfectious	Chronic (without treatment), possibly fatal
Benign	Gummas (chronic, destructive lesions affecting any organ of body, especially skin, bone, liver, mucous membranes)	Spinal fluid possibly containing organism	
Cardiovascular	Aortic valve insufficiency or saccular aneurysm of thoracic aorta, aortitis		
Neurosyphilis	General paresis (personality changes from minor to psychotic, tremors, physical and mental deterioration)		
	Tabes dorsalis (ataxia, areflexia, paresthesias, lightning pains, damaged joints [Charcot's joints])		

*Several forms such as cardiovascular and neurosyphilis occur together in approximately 25% of untreated cases.

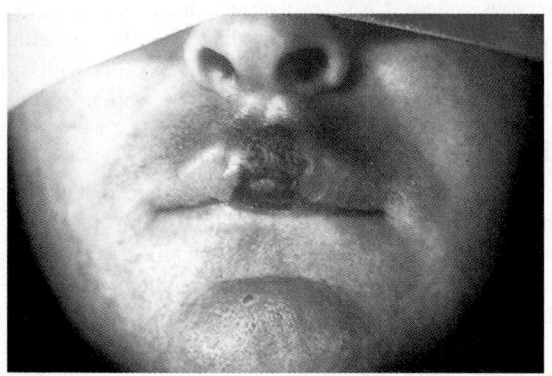

FIG. 51-4 Primary syphilis chancre on upper lip.

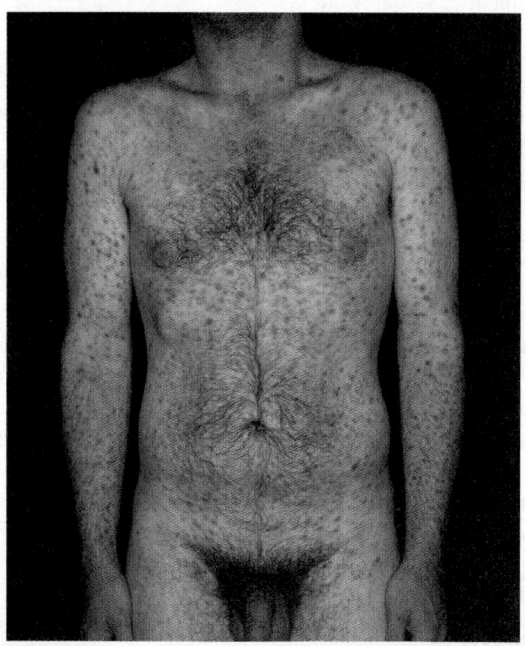

FIG. 51-5 Secondary syphilis. Bilateral, symmetric cutaneous lesions.

agnosis is established by a positive specific treponemal antibody test for syphilis together with a normal cerebrospinal fluid (CSF) examination and the absence of clinical manifestations on physical examination and chest x-rays. About 70% of untreated patients with latent syphilis never develop clinically evident, third-stage syphilis, but the occurrence of a spontaneous cure of syphilis is doubtful.[11]

The *third stage* of syphilis (also called *late* or *tertiary* syphilis) is the most severe stage of the disease. Because antibiotics can cure syphilis, manifestations of late syphilis are rare. However, when it does occur, it is responsible for significant morbidity and mortality rates. The pathogenesis of the manifestations of this stage is unclear. **Gummas** (destructive skin, bone, and soft tissue nodular lesions associated with late syphilis) are probably caused by a severe hypersensitivity reaction to the microorganism. Within the cardiovascular system late syphilis may cause aneurysms, heart valve insufficiency, and heart failure. Within the CNS the presence of *T. pallidum* in CSF may cause manifestations of *neurosyphilis* (general paresis) (see Table 51-3).

Complications

Complications of the disease occur mostly in late syphilis. The gummas of benign late syphilis may produce irreparable damage to bone, liver, or skin but seldom result in death. In cardiovascular syphilis, the resulting aneurysm may press on structures such as the intercostal nerves, causing pain. The possibility of a rupture exists as the aneurysm increases in size. Scarring of the aortic valve results in aortic valve insufficiency and eventually heart failure.

Neurosyphilis is responsible for degeneration of the brain with mental deterioration. Evidence of other neurologic deficits may be present. Problems related to sensory nerve involvement are a result of **tabes dorsalis** (progressive locomotor ataxia). There may be sudden attacks of pain anywhere in the body, which can confuse the diagnosis with other conditions. Loss of vision and sense of position in the feet and legs can also occur. Walking may become even more difficult as joint stability is lost. (Late syphilis is also discussed in Chapter 57.)

Diagnostic Studies

The first step in diagnosis is to obtain a detailed and accurate sexual history. A physical examination should be done to identify any suspicious lesions, as well as to note other significant signs and symptoms.

The presence of spirochetes on dark-field microscopy and direct fluorescent antibody tests of lesion exudate or tissue can confirm a clinical diagnosis of syphilis. However, syphilis is more commonly diagnosed by a serologic test. Tests for syphilis may be classified as those performed for screening and those performed for confirmation of a positive screening test. Nonspecific antitreponemal antibodies can be detected by tests such as the Venereal Disease Research Laboratory (VDRL) test and the rapid plasma reagin (RPR) test. These nontreponemal tests are suitable for screening purposes and usually become positive 10 to 14 days after the appearance of a chancre. The fluorescent treponemal antibody absorption (FTA-ABS) test and the microhemagglutination (MHA) test detect specific antitreponemal antibodies and are suitable for confirming the diagnosis.

False-negative and false-positive test results do occur with the nontreponemal tests (VDRL, RPR). A false-negative result may be obtained during primary syphilis if the test is done before the individual has had time to produce antibodies. A false-positive finding may occur with other diseases or conditions such as hepatitis, infectious mononucleosis, after smallpox vaccination, collagen diseases (e.g., systemic lupus erythematosus), pregnancy, or aging. Positive nontreponemal test results should be confirmed by more specific treponemal tests to rule out other causes. In the CSF, changes such as increased white blood cell count, increased total protein, and a positive treponemal antibody test are diagnostic of asymptomatic neurosyphilis.

If a patient is treated with antibiotics early in the course of the disease on the basis of the history and the symptoms, the serologic testing may not indicate the presence of syphilis. Once a person has positive serologic findings for syphilis, indicating the presence of antibodies, these findings may remain positive for an indefinite period in spite of successful treatment.

Collaborative Care

Drug Therapy. Management of syphilis is aimed at eradication of all syphilitic organisms (Table 51-4). However, treatment cannot reverse damage that is already present in the late stage of the disease. Benzathine penicillin G (Bicillin) or aqueous procaine penicillin G remains the treatment of choice for all stages of syphilis. To date, after four decades of use, there is no evidence to suggest a decrease in the effectiveness of penicillin against *T. pallidum*. Table 51-5 describes therapy for the various stages of syphilis and is in accordance with U.S. Public Health Service recommendations. All stages of syphilis should be

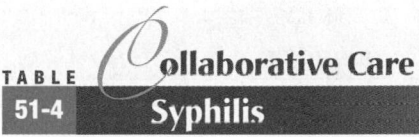

TABLE 51-4   Collaborative Care   Syphilis

Diagnostic
History and physical examination
Dark-field microscopy
Nontreponemal or treponemal serologic testing
Testing for other STDs (HIV, gonorrhea, chlamydia)

Collaborative Therapy
Appropriate drug therapy (see Table 51-5)
Confidential counseling and testing for HIV infection
Case finding
Surveillance
   Repeat of quantitative nontreponemal tests at 3, 6, and 12 mo
   Examination of cerebrospinal fluid at 1 year if treatment
      involves alternative antibiotics or treatment failure has
      occurred

HIV, Human immunodeficiency virus; *STD*, sexually transmitted disease.

TABLE 51-5   Drug Therapy   Syphilis

STAGE	TYPE OF PENICILLIN	OTHER ANTIBIOTICS*
Early syphilis (primary, secondary, and early latent)	2.4 million U IM of penicillin G benzathine (Bicillin) in a single dose	doxycycline (Vibramycin) 100 mg orally twice a day for 2 wk, or tetracycline 500 mg orally four times a day for 2 wk
Re-treatment, if needed	7.2 million U of Bicillin total, given as 3 doses of 2.4 million U IM of Bicillin each, at 1 wk intervals	
Late latent syphilis	7.2 million U total of Bicillin given as 3 doses of 2.4 million U IM of Bicillin each at 1 wk intervals	doxycycline or tetracycline given for 4 wk at same dosage/routes as early syphilis
Tertiary syphilis		
Gumma, cardiovascular	Same as for re-treatment and late latent stage	Same as for late latent stage
Neurosyphilis	Aqueous crystalline penicillin G 18-24 U IV daily, given as 3-4 million U every 4 hr for 10-14 days	procaine penicillin 2.4 million U IM once daily plus probenecid (Benemid) 500 mg orally 4 times a day; both drugs given for 10-14 days

Modified from Centers for Disease Control and Prevention: STD treatment guidelines, *MMWR* 51(RR-6):1, 2002.
*Given when penicillin is contraindicated.
IM, Intramuscular; *IV*, intravenous.

treated. Patients having persistent or recurring symptoms after drug therapy has ended should be re-treated. All patients with neurosyphilis must be carefully monitored, with periodic serologic testing, clinical evaluation at 6-month intervals, and repeat CSF examinations for at least 3 years. Specific management is based on the symptoms.

Appropriate penicillin treatment according to the stage of syphilis before the eighteenth week of pregnancy prevents maternal transmission to the fetus. Appropriate treatment after 18 weeks of pregnancy usually cures both mother and fetus because the antibiotics can cross the placental barrier. Treatment administered in the second half of pregnancy may pose a risk of premature labor and fetal distress. Some authorities recommend hospitalization and fetal monitoring of women at 20 weeks of gestation or greater.[12]

CHLAMYDIAL INFECTIONS

Chlamydial infections are the most prevalent bacterial STDs in the United States today. More than 650,000 cases are reported annually, and three of every four cases reported occurred in persons under age 25.[13] As many as 3 million Americans per year may be infected with chlamydia. Underreporting is substantial because most people are asymptomatic and do not seek testing. Chlamydial infections are a major contributor to PID, ectopic pregnancy, infertility among women, and nongonococcal urethritis in men.

Etiology and Pathophysiology

Chlamydial infections are caused by *Chlamydia trachomatis,* a gram-negative bacterium. Chlamydia can be transmitted during vaginal, anal, or oral sex. Numerous different serotypes, or strains, of *C. trachomatis* cause urogenital infections (e.g., nongonococcal urethritis [NGU] in men and cervicitis in women), ocular trachoma, and lymphogranuloma venereum. Women with chlamydial infections during the second week of pregnancy are two to three times more likely to have a preterm birth.[14]

Chlamydia is largely underreported because most people infected are asymptomatic and do not seek health care.[5] By age 30, it is estimated that at sometime during their lives 50% of all sexually active women have had a chlamydial infection. Women with chlamydia may also be at high risk for acquiring HIV from an infected partner.

Because chlamydial infections are closely associated with gonococcal infections, clinical differentiation may be difficult (Table 51-6). Therefore both infections are usually treated concurrently even without diagnostic evidence. The incubation period of 1 to 3 weeks for chlamydial infection is longer than that for gonorrhea, and the symptoms are often milder. The high incidence of recurrence may be because of failure to treat the sexual partners of infected persons. Table 51-7 lists the risk factors for chlamydial infection. Because of the high prevalence of asymptomatic infections, screening of high risk populations is needed to identify those infected.

Clinical Manifestations and Complications

Chlamydia is known as a silent disease because symptoms may be absent or minor in most infected women and in many men. As with gonorrhea, chlamydial infections result in a superficial mucosal infection that can become more invasive. Signs and symptoms in men include urethritis (dysuria, urethral dis-

charge), epididymitis (unilateral scrotal pain, swelling, tenderness, fever), and proctitis (rectal discharge and pain during defecation) (Fig. 51-6). Signs and symptoms in women include cervicitis (mucopurulent discharge and hypertrophic ectopy [area that is edematous and bleeds easily]), urethritis (dysuria, frequent urination, and pyuria), bartholinitis (purulent exudate), PID (abdominal pain, nausea, vomiting, fever, malaise, abnormal vaginal bleeding, and menstrual abnormalities), and perihepatitis (fever, nausea, vomiting, and right upper quadrant pain). A large number of women with chlamydial cervicitis have been found to have a male partner with NGU.

Complications often develop from poorly managed, inaccurately diagnosed, or undiagnosed chlamydial infections. The infection is often not diagnosed until complications appear. Complications in men may result in epididymitis, with possible

TABLE 51-6 Comparison of Gonorrhea and Chlamydia

SITE OF INFECTION	N. GONORRHOEAE	C. TRACHOMATIS
Men		
Urethra	Urethritis	Nongonococcal urethritis; post-gonococcal urethritis
Epididymis	Epididymitis	Epididymitis
Rectum	Proctitis	Proctitis
Conjunctiva	Conjunctivitis	Conjunctivitis
Systemic	Disseminated gonococcal infection	Reiter syndrome
Women		
Urethra	Acute urethral syndrome	Acute urethral syndrome
Bartholin's gland	Bartholinitis	Bartholinitis
Cervix	Cervicitis	Cervicitis; atypical cervical cells
Fallopian tube	Salpingitis	Salpingitis
Conjunctiva	Conjunctivitis	Conjunctivitis
Liver capsule	Perihepatitis	Perihepatitis
Systemic	Disseminated gonococcal infection	Arthritis-dermatitis syndrome

Data from Holmes KK, et al, editors: *Sexually transmitted diseases,* ed 2, New York, 1990 McGraw-Hill. In McCance KL, Huether SE: *Pathophysiology: the biologic basis for disease in adults and children,* ed 4, St Louis, 2002, Mosby.

TABLE 51-7 Risk Factors for Chlamydial Infection

- Women and adolescents
- New or multiple sex partners
- Sex partners who have had multiple partners
- History of STDs and cervical ectopy
- Patients with other STDs
- Lack of barrier contraception

Data from United States Preventive Services Task Force: Screening for chlamydial infection: recommendations and rationale, *Am J Prev Med* 20(3 suppl):90, 2001. *STDs,* Sexually transmitted diseases.

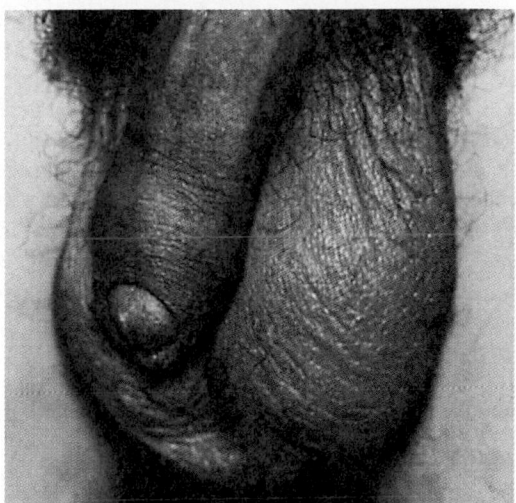

FIG. 51-6 Chlamydial epididymitis. Red, swollen scrotum.

infertility and Reiter's disease (a systemic condition characterized by urethritis, conjunctivitis, arthritis, and mucocutaneous lesions). Complications from chlamydial infections in women may result in PID, which can lead to chronic pelvic pain and infertility. For this reason the CDC recommends that all females younger than 20 years of age be routinely screened for chlamydia at their annual gynecologic examination. They further advise annual screening of all sexually active women older than 20 years of age with one or more risk factors for the disease.[15]

Diagnostic Studies and Collaborative Care

Chlamydial infections in men can be diagnosed by excluding gonorrhea. The cervical or urethral discharge appears to be less purulent, watery, and painful in chlamydial infections than in gonorrhea. If no gram-negative diplococci are found on the Gram-stained smear of male urethral discharge or the sediment of a first-catch urine specimen, a culture for both *C. trachomatis* and *N. gonorrhoeae* may be appropriate. If both cultures are negative and signs of inflammation are present (e.g., polymorphonuclear leukocytes [PMNs] on the Gram-stained smear), a diagnosis of NGU chlamydia infection can be made.

The availability of nonculture tests has allowed for the screening and confirmation of diagnoses in both men and women. Direct fluorescent antibody (DFA) tests, enzyme immunoassay (EIA), and DNA amplification do not require special handling of specimens and are easier to perform than cell cultures. DNA amplification tests are the most sensitive diagnostic methods available. In addition, they can be used with urine samples rather than urethral and cervical swabs.

Drug Therapy. When diagnosed, chlamydia can be easily treated and cured. Chlamydial infections respond to treatment with doxycycline (Vibramycin) or azithromycin (Zithromax).[16] For doxycycline, the dosage is 100 mg two times a day for 7 days. Azithromycin (1 g in a single dose) offers the advantage of ease of administration. Alternative regimens include erythromycin, ofloxacin (Floxin), or levofloxacin (Levaquin). Follow-up care should include advising the patient to return if the symptoms persist or recur, treatment of sex partners, and encouraging the use of condoms during all sexual contacts.

ETHICAL DILEMMAS
Confidentiality

Situation

A nurse in a clinic gives the positive results of a test for chlamydia to a patient and advises her to tell her sexual partners that she has this disease. The patient refuses to tell her boyfriend because he will know that she has had sex with another partner. Should the nurse contact the boyfriend?

Important Points for Consideration

- Nurses and other health care professionals have both a legal and an ethical obligation to maintain confidentiality of patient information. If confidentiality is violated, trust is eroded and patients may not share privileged information that is essential to plan effective care.
- Health care providers have an obligation to maintain confidentiality unless there is a risk to the health or life of innocent third parties. Each state has requirements for reporting communicable diseases and other health-related data.
- The nurse's primary obligation is to the patient seeking care. However, there are long-term health consequences for this patient, as well as the public in general.
- Patient teaching is one way to establish a partnership with this woman. Information should be shared about the effects of the disease being untreated, the consequences of reinfection, and the results that the disease may have on others who may not know they are infected. The patient can then be encouraged to inform her partners of the diagnosis for the good of everyone.

Critical Thinking Questions

1. What are your state's requirements for reportable conditions?
2. Should the nurse contact the boyfriend?
3. In your opinion, what is the best way to balance the needs of an individual patient with those of the general public?

Lymphogranuloma Venereum

Lymphogranuloma venereum (LGV) is an STD caused by specific strains of *C. trachomatis*. LGV is rare in the United States, but it is endemic in other areas of the world, including Africa, India, Southeast Asia, South America, and the Caribbean.

The strain of *C. trachomatis* that causes LGV is transmitted through intercourse or through contact with exudate from active lesions. LGV begins as a genital lesion and spreads via the lymph nodes of the genital-rectal areas. It may also spread systemically through the bloodstream and enter the CNS. Penile, vulvar, and anal infection can lead to inguinal and femoral lymphadenopathy. Marked inflammation occurs, resulting in necrosis, *buboes* (greatly enlarged, inflamed lymph nodes), abscesses of inguinal lymph nodes, and infection of surrounding tissue. Healing occurs by fibrosis after several weeks or months and can result in chronic scarring, which damages the lymph nodes and disrupts nodal function.

Constitutional symptoms that occur during the stage of regional lymphadenopathy include fever, chills, headache, *meningismus* (meningitis-like symptoms), anorexia, myalgia, and arthralgia. Complications of untreated anorectal infection include strictures, fissures, constipation, perirectal abscesses, and rectovaginal and perianal fistulas. LGV is generally treated with doxycycline (Vibramycin), 100 mg orally twice a day, for 21 days. Also effective is erythromycin 500 mg orally four times a day for

21 days. Buboes may require aspiration to prevent inguinal and femoral ulcerations from occurring. Sex partners should also be treated.

Viral Infections

GENITAL HERPES

Because **genital herpes** is not a reportable disease in most states, its true incidence is difficult to determine. It is estimated that more than 45 million people in the United States are infected with genital herpes.[3] Since the late 1970s the prevalence of herpes simplex virus type 2 (HSV-2) has risen by 30%.

Etiology and Pathophysiology

The herpes simplex virus (HSV) enters through the mucous membranes or breaks in the skin during contact with an infected person (Fig. 51-7). HSV then reproduces inside the cell and spreads to the surrounding cells. The virus next enters the peripheral or autonomic nerve endings and ascends to the sensory or autonomic nerve ganglion, where it often becomes dormant. Viral reactivation (recurrence) may occur when the virus descends down to the initial site of infection, either the mucous membranes or skin. When a person is infected with HSV, the virus usually persists within the individual for life. Shedding of the virus even in the absence of an identifiable lesion is a well-established phenomenon.

Two different strains of HSV cause infection. In general, HSV type 1 (HSV-1) causes infection above the waist, involving the gingivae, the dermis, the upper respiratory tract, and the CNS. HSV type 2 (HSV-2) most frequently infects the genital tract and the perineum (i.e., locations below the waist). However, either strain can cause disease on the mouth or the genitals. Because HSV is readily inactivated at room temperature and by drying, airborne and fomitic (nonliving objects) spread have not been documented as significant means of transmission. Most people infected with HSV-1 or HSV-2 are asymptomatic or unaware of their infection.[17]

Clinical Manifestations

In the *primary (initial) episode* of genital herpes the patient may complain of burning or tingling at the site of inoculation. Vesicular lesions, which may occur on the penis, scrotum, vulva, perineum, perianal region, vagina, or cervix, contain large quantities of infectious viral particles (Fig. 51-8). The lesions rupture and form shallow, moist ulcerations. Finally, crusting and epithelialization of the erosions occur. Primary infections tend to be associated with local inflammation and pain, accompanied by sys-

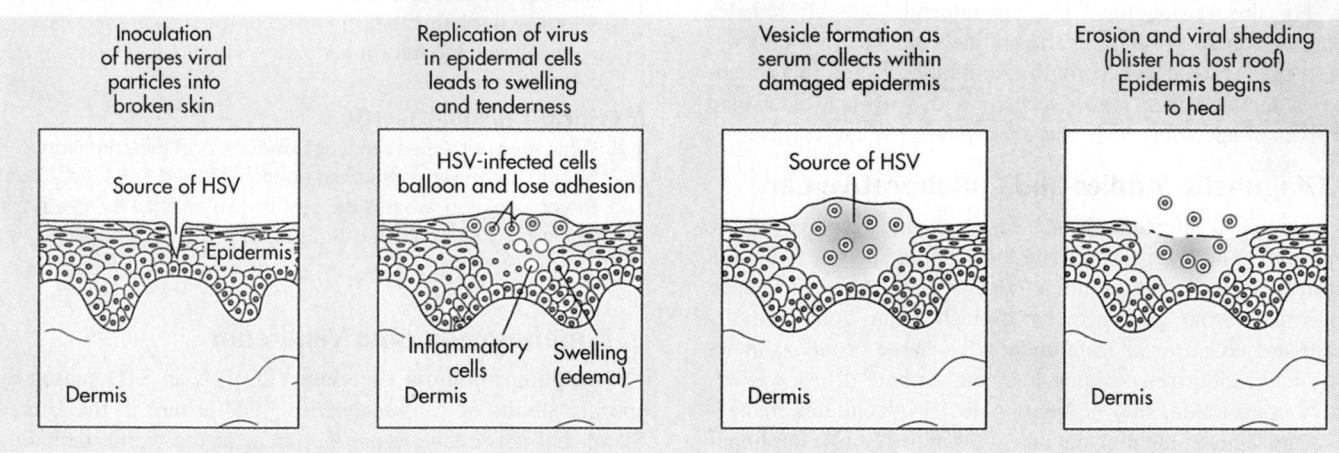

FIG. 51-7 Infection with herpes simplex virus (HSV).

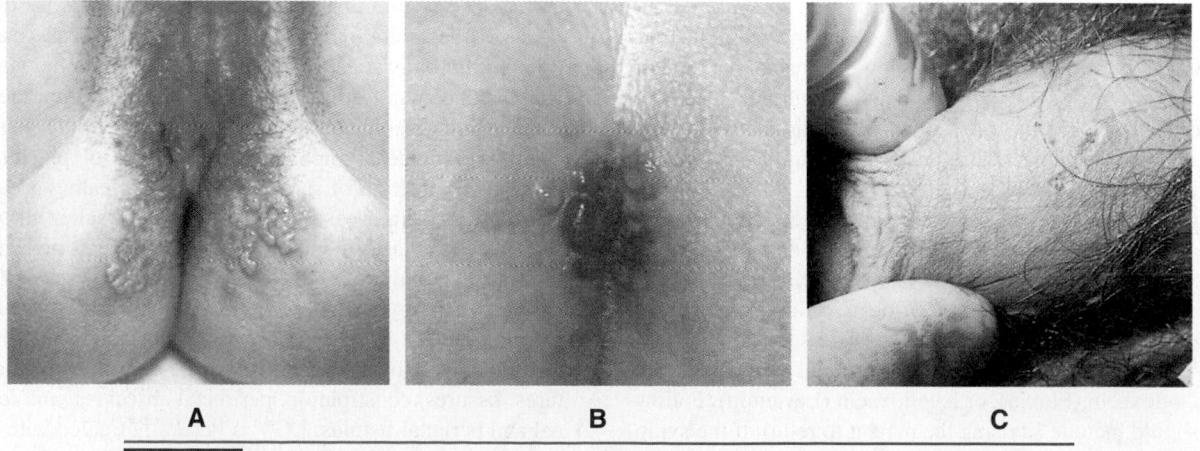

FIG. 51-8 Unruptured vesicles of herpes simplex virus (HSV) type 2. **A,** Vulvar area. **B,** Perianal area. **C,** Penile herpes simplex, ulcerative stage.

temic manifestations of fever, headache, malaise, myalgia, and regional lymphadenopathy.

Urination may be painful from the urine touching active lesions. Urinary retention may occur as a result of HSV urethritis or cystitis. A purulent vaginal discharge may develop with HSV cervicitis. The duration of symptoms is longer and the frequency of complications is greater in women. Primary lesions are generally present for 17 to 20 days, but new lesions sometimes continue to develop for 6 weeks. The lesions heal spontaneously unless secondary infection occurs.

Recurrent genital herpes occurs in about 50% to 80% of individuals during the year following the primary episode. Stress, fatigue, sunburn, and menses are commonly noted trigger factors. Many patients can predict a recurrence by noticing the early prodromal symptoms of tingling, burning, and itching at the site where the lesions will eventually appear. The symptoms of recurrent episodes are less severe, and the lesions usually heal within 8 to 12 days. With time the recurrent lesions will generally occur less frequently.

Women with recurrent symptomatic genital herpes can shed the virus up to 1% of the time even when no visible lesions are present. Suppressive therapy with antiviral agents can reduce but not eradicate asymptomatic shedding.[18] Barrier forms of contraception, especially condoms, used during asymptomatic periods may decrease transmission of the virus. When lesions are present, the patient should avoid sexual activity altogether because even barrier protection is not satisfactory in eliminating disease transmission.

Complications

Although most infections are of a relatively benign nature, complications of genital herpes may involve the CNS, causing aseptic meningitis and lower motor neuron damage. Neuron damage may result in atonic bladder, impotence, and constipation. Another complication is *autoinoculation* of the virus to extragenital sites such as the lips, breasts, and, most commonly, the fingers (herpetic whitlow) (Fig. 51-9).

Herpes Simplex Virus Infection in Pregnancy. Studies indicate no difference in the length or severity of symptoms between pregnant and nonpregnant women. Women with a primary

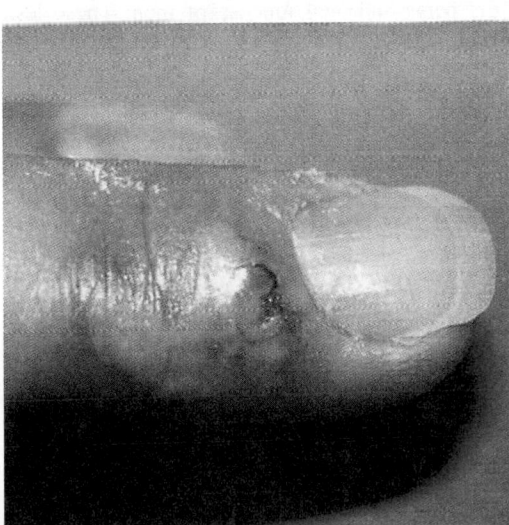

FIG. 51-9 Autoinoculation of herpes simplex virus (HSV), herpetic whitlow.

episode of HSV near the time of delivery have the highest risk of transmitting genital herpes to the neonate. The risk of transmission is lowest for women who acquire HSV early in the pregnancy or have a history of recurrent HSV. Although women with recurrent HSV infections are not at higher risk for transmitting the virus to their infants, an active genital lesion at the time of delivery is usually an indication for cesarean section delivery, because most infections to neonates occur during birth.[19]

Diagnostic Studies

A diagnosis of genital herpes is usually based on the patient's symptoms and history. The diagnosis can be confirmed through isolation of the virus from active lesions by means of tissue culture. Tzanck- or Pap-stained smears from lesions may show the cellular characteristics of viral infection, including multinucleated giant cells and intranuclear inclusions. HSV infection can be confirmed by isolation of the virus in culture. Other techniques to detect HSV include direct immunofluorescence and EIA. In addition, DNA amplification can be performed to detect HSV. These tests permit more rapid identification of HSV than a culture. Highly accurate serologic methods for detecting the HSV type are available.

Collaborative Care

Drug Therapy. Three antiviral agents are available for the treatment of HSV: acyclovir (Zovirax), valacyclovir (Valtrex), and famciclovir (Famvir). These drugs inhibit herpetic viral replication and are prescribed for primary and recurrent infections (Table 51-8). Acyclovir, valacyclovir, and famciclovir are also used to suppress frequent recurrences (more than six episodes per year). Although not a cure, these drugs shorten the duration of viral shedding and the healing time of genital lesions and reduce outbreaks by 75%.[15] Continued use of oral acyclovir as suppressive therapy for up to 5 years is safe and effective. Adverse reactions are mild and include headache, occasional nausea and vomiting, and diarrhea. The safety of these drugs for treatment of pregnant women has not been established. Acyclovir ointment appears to have no clinical benefit in the treatment of recurrent lesions, either in speed of healing or in resolution of pain, and is not commonly recommended. IV acyclovir is reserved for severe or life-threatening infections in which hospitalization is required for the treatment of disseminated infections, CNS infections (meningitis), or pneumonitis. Nephrotoxicity has been observed with high-dose IV use.

Symptomatic Care. Symptomatic treatment such as good genital hygiene and the wearing of loose-fitting cotton undergarments should be encouraged. The lesions should be kept clean and dry. To ensure complete drying of the perineal area, women may use a hair dryer set on a cool setting. Frequent sitz baths may soothe the area and reduce inflammation. Drying agents such as colloidal oatmeal (Aveeno) and aluminum salts (Burow's solution) may provide some relief from the burning and itching. Techniques to reduce pain on urination include pouring a pitcher of water onto the perineal area while voiding to dilute the urine, and voiding in a warm tub of water or shower. Pain may require a local anesthetic such as lidocaine (Xylocaine) or systemic analgesics such as codeine and aspirin. Sexual transmission of HSV has been documented during asymptomatic periods, and the use of barrier methods, especially condoms, should be encouraged.

TABLE 51-8 Collaborative Care — Genital Herpes

Diagnostic
History and physical examination
Viral isolation by tissue culture
Antibody assay for specific HSV viral type

Collaborative Therapy

Primary Infection
acyclovir (Zovirax) 400 mg three times a day or acyclovir 200 mg five times a day or famciclovir (Famvir) 250 mg three times a day or valacyclovir (Valtrex) 1 g twice a day. All drugs are given orally for 7 to 10 days.

Recurrent Episodic Infection
acyclovir 400 mg three times a day or acyclovir 200 mg five times a day or acyclovir 800 mg two times a day or famciclovir 125 mg twice a day or valacyclovir 500 mg twice a day or valacyclovir 1 g once a day. Drugs are given orally for 5 days.
Attempt to identify trigger mechanisms.
Yearly Pap smear.
Abstinence from sexual contact while lesions are present; however, virus may be shed without lesions.
Symptomatic care.
Confidential counseling and testing for HIV.

Suppressive Therapy for Frequent Recurrence
acyclovir 400 mg two times a day or famciclovir 250 mg two times a day or valacyclovir 500 mg twice a day or valacyclovir 1 g once a day.

Severe Infection
acyclovir 5 to 10 mg/kg IV every 8 hours for 2 to 7 days or until clinical improvement, followed by oral antiviral therapy to complete at least 10 days of treatment.

Modified from Centers for Disease Control and Prevention: STD treatment guidelines, *MMWR* 51(RR-6):1, 2002.
HIV, Human immunodeficiency virus; *HSV,* herpes simplex virus.

GENITAL WARTS

Genital warts (*condylomata acuminata*) are caused by the human papillomavirus (HPV). Visible genital warts are usually caused by HPV types 6 and 11. These types can also cause warts on the anus, urethra, and vagina. Other HPV types in the genital region (e.g., types 16, 18, 31, 33, and 35) are associated with vaginal, anal, and cervical dysplasia. HPV is a highly contagious STD seen frequently in young, sexually active adults. An estimated 20 million people are currently infected with HPV.[1] It is found 25% of the time in conjunction with other STDs.[20]

Minor trauma during intercourse can cause abrasions that allow HPV to enter the body. The epithelial cells infected with HPV undergo transformation and proliferation to form a warty growth. The incubation period of the virus is generally 1 to 6 months, but may be longer. Prevention is hampered by a high proportion of asymptomatic infections and lack of curative treatment. In most states, genital warts is not a reportable disease.

Clinical Manifestations and Complications

Genital warts are discrete single or multiple papillary growths that are white to gray and pink-flesh colored. They may grow and coalesce to form large, cauliflower-like masses. Most patients have from 1 to 10 genital warts. In men, the warts may occur on the penis and scrotum, around the anus, or in the urethra. In women, the warts may be located on the vulva, vagina, or cervix and in the perianal area (Fig. 51-10). There are usually no other signs or symptoms. Itching may occur with anogenital warts. Bleeding on defecation may occur with anal warts.

During pregnancy, genital warts tend to grow rapidly. An infected mother may transmit the condition to her newborn. Cesarean delivery is not routinely indicated unless the birth canal becomes blocked by massive warts.

Subclinical Human Papillomavirus Infections. HPV infection has been linked with cervical and vulvar cancer in women and with anorectal and squamous cell carcinoma of the penis in men. To date more than 100 types of HPV have been identified, at least 33 of which invade the genital tract.[21] Some of these types appear to be harmless and self-limiting (e.g., types 6 and 11 commonly found in genital warts), whereas others are thought to have oncogenic (cancer-causing) potential (e.g., types 16 and 18). Up to two thirds of the early lesions caused by HPV are undetectable by visual examination. Flat subclinical lesions are commonly found on the cervix and anal mucosa of women and on the penis and anal mucosa of men. These lesions are strongly associated with the development of dysplasia and neoplasia at these sites.

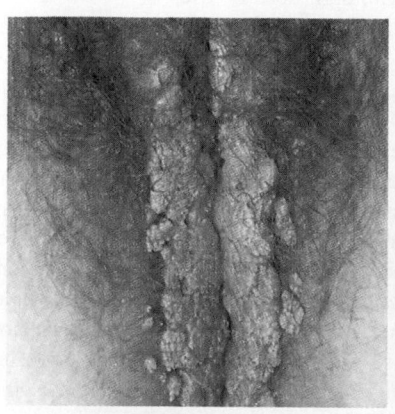 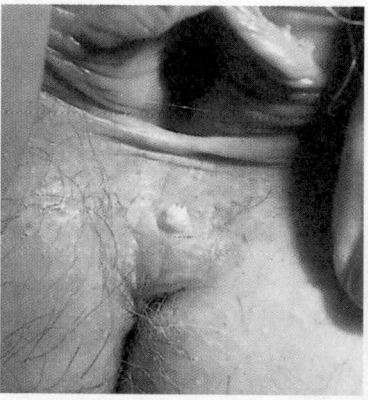 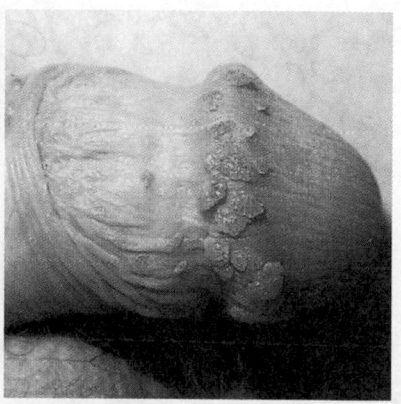

A   B   C

FIG. 51-10 Genital warts. **A,** Severe vulvular warts. **B,** Perineal wart. **C,** Multiple genital warts of the glans penis.

Diagnostic Studies and Collaborative Care

A diagnosis of genital warts can be made on the basis of the gross appearance of the lesions. However, the warts may be confused with condylomata lata of secondary syphilis, carcinoma, or benign neoplasms. Serologic and cytologic testing should be done to rule out these conditions. If dysplasia is confirmed by the Papanicolaou (Pap) smear, a colposcopic examination and biopsies should be performed. Virapap, a test that uses DNA amplification techniques, can be used to determine some molecular types of HPV present in a lesion. Currently, HPV cannot be confirmed by culture.

The primary goal when treating visible genital warts is the removal of symptomatic warts. The removal may or may not decrease infectivity. Genital warts are difficult to treat and often require multiple office visits with a variety of treatment modalities. None of the treatments are superior to other treatments. Many patients will have a course of therapy rather than one treatment. The therapy should be modified if a patient has not improved after three treatments or if after six treatments the warts have not completely disappeared. One common treatment is the use of 80% to 90% trichloroacetic acid (TCA) or bichloroacetic acid (BCA) applied directly to the wart surface. Petroleum jelly is applied to the surrounding normal skin to minimize irritation before a small amount of TCA is applied to the wart with a cotton swab. A sharp stinging pain is often felt with initial acid contact, but this quickly subsides. TCA is not washed off after treatment. It can be used in pregnant women.

Podophyllin resin (10% to 25%), a cytotoxic agent, is recommended therapy for small external genital warts. When podophyllin is used, it is applied carefully to each wart, with normal tissue being avoided, and is then thoroughly washed off in 1 to 4 hours. This substance encourages the sloughing off of skin containing viral particles. Podophyllin has local (e.g., pain, burning) and systemic (e.g., nausea, dizziness, leukopenia, respiratory distress) toxic symptoms. It is contraindicated in pregnant women. In general, warts located on moist surfaces respond better to topical treatment (e.g., TCA, podophyllin) than do warts on drier surfaces.

Patient-managed treatment is also an option. Podofilox liquid and gel are available by prescription (Condylox and Condylox Gel). The patient applies the solution or gel for 3 successive days followed by 4 days of no treatment. Treatment can be repeated for up to 4 weeks or until resolution of the lesions. Imiquimod cream (Aldara) is an immune response modifier that is applied once daily at bedtime, three times a week for up to 16 weeks. None of these treatments is recommended for use during pregnancy or lactation.

If the warts do not regress with any of these therapies, treatments such as cryotherapy with liquid nitrogen, electrocautery, laser therapy, intralesional use of interferon, and surgical excision may be indicated.[22] Because treatment does not destroy the virus, merely the infected tissue, recurrences and reinfection are possible, and careful long-term follow-up is advised.

NURSING MANAGEMENT
SEXUALLY TRANSMITTED DISEASES

■ Nursing Assessment

Subjective and objective data that should be obtained from a person with an STD are presented in Table 51-9.

■ Nursing Diagnoses

Nursing diagnoses for the patient with an STD include, but are not limited to, the following:

- Risk for infection *related to* lack of knowledge about mode of transmission, inadequate personal and genital hygiene, and failure to practice precautionary measures
- Anxiety *related to* impact of condition on relationships, disease outcome, and lack of knowledge of disease
- Ineffective health maintenance *related to* lack of knowledge about disease process, appropriate follow-up measures, and possibility of reinfection

TABLE 51-9	Nursing Assessment Sexually Transmitted Disease

Subjective Data
Important Health Information
Past health history: Contact with individuals with STDs, multiple sexual partners, pregnancy
Medications: Use of oral contraceptives; allergy to any antibiotics, especially penicillin
Functional Health Patterns
Health perception–health management: Shared needles during IV drug use; malaise
Nutritional-metabolic: Nausea, vomiting, anorexia; pharyngitis, oral lesions, itching at infected site; chills; alopecia
Elimination: Dysuria, urinary frequency, retention; urethral discharge; tenesmus, proctitis
Cognitive-perceptual: Arthralgia; headache; painful, burning lesions
Sexuality-reproductive: Dyspareunia; vaginal discharge, menstrual abnormalities; presence of genital or perianal lesions

Objective Data
General
Fever, lymphadenopathy (generalized or inguinal)
Integumentary
Syphilis: Primary: painless, indurated genital, oral, or perianal lesions; secondary: bilateral, symmetric rash on palms, soles, or entire body, mucous patches on mouth or tongue, alopecia
Genital herpes: Painful genital or anal vesicular lesions
Genital warts: Single or multiple gray or white genital or anal warts (possibly becoming massive)
Gastrointestinal
Purulent rectal discharge (indicator of gonorrhea), rectal lesions, proctitis
Urinary
Urethral discharge, erythema
Reproductive
Cervical discharge, lesions, inflamed Bartholin's glands
Possible Findings
Gonorrhea: Positive Gram stain, smears, cultures, and DNA amplification for *N. gonorrhoeae*
Syphilis: Positive findings on VDRL and RPR, spirochetes on dark-field microscopy
Chlamydia: Positive culture or DNA amplification for *Chlamydia* organism
Genital herpes: Positive tissue culture for HSV-2 or anti–HSV-2 antibody assay

HSV-2, Herpes simplex virus type 2; *IV,* intravenous, *RPR,* rapid plasma reagin; *STD,* sexually transmitted disease; *VDRL,* Venereal Disease Research Laboratory.

■ Planning

The overall goals are that the patient with an STD will (1) demonstrate understanding of the mode of transmission of STDs and the risk posed by STDs, (2) complete treatment and return for appropriate follow-up, (3) notify or assist in notification of sexual contacts about their need for testing and treatment, (4) abstain from intercourse until infection is resolved, and (5) demonstrate knowledge of safer sex practices.

■ Nursing Implementation

Health Promotion. Many approaches to curtailing the spread of STDs have been advocated and have met with varying degrees of success. Nurses should be prepared to discuss practices with all patients, not only those who are perceived to be at risk. These "safe" sex practices include abstinence, monogamy with an uninfected partner, avoidance of certain high risk sexual practices, and use of condoms and other barriers to limit contact with potentially infectious body fluids or lesions. Sexual abstinence is a certain method of avoiding all STDs, but few adults consider this a feasible alternative to sexual expression. Limiting sexual intimacies outside of a well-established monogamous relationship can reduce the risk of contracting an STD. A patient and family teaching guide related to the patient with an STD is presented in Table 51-10.

All sexually active women should be screened for cervical cancer. Women with a history of STDs are at greater risk for cervical cancer than women without this history. Pap smears are discussed in Chapter 52.

Measures to prevent infection. An inspection of the sexual partner's genitals before coitus is recommended. The presence of discharge, sores, blisters, or rash should be viewed with concern. A patient who is aware of specific signs and symptoms of infection can intelligently make the decision to continue the sexual interaction with modifications or elect not to have sexual relations. The patient should remember that, when engaging in sex, there is exposure to the infections of everyone with whom the partner has ever had sex. Men should be told that some protection is provided if they void immediately following intercourse and wash their genitalia and the adjacent areas with soap and water. Women may also benefit from postcoital voiding and washing. However, it should not be assumed that this provides adequate protection against STDs after exposure to infection. Although spermicidal jellies and creams have a mild detergent effect that may reduce the risk of contracting STDs, this has not been proven. These same barriers can serve as supplementary lubrication, thereby decreasing irritation and friction and chances for development of a minor laceration that could serve as an entry point for the organism.

Proper use of a latex condom provides a highly effective mechanical barrier to infection. The condom should be undamaged and correctly in place throughout all phases of sexual activity. It is unknown if a condom lubricated with a spermicide such as nonoxynol-9 further reduces the risk of STDs. Vaginal spermicides, when used alone without a condom, reduce the risk for chlamydia and gonorrhea.[15] A deterrent to condom usage is alcohol and drug use. Studies continue to document that IV drug users do not consistently use condoms.[23] Use of barrier contraceptives requires planning and motivation, both of which are impaired with alcohol or drug ingestion. The patient should be

---

TABLE 51-10 ◢atient & Family Teaching Guide
Sexually Transmitted Disease

1. Instruct patient in hygienic measures, such as washing and urinating after intercourse to destroy many causative organisms.
2. Explain the importance of taking all antibiotics as prescribed. Symptoms will improve after 1-2 days of therapy, but organisms may still be present.
3. Teach patient about the need for treatment of sexual partners with antibiotics to prevent transmission of disease.
4. Instruct patient to abstain from sexual intercourse during treatment and to use condoms when sexual activity is resumed to prevent spread of infection and prevent reinfection.
5. Explain the importance of follow-up examination and reculture at least once after treatment if appropriate to confirm complete cure and prevent relapse.
6. Allow patient and partner to verbalize concerns to clarify areas that need explanation.
7. Instruct patient about symptoms of complications and need to report problems to ensure proper follow-up and early treatment of reinfection.
8. Explain precautions to take, such as being monogamous; asking potential partners about sexual history; avoiding sex with partners who use IV drugs or who have visible oral, inguinal, genital, perineal, or anal lesions; using condoms; voiding and washing genitalia after coitus to reduce the occurrence of reinfection.
9. Inform patient regarding state of infectivity to prevent a false sense of security, which might result in careless sexual practices and poor personal hygiene.

---

given specific verbal and written instructions on the proper use of condoms (see Chapter 14, Figs. 14-6 and 14-7). The objections to condom usage, such as interference with spontaneity and the presence of a barrier, should be discussed by the partners. Information about the mechanics of sexual arousal and incorporating a condom into lovemaking can help in overcoming patient or partner resistance to its use. Female condoms are lubricated polyurethane sheaths with a ring at each end designed for vaginal wear (see Chapter 14, Fig. 14-7). Laboratory studies indicate that it is an effective barrier to microorganisms, including viruses, but clinical trials are currently lacking for STDs.

Sexual contact with persons known or suspected to have HIV infection should be avoided (see Chapter 14). Among couples with one infected partner, consistent and scrupulous condom use can reduce transmission to the uninfected partner. A sexually active homosexual man can reduce risk by minimizing the number of sexual contacts. Unprotected anal intercourse and other high risk behaviors should be eliminated, and condoms should be used if sexual contact continues.

The nurse can initiate an interview to establish the patient's risk for contracting an STD. Questions to ask include number of partners, type of birth control used, use of condoms, use of IV drugs, and sexual preference. Patient education can be planned based on the response to these questions. Interpersonal skills necessary for this interview include respect, compassion, and a nonjudgmental attitude. Counseling should be tailored to the individual patient.

Screening programs. Screening programs that are used to detect infected patients can also help prevent certain STDs. For many years, there have been various screening programs to find cases of syphilis. With the decline of infection rates across the United States, many states have eliminated laws requiring premarital testing for syphilis. Many institutions offer voluntary prenatal HIV and syphilis testing and counseling for pregnant women.

Screening programs have been developed and implemented for detection of gonorrhea and chlamydia. These programs are targeted to women because women are more likely to have asymptomatic gonorrhea and thereby serve as sources of infection. Routine gonorrheal and chlamydial testing during pelvic examinations and prenatal visits are being performed as a major part of these programs. Their effectiveness is well documented.[24] Mass application of screening programs for genital chlamydial infections, genital herpes, and HPV infections (warts) may also be possible with the advent of rapid, cost-effective tests.

Case finding. Interviewing and case finding are other processes used to control STDs. These activities are directed toward locating and examining all contacts of each known patient with an STD as soon after sexual exposure as possible, so that effective treatment can be initiated. Trained interviewers may often find cases even if they are supplied with only limited information. The caseworkers, who are often nurses, are aware of the social implications of these diseases and the need for discretion. Sexual contacts are often not informed about the origin of the information naming them as a contact so that greater cooperation and privacy is ensured.

Educational and research programs. Nurses can actively encourage their communities to provide better education about STDs for their citizens. Teenagers, who are known to have a high incidence of infection, should be a prime target for such educational programs. Hot-line services, school nurses, nurse practitioners, nurse midwives, and outreach programs sponsored by the CDC in the United States and Canada's Health Protection Branch are effective. The National Gay Task Force and the Herpes Resource Center were established to provide education and support. Knowledge and understanding can decrease the STD epidemic. Currently, efforts are being made to develop vaccines for syphilis, gonorrhea, genital herpes, HPV, and HIV. The development of effective vaccines is viewed by many clinicians as a prerequisite for eradication of STDs.

Acute Intervention

Psychologic support. The diagnosis of an STD may be met with a variety of emotions, such as shame, guilt, anger, and a desire for vengeance. The nurse should provide counseling and try to help the patient verbalize feelings. Couples in marital or committed relationships are confronted with an added problem when an STD is diagnosed. The implication of sexual activity by one of the partners with a person outside the relationship must be faced. Other concerns relative to their relationship are present, and the acute problem may serve as an incentive for further problem solving. Support and counseling for the couple are needed. A referral for professional counseling to explore the ramifications of an STD in their relationship may be indicated.

EVIDENCE-BASED PRACTICE
Sexually Transmitted Diseases and Cervical Cancer

Clinical Problem
What is the effectiveness of health education interventions to promote sexual risk reduction behaviors among women in order to reduce the transmission of human papillomavirus (HPV)?

Best Clinical Practice
- Evidence summarized from 30 studies showed a positive effect of educational interventions on sexual risk reduction behavior, typically with increased use of condoms for vaginal intercourse.
- The positive effects of the interventions lasted up to 3 months after the intervention.

Implications for Nursing Practice
- Educational interventions can promote sexual risk reduction behavior.
- These interventions have the potential to reduce the transmission of HPV and possibly reduce the incidence of cervical carcinoma.

Reference for Evidence
Sheperd J et al: Interventions for encouraging sexual lifestyles and behaviors intended to prevent cervical cancer, *Cochrane Database of Systematic Reviews* (2), CD001035, 2000.

A patient who has genital herpes is faced with the fact that repeated infections can occur and that no cure is available. This can be frustrating and disruptive to the patient's physical, emotional, social, and sexual lives. Helping the patient identify and avoid any factors that may precipitate the condition is indicated. Informing the patient that the incidence and severity of recurrences will decrease over time may provide some support.

HPV infections involve a prolonged course of treatment. The patient can become frustrated and distressed because of frequent office visits, associated costs, potential for unpleasant side effects as a result of treatment, and effects of the infection on future health and sexual relationships. Tremendous support and a willingness to listen to the patient's concerns are needed.

Compliance and follow-up. A nurse working in public health facilities, clinics, or other outpatient settings may care for a patient with an STD more often than a nurse in a hospital. This nurse is in a position to explain and interpret treatment measures such as the purpose and possible side effects of prescribed drugs and the need for follow-up care.

Frequently, single-dose treatment for gonorrhea, chlamydial infection, and syphilis helps prevent the problems associated with noncompliance with drug therapy. The patient requiring multiple-dose therapy should be given special instructions in completing the prescribed regimen and should be informed about problems resulting from noncompliance. All patients should return to the treatment center for a repeat culture from the infected sites or for serologic testing at designated times to determine the effectiveness of the treatment. Informing the patient that cures are not always obtained on the first treatment can reinforce the need for a follow-up visit. The patient should also be advised to inform sexual partners of the need for testing and treatment, regardless of whether they are free of symptoms or experiencing symptoms.

Hygiene measures. The patient with an STD should have certain hygiene measures emphasized. An important measure is frequent hand washing and bathing. Bathing and cleaning of the involved areas can provide local comfort and prevent secondary infection. Douching may spread the infection or undermine local immune responses and is therefore contraindicated. The synthetic materials used in most undergarments frequently increase or exacerbate local irritations by trapping moisture. Cotton undergarments provide better absorption and are cooler and more comfortable for the patient with an STD.

Sexual activity. Sexual abstinence is indicated during the communicable phase of the disease. If sexual activity occurs before treatment of the patient has been completed, the use of condoms may prevent the spread of infection and reinfection. Condom usage after treatment should be encouraged to prevent future exposure to infection. The patient can also choose to relate to a partner in an intimate way that avoids both coitus and oral-genital contact. It is important to note that even single-dose treatments can take up to 1 week to be effective and thus the patient is infective during this period.

Ambulatory and Home Care. Because many STDs are cured with a single dose or short course of antibiotic therapy, many persons are casual about the outcome of these diseases. The consequences of this attitude can include delays in treatment, noncompliance with instructions, and subsequent development of complications. The complications are serious and costly; they can result in disfigurement and destruction of important tissues and organs.

Surgery and prolonged therapy are indicated for many patients with disease-related complications. Major surgical procedures such as resection of an aneurysm or aortic valve replacement may be necessary to treat cardiovascular problems caused by syphilis. Pelvic surgery and procedures to correct fertility problems secondary to an STD may include lysis of adhesions, dilation of strictures, reconstructive tuboplasty, and in vitro fertilization.

■ Evaluation

Expected outcomes for the patient with an STD are that the patient will
- describe modes of transmission
- use appropriate hygienic measures
- experience no reinfection
- demonstrate compliance with follow-up protocol

CRITICAL THINKING EXERCISES

Case Study
Chlamydia
Patient Profile. Jade K. is a 17-year-old female who visits the outpatient Teen Clinic seeking birth control pills.

Subjective Data
- Had first-time intercourse with boyfriend 2 weeks ago
- Did not use condom or spermicide
- Has not asked boyfriend about his sexual practices
- Denies any symptoms

Objective Data
- Has cervical ectopy noted during Pap test
- Tests positive for *Chlamydia*
- Crying and very upset when informed of positive test result

Collaborative Care
- Doxycycline 100 mg bid for 7 days

CRITICAL THINKING QUESTIONS
1. What were Jade's risk factors for acquiring chlamydial infection?
2. What complications could have occurred if Jade's infection had not been detected?
3. What impact is her diagnosis likely to have on Jade's self-image? On her relationship with her boyfriend?
4. What instructions should Jade receive to ensure successful treatment? To prevent reinfection? To prevent further transmission of the infection?
5. What does she need to know about other STDs? What other testing would you recommend?
6. Based on the assessment data presented, write one or more nursing diagnoses. Are there any collaborative problems?

Nursing Research Issues
1. What are the best strategies for encouraging safer sex practices and condom use among high risk populations?
2. What is the level of teens' knowledge of risk, transmission, and impact of STDs? How can teaching about STDs best be adapted to their developmental level?
3. Does education about safer sex practices increase preventive behaviors?

REVIEW QUESTIONS

The number of the question corresponds to the same-numbered objective at the beginning of the chapter.

1. The individual with the lowest risk for sexually transmitted pelvic inflammatory disease is a woman who
   a. uses oral contraceptives.
   b. uses barrier methods of contraception.
   c. uses an intrauterine device for contraception.
   d. uses a Norplant implant or injectible Depo-Provera for contraception.

2. While obtaining subjective assessment data from a woman reported as a sexual contact of a man with chlamydia, the nurse understands that symptoms of chlamydial infections in women
   a. are frequently absent.
   b. mimic those of genital herpes.
   c. include a macular palmar rash in later stages.
   d. may involve chancres hidden inside the vagina.

REVIEW QUESTIONS—cont'd

3. A primary HSV infection differs from recurrent episodes in that
   a. it is of shorter duration than recurrent episodes.
   b. only primary infections are sexually transmissible.
   c. systemic manifestations such as fever and myalgia are more common.
   d. transmission of the virus to a fetus is less likely during primary infection.

4. The nurse explains to a patient with gonorrhea that treatment will include both ceftriaxone and doxycycline because
   a. most patients do not respond to ceftriaxone alone.
   b. coverage with more than one antibiotic prevents reinfection.
   c. no single agent successfully eradicates all strains of gonorrhea.
   d. the high rate of coexisting chlamydia and gonorrhea indicates dual coverage.

5. A patient with an STD who is most likely to have a nursing diagnosis of disturbed body image that hinders future sexual relationships is the patient with
   a. syphilis.
   b. gonorrhea.

c. genital warts.
d. chlamydial infection.

6. Teaching by the nurse to prevent infection and transmission of STDs includes explanations of
   a. the appropriate use of birth control pills.
   b. sexual positions used to avoid infection.
   c. sexual practices that are considered high risk.
   d. the necessity of annual Pap smears for patients with HPV.

7. An appropriate nursing intervention to provide emotional support to a patient with an STD is to
   a. use concerned listening when the patient expresses negative feelings.
   b. reassure the patient that the disease is curable with appropriate treatment.
   c. offer many alternatives that the patient can use to change sexual relationships.
   d. help the patient who is an innocent sexual partner forgive the infecting partner.

REFERENCES

1. Centers for Disease Control and Prevention, Division of STD Prevention: *Tracking the hidden epidemics, 2000,* Atlanta, 2000, Centers for Disease Control and Prevention.
2. Centers for Disease Control and Prevention, Divisions of HIV/AIDS Prevention: *Prevention and treatment of sexually transmitted diseases as an HIV prevention strategy. Fact sheet,* Atlanta, 1998, Centers for Disease Control and Prevention.
3. Sarma SP, Garafalo K, Graves WL: Use of intrauterine device by inner city women, *Arch Fam Med* 7:130, 1998.
4. Cushman L et al: Condom use among women choosing long-term hormonal contraception, *Fam Plann Perspect* 30:240, 1998.
5. Centers for Disease Control and Prevention, Division of STD Prevention: *Sexually transmitted disease surveillance, 1999,* Atlanta, 2000, Centers for Disease Control and Prevention.
6. Bignell C et al: National guidelines for the management of gonorrhea in adults, *Sex Transm Dis* (suppl 1):S13, 1999.
7. Centers for Disease Control and Prevention: Primary and secondary syphilis—United States, 1999, *MMWR* 50:7, 2001.
8. Centers for Disease Control and Prevention, Division of STD Prevention: *National plan to eliminate syphilis from the United States,* Atlanta, 1999, National Center for HIV, STD and TB Prevention.
9. Jacobs R: Infectious diseases—spirochetal. In Tierney L et al, editors: *Current medical diagnosis and treatment,* ed 40, New York, 2001, Lange/McGraw-Hill.
10. Centers for Disease Control and Prevention, Division of Sexually Transmitted Diseases: *Syphilis elimination—history in the making,* media release, Atlanta, Nov 28, 2001.
11. Lukehart SA, Holmes KK: Syphilis. In Fauci AS et al, editors: *Harrison's principles of internal medicine,* ed 15, New York, 2000, McGraw-Hill.
12. Centers for Disease Control and Prevention, Division of Sexually Transmitted Diseases: *Syphilis elimination—history in the making. Fact sheets,* Atlanta, May 2001, Centers for Disease Control and Prevention.
13. Centers for Disease Control and Prevention: *Chlamydia trachomatis* genital infections—United States, 1999, *MMWR* 48:1, 2001.
14. Andrews W et al: The preterm prediction study: association of second trimester genitourinary chlamydia infection with subsequent spontaneous birth, *Am J Obstet Gynecol* 183:662, 2000.
15. Centers for Disease Control and Prevention: *1998 guidelines for treatment of sexually transmitted diseases,* Atlanta, 1998, Centers for Disease Control and Prevention.
16. Centers for Disease Control and Prevention: STD treatment guidelines, *MMWR* 51(RR-6):1, 2002.
17. Sacks S: Improving the management of genital herpes, *Hosp Pract* 34:41, 1999.
18. Herpes Simplex Advisory Panel: National guidelines for the management of genital herpes, *Sex Transm Infect* (suppl 1):S24, 1999.
19. Thomas D: Sexually transmitted viral infections: epidemiology and treatment, *JOGNN* 30:316, 2001.
20. Wright T: Genital warts: their etiology and treatment, *Nurs Times* 94:52, 1998.
21. Centers for Disease Control and Prevention, Division of STD Prevention: *Prevention of genital HPV infection and sequelae,* Atlanta, 1999, Centers for Disease Control and Prevention.
22. McKay S: Why we need to worry about warts, *RN* 63:68, 2000.
23. Metsch L et al: Alternative strategies for sexual risk reduction used by active drug users, *AIDS and Behavior* 5:75, 2001.
24. Centers for Disease Control and Prevention: *Recommendations for the prevention and management of* Chlamydia trachomatis *infections, 1998,* Atlanta, 1998, Centers for Disease Control and Prevention.

RESOURCES

Herpes Resource Center
American Social Health Association
P.O. Box 13827
Research Triangle Park, NC 27709
919-361-8400
Fax: 919-361-8425
www.ashastd.org
www.iwannaknow.org (for teens)
National STD/AIDS Hotline
800-342-2437 (800-342-AIDS)
Sexuality Information and Education Council of the United States
130 West 42nd Street, Suite 350
New York, NY 10036-7802
212-819-9770
Fax: 212-819-9776
www.siecus.org

For additional Internet resources, see the website for this book at *http://evolve.elsevier.com/Lewis/medsurg/.*

CHAPTER 52

NURSING MANAGEMENT
Female Reproductive Problems

Nancy J. MacMullen
Laura Dulski

LEARNING OBJECTIVES

1. Identify causes of infertility and the strategies for diagnosis and treatment of infertility.
2. Discuss the nursing management of women who miscarry or terminate a pregnancy.
3. Describe the etiology, clinical manifestations, and collaborative and nursing management of menstrual problems and irregular vaginal bleeding.
4. Identify the risk factors, clinical manifestations, and collaborative care of ectopic pregnancy.
5. Discuss the changes related to menopause and the collaborative and nursing management of the patient with menopausal symptoms.
6. Identify the clinical manifestations of sexual assault and the appropriate collaborative and nursing management of the patient who has been sexually assaulted.
7. Differentiate among the common problems that affect the vulva, vagina, and cervix and the related collaborative care and nursing management.

8. Describe the assessment, collaborative care, and nursing management of women with pelvic inflammatory disease.
9. Describe the clinical manifestations, complications, collaborative care, and nursing management of endometriosis.
10. Describe the clinical manifestations and collaborative care of benign tumors of the female reproductive system.
11. Identify the clinical manifestations, diagnostic studies, collaborative care, and surgical therapy for cervical, endometrial, ovarian, and vulvar cancers.
12. Describe the preoperative and postoperative nursing management for the patient requiring surgery of the female reproductive system.
13. Describe common problems that occur with cystoceles, rectoceles, and fistulas and the related collaborative and nursing management.

KEY TERMS

abortion, p. 1402
amenorrhea, p. 1406
cystocele, p. 1431
dysmenorrhea, p. 1405
ectopic pregnancy, p. 1408
endometriosis, p. 1418
hysterectomy, p. 1419
infertility, p. 1400
leiomyomas, p. 1419
menopause, p. 1409
menorrhagia, p. 1406

metrorrhagia, p. 1406
pelvic inflammatory disease, p. 1416
perimenopause, p. 1409
postmenopause, p. 1409
premenstrual syndrome (PMS), p. 1404
rectocele, p. 1431
sexual assault, p. 1412
uterine prolapse, p. 1430

INFERTILITY

Infertility is the inability to achieve a pregnancy after at least 1 year of regular intercourse without contraception.[1] Approximately 15% of couples in North America are infertile. Assessment and therapy measures can be invasive, expensive, and lengthy. Understandably, infertility can constitute a physical and emotional crisis.

Reviewed by Susan K. Goebel, RNC, MS, WHNP, SANE, Assistant Professor of Nursing, Mesa State College, Grand Junction, Colo.; Nurse Practitioner, Mesa County Health Department.

Etiology and Pathophysiology

Infertility may be caused by either female, male, or combined factors. Conditions that cause male infertility are discussed in Chapter 53. In up to 20% of the couples evaluated, the cause of infertility may not be identified.[1] The most frequent female causes of infertility include factors associated with ovulation (anovulation or inadequate corpus luteum), tubal obstruction or dysfunction (endometriosis or damage from pelvic infection), and uterine or cervical factors (fibroid tumors or structural anomalies). Risk factors for infertility include tobacco and illicit drug use, infection of the reproductive tract, and specific occupational and environmental exposures. In women the risk for infertility increases with age.[1]

Diagnostic Studies

A detailed history and general physical examination of the woman and her partner provide the basis for selecting diagnostic studies (Table 52-1). The possibility of medical or gynecologic diseases is explored before tests are performed to determine problems affecting general health, as well as fertility. These tests include ovulatory studies, tubal patency studies, and postcoital studies.

Ovulatory Studies. A basal body temperature record is kept to determine whether there is regular ovulation (Fig. 52-1). The woman is instructed to take and graph her temperature, referred to as *basal body temperature*, on awakening before any ac-

TABLE
52-1

Collaborative Care
Infertility

Diagnostic
History and physical examination of both partners, including psychosocial functioning
Review of menstrual history
Assessment of possible sexually transmitted diseases
Basal body temperature record
Serum hormone levels (e.g., FSH, LH, prolactin)
Urinary LH
Sperm penetration assay
Papanicolaou test
Semen analysis
Postcoital test
Endometrial biopsy
Hysterosalpingogram
Pelvic ultrasound

Collaborative Therapy
Hormone supplement therapy
Drug therapy (see Table 52-2)
Intrauterine insemination
Assisted reproductive technologies (ARTs)

FSH, Follicle-stimulating hormone; *LH,* luteinizing hormone.

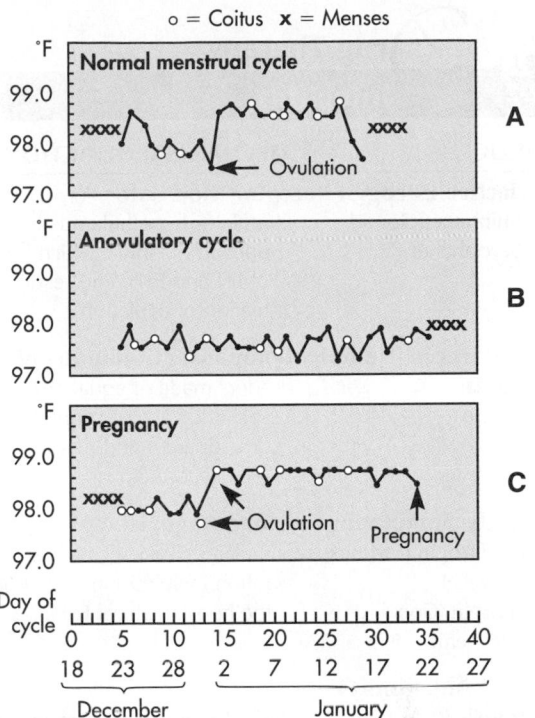

o = Coitus   x = Menses

FIG. 52-1 Basal body temperature chart. A, Typical biphasic temperature curve indicative of ovulation and normal progesterone effect. B, Irregular monophasic curve characteristic of anovulatory cycles. C, Ovulatory curve with sustained temperature elevation following conception and the first missed period.

tivity. The same site (e.g., oral, rectal) for taking the temperature should be used each time. Any cause for variation, such as sleeplessness or illness, should be noted. As ovulation approaches, the production of estrogen increases. This may cause a drop in temperature. When ovulation occurs, progesterone is produced, causing a rise in temperature. The temperature graph thus helps detect ovulation and suggests the timing of intercourse if pregnancy is desired. Rigid adherence to a schedule for intercourse can produce psychologic stress sufficient to inhibit sexual relations.

Ovulation prediction kits are now available for use by women at home. These kits are generally used daily to measure luteinizing hormone (LH) levels in urine samples. Ovulation occurs about 28 to 36 hours after the first rise of LH, so intercourse can be timed accordingly. Other tests for ovulation include cervical and vaginal smears, endometrial biopsy, and plasma progesterone levels.

Tubal Patency Studies. Tubal factors (occlusion or deformity) are assessed most commonly by means of hysterosalpingogram. This procedure consists of the radiographic visualization of the uterus and tubes by injecting a radiopaque dye through the cervix. Tubal patency, shape, position, and any distortions of the endometrial cavity can be determined. Laparoscopy may be used when hysterosalpingogram is contraindicated or other pelvic pathology appears likely.

Postcoital Studies. Examination of the cervical mucus can reveal whether it undergoes favorable changes at ovulation, enabling penetration, survival, and normal motility of the sperm. A postcoital test can determine whether the cervical environment is favorable for the sperm. The couple is asked to have intercourse about the time ovulation is expected and 2 to 12 hours before the office visit. Douching or bathing should be avoided before the

test. The cervical and vaginal secretions are aspirated and examined for the number and motility of sperm present. Other screening tests for infertility include semen analysis, endometrial biopsy, and laser laparoscopy.

NURSING *and* COLLABORATIVE MANAGEMENT
INFERTILITY

The management of infertility problems depends on the cause. If infertility is secondary to an alteration in ovarian function, supplemental hormone therapy to restore and maintain ovulation may be attempted.[2] Drug therapy used to treat infertility is presented in Table 52-2. Chronic cervicitis and inadequate estrogenic stimulation are cervical factors causing infertility. Antibiotic therapy is indicated for cervicitis. Inadequate estrogenic stimulation is treated by the administration of estrogens.

When a couple has not succeeded in conceiving while under infertility management, an option is intrauterine insemination with sperm from the partner or a donor. If this technique does not succeed, assisted reproductive technologies (ARTs) may be used. ARTs include in vitro fertilization (IVF), gamete intrafallopian transfer (GIFT), zygote intrafallopian transfer (ZIFT), donor gametes, and embryo cryopreservation. IVF is the removal of mature oocytes from the woman's ovarian follicle via laparoscopy, followed by in vitro fertilization of the ova with the partner's sperm. When fertilization and cleavage have occurred, the resulting embryos are transferred into the woman's uterus. The procedure requires 2 to 3 days to complete and is used in cases of fallopian tube obstruction, diminished sperm count, and unexplained

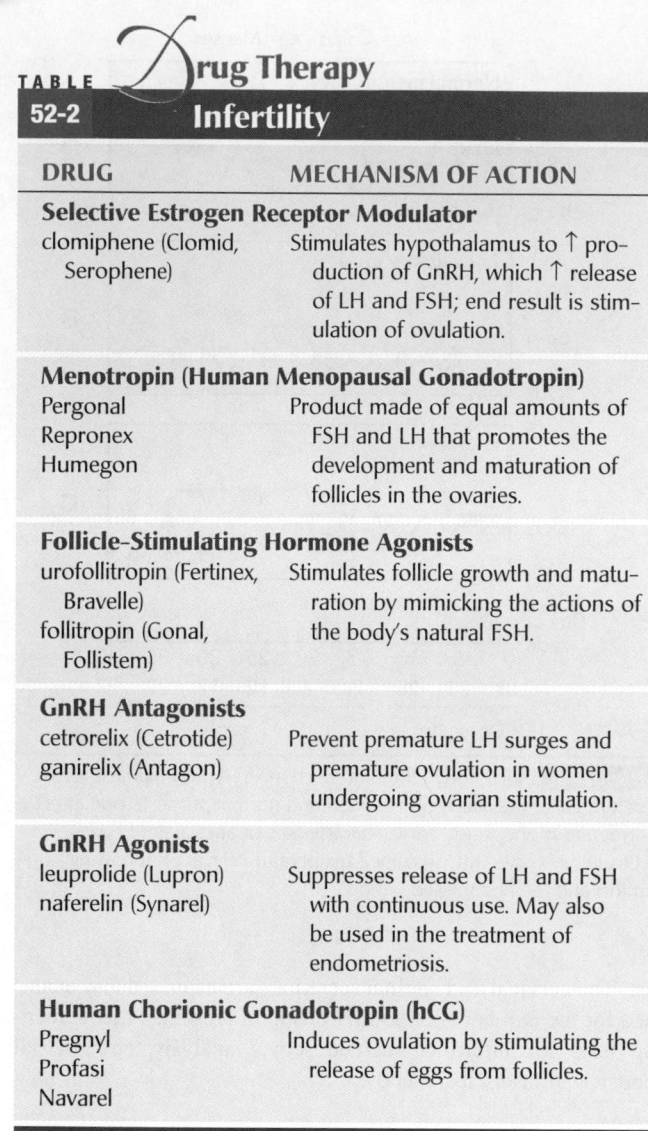

DRUG	MECHANISM OF ACTION
Selective Estrogen Receptor Modulator	
clomiphene (Clomid, Serophene)	Stimulates hypothalamus to ↑ production of GnRH, which ↑ release of LH and FSH; end result is stimulation of ovulation.
Menotropin (Human Menopausal Gonadotropin)	
Pergonal Repronex Humegon	Product made of equal amounts of FSH and LH that promotes the development and maturation of follicles in the ovaries.
Follicle-Stimulating Hormone Agonists	
urofollitropin (Fertinex, Bravelle) follitropin (Gonal, Follistem)	Stimulates follicle growth and maturation by mimicking the actions of the body's natural FSH.
GnRH Antagonists	
cetrorelix (Cetrotide) ganirelix (Antagon)	Prevent premature LH surges and premature ovulation in women undergoing ovarian stimulation.
GnRH Agonists	
leuprolide (Lupron) naferelin (Synarel)	Suppresses release of LH and FSH with continuous use. May also be used in the treatment of endometriosis.
Human Chorionic Gonadotropin (hCG)	
Pregnyl Profasi Navarel	Induces ovulation by stimulating the release of eggs from follicles.

FSH, Follicle-stimulating hormone; *GnRH,* gonadotropin-releasing hormone; *LH,* luteinizing hormone.

infertility. IVF is costly and emotionally stressful, but it has become a recognized and accepted method of therapy for infertile couples.

With the increasing sophistication of ART, couples will have an increased potential for pregnancy. However, the use of ART poses many ethical, legal, and social concerns.

Nurses can assist women experiencing infertility by providing information about the physiology of reproduction, infertility evaluation, and addressing the psychologic and social distress that can accompany infertility. Reducing psychologic stress can improve the emotional climate, making it more conducive to achieving a pregnancy.

The nurse has a major responsibility for teaching and providing emotional support throughout infertility testing and treatment. Feelings of anger, frustration, grief, and helplessness may heighten as additional diagnostic tests are performed. Infertility can generate great tension in a marriage as the couple exhausts financial and emotional resources. Few insurance carriers cover the high cost of infertility testing or expensive in-

fertility treatment. Recognizing and taking steps to deal with the psychologic factors that surface can assist the couple to better cope with the situation. Couples should be encouraged to participate in a support group for infertile couples, as well as individual therapy.

ABORTION

An **abortion** is the loss or termination of a pregnancy before the fetus has developed to a state of viability. Abortions are classified as *spontaneous* (those occurring naturally) or *induced* (those occurring as a result of mechanical or medical intervention). *Miscarriage* is the common term for the unintended loss of a pregnancy. *Habitual abortion* is defined as a history of three or more abortions.

Spontaneous Abortion

Spontaneous abortion is the natural loss of pregnancy before 20 weeks of gestation. Fetal chromosomal anomalies account for 50% of miscarriages before 8 weeks of gestation. Other causes of spontaneous abortions include endocrine abnormalities, maternal infection, acquired anatomic abnormalities (e.g., uterine fibroids, endometriosis), immunologic factors, and environmental factors. About 10% to 15% of all pregnancies end as a result of spontaneous abortion.[3]

Uterine cramping coupled with vaginal bleeding often indicates a spontaneous abortion. Cramping is usually absent if the vaginal bleeding is caused by other conditions, such as polyps. Serial serum β–human chorionic gonadotropin hormone (hCG) and vaginal ultrasound examination of the pelvis are the most reliable indicators of pregnancy with an early abortion. The gestational sac can be visualized using ultrasound as early as 6 weeks of gestation.

Treatment for a possible spontaneous abortion is limited. Although bed rest and avoiding vaginal intercourse are often recommended, there is no evidence that these measures improve the outcome. The woman is advised to report any bleeding to her health care provider. An estimated 80% of patients proceed to abortion regardless of treatment. If the products of conception do not pass completely or bleeding becomes excessive, a *dilation and curettage* (D&C) procedure is generally performed. The D&C involves dilating the uterine cervix and scraping the endometrium of the uterus to empty the uterus of the products of conception.

Women who are experiencing bleeding and cramping during pregnancy may be admitted to the hospital. Nurses need to attend to both the physical and the emotional needs of patients. Vital signs and estimated blood loss are monitored. Any tissue or blood clots that might contain tissue are examined for products of conception. Women are very distressed and experience both physical and emotional pain. Nurses should use comfort measures to provide the needed physical and mental rest. Arranging for someone to stay with the patient provides important emotional support. The nurse should be aware of the grieving process that results from pregnancy loss. Support of the patient and her family is essential.

Induced Abortion

Induced abortion is an intentional termination of a pregnancy. Induced abortion is done for personal reasons (at the request of the woman) and for medical reasons. Several techniques are used to induce abortion, including menstrual extraction, suction curettage, dilation and evacuation (D&E), and drug therapy. Deciding which technique to use to terminate a pregnancy depends on the gestational length of the pregnancy and the woman's condition. Suction curettage may be performed up to 14 weeks of gestation and accounts for more than 90% of abortion procedures.[3] Table 52-3 lists current techniques for abortion.

Drug therapy to induce abortion (medical abortion) early in pregnancy is also available. These agents must be given within the first 49 days of pregnancy (day 1 being the first day of the last menstrual period). Mifepristone (Mifeprex) (also known as

TABLE 52-3 Methods for Inducing Abortion

METHOD	LENGTH OF PREGNANCY	PROCEDURE	ADVANTAGES	DISADVANTAGES
Early Abortion				
Menstrual extraction	Usually up to 2 wk after first missed period	Catheter is inserted through cervix into uterus, and suction is applied. Endometrium and contents of uterus are aspirated.	Low cost, simple, done at outpatient facility without anesthesia or cervical dilation, minimally traumatic	Continuation of pregnancy possible, potential for uterine injury and bleeding
Suction curettage	Up to 14 wk	Cervix is usually dilated, uterine aspirator is introduced, and suction is applied, removing endometrial tissue and implanted pregnancy.	Outpatient procedure, most often involving local anesthesia, 1- to 2-day recovery period	Infection, uterine perforation possible
Dilation and evacuation (D&E)	10-16 wk (approximate)	Cervix is dilated, and products of conception are removed by vacuum cannula and the use of other instruments as needed.	Safe and effective procedure for more advanced pregnancy, outpatient procedure with general anesthesia, 2-day recovery period	More psychologic trauma, more expensive, greater risk with general anesthesia and more invasive procedure
mifepristone (Mifeprex) (RU 486) with misoprostol (Cytotec)	Up to 7 wk	Mifepristone is administered orally. Misoprostol is administered orally or intravaginally 2 days later.	Safe, effective, does not require surgical procedure	Very expensive; prolonged bleeding possible
methotrexate with misoprostol	Up to 7 wk	Methotrexate is administered intramuscularly. Misoprostol is given intravaginally 5-7 days later.	Safe, effective, does not require surgical procedure	Not considered as effective as mifepristone; prolonged bleeding possible
Late Abortion				
Instillation of drugs • Hypertonic saline solution	After 16 wk	About 200 ml of amniotic fluid is withdrawn, and a similar amount of 20% normal saline solution is injected. Uterus is irritated and begins to contract within 12-36 hr. Contractions may be assisted with IV oxytocin.	Inexpensive, readily available, feticidal	Hypernatremia, infection, hemorrhage, disseminated intravascular coagulation, more emotional trauma because of time required
• Prostaglandins	After 16 wk	Amniocentesis is done, and 8 ml of prostaglandin is inserted into amniotic sac, resulting in stimulation of smooth muscle of uterus. Expulsion of uterine contents occurs within 24 hr.	Fast induction, no need for surgery	Nausea and vomiting, abdominal cramps, cervical laceration, possible delivery of live fetus, high cost
Hysterotomy	16-20 wk	Miniature cesarean section is performed. Incision is made into uterus and contents are removed.	Concurrent sterilization procedure possible	More difficult and expensive in time and money, surgical incision with possible complications

IV, Intravenous.

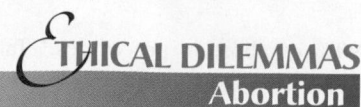

ETHICAL DILEMMAS
Abortion

Situation
A recently married, 39-year-old woman is informed that the results of her amniocentesis indicate that her fetus has major chromosomal abnormalities and is expected to have severe physical and mental disabilities. The patient has no children, but her husband has three children from a previous marriage. She asks the nurse what she should do. How would the nurse respond?

Important Points for Consideration
- Decisions about whether to continue a pregnancy with a child who has severe disabilities are extremely personal and emotional. The woman and her husband will need support and information to explore their options and their values.
- Pregnancy counseling is warranted about the woman's choices, her feelings about the pregnancy, her desire to have a child with her husband, her concerns about raising a child with severe disabilities, her feelings about abortion, and concerns about possible future pregnancies.
- Patient autonomy ensures that a woman decide for herself whether or not to continue a pregnancy.
- The Supreme Court decision in 1973, *Roe v. Wade*, legalized abortion in the United States. In the first trimester, abortion is a private matter between a woman and her physician. In the second trimester, the state may regulate abortion services for safety reasons. In the third trimester, abortions may only be performed when the life or health of the woman is endangered by the pregnancy.
- The role of the health care professional in these difficult situations is to provide education and support, to facilitate a decision consistent with the patient's values.

Critical Thinking Questions
1. How would your feelings about abortion affect your ability to care for this patient?
2. How would you proceed in this case?

RU 486) works by blocking progesterone, a hormone needed for pregnancy to continue. It is given in combination with misoprostol (Cytotec), an agent that produces uterine contractions resulting in expulsion of the products of conception.[4]

Methotrexate, also given in combination with misoprostol, is another option for medically induced abortions. Methotrexate induces abortion because of its toxicity to trophoblastic tissue; misoprostol induces uterine contractions.

Once the decision is made to have an abortion, the woman and her significant others need support and acceptance. The patient should be prepared for what to expect both emotionally and physically. Grief and sadness are normal emotions after an abortion. The patient needs to understand the procedure, including instructions for preprocedure and postprocedure care. The nurse's caring attitude can be a positive factor in the patient's experience.

Follow-up care includes instructions on signs and symptoms of possible complications, including abnormal vaginal bleeding, severe abdominal cramping, fever, and foul drainage. Avoiding intercourse, tampons, and douching until reexamination should be stressed. The patient needs to return for reexamination in 2 weeks. Contraception can be started the day of the procedure or during the patient's return visit in accordance with her needs and desires.

Problems Related to Menstruation

The normal menstrual cycle is discussed in Chapter 49. The hormonal influences related to the menstrual cycle are shown in Fig. 49-9. Menstruation may be irregular during the first few years after menarche and the years preceding menopause. Once established, a woman's menstrual cycles usually have a predictable pattern. However, considerable normal variation exists among women in cycle length, as well as in the duration, amount, and character of the menstrual flow (see Table 49-2).

PREMENSTRUAL SYNDROME

Premenstrual syndrome (PMS) is a common disorder in women in which a group of physical and psychologic symptoms occur during the last few days of the menstrual cycle and before the onset of menstruation. The symptoms can be severe enough to impair interpersonal relationships or interfere with usual activities. Because many symptoms are associated with PMS, it is difficult to concisely define it. However, PMS symptoms always occur cyclically during the luteal phase before the onset of menstruation and are not present at other times of the month.

Etiology and Pathophysiology

The etiology and pathophysiology are not well understood. PMS is thought to have a biologic trigger with compounding psychosocial factors. Some women may have a genetic predisposition to PMS. Other proposed causes of PMS include estrogen and progesterone imbalances and nutritional deficiencies of pyridoxine (vitamin B_6) or magnesium.[5] *Premenstrual dysphoric disorder* (PMD-D) is the term applied to a type of PMS. Women with PMD-D have a severe mood disorder in addition to PMS.

Clinical Manifestations

PMS is extremely variable in its clinical manifestation. Variation is common between women and, for an individual woman, from one cycle to another. Commonly occurring physical symptoms include breast discomfort, peripheral edema, abdominal bloating, sensation of weight gain, episodes of binge eating, and headache. Abdominal bloating and breast swelling are caused by fluid shifts because total body weight does not generally change. Symptoms of autonomic nervous system arousal (e.g., heart palpitations, dizziness) have been reported by women with PMS. Anxiety, depression, irritability, and mood swings are some of the emotional symptoms that women may experience.

Diagnostic Studies and Collaborative Care

PMS can be diagnosed only when other possible causes for the symptoms have been eliminated. A focused health history and physical examination are done to identify any underlying conditions, such as thyroid dysfunction, uterine fibroids, or depression, that may account for the symptoms. No definitive diagnostic test is available for PMS. When PMS or PMD-D is a possible diagnosis, a woman is given a symptom diary to record her symptoms prospectively for two or three menstrual cycles. Diagnosis is based on an evaluation of the woman's symptoms.

Nonpharmacologic and pharmacologic strategies can relieve some PMS symptoms (Table 52-4). However, no single treatment

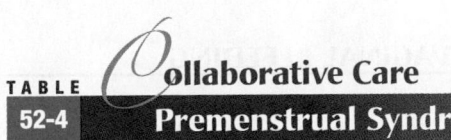

TABLE 52-4	Collaborative Care
Premenstrual Syndrome	

Diagnostic
History and physical examination
Symptom diary

Collaborative Therapy
Stress management and relaxation therapy
Nutritional therapy
- Avoid caffeine and alcohol
- Reduce refined carbohydrates
- Vitamin B_6
- Limit salt intake before menstruation

Aerobic exercise

Drug therapy
- Diuretics
- Prostaglandin inhibitors (e.g., ibuprofen [Advil, Motrin])
- buspirone (Buspar)
- Tricyclic antidepressants (e.g., amitriptyline [Elavil])
- fluoxetine (Sarafem)
- Selective serotonin reuptake inhibitors (e.g., sertraline [Zoloft])
- Combined oral contraceptives

is available. The goal of treatment is to reduce the severity of symptoms and enhance the woman's sense of control and quality of life.

Several conservative approaches to managing PMS symptoms are considered helpful, including stress management, diet changes, exercise, education, and counseling.[5] Techniques for stress reduction include yoga, meditation, imagery, and biofeedback training. To decrease autonomic nervous system arousal, women should avoid caffeine, reduce refined carbohydrates, exercise on a regular basis, and practice relaxation techniques. Eating complex carbohydrates with high fiber, foods rich in vitamin B_6, and sources of tryptophan (dairy and poultry) are thought to promote serotonin production, which improves the symptoms. Vitamin B_6 may be found in such foods as pork, milk, egg yolk, and legumes. Although no strongly supportive data exist, limiting salt intake before menstruation and increasing calcium intake have been proposed to alleviate fluid retention, weight gain, bloating, breast swelling, and tenderness.

Exercise results in a release of endorphins, leading to mood elevation. Aerobic exercise can also have a relaxing effect. Because fatigue tends to exaggerate the symptoms of PMS, adequate rest in the premenstrual period is a priority.

Explanations about PMS help the woman understand the complexity of the disorder and ways that she can regain a better sense of control. The patient needs to be assured that her symptoms are real, PMS exists, and she is not "crazy." Acknowledgment of having PMS can itself be therapeutic. Teaching the woman's partner about the nature of PMS assists the partner to better understand PMS and to provide support to the woman in making lifestyle changes to reduce the symptoms of PMS.

Drug Therapy. Drug therapy is considered when symptoms persist. Presently, no single drug can treat PMS symptoms. One therapy may be tried for a time, and if no improvement is ob-

served, another approach is tried. Some treatments are symptom specific. For fluid retention, diuretics such as spironolactone (Aldactone) are used. For reducing cramps, backache, and headache, prostaglandin inhibitors such as ibuprofen (Motrin, Advil) are used. To improve negative mood, vitamin B_6 supplementation (50 mg daily) may be used. For anxiety, buspirone (Buspar) taken during the luteal phase has helped some women. Women with PMD-D may benefit from antidepressants, including fluoxetine (Sarafem) and tricyclic antidepressants (e.g., amitriptyline [Elavil]).

Other pharmacologic treatments are directed at PMS in general. Selective serotonin reuptake inhibitors (SSRIs) (e.g., sertraline [Zoloft]) have provided significant relief to women with severe PMS. Other general treatments include oral contraceptives containing estrogen and progesterone. Evening primrose oil, an herb, may help some women.

DYSMENORRHEA

Dysmenorrhea is abdominal cramping pain or discomfort associated with menstrual flow. The degree of pain and discomfort varies with the individual. The two types of dysmenorrhea are primary, when no pathology exists, and secondary, when pelvic disease is the underlying cause. Dysmenorrhea is one of the most common gynecologic problems, affecting approximately 50% of all women.[6]

Etiology and Pathophysiology

Primary dysmenorrhea is not a disease; rather it is caused by an excess of prostaglandin $F_2\alpha$ ($PGF_2\alpha$) and/or an increased sensitivity to it. The sequential stimulation of the endometrium by estrogen, followed by progesterone, results in a dramatic increase in prostaglandin production by the endometrium. With the onset of menses, degeneration of the endometrium releases prostaglandin. Locally, prostaglandins increase myometrial contractions and constriction of small endometrial blood vessels with consequent tissue ischemia and increased sensitization of the pain receptors, resulting in menstrual pain. Prostaglandins absorbed into the circulatory system may be responsible for symptoms of headache, diarrhea, and vomiting. Primary dysmenorrhea begins in the few years after menarche, typically with the onset of regular ovulatory cycles.

Secondary dysmenorrhea is usually acquired after adolescence, occurring most commonly at 30 to 40 years of age. Common pelvic conditions that cause secondary dysmenorrhea include endometriosis, chronic pelvic inflammatory disease, and uterine fibroids. Because secondary dysmenorrhea is caused by multiple conditions, symptoms vary. However, painful menses is present in all situations.[6]

Clinical Manifestations

Primary dysmenorrhea starts 12 to 24 hours before the onset of menses. The pain is most severe the first day of menses and rarely lasts more than 2 days. Characteristic manifestations include lower abdominal pain that is colicky in nature, frequently radiating to the lower back and upper thighs. The abdominal pain is often accompanied by nausea, diarrhea, loose stools, fatigue, headache, and light-headedness.

Secondary dysmenorrhea usually occurs after the woman has experienced problem-free periods for some time. The pain, which may be unilateral, is generally more constant in nature and usually continues longer than in primary dysmenorrhea. Depending on the cause, symptoms such as *dyspareunia* (painful intercourse), painful defecation, or irregular bleeding may occur at times other than menstruation.

Collaborative Care

Evaluation begins with distinguishing primary from secondary dysmenorrhea. A complete health history with special attention to menstrual and gynecologic history should be obtained. A pelvic examination is also performed. If the history reveals an onset shortly after menarche and symptoms only associated with menses in addition to normal pelvic examination findings, the probable diagnosis is primary dysmenorrhea. If any specific cause of dysmenorrhea is evident, the diagnosis is secondary dysmenorrhea.

Treatment for primary dysmenorrhea includes heat, exercise, and drug therapy. Heat is applied to the lower abdomen or back. Regular exercise is thought to be beneficial because it may reduce endometrial hyperplasia and subsequently reduce prostaglandin production. The primary drug therapy is nonsteroidal antiinflammatory drugs (NSAIDs) such as ibuprofen, which has antiprostaglandin activity. NSAIDs should be started at the first sign of menses and continued every 4 to 8 hours to maintain a sufficient level of the drug to inhibit prostaglandin synthesis for the usual duration of discomfort. Birth control pills may also be used. They decrease dysmenorrhea by reducing endometrial hyperplasia.

Acupuncture and transcutaneous nerve stimulation also provide varying degrees of relief. (See Chapter 7 for a discussion of acupuncture.) These methods may be used for women who obtain inadequate relief from medications or who prefer not to take medications. Patients who are unresponsive to these treatments should be evaluated for chronic pelvic pain.

Treatment of secondary dysmenorrhea depends on the cause. Some individuals with secondary dysmenorrhea will be helped by the approaches used for primary dysmenorrhea. Depending on the underlying causes of dysmenorrhea, additional drug or surgical interventions are used.

NURSING MANAGEMENT
DYSMENORRHEA

One of the primary roles of the nurse is teaching. Women should be taught why dysmenorrhea occurs, as well as how to treat it. Teaching and supportive therapy can provide women with a foundation for coping with this common occurrence and increase feelings of control and self-reliance.

Women often ask the nurse what can be done for minor discomforts associated with menstrual cycles. Women should be advised that during acute pain, relief may be obtained by lying down for short periods, drinking hot beverages, applying heat to the abdomen or back, and taking an antiinflammatory drug for analgesia. The nurse can also suggest noninvasive pain-relieving practices such as distraction and guided imagery.

Other health care measures can reduce the discomfort of dysmenorrhea. These include regular exercise and proper nutritional habits. Avoiding constipation, maintaining good body mechanics, and eliminating stress and fatigue, particularly during the time preceding menstrual periods, can also decrease discomfort. Staying active and interested in activities may also help.

IRREGULAR VAGINAL BLEEDING

Irregular vaginal bleeding is a common gynecologic concern. Irregularities include *oligomenorrhea* (long intervals between menses), **amenorrhea** (absence of menstruation), **menorrhagia** (excessive menstrual bleeding), and **metrorrhagia** (irregular bleeding or bleeding between menses). The cause of irregular bleeding may vary from anovulatory menstrual cycles to more serious causes such as ectopic pregnancy or endometrial cancer. The age of the woman provides direction for identifying the cause of bleeding. For example, a postmenopausal woman with irregular bleeding must always be evaluated for endometrial cancer but does not need to be evaluated for possible pregnancy. For a 20-year-old woman with irregular bleeding, the possibility of pregnancy must always be considered and the possibility of endometrial cancer would be unlikely.

Irregular bleeding may be caused by dysfunction of the hypothalamic-pituitary-ovarian axis such as a pituitary adenoma. Another cause may be infection. Changes in lifestyle such as marriage, recent moves, a death in the family, financial stress, and other emotional crises can also cause irregular bleeding. Because psychologic factors can influence endocrine function, they should be considered when the patient is evaluated.

Types of Irregular Bleeding

Oligomenorrhea and Secondary Amenorrhea. Anovulation is the most common cause for missing menses once pregnancy has been ruled out. Additional causes of amenorrhea are listed in Table 52-5. *Primary amenorrhea* refers to the failure of menstrual cycles to begin by age 16 years or by age 14 years if secondary sex characteristics are present. *Secondary amenorrhea,* on the other hand, refers to cessation of menstrual cycles once established.

Ovulation is often erratic for several years following menarche and before menopause. Thus oligomenorrhea due to anovulation is common for women at the beginning and end of menstruation. In anovulatory cycles, the corpus luteum that produces progesterone does not form. This may result in a situation referred to as *unopposed estrogen.* When unopposed by progesterone, estrogen can cause excessive buildup of the endometrium. Persistent overgrowth of the endometrium increases a woman's risk for endometrial cancer. To reduce this risk, progesterone or birth control pills are prescribed to ensure that the patient's endometrial lining will be shed at least four to six times per year.

Menorrhagia. Excessive bleeding associated with menorrhagia may be an increased duration (more than 7 days), increased amount (more than 80 ml), or both. Anovulatory uterine bleeding is the most common cause of menorrhagia. An unopposed estrogen state continues to build up the endometrium until it becomes unstable, resulting in menorrhagia. For young women with excessive bleeding, clotting disorders must be considered. Uterine fibroids (also called *leiomyomas*) are a common cause of menorrhagia for women in their thirties and forties.

Metrorrhagia. Metrorrhagia, also referred to as *spotting* or *breakthrough bleeding,* is bleeding between menstrual periods. For all reproductive-age women, pregnancy complications such as spontaneous abortion or ectopic pregnancy must be considered as a possible cause. Other causes include cervical or endometrial polyps, infection, and carcinoma. Spotting is common during the first three cycles of birth control pills. If spotting continues past

TABLE 52-5	Causes of Amenorrhea

Hypothalamic-Pituitary Axis

Reversible CNS-mediated causes (e.g., emotional stress, anorexia nervosa or severe dieting, strenuous exercise, post-pill syndrome, chronic or acute illness)
Prolactinoma and other causes of hyperprolactinemia (e.g., drugs)
Craniopharyngioma and other brainstem or parasellar tumors
Congenital conditions (e.g., isolated gonadotropin deficiency)*
Trauma (e.g., head injury with hypothalamic contusion)
Infiltrative processes (e.g., sarcoidosis)
Vascular disease (e.g., hypothalamic vasculitis)
Pituitary tumors
Sheehan syndrome

Ovaries

Autoimmune disease (often involving thyroid, adrenal, and islet cells)
Premature menopause (idiopathic) or resistant-ovary syndrome
Polycystic ovary disease
Tumors
Congenital or genetic conditions (e.g., Turner syndrome)*
Infection (e.g., mumps oophoritis)
Toxins (especially alkylating chemotherapeutic agents)
Radiation
Trauma, torsion (rare)

Uterovaginal Outflow Tract

Asherman syndrome (postcurettage loss of endometrium)
Müllerian dysgenesis*

Hormonal Synthesis and Action

Male pseudohermaphroditism (e.g., testicular feminization)*
17-Hydroxylase deficiency*

*Usually manifests as primary amenorrhea.
CNS, Central nervous system.

the woman's third cycle using birth control pills, a different pill formulation can be prescribed when other causes of metrorrhagia have been ruled out. Spotting with long-acting progestin therapy, such as Depo-Provera or Norplant, is also common. For post-menopausal women, endometrial cancer must be considered whenever spotting is experienced. In postmenopausal women, exogenous estrogen administration during hormone replacement therapy is a common cause of metrorrhagia. *Menometrorraghia* is excessive bleeding that occurs at irregular intervals. It may be caused by endometrial cancer or uterine fibroids.

Diagnostic Studies and Collaborative Care

Because irregular vaginal bleeding has multiple causes, diagnostic and collaborative care vary as well. A health history and physical examination directed at the most likely causes of vaginal bleeding for the woman's age-group is the first step. These findings will provide the basis for selecting the necessary laboratory tests and diagnostic procedures. Treatment depends on the nature of the problem (e.g., menorrhagia, amenorrhea), degree of threat to the patient's health, and whether children are desired in the future.

Combined oral contraceptives may be prescribed for a woman with amenorrhea to ensure regular shedding of endome-trium if she also wants contraception. If she does not need birth control, progesterone may be prescribed to ensure a shedding of the endometrial lining four to six times per year. On the other hand, if she wants to become pregnant, a fertility drug may be prescribed.

The treatment goal for women with menorrhagia is to minimize further blood loss. If menorrhagia is the result of anovulatory cycles, the endometrium must be stabilized by a combination of oral estrogen and progesterone.

A new therapy for treating menorrhagia has recently become available. Balloon therapy is a technique that involves the introduction of a soft, flexible balloon into the uterus; the balloon is then inflated with sterile fluid (Fig. 52-2). The fluid in the balloon is heated and maintained for 8 minutes, thus causing ablation (removal) of the uterine lining. When the treatment is completed, the fluid is withdrawn from the balloon and the catheter is removed from the uterus. The uterine lining sloughs off in the following 7 to 10 days. Uterine balloon therapy is contraindicated for women desiring future fertility and for women with any suspected uterine abnormalities such as fibroids, suspected endometrial carcinoma, previous classical cesarean section, or myomectomy.[7] With severe bleeding, hospitalization is indicated. All patients with menorrhagia should be evaluated for anemia and treated as indicated.

Surgical Therapy. Surgery may be indicated depending on the underlying cause of the irregular vaginal bleeding. Dilation and curettage (D&C) was once a common therapy for excessive bleeding or for spotting in perimenopausal women. Now D&C is used only in extreme cases of bleeding or for older women when endometrial biopsy and ultrasonography have not provided the necessary diagnostic information. Endometrial ablation done by laser or electrosurgical technique has been successful with many patients with uncontrolled menorrhagia. If menorrhagia is caused by uterine fibroids, a hysterectomy may be performed. A *myomectomy* (removal of fibroids without removal of the uterus) may be performed if the patient wants to preserve her uterus. Hormonal regimens, ablative techniques, and embolization of blood vessels supplying the fibroid are newer options.[8]

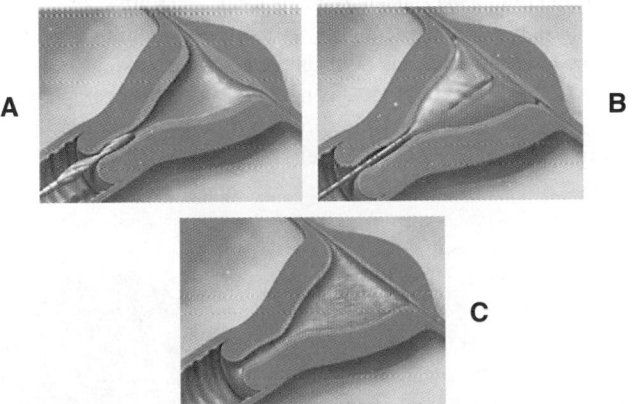

FIG. 52-2 Balloon thermotherapy for treatment of menorrhagia. **A,** Balloon-tipped catheter is inserted into the uterus through the vagina and cervix. **B,** The balloon is inflated with a sterile fluid that expands to fit the size and shape of the uterus. The fluid is heated to 188° F (87° C) and maintained for 8 minutes while the uterine lining is treated. **C,** Fluid is withdrawn from the balloon and the catheter is removed.

NURSING MANAGEMENT
IRREGULAR VAGINAL BLEEDING

For some women, infrequent or no menses might seem a desirable state. Teaching women about the characteristics of the menstrual cycle will assist them to identify normal variations.

Table 49-2 includes characteristics of the menstrual cycle and related patient teaching. This knowledge can diminish apprehension and dispel misconceptions about the menstrual cycle. If the patient's menstrual cycle pattern does not fall within the normal range, the nurse should urge her to visit her health care provider. Myths concerning activities allowed during menstruation are common. The nurse should be prepared to clarify the facts. The patient should be assured that bathing and hair washing are safe. A daily warm tub bath may actually relieve some of the associated pelvic discomfort. Women can swim, exercise, have intercourse, and basically continue their usual daily activities.

Frequent changing of tampons or pads meets comfort and hygiene needs during menstruation. The selection of internal or external sanitary protection is a matter of personal preference. Tampons are convenient and make menstrual hygiene easier, whereas pads may provide better protection. Using a combination of tampons and pads and avoiding prolonged use of superabsorbent tampons may decrease the risk of *toxic shock syndrome* (TSS).[8] TSS is an acute condition caused by a toxin from *Staphylococcus aureus*. TSS causes high fever, vomiting, diarrhea, weakness, myalgia, and a sunburn-like rash.

Whenever excessive, the amount of the patient's vaginal bleeding should be assessed as accurately as possible. The number and size of pads or tampons used and the degree of saturation should be reported and recorded. The patient's fatigue level, along with variations in blood pressure and pulse, should be monitored because anemia and hypovolemia may be present. If a surgical procedure is indicated, the nurse should provide appropriate preoperative and postoperative care.

ECTOPIC PREGNANCY

An **ectopic pregnancy** is the implantation of the fertilized ovum anywhere outside the uterine cavity (Fig. 52-3). Between 97% and 98% of ectopic pregnancies occur in the fallopian tube. The remaining 2% to 3% may be ovarian, abdominal, or cervical (Fig. 52-4). Ectopic pregnancy is a life-threatening condition. Earlier identification has contributed to a decrease in mortality rates. However, 40 to 50 deaths occur as a result of ectopic pregnancy each year in the United States. Ectopic pregnancy is the leading cause of maternal death among African American women.[9]

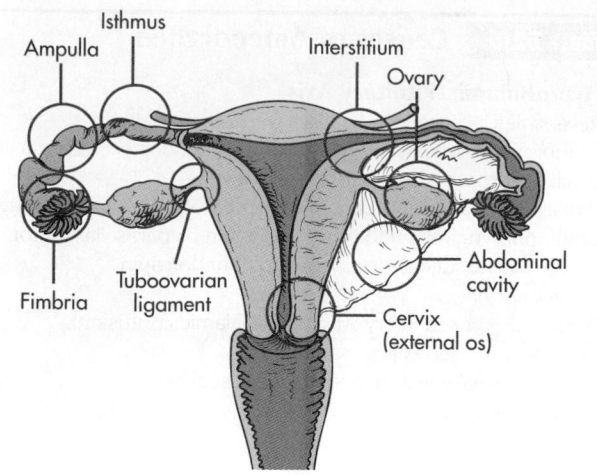

FIG. 52-4 Sites of implantation of ectopic pregnancies. Order of frequency of occurrence is ampulla, isthmus, interstitium, fimbria, tuboovarian ligament, ovary, abdominal cavity, and cervix (external os).

Etiology and Pathophysiology

Any blockage of the tube or reduction of tubal peristalsis that impedes or delays the zygote passing to the uterine cavity can result in tubal implantation. After implantation, the growth of the gestational sac expands the tubal wall. Eventually the tube ruptures, causing acute peritoneal symptoms. Less acute symptoms usually begin within 6 to 8 weeks after the last normal menstrual period and weeks before rupture would occur.

Risk factors for ectopic pregnancy include a history of pelvic inflammatory disease, prior ectopic pregnancy, current progestin-releasing intrauterine device (IUD), progestin-only birth control failure, and prior pelvic or tubal surgery. Additional risk factors for ectopic pregnancy include procedures used in infertility treatment, including in vitro fertilization procedures, embryo transfer, and ovulation induction.

Clinical Manifestations

The classic symptoms of ectopic pregnancy are abdominal or pelvic pain, missed menses, and irregular vaginal bleeding. Other symptoms include amenorrhea, morning sickness, breast tenderness, gastrointestinal disturbance, malaise, and syncope. Pain is almost always present and is caused by distention of the fallopian tube. It may start unilaterally and then spread to become bilateral. The character of the pain varies among women and can be colicky or vague. If tubal rupture occurs, the pain is intense and may be referred to the shoulder as a result of irritation of the

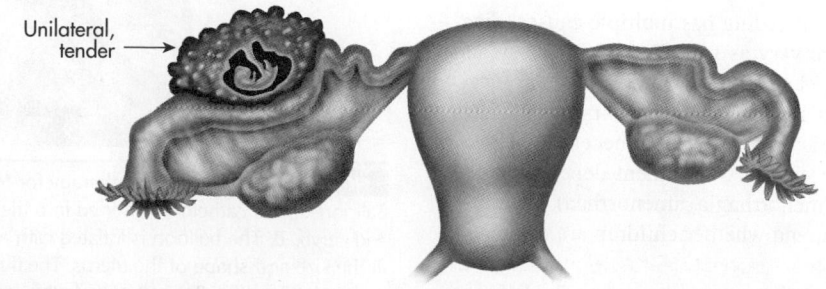

FIG. 52-3 Ruptured tubal pregnancy.

diaphragm by blood released into the abdominal cavity. Symptom severity does not necessarily correlate with the extent of external bleeding present. With rupture, the risk of hemorrhage and hypovolemic shock is present. Suspected rupture is treated as an emergency.

The vaginal bleeding that may accompany ectopic pregnancy is usually described as spotting. However, it is also possible that bleeding may be heavier and can be confused with menses. The woman may also experience irregular bleeding.

Diagnostic Studies

Because of the life-threatening nature of ectopic pregnancy, it should be considered whenever pregnancy is even remotely possible. Ectopic pregnancy can be a diagnostic challenge because of its similarity to other pelvic and abdominal disorders, such as salpingitis, spontaneous abortion, ruptured ovarian cyst, appendicitis, and peritonitis. A sensitive serum pregnancy test should be performed. If the test is negative, an ectopic pregnancy is not likely. If ectopic pregnancy cannot be excluded by the pregnancy test, further evaluation is warranted. If the patient is in a stable condition, a combination of serial β–human chorionic gonadotropin (β-hCG) and vaginal ultrasonography is used. β-hCG is expected to double about every 48 hours in a normal pregnancy. If the hCG level fails to double, the patient may have an ectopic pregnancy. Ultrasound can be used to confirm the presence of an intrauterine pregnancy once the β-hCG level has reached 2000 mIU/ml.

Absence of a normal intrauterine pregnancy means that the diagnosis is probably spontaneous abortion or ectopic pregnancy. With a spontaneous abortion, serial β-hCG levels will decrease over time. A complete blood count is obtained when there is any concern regarding the amount of blood loss or if surgery is contemplated. A gradually decreasing hematocrit may indicate internal bleeding.

NURSING and COLLABORATIVE MANAGEMENT
ECTOPIC PREGNANCY

Surgery remains the primary approach for treating ectopic pregnancies and should be performed immediately. However, medical management with methotrexate (Folex) is being used with increasing success with patients who are hemodynamically stable and have a mass less than 3 cm in size. A conservative surgical approach limits damage to the reproductive system as much as possible. Removal of the pregnancy from the tube is preferred to removing the tube. Laparoscopy is preferable to laparotomy, because it decreases blood loss and the length of the hospital stay. If the tube ruptures, conservative surgical approaches may not be possible. The patient may need a blood transfusion and supplemental intravenous (IV) fluid therapy to relieve shock and restore a satisfactory blood volume for safe anesthesia and surgery. The use of microsurgery techniques has resulted in fewer repeated ectopic pregnancies and a higher rate of future successful pregnancies.

Nursing care depends on the condition of the patient. Before the diagnosis has been confirmed, the nurse should be alert to signs of increasing pain and vaginal bleeding, which may indicate that rupture of the tube has occurred. Vital signs are monitored closely, along with observation for signs of shock. Explanations and preparation for diagnostic procedures are given when

appropriate. Preparation of the patient for abdominal surgery may follow rapidly. The patient's emotional status should be assessed. Reassurance and support for the surgery should be given to the patient and her family. Postoperatively, the patient may express a fear of future ectopic pregnancies and have many questions about the impact of this experience on her future fertility.

PERIMENOPAUSE AND POSTMENOPAUSE

The **perimenopause** is a normal life transition that begins with the first signs of change in menstrual cycles and ends after cessation of menses. **Menopause** is the physiologic cessation of menses associated with declining ovarian function. It is usually considered complete after 1 year of *amenorrhea* (absence of menstruation). Menopause starts gradually and is usually associated with changes in menstruation, including menstrual flows that are increased, decreased, and/or irregular. Cessation of menses finally occurs. **Postmenopause** is a term that refers to the time in a woman's life after menopause.

The age at which menopause occurs ranges from 45 to 55 years but may occur earlier due to illness, surgical removal of the uterus or both ovaries, side effects of radiation therapy or chemotherapy, or drugs. The age at which menopause occurs is not affected by age at menarche, race, physical characteristics, number of pregnancies, date of last pregnancy, socioeconomic status, or oral contraceptive use. However, cigarette smoking, chemotherapy, and radiation have been linked to acceleration of menopause.[10]

Changes in the ovary start the cascade of events that finally result in menopause. The regression of the follicles within each ovary begins with puberty and accelerates after age 35. With age, fewer and fewer follicles remain that are responsive to follicle-stimulating hormone (FSH). FSH normally stimulates the dominant follicle to secrete estrogen. When the follicles can no longer respond to FHS, ovarian production of estrogen and progesterone declines. However, perimenopausal women can get pregnant until menopause has occurred.

With decreased ovarian function there are decreased levels of estrogen that cause a gradual increase in FSH and LH as a result of the negative feedback process. By the time menopause occurs, there is a tenfold to twentyfold increase in FSH. The elevated FSH level may take several years to return to the premenopausal level. The reduced estrogen level also causes a decrease in the frequency of ovulation and results in changes in the secondary sex characteristics (e.g., decreased skin elasticity).

Clinical Manifestations

Clinical manifestations of perimenopause and postmenopause are presented in Table 52-6. The perimenopause is a time of erratic hormonal fluctuation. Irregular vaginal bleeding is common. With decreasing estrogen, hot flashes and other symptoms begin. The signs and symptoms of diminished estrogen are listed in Table 52-7. The loss of estrogen plays a significant role in the cause of age-related alterations. Changes most critical to a woman's well-being are the increased risks for coronary artery disease and osteoporosis secondary to bone density loss. Other changes include a redistribution of fat, a tendency to gain weight more easily, muscle and joint pain, loss of skin elasticity, changes in hair amount and distribution, and atrophy of external genitalia and breast tissue.

Hallmarks of the perimenopause include *vasomotor instability* (hot flashes) and irregular menses. A hot flash is described as a

TABLE 52-6   Clinical Manifestatons of Perimenopause and Postmenopause

PERIMENOPAUSE	POSTMENOPAUSE
Irregular menses	Cessation of menses
Vasomotor instability (hot flashes and night sweats)	Occasional vasomotor symptoms
Atrophy of genitourinary tissue (e.g., vaginal epithelium)	Atrophy of genitourinary tissue with decreased support
Stress and urge incontinence	Stress and urge incontinence
Breast tenderness	Osteoporosis
Mood changes	

TABLE 52-7   Signs and Symptoms of Estrogen Deficiency

Vasomotor
Hot flashes
Night sweats
Genitourinary
Atrophic vaginitis
Dyspareunia secondary to poor lubrication
Incontinence
Psychologic
Emotional lability
Change in sleep pattern
Decreased REM sleep
Skeletal
Increased fracture rate, particularly of vertebral bodies but also of humerus, distal radius, and upper femur
Cardiovascular
Decreased high-density lipoproteins (HDL)
Increased low-density lipoproteins (LDL)
Dermatologic
Diminished collagen content of skin
Breast tissue changes

REM, Rapid eye movement.

sensation of warmth in the upper part of the chest, neck, and face followed by profuse perspiration and sometimes chilling. These sensations last from several seconds to 5 minutes and occur most often at night, thereby disturbing sleep. The cause of hot flashes, or vasomotor instability, is not clearly understood. It has been theorized that temperature regulators in the brain are in proximity to the area where gonadotropin-releasing hormone (GnRH) is released. However, lowered estrogen levels are correlated with dilation of cutaneous blood vessels resulting in hot flashes and increased sweating. The more sudden the withdrawal of estrogen (e.g., surgical removal of the ovaries), the more likely the symptoms will be severe if no hormone replacement is provided. These symptoms subside over time with or without hormone replacement therapy. Hot flashes can be triggered by situations that affect body temperature, such as eating a hot meal, hot weather, drinking an alcoholic beverage, stress, or warm clothing.

Atrophic vaginal changes secondary to decreased estrogen include thinning of the vaginal mucosa and disappearance of rugae. Vaginal secretions also decrease and become more alkaline. As a result of these changes, the vagina is easily traumatized and susceptible to infection. *Dyspareunia* (painful intercourse) may also occur. This can lead to unnecessary and premature cessation of sexual activity. Dryness is a problem that can be easily corrected with water-soluble lubricants or, if needed, with hormonal creams or systemic hormone replacement therapy. In general, the extent and severity of the symptoms of menopause vary and are not easily predicted, even with a detailed history of family patterns.

Atrophic changes in the lower urinary tract also occur with a decrease in estrogen. Bladder capacity decreases and the bladder and urethral tissue lose tone. These changes can cause symptoms that mimic a bladder infection (e.g., dysuria, urgency, frequency) when no infection is present.

Whether decreasing estrogen is responsible for the psychologic changes associated with perimenopause is unclear. The attributed depression, irritability, and cognitive problems could result from life stressors or sleep deprivation from hot flashes. Research has not found a statistically significant relationship between perimenopause and depression.[11] Women who are most likely to be depressed believe that depression is related to menopause, are concerned about menopause and aging, or have a previous history of depression or unemployment.[11]

Collaborative Care

The diagnosis of perimenopause should be made only after careful consideration of other possible causes for the woman's symptoms. Depression, thyroid dysfunction, anemia, or anxiety reactions could be responsible for the same symptoms. Because of the hormonal fluctuations that occur before menopause, routine testing of the serum FSH level is not indicated. After age 50, postmenopause can be diagnosed by an FSH of 30 mIU/ml or greater if the woman is not on any hormonal medication.

Nonhormonal Therapy. The frequency and severity of hot flashes can be reduced by avoiding things that increase heat production and by promoting heat loss. Keeping a cool environment and reducing caffeine and alcohol intake reduce heat production. Behavioral changes, such as relaxation techniques, also help. To promote heat loss at night when hot flashes can disrupt sleep, increasing air circulation in the room and avoiding bedding that traps the heat (e.g., heavy quilts) may help. Loose-fitting clothes do not retain body heat, as do clothes with tight necks and wrists. Cool cloths applied to flushed areas also aid heat loss. Daily intake of vitamin E in doses up to 600 IU may help reduce hot flashes.[12]

Dry skin can be improved by the use of moisturizing soaps and body lotions. Kegel exercises can decrease stress incontinence. Dyspareunia related to vaginal dryness can be managed with a water-soluble lubricant.

Improving nutrition, exercise, and sleep can improve anxiety and depression. Sleep may be improved by avoiding alcohol and controlling hot flashes. Stress reduction techniques can improve sleep by decreasing anxiety.

Hormonal Therapy. Hormone replacement therapy (HRT) includes estrogen for women without a uterus or estrogen and progesterone for women with a uterus. Some HRT regimens include low-dose testosterone to increase libido. HRT helps retard bone loss and may help prevent osteoporosis. HRT also minimizes atrophic changes to the genitourinary tissues. Although observational studies have suggested that estrogen replacement in women may reduce the risk of Alzheimer's disease, there are no definitive research findings to support the use of estrogen to prevent Alzheimer's disease.[13]

Known or suspected breast cancer is generally a contraindication to estrogen use.[14] In addition to known or suspected breast cancer, other absolute contraindications to HRT include abnormal vaginal bleeding, pregnancy, active thrombophlebitis, thromboembolic disorder, and liver dysfunction. Long-term use of HRT increases the risk for endometrial cancer, but this increased risk is decreased with 12 or more days of progesterone per month. The risk for endometrial cancer is present only in those women who still have a uterus. Some women will have an increase in hyperlipidemia with progesterone. However, this is not a contraindication to HRT. The lowest dose of progesterone is used, and serum lipid levels are monitored.

Many different regimens of HRT are available, from continuous combined estrogen-progesterone therapy to various sequential and cyclic patterns. The choice of using HRT or not, and if using, which regimen to use, is tailored to the individual woman. Factors for consideration include concern about cancer, previously used regimens, tolerance of hormonal side effects, and presence of perimenopausal symptoms (see Evidence-Based Practice box).

EVIDENCE-BASED PRACTICE
Hormone Replacement Therapy (HRT) and Coronary Artery Disease

Clinical Problem

Does long-term use of estrogen therapy prevent coronary artery disease?

Best Clinical Practice

- Combination estrogen-medroxyprogesterone (Prempro) does not have a protective effect for coronary artery disease.
- Prempro should not be prescribed to postmenopausal women for prevention of cardiovascular problems.
- Women taking Prempro have an increased risk of breast cancer and cardiovascular disease (myocardial infarction and stroke) but lower risk of fractures and colorectal cancer.
- Because of the differences in estrogen potency and product composition, the extent to which these findings can be generalized to other combination estrogen-progesterone products is not known.

Implications for Nursing Practice

- Based on their individual risk factors and health care needs, women should discuss the benefits and risks of using HRT with their health care provider.
- If a woman and her health care provider believe that the use of HRT is important to manage symptoms of menopause, the best recommendation is to use HRT on a short-term basis.
- Herb and dietary supplements may be used to reduce the symptoms of menopause (see Complementary and Alternative Therapies box on p. 1412).

Reference for Evidence

Writing Group for the Women's Health Initiative Investigators: Risks and benefits of estrogen plus progestin in healthy postmenopausal women: principal results from the Women's Health Initiative randomized controlled trial, *JAMA* 288:321, 2002.

The side effects of estrogen include nausea, fluid retention, headache, and breast enlargement. Side effects of progesterone include increased appetite, weight gain, irritability, depression, spotting, and breast tenderness. To minimize these unwanted side effects, the lowest possible dose of each should be used.

A commonly used estrogen preparation is 0.625 mg of conjugated estrogen (Premarin) daily. For symptom relief, a higher dose may be needed. To receive the protective benefit of progesterone, 5 to 10 mg of medroxyprogesterone (Provera) is indicated for 12 days of each month on a cyclic regimen or 2.5 mg if on a continuous regimen. If the estrogen is to be increased for symptom relief, the progesterone should also be increased. Other forms of progesterone include norethindrone (Aygestin) and micronized progesterone (Prometrium). Estrogen comes in a variety of forms including oral tablets, vaginal creams, dermal patches, rings placed around the cervix, and subcutaneous pellets. Vaginal creams are especially useful for urogenital symptoms (e.g., dryness). Transdermal (skin patch) estrogen has the advantage of bypassing the liver, but has the disadvantage of causing skin irritation.

Selective estrogen receptor modulators (SERMs) are also used in treating menopausal problems. These drugs have some of the positive benefits of estrogen, such as preventing bone loss, without the negative effects such as endometrial hyperplasia. Raloxifene (Evista) competes with estrogen for estrogen receptor sites. It decreases bone loss and serum cholesterol but has minimal effects on breast and uterine tissue. SERMs are also discussed, with respect to their role in the management of osteoporosis, in Chapter 62.

Nutritional Therapy. Good nutrition can decrease the risk of cardiovascular disease and osteoporosis in addition to assisting with vasomotor symptoms. A daily intake of about 30 kcal/kg of body weight with maintenance of sound nutrition is recommended. A decrease in metabolic rate and careless eating habits can cause the weight gain and fatigue often attributed to menopause. An adequate intake of calcium and vitamin D helps maintain healthy bones and counteracts loss of bone density. Postmenopausal women who are not receiving supplemental estrogen should have a daily calcium intake of at least 1500 mg; those who are taking estrogen replacement need at least 1000 mg per day. Calcium supplements are best absorbed when taken with meals. Either dietary calcium or calcium supplements may be used (see Chapter 62, Tables 62-12 and 62-13).

The diet should be high in complex carbohydrates and vitamin B complex, especially B$_6$. Phytoestrogens from plant sources have been shown to be beneficial in some women.[15] Examples of foods containing phytoestrogens include soy, tofu, chick peas, and sunflower seeds. Herbal remedies have become popular in treating menopausal symptoms (see Complementary and Alternative Therapies box). Consultation with an experienced herbal practitioner is recommended before initiating therapy. Many herbs can cause serious adverse effects.[11]

■ Culturally Competent Care: Menopause

Nurses must be aware of the differences in attitudes and beliefs regarding menopause among women from various ethnic backgrounds. Menopause is a significant milestone in a woman's life. The way in which she approaches this life change is embedded in her own personality and her culture. American culture is

COMPLEMENTARY & ALTERNATIVE THERAPIES
Herbs and Supplements for Menopause

Phytoestrogens

Phytoestrogens are found in plants and may act similar to estrogen produced naturally in the body. The food that is richest in phytoestrogens is soybeans.

Clinical Uses

Menopausal symptoms such as hot flashes, night sweats, insomnia, mood swings, dry skin, and vaginal mucosa

Effects

Soy: May lower cholesterol, decrease hot flashes, and promote bone strength.

Black cohosh: Reduces hot flashes; possible positive effect on bone and cardiovascular health and mood. Can cause minor upset stomach. May interact with antihypertensive medication. Large amounts may cause toxicity.

Dong quai: Chinese herb promoted as being able to reduce hot flashes and improve cardiovascular health. May be toxic. Increases the effects of oral anticoagulants. Can cause photosensitivity.

Nursing Implications

- Women who have had a history of breast cancer should consult with their health care provider before using any of these herbs and supplements.
- Increasing consumption of soy products in the diet appears to be an effective treatment modality for postmenopausal women.

COMPLEMENTARY & ALTERNATIVE THERAPIES
Valerian

Clinical Uses

Insomnia, anxiety, restlessness, urinary tract disorders

Effects

Mild tranquilizer, muscle relaxant, sedative, or sleep aid. May cause hepatotoxicity when combined with other herbs such as skullcap or mistletoe.

Nursing Implications

Valerian should not be taken with alcohol, drugs that depress the central nervous system, or Antabuse. Valerian should not be used on a regular basis. Liver function should be assessed if used on a long-term basis.

---

generally negative toward aging and places a high value on youth. Many ethnic groups have their traditions and beliefs regarding childbirth and menopause. Research has found that African American women are more positive in attitude toward menopause than other ethnic groups.[16] African American women are more likely than white American women to experience hot flashes.[17] ■

NURSING MANAGEMENT
PERIMENOPAUSE AND POSTMENOPAUSE

Nurses can play a key role in helping women to understand perimenopausal changes and options to minimize unwanted symptoms. Women can decrease their risk for cardiovascular disease and osteoporosis. Nurses can foster a positive image of perimenopause as a time of vitality and attractiveness. Perimenopause can provide women with an incentive to enhance self-care.

Nurses should provide teaching and reassurance to perimenopausal women distraught by their symptoms. They should be taught that the symptoms are normal and only temporary. Nonpharmacologic approaches to managing symptoms should be discussed. The nurse should dispel misconceptions about menopause. This can reduce unnecessary anxiety.

A regular program of exercise and physical activity can improve circulation, maintain good muscle tone, and delay some aspects of aging for postmenopausal women. Regular aerobic exercise stimulates osteoblastic activity, thereby stimulating calcium deposition into bone and delaying osteoporosis.

Sexual function can continue with little change in the vast majority of postmenopausal women. Cessation of menstruation and ability to bear children should not be equated with cessation of sexual capability; in fact it may be liberating. Femininity and libido do not disappear with menopause. Atrophic changes in vaginal epithelium associated with decreased estrogen may lead to dyspareunia. A water-soluble lubricant (e.g., Replens, Astroglide, K-Y jelly) is often effective in managing this problem. An active sex life helps increase lubrication and maintains the pliability of vaginal tissues. The patient should be given an opportunity to candidly discuss concerns related to sexual functioning.

SEXUAL ASSAULT

Sexual assault is defined as the forcible perpetration of a sexual act on a person without his or her consent. It can include any of the following actions: sodomy, forced anal intercourse, oral copulation, forced copulation of mouth or anus of another, assault with a foreign object, and serial battery. Sexual assault can dramatically disrupt the roles normally performed by the adult woman.

Clinical Manifestations

Physical. Of the women who seek help immediately after the assault, between one half and two thirds will not have any evidence of physical trauma. Evidence of trauma may be limited because women do not resist for fear of physical danger and injury. When present, physical injuries may include bruising and lacerations to the perineum, hymen, vulva, vagina, cervix, and anus. Fractures, subdural hematomas, cerebral concussions, and intraabdominal injuries have resulted in the need for hospitalization. Sexual assault also places women at risk for sexually transmitted diseases (STDs) and pregnancy.

Psychologic. Immediately after the assault, women may show shock, numbness, denial, or withdrawal. Some women may seem unnaturally calm; others may cry or express anger. Feelings of humiliation, degradation, embarrassment, anger, self-blame, and fear of another assault are commonly expressed. These symptoms usually decrease after 2 weeks, and victims may appear to have adjusted. Yet any time from 2 to 3 weeks to months to years after the assault, symptoms may return and become more severe. The rape-trauma syndrome is a classification of posttraumatic stress disorder. Flashbacks, intrusive recall, sleep disturbances, and numbing of feelings are common initial symptoms. Women will feel embarrassment, self-blame, and powerlessness.

Later symptoms include mood swings, irritability, and anger. Feelings of despair, shame, and hopelessness are often the cause of the anger. These feelings may be internalized and expressed as depression. Suicidal ideations may also occur.

Collaborative Care

In the acute care of an assault survivor, ensuring the woman's emotional and physical safety has the highest priority. Table 52-8 outlines the emergency management of the patient who has been sexually assaulted. Most emergency departments (EDs) have identified personnel who have received special training in order to work with women who have been assaulted. Many crime-fighting agencies within communities have created the position of the Sexual Assault Nurse Examiner (SANE).[18] The SANE is a registered nurse who is certified to provide care to victims of sexual assault, while ensuring evidence is safeguarded. Special procedures are followed in taking the history and conducting the examination in order to preserve all evidence in case of future prosecution.

When the survivor of an assault is admitted to the ED or clinic, a specific chain of events occurs (Table 52-9). A signed informed consent is obtained from the woman before any data are collected. All materials gathered are well documented, labeled, and given to the appropriate person, such as the pathologist or a police officer. The materials are handled by as few people as possible, and signatures of all responsible for keeping and handling the data are obtained. Many items can be used as evidence if the victim chooses to file a complaint. Consequently, the integrity of the material must be maintained. The nurse's involvement in the medicolegal process depends on the policies of the individual institution and state law.

A gynecologic and sexual history and an account of the assault (who, what, when, and where), as well as a general physical and pelvic examination, add further information about the rape incident. Laboratory tests are done primarily to determine the presence of sperm in the vagina and to identify any existing STDs or pregnancy.

Follow-up physical and psychologic care is essential. Women should return weekly for the first month following the assault. This includes the time period when women's psychologic reactions may be the most severe. Providers should have the telephone numbers and names of contact persons for local resources for sexual assault survivors, including rape crisis centers, legal and law enforcement authorities, and human services.

NURSING MANAGEMENT
SEXUAL ASSAULT

Nurses can assist all women in becoming aware of prevention tactics (Table 52-10). They should also be encouraged to learn some basic techniques of self-defense. Local high schools and the

TABLE 52-8	Emergency Management — Sexual Assault	
ETIOLOGY	**ASSESSMENT FINDINGS**	**INTERVENTIONS**
Sexual molestation Sodomy Assault involving genitalia (male or female) without consent	• Emotional or physical manifestations of shock • Hysteria • Crying • Anger • Silence • Decreased level of consciousness • Hyperventilation • Oral, vaginal, and rectal injuries • Extragenital injuries • Pain in genital area or extragenital area	**Initial** • Treat shock and other urgent medical problems, (e.g., head injury, hemorrhage, wounds, fractures). • Assess emotional state. • Contact support person (i.e., social worker, rape advocate, sexual assault nurse examiner). • Do *not* clean the patient until all evidence is collected. Make sure the patient does not wash, douche, urinate, brush teeth, or gargle. • Place sheet on floor. Then have patient stand on sheet to remove clothing. Place sheet with clothing in paper bag. • Obtain forensic evidence per local protocol (i.e., body hair, nail scrapings, tissue, dried semen, vaginal washing, blood samples). • Maintain chain of evidence for all legal specimens. Clearly label evidence and keep in locked cabinet until given to law enforcement agency. • Obtain baseline HIV, syphilis, and other STD screening. • Determine method of contraception, date of last menstrual period, and date of last tetanus immunization. • Consider tetanus prophylaxis if lacerations contain soil/dirt. • Vaccinate with hepatitis B if not immunized. **Ongoing Monitoring** • Monitor vital signs and emotional status. • Provide clothing as needed. • Counsel patient regarding confidential HIV and STD testing.

HIV, Human immunodeficiency virus; *STD,* sexually transmitted disease.

TABLE 52-9   Evaluation of Alleged Sexual Assault

1. Medicolegal
Valid written consent for examination, photographs, laboratory tests, release of information, and laboratory samples
Appropriate "chain of evidence" documentation

2. History
History of assault (who, what, when, where)
Penetration, ejaculation, extragenital acts
Activities since assault (e.g., changed clothes, bathed, douched)
Inquire about safety
Menstrual and contraceptive history
Medical history
Emotional status
Current symptoms

3. General Physical Examination
Vital signs and general appearance
Extragenital trauma—mouth, breasts, neck
Cuts, bruises, scratches (photograph taken)

4. Pelvic Examination
Vulvar trauma, erythema; hymen, anal, and rectal status
Matted hairs or free hairs
Vaginal examination with unlubricated speculum for discharge, blood, lacerations
Uterine size
Adnexa, especially hematomas

5. Laboratory Samples
Vaginal vault content sampling
Vaginal smears—microscope evaluation for trichomonads and semen
Oral or rectal swabs and smears, if indicated
Blood samples—VDRL serology, pregnancy test; serologic testing for HIV and hepatitis B infection
Freeze serum sample for later testing
Cultures—cervix and other areas (if indicated) for gonorrhea and chlamydia
Fingernail scrapings
Pubic hair scrapings
Clipping of matted pubic hairs

6. Treatment
Care of injuries and emotional trauma
Prophylaxis for STDs, tetanus, and hepatitis B (see appropriate chapters)
Follow-up for pregnancy test in 2-3 wk (if appropriate)
Testing for HIV, syphilis, and hepatitis B may be done at 6-8 wk
Protection of legal rights
Recommendation of continued follow-up and services of rape crisis center

HIV, Human immunodeficiency virus; *STDs,* sexually transmitted diseases; *VDRL,* Venereal Disease Research Laboratory.

TABLE 52-10   Patient & Family Teaching Guide — Sexual Assault Prevention

1. See that there are lights at all entrances to your home.
2. Keep your doors locked and do not open them to a stranger; ask for identification if a service person comes to the door.
3. Do not advertise that you live alone; list only your initials with your last name in the telephone directory or on the mailbox; never reveal to a caller that you are home alone.
4. Avoid walking alone in deserted areas; walk to the parking lot with a friend; be sure you see each other leave.
5. Have your keys ready as you approach your car or home.
6. Keep all doors locked and windows up when driving.
7. Never get on an elevator with a suspicious person; pretend you have forgotten something and get off.
8. Say what you mean in social situations; be sure your voice and body language reflect your response.
9. Carry a loud whistle and use it when you think you are in danger.
10. Yell "fire" if you are attacked and run toward a lighted area.

the examinations that follow. The patient should not be left alone. Whenever possible, the same nurse should remain with her throughout her stay and provide needed emotional support. The patient's actions and words as she describes the incident may be inconsistent, confused, and inappropriate. The nurse should maintain a nonjudgmental attitude.

The patient usually has many feelings and thoughts about the assault and generally wants to talk about them to an interested listener. Talking may help the patient feel better and gain understanding of her reactions to the incident. When the nurse listens carefully, the patient feels that she is not alone and is better able to gain control over the situation.

The nurse should assess the patient's stress level before preparing her for the various procedures that will follow. The patient's coping mechanisms are supported when she knows what to expect and what is expected of her, as well as why the particular procedure must be done. Because the pelvic examination may trigger a flashback of the attack, the nurse should answer all related questions before the examination and be a supportive presence during the examination.

Following the examinations, the patient's physical comfort needs should be considered. She will need a change of clothing, because her original garments may be torn or soiled, or kept as evidence. Most women who have been sexually assaulted feel dirty and would appreciate a place to wash, as well as use a mouthwash, especially if oral sex was involved. Food and drink may also provide comfort to the victim.

Many sexual assault survivors are unaware of the availability of financial compensation (a law in most states) and appreciate information about the application process. This compensation is to assist them in paying for emergency services and for emotional injuries that may temporarily interfere with their ability to work.

When the patient is discharged, the nurse should make certain the patient has transportation home. If friends or family members

YWCA usually have self-defense classes in which formal instruction is given. Practicing the various techniques with a friend builds up a woman's confidence in her ability to fight back. Learning self-defense can make the woman less vulnerable and more self-reliant.

When a sexual assault survivor is brought to the clinic or ED, a quiet, private area should be used for the initial assessment and

are not available, the hospital or clinic should make arrangements with an appropriate community resource. The patient should not be sent home alone. The victim's partner and family have a tremendous potential for both negative and positive influence. They can "revictimize" her and increase her burden in resolving the sexual assault, or they can provide her with support and find support themselves in resolving a shared crisis.

Many communities today have crisis centers. These public service organizations have trained professional and nonprofessional volunteers who provide an emotional support system for survivors on request. Their programs provide advocacy to ensure dignified treatment throughout the medical and police procedures, short-term counseling for the woman and her family, and court assistance and public education on rape-related issues. The nurse should be able to give the patient the names and local telephone numbers of such organizations.

CONDITIONS OF THE VULVA, VAGINA, AND CERVIX

Etiology and Pathophysiology

Infection and inflammation of the vagina, cervix, and vulva tend to occur when the natural defenses of the acid vaginal secretions (maintained by sufficient estrogen levels) and the presence of *Lactobacillus* are disrupted. The woman's resistance may also be decreased as a result of aging, poor nutrition, and the use of drugs (e.g., antibiotics) that alter the bacterial flora or mucosa. Organisms gain entrance to the areas through contaminated hands, clothing, and douche tips and during intercourse, surgery, and childbirth. Table 52-11 relates the specific etiologic factors, clinical manifestations and diagnostic methods, and collaborative care of common inflammations and infections.

Most lower genital tract infections are related to sexual intercourse. Intercourse can transmit organisms, injure tissues, and alter the acid-base balance of the vagina. Vulvar infections caused by viruses such as herpes and genital warts can be sexually transmitted when no lesions are apparent. Oral contraceptives, antibiotics, and corticosteroids may produce changes in the vaginal pH and trigger an overgrowth of the organisms present. For example, *Candida albicans* may be present in small numbers in the vagina. An overgrowth of this organism causes vulvovaginitis.

Clinical Manifestations

Abnormal vaginal discharge and vulvar lesions are the two main clinical manifestations. In addition to a thick white curdy discharge, women with vulvovaginal candidiasis (VVC) often experience intense itching and dysuria, which is the result of urine coming into contact with fissures and irritated areas on the vulva. The hallmark of bacterial vaginosis is the fishy odor of

---

TABLE 52-11   Infections of the Lower Genital Tract

INFECTION/ETIOLOGY	CLINICAL MANIFESTATIONS AND DIAGNOSTIC METHODS	DRUG THERAPY
Vulvovaginal Candidiasis (VVC) (Monilial Vaginitis)		
Candida albicans (fungus)	Commonly found in mouth, gastrointestinal tract, and vagina; pruritus, thick white curdy discharge; KOH microscopic examination—pseudohyphae; pH 4.0-4.7	Antifungal agents (e.g., Monistat, Gyne-Lotrimin, Myclex [available over the counter]) available in cream or suppository
Trichomoniasis		
Trichomonas vaginalis (protozoa)	Sexually transmitted; pruritus; frothy greenish or gray discharge; hemorrhagic spots on cervix or vaginal walls; saline microscopic examination—swimming trichomonads; pH 5.0-7.0	Metronidazole (Flagyl) orally in single dose for patient and partner
Bacterial Vaginosis		
Gardnerella vaginalis *Corynebacterium vaginale*	Watery discharge with fishy odor; may or may not have other symptoms; saline microscopic examination—epithelial cells; pH 5.0-5.5	Sexually transmitted; metronidazole (Flagyl) 500 mg orally or clindamycin (Cleocin) 300 mg orally bid for 7 days; examine and treat partner
Cervicitis		
Chlamydia trachomatis *Neisseria gonorrhoeae* *Staphylococcus aureus*	Sexually transmitted; mucopurulent discharge with postcoital spotting from cervical inflammation; culture for chlamydia and gonorrhea	Azithromycin (Zithromax) PO single dose or doxycycline PO bid for 7 days and ciprofloxacin (Cipro) PO single dose or ceftriaxone (Rocephin) IM in single dose; treat partners with same drugs
Severe Recurrent Vaginitis		
Candida albicans (most often)	May be indication of HIV infection; all women who are unresponsive to first-line treatment should be counseled and offered HIV testing	Drug appropriate to opportunistic organism

HIV, Human immunodeficiency virus; *IM*, intramuscular.

the discharge. Women with cervicitis may notice spotting after intercourse.

Common vulvar lesions include herpes infection and genital warts. Initial or primary herpes infections may be extremely painful. Herpes begins as a small vesicle followed by a superficial red ulcer. Most herpes lesions are painful. Dysuria is common when urine touches the lesion. Genital warts, caused by the human papillomavirus, vary in appearance. Irregularly shaped "cauliflower" lesions are common. Genital warts are painless unless traumatized. (Herpes infection and genital warts are discussed in Chapter 51.)

Older women may develop gynecologic problems such as lichen sclerosis.[19] This condition is associated with intense itching. The lesions are white initially, although scratching produces changes in the appearance.

Collaborative Care

Genital problems are evaluated by taking a history, performing a physical examination, and obtaining the appropriate laboratory and diagnostic studies. Because many problems relate to sexual activity, a sexual history is essential. The nature of the problem directs specific aspects of the evaluation. Ulcerative lesions should be cultured for herpes. A blood test for syphilis may be done when ulcerative lesions are present. Genital warts are usually identified by their clinical appearance. Vulva dystrophies may be examined via colposcopy. A biopsy is taken for diagnosis.

Problems involving vaginal discharge are evaluated by microscopy and cultures. The most common vaginal conditions (bacterial vaginosis, VVC, and trichomoniasis) are diagnosed by a procedure called a *wet mount*. The findings characteristic of each condition are shown in Table 52-11. To assess for cervicitis, endocervical cultures are obtained for chlamydia and gonorrhea. If purulent discharge is observed coming from the cervix, a sample of endocervical cells may be taken to conduct a Gram stain. The Gram-stained slide is examined on high power to identify white blood cells and gram-negative diplococci (indicative of gonorrhea). (STDs are discussed in Chapter 51.)

Drug therapy is based on the diagnosis and is shown in Table 52-11.[20] Antibiotics taken as directed will cure bacterial infections. Antifungal preparations, usually creams, are indicated for VVC. Women with vaginal conditions or cervical infection should abstain from intercourse for at least 1 week. Douching should be avoided. Douching disrupts the normal protective mechanisms within the vagina and may force the pathogens higher into the genital tract. Sexual partners must be evaluated and treated if the patient is diagnosed with trichomoniasis, chlamydia, gonorrhea, or syphilis.

Treatment of vulvar dystrophies is symptomatic because no cures are available. Treatment involves controlling the itching and hence the scratching. Interrupting the "itch-scratch cycle" prevents further secondary damage to the skin.

NURSING MANAGEMENT
CONDITIONS OF THE VULVA, VAGINA, AND CERVIX

Nurses have the opportunity to teach women about common genital conditions and how to reduce their risks. Recognizing symptoms that indicate a problem helps women seek care in a timely manner. Discussing problems concerning one's genitals or sexual intercourse is frequently difficult. The nurse's nonjudgmental attitude makes women feel more comfortable and empowers them to ask questions seeking accurate information.

When a woman is diagnosed with a genital condition, the nurse should ensure that she fully understands the directions for treatment. Taking the full course of medication is especially important to decrease the chance of relapse. Because genitalia are such a private area, use of graphs and models is especially helpful for patient teaching. When a woman will be using a vaginal medication for the first time, showing her the applicator and how to fill it is important. The woman should be taught where and how the applicator should be inserted using visual aids or models. Vaginal creams should be inserted before going to bed so that the medication will remain in the vagina for a long period of time. Women using vaginal creams or suppositories may wish to use panty liners during the day, when the residual medication may drain out.

PELVIC INFLAMMATORY DISEASE

Pelvic inflammatory disease (PID) is an infectious condition of the pelvic cavity that may involve infection of the fallopian tubes (salpingitis), ovaries (oophoritis), and pelvic peritoneum (peritonitis). A tubo-ovarian abscess may also form. PID is referred to as "silent" when women do not perceive any symptoms. Other women with PID will be in acute distress.

Etiology and Pathophysiology

PID is often the result of untreated cervicitis. The organism infecting the cervix ascends higher into the uterus, fallopian tubes, ovaries, and peritoneal cavity (Fig. 52-5). *Chlamydia tra-*

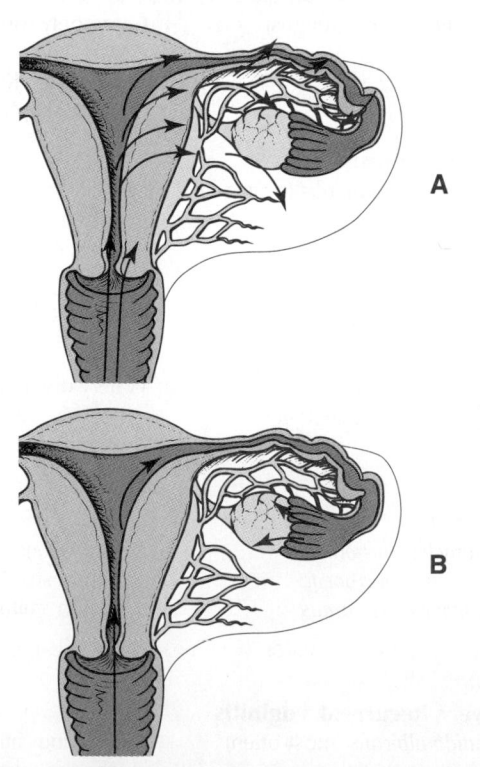

FIG. 52-5 Common routes of the spread of pelvic inflammatory disease. **A,** Direct spread of bacterial infection other than *Neisseria gonorrhoeae*. **B,** Direct spread of *Neisseria gonorrhoeae*.

chomatis and *Neisseria gonorrhoeae* are the most common causative organisms of PID. These organisms, as well as mycoplasma, streptococci, and anaerobes, gain entrance during sexual intercourse or after pregnancy termination, pelvic surgery, or childbirth. It is important to remember that not all cases of PID are the result of an STD.

Women at increased risk for chlamydia infections (younger than 24 years of age, have multiple sex partners, or a new sex partner) should be routinely tested for chlamydia. Chlamydial infections can be asymptomatic and unknowingly transmitted during intercourse. Silent PID can cause damage that cannot be reversed. PID remains a major cause of female infertility.

Clinical Manifestations

Women with PID usually go to a health care provider because they are experiencing lower abdominal pain. The pain typically starts gradually and is constant. The intensity may vary from mild to severe. Movement such as walking can increase the pain; pain is also frequently associated with intercourse. Spotting after intercourse and abnormal vaginal discharge are common. Fever and chills may also be present. Women with less acute symptoms notice increased cramping pain with menses, irregular bleeding, and some pain with intercourse. Women who have mild symptoms may go untreated either because they did not seek care or the health care provider misdiagnosed their complaints.

PID is a clinical diagnosis based on the patient's signs and symptoms. The diagnosis of PID is based on data obtained during the bimanual portion of the pelvic examination.[20] Women with PID have lower abdominal tenderness, bilateral adnexal tenderness, and positive cervical motion tenderness. Additional criteria useful for diagnosis include fever and abnormal discharge (vaginal or cervical). Cultures for gonorrhea and chlamydia are obtained from the endocervix. A pregnancy test should be done. Drug therapy begins when minimal diagnostic criteria are met, thus treatment is not delayed for culture results. When the patient's pain or obesity compromises the pelvic examination and a tubo-ovarian abscess may be present, a vaginal ultrasound is indicated. This patient meets the minimal criteria for diagnosing and treating PID. If a tubo-ovarian abscess is present, hospitalization is necessary.

Complications

Immediate complications of PID include septic shock and *Fitz-Hugh–Curtis syndrome,* which occurs when PID spreads to the liver and causes acute perihepatitis. The patient will have symptoms of right upper quadrant pain, but liver function tests will be normal. Pelvic and tubo-ovarian abscesses may "leak" or rupture, resulting in pelvic or generalized peritonitis. As the general circulation is flooded with bacterial endotoxins from the infected areas, septic shock may result. Embolisms may occur as the result of thrombophlebitis of the pelvic veins.

Long-term complications include ectopic pregnancy, infertility, and chronic pelvic pain. PID can cause adhesions and strictures to develop in the fallopian tubes. Ectopic pregnancy may result when a tube is partially obstructed because the sperm can pass through the stricture but the fertilized ovum cannot reach the uterus. After one episode of PID, the risk of having an ectopic pregnancy increases tenfold. Further damage can obstruct the fallopian tubes and cause infertility.

Collaborative Care

PID is usually treated on an outpatient basis. The patient is given a combination of antibiotics such as cefoxitin (Mefoxin) and doxycycline (Vibramycin) to provide broad coverage against the causative organisms. With effective antibiotic therapy, the pain should subside. The patient must have no intercourse for 3 weeks. Her partner(s) must be examined and treated. An important part of care is physical rest and oral fluids. Reevaluation in 48 to 72 hours, even if symptoms are improving, is an essential part of outpatient care.

If outpatient treatment is unsuccessful or if the patient is acutely ill or in severe pain, admission to the hospital is indicated. Maximum doses of parenteral antibiotics are given in the hospital. Some providers believe that the addition of corticosteroids to the antibiotic regimen reduces the inflammation, allowing for faster recovery and improvement in subsequent fertility. Application of heat to the lower abdomen or sitz baths may be used to improve circulation and decrease pain. Bed rest in the semi-Fowler position promotes drainage of the pelvic cavity by gravity and may prevent the development of abscesses high in the abdomen. Analgesics to relieve pain and IV fluids to prevent dehydration are also prescribed.

An indication for surgery is the presence of abscesses that fail to resolve with IV antibiotics. The abscess may be drained by laparoscopy or laparotomy. In extreme cases, a hysterectomy may be performed. When surgery is necessary, the capacity for childbearing is preserved whenever possible.

NURSING MANAGEMENT
PELVIC INFLAMMATORY DISEASE

Subjective and objective data that should be obtained from the woman with PID are presented in Table 52-12. Prevention, early recognition, and prompt treatment of vaginal and cervical infections can help prevent PID and its serious complications. Nurses can provide accurate information about factors that place a woman at increased risk for PID. Nurses should urge women to seek medical attention for any unusual vaginal discharge or possible infection of their reproductive organs. Women should be helped to understand that not all discharge is indicative of infection, but that early diagnosis and treatment of an infection, if present, can prevent serious complications. Women should be informed of the methods to decrease the risk of getting STDs and to recognize the signs of infection in their partner(s).

The patient may have guilt feelings about having PID, especially if it was associated with an STD. She may also be concerned about the complications associated with PID, such as adhesions and strictures of the fallopian tubes, infertility, and the increased incidence of ectopic pregnancy. Discussion with the patient regarding her feelings and concerns can assist her to cope more effectively with them.

For patients requiring hospitalization, nurses have an important role in implementing drug therapy, monitoring the patient's health status, and providing symptom relief and patient teaching. Vital signs and the character, amount, color, and odor of the vaginal discharge should be recorded. Explanations about the need for limited activity, being in a semi-Fowler position, and increased fluid intake should increase patient cooperation. Assessing the degree of abdominal pain will provide information about the effectiveness of drug therapy.

TABLE 52-12	Nursing Assessment
	Pelvic Inflammatory Disease

Subjective Data

Important Health Information

Past health history: Use of IUD; previous PID, gonorrhea, or chlamydia; multiple sexual partners; exposure to partner with urethritis; infertility

Medications: Use of and allergy to any antibiotics

Surgery or other treatments: Recent abortion or pelvic surgery

Functional Health Patterns

Health perception-health management: Malaise

Nutritional-metabolic: Nausea, vomiting; chills

Elimination: Urinary frequency, urgency

Cognitive-perceptual: Lower abdominal and pelvic pain; low back pain; pain on fundal palpation and cervical motion; onset of pain just after a menstrual cycle; dysmenorrhea, dyspareunia, dysuria, vulvar pruritus

Sexuality-reproductive: Abnormal vaginal bleeding and menstrual irregularity; vaginal discharge

Objective Data

General

Fever

Reproductive

Mucopurulent cervicitis, vulvar maceration, vaginal discharge (heavy and purulent to thin and mucoid), tenderness on motion of cervix and uterus; presence of inflammatory masses on palpation

Possible Findings

Leukocytosis; ↑ erythrocyte sedimentation rate; positive culture of secretions or endocervical fluid; pelvic inflammation and positive endometrial biopsy on laparoscopic examination; abscess or inflammation on ultrasonography

IUD, Intrauterine device; *PID,* pelvic inflammatory disease.

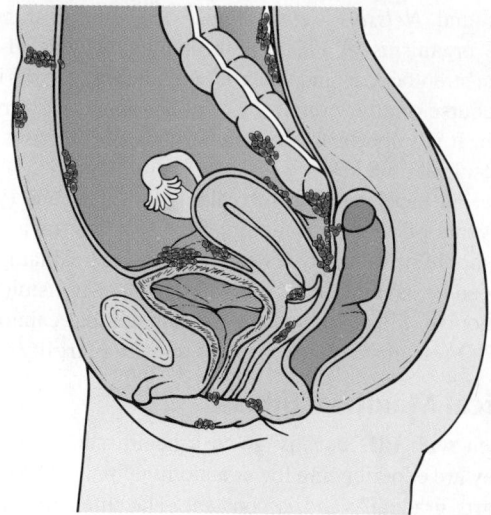

FIG. 52-6 Common sites of endometriosis.

ENDOMETRIOSIS

Endometriosis is the presence of normal endometrial tissue in sites outside the endometrial cavity. The most frequent sites are in or near the ovaries, the uterosacral ligaments, and the uterovesical peritoneum (Fig. 52-6). However, endometrial tissues can be in many other locations such as the stomach, lungs, intestines, and spleen. The tissue responds to the hormones of the ovarian cycle and undergoes a "mini–menstrual cycle" similar to the uterine endometrium.

Endometriosis is found equally among whites and African Americans, but is slightly more prevalent in Asian women. It occurs across all socioeconomic groups. However, most typically, the patient with endometriosis will be in her late twenties or early thirties, white, and never had a full-term pregnancy. Although it is not a life-threatening condition, endometriosis is responsible for considerable pain and loss of work time. Endometriosis is found in 5% to 10% of women of reproductive age.[21]

Etiology and Pathophysiology

The etiology is not well understood, and many theories about the cause of endometriosis have been proposed. A widely held view is that retrograde menstrual flow passes through the fallopian tubes carrying viable endometrial tissues into the pelvis. The tissue attaches to various sites shown in Fig. 52-6. Another theory suggests that undifferentiated embryonic peritoneal cavity cells remain dormant in the pelvic tissue until the ovaries produce sufficient hormones to stimulate their growth. Other proposed causes are a genetic predisposition and altered immune function.

Clinical Manifestations

In patients with endometriosis a wide range of clinical manifestations and severity exists. The magnitude of a woman's symptoms does not necessarily correlate with the clinical extent of her endometriosis. Dysmenorrhea after years of relatively pain-free menses and infertility may serve as clues to the presence of endometriosis. The most common manifestations are secondary dysmenorrhea, infertility, pelvic pain, dyspareunia, and irregular bleeding. Less common manifestations include backache, painful bowel movements, and dysuria. These symptoms may or may not correspond to the woman's menstrual cycles. With menopause, estrogen is no longer produced in the ovaries. This may lead to the disappearance of the symptoms.

When the ectopic endometrial tissues "menstruate," the blood collects in cystlike nodules that have a characteristic bluish black color. Nodules in the ovaries are sometimes called *chocolate cysts* because of the thick, chocolate-colored material they contain. When a cyst ruptures, the pain may be acute and the resulting irritation promotes the formation of adhesions, which fix the affected area to another pelvic structure. The adhesions may become severe enough to cause a bowel obstruction or painful micturition. Adhesions involving the uterus, tubes, or ovaries may result in infertility.

Collaborative Care

Endometriosis may be suspected from a woman's history of the characteristic symptoms and the health care provider's palpation of firm nodular lumps in the adnexa on bimanual examination. However, laparoscopy is necessary for a definitive diagnosis. The treatment of endometriosis is influenced by the patient's age, desire for pregnancy, symptom severity, and extent and location of the disease. When symptoms are not disruptive, a watch and wait approach is used. When endometriosis is identified as a probable cause of infertility, therapy proceeds more rapidly.

Surgical Therapy. The only cure for endometriosis is surgical removal of all the endometrial implants. Surgical therapy may be conservative or definitive. Conservative surgery is done to confirm the diagnosis or to remove implants. It involves removal or destruction of endometrial implants and lysing or excision of adhesions by means of laparoscopic laser surgery or laparotomy. Gonadotropin-releasing hormone (GnRH) agonist therapy (e.g., leuprolide [Lupron]) can be administered for 4 to 6 months to reduce the size of the lesions before surgery. By reducing the extent of the surgery, this preoperative drug treatment helps reduce the development of adhesions that may further threaten fertility.

For women wishing to get pregnant, conservative surgical therapy is used to remove implants blocking the fallopian tube. Adhesions are removed from the tubes, ovaries, and pelvic structures. Efforts are made to conserve all tissues necessary to maintain fertility.

Definitive surgery involves removal of the uterus, tubes, ovaries, and as many endometrial implants as possible. The individual woman should be actively involved in making the decision about preserving part or all of her ovaries, if surgically possible. Her feelings about maintaining her cyclic ovarian function need to be explored. The health care provider should assess the woman's risk for ovarian cancer and provide this information for her consideration.

Drug Therapy. Drug therapy is used to reduce symptoms. Drugs are selected to inhibit estrogen production by the ovary so that the endometrial tissue will shrink. The various drugs used imitate a state of pregnancy or menopause. Continuous use (for 9 months) of combined oral contraceptives causes regression of endometrial tissue. Ovulation is suppressed and *pseudopregnancy* (hyperhormonal amenorrhea) is produced by progestin agents such as Depo-Provera. Another approach to hormonal treatment is danazol (Danocrine), a synthetic androgen that inhibits the anterior pituitary. This drug produces a *pseudomenopause* (ovarian suppression) with atrophy of ectopic endometrial tissue. Subjective relief of symptoms is noted within 6 weeks of danazol use. Side effects include weight gain, acne, hot flashes, and hirsutism. These side effects and the expense of this drug restrict its use.

Another class of drugs used is GnRH agonists (e.g., leuprolide [Lupron], nafarelin [Synarel]). These drugs cause a hypoestrogenic state resulting in amenorrhea. The side effects reported by patients are usually the same as menopause (hot flashes, vaginal dryness, and emotional lability). Loss of bone density has also been reported in women who remain on the therapy longer than 6 months. Endometriosis is controlled but not cured by hormonal therapy. Persistent lesions give rise to subsequent recurrences once the menstrual cycle is reestablished.

NURSING MANAGEMENT
ENDOMETRIOSIS

Education of the patient and reassurance that a life-threatening situation does not exist may permit her to accept a conservative and progressive treatment. When the symptoms are less severe, teaching about nondrug comfort measures may be helpful. Nurses need to assist patients to understand the drugs that have been ordered to treat their condition. The action of the prescribed drug should be explained, as well as the possible side effects. Psychologic support may be needed for women experiencing severe disabling pain, sexual difficulties secondary to dyspareunia, and infertility.

If conservative surgery is the treatment selected, the nursing care is similar to the general preoperative and postoperative care of a patient undergoing laparotomy (see Chapter 41, p. 1063). If definitive surgery is planned, the nursing care is similar to the patient undergoing an abdominal **hysterectomy** (surgical removal of the uterus) (NCP 52-1). The nurse must know the extent of the procedure so that appropriate preoperative teaching can be done.

Benign Tumors of the Female Reproductive System

LEIOMYOMAS

Etiology and Pathophysiology

Leiomyomas (uterine fibroids) are benign smooth-muscle tumors that occur within the uterus. Leiomyomas are the most common benign tumors of the female genital tract (Fig. 52-7). By 30 years of age, 10% of white women and 30% of African American women have uterine leiomyomas. The cause of leiomyomas is unknown. They appear to depend on ovarian hormones because they grow slowly during the reproductive years and undergo atrophy after menopause.

Clinical Manifestations

The majority of women with leiomyomas do not have any symptoms. Of the women who develop symptoms, the most common include abnormal uterine bleeding, pain, and symptoms associated with pelvic pressure. Increased bleeding is thought to be associated with increased endometrial surface area that is associated with leiomyomas. Pain is thought to be associated with infection or twisting of the pedicle from which the tumor is growing. Devascularization and blood vessel compression are also thought to contribute to pain. Pressure on surrounding organs may result in rectal, bladder, and lower abdominal discomfort. Large tumors may

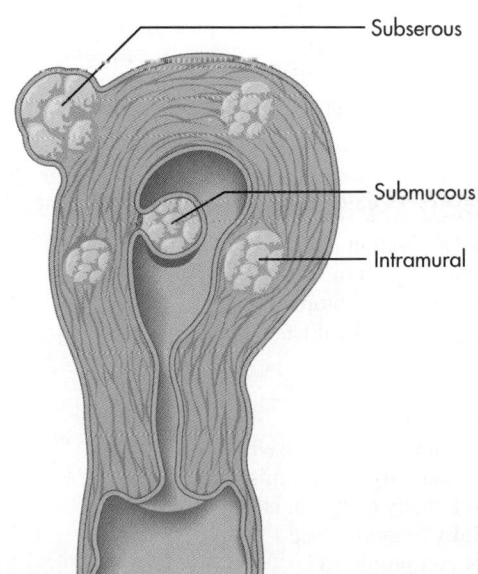

FIG. 52-7 Leiomyomas. Uterine section showing whorl-like appearance and locations of leiomyomas, which are also called *uterine fibroids*.

NURSING CARE PLAN 52-1

Patient with Abdominal Hysterectomy

NURSING DIAGNOSIS **Acute pain** *related to* incision and manipulation of internal organs *as manifested by* statements about pain, guarding of incision, reluctance to ambulate, and facial grimacing.

OUTCOMES–NOC	INTERVENTIONS–NIC and *RATIONALES*
Pain Control (1605)	*Pain Management (1400)*
• Reports pain control _____	• Perform a compressive assessment of pain to include location, characteristics, onset/duration, frequency, quality, intensity or severity, and precipitating factors *to plan appropriate interventions and establish a baseline pain level.*
• Uses preventive measures _____	
• Uses analgesics appropriately _____	• Use therapeutic communication strategies *to acknowledge the pain experience and convey acceptance of the patient's response to pain.*
	• Use pain control measures before pain becomes severe by providing medication at a given intensity level that has been decided with the patient before having pain *so that appropriate medications and dosages can be used.*
Outcome Scale	• Teach the use of nonpharmacologic techniques, such as splinting the incision with a pillow when coughing or moving and/or relaxation techniques, *to help minimize pain.*
1 = Never demonstrated	*Medication Administration (2300)*
2 = Rarely demonstrated	
3 = Sometimes demonstrated	• Give medication using appropriate technique and route *to provide the appropriate relief of pain.*
4 = Often demonstrated	
5 = Consistently demonstrated	• Document medication administration and patient responsiveness.

NURSING DIAGNOSIS **Disturbed body image** *related to* perceived loss of femininity and future inability to conceive *as manifested by* crying, weeping, depression; verbalization of perceived loss of femininity and/or ability to conceive.

OUTCOMES–NOC	INTERVENTIONS–NIC and *RATIONALES*
Sexual Identify: Acceptance (1207)	*Body Image Enhancement (5220)*
• Affirmation of self as a sexual being _____	• Determine patient's body image expectations based on developmental stage *to establish need and plan for interventions.*
• Challenges negative images of sexual self _____	• Assist patient to discuss changes caused by surgery, as appropriate, *to clarify any misunderstandings.*
	• Determine patient's and family's perceptions of the alteration in body image versus reality *to provide accurate facts and decrease fear of consequences of hysterectomy.*
Outcome Scale	• Identify support groups available to patient *to minimize emotional impact of hysterectomy through open discussion.*
1 = Never demonstrated	
2 = Rarely demonstrated	
3 = Sometimes demonstrated	• Assist the patient to discuss stressors affecting body image due to surgery (e.g., surgical menopause) *so patient is informed about possible treatment* (e.g., hormone replacement therapy).
4 = Often demonstrated	
5 = Consistently demonstrated	

NURSING DIAGNOSIS **Urinary retention** *related to* loss of bladder tone, uncomfortable urinating position, and pain *as manifested by* patient's statement, "I can't pass my water when I feel I need to," distention of bladder, and voiding small amounts.

OUTCOMES–NOC	INTERVENTIONS–NIC and *RATIONALES*
Urinary Elimination (0503)	*Urinary Retention Care (0620)*
• Elimination pattern IER _____	• Monitor intake and output *to determine if satisfactory fluid balance is maintained.*
• Empties bladder completely _____	
• Urine passes without hesitancy _____	• Monitor degree of bladder distention by palpation and percussion *to detect distention.*
	• Provide time for bladder emptying while providing patient's privacy *to assist urinary flow.*
Outcome Scale	• Catheterize *to determine amount of residual,* as appropriate.
1 = Extremely compromised	• Provide Credé maneuver, as necessary, *to help flow of urine.*
2 = Substantially compromised	• Stimulate the bladder by applying cold to the abdomen, stroking the inner thigh, running water, and providing the patient with an upright position to void, as appropriate, *to allow for bladder emptying.*
3 = Moderately compromised	
4 = Mildly compromised	
5 = Not compromised	

IER, In expected range.

cause a general enlargement of the lower abdomen. These tumors are sometimes associated with miscarriage and infertility.

Collaborative Care

Clinical diagnosis is based on the characteristic pelvic findings of an enlarged uterus distorted by nodular masses. Treatment depends on the symptoms, the age of the patient, her desire to bear children, and the location and size of the tumor or tumors. If the symptoms are minor, the provider may elect to follow the patient closely for a time. If the woman is experiencing menorrhagia, the use of aspirin is discouraged because of its effect on platelets.

Persistent heavy menstrual bleeding causing anemia and large or rapidly growing tumors are indications for surgery. The leiomyomas are removed by hysterectomy or myomectomy. A myomectomy is performed for women who wish to have children. In this case, only the fibroids are removed to preserve the uterus. Small tumors may be removed using a hysteroscope and laser resection instruments.[22] Embolization of the fibroid blood supply and cryosurgery are other options. In cases of large leiomyomas, a GnRH agonist (e.g., leuprolide [Leupron]) may be used preoperatively to shrink the size of the tumor. However, the risks and benefits of this drug should be fully discussed, including the potential for irreversible loss of bone mass.

CERVICAL POLYPS

Cervical polyps are benign pedunculated lesions that generally arise from the endocervical mucosa and are seen protruding through the cervical os during a speculum examination. Polyps are a characteristic bright cherry red and are soft and fragile in consistency. They are generally small, measuring less than 3 cm in length, and may be single or multiple. Their cause is unknown. Symptoms are usually not present, but metrorrhagia and bleeding after straining and coitus can occur. Polyps are prone to infection. When the polyp is small, it can be excised in an outpatient procedure. If the point of attachment of the polyp cannot be identified and is not accessible to cautery, a polypectomy is performed in an operating room. All tissue removed is sent for pathologic review because polyps occasionally undergo malignant changes.

BENIGN OVARIAN TUMORS

There are many different types of benign tumors. The cause of most of them is unknown. They can be divided into cysts and neoplasms. *Cysts* are usually soft, surrounded by a thin capsule, and may be detected during the reproductive years (Fig. 52-8). Follicle and corpus luteum cysts are common ovarian cysts. Multiple small ovarian follicles may occur in a condition called *polycystic ovary syndrome* (PCOS) (discussed in the next section). Epithelial ovarian neoplasms may be cystic or solid, small or extremely large. Cystic teratomas, or dermoid cysts, originate from germ cells and can contain bits of any type of body tissue, such as hair or teeth.

Ovarian masses are often asymptomatic until they are large enough to cause pressure in the pelvis. Constipation, menstrual irregularities, urinary frequency, a full feeling in the abdomen, anorexia, and peripheral edema may occur, depending on the size and location of the tumor. There may be an increase in abdominal girth. Pelvic pain may be present if the tumor is growing rapidly. Severe pain results when the cyst twists on its pedicle (ovarian torsion).

Pelvic examination reveals a mass or an enlarged ovary that demands further investigation. If the mass is cystic and smaller

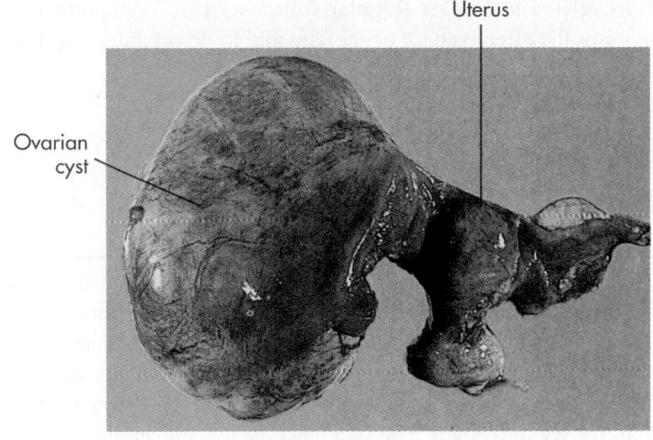

FIG. 52-8 Large ovarian cyst.

than 8 cm, the patient is asked to return for reexamination in 4 to 6 weeks. If the mass is cystic and greater than 8 cm or is solid, laparoscopic surgery or laparotomy is performed. Immediate surgery is necessary if ovarian torsion occurs, causing the ovary to rotate and cutting off circulation. Surgical techniques are used to save as much of the ovary as possible.

Polycystic Ovary Syndrome

Polycystic ovary syndrome (PCOS), also known as Stein-Leventhal syndrome, is a chronic disorder in which many benign cysts form on the ovaries. It most commonly occurs in women under 30 years old. It affects about 5% of women of reproductive age. PCOS is caused by increased production of LH and decreased FSH. This imbalance prevents the ovaries from releasing an egg each month. The ovaries produce estrogen and excess testosterone but not progesterone. Small cysts develop in the ovaries related to chronic failure of the ovaries to release eggs. Recent research suggests a familial or genetic basis and a close association with obesity.[23]

Clinical manifestations include irregular menstrual periods (particularly long cycles), amenorrhea or oligomenorrhea, dysfunctional uterine bleeding, infertility, hirsutism, obesity, and acne. Many start with normal menstrual periods and then, after 1 to 2 years, the periods become irregular and then infrequent. If left untreated, cardiovascular disease, abnormal insulin metabolism with type 2 diabetes mellitus, and ovarian and endometrial cancers may develop.

Successful management includes early diagnosis and treatment to improve quality of life and decrease the risk of complications. Pelvic ultrasound will reveal enlarged ovaries with multiple small cysts. Oral contraceptives are useful in regulating menstrual cycles.

Hyperandrogenism can be treated with flutamide (Eulexin) and a GnRH agonist such as leuprolide (Lupron). Metformin (Glucophage) has been shown to improve hyperandrogenism and restore ovulation. For women desiring to become pregnant, fertility drugs (e.g., clomiphene [Clomid]) may be used to induce ovulation. If all other treatments are unsuccessful, a hysterectomy with bilateral salpingectomy and oophorectomy may be performed.

Patient teaching for the patient with PCOS includes the importance of weight management. Obesity exacerbates the problems related to PCOS. Regular follow-up care is important to monitor the effectiveness of therapy and to detect any complications such as ovarian or endometrial cancer.

Cancer of the Female Reproductive System

CERVICAL CANCER

In 2002 approximately 13,000 women in the United States had invasive cervical cancer and 4100 women died from cervical cancer. Noninvasive cervical cancer is about four times more common than invasive cervical cancer.[24] The mortality rate for cervical cancer is twice as high for African American women than for white women. The incidence is also higher among Hispanic women than white women. An increased risk of cervical cancer is associated with low socioeconomic status, early sexual activity (before 17 years of age), multiple sexual partners, infection with human papillomavirus, and smoking.[25]

The number of deaths from cervical cancer has fallen steadily over the past 40 years. This is attributable to better and earlier diagnosis with the widespread use of the Papanicolaou (Pap) test. In addition to cancer, the Pap test detects precancerous changes. By treating precancerous lesions, progression to cervical cancer can be prevented. The American Cancer Society recommends annual Pap tests beginning with the onset of sexual activity. After three negative Pap tests, less frequent tests may be recommended by the health care provider.

Etiology and Pathophysiology

The progression from normal cervical cells to dysplasia and then to cervical cancer appears to be related to repeated injuries to the cervix. The progression occurs slowly over years rather than months. There is a relationship between certain subtypes of human papillomavirus (HPV) and cervical cancer.[25] However, a cofactor such as smoking is thought to be needed in addition to the specific subtype of HPV. Women who smoke have a 50% higher risk for developing cervical cancer than nonsmokers. This risk is greatest in those with longer duration of smoking, increased number of cigarettes smoked, and use of unfiltered cigarettes.[24]

CULTURAL & ETHNIC CONSIDERATIONS
Cancer of the Female Reproductive System

- Japanese women have a low incidence of ovarian cancer. However, second- and third-generation Japanese women in the United States have much higher rates, similar to those of white women born in the United States. Dietary practices may explain this difference.
- Although the incidence of endometrial cancer is higher for white women and African American women, the mortality rate for African American women is nearly twice as high as that for white women.
- Cervical cancer has a higher incidence among Hispanic, African American, and Native American women than white women.
- Mortality rates from cervical cancer are more than twice as high among African American women as among white women.

Clinical Manifestations

Precancerous changes are asymptomatic. This highlights the importance of routine screening. The peak incidence of noninvasive cervical cancer is in women in their early thirties. The average age for women with invasive cervical cancer is 50. Early cervical cancer is generally asymptomatic, but leukorrhea and intermenstrual bleeding eventually occur. The discharge is usually thin and watery but becomes dark and foul smelling as the disease advances, suggesting the presence of an infection. The vaginal bleeding is initially only spotting, but as the tumor enlarges, it becomes heavier and more frequent. Pain is a late symptom and is followed by weight loss, anemia, and cachexia.

Diagnostic Studies

The Pap test, the Schiller iodine test, colposcopy, and biopsy are used to diagnose cervical cancer. These diagnostic tests are described in Chapter 49. Various classification systems are used to interpret the cytologic findings. The current trend is to use the Bethesda system because it improves accuracy and quality of diagnosis by standardizing diagnostic reports (Table 52-13). Pap tests are less than 100% accurate. There are problems with both

---

TABLE 52-13 Bethesda Classification System for Reporting Pap Test Results

Negative for Intraepithelial Lesion or Malignancy
Organisms
- *Trichomonas vaginalis*
- Fungal organisms morphologically consistent with *Candida* species
- Shift in flora suggestive of bacterial vaginosis
- Bacteria morphologically consistent with *Actinomyces* species
- Cellular changes consistent with herpes simplex virus
Other nonneoplastic findings
- Reactive cellular changes associated with inflammation, radiation, or intrauterine contraceptive device
- Glandular cells status posthysterectomy
- Atrophy

Epithelial Cell Abnormalities
Squamous cell
- Atypical squamous cells (ASC) of undetermined significance (ASC-US) cannot exclude HSIL (ASC-H)
- Low-grade squamous intraepithelial lesion (LSIL) encompassing: human papillomavirus/mild dysplasia/cervical intraepithelial neoplasia (CIN) 1
- High-grade squamous intraepithelial lesion (HSIL) encompassing: moderate and severe dysplasia, carcinoma in situ; CIN 2 and CIN 3
- Squamous cell carcinoma
Glandular cell
- Atypical glandular cells (AGC)
- Atypical glandular cells, favor neoplastic
- Endocervical adenocarcinoma in situ (AIS)
- Adenocarcinoma

Other
Endometrial cells in a woman ≥40 years of age

Source: Solomon D et al: The 2001 Bethesda System: terminology for reporting results of cervical cytology, *JAMA* 287:2114, 2002.

false-positive and false-negative reports. New techniques for cervical cancer screening are being explored. A new technique for Pap smears, Thin Prep, has reduced the amount of equivocal or limited Pap smear results. Recent research indicates that HPV testing may be more effective than the Pap test in identifying patients at risk for cervical cancer.[26]

Collaborative Care

The finding of an abnormal Pap smear indicates the need for follow-up. The type of follow-up depends on the findings. Women with minor changes may be followed with a repeated Pap test in 3 to 4 months. Up to 80% may revert to normal spontaneously. Women with more prominent changes will receive additional procedures, such as colposcopy and biopsy, before a definitive diagnosis can be made. Colposcopy involves examination of the cervix with a binocular microscope with low levels of magnification (10× to 40×). The procedure helps in the identification of possible epithelial abnormalities and suggests areas for biopsy. Biopsies are sent to pathology for evaluation. Colposcopy and biopsy have improved diagnosis and allow more focused treatments to be selected.

The type and extent of the biopsy vary with the abnormality seen. A punch biopsy may be done on an outpatient basis with special punch biopsy forceps. The excision of a cone-shaped section of the cervix may be used for both diagnosis and treatment. Conization is accomplished using one of several techniques. The choice of procedure is determined by the health care provider's experience and the availability of equipment. Cryotherapy (freezing) and laser cone vaporization destroy the tissue. Laser cone excision and loop electrosurgery excision procedure (LEEP) remove the identified tissue and allow for histologic examination to ensure that all microinvasive tissue has been removed. These procedures can be performed in the office with mild analgesics or sedation. Complications of these procedures include excessive bleeding and possible cervical stenosis after healing.

Treatment of cancer of the cervix is guided by the stage of the tumor and the patient's age and general state of health (Table 52-14). There are four procedures in which fertility can be preserved. Conization may be the only type of therapy needed for noninvasive cervical cancer if analysis of removed tissue demonstrates that a wide area of normal tissue surrounds the excised tissue. Laser treatments can be used in which a directed infrared beam is employed to destroy abnormal tissue. Alternatively, cautery and cryosurgery may also be used.

Invasive cancer of the cervix is treated with surgery, radiation, or a combination of the two. Surgical procedures include hysterectomy, radical hysterectomy (involving adjacent structures), and, rarely, pelvic exenterations. (Surgical therapy is discussed on pp. 1426-1428.) Radiation may be external (e.g., cobalt) or internal (e.g., cesium, radium). Standard radiation treatment is 4 to 6 weeks of external radiation followed with one or two treatments with internal implants. (Radiation therapy is discussed in Chapter 15.)

ENDOMETRIAL CANCER

Cancer of the endometrium is the most common gynecologic malignancy, accounting for nearly 50% of female genital tract neoplasms. Approximately 39,300 newly diagnosed cases of endometrial cancer and 6600 deaths occur each year. Endometrial cancer has a relatively low mortality rate, with a survival rate of 94% if the cancer has not spread at the time of diagnosis.[27] About 25% of the cases of endometrial cancer are diagnosed before women reach menopause. The average age at the time of diagnosis is 61 years old.[27]

TABLE 52-14	International Classification of Clinical Stages of Cervical Cancer	
STAGE	**EXTENT**	**TREATMENT**
Stage 0	In situ, intraepithelial	Cervical conization, total hysterectomy, cryosurgery, laser surgery
Stage I	Strict confinement to cervix (no consideration of extension to corpus)	
Stage IA	Microinvasive (early stromal invasion)	Radiation or surgery
Stage IB	All other cases of stage I	Radiation, Wertheim's hysterectomy
Stage II	Extension beyond cervix but not to pelvic wall, involvement of vagina, but not as far as lower third	
Stage IIA	No obvious parametrial involvement	Radiation, Wertheim's hysterectomy
Stage IIB	Obvious parametrial involvement	Radiation; if this fails, pelvic exenteration may be required
Stage III	Extension to pelvic wall, no cancer-free space between tumor and pelvic wall on rectal examination, involvement of lower third of vagina, hydronephrosis or nonfunctioning kidney	Radiation
Stage IIIA	No extension to pelvic wall	
Stage IIIB	Extension to pelvic wall or hydronephrosis or nonfunctioning kidney	
Stage IV	Extension beyond true pelvis or clinical involvement of the mucosa of bladder or rectum, no stage IV classification with bullous edema alone	Radiation, surgery (e.g., exenteration)
Stage IVA	Spread to adjacent organs	
Stage IVB	Spread to distant organs	

Etiology and Pathophysiology

The major risk factor for endometrial cancer is estrogen, especially unopposed estrogen. Additional risk factors include increasing age, nulliparity, obesity, hypertension, diabetes mellitus, and having a personal or family history of hereditary nonpolyposis colorectal cancer. Obesity is a risk factor because adipose cells store estrogen. This increases endogenous estrogen and increases its availability. Pregnancy and birth control pills are protective factors.

Endometrial cancer arises from the lining of the endometrium. Most tumors are adenocarcinomas. The precursor may be a hyperplasic state that progresses to invasive carcinoma. Hyperplasia occurs when estrogen is not counteracted by progesterone. The cancer directly extends into the cervix and through the uterine serosa. As invasion of the myometrium occurs, regional lymph nodes, including the paravaginal and paraaortic, become involved. Hematogenous metastases develop concurrently. The usual sites of metastases are lung, bone, liver, and eventually the brain. Malignant cells can be found in the peritoneal cavity, presumably by tubal transport, and their presence is included in staging. Prognostic factors include histologic differentiation, uterine size at time of diagnosis, myometrial invasion, peritoneal cytology, lymph node and adnexal metastases, and tumor size. Endometrial cancer grows slowly, metastasizes late, and is amenable to therapy if diagnosed early.

Clinical Manifestations

The first sign of endometrial cancer is abnormal uterine bleeding, usually in postmenopausal women. Because perimenopausal women have sporadic periods for a time, it is important that this sign not be ignored or attributed to menopause. Pain occurs late in the disease process, and other symptoms that may arise are related to metastasis to other organs.

Collaborative Care

Endometrial biopsy is the primary diagnostic procedure for endometrial cancer. Endometrial biopsy, which is done on an outpatient basis, involves obtaining endometrial tissue from the uterus. Any occurrence of spotting or unexpected bleeding in a postmenopausal woman mandates obtaining a tissue sample to exclude endometrial cancer. The American Cancer Society recommends that an endometrial biopsy be performed at menopause and then periodically in women who are at risk. The Pap test is not a reliable diagnostic tool for endometrial cancer, but it can rule out cervical cancer.

Treatment of endometrial cancer is a total hysterectomy and bilateral salpingo-oophorectomy with lymph node biopsies. Although they are not in widespread use, molecular markers help identify high risk groups that could benefit from postoperative adjuvant therapy. These markers include p53 and p16 overexpression, markers of high proliferative activity, and the expression of estrogen and/or progesterone receptors by the tumor cells. The absence of estrogen and progesterone receptors is a poor prognostic indicator.

Most cases of endometrial cancer are diagnosed at an early stage when surgery alone may result in cure. Surgery may be followed by radiation, either to the pelvis or abdomen externally or intravaginally, to decrease local recurrence. Treatment of advanced or recurrent disease is difficult. Progesterone hormonal therapy (e.g., megestrol [Megace]) is the treatment of choice when the progesterone receptor status is positive and the tumor is well differentiated. Tamoxifen (Novaldex), either alone or in combination with progesterone therapy, is also effective in women with advanced or recurrent endometrial cancer. Chemotherapy is considered when progesterone therapy is unsuccessful. The most common agents used are doxorubicin (Adriamycin), cisplatin (Platinol), carboplatin (Paraplatin), and paclitaxel (Taxol).[25]

OVARIAN CANCER

Ovarian cancer is a malignant neoplasm of the ovaries. In 2002 there were 23,300 new cases of ovarian cancer in the United States, and 13,900 women died from the disease.[28] It is the fifth leading cause of cancer deaths in the United States. Because most women with ovarian cancer have advanced disease at diagnosis, it causes more deaths than any other cancer of the female reproductive system. It occurs most frequently in women between 55 and 65 years of age. White women of North American or European descent are at greater risk for ovarian cancer as compared with African American women.

Etiology and Pathophysiology

The cause of ovarian cancer is not known. Women who have mutations of the BRCA genes have increased susceptibility for ovarian cancer.[28] The BRCA genes are tumor suppressor genes that inhibit tumor growth when functioning normally. When they mutate, they lose their tumor suppressor ability, and hence there is increased risk for women to develop ovarian or breast cancer (see the Genetics in Clinical Practice box).

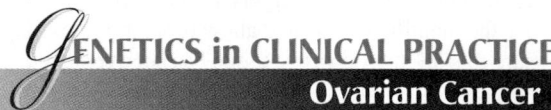

GENETICS in CLINICAL PRACTICE
Ovarian Cancer

Genetic Basis
- Mutations in genes BRCA-1 and BRCA-2
- Autosomal dominant transmission
- Mutations can be passed down from either mother or father

Incidence
- About 10% of cases of ovarian cancer are genetically related.
- Women with BRCA-1 mutations have a 25% to 40% lifetime risk of developing ovarian cancer.
- Women with BRCA-2 mutations have a 10% to 20% lifetime risk of developing ovarian cancer.
- Family history of both breast and ovarian cancer increases the risk of having a BRCA mutation.
- BRCA mutations occur in 10% to 20% of patients with ovarian cancer who have no family history of breast or ovarian cancer.
- Family of genes associated with hereditary nonpolyposis colorectal cancer accounts for 10% of ovarian cancers.

Genetic Testing
- DNA testing is available for BRCA-1 and BRCA-2.

Clinical Implications
- Bilateral oophorectomy reduces the risk of ovarian cancer in women with BRCA-1 and BRCA-2 mutations.
- Genetic counseling and testing for BRCA mutations should be considered for women whose personal or family history puts them at high risk for a genetic predisposition to ovarian cancer.

The greatest risk factor for ovarian cancer is family history (one or more first-degree relatives). Having a family history of breast or colon cancer is also a risk factor. Other risk factors include a personal history of breast or colon cancer and hereditary nonpolyposis colorectal cancer. Women who have never been pregnant (nulliparity) are also at higher risk. Other risk factors include increasing age, high-fat diet, increased number of ovulatory cycles (usually associated with early menarche and late menopause), hormone replacement therapy, and use of infertility drugs. The use of oral contraceptives is associated with lower ovarian cancer risk.

Breast-feeding, multiple pregnancies, oral contraceptive use (greater than 5 years), and early age at first birth seem to reduce the risk of ovarian cancer. It is thought that these factors have a protective effect because they reduce the number of ovulatory cycles, and thus reduce the exposure to estrogen.[29]

About 90% of ovarian cancers are epithelial carcinomas that arise from malignant transformation of the surface epithelial cells. Germ cell tumors account for another 10%. Histologic grading is an important prognostic determinant. Tumors are graded according to how well differentiated they are. These include well differentiated (grade I), moderately well differentiated (grade II), and poorly differentiated (grade III). Grade III lesions carry a poorer prognosis than the other grades.

Ovarian cancer can metastasize directly by shedding malignant cells, which frequently implant on the uterus, bladder, bowel, and omentum. In addition, ovarian cancer can metastasize by lymphatic spread. Primary lymphatic drainage of the ovary is through the retroperitoneal lymph nodes, but drainage also can occur through the iliac and inguinal lymph nodes.

Clinical Manifestations

In its early stages, ovarian cancer is usually asymptomatic. Clinical manifestations may include general abdominal discomfort (gas, indigestion, pressure, bloating, cramps), sense of pelvic heaviness, loss of appetite, feeling of fullness, and change in bowel habits. Pain is not an early symptom. As the malignancy grows, a variety of manifestations, such as an increase in abdominal girth, bowel and bladder dysfunction, persistent pelvic or abdominal pain, menstrual irregularities, and ascites, can occur. An ovarian malignancy should be considered when abnormal vaginal bleeding occurs.

Diagnostic Studies

Unlike the Pap test used to screen for cervical cancer, no screening test exists for ovarian cancer. Because early ovarian cancer is usually asymptomatic, yearly bimanual pelvic examinations should be performed to identify the presence of an ovarian mass. Postmenopausal women should not have palpable ovaries, so a mass of any size should be suspected as possible ovarian cancer. An abdominal or vaginal ultrasound can be used to detect ovarian masses. Color Doppler imaging, in conjunction with ultrasonography, can be used to visualize vascular changes associated with malignancy.

For women with a high risk for ovarian cancer, screening using a combination of the tumor marker, CA-125, and ultrasound is recommended in addition to a yearly pelvic examination. CA-125 is positive in 80% of women with epithelial ovarian cancer and is used to monitor the course of the disease.[25] However, levels of CA-125 may be elevated with other non-

ovarian malignancies or with benign conditions such as fibroids or endometriosis.

Collaborative Care

Women identified as being at high risk based on family and health history may require counseling regarding options such as prophylactic oophorectomy and birth control pills. It is important to note that although oophorectomy will significantly reduce the risk of ovarian cancer, it will not completely eliminate the possibility of disease.

If a diagnosis of ovarian cancer is made, staging is critical for guiding treatment decisions. Because of the numerous metastatic pathways for ovarian cancer, accurate staging usually involves multiple biopsies. Stage I describes disease limited to the ovaries; stage II, disease limited to the true pelvis; stage III, disease limited to the abdominal cavity; and stage IV, distant metastatic disease. The usual treatment for stage I malignancies is a total abdominal hysterectomy and bilateral salpingo-oophorectomy with removal of as much of the tumor as possible (i.e., tumor debulking). The remaining tissues in the abdomen and pelvis are carefully scruti-

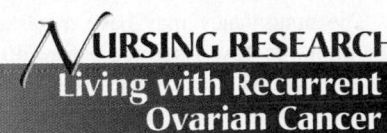

NURSING RESEARCH
Living with Recurrent Ovarian Cancer

Citation
Fitch MI, Gray RE, Frannsen EM: Women's perspectives regarding the impact of ovarian cancer: implications for nursing practice, *Cancer Nurs* 23:359, 2000.

Purpose
The purpose of this study was to gain knowledge about the experiences of women living with recurrent ovarian cancer.

Methods
The study was conducted using a survey instrument developed by the authors. Surveys were distributed to 1068 women with ovarian cancer. Respondents were divided into two groups: those with recurrent disease ($n = 93$) and those without recurrent disease ($n = 170$).

Results and Conclusions
A greater proportion of women with recurrent ovarian cancer reported bowel problems, fear of dying, pain, mobility problems, and self-blame than women without recurrent disease. These women did not feel that they were receiving adequate help for bowel problems and problems with sexual function. They rated their quality of life lower than women without recurrent disease and indicated a greater need to talk about their problems. Women with recurrent disease reported dissatisfaction with the information they received regarding emotional reactions to their disease and treatment. Nurses were identified as helpful by women with recurrent ovarian cancer.

Implications for Nursing Practice
This study identified a patient population whose needs are not being met. Nurses working with ovarian cancer patients need to assess them carefully and plan educational interventions based on their needs. Referrals to community resources are important. Further research is needed to find ways to identify methods to meet the unmet needs of patients with ovarian cancer.

nized. Ascitic fluid is submitted for cytologic study, and appropriate biopsies are performed to determine the stage of the disease.

The addition of chemotherapy or the instillation of intraperitoneal radioisotopes is usually suggested for stage I disease. The patient with stage II disease may receive external abdominal and pelvic radiation, intraperitoneal radiation, or systemic combined chemotherapy after tumor-reducing surgery. After completion of systemic chemotherapy in the patient who is clinically free of symptoms, a "second-look" surgical procedure is often performed to determine whether there is any evidence of disease. This option does not necessarily improve the outcome. If no disease is found, the patient is monitored for recurrent disease.

Chemotherapy (e.g., cisplatin [Platinol], carboplatin [Paraplatin]) is used for the treatment of stage III and stage IV diseases. Altretamine (Hexalen) is used for palliative treatment of persistent, recurrent ovarian cancer. Paclitaxel (Taxol) and topotecan (Hycamtin) are used to treat metastatic ovarian cancer. Surgical debulking is often done in conjunction with chemotherapy for advanced disease. Intraperitoneal chemotherapy, although associated with substantial side effects, is coming into wider use for the patient who has minimum residual disease after surgery.

The malignancy may have metastasized to the peritoneum, omentum, or bowel surface before discovery of the tumors. In these situations the prognosis is poor. Recurrent pleural effusion causing shortness of breath and discomfort may require frequent paracentesis, but the fluid accumulates again. Radiation and chemotherapy may be used to shrink the size of the tumor, relieving pressure and pain.

VAGINAL CANCER

Primary vaginal cancers are rare, with 2000 new cases reported in 2002.[27] The peak incidence is between 50 and 70 years of age. Vaginal tumors are usually secondary sites or metastases of other cancers such as cervical or endometrial cancer. The most common type of vaginal cancer is squamous cell carcinoma. Intrauterine exposure to diethylstilbestrol (DES) places a woman at risk for clear cell adenocarcinoma of the vagina. Treatment of vaginal cancer depends on the type of cells involved and the stage of the disease, the size of the tumor, and the location of the tumor. Squamous cell carcinomas can be treated with both surgery and radiation.

VULVAR CANCER

Cancer of the vulva is relatively rare, with 3800 new cases reported in 2002.[27] Similar to cervical cancer, preinvasive lesions referred to as vulvar intraepithelial neoplasia (VIN) precede invasive vulvar cancer (Fig. 52-9). The invasive form occurs mainly in women over 60 years of age with the highest incidence being in women in their seventies.[25] Patients with vulvar neoplasia may have symptoms of vulvar itching or burning, pain, bleeding, or discharge. Women who are immunosuppressed and/or have diabetes mellitus, hypertension, or chronic vulvar dystrophies are at a higher risk for developing vulvar cancers. Several subtypes of human papillomavirus have been identified in some but not all vulvar cancers.[22]

Diagnosis of vulvar cancer is determined by the pathology report on the biopsy of the suspicious lesion. VIN is managed by eradicating the lesion medically with 5-fluorouracil (5-FU) or surgical excision. Larger lesions may require more extensive surgery and skin graft. The traditional treatment for vulvar can-

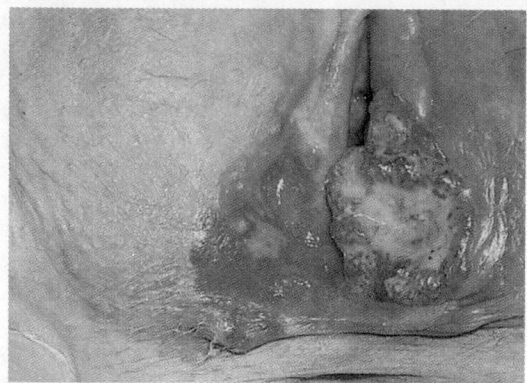

FIG. 52-9 Ulcerative squamous cell carcinoma of the vulva.

cer has been radical vulvectomy. However, the procedure results in extensive morbidity related to scarring and wound breakdown. For this reason, more conservative surgical techniques such as radical hemivulvectomy are being used. Cure rates are comparable between the radical vulvectomy and hemivulvectomy. Morbidity and loss of function have been significantly decreased with the hemivulvectomy.

SURGICAL PROCEDURES: FEMALE REPRODUCTIVE SYSTEM

A variety of surgical procedures are performed when benign or malignant tumors of the genital tract are found (Table 52-15). A hysterectomy may be done either vaginally or abdominally. A

TABLE 52-15 Surgical Procedures Involving the Female Reproductive System

TYPE OF SURGERY	DESCRIPTION
Subtotal hysterectomy	Removal of uterus without cervix (rarely done today)
Total hysterectomy	Removal of uterus and cervix
Panhysterectomy (TAH-BSO)	Removal of uterus, cervix, fallopian tubes, and ovaries
Simple vulvectomy	Excision of vulva and wide margin of skin
Radical vulvectomy	Excision of tissue from anus to few cm above symphysis pubis (skin, labia majora and minora, and clitoris) with superficial and deep lymph node dissection
Vaginectomy	Removal of vagina
Radical hysterectomy (Wertheim)	Panhysterectomy, partial vaginectomy, and dissection of lymph nodes in pelvis
Pelvic exenteration	Radical hysterectomy, total vaginectomy, removal of bladder with diversion of urinary system and resection of bowel with colostomy
Anterior pelvic exenteration	Above operation without bowel resection
Posterior pelvic exenteration	Above operation without bladder removal

TAH-BSO, Total abdominal hysterectomy and bilateral salpingo-oophorectomy.

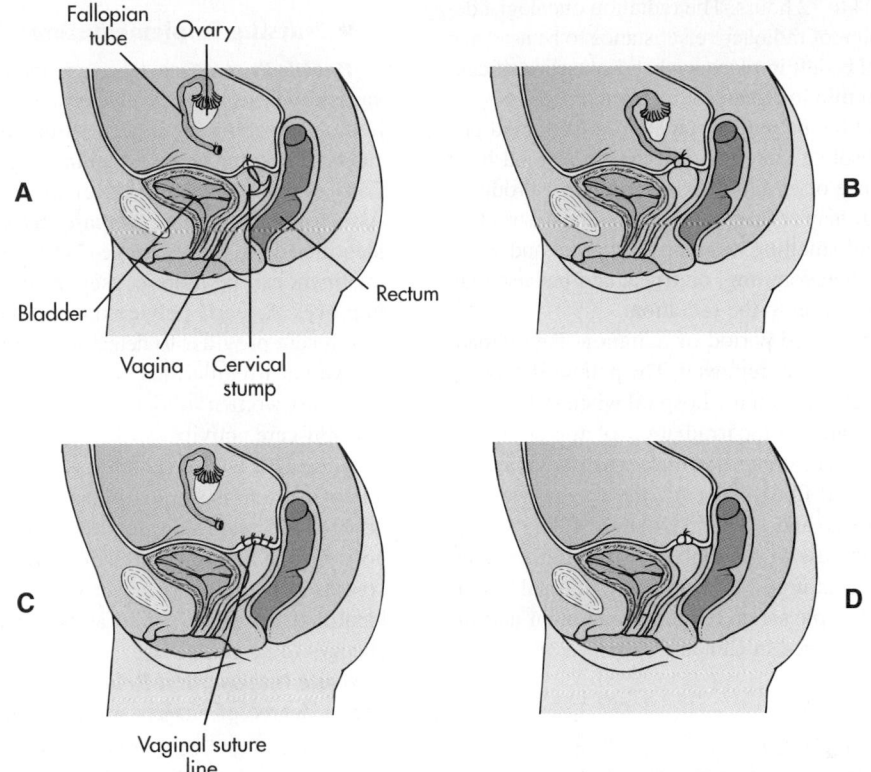

FIG. 52-10 **A**, Cross section of subtotal hysterectomy. Note that cervical stump, fallopian tubes, and ovaries remain. **B**, Cross section of total hysterectomy. Note that fallopian tubes and ovaries remain. **C**, Cross section of vaginal hysterectomy. Note that fallopian tubes and ovaries remain. **D**, Total hysterectomy, salpingectomy, and oophorectomy. Note that uterus, fallopian tubes, and ovaries are completely removed.

vaginal route is often used when vaginal repair is to be done in addition to removal of the uterus. The abdominal route is used when large tumors are present and the pelvic cavity is to be explored or when the tubes and ovaries are to be removed at the same time (Fig. 52-10). The abdominal route can present more postoperative problems because it involves an incision and the opening of the abdominal cavity. In both vaginal and abdominal hysterectomies, the ligaments that support the uterus are attached to the vaginal cuff so that normal depth of the vagina is maintained. A combined approach using laparoscopy with vaginal hysterectomy is becoming more common. This surgical technique decreases morbidity associated with abdominal hysterectomy.

RADIATION THERAPY: CANCERS OF THE FEMALE REPRODUCTIVE SYSTEM

Radiation is used to cure, control, or act as a palliative measure for cancers of the female reproductive system either alone or in combination with other treatments. The goal of radiation therapy is to deliver a specific amount of high-energy (or ionizing) radiation to the cancer and with minimal damage to the normal surrounding tissue.[25] Radiation therapy may be external or internal.

External Radiation Therapy

With external radiation therapy, a source outside of the body delivers electromagnetic radiation in the form of waves. (External radiation therapy is discussed in Chapter 15.)

Internal Radiation Therapy

Use of internal radiation therapy allows the radiation to be placed near or into the tumor. This method can deliver a high dose of radiation directly to the tumor. The dose decreases sharply the farther away from the source, causing less damage to the surrounding normal tissue. A variety of forms are used to deliver internal radiation, including wires, capsules, needles, tubes, and seeds. Internal radiation is used in the management of cervical and endometrial cancer because of the accessibility of these body parts and the favorable results obtained. Radium and cesium are two commonly used isotopes. In preparation of the patient for the treatment, a cleansing enema is given to prevent straining at stool, which could cause displacement of the isotope. An indwelling catheter is inserted to prevent a distended bladder from coming into contact with the radioactive source.

A variety of applicators have been developed for intrauterine treatment. Applicators are inserted into the endometrial cavity and vagina of an anesthetized patient in the operating room. When the applicator contains the radioactive material, this is known as preloading. In afterloading, the applicator is implanted in the operating room but is not loaded with the radioactive material until its correct placement is verified and the patient has been returned to her room. Radiation exposure to the patient is precisely controlled. The radiation exposure to the physician and other personnel involved in the implantation is reduced when the afterload technique is used. The applicator is secured with vaginal packing and is left in place for 24 to 72 hours. The radiation oncologist determines the exact amount of radioactive substance to be used and the length of time it will be left in place so that destruction of cancer cells can occur with minimal damage to normal cells.

During the treatment the patient is placed in a lead-lined private room and is on absolute bed rest. She may be turned from side to side. The presence of an intrauterine applicator produces uterine contractions that may require analgesics. The destruction of cells results in a foul-smelling vaginal discharge, and a deodorizer is helpful. Nausea, vomiting, diarrhea, and malaise may develop as a systemic reaction to the radiation.

At the end of the prescribed period of radiation, the radioactive material and the catheter are removed. The patient is allowed off bed rest and is discharged from the hospital when stable. Late complications that may arise after irradiation of the uterus include fistulas (vesicovaginal, ureterovaginal), cystitis, phlebitis, hemorrhage, and fibrosis. If fibrosis occurs, the vaginal wall becomes smaller in diameter and shorter. Dilation of the vagina through intercourse or the use of sequentially sized dilators may be indicated. The patient is urged to report any unusual symptoms or complaints to her physician. (Internal radiation and related nursing care are discussed in Chapter 15.)

NURSING MANAGEMENT
CANCERS OF THE FEMALE REPRODUCTIVE SYSTEM

■ Nursing Assessment

Malignant tumors of the female reproductive system can be found in the cervix, endometrium, ovaries, vagina, and vulva. The patient with any of these malignant tumors may experience a variety of clinical manifestations, including leukorrhea, irregular vaginal bleeding, vaginal discharge, increase in abdominal pain and pressure, bowel and bladder dysfunction, and vulvar itching and burning. Assessment for these signs and symptoms is an important nursing responsibility.

■ Nursing Diagnoses

Nursing diagnoses for the female patient with cancer of the reproductive system include, but are not limited to, the following:
- Anxiety *related to* threat of a malignancy and lack of knowledge about the disease process and prognosis
- Acute pain *related to* pressure secondary to enlarging tumor
- Disturbed body image *related to* loss of body part and loss of good health
- Ineffective sexuality patterns *related to* physiologic limitations and fatigue
- Ineffective breathing pattern *related to* presence of ascites and effusions
- Anticipatory grieving *related to* poor prognosis of advanced disease

■ Planning

The overall goals are that the patient with a malignant tumor of the female reproductive system will (1) actively participate in treatment decisions, (2) achieve satisfactory pain and symptom management, (3) recognize and report problems promptly, (4) maintain preferred lifestyle as long as possible, and (5) continue to practice cancer detection strategies.

■ Nursing Implementation

Health Promotion. Through their contact with women in a variety of settings, nurses can teach women the importance of routine screening for cancers of the reproductive system. Cancer can be prevented when screening can reveal precancerous conditions of the vulva, cervix, endometrium, and, rarely, ovaries. Also, routine screening increases the chance that a cancer will be identified in its early stage. When cancer is identified earlier, treatment can be more conservative and the woman's prognosis improves. A yearly pelvic examination and Pap test will allow the health care provider to detect lesions on the vulva or any uterine or ovarian irregularities and screen for cervical cancer. Nurses can assist women to view routine cancer screening as an important self-care activity.

Educating women about risk factors for cancers of the reproductive system is also important. Limiting sexual activity during adolescence, using condoms, having fewer sexual partners, and not smoking reduce the risk of cervical cancer. A high-fat diet increases risk for ovarian cancer. When high risk behaviors are identified, nurses should assist women to identify lifestyle changes to decrease risk.

Acute Intervention Related to Surgery. All patients experience a degree of anxiety when surgery is contemplated, but the prospect of major gynecologic surgery may heighten these concerns. Some women may fear a loss of femininity and worry about possible changes in their secondary sex characteristics. Others may experience feelings of guilt, anger, or embarrassment. Still others may focus on the effect the surgery will have on their reproductive and sexual functions. Some women view the whole process as annoying, whereas others are relieved by the thought of no longer having menstrual periods or becoming pregnant. Each patient must be understood in light of her fears and concerns and must be approached and evaluated individually. The nurse who exhibits interest and a willingness to listen can provide considerable psychologic support.

Hysterectomy. Preoperatively, the patient is prepared physically for surgery with the standard perineal or abdominal preparation. A vaginal douche and enemas may be given, according to the preference of the surgeon. The bladder should be emptied before the patient is sent to the operating room. An indwelling catheter is commonly inserted preoperatively.

After surgery the patient who has had a hysterectomy will have an abdominal dressing (abdominal hysterectomy) or a sterile perineal pad (vaginal hysterectomy). (See NCP 52-1 for care of the patient after a total abdominal hysterectomy.) The dressing should be observed frequently for any sign of bleeding during the first 8 hours after surgery. A moderate amount of serosanguineous drainage on the perineal pad is expected following a vaginal hysterectomy.

The patient may experience urinary retention postoperatively because of temporary bladder atony resulting from edema or nerve trauma. This problem is more acute when a radical hysterectomy has been performed. At times an indwelling catheter is used for 1 to 2 days postoperatively to maintain constant drainage of the bladder and prevent strain on the suture line. If an indwelling catheter is not used, catheterization may be necessary if the patient has not urinated for 8 hours postoperatively. If residual urine is suspected after the removal of an indwelling catheter, catheterization is done to prevent bladder infection caused by pooling of urine. Accidental ligation of a ureter is a serious surgical complication. Any complaint of backache or decreased urine output should be reported to the surgeon.

Abdominal distention may develop from the sudden release of pressure on the intestines when a large tumor is removed or from paralytic ileus secondary to anesthesia and pressure on the bowel. Food and fluids may be restricted if the patient is nauseated. A rectal tube may be prescribed to relieve abdominal flatus, and ambulation is encouraged. A Fleet enema or suppository is frequently given on the third postoperative day.

Special care must be taken to prevent the development of deep vein thrombosis (DVT). Frequent changes of position, avoidance of the high Fowler position, and avoidance of pressure under the knees minimize stasis and pooling of blood. Special attention must be given to patients with varicosities. Leg exercises to promote circulation and the use of elastic gradient compression stockings or elastic bandages can be helpful.

The loss of the uterus may bring about grief responses similar to any great personal loss. The ability to bear children is central to society's image of being a woman. Although not experienced by all women, grief over this loss is normal. Eliciting the woman's feelings and concerns about her surgery will provide the needed information to give understanding care. When surgery removes the ovaries as well, women experience surgical menopause. Estrogen is no longer available from the ovaries, so symptoms of estrogen deficiency will arise. To counter this, hormone replacement therapy may be initiated in the early postoperative period.

Discharge teaching should prepare the patient for what to expect following surgery (e.g., she will not menstruate). Teaching should include specific activity restrictions. Intercourse should be avoided until the wound is healed (about 4 to 6 weeks). However, intercourse is not contraindicated once healing is complete. If a vaginal hysterectomy is performed, the woman needs to know that there may be a temporary loss of vaginal sensation. She should be reassured that sensation will return in several months.

Physical restrictions are limited for a short time. Heavy lifting should be avoided for 2 months. Activities that may increase pelvic congestion, such as dancing and walking swiftly, should be avoided for several months, whereas activities such as swimming may be both physically and mentally helpful. Wearing a girdle is allowed and may provide comfort. Once the patient has been assured that healing is complete, all previous activity can be resumed.

Salpingectomy and oophorectomy. Postoperative care of the woman who has undergone removal of a fallopian tube (salpingectomy) or an ovary (oophorectomy) is similar to that for any patient having abdominal surgery. One exception is that if a large ovarian cyst is removed, there may be abdominal distention caused by the sudden release of pressure in the intestines. An abdominal binder may provide relief until the distention subsides.

When both ovaries are removed (bilateral oophorectomy), surgical menopause results. The symptoms are similar to those of regular menopause but may be more severe because of the sudden withdrawal of hormones. Attempts may be made to leave at least a portion of an ovary.

Vulvectomy. Although cancer of the vulva is relatively uncommon, it is important that the nurse recognize the extent of the vulvectomy and the significant effect it is likely to have on the patient's life. An honest, open attitude with the patient and her partner preoperatively can be most helpful in the postoperative period.

After a vulvectomy the patient returns to the unit with a wound in the perineal area extending to the groin. The wound may be covered or left exposed and frequently has drains attached to portable suction (e.g., Hemovac). A heavy pressure dressing is often in place for the first 24 to 48 hours. The wound is cleaned with normal saline solution or an antiseptic twice daily. Solutions can be applied with an aseptic bulb syringe or a Water Pik machine. A heat lamp or a hair dryer is then used to dry the area. Wound care must be meticulous to prevent infection, which results in delayed healing.

Special attention to bowel and bladder care is needed. A low-residue diet and stool softeners prevent straining and wound contamination. An indwelling catheter is used to provide urinary drainage. Great care is taken not to dislodge the catheter because extensive edema makes its reinsertion difficult. Heavy, taut sutures are often used to close the wounds, resulting in severe discomfort for the patient. In other instances the wound may be allowed to heal by granulation. Analgesics may be required frequently to control pain. Careful positioning of the patient through the use of strategically placed pillows provides comfort. Ambulation is usually begun on the second postoperative day, but this varies with the preference of the surgeon. Anticoagulant therapy to prevent DVTs is common.

Because the surgery causes mutilation of the perineal area and the healing process is slow, the patient is likely to become discouraged. Opportunities for the patient to express her feelings and concerns about the operation should be provided. The patient needs specific instructions in self-care before she is discharged. She should be told to report any unusual odor, fresh bleeding, breakdown of incision, or perineal pain. Home care nursing can benefit the patient during her adjustment period. Sexual function is often retained. Whether clitoral sensation is retained may be critical to some women, particularly if it was a primary source of orgasmic satisfaction. A discussion of alternative methods of achieving sexual satisfaction may also be indicated.

Pelvic exenteration. When other forms of therapy are ineffective in controlling the spread of cancer and no metastases have been found outside of the pelvis, pelvic exenteration may be performed. Although different types are done, this radical surgery usually involves removal of the uterus, ovaries, fallopian tubes, vagina, bladder, urethra, and pelvic lymph nodes (Fig. 52-11). In

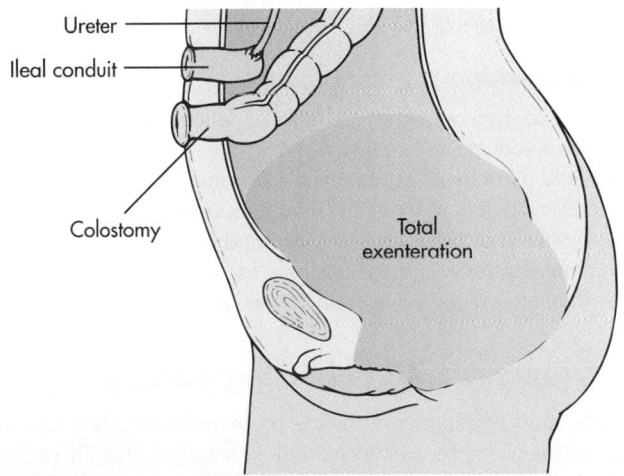

Ureter

Ileal conduit

Colostomy

Total
exenteration

FIG. 52-11 Total exenteration is removal of all pelvic organs with creation of an ileal conduit and colostomy.

some situations, the descending colon, rectum, and anal canal may also be removed. Candidates for this procedure are selected on the basis of their likelihood of surviving the surgery and their ability to adjust to and accept the resulting limitations.

The postoperative care involves that of a patient who has had a radical hysterectomy, an abdominal perineal resection, and an ileostomy or colostomy. The physical, emotional, and social adjustments to life on the part of the woman and her family are great. There are urinary or fecal diversions in the abdominal wall, a reconstructed vagina, and the onset of menopausal symptoms.

The patient's rehabilitative process should keep pace with her acceptance of the situation. Much understanding and support is needed from the nursing staff during a long recovery period. The patient should be gently encouraged to regain her independence. She needs to verbalize her feelings about her altered body structure. Inclusion of the family in the plan of care is important.

The patient will need to return to her health care provider at specified intervals. Early recurrence of the cancer may be identified and treated. At this time the patient's physical and emotional adjustment to the changes in body image produced by the surgery and her ability to carry out any treatment measures can also be assessed. Additional teaching and counseling can then be provided.

Acute Intervention with Radiation Therapy. Nursing management of the patient receiving internal radiation therapy requires special considerations. The nurse should not stay in the immediate area any longer than is necessary to give proper care and attention. No individual nurse should attend the patient for more than 30 minutes per day. The nurse should stay at the foot of the bed or at the entrance to the room to minimize radiation exposure. Visitors need to be told to stay 6 feet away from the bed and limit visits to less than 3 hours a day. Efficient organization of nursing care is essential, so that the nurse does not stay in the immediate area of the patient any longer than is necessary. The reasons for these precautions must be explained fully to the patient and her visitors. (A more detailed discussion of nursing care of the patient with an internal implant is given in Chapter 15.)

When the patient is to receive external radiation, she should be told to urinate immediately before the treatment to minimize radiation exposure to the bladder. She should be advised about radiation side effects, including enteritis and cystitis. These are natural reactions to radiotherapy and do not indicate an overdose. The patient should be fully informed of the possible side effects and measures to use to reduce their impact.

■ Evaluation

The expected outcomes are that the patient with cancer of the female reproductive system will
- actively participate in treatment decisions
- achieve satisfactory pain and symptom management
- recognize and report problems promptly
- maintain preferred lifestyle as long as possible
- continue to practice cancer detection strategies

Problems with Pelvic Support

The most commonly occurring problems with pelvic support are uterine prolapse, cystocele, and rectocele. Although vaginal birth increases the risk for these problems, these conditions can occur in women who have never experienced childbirth. Obesity, chronic coughing, and straining during bowel movements can in-

crease the likelihood of these problems. The decreased estrogen that normally accompanies the perimenopause also reduces some connective tissue support.

UTERINE PROLAPSE

Uterine prolapse is the downward displacement of the uterus into the vaginal canal (Fig. 52-12). Prolapse is rated by degrees. In first-degree prolapse, the cervix rests in the lower part of the vagina. Second-degree prolapse means the cervix is at the vaginal opening. A third-degree prolapse means the uterus protrudes through the introitus. Symptoms vary with the degree of prolapse. The patient may describe a feeling of "something coming down." She may have dyspareunia, a dragging or heavy feeling in the pelvis, backache, and bowel or bladder problems if cystocele or rectocele is also present. Stress incontinence is a common and troubling problem. When third-degree uterine prolapse occurs, the protruding cervix and vaginal walls are subjected to constant irritation, and tissue changes may occur.

Therapy depends on the degree of prolapse and how much the woman's daily activities have been affected. Pelvic muscle strengthening exercises (Kegel exercises) may be effective for some women. If not, a pessary may be used. A *pessary* is a device that is placed in the vagina to help support the uterus. A wide variety of shapes exist, including rings, arches, and balls. Most are made of plastic or wire coated with plastic. When a woman first receives a pessary, she needs instructions for its cleaning and follow-up. Pessaries that are left in place for long periods are associated

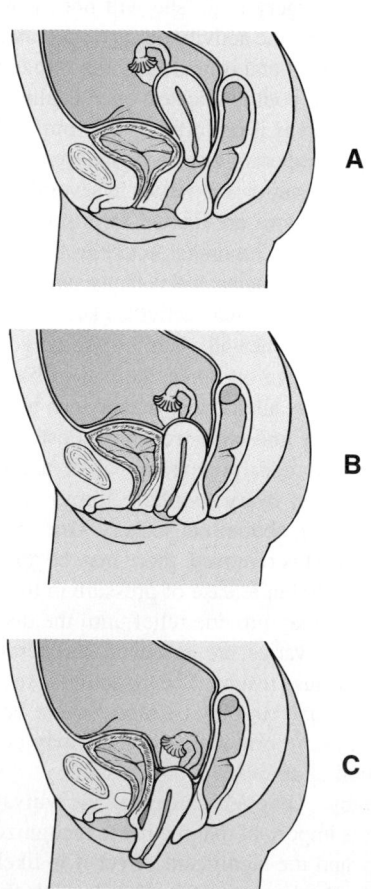

FIG. 52-12 Uterine prolapse. A, First-degree prolapse. B, Second-degree prolapse. C, Third-degree prolapse.

with erosion, fistulas, and an increased incidence of vaginal carcinoma. If more conservative measures are not successful, surgery is indicated. Surgery generally involves a vaginal hysterectomy with anterior and posterior repair of the vagina and underlying fascia.

CYSTOCELE AND RECTOCELE

Cystocele occurs when support between the vagina and bladder is weakened (Fig. 52-13). Similarly, a **rectocele** results from weakening between the vagina and rectum. These problems are common and asymptomatic in many women. With large cystoceles, complete emptying of the bladder can be difficult, predisposing women to bladder infections. A woman with a large rectocele may not be able to completely empty her rectum when defecating unless she helps push the stool out by putting her fingers in her vagina.

As with uterine prolapse, Kegel exercises may be used to strengthen the weakened perineal muscles if the cystocele or rectocele is not too problematic. A pessary may be helpful for cystoceles. Surgery designed to tighten the vaginal wall is generally the method of treatment. A cystocele is corrected with a procedure called an anterior colporrhaphy, whereas a posterior colporrhaphy is done for a rectocele. If further surgery is needed to relieve stress incontinence, procedures to support the urethra and restore the proper angle between the urethra and the posterior bladder wall are used.

NURSING MANAGEMENT
PROBLEMS WITH PELVIC SUPPORT

Nurses can assist women to avoid or decrease problems with pelvic support by teaching them how to do Kegel exercises. Women of all ages can benefit from these exercises. However, Kegel exercises are especially important following childbirth or whenever women begin to have incontinence. To instruct a patient in this exercise, she should be told to pull in or contract her muscles as if she were trying to stop the flow of urine. She should hold the contraction for several seconds and then relax. Sets of 5 to 10 contractions each should be done several times daily.

If vaginal surgery is necessary, the preoperative preparation usually includes a cleansing douche the morning of surgery. A cathartic and a cleansing enema are usually given when a rectocele repair is scheduled. A perineal shave is done.

In the postoperative period, the goals of care are to prevent wound infection and pressure on the vaginal suture line. This necessitates perineal care at least twice a day and after each urination or defecation. An ice pack applied locally may relieve the initial perineal discomfort and swelling. A disposable glove filled with ice and covered with a cloth works well in these instances. Later, sitz baths may be used.

After an anterior colporrhaphy, an indwelling catheter is usually left in the bladder for 4 days to allow the local edema to subside. The catheter keeps the bladder empty, preventing strain on the sutures. Catheter care with an antiseptic is generally done twice daily. After posterior colporrhaphy, straining at stool is avoided by means of a low-residue diet and the prevention of constipation. A stool softener is usually given each night.

Discharge instructions should be reviewed before the patient leaves the hospital. They include the use of douches or a mild laxative as needed; restriction of heavy lifting and prolonged standing, walking, or sitting; and avoidance of intercourse until the physician gives permission. There may be a loss of vaginal sensation, which can last for several months. The patient needs to be reassured that this situation is temporary.

FISTULA

A *fistula* is an abnormal opening between internal organs or between an organ and the exterior of the body (Fig. 52-14). Gynecologic procedures cause 75% of urinary tract fistulas.[22] Other causes include injury during childbirth and disease processes, such as carcinoma. They may develop between the vagina and the bladder, urethra, ureter, or rectum. When vesicovaginal fistulas (between the bladder and the vagina) develop, some urine leaks into the vagina, whereas with rectovaginal fistulas (between

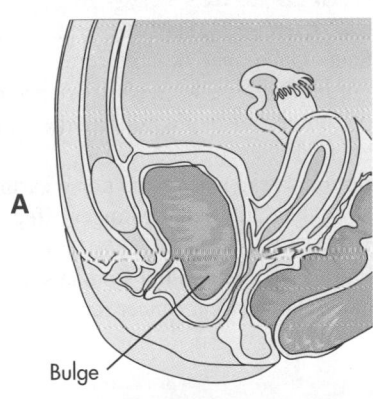

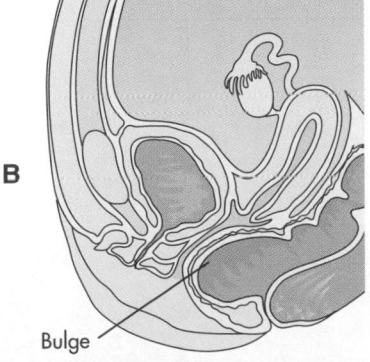

FIG. 52-13 A, Cystocele. B, Rectocele.

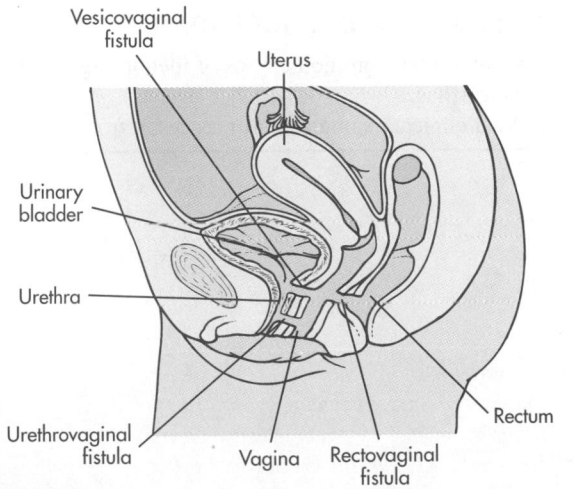

FIG. 52-14 Common fistulas involving the vagina.

the rectum and the vagina), flatus and feces escape into the vagina. In both instances, excoriation and irritation of the vaginal and vulvar tissues occur and may lead to severe infections. In addition to wetness, offensive odors may develop, causing embarrassment and severely limiting socialization.

Because small fistulas may heal spontaneously within a matter of months, treatment may not be needed. If the fistula does not heal, surgical excision is required. Inflammation and tissue edema must be eliminated before surgery is attempted. This may involve a wait of up to 6 months for the surgery. The fistulectomy may result in the patient's having an ileal conduit or temporary colostomy.

NURSING MANAGEMENT
FISTULA

Perineal hygiene is of great importance, both preoperatively and postoperatively. The perineum should be cleansed every 4 hours. Warm sitz baths should be taken three times daily if pos-

sible. Perineal pads should be changed frequently. The patient should be encouraged to maintain an adequate fluid intake. Encouragement and reassurance are needed in helping the patient cope with her problems.

Postoperatively, nursing care emphasis is on avoidance of stress on the repaired areas and prevention of infection. Care should be taken so that the indwelling catheter, usually in place for 7 to 10 days, is draining at all times. Oral fluids should be urged to provide for internal catheter irrigation. Minimal pressure and strict asepsis are used if catheter irrigation becomes necessary. The first stool after bowel surgery may be purposely delayed to prevent contamination of the wound. Later, stool softeners or mild laxatives may be given. See Chapter 44 for care of a patient with an ileal conduit and Chapter 41 for care of a patient with a colostomy. Surgical repair of fistulas is not always effective, even in the best conditions. Therefore supportive nursing care for the patient and her significant others is especially important.

CRITICAL THINKING EXERCISES

Case Study
Total Abdominal Hysterectomy
Patient Profile. Marion P., a 40-year-old Hispanic woman with two children, consulted her health care provider about experiencing menorrhagia and occasionally metrorrhagia for the past 5 months. She was diagnosed with leiomyomas, and a total abdominal hysterectomy was recommended.

Subjective Data
- Was initially reluctant about surgery
- States she wants no more children
- Concerned that she may have uterine cancer

Objective Data

Physical Examination
- Has several large, firm masses in body of uterus thought to be leiomyomas
- Had otherwise normal physical examination

Postoperative Status
- Returned to room with indwelling urinary catheter in place
- Legs wrapped in full-length elastic compression gradient stockings

CRITICAL THINKING QUESTIONS

1. What are the common causes of menorrhagia and metrorrhagia?
2. What clinical manifestations may result from leiomyomas?

3. What physical and psychologic preoperative preparation should be given to this patient?
4. What observation should be made in the patient's immediate postoperative period?
5. What possible complications, including their basis for development, can arise after abdominal hysterectomy?
6. Based on the assessment data, write one or more appropriate nursing diagnoses. Are there any collaborative problems?

Nursing Research Issues
1. Do women who exercise regularly experience less dysmenorrhea than women who do not exercise regularly?
2. Do working or nonworking women experience more episodes of vasomotor instability during the perimenopausal period?
3. Does the emotional response of the nurse caring for a victim of sexual assault help or hinder effective intervention?
4. What factors are associated with a woman's decision to participate in regular cervical cancer screening?

REVIEW QUESTIONS

The number of the question corresponds to the same-numbered objective at the beginning of the chapter.

1. In telling a patient with infertility what she and her partner can expect, the nurse explains that
   a. the cause should be diagnosed by the second visit.
   b. a hysterosalpingogram is a common diagnostic study.
   c. the cause will remain unexplained for 50% of couples.
   d. if postcoital studies are normal, infection tests will be done.

2. A patient with a spontaneous abortion is more likely than a patient with an induced abortion to have
   a. a D&C.
   b. feelings of loss and grief.
   c. physical complications such as infection.
   d. emotional support from family and friends.

3. An appropriate question to ask the patient with painful menstruation to differentiate primary from secondary dysmenorrhea is,
   a. "Does your pain become worse with activity or overexertion?"
   b. "Have you had a recent personal crisis or change in your lifestyle?"
   c. "Is your pain relieved by nonsteroidal antiinflammatory medications?"
   d. "When in your menstrual history did the pain with your period begin?"

4. In caring for a patient after an ectopic pregnancy was surgically removed, the nurse advises the patient that
   a. most ectopic pregnancies attach to the ovary.
   b. she will not be able to get pregnant in the future.
   c. bed rest must be maintained for 24 hours to assist healing.
   d. having one ectopic pregnancy increases her risk for another.

5. To prevent or decrease age-related changes that occur after menopause in a patient who chooses not to take hormone therapy, the nurse teaches the patient that the most important self-care measure is
   a. maintaining usual sexual activity.
   b. increasing the intake of dairy products.
   c. performing regular aerobic, weight-bearing exercise.
   d. taking vitamin E and B-complex vitamin supplements.

6. The first nursing intervention for the patient who has been sexually assaulted is to
   a. treat urgent medical problems.
   b. contact support person for the patient.
   c. provide supplies for the patient to cleanse self.
   d. document bruises and lacerations of the perineum and cervix.

7. The patient's history indicating thick, white, and curd-like vaginal discharge and vulvar pruritus is most consistent with
   a. trichomoniasis.
   b. monilial vaginitis.
   c. bacterial vaginosis.
   d. chlamydial cervicitis.

8. The nurse caring for a patient with pelvic inflammatory disease places her in semi-Fowler position. The rationale for this measure is to
   a. relieve pain.
   b. prevent the complication of sterility.
   c. promote drainage to prevent abscesses.
   d. improve circulation and promote healing.

9. In planning care for the patient receiving medical management of endometriosis, the nurse includes teaching regarding the side effect of
   a. estrogen supplementation.
   b. long-term use of an NSAID.
   c. large doses of vitamins A and E.
   d. hormonal suppression of ovulation.

10. A 31-year-old woman who wishes to have children is diagnosed with leiomyoma. The nurse plans care for the patient based on the knowledge that
    a. a hysterectomy will be necessary to treat the tumor.
    b. a myomectomy may be performed to maintain fertility.
    c. aspirin and other NSAIDs used to control pain may cause fetal defects.
    d. hormonal therapy to shrink the tumor and increase fertility can be used.

11. A 52-year-old woman who has not had a menstrual period for 18 months tells the nurse that she has recently had some spotting. The nurse advises the patient that
    a. she should keep a menstrual calendar for the next 6 months.
    b. this problem should be further investigated by an endometrial biopsy.
    c. this is a common, but not serious, problem that can occur after menopause.
    d. warm douching is recommended to promote healing of fragile vaginal tissue.

12. The nurse plans early and frequent ambulation for the patient who has undergone an abdominal hysterectomy in order to
    a. prevent urinary retention.
    b. promote pelvic circulation.
    c. relieve abdominal distention.
    d. maintain a sense of normalcy.

13. Nursing responsibilities related to the patient receiving internal radiation for endometrial cancer include
    a. maintaining absolute bed rest.
    b. allowing the patient bathroom privileges only.
    c. limiting an individual nurse's contact with the patient to 1 hour per day.
    d. allowing visitors to stay as long as desired if they stay 6 feet (2 meters) from the bed.

REFERENCES

1. McKinney ES et al: *Maternal-child nursing,* ed 2, Philadelphia, 2000, WB Saunders.
2. Leibowitz D, Hoffman J: Fertility drug therapies: past, present and future, *JOGNN* 29:201, 2000.
3. Henshaw SK, Singh D, Haas T: The incidence of abortion worldwide, *Fam Plann Perspect Digest* 25(suppl):S30, 1999.
4. Papp D et al: Biological mechanisms underlying the clinical effects of mifepristone (RU 486) on the endometrium, *Early Pregnancy* 4:230, 2000.
5. Moline M, Zendell SM: Evaluating and managing premenstrual syndrome, *Medscape Women's Health* 5:1, 2000.
6. Proctor M, Farquhar D: Dysmenorrhoea, *Clinical Evidence* 7:1639, 2002.
7. Excessive menstrual bleeding: what you can expect. Available at *www.ethiconinc.com* (accessed Feb 18, 2003).
8. Shoupe D: Hysterectomy or an alternative? *Hosp Pract* 35:52, 2000.
9. Soriano D et al: Diagnosis and treatment of heterotopic pregnancy compared with ectopic pregnancy, *Journal of the American Association of Gynecologic Laparoscopists* 9:352, 2002.
10. McCoy NL: Longitudinal study of menopause and sexuality, *Acta Obstet Gynecol Scand* 81:617, 2002.
11. Kass-Annese B: *Management of the perimenopausal and postmenopausal woman: a total wellness program,* Philadelphia, 1999, Lippincott Williams & Wilkins.
12. Warren MP, Shortle B, Dominguez JE: Use of alternative therapies in menopause, *Best Practice and Research in Clinical Obstetrics and Gynaecology* 16:411, 2002.
13. Mayhew MS, Hersey LC, McMullen PC: Hormone replacement therapy. In Edmunds MW, Mayhew MS, editors: *Pharmacology for the primary care provider,* St Louis, 2000, Mosby.
14. Arcangelo VP, Nichols A: Menopause and hormone replacement therapy. In Arcangelo VP, Peterson AM, editors: *Pharmacotherapeutics for advanced practice: a practical approach,* Philadelphia, 2001, Lippincott.
15. Ewiss AA: Phytoestrogens in the management of the menopause: up-to-date, *Obstet Gynecol Surv* 57:306, 2002.
16. Sommer B et al: Attitudes toward menopause and aging across ethnic/racial groups, *Psychosom Med* 61:868, 1999.
17. Grisso JA et al: Racial differences in menopause information and the experiences of hot flashes, *J Gen Intern Med* 14:98, 1999.
18. The Mamouth County S.A.N.E. program. Available at *www.wcmcnj.org* (accessed Nov 10, 2002).
19. Staats DO: Geriatric gynecology in long-term care settings, *Ann Long Term Care* 8:52, 2000.
20. Centers for Disease Control and Prevention: 2002 guidelines for treatment of sexually transmitted diseases, *MMWR* 47, 2002.
21. Attaran M, Falcone T, Goldberg J: Endometriosis: still tough to diagnose and treat, *Cleve Clin J Med* 69:647, 2002.
22. MacKay H, Trent MD: Gynecology. In Tierney LM, McPhee SJ, Papadakis M, editors: *Current medical diagnosis and treatment,* ed 41, Stamford, CT, 2002, Appleton & Lange.
23. Markle ME: Polycystic ovary syndrome: implications for the advanced practice nurse in primary care, *J Am Acad Nurse Pract* 13:160, 2001.
24. Reproductive Health Outlook: Cervical cancer. Available at *www.rho.org* (accessed Feb 18, 2003).
25. Moore-Higgs GJ et al: *Women and cancer: a gynecologic oncology nursing perspective,* ed 2, Boston, 2000, Jones & Bartlett.
26. Mandelblatt JS et al: Benefits and costs of using HPV testing to screen for cervical cancer, *JAMA* 287:2372, 2002.
27. American Cancer Society: *Cancer facts and figures: 2002,* Atlanta, 2002, American Cancer Society.
28. Harris LL: Ovarian cancer: screening for early detection, *Am J Nurs* 102:46 2002.
29. Tiedeman D: Oncology today: ovarian cancer, *RN* 63:36, 2000.

RESOURCES

American Cancer Society
    1599 Clifton Road, NE
    Atlanta, GA 30329
    800-ACS-2345 or 404-320-3333
    www.cancer.org

American College of Obstetricians and Gynecologists
    409 12th Street SW
    P.O. Box 96920
    Washington, DC 20090-6920
    202-863-2518
    Fax: 202-484-1595
    www.acog.org

American Urological Association
    1120 North Charles Street
    Baltimore, MD 21201
    410-727-1100
    Fax: 410-223-4370
    www.auanet.org

Hysterectomy Educational Resources and Services (HERS) Foundation
    422 Bryn Mawr Avenue
    Bala Cynwyd, PA 19004
    888-750-HERS (4377)
    610-667-7757
    Fax: 610-667-8096
    www.hersfoundation.com

Sexuality Information and Education Council of the United States (SIECUS)
    130 West 42nd Street, Suite 350
    New York, NY 10036-7802
    212-819-9770
    Fax: 212-819-9776
    www.siecus.org

For additional Internet resources, see the website for this book at *http://evolve.elsevier.com/Lewis/medsurg/*.

CHAPTER 53
NURSING MANAGEMENT
Male Reproductive Problems

Jean Foret Giddens

LEARNING OBJECTIVES

1. Describe the pathophysiology, clinical manifestations, and collaborative care of benign prostatic hyperplasia.
2. Discuss the nursing management of benign prostatic hyperplasia.
3. Describe the pathophysiology, clinical manifestations, and collaborative care of prostate cancer.
4. Discuss the nursing management of prostate cancer.

5. Describe the pathophysiology, clinical manifestations, and collaborative and nursing management of problems of the penis, problems of the scrotum, and prostatitis.
6. Discuss the nursing management of problems related to male sexual functioning.
7. Identify the psychologic and emotional implications related to male reproductive problems.

KEY TERMS

benign prostatic hyperplasia, p. 1435	prostate cancer, p. 1444
epididymitis, p. 1452	prostate-specific antigen, p. 1444
epispadias, p. 1451	prostatitis, p. 1450
erectile dysfunction, p. 1456	radical prostatectomy, p. 1446
hydrocele, p. 1453	spermatocele, p. 1453
hypospadias, p. 1451	testicular torsion, p. 1453
orchitis, p. 1453	transurethral resection of the prostate, p. 1438
paraphimosis, p. 1451	varicocele, p. 1453
phimosis, p. 1451	vasectomy, p. 1455

Problems of the male reproductive system can involve a variety of structures, including the prostate, penis, urethra, ejaculatory duct, scrotum, testes, epididymis, vas deferens, and rectum (Fig. 53-1).

Problems of the Prostate Gland

BENIGN PROSTATIC HYPERPLASIA

Benign prostatic hyperplasia (BPH) is an enlargement of the prostate gland resulting from an increase in the number of epithelial cells and stromal tissue. It is the most common problem of the adult male reproductive system. BPH occurs in about 50% of men over 50 years of age and in over 80% of men over 80 years of age. Approximately 25% of men require some form of treatment by the time they reach age 80.[1] Prostate hyperplasia does not predispose to the development of prostate cancer.

Etiology and Pathophysiology

Although the cause of BPH is not completely understood, it is thought that BPH results from endocrine changes associated with the aging process. Possible causes include excessive accumulation of dihydroxytestosterone (the principal intraprostatic androgen), stimulation by estrogen, and local growth hormone action.[1]

Typically BPH develops in the inner part of the prostate. (Prostate cancer is most likely to develop in the outer part.) This enlargement gradually compresses the urethra, eventually leading to partial or complete obstruction (Fig. 53-2). It is the compression of the urethra that ultimately leads to the development of clinical symptoms. There is no direct relationship between the size of the prostate and degree of obstruction. It is the location of the enlargement that is most significant in the development of obstructive symptoms. For example, it is possible for mild hyperplasia to cause severe obstruction; likewise, it is possible for extreme hyperplasia to cause few obstructive symptoms.

Risk factors for BPH include a family history (particularly involving first-degree relatives), environment, and diet. Although men from both Western and Eastern cultures develop BPH disease at about the same rates, men from Western cultures are

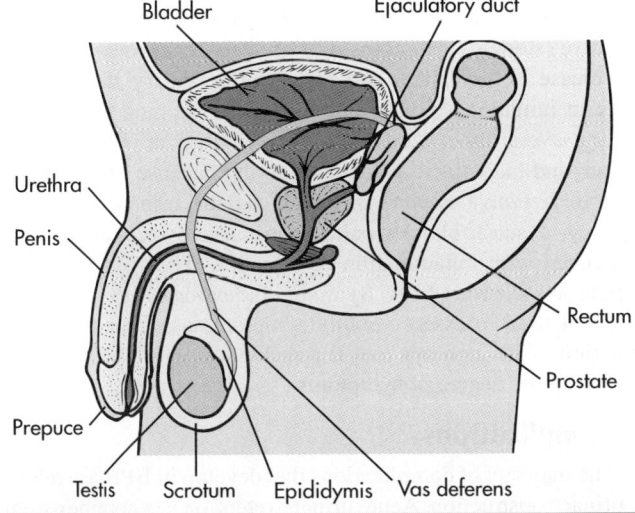

FIG. 53-1 Areas of the male reproductive system in which problems are likely to develop.

Reviewed by Judy L. Goodhart, RN, MSN, Professor of Nursing, Mesa State College, Grand Junction, Colo.

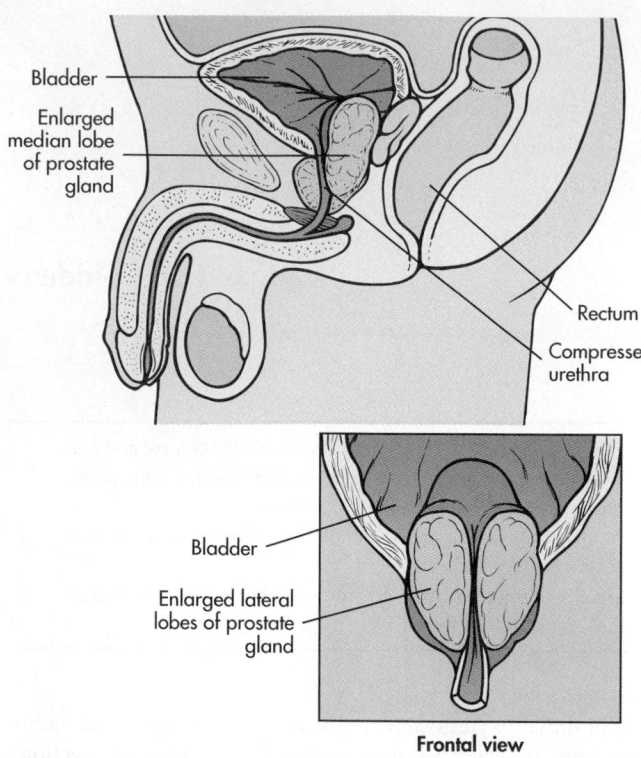

Bladder

Enlarged median lobe of prostate gland

Rectum

Compressed urethra

Bladder

Enlarged lateral lobes of prostate gland

Frontal view

FIG. 53-2 Benign prostatic hyperplasia.

much more likely to develop obstructive problems. Higher risk for BPH has been found in association with a diet high in zinc, butter, and margarine, whereas individuals who eat lots of fruits are thought to have a lower risk for BPH.

Clinical Manifestations

The symptoms of BPH experienced by the patient result from urinary obstruction. Symptoms are usually gradual in onset and may not be noticed until prostatic enlargement has been present for some time. Early symptoms are usually minimal because the bladder can compensate for a small amount of resistance to urine flow. The symptoms gradually worsen as the degree of urethral obstruction increases.

Symptoms fall into one of two groups: voiding symptoms and irritative (storage) symptoms. *Classic voiding symptoms* include a decrease in the caliber and force of the urinary stream, difficulty in initiating voiding, intermittency (stopping and starting stream several times while voiding), dribbling at the end of urination, and incomplete bladder emptying because of urinary retention. *Irritative symptoms,* which include urinary frequency, urgency, dysuria, bladder pain, nocturia, and incontinence, are associated with inflammation or infection. The American Urological Association (AUA) Symptom Index for BPH (Table 53-1) is a tool used to assess voiding symptoms associated with obstruction.[2] Although this tool is not diagnostic, it is useful in determining the degree of symptoms.

Complications

The majority of complications that develop in BPH are related to urinary obstruction. Acute urinary retention is a common complication and is an indication for surgical intervention in about

25% to 30% of patients.[3] Another common complication is urinary tract infection (UTI) and potentially sepsis secondary to UTI. Incomplete bladder emptying (associated with partial obstruction) results in residual urine, providing a favorable environment for bacterial growth. Calculi may develop in the bladder because of the alkalinization of the residual urine. Although bladder stones are eight times more common in men with BPH, risk of renal calculi is not significantly increased.[3] Other less common but potential complications include renal failure caused by *hydronephrosis* (distention of pelvis and calyces of kidney by urine that cannot flow through the ureter to the bladder), pyelonephritis, and bladder damage if treatment for acute urinary retention is delayed.

Diagnostic Studies

The primary methods used to diagnose BPH include a history and physical examination. The prostate can be palpated by digital rectal examination (DRE). Using DRE, the health care provider can estimate the size, symmetry, and consistency of the prostate gland. In BPH the prostate is symmetrically enlarged, firm, and smooth.

Additional diagnostic tests may be indicated, depending on the type and severity of symptoms and clinical findings. Diagnostic tests are typically done to determine the presence of complications or for differential diagnosis. A urinalysis with culture is routinely done to determine the presence of infection. The presence of bacteria, white blood cells, or microscopic hematuria is an indication of infection or inflammation. The prostate-specific antigen (PSA) blood level is usually measured to rule out prostate cancer. However, PSA levels may be slightly elevated in patients with BPH. Serum creatinine may be ordered to rule out renal insufficiency.

In patients with an abnormal DRE and elevated PSA, a *transrectal ultrasound* (TRUS) scan is typically indicated. This examination allows for accurate assessment of prostate size and is helpful in differentiating BPH from prostate cancer.[4] Biopsies can be taken during the ultrasound procedure. *Uroflometry,* a study that measures the volume of urine expelled from the bladder per second, is helpful in determining the extent of uretheral blockage and thus the type of treatment needed. Postvoid residual urine volume is often measured to determine the degree of urine flow obstruction. Cystourethroscopy, a procedure allowing internal visualization of the urethra and bladder, is performed if the diagnosis is uncertain and in patients who are scheduled for prostatectomy.[5] Diagnostic studies are outlined in Table 53-2.

Collaborative Care

The goals of collaborative care are to restore bladder drainage, relieve the patient's symptoms, and prevent or treat the complications of BPH. Treatment is generally based on the degree to which the symptoms bother the patient or the presence of complications rather than the size of the prostate. The numerous treatment options for BPH can be categorized as conservative (including drug therapy) and invasive therapy.

The most conservative initial treatment for BPH is referred to as "watchful waiting." When there are no symptoms or only mild ones (AUA symptom scores less than 7), a wait-and-see approach is taken. Because symptoms may come and go, a con-

| TABLE 53-1 | American Urological Association Symptom Index to Determine Severity of Prostatic Problems |

QUESTIONS TO BE ANSWERED	AMERICAN UROLOGICAL ASSOCIATION (AUA) SYMPTOM SCORE* (CIRCLE 1 NUMBER ON EACH LINE)					
	NOT AT ALL	LESS THAN 1 TIME IN 5	LESS THAN HALF THE TIME	ABOUT HALF THE TIME	MORE THAN HALF THE TIME	ALMOST ALWAYS
Over the past month, 1. How often have you had a sensation of not emptying your bladder completely after you finished urinating?	0	1	2	3	4	5
2. How often have you had to urinate again, less than 2 hr after you finished urinating?	0	1	2	3	4	5
3. How often have you found you stopped and started again several times when you urinated?	0	1	2	3	4	5
4. How often have you found it difficult to postpone urination?	0	1	2	3	4	5
5. How often have you had a weak urinary stream?	0	1	2	3	4	5
6. How often have you had to push or strain to begin urination?	0	1	2	3	4	5
7. How many times did you most typically get up to urinate from the time you went to bed at night until the time you got up in the morning?	0 (None)	1 (1 time)	2 (2 times)	3 (3 times)	4 (4 times)	5 (5 times or more)
Sum of circled numbers (AUA Symptom Score):* _____						

From Barry B et al: The American Urological Association symptom index for benign prostatic hyperplasia, *J Urol* 148:1547, 1992. Used with permission.
*Score is interpreted as: 0-7, mild; 8-19, moderate; 20-35, severe.

servative approach has value. Dietary changes (decreasing intake of caffeine and artificial sweeteners, limiting spicy or acidic foods), avoiding medication such as decongestants and anticholinergics, and restricting evening fluid intake may result in improvement of symptoms. A timed voiding schedule may reduce or eliminate symptoms, thus negating the need for further intervention. If the patient begins to have signs or symptoms that indicate an increase in obstruction, further treatment is indicated.

Drug Therapy. Drugs that have been used to treat BPH with variable degrees of success include 5α-reductase inhibitors and α-adrenergic receptor blockers.

5α-Reductase inhibitors. These drugs work by reducing the size of the prostate gland. Finasteride (Proscar) blocks the enzyme 5α-reductase, which is necessary for the conversion of testosterone to dihydroxytestosterone, the principal intraprostatic androgen. This drug results in regression of hyperplastic tissue through suppression of androgens. Finasteride is an appropriate treatment option for individuals who score between 12 and 26 on the AUA Symptom Index for BPH (see Table 53-1).

Although 40% to 50% of those treated show improvement, it takes between 3 and 6 months to be effective, and the medication must be taken on a continuous basis to maintain therapeutic results. Duasteride (Duagen) is a dual inhibitor of 5α-reductase type 1 and 2 isoenzymes. (Finasteride inhibits only the type 2 isoenzyme.) Side effects of 5 α-reductase inhibitors include decreased libido, decreased volume of ejaculate, and erectile dysfunction.

α-Adrenergic receptor blockers. Another drug treatment option for BPH is agents that block α₁-adrenergic receptors. Although this group of drugs is more commonly used for treatment of hypertension, these drugs promote smooth muscle relaxation in the prostate. α₁-Adrenergic receptors are abundant in the prostate and are increased in hyperplastic prostate tissue. Relaxation of the smooth muscle ultimately facilitates urinary flow through the urethra. Currently, the α-adrenergic blockers are the most widely prescribed drug for the patient with BPH who is experiencing moderate symptoms without the presence of other complications. These agents demonstrate a 50% to 60% efficacy in improvement of symptoms. Improvement of symptoms occurs

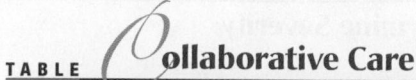

TABLE
53-2

Collaborative Care
Benign Prostatic Hyperplasia

Diagnostic

History and physical examination
Digital rectal examination (DRE)
Urinalysis with culture
Serum creatinine
Prostate-specific antigen (PSA)
Postvoid residual
Uroflowmetry
Transrectal ultrasound (TRUS)
Cystourethroscopy

Collaborative Therapy

Conservative therapy ("watchful waiting")
Drug therapy
- 5α-Reductase inhibitors
- α-Adrenergic receptor blockers
- Herb therapy
Invasive therapy
- Transurethral resection of the prostate (TURP)
- Simple open prostatectomy
- Transurethral incision of the prostate (TUIP)
- Transurethral microwave thermotherapy (TUMT)
- Transurethral needle ablation (TUNA)
- Laser prostatectomy
- Transurethral electrovaporization of the prostate (TUVP)
- Urethral stents.

COMPLEMENTARY & ALTERNATIVE THERAPIES
Saw Palmetto

Clinical Uses

Benign prostatic hyperplasia (BPH), urinary tract infections.

Effects

Extract of saw palmetto *(Serenoa repens)* is considered an antiandrogen herb. Improves urinary symptoms and urinary flow measures. Side effects are mild and infrequent. May cause gastrointestinal disturbances (e.g., diarrhea) and headache or dizziness. May cause increase in blood pressure in some people.

Nursing Implications

Men should see a physician for the correct diagnosis of BPH. Self-treatment is not recommended. Prostate-specific antigen levels should be done before starting this herb. The long-term effectiveness and ability to prevent complications are not currently known. Should not take if on hormonal replacement therapy.

---

within 2 to 3 weeks. The most important side effects are orthostatic hypotension and dizziness.

Several α-adrenergic blockers, including doxazosin (Cardura), terazosin (Hytrin), and tamsulosin (Flomax), are currently being used. Side effects, including postural hypotension, dizziness, and fatigue, can be problematic, especially if the patient is also taking cardiac or other antihypertensive medication. It must be pointed out that although these drugs offer symptomatic relief of BPH, they do not treat hyperplasia.

Herbal therapy. Herbs extracted from plants have been used in the management of BPH. In particular, plant extracts, such as saw palmetto *(Serenoa repens),* have been used. Saw palmetto has been shown to improve urinary symptoms and urinary flow measures. However, the long-term effectiveness and ability to prevent complications are currently unknown (see the Complementary and Alternative Therapies box on this page).

Invasive Therapy. Invasive therapy is indicated when there is a decrease in urine flow sufficient to cause discomfort, persistent residual urine, acute urinary retention because of obstruction with no reversible precipitating cause, or hydronephrosis. Intermittent catheterization or insertion of an indwelling catheter can temporarily reduce symptoms and bypass the obstruction. However, long-term catheter use should be avoided because of the increased risk of infection.

Invasive treatment of symptomatic BPH primarily involves resection or ablation of the prostate. The choice of the treatment approach depends on the size and location of the prostatic en-

largement, as well as patient factors such as age and surgical risk. Various invasive treatments are summarized in Table 53-3.

Transurethral resection of the prostate. Transurethral resection of the prostate (TURP) is a surgical procedure involving the removal of prostate tissue using a resectoscope inserted through the urethra. TURP has long been considered the "gold standard" surgical treatment for obstructing BPH. Although this procedure remains by far the most common operation performed, there has been a decrease in the number of TURP procedures done in recent years due to the development of less invasive technologies.[6]

The TURP is performed under a spinal or general anesthetic. No external surgical incision is made. A resectoscope is inserted through the urethra to excise and cauterize obstructing prostatic tissue (Fig. 53-3). A large three-way indwelling catheter with a 30 ml balloon is inserted into the bladder after the procedure to provide hemostasis and to facilitate urinary drainage. The bladder is irrigated, either continuously or intermittently, usually for the first 24 hours to prevent obstruction from mucus and blood clots.

The outcome for 80% to 90% of patients is excellent, with marked improvements in symptoms and urinary flow rates. TURP is a surgical procedure with relatively low risk. Some of the postoperative complications include bleeding, clot retention, and dilutional hyponatremia associated with irrigation. Because bleeding is a common complication, patients taking aspirin or warfarin (Coumadin) must discontinue these medications several days before surgery.

Transuretheral microwave thermotherapy. Transuretheral microwave thermotherapy (TUMT) is an outpatient procedure that involves the delivery of microwaves directly to the prostate through a transurethral probe in order to raise the temperature of the prostate tissue to about 113° F (45° C).[7] The heat causes necrosis and death of tissue, thus relieving the obstruction. A rectal temperature probe is used during the procedure to ensure that the rectal temperature is kept below 110° F (43.5° C) to prevent rectal tissue damage. Although infrequent, serious thermal injuries can occur as a consequence of TUMT as a result of incor-

TABLE 53-3	Invasive Treatment Options for Benign Prostatic Hyperplasia		
TREATMENT	**DESCRIPTION**	**ADVANTAGES**	**DISADVANTAGES**
Transurethral resection of the prostate (TURP)	Use of excision and cauterization to remove prostate tissue cystoscopically. Considered the most effective treatment of BPH.	Best long-term relief of prostatic obstruction Erectile dysfunction unlikely	Bleeding Retrograde ejaculation
Open prostatectomy	Surgery of choice for men with large prostates. Involves external incision with three possible approaches (see Fig. 53-4).	Complete visualization of prostate and surrounding tissue Usually only indicated if prostate gland is very large	Erectile dysfunction Bleeding Postoperative pain Risk of infection
Transurethral incision of the prostate (TUIP)	Involves making transurethral slits or incisions into prostatic tissue to relieve obstruction. Effective for men with relatively little prostatic enlargement.	Outpatient procedure Minimal complications Good for high risk patients No erectile dysfunction or retrograde ejaculation	Considered temporary solution to obstructive problem Urinary catheter needed after procedure
Transurethral microwave thermotherapy (TUMT)	Use of microwave radiating heat to produce coagulative necrosis of the prostate.	Outpatient procedure Short procedure Erectile dysfunction and retrograde ejaculation are rare	Potential for damage to surrounding tissue Urinary catheter needed after procedure
Transurethral needle ablation of the prostate (TUNA)	Low-wave radiofrequency used to heat the prostate causing necrosis.	Short outpatient procedure Erectile dysfunction and retrograde ejaculation are rare Precise delivery of heat to desired area Very little pain experienced by patient	Urinary retention common Irritative voiding symptoms Hematuria
Laser prostatectomy	Procedure uses a laser beam to cut or destroy part of the prostate. Different techniques are available: Visual laser ablation of prostate (VLAP) Contact laser technique Interstitial laser coagulation (ILC)	Short procedure Minimal bleeding Fast recovery time Very effective	Postprocedure catheterization (up to 7 days) needed because of edema and urinary retention Delayed sloughing of tissue Takes several weeks to reach optimal effect Retrograde ejaculation
Transurethral electrovaporization of prostate (TUVP)	Electrosurgical vaporization and desiccation are used together to destroy prostatic tissue.	Minimal risks Minimal bleeding and sloughing	Retrograde ejaculation Intermittent hematuria
Urethral stents	Insertion of self-expandable metallic stent into the urethra where enlarged area of prostate occurs.	Safe and effective Low risk	Stent may move Long-term experience is limited

rect placement of the transurethral probe or rectal temperature probe.[8]

Postoperative urinary retention is a common complication. Thus the patient is generally sent home with an indwelling catheter for 2 to 7 days to maintain urinary flow and to facilitate the passing of small clots or necrotic tissue. Antibiotics, pain medication, and bladder antispasmodic medications are used to treat and prevent postprocedure problems. The procedure is not appropriate for men with rectal problems. Anticoagulant therapy should be stopped 10 days before treatment. Mild side effects include occasional problems of bladder spasm, hematuria, dysuria, and retention.

Transuretheral needle ablation. Transuretheral needle ablation (TUNA) is another procedure that increases the tempera-

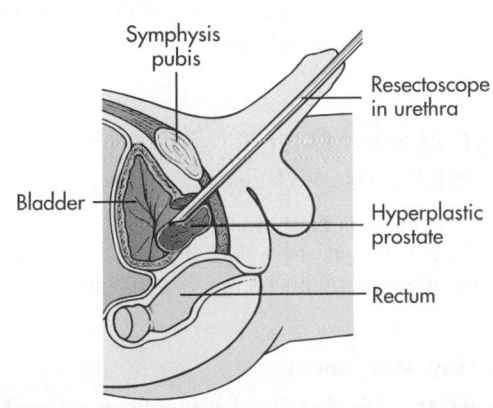

FIG. 53-3   Transurethral resection of the prostate.

ture of prostate tissue, thus causing localized necrosis. TUNA differs from TUMT in that low-wave radiofrequency is used to heat the prostate, and only prostate tissue in direct contact with the needle is affected, allowing greater precision in removal of the target tissue. The extent of tissue removed by this process is determined by the amount of tissue contact (needle length), amount of energy delivered, and duration of treatment. Seventy percent of patients undergoing TUNA report an improvement in symptoms, making this an attractive treatment option for men with BPH.[9]

This procedure is performed in an outpatient unit or physician's office using local anesthesia and intravenous or oral sedation. The TUNA procedure typically lasts only 30 minutes. The patient typically experiences little pain and an early return to regular activities. Complications include urinary retention, urinary tract infection, and irritative voiding symptoms (e.g., frequency, urgency, dysuria). Some patients require a urinary catheter for a short duration. Patients typically have hematuria for up to a week.

Laser prostatectomy. The use of laser therapy has recently been developed to treat BPH. The laser beam is delivered transurethrally through a fiber instrument and is used for cutting, coagulation, and vaporization of prostatic tissue. There are a variety of laser procedures using different sources, wavelengths, and delivery systems. A common laser procedure is laser coagulation of the prostate, often referred to as visual laser ablation of the prostate (VLAP). VLAP uses the laser beam to produce deep coagulation necrosis of the prostate. The affected prostate tissue gradually sloughs in the urinary stream. It takes several weeks before the patient reaches optimal results following this type of laser therapy. At the completion of VLAP, a urinary catheter is inserted to allow for drainage.

Contact laser technique involves the direct contact of the laser to the prostate tissue. This produces an immediate vaporization of the prostate tissue. Blood vessels near the laser tip immediately are cauterized, thus bleeding during the procedure is rare. A three-way catheter with slow-drip irrigation is placed immediately after the procedure for a short time. Typically the catheter is removed within 6 to 8 hours after the procedure. Advantages of this procedure over TURP include minimal bleeding both during and after the procedure, faster recovery time, and ability to perform the surgery on patients taking anticoagulants.

Another approach to laser prostatectomy is interstitial laser coagulation (ILC). The prostate is viewed through a cytoscope. A laser is used to quickly treat precise areas of the enlarged prostate by placement of interstitial light guides directly into the prostate tissue.

NURSING MANAGEMENT
BENIGN PROSTATIC HYPERPLASIA

Because the nurse is most directly involved with care of patients with BPH having invasive procedures, the focus of nursing management in this section is on preoperative and postoperative care.

■ Nursing Assessment

Subjective and objective data that should be obtained from a patient with BPH are presented in Table 53-4.

TABLE 53-4	Nursing Assessment — Benign Prostatic Hyperplasia

Subjective Data
Important Health Information
Medications: Estrogen or testosterone supplementation
Surgery or other treatments: Previous treatment for BPH
Functional Health Patterns
Health perception–health management: Knowledge of the condition
Nutritional-metabolic: Voluntary fluid restriction
Elimination: Urinary urgency, diminution in caliber and force of urinary stream; hesitancy in initiating voiding; postvoiding dribbling; urinary retention; incontinence
Sleep: Nocturia
Cognitive-perceptual: Dysuria, sensation of incomplete voiding; bladder discomfort
Sexuality-reproductive: Anxiety about sexual dysfunction

Objective Data
General
Older adult male
Urinary
Distended bladder on palpation; smooth, firm, elastic enlargement of prostate on rectal examination
Possible Findings
Enlarged prostate on ultrasonography; vesicle neck obstruction on cystourethroscopy; residual urine with postvoiding catheterization; presence of white blood cells, bacteria, or microscopic hematuria with infection; ↑ serum creatinine levels with renal involvement

BPH, Benign prostatic hyperplasia.

■ Nursing Diagnoses

Nursing diagnoses for the patient with BPH may include, but are not limited to, those presented in NCP 53-1.

■ Planning

The overall preoperative goals for the patient having invasive procedures are to have (1) restoration of urinary drainage, (2) treatment of any urinary tract infection, and (3) understanding of the upcoming procedure, implications for sexual functioning, and urinary control. The overall postoperative goals are to have (1) no complications, (2) restoration of urinary control, (3) complete bladder emptying, and (4) satisfying sexual expression.

■ Nursing Implementation

Health Promotion. The cause of BPH is largely attributed to the aging process. The focus of health promotion is on early detection and treatment. The American Cancer Society, along with the AUA, recommends a yearly medical history and DRE for men over 50 years of age in an effort to provide early detection of prostate problems. When symptoms of prostatic hyperplasia become evident, further diagnostic screening may be necessary (see Table 53-2).

Some men find that the ingestion of alcohol and caffeine tends to increase prostatic symptoms because the diuretic effect of these substances increases bladder distention. Compounds found in common cough and cold remedies such as pseudoephedrine (in Sudafed) and phenylephrine (in Allerest and Coricidin prepa-

NURSING CARE PLAN 53-1

Patient Undergoing Prostate Surgery*

EXPECTED PATIENT OUTCOMES	NURSING INTERVENTIONS and *RATIONALES*

PREOPERATIVE

NURSING DIAGNOSIS **Acute pain** *related to* bladder distention secondary to enlarged prostate *as manifested by* complaints of discomfort caused by inability to void, palpable bladder, no urine output, diaphoresis, restlessness.

- No complaints of pain

- Assist with insertion of indwelling catheter (usually done by urologist) *to reduce pain by providing urinary drainage of urine from bladder.*
- Monitor intake and output *to evaluate fluid balance.*
- Percuss bladder for distention *to validate adequate emptying of the bladder.*
- Maintain patency of catheter *to ensure continuous flow of urine from the bladder.*
- Assess comfort status *to continue or revise plan as necessary.*

NURSING DIAGNOSIS **Risk for infection** (urinary tract) *related to* indwelling catheter, environmental pathogens, and urinary stasis.

- No evidence of urinary tract infection

- Assess for elevated temperature and cloudy, foul-smelling urine *to identify manifestations of infection and initiate appropriate interventions.*
- Obtain urinalysis for culture (if ordered) *to determine presence and cause of infection.*
- Give patient 8 oz of water every waking hour *to prevent urinary stasis and dilute the urine.*
- Observe strict aseptic technique for catheter care *to minimize the risk of introducing an infectious organism.*

NURSING DIAGNOSIS **Fear** *related to* actual or potential sexual dysfunction, possible diagnosis of cancer, and lack of knowledge regarding surgical procedure and postoperative care *as manifested by* verbalization of fear about impact of surgery on sexuality; questioning or inaccurate comments about surgical course.

- Decreased fear about effect of surgery on sexuality and surgical course
- Correct responses to questions
- Calm demeanor

- Perform preoperative teaching *to provide information regarding the preoperative and postoperative routines.*
- Assess patient's concerns related to sexual functioning and correct misconceptions and inaccuracies *to plan appropriate interventions that address unique concerns.*
- Provide opportunity for private conversation for patient to ask personal questions *because a private setting facilitates open discussion.*

POSTOPERATIVE

NURSING DIAGNOSIS **Acute pain** *related to* irrigations and clots, presence of catheter, and surgical procedure *as manifested by* expression of pain; nonverbal signs of pain such as moaning, crying, legs drawn to abdomen.

- Decreased or no pain

- Maintain patency of catheter *because clots cause obstruction of urine flow resulting in bladder spasms.*
- Irrigate catheter if occluded with clots (according to aseptic technique and institution protocols) *so urine can flow freely.*
- Instruct patient to try not to urinate around catheter *because this increases the occurrence of spasm.*
- Give belladonna and opium suppository as needed; instruct patient in relaxation techniques such as deep breathing exercises, distraction therapy, and visual imagery *to relieve pain and decrease spasm.*

NURSING DIAGNOSIS **Ineffective therapeutic regimen management** *related to* lack of knowledge regarding need for follow-up care and activity restriction postoperatively *as manifested by* questioning or inaccurate comments about postoperative activity.

- No postoperative bleeding because of performing activities that increase intraabdominal pressure

- Teach patient to avoid heavy lifting (>10 lb [45 kg]), straining during defecation, prolonged periods of travel, stair climbing, driving, and sexual activity until surgeon approves such activity *to prevent increases in intraabdominal pressure and the possibility of bleeding.*
- Teach patient about the need for follow-up care *to evaluate prostate (if present) and overall health.*

*The specific nursing management will vary depending on the type of surgical intervention for BPH or prostate cancer.

Continued

NURSING CARE PLAN 53-1

Patient Undergoing Prostate Surgery—cont'd

POSTOPERATIVE—cont'd

EXPECTED PATIENT OUTCOMES	NURSING INTERVENTIONS and *RATIONALES*
NURSING DIAGNOSIS	**Urge urinary incontinence** *related to* poor sphincter control *as manifested by* inappropriate leakage of urine.
• Absence of or satisfactory control of dribbling	• Teach patient Kegel exercises *to strengthen sphincter tone.* • Advise patient about devices to control dribbling *so patient is aware of various devices and can make an informed decision among alternatives.*
NURSING DIAGNOSIS	**Risk for infection** *related to* indwelling catheter, bladder irrigations, environmental pathogens, inadequate oral intake, and poor catheter care.
• No evidence of infection	• Assess for fever, diaphoresis, self-restriction of fluid intake, cloudy urine *to determine if risk factors and/or signs and symptoms of infection are present.* • Monitor temperature q4hr first 48 hr postoperatively *because fever is an indicator of infection.* • Give patient 8 oz of water hourly while awake *to maintain good urine flow and dilute the urine.* • Observe strict aseptic technique for catheter care and bladder irrigations *to prevent introducing infectious organisms.*

COLLABORATIVE PROBLEM

NURSING GOALS	NURSING INTERVENTIONS and *RATIONALES*
POTENTIAL COMPLICATION	**Hemorrhage** *related to* surgical procedure.
• Monitor for and report signs of hemorrhage • Carry out appropriate medical and nursing interventions	• Observe urinary drainage and report bright red bleeding in larger than expected quantities *because this could indicate hemorrhage and the need for immediate intervention.* • Monitor blood pressure, pulse, and respirations and report abnormalities *because increasing pulse and respirations and decreasing blood pressure can indicate hemorrhage and possible shock.* • Maintain catheter drainage *to prevent obstruction and allow monitoring of bleeding and urine flow.* • Do not perform rectal treatments such as enemas or rectal temperatures (except belladonna and opium suppositories for bladder spasms) *because bleeding could be initiated.*

rations) often worsen the symptoms of BPH. These drugs are α-adrenergic agonists that cause smooth muscle contraction. If this happens, the patient should avoid these drugs.

The patient with obstructive symptoms should be advised to urinate every 2 to 3 hours and when first feeling the urge. This will minimize urinary stasis and acute urinary retention. Fluid intake should be maintained at a normal level to avoid dehydration or fluid overload. The patient may believe that if he restricts his fluid intake, symptoms will be less severe, but this only increases the chances of an infection. However, if the patient increases his intake too rapidly, bladder distention can develop because of the prostatic obstruction.

Acute Intervention

Preoperative care. Urinary drainage must be restored before surgery. Prostatic obstruction may result in acute retention or inability to void. A urethral catheter such as a Coudé (curved-tip) catheter may be needed to restore drainage. In many health care settings, 10 ml of sterile 2% lidocaine gel is injected into the urethra before insertion of the catheter. The lidocaine gel not only acts as a lubricant, but also provides local anesthesia and helps open the urethral lumen.[10] If a sizable obstruction of the urethra exists, a urologist may insert a filiform catheter with sufficient rigidity to pass the obstruction. Aseptic technique is important at all times to avoid introducing bacteria into the bladder. (Urinary catheters are discussed in Chapter 44.)

Antibiotics are usually administered before any invasive procedure. Any infection of the urinary tract must be treated before surgery. Restoring urine drainage and encouraging a high fluid intake (2 to 3 L/day unless contraindicated) are also helpful in managing the infection.

The patient is often concerned about the impact of the impending surgery on his sexual functioning. Data gathered from the health history relating to sexual activities will identify possible problem areas. The nurse should provide an opportunity for the patient and partner to express their concerns. The patient needs to know how the surgery may affect sexual functioning. All types of prostatic surgery generally result in some degree of retrograde ejaculation. The patient should be informed that the ejaculate may be decreased in amount or totally absent. This may decrease orgasmic sensations felt during ejaculation. Retrograde ejaculation is not harmful because the semen is eliminated during the next urination.

Postoperative care. The main complications following surgery are hemorrhage, bladder spasms, urinary incontinence, and infection. The plan of care should be adjusted to the type of surgery, the reasons for surgery, and the patient's response to surgery.

After surgery the patient will have a standard catheter or a triple-lumen catheter. Bladder irrigation is typically done to remove clotted blood from the bladder and ensure drainage of urine. The bladder is irrigated either manually on an intermittent basis or more commonly as a continuous bladder irrigation (CBI) with sterile normal saline solution or another prescribed solution. If the bladder is manually irrigated (if ordered), 50 ml of irrigating solution should be instilled and then withdrawn with a syringe to remove clots that may be in the bladder and catheter. Painful bladder spasms often occur as a result of manual irrigation. With CBI, irrigating solution is continuously infused and drained from the bladder. The rate of infusion is based on the color of drainage. Ideally the urine drainage should be light pink without clots. The inflow and outflow of irrigant must be continuously monitored. If outflow is less than inflow, the catheter patency should be assessed for kinks or clots. If the outflow is blocked and patency cannot be reestablished by manual irrigation, the CBI is stopped and the physician notified.

Careful aseptic technique should be used when irrigating the bladder because bacteria can easily be introduced into the urinary tract. Proper care of the catheter is important. To prevent urethral irritation and minimize the risk of bladder infection, the catheter must be secured to the leg or abdomen with tape or catheter strap. The catheter should be connected to a closed-drainage system and should not be disconnected unless it is being removed, changed, or irrigated. The secretions that accumulate around the meatus can be cleansed daily with soap and water.

Blood clots are expected after prostate surgery for the first 24 to 36 hours. However, large amounts of bright red blood in the urine can indicate hemorrhage. Postoperative hemorrhage may occur from displacement of the catheter, dislodging a large clot, or increases in abdominal pressure. Release or displacement of the catheter dislodges the balloon that provides counterpressure on the operative site. Traction on the catheter may be applied to provide counterpressure (tamponade) on the bleeding site in the prostate, thereby decreasing bleeding. Such traction can result in local necrosis if pressure is applied for too long. Pressure should therefore be relieved on a scheduled basis by qualified personnel. Activities that increase abdominal pressure, such as sitting or walking for prolonged periods and straining to have a bowel movement (Valsalva maneuver), should be avoided in the postoperative recovery period.

Bladder spasms are a distressing complication for the patient after transurethral procedures. They occur as a result of irritation of the bladder mucosa from the insertion of the resectoscope, presence of a catheter, or clots leading to obstruction of the catheter. The patient should be instructed not to urinate around the catheter because this increases the likelihood of spasm. If bladder spasms develop, the catheter should be checked for clots. If present, the clots should be removed by irrigation so that urine can flow freely. Belladonna and opium suppositories, or other antispasmodics (e.g., oxybutynin [Ditropan]) along with relaxation techniques, are used to relieve the pain and decrease spasm. The catheter is often removed 2 to 4 days after surgery. The patient should urinate within 6 hours after catheter removal. If he cannot, a catheter is reinserted for a day or two. If the problem continues, the nurse may need to instruct the patient in clean intermittent self-catheterization (see Chapter 44).

Sphincter tone may be poor immediately after catheter removal, resulting in urinary incontinence or dribbling. This is a common but distressing situation for the patient. Sphincter tone can be strengthened by having the patient practice Kegel exercises (pelvic floor muscle technique) 10 to 20 times per hour while awake. The patient should be encouraged to practice start-

ing and stopping the stream several times during urination. This facilitates learning the pelvic floor exercises. It usually takes several weeks to achieve urinary continence. In some instances, control of urine may never be fully regained. Continence can improve for up to 12 months. If continence has not been achieved by that time, the patient may be referred to a continence clinic. A variety of methods, including biofeedback, have been used to achieve positive results. The patient can also be instructed to use a penile clamp, condom catheter, or incontinence pads or briefs to avoid embarrassment from dribbling. In severe cases, an occlusive cuff that serves as an artificial sphincter can be surgically implanted to restore continence. The nurse should assist the patient in finding ways to manage the problem that will allow him to continue socializing and interacting with others.

The patient should be observed for signs of postoperative infection. If an external wound is present (from an open prostatectomy), the area should be observed for redness, heat, swelling, and purulent drainage. Special care must be taken if a perineal incision is present because of the proximity of the anus. Rectal procedures, such as taking rectal temperatures and administering enemas, should be avoided. The insertion of well-lubricated belladonna and opium suppositories is acceptable.

Dietary intervention and stool softeners are important in the postoperative period to prevent the patient from straining while having bowel movements. Straining increases the intraabdominal pressure, which can lead to bleeding at the operative site. A diet high in fiber facilitates the passage of stool.

Ambulatory and Home Care. Discharge planning and home care issues are important aspects of care after prostate surgery. Instructions include (1) caring for an indwelling catheter (if one is left in place); (2) managing urinary incontinence; (3) maintaining oral fluids between 2000 and 3000 ml per day; (4) observing for signs and symptoms of urinary tract and wound infection; (5) preventing constipation; (6) avoiding heavy lifting (more than 10 lb [4.5 kg]); and (7) refraining from driving or intercourse after surgery as directed by the physician.

The patient may experience a change in sexual functioning following surgery. Many men experience retrograde ejaculation because of trauma to the internal sphincter. Semen is discharged into the bladder at orgasm and may produce cloudy urine when the patient urinates after orgasm. Physiologic erectile dysfunction (ED) may occur if the nerves are cut or damaged during surgery. The patient may experience anxiety over the change due to a perceived loss of his sex role, self-esteem, or quality of sexual interaction with his partner. The nurse should discuss these changes with the patient and his partner and allow them to ask questions and express their concerns. Sexual counseling and treatment options may be necessary if ED becomes a chronic or permanent problem. ED is discussed later in the chapter. It should be pointed out that although some patients experience concerns regarding change in sexual function, this is not a universal concern. Many men are comfortable with such changes and view them as appropriate for their age. If this is the case, nurses should be careful not to impose concern in their enthusiastic attempts to pursue such problems.[11]

The bladder may take up to 2 months to return to its normal capacity. The patient should be instructed to drink at least 2 L of fluid per day and urinate every 2 to 3 hours to flush the urinary tract. Bladder irritants such as caffeine products, citrus juices, and alcohol should be avoided or limited to small amounts.

Because the patient may be experiencing incontinence or dribbling, he may incorrectly believe that decreasing fluid intake will relieve this problem. Urethral strictures may result from instrumentation or catheterization. Treatment may include teaching the patient intermittent clean catheterization or having a urethral dilation.

The patient must be advised that he should continue to have a yearly DRE if he has had any procedure other than complete removal of the prostate. Hyperplasia or cancer can occur in the remaining prostatic tissue.

■ Evaluation

Expected outcomes for the patient with BPH are presented in NCP 53-1.

PROSTATE CANCER

Prostate cancer is a malignant tumor of the prostate gland. It is estimated that 189,000 new cases of prostate cancer were diagnosed in 2002, and 30,200 men died from the disease.[12] One of every five men will develop prostate cancer at some point during their lives. Prostate cancer is the most common cancer among men, excluding skin cancer. It is the second leading cause of cancer death in men (exceeded only by lung cancer). The majority (more than 75%) of cases occur in men over age 65. However, many cases occur in younger men who sometimes have a more aggressive type of cancer. There was a large increase in the incidence of newly diagnosed cases of prostate cancer between 1988 and 1992. This increase in number was attributed to the widespread use of prostate-specific antigen (PSA) as a screening procedure, allowing early detection of prostate cancer. The incidence of prostate cancer appears to have peaked and has now leveled off.[12]

Etiology and Pathophysiology

Prostate cancer is an androgen-dependent adenocarcinoma. The majority of tumors occur in the outer aspect of the prostate gland. Prostate cancer is usually slow growing. It can spread by three routes: direct extension, through the lymph system, or through the bloodstream. Spread by direct extension involves the seminal vesicles, urethral mucosa, bladder wall, and external sphincter. The cancer later spreads through the lymphatic system to the regional lymph nodes. The veins from the prostate seem to be the mode of spread to the pelvic bones, head of the femur, lower lumbar spine, liver, and lungs.

Age, ethnicity, and family history are three nonmodifiable risk factors for prostate cancer. The incidence of prostate cancer rises markedly after age 50; more than 80% of men diagnosed are older than 65.[13] African Americans have the highest incidence of prostate cancer of any ethnic group, with a rate twice that of white men. In addition, they are more likely to have prostate cancer at a younger age, have more aggressive tumors at diagnosis, and have higher mortality rates.[14] A family history of prostate cancer, especially first-degree relatives (fathers, brothers), is also associated with an increased risk. Genetic mutations in certain genes may contribute to the risk of prostate cancer in susceptible men.

A high-fat diet is thought to be associated with an increased risk of prostate cancer.[15,16] Although occupational exposure to chemicals (e.g., cadmium) may be associated with higher prostate cancer risk, this possible risk continues to be studied.[13,14] A history of BPH is not a risk factor for prostate cancer.

Clinical Manifestations and Complications

Prostate cancer is usually asymptomatic in the early stages. Eventually the patient may have symptoms similar to those of BPH, including dysuria, hesitancy, dribbling, frequency, urgency, hematuria, nocturia, retention, interruption of urinary stream, and inability to urinate. Pain in the lumbosacral area that radiates down to the hips or legs, when coupled with urinary symptoms, may indicate metastasis.

Early recognition and treatment is required to control growth, prevent metastasis, and preserve quality of life. The tumor can spread to pelvic lymph nodes, bones, bladder, lungs, and liver. Once the tumor has spread to distant sites, the major problem becomes the management of pain. As the cancer spreads to the bones (a common site of metastasis), pain can become severe, especially in the back and the legs because of compression of the spinal cord and destruction of bone.

Diagnostic Studies

Improved diagnostic techniques have greatly enhanced the detection of prostate cancer. The two primary screening tools are DRE and a blood test for **prostate-specific antigen** (PSA), a glycoprotein produced by the prostate. On DRE the prostate may feel hard and have asymmetric enlargement with areas of induration or nodules.

Elevated levels of PSA (normal level, 0 to 4 ng/ml [0 to 4 μg/L]) indicate prostatic pathology, although not necessarily prostate cancer. Mild elevations in PSA may occur in BPH, acute or chronic prostatitis, or urinary retention, or after long bike rides. In addition, cystoscopy, indwelling urethral catheters, and prostate biopsies may produce an elevation. When prostate cancer exists, serum PSA levels are a useful marker of tumor volume (i.e., the higher the PSA level, the greater the tumor mass). Some men with prostate cancer have normal PSA levels.

PSA is not only used to detect prostate cancer, but it is also used to monitor the success of treatment. When the treatment has been successful in removing prostate cancer, PSA levels should fall to undetectable levels. Regular measurement of PSA levels following treatment is important to evaluate the effectiveness of treatment and possible recurrence of prostate cancer.

CULTURAL & ETHNIC CONSIDERATIONS
Cancer of the Male Reproductive System

- Prostate cancer occurs twice as frequently among African American men as among white men.
- African American men tend to be diagnosed with prostate cancer at an earlier age, have more advanced disease at the time of diagnosis, and have a higher mortality rate than do white men. Although the mortality rate among African American men is higher than that among whites, the mortality rate is declining.
- Hispanic and Asian American men have a lower incidence of prostate cancer and lower mortality rates as compared with white men.
- Testicular cancer occurs most frequently among whites compared with other ethnic groups and is rare in African Americans.

Elevated levels of prostatic isoenzyme of serum acid phosphatase (prostatic acid phosphatase [PAP]) is another indication of prostate cancer, especially if there is extracapsular spread. With advanced prostate cancer, serum alkaline phosphatase is increased as a result of bone metastasis. Investigation is now under way to locate a serum marker for prostate cancer similar to CA-125, which is a useful marker in ovarian cancer. (Ovarian cancer is discussed in Chapter 52.)

Neither PSA nor DRE is a definitive diagnostic test for prostate cancer. If PSA levels are elevated or if the DRE is abnormal, biopsy of the prostate tissue is indicated. Biopsy of prostate tissue is necessary to confirm the diagnosis of prostate cancer. The biopsy is typically done using TRUS because it allows the physician to visualize the prostate and pinpoint abnormalities. When a suspicious area is located, a special biopsy needle is inserted into the prostate to obtain a tissue sample. A pathologic examination of the tissue specimen is done to assess for malignant changes. Other tests used to determine the location and extent of the spread of the cancer may include bone scan, computed tomography (CT), magnetic resonance imaging (MRI) using an endorectal probe, and TRUS.

The Prostascint scan is a single-photon emission computed tomography (SPECT) imaging technique that uses a monoclonal antibody to target prostate-specific membrane antigens. This procedure is able to detect spread of prostate cancer to the pelvic lymph nodes.

Collaborative Care

Early-stage prostate cancer is a curable disease in the majority of men. Based on findings from diagnostic studies, the prostate cancer is staged and graded. Two common classification systems used for staging prostate cancer, the Whitmore-Jewett and tumor, node, metastasis (TNM) systems, are both based on the size (volume) of the tumor and spread (Table 53-5). It is estimated that 80% of patients with prostate cancer are initially diagnosed when the cancer is in either a local or regional stage. The 5-year survival rate with an initial diagnosis at this stage is 100%.[12]

Grading of the tumor is done based on tumor histology using the Gleason scale. With this scale, tumors are graded from 1 to 5 based on the degree of glandular differentiation. Grade 1 represents the most well differentiated (most like the original cells) and grade 5 represents the most poorly differentiated (undifferentiated). Gleason grades are given to the two most commonly occurring patterns of cells and added together. The Gleason score is a number from 2 to 10. This scale is used to predict how quickly the cancer will progress.

The collaborative care of the patient with prostate cancer depends on the stage of the cancer and the overall health of the patient. At all stages, there is more than one possible treatment option. The decision of which treatment course to pursue is made jointly by the patient and the physician based on a careful analysis of the facts and the patient's preference.[17] Table 53-6 summarizes the various treatment options available.

Conservative Therapy. Prostate cancer is relatively slow growing. Therefore a conservative approach to management of prostate cancer is "watchful waiting" (also known as "deferred treatment"). The decision to adopt a strategy of watchful waiting is appropriate when there is (1) a life expectancy of less than 10 years, (2) presence of significant comorbid disease, and (3) presence of a low-grade, low-stage tumor. These patients are

---

TABLE 53-5 Whitmore-Jewett Staging Classification of Prostate Cancer

Stage A: Clinically Unrecognized

A1	<5% of prostatic tissue neoplastic
A2	>5% of prostatic tissue neoplastic, all high-grade tumors

Stage B: Clinically Intracapsular

B1	Nodule <2 cm and surrounded by palpably normal tissue
B2	Nodule >2 cm or multiple nodules

Stage C: Clinically Extracapsular, Localized to Periprostatic Area

C1	Minimal extracapsular extension
C2	Large tumors involving seminal vesicles, adjacent structures, or both

Stage D: Metastatic Disease

D1	Pelvic lymph node metastases or ureteral obstruction causing hydronephrosis
D2	Distant metastases to bone, viscera, or other soft tissue structures

---

TABLE 53-6 Collaborative Care — Prostate Cancer

Diagnostic
History and physical examination
Digital rectal examination (DRE)
Prostate-specific antigen (PSA)
Prostatic acid phosphatase (PAP)
Transrectal ultrasound
Biopsy of prostate and lymph nodes
Computed tomography (CT), magnetic resonance imaging (MRI), bone scan (to evaluate for metastatic disease)

Collaborative Therapy
Stage A
Watchful waiting with annual PSA and DRE
Radical prostatectomy
Radiation therapy
• External beam
• Brachytherapy
Stage B
Radical prostatectomy
Radiation therapy
Stage C
Radical prostatectomy
Radiation therapy
Hormone therapy
Orchiectomy
Stage D
Hormone therapy
Orchiectomy
Chemotherapy
Radiation therapy to metastatic bone areas

typically followed with frequent PSA measurements, along with DRE, to monitor the progress of the disease. Significant changes in either PSA, DRE, or the development of symptoms warrant a reevaluation of treatment options, whether they be definitive or palliative.

Surgical Therapy

Radical prostatectomy. With **radical prostatectomy,** the entire prostate gland, seminal vesicles, and part of the bladder neck (ampulla) are removed. The entire prostate is removed because the cancer tends to be in many different locations within the gland. In addition, a retroperitoneal lymph node dissection is usually done. A radical prostatectomy is the surgical procedure considered the most effective treatment for long-term survival. Thus it is the preferred treatment for men younger than 70 years of age who are in good health and with the cancer confined to the prostate (stages A and B).[17] Surgery is usually not considered an option for stage D cancer (except to relieve symptoms associated with obstruction) because metastasis has already occurred. The two most common approaches for radical prostatectomy are retropubic and perineal resection (Fig. 53-4). With the *retropubic*

approach, a low midline abdominal incision is made to access the prostate gland, and the pelvic lymph nodes can be dissected. With the *perineal* resection, an incision is made between the scrotum and anus. This procedure cannot remove lymph nodes. A laparoscopic approach to prostatectomy is being used in some settings. It has the potential to offer technologic improvement, less bleeding, less pain, and faster recovery compared with traditional approaches, but the long-term benefits are still being investigated.[18]

After surgery, the patient has a large indwelling catheter with a 30 ml balloon placed in the bladder via the urethra. This catheter is typically left in place for 1 to 2 weeks. A drain is left in the surgical site to aid in the removal of drainage from the area. This drain is typically removed after a couple of days. Because the perineal approach has a higher risk of postoperative infection (due to of the location of the incision related to the anus), careful dressing changes and perineal care after each bowel movement are important for comfort and to prevent infection. The typical length of hospital stay postoperatively is 3 days.

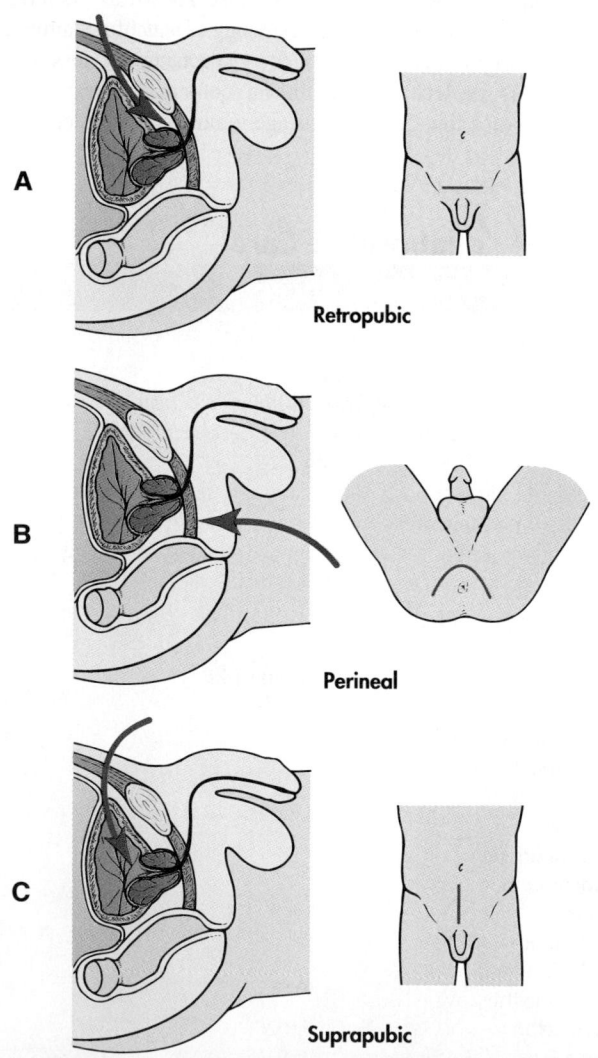

Retropubic

Perineal

Suprapubic

FIG. 53-4 Three approaches used to perform a prostatectomy. **A,** Retropubic approach involves a midline abdominal incision. **B,** Perineal approach involves an incision between the scrotum and anus. **C,** Suprapubic approach involves an abdominal incision.

NURSING RESEARCH

Incontinence and Impotence after Prostatectomy for Prostate Cancer

Citation
Maliski SL, Heilemann MV, McCorkle R: Mastery of post-prostatectomy incontinence and impotence: his work, her work, our work, *Oncol Nurs Forum* 28:985, 2001.

Purpose
To describe couples' experiences of incontinence and impotence following prostatectomy for prostate cancer.

Method
This qualitative design involved a sample of 20 couples from a clinical trial of a Standardized Nursing Intervention Protocol Postprostatectomy. The couples were interviewed using a semistructured guide to discuss their experiences with incontinence and impotence as a result of prostatectomy. Data were analyzed using grounded theory techniques.

Results and Conclusions
The men focused on gaining an understanding of incontinence, mastering incontinence, networking, confronting impotency, and putting these issues in perspective. Wives were supportive by managing anxiety, encouraging mastery, putting impotence into perspective, and reassuring their spouses. The couples found nurses to be a source of information, support, and affirmation. Both men and women worked through incontinence and impotence in the context of surviving cancer and maintaining a loving relationship. Mastery emerged as a key concept from the findings.

Implications for Nursing Practice
Incontinence and impotence that result from prostectomy affect both the man and his wife. The wife can play a key role in dealing with these issues. Nursing interventions that promote mastery, as well as helping couples place these issues in the context of cancer survival, are an important aspect of helping couples cope with incontinence and impotence. Nurses can help couples regain a sense of mastery by providing information, encouraging the attainment of self-care skills, confirming progress, and providing emotional support.

The two major complications following a radical prostatectomy are erectile dysfunction and incontinence.[19] Because this procedure destroys the nerves needed for erection, erectile dysfunction occurs. The incidence of erectile dysfunction is dependent on the patient's age, preoperative sexual functioning, whether nerve-sparing surgery was performed, and the expertise of the surgeon. Problems with urinary control occur in nearly all men for the first few months following surgery because the bladder must be reattached to the urethra after the prostate is removed. Over time, the bladder adjusts and most men regain control. One study reported that only 6.4% were incontinent 18 months after surgery.[20] Other common complications associated with surgery include hemorrhage, urinary retention, infection, wound dehiscence, deep vein thrombosis, and pulmonary emboli.

Nerve-sparing procedure. Many men desire to retain sexual function following radical prostatectomy. In such cases a nerve-sparing procedure that spares the nerves responsible for erection may be possible. This procedure is the preferred choice for most men undergoing prostatectomy in the early stage of the disease. Nerve-sparing prostatectomy is indicated only for patients with cancer confined within the prostate gland. Although the risk of erectile dysfunction is significantly reduced with this procedure, there is no guarantee that potency will be maintained. Because the nerves lie directly beneath the prostate gland, the risk of damage is very high. The percent of success reported varies.[20]

Cryosurgery. Prostatic cryosurgery is a surgical technique that destroys cancer cells by freezing the tissue. It has been used both as an initial treatment and as a second-line treatment after radiation treatment failures. A transrectal ultrasound probe is inserted to visualize the prostate gland. Probes containing liquid nitrogen are then inserted into the prostate. Liquid nitrogen delivers freezing temperatures, destroying the tissue. The treatment takes about 2 hours under general or spinal anesthesia and does not involve an abdominal incision. Possible complications of prostatic cryosurgery include damage to the urethra, and, in rare cases, a urethrorectal fistula (an opening between the urethra and the rectum) or a urethrocutaneous fistula (an opening between the urethra and the skin). Tissue sloughing, erectile dysfunction, urinary incontinence, prostatitis, and hemorrhage have also been reported.

Radiation Therapy. Radiation therapy is a common treatment option for prostate cancer, especially for men over 70, patients who are poor surgical risks, or those who wish to avoid surgery. The long-term outcome of radiation therapy is dependent on the stage of the cancer. Because many of the men choosing radiation therapy are older and perhaps not in as good health as those undergoing prostatectomy, comparisons are difficult.[21] Radiation therapy may be offered as the only treatment, or it may be offered in combination with surgery or with hormonal therapy.

External beam radiation. External beam is the most widely used method of delivering radiation treatments for those with prostate cancer. This therapy can be used to treat patients with prostate cancer confined to the prostate and/or surrounding tissue (stages A, B, and C). Patients are treated on an outpatient basis 5 days a week for 6 to 8 weeks. Each treatment lasts only a few minutes. Side effects from radiation can be acute (occurring during treatment or within 90 days that follow) or delayed (occurring months or years after treatment). Common side effects involve the skin (dryness, redness, irritation, pain), gastrointestinal tract (diarrhea, abdominal cramping, bleeding), urinary tract (dysuria, frequency, hesitancy, urgency, nocturia), sexual functioning (erectile dysfunction), fatigue, and bone marrow suppression.[21] These problems usually resolve 2 to 3 weeks after the completion of radiation therapy. In patients with clinically localized disease, cure rates with external beam radiation are comparable to those with radical prostatectomy.

Brachytherapy. Brachytherapy involves the implantation of radioactive seed implants into the prostate gland, allowing higher radiation doses directly in the tissue while sparing the surrounding tissue (rectum and bladder). The radioactive seeds are placed in the prostate gland with a needle through a grid template guided by transrectal ultrasound (Fig. 53-5). The grid template and ultrasound ensure accurate placement of the seeds.[21] Because brachytherapy is a one-time outpatient procedure, many patients find this more convenient than external beam radiation treatment. Brachytherapy is best suited for patients with stage A or B prostate cancer.[17] The most common side effect is the development of urinary irritative or obstructive problems. The AUA Symptom Index (see Table 53-1) can be used to measure urinary function for patients undergoing brachytherapy and can be incorporated into postoperative nursing management.[22] For those with more advanced tumors, brachytherapy may be offered in combination with external beam radiation treatment. Brachytherapy is discussed further in Chapter 15.

Drug Therapy. The forms of drug therapy available for the treatment of prostate cancer are hormonal therapy, chemotherapy, or a combination of both.

Hormonal therapy. Prostate cancer growth is largely dependent on the presence of androgens. Therefore androgen deprivation is the primary therapeutic approach for men with prostatic cancer. Hormone therapy is focused on reducing the levels of circulating androgens in order to reduce the tumor growth. Hormone or antiandrogen therapy can also be used as adjunct therapy before surgery or radiation therapy to reduce tumor size, and in men with locally advanced disease (stage C). One of the biggest challenges with hormonal therapy is the development of hormone-refractory disease. The duration of response to initial hormonal therapy averages from 18 to 24 months.[23] Androgen ablation can be produced by interference with androgen production (e.g.,

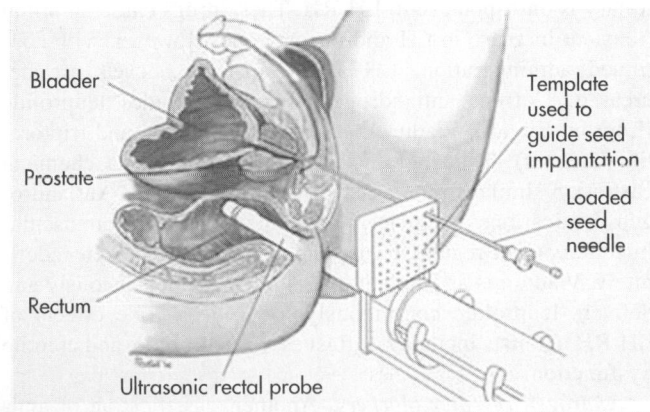

FIG. 53-5 Prostate brachytherapy. Radioactive seeds are implanted with a needle guided by ultrasound and a template grid.

Bladder

Template used to guide seed implantation

Prostate

Loaded seed needle

Rectum

Ultrasonic rectal probe

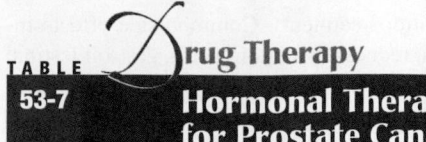

TABLE 53-7	Drug Therapy — Hormonal Therapy for Prostate Cancer	
THERAPY	**MECHANISM OF ACTION**	
Luteinizing Hormone–Releasing Hormone (LH-RH) Agonists		
leuprolide (Lupron, Eligard, Viadur subcutaneous implant) goserelin (Zoladex) buserelin (Suprefact) triptorelin (Trelstar)	• Suppress release of LH-RH • Prevent release of LH • Decrease testosterone production	
Androgen Receptor Blockers		
bicalutamide (Casodex) flutamide (Eulexin) nilutamide (Nilandron)	• Block the action of testosterone by competing with receptor sites	
Estrogen		
diethlystilbestrol (DES)	• Inhibits LH secretion • Decreases testosterone production • Blocks circulating testosterone	
Orchiectomy		
Surgical removal of testicles	• Removes 95% of testosterone source	

LH, Luteinizing hormone.

luteinizing hormone–releasing hormone [LH-RH] agonists, orchiectomy) or androgen receptor blockers (Table 53-7).

Luteinizing hormone–releasing hormone agonists. Luteinizing hormone–releasing hormone (LH-RH) is released from the hypothalamus to stimulate the anterior pituitary to produce luteinizing hormone (LH) and follicle-stimulating hormone (FSH). LH stimulates the testicular Leydig cells to produce testosterone. The LH-RH agonists superstimulate the pituitary. This ultimately results in downregulation of the LH-RH receptors, leading to a refractory condition in which the anterior pituitary is unresponsive to LH-RH. These drugs cause an initial transient increase in LH and testosterone. However, with continued administration, LH and testosterone levels are decreased. Current antiandrogen therapy includes leuprolide (Lupron, Eligard, Viadure), goserelin (Zoladex), and triptorelin (Trelstar). This therapy essentially produces a chemical castration similar to the effects of an orchiectomy. Antiandrogen medications are given by subcutaneous or intramuscular injections on a regular basis, and they must be taken indefinitely. Viadure is an implant that is placed subcutaneously and delivers leuprolide continuously for 1 year. Side effects of LH-RH agonists include hot flashes, loss of libido, and erectile dysfunction.

Androgen receptor blockers. Another classification of antiandrogens are drugs that compete with circulating androgens at the receptor sites. Flutamide (Eulexin), nilutamide (Nilandron),

and bicalutamide (Casodex) are nonsteroidal androgen receptor blockers. They can be used in combination with goserelin or leuprolide. The combination has been found to be safe and well tolerated as a potency-sparing, androgen-ablative therapy. Adverse effects of androgen receptor blockers include loss of libido, erectile dysfunction, and hot flashes. Breast pain and gynecomastia may also occur in men treated with androgen receptor blockers.

Estrogen. Estrogen (e.g., diethylstilbestrol) has been used as a form of androgen deprivation therapy. However, estrogen treatment is declining in popularity because of cardiovascular complications (e.g., myocardial infarction, deep vein thrombosis, cerebrovascular disease), and the development of more effective hormone therapies.

Orchiectomy. A bilateral orchiectomy is the surgical removal of the testes that may be done alone or in combination with prostatectomy. For advanced stages of prostate cancer (stage D) an orchiectomy is one treatment option for cancer control. Testosterone, produced by the testes, stimulates growth of the prostate cancer. An orchiectomy reduces the circulating testosterone levels by 90%.[18] Another possible benefit of this procedure is the rapid relief of bone pain associated with advanced tumors. Orchiectomy may also induce sufficient shrinkage of the prostate to relieve urinary obstruction in later stages of disease when surgery is not an option.

Side effects of orchiectomy include hot flashes, erectile dysfunction, loss of sex drive, and irritability. Weight gain and loss of muscle mass, which are also common, can alter a man's physical appearance. Osteoporosis has also been reported as a consequence of orchiectomy. These physical changes can affect self-esteem, leading to grief and depression. Although this procedure is permanent and cost effective (compared with chemical hormone manipulation using LH-RH agonists), many men prefer drug therapy to orchiectomy.

Chemotherapy. The use of chemotherapeutic agents has primarily been limited to treatment for those with hormone-resistant prostate cancer (HRPC) in late-stage disease. In HRPC the cancer is progressing despite treatment. This occurs in patients who have taken an antiandrogen for a certain period of time. Historically, prostate cancer has been poorly responsive to chemotherapy and has not been shown to improve survival. Thus the goal of chemotherapy is palliation.[24] Some of the more commonly used chemotherapy drugs include mitoxantrone (Novantrone), cyclosphophamide (Cytoxan), idarubicin (Idamycin), epirubicin (Ellence), and estramustine (Emcyt).

Bisphosphonates. Patients with advanced prostate cancer have a high risk of developing bone complication such as pain, fractures, and spinal cord compression. Bisphosphonates can be used to prevent and treat bone complications in advanced prostate cancer. Bisphosphonates include zolendronate (Zomex), risendronate (Actonel), etidronate (Didronel), and alendronate (Fosamax).

■ Culturally Competent Care: Prostate Cancer

Nurses must be aware of not only the epidemiologic differences that occur with prostate cancer, but also the differences that exist in health promotion practice. Demographic characteristics should be considered when providing information about the risk for prostate cancer and screening recommendations.

African American men suffer higher mortality rates than white men, in part because their prostate cancer often is more advanced at the time of diagnosis. Despite the availability of early screening measures (PSA and DRE), African American men and those in lower socioeconomic groups frequently do not use such services. This is partially related to actual and perceived knowledge levels of prostate cancer.[25] One study found that men are most likely to take part in regular screenings when a health care provider informed them of their risk of prostate cancer and screening options.[26] Although exposure to electronic and print media is successful in informing some men about prostate cancer, significant differences of effectiveness exist based on demographic variables such as ethnicity, age, education level, and socioeconomic level. Ideally, no man should be unaware of the risks associated with prostate cancer and screening methods available. The nurse must consider the best method to communicate this information to men of all cultures that will result in the greatest degree of understanding and participation in prostate cancer screening. ■

NURSING MANAGEMENT
PROSTATE CANCER

■ Nursing Assessment

Subjective and objective data that should be obtained from a patient with prostate cancer are presented in Table 53-8.

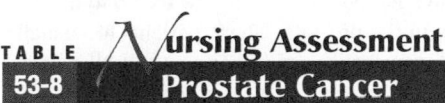

TABLE 53-8	Nursing Assessment Prostate Cancer

Subjective Data
Important Health Information
Medications: Testosterone supplements; use of any medications affecting urinary tract such as morphine, anticholinergics, monoamine oxidase inhibitors, and tricyclic antidepressants
Functional Health Patterns
Health perception–health management: Positive family history; increasing fatigue and malaise
Nutritional-metabolic: High-fat diet; anorexia, weight loss (possible indicators of metastasis)
Elimination: Hesitancy or straining to start stream, urinary urgency, frequency, retention with dribbling, weak stream, hematuria
Sleep: Nocturia
Cognitive-perceptual: Dysuria; low back pain radiating to legs or pelvis, bone pain (possible indicators of metastasis)
Self-perception–self-concept: Anxiety regarding self-concept

Objective Data
General
Older adult male; pelvic lymphadenopathy (late sign)
Urinary
Distended bladder on palpation; unilaterally hard, enlarged, fixed prostate on rectal examination
Musculoskeletal
Pathologic fractures (metastasis)
Possible Findings
↑ Serum PSA; ↑ serum PAP (metastasis); nodular and irregular prostate on ultrasonography, positive biopsy results; anemia

PAP, Prostatic acid phosphatase; *PSA,* prostate-specific antigen.

■ Nursing Diagnoses

Nursing diagnoses for the patient with prostate cancer depend on the stage of the cancer. General nursing diagnoses, which may or may not apply to every patient with cancer of the prostate, may include, but are not limited to, the following:
- Decisional conflict *related to* numerous alternative treatment options
- Acute pain *related to* surgery, prostatic enlargement, bone metastasis, and bladder spasms
- Urinary retention *related to* obstruction of urethra or bladder neck by the prostate, blood clots, and loss of bladder tone
- Impaired urinary elimination *related to* bladder neck sphincter damage
- Constipation or diarrhea *related to* treatment interventions
- Sexual dysfunction *related to* effects of treatment
- Anxiety *related to* uncertain outcome of disease process on life and lifestyle and effect of treatment on sexual functioning

■ Planning

The overall goals are that the patient with prostate cancer will (1) be an active participant in the treatment plan, (2) have satisfactory pain control, (3) follow the therapeutic plan, (4) accept the effect of the therapeutic plan on sexual function, and (5) find a satisfactory way to manage the impact on bladder or bowel function.

■ Nursing Implementation

Health Promotion. One of the most important roles for nurses in relation to prostate cancer is to encourage patients to have an annual prostate screening (PSA and DRE) starting at age 50 or younger if risk factors are present. Because of their increased risk of prostate cancer, African American men and other men with a family history of prostate cancer should have an annual PSA and DRE beginning at age 45.[27]

Acute Intervention. Preoperative and postoperative phases of radical prostatectomy are similar to surgical procedures for BPH (see pp. 1441-1443). Nursing interventions for the patient who undergoes radiation therapy and chemotherapy are discussed in Chapter 15. An additional consideration is the psychologic response of the patient to a diagnosis of cancer. The nurse should provide sensitive, caring support for the patient and his family to help them cope with the diagnosis of cancer. Prostate support groups are available for men and their families to encourage them to be active, informed participants in their own care.

Ambulatory and Home Care. If the patient is discharged with an indwelling catheter in place, the nurse must teach appropriate catheter care. The patient should be instructed to clean the urethral meatus with soap and water once a day; maintain a high fluid intake; keep the collecting bag lower than the bladder at all times; keep the catheter securely anchored to the inner thigh or abdomen; and report any signs of bladder infection, such as bladder spasms, fever, or hematuria. If urinary incontinence is a problem, patients should be encouraged to practice pelvic floor muscle exercises (Kegel exercises) at every urination and throughout the day. Continuous practice during the 4- to 6-week healing process improves the success rate. Products used for incontinence specifically designed for men are available through home care product catalogs and many retail stores.

Although prostate cancer has a high cure rate if detected and treated early, prognosis for stage D prostate cancer is very unfavorable. Hospice care is often appropriate and beneficial to the patient and family. (Hospice care is discussed in Chapter 6.) Common problems experienced by the patient with advanced prostate cancer include fatigue, bladder outlet obstruction and ureteral obstruction (caused by compression of the urethra and/or ureters from tumor mass or lymph node metastasis), severe bone pain and fractures (caused by bone metastasis), spinal cord compression (from spinal metastasis), and leg edema (caused by lymphedema, deep vein thrombosis, and other medical conditions). Nursing interventions must focus on all of these problems. However, management of pain is one of the most important aspects of nursing care for these patients. Pain control is managed through ongoing pain assessment, administration of prescribed medications (both narcotic and non-narcotic agents), and the use of nonpharmacologic methods of pain relief. (Pain management is discussed further in Chapter 9.)

■ Evaluation

Evaluation is based on expected outcomes. The outcomes are that the patient with prostate cancer will
- be an active participant in the treatment plan
- have satisfactory pain control
- follow the therapeutic plan
- accept the effect of the treatment on sexual function
- find a satisfactory way to manage the impact on bladder or bowel function

PROSTATITIS

Etiology and Pathophysiology

Prostatitis is a broad term that describes a group of inflammatory conditions affecting the prostate gland. It is the most common urologic problem in men younger than 50 years of age.

Nearly 2 million men are treated for prostatitis each year.[28] Historically, this condition has lacked a strong agreement regarding the cause, diagnosis, and optimal treatment. To bring greater consistency in approaching this common condition, the National Institutes of Health established consensus classifications of prostatitis syndromes. The consensus classifications include four categories: (1) acute bacterial prostatitis, (2) chronic bacterial prostatitis, (3) chronic prostatitis/chronic pelvic pain syndrome, and (4) asymptomatic inflammatory prostatitis.[29]

Both acute and chronic bacterial prostatitis generally result from organisms reaching the prostate gland by one of the following routes: ascending from the urethra, descending from the bladder, and invasion via the bloodstream or the lymphatic channels. Common causative organisms are *Escherichia coli, Klebsiella, Pseudomonas, Enterobacter, Proteus, Chlamydia trachomatis, Neisseria gonorrhoeae,* and group D streptococci. Chronic bacterial prostatitis differs from acute prostatitis in that it involves recurrent episodes of infection.[29]

Chronic prostatitis/chronic pelvic pain syndrome is a new term that describes the syndrome with prostate and urinary pain in the absence of an obvious infectious process. The etiology of chronic prostatitis/chronic pelvic pain syndrome is unclear. It may occur after a viral illness, or it may be associated with sexually transmitted diseases (STDs), particularly in a younger adult. The etiology is not known, and a culture reveals no causative organisms. However, leukocytes may be found in prostatic secretions.

Asymptomatic inflammatory prostatitis is usually diagnosed in individuals who have no symptoms, but are found to have an inflammatory process in the prostate. These patients are usually diagnosed during the evaluation of other genitourinary tract problems. Leukocytes are present in the seminal fluid from the prostate, but the cause of this process is unclear.

Clinical Manifestations and Complications

Common clinical manifestations of acute bacterial prostatitis include fever, chills, back pain, and perineal pain, along with acute urinary symptoms such as dysuria, urinary frequency, urgency, and cloudy urine. The patient may also have acute urinary retention caused by prostatic swelling. With DRE, the prostate is extremely swollen, very tender, and firm. The complications of prostatitis are epididymitis and cystitis. Sexual functioning may be affected as manifested by postejaculation pain, libido problems, and erectile dysfunction. Prostatic abscess is also a potential, but uncommon, complication.

Chronic bacterial prostatitis and chronic prostatitis/pelvic pain syndrome manifest with similar symptoms that are generally milder than those associated with acute bacterial prostatitis. These include irritative voiding symptoms (frequency, urgency, dysuria), backache, perineal/pelvic pain, and ejaculatory pain. Obstructive symptoms are uncommon unless the patient has coexisting BPH. With DRE, the prostate feels enlarged and firm (often described as boggy) and is slightly tender with palpation. Chronic prostatitis can predispose the patient to recurrent urinary tract infections.

The clinical features of prostatitis can be mimicked by urinary tract infection. However, acute cystitis is not common in men.

Diagnostic Studies

Because patients with prostatitis have urinary symptoms, a urinalysis (UA) and urine culture are indicated; often white blood cells (WBCs) and bacteria are present. If the patient has a fever,

WBC count and blood cultures are also indicated. The PSA test may be done to rule out prostate cancer. However, PSA levels are often elevated with prostatic inflammation. Thus it is not considered diagnostic in itself.

Microscopic evaluation and culture of expressed prostate secretion (EPS) is considered useful in the diagnosis of prostatitis. EPS is obtained using a premassage and postmassage test. The patient is asked to void into a specimen cup just before and just after a vigorous prostate massage. Prostatic massage (for EPS) should be avoided if acute bacterial prostatitis is suspected, because compression is extremely painful and can increase the risk of bacteria spread.[30] TRUS has not been particularly useful in the diagnosis of prostatitis. However, transabdominal ultrasound or MRI may be done to rule out an abscess on the prostate.

NURSING *and* COLLABORATIVE MANAGEMENT
PROSTATITIS

Antibiotics commonly used for acute and chronic bacterial prostatitis include trimethoprim-sulfamethoxazole (Bactrim), ciprofloxacin (Cipro), and floxacin (Floxin). Doxycycline (Vibramycin) or tetracycline may be prescribed for those patients with multiple sex partners. Antibiotics are usually given orally for up to 4 weeks for acute bacterial prostatitis. However, if the patient has high fever or other signs of impending sepsis, hospitalization and intravenous antibiotics are prescribed. Patients with chronic bacterial prostatitis are given oral antibiotic therapy for 4 to 16 weeks. A short course of oral antibiotics is usually prescribed for those with chronic prostatitis/chronic pelvic pain syndrome. However, antibiotic therapy often is ineffective for these patients.

Although patients with acute and chronic bacterial prostatitis tend to experience a great amount of discomfort, the pain resolves as the infection is treated. Pain management for patients with chronic prostatitis/chronic pelvic pain syndrome is more difficult because the pain persists for weeks to months. Antiinflammatory agents are the most common agents used for pain control in prostatitis, but these provide only moderate pain relief. Narcotic pain medications can be used, but because this pain is chronic in nature, the use of narcotics should be approached cautiously.

Acute urinary retention can develop in acute prostatitis requiring bladder drainage with suprapubic catheterization. Passage of a catheter through an inflamed urethra is contraindicated in acute prostatitis. Repetitive prostatic massage is thought to be therapeutic for most types of prostatitis, but it is not an appropriate measure for acute bacterial prostatitis. This measure relieves congestion within the prostate by squeezing out excess prostatic secretions, thus providing pain relief. Prostatic massage is performed by using the index finger of a gloved hand and pressing down on the prostate, covering the entire gland's surface in longitudinal strokes. This is done two to three times a week for 6 weeks.[30] Measures to stimulate ejaculation (masturbation and intercourse) help drain the prostate as well and are encouraged.

Because the prostate can serve as a source of bacteria, fluid intake should be kept at a high level for all patients experiencing prostatitis. Nursing interventions are aimed at encouraging the patient to drink plenty of fluids. This is especially important for those with acute bacterial prostatitis because of the increased fluid needs associated with fever and infection. Management of fever is also an important nursing intervention.

Problems of the Penis

Health problems of the penis are rare if sexually transmitted infectious diseases are excluded (see Chapter 51). Problems of the penis may be classified as congenital, problems of the prepuce, problems with the erectile mechanism, and cancer.

CONGENITAL PROBLEMS

Hypospadias is a urologic abnormality in which the urethral meatus is located on the ventral surface of the penis anywhere from the corona to the perineum. Hormonal influences in utero, environmental factors, and genetic factors are possible causes. Surgical repair of hypospadias may be necessary if it is associated with *chordee* (a painful downward curvature of the penis during erection) or if it prevents intercourse or normal urination. Surgery may also be done for cosmetic reasons or emotional well-being.

Epispadias, an opening of the urethra on the dorsal surface of the penis, is a complex birth defect that is usually associated with other genitourinary tract defects. Corrective surgery to place the urethra in a normal position in the penis is usually done in early childhood.

PROBLEMS OF THE PREPUCE

Problems of the prepuce in the United States are rare because circumcision has been a routine procedure for most male infants for many years. Circumcision, the surgical removal of the foreskin of the penis, is a procedure done to male infants for religious or cultural reasons. It is believed to prevent problems such as *phimosis* (tightness of the foreskin resulting in the inability to retract it), *paraphimosis* (tightness of the foreskin resulting in the inability to pull it forward from a retracted position), and cancer of the penis. A recent trend is that fewer parents are having their infants circumcised, which may result in an increased incidence of problems in the future.

Phimosis is a constriction of the uncircumcised foreskin around the head of the penis, making retraction difficult. It is caused by edema or inflammation of the foreskin, usually associated with poor hygiene techniques that allow bacterial and yeast organisms to become trapped under the foreskin.

Paraphimosis is edema of the retracted uncircumcised foreskin, preventing normal return over the glans. This can occur when the foreskin is pulled back during bathing, use of urinary catheters, or intercourse and is not placed back in the forward position. Antibiotics, warm soaks, and sometimes circumcision or dorsal slit of the prepuce may be required. Careful cleaning followed by replacement of the foreskin generally prevents these problems.

PROBLEMS OF THE ERECTILE MECHANISM

Priapism is a painful erection lasting longer than 6 hours. Causes of priapism include thrombosis of the corpus cavernosal veins, leukemia, sickle cell anemia, diabetes mellitus, degenerative lesions of the spine, neoplasms of the brain or spinal cord, prolonged foreplay, injection of vasoactive medications into the corpus cavernosa, and cocaine use. Treatment may include sedatives, injection of smooth muscle relaxants directly into the penis, aspiration and irrigation of the corpora cavernosa with a large-bore needle, or the surgical creation of a shunt to drain the corpora. Prolonged priapism constitutes a medical emergency. Complications may include penile tissue necrosis caused by lack of blood flow or hydronephrosis from bladder distention. After an episode of priapism, the patient may be unable to achieve a normal erection.

Peyronie's disease, sometimes referred to as curved or crooked penis, is caused by plaque formation in one of the corpora cavernosa of the penis. The palpable, nontender, hard plaque formation is usually found on the posterior surface. It may result from trauma to the penile shaft or may occur spontaneously. The plaque prevents adequate blood flow into the spongy tissue, which results in a curvature during erection. The condition is not dangerous but can result in painful erections, erectile dysfunction, or embarrassment. If conservative measures do not correct the problem, surgery may be necessary.

CANCER OF THE PENIS

Cancer of the penis is rare apart from cancers associated with the STD human papillomavirus (HPV) and in men who were not circumcised as infants.[31] The tumor may appear as a superficial ulceration or a pimple-like nodule. The nontender warty lesion may be mistaken for a venereal wart. The majority of malignancies (95%) are well-differentiated squamous cell carcinomas. Treatment in the early stages is laser removal of the growth. A radical resection of the penis may be done if the cancer has spread. Surgery, radiation, or chemotherapy may be tried depending on the extent of the disease, lymph node involvement, or metastasis.

Problems of the Scrotum and Testes
INFLAMMATORY AND INFECTIOUS PROBLEMS
Skin Problems

The skin of the scrotum is susceptible to a number of common skin diseases. The most common conditions of the scrotal skin are fungal infections, dermatitis (neurodermatitis, contact dermatitis, seborrheic dermatitis), and parasitic infections (scabies, lice). These conditions involve discomfort for the patient but are associated with few, if any, severe complications (see Chapter 23).

Epididymitis

Epididymitis is an inflammatory process of the epididymis (Fig. 53-6), usually secondary to an infectious process (sexually or nonsexually transmitted), trauma, or urinary reflux down the vas deferens. When the problem is associated with prostatitis, it is usually painful. Swelling may progress to the point that the epididymis and testis are indistinguishable. In men younger than 35 years of age, the most common cause is through sexual transmission of either gonorrhea or chlamydia. The use of antibiotics is important for both partners if the transmission is through sexual contact. Patients should be encouraged to refrain from sexual intercourse during the acute phase. If they do engage in intercourse, a condom should be used. Conservative treatment consists of bed rest with elevation of the scrotum, use of ice packs, and analgesics. Ambulation places the scrotum in a dependent position and increases pain. Most tenderness subsides within 1 week, although swelling may last for weeks or months.

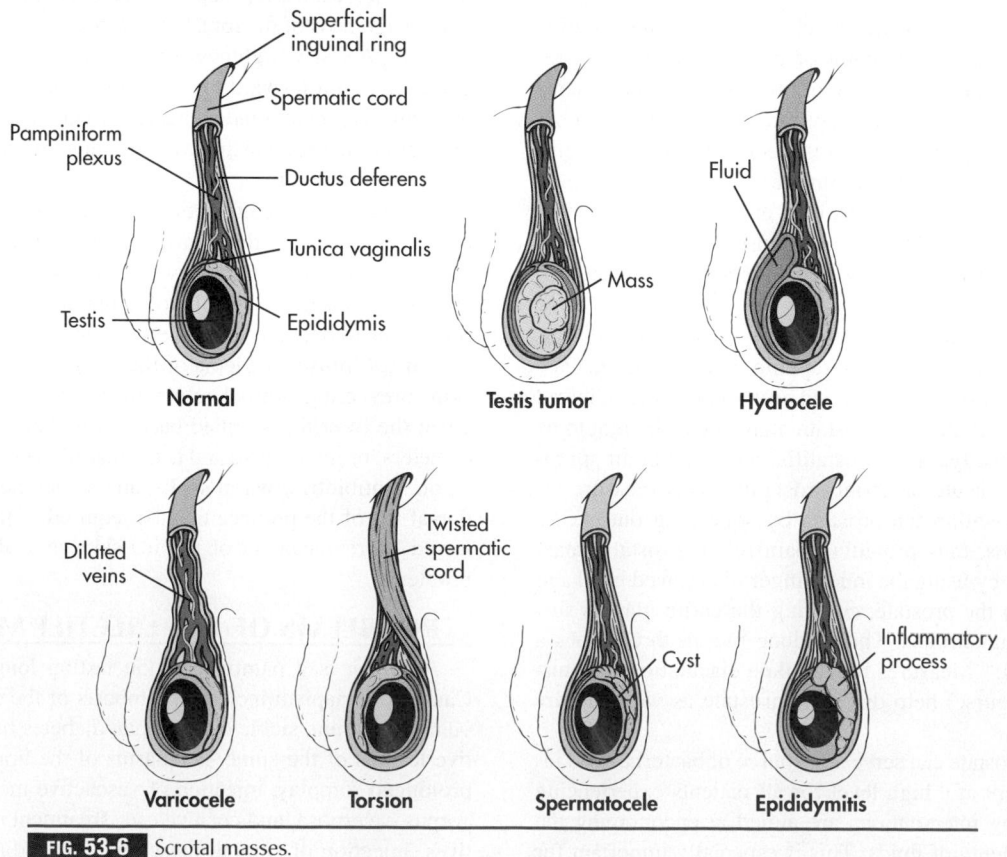

FIG. 53-6 Scrotal masses.

Orchitis

Orchitis refers to an acute inflammation of the testis. In orchitis, the testis is painful, tender, and swollen. It generally occurs after an episode of bacterial or viral infections such as mumps, pneumonia, tuberculosis, or syphilis. It can also be a side effect of epididymitis, prostatectomy, trauma, infectious mononucleosis, influenza, catheterization, or complicated urinary tract infection. Mumps orchitis is a condition contributing to infertility and could easily be decreased by childhood vaccination against mumps. Treatment involves the use of antibiotics (if the organism is known), pain medications, or bed rest with the scrotum elevated on an ice pack.

CONGENITAL PROBLEMS

Cryptorchidism (undescended testes) is failure of the testes to descend into the scrotal sac before birth. It is the most common congenital testicular condition. It may occur bilaterally or unilaterally and may be the cause of infertility if corrective surgery is not done by 2 years of age. The incidence of testicular cancer is also higher if the condition is not corrected before puberty. Surgery is performed to locate and suture the testis or testes to the scrotum.

Absence of the vas deferens is a rare condition associated most often with cystic fibrosis. With the advent of advanced techniques to treat infertility, this defect can be circumvented by aspirating the sperm directly from the testis.

"DES sons" are the male children of women who took diethylstilbestrol (DES) during pregnancy. The effects of DES on males can include undescended or underdeveloped testes, small penis, varicocele, or epididymal cysts. These males also have an increased risk of infertility and testicular cancer.[32]

ACQUIRED PROBLEMS

Hydrocele

A **hydrocele** is a nontender, fluid-filled mass that results from interference with lymphatic drainage of the scrotum and swelling of the tunica vaginalis that surrounds the testis (Figs. 53-6 and 53-7). Diagnosis is fairly simple because the mass can be seen by shining a flashlight through the scrotum (transillumination). No treatment is indicated unless the swelling becomes very large and uncomfortable, in which case aspiration or surgical drainage of the mass is performed.

Spermatocele

A **spermatocele** is a firm, sperm-containing, painless cyst of the epididymis that may be visible with transillumination (see Fig. 53-6). The cause is unknown, and surgical removal is the treatment. It is important for the patient to see his doctor if he feels any scrotal lumps. He would be unable to distinguish this cyst from cancer when performing self-examination.

Varicocele

A **varicocele** is a dilation of the veins that drain the testes (Figs. 53-6 and 53-8). The scrotum feels wormlike when palpated. The cause of the problem is unknown. The varicocele is usually located on the left side of the scrotum as a consequence of retrograde blood flow from the left renal vein. Surgery is indicated if the patient is infertile, because persistent varicoceles are

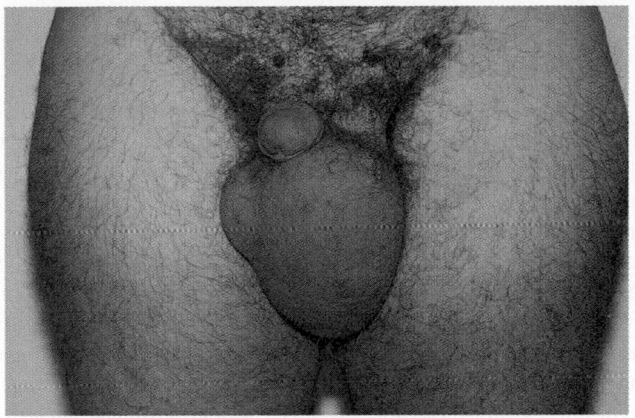

FIG. 53-7 Hydrocele.

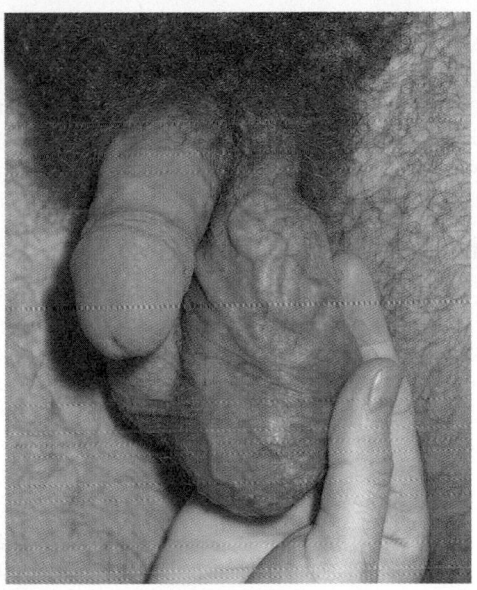

FIG. 53-8 A large varicocele.

associated with 40% to 50% of cases of infertility. Repair of the varicocele may be through injection of a sclerosing agent or by surgical ligation of the spermatic vein.

Testicular Torsion

Testicular torsion involves a twisting of the spermatic cord that supplies blood to the testes and epididymis (see Fig. 53-6). It is most commonly seen in males younger than age 20. The patient experiences severe scrotal pain, tenderness, swelling, nausea, and vomiting. Urinary symptoms, fever, and WBCs or bacteria in the urine are absent. The pain does not usually subside with rest or elevation of the scrotum. Nuclear technetium scan of the testes or Doppler ultrasound is typically performed to assess blood flow within the testicle. A decrease or absence in blood flow confirms the diagnosis.[33] Unless it resolves spontaneously, surgery to untwist the cord and restore the blood supply must be performed immediately. Torsion constitutes a surgical emergency because if the blood supply to the affected testicle is not restored within 4 to 6 hours, ischemia to the testis will occur, leading to necrosis and the possible need for removal.

TESTICULAR CANCER

Etiology and Pathophysiology

Testicular cancer is relatively rare, accounting for less than 1% of all cancers found in males. However, testicular cancer is the most common type of cancer in young men between 15 and 35 years of age. In the United States in 2002, 7500 new cases of and 400 deaths from testicular cancer occurred. The incidence of testicular cancer is four times higher in white males than in African American males, and it occurs more commonly in the right testicle than the left.[31] Testicular tumors are also more common in males who have had undescended testes (cryptorchidism) or a family history of testicular cancer or anomalies. Other predisposing factors include orchitis, human immunodeficiency virus infection, maternal exposure to DES, and testicular cancer in the contralateral testis.

Most testicular cancers develop from embryonic germ cells. The two types of germ cell cancers are seminomas and nonseminomas. Although seminoma germ cell cancers are the most common, they are the least aggressive. Nonseminoma testicular germ cell tumors are rare, but are very aggressive. Non–germ cell tumors arise from other testicular tissue and include Leydig cell and Sertoli cell tumors. These account for less than 10% of testicular cancers.

Clinical Manifestations and Complications

Testicular cancer may have a slow or rapid onset depending on the type of tumor. The patient may notice a lump in his scrotum, as well as scrotal swelling and a feeling of heaviness. The scrotal mass usually is nontender and is very firm. Some patients complain of a dull ache or heavy sensation in the lower abdomen, perianal area, or scrotum. Acute pain is the presenting symptom in about 10% of patients. Manifestations associated with metastasis to other systems are varied and include back pain, cough, dyspnea, hemoptysis, dysphagia (difficulty swallowing), alterations in vision or mental status, papilledema, and seizures.

Diagnostic Studies

Palpation of the scrotal contents is the first step in diagnosing testicular cancer. A cancerous mass is firm and does not transilluminate. Ultrasound of the testes is indicated whenever testicular cancer is suspected (e.g., palpable mass) or when persistent or painful testicular swelling is present. If a testicular neoplasm is suspected, blood is obtained to determine the serum levels of α-fetoprotein (AFP) and human chorionic gonadotropin (hCG). (These tumor markers are discussed in Chapter 15.) A chest x-ray and CT scan of the abdomen and pelvis are done to detect metastasis.

NURSING *and* COLLABORATIVE MANAGEMENT
TESTICULAR CANCER

■ Testicular Self-Examination

As with many forms of cancer, the survival of the patient is closely associated with early recognition of the tumor. The scrotum is easily examined, and beginning tumors are usually palpable. Every male at puberty should be taught and encouraged to perform a monthly testicular self-examination for the purpose of detecting testicular tumors or other scrotal abnormalities such as varicoceles. The nurse should teach the patient how to perform

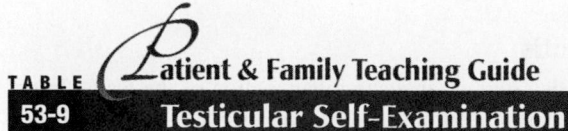

| TABLE 53-9 | Patient & Family Teaching Guide — Testicular Self-Examination |

1. During a shower or bath is the easiest time to examine the testes. Warm temperatures make the testes hang lower in the scrotum (see Fig. 53-9).
2. Use both hands to feel each testis. Roll the testis between the thumb and first three fingers until the entire surface has been covered. Palpate each one separately.
3. Identify the structures. The testis should feel round and smooth, like a hard-boiled egg. Differentiate the testis from the epididymis. The epididymis is not as smooth as the egg-shaped testis. One testis may be larger than the other. Size is not as important as texture. Check for lumps, irregularities, pain in the testes, or a dragging sensation. Locate the spermatic cord, which is usually firm and smooth and goes up toward the groin.
4. Choose a consistent day of the month, such as a birth date, that is easy to remember to examine the testes. The examination can be performed more frequently if desired.
5. Notify the health care provider at once if any abnormalities are found.

self-examination with a particular emphasis on males with a history of an undescended testis or a previous testicular tumor.

The procedure for self-examination is not difficult. The man may indicate some reluctance to examine his own genitals, but with encouragement he can learn this simple procedure. He should be encouraged to perform self-examinations frequently until he is comfortable with the procedure. The scrotum should then be examined once a month. Videotapes and illustrations on shower hangers are available as teaching aids and ideally should be introduced during high school or college physical education classes. Free information is available through the American Cancer Society and on various medical websites.

Guidelines for self-examination of the scrotum are presented in Table 53-9 and Fig. 53-9. The nurse should make this procedure as simple and uncomplicated for the man as possible. The man should choose a technique that is comfortable and consistent for him.

■ Collaborative Care

Collaborative care of testicular cancer generally involves an orchiectomy or a radical orchiectomy (surgical removal of the affected testis, spermatic cord, and regional lymph nodes). Postorchiectomy treatment involves surveillance, radiation therapy, or chemotherapy, depending on the stage of the cancer. Chemotherapy protocols use combination therapy including cisplatin (Platinol), etoposide (VePesid), and/or bleomycin (Blenoxane). (Testicular germ cell tumors are more sensitive to systemic chemotherapy than any other adult solid tumor.)

The prognosis for patients with testicular cancer has improved, and 95% of the patients obtain complete remission if the disease is detected in the early stages. As a result of treatment successes, the majority of men with testicular cancer are long-term survivors and treatment-related toxicity is a significant issue. All patients with testicular cancer, regardless of pathology or stage, require meticulous follow-up and regular physical exami-

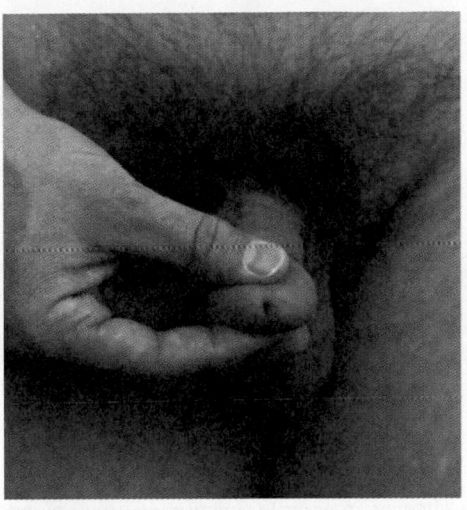
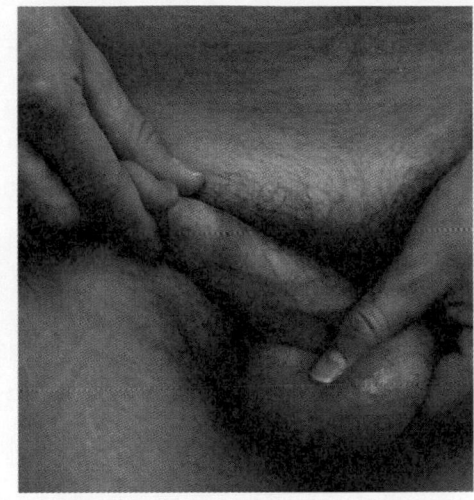

FIG. 53-9 Testicular self-examination.

nations, chest x-rays, CT scans, and assessment of hCG and AFP. The goal is to detect relapse when the tumor burden is minimal. Secondary malignancies that occur as a result of chemotherapy and radiation are described in Chapter 15.

The man with testicular cancer should have the opportunity to discuss fertility and sperm banking before any treatment. The nurse should be sensitive to any psychosocial problems this type of cancer can have on a man's feelings of maleness or self-worth.[34] Treatment has the potential to interfere with both erections and fertility.

Sexual Functioning

VASECTOMY

Vasectomy is the bilateral surgical ligation or resection of the vas deferens performed for the purpose of sterilization (Fig. 53-10). The procedure requires only 15 to 30 minutes and is usually performed with the patient under local anesthesia on an outpatient

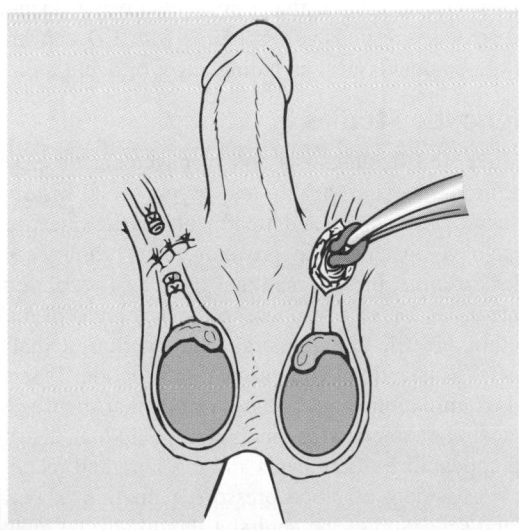

FIG. 53-10 Vasectomy procedure. The vas deferens is ligated or resected for the purpose of sterilization.

ETHICAL DILEMMAS
Sterilization

Situation

A 43-year-old male patient is requesting a vasectomy and informs the nurse that he does not wish to discuss this with his wife. The physician's policy is to have the spouse or partner sign a form acknowledging the patient's desire to be sterilized. This patient explains that although his wife wants to have more children, the one they already have is all he wants.

Important Points for Consideration

- Patient autonomy suggests that matters of reproduction are left to the privacy and discretion of the individual. Competent adults may legally choose to be sterilized for medical reasons or convenience.
- To prevent possible future harm, this man should include his wife in the decision to permanently eliminate his ability to procreate.
- In most states, women can terminate a pregnancy without proof that their husbands are aware of their intentions. Sterilization, on the other hand, is a more permanent decision that has consequences for both parties in the relationship.
- This physician's standard is to have evidence of the spouse's or significant other's knowledge of the intent for sterilization. This is not a state requirement. The nurse should inform the man of the standard in this particular physician's practice and the benefits to the integrity of his marriage.
- If the patient is still unwilling to discuss the matter with his wife, either the nurse or the physician should inform the man that they will not participate in deception and he is free to select another physician to perform the procedure.

Critical Thinking Questions

1. How would you approach this situation?
2. Should the nurse tell the wife of her husband's plans?
3. Are there ever circumstances in which deception of a patient or family would be justified?

basis. Vasectomy is considered a permanent form of sterilization, although some successful reversals (vasovasotomy) have been reported.

After vasectomy, the patient should not notice any difference in the look or feel of the ejaculate, because its major component is seminal and prostatic fluid. The patient will need to use an alternative form of contraception until semen examination reveals no sperm. This usually requires at least 10 ejaculations or 6 weeks to evacuate sperm distal to the surgical site. Sperm cells continue to be produced by the testes but are absorbed by the body rather than being passed through the vas deferens. Occasionally postoperative hematoma and swelling of the scrotum occur.

Vasectomy does not affect the production of hormones, ability to ejaculate, or physiologic mechanisms related to erection or orgasm. Psychologic adjustment may be a problem after surgery. It may be difficult for the patient to separate vasectomy from castration at a subconscious level. Some men may develop erectile dysfunction or may feel the need to become much more sexually active than they were in the past to prove their masculinity. Careful discussion of the procedure and its outcome before the surgery can be helpful in detecting patients who may have problems with psychologic adjustment. Surgery should be delayed for these patients.

ERECTILE DYSFUNCTION

Erectile dysfunction (ED) is the inability to attain or maintain an erect penis that allows satisfactory sexual performance. Although sexual function is a topic that many individuals are uncomfortable discussing, health care providers must be able and willing to address ED. This topic has been more visible in recent years, partially due to the improvements in treatment with the introduction of sildenafil (Viagra).

The effects of ED potentially interfere with a man's self-esteem, confidence, relationships, and overall sense of well-being. ED is a condition that is significant because of its prevalence; it is estimated that 20 million to 30 million men in the United States experience ED.[35] ED can occur at any age, although the incidence increases with age. In fact, it is estimated that about 50% of all men between ages 40 and 70 have at least some degree of ED.[35] The problem is increasing in all segments of the sexually active male population and affects both the man and his partner. In younger men the increase is attributed to substance abuse, such as recreational drugs and alcohol. Middle-aged men are affected by medical conditions such as diabetes, hypertension, renal disease, organ transplants, coronary artery bypass surgeries, and cancer, or the therapy for these problems. The older population (men over 70 years of age) are living longer, fuller lives and expect to remain sexually active, regardless of any existing medical conditions. Stress factors associated with modern lifestyles are affecting men of all ages and contribute greatly to the overall causes of erectile failure.

Etiology and Pathophysiology

Normal erectile function is a parasympathetic reflex initiated mainly by certain tactile, visual, and mental stimuli. It consists of dilation of the arteries and arterioles of the penis, which in turn fills and distends spaces in its erectile tissue and compresses veins. When this occurs, more blood enters the penis through the dilated arteries than leaves it through the constricted veins. The penis then becomes larger and rigid, or, in other words, erection occurs. Problems occur when these spaces (corporeal bodies) fail to fill when desired or when they empty before orgasm. A functional erection requires not only the desire but also adequate blood supply, nerve innervation, and hormone balance.

ED can result from a number of factors in two general categories: physiologic (organic) and psychogenic. From 80% to 90% of cases of ED are attributed to physiologic causes.[36] *Physiologic ED* can result from a number of etiologic factors (Table 53-10). Common causes include diabetes mellitus, vascular disease, side effects from medications, result of surgery (such as prostatectomy), trauma, chronic illness, and Peyronie's disease. *Psychologic ED* can be caused by a number of issues but is most often associated with stress, difficulty in a relationship, depression, or low self-esteem.

Normal physiologic age-related changes are associated with changes in erectile function and may be an underlying cause of ED for some men. Table 53-11 lists normal age-related changes in sexual performance. Explanation of these age-related changes may be necessary to reassure an anxious older man regarding normal changes in his sexual abilities.

Clinical Manifestations and Complications

A patient's self-report of problems associated with sexual performance is the typical symptom of ED. The patient usually describes an inability to attain or maintain an erection. The symptoms may occur only occasionally, or may be constant with an onset occurring gradually over time, or very rapidly. A gradual onset of symptoms usually is associated with physiologic ED, whereas sudden or rapid onset of symptoms is typically associated with ED caused by psychologic issues.

Although the patient may specifically seek help to alleviate the problem, many men have misconceptions about ED that make them less likely to present this as their chief complaint. More often ED is identified from the history-taking process. This underscores the need for nurses to conduct interviews that address sexuality with men of all ages.

The major complication of ED is that the man's inability to perform sexually can cause great distress in his interpersonal relationships and may interfere with his concept of himself as a man. Our society promotes images of a man being strong, capable, and sexually responsive. Problems with ED can lead to a number of personal issues, including anger or depression.

Diagnostic Studies

The first step in diagnosis and management of ED begins with a thorough sexual, health, and psychosocial history. Self-administered assessment and treatment-related questionnaires have been developed and may prove useful as primary screening tools. For example, the International Index of Erectile Function (IIEF) identifies a man's response to five key areas of male sexual function: erectile function, orgasmic function, sexual desire, intercourse satisfaction, and overall satisfaction.[37] Second, a physical examination should be performed that focuses on secondary sexual characteristics, including pubic hair distribution, size and appearance of the penis and scrotum, and rectal examination. Assessment of blood pressure, palpation of peripheral pulses, and sensation of the genitalia should also be included.

Further examination or diagnostic testing is typically based on findings from the history and physical examination. A serum glu-

TABLE 53-10 **Risk Factors for Erectile Dysfunction**

Anatomic
Congenital deformities of the penis (e.g., hypospadias)
Peyronie's disease

Cardiorespiratory
Angina pectoris
Atherosclerosis
Emphysema
Hypertension
Myocardial infarction
Post-cardiac surgery

Drug Induced
5α-Reductase inhibitors (finasteride [Proscar])
Alcohol
Antiandrogens
Antilipidemic agents
Antihypertensives
Caffeine
Diuretics (chlorothiazide [Diuril]; spironolactone [Aldactone])
Drugs for Parkinson's disease (carbidopa-levodopa [Sinemet])
Estrogens
Major tranquilizers (diazepam [Valium]; alprazolam [Xanax])
Marijuana, cocaine, LSD
Narcotics
Nicotine
Tricyclic antidepressants (amitriptyline [Elavil])

Endocrine
Addison's disease
Diabetes mellitus
High levels of prolactin
Obesity
Pituitary tumor
Testosterone deficiency
Thyrotoxicosis

Genitourinary
Cystectomy
Hydrocele
Perineal or suprapubic prostatectomy
Phimosis
Post–kidney transplant
Postpriapism
Prostatitis
Renal failure
Varicocele

Neurologic and Nerve Conduction
Central nervous system disorders
Electroshock therapy
Multiple sclerosis
Parkinson's disease
Peripheral neuropathic conditions
Spina bifida
Stroke
Sympathectomy
Trauma to the spinal cord
Tumors or transection of spinal cord

Psychogenic
Depression
Excessive stress in family, work, or interpersonal relationships
Fatigue
Fear of failure to perform

Vascular
Aortic aneurysm
Aortofemoral bypass surgery
Atherosclerosis of pelvic blood vessels

cose and lipid profile is recommended to rule out diabetes mellitus. Hormonal levels for testosterone, prolactin, and thyroid may help identify endocrine-related problems, and other blood chemistries and complete blood count may be helpful in identifying unrecognized systemic diseases.

Other diagnostic tests may be conducted to diagnose ED. Nocturnal penile tumescence and rigidity testing is a noninvasive method that involves the continuous measurement of penile circumference and axial rigidity during sleep. Such measurements are used to differentiate between physiologic or psychogenic causes of ED, as well as to evaluate the effectiveness of drug therapy. Vascular studies including penile arteriography, penile blood flow study, and duplex Doppler ultrasound studies are used to assess penile blood inflow and outflow. Such studies help assess vascular problems interfering with erection.

Collaborative Care

The goal of ED therapy is for the patient and his partner to achieve a satisfactory sexual relationship. The treatment for ED is based on the underlying cause. A step-wise treatment approach with a ranking of treatment options is advocated (Table 53-12).[37]

TABLE 53-11 **Effects of Aging on Sexual Performance**

- Time lag between perceiving sexual opportunity and full erection
- Diminished size and rigidity of the penis at full erection
- Increased time interval to ejaculation
- Changed nature of ejaculation with less spurting and lessened intensity of feeling
- Shortened period between ejaculation and flaccidity
- Increase in time to next reaction to sexual stimulation

The results of these interventions are usually most satisfactory when both partners are involved in the decision-making process and have realistic expectations of the treatment.

It is important to determine if ED is reversible before treatment is started. For example, if ED appears to be a side effect of prescribed drugs, alternative agents and/or treatments should be explored. When there is an established diagnosis of testicular

TABLE 53-12	Collaborative Care
Erectile Dysfunction	

Diagnostic
History and physical examination
Sexual history
Serum glucose and lipid profile
Testosterone, prolactin, and thyroid hormone levels
Nocturnal penile tumescence and rigidity testing
Vascular studies

Collaborative Therapy
Modify reversible causes
First-line interventions
- sildenafil (Viagra), vardenafil (Nuviva), tadalafil (Cialis)
- Vacuum constriction device (VCD)
- Sexual therapy
Second-line interventions
- Intraurethral medication pellet
- Intracavernosal self-injection
- Topical gels
Third-line interventions
- Penile implants

failure (hypogonadism), androgen replacement therapy may sometimes be effective in improving erectile function. For individuals who have ED that is psychogenic in nature, counseling for the patient (and possibly his partner) is recommended.[38] This counseling should be carried out by a qualified therapist.

First-Line Interventions

Oral drug therapy. Sildenafil (Viagra), tadalafil (Cialis), and vardenafil (Nuviva) are erectogenic drugs. Because these drugs have been found to be safe and effective for the treatment of most types of ED, they are considered first-line treatment. These drugs cause smooth muscle relaxation and increased arterial inflow with corporal venoocclusion resulting in an erection. They are taken orally about 1 hour before sexual activity, but not more than once a day. Because they potentiate the hypotensive effect of nitrates, they are contraindicated for individuals taking nitrates (such as nitroglycerin). The success of these drugs has had a revolutionary

impact on drug therapy for ED, resulting in an explosive area for further research.[39]

Vacuum constriction device. A second option that is considered a first-line intervention is the vacuum constriction device (VCD). Suction devices applied to the flaccid penis produce an erection by pulling blood up into the corporeal bodies. A penile ring or constrictive band is placed around the base of the penis to retain venous blood, thereby preventing the erection from subsiding (Fig. 53-11). Special care must be taken in using these devices to prevent tissue bruising.

Sexual therapy. Treatment of ED may include sexual therapy. This therapy addresses psychologic or interpersonal factors that may enhance sexual expression, as well as other factors that are of concern. The therapy can be effective for the individual patient, but it is typically preferred to include his partner, particularly if he is involved in a long-term relationship.

Second-Line Interventions.
The second-line therapies are indicated for patients for whom first-line interventions fail, or based on patient preference. These interventions include the use of vasoactive drugs administered as topical gel, an injection into the penis (intracavernosal self-injection) (Fig. 53-12, B), or insertion of a medication pellet (alprostadil) into the urethra (intraurethral) using a medicated urethral system for erection (MUSE) device (Fig. 53-12, A). These vasoactive drugs enhance blood flow into the penile arteries. Current vasoactive medications include papaverine (topical gel or injection), alprostadil

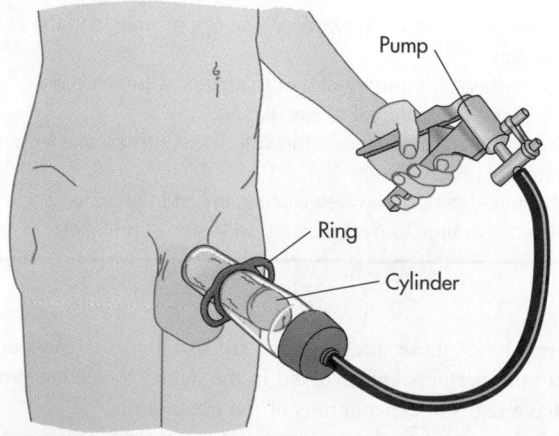

FIG. 53-11 Vacuum constriction device. With the vacuum device in place, blood can be drawn into the penis by means of a hand pump. This creates an erection. For intercourse, the ring is slipped to the base of the penis and the cylinder removed.

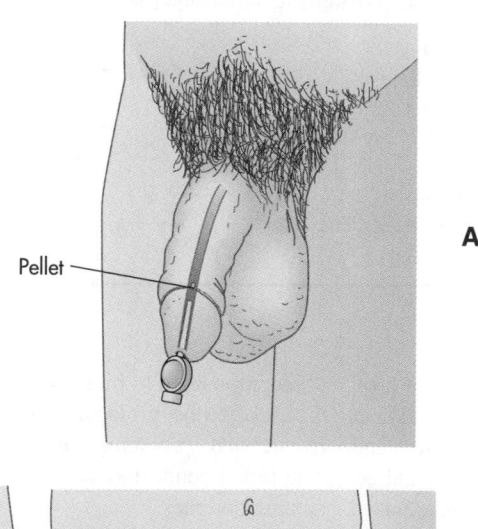

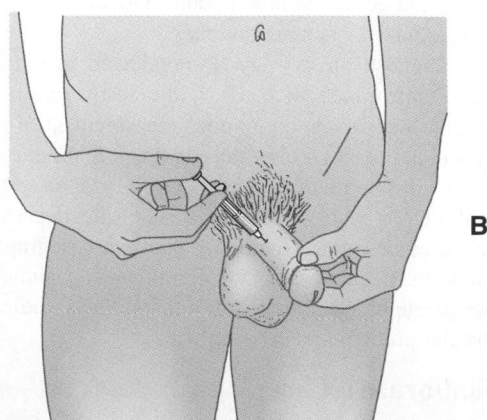

FIG. 53-12 A, Intraurethral insertion of medicated pellet (alprostadil) using a medicated urethral system for erection (MUSE) device. B, Intracavernosal self-injection. Self-injection therapy involves injecting a medication directly into the penis. This increases blood flow and causes an erection.

(Caverject) (topical gel, transurethral pellet, or injection), and phentolamine (Vasomax).

The vasoactive medication dose is regulated on an individual basis to prevent side effects. Side effects may include penile pain, priapism, corporal fibrosis, fibrotic nodules, and hypotension. It is important to instruct patients carefully on the specific administration techniques and precautions for any of the vasoactive medications.

Home injection therapy instruction is given to those men who are suitable candidates for the therapy. The injection is nearly painless and generally begins to work in 20 to 30 minutes. Success rates have been high when there is adequate patient teaching and follow-up. This treatment is not suitable for men with severe vascular problems, intolerance for transient hypotension, severe psychiatric disease, poor manual dexterity, or poor vision or those receiving anticoagulant therapy. The man may discontinue treatment if he perceives a lack of spontaneity, has a needle phobia, or wants a more permanent treatment option.

Third-Line Interventions. Surgical implantation of semirigid or inflatable penile prostheses are third-line interventions (Fig. 53-13). These surgical procedures are highly invasive and associated with many potential complications. Thus they are usually indicated for men with severe ED in which first- and second-line interventions are ineffective.

Penile implants have provided surgical management of ED for more than 25 years. The devices are implanted into the corporeal bodies to provide an erection firm enough for penetration. All implants provide a usable erection and should be chosen carefully based on the man's mental and physical capabilities, surgical risk factors, personal lifestyle, insurance, and financial resources.

The semirigid malleable implant is displayed in Fig. 53-13, A. The inflatable implant consists of cylinders in the penis, a small pump in the scrotum, and a reservoir in the lower abdomen (Fig. 53-13, B). The main problems associated with penile prostheses are mechanical failure, infection, and erosions.

For essentially healthy men the surgical procedure may be performed on an outpatient basis, with patients also being monitored on an outpatient basis. Complete recovery time varies from 4 to 6 weeks. Patients considered to be at high risk for complications include those with uncontrolled diabetes mellitus and those with severe circulatory problems.

Patients should be advised that none of the options will restore ejaculation or tactile sensations if they were absent before treatment. Sexual counseling is often recommended before and after treatment. The ability to please both partners enhances satisfaction levels.

NURSING MANAGEMENT
ERECTILE DYSFUNCTION

The man experiencing ED requires a great deal of emotional support for both himself and his partner. Men often do not feel comfortable discussing their problems with others because of society's expectations of a man's sexual abilities. The man may experience and demonstrate isolation from support systems, and he may also lose self-esteem.

The patient needs reassurance that confidentiality will be maintained. In conjunction with medical treatment, it often becomes necessary to provide counseling and therapy for the couple to establish realistic expectations and develop meaningful communication patterns. The majority of men delay seeking medical assistance. They are often highly motivated and expect immediate solutions to their problems. The health care team should provide a support system and accurate information as soon as possible.

Nurses are in a unique position of conducting routine health assessments on men seeking any form of medical treatment. It provides an opportunity to ask questions pertaining to general health, as well as sexual health and function. Given the opportunity, men will be less hesitant to answer these questions when they know that someone cares and can provide them with answers.

INFERTILITY

Infertility in a couple is defined as the inability to achieve conception despite 1 year of frequent unprotected intercourse. Infertility is a disorder of a couple, not of one individual. For this reason, both partners must be involved in determining the cause of infertility. The primary cause of infertility is due to factors involving the man in about 33% of the cases. Male infertility can

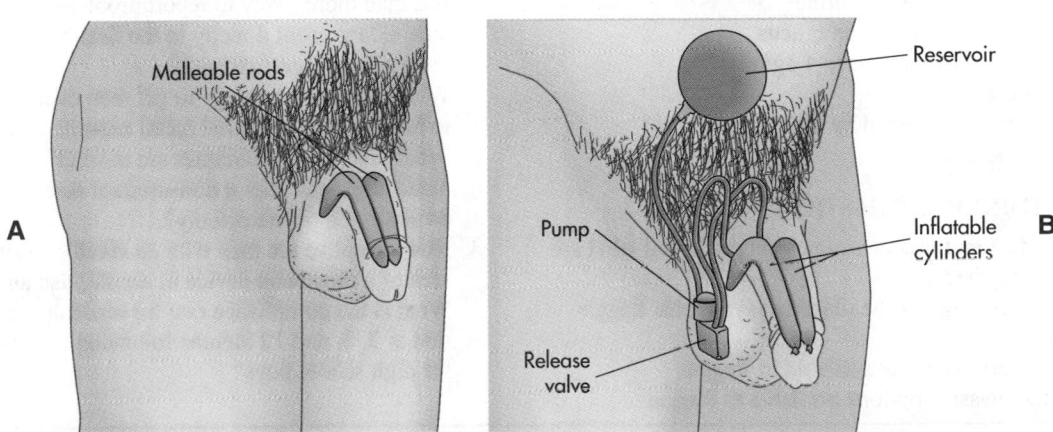

FIG. 53-13 Penile implants. **A,** Malleable implant is always erect but can be bent close to body for concealment. **B,** Inflatable implant consists of cylinders in the penis, a small pump in the scrotum, and a reservoir in the lower abdomen. When activated, the pump fills the cylinders with fluid from the reservoir. A small release valve permits the fluid to drain back into the reservoir after intercourse.

be caused by disorders of the hypothalamic-pituitary system, disorders of the testes, and abnormalities of the ejaculatory system.

The physical causes are generally divided into three categories: pretesticular, testicular, and posttesticular. The pretesticular or endocrine causes occur only in about 3% of the cases and can generally be treated with medication or surgery. Testicular problems make up 50% of the cases. The most common cause of male infertility is a varicocele. Other factors that influence the testes include infection (e.g., mumps virus, STDs, bacterial infections), congenital anomalies, medications, radiation, substance abuse (alcohol, nicotine, drugs), and environmental hazards. Posttesticular causes account for approximately 5% to 7% of the cases, with obstruction, infection, or the result of a surgical procedure being the primary causes. The remaining 40% are classified as *idiopathic,* or of unknown causes.

A careful health history and examination may reveal the cause of a patient's infertility. Thus the history is a starting point for determining cause and treatment. The history should include age; occupation; past injury, surgery, or infections to the genital tract; lifestyle issues such as hot tubs, weight training, or wearing tight undergarments; sexual practices; frequency of intercourse; and emotional factors such as stress levels and the desire for children. The use of drugs, such as chemotherapeutic agents, anabolic steroids (testosterone), sulfasalazine (Azulfidine), cimetidine (Tagamet), and recreational drugs, should be documented because these can reduce sperm count. A physical examination can disclose a varicocele, Peyronie's disease, or other physical abnormalities.

The first test in an infertility study is a semen analysis. The test determines the sperm concentration (count greater than 20 million/ml), forward progressive motility (at least 60% with a grade greater than 2), and morphology (at least 60% have normal oval head and long tail).[40] Additional tests that may be helpful in determining the etiology include plasma testosterone and serum LH and FSH measurements. A test for sperm penetration abilities may also be done. The specific cause of infertility is often not determined.

The nurse should be concerned and tactful in dealing with the male patient undergoing infertility studies. For many men, fertility and masculinity are equated. The nurse must be sensitive to the problem of gender identity in the infertile man.

Treatment options for the man include medications, conservative lifestyle changes (e.g., avoidance of scrotal heat, substance abuse, high stress), in vitro fertilization techniques, and corrective surgery. Achievement of pregnancy varies from 8% to 60% and ranges in cost from several hundred to several thousand dollars. Infertility can seriously strain a marriage, and the couple may require counseling and discussion of alternatives if conception is not achieved. (Female infertility is discussed in Chapter 52.)

CRITICAL THINKING EXERCISES

Case Study
Benign Prostatic Hyperplasia

Patient Profile. Reggie Keller, a 71-year-old African American married man, comes to the emergency department because of an inability to void for the past 12 hours.

Subjective Data

- Complains of severe bladder pain and pressure
- Is very restless and agitated
- Relates history of three cans of beer the previous evening; has not voided since then

Objective Data

- Has prostate enlargement on digital rectal examination
- Has hematuria and WBCs in urine
- Has palpable bladder above umbilicus
- PSA test: 6 ng/ml (normal: 0 to 4 ng/ml)

Collaborative Care

- Indwelling catheter inserted by a urology resident
- Admitted to the hospital

CRITICAL THINKING QUESTIONS

1. What risk factors for acute urinary retention and BPH are present in Reggie?
2. Explain the etiology of the objective symptoms Reggie exhibited.
3. Discuss the drug options available to Reggie.
4. Discuss the invasive options available to Reggie.

5. Reggie asks you about the effect of the various treatment options on his ability to have sex. How would you respond?
6. Write one or more appropriate nursing diagnoses based on the assessment data presented. Are there any collaborative problems?
7. On further assessment, you note that Reggie has a nursing diagnosis of decisional conflict. How would you help him resolve this conflict related to treatment options?

Nursing Research Issues

1. Is a man more likely to report problems related to prostatic enlargement directly to the health care provider or via a printed questionnaire?
2. What is the best strategy to get men over 50 years of age to have an annual digital rectal examination?
3. What relaxation techniques are most effective in relieving bladder spasms after a transurethral resection of the prostate or a prostatectomy?
4. How receptive are men with an erectile dysfunction to the idea of a prosthetic device to accomplish an erection?
5. What is the compliance rate for testicular self-examination at 3, 6, and 12 months following a training program for high school boys?

REVIEW QUESTIONS

The number of the question corresponds to the same-numbered objective at the beginning of the chapter.

1. A patient with BPH experiences hesitancy in initiating voiding and a feeling of incomplete bladder emptying. In assessing for complications related to these symptoms, the nurse asks specifically about the presence of
   a. constipation.
   b. dysuria and urgency.
   c. gross blood in the urine.
   d. decreased force of the urinary stream.

2. Postoperatively, a patient who has had a transurethral prostatectomy has continuous bladder irrigation with a three-way Foley with a 30 ml balloon and traction applied. The patient complains that he feels the urge to void even with the catheter in place. The nurse should
   a. hand-irrigate the catheter to ensure that it is patent.
   b. deflate the catheter balloon to 10 ml to decrease bulk in the bladder.
   c. encourage the patient to try to have a bowel movement to relieve colon pressure.
   d. explain that this feeling is normal and that he should not try to urinate around the catheter.

3. In teaching health promotion related to early detection of prostate cancer, the nurse advises that beginning at middle age men should have an annual
   a. urinalysis.
   b. prostatic ultrasound.
   c. digital rectal examination.
   d. prostatic acid phosphatase (PAP).

4. A patient scheduled for a prostatectomy for prostate cancer expresses the fear that he will be impotent. In responding to the patient, the nurse must keep in mind that
   a. impotence is a possibility even with a nerve-sparing procedure.
   b. the most common complication of this surgery is postoperative urinary retention.
   c. pain control will be a more important factor than sexual function or the long-term consideration of his condition.
   d. a penile implant is the best method to treat erectile dysfunction and should be considered after he has recovered from his surgery.

5. The nurse advises the patient with chronic prostatitis that management includes
   a. a permanent indwelling catheter.
   b. regular injection of sclerosing agents.
   c. sexual activities that result in ejaculation.
   d. aspiration or surgical drainage of abscesses.

6. Discharge teaching for the patient who has had a vasectomy includes explaining that
   a. the procedure blocks the production of sperm.
   b. the ejaculate will be about half the volume it was before the procedure.
   c. an alternative form of contraception will be necessary for 6 to 8 weeks.
   d. erectile dysfunction is temporary and will return with continued sexual activity.

7. A nursing measure that can decrease the patient's discomfort over care involving his reproductive organs includes
   a. relating his sexual concerns to his sexual partner.
   b. arranging to have only male nurses care for the patient.
   c. maintaining a nonjudgmental attitude toward his sexual practices.
   d. using only technical terminology when discussing reproductive function.

REFERENCES

1. Partin AW: Benign prostatic hyperplasia. In Lepor H, editor: *Prostatic diseases,* Philadelphia, 2000, WB Saunders.
2. Barry B et al: The American Urologic Association symptom index for benign prostatic hyperplasia, *J Urol* 148:1549, 1992.
3. Barry MJ, Meigo JB: The natural history of benign prostatic hyperplasia. In Lepor H, editor: *Prostatic diseases,* Philadelphia, 2000, WB Saunders.
4. Hamper UM: Elevated PSA and/or abnormal prostate physical exam. In Bluth EI et al, editors: *Ultrasonography in urology,* New York, 2001, Thieme.
5. Nelson DA, Schumann L. Continuing education forum. Differentiating prostate disorders, *J Am Acad Nurse Pract* 10:415, 1998.
6. Nobel MJ, Mebust WK: Transurethral resection of the prostate. In Resnick MI, Thomson IM, editors: *Advanced therapy of prostate disease,* Hamilton, Ontario, 2000, Decker.
7. DeWildt M, DeLa Rosette J: Transurethral microwave thermotherapy. In Koshiba K et al, editors: *Treatment of benign prostatic hyperplasia,* Toyko, 2000, Springer.
8. Henney JE: Microwave therapy warning, *JAMA* 284:2711, 2000.
9. Schulman CC, Zlotta AR: Transurethral needle ablation of the prostate for treatment of benign prostate hyperplasia. In Resnick MI, Thomson IM, editors: *Advanced therapy of prostate disease,* Hamilton, Ontario, 2000, Decker.
10. Gray M: Urinary retention: management in the acute care setting, *Am J Nurs* 100:36, 2000.
11. Pateman B, Johnson M: Men's lived experiences following transuretheral prostatectomy for benign prostatic hypertrophy, *J Adv Nurs* 31:51, 2000.
12. *Cancer facts and figures,* Atlanta, 2002, American Cancer Society.
13. *Prostate cancer,* Rochester, 2000, Mayo Foundation for Medical Education and Research.
14. Brawley OW, Barnes S: The epidemiology of prostate cancer in the United States, *Semin Oncol Nurs* 17:72, 2001.
15. Kolonel LN, Nomura MNY, Cooney RV: Dietary fat and prostate cancer: current status, *J Natl Cancer Inst* 91:414, 1999.
16. Hayes RB et al: Dietary factors and risk for prostate cancer among blacks and whites in the United States, *Cancer Epidemiol Biomarkers Prev* 8:25, 1999.
17. Hines S: Treating early prostate cancer: difficult decisions abound, *Patient Care for the Nurse Practitioner* 2:18,1999.
18. Marschke PS: The role of surgery in the treatment of prostate cancer, *Semin Oncol Nurs* 17:85, 2001.
19. Moore KN, Estey A: The early postoperative concerns of men after radical prostatectomy, *J Adv Nurs* 29:1121, 1999.
20. Stanford JL et al: Urinary and sexual function after radical prostatectomy for clinically localized prostate cancer, *JAMA* 283:354, 2000.
21. Iwamoto RR, Maher KE: Radiation therapy for prostate cancer, *Semin Oncol Nurs* 17:90, 2001.
22. Abel LJ et al: The role of urinary assessment scores in the nursing management of patients receiving prostate brachytherapy, *Clin J Oncol Nurs* 4:126, 2000.
23. Stempkowski L: Hormonal therapy. In Held-Warmkessel J, editor: *Contemporary issues in prostate cancer: a nursing perspective,* Boston, 2000, Jones & Bartlett.
24. Held-Warmkessel J: Treatment of advanced prostate cancer, *Semin Oncol Nurs* 17:118, 2001.
25. Agho AO, Lewis MA: Correlates of actual and perceived knowledge of prostate cancer among African Americans, *Cancer Nurs* 24:165, 2001.
26. Nivens AS et al: Cues to participation in prostate cancer screening: a theory for practice, *Oncol Nurs Forum* 28:1449, 2001.
27. McDougall GJ: The controversy of prostate screening, *Geriatr Nurs* 21:245, 2000.
28. Ridner SL: Prostatitis: an advanced nursing practice guideline, *Geriatr Nurs* 21:49, 2000.
29. Krieger JN, Nyberg L, Nickel JC: NIH consensus definition and classification of prostatitis, *JAMA* 282:236, 1999.
30. Gleich P: Prostatitis: a state-of-the-art review of diagnosis and therapy, *Consultant* 38:345, 1998.
31. Epperson WJ, Frank WL: Male genital cancers, *Prim Care* 25:459, 1998.
32. McLachlan JA et al: Are estrogens carcinogenic during development of the testes? *AOMIS* 106:240, 1998.
33. Blaivas M, Batts M, Lambert M: Ultrasonographic diagnosis of testicular torsion by emergency physicians, *J Emerg Med* 18:198, 2000.
34. Arai Y et al: Psychosocial aspects in long-term survivors of testicular cancer, *J Urol* 155:574, 1996.
35. Laumann EO, Paik A, Rosen C: Sexual dysfunction in the United States. Prevalence and predictors, *JAMA* 281:537, 1999.
36. Althof S: The patient with erectile dysfunction: psychological issues, *Nurse Pract* 25(suppl):11, 2000.
37. Rosen RC et al: The international index of erectile function (IIEF): a multidimensional scale for assessment of erectile dysfunction, *Urology* 49:822, 1997.
38. Padma-Nathan H, Forrest C: Diagnosis and treatment of erectile dysfunction: the process of care model, *Nurse Pract* 25(suppl):4, 2000.
39. Padma-Nathan H, Giuliano F: Oral pharmacotherapy. In Mulcahy JJ, editor: *Current clinical urology: male sexual function: a guide to clinical management,* Totowa, NJ, 2001, Humana Press.
40. Jequier AM: *Male infertility: a guide for the clinician,* London, 2000, Blackwell Science.

RESOURCES

American Cancer Society
1599 Clifton Road NE
Atlanta, GA 30329-4251
800-ACS-2345
www.cancer.org

American Urological Association
1120 North Charles Street
Baltimore, MD 21201
410-727-1100
Fax: 410-223-4370
www.auanet.org

National Prostate Cancer Coalition
1158 15th Street NW
Washington, DC 20005
888-245-9455 or 202-463-9455
Fax: 202-463-9456
www.4npcc.org

Sexuality Information and Education Council of the United States
130 West 42nd Street, Suite 350
New York, NY 10036-7802
212-819-9770
Fax: 212-819-9776
www.siecus.org

Urologic Oncology Program
University of Michigan Comprehensive Cancer Center
1500 East Medical Center Drive
Ann Arbor, MI 48109-0944
Cancer Information Line: 800-865-1125
www.cancer.med.umich.edu/prostcan/prostcan.html

For additional Internet resources, see the website for this book at *http://evolve.elsevier.com/Lewis/medsurg.*

Problems Related to Movement and Coordination

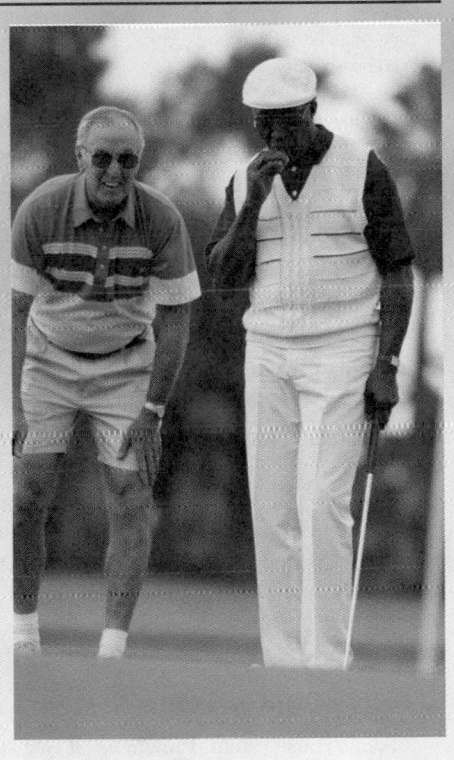

SECTION OUTLINE

CHAPTER 54

NURSING ASSESSMENT
Nervous System

Judith M. Ozuna

LEARNING OBJECTIVES

1. Describe the functions of neurons and neuroglia.
2. Explain the electrochemical aspects of nerve impulse transmission.
3. Explain the anatomic location and functions of the cerebrum, brainstem, cerebellum, spinal cord, peripheral nerves, and cerebrospinal fluid.
4. Identify the major arteries supplying the brain.
5. Describe the functions of the 12 cranial nerves.
6. Compare the functions of the two divisions of the autonomic nervous system.
7. Describe age-related changes in the neurologic system and differences in assessment findings.
8. Identify the significant subjective and objective data related to the nervous system that should be obtained from a patient.
9. Describe the techniques used in the physical assessment of the nervous system.
10. Differentiate normal from common abnormal findings of a physical assessment of the nervous system.
11. Describe the purpose, significance of results, and nursing responsibilities related to diagnostic studies of the nervous system.

KEY TERMS

autonomic nervous system, p. 1473	neuroglia, p. 1464
blood-brain barrier, p. 1475	neuron, p. 1464
central nervous system, p. 1464	neurotransmitter, p. 1466
cerebrospinal fluid, p. 1470	peripheral nervous system, p. 1464
cranial nerves, p. 1473	reflex, p. 1468
dermatome, p. 1472	synapse, p. 1466
lower motor neurons, p. 1468	upper motor neurons, p. 1468
meninges, p. 1476	

STRUCTURES AND FUNCTIONS OF THE NERVOUS SYSTEM

The human nervous system is a highly specialized system responsible for the control and integration of the body's many activities. The nervous system can be divided into the central nervous system (CNS) and the peripheral nervous system (PNS). The **central nervous system** consists of the brain and spinal cord. The **peripheral nervous system** consists of the cranial and spinal nerves and the peripheral components of the autonomic nervous system (ANS). Before considering higher-order structures and their functions, cellular elements and nerve impulse transmission are discussed.

Cells of the Nervous System

The nervous system is made up of two types of cells: neurons and neuroglia. Although neuroglial cells are more numerous, they are mainly supportive to the **neuron** (the primary functional unit of the nervous system). Neurons are generally nonmitotic; that is, they do not replicate and cannot replace themselves if they are irreversibly damaged. However, the brain is capable of generating new neurons from stem cells located in certain regions of the brain.[1] Neuroglia are mitotic and can replicate themselves.

Neurons. The neurons of the nervous system come in many different shapes and sizes, but they all share common characteristics: (1) excitability, or the ability to generate a nerve impulse; (2) conductivity, or the ability to transmit the impulse to other portions of the cell; and (3) the ability to influence other neurons, muscle cells, and glandular cells by transmitting nerve impulses to them.

A typical neuron consists of a cell body, an axon, and several dendrites (Fig. 54-1). The cell body containing the nucleus and cytoplasm is the metabolic center of the neuron. Dendrites are short processes extending from the cell body. They receive nerve impulses from the axons of other neurons and conduct impulses toward the cell body. The nerve axon projects varying distances from the cell body, ranging from several micrometers to more than a meter. Its function is to carry nerve impulses to other neurons or to end organs. The end organs are smooth and striated muscles and glands. Axons may be myelinated or unmyelinated. Many axons present in the CNS and the PNS are covered by a segmentally interrupted myelin sheath composed of a white, lipid substance that acts as an insulator for the conduction of impulses. Generally, the smaller fibers are unmyelinated.

Neuroglia. Neuroglia, or glial cells, provide support, nourishment, and protection to neurons. They constitute almost half the brain and spinal cord mass and are 5 to 10 times more numerous than neurons. Different types of glial cells, including oligodendrocytes, astrocytes, ependymal cells, and microglia, have specific functions. *Oligodendrocytes* are specialized cells that produce the myelin sheath of nerve fibers in the CNS (Schwann cells myelinate the nerve fibers in the periphery) and are primarily found in the white matter of the CNS.

Astrocytes provide structural support to neurons and their delicate processes, form the blood-brain barrier with the endothelium of the blood vessels, and play a role in synaptic transmission (conduction of impulses between neurons). They are found primarily in gray matter. When the brain is injured, astrocytes act

---

Reviewed by Mary S. Baird, RN, MN, CNRN, ARNP, Nurse Practitioner, Northwest Neuromuscular Association, Olympia, Wash.

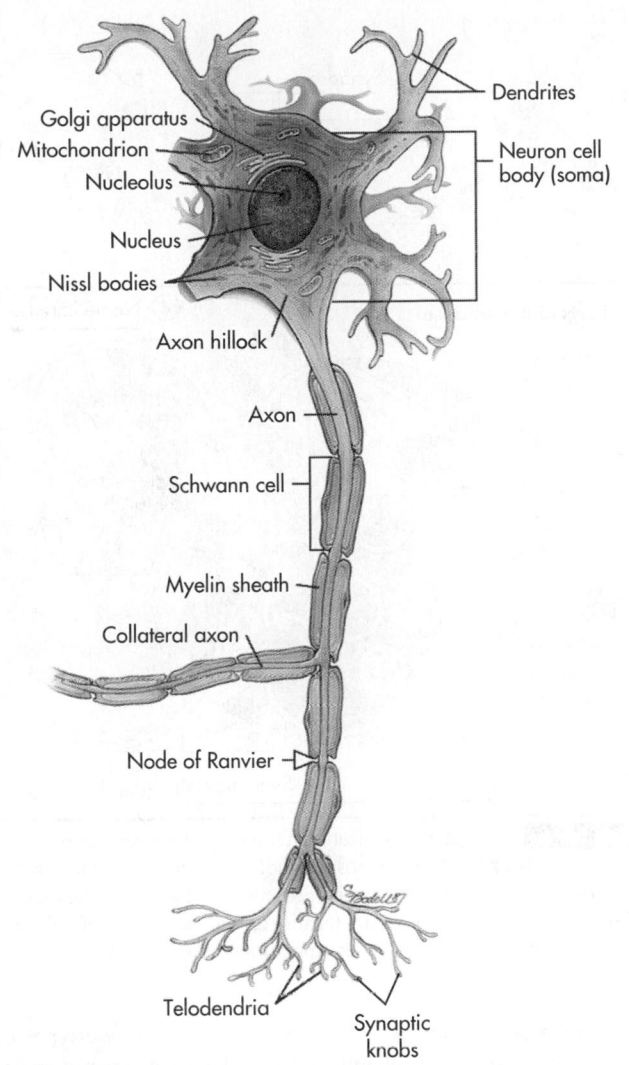

FIG. 54-1 Structural features of neurons: dendrites, cell body, and axons.

Labels: Dendrites, Neuron cell body (soma), Golgi apparatus, Mitochondrion, Nucleolus, Nucleus, Nissl bodies, Axon hillock, Axon, Schwann cell, Myelin sheath, Collateral axon, Node of Ranvier, Telodendria, Synaptic knobs

as phagocytes for neuronal debris. They help restore the neurochemical milieu and provide support for repair. Proliferation of astrocytes contributes to the formation of scar tissue (gliosis) in the CNS. *Ependymal cells* line the brain ventricles and aid in the secretion of cerebrospinal fluid (CSF). *Microglia*, a type of macrophage, are relatively rare in normal CNS tissue. They are phagocytes and are important in host defense.

Most primary CNS tumors involve neuroglia. Primary malignancies involving neurons are rare because these cells are not usually mitotic.

Nerve Regeneration

If the axon of the nerve cell is damaged, the cell attempts to repair itself. When damaged, all nerve cells attempt to grow back to their original destinations by sprouting many branches from the damaged ends of their axons. Unfortunately, axons in the CNS are less successful than peripheral axons in regenerating. This difference may be because of scar formation and lack of trophic factors within the CNS.[2] Regenerating nerve fibers grow 4 mm per day.

In the PNS (outside the brain and the spinal cord), injured nerve fibers can successfully regenerate by growing within the

protective myelin sheath of the supporting Schwann cells if the cell body is intact. The final result of nerve regeneration depends on the number of axon sprouts that join with the appropriate Schwann cell columns and reinnervate appropriate end organs.

Nerve Impulse

The purpose of a neuron is to initiate, receive, and process messages about events both within and outside the body. The initiation of a neuronal message (nerve impulse) involves the generation of an action potential. Once an action potential is initiated, a series of action potentials travel along the axon. When the impulse reaches the end of the nerve fiber, it is transmitted across the junction between nerve cells (synapse) by a chemical interaction involving neurotransmitters. This chemical interaction generates another set of action potentials in the next neuron. These events are repeated until the nerve impulse reaches its destination.

Action Potential. When nerve cells are in a resting (nonactive) state, the inside of the cell carries a negative electric charge relative to the outside of the cell. Sodium ions (Na^+) are in high concentration outside the cell, and potassium ions (K^+) are in high concentration inside the cell. The difference in electric charge across the cell membrane is termed the *resting membrane potential* (Fig. 54-2). An action potential occurs when a stimulus is of sufficient magnitude to alter the membrane potential.

During the action potential, the cell membrane becomes more permeable to Na^+, allowing the Na^+ to move readily into the cell. The resulting change in the voltage across the cell membrane is called *depolarization*. The inside of the cell temporarily becomes positive relative to the outside. After rapid depolarization, repo-

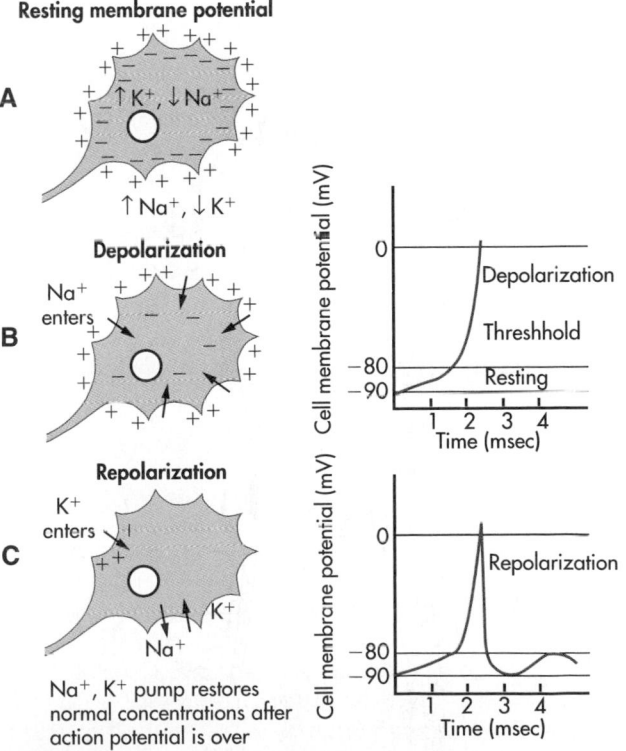

FIG. 54-2 A, Resting membrane potential. B, Depolarization. C, Repolarization.

larization (the inside of the cell becoming negative relative to the outside) is facilitated by a slower increase in K^+ permeability, which in turn is caused by the depolarization associated with entry of Na^+ into the cell. The whole process of depolarization and repolarization of the nerve cell membrane takes only 1 to 2 milliseconds. With repeated action potentials the cells accumulate Na^+. An active metabolic process within the cell is required to move Na^+ out of and K^+ back into the cell. This metabolic process is accomplished by the Na^+-K^+ pump, which requires energy from the breakdown of adenosine triphosphate (ATP).

The action potential has an all-or-none quality; that is, once the cell depolarizes enough to cause an action potential, the size of the action potential is independent of the strength of the stimulus. When an action potential is initiated at one point of a neuron, it is transmitted along the axon without losing its intensity.

Because of its insulating capacity, myelination of nerve axons facilitates the conduction of an action potential. Many peripheral nerve axons have gaps, termed *nodes of Ranvier,* at regular intervals in the myelin sheath surrounding them. An action potential traveling down one of these axons hops from node to node without traversing the insulated membrane segment between nodes, making the action potential travel much faster than it would otherwise. This is called *saltatory* (hopping) conduction. In an unmyelinated fiber the wave of depolarization traverses the entire length of the axon, with each portion of the membrane becoming depolarized in turn. Fig. 54-3 compares nerve impulse transmission of myelinated and unmyelinated fibers.

Synapse. A **synapse** is the structural and functional junction between two neurons. It is the point at which the nerve impulse is transmitted from one neuron to another or from neuron to glands or muscles. The essential structures of synaptic transmission are a presynaptic terminal, a synaptic cleft, and a receptor

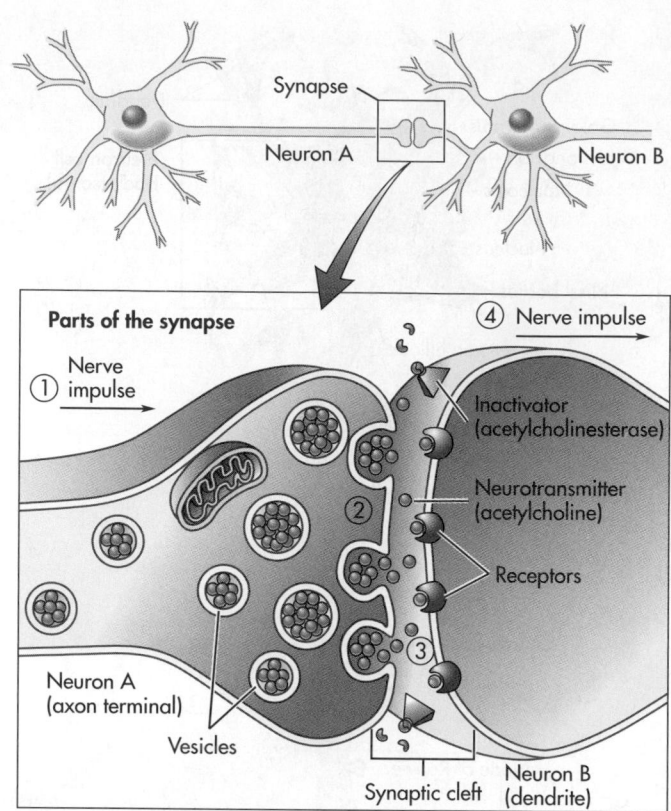

FIG. 54-4   The synapse is located in the space between neuron A and neuron B. Parts of the synapse include the neurotransmitters, inactivators, and receptors. The neurotransmitters are located in the vesicles of neuron A. The inactivators are located on the membrane of neuron B. The receptors are located on the membrane of neuron B.

site on the postsynaptic cell (Fig. 54-4). There are two types of synapses: electrical and chemical. In an electrical synapse an action potential moves from neuron to neuron directly by allowing electrical current to flow between neurons. In a chemical synapse an action potential reaches the end of the axon (presynaptic terminal); then it causes release of a chemical substance (neurotransmitter) from tiny vesicles within the axon terminal. This release depends on influx of calcium, initiated by depolarization of the nerve terminal. The neurotransmitter then crosses the microscopic space (synaptic cleft) between the two neurons and attaches to receptor sites of the receiving (postsynaptic) neuron. This causes a change in the permeability of the postsynaptic cell membrane to specific ions such as Na^+ and K^+ and a change in the electric potential of the membrane.

Neurotransmitters. A **neurotransmitter** is a chemical agent involved in the transmission of an impulse across the synaptic cleft. Some neurotransmitters are excitatory: they cause an increase in Na^+ permeability at the postsynaptic cell membrane, increasing the likelihood that an action potential will be generated. This type of synaptic input results in an excitatory postsynaptic potential. Other neurotransmitters are inhibitory: they cause an increase in permeability of K^+ and chloride (Cl^-) ions, decreasing the likelihood that an action potential will be generated. This type of synaptic input results in an inhibitory postsynaptic potential.

Each of the hundreds to thousands of synaptic connections of a single neuron has an influence on that neuron. The net effect of

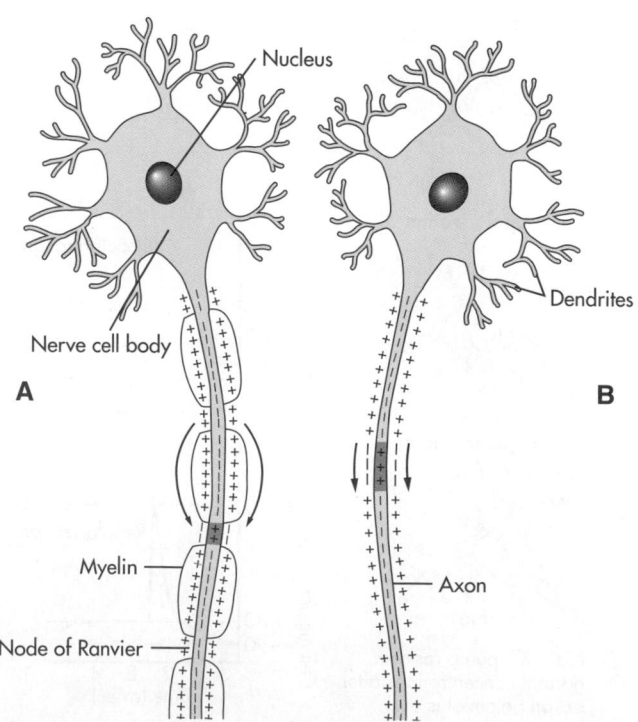

FIG. 54-3   **A,** Saltatory conduction in a myelinated nerve. **B,** Depolarization in an unmyelinated fiber.

the input is sometimes excitatory and sometimes inhibitory. In general, the net effect depends on the number of presynaptic neurons that are releasing neurotransmitters on the postsynaptic cell. A presynaptic cell that releases an excitatory neurotransmitter does not always cause the postsynaptic cell to depolarize enough to generate an action potential. However, when many presynaptic cells release excitatory neurotransmitters on a single neuron, the sum of their input is enough to generate an action potential. The presynaptic input can be summed by the number of presynaptic cells firing *(spatial summation)* or by the frequency of firing of a single presynaptic cell *(temporal summation)*. Summation usually occurs by both events.

The effect of an excitatory or inhibitory neurotransmitter depends on which ion channels in the postsynaptic membrane are influenced by that neurotransmitter. The neurotransmitters that are known to generally have an excitatory influence are acetylcholine, norepinephrine, serotonin, dopamine, glutamate, and histamine. The neurotransmitters that generally have an inhibitory influence are gamma-aminobutyric acid (GABA) and glycine.

Neurotransmitters continue to combine with the receptor sites at the postsynaptic membrane until they are inactivated by enzymes, are taken up by the presynaptic endings, or diffuse away from the synaptic region. In addition, neurotransmitters can be affected by drugs and toxins, which can modify their function or block their attachment to receptor sites on the postsynaptic membrane. Enkephalins and endorphins are also considered neurotransmitters. These substances have opiate-like properties. They are found in multiple areas of the CNS and PNS and act to inhibit pain perception (see Chapter 9).

Central Nervous System

Major structural components of the CNS are the spinal cord and brain. The brain consists of the cerebral hemispheres, cerebellum, and brainstem.

Spinal Cord. The spinal cord is continuous with the brainstem and exits from the cranial cavity through the foramen magnum. A cross section of the spinal cord reveals gray matter that is centrally located in an H shape and is surrounded by white matter (Fig. 54-5). The gray matter contains the cell bodies of

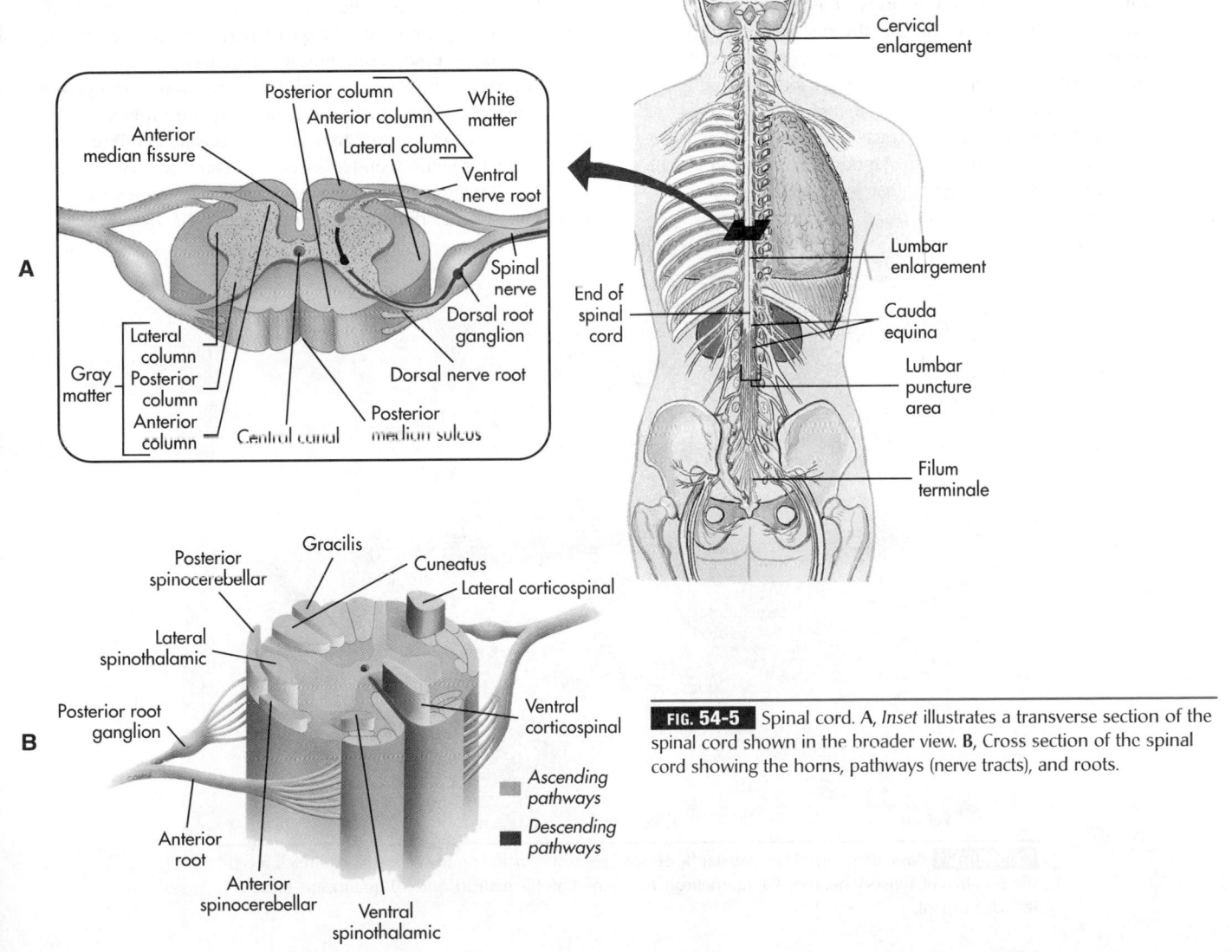

FIG. 54-5 Spinal cord. **A,** *Inset* illustrates a transverse section of the spinal cord shown in the broader view. **B,** Cross section of the spinal cord showing the horns, pathways (nerve tracts), and roots.

voluntary motor neurons and preganglionic autonomic motor neurons, as well as cell bodies of association neurons (interneurons). The white matter contains the axons of the ascending sensory and the descending (suprasegmental) motor fibers. The myelin surrounding these fibers gives them their white appearance. Specific ascending and descending pathways in the white matter can be identified. The spinal pathways or tracts are named for the point of origin and the point of destination (e.g., spinocerebellar tract [ascending], corticospinal tract [descending]). The major spinal pathways are presented in Fig. 54-5.

Ascending tracts. In general, the ascending tracts carry specific sensory information to higher levels of the CNS. This information comes from special sensory endings (receptors) in the skin, muscles and joints, viscera, and blood vessels and enters the spinal cord by way of the dorsal roots of the spinal nerves. The fasciculus gracilis and the fasciculus cuneatus (commonly called the dorsal or posterior columns) carry information and transmit impulses concerned with touch, deep pressure, vibration, position sense, and kinesthesia (appreciation of movement, weight, and body parts). The *spinocerebellar tracts* carry subconscious information about muscle tension and body position to the cerebellum for coordination of movement. This information is not consciously perceived. The *spinothalamic tracts* carry pain and temperature sensations. Therefore the ascending tracts are organized by sensory modality, as well as by anatomy.

Although the functions of these pathways are generally accepted, other ascending tracts may also carry sensory modalities. The symptoms of various neurologic diseases suggest that additional pathways for touch, position sense, and vibration exist.

Descending tracts. Descending tracts carry impulses that are responsible for muscle movement. Among the most important descending tracts are the corticobulbar and corticospinal tracts, collectively termed the *pyramidal tract.* These tracts carry voli-

tional (voluntary) impulses from the cortex to the cranial and peripheral nerves, respectively. Another group of descending motor tracts carries impulses from the extrapyramidal system, which includes all motor systems (except the pyramidal system) concerned with voluntary movement. It includes descending pathways originating in the brainstem, basal ganglia, and cerebellum. The motor output exits the spinal cord by way of the ventral roots of the spinal nerves.

Lower and upper motor neurons. Lower motor neurons (LMNs) are the final common pathway through which descending motor tracts influence skeletal muscle, the effector organ for movement. The cell bodies of LMNs, which send axons to innervate the skeletal muscles of the arms, trunk, and legs, are located in the anterior horn of the corresponding segments of the spinal cord (e.g., cervical segments contain LMNs for the arms). LMNs for skeletal muscles of the eyes, face, mouth, and throat are located in the corresponding segments of the brainstem. These cell bodies and their axons make up the somatic motor components of the cranial nerves. LMN lesions generally cause weakness or paralysis, denervation atrophy, hyporeflexia or areflexia, and decreased muscle tone (flaccidity).

Upper motor neurons (UMNs) originate in the cerebral cortex and project downward. The corticobulbar tract ends in the brainstem, and the corticospinal tract descends into the spinal cord. These neurons influence skeletal muscle movement. UMN lesions generally cause weakness or paralysis, disuse atrophy, hyperreflexia, and increased muscle tone (spasticity).

Reflex arc. A **reflex** is defined as an involuntary response to a stimulus. The components of a monosynaptic reflex arc (the simplest kind of reflex arc) are a receptor organ, an afferent neuron, an effector neuron, and an effector organ (e.g., skeletal muscle). The afferent neuron synapses with the efferent neuron in the gray matter of the spinal cord. A reflex arc is shown in Fig. 54-6.

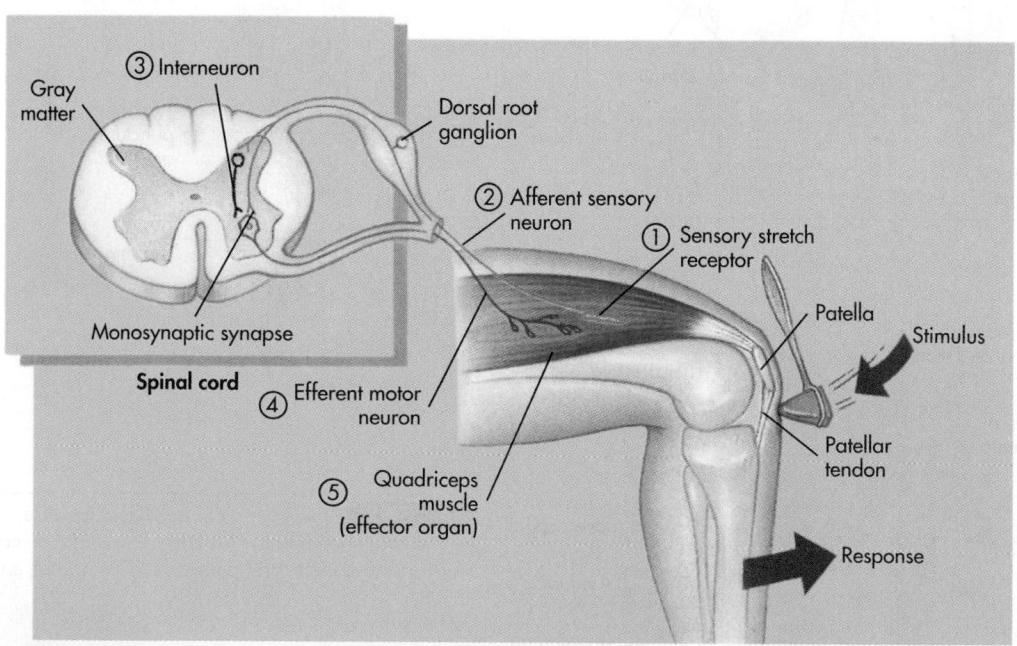

FIG. 54-6 Basic diagram of the patellar "knee-jerk" reflex arc, including the *(1)* sensory stretch receptor, *(2)* afferent sensory neuron, *(3)* interneuron, *(4)* efferent motor neuron, and *(5)* quadriceps muscle (effector organ).

More complex reflex arcs have other neurons (interneurons) in addition to the afferent neuron influencing the effector neuron. In the spinal cord, reflex arcs play an important role in maintaining muscle tone, which is essential for body posture.

Brain. The brain can be divided into three major components: cerebrum, brainstem, and cerebellum.

Cerebrum. The *cerebrum* is composed of the right and left hemispheres. Both hemispheres can be further divided into four major lobes: frontal, temporal, parietal, and occipital (Fig. 54-7). These divisions are useful to delineate portions of the neocortex (gray matter), which makes up the outer layer of the cerebral hemispheres. Neurons in specific parts of the neocortex are essential for various highly complex and sophisticated aspects of mental functioning, such as language, memory, and appreciation of visual-spatial relationships.

The functions of the cerebrum are multiple and complex. Specific areas of the cerebral cortex are associated with specific functions. Table 54-1 summarizes the location and function of the parts of the cerebrum.

The basal ganglia, thalamus, hypothalamus, and limbic system are also located in the cerebrum. The basal ganglia are a group of paired structures located centrally in the cerebrum and midbrain; most of them are on both sides of the thalamus. The function of the basal ganglia is to modulate the initiation, execution, and completion of voluntary movements and automatic movements associated with skeletal muscle activity, such as swinging of the arms while walking, swallowing saliva, and blinking.

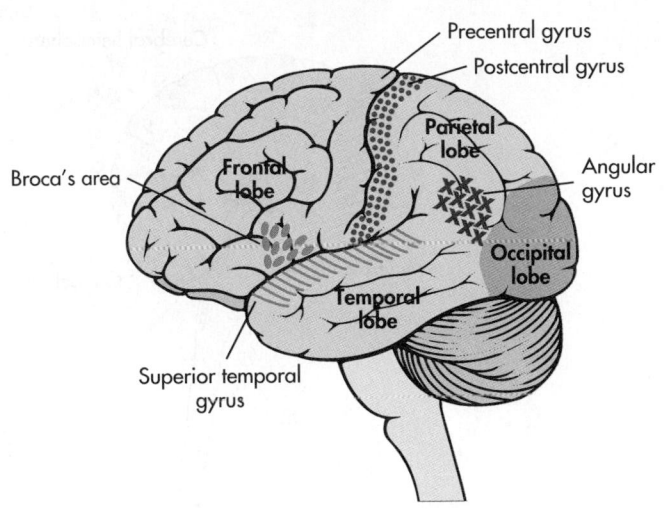

FIG. 54-7 Left hemisphere of cerebrum, lateral surface, showing major lobes and areas of the brain.

The thalamus (part of the diencephalon) lies directly above the brainstem (Fig. 54-8) and is the major relay center for sensory and other afferent (i.e., cerebellar) inputs to the cerebral cortex. The hypothalamus is located just inferior to the thalamus and slightly in front of the midbrain. It regulates the ANS and the endocrine system. The limbic system is, phylogenetically, an old part of the human cerebrum. It is located near the inner surfaces

TABLE 54-1	**Location and Function of the Parts of the Cerebrum**	
PART	**LOCATION**	**FUNCTION**
Cortical areas		
Motor		
Primary	Precentral gyrus	Controls initiation of movement on opposite side of body
Supplemental	Anterior to precentral gyrus	Facilitates proximal muscle activity, including activity for stance and gait, and spontaneous movement and coordination
Sensory		
Somatic	Postcentral gyrus	Registers body sensations (e.g., temperature, touch, pressure, pain) from opposite side of body
Visual	Occipital lobe	Registers visual images
Auditory	Superior temporal gyrus	Registers auditory inputs
Association areas	Parietal lobe	Integrates somatic and special sensory inputs
	Posterior temporal lobe	Integrates visual and auditory inputs for language comprehension
	Anterior temporal lobe	Integrates past experiences
	Anterior frontal lobe	Controls higher-order processes (e.g., judgment, insight, reasoning, problem solving, planning)
Language		
Comprehension	Wernicke's area	Integrates auditory language (understanding of spoken words)
Expression	Broca's area	Regulates verbal expression
Basal ganglia	Near lateral ventricles of both cerebral hemispheres	Controls and facilitates learned and automatic movements
Thalamus	Below basal ganglia	Relays sensory and motor inputs to cortex and other parts of cerebrum
Hypothalamus	Below thalamus	Regulates endocrine and autonomic functions (e.g., feeding, sleeping, emotional and sexual responses)
Limbic system	Lateral to hypothalamus	Influences affective (emotional) behavior and basic drives such as feeding and sexual behavior

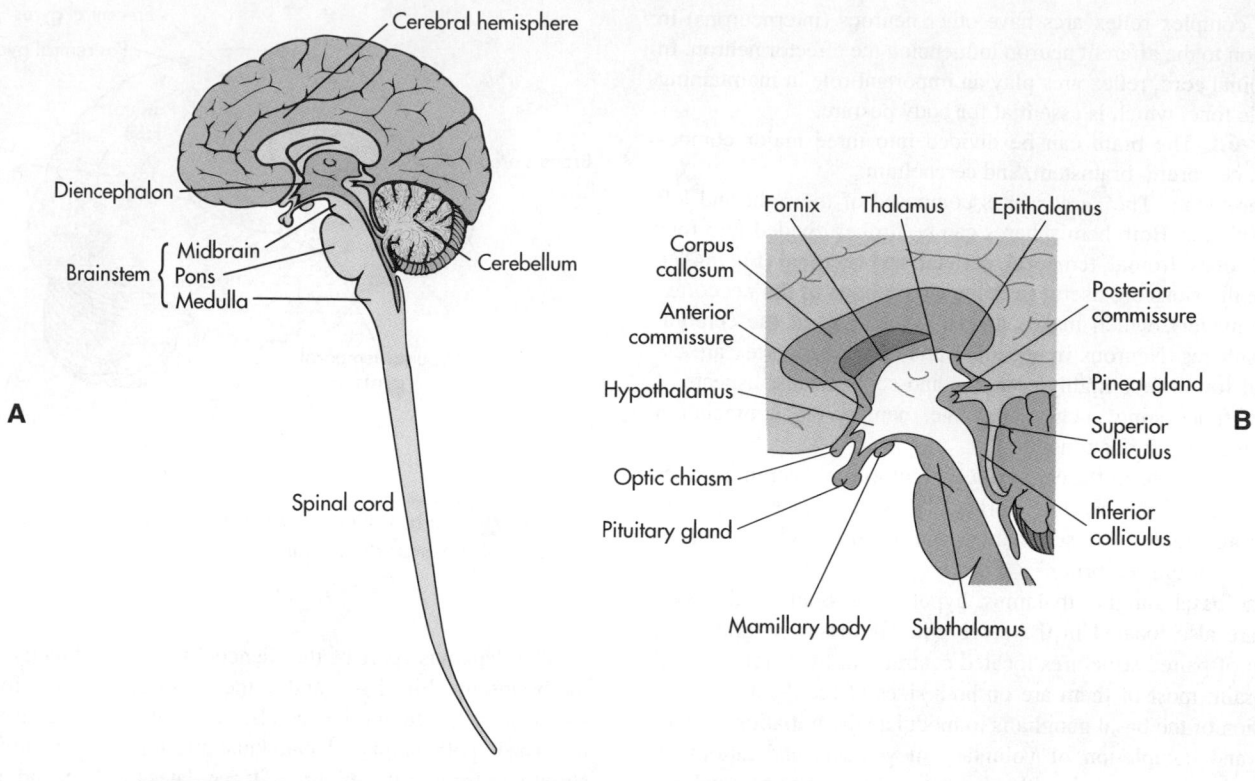

FIG. 54-8 **A,** Major divisions of the central nervous system (CNS). **B,** Diencephalon (thalamus and hypothalamus).

of the cerebral hemispheres (Fig. 54-9) and is concerned with emotion, aggression, feeding behavior, and sexual response.

Brainstem. The *brainstem* includes the midbrain, pons, and medulla (see Fig. 54-8). Ascending and descending fibers pass through the brainstem going to and from the cerebrum and cerebellum. The cell bodies, or nuclei, of cranial nerves III through XII are in the brainstem. Also located in the brainstem is the *reticular formation,* a diffusely arranged group of neurons and their axons that extends from the medulla to the thalamus and hypothalamus. The functions of the reticular formation include relaying sensory information, influencing excitatory and inhibitory control of spinal motor neurons, and controlling vasomotor and respiratory activity. The reticular activating system is part of the reticular formation and is the regulatory system for arousal, a component of consciousness.

The vital centers concerned with respiratory, vasomotor, and cardiac function are located in the medulla. The brainstem also contains the centers for sneezing, coughing, hiccupping, vomiting, sucking, and swallowing.

Cerebellum. The cerebellum is located in the posterior part of the cranial fossa, along with the brainstem, under the occipital lobe of the cerebrum. The function of the cerebellum is to coordinate voluntary movement and to maintain trunk stability and equilibrium. It influences motor activity through its axonal connections to the motor cortex, brainstem nuclei, and their descending pathways. To perform these functions, the cerebellum receives information from the cerebral cortex, muscles, joints, and inner ear.

Ventricles and cerebrospinal fluid. Several supporting structures located within the CNS are important in regulating neuronal

function and physical support of the brain. The ventricles are four fluid-filled cavities within the brain that connect with one another and with the spinal canal. The lower portion of the fourth ventricle becomes the central canal in the lower part of the brainstem. The spinal canal is located in the center and extends the full length of the spinal cord. Fig. 54-10 shows the ventricles and the flow of CSF in the CNS.

Cerebrospinal fluid (CSF) circulates within the subarachnoid space that surrounds the brain, brainstem, and spinal cord. This fluid provides cushioning for the brain and spinal cord, allows fluid shifts from the cranial cavity to the spinal cavity, and carries nutrients. The formation of CSF in the choroid plexus in the ventricles involves both passive diffusion and active transport of substances. CSF resembles an ultrafiltrate of blood. Although CSF is continually being formed, many physiologic factors influence its rate of absorption and formation. The ventricles and central canal are normally filled with an average of 135 ml of CSF.

The CSF circulates throughout the ventricles and seeps into the subarachnoid space surrounding the brain and spinal cord. It is absorbed primarily through the *arachnoid villi* (tiny projections into the subarachnoid space), into the intradural venous sinuses, and eventually into the venous system. The analysis of CSF composition provides useful diagnostic information relating to certain nervous system diseases. CSF pressure is sometimes measured in patients with actual or suspected intracranial diseases. Increases in intracranial pressure, indicated by increased CSF pressure, can lead to herniation of the brain and compression of vital brainstem structures. The

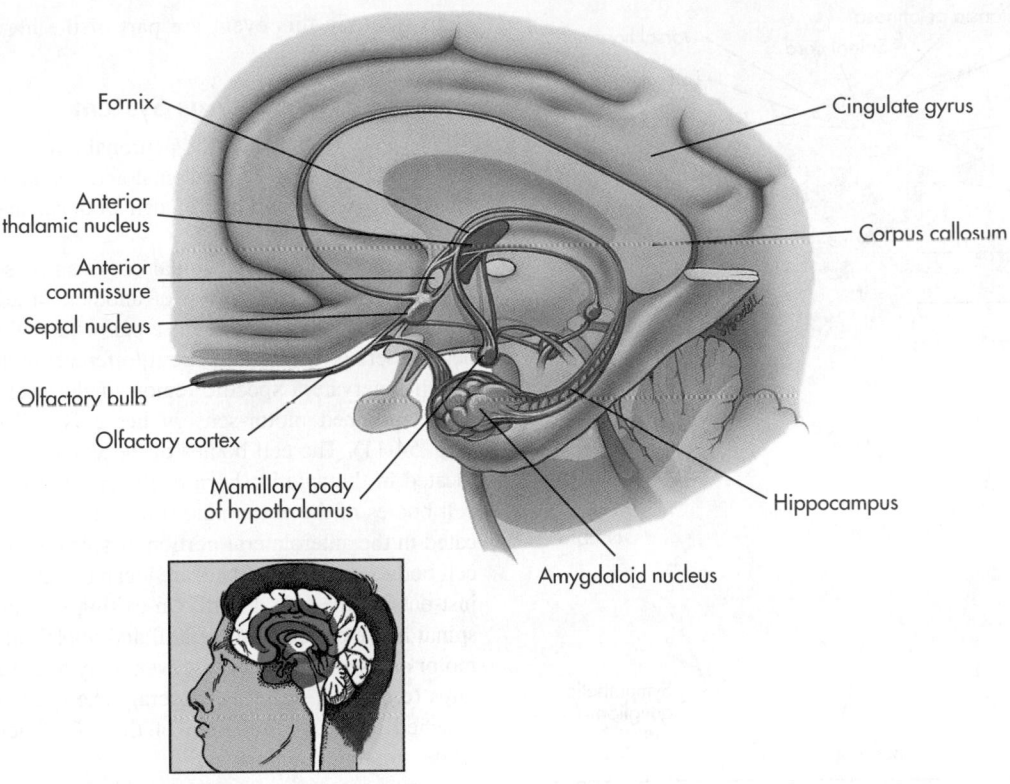

Fornix

Anterior
thalamic nucleus

Anterior
commissure

Septal nucleus

Olfactory bulb

Olfactory cortex

Mamillary body
of hypothalamus

Cingulate gyrus

Corpus callosum

Hippocampus

Amygdaloid nucleus

FIG. 54-9 Structures of the limbic system.

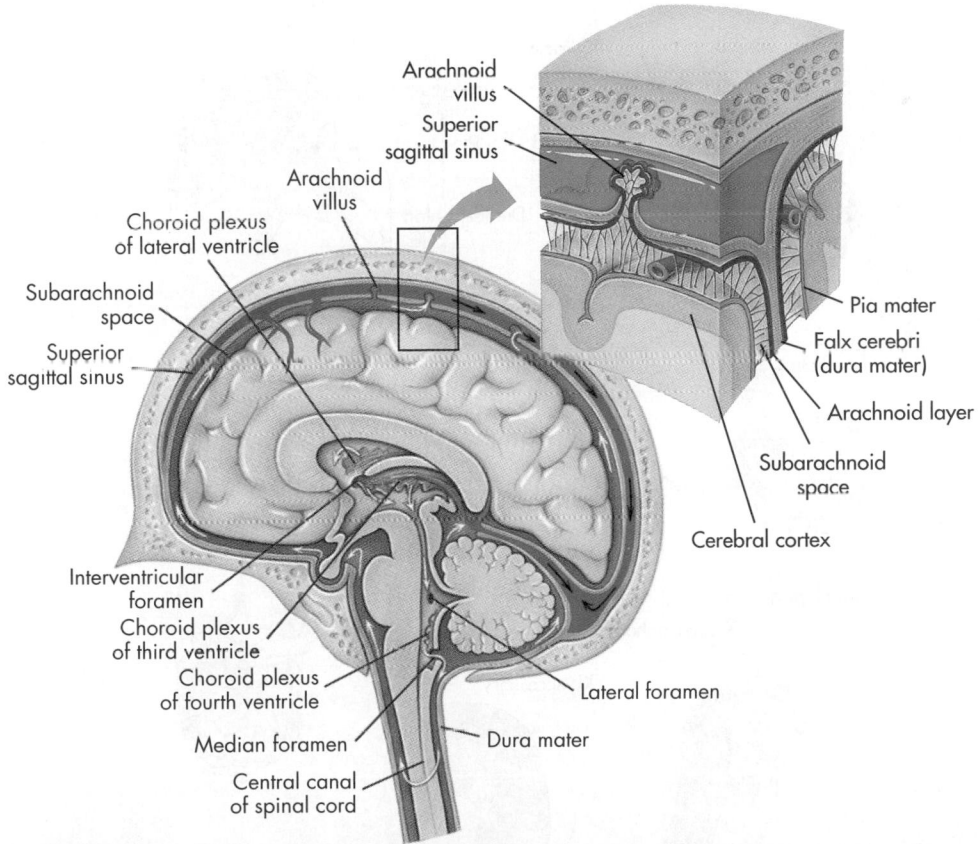

Arachnoid
villus

Superior
sagittal sinus

Arachnoid
villus

Choroid plexus
of lateral ventricle

Subarachnoid
space

Superior
sagittal sinus

Interventricular
foramen

Choroid plexus
of third ventricle

Choroid plexus
of fourth ventricle

Median foramen

Central canal
of spinal cord

Dura mater

Lateral foramen

Pia mater

Falx cerebri
(dura mater)

Arachnoid layer

Subarachnoid
space

Cerebral cortex

FIG. 54-10 Flow of cerebrospinal fluid (CSF). The fluid produced by filtration of blood by the choroid plexus of each ventricle flows inferiorly through the lateral ventricles, interventricular foramen, third ventricle, cerebral aqueduct, fourth ventricle, and subarachnoid space and to the blood.

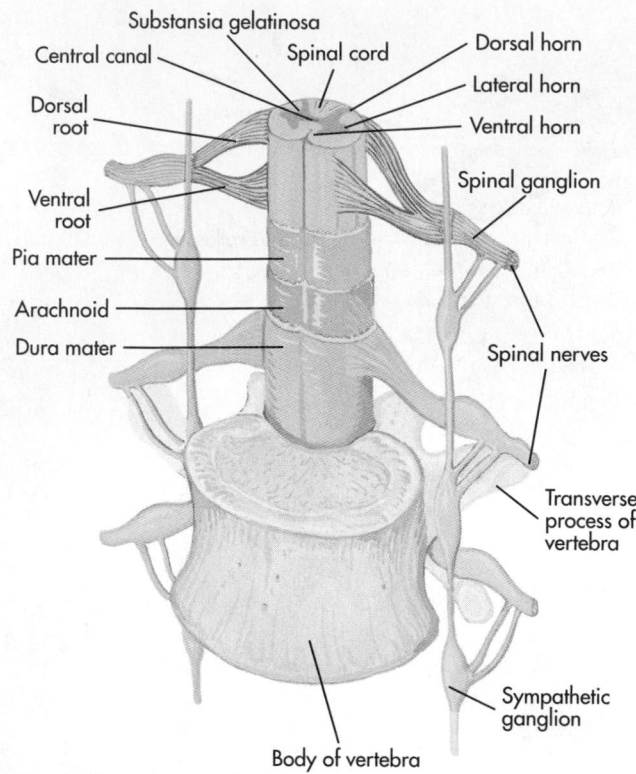

FIG. 54-11 Cross section of spinal cord showing attachments of spinal nerves and coverings of the spinal cord.

signs marking this event are part of the herniation syndrome (see Chapter 55).

Peripheral Nervous System

The PNS includes all the neuronal structures that lie outside the CNS. It consists of the spinal and cranial nerves, their associated ganglia (groupings of cell bodies), and portions of the ANS.

Spinal Nerves. The spinal cord can be seen as a series of spinal segments, one on top of another. In addition to the cell bodies, each segment contains a pair of dorsal (afferent) sensory nerve fibers or roots and ventral (efferent) motor fibers or roots, which innervate a specific region of the neck, trunk, or limbs. This combined motor-sensory nerve is called a *spinal nerve* (Fig. 54-11). The cell bodies of the voluntary motor system are located in the anterior horn of the spinal cord gray matter. The cell bodies of the autonomic (involuntary) motor system are located in the anterolateral portion of spinal cord gray matter. The cell bodies of sensory fibers are located in the dorsal root ganglia just outside the spinal cord. On exiting the spinal column, each spinal nerve divides into ventral and dorsal rami, a collection of motor and sensory fibers that eventually goes to peripheral structures (e.g., skin, muscles, viscera). The sympathetic ganglia are attached to the ventral rami of the spinal nerves by gray and white rami communicantes.

A **dermatome** is the area of skin innervated by the sensory fibers of a single dorsal root of a spinal nerve. The dermatomes

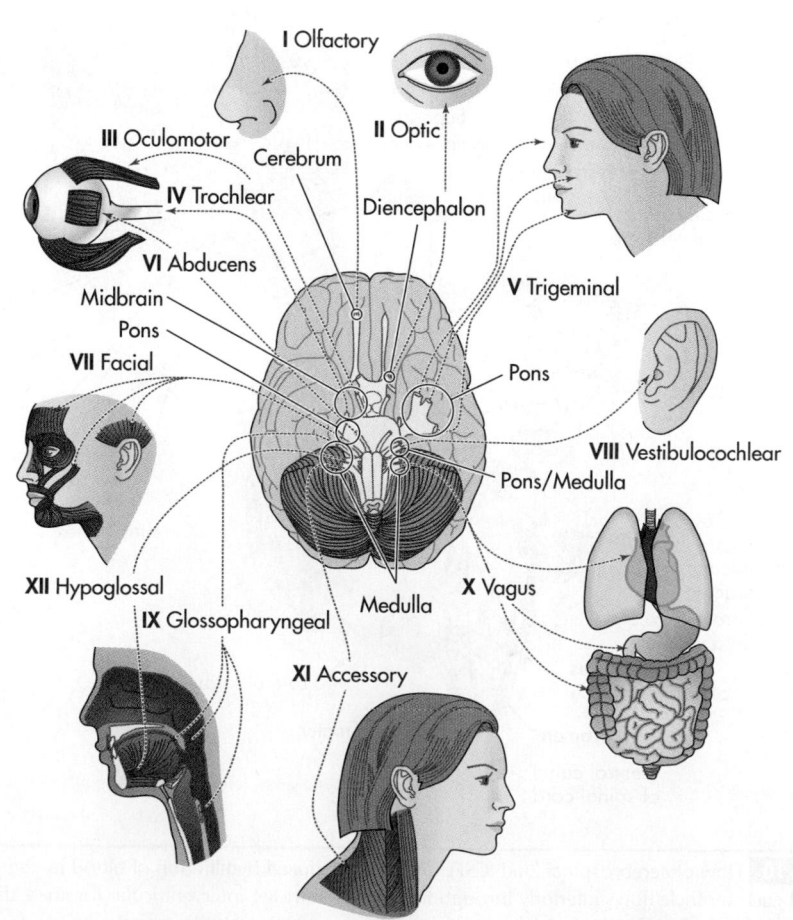

FIG. 54-12 The cranial nerves are numbered according to the order in which they leave the brain.

give a general picture of somatic sensory innervation by spinal segments. A *myotome* is a muscle group innervated by the primary motor neurons of a single ventral root. These are simple components in the embryonic stage of human development. However, the dermatomes and myotomes of a given spinal segment overlap with those of adjacent segments because of the development of ascending and descending collateral branches of nerve fibers.

Cranial Nerves. The **cranial nerves** (CNs) are the 12 paired nerves composed of cell bodies with fibers that exit from the cranial cavity. Unlike the spinal nerves, which always have both afferent sensory and efferent motor fibers, some CNs have only afferent and some only efferent fibers; others have both. Table 54-2 summarizes the motor and sensory components of the CNs. Fig. 54-12 shows the position of the CNs in relation to the brain and spinal cord. Just as the cell bodies of the spinal nerves are located in specific segments of the spinal cord, so are the cell bodies (nuclei) of the CNs located in specific segments of the brain. Exceptions are the nuclei of the olfactory and optic nerves. The primary cell bodies of the olfactory nerve are located in the nasal epithelium, and those of the optic nerve are in the retina. CN XI is a spinal nerve, and its efferent fibers migrate upward before exiting the neuroaxis at the level of the medulla.

Autonomic Nervous System. The **autonomic nervous system** (ANS) governs involuntary functions of cardiac muscle, smooth (involuntary) muscle, and glands.

The ANS is divided into two components, sympathetic and parasympathetic, which are anatomically and functionally different. These two systems function together to maintain a relatively balanced internal environment. The ANS is both an efferent and afferent system. It consists of preganglionic nerves and postganglionic nerves.

The preganglionic cell bodies of the *sympathetic nervous system* (SNS) are located in spinal segments T1 through L2. The sympathetic ganglia, which contain the cell bodies of the postganglionic neurons, lie close to the spinal column, along the vertebral bodies in the rami communicantes. These ganglia and the connecting nerves are called the paravertebral chain. The major neurotransmitter released by the postganglionic fibers of the SNS is norepinephrine, and the neurotransmitter released by the preganglionic fibers is acetylcholine.

In contrast, the preganglionic cell bodies of the *parasympathetic nervous system* (PSNS) are located in the brainstem and in the sacral spinal segments (S2 through S4). The parasympathetic ganglia are located in or near the structures that they innervate. Acetylcholine is the neurotransmitter released at both preganglionic and postganglionic nerve endings.

The ANS provides dual and often reciprocal innervation to many structures. For example, the SNS increases the rate and force of the heart contraction, and the PSNS decreases the rate and force. The SNS dilates bronchi and bronchioles of the lungs, and the PSNS constricts them. Some structures are innervated by only one system (e.g., the hair follicles and the sweat glands,

---

TABLE 54-2   Cranial Nerves

NERVE	CONNECTION WITH BRAIN	FUNCTION
I Olfactory nerves and tract	Anterior ventral cerebrum	*Sensory:* from olfactory epithelium of superior nasal cavity
II Optic nerve	Lateral geniculate body of the thalamus	*Sensory:* from retina of eyes
III Oculomotor nerve	Midbrain	*Motor:* to four eye movement muscles and levator palpebrae Parasympathetic: smooth muscle in eyeball
IV Trochlear nerve	Midbrain	*Motor:* to one eye movement muscle, the superior oblique
V Trigeminal nerve		
Ophthalmic branch	Pons	*Sensory:* from forehead, eye, superior nasal cavity
Maxillary branch	Pons	*Sensory:* from inferior nasal cavity, face, upper teeth, mucosa of superior mouth
Mandibular branch	Pons	*Sensory:* from surfaces of jaw, lower teeth, mucosa of lower mouth, and anterior tongue *Motor:* to muscles of mastication
VI Abducens nerve	Pons	*Motor:* to one eye movement muscle, the lateral rectus
VII Facial nerve	Junction of pons and medulla	*Motor:* to facial muscles of expression and cheek muscle, the buccinator *Sensory:* taste from anterior two thirds of tongue
VIII Vestibulocochlear nerve		
Vestibular branch	Junction of pons and medulla	*Sensory:* from equilibrium sensory organ, the vestibular apparatus
Cochlear branch	Junction of pons and medulla	*Sensory:* from auditory sensory organ, the cochlea
IX Glossopharyngeal nerve	Medulla	*Sensory:* from pharynx and posterior tongue, including taste *Motor:* superior pharyngeal muscles
X Vagus nerve	Medulla	*Sensory:* much of viscera of thorax and abdomen *Motor:* larynx and middle and inferior pharyngeal muscles Parasympathetic: heart, lungs, most of digestive system
XI Accessory nerve	Medulla and superior spinal segments	*Motor:* to several neck muscles, sternocleidomastoid and trapezius
XII Hypoglossal nerve	Medulla	*Motor:* to intrinsic and extrinsic muscles of tongue

TABLE 54-3   Effect of Sympathetic and Parasympathetic Nervous Systems

VISCERAL EFFECTOR	EFFECT OF SYMPATHETIC NERVOUS SYSTEM*	EFFECT OF PARASYMPATHETIC NERVOUS SYSTEM†
Heart	Increase in rate and strength of heartbeat (β-receptors)	Decrease in rate and strength of heartbeat
Smooth muscle of blood vessels		
Skin blood vessels	Constriction (α-receptors)	No effect
Skeletal muscle blood vessels	Dilation (β-receptors)	No effect
Coronary blood vessels	Dilation (β-receptors), constriction (α-receptors)	Dilation
Abdominal blood vessels	Constriction (α-receptors)	No effect
Blood vessels of external genitals	Ejaculation (contraction of smooth muscle in male ducts [e.g., epididymis, ductus deferens])	Dilation of blood vessels causing erection in male
Smooth muscle of hollow organs and sphincters		
Bronchi	Dilation (β-receptors)	Constriction
Digestive tract, except sphincters	Decrease in peristalsis (β-receptors)	Increase in peristalsis
Sphincters of digestive tract	Contraction (α-receptors)	Relaxation
Urinary bladder	Relaxation (β-receptors)	Contraction
Urinary sphincters	Contraction (α-receptors)	Relaxation
Eye		
Iris	Contraction of radial muscle, dilation of pupil	Contraction of circular muscle, constriction of pupil
Ciliary	Relaxation, accommodation for far vision	Contraction, accommodation for near vision
Hairs (pilomotor muscles)	Contraction producing goose pimples or piloerection (α-receptors)	No effect
Glands		
Sweat	Increase in sweat (neurotransmitter, acetylcholine)	No effect
Digestive (e.g., salivary, gastric)	Decrease in secretion of saliva; not known for others	Increase in secretion of saliva and gastric HCl acid
Pancreas, including islets	Decrease in secretion	Increase in secretion of pancreatic juice and insulin
Liver	Increase in glycogenolysis (β-receptors), increase in blood glucose level	No effect
Adrenal medulla‡	Increase in epinephrine secretion	No effect

Modified from Thibodeau GA, Patton KT: *Anatomy and physiology*, ed 5, St Louis, 2003, Mosby.
*Neurotransmitter is norepinephrine unless otherwise stated.
†Neurotransmitter is acetylcholine unless otherwise stated.
‡Sympathetic preganglionic axons terminate in contact with secreting cells of the adrenal medulla. Thus the adrenal medulla functions as a "giant sympathetic postganglionic neuron."

which are innervated only by the SNS). Table 54-3 compares the SNS and PSNS.

The result of SNS stimulation is activation of mechanisms required for the "fight or flight" response that occurs throughout the body. In contrast, the PSNS is geared to act in localized and discrete regions. It serves to conserve and restore the energy stores of the body.

Cerebral Circulation

The blood supply of the brain arises from the internal carotid arteries (anterior circulation) and the vertebral arteries (posterior circulation), which are shown in Fig. 54-13. Knowledge of the distribution of the major arteries of the brain and the area supplied is essential for understanding and evaluating the signs and symptoms of cerebrovascular disease and trauma.

Each internal carotid artery supplies the ipsilateral hemisphere, whereas the basilar artery, formed by the junction of the two vertebral arteries, supplies structures within the posterior fossa (cerebellum and brainstem). The *circle of Willis* arises from the basilar artery and the two internal carotid arteries (Fig. 54-14). This vascular circle may act as a safety valve when differential pressures are present in these arteries. It also may function as an anastomotic pathway when occlusion of a major artery on one side of the brain occurs. In general, the two anterior cerebral arteries supply the medial portion of the frontal lobes. The two middle cerebral arteries supply the outer portions of the frontal, parietal, and superior temporal lobes. The two posterior cerebral arteries supply the medial portions of the occipital and inferior temporal lobes. Fig. 54-13 shows the major cerebral arteries. Venous blood drains from the brain through the

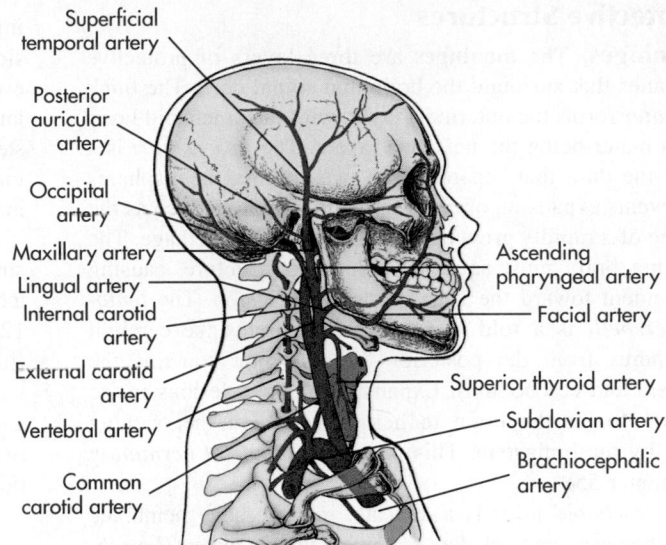

FIG. 54-13 Arteries of the head and neck. **A,** Brachio-cephalic artery, right common carotid artery, right subclavian artery, and their branches. The major arteries to the head are the common carotid and vertebral arteries. **B,** Inferior view of the brain showing the vertebral, basilar, and internal carotid arteries and their branches.

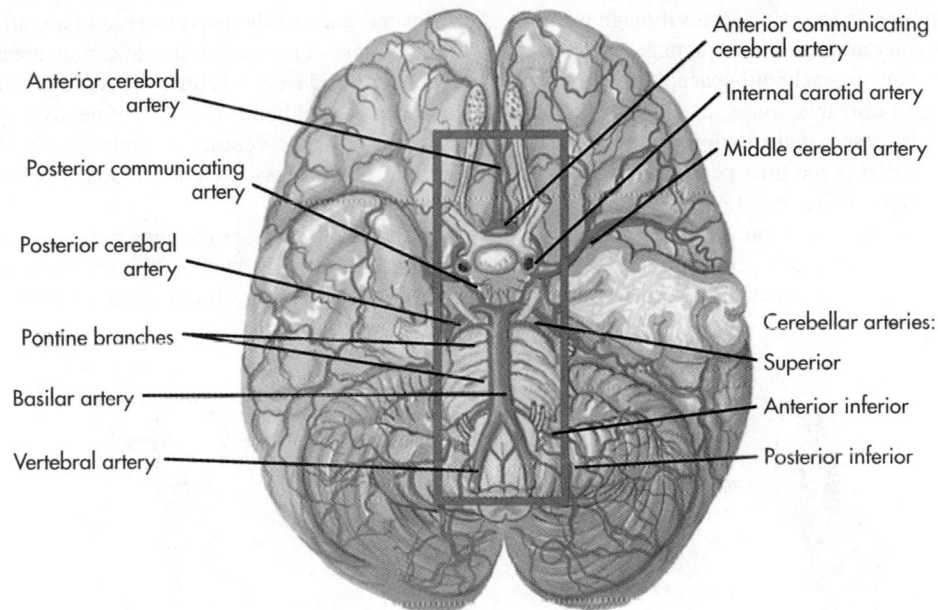

dural sinuses, which form channels that drain into the two jugular veins.

Blood-Brain Barrier. The **blood-brain barrier** is a physiologic barrier between blood capillaries and brain tissue. The structure of brain capillaries differs from that of other capillaries. Some substances that normally pass readily into most tissues are prevented from entering brain tissue. This barrier protects the brain from certain potentially harmful agents, while allowing nutrients and gases to enter. Because the blood-brain barrier affects the penetration of drugs, only certain ones can enter the CNS from the bloodstream. Lipid-soluble compounds enter the brain easily, whereas water-soluble and ionized drugs enter the brain and spinal cord slowly. Damage to the blood-brain barrier results in the penetration of drugs and other substances into brain tissue.

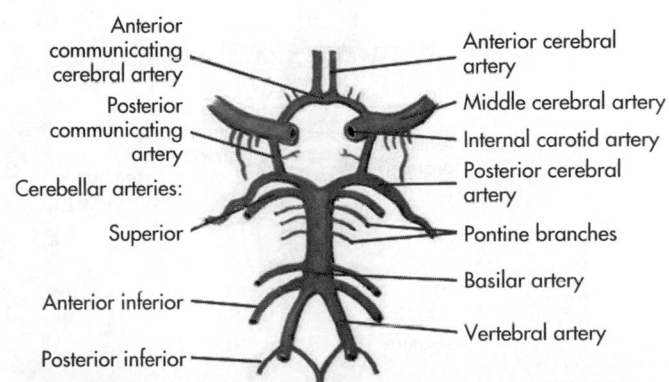

FIG. 54-14 Arteries at the base of the brain. The arteries that compose the circle of Willis are the two anterior cerebral arteries joined to each other by the anterior communicating cerebral artery and to the posterior cerebral arteries by the posterior communicating arteries.

Protective Structures

Meninges. The **meninges** are three layers of protective membranes that surround the brain and spinal cord. The thick *dura mater* forms the outermost layer, with the arachnoid layer and pia mater being the next two layers. The *falx cerebri* is a fold of the dura that separates the two cerebral hemispheres and prevents expansion of brain tissue in situations such as the presence of a rapidly growing tumor or acute hemorrhage. The expanding brain must squeeze under this structure, causing displacement toward the side opposite the lesion. The *tentorium cerebelli* is a fold of dura that separates the cerebral hemispheres from the posterior fossa (which contains the brainstem and cerebellum). Expansion of mass lesions in the cerebrum forces the brain to herniate through the opening created by the brainstem. This is termed *tentorial herniation* (see Chapter 55).

The *arachnoid* layer is a delicate, impermeable membrane that lies between the thick dura mater and the pia mater. The *subarachnoid space* lies between the arachnoid layer and the pia mater. This space is filled with CSF. Structures passing to and from the brain and the skull or its foramina (holes through which blood vessels and nerves enter and exit the intracranial compartment) must pass through the subarachnoid space. Therefore all cerebral arteries and veins lie in this space, as do the CNs. A larger subarachnoid space is present in the region of the third and fourth lumbar vertebrae, which is the area penetrated to obtain CSF during a lumbar puncture. (The spinal cord itself ends between the first and second lumbar vertebrae.)

Skull. The bony skull protects the brain from external trauma. It is composed of 8 cranial bones and 14 facial bones.

The structure of the skull cavity explains the physiology of head injuries (see Chapter 55). Although the top and sides of the inside of the skull are relatively smooth, the bottom surface is uneven. It has many ridges, prominences, and foramina. The largest hole is the foramen magnum, through which the brainstem extends to the spinal cord. This foramen offers the only major space for the expansion of brain contents when increased intracranial pressure occurs.

Vertebral Column. The vertebral column protects the spinal cord, supports the head, and provides flexibility. The vertebral column is made up of 33 individual vertebrae: 7 cervical, 12 thoracic, 5 lumbar, 5 sacral (fused into one), and 4 coccygeal (fused into one). Each vertebra has a central opening through which the spinal cord passes. The vertebrae are held together by a series of ligaments. Intervertebral disks occupy the spaces between vertebrae. Fig. 54-15 shows the vertebral column in relation to the trunk.

▪ Gerontologic Considerations: Effects of Aging on the Nervous System

Several parts of the nervous system are affected by aging. In the CNS, loss of neurons occurs in certain areas of the brainstem, cerebellum, and cerebral cortex. This is a gradual process that begins in early adulthood. With loss of neurons there is widening or enlargement of the ventricles. Brain weight also decreases as a result of neuron loss. Cerebral blood flow decreases, and CSF production declines.

In the PNS there are changes in the anterior horn cells and peripheral nerves, as well as the target organ, muscle. Degenerative changes in myelin cause a decrease in nerve conduc-

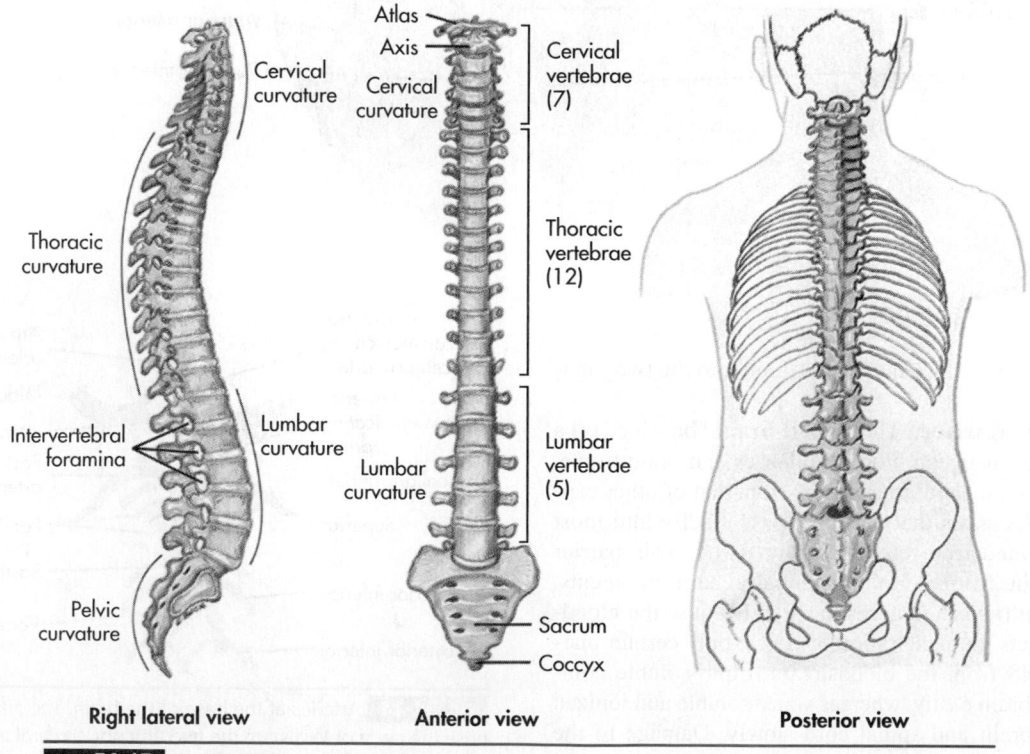

Right lateral view   **Anterior view**   **Posterior view**

FIG. 54-15 Vertebral column (three views).

tion. Coordinated neuromuscular activity, such as the maintenance of blood pressure in response to changing from a lying to a standing position, is altered with aging. As a result, older adults are more vulnerable to problems with orthostatic hypotension. Similarly, coordination of neuromuscular activity to maintain body temperature is also less efficient with aging. Older adults are less able to adapt to extremes in environmental temperature and are more vulnerable to both hypothermia and hyperthermia.

Additional relevant changes associated with aging include decreases in memory, vision, hearing, taste, smell, vibration and position sense, muscle strength, and reaction time.[3] Sensory changes including decreases in taste and smell perception may result in decreased dietary intake in the older adult. Reduced hearing and vision can result in perceptual confusion. Problems with balance and coordination can put the older adult at risk for falls and subsequent fractures.

Changes in assessment findings result from age-related alterations in the various components of the nervous system. Age-related changes in the nervous system and differences in assessment findings are presented in Table 54-4. ∎

ASSESSMENT OF THE NERVOUS SYSTEM

Subjective Data

Important Health Information

Past health history. Three points should be considered in taking the history of a patient with neurologic problems. First, avoid suggesting certain symptoms to the patient or asking leading questions such as, "Is your headache throbbing?" or

---

TABLE 54-4   Gerontologic Differences in Assessment — Nervous System

COMPONENT	CHANGES	DIFFERENCES IN ASSESSMENT FINDINGS
Central Nervous System		
Brain	Reduction in cerebral blood flow and metabolism	Alterations in selected mental functioning
	Decrease in efficiency of temperature-regulating mechanism	Decrease in body temperature, impairment of ability to adapt to environmental temperature
	Decrease in neurotransmitter content, disruption in integration as result of loss of neurons	Repetitive movements, tremors
	Decrease in oxygen supply, changes in basal ganglia caused by vascular changes	Changes in gait and ambulation (e.g., extrapyramidal, Parkinson-like gait); diminished kinesthetic sense
Peripheral Nervous System		
Cranial and spinal nerves	Loss of myelin and decrease in conduction time in some nerves	Decrease in reaction time in specific nerves
	Cellular degeneration, death of neurons	Decrease in speed and intensity of neuronal reflexes
Functional Divisions		
Motor	Decrease in muscle bulk	Diminished strength and agility
	Decrease in electrical activity	Decrease in reactions and movement time
Sensory*	Decrease in sensory receptors caused by degenerative changes and involution of fine corpuscles of nerve endings	Diminished sense of touch; inability to localize stimuli; decrease in appreciation of touch, temperature, and peripheral vibrations
	Decrease in electrical activity	Slowing of or alteration in sensory reception
	Atrophy of taste buds	Signs of malnutrition, weight loss
	Degeneration and loss of fibers in olfactory bulb	Diminished sense of smell
	Degenerative changes in nerve cells in vestibular system of inner ear, cerebellum, and proprioceptive pathways in nervous system	Poor ability to maintain balance, widened gait
Reflexes	Possible decrease in deep tendon reflexes	Below-average reflex score
	Decrease in sensory conduction velocity as result of myelin sheath degeneration	Sluggish reflexes, slowing of reaction time
Reticular Formation		
Reticular activating system	Modification of hypothalamic function, reduction in stage IV sleep	Increase in frequency of spontaneous awakening together with tiredness, interrupted sleep, insomnia
Autonomic Nervous System		
SNS and PSNS	Morphologic features of ganglia, slowing of ANS responses	Orthostatic hypotension, systolic hypertension

*Specific changes related to the eye are in Table 20-1 and specific changes related to the ear are in Table 20-7.
ANS, Autonomic nervous system; *PSNS*, parasympathetic nervous system; *SNS*, sympathetic nervous system.

"Are you weak on the right side?" It is better to ask open-ended questions such as, "What is your headache like?" or "Is there anything about your right side that bothers you?" Second, the mode of onset and the course of the illness are especially important aspects of the history. Often the nature of a neurologic disease process can be described by these facts alone, and the nurse should obtain all pertinent data in the history of the present illness, especially data related to the characteristics and progression of the symptoms. Third, because many neurologic diseases affect a patient's mental functioning, mental status must be assessed accurately before assuming that the history is factual. If the patient is not considered a reliable historian, obtain the history from a person who has firsthand knowledge of the patient's problems and complaints. Many times a health history cannot be obtained, and the nurse must proceed with only objective data.

The health history helps guide the approach for the neurologic examination; that is, it can direct the health care provider toward the parts of the nervous system that need to be closely assessed. If the patient's primary complaint is dizziness, the examination may be focused on visual, vestibular, and cerebellar functions rather than on somatic motor and sensory functions.

Medications. Special attention should be given to obtaining a careful medication history, especially the use of sedatives, narcotics, tranquilizers, and mood-elevating drugs. Many other drugs can also cause neurologic adverse effects.

Surgery or other treatments. The nurse should inquire about any surgery involving any part of the nervous system, such as the head, spine, or sensory organs. If a patient had surgery, the date, cause, procedure, recovery, and current status should be investigated.

The perinatal history may reveal exposure to toxic agents such as viruses, alcohol, tobacco, drugs, and radiation, which are known to adversely influence the development of the nervous system. The history may reveal a difficult labor and delivery, which can cause brain damage as a result of hypoxia, forceps delivery, or Rh incompatibility.

Growth and developmental history can be important in ascertaining whether nervous system dysfunction was present at an early age. The nurse should specifically inquire about major developmental tasks such as walking and talking. Successes at school or identified problems in an educational setting are other important developmental data to gather. Often this information is not available when the older patient is interviewed.

Functional Health Patterns. Key questions to ask a patient with a neurologic problem are presented in Table 54-5.

Health perception–health management pattern. The nurse should ask about the patient's health practices related to the nervous system, such as avoidance of substance abuse and smoking, maintenance of adequate nutrition, safe participation in physical and recreational activities, use of seat belts and helmets, and control of hypertension. The nurse should ask about previous hospitalizations for neurologic problems. A careful family history may determine whether the neurologic problem has a hereditary or congenital background.

If the patient has an existing neurologic problem, the nurse should ask about how it affects daily living and the ability to carry out self-care. After a careful review of information, the nurse should ask someone who knows the patient well whether any mental or physical changes have been noticed in the patient. The patient with a neurologic problem may not be aware of it or may be unable to provide enough specific data to aid in the diagnosis.[4]

Nutritional-metabolic pattern. Neurologic problems can result in problems of inadequate nutrition. Problems related to chewing, swallowing, facial nerve paralysis, and muscle coordination could make it difficult for the patient to ingest adequate nutrients. Also, certain vitamins such as thiamine (B_1), niacin, and pyridoxine (B_6) are essential for the maintenance and health of the CNS. Deficiencies in one or more of these vitamins could result in such nonspecific complaints as depression, apathy, neuritis, weakness, mental confusion, and irritability.

Elimination pattern. Bowel and bladder problems are often associated with neurologic problems, such as stroke, head injury, spinal cord injury, multiple sclerosis, and dementia. It is important to determine if the bowel or bladder problem was present before or after the neurologic event to plan appropriate interventions. Incontinence of urine and feces and urinary retention are the most common elimination problems associated with a neurologic problem. Careful documentation of the details of the problem, such as number of episodes, accompanying sensations or lack of sensations, and measures to control the problem, is important.

Activity-exercise pattern. Many neurologic disorders can cause problems in the patient's mobility, strength, and coordination. These problems can result in changes in the patient's usual activity and exercise patterns. Falls can also result from such problems. Many aspects of daily living such as getting out of a bed or chair, ambulating, preparing meals, and performing personal hygiene can be affected and should be assessed. The ability to perform fine motor tasks may be affected, which increases the possibility of personal injury.

Sleep-rest pattern. Sleep can be disrupted by many neurologically related factors. Discomfort from pain and inability to move and change to a position of comfort because of muscle weakness and paralysis could interfere with sound sleep. Hallucinations resulting from dementia or drugs can also interrupt sleep. The nurse should carefully document the sleep problem and the patient's methods of dealing with the problem.

Cognitive-perceptual pattern. Because the nervous system controls cognition and sensory integration, many neurologic disorders affect these functions. The nurse should assess memory, language, calculation ability, problem-solving ability, insight, and judgment. Often a structured mental status questionnaire is used to evaluate these functions and provide baseline data.

Information about sensory changes related to hearing, sight, and touch should be sought. In addition, the patient should be questioned about problems with vertigo and sensitivity to heat and cold.

Ability to both use and understand language is a cognitive function that the nurse should also assess. Appropriateness of responses is a useful indicator of cognitive and perceptual ability.

Pain is a common event associated with many health problems. It is often the reason a patient seeks health care. A careful assessment of the patient's pain should be carried out (see Chapter 9).

Neurologic problems and their treatment can be complex and confusing. The patient's understanding and ability to carry out necessary treatments should be determined. Cognitive changes

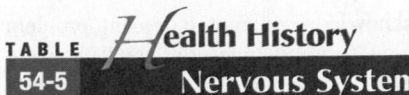

TABLE 54-5	Health History: Nervous System

Health Perception–Health Management Pattern
- What are your usual daily activities?
- Do you use any recreational drugs?*
- What safety practices do you perform in a car? On a motorcycle? On a bicycle?
- Do you have hypertension? If so, is it controlled?
- Have you ever been hospitalized for a neurologic problem?*
- How does it affect your daily living?

Nutritional-Metabolic Pattern
- Give a 24-hour dietary recall.
- Do you have any problems getting adequate nutrition because of chewing or swallowing difficulties, facial nerve paralysis, or poor muscle coordination?*
- Are you able to feed yourself?

Elimination Pattern
- Do you have incontinence of bowel or bladder? If yes, explain in detail the onset and pattern of the problem.
- What measures have you used to control the incontinence?
- Do you ever experience problems with hesitancy, urgency, retention?*
- Do you postpone defecation?*
- Does a neurologic problem make it difficult to reach a toilet when needed?
- Do you take any medication to manage neurologic problems? If so, what?

Activity-Exercise Pattern
- Describe any problems you experience with usual activities and exercise as a result of a neurologic problem.
- Do you have weakness or lack of coordination caused by a neurologic problem?*
- Does a neurologic problem keep you from performing your personal hygiene needs independently?*

Sleep-Rest Pattern
- Describe any problems you have with sleep.
- If you have trouble falling asleep, what do you do about it? (Ask specifically about use of sleep-inducing drugs.)

Cognitive-Perceptual Pattern
- Have you noticed any changes in your memory?*
- Do you experience vertigo, heat or cold sensitivity, numbness, or tingling?*
- Describe any pain you have experienced during the past 6 months.
- Do you have any difficulty with verbal or written communication?*

Self-Perception–Self-Concept Pattern
- What effect has your neurologic problem had on how you feel about yourself? Your abilities? Your body?
- Describe your general emotional pattern.

Role-Relationship Pattern
- Have you experienced changes in roles such as spouse, parent, or breadwinner because of neurologic disease?*
- How do you feel about these changes?

Sexuality-Reproductive Pattern
- Are you satisfied with sexual functioning? Describe any problems you experience related to your sexuality and sexual functioning.
- Are problems related to sexual functioning causing tension in an important relationship?*
- Do you feel the need for professional counseling related to your sexual functioning?*
- Do you use alternative methods of achieving sexual satisfaction?

Coping–Stress Tolerance Pattern
- Describe your usual coping pattern.
- Do you think your present coping pattern is adequate to meet the stressors of your neurologic problem?*
- Is your support system adequate to meet your needs? If not, what needs are unmet?

Value-Belief Pattern
- Describe any culturally specific beliefs and attitudes that may influence the treatment of this neurologic problem.

*If yes, describe.

---

associated with the problem can also interfere with understanding and compliance.[5]

Self-perception–self-concept pattern. Neurologic disease can drastically alter control over one's life and create dependency on others for daily needs. Also, the patient's physical appearance and emotional control can be affected. The nurse should ask about the patient's evaluation of self-worth, perception of abilities, body image, and general emotional pattern.

Role-relationship pattern. The patient should be asked if changes in roles, such as spouse, parent, or breadwinner, resulting from a neurologic problem have occurred. Physical impairments such as weakness and paralysis can alter or limit participation in usual roles and activities. Cognitive changes, however, can permanently change a person's ability to maintain previous roles. These changes can dramatically affect both the patient and significant others. Dependent relationships can develop.

Sexuality-reproductive pattern. The ability to participate in sexual activity should be assessed because many nervous system disorders can affect sexual response. Cerebral lesions may inhibit the desire phase or the reflex responses of the excitement phase. Brainstem and spinal cord lesions may partially or completely interrupt the connections between the brain and effector systems necessary for intercourse.

Neuropathies and spinal cord lesions that affect sensation, especially in the erotic zones, may decrease desire. Autonomic neuropathies and lesions of the sacral cord and cauda equina may prevent reflex activities of the sexual response. The nurse should determine if the patient and the spouse or significant other are satisfied with their sexual activity. The use or need for alternative methods of achieving sexual satisfaction should be explored. Despite neurologic-related changes in sexual functioning, many persons can achieve satisfying expression of intimacy and affection.

Coping–stress tolerance pattern. The physical sequelae of a neurologic problem can seriously strain a patient's coping patterns. Often the problem is chronic and may require that the patient learn new coping skills. The nurse should assess the patient's usual coping pattern to determine if coping skills are adequate to meet the stress of a problem.

When the problem is a decrease in cognitive functioning, both the patient and the caregiver can be seriously stressed. The nurse should assess for the potential for suicide, abuse, and burnout. The presence of an adequate support system in this type of situation should be assessed.

Value-belief pattern. Many neurologic problems have serious, long-term, life-changing effects. These effects can strain the patient's belief system and should be assessed. The nurse should also determine if any religious or cultural beliefs could interfere with the planned treatment regimen.

Objective Data

Physical Examination. The standard neurologic examination helps determine the presence, location, and nature of disease of the nervous system. The examination assesses six categories of functions: mental status, function of CNs, motor function, cerebellar function, sensory function, and reflex function. The choice of particular parts of the examination depends on the purpose for which it is done. If a comprehensive baseline assessment of neurologic functioning is desired, all components of the examination are done. However, if a specific problem is to be evaluated, only certain components may be assessed. For example, if a patient's primary complaint is lack of feeling in the feet, the examination may be focused only on movement and sensation of the lower limbs. Similarly, if a patient comes into the emergency department after a head injury and is unconscious, a limited examination is conducted because the patient is not able to respond to verbal instructions.[6]

A different approach to the neurologic examination has been proposed for nursing purposes.[7] The primary purposes of the nursing neurologic examination are to determine the effects of neurologic dysfunction on daily living in relation to the patient's and the family's ability to cope with the neurologic deficits. Although the method of gathering data may be the same, the interpretation of the data differs from the medical model. The standard medical model of the neurologic examination can also be used for nursing purposes. Health care providers share the responsibility for assessing life-threatening neurologic dysfunction.

Mental status. Assessment of mental status (cerebral functioning) gives an indication of how the patient is functioning as a whole and how the patient is adapting to the environment. It involves determination of complex and high-level cerebral functions that are governed by many areas of the cerebral cortex. Much of the area covered in this part of the examination is assessed during the history and therefore does not need to be evaluated further. For example, language and memory can be assessed when the patient is asked for details of the illness and significant past events. The patient's cultural and educational background should be taken into account when evaluating mental status.

The components of the mental status examination are as follows:

- *General appearance and behavior.* This component includes motor activity, body posture, dress and hygiene, facial expression, and speech.
- *State of consciousness.* The patient must be conscious before other functions can be determined. The nurse should note orientation to time, place, person, and situation, as well

as memory, general knowledge, insight, judgment, problem solving, and calculation. Common questions are "Who were the last three presidents?" "What does 'a stitch in time saves nine' mean?" "Subtract 7 from 100, and keep subtracting 7." The nurse should consider whether the patient's plans and goals match the physical and mental capabilities. Problems with memory may have implications for the ability to retain patient education.

- *Mood and affect.* The nurse should note agitation, anger, depression, or euphoria and the appropriateness of these states. Questions should be directed to bring out the feelings of the patient.
- *Thought content.* The nurse should note illusions, hallucinations, delusions, or paranoia.
- *Intellectual capacity.* The nurse should note retardation, dementia, and intelligence.

Cranial nerves. Testing of each CN is an essential component of the neurologic examination (see Table 54-2).

Olfactory nerve. After determining that both nostrils are patent, the olfactory nerve (CN I) is tested by asking the patient to close one nostril, close both eyes, and sniff from a bottle containing coffee, spice, soap, or some other readily recognized odor. The same is done for the other nostril. Generally, olfaction is not tested unless the patient has some disturbance with smell. Chronic rhinitis, sinusitis, and heavy smoking can often decrease the sense of smell. Disturbance in ability to smell may be associated with a tumor involving the olfactory bulb, or it may be the result of a basilar skull fracture that has damaged the olfactory fibers as they pass through the delicate cribriform plate of the skull.

Optic nerve. Visual fields and visual acuity are assessed to test the function of the optic nerve (CN II). Visual fields are assessed by confrontation. The examiner, positioned directly opposite the patient, asks the patient to close one eye, look directly at the bridge of the examiner's nose, and indicate when an object (finger, pencil tip, head of pin) presented from the periphery of each of the four visual field quadrants is seen (Fig. 54-16). The same test is repeated for the other eye. The examiner is used as a control because both examiner and patient are sharing the same visual field. It is important to remember that the nasal side of the visual field is narrower because of the nasal bridge. Visual field defects may arise from lesions of the optic nerve, optic chiasm, or tracts that extend through the temporal, parietal, or occipital lobes. Visual field changes resulting from brain lesions are usually either a *hemianopsia* (one half of the visual field is affected), a *quadrantanopsia* (one fourth of the visual field is affected), or monocular.

Visual acuity is tested by asking the patient to read a Snellen chart from 20 feet away. The number on the lowest line that the patient can read with 50% accuracy is recorded. The patient who wears glasses should wear them during testing, unless they are used only for reading. The eyes should be tested individually and together. If a Snellen chart is not available, the patient should be asked to read newsprint for a gross assessment of acuity. The distance from the patient to the newsprint required for accurate reading should be recorded. Acuity may not be testable by these means if the patient does not read English or is aphasic.

Funduscopy reveals the physical condition of the optic disc (head of the optic nerve), as well as the retina and blood vessels. This procedure is routinely performed when the optic nerve is tested. Optic nerve atrophy and papilledema can be detected by this method.

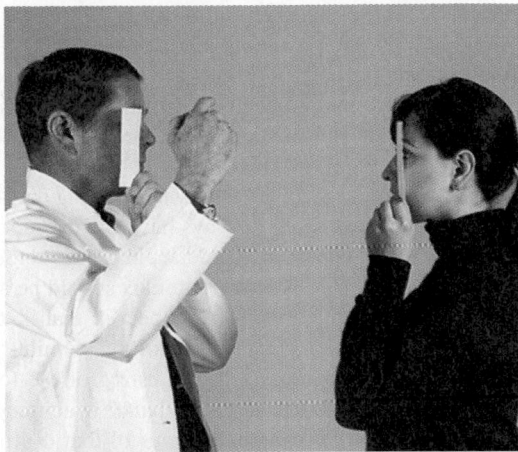

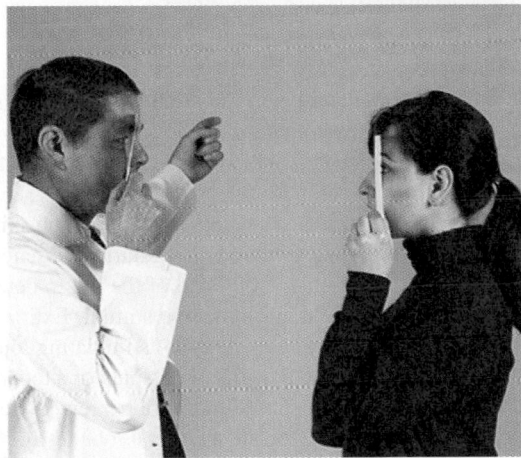

FIG. 54-16 Assessment of visual fields by gross confrontation.

Oculomotor, trochlear, and abducens nerves. Because the oculomotor (CN III), trochlear (CN IV), and abducens (CN VI) nerves all help move the eye, they are tested together. The patient is asked to follow the examiner's finger as it moves horizontally and vertically (making a cross) and diagonally (making an X). If there is weakness or paralysis of one of the eye muscles, the eyes do not move together, and the patient has a *disconjugate gaze.* The presence and direction of *nystagmus* (fine, rapid jerking movements of the eyes) are observed at this time, even though this condition most often indicates vestibulocerebellar problems.

Other functions of the oculomotor nerve are tested by checking for pupillary constriction and for *convergence* (eyes turning inward) and *accommodation* (pupils constricting with near vision). To test pupillary constriction, the examiner shines a light into the pupil of one eye and looks for ipsilateral constriction of the same pupil and contralateral (consensual) constriction of the opposite eye. The size and shape of the pupils are also noted. The optic nerve must be intact for this reflex to occur. Testing for pupillary constriction is an important component of the neurologic assessment of patients at risk for herniation syndrome (see Chapter 55). Because the oculomotor nerve exits at the top of the brainstem at the tentorial notch, it can be easily compressed by expanding mass lesions in the cerebral hemispheres. The result is a pupil that does not constrict to light; it may become dilated because the sympathetic input to the pupil acts unopposed. Convergence and accommodation are tested by having the patient focus

on the examiner's finger as it moves toward the patient's nose. Another function of the oculomotor nerve is to keep the eyelid open. Damage to the nerve can cause *ptosis* (drooping eyelid), pupillary abnormalities, and eye muscle weakness.

Trigeminal nerve. The sensory component of the trigeminal nerve (CN V) is tested by having the patient identify light touch (cotton) and pinprick in each of the three divisions (ophthalmic, maxillary, and mandibular) of the nerve on both sides of the face. The patient's eyes should be closed during this part of the examination. The motor component is tested by asking the patient to clench the teeth and palpating the masseter muscles just above the mandibular angle. The corneal reflex test evaluates CN V and CN VII simultaneously. It involves applying a cotton wisp strand to the cornea. The sensory component of this reflex (corneal sensation) is innervated by the ophthalmic division of CN V. The motor component (eye blink) is innervated by the facial nerve (CN VII). This reflex is not normally tested in patients who are awake and alert because other tests evaluate these two nerves. However, for patients with a decreased level of consciousness, the corneal reflex test provides an opportunity to evaluate the integrity of the brainstem at the level of the pons because the fibers of CN V and CN VII have connections in this area.

Facial nerve. The facial nerve (CN VII) innervates the muscles of facial expression. Its function is tested by asking the patient to raise the eyebrows, close the eyes tightly, purse the lips, draw back the corners of the mouth in an exaggerated smile, and frown. The examiner should note any asymmetry in the facial movements because they can indicate damage to the facial nerve. Although taste discrimination of salt and sugar in the anterior two thirds of the tongue is a function of this nerve, it is not routinely tested unless a peripheral nerve lesion is suspected.

Acoustic nerve. The cochlear portion of the acoustic (vestibulocochlear) nerve (CN VIII) is tested by having the patient close the eyes and indicate when a ticking watch or the rustling of the examiner's fingertips is heard as the stimulus is brought closer to the ear. Each ear is tested individually, and the distance from the patient's ear to the sound source when first heard is recorded. This test identifies only gross deficits in hearing. For more precise assessment of hearing, an audiometer is used (see Chapter 20). The vestibular portion of this nerve is not routinely tested unless the patient complains of dizziness, vertigo, or unsteadiness or has auditory dysfunction. If this is the case, caloric testing, which is beyond the scope of routine testing, may be done.

Glossopharyngeal and vagus nerves. The glossopharyngeal and vagus nerves are tested together because both innervate the pharynx. The glossopharyngeal nerve (CN IX) is primarily sensory. In the gag reflex (bilateral contraction of the palatal muscles initiated by stroking or touching either side of the posterior pharynx or soft palate with a tongue blade), the sensory component is mediated by CN IX and the major motor component by the vagus nerve (CN X). It is important to assess the gag reflex in patients who have a decreased level of consciousness, a brainstem lesion, or a disease involving the throat musculature. If the reflex is weak or absent, the patient is in danger of aspirating food or secretions. The strength and efficiency of swallowing are important to test in these patients for the same reason. Another test for the awake, cooperative patient is to have the patient phonate by saying "ah" and to note the bilateral symmetry of elevation of the soft palate. Any asymmetry can indicate weakness or paralysis. Swallowing is also assessed by lightly holding the examiner's hands on either side of the patient's throat and asking the patient to swallow. Any asymmetry is noted.

Spinal accessory nerve. The spinal accessory nerve (CN XI) is tested by asking the patient to shrug the shoulders against resistance and to turn the head to either side against resistance. There should be smooth contraction of the sternomastoid and trapezius muscles. Symmetry, atrophy, or fasciculation of the muscle should also be noted.

Hypoglossal nerve. The hypoglossal nerve (CN XII) is tested by asking the patient to protrude the tongue. It should protrude in the midline. The patient should also be able to push the tongue to either side against the resistance of a tongue blade. Again, any asymmetry, atrophy, or fasciculation should be noted.

Motor system. The motor system examination includes assessment of bulk, tone, and power of the major muscle groups of the body, as well as assessment of balance and coordination. The examiner tests strength by asking the patient to push and pull against the resistance of the examiner's arm as it opposes flexion and extension of the patient's muscle. The patient should be asked to offer resistance at the shoulder, elbow, wrist, hips, knees, and ankles. The patient's grip strength can also be tested. Mild weakness of the upper extremities may be tested by having the patient extend both arms forward at shoulder height with palms up while the eyes are closed. Mild weakness of the arm is demonstrated by downward drifting of the arm or pronation of the palm *(pronator drift)*. Any weakness or asymmetry of strength between the same muscle groups of the right and left side should be noted.[8]

Tone is tested by passively moving the limbs through their range of motion; there should be a slight resistance to these movements. Abnormal tone is described as *hypotonia* (flaccidity) or *hypertonia* (spasticity). Involuntary movements (e.g., tics, tremor, *myoclonus* [spasm of muscles], *athetosis* [slow, writhing, involuntary movements of extremities], *chorea* [involuntary, purposeless, rapid motions], *dystonia* [impairment of muscle tone]) should be noted.

Cerebellar function is tested by assessing balance and coordination. A good screening test for both balance and muscle strength is to observe the patient's stature (posture while standing) and gait. The examiner should note the pace and rhythm of the gait and observe the arm swing. (The arms should move symmetrically and in the opposite direction of the leg on the same side.) The patient's ability to ambulate is a key factor in determining the amount of nursing care that is needed and the risk of injury from falling. A patient with cerebellar disease may have an ataxic or staggering gait, in which the feet are placed wide apart and the steps are unsteady.

Coordination can be easily tested in several ways. The finger-to-nose test involves having the patient alternately touch the nose with the index finger, then touch the examiner's finger. The examiner repositions the finger while the patient is touching the nose so that the patient must adjust to a new distance each time the examiner's finger is touched. These movements should be performed smoothly and accurately. Other tests include asking the patient to pronate and supinate both hands rapidly and to do a shallow knee bend, first on one leg and then on the other. Dysarthria or slurred speech should be noted because it is a sign of incoordination of the speech muscles.

The heel-to-shin test involves having the patient place one heel on the opposite shin below the knee and moving the heel down the shin to the ankle. This is repeated for the other leg. These movements should flow smoothly without jerking or hesitation.

Sensory system. Several modalities are tested in the somatic sensory examination. Each modality is carried by a specific ascending pathway in the spinal cord before it reaches the sensory cortex.

There are some general guidelines for performing the sensory examination. The patient should always have the eyes closed to avoid visual clues. The examiner should avoid giving verbal cues such as, "Is this sharp?" The sensory stimulus should be applied in such a way that the patient does not expect it; that is, the examiner should avoid rhythmic application of the stimulus. In the routine neurologic examination, sensory testing of the four extremities is sufficient. However, if a disturbance in sensory function of the skin is identified, the boundaries of that dysfunction should be carefully delineated.

Light touch. Light touch is usually tested first. The examiner gently strokes a cotton wisp over each of the four extremities and asks the patient to indicate when the stimulus is felt by saying "touch." (The sensory examination of the trigeminal nerve may be delayed until this time because the same material for testing sensation is used.)

Pain and temperature. Pain is tested by touching the skin with the sharp end of a pin. This stimulus is irregularly alternated with a simple touch stimulus with the dull end of the pin to determine whether the patient can distinguish the two stimuli. Extinction or inhibition is assessed by simultaneously stimulating opposite sides of the body symmetrically with either a pain or a touch stimulus. Normally, the simultaneous stimuli are perceived (sensed); perception of only one may indicate a parietal lobe lesion.

The sensation of temperature is tested by applying tubes of warm and cold water to the skin and asking the patient to identify the stimuli with the eyes closed. If pain sensation is intact, assessment of temperature sensation may be omitted because both sensations are carried by the same ascending pathways.

Vibration sense. Vibration sense is assessed by applying a vibrating C128 tuning fork to the fingernails and the bony prominences of the hands, legs, and feet with the patient's eyes closed. The examiner asks the patient if the vibration or "buzz" is felt. The examiner then asks the patient to indicate when the vibration ceases. The examiner stops the vibration with the hand as desired.

Position sense. Position sense is assessed by placing the thumb and forefinger on either side of the patient's forefinger or great toe and gently moving the finger up or down. The patient is asked to indicate the direction in which the digit is moved.

Another test of position sense of the lower extremities is the Romberg test. The patient is asked to stand with the feet together and then close his or her eyes. If the patient is able to maintain balance with the eyes open but sways or falls with the eyes closed (i.e., a positive Romberg test), this may indicate disease in the posterior columns of the spinal cord. It is important that the nurse be aware of patient safety during this test.

Cortical sensory functions. Several tests evaluate cortical integration of sensory perceptions (which occurs in the parietal lobes). Two-point discrimination is assessed by placing the two points of a calibrated compass on the tips of the fingers and toes. The minimum recognizable separation is 4 to 5 mm in the fingertips and a greater degree of separation elsewhere. This test is important in diagnosing diseases of the sensory cortex and peripheral nervous system.

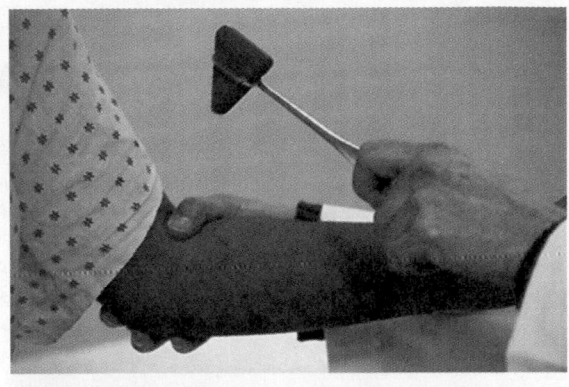

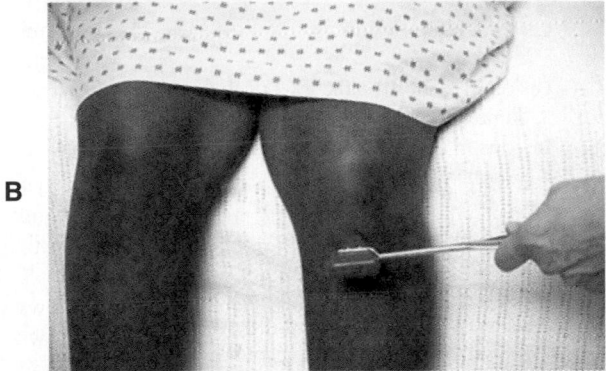

FIG. 54-17 The examiner strikes a swift blow over a stretched tendon to elicit a stretch reflex. **A,** Biceps reflex. **B,** Patellar reflex.

TABLE 54-6	Normal Physical Assessment of the Nervous System*

Mental Status
Alert and oriented, orderly thought processes, appropriate mood and affect

Cranial Nerves†
Smell intact to soap and coffee; visual fields full to confrontation; visual acuity 20/20 in both eyes; intact extraocular movements; no nystagmus; pupils equal, round, reactive to light and accommodation; intact facial sensation to touch and pinprick; facial movements full; intact gag and swallow reflexes; symmetric elevation of soft palate; full strength with head turning and shrugging of shoulders against resistance; midline protrusion of tongue

Motor System
Normal gait and station; normal tandem walk; negative Romberg test; normal and symmetric muscle bulk, tone, strength; smooth performance of finger-nose, heel-shin movements

Sensory System
Intact sensation to light touch, position sense, vibration, pinprick, heat and cold, two-point discrimination; intact stereognosis and graphesthesia

Reflexes‡
Biceps, triceps, brachioradialis, patellar, and Achilles tendon reflexes 2+ bilaterally; downgoing toes with plantar stimulation

*If some portion of the neurologic examination was not done, this should be indicated (e.g., "Smell not tested").
†May also be recorded as "CN I to XII intact."
‡May also be recorded as drawing of stick figure indicating reflex strength at appropriate sites.

Graphesthesia (ability to feel writing on skin) is tested by having the patient identify numbers traced on the palm of the hands. *Stereognosis* (ability to perceive the form and nature of objects) is tested by having the patient identify the size and shape of easily recognized objects (e.g., coins, keys, a safety pin) placed in the hands. Sensory extinction or inattention is evaluated by touching both sides of the body simultaneously. An abnormal response occurs when the patient perceives the stimulus only on one side. The other stimulus is "extinguished."

Reflexes. Tendons attached to skeletal muscles have receptors that are sensitive to stretch. A reflex contraction of the skeletal muscle occurs when the tendon is stretched. A simple muscle stretch reflex is initiated by briskly tapping the tendon of a stretched muscle, usually with a reflex hammer (Fig. 54-17). The response (muscle contraction of the corresponding muscle) is measured as follows: 0/5 absent, 1/5 weak response, 2/5 normal response, 3/5 exaggerated response, 4/5 hyperreflexia with clonus. *Clonus,* an abnormal response, is a continued rhythmic contraction of the muscle with continuous application of the stimulus.

In general, the biceps, triceps, brachioradialis, and patellar and Achilles tendon reflexes are tested. The examiner elicits the biceps reflex by placing the thumb over the biceps tendon in the antecubital space and striking the thumb with a hammer. The patient should have the arms partially flexed at the elbow with the palms up. The normal response is flexion of the arm at the elbow or contraction of the biceps muscle that can be felt by the examiner's thumb.

The triceps reflex is elicited by striking the triceps tendon above the elbow while the patient's arm is flexed. The normal response is extension of the arm or visible contraction of the triceps.

The brachioradialis reflex is elicited by striking the radius 3 to 5 cm above the wrist while the patient's arm is relaxed. The normal response is flexion and supination at the elbow or visible contraction of the brachioradialis muscle.

The patellar reflex is elicited by striking the patellar tendon just below the patella. The patient can be sitting or lying as long as the leg being tested hangs freely. The normal response is extension of the leg with contraction of the quadriceps.

The Achilles tendon reflex is elicited by striking the Achilles tendon while the patient's leg is flexed at the knee and the foot is dorsiflexed at the ankle. The normal response is plantar flexion at the ankle.

Table 54-6 is an example of a normal neurologic assessment. Common abnormal assessment findings of the neurologic system are presented in Table 54-7.

DIAGNOSTIC STUDIES OF THE NERVOUS SYSTEM

Diagnostic studies provide important information to the nurse in monitoring the patient's condition and planning appropriate interventions. These studies are considered to be objective data. Diagnostic studies used to assess the nervous system are presented in Table 54-8.

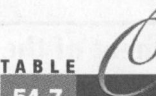

TABLE 54-7	Common Assessment Abnormalities	
Nervous System		

FINDING	DESCRIPTION	POSSIBLE ETIOLOGY AND SIGNIFICANCE
Altered consciousness	Inability to speak, obey commands, open eyes appropriately with verbal or painful stimulus	Intracranial lesions, metabolic disorder, psychiatric disorders
Anisocoria	Inequality of pupil size	Lesion, injury, or intracranial pressure in area of midbrain
Agnosia	Inability to determine meaning or significance of sensory stimulus	Cerebral cortex lesion
Apraxia	Inability to perform learned movements, defect in motor planning	Cerebral cortex lesion
Aphasia	Loss of language faculty (language comprehension, language expression, or both)	Cerebral cortex lesion
Analgesia	Loss of pain sensation	Lesion in spinothalamic tract or thalamus, lack of or damage to sensory nerve endings
Anesthesia	Absence of sensation	Lesions in spinal cord, thalamus, sensory cortex, or peripheral sensory nerve
Hyperesthesia	Increase in sensation	
Hypoesthesia	Decrease in sensation	
Anosognosia	Inability to recognize bodily defect or disease	Lesions in right parietal cortex, common in right-brain stroke
Astereognosis	Inability to recognize form of object by touch	Lesions in parietal cortex
Ataxia	Lack of coordination of movement	Lesions of sensory or motor pathways, cerebellum; antiseizure drugs, sedative, hypnotic drug toxicity (including alcohol)
Muscle atrophy (disuse or denervation atrophy)	Wasting away or diminution in size of muscle	Suprasegmental (upper motor neuron) lesions, segmental (lower motor neuron) lesions
Bladder dysfunction		
Atonic (autonomous)	Absence of muscle tone and contractility, enlargement of capacity, no sensation of discomfort, overflow with large residual, inability to voluntarily empty or empty by reflex	Early stage of spinal cord injury
Hypotonic	More ability than atonic bladder but less than normal	Interruption of afferent pathways from bladder
Hypertonic	Increase in muscle tone, diminished capacity, reflex emptying, dribbling, incontinence	Lesions in pyramidal tracts (efferent pathways)
Diplopia	Double vision	Lesions affecting nerves of extraocular muscles, cerebellar damage
Dysarthria	Lack of coordination in articulating speech	Lesions in cerebellum or pathway of cranial nerves (including brainstem); antiseizure drug, sedative, or hypnotic drug toxicity (including alcohol)
Dyskinesia	Impairment of power of voluntary movement, resulting in fragmentary or incomplete movements	Disorders of basal ganglia, idiosyncratic reaction to psychotropic drugs
Dysphagia	Difficulty in swallowing	Lesions involving motor pathways of CN IX, X (including lower brainstem)
Extensor plantar response (Babinski's sign)	Upgoing toes with plantar stimulation	Suprasegmental or upper motor neuron lesion
Homonymous hemianopsia	Loss of vision in one side of visual field	Injury or lesions in area of optic tract or its radiations to occipital cortex
Hemiplegia	Paralysis on one side	Stroke and other lesions involving motor cortex
Nystagmus	Jerking or bobbing of eyes as they track moving object	Lesions in cerebellum, brainstem, vestibular system; antiseizure, sedative, hypnotic toxicity (including alcohol)
Ophthalmoplegia	Paralysis of eye muscles	Lesions in brainstem or CN III, IV, VI
Opisthotonus	Extreme arching of back with retraction of head	Meningitis, tonic phase of grand mal seizure
Papilledema	"Choked disc," swelling of optic nerve head	Increase in intracranial pressure
Paraplegia	Paralysis of lower extremities	Spinal cord transection or mass lesion (thoracolumbar region)
Tetraplegia (quadriplegia)	Paralysis of all extremities	Spinal cord transection or mass lesion (cervical region) or brainstem

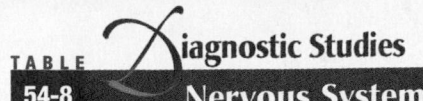
STUDY	DESCRIPTION AND PURPOSE	NURSING RESPONSIBILITY
Cerebrospinal Fluid Analysis		
▪ Lumbar puncture	CSF is aspirated by needle insertion in L3–4 or L4–5 interspace to assess many CNS diseases. (See Table 54-9.)	Assist patient to assume and maintain lateral recumbent position with knees flexed. Ensure maintenance of strict aseptic technique. Ensure labeling of CSF specimens in proper sequence. Keep patient flat for at least a few hours depending on physician preference. Encourage fluids. Monitor neurologic and VS. Administer analgesia as needed.
Radiologic		
▪ Skull and spine x-rays	Simple x-ray of skull and spinal column is done to detect fractures, bone erosion, calcifications, abnormal vascularity.	Explain that procedure is noninvasive. Explain positions to be assumed.
▪ Cerebral angiography	Serial x-ray visualization of intracranial and extracranial blood vessels is performed to detect vascular lesions and tumors of brain. Contrast medium is used.	Withhold preceding meal. Explain that patient will have hot flush of head and neck when contrast medium is injected. Administer premedication. Explain need to be absolutely still during procedure. Monitor neurologic and VS every 15–30 min first 2 hr, every hour next 6 hr, then every 2 hr for 24 hr. Maintain pressure dressing and ice to injection site. Maintain bed rest until patient is alert and VS are stable. Report any signs of change in neurologic status.
▪ Computed tomography (CT) scan	Computer-assisted x-ray of several levels or thin cross sections of body parts are done to detect problems such as hemorrhage, tumor, cyst, edema, infarction, brain atrophy, and other abnormalities.	Explain that procedure is noninvasive (if no contrast medium used). Observe for allergic reaction and note puncture site (if contrast medium used). Explain appearance of scanner. Instruct patient on need to remain absolutely still during procedure.
▪ Magnetic resonance imaging (MRI)	Imaging of brain, spinal cord, and spinal canal by means of magnetic energy. Used in detection of strokes, multiple sclerosis, tumors, trauma, herniation, and seizures. No invasive procedures are required. Gadolinium contrast media may be used to enhance visualization.	Screen patient for metal parts and pacemaker in body. Instruct patient on need to lie very still for up to 1 hr. Sedation may be necessary if patient is claustrophobic.
▪ Magnetic resonance angiography (MRA)	Uses differential signal characteristics of flowing blood to evaluate extracranial and intracranial blood vessels. Provides both anatomic and hemodynamic information. Can be used in conjunction with contrast media (contrast-enhanced MRA [cMRA]). Rapidly replacing cerebral angiography for use in diagnosing cerebrovascular diseases.	Similar to MRI (see above).
▪ Magnetic resonance spectroscopy (MRS)	Provides information about chemical composition of tissue. Used to study brain diseases, including brain tumors, Alzheimer's disease, strokes, acquired immunodeficiency syndrome, seizure disorders, and multiple sclerosis. Markers of neuronal integrity (e.g., N-acetyl aspartate) used to determine loss of neurons.	Similar to MRI (see above).
▪ Functional MRI (fMRI)	Use of MRI to detect changes in cerebral metabolism or blood flow, volume, or oxygenation response to specific tasks, consisting of periods of activity and periods of rest. Can functionally map brain.	Similar to MRI (see above).
▪ Myelography	X-ray of spinal cord and vertebral column after injection of contrast medium into subarachnoid space is used to detect spinal lesions (e.g., ruptured disk, tumor).	Administer preprocedure sedation as ordered. Instruct patient to empty bladder. Inform patient that test is performed with patient on tilting table that is moved during test. Encourage fluids. Monitor neurologic and VS.

CSF, Cerebrospinal fluid; *CNS*, central nervous system; *IV*, intravenous; *VS*, vital signs.

Continued

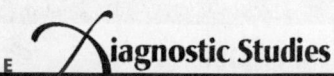

TABLE
54-8   Diagnostic Studies
Nervous System—cont'd

STUDY	DESCRIPTION AND PURPOSE	NURSING RESPONSIBILITY
Radiologic—cont'd		
▪ Positron emission tomography (PET)	Measures metabolic activity of brain regions to assess cell death or damage. Uses radioactive material that shows up as a bright spot on the image.	Explain procedure to patient. Explain that two IV lines will be inserted. Instruct patient not to take sedatives or tranquilizers. Empty bladder before procedure. May be asked to perform different activities during test.
▪ Single-photon emission computed tomography (SPECT)	A method of scanning similar to PET, but it uses more stable substances and different detectors. Radiolabeled compounds are injected and their photon emissions can be detected. Images made are accumulation of labeled compound. Used to visualize blood flow or oxygen or glucose metabolism in the brain. Useful in diagnosing strokes, brain tumors, and seizure disorders.	Similar to PET (see above)
Electrographic		
▪ Electroencephalography (EEG)	Electrical activity of brain is recorded by scalp electrodes to evaluate cerebral disease, CNS effects of systemic diseases, brain death.	Inform patient that procedure is painless and without danger of electric shock. Withhold stimulants. Inform that patient may be asked to perform various activities such as hyperventilation during test. Determine whether any medications (e.g., tranquilizers, antiseizure drugs) should be withheld. Resume medications after test. Assist patient to wash electrode paste out of hair.
▪ Magnetoencephalography (MEG)	Uses a sensitivity machine called a biomagnetometer, which detects very small magnetic fields generated by neural activity. It can accurately pinpoint the part of the brain involved in a stroke, seizure, or other disorder or injury. Measures extracranial magnetic fields, as well as scalp electric field (EEG).	MEG, a passive sensor, does not make physical contact with patient. Explain procedure to patient.
▪ Electromyography (EMG) and nerve conduction	Electrical activity associated with nerve and skeletal muscle is recorded by insertion of needle electrodes to detect muscle and peripheral nerve disease.	Inform patient of slight discomfort associated with insertion of needles.
▪ Evoked potentials	Electrical activity associated with nerve conduction along sensory pathways is recorded by electrodes placed on skin and scalp. Stimulus generates the impulse. Procedure is used to diagnose disease, locate nerve damage, and monitor function intraoperatively.	Explain procedure to patient.
Visual evoked potentials	Electrical activity in visual pathway is recorded with rapidly reversing checkerboard pattern on television screen. One eye is tested at a time.	Explain procedure to patient.
Brainstem auditory evoked potentials	Electrical activity in auditory pathway is recorded with earphones that produce clicking sounds. One ear is tested at a time.	Explain procedure to patient.
Somatosensory evoked potentials	Electrical activity in certain nerve pathways is recorded with mild electrical pulse (several per second).	Inform patient that stimulus may cause mild discomfort or muscle twitch.
Ultrasound		
▪ Carotid duplex studies	Sound waves determine blood flow velocity, which indicates presence of occlusive vascular disease.	Explain procedure to patient.
▪ Transcranial Doppler	Same technology as carotid duplex, but evaluates intracranial vessels.	Explain procedure to patient.

TABLE 54-9	Normal Cerebrospinal Fluid Values
PARAMETER	**NORMAL VALUE**
Specific gravity	1.007
pH	7.35
Appearance	Clear, colorless
RBCs	None
WBCs	0-8/μl (0-0.008/L)
Protein	
Lumbar	15-45 mg/dl (0.15-0.45 g/L)
Cisternal	15-25 mg/dl (0.15-0.25 g/L)
Ventricular	5-15 mg/dl (0.05-0.15 g/L)
Glucose	45-75 mg/dl (2.5-4.2 mmol/L)
Microorganisms	None
Opening pressure with lumbar puncture	60-150 mm H_2O

RBCs, Red blood cells; *WBCs*, white blood cells.

Cerebrospinal Fluid Analysis. CSF analysis provides information about a variety of CNS diseases. Normal CSF fluid is clear, colorless, and free of red blood cells and contains little protein. Normal CSF values are listed in Table 54-9.

Lumbar Puncture. Lumbar puncture is the most common method of obtaining CSF for analysis. It is contraindicated in the presence of increased intracranial pressure or infection at the site of puncture.

Nurses often assist in this procedure because it is usually performed in the patient's room. Before the procedure, the nurse should have the patient empty the bladder. The patient should lie in the lateral recumbent position, with the back as near as possible to the edge of the bed. The nurse should assist the patient to draw up the knees to the abdomen and flex the head to the chest. This helps separate the vertebrae so that the needle can be inserted more easily.

Using strict sterile technique, the physician inserts a long needle below the third lumbar vertebra. This may cause some local discomfort. There is no danger of injuring the spinal cord because the cord terminates between the first and second lumbar vertebrae. However, the patient may have some pain radiating down the leg or muscle twitching if the needle irritates the spinal root. The nurse can assure the patient that this is temporary and that the patient is not in danger of being paralyzed.

A manometer is attached to the needle, and CSF pressure is determined after the patient is asked to relax and extend the legs. If this is not done, the pressure appears abnormally high. CSF is withdrawn in a series of tubes and sent for analysis. Some examiners believe that the patient should be kept lying flat for at least a few hours after the procedure to avoid a spinal headache, which is presumably caused by loss of the cushioning effect of CSF as a result of leakage of CSF at the puncture site. The prone position may be effective in preventing CSF leakage. Others do not believe that the lying position is necessary because headache seems to develop in some patients despite precautions. Meningeal irritation (nuchal rigidity) or signs and symptoms of local trauma (e.g., hematoma, pain) may develop in some patients.

Radiologic Studies

Cerebral Angiography. Cerebral angiography is indicated when vascular lesions or tumors are suspected. A catheter is inserted into the femoral (sometimes brachial) artery. It is then passed up the artery to the aortic arch and into the base of a carotid or a vertebral artery for injection of radiopaque contrast medium. A series of x-rays is taken in a timed sequence so that pictures of the arteries, smaller vessels, and veins can be obtained (Fig. 54-18). This study can help to localize and determine the presence of abscesses, aneurysms, hematomas, arteriovenous malformations, arterial spasm, and certain tumors.

Because this is an invasive procedure, adverse reactions may occur. The patient may have an allergic (anaphylactic) reaction to the contrast medium. This reaction usually occurs immediately after injection of the contrast medium and may require emergency resuscitation measures in the procedure room. The most common precaution for nurses to take in caring for the patient after the return to the room is observation for bleeding at the catheter puncture site (usually the groin). A pressure dressing and ice are usually placed on the site to promote hemostasis and prevent swelling.

Computed Tomography. Computed tomography (CT) is a noninvasive procedure, although intravenous injection of contrast medium may be used to enhance visualization of the blood vessels and identify disruptions in the blood-brain barrier. CT scans can be done on an outpatient basis. A number of x-rays scanning different levels of the brain are compiled with computer assistance and presented in a series of black-and-white pictures. These pictures, which illustrate "slices" of the brain, can show hemorrhages, tumors, cysts, edema, infarction, brain atrophy, and hydrocephalus. CT scans do not illustrate structures in the posterior fossa and the base of the brain as clearly as does magnetic resonance imaging (MRI).

Magnetic Resonance Imaging. Rather than using x-rays, MRI involves two kinds of magnetism. The patient is placed within a giant magnetic field that aligns the protons of the hydrogen ions in the cells of the body (Fig. 54-19). Bursts of radiofrequency magnetism are introduced to flip the protons out of

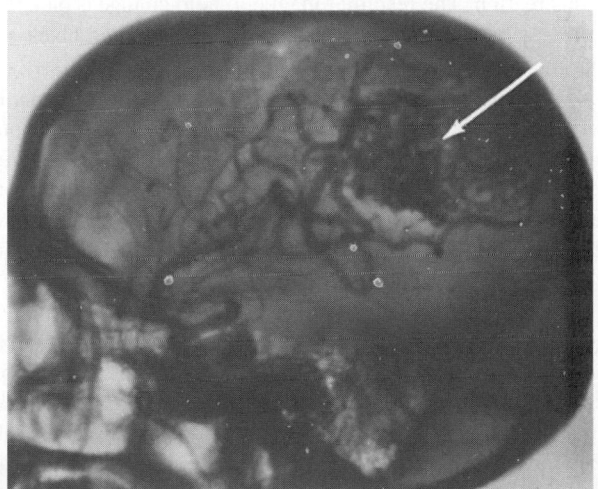

FIG. 54-18 Cerebral angiogram illustrating an arteriovenous malformation (*arrow*).

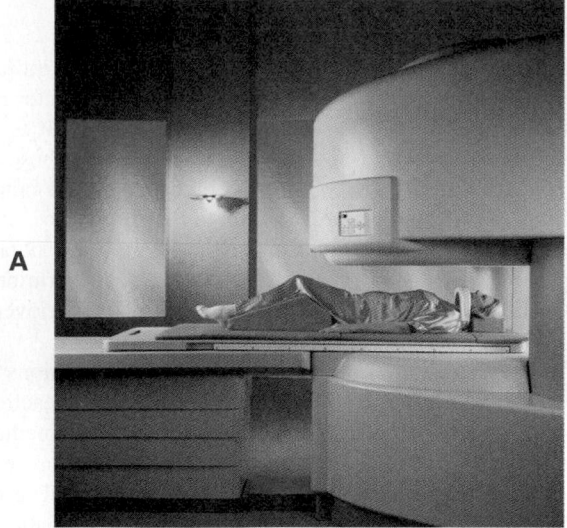

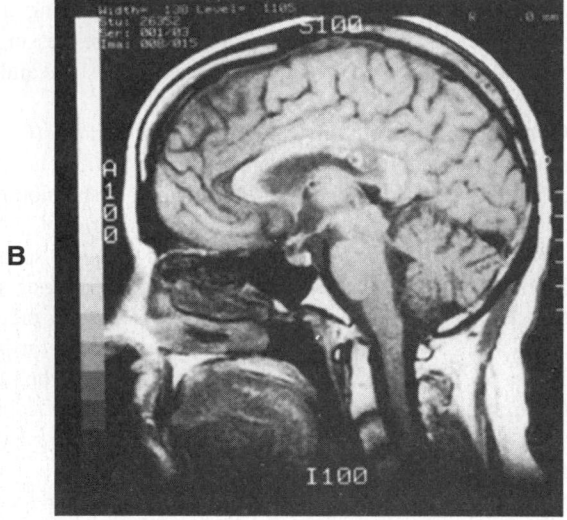

FIG. 54-19 A, Clinical setting for magnetic resonance imaging (MRI). B, Midline sagittal view of the brain using MRI.

alignment. When the radiofrequency magnetism is turned off, the protons realign. The resulting magnetic field change is picked up by the machine and processed by a computer. Vivid black-and-white pictures are then produced.

MRI is useful in evaluating brain and spinal cord edema, hemorrhage, infarction, blood vessels, tumors, herniation, and bone lesions. It is used in the detection of early strokes and multiple sclerosis. Intravenous injection of gadolinium can enhance the images obtained with MRI. Because MRI yields greater contrast in the images of soft tissue structures than does the CT scan, it is the diagnostic test of choice for many neurologic diseases.

Positron Emission Tomography. *Positron emission tomography* (PET) is used to determine regional metabolism in the brain. PET provides a noninvasive means of determining biochemical processes that occur in the brain. There is increasing clinical use of PET scanning to monitor patients with stroke, Alzheimer's disease, seizure disorders, epilepsy, tumors, and Parkinson's disease.

Myelography. *Myelography* is used to visualize the spinal column and the subarachnoid space when a spinal lesion is sus-

pected. The most common lesion for which this test is used is a herniated or protruding intervertebral disk. Other lesions include spinal tumors, adhesions, syringomyelia, bony deformations, and arteriovenous malformations. The test involves x-rays of the spinal column after injection of the contrast medium into the subarachnoid space via a catheter. Water-soluble iodine contrast materials such as iopamidol (Isovue) are used most often because they are absorbed into the bloodstream and excreted by the kidneys.

Preparation for this procedure is the same as for lumbar puncture. Before the contrast material is injected, patients must be asked whether they have any allergies, specifically whether they have had any anaphylactic or hypotensive episodes from other contrast media. After myelography the patient should lie flat for a few hours.

Headache is the most common complaint after myelography. It may be accompanied by nausea and occasionally by vomiting. The nurse should observe the patient for any changes in neurologic status and provide a quiet, comfortable environment after the procedure.

Electrographic Studies

Electroencephalography. The technique of *electroencephalography (EEG)* involves the recording of the electrical activity of the surface cortical neurons of the brain by 8 to 16 electrodes placed on specific areas of the scalp. This test is done to evaluate not only cerebral disease but also the CNS effects of many metabolic and systemic diseases and to determine brain death. Among the cerebral diseases assessed by EEG are epilepsy, mass lesions (e.g., tumor, abscess, hematoma), cerebrovascular lesions, and brain injury (Fig. 54-20). The procedure is noninvasive. Patients sometimes have the misconception that the recording electrodes will give them an electric shock. They should be assured that this is not true and that the procedure is similar to electrocardiography.

Electromyography and Nerve Conduction Studies. *Electromyography (EMG)* is the recording of electrical activity associated with innervation of skeletal muscle. The recording is displayed on a computer screen and may be played on a loudspeaker for simultaneous analysis. Needle electrodes are inserted into the muscle to record specific motor units because recording from the skin is not sufficient. Normal muscle at rest shows no electrical activity. Typical electrical activity occurs when the muscle contracts. This activity may be altered in diseases of muscle itself (e.g., myopathic conditions) or in disorders of muscle innervation (e.g., segmental or LMN lesions, peripheral neuropathic conditions). Fibrillations are spontaneous, independent contractions of individual muscle fibers that can be detected only by EMG. They appear on EMG 1 to 3 weeks after a muscle has lost its nerve supply.

Nerve conduction studies involve application of a brief electrical stimulus to a distal portion of a sensory or mixed nerve and recording the resulting wave of depolarization at some point proximal to the stimulation. For example, a stimulus can be applied to the forefinger and a recording electrode placed over the median nerve at the wrist. The time between the onset of the stimulus and the initial wave of depolarization at the recording electrode is measured. This is termed *nerve conduction velocity.* Damaged nerves have slower conduction velocities.

Evoked Potentials. *Evoked potentials* are recordings of electrical activity associated with nerve conduction along sen-

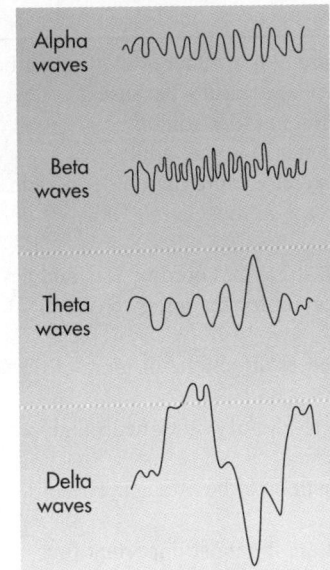
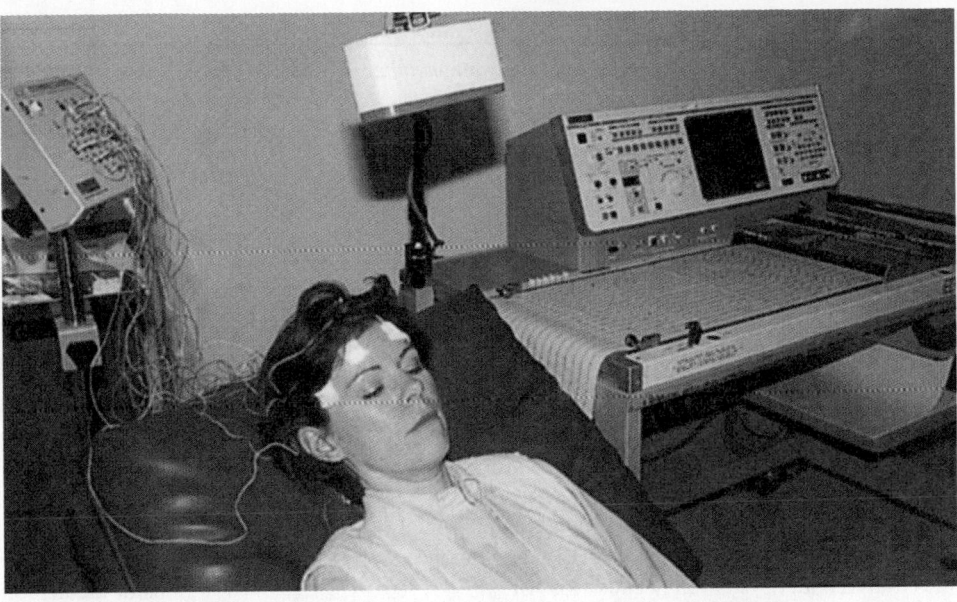

FIG. 54-20 Electroencephalogram (EEG). **A**, Examples of alpha, beta, theta, and delta waves seen on an EEG. **B**, Photograph showing a person undergoing an EEG test. Notice the scalp electrodes that detect voltage fluctuations within the cranium.

sory pathways. The activity is generated by a specific sensory stimulus related to the type of study (e.g., checkerboard patterns for visual evoked potentials, clicking sounds for auditory evoked potentials, mild electrical pulses for somatosensory evoked potentials). Electrodes placed on specific areas of the skin and scalp record the electrical activity, which is stored and averaged by a computerized instrument. A wave pattern appears on a screen and is printed on paper. Peaks in the wave pattern correspond to conduction of the stimulus through certain points along the sensory pathway (e.g., peripheral nerve, brainstem, cortical areas). Increases in the normal time from stimulus onset to a given peak (latency) indicate slowed nerve conduction or nerve damage. This technique is useful in diagnosing abnormalities of the visual or auditory systems because it reveals whether a sensory impulse is reaching the appropriate part of the brain. Indications for these tests include evaluation of the optic nerve in conditions such as multiple sclerosis (optic neuritis) and the vestibulocochlear nerve in acoustic neuroma.

Combined Doppler and Ultrasound (Duplex) Studies

Carotid Duplex. A duplex study uses combined ultrasound and pulsed Doppler technology. A technician places a probe on the skin over the carotid artery and slowly moves the probe along the course of the common carotid to the bifurcation of the external and internal carotid arteries. The ultrasound signal emitted from the probe reflects off the moving blood cells within the vessel. The frequency of the reflected signal corresponds to the blood velocity. This response is amplified and is registered on a graphic record and also as sound. The graphic record registers blood velocity. Increased blood flow velocity can indicate stenosis of a vessel. Duplex scanning is a noninvasive study that evaluates the degree of stenosis of the carotid and vertebral arteries.

Transcranial Doppler Sonography. Transcranial Doppler (TCD) sonography uses the same technology as duplex studies, except that it records blood flow velocities of the intracranial blood vessels. The probe is placed on the skin at various "windows" in the skull (areas in the skull that have only a thin bony covering) to register velocities of the middle cerebral artery, anterior cerebral artery, posterior cerebral artery, terminal carotid artery, and occasionally the anterior and posterior communicating arteries. The temporal, orbital, and suboccipital sites are used. The ultrasound signal received is recorded graphically as a waveform. Peak blood flow velocities and systolic-diastolic ratios can be calculated from this information. TCD sonography is a noninvasive technique that is useful in assessing vasospasm associated with subarachnoid hemorrhage, altered intracranial blood flow dynamics associated with occlusive vascular disease, presence of emboli, and cerebral autoregulation.

REVIEW QUESTIONS

The number of the question corresponds to the same-numbered objective at the beginning of the chapter.

1. In a patient with a disease that affects the myelin sheath of nerves, such as multiple sclerosis, the glial cells that are affected are the
   a. microglia.
   b. astrocytes.
   c. oligodendrocytes.
   d. ependymal cells.

2. A state of hypoxia alters the repeated action potentials necessary for transmission of nerve impulses because energy is required for
   a. repolarization of the cell membrane.
   b. creation of cell membrane permeability.
   c. movement of sodium into the nerve cell.
   d. maintenance of the resting membrane potential.

3. Drugs or diseases that impair the function of the extrapyramidal system may cause loss of
   a. sensations of pain and temperature.
   b. regulation of the autonomic nervous system.
   c. integration of somatic and special sensory inputs.
   d. automatic movements associated with skeletal muscle activity.

4. An obstruction of the anterior cerebral arteries will affect functions of
   a. visual imaging.
   b. balance and coordination.
   c. judgment, insight, and reasoning.
   d. visual and auditory integration for language comprehension.

5. Paralysis of lateral gaze indicates a lesion of cranial nerve
   a. II.
   b. III.
   c. IV.
   d. VI.

6. A result of stimulation of the parasympathetic nervous system is
   a. dilation of skin blood vessels.
   b. increased secretion of insulin.
   c. increased blood glucose levels.
   d. relaxation of the urinary sphincters.

7. Assessment of muscle strength of older adults cannot be compared with that of younger adults because
   a. stroke is more common in older adults.
   b. nutritional status is better in young adults.
   c. most young people exercise more than older people.
   d. aging leads to a decrease in muscle bulk and strength.

8. Data regarding mobility, strength, coordination, and activity tolerance are important for the nurse to obtain because
   a. many neurologic diseases affect one or more of these areas.
   b. patients are less able to identify other neurologic impairments.
   c. these are the first functions to be affected by neurologic disease.
   d. aspects of movement are the most important functions of the nervous system.

9. During neurologic testing the patient is able to perceive pain elicited by pinprick. Based on this finding, the nurse may omit testing for
   a. position sense.
   b. patellar reflexes.
   c. temperature perception.
   d. heel-to-shin movements.

10. A patient's eyes jerk as they follow the nurse's moving finger. The nurse records this finding as
   a. nystagmus.
   b. normal tracking.
   c. ophthalmoplegia.
   d. ophthalmic dyskinesia.

11. Nursing responsibilities for lumbar puncture include
   a. ensuring the patient has a full bladder.
   b. placing the patient in the lateral recumbent position.
   c. straightening the patient's legs just before the puncture.
   d. having the patient cough when the needle has been inserted.

REFERENCES

1. Kempermann G, Gage FH: Neurogenesis in the adult hippocampus, *Novartis Found Symp* 231:231, 2000.
2. Kandel ER, Schwartz JH, Jessell TM, editors: *Principles of neural science*, New York, 2000, McGraw-Hill.
3. Odenheimer GL: Geriatric neurology, *Neurol Clin* 16:561, 1998.
4. Motyka KM, Yanuck SF: Expanding the neurological examination using functional neurologic assessment: part 1: methodological considerations, *International Journal of Applied Kinesiology & Kinesiologic Medicine* 7:28, 2000.
5. Lower J: Facing neuro assessment fearlessly, *Nursing* 32:58, 2002.
6. Beckerman B: Nervous energy: conducting a neurologic assessment in the field, *Emerg Med Serv* 29:45, 2000.
7. Mitchell PH et al: *Neurologic assessment for nursing practice,* Reston, Va, 1984, Reston.
8. Baker RA, Andrew MJ, Knight JL: Evaluation of neurologic assessment and outcomes in cardiac surgical patients, *Semin Thorac Cardiovasc Surg* 13:149, 2001.

RESOURCES

Resources for this chapter are listed after Chapter 55 on page 1524, Chapter 56 on page 1548, Chapter 57 on pages 1579 and 1580, Chapter 58 on page 1600, and Chapter 59 on page 1634.

CHAPTER 55

NURSING MANAGEMENT
Acute Intracranial Problems

Mary Kerr
Elizabeth A. Crago

LEARNING OBJECTIVES

1. Identify the physiologic mechanisms that maintain normal intracranial pressure.
2. Identify the common etiologies, clinical manifestations, and collaborative care of the patient with increased intracranial pressure.
3. Describe the collaborative and nursing management of the patient with increased intracranial pressure.
4. Differentiate types of head injury by mechanism of injury and clinical manifestations.
5. Describe the collaborative care and nursing management of the patient with a head injury.
6. Compare the types, clinical manifestations, and collaborative care of brain tumors.
7. Discuss the nursing management of the patient with a brain tumor.
8. Describe the nursing management of the patient undergoing cranial surgery.
9. Compare the primary causes, collaborative care, and nursing management of meningitis, encephalitis, and brain abscess.

KEY TERMS

brain abscess, p. 1522	Glasgow Coma Scale, p. 1500
cerebral edema, p. 1493	head injury, p. 1505
coma, p. 1494	intracerebral hematoma, p. 1508
concussion, p. 1507	intracranial pressure, p. 1491
contusion, p. 1507	meningitis, p. 1518
diffuse axonal injury, p. 1507	nuchal rigidity, p. 1518
encephalitis, p. 1521	subdural hematoma, p. 1507
epidural hematoma, p. 1507	unconsciousness, p. 1495

Acute intracranial problems include diseases and disorders that can increase intracranial pressure (ICP). This chapter discusses the mechanisms that maintain normal ICP, increased ICP, head injury, brain tumors, and cerebral inflammatory disorders.

INTRACRANIAL PRESSURE

Understanding the mechanisms associated with ICP is important in caring for patients with many different neurologic problems. The skull is like a closed box with three essential volume components: brain tissue, blood, and cerebrospinal fluid (CSF) (Fig. 55-1). The total volume in the skull is 1900 ml. The intracellular and extracellular fluids of brain tissue make up approximately 78% of this volume. Blood in the arterial, venous, and capillary network makes up 12% of the volume, and the remaining 10% is the volume of the CSF. Under normal conditions, in which intracranial volume remains relatively constant, the balance among these components maintains the ICP. Factors that influence ICP under normal circumstances are changes in (1) arterial pressure, (2) venous pressure, (3) intraabdominal and intrathoracic pressure, (4) posture, (5) temperature, and (6) blood gases, particularly CO_2 levels. The degree to which these factors increase

Reviewed by Sherry Garrett Hendrickson RN, PhD, CNS, Assistant Professor of Clinical Nursing, University of Texas at Austin School of Nursing, Austin, Tex.

or decrease the ICP depends on the ability of the brain to accommodate to the changes.

Regulation and Maintenance of Intracranial Pressure

Normal Intracranial Pressure. Intracranial pressure (ICP) is the hydrostatic force measured in the brain CSF compartment. Normal ICP is the pressure exerted by the total volume from the three components within the skull: brain tissue, blood, and CSF. The modified Monro-Kellie doctrine describes the relatively constant volume of these three components within the rigid skull structure. If the volume in any one of the three components increases within the cranial vault and the volume from another component is displaced, the total intracranial volume will not change.[1] This hypothesis is not applicable in situations in which the skull is not rigid (e.g., in neonates, in adults with unfused skull fractures).

Normal Compensatory Adaptations. In applying the modified Monro-Kellie doctrine, the body can adapt to changes

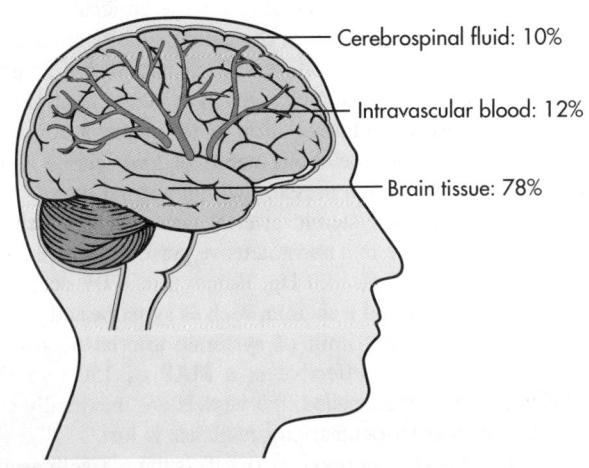

Cerebrospinal fluid: 10%

Intravascular blood: 12%

Brain tissue: 78%

FIG. 55-1 Components of the brain.

in the volume of components of the skull to maintain a normal ICP. Initial compensatory mechanisms include changes in the CSF volume by altering CSF absorption or production and displacement of CSF into the spinal subarachnoid space. Alterations in intracranial blood volume occur through the collapse of cerebral veins and dural sinuses, regional cerebral vasoconstriction or dilation, and changes in venous outflow. Tissue brain volume compensates through dispensability of the dura or compression of brain tissue. Initially, an increase in volume produces no increase in ICP as a result of these compensatory mechanisms. However, these compensatory adaptations to changes in volume are limited; as the volume increase continues, the ICP rises and decompensation occurs, resulting in compression and ischemia.[1]

Measuring ICP. ICP can be measured in the ventricles, subarachnoid space, subdural space, epidural space, or brain parenchymal tissue using a water manometer or a pressure transducer. Normal intracranial ICP ranges from 0 to 15 mm Hg with the use of the pressure transducer. A sustained pressure above the upper limit is considered abnormal. ICP may become elevated because of head trauma, stroke, subarachnoid hemorrhage, brain tumor, inflammation, hydrocephalus, or brain tissue damage from other causes. Any patient who becomes acutely unconscious, regardless of the cause, is managed as if there were actual or potential elevations in the ICP. Patients with or at risk for elevated ICP usually receive invasive ICP monitoring in an intensive care unit (ICU), except those with irreversible problems or advanced neurologic disease. Goals for nursing management of an elevated ICP include preservation of cerebral perfusion, early identification of neurologic changes, and prevention of complications.

Cerebral Blood Flow

Cerebral blood flow (CBF) is the amount of blood in milliliters passing through 100 g of brain tissue in 1 minute. The global CBF is approximately 50 ml per minute per 100 g of brain tissue. There is a difference in flow between the white and gray matter of the brain. The white matter has a slower blood flow, approximately 25 ml per minute per 100 g, and the gray matter has a faster blood flow, approximately 75 ml per minute per 100 g.[2] The maintenance of blood flow to the brain is critical because the brain requires a constant supply of oxygen and glucose. The brain uses 20% of the body's oxygen and 25% of its glucose.

Autoregulation of Cerebral Blood Flow. The brain has the ability to regulate its own blood flow in response to its metabolic needs in spite of wide fluctuations in systemic arterial pressure. *Autoregulation* is defined as the automatic alteration in the diameter of the cerebral blood vessels to maintain a constant blood flow to the brain during changes in systemic arterial pressure.[3] The purpose of autoregulation is to ensure a consistent CBF to provide for the metabolic needs of brain tissue and to maintain cerebral perfusion pressure within normal limits.

The lower limit of systemic arterial pressure at which autoregulation is effective in a normotensive person is a mean arterial pressure (MAP) of 50 mm Hg. Below this, CBF decreases, and symptoms of cerebral ischemia, such as syncope and blurred vision, occur. The upper limit of systemic arterial pressure at which autoregulation is effective is a MAP of 150 mm Hg.[2] When this pressure is exceeded, the vessels are maximally constricted, and further vasoconstrictor response is lost.

The *cerebral perfusion pressure* (CPP) is the pressure needed to ensure blood flow to the brain. CPP is equal to the MAP mi-

TABLE 55-1	**Calculation of Cerebral Perfusion Pressure**

$$CPP = MAP - ICP$$

$$MAP = DBP + \tfrac{1}{3}(SBP - DBP) \text{ or } \frac{SBP + 2(DBP)}{3}$$

Example: Systemic blood pressure = 122/84
  MAP = 97
  ICP = 12 mm Hg
  CPP = 85 mm Hg

CPP, Cerebral perfusion pressure; *DBP,* diastolic blood pressure; *ICP,* intracranial pressure; *MAP,* mean arterial pressure; *SBP,* systolic blood pressure.

nus the ICP (CPP = MAP − ICP) (see example in Table 55-1). This formula is clinically useful, although it does not consider the effect of systemic vascular resistance. Cerebral vascular resistance, generated by the arterioles within the cranium, links CPP and blood flow as follows:

$$CPP = Flow \times Resistance$$

Noninvasive techniques used in intensive care to monitor changes in cerebrovascular resistance include transcranial Doppler.

As the CPP decreases, autoregulation fails and CBF decreases. Normal CPP is 70 to 100 mm Hg. At least 50 to 60 mm Hg is necessary for adequate cerebral perfusion. CPP less than 50 mm Hg is associated with ischemia and neuronal death. A CPP below 30 mm Hg results in cellular ischemia and is incompatible with life. Under normal circumstances, autoregulation maintains an adequate CBF and perfusion pressure primarily by cerebral vasoreactivity and metabolic adjustments that impact ICP. It is of paramount importance to maintain MAP when ICP is elevated. It should be remembered that CPP does not reflect perfusion pressure in all parts of the brain. There may be local areas of swelling and compression limiting regional perfusion pressure. Thus a higher CPP may be needed for these patients to prevent localized tissue damage.

Pressure Changes. The relationship of pressure to volume is depicted in the pressure-volume curve. The curve is affected by the brain's elastance and compliance. *Elastance* is the brain's ability to accommodate changes in volume. It represents the stiffness of the brain. With high elastance, large increases in pressure occur with small increases in volume.

$$Elastance = Pressure/Volume$$

Compliance is the inverse of elastance and is the expandability of the brain. It is represented as the volume increase for each unit increase in pressure. Low compliance is the same as high elastance. With low compliance, high changes in pressure result from small changes in volume.

$$Compliance = Volume/Pressure$$

The concept of the pressure-volume curve can be used to represent the stages of increased ICP (intracranial hypertension) (Fig. 55-2). At stage 1 on the curve, there is high compliance and low elastance. The brain is in total compensation, with accommodation and autoregulation intact. An increase in volume (in any of the three volume components) does not increase the ICP. At stage 2, the compliance is lower and elastance is increasing. An increase in volume places the patient at risk of increased ICP.

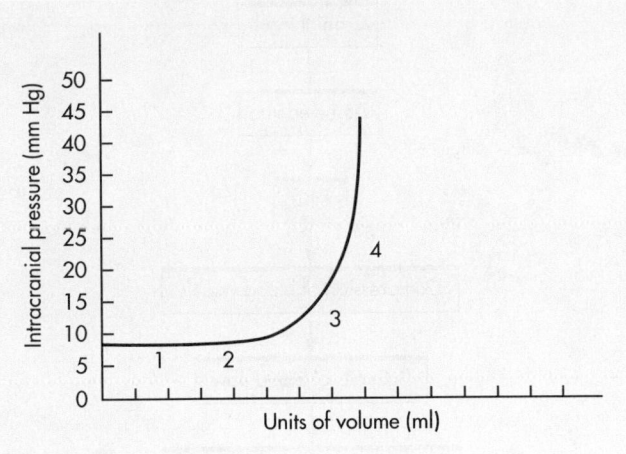

FIG. 55-2 Intracranial volume-pressure curve. (See text for descriptions of *1, 2, 3,* and *4.*)

At stage 3, there is high elastance and low compliance. Any small addition of volume causes a great increase in pressure. Compensatory mechanisms fail, there is a loss of autoregulation, and the patient may exhibit symptoms indicating increased ICP, such as changes in mentation or level of consciousness, headache, or pupillary responsiveness.

With a loss of autoregulation and a rise in systolic blood pressure as a result of the Cushing response, decompensation occurs. The Cushing triad includes systolic hypertension with an increased pulse pressure, bradycardia, and irregular respiratory rate.

As the patient enters stage 4, the ICP rises to terminal levels with little increase in volume. Herniation occurs as the brain tissue shifts from the compartment of greater pressure to a compartment of lesser pressure.

Factors Affecting Cerebral Blood Flow. Carbon dioxide, oxygen, and hydrogen ion concentration affect cerebral vessel tone. The partial pressure of arterial carbon dioxide ($PaCO_2$) is a potent vasoactive agent. An increase in $PaCO_2$ relaxes smooth muscle, dilates cerebral vessels, decreases cerebrovascular resistance, and increases CBF. Alternately, a decrease in $PaCO_2$ reverses this process and decreases CBF. Cerebral oxygen tension below 50 mm Hg results in cerebral vascular dilation. This dilation decreases cerebral vascular resistance, increases CBF, and raises oxygen tension. However, if oxygen tension is not raised, anaerobic metabolism begins, resulting in an accumulation of lactic acid. As lactic acid increases and hydrogen ions accumulate, the environment becomes more acidic. Within this acidic environment, further vasodilation occurs in a continued attempt to increase blood flow. The combination of a severely low arterial oxygen pressure ($PaCO_2$) and an elevated hydrogen ion concentration (acidosis), which are both potent cerebral vasodilators, may produce a state wherein autoregulation is lost and compensatory mechanisms fail to meet tissue metabolic demands.[1]

CBF can be globally affected by cardiac or respiratory arrest, systemic hemorrhage, and other pathophysiologic states (e.g., diabetic coma, encephalopathies, infections, toxicities). Regional CBF can also be affected by trauma, tumors, cerebral hemorrhage, or stroke. When regional or global autoregulation is lost, CBF is no longer maintained at a constant level but is directly in-

fluenced by changes in systemic blood pressure, hypoxia, or catecholamines.

INCREASED INTRACRANIAL PRESSURE

Increased ICP is a life-threatening situation that results from an increase in any or all of the three components (brain tissue, blood, CSF) of the skull. Cerebral edema is an important factor contributing to increased ICP.

Cerebral Edema

As shown in Table 55-2 there are a variety of causes of **cerebral edema** (increased accumulation of fluid in the extravascular spaces of brain tissue). Regardless of the cause, cerebral edema results in an increase in tissue volume that carries the potential for increased ICP. The extent and severity of the original insult are factors that determine the degree of cerebral edema.

Three types of cerebral edema have been distinguished: vasogenic, cytotoxic, and interstitial edema.[3] More than one type may result from a single insult in the same patient.

Vasogenic Cerebral Edema. *Vasogenic cerebral edema,* the most common type of edema, occurs mainly in the white matter and is attributed to changes in the endothelial lining of cerebral capillaries. These changes allow leakage of macromolecules from the capillaries into the surrounding extracellular space, resulting in an osmotic gradient that favors the flow of water from the intravascular to the extravascular space. A variety of insults, such as brain tumors, abscesses, and ingested toxins, may cause an increase in the permeability of the blood-brain barrier and produce an increase in the extracellular fluid volume. The speed and extent of the spread of the edema fluid are influenced by the systemic blood pressure, the site of the brain injury, and the extent of the blood-brain barrier defect. This edema may produce a con-

TABLE 55-2	Causes of Cerebral Edema

Mass Lesions
Brain abscess
Brain tumor (primary or metastatic)
Hematoma (intracerebral, subdural, epidural)
Hemorrhage (intracerebral, cerebellar, brainstem)

Head Injuries
Contusion
Hemorrhage
Posttraumatic brain swelling

Brain Surgery

Cerebral Infections
Meningitis
Encephalitis

Vascular Insult
Anoxic and ischemic episodes
Cerebral infarction (thrombotic or embolic)
Venous sinus thrombosis

Toxic or Metabolic Encephalopathic Conditions
Lead or arsenic intoxication
Hepatic encephalopathy
Uremia

tinuum of symptoms ranging from focal neurologic deficits to disturbances in consciousness, including **coma** (profound state of unconsciousness).

Cytotoxic Cerebral Edema. *Cytotoxic cerebral edema* results from local disruption of the functional or morphologic integrity of cell membranes and occurs most often in the gray matter. Cytotoxic cerebral edema develops from destructive lesions or trauma to brain tissue resulting in cerebral hypoxia or anoxia, sodium depletion, and syndrome of inappropriate antidiuretic hormone (SIADH). Cerebral edema results as fluid and protein shift from the extracellular space directly into the cells, with subsequent swelling and loss of cellular function.

Interstitial Cerebral Edema. *Interstitial cerebral edema* is the result of periventricular diffusion of ventricular CSF in a patient with uncontrolled hydrocephalus. It can also be caused by enlargement of the extracellular space as a result of systemic water excess (hyponatremia). Fluid moves into the cells to equilibrate with the hypoosmotic interstitial fluid. Regardless of the cause of cerebral edema, manifestations of increased ICP result, unless compensation is adequate.

Mechanisms of Increased Intracranial Pressure

Elevated ICP (above the threshold of 20 mm Hg) is clinically significant because it diminishes CPP, increases risks of brain ischemia and infarction, and is associated with a poor prognosis.[4] Increased ICP can be caused by several clinical problems, including a mass lesion (e.g., hematoma, contusion, abscess, tumor), cerebral edema (associated with brain tumors, hydrocephalus, head injury, or brain inflammation), or metabolic insult. These cerebral insults may result in hypercapnia, cerebral acidosis, impaired autoregulation, and systemic hypertension, which promote the formation and spread of cerebral edema. This edema distorts brain tissue, further increasing the ICP, which leads to even more tissue hypoxia and acidosis. Fig. 55-3 illustrates the progression of increased ICP.

Crucial to preservation of tissue is maintenance of CBF. Elevations in pressure that are more evenly distributed throughout the brain or slow increases in ICP (e.g., an enlarging brain lesion) preserve blood flow better than a rapid increase, as in primary brain injury. Sustained increases in ICP result in brainstem compression and herniation of the brain from one compartment to another.

Displacement and herniation of brain tissue cause a potentially reversible pathophysiologic process to become irreversible. Ischemia and edema are further increased, compounding the pre-existing problem. Compression of the brainstem and cranial nerves may be fatal. Fig. 55-4 illustrates herniation. Herniations force the cerebellum and brainstem downward through the foramen magnum. If compression of the brainstem is unrelieved, respiratory arrest may occur.

Clinical Manifestations

The clinical manifestations of increased ICP can take many forms, depending on the cause, location, and rate at which the pressure increase occurs (Fig. 55-5). The earlier the condition is recognized and treated, the better the prognosis. The clinical manifestations of increased ICP are discussed below.

Change in Level of Consciousness. The *level of consciousness* (LOC) is a sensitive and important indicator of the pa-

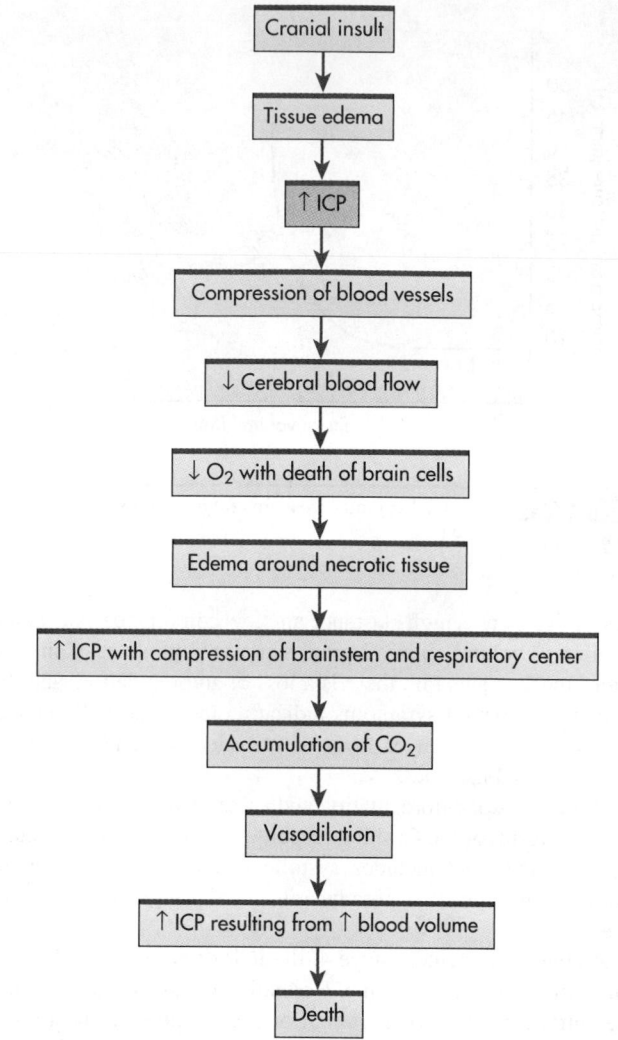

FIG. 55-3 Progression of increased intracranial pressure.

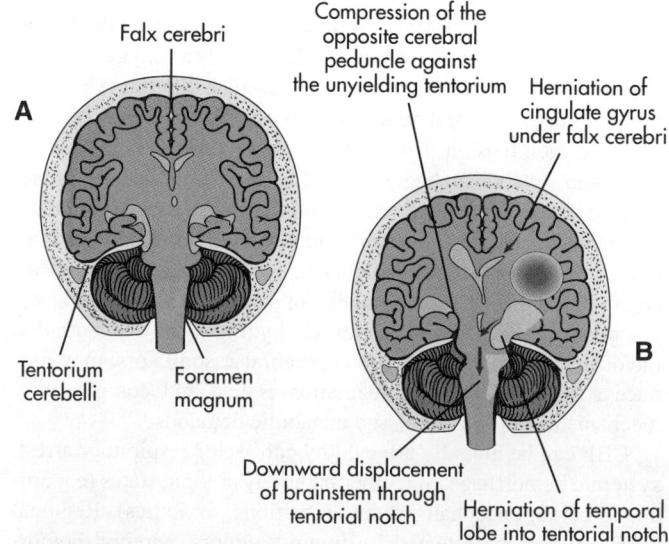

FIG. 55-4 Herniation. A, Normal relationship of intracranial structures. B, Shift of intracranial structures.

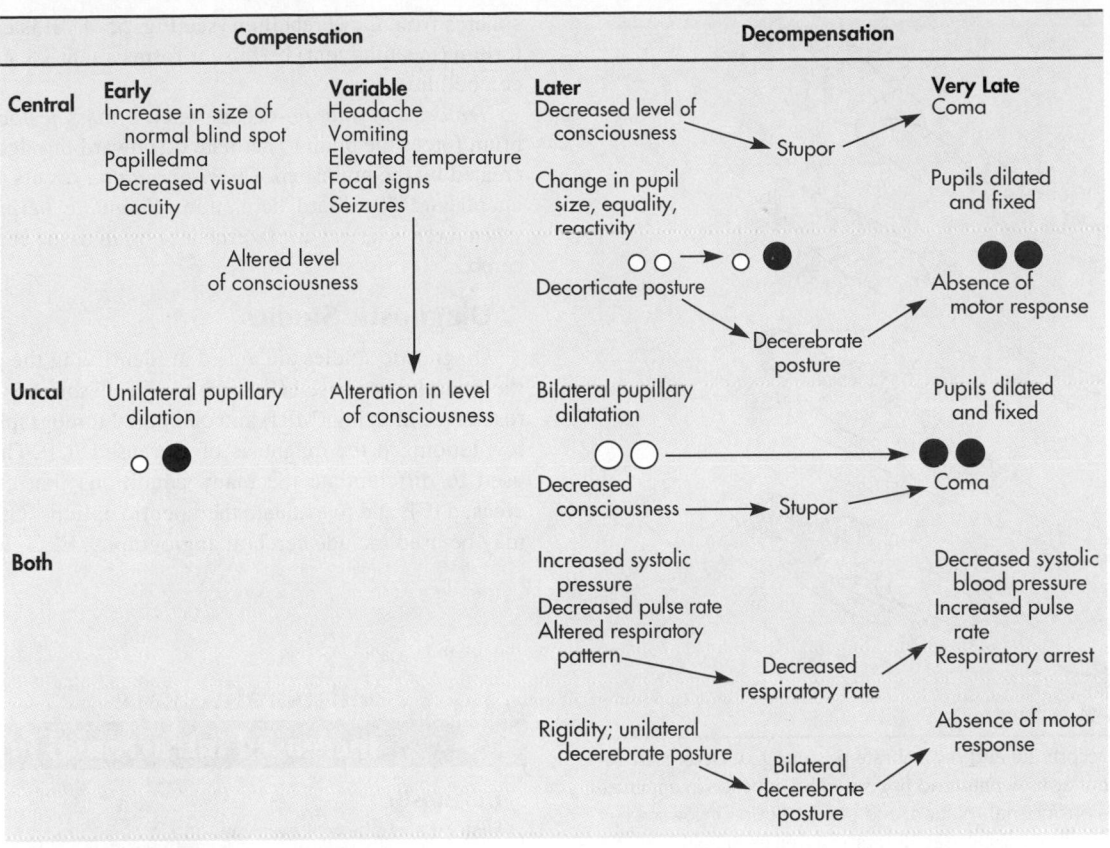

FIG. 55-5 Clinical manifestations of increased intracranial pressure.

tient's neurologic status. Changes in LOC are a result of impaired CBF, which affects the cells of the cerebral cortex and the reticular activating system (RAS). The RAS is located in the brainstem with neural connections to many parts of the nervous system. An intact RAS can maintain a state of wakefulness even in the absence of a functioning cerebral cortex.

Interruptions of impulses from the RAS or alteration of the functioning of the cerebral hemispheres can cause **unconsciousness** (abnormal state of complete or partial unawareness of self or environment).

The patient's state of consciousness is defined by both the behavior and the pattern of brain activity recorded by an electroencephalogram (EEG). The change in consciousness may be dramatic, as in coma, or subtle, such as a flattening of affect, change in orientation, or decrease in level of attention. In the deepest state of unconsciousness (i.e., coma), the patient does not respond to painful stimuli. Corneal and pupillary reflexes are absent. The patient cannot swallow or cough and is incontinent of urine and feces. The EEG pattern demonstrates decreased or absent neuronal activity.

Changes in Vital Signs. Changes in vital signs are caused by increasing pressure on the thalamus, hypothalamus, pons, and medulla. Manifestations such as Cushing triad consisting of increasing systolic pressure (widening pulse pressure), bradycardia with a full and bounding pulse, and irregular respiratory pattern may be present but often do not appear until ICP has been increased for some time or markedly increased suddenly (e.g., head trauma). A change in body temperature may also be noted.

Ocular Signs. Compression of the oculomotor nerve (cranial nerve [CN] III) results in dilation of the pupil ipsilateral to the mass or lesion, sluggish or no response to light, inability to move the eye upward, and ptosis of the eyelid. These signs can be the result of a shifting of the brain from the midline, a process that compresses the trunk of CN III, paralyzing the pupil sphincter. A fixed, unilaterally dilated pupil is a neurologic emergency that indicates herniation of the brain. Other cranial nerves may also be affected, such as the optic (CN II), trochlear (CN IV), and abducens (CN VI) nerves. Signs of dysfunction of these cranial nerves include blurred vision, diplopia, and changes in extraocular eye movements. Central herniation may initially manifest as sluggish but equal pupil response. Uncal herniation may cause a dilated unilateral pupil. *Papilledema*, a choked optic disc seen on retinal examination, is also noted and is a nonspecific sign associated with long-standing increased ICP.

Decrease in Motor Function. As the ICP continues to rise, the patient manifests changes in motor ability. A contralateral hemiparesis or hemiplegia may be seen, depending on the location of the source of the increased ICP. If painful stimuli are used to elicit a motor response, the patient may exhibit localization to the stimuli or a withdrawal from the stimuli. *Decorticate* (flexor) and *decerebrate* (extensor) posturing may also be elicited by noxious stimuli (Fig. 55-6). Decorticate posture consists of internal rotation and adduction of the arms with flexion of the elbows, wrists, and fingers as a result of interruption of voluntary motor tracts. Extension of the legs may also be seen. A decerebrate posture may indicate more serious damage and results from

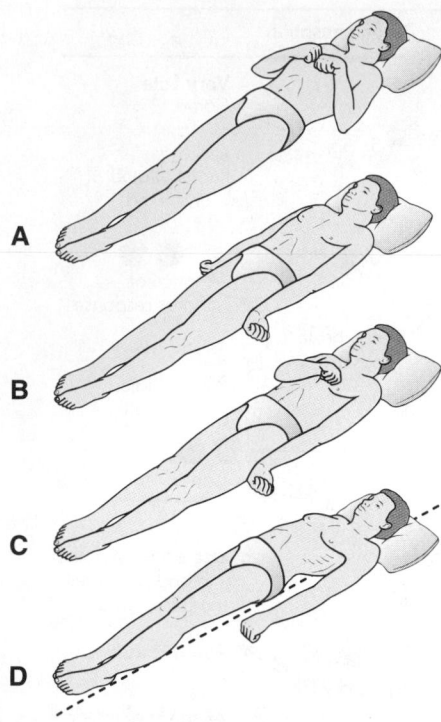

FIG. 55-6 Decorticate and decerebrate posturing. **A**, Decorticate response. Flexion of arms, wrists, and fingers with adduction in upper extremities. Extension, internal rotation, and plantar flexion in lower extremities. **B**, Decerebrate response. All four extremities in rigid extension, with hyperpronation of forearms and plantar flexion of feet. **C**, Decorticate response on right side of body and decerebrate response on left side of body. **D**, Opisthotonic posturing.

disruption of motor fibers in the midbrain and brainstem. In this position, the arms are stiffly extended, adducted, and hyperpronated. There is also hyperextension of the legs with plantar flexion of the feet.

Headache. Although the brain itself is insensitive to pain, compression of other intracranial structures, such as the walls of arteries and veins and the cranial nerves, can produce headache. The headache is often continuous but worse in the morning. Straining or movement may accentuate the pain.

Vomiting. Vomiting, usually not preceded by nausea, is often a nonspecific sign of increased ICP. This is called unexpected vomiting and is related to pressure changes in the cranium. Projectile vomiting may also be seen and is related to increased ICP.

It is often difficult to identify increased ICP as the cause of coma. Loss of consciousness also confuses the interpretation of clinical signs, making it difficult to follow the progression of the increasing ICP.

Complications

The major complications of uncontrolled increased ICP are inadequate cerebral perfusion and cerebral herniation (see Fig. 55-4). To better understand cerebral herniation, two important structures in the brain must be described. The *falx cerebri* is a thin wall of dura that folds down between the cortex, separating the two cerebral hemispheres. The *tentorium cerebelli* is a rigid fold of dura that separates the cerebral hemi-

spheres from the cerebellum (see Fig. 55-4). It is called the tentorium (meaning tent) because it forms a tentlike cover over the cerebellum.

Tentorial herniation occurs when a mass lesion in the cerebrum forces the brain to herniate downward through the opening created by the brainstem. *Uncal herniation* occurs when there is lateral and downward herniation. *Cingulate herniation* occurs when there is lateral displacement of brain tissue beneath the falx cerebri.

Diagnostic Studies

Diagnostic studies are aimed at identifying the presence and the underlying cause of increased ICP (Table 55-3). Magnetic resonance imaging (MRI) and computed tomography (CT) have revolutionized the diagnosis of increased ICP. These tests are used to differentiate the many conditions that can cause increased ICP and to evaluate therapeutic options. Other tests that may be used include cerebral angiography, EEG, ICP measure-

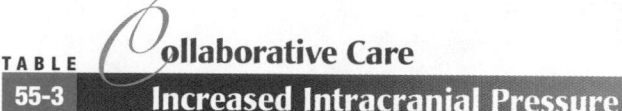

TABLE 55-3	Collaborative Care Increased Intracranial Pressure

Diagnostic
History and physical examination
Vital signs, neurologic assessments, ICP measurements
Skull, chest, and spinal x-ray studies
MRI, CT scan, PET, EEG, angiography
Transcranial Doppler studies
Laboratory studies, including CBC, coagulation profile, electrolytes, creatinine, ABGs, ammonia level, general drug and toxicology screen, CSF analysis for protein, cells, glucose
ECG

Collaborative Therapy
Elevation of head of bed to 30 degrees with head in a neutral position
ICP monitoring
Intubation and mechanical ventilation
Maintenance of PaO₂ at 100 mm Hg or greater
Maintenance of fluid balance and assessment of osmolality
Maintenance of systolic arterial pressure between 100 and 160 mm Hg
Maintenance of CPP >70 mm Hg
Reduction of cerebral metabolism (e.g., high-dose barbiturates)
Drug therapy
   Osmotic diuretics (mannitol)
   Loop diuretics (e.g., furosemide [Lasix], ethacrynic acid [Edecrin])
   Antiseizure drugs (e.g., phenytoin [Dilantin])
   Corticosteroids (dexamethasone [Decadron])
   Histamine H₂-receptor antagonist (e.g., cimetidine [Tagamet]) or proton pump inhibitor (e.g., omeprazole [Prilosec]) to prevent GI ulcers and bleeding

ABGs, Arterial blood gases; *CBC,* complete blood count; *CPP,* cerebral perfusion pressure; *CSF,* cerebrospinal fluid; *CT,* computed tomography; *ECG,* electrocardiogram; *EEG,* electroencephalogram; *GI,* gastrointestinal; *ICP,* intracranial pressure; *MRI,* magnetic resonance imaging; *PaO₂,* partial pressure of arterial oxygen; *PET,* positron emission tomography.

ment, transcranial Doppler studies, near-infrared spectroscopy for regional cerebral oxygenation, and evoked potential studies. Positron emission tomography (PET) is also used to diagnose the cause of increased ICP. In general, a lumbar puncture is not performed when increased ICP is suspected because of the possibility of cerebral herniation from the sudden release of the pressure in the skull from the area above the lumbar puncture.

Measurement of ICP

Indications for ICP Placement. ICP monitoring is used to guide clinical care when the patient is at risk for or has elevations in ICP. It may be used in patients with a variety of neurologic insults, including hemorrhage, stroke, tumor, infection, or traumatic brain injury. ICP should be monitored if patients are admitted with a Glasgow Coma Scale (GCS) score of 8 or less and an abnormal CT scan (hematomas, contusion, edema, or compressed basal cisterns).[5]

Methods of Measuring ICP. Multiple methods and devices are available to monitor ICP (Fig. 55-7).

The "gold standard" for monitoring ICP is the ventriculostomy, whereby a catheter is inserted into the lateral ventricle and coupled to an external transducer. This technique directly measures the pressure within the ventricles, facilitates removal and/or sampling of CSF, and allows for intraventricular drug administration. As with fluid-coupled blood pressure monitoring systems, signals can be distorted by excessive tube length or bubbles in the line. In these systems, the transducer is external, and its position must remain constant with respect to the patient's head to produce comparable pressures. An alternative technology, the fiberoptic catheter, uses a sensor transducer located within the catheter tip. The sensor tip is placed within the ventricle or the brain tissue and provides a direct measurement of brain pressure. Other less commonly used transducers include pneumatic systems and intracranial strain gauges. Similar to the fiberoptic system, these systems produce excellent quality waveforms, do not require repositioning with patient movement, and usually cannot be rezeroed.

Infection is a serious consideration with ICP monitoring. Infection rates are highest in fluid-coupled systems, with incidence rates ranging from 1% to 30%.[6] Prophylactic systemic antibiotics may be administered to reduce the chances of infection. Factors that contribute to the development of infection include ICP monitoring greater than 5 days, use of a ventriculostomy, the presence of a CSF leak, and a concurrent systemic infection. Routine care may include regular diagnostic testing for CSF organism growth.

ICP should be measured as a mean pressure at the end of expiration. If a CSF drainage device is in place, the drain must be closed for at least 6 minutes to ensure an accurate reading. The waveform strip should be recorded along with other pressure monitoring waveforms. The normal ICP waveform is shaped somewhat like an arterial pressure trace (Fig. 55-8, *A*), although the pressures are in a much lower range. This is because arterial pressure is transmitted to the choroid plexus and then to the CSF in the ventricular and subarachnoid spaces. When the waveform is monitored so that components in synchrony with the cardiac cycle can be visualized, the normal ICP waveform has three phases (Table 55-4).

It is important that the nurse monitor the ICP waveform, as well as mean CPP. It has been noted that when the height of P2 is higher than P1, the intracranial space may be noncompliant and the patient is at risk for development of elevated ICP (see Fig. 55-8, *B*). It is important to consider the rate at which changes occur and the patient's clinical condition. Neurologic deterioration might not occur until ICP elevation is pronounced and sustained. Any indication of ICP elevation, either as a mean increase in pressure or as an abnormal waveform configuration, should be reported to the health care provider immediately.

Inaccurate ICP readings can be caused by CSF leaks around the monitoring device, obstruction of the intraventricular catheter or bolt (from tissue or blood clot), difference between the height of the bolt and the transducer, and kinks in the tubing. In fluid-coupled systems, bubbles or air in the tubing also dampens the waveform.

CSF Drainage. With the ventricular catheter and certain fiberoptic systems, it is possible to control ICP by removing CSF.

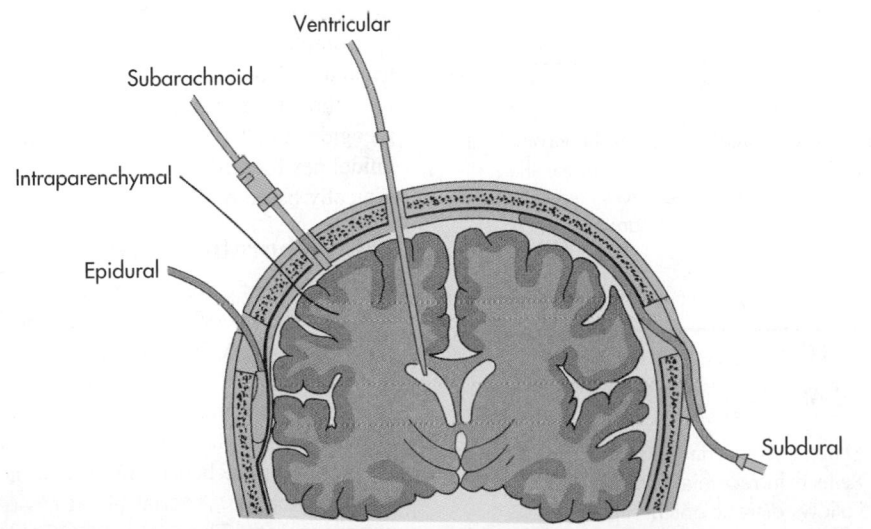

FIG. 55-7 Coronal section of brain showing potential sites for placement of ICP monitoring devices.

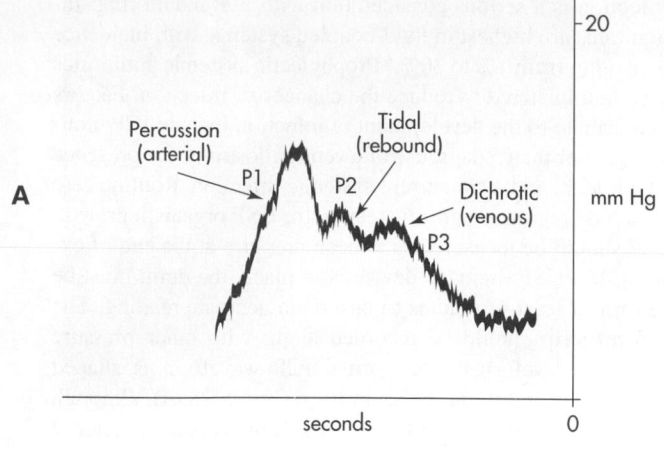

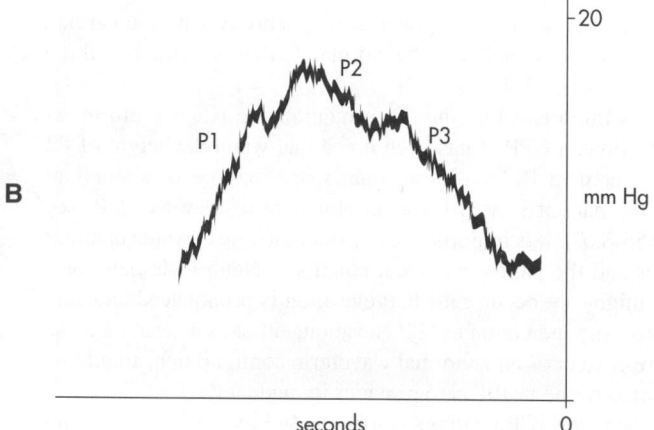

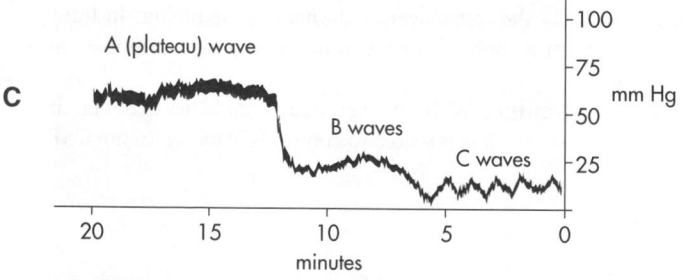

FIG. 55-8 A, Normal intracranial pressure (ICP) waveform as noted on a fast time scale recording indicating P1, P2, P3 (see Table 55-4). B, Abnormal ICP waveform indicating high pressure and noncompliant brain. C, Pathologic ICP waveforms. A (plateau) waves indicate sharp increases in ICP. B waves often precede A waves. C waves are related to normal fluctuations in respirations and blood pressure.

TABLE 55-4   Normal ICP Waveforms*

WAVEFORM	MEANING
P1 percussion wave	Represents arterial pulsations
P2 rebound wave	Reflects intracranial compliance
P3 dicrotic wave	Follows dicrotic notch; represents venous pulsations

*See Fig. 55-8.

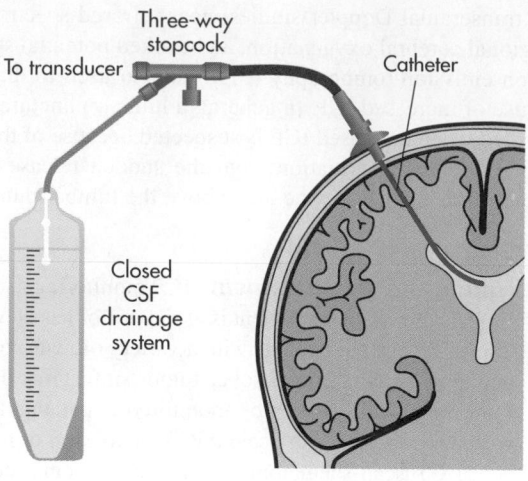

Intraventricular catheter

FIG. 55-9 Intermittent drainage system. CSF is drained via a ventriculostomy when ICP exceeds the upper pressure parameter set by the physician. The three-way stopcock is opened to allow CSF to flow into the draining bag for brief periods (30 to 120 seconds) until the pressure is below the upper pressure parameters.

To do this, a Y connector is inserted in the line (Fig. 55-9). Using a closed system, elevations in ICP are controlled by removal of CSF by gravity drainage and by adjusting the height of the drip chamber and drainage bag relative to the patient's ventricular reference point. Typically a point 15 cm above the ear canal (foramen of Monroe) is selected. Raising the system diminishes drainage, whereas lowering the system increases drainage volume. Careful monitoring of the volume of CSF drained is essential, keeping in mind that normal adult CSF production is about 20 to 30 ml per hour, with a total CSF volume of 90 to 150 ml within the ventricles and subarachnoid space. The level of the ICP to initiate drainage, amount of fluid to be drained, height of the system, and frequency of drainage are ordered by the physician. Prevention of infection by use of strict aseptic technique during dressing changes or sampling of CSF is imperative. The system must remain intact to ensure that the ICP readings are accurate because treatment is initiated on the basis of the level of the pressures.

Complications of this type of drainage system include ventricular collapse, infection, and herniation or subdural hematoma formation from rapid decompression. Although it is generally recognized that CSF removal decreases ICP and improves CPP, guidelines for CSF removal are not universally accepted but are typically based on institution or physician preference.[7]

Collaborative Care

The goals of collaborative care (see Table 55-3) are to identify and treat the underlying cause of increased ICP and to support brain function. A careful history is an important diagnostic aid that can direct the search for the underlying cause.

Ensuring adequate oxygenation to support brain function is the first step in the management of increased ICP. An endotracheal tube or tracheostomy may be necessary to maintain adequate ventilation. Arterial blood gas (ABG) analysis guides the oxygen therapy. The goal is to maintain the PaO_2 at 100 mm Hg or greater. It may be necessary to maintain the patient on a mechanical ventilator to ensure adequate oxygenation.

If the condition is caused by a mass lesion, such as a tumor or hematoma, surgical removal of the mass is the best management (see Brain Tumors and Cranial Surgery later in this chapter). Nonsurgical intervention for the reduction of tissue volume related to cerebral tissue swelling and cerebral edema includes the use of diuretics and corticosteroids.

Drug Therapy. Drug therapy plays an important part in the management of increased ICP. Mannitol (Osmitrol), glycerol, and urea are used as osmotic diuretics. Mannitol (25%) is the most widely used agent and is given intravenously. Mannitol acts to decrease the ICP in two ways: plasma expansion and osmotic effect. There is an immediate plasma-expanding effect that reduces the hematocrit and blood viscosity, thereby increasing CBF and cerebral oxygen delivery. A vascular osmotic gradient is created by mannitol. Thus fluid moves from the tissues into the blood vessels. Therefore the ICP is reduced by a decrease in the total brain fluid content. Fluid and electrolyte status must be monitored when osmotic diuretics are used. Mannitol may be contraindicated if renal disease is present and if serum osmolality is elevated.[8]

Loop diuretics such as furosemide (Lasix), bumetanide (Bumex), and ethacrynic acid (Edecrin) may also be used in the management of increased ICP. These diuretics inhibit sodium and chloride reabsorption in the ascending limb of the loop of Henle and thus reduce blood volume and, ultimately, tissue volume. In addition, these agents cause a reduction in the rate of CSF production, which also contributes to the reduction in ICP.[3]

Corticosteroids (e.g., dexamethasone [Decadron]) are thought to control the vasogenic edema surrounding tumors and abscesses but appear to have limited value in the management of head-injured patients. The mode of action of corticosteroids is not completely known. It is theorized that they act by their stabilizing effect on the cell membrane and by inhibiting the synthesis of prostaglandins (see Chapter 12, Fig. 12-7), thus preventing the formation of proinflammatory mediators. Corticosteroids are also thought to improve neuronal function by improving CBF and restoring autoregulation.

Complications associated with the use of corticosteroids include hyperglycemia, increased incidence of infections, gastrointestinal (GI) bleeding, and hyponatremia. Fluid intake and sodium and glucose levels should be monitored regularly. Patients receiving corticosteroids should concurrently be given antacids or histamine H_2 receptor blockers (e.g., cimetidine [Tagamet]) or proton pump inhibitors (e.g., omeprazole [Prilosec]) to prevent GI ulcers and bleeding.

Drug therapy for reducing cerebral metabolism may be an effective strategy to control ICP. The reduction in the metabolic rate decreases the CBF and therefore the ICP. High-dose barbiturates (e.g., pentobarbital [Nembutal], thiopental [Pentothal]) are used in patients with increased ICP refractory to treatment. Barbiturates produce a decrease in cerebral metabolism and a subsequent decrease in ICP. A secondary effect is a reduction in cerebral edema and production of a more uniform blood supply to the brain.[3] Capabilities to monitor the patient's ICP, blood flow, EEG, and metabolism should be available when this treatment is used. Antiseizure drugs such as phenytoin (Dilantin) may be used because seizures can further increase ICP.

Hyperventilation Therapy. In the past, aggressive hyperventilation (PaCO$_2$ <25 mm Hg) had been a mainstay treatment of elevated ICP. The lowering of the PaCO$_2$ leads to constriction of the cerebral blood vessels, reducing CBF and thereby decreasing the ICP. More recent evidence suggests that aggressive hyperventilation increases the risk of focal cerebral ischemia and may adversely affect outcomes.[3] Prolonged aggressive hyperventilation therapy should be avoided in the absence of increased ICP, particularly during the first 24 hours following a head injury or when CBF is low. Brief periods of hyperventilation therapy may be useful for refractory intracranial hypertension.[3,5]

Nutritional Therapy. All patients must have their nutritional needs met, regardless of their state of consciousness or health. Early feeding following brain injury improves outcomes[9] (see the Evidence-Based Practice box). The patient with increased ICP is in a hypermetabolic and hypercatabolic state that increases the need for glucose to provide the necessary fuel for metabolism of the injured brain. If the patient cannot maintain an adequate oral intake, other means of meeting the nutritional requirements, such as enteral feedings or total parenteral nutrition, should be initiated. Nutritional replacements should begin within 3 days after injury to reach full nutritional replacement within 7 days after injury.[9] Because malnutrition promotes continued cerebral edema, maintenance of optimal nutrition is imperative. (Nutritional therapy is discussed in Chapter 39.) Feedings or supplements should be guided by the patient's fluid and electrolyte status, as well as the patient's metabolic needs.

It is controversial as to whether patients should be maintained in a state of moderate dehydration. On one hand, moderate dehydration is thought to be effective in reducing cerebral edema; in this case, fluids are restricted to 65% to 75% of normal requirements. However, the concern is that hypovolemia may result in a decrease in cardiac output and blood pressure, which may affect cerebral perfusion and the amount of oxygen delivered to the brain. There is additional concern that dehydrated patients do not respond well to vasoactive drugs. Because of this, the current therapy is directed at keeping patients normovolemic. The use of

EVIDENCE-BASED PRACTICE

Nutritional Support Following Head Injury

Clinical Problem

Does nutritional support following head injury affect mortality and morbidity?

Best Clinical Practice

- Early feeding is associated with better outcomes in terms of survival and disability.
- Nutritional support can include parenteral nutrition or enteral nutrition (nasogastric or nasojejunal), depending on the condition of the patient and presence of bowel sounds.

Implications for Nursing Practice

- Head injury increases the body's metabolic responses and therefore nutritional demands.
- Provision of an adequate supply of nutrients is associated with improved outcome.
- The nurse must assess the nutritional status of the patient with a head injury and ensure that the patient receives adequate nutrition.

Reference for Evidence

Yanagawa T et al: Nutritional support for head-injured patients, *Cochrane Database Syst Rev*, Issue 3, 2002.

fluid restriction to reduce tissue volume should be evaluated on the basis of clinical factors such as urine output, insensible fluid loss, serum and urine osmolality, and the condition of the patient. Intravenous (IV) 0.45% or 0.9% sodium chloride is the preferred solution for administration of piggyback medications because a lowering of serum osmolarity and an increase in cerebral edema occur if 5% dextrose in water is used.

NURSING MANAGEMENT
INCREASED INTRACRANIAL PRESSURE

■ Nursing Assessment

Subjective data about the patient with increased ICP can be obtained from the patient or family members or other persons who are familiar with the patient. The nurse must learn appropriate assessment techniques and describe the LOC by noting the specific behaviors observed. When a deviation from the normal state of consciousness occurs, a more structured method of observation should be initiated. This type of systematic approach to nursing assessment is illustrated in Fig. 55-10 and consists of assessing the LOC by the GCS (Table 55-5) and by body functions. Adequate circulation and respiration are the most vital and should always be the first body functions assessed.

Glasgow Coma Scale. Because of the confusion and ambiguity that surround terms describing altered states of consciousness, the GCS was developed in 1974. The **Glasgow Coma Scale** is a quick, practical, and standardized system for assessing the degree of consciousness impairment. The three areas assessed in the GCS correspond to the definition of coma as the inability of a patient to speak, obey commands, or open the eyes when a verbal or painful stimulus is applied.[10] Specific assessments evaluate the patient's response to varying degrees of stimuli. Three indicators of response are evaluated: (1) opening of the eyes, (2) the best verbal response, and (3) the best motor response (see Table 55-5). Specific behaviors that are seen as responses to the testing stimulus in each of these three areas are given a numeric value and can be plotted on a graph. The nurse's responsibility is to elicit the best response on each of the scales: the higher the scores, the higher the level of brain functioning. A graph can be used to determine whether the patient is stable, improving, or deteriorating. The subscale scores are particularly important if a patient is untestable in one area. For example, severe periorbital edema may make eye opening impossible. The total GCS score is a sum of the numeric values assigned to each of the three areas evaluated. The highest GCS score is 15 for a fully alert person, and the lowest possible score is 3. A GCS score of 8 or less is generally indicative of coma.[11]

The GCS offers several advantages in the assessment of the unconscious patient. It is specific and structured, allowing different health care professionals to arrive at the same conclusion regarding the patient's status. It saves time for the assessor because the ratings are done with numbers rather than with lengthy descriptions.

The GCS is also specific enough to discriminate between different or changing states. The GCS is used to assess the arousal aspect of consciousness. Other components of the neurologic assessment include pupillary checks, extremity strength testing, and, if appropriate, corneal reflex testing.

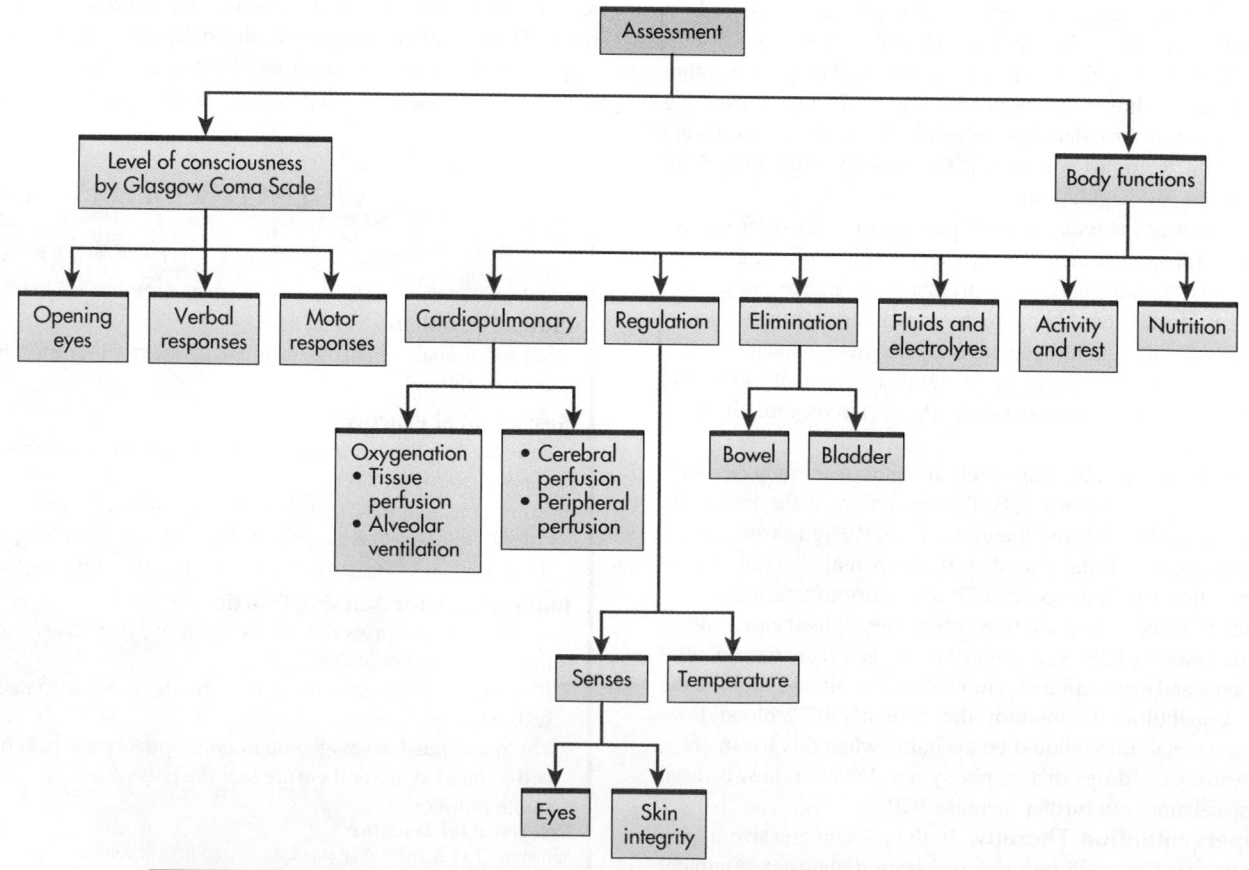

FIG. 55-10 Systematic approach to nursing assessment of the unconscious patient.

TABLE 55-5	Glasgow Coma Scale		
CATEGORY OF RESPONSE	APPROPRIATE STIMULUS	RESPONSE	SCORE
Eyes Open	• Approach to bedside • Verbal command • Pain	Spontaneous response	4
		Opening of eyes to name or command	3
		Lack of opening of eyes to previous stimuli but opening to pain	2
		Lack of opening of eyes to any stimulus	1
		Untestable	U
Best Verbal Response	• Verbal questioning with maximum arousal	Appropriate orientation, conversant, correct identification of self, place, year, and month	5
		Confusion, conversant, but disorientation in one or more spheres	4
		Inappropriate or disorganized use of words (e.g., cursing), lack of sustained conversation	3
		Incomprehensible words, sounds (e.g., moaning)	2
		Lack of sound, even with painful stimuli	1
		Untestable	U
Best Motor Response	• Verbal command (e.g., "raise your arm, hold up two fingers") • Pain (pressure on proximal nailbed)	Obedience of command	6
		Localization of pain, lack of obedience but presence of attempts to remove offending stimulus	5
		Flexion withdrawal,* flexion of arm in response to pain without abnormal flexion posture	4
		Abnormal flexion, flexing of arm at elbow and pronation, making a fist	3
		Abnormal extension, extension of arm at elbow usually with adduction and internal rotation of arm at shoulder	2
		Lack of response	1
		Untestable	U

*Added to the original scale by many centers.

Neurologic Assessment. The pupils are compared to one another for size, movement, and response (Fig. 55-11). If the oculomotor nerve is compressed, the pupil on the affected side (ipsilateral) becomes larger until it fully dilates. If ICP continues to increase, both pupils dilate.

Pupillary reaction is tested with a flashlight. The normal reaction is brisk constriction when the light is shone directly into the eye. A consensual response (a slight constriction in the opposite pupil) should also be noted at the same time. A sluggish reaction can indicate early pressure on cranial nerve III. A fixed pupil shows no response to light stimulus, which usually indicates increased ICP.

Evaluation of other cranial nerves can be included in the neurologic check. Eye movements controlled by cranial nerves III, IV, and VI can be examined in the patient who is awake and can be used to assess the function of the brainstem. In the unconscious patient, extraocular eye movements are not specifically tested. Testing the corneal reflex gives information on the functioning of cranial nerves V and VII. If this reflex is absent, routine eye care should be initiated to prevent corneal abrasion (see Chapters 20 and 21).

Eye movements of the uncooperative or unconscious patient can be elicited by reflex with the use of head movements (oculocephalic) and caloric stimulation (oculovestibular) (see Chapters 20 and 21). To test the oculocephalic reflex (doll's head or doll's

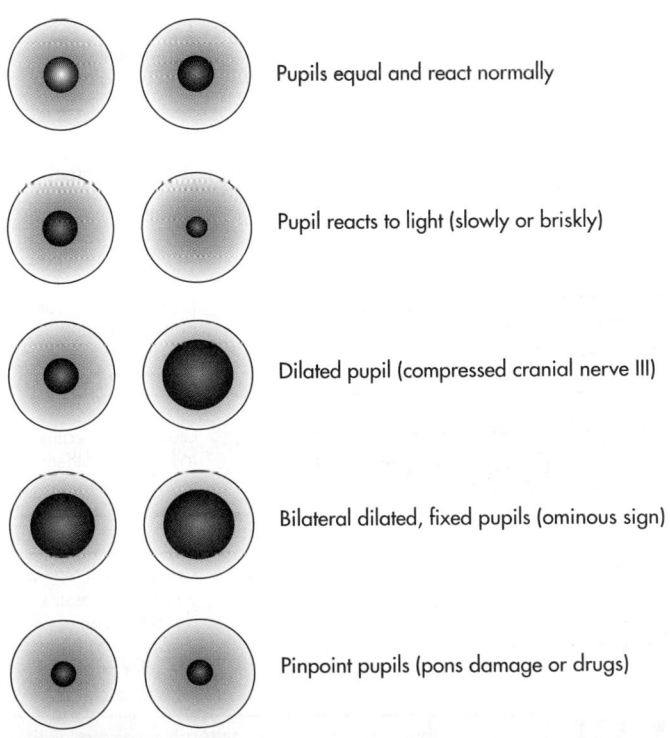

Pupils equal and react normally

Pupil reacts to light (slowly or briskly)

Dilated pupil (compressed cranial nerve III)

Bilateral dilated, fixed pupils (ominous sign)

Pinpoint pupils (pons damage or drugs)

FIG. 55-11 Pupillary check for size and response.

eyes phenomenon), the nurse rotates the patient's head briskly while holding the eyelids open. A positive response is movement of the eyes across the midline in the direction opposite that of the rotation. Next, the nurse quickly flexes and then extends the neck. Eye movement should be opposite to the direction of head movement—up when the neck is flexed and down when it is extended. Abnormal responses can aid in locating the intracranial lesion. This test should not be attempted if a cervical spine problem is suspected. (The oculovestibular reflex is discussed in Chapter 20.)

Motor strength is tested by asking the awake patient to squeeze the nurse's hands to compare strength in the hands. The palmar drift test is an excellent measure of strength in the upper extremities. The patient raises the arms in front of the body with the palmar surface facing upward. If there is any weakness in the upper extremity, the palmar surface turns downward and the arm drifts downward. Asking the patient to raise the foot from the bed or to bend the knees up in bed is a good assessment of lower extremity strength. All four extremities should be tested for strength and evaluated for any asymmetry in strength or movement.

The motor strength of the unconscious or uncooperative patient can be assessed by observation of spontaneous movement. If no spontaneous movement is possible, a pain stimulus should be applied to the patient, and the response should be noted. Resistance to movement during passive range-of-motion exercises is another measure of strength.

The vital signs, including blood pressure, pulse, respiratory rate, and temperature, should also be systematically recorded. The nurse must be aware of Cushing triad because this indicates severe increased ICP. Besides recording respiratory rate, the nurse should also note the respiratory pattern (Fig. 55-12).

Pattern	Location of Lesion	Description
1. Cheyne-Stokes 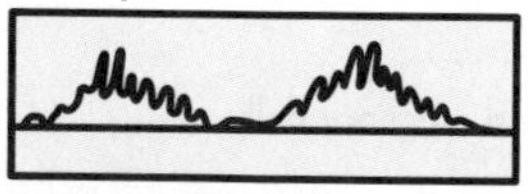	Bilateral hemispheric disease or metabolic brain dysfunction	Cycles of hyperventilation and apnea
2. Central neurogenic hyperventilation 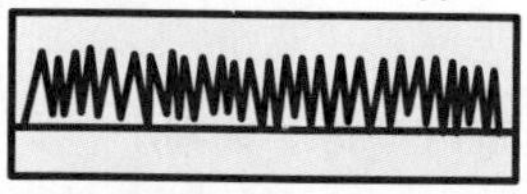	Brainstem between lower midbrain and upper pons	Sustained, regular rapid and deep breathing
3. Apneustic breathing 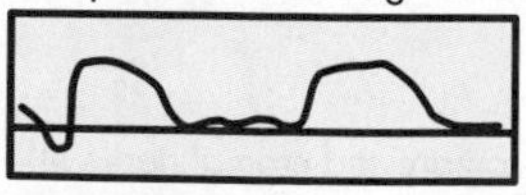	Mid or lower pons	Prolonged inspiratory phase or pauses alternating with expiratory pauses
4. Cluster breathing 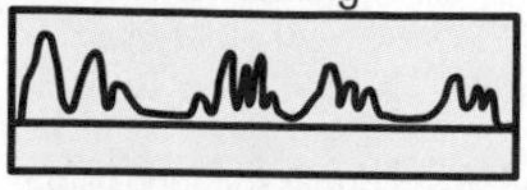	Medulla or lower pons	Clusters of breaths follow each other with irregular pauses between
5. Ataxic breathing 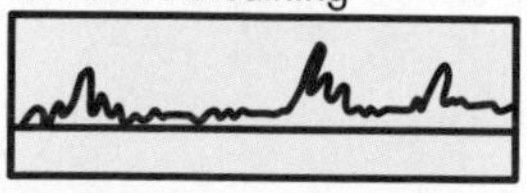	Reticular formation of the medulla	Completely irregular with some breaths deep and some shallow. Random, irregular pauses, slow rate

FIG. 55-12 Common abnormal respiratory patterns associated with coma.

■ Nursing Diagnoses

Nursing diagnoses for the patient with increased ICP include, but are not limited to, those presented in NCP 55-1.

■ Planning

The overall goals are that the patient with increased ICP will (1) have ICP within normal limits, (2) maintain a patent airway, (3) demonstrate normal fluid and electrolyte balance, and (4) have no complications secondary to immobility and decreased LOC.

■ Nursing Implementation

Acute Intervention

Respiratory function. Maintenance of a patent airway is critical in the patient with increased ICP and is a primary nursing responsibility. As the LOC decreases, the patient is at increased risk of airway obstruction from the tongue dropping back and occluding the airway or from accumulation of secretions. Altered breathing patterns may become evident. Airway patency can be aided by keeping the patient lying on one side, with frequent position changes. Snoring sounds, which may indicate obstruction, should be noted. Accumulated secretions should be removed by suctioning, as needed. An oral airway facilitates breathing and provides an easier suctioning route in the comatose patient.

The nurse must use measures to prevent hypoxia and hypercapnia. Proper positioning of the head is important. Elevation of the head of the bed by 30 degrees enhances respiratory exchange and aids in decreasing cerebral edema. Suctioning and coughing can cause transient decreases in the PaO_2 and increases in the ICP. Suctioning should be kept to a minimum and should be less than 10 seconds in duration, with administration of 100% oxygen before and after to prevent decreases in the PaO_2.[12] To avoid cumulative increases in the ICP with suctioning, suctioning should be limited to two passes per suction procedure. Patients with elevated ICP are at risk for lower CPP during suctioning.[13]

Abdominal distention can interfere with respiratory function and should be prevented. Insertion of a nasogastric tube to aspirate the stomach contents can prevent distention, vomiting, and possible aspiration. However, in patients with facial and skull fractures, a nasogastric tube is contraindicated, and oral insertion of a gastric tube is preferred.

Pain, anxiety, and fear from the initial injury, therapeutic procedures, or noxious stimuli can increase ICP and blood pressure, complicating the management and recovery of the brain-injured patient. The appropriate choice or combination of sedatives, paralytics, and analgesics for symptom management presents a challenge to the ICU team. Administration of these agents may alter the neurologic state, masking true neurologic changes. It may be necessary to temporarily suspend pharmacologic therapy to appropriately assess neurologic status. The choice, dose, and combination of agents may vary depending on the patient's history, neurologic state, and overall clinical presentation.

Narcotics, such as morphine sulfate, fentanyl (Actiq, Duragesic), and sufentanil (Sufenta), are rapid-onset analgesics with minimal effect on CBF or oxygen metabolism. The IV anesthetic sedative propofol (Diprivan) has gained popularity in the management of pain and anxiety in the ICU because of its rapid onset, short half-life, and oxygen-saving properties. Unlike narcotics, it decreases the ICP, CBF, and oxygen metabolism. Nondepolarizing

NURSING CARE PLAN 55-1

Patient with Increased Intracranial Pressure

EXPECTED PATIENT OUTCOMES	NURSING INTERVENTIONS and *RATIONALES*
NURSING DIAGNOSIS	**Ineffective airway clearance** *related to* decreased level of consciousness (LOC), immobility, and inability to mobilize secretions *as manifested by* ineffective cough, inability to clear secretions, crackles on auscultation, thick secretions.
• Demonstration of increased air exchange as measured by ABGs within normal limits • Normal breath sounds in all lobes of the lungs	• Maintain patient's side-lying position, keeping head of bed elevated *to prevent aspiration and tongue from blocking airway.* • Suction frequently *to remove accumulated secretions, reduce risk of aspiration, and ensure patent airway.* • Perform chest physical therapy at least q4hr *to improve ventilation and prevent pulmonary complications.* • Monitor patient for signs of decreased oxygenation, including changes in LOC, decreased PaO_2 or SaO_2, and increased respiratory rate *as low as PaO_2 and a high hydrogen ion concentration (acidosis) are potent cerebral blood vasodilators that increase cerebral blood flow and may increase ICP.*
NURSING DIAGNOSIS	**Ineffective tissue perfusion (cerebral)** *related to* cerebral edema *as manifested by* Glasgow Coma Scale <8; agitation; elevated systolic blood pressure, bradycardia, and widened pulse pressure; intracranial pressure >20 mm Hg, CPP <60 mm Hg.
• No further deterioration in LOC • ICP <20 mm Hg, CPP >60 mm Hg • Stable vital signs	• Monitor patient's neurologic status at least every hour initially; assess LOC and document *to evaluate patient's response to treatment and modify if necessary.* • Monitor ICP and calculate CPP *to evaluate adequacy of cerebral blood perfusion and detect patient's response to treatment.* • Limit care activities that increase ICP (e.g., suctioning) *to prevent increases in ICP.* • Provide comfort measures *as pain or agitation increase ICP.* • Elevate head of bed 30 to 45 degrees *to facilitate reduction of cerebral edema.* • Monitor reactions to all medications (especially diuretics and sedatives) *to evaluate for signs (e.g., change in LOC) of reduced cerebral edema.* • Calibrate and maintain intracranial monitoring device *to provide an accurate indicator of ICP.*
NURSING DIAGNOSIS	**Impaired skin integrity** *related to* nutritional deficit, self-care deficit, and immobility *as manifested by* inability to move or change position, dry skin, weight loss >10 lb (4.5 kg), abrasions or lacerations.
• Absence of skin breakdown • Intact skin	• Assess skin frequently, especially over bony prominences and around genitalia and buttocks *to identify potential or actual skin problems and initiate a plan of care.* • Turn patient at least q2hr as indicated *as prolonged pressure decreases circulation and leads to tissue ischemia and necrosis.* • Use low-air-loss beds as indicated *to reduce pressure to bony prominences by distributing body weight evenly.* • Cleanse all abrasions and lacerations *to reduce risk of infection;* massage skin as indicated *to stimulate circulation.*
NURSING DIAGNOSIS	**Self-care deficit (total)** *related to* altered LOC *as manifested by* inability to follow commands or move purposefully, inability to perform ADLs.
• All ADLs met by caregivers until self-care is possible	• Assess level of motor and sensory abilities at least q4hr *to determine level of care needed.* • Bathe patient daily *to maintain hygienic needs.* • Perform ROM exercises at least q4hr as tolerated *to maintain joint ROM and muscle strength.* • Begin bowel program as soon as possible *to resume usual bowel elimination pattern and prevent constipation and impaction.* • Provide urinary catheter care *to reduce risk of infection.*

Continued

NURSING CARE PLAN 55-1

Patient with Increased Intracranial Pressure—cont'd

EXPECTED PATIENT OUTCOMES	NURSING INTERVENTIONS and *RATIONALES*
NURSING DIAGNOSIS	**Interrupted family processes** *related to* comatose family member *as manifested by* inability to adapt to health crisis of family member, lack of communication or miscommunication among family members.
▪ Verbalization of feelings by family members ▪ Participation in care of ill member by family members ▪ Use of appropriate referrals	▪ Assess effect of ill family member on family as a whole *to determine extent of problems and to plan appropriate interventions.* ▪ Teach and assist family members to provide care to ill family members *to enable the family to be an integral part of patient's care.* ▪ Facilitate family communication and realistic planning for needs of ill family member *so patient's care needs are met with minimal disruption to lives of other family members.* ▪ Provide accurate information to family regarding patient's situation *to promote understanding and facilitate effective coping.* ▪ Initiate referrals as indicated *so specialized care and instruction are provided as needed.*

COLLABORATIVE PROBLEM

NURSING GOALS	NURSING INTERVENTIONS and *RATIONALES*
POTENTIAL COMPLICATION	**Increased ICP** *related to* cerebral edema.
▪ Monitor for signs of increased ICP ▪ Report deviations from acceptable parameters ▪ Carry out appropriate medical and nursing interventions	▪ Assess for signs of increased ICP (e.g., altered LOC, headache, pupil inequality, decreased respirations and pulse rate, elevated systolic blood pressure with widened pulse pressure *to enable immediate reporting and initiation of treatment.* ▪ Report significant changes *to enable prompt intervention and to prevent serious complications.* ▪ Calibrate and maintain ICP monitoring equipment in functioning condition *to ensure accurate readings.* ▪ Administer diuretics and corticosteroids as ordered *to reduce cerebral edema.* ▪ Position patient with head of bed elevated to 30 degrees *to promote venous drainage from head, reducing cerebral edema.* ▪ Manage elevated temperature *as elevated temperature increases cerebral metabolism and causes increased ICP.* ▪ Use measures to decrease agitation and hyperactivity *to reduce risk of self-injury and to prevent increased ICP.*

neuromuscular blocking agents (e.g., vecuronium [Norcuron], pancuronium [Pavulon]) are useful for ventilatory management and treatment of refractory intracranial hypertension. Because these agents paralyze muscles without blocking pain or noxious stimuli, they are used in combination with sedatives, analgesics, or benzodiazepines. Benzodiazepines, although useful for symptom management and ventilatory support, are usually avoided in the management of the patient with increased ICP because of the hypotension effect and long half-life, unless used as an adjunct to neuromuscular blocking agents.

ABGs should be measured and evaluated regularly (see Chapter 25). The nurse should frequently monitor the ABG values and maintain the levels within prescribed or acceptable parameters. The appropriate ventilatory support can be ordered on the basis of the PaO_2 and $PaCO_2$ values.

Fluid and electrolyte balance. Fluid and electrolyte disturbances can have an adverse effect on ICP. IV fluids should be closely monitored with the use of a limited-volume device or a volume-control apparatus for accuracy. Intake and output, with insensible losses and daily weights taken into account, are important parameters in the assessment of fluid balance.

Electrolyte determinations should be made daily, and any abnormal values should be discussed with the physician. It is especially important to monitor serum glucose, sodium, potassium, and osmolality. Urinary output is monitored to detect problems related to *diabetes insipidus* (e.g., increased urinary output related to a decrease in antidiuretic hormone secretion) and SIADH (syndrome of inappropriate antidiuretic hormone), which results in decreased urinary output. Besides urinary output, the serum sodium and osmolality are also used to diagnose diabetes insipidus and SIADH. Diabetes insipidus may result in severe dehydration unless treated. The usual treatment is fluid replacement, vasopressin (Pitressin), or desmopressin acetate (DDAVP) (see Chapter 48). SIADH results in a dilutional hyponatremia that may produce cerebral edema, changes in LOC, seizures, and coma. (Treatment of SIADH is described in Chapter 48.)

Monitoring intracranial pressure. The measurement of ICP enhances clinical decision-making by detecting early signs of intracranial hypertension and response to therapy. ICP monitoring is used in combination with other physiologic parameters to guide the care of the patient and assess the patient's response to routine care. Valsalva maneuver, coughing, sneezing, hypoxemia, and arousal from sleep are factors that can increase ICP. Nurses should be alert to these factors and should attempt to minimize them. Nursing management of the patient with increased ICP is one of the most important aspects of the care provided these patients.

Body position. The patient with increased ICP should be maintained in the head-up position. The nurse must take care to prevent extreme neck flexion, which can cause venous obstruction and contribute to elevated ICP. The body position should be adjusted to decrease the ICP maximally and to improve the CPP. Traditional practice has been to elevate the head of the bed to 30 degrees, unless a concurrent cervical neck injury has been identified. Research now suggests there is an inconsistent response of the ICP and the CPP to head elevation.[3,14] Elevation of the head of the bed reduces sagittal sinus pressure, promotes venous drainage from the head via the valveless jugular system, and decreases the vascular congestion that can produce cerebral edema. However, raising the head of the bed above 30 degrees may decrease the CPP. There is no evidence, however, that head-of-bed elevation decreases cerebral tissue oxygenation.[3] Careful evaluation of the effects of elevation of the head of the bed on both the ICP and the CPP is required. The bed should be positioned so that it lowers the ICP while maintaining the CPP and other indices of cerebral oxygenation.

Care should be taken to turn the patient with slow, gentle movements because rapid changes in position may increase the ICP. Caution should be used to prevent discomfort in turning and positioning the patient because pain or agitation also increases pressure. Increased intrathoracic pressure contributes to increased ICP by impeding the venous return. Thus coughing, straining, and the Valsalva maneuver should be avoided. Extreme hip flexion should be avoided to decrease the risk of raising the intraabdominal pressure, which can restrict movement of the diaphragm and cause respiratory distress. The patient should be turned at least every 2 hours.

Decorticate or decerebrate posturing is a reflex response in some patients with increased ICP. Turning, skin care, and even passive range of motion can elicit the posturing reflexes. Attempts should be made to provide needed physical care activities to minimize complications of immobility, such as atelectasis and contractures. In cases of severe posturing reflexes, these activities may have to be done less frequently because posturing can cause increases in ICP.

Protection from injury. The patient with increased ICP and a decreased LOC needs protection from self-injury. Confusion, agitation, and the possibility of seizures can put the patient at risk for injury. Restraints should be used judiciously in the agitated patient. If restraints are absolutely necessary to keep the patient from removing tubes or falling out of bed, they should be secure enough to be effective, and the skin area under the restraints should be observed regularly for irritation. Agitation may increase with the use of restraints, which indicates the need for other measures to protect the patient from injury. Light sedation with agents such as haloperidol (Haldol) or lorazepam (Ativan) may be needed. Having a family member stay with the patient may have a calming effect. For the patient with seizures or the patient at risk for seizure activity, seizure precautions should be instituted. These include padded side rails, an airway at the bedside, accurate and timely administration of antiseizure drugs, and close observation.

The patient can benefit from a quiet, nonstimulating environment. The nurse should always use a calm, reassuring approach.

Touching and talking to the patient, even one who is in a coma, is always appropriate care. The nurse must create a balance between sensory deprivation and overload for the patient with increased ICP.

Psychologic considerations. Besides the carefully planned physical care provided patients with increased ICP, the nurse must also be aware of the psychologic well-being of the patients and their families. Anxiety over the diagnosis and the prognosis for the patient with neurologic problems can be distressing to the patient, the family, and the nursing staff. The nurse's competent and assured manner in performing the care needed by the patient is reassuring to everyone involved. Short, simple explanations are appropriate and allow the patient and the family to acquire the amount of information they desire. There is a need for support, information, and education of both patients and families. The nurse should assess the family members' desire and need to assist in providing care for the patient and allow for their participation as appropriate.

■ **Evaluation**

The expected outcomes for the patient with ICP are addressed in NCP 55-1.

HEAD INJURY

Head injury includes any trauma to the scalp, skull, or brain. The term *head trauma* is used primarily to signify craniocerebral trauma, which includes an alteration in consciousness, no matter how brief.

Statistics regarding the occurrence of head injuries are incomplete because many victims die at the scene of the accident or because the condition is considered minor and health care services are not sought. In the United States an estimated 1 million persons are treated and released with traumatic brain injury (TBI) in hospital emergency departments. Fifty thousand people die and 230,000 persons are hospitalized with TBI. Of individuals hospitalized, 22% of the patients die.[15] It is estimated that there has been a 21% decline in fatalities related to head injury since 1976.[16] In the past, motor vehicle accidents and falls were the most common causes of head injury in both Canada and the United States. More recently, in the United States, deaths from motor vehicle accidents and falls have decreased, whereas firearm-related head injury death rates have increased.[16] Other causes of head injury include assaults, sports-related injuries, and recreational accidents.

Head trauma has a high potential for poor outcome.[16] Deaths from head trauma occur at three time points after injury: immediately after the injury, within 2 hours after injury, and approximately 3 weeks after injury. Factors that predict a poor outcome include the presence of an intracranial hematoma, increasing age of the patient, abnormal motor responses, impaired or absent eye movements or pupil light reflexes, early sustained hypotension, hypoxemia or hypercapnia, and ICP levels higher than 20 mm Hg.[17] The majority of deaths after a head injury occur immediately after the injury, either from the direct head trauma or from massive hemorrhage and shock. Deaths occurring within a few hours of the trauma are caused by progressive worsening of the head injury or from internal bleeding. An immediate note of changes in neurologic status and surgical intervention are critical in the prevention of deaths at this point. Deaths occurring 3 weeks or more after injury result from multisystem failure. Expert nursing care in the weeks following the injury is crucial in decreasing mortality.

Types of Head Injuries

Scalp Lacerations. *Scalp lacerations* are the most minor type of head trauma. Because the scalp contains many blood vessels with poor constrictive abilities, most scalp lacerations are associated with profuse bleeding. The major complication associated with scalp laceration is infection.

TABLE 55-6	Types of Skull Fractures	
DESCRIPTION	**CAUSE**	
Linear Break in continuity of bone without alteration of relationship of parts	Low-velocity injuries	
Depressed Inward indentation of skull	Powerful blow	
Simple Linear or depressed skull fracture without fragmentation or communicating lacerations	Low-to-moderate impact	
Comminuted Multiple linear fractures with fragmentation of bone into many pieces	Direct, high-momentum impact	
Compound Depressed skull fracture and scalp laceration with communicating pathway to intracranial cavity	Severe head injury	

TABLE 55-7	Clinical Manifestations of Different Types of Skull Fractures
LOCATION	**SYNDROME OR SEQUELAE**
Frontal fracture	Exposure of brain to contaminants through frontal air sinus, possible association with air in forehead tissue, CSF rhinorrhea, or pneumocranium
Orbital fracture	Periorbital ecchymosis (raccoon eyes)
Temporal fracture	Boggy temporal muscle because of extravasation of blood, oval-shaped bruise behind ear in mastoid region (Battle's sign), CSF otorrhea
Parietal fracture	Deafness, CSF or brain otorrhea, bulging of tympanic membrane caused by blood or CSF, facial paralysis, loss of taste, Battle's sign
Posterior fossa fracture	Occipital bruising resulting in cortical blindness, visual field defects; rare appearance of ataxia or other cerebellar signs
Basilar skull fracture	CSF or brain otorrhea, bulging of tympanic membrane caused by blood or CSF, Battle's sign, tinnitus or hearing difficulty, facial paralysis, conjugate deviation of gaze, vertigo

CSF, Cerebrospinal fluid.

Skull Fractures. *Skull fractures* frequently occur with head trauma. There are several ways to describe skull fractures: (1) linear or depressed; (2) simple, comminuted, or compound; and (3) closed or open (Table 55-6). Fractures may be closed or open, depending on the presence of a scalp laceration or extension of the fracture into the air sinuses or dura. The type and severity of a skull fracture depend on the velocity, the momentum, the direction of injuring agent, and the site of impact.

The location of the fracture alters the presentation of the manifestations (Table 55-7). For example, a specialized type of linear fracture is seen when the fracture occurs at the base of the skull, a basilar skull fracture. Manifestations include facial paralysis, Battle's sign (Fig. 55-13), and conjugate deviation of gaze. This fracture generally crosses a sinus and tears the dura (e.g., the frontal or the temporal) and is associated with leakage of CSF. Rhinorrhea (CSF leakage from the nose) or otorrhea (CSF leakage from the ear) generally confirms that the fracture has traversed the dura (Fig. 55-14).

Two methods of testing can be used to determine whether the fluid leaking from the nose or ear is CSF. The first method is to

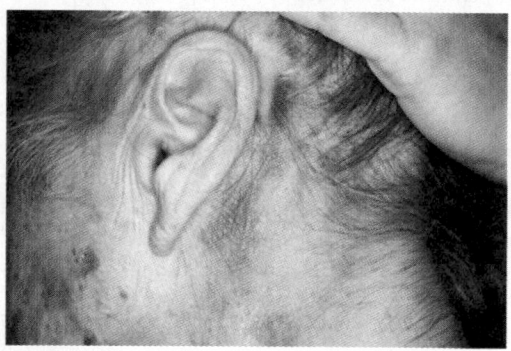

FIG. 55-13 Battle's sign.

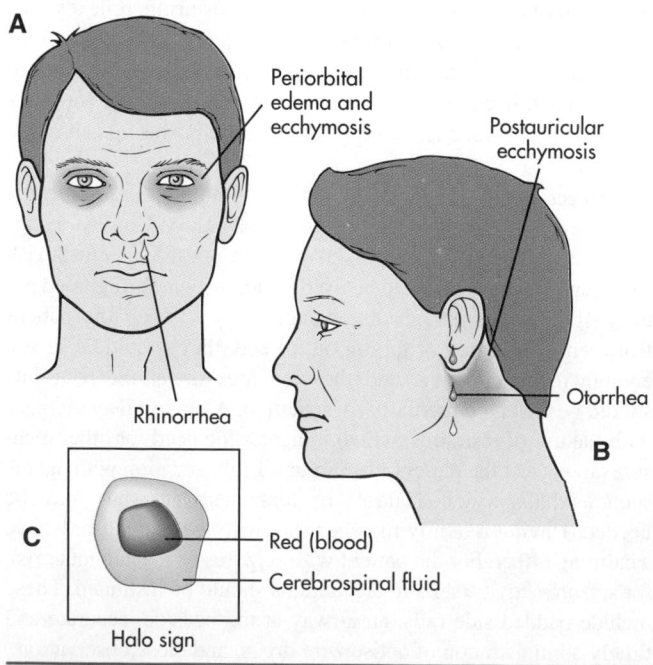

FIG. 55-14 A, Raccoon eyes and rhinorrhea. B, Battle's sign (postauricular ecchymosis) with otorrhea. C, Halo or ring sign (see text).

test the leaking fluid with a Dextrostix or Tes-Tape strip to determine whether glucose is present. CSF gives a positive reading for glucose. If blood is present in the fluid, testing for the presence of glucose is unreliable because blood contains glucose. In this event, the nurse should look for the "halo" or "ring" sign (see Fig. 55-14, *C*). To perform this test, the nurse allows the leaking fluid to drip onto a white pad (4 x 4) or towel and observes the drainage. Within a few minutes the blood coalesces into the center, and a yellowish ring encircles the blood if CSF is present. The color, appearance, and amount of leaking fluid must be noted because both tests can give false-positive results.

The major potential complications of skull fractures are intracranial infections and hematoma, as well as meningeal and brain tissue damage.

Minor Head Trauma. Brain injuries are categorized as being minor or major. **Concussion** (a sudden transient mechanical head injury with disruption of neural activity and a change in the LOC) is considered a minor head injury. The patient may not lose total consciousness with this injury.

Signs of concussion include a brief disruption in LOC, amnesia regarding the event (retrograde amnesia), and headache. The manifestations are generally of short duration. If the patient has not lost consciousness, or if the loss of consciousness lasts less than 5 minutes, the patient is usually discharged from the care facility with instructions to notify the health care provider if symptoms persist or if behavioral changes are noted.

The *postconcussion* syndrome is seen anywhere from 2 weeks to 2 months after the concussion. Symptoms include persistent headache, lethargy, personality and behavioral changes, shortened attention span, decreased short-term memory, and changes in intellectual ability. This syndrome can significantly affect the patient's abilities to perform the activities of daily living.

Although concussion is generally considered benign and usually resolves spontaneously, the symptoms may be the beginning of a more serious, progressive problem. At the time of discharge, it is important to give the patient and the family instructions for observation and accurate reporting of symptoms or changes in neurologic status.

Major Head Trauma. Major head trauma includes cerebral contusions and lacerations. Both injuries represent severe trauma to the brain. Contusions and intracerebral lacerations are generally associated with closed injuries.

A **contusion** is the bruising of the brain tissue within a focal area that maintains the integrity of the pia mater and arachnoid layers. A contusion develops areas of hemorrhage, infarction, necrosis, and edema. A contusion frequently occurs at the site of a fracture. With contusion, the phenomenon of *coup-contrecoup injury* is often noted. Damage from coup-contrecoup injury occurs because of mass movement of the brain inside the skull. Contusions or lacerations occur both at the site of the direct impact of the brain on the skull (*coup*) and at a secondary area of damage on the opposite side away from injury (*contrecoup*), leading to multiple contused areas. Bleeding around the contusion site is generally minimal, and the blood is reabsorbed slowly. Neurologic assessment demonstrates focal findings and a generalized disturbance in the LOC. Seizures are a common complication of brain contusion.

Lacerations involve actual tearing of the brain tissue and often occur in association with depressed and compound fractures and penetrating injuries. Tissue damage is severe, and surgical

repair of the laceration is impossible because of the texture of the brain tissue. If bleeding is deep into the brain parenchyma, focal and generalized signs are noted.

When major head trauma occurs, many delayed responses are seen, including hemorrhage, hematoma formation, seizures, and cerebral edema. Intracerebral hemorrhage is generally associated with cerebral laceration. This hemorrhage manifests as a space-occupying lesion accompanied by unconsciousness, hemiplegia on the contralateral side, and a dilated pupil on the ipsilateral side. As the hematoma expands, symptoms of increased ICP become more severe. Prognosis is generally poor for the patient with a large intracerebral hemorrhage. Subarachnoid hemorrhage and intraventricular hemorrhage can also occur secondary to head trauma.

Pathophysiology

Diffuse axonal injury (DAI) is widespread axonal damage occurring after a mild, moderate, or severe TBI. The damage occurs primarily around axons in subcortical white matter of the cerebral hemispheres, basal ganglia, thalamus, and brainstem.[18] Initially, DAI was believed to occur from the tensile forces of trauma that sheared axons, resulting in axonal disconnection. There is increasing evidence that axonal damage is not preceded by an immediate tearing of the axon from the traumatic impact, but rather the trauma changes the function of the axon, resulting in axon swelling (axonal ballooning) and disconnection. This process takes approximately 12 to 24 hours to develop and may persist longer. The clinical signs and symptoms include a decreased LOC, increased ICP, decerebration or decortication, and global cerebral edema.

Complications

Epidural Hematoma. An **epidural hematoma** results from bleeding between the dura and the inner surface of the skull. An epidural hematoma is a neurologic emergency and is usually associated with a linear fracture crossing a major artery in the dura, causing a tear. It can have a venous or an arterial origin. Venous epidural hematomas are associated with a tear of the dural venous sinus and develop slowly. With arterial hematomas, the middle meningeal artery lying under the temporal bone is often torn. Hemorrhage occurs into the epidural space, which lies between the dura and the inner surface of the skull (Fig. 55-15, *A*). Because this is an arterial hemorrhage, the hematoma develops rapidly and under high pressure. Symptoms typically include unconsciousness at the scene, with a brief lucid interval followed by a decrease in LOC. Other symptoms may be a headache, nausea and vomiting, or focal findings. Rapid surgical intervention to prevent cerebral herniation dramatically improves outcomes.[19] Patients over 65 years of age with increased ICP have a higher mortality rate than younger patients.[15]

Subdural Hematoma. A **subdural hematoma** occurs from bleeding between the dura mater and the arachnoid layer of the meningeal covering of the brain. A subdural hematoma usually results from injury to the brain substance and its parenchymal vessels (see Fig. 55-15, *B*). The veins that drain from the surface of the brain into the sagittal sinus are the source of most subdural hematomas. Because a subdural hematoma is usually venous in origin, the hematoma is much slower to develop into a mass large enough to produce symptoms. However, a subdural hematoma may be caused by an arterial hemorrhage, in which

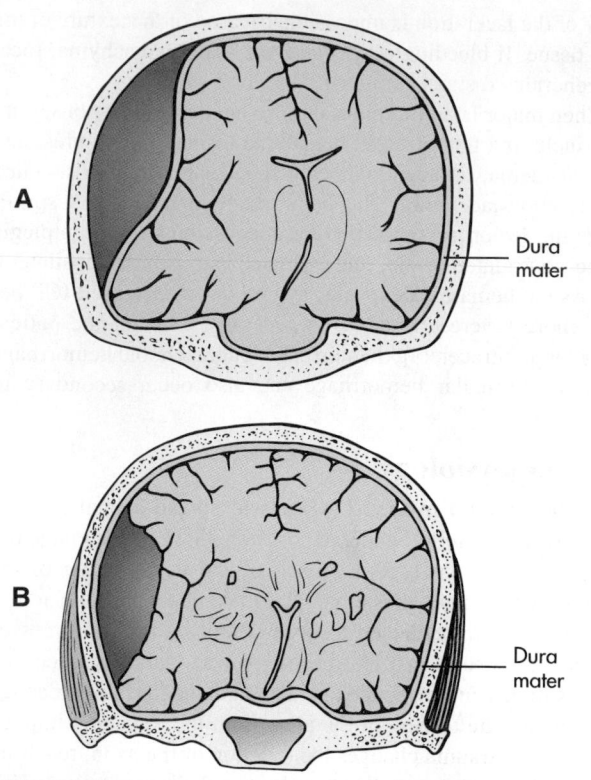

A, Epidural hematoma in the temporal fossa, usually a result of laceration of the middle meningeal artery. B, Subdural hematoma, usually a result of laceration of the subdural veins.

FIG. 55-15 A, Epidural hematoma in the temporal fossa, usually a result of laceration of the middle meningeal artery. **B,** Subdural hematoma, usually a result of laceration of the subdural veins.

case it develops more rapidly. Subdural hematomas may be acute, subacute, or chronic (Table 55-8).

An *acute subdural hematoma* manifests signs within 48 hours of the injury. The signs and symptoms are similar to those associated with brain tissue compression in increased ICP and include decreasing LOC and headache. The patient appears drowsy and confused. The ipsilateral pupil dilates and becomes fixed.

A *subacute subdural hematoma* usually occurs within 2 to 14 days of the injury. Failure to regain consciousness may point to this possibility. After the initial bleeding, a subdural hematoma may appear to enlarge over time as the breakdown products of the blood draw fluid into the subdural space to reach isotonicity.

A *chronic subdural hematoma* develops over weeks or months after a seemingly minor head injury. The peak incidence of chronic subdural hematoma is in the sixth and seventh decades of life when a potentially larger subdural space is available as a result of brain atrophy. With atrophy, the brain remains attached to the supportive structures, but tension is increased, and it is subject to tearing. The larger size of the subdural space also accounts for the presenting complaint to be the focal symptoms, rather than the signs of increased ICP. Chronic alcoholics are also prone to cerebral atrophy and subsequent development of subdural hematoma.

Delay in diagnosis of a subdural hematoma in the older adult can be attributed to symptoms that mimic other health problems in persons of this age-group, such as vascular disease and senile dementia. Somnolence, confusion, lethargy, and memory loss are associated with health problems other than subdural hematoma.

Intracerebral Hematoma. Intracerebral hematoma occurs from bleeding within the parenchyma and occurs in approximately 16% of head injuries. It usually occurs within the frontal and temporal lobes, possibly from the rupture of intracerebral vessels at the time of injury. A "burst" lobe is an intracerebral or intracerebellar hematoma that is an extension of a subarachnoid hemorrhage. This type of intracerebral hematoma is thought to result from hemorrhage of supracortical vessels.

Diagnostic Studies and Collaborative Care

CT scan is considered the best diagnostic test to determine craniocerebral trauma because it allows for rapid diagnosis and intervention. MRI, PET, and evoked potential studies may also be used in the diagnosis and differentiation of head injuries. An MRI scan is more sensitive in detecting small DAI lesions than the CT scan because of the lack of gross pathologic changes in brain tissue. Transcranial Doppler studies allow for the measurement of CBF velocity. A cervical spine x-ray may also be indicated. In general, the diagnostic studies are similar to those used for a patient with increased ICP (see Table 55-3). The GCS can be used to classify head injury as mild (score of 13 to 15), moderate (score of 9 to 12), or severe (score of 3 to 8).

Emergency management of the patient with a head injury is presented in Table 55-9. In addition to measures to prevent secondary injury by treating cerebral edema and managing increased ICP, the principal treatment of head injuries is timely diagnosis and surgery if necessary. For the patient with concussion and contusion, observation and management of increased ICP are the primary management strategies.

The treatment of skull fractures is usually conservative. For depressed fractures and fractures with loose fragments, a craniotomy is necessary to elevate the depressed bone and remove the free fragments. If large amounts of bone are destroyed, the bone

TABLE 55-8	Types of Subdural Hematomas		
TYPE	**OCCURRENCE AFTER INJURY**	**PROGRESSION OF SYMPTOMS**	**TREATMENT**
Acute	24–48 hr after severe trauma	Immediate deterioration	Craniotomy, evacuation and decompression
Subacute	48 hr–2 wk after severe trauma	Initial unconsciousness, gradual improvement, deterioration over hours, dilation of pupils, ptosis	Evacuation and decompression
Chronic	Weeks, months, usually >20 days after injury; often injury seemed trivial or forgotten by patient	Nonspecific, nonlocalizing progression; progressive alteration in LOC	Evacuation and decompression, membranectomy

LOC, Level of consciousness.

may be removed (craniectomy) and a cranioplasty will be needed at a later time (see Cranial Surgery later in this chapter).

In cases of acute subdural and epidural hematomas, the blood must be removed. A craniotomy is generally performed to visualize the bleeding vessels so that the bleeding can be controlled. Burr-hole openings may be used in an extreme emergency for a more rapid decompression, followed by a craniotomy to stop all bleeding. A drain is generally placed postoperatively for several days to prevent any reaccumulation of blood.

NURSING MANAGEMENT
HEAD INJURY

■ Nursing Assessment

The patient with a head injury is always considered to have the potential for developing increased ICP. Increased ICP is associated with higher mortality rates and poorer functional outcomes.[6] The most important aspects of the objective data are noting the GCS score (see Table 55-5), assessing and monitoring the neurologic status (see Fig. 55-10), and determining whether a CSF leak has occurred. (Nursing assessment related to increased ICP is on pp. 1500-1502.)

■ Nursing Diagnoses

Nursing diagnoses and potential complication for the patient who has sustained a head injury may include, but are not limited to, the following:

- Ineffective tissue perfusion (cerebral) *related to* interruption of CBF associated with cerebral hemorrhage, hematoma, and edema
- Hyperthermia *related to* increased metabolism, infection, and loss of cerebral integrative function secondary to possible hypothalamic injury
- Acute pain (headache) *related to* trauma and cerebral edema
- Impaired physical mobility *related to* decreased LOC and treatment-imposed bed rest
- Anxiety *related to* abrupt change in health status, hospital environment, and uncertain future
- Potential complication: increased ICP *related to* cerebral edema and hemorrhage

■ Planning

The overall goals are that the patient with an acute head injury will (1) maintain adequate cerebral perfusion; (2) remain normothermic; (3) be free from pain, discomfort, and infection; and (4) attain maximal cognitive, motor, and sensory function.

■ Nursing Implementation

Health Promotion. One of the best ways to prevent head injuries is to prevent car and motorcycle accidents. The nurse can be active in campaigns that promote driving safety and can speak to driver education classes regarding the dangers of unsafe driving and of driving after drinking alcohol. The use of seat belts in cars and the use of helmets for riding on motorcycles are the most effective measures for increasing survival after accidents. Increasingly, individual states are passing legislation requiring the use of automobile safety devices for both children and adults. The wearing of protective helmets by lumberjacks, construction workers, miners, horseback riders, bicycle riders, snowboarders, and skydivers is also recommended. The nurse should be familiar with data on outcomes with and without safety devices in working with groups who oppose safety legislation as an infringement of personal freedom.

Acute Intervention. Management at the scene of the accident can have a significant impact on the outcome of the head injury. Emergency management of head injury is discussed in Table 55-9. The general goal of nursing management of the head-injured patient is to maintain cerebral perfusion and prevent secondary cerebral ischemia. Surveillance or monitoring for changes in neurologic status is critically important because the patient's condition may deteriorate rapidly, necessitating emergency surgery. Appropriate preoperative and postoperative nursing interventions are initiated if surgery is anticipated. Because of the close association between hemodynamic status and cerebral perfusion, the nurse must be aware of any coexisting injuries or conditions. In the acute injury period, treating other life-threatening conditions (i.e., hemorrhage, hypoxia) may take initial priority in nursing care.

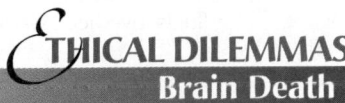

ETHICAL DILEMMAS
Brain Death

Situation

The emergency nurse receives a radio call from emergency medical service (EMS) personnel about a young man who has been involved in a motorcycle crash. The patient was not wearing a helmet and has a large open skull fracture with obvious gray matter oozing from the area. Transport from the accident scene was delayed by 45 minutes as a result of a severe thunderstorm and traffic congestion. On the way to the hospital the patient has fixed, dilated pupils and a cardiac arrest. Estimated arrival at the hospital is still an additional 45 minutes as a result of the severe weather. EMS personnel request permission to stop cardiopulmonary resuscitation (CPR) efforts.

Important Points for Consideration

- Brain death occurs when the cerebral cortex stops functioning or is irreversibly destroyed.
- Since technology has been developed that assists in supporting life, controversies have arisen related to an exact definition of death.
- Criteria for brain death include coma or unresponsiveness, absence of brainstem reflexes, and apnea (see Chapter 10). Specific assessments by a physician are required to validate each of the criteria.
- The patient's clinical manifestations indicate that brain death has occurred.
- Although there is a slight chance that the patient's heart function could be resuscitated and supported with mechanical ventilation, there is no obligation to provide medically futile care for a patient with brain death.
- Brain death criteria do not address patients in permanent vegetative state because the brainstem activity in these patients is adequate to maintain heart and lung function.

Critical Thinking Questions

1. What are your feelings about cessation of brain function versus cessation of heart and lung function as the criteria for death of a patient?
2. What are your state's laws or practices about stopping CPR efforts by EMS personnel in the field?

TABLE 55-9   Emergency Management — Head Injury

ETIOLOGY	ASSESSMENT FINDINGS	INTERVENTIONS
Blunt Motor vehicle collision Pedestrian event Fall Assault Sports injury **Penetrating** Gunshot wound Arrow	**Surface Findings** • Scalp lacerations • Fracture or depressions in skull • Bruises or contusions on face, Battle's sign (bruising behind ears) • Raccoon eyes (dependent bruising around eyes) **Respiratory** • Central neurogenic hyperventilation • Cheyne-Stokes respirations • Decreased O_2 saturation • Pulmonary edema **Central Nervous System** • Unequal or dilated pupils • Asymmetric facial movements • Garbled speech, abusive speech • Confusion • Decreased level of consciousness • Combativeness • Involuntary movements • Seizures • Bowel and bladder incontinence • Flaccidity • Depressed or hyperactive reflexes • Decerebrate or decorticate posturing • Glasgow Coma Scale score <12 • CSF leaking from ears or nose	**Initial** • Ensure patent airway. • Stabilize cervical spine. • Administer O_2 via nasal cannula or non-rebreather mask. • Establish IV access with two large-bore catheters to infuse normal saline or lactated Ringer's solution. • Control external bleeding with sterile pressure dressing. • Assess for rhinorrhea, otorrhea, scalp wounds. • Remove patient's clothing. **Ongoing Monitoring** • Maintain patient warmth using blankets, warm IV fluids, overhead warming lights, warm humidified O_2. • Monitor vital signs, level of consciousness, O_2 saturation, cardiac rhythm, Glasgow Coma Scale score, pupil size and reactivity. • Anticipate need for intubation if gag reflex is absent. • Assume neck injury with head injury. • Administer fluids cautiously to prevent fluid overload and increasing ICP.

CSF, Cerebrospinal fluid; *ICP,* intracranial pressure; *IV,* intravenous.

TABLE 55-10   Patient & Family Teaching Guide — Head Injury

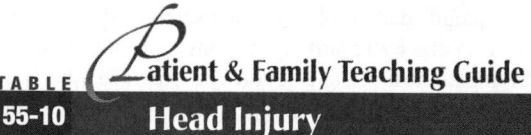

Teaching guidelines for the patient and family during the initial 2 to 3 days after a head injury include the following:

1. Notify your health care provider immediately if experiencing signs and symptoms that may indicate complications. These include:
   • Increased drowsiness (e.g., difficulty arousing, confusion)
   • Nausea and/or vomiting
   • Worsening headache or stiff neck
   • Seizures
   • Vision difficulties (e.g., blurring)
   • Behavioral changes (e.g., irritability, anger)
   • Motor problems (e.g., clumsiness, difficulty walking, slurred speech, weakness in arms or legs)
   • Sensory disturbances (e.g., numbness)
   • Decreased heart rate
2. Have someone stay with the patient.
3. Abstain from alcohol.
4. Check with your health care provider before taking drugs that may increase drowsiness, including muscle relaxants, tranquilizers, and narcotic pain medications.
5. Avoid driving, using heavy machinery, playing contact sports, and taking warm baths.

The nurse should explain the need for frequent neurologic assessments to both the patient and the family. Behavioral manifestations associated with head injury can result in a frightened, disoriented patient who is combative and resists help. The nurse's approach should be calm and gentle. A family member may be available to stay with the patient and thus prevent increasing anxiety and fear. Other teaching points are presented in Table 55-10.

The nurse should perform neurologic assessments at intervals based on the patient's condition. The GCS is useful in assessing the level of arousal (see Table 55-5). Indications of a deteriorating neurologic state, such as a decreasing LOC or a lessening of motor strength, should be reported to the health care provider, and the patient's condition should be closely monitored.

The major focus of nursing care for the brain-injured patient relates to increased ICP (see NCP 55-1). However, there may be specific problems that require nursing intervention.

Eye problems may include loss of the corneal reflex, periorbital ecchymosis and edema, and diplopia. Loss of the corneal reflex may necessitate administering lubricating eye drops, taping the eyes shut, or suturing the eyelids to prevent abrasion. Periorbital ecchymosis and edema disappear spontaneously, but cold and, later, warm compresses provide comfort and hasten the process. Diplopia can be relieved by use of an eye patch.

Hyperthermia may occur from injury to or inflammation of the hypothalamus. Elevations in body temperature can result in increased CBF, cerebral blood volume, and ICP.[3] Increased metabolism secondary to hyperthermia increases metabolic waste, which in turn produces further cerebral vasodilation. The nurse should attempt to control hyperthermia and maintain normothermia in the head-injured patient. There is some evidence to suggest that therapeutic hypothermia (32° to 35° C) may be beneficial during the first 24 hours following injury.[3]

If CSF rhinorrhea or otorrhea occurs, the nurse should inform the physician immediately. The patient should lie flat in bed unless this is contraindicated because of increased ICP. The head of the bed may be raised to decrease the CSF pressure so that a tear can seal. A loose collection pad may be placed under the nose or over the ear. No dressing should be placed into the nasal or ear cavities. The patient should be cautioned not to sneeze or blow the nose. Nasogastric tubes should not be used, and nasotracheal suctioning should not be performed on these patients.

Nursing measures specific to the care of the immobilized patient, such as those related to bladder and bowel function, skin care, and infection, are also indicated. Nausea and vomiting may be a problem and can be alleviated by antiemetic drugs. Headache can usually be controlled with acetaminophen or small doses of codeine.

If the patient's condition deteriorates, intracranial surgery may be necessary (see Cranial Surgery later in this chapter). A burr-hole opening or craniotomy may be indicated, depending on the underlying injury that is causing the symptoms. The emergency nature of the surgery may hasten the usual careful preoperative preparation. The nurse should consult with the neurosurgeon to determine specific preoperative nursing measures.

The patient is often unconscious before surgery, making it necessary for a family member to sign the consent form for surgery. This is a difficult and frightening time for the patient's family and requires sensitive nursing management. The suddenness of the situation makes it especially difficult for the family to cope.

Ambulatory and Home Care. Once the condition has stabilized, the patient is usually transferred for acute rehabilitation management to prepare the patient for reentry into the community. As with any craniocerebral problem, there may be chronic problems related to motor and sensory deficits, communication, memory, and intellectual functioning. Many of the principles of nursing management of the patient with a stroke are appropriate (see Chapter 56). Conditions that may require nursing and collaborative management include poor nutritional status, bowel and bladder management, spasticity, dysphagia, neurogenic heterotopic ossification (overgrowth of bone), deep vein thrombosis, and hydrocephalus. With time and patience, many of the chronic problems subside or disappear. The patient's outward appearance is not a good indicator of how well the patient will function in the home or work environment.

Seizure disorders are seen in approximately 5% of patients with a nonpenetrating head injury. The most vulnerable time for seizures to develop is during the first week after the head injury. Some patients may not develop a seizure disorder until years after the initial injury. Some health care providers recommend that antiseizure drugs be used prophylactically. Others may not institute treatment until a seizure is witnessed or an EEG demonstrates seizure activity. Phenytoin (Dilantin) is the antiseizure drug of choice in posttraumatic seizure activity.

The mental and emotional sequelae of brain trauma are often the most incapacitating problems. Many of the patients with head injuries who have been comatose for more than 6 hours undergo some personality change. They may suffer loss of concentration and

memory and defective memory processing. Personal drive may decrease; apathy and apparent laziness may increase. Euphoria and mood swings, along with a seeming lack of awareness of the seriousness of the injury, may occur. The patient's behavior may indicate a loss of social restraint, judgment, tact, and emotional control.

Progressive recovery may continue for 6 months or more before a plateau is reached and a prognosis for recovery can be made. Specific nursing management in the posttraumatic phase depends on specific residual deficits.

In all cases the family must be given special consideration. They need to understand what is happening and taught appropriate interaction patterns. The nurse must give guidance and referrals for financial aid, child care, and other personal needs and must assist the family in involving the patient in family activities whenever possible. Assisting the patient and family in developing and maintaining hope and keeping communication open are strategies perceived as supportive by families.[20,21]

The family often has unrealistic expectations of the patient as the coma begins to recede. The family expects full return to pretrauma status. In reality, the patient experiences a reduced awareness and ability to interpret environmental stimuli. The nurse must prepare the family for the emergence of the patient from coma and must explain that the process of awakening often takes several weeks.

When the time for discharge planning arrives, the family and the patient may benefit from very specific posthospital instructions to avoid family-patient friction.[22] Special "no" policies that may be appropriately suggested by the neurosurgeon, neuropsychologist, and nurse include no drinking of alcoholic beverages, no driving, no use of firearms, no work with hazardous implements and machinery, and no unsupervised smoking.[16] Family members, particularly spouses, go through role transition as the role changes from one of spouse to that of caregiver.

■ **Evaluation**

The expected outcomes are that the patient with a head injury will

- maintain normal cerebral perfusion pressure
- achieve maximal cognitive, motor, and sensory function
- experience no infection, hyperthermia, or pain

BRAIN TUMORS

The annual rate of newly diagnosed brain tumors in the United States is 17,000, with an estimated 13,100 deaths related to brain tumors.[22] The brain is also a frequent site for metastasis from other sites. Brain tumors rank fourth as cause of death from cancer in individuals 35 to 54 years of age. The incidence of

CULTURAL & ETHNIC CONSIDERATIONS
Brain Tumors

- Whites have a higher incidence of malignant brain tumors compared with African Americans.
- White males have the highest incidence of malignant brain tumors.
- African Americans have a higher incidence of benign brain tumors (e.g., meningiomas) compared with whites.
- Meningiomas are the most common brain tumor in many areas of Africa.

brain tumors has increased in the past 20 years, especially in older adults.[23]

Types

Brain tumors can occur in any part of the brain or spinal cord. Tumors of the brain may be *primary,* arising from tissues within the brain, or *secondary,* resulting from a metastasis from a malignant neoplasm elsewhere in the body. Secondary brain tumors are the most common type. Brain tumors are generally classified according to the tissue from which they arise. The most common primary brain tumors originate in astrocytes. These tumors are called gliomas (astrocytoma, glioblastoma multiforme) and account for 65% of primary brain tumors (Table 55-11). Glioblastoma multiforme is the most common primary brain tumor, followed by meningioma and astrocytoma. More than half of the brain tumors are malignant; they infiltrate the brain parenchyma and are not amenable to complete surgical removal. Other tumors may be histologically benign but are located such that complete removal is not possible. Brain tumors are more commonly seen in middle-aged persons, but they may occur at any age.

Unless treated, all brain tumors eventually cause death from increasing tumor volume leading to increased ICP. Brain tumors rarely metastasize outside the central nervous system (CNS) because they are contained by structural (meninges) and physiologic (blood-brain) barriers. Table 55-11 compares the major brain tumors. A glioblastoma and meningioma are depicted in Fig. 55-16.

Clinical Manifestations

The clinical manifestations of brain tumors depend mainly on the location and size of the tumor. The rate of growth and the appearance of manifestations depend on the location, size, and mitotic rate of the cells of tissue of origin. Fig. 55-17 illustrates the functional areas of the cerebral cortex and can be used as a guide to correlate manifestations with the location of the tumor.

Wide ranges of possible clinical manifestations are associated with brain tumors. Headache is a common problem. Tumor-related headaches tend to be worse at night and may awaken the patient. The headaches are usually dull and constant but occasionally throbbing. Seizures are common in gliomas and brain metastases. Brain tumors can cause nausea and vomiting from increased ICP. Cognitive dysfunction, including memory problems and mood or

TABLE 55-11   Types of Brain Tumors

TYPE	TISSUE OF ORIGIN	CHARACTERISTICS
Gliomas		
• Astrocytoma	Supportive tissue, glial cells and astrocytes	Can range from low-grade to moderate-grade malignancy
• Glioblastoma multiforme	Primitive stem cell (glioblast)	Highly malignant and invasive; among the most devastating of primary brain tumors
• Oligodendroglioma	Oligodendrocytes	Benign (encapsulation and calcification)
• Ependymoma	Ependymal epithelium	Range from benign to highly malignant; most are benign and encapsulated
• Medulloblastoma	Primitive neuroectodermal cell	Highly malignant and invasive; metastatic to spinal cord and remote areas of brain
Meningioma	Meninges	Can be benign or malignant; most are benign
Acoustic neuroma (Schwannoma)	Cells that form myelin sheath around nerves; commonly affects cranial nerve VIII	Many grow on both sides of the brain; usually benign or low-grade malignancy
Pituitary adenoma	Pituitary gland	Usually benign
Hemangioblastoma	Blood vessels of brain	Rare and benign; surgery is curative
Primary central nervous system lymphoma	Lymphocytes	Increased incidence in transplant recipients and acquired immunodeficiency syndrome (AIDS) patients
Metastatic tumors	Lungs, breast, kidney, thyroid, prostate	Malignant

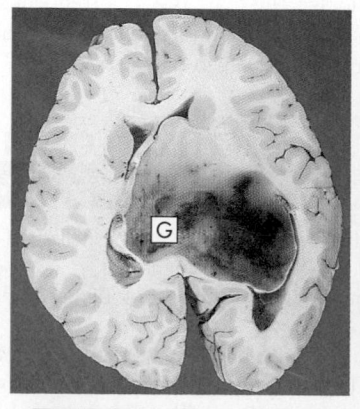
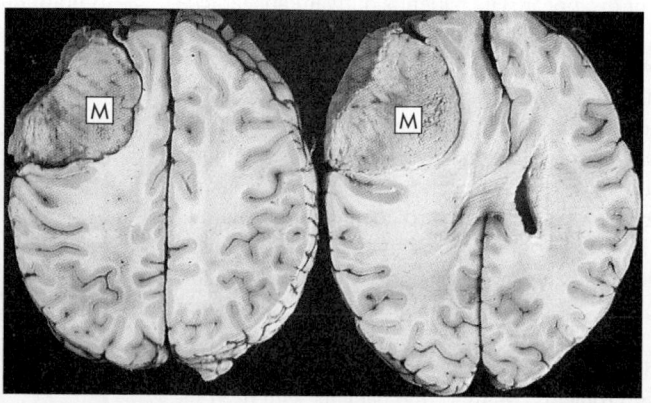

FIG. 55-16 A, Glioblastoma. A large glioblastoma *(G)* arises from one cerebral hemisphere and has grown to fill the ventricular system. B, Meningioma. These two different sections from different levels in the same brain show a meningioma *(M)* compressing the frontal lobe and distorting underlying brain.

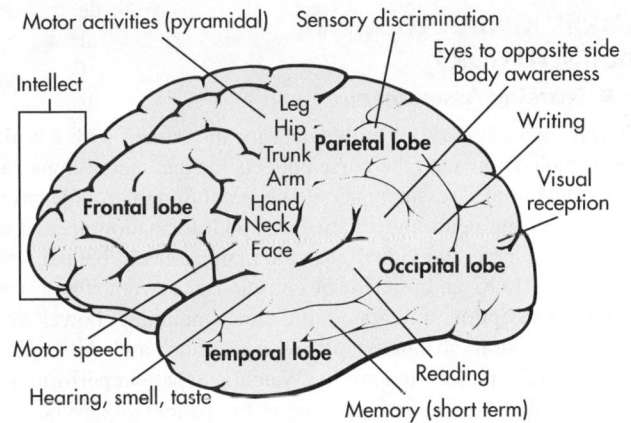

Motor activities (pyramidal)   Sensory discrimination

Eyes to opposite side
Body awareness

Intellect

Writing

Leg
Hip
Trunk   **Parietal lobe**
Arm
Hand
Neck
Face

Frontal lobe

Visual
reception

Occipital lobe

Motor speech   **Temporal lobe**

Hearing, smell, taste   Reading

Memory (short term)

FIG. 55-17 Each area of the brain controls a particular activity.

personality changes, is another common manifestation, especially in patients with brain metastases. Muscle weakness, sensory losses, aphasia, and visuospatial dysfunction are also manifestations of brain tumors. As the brain tumor expands, it may also produce manifestations of increased ICP, cerebral edema, or obstruction of the CSF pathways. Manifestations may clearly indicate the location of the tumor by an alteration in the function controlled by the affected area (Table 55-12).

Complications

If the tumor mass obstructs the ventricles or occludes the outlet, ventricular enlargement (hydrocephalus) can occur. Surgical treatment is necessary to relieve the pressure and involves placement of a ventriculoatrial or a ventriculoperitoneal shunt. A catheter with one-way valves is placed in the lateral ventricle and then tunneled through the skin to drain CSF into the right atrium or the peritoneum. Rapid decompression of ICP can cause prostration and headache that may be prevented by gradually introducing the patient to the upright position. The patient should be instructed to avoid contact sports that may result in a blow to the valve or shearing of the catheter. The health care provider should

be notified if signs of increased ICP occur, such as decreasing LOC, restlessness, headache, blurred vision, or vomiting without nausea. Signs of an infected shunt, such as high fever, persistent headache, and stiff neck, warrant investigation.

Diagnostic Studies

An extensive history and a comprehensive neurologic examination must be done in the workup of a patient with a suspected brain tumor. A careful history and physical examination may provide data with respect to location. Diagnostic studies are similar to those used for a patient with increased ICP (see Table 55-3). The sensitivity of techniques such as MRI and PET allows for detection of very small tumors and may provide more reliable diagnostic information. CT and brain scanning are used to diagnose the location of the lesion. Other tests include magnetic resonance spectroscopy, functional MRI, PET scans, and single photon emission computed tomography (SPECT). The EEG is useful but of less importance. A lumbar puncture is seldom diagnostic and carries with it the risk of cerebral herniation. Angiography can be used to determine blood flow to the tumor and further localize the tumor. Other studies are done to rule out a primary lesion elsewhere in the body. Endocrine studies are helpful when a pituitary adenoma is suspected (see Chapter 48).

The correct diagnosis of a brain tumor can be made by obtaining tissue for histologic study. In most patients, tissue is obtained at the time of surgery. A smear or frozen section can be performed in the operating room for a preliminary interpretation of the histologic type. With this information, the neurosurgeon can make a better decision about the extent of surgery. In some cases, immunohistochemical stains or electron microscopy may be necessary to ascertain the correct diagnosis. Determination of the MIB-1 index, a measure of mitotic rate, is often helpful in assessing the mitotic activity of a given tumor.

Collaborative Care

Treatment goals are aimed at (1) identifying the tumor type and location, (2) removing or decreasing tumor mass, and (3) preventing or managing increased ICP.

TABLE 55-12 Brain Tumor Locations and Presenting Manifestations	
TUMOR LOCATION	**PRESENTING MANIFESTATIONS**
Cerebral hemisphere	
• Frontal lobe (unilateral)	Unilateral hemiplegia, seizures, memory deficit, personality and judgment changes, visual disturbances
• Frontal lobe (bilateral)	Symptoms associated with unilateral frontal lobe tumors; ataxic gait
• Parietal lobe	Speech disturbance (if tumor is in the dominant hemisphere: inability to write, spatial disorders, unilateral neglect)
• Occipital lobe	Blindness and seizures
• Temporal lobe	Few symptoms; seizures, dysphagia
Subcortical	Hemiplegia; other symptoms may depend on area of infiltration
Meningeal tumors	Symptoms are associated with compression of the brain and depend on tumor location
Metastatic tumors	Headache, nausea, or vomiting because of ↑ ICP; other symptoms depend on tumor location
Thalamus and sellar tumors	Headache, nausea, vision disturbances, papilledema, and nystagmus occur from ↑ ICP; diabetes insipidus may occur
Fourth ventricle and cerebellar tumors	Headache, nausea, and papilledema from ↑ ICP; ataxic gait and changes in coordination
Cerebellopontine tumors	Tinnitus and vertigo, deafness
Brainstem tumors	Headache on awakening, drowsiness, vomiting, ataxic gait, facial muscle weakness, hearing loss, dysphagia, dysarthria, "crossed eyes" or other visual changes, hemiparesis

ICP, Intracranial pressure.

Surgical Therapy. Surgical removal is the preferred treatment for brain tumors (see Cranial Surgery later in this chapter). Stereotactic surgical techniques are used with greater frequency to perform a biopsy and remove small brain tumors. The outcome of surgical therapy depends on the type, size, and location of the tumor. Meningiomas and oligodendrogliomas can usually be completely removed, whereas the more invasive gliomas and medulloblastomas can be only partially removed. Computer-guided stereotactic biopsy, ultrasound, functional MRI, and cortical mapping can be used to localize brain tumors intraoperatively. Complete surgical removal is not always possible because the tumor is not always accessible or it has involved vital parts of the brain. Surgery can reduce tumor mass, which decreases ICP and provides relief of symptoms with an extension of survival time. Tumors located in the deep central areas of the dominant hemisphere, the posterior corpus callosum, or the upper brain-stem cause extensive neurologic damage and are considered probably inoperable.

Radiation Therapy and Radiosurgery. Radiation therapy is commonly used as a follow-up measure after surgery. Radiation seeds can also be implanted into the brain. Cerebral edema and rapidly increasing ICP may be a complication of radiation therapy, but they can be managed with high doses of corticosteroids (dexamethasone [Decadron], prednisone, or methylprednisolone [Solu-Medrol]). (Radiation therapy is discussed in Chapter 15.)

Stereotactic radiosurgery is a method of delivering a high concentrated dose of radiation precisely directed at a location within the brain. Stereotactic radiosurgery may be used when conventional surgery has failed or is not an option because of the tumor location. (Radiosurgery is discussed on p. 1516.)

Chemotherapy. The effectiveness of chemotherapy has been limited by difficulty getting drugs across the blood-brain barrier, tumor cell heterogeneity, and tumor cell drug resistance. A group of chemotherapeutic drugs called the nitrosoureas (e.g., carmustine [BCNU], lomustine [CCNU]) are particularly effective in treating brain tumors. Normally the blood-brain barrier prohibits the entry of most drugs into the brain. The most malignant tumors cause a breakdown of the blood-brain barrier in the area of the tumor, allowing chemotherapeutic agents to be used to treat the malignancy. Chemotherapy-laden biodegradable wafers (e.g., Gliadel wafer [polifeprosan with carmustine implant]) implanted at the time of surgery can deliver chemotherapy directly to the tumor site. Other drugs being used include methotrexate and procarbazine (Matulane). Two methods used to deliver chemotherapeutic drugs directly to the CNS are via an Ommaya reservoir (see Chapter 15) and intrathecal administration.

Temozolomide (Temodar) is the first oral chemotherapeutic agent found to cross the blood-brain barrier. In contrast with many traditional chemotherapies, which require metabolic activation to exert their effects, temozolomide has the ability to convert spontaneously to a reactive agent that directly interferes with tumor growth. It does not interact with other drugs commonly taken by patients with brain tumors such as antiseizure medications, corticosteroids, and antiemetics.

Many techniques to control and treat brain tumors are currently under investigation. These include local hyperthermia and biologic therapy. Although progress in treatment has increased length and quality of survival of patients with gliomas, outcomes still remain poor.[24]

NURSING MANAGEMENT
BRAIN TUMORS

■ Nursing Assessment

The subjective and objective data for the patient with a brain tumor include the data the nurse collects for the unconscious patient. The initial assessment should be structured to provide baseline data of the neurologic status and the information needed to design a realistic, individualized care plan. Areas to be assessed include the LOC and content of consciousness, motor abilities, sensory perception, integrated function (including bowel and bladder function), balance and proprioception, and the coping abilities of the patient and family. Watching a patient perform activities of daily living and listening to the patient's conversation are convenient ways to perform part of the neurologic assessment. Having the patient or the family explain the problem can be helpful in determining the patient's limitations and can also provide the nurse with information about the patient's insight into the problems. All initial data should be accurately recorded to provide a baseline for comparison to determine whether the patient's condition is improving or deteriorating.

Interview data are as important as the actual physical assessment. Questions concerning medical history, intellectual abilities and educational level, and history of nervous system infections and trauma should be asked. Determination of the presence of seizures, syncope, nausea and vomiting, pain, and headaches or other pain is important in planning care for the patient.

■ Nursing Diagnoses

Nursing diagnoses for the patient with a brain tumor may include, but are not limited to, the following:

- Impaired tissue perfusion (cerebral) *related to* cerebral edema
- Acute pain (headache) *related to* cerebral edema and increased ICP
- Self-care deficits *related to* altered neuromuscular function secondary to tumor growth and cerebral edema
- Anxiety *related to* diagnosis and treatment
- Potential complication: seizures *related to* abnormal electrical activity of the brain
- Potential complication: increased ICP *related to* presence of tumor and failure of normal compensatory mechanisms

■ Planning

The overall goals are that the patient with a brain tumor will (1) maintain normal ICP, (2) maximize neurologic functioning, (3) be free from pain and discomfort, and (4) be aware of the long-term implications with respect to prognosis and cognitive and physical functioning.

■ Nursing Implementation

A primary or metastatic tumor of the frontal lobe can cause behavioral and personality changes. Loss of emotional control, confusion, disorientation, memory loss, and depression may be signs of a frontal lobe lesion. These behavioral changes are often not perceived by the patient but can be disturbing and even frightening to the family. These changes can also cause a distancing to occur between the family and the patient. Assisting the family in understanding what is happening to the patient and supporting the family through this diagnostic phase are important roles for the nurse.

The confused patient with behavioral instability can be a challenge. Protecting the patient from self-harm is an important part of nursing care. At times when the patient manifests rage and aggression, the nurse must also be concerned about self-protection. Close supervision of activity, use of side rails, judicious use of restraints, padding of the rails and the area around the bed, and a calm, reassuring approach to care are all essential techniques in the care of these patients.

Perceptual problems associated with frontal lobe and parietal lobe tumors contribute to a patient's disorientation and confusion. Minimization of environmental stimuli, creation of a routine, and use of reality orientation can be incorporated into the care plan for the confused patient.

Seizures often occur with brain tumors. These are managed with antiseizure drugs. Seizure precautions should be instituted for the protection of the patient. Some behavioral changes seen in the patient with a brain tumor are a result of seizure disorders and can improve with control of the seizures by means of drugs (see Chapter 57).

Motor and sensory dysfunctions are problems that interfere with the activities of daily living. Alterations in mobility must be managed, and the patient should be encouraged to provide as much self-care as physically possible. Self-image often depends on the patient's ability to participate in care within the limitations of the physical deficits.

Language deficits can also occur in patients with brain tumors. Motor (expressive) or sensory (receptive) dysphasia may occur. The disturbance in communication can be frustrating for the patient and may interfere with the nurse's ability to meet the patient's needs. Attempts should be made to establish a communication system that can be used by both the patient and the staff.

Nutritional intake may be decreased because of the patient's inability to eat, loss of appetite, or loss of desire to eat. Assessing the nutritional status of the patient and ensuring adequate nutritional intake are important aspects of care. The patient may need encouragement to eat or, in some cases, may have to be fed orally, by gastrostomy or nasogastric tube, or by total parenteral nutrition. The patient with a brain tumor who undergoes cranial surgery requires complex nursing care. This is discussed in the next section.

■ Evaluation

The expected outcomes are that the patient with a brain tumor will

- be free of pain, vomiting, and other discomforts
- maintain ICP within normal limits
- demonstrate maximal neurologic function (cognitive, motor, sensory) with regard to the location and extent of the tumor
- maintain optimal nutritional status
- accept the long-term consequences of the tumor and its treatment

CRANIAL SURGERY

The cause or indication for cranial surgery may be related to a brain tumor, CNS infection (e.g., abscess), vascular abnormalities, craniocerebral trauma, epilepsy, or intractable pain (Table 55-13).

TABLE 55-13 Indications for Cranial Surgery

INDICATION	CAUSE	MANIFESTATIONS	PROCEDURE
Intracranial infection	Bacteria	*Early findings:* stiff neck, headache, fever, weakness, seizures *Later findings:* seizures, hemiplegia, speech disturbances, ocular disturbances, change in LOC	Excision or drainage of abscess
Hydrocephalus	Overproduction of CSF, obstruction to flow, defective reabsorption	*Early findings:* mental changes, disturbances in gait *Later findings:* memory impairment, urinary incontinence, increased tendon reflexes	Placement of ventriculoatrial or ventriculoperitoneal shunt
Brain tumors	Benign or malignant cell growth	Change in LOC, pupillary changes, sensory or motor deficit, papilledema, seizures, personality changes	Excision or partial resection of tumor
Intracranial bleeding	Rupture of cerebral vessels because of trauma or stroke	*Epidural:* momentary unconsciousness; lucid period, then rapid deterioration *Subdural:* headache, seizures, pupillary changes	Surgical evacuation through burr holes or craniotomy
Skull fractures	Trauma to skull	Headache, CSF leakage, cranial nerve deficit	Debridement of fragments and necrotic tissue, elevation and realignment of bone fragments
Arteriovenous (AV) malformation	Congenital tangle of arteries and veins (frequently in middle cerebral artery)	Headache, intracranial hemorrhage, seizures, mental deterioration	Excision of malformation
Aneurysm repair	Dilation of weak area in arterial wall (usually near anterior portion of circle of Willis)	*Before rupture:* headache, lethargy, visual disturbance *After rupture:* violent headache, decreased LOC, visual disturbances, motor deficit	Dissection and clipping or coiling of aneurysm

CSF, Cerebrospinal fluid; *LOC,* level of consciousness.

Types

Various types of cranial surgical procedures are presented in Table 55-14.

Stereotactic Surgery. Stereotactic surgery is neurosurgery using a precision apparatus (often computer-guided) to assist the surgeon to precisely target an area of the brain (Fig. 55-18). Stereotactic biopsy can be performed to obtain tissue samples

TABLE 55-14 Types of Cranial Surgery

TYPE	DESCRIPTION
Burr hole	Opening into the cranium with a drill; used to remove localized fluid and blood beneath the dura
Craniotomy	Opening into the cranium with removal of a bone flap and opening the dura to remove a lesion, repair a damaged area, drain blood, or relieve increased ICP
Craniectomy	Excision into the cranium to cut away a bone flap
Cranioplasty	Repair of a cranial defect resulting from trauma, malformation, or previous surgical procedure; artificial material used to replace damaged or lost bone
Stereotaxis	Precision localization of a specific area of the brain using a frame or a frameless system based on three-dimensional coordinates; procedure is used for biopsy, radiosurgery, or dissection
Shunt procedures	Alternate pathway to redirect cerebrospinal fluid from one area to another using a tube or implanted device; examples include ventriculoperitoneal shunt and Ommaya reservoir

ICP, Intracranial pressure.

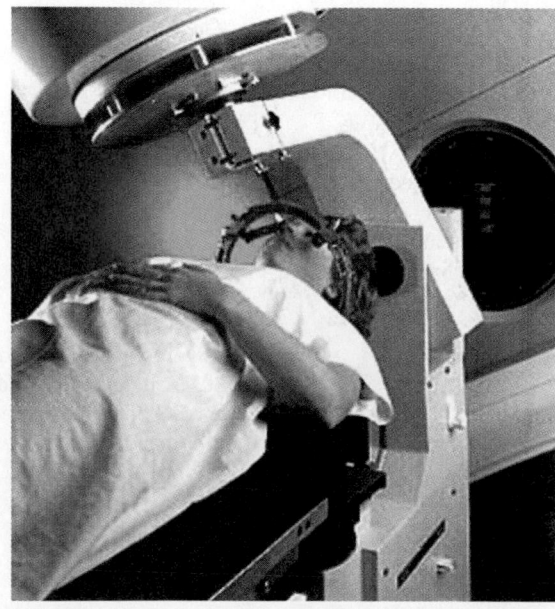

FIG. 55-18 Stereotactic frame.

for histologic examination. CT scanning and MRI are used to image the targeted tissue. With the patient under general or local anesthesia, the surgeon drills a burr hole or creates a bone flap for an entry site and then introduces a probe and biopsy needle. Stereotactic procedures are used for removal of small brain tumors and abscesses, drainage of hematomas, ablative procedures for extrapyramidal diseases (e.g., Parkinson's disease), and repair of arteriovenous malformations. A major advantage of the stereotactic approach is a reduction in damage to surrounding tissue.

Stereotactic radiosurgery is a procedure that involves closed-skull destruction of an intracranial target using ionizing radiation focused with the assistance of an intracranial guiding device. A sophisticated computer program is used while the patient's head is held still in a stereotactic frame. Radiosurgical techniques can use linear accelerator or a gamma knife. In the gamma knife procedure, a high dose of cobalt radiation is delivered to precisely targeted tumor tissue. The dose of radiation can be delivered over a single 4- to 6-hour treatment time. In some situations, some tumors are treated over several weeks.

In combination with stereotactic procedures to identify and localize tumor sites, surgical lasers can be used to destroy tumors. Stereotactic procedures are used to identify the tumor site. Three surgical lasers currently used include the carbon dioxide, argon, and neodymium: yttrium-aluminum-garnet (Nd:YAG) lasers. All three work by creating thermal energy, which destroys the tissue on which it is focused. Laser therapy also provides the benefit of reducing damage to surrounding tissue.

Craniotomy. Depending on the location of the pathologic condition, a craniotomy may be frontal, parietal, occipital, temporal, or a combination of any of these. A set of burr holes is drilled, and a saw is used to connect the holes to remove the bone flap. Sometimes operating microscopes are used to magnify the site. After surgery the bone flap is wired or sutured. Sometimes drains are placed to remove fluid and blood. Patients are usually cared for in an ICU until stable.

NURSING MANAGEMENT
CRANIAL SURGERY

■ Nursing Assessment

The nursing assessment of the patient undergoing cranial surgery would be similar to that for the patient with increased ICP (see pp. 1500-1502).

■ Nursing Diagnoses

Nursing diagnoses for the patient with cranial surgery are similar to that for the patient with increased ICP and may include, but are not limited to, those presented in NCP 55-1.

■ Planning

The overall goals are that the patient with cranial surgery will (1) return to normal consciousness, (2) be free from pain and discomfort, (3) maximize neuromuscular functioning, and (4) be rehabilitated to maximum ability.

■ Nursing Implementation

Acute Intervention. The general preoperative and postoperative nursing care for the patient undergoing cranial surgery is similar regardless of the cause. Nursing management is presented in NCP 55-1. The patient (if conscious and coherent) and the family will be gravely concerned about the potential physical and emotional problems that can result from surgery. The uncertainty regarding prognosis and outcome requires compassionate nursing care in the preoperative period.

Preoperative teaching is important in allaying the fears of the patient and the family and also in preparing them for the postoperative period. The patient and the family should be given general information concerning the type of operation that will be performed and what can be expected immediately after the operation. Explaining that some hair is shaved to allow for better exposure and prevention of contamination may prevent unnecessary concern over this task. The hair is usually removed in the operating room after induction of anesthesia. The family should also be informed that the patient will be taken to an ICU or to a special care unit after the operation.

The primary goal of care after cranial surgery is prevention of increased ICP. (Nursing management of the patient with increased ICP is presented on pp. 1502-1505.) Frequent assessment of the neurologic status of the patient is essential during the first 48 hours. In addition to the neurologic functions, fluids, electrolyte levels, and osmolality are monitored closely to detect changes in sodium regulation, the onset of diabetes insipidus, or severe hypovolemia. The turning and positioning of the patient sometimes depend on the site of the operation. If the surgical approach is in the posterior fossa, the patient is generally kept flat or at a slight elevation (10 to 15 degrees). Lying on the back will be prevented as much as possible, and flexion of the neck will be avoided to protect the suture line. The maximum swelling in the operative area occurs within 24 to 48 hours after the surgery.

The dressing is usually in place for 3 to 5 days. With an incision over the skull in the anterior or middle fossa, the patient will return from the operating room with the head elevated at an angle of 30 to 45 degrees. If a bone flap has been removed (craniectomy), care should be taken not to have the patient positioned on the operative side. The dressing should be observed for color, odor, and amount of drainage. The health care provider should be notified immediately of any excessive bleeding or clear drainage. Checking drains for placement and assessing the area around the dressing are also important. Scalp care should include meticulous care of the incision to prevent wound infection. The area should be cleansed with povidone iodine (Betadine) or a similar antiseptic disinfectant. Cleansing should be followed by application of an antibiotic ointment according to procedure. Once the dressing is removed, use of an antiseptic soap for washing the scalp may also be beneficial. The psychologic impact of hair removal can be alleviated by the use of a wig, turban, scarves, or cap after the incision has completely healed. For the patient who is receiving radiation, use of a sunblock and head covering should be advocated if any exposure to the sun is anticipated.

Ambulatory and Home Care. The rehabilitative potential for a patient after cranial surgery depends on the reason for the surgery, the postoperative course, and the patient's general state of health. Nursing interventions must be based on a realistic appraisal of these factors. An overall goal for the nurse is to foster independence for as long as possible and to the highest degree possible.

Specific rehabilitation potential cannot be determined until cerebral edema and increased ICP subside postoperatively. Care must be taken to maintain as much function as possible through measures such as careful positioning, meticulous skin and mouth care, regular range-of-motion exercises, bowel and bladder care, and adequate nutrition.

Referrals may be made to other specialists on the health care team. For example, the speech therapist may be helpful to the patient who has a speech problem, or the physical therapist may provide an exercise plan to regain functional deficits. The needs and problems of each patient should be addressed individually because many variables affect the plan.

The mental and physical deterioration of the patient, including seizures, personality disorganization, apathy, and wasting, is difficult for both family and health professionals to endure. Mental and emotional residual deficits are often more difficult for the patient and the family to accept than are motor and sensory losses. Although progress is continually being made to help the patient with a brain tumor by means of chemotherapy, conventional and interstitial radiation, and biologic therapies, the prognosis remains grim. The nurse can provide much help and support during the adjustment phase and in long-range planning.

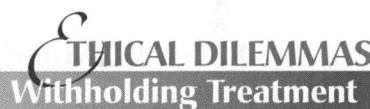

ETHICAL DILEMMAS
Withholding Treatment

Situation

A 26-year-old patient in a permanent vegetative state is diagnosed with her fifteenth bladder infection. Her home care nurse must determine whether or not to seek antibiotics for this infection. The family members have expressed a concern that no heroic measures be used to extend the biologic life of the patient, but they have been unwilling to withdraw the existing treatment, which is enteral nutrition through a gastrostomy tube. Should antibiotics be withheld?

Important Points for Consideration

- Patients in persistent vegetative state do not recover.
- Providing nutrition and hydration, even if by artificial means, can have significant cultural, religious, and psychologic meaning to patients and families.
- Clarification with the family about the goals of treatment and the patient's wishes, when she was competent and if they are known, is imperative. It is important to know whether treatment for an infection would be considered heroic based on the family's perspective of what the patient would want.
- The family's concerns about pain, suffering, and quality of life for the patient must be explored within the context of the overall plan of care.
- Withholding treatment is morally acceptable when a competent patient consents to it, if there is no medical benefit to the patient, if the treatment merely prolongs life, or if the burden of treatment outweighs the benefit to the patient.

Critical Thinking Questions

1. How would you approach the patient's family?
2. What are your feelings about providing nutrition, hydration, and treatments that will prolong life in a patient for whom there is no hope of recovery?

■ Evaluation

The expected outcomes are that the patient who has had cranial surgery will

- regain maximal cognitive, motor, and sensory function possible
- be free of infection
- have pain and discomfort alleviated
- be free of seizures
- have optimal nutritional intake

Inflammatory Conditions of the Brain

Meningitis, encephalitis, and brain abscesses are the most common inflammatory conditions of the brain and spinal cord. Inflammation can be caused by bacteria, viruses, fungi, and chemicals (e.g., contrast media used in diagnostic tests or blood in the subarachnoid space) (Table 55-15). CNS infections may occur via the bloodstream, by extension from a primary site, or along cranial and spinal nerves. The mortality rate is approximately 15% in the general population, with higher rates in elderly patients. Up to 15% of those who recover have long-term neurologic deficits.[25]

BACTERIAL MENINGITIS

Etiology and Pathophysiology

Meningitis is an acute inflammation of the pia mater and the arachnoid membrane surrounding the brain and the spinal cord. Therefore meningitis is always a cerebrospinal infection. Bacterial meningitis is considered a medical emergency. Untreated bacterial meningitis has a mortality rate approaching 100%. The organisms usually gain entry to the CNS through the upper respiratory tract or the bloodstream, but they may enter by direct extension from penetrating wounds of the skull or through fractured sinuses in basal skull fractures.

Meningitis usually occurs in the fall, winter, or early spring and is often secondary to viral respiratory disease. Older adults and persons who are debilitated are more often affected than is the general population. *Streptococcus pneumoniae* and *Neisseria meningitidis* are the leading causes of bacterial meningitis. *Haemophilus influenzae* was once the most common cause. However, the use of *H. influenzae* vaccine has resulted in a significant decrease in meningitis related to this organism.

The inflammatory response to the infection tends to increase CSF production, with a moderate increase in ICP. In bacterial meningitis the purulent secretions produced quickly spread to other areas of the brain through the CSF. If this process extends into the brain parenchyma or if concurrent encephalitis is present, cerebral edema and increased ICP become more of a problem. All patients with meningitis must be observed closely for manifestations of increased ICP, which is thought to be a result of swelling around the dura, and increased CSF volume.

Clinical Manifestations

Fever, severe headache, nausea, vomiting, and **nuchal rigidity** (resistance to flexion of the neck) are key signs of meningitis. A positive Kernig sign, a positive Brudzinski sign (see Chapter 54), photophobia, a decreased LOC, and signs of increased ICP may also be present. Coma is associated with a poor prognosis and occurs in 5% to 10% of patients with bacterial meningitis. Seizures occur in 20% of all cases.[26] With meningitis the headache be-

TABLE 55-15	Comparison of Cerebral Inflammatory Conditions		
	MENINGITIS	**ENCEPHALITIS**	**BRAIN ABSCESS**
Causative Organisms	Bacteria (*Streptococcus pneumoniae, Neisseria meningitidis*, group B streptococcus, viruses, fungi)	Bacteria, fungi, parasites, herpes simplex virus (HSV), other viruses (e.g., West Nile virus)	Streptococci, staphylococci through bloodstream
CSF			
Pressure (normal, 60-150 mm H$_2$O)	Increased	Normal to slight increase	Increased
WBC count (normal, 0-8/μl)	*Bacterial:* >1000/μl (mainly PMN) *Viral:* 25-500/μl (mainly lymphocytes)	500/μl, PMN (early), lymphocytes (later)	25-300/μl (PMN)
Protein (normal, 15-45 mg/dl [0.15-0.45 g/L])	*Bacterial:* >500 mg/dl *Viral:* 50-500 mg/dl	Slight increase	Normal
Glucose (normal, 45-75 mg/dl [2.5-4.2 mmol/L])	*Bacterial:* decreased *Viral:* normal or low	Normal	Low or absent
Appearance	*Bacterial:* turbid, cloudy *Viral:* clear or cloudy	Clear	Clear
Diagnostic Studies	Gram stain, smear, culture, PCR*	EEG, MRI, PET, PCR, IgM antibodies to virus in serum or CSF	CT scan, EEG, skull x-ray
Treatment	Antibiotics, supportive care, prevention of ↑ ICP	Supportive care, prevention of ↑ ICP, acyclovir (Zovirax) for HSV	Antibiotics, incision and drainage Supportive care

*PCR is used to detect viral RNA or DNA.

CSF, Cerebrospinal fluid; *CT*, computed tomography; *EEG*, electroencephalogram; *ICP*, intracranial pressure; *MRI*, magnetic resonance imaging; *PCR*, polymerase chain reaction; *PET*, positron emission tomography; *PMN*, polymorphonuclear cells; *WBC*, white blood cell.

comes progressively worse and may be accompanied by vomiting and irritability. If the infecting organism is a meningococcus, a skin rash is common and petechiae may be seen.

Complications

The most common acute complication of bacterial meningitis is increased ICP. More than 90% of patients will have increased ICP, and it is the major cause of unconsciousness. Another complication of bacterial meningitis is residual neurologic dysfunction. Cranial nerve dysfunction often occurs with cranial nerves III, IV, VI, VII, or VIII in bacterial meningitis. The dysfunction usually disappears within a few weeks. However, hearing loss may be permanent after bacterial meningitis.

Cranial nerve irritation can have serious sequelae. The optic nerve (CN II) is compressed by increased ICP. Papilledema is often present, and blindness may occur. When the oculomotor (CN III), trochlear (CN IV), and abducens (CN VI) nerves are irritated, ocular movements are affected. Ptosis, unequal pupils, and diplopia are common. Irritation of the trigeminal nerve (CN V) is evidenced by sensory losses and loss of the corneal reflex, and irritation of the facial nerve (CN VII) results in facial paresis. Irritation of the vestibulocochlear nerve (CN VIII) causes tinnitus, vertigo, and deafness.

Hemiparesis, dysphasia, and hemianopsia may also occur. These signs usually resolve over time. If resolution does not occur, a cerebral abscess, subdural empyema, subdural effusion, or persistent meningitis is suggested. Acute cerebral edema may occur with bacterial meningitis, causing seizures, CN III palsy, bradycardia, hypertensive coma, and death.

A noncommunicating hydrocephalus may occur if the exudate causes adhesions that prevent the normal flow of the CSF from the ventricles. CSF reabsorption by the arachnoid villi may also be obstructed by the exudate. Surgical implantation of a shunt is the only treatment.

A complication of meningococcal meningitis is the Waterhouse-Friderichsen syndrome. The syndrome is manifested by petechiae, disseminated intravascular coagulation (DIC), and adrenal hemorrhage. DIC is a serious complication of meningitis. (DIC is discussed in Chapter 30.) DIC is the cause of death in about 1% of patients with meningitis.

Diagnostic Studies

When a patient presents with manifestations suggestive of bacterial meningitis, a blood culture should be done. Diagnosis is usually verified by doing a lumbar puncture and analysis of the CSF. Variations in the CSF depend on the causative organism. Protein levels in the CSF are usually elevated and are higher in bacterial than in viral meningitis. Decreased CSF glucose concentration is common in bacterial meningitis and may be normal in viral meningitis. The CSF is purulent and turbid in bacterial meningitis; it may be the same or clear in viral meningitis. The predominant white blood cell type in the CSF during bacterial meningitis is polymorphonuclear cells (see Table 55-15). Specimens of the CSF, sputum, and nasopharyngeal secretions are taken for culture before the start of antibiotic therapy to identify the causative organism. A Gram stain is done to detect bacteria.

X-rays of the skull may demonstrate infected sinuses. CT scans and MRI may be normal in uncomplicated meningitis. In other cases, CT scans may reveal evidence of increased ICP or hydrocephalus.

Collaborative Care

Bacterial meningitis is a medical emergency. Rapid diagnosis based on history and physical examination is crucial because the patient is usually in a critical state when health care is sought. When meningitis is suspected, antibiotic therapy is instituted after the collection of specimens for cultures, even before the diagnosis is confirmed (Table 55-16). The fundus of the eye should be examined via ophthalmoscope for papilledema before lumbar puncture for identification of possible increased ICP.

Ampicillin, penicillin, cefuroxime (Ceftin), cefotaxime (Claforan), ceftriaxone (Rocephin), ceftizoxime (Cefizox), and ceftazidime (Ceptaz) are the drugs of choice for treating meningitis. These drugs are effective because of their ability to penetrate the blood-brain barrier.

NURSING MANAGEMENT
BACTERIAL MENINGITIS

■ Nursing Assessment

Initial assessment should include vital signs, neurologic evaluation, fluid intake and output, and evaluation of the lungs and skin (see Fig. 55-10).

■ Nursing Diagnoses

Nursing diagnoses for the patient with bacterial meningitis may include, but are not limited to, those presented in NCP 55-2.

■ Planning

The overall goals are that the patient with bacterial meningitis will have (1) return to maximal neurologic functioning, (2) resolution of infection, and (3) decreased pain and discomfort.

TABLE 55-16	*Collaborative Care* **Bacterial Meningitis**

Diagnostic
History and physical examination
Analysis of CSF for protein, glucose, WBC, Gram stain, and culture
CBC, coagulation profile, electrolyte levels, glucose, platelet count
Blood culture
CT scan, MRI, PET scan
Skull x-ray studies

Collaborative Therapy
Bed rest
IV fluids
Antibiotics IV
  ampicillin, penicillin
  cephalosporin (e.g., cefotaxime [Claforan], ceftriaxone [Rocephin])
Codeine for headache
Acetaminophen or aspirin for temperature above 100.4° F (38° C)
Hypothermia
Clear liquids as desired or tolerated
phenytoin (Dilantin) IV
furosemide (Lasix) or mannitol IV for diuresis

CBC, Complete blood count; *CSF,* cerebrospinal fluid; *CT,* computed tomography; *IV,* intravenous; *MRI,* magnetic resonance imaging; *PET,* positron emission tomography; *WBC,* white blood cell.

NURSING CARE PLAN 55-2

Patient with Bacterial Meningitis

EXPECTED PATIENT OUTCOMES	NURSING INTERVENTIONS and *RATIONALES*
NURSING DIAGNOSIS	**Disturbed sensory perception** *related to* decreased LOC *as manifested by* inaccurate interpretation of environment, signs of fear or anxiety, disorientation, and restlessness.
▪ Minimal disorientation ▪ Lack of evidence of agitation	▪ Assess LOC *to determine extent of the problem.* ▪ Administer sedative medication as ordered *to reduce fear and anxiety.* ▪ Keep room quiet and lights dim; use calm, reassuring approach *to avoid stimulating or frightening the patient.* ▪ Assist and support patient during uncomfortable or frightening diagnostic procedures; have family member at bedside when possible *to assist with orientation and reduce anxiety.*
NURSING DIAGNOSIS	**Acute pain** *related to* headache and muscle and joint aches *as manifested by* general discomfort of head, joints, and muscles; apathy; grimacing on movement.
▪ Satisfaction with pain relief ▪ Increased participation in treatment plan	▪ Administer mild analgesia as needed; assist patient to position of comfort in bed *to relieve pain.* ▪ Encourage gentle range-of-motion and leg exercises *to reduce joint stiffness and promote circulation.* ▪ Massage muscles as needed or requested *to promote comfort and show a caring attitude.* ▪ Control environment to encourage rest *because pain can be exhausting to the patient.*
NURSING DIAGNOSIS	**Hyperthermia** *related to* infection and abnormal temperature regulation by hypothalamus from increased ICP *as manifested by* increased temperature and chills.
▪ Normal body temperature	▪ Carry out general measures of care for patient with a fever.* ▪ If prescribed, use hypothermia blanket to reduce temperature *because an elevated temperature increases brain metabolism and increases the risk of seizures or increased ICP.* ▪ Reduce temperature gradually *to prevent shivering, which can cause a rebound effect and raise rather than lower the temperature.*
NURSING DIAGNOSIS	**Ineffective therapeutic regimen management** *related to* possible sequelae of condition *as manifested by* motor or sensory problems and activity limitations.
▪ Satisfactory management of condition by self or others	▪ Monitor for residual effects of condition such as vision, hearing, activity, and cognitive problems *to determine appropriate referrals.* ▪ Inform patient and others that residual problems often improve over time *to reduce anxiety.* ▪ Arrange for post-discharge care if required *so that patient's needs are met.*

COLLABORATIVE PROBLEMS

NURSING GOALS	NURSING INTERVENTIONS and *RATIONALES*
POTENTIAL COMPLICATION	**Seizure activity** *related to* cerebral irritation.
▪ Monitor for seizure activity ▪ Carry out appropriate medical and nursing interventions ▪ Report and record any seizure activity	▪ Monitor for seizure activity *so that interventions can be initiated immediately.* ▪ Keep side rails up and padded *to protect patient if a seizure occurs.* ▪ Administer sedative and antiseizure drugs as ordered *to control or prevent seizure activity.* ▪ Reduce fever *to decrease brain's oxygen demand.* ▪ Carry out interventions to treat underlying causes of inflammatory brain condition *to prevent seizure activity.*
POTENTIAL COMPLICATION	**Increased ICP** *related to* presence of infectious exudate, increased production of CSF.†

*See the Nursing Care Plan for the Patient with a Fever (NCP 12-1) on p. 219.
†See NCP 55-1 on p. 1503.
CSF, Cerebrospinal fluid; *ICP,* intracranial pressure; *LOC,* level of consciousness.

▪ Nursing Implementation

Health Promotion. Prevention of respiratory infections through vaccination programs for pneumococcal pneumonia and influenza should be supported by nurses.[27] In addition, early and vigorous treatment of respiratory and ear infections is important. Persons who have close contact with anyone who has bacterial meningitis should be given prophylactic antibiotics.

Acute Intervention. The patient with bacterial meningitis is usually acutely ill. The fever is high, and head pain is severe. Irritation of the cerebral cortex may result in seizures. The changes in mental status and LOC depend on the degree of increased ICP. Assessment of vital signs, neurologic evaluation, fluid intake and output, and evaluation of lung fields and skin should be performed at regular intervals based on the patient's condition and recorded carefully.

Head pain and neck pain secondary to movement require attention. Codeine provides some pain relief without undue sedation for most patients. The patient should be assisted to a position of comfort, often curled up with the head slightly extended. The head of the bed should be slightly elevated, when permitted after lumbar puncture. A darkened room and a cool cloth over the eyes relieve the discomfort of photophobia.

For the delirious patient, additional low lighting may be necessary to decrease hallucinations. All patients suffer some degree of mental distortion and hypersensitivity and may be frightened and misinterpret the environment. Every attempt should be made to minimize environmental stimuli and prevent injury. Restraints should be avoided. Armboards, secured with multiple layers of stretch gauze (e.g., Kerlix), protect the IV infusion site. The presence of a familiar person at the bedside has a calming effect. The nurse must be efficient with care but also should project an attitude of caring and of unhurried gentleness. The use of touch and a soothing voice to give simple explanations of activities is helpful. If seizures occur, appropriate observations should be made and protective measures should be taken. Antiseizure drugs such as phenytoin (Dilantin) are administered as ordered. Problems associated with increased ICP are also managed (see Increased ICP earlier in this chapter).

Fever must be vigorously managed because it increases cerebral edema and the frequency of seizures. In addition, neurologic damage may result from an extremely high temperature over a prolonged time. Acetaminophen or aspirin may be used to reduce fever. However, if the fever is resistant to aspirin or acetaminophen, more vigorous means are necessary, such as an automatic cooling blanket. Care should be taken not to reduce the temperature too rapidly because shivering may result, causing a rebound effect and increasing the temperature. The extremities should be wrapped in sheepskin, soft towels, or a blanket covered with a sheet to protect them from "frostbite." Care of the skin should be frequent to prevent breaks in the skin. If a cooling blanket is not available or desirable, tepid sponge baths with water may be effective in lowering the temperature. The skin must be protected from excessive drying and injury.

Because high fever greatly increases the metabolic rate and thus insensible fluid loss, the patient should be assessed for dehydration and adequacy of fluid intake. Diaphoresis further increases fluid losses, which should be estimated and included in an intake and output record. Replacement fluids should be calculated as 800 ml per day for respiratory losses and 100 ml for each degree of temperature above 100.4° F (38° C). Supplemental feeding to maintain adequate nutritional intake via tube or oral feedings may be necessary. The designated antibiotic schedule must be followed to maintain therapeutic blood levels. Observations should be made for side effects of the drugs used.

In most cases, meningitis does not require isolation, with the exception of meningococcal meningitis. However, good aseptic technique is essential to protect the patient and the nurse.

Ambulatory and Home Care. After the acute period has passed, the patient requires several weeks of convalescence before normal activities can be resumed. In this period, good nutrition should be stressed, with an emphasis on a high-protein, high-calorie diet in small, frequent feedings.

Muscle rigidity may persist in the neck and the backs of the legs. Progressive range-of-motion exercises and warm baths are useful. Activity should be gradually increased as tolerated, but adequate bed rest and sleep should be encouraged.

Residual effects are uncommon in meningococcal meningitis, but pneumococcal meningitis can result in sequelae such as dementia, seizures, deafness, hemiplegia, and hydrocephalus. Vision, hearing, cognitive skills, and motor and sensory abilities should be assessed after recovery, with appropriate referrals as indicated. Meningitis in infancy may have "silent" neurologic sequelae, which are manifested as learning and behavioral problems when the child reaches school age.

Throughout the acute and convalescent periods the nurse should be aware of the anxiety and stress experienced by individuals close to the patient.

■ Evaluation

The expected outcomes for the patient with bacterial meningitis are addressed in NCP 55-2.

VIRAL MENINGITIS

The most common causes of viral meningitis are enteroviruses, arboviruses, human immunodeficiency virus, and herpes simplex virus (HSV). Viral meningitis usually presents as a headache, fever, photophobia, and stiff neck. The fever may be moderate or high. There are usually no symptoms of brain involvement.

The most important diagnostic test is examination of the CSF. The typical finding is lymphocytosis (see Table 55-15). Organisms are not seen on Gram stain or acid-fast smears. Polymerase chain reaction (PCR) used to detect viral-specific DNA or RNA is the most important method for diagnosing CNS viral infections.

Viral meningitis is managed symptomatically because the disease is self-limiting. Antiviral therapy is not used. Full recovery from viral meningitis is expected. Rare sequelae include persistent headaches, mild mental impairment, and incoordination.

ENCEPHALITIS

Encephalitis, an acute inflammation of the brain, is a serious, and sometimes fatal, disease. In the United States, encephalitis is responsible for about 20,000 cases and 1400 deaths annually.[28]

Etiology and Pathophysiology

Encephalitis is usually caused by a virus. Many different viruses have been implicated in encephalitis, some of them associated with certain seasons of the year and endemic to certain geographic areas. Ticks and mosquitoes transmit epidemic encephalitis. Examples include Eastern equine encephalitis, Japanese encephalitis (rarely seen in the United States at this time), LaCrosse encephalitis, St. Louis encephalitis, West Nile virus, and Western equine encephalitis. Nonepidemic encephalitis may occur as a complication of measles, chickenpox, or mumps. HSV encephalitis is the most common cause of acute nonepidemic viral encephalitis. Cytomegalovirus encephalitis is one of the common complications in patients with acquired immunodeficiency syndrome (AIDS).

The West Nile virus was first identified in North America in New York City in the summer of 1999. Advanced age is the primary risk factor for encephalitis and mortality associated with this virus. The incubation period of West Nile Virus is from 3 to 14 days. Most cases are mild flulike symptoms. However, about 1 in 150 infections will result in severe neurologic disease, with encephalitis more commonly seen than meningitis.[29]

Clinical Manifestations and Diagnostic Studies

The onset of infection is typically nonspecific with fever, headache, nausea, and vomiting. It can be acute or subacute. Signs of encephalitis appear on day two or three and may vary from minimal alterations in mental status to coma. Virtually any CNS abnormality can occur, including hemiparesis, tremors, seizures, cranial nerve palsies, personality changes, memory impairment, amnesia, and dysphasia.

Early diagnosis and treatment of viral encephalitis are essential for favorable outcomes. Diagnostic findings related to viral encephalitis are shown in Table 55-15. Brain imaging techniques include MRI and PET. PCR tests for HSV DNA and RNA levels in CSF allow for early detection of HSV viral encephalitis.[30] West Nile virus should be strongly considered in adults over 50 years old who develop encephalitis or meningitis in summer or early fall. The best diagnostic test for West Nile virus is IgM antibody to the virus in serum or CSF collected within 8 days of illness onset. Because IgM dose not cross the blood-brain barrier, IgM antibody in the CSF strongly suggests CNS infection.

The clinical distinction between meningitis and encephalitis is based on brain function. Patients with meningitis may be uncomfortable, lethargic, or distracted by headache, but their cerebral function remains normal. In encephalitis, however, abnormalities in brain function are common, including altered mental status, motor or sensory deficits, and speech or movement disorders.

NURSING and COLLABORATIVE MANAGEMENT VIRAL ENCEPHALITIS

To prevent encephalitis, mosquito control should be practiced, including cleaning rain gutters, removing old tires, draining bird baths, and removing water where mosquitoes can breed. In addition, insect repellant should be used during mosquito season.

Collaborative and nursing management of encephalitis is symptomatic and supportive. Cerebral edema is a major problem, and diuretics (mannitol) and corticosteroids (dexamethasone [Decadron]) are used to control it. In the initial stages of encephalitis, many patients require intensive care.

Acyclovir (Zovirax) and vidarabine (Vira-A) are used to treat encephalitis caused by HSV infection. Acyclovir has fewer side effects than vidarabine and is often the preferred treatment. Use of these antiviral agents has been shown to reduce mortality rates although neurologic complications may not be reduced. For maximal benefit, antiviral agents should be started before the onset of coma. Seizure disorders should be treated with antiseizure drugs (see Table 57-9). Prophylactic treatment with antiseizure drugs may be used in severe cases of encephalitis. Treatment of cytomegalovirus encephalitis in AIDS patients is discussed in Chapter 14.

BRAIN ABSCESS

Brain abscess is an accumulation of pus within the brain tissue that can result from a local or a systemic infection. Direct extension from ear, tooth, mastoid, or sinus infection is the primary cause. Other causes for brain abscess formation include spread from a distant site (e.g., pulmonary infection, bacterial endocarditis) skull fracture, and a prior brain trauma or surgery. Streptococci and *Staphylococcus aureus* are the primary infective organisms.

Manifestations are similar to those of meningitis and encephalitis and include headache, fever, and nausea and vomiting. Signs of increased ICP may include drowsiness, confusion, and seizures. Focal symptoms may be present and reflect the local area of the abscess. For example, visual field defects or psychomotor seizures are common with a temporal lobe abscess, whereas an occipital abscess may be accompanied by visual impairment and hallucinations. Computed tomography (CT) and MRI are used to diagnose a brain abscess.

Antimicrobial therapy is the primary treatment for brain abscess. Other manifestations are treated symptomatically. If drug therapy is not effective, the abscess may need to be drained, or removed if it is encapsulated. In untreated cases, the mortality rate approaches 100%. Nursing measures are similar to those for management of meningitis or increased ICP. If surgical drainage or removal is the treatment of choice, nursing care is similar to that described under cranial surgery.

Other infections of the brain include subdural empyema, osteomyelitis of the cranial bones, epidural abscess, and venous sinus thrombosis after periorbital cellulitis.

CRITICAL THINKING EXERCISES

Case Study
Head Injury

Patient Profile. T.J. is a 43-year-old white man who was the driver of a motorcycle that ran into an automobile. He was sedated, paralyzed, and intubated by paramedics at the scene before transport by helicopter. He was brought to the emergency department with a diagnosis of closed head injury with skull fracture.

Subjective Data

He was reportedly unresponsive at the scene with a Glasgow Coma Scale score = 3, hypotension, tachycardia, and shallow irregular respirations.

Objective Data

At the Scene

- Unresponsive with obvious deformity to the left side of the skull
- Respirations were shallow and irregular

- O_2 saturations ranged from 90% to 95%
- Systolic blood pressure ranged from 50 to 80 mm Hg
- Heart rate ranged from 100 to 130 beats/min

In the ED

- Right pupil, 4 mm nonreactive; left pupil, 3 mm nonreactive
- Glasgow Coma Scale score = 3
- Hypotension and tachycardia continued in spite of fluid resuscitation

Diagnostic Studies

- CT of the head was positive for left skull fracture, left subdural hematoma, bilateral intraventricular and subarachnoid hemorrhage, and cerebral edema.
- CT of the abdomen/pelvis showed a lacerated liver, multiple infarcts to the right kidney, fluid around the duodenum and pancreas, and multiple left pelvic fractures.
- C-spine series was negative.

CRITICAL THINKING EXERCISES—cont'd

- Chest x-ray showed a right lung contusion and pneumo-mediastinum and subcutaneous emphysema.

CRITICAL THINKING QUESTIONS

1. What could be the cause of T.J.'s hypoxia, hypotension, and tachycardia?
2. How could the injuries impact his neurologic condition?
3. What area of the brain do T.J.'s clinical manifestations suggest may be injured?
4. What nursing interventions should be implemented? What are the priorities?
5. Based on the assessment data presented, write one or more nursing diagnoses. Are there any collaborative problems?

Nursing Research Issues

1. What type of information and education do families need at each stage of recovery for the head-injured patient?
2. What is the effect of nursing activities or interventions on intracranial pressure, cerebral perfusion pressure, cerebral blood flow, and cerebral tissue oxygenation?
3. What is the most valid noninvasive or continuous method for real-time monitoring of cerebral tissue perfusion and oxygenation?
4. Do cognitive stimulation programs decrease the frequency of cognitive and behavioral changes that occur after minor head injury?

REVIEW QUESTIONS

The number of the question corresponds to the same-numbered objective at the beginning of the chapter.

1. Vasogenic cerebral edema increases intracranial pressure by
   a. shifting fluid in the gray matter.
   b. altering the endothelial lining of cerebral capillaries.
   c. leaking molecules from the intracellular fluid to the capillaries.
   d. altering the osmotic gradient flow into the intravascular component.

2. A patient with intracranial pressure monitoring has pressure of 12 mm Hg. The nurse understands that this pressure reflects
   a. a severe decrease in cerebral perfusion pressure.
   b. an alteration in the production of cerebrospinal fluid.
   c. the loss of autoregulatory control of intracranial pressure.
   d. a normal balance between brain tissue, blood, and cerebrospinal fluid.

3. The nurse plans care for the patient with increased intracranial pressure with the knowledge that the best way to position the patient is to
   a. keep the head of the bed flat.
   b. elevate the head of the bed to 30 degrees.
   c. maintain patient on left side with head supported on pillow.
   d. use a continuous-rotation bed to continuously change patient position.

4. The nurse is alerted to a possible acute subdural hematoma in the patient who
   a. has a linear skull fracture crossing a major artery.
   b. has focal symptoms of brain damage with no recollection of a head injury.
   c. develops decreased level of consciousness and a headache within 48 hours of a head injury.
   d. has an immediate loss of consciousness with a brief lucid interval followed by decreasing level of consciousness.

5. During admission of a patient with a severe head injury to the emergency department, the nurse places the highest priority on assessment for
   a. patency of airway.
   b. presence of a neck injury.
   c. neurologic status with the Glasgow Coma Scale.
   d. cerebrospinal fluid leakage from the ears or nose.

6. A patient is suspected of having a cranial tumor. The signs and symptoms include memory deficits, visual disturbances, weakness of right upper and lower extremities, and personality changes. The nurse recognizes that the tumor is most likely located in the
   a. frontal lobe.
   b. parietal lobe.
   c. occipital lobe.
   d. temporal lobe.

7. Nursing management of a patient with a brain tumor includes
   a. discussing with the patient methods to control inappropriate behavior.
   b. using diversion techniques to keep the patient stimulated and motivated.
   c. assisting and supporting the family in understanding any changes in behavior.
   d. limiting self-care activities until the patient has regained maximum physical functioning.

8. The primary goal of nursing care after a craniotomy is
   a. preventing infection.
   b. ensuring patient comfort.
   c. avoiding the need for secondary surgery.
   d. preventing increased intracranial pressure.

9. A nursing measure that is indicated to reduce the potential for seizures and increased intracranial pressure in the patient with bacterial meningitis is
   a. administering codeine for relief of head and neck pain.
   b. controlling fever with prescribed drugs and cooling techniques.
   c. keeping the room darkened and quiet to minimize environmental stimulation.
   d. maintaining the patient on strict bed rest with the head of the bed slightly elevated.

REFERENCES

1. Cushing H: *Studies in intracranial physiology and surgery,* London, 1925, Oxford University Press.
2. Cold GE: Measurement of cerebral blood flow and oxygen consumption, and the regulation of cerebral circulation, *ACTA Neurochir Suppl* 49:1, 1990.
3. Wong FWH: Prevention of secondary brain injury, *Crit Care Nurs* 20:18, 2000.
4. Juul N et al: Intracranial hypertension and cerebral perfusion pressure: influence on neurological deterioration and outcome in severe head injury, *J Neurosurg* 92:1, 2000.
5. Bullock R et al: The Brain Trauma Foundation. The American Association of Neurological Surgeons. The Joint Section on Neurotrauma and Critical Care. Recommendations for intracranial pressure monitoring technology, *J Neurotrauma* 17:497, 2000.
6. Rebuck JA et al: Infection related to intracranial pressure monitors in adults: analysis of risk factors and antibiotic prophylaxis, *J Neurol Neurosurg Psychiatry* 69:381, 2000.
7. Kerr ME et al: Dose response to cerebrospinal fluid drainage on cerebral perfusion in traumatic brain-injured adults, *Neurosurg Focus* 11:Article 2, 2001.
8. Nau R: Osmotherapy for elevated intracranial pressure: a critical reappraisal, *Clin Pharmacokin* 38:23, 2000.
9. Yanagawa T et al: Nutritional support for head-injured patients (Cochrane Review), *Cochrane Database Syst Rev* 3:CD001530, 2002.
10. Jennett B, Teasdale G: Aspects of coma after severe head injury, *Lancet* 23:878, 1977.
11. Plum F, Posner J: *The diagnosis of stupor and coma,* ed 3, Philadelphia, 1980, FA Davis.
*12. Kerr ME et al: Effect of short-duration hyperventilation during endotracheal suctioning on intracranial pressure in severe head injured adults, *Nurs Res* 48:195, 1997.
13. Gemma M et al: Intracranial effects of endotracheal suctioning in the acute phase of head injury, *J Neurosurg Anesthesiol* 14:50, 2002.
14. Moraine JJ, Berre J, Melot C: Is cerebral perfusion pressure a major determinant of cerebral blood flow during head elevation in comatose patients with severe intracranial lesions? *J Neurosurg* 92:606, 2000.
15. Traumatic brain injury in the United States: a report to congress, 1999, Centers for Disease Control.
16. Traumatic brain injury in the United States, Centers for Disease Control. Available at www.cdc.gov/ncipc/didop/tbi (accessed August 22, 2002).
17. Marmarou A et al: Impact of ICP instability and hypotension on outcome in patients with severe head trauma, *J Neurosurg* 75:S59, 1991.
18. Meythaler JM et al: Current concepts: diffuse axonal injury-associated traumatic brain injury, *Arch Phys Med Rehabil* 82:1461, 2001.
19. Walleck C: Patients with head injury and brain dysfunction. In Clochesy JM et al, editors: *Critical Care Nursing,* ed 2, Philadelphia, 1996, WB Saunders.
20. Machamer J, Temkin N, Dikmen S: Significant other burden and factors related to it in traumatic brain injury, *J Clin Exp Neuropsychol* 24:420, 2002.
21. Boyle GJ, Haines S: Severe traumatic brain injury: some effects on family caregivers, *Psychol Rep* 90:415, 2002.

22. Paterson B, Kieloch B, Gmiterek J: "They never told us anything": postdischarge instruction for families of persons with brain injuries, *Rehabil Nurs* 26:48, 2001.
23. *Cancer Facts and Figures 2002,* Atlanta, 2002, American Cancer Society.
24. Stafford SI et al: Meningioma radiosurgery: tumor control, outcomes, and complications among 190 consecutive patients, *Neurosurgery* 49:1029, 2001.
25. Miner JR et al: Presentation, time to antibiotics, and mortality of patients with bacterial meningitis at an urban county medical center, *J Emerg Med* 21:387, 2001.
26. Choi C: Bacterial meningitis in aging adults, *Clin Infect Dis* 33:1380, 2001.
27. Patel M, Lee CK: Polysaccharide vaccines for preventing serogroup A meningococcal meningitis, *Cochrane Database Syst Rev* 3:CD001093, 2001.
28. Khetsuriani N, Holman RC, Anderson LJ: Burden of encephalitis-associated hospitalizations in the United States, 1988-1997, *Clin Infect Dis* 15; 35:175, 2002.
29. West Nile virus encephalitis, *N Engl J Med* 347:1225, 2002.
30. Simko JP et al: Differences in laboratory findings for cerebrospinal fluid specimens obtained from patients with meningitis or encephalitis due to herpes simplex virus (HSV) documented by detection of HSV DNA, *Clin Infect Dis* 35:414, 2002.

*Nursing research–based reference.

RESOURCES

American Brain Tumor Association
2720 River Road
Des Plaines, IL 60018
800-886-2282 or 847-827-9910
Fax: 847-827-9918
www.abta.org

Brain Injury Association of America
105 North Alfred Street
Alexandria, VA 22314
800-444-6443 (family helpline) or 703-236-6000
Fax: 703-236-6001
www.biausa.org

Brain Tumor Center
Massachusetts General Hospital/Harvard Medical School
Cox-315, 100 Blossom Street
Boston, MA 02114
617-724-8770
Fax: 617-724-8769
http://btc.mgh.harvard.edu

National Brain Tumor Foundation
414 Thirteenth Street, Suite 700
Oakland, CA 94612-2603
800-934-CURE (2873) (Brian Tumor Information Line) or
   510-839-9777
Fax: 510-839-9779
www.braintumor.org

For additional Internet resources, see the website for this book at *http://evolve.elsevier.com/Lewis/medsurg/.*

CHAPTER 56
NURSING MANAGEMENT
Stroke

Catherine Kirkness

LEARNING OBJECTIVES

1. Describe the incidence of and risk factors for stroke.
2. Explain mechanisms that affect cerebral blood flow.
3. Compare and contrast the etiology and pathophysiology of ischemic and hemorrhagic strokes.
4. Correlate the clinical manifestations of stroke with the underlying pathophysiology.
5. Identify diagnostic studies performed for patients with strokes.
6. Describe the collaborative care, drug therapy, and nutritional therapy for a patient with a stroke.
7. Describe the acute nursing management of the patient with a stroke.
8. Describe the rehabilitative nursing management of the patient with a stroke.
9. Explain the psychosocial impact of a stroke on the patient and family.

KEY TERMS

aneurysm, p. 1529	ischemic strokes, p. 1528
aphasia, p. 1531	lacunar stroke, p. 1529
dysarthria, p. 1531	stroke, p. 1525
dysphasia, p. 1531	subarachnoid hemorrhage, p. 1529
embolic stroke, p. 1529	
hemorrhagic strokes, p. 1529	thrombotic stroke, p. 1528
intracerebral hemorrhage, p. 1529	transient ischemic attack, p. 1527

Stroke occurs when there is *ischemia* (inadequate blood flow) to a part of the brain or hemorrhage into the brain that results in death of brain cells. Functions, such as movement, sensation, or emotions, that were controlled by the affected area of the brain are lost or impaired. The severity of the loss of function varies according to the location and extent of the brain involved.

Stroke is a major public health concern. An estimated 700,000 to 750,000 persons in the United States and 50,000 in Canada suffer a stroke annually.[1,2] Stroke is the third most common cause of death in the United States and Canada, behind cancer and heart disease.[2,3] Stroke is also a leading cause of serious, long-term disability. There are an estimated 4.5 million stroke survivors in the United States and up to 300,000 in Canada.[2,3] With an aging population, a further increase in stroke incidence can be expected.

Approximately 25% of individuals who have an initial stroke die within 1 year.[3] The percentage is higher for people age 65 and older. Of those who survive, 50% to 70% will be functionally independent, and 15% to 30% will live with permanent disability.[3] Common long-term disabilities include hemiparesis, inability to walk, complete or partial dependence in activities of daily living (ADLs), and aphasia. Over a lifetime, four out of five families will be affected by stroke.[4]

In addition to the physical, cognitive, and emotional impact of stroke on stroke survivors and their families, stroke also has an enormous financial impact. The direct and indirect costs of strokes are estimated to be greater than $51 billion per year in the United States and $2.7 billion per year in Canada.[1,2]

ETIOLOGY AND PATHOPHYSIOLOGY

Risk Factors for Stroke

The most effective way to decrease the burden of stroke is prevention. Awareness and control of modifiable risk factors can contribute to reducing the incidence and burden of stroke. Risk factors can be divided into nonmodifiable and modifiable. Stroke risk increases several-fold with multiple risk factors.

Nonmodifiable risk factors include age, gender, race, and heredity. Stroke risk increases with age, doubling each decade after 55 years of age. Two thirds of all strokes occur in individuals over 65 years, but stroke can occur at any age. The overall incidence and prevalence of stroke are almost equal for men and women, but women die more often from stroke than men.[3] Because women tend to live longer than men, they have more opportunity to suffer a stroke. African Americans have a higher incidence of stroke, as well as a higher death rate from stroke, than whites.[1] This may be related in part to a higher incidence of hypertension, obesity, and diabetes mellitus in African Americans. Hispanics, American Indians/Alaska Natives, and Asian Americans also have a higher stroke incidence than whites. A family history of stroke, a prior transient ischemic attack, or a prior stroke also increases the risk of stroke.[1]

CULTURAL & ETHNIC CONSIDERATIONS
Cerebrovascular Disease

- African Americans have a higher incidence of stroke and higher death rates from strokes than whites. This may be related to a higher incidence of hypertension, obesity, and diabetes mellitus in African Americans.
- Hispanics, Native Americans, and Asian Americans have a higher stroke incidence than whites.

Reviewed by Patricia A. Blissitt, RN, PhD, CCRN, CNRN, CCM, CS, Staff Nurse, Neurosurgical Intensive Care Unit, Harborview Medical Center, Seattle, Wash.

TABLE 56-1 Modifiable Risk Factors for Stroke

- Asymptomatic carotid stenosis
- Diabetes mellitus
- Heart disease, atrial fibrillation
- Heavy alcohol consumption
- Hypercoagulability
- Hyperlipidemia
- Hypertension
- Obesity
- Oral contraceptive use
- Physical inactivity
- Sickle cell disease
- Smoking

Modifiable risk factors are those that can potentially be altered through lifestyle changes and medical treatment, thus reducing the risk of stroke (Table 56-1). Hypertension is the single most important modifiable risk factor, but it is still often undetected and inadequately treated.[4] Increases in systolic and diastolic blood pressure independently increase the risk of stroke. Stroke risk can be reduced by up to 42% with appropriate treatment of hypertension.[5]

Heart disease, including atrial fibrillation, myocardial infarction, cardiomyopathy, cardiac valve abnormalities, and cardiac congenital defects, is also a risk factor for stroke. Of these, atrial fibrillation is the most important treatable cardiac-related risk factor.[6] The incidence of atrial fibrillation increases with age. Approximately 25% of strokes in patients over 80 years of age are due to atrial fibrillation.[7] Following myocardial infarction, nearly 8% of men and 11% of women will have a stroke within 6 years. Diabetes mellitus is a significant risk for stroke.[8,9] Although tight control of hypertension in diabetics significantly decreases stroke risk, tight control of blood glucose has not been shown to reduce stroke risk.[9]

Increased serum cholesterol is another risk factor for stroke.[10,11] Smoking nearly doubles the risk of stroke.[1,12] Fortunately, the risk associated with smoking decreases over time after quitting smoking and is reduced to that of nonsmokers by 5 years.[12] Asymptomatic carotid stenosis, which can be detected by the presence of a cervical bruit or by ultrasound testing, is another risk factor.[13]

Other modifiable risk factors include lifestyle habits such as excessive alcohol consumption, obesity, physical inactivity, poor diet, and drug abuse. The effect of alcohol on stroke risk appears to depend on the amount consumed. Moderate alcohol consumption (≤2 drinks/day) may be protective, but heavy alcohol consumption (>2 drinks/day) is associated with increased risk.[14,15] Abdominal obesity in men increases stroke risk, and obesity and weight gain in women increase the risk of ischemic stroke but not hemorrhagic stroke.[16] In addition, obesity is also associated with conditions such as hypertension, high blood glucose, and elevated blood lipid levels, which also increase stroke risk.

An association of physical inactivity and increased stroke risk is present in both men and women, regardless of ethnicity. Benefits of physical activity can occur with even light-to-moderate regular activity and may be in part related to the beneficial effect of exercise on other risk factors. The effect of diet on stroke risk is not clear, although a diet high in saturated fat and low in fruits and vegetables may increase stroke risk. Illicit drug use, commonly cocaine, has been associated with stroke risk.[17,18]

Older, high-dose estrogen oral contraceptives are strongly associated with increased stroke risk. A meta-analysis of studies looking at the relationship between low-dose (<50 μg) estrogen oral contraception and ischemic stroke concluded that low-dose estrogen use is associated with an increased risk of ischemic stroke, but the absolute risk is low, given a low incidence of stroke in this group of individuals.[19] The presence of other risk factors, particularly smoking and hypertension, in women taking oral contraceptives can increase stroke risk.[20] In 2002, data from the Women's Health Initiative (longitudinal intervention trial in middle-aged women) showed an increased risk of strokes in women taking estrogen plus progestin compared with those not receiving hormone replacement therapy. These data suggest that postmenopausal hormone replacement therapy does not protect against stroke.[21] Other conditions that may increase stroke risk include migraine headaches, inflammatory states, and hyperhomocysteinemia.

Hypercoagulation disorders predispose to vascular occlusive diseases including ischemic strokes, especially in younger adults.[22] Sickle cell disease is another known stroke risk factor for stroke.[1]

Pathophysiology

Anatomy of Cerebral Circulation. Blood is supplied to the brain by two major pairs of arteries: the internal carotid arteries (anterior circulation) and the vertebral arteries (posterior circulation). The carotid arteries branch to supply most of the frontal, parietal, and temporal lobes; the basal ganglia; and part of the diencephalon (thalamus and hypothalamus). The major branches of the carotid arteries are the middle cerebral and the anterior cerebral arteries. The vertebral arteries join to form the basilar artery, which branches to supply the middle and lower part of the temporal lobes, the occipital lobes, cerebellum, brainstem, and part of the diencephalon. The main branch of the basilar artery is the posterior cerebral artery. The anterior and posterior cerebral circulation is connected at the circle of Willis by the anterior and posterior communicating arteries (Fig. 56-1). Anomalies in this area are common, and all connecting vessels may not be present.

Regulation of Cerebral Blood Flow. The brain requires a continuous supply of blood to provide the oxygen and glucose that neurons need to function. Blood flow must be maintained at 750 to 1000 ml per minute (55 ml per 100 g of brain tissue), or 20% of the cardiac output, for optimal brain functioning. If blood flow to the brain is totally interrupted (e.g., cardiac arrest), neurologic metabolism is altered in 30 seconds, metabolism stops in 2 minutes, and cellular death occurs in 5 minutes.

The brain is normally well protected from changes in mean systemic arterial blood pressure over a range from 50 and 150 mm Hg by a mechanism known as *cerebral autoregulation*. This involves changes in the diameter of cerebral blood vessels in response to changes in pressure so that the blood flow to the brain stays constant. Cerebral autoregulation may be impaired following cerebral ischemia, and cerebral blood flow then changes directly in response to changes in blood pressure. Carbon dioxide is a potent cerebral vasodilator, and changes in arterial carbon dioxide levels have a dramatic effect on cerebral blood flow (increased carbon dioxide levels increase cerebral blood flow and vice versa). Very low arterial oxygen levels (partial pressure of arterial oxygen <50 mm Hg) or an increase in hydrogen ion concentration also increase cerebral blood flow.

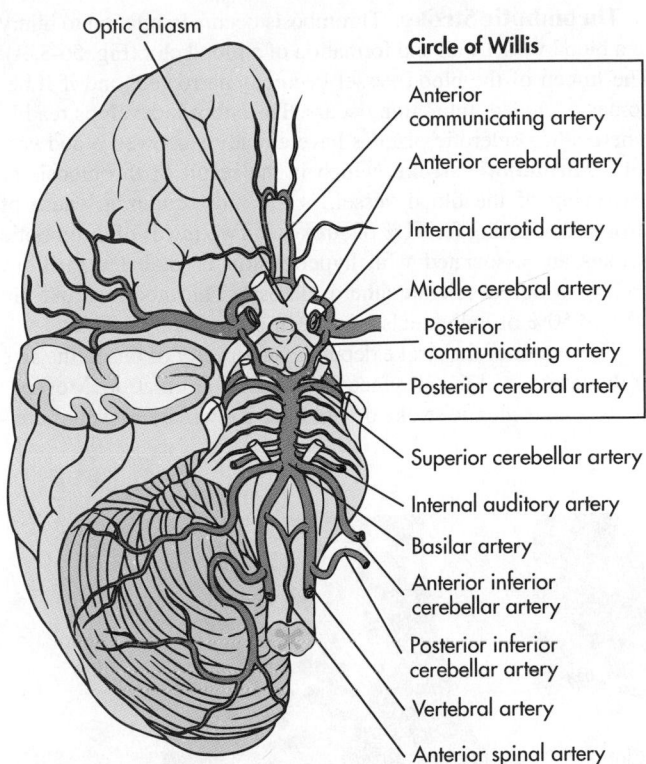

FIG. 56-1 Cerebral arteries and the circle of Willis. The tip of the temporal lobe has been removed to show the course of the middle cerebral artery.

Optic chiasm

Circle of Willis

Anterior communicating artery

Anterior cerebral artery

Internal carotid artery

Middle cerebral artery

Posterior communicating artery

Posterior cerebral artery

Superior cerebellar artery

Internal auditory artery

Basilar artery

Anterior inferior cerebellar artery

Posterior inferior cerebellar artery

Vertebral artery

Anterior spinal artery

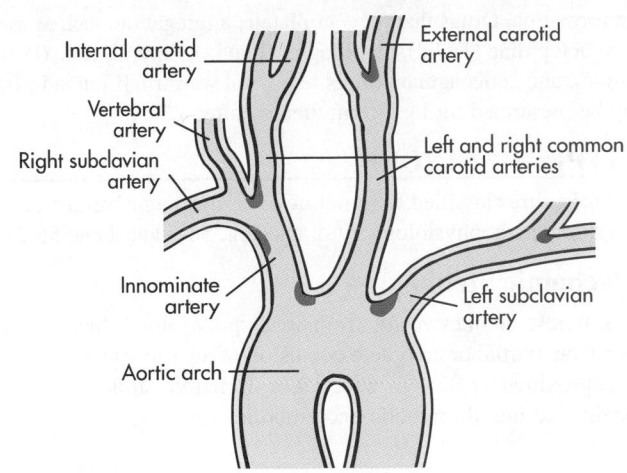

Internal carotid artery

External carotid artery

Vertebral artery

Right subclavian artery

Left and right common carotid arteries

Innominate artery

Left subclavian artery

Aortic arch

FIG. 56-2 Common sites for the development of atherosclerosis in extracranial and intracranial arteries. The main locations are just above the common carotid bifurcation (most common site) and the start of the branches from the aorta, innominate, and subclavian arteries.

Factors that affect blood flow to the brain include systemic blood pressure, cardiac output, and blood viscosity. During normal activity, oxygen requirements vary considerably, but changes in cardiac output, vasomotor tone, and distribution of blood flow normally maintain adequate blood flow to the head. Cardiac output has to be reduced by one third before cerebral blood flow is reduced. Changes in blood viscosity affect cerebral blood flow, with decreased viscosity increasing flow.

Collateral circulation may develop to compensate for a decrease in cerebral blood flow. Because of the connections between arteries at the circle of Willis, an area of the brain can potentially receive blood supply from another blood vessel if its original blood supply is cut off (e.g., because of thrombosis). Individual differences in collateral circulation partly determine the degree of brain damage and functional loss when a stroke occurs.

Intracranial pressure (ICP) also influences cerebral blood flow (see Chapter 55). Increased ICP causes brain compression and reduced cerebral blood flow.

Atherosclerosis. Atherosclerosis (hardening and thickening of arteries) is a major cause of stroke. It can lead to thrombus formation and contribute to emboli. (The role of atherosclerosis in thrombosis and emboli development is discussed in Chapter 33 and shown in Fig. 33-4.) Initially there is abnormal infiltration of lipids in the intimal layer of the artery. This fatty streak further develops into a plaque. Plaques often develop in areas of increased turbulence of the blood, such as at the bifurcation of an artery or a tortuous area (Fig. 56-2). Calcified, brittle plaques may rupture or fissure. Platelet and fibrin stick to the roughened plaque surface. Plaques lead to narrowing or occlusion of the artery. Also, parts of the plaque or thrombus can break off and travel to a nar-

rower distal artery. Cerebral infarction occurs when an artery becomes blocked and blood supply to the brain beyond the blockage is cut off.

In response to ischemia a series of metabolic events, termed the *ischemic cascade,* occur, including inadequate adenosine triphosphate (ATP) production, loss of ion homeostasis, release of excitatory amino acids (e.g., glutamate), free radical formation, and cell death.[23] Around the core area of ischemia is a border zone of reduced blood flow where ischemia is potentially reversible. If adequate blood flow can be restored early (e.g., within 3 hours) and the ischemic cascade can be interrupted, there may be less brain damage and less neurologic function lost. Research is ongoing to identify thrombolytic and neuroprotective therapies to reestablish blood flow and protect neurons from further ischemic damage.

Transient Ischemic Attack

A **transient ischemic attack** (TIA) is a temporary focal loss of neurologic function caused by ischemia of one of the vascular territories of the brain, lasting less than 24 hours and often lasting less than 15 minutes. Most TIAs resolve within 3 hours. TIAs may be due to microemboli that temporarily block the blood flow. TIAs are a warning sign of progressive cerebrovascular disease. The signs and symptoms of a TIA depend on the blood vessel that is involved and the area of the brain that is ischemic. If the carotid system is involved, patients may have a temporary loss of vision in one eye *(amaurosis fugax),* a transient hemiparesis, numbness or loss of sensation, or a sudden inability to speak. Signs of a TIA involving the vertebrobasilar system may include tinnitus, vertigo, darkened or blurred vision, diplopia, ptosis, dysarthria, dysphagia, ataxia, and unilateral or bilateral numbness or weakness.

Evaluation must be done to confirm that the signs and symptoms of a TIA are not related to other brain lesions, such as a developing subdural hematoma or an increasing tumor mass. Computed tomography (CT) of the brain without contrast is the most important initial diagnostic study. Cardiac monitoring and tests may reveal an underlying cardiac condition that is responsible for clot formation. Drugs that prevent platelet aggregation, such as aspirin, ticlopidine (Ticlid), clopidogrel (Plavix), dipyridamole (Persantine), and anticoagulant drugs (e.g., oral warfarin [Coumadin]), may be prescribed for long-term therapy after a TIA.

TYPES OF STROKE

Strokes are classified as ischemic or hemorrhagic based on the underlying pathophysiologic findings (Fig. 56-3 and Table 56-2).

Ischemic Stroke

Ischemic strokes result from inadequate blood flow to the brain from partial or complete occlusion of an artery and account for approximately 85% of all strokes. Ischemic strokes are further divided into thrombotic and embolic.

Thrombotic Stroke. Thrombosis occurs in relation to injury to a blood vessel wall and formation of a blood clot (Fig. 56-3, *A*). The lumen of the blood vessel becomes narrowed, and if it becomes occluded, infarction occurs. Thrombosis develops readily where atherosclerotic plaques have already narrowed blood vessels. **Thrombotic stroke,** which is the result of thrombosis or narrowing of the blood vessel, is the most common cause of stroke, accounting for 61% of strokes.[24] Two thirds of thrombotic strokes are associated with hypertension or diabetes mellitus, both of which accelerate atherosclerosis. Thrombotic strokes in 30% to 50% of individuals have been preceded by a TIA.

The extent of the stroke depends on rapidity of onset, the size of the lesion, and the presence of collateral circulation. Most patients with ischemic stroke do not have a decreased level of con-

A

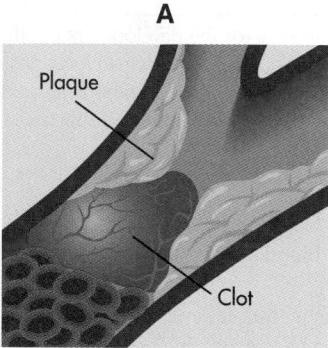

Thrombotic stroke. Cerebral thrombosis is a narrowing of the artery by fatty deposits called *plaque*. Plaque can cause a clot to form, which blocks the passage of blood through the artery.

B

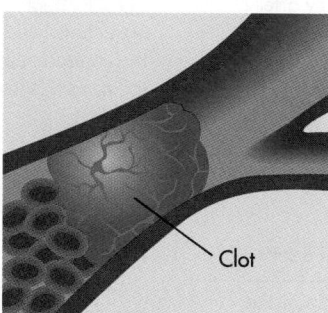

Embolic stroke. An embolus is a blood clot or other debris circulating in the blood. When it reaches an artery in the brain that is too narrow to pass through, it lodges there and blocks the flow of blood.

C

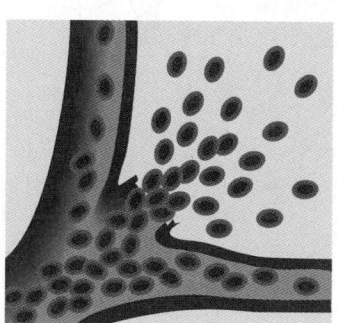

Hemorrhagic stroke. A burst blood vessel may allow blood to seep into and damage brain tissues until clotting shuts off the leak.

FIG. 56-3   Major types of stroke.

TABLE 56-2   Types of Stroke

TYPE	GENDER/AGE	WARNING	TIME OF ONSET	COURSE/PROGNOSIS
Ischemic				
Thrombotic	Men more than women, oldest median age	TIA (30%-50% of cases)	During or after sleep	Stepwise progression, signs and symptoms develop slowly, usually some improvement, recurrence in 20%-25% of survivors
Embolic	Men more than women	TIA (uncommon)	Lack of relationship to activity, sudden onset	Single event, signs and symptoms develop quickly, usually some improvement, recurrence common without aggressive treatment of underlying disease
Hemorrhagic				
Intracerebral	Slightly higher in women	Headache (25% of cases)	Activity (often)	Progression over 24 hr; poor prognosis, fatality more likely with presence of coma
Subarachnoid	Slightly higher in women, youngest median age	Headache (common)	Activity (often), sudden onset; Most commonly related to head trauma	Single sudden event usually, fatality more likely with presence of coma

TIA, Transient ischemic attack.

sciousness in the first 24 hours, unless it is due to a brainstem stroke or other conditions such as seizures, increased ICP, or hemorrhage. Ischemic stroke symptoms may progress in the first 72 hours as infarction and cerebral edema increase.

A **lacunar stroke** refers to a stroke from occlusion of a small penetrating artery with development of a cavity in the place of the infarcted brain tissue. This most commonly occurs in the basal ganglia, thalamus, internal capsule, or pons. Although a large percentage of lacunar strokes are asymptomatic, when present, symptoms can cause considerable deficits. These include pure motor hemiplegia, pure sensory stroke (contralateral loss of all sensory modalities), contralateral leg and face weakness with arm and leg ataxia, and isolated motor or sensory stroke. Multiple small vessel infarcts may also result in a decrease in cognitive function (i.e., multiinfarct dementia) (see Chapter 58).[25]

Embolic Stroke. **Embolic stroke** occurs when an embolus lodges in and occludes a cerebral artery, resulting in infarction and edema of the area supplied by the involved vessel (Fig. 56-3, *B*). Embolism is the second most common cause of stroke, accounting for about 24% of strokes.[24] The majority of emboli originate in the endocardial (inside) layer of the heart, with plaque breaking off from the endocardium and entering the circulation. The embolus travels upward to the cerebral circulation and lodges where a vessel narrows or bifurcates. Heart conditions associated with emboli include atrial fibrillation, myocardial infarction, infective endocarditis, rheumatic heart disease, valvular prostheses, and atrial septal defects. Less common causes of emboli include air and fat from long bone (femur) fractures.

The patient with an embolic stroke commonly has a rapid occurrence of severe clinical symptoms. Embolic strokes can affect any age group. Rheumatic heart disease is one cause of embolic stroke in young to middle-aged adults. An embolus arising from an atherosclerotic plaque is more common in older adults. Warning signs are less common with embolic than with thrombotic stroke. The onset of an embolic stroke is usually sudden and may or may not be related to activity. The patient usually remains conscious although may have a headache. Prognosis is related to the amount of brain tissue deprived of its blood supply. The effects of the emboli are initially characterized by severe neurologic deficits, which can be temporary if the clot breaks up and allows blood to flow. Smaller emboli then continue to obstruct smaller vessels, which in turn involve smaller portions of the brain with fewer deficits noted. The embolic stroke often occurs rapidly, and the body does not have time to accommodate by developing collateral circulation. Recurrence of embolic stroke is common unless the underlying cause is aggressively treated.

Hemorrhagic Stroke

Hemorrhagic strokes account for approximately 15% of all strokes and result from bleeding into the brain tissue itself (intracerebral or intraparenchymal hemorrhage) or into the subarachnoid space or ventricles (subarachnoid hemorrhage or intraventricular hemorrhage).

Intracerebral Hemorrhage. **Intracerebral hemorrhage** is bleeding within the brain caused by a rupture of a vessel (Fig. 56-3, *C*). Hypertension is the most important cause of intracerebral hemorrhage. Other causes include cerebral amyloid angiopathy, vascular malformations, coagulation disorders, anticoagulant and thrombolytic drugs, trauma, brain tumors, and ruptured aneurysms. Hemorrhage commonly occurs during periods of activity. There is most often a sudden onset of symptoms, with progression over minutes to hours because of ongoing bleeding. Symptoms include neurologic deficits, headache, nausea, vomiting, decreased level of consciousness (in about 50% of patients), and hypertension. The extent of the symptoms varies depending on the amount and duration of the bleeding. A blood clot within the closed skull can result in a mass that causes pressure on brain tissue, displaces brain tissue, and decreases cerebral blood flow, leading to ischemia and infarction.

Approximately half of intracerebral hemorrhages occur in the putamen and internal capsule, central white matter, thalamus, cerebellar hemispheres, and pons. Initially, patients experience a severe headache with nausea and vomiting. Clinical manifestations of putaminal and internal capsule bleeding include weakness of one side (including the face, arm, and leg) slurred speech, and deviation of the eyes. Progression of symptoms related to a severe hemorrhage includes hemiplegia, fixed and dilated pupils, abnormal body posturing, and coma. Thalamic hemorrhage results in hemiplegia with more sensory than motor loss. Bleeding into the subthalamic areas of the brain leads to problems with vision and eye movement. Cerebellar hemorrhages are characterized by severe headache, vomiting, loss of ability to walk, dysphagia, dysarthria, and eye movement disturbances. Hemorrhage in the pons is the most serious because basic life functions (e.g., respiration) are rapidly affected. Hemorrhage in the pons can be characterized by hemiplegia leading to complete paralysis, coma, abnormal body posturing, fixed pupils, hyperthermia, and death. The prognosis of patients with intracerebral hemorrhage is poor, with over 50% of patients dying soon after the hemorrhage occurs and only about 20% being functionally independent at 6 months.[26]

Subarachnoid Hemorrhage. **Subarachnoid hemorrhage** occurs when there is intracranial bleeding into the cerebrospinal fluid–filled space between the arachnoid and pia mater membranes on the surface of the brain. Subarachnoid hemorrhage is commonly caused by rupture of a cerebral **aneurysm** (congenital or acquired weakness and ballooning of vessels). Aneurysms may be saccular or berry aneurysms ranging from a few millimeters to 20 to 30 mm in size or fusiform atherosclerotic aneurysms. The majority of aneurysms are in the circle of Willis. Other causes of subarachnoid hemorrhage include arteriovenous malformations (AVMs), trauma, and illicit drug (cocaine) abuse. The annual incidence of subarachnoid hemorrhage caused by ruptured aneurysm is 6 to 16 per 100,000.[27] The incidence increases with age and is higher in women than men.

The patient may have warning symptoms if the ballooning artery applies pressure to brain tissue or minor warning symptoms from leaking of an aneurysm before major rupture. The characteristic presentation of a ruptured aneurysm is the sudden onset of a severe headache that is different from a previous headache and typically the "worst headache of one's life." Loss of consciousness may or may not occur, and the patient's level of consciousness may range from alert to comatose, depending on the severity of the bleed. Other symptoms include focal neurologic deficits (including cranial nerve deficits), nausea, vomiting, seizures, and stiff neck. Despite improvements in surgical techniques and management, many patients with subarachnoid hemorrhage die, and many are left with significant morbidity, including cognitive difficulties.[27]

Complications of aneurysmal subarachnoid hemorrhage include rebleeding before surgery or other therapy is initiated and cerebral vasospasm (narrowing of the large blood vessels at the base of the brain), which can result in cerebral infarction. Cerebral vasospasm is most likely due to an interaction between the metabolites of blood and the vascular smooth muscle. During the lysis of subarachnoid blood clots, metabolites are released. These metabolites can cause endothelial damage and vasoconstriction. In addition, release of *endothelin* (a potent vasoconstrictor) may play a major role in the induction of cerebral vasospasm after subarachnoid hemorrhage.

The most frequent surgical procedure to prevent rebleeding is clipping of the aneurysm (Fig. 56-4). Endovascular techniques may also be used. In the procedure known as *coiling,* a metal coil can be inserted into the lumen of the aneurysm via interventional neuroradiology (Fig. 56-5). This results in thrombus formation around the coil, resulting in blockage of the aneurysmal sac. Interventions to treat cerebral vasospasm either before or following aneurysm clipping or coiling include administration of the calcium channel blocker nimodipine (Nimotop). Following aneurysmal occlusion, hyperdynamic therapy, including hemodilution, induced hypertension using vasoconstricting agents (e.g., phenylephrine or dopamine [Intropin]), and hypervolemia, may be instituted in an effort to increase the mean arterial pressure and increase cerebral perfusion. Volume expansion is achieved via crystalloid or colloid solution.

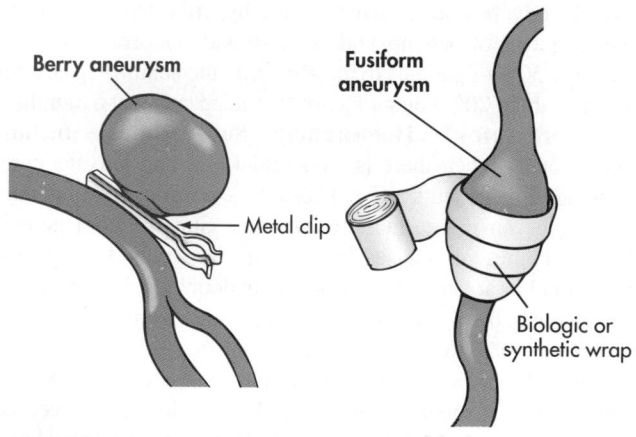

FIG. 56-4 Clipping and wrapping of aneurysms.

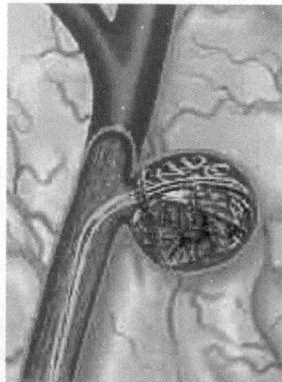

FIG. 56-5 Coil is used to occlude an aneurysmal sac. Soft platinum coil is attached to a stainless steel delivery wire. The softness allows the coil to conform to the often irregular shape of intracranial aneurysms.

Clinical Manifestations

A stroke can have an effect on many body functions, including motor activity, elimination, intellectual function, spatial-perceptual alterations, personality, affect, sensation, and communication. The functions affected are directly related to the artery involved and area of the brain it supplies (Table 56-3). Manifestations related to right- and left-brain damage differ somewhat and are shown in Fig. 56-6.

The term *brain attack* is increasingly being used to describe stroke and communicate the urgency of recognizing stroke symptoms and treating their onset as a medical emergency, similar to what would be done with a *heart attack.* Following the onset of stroke symptoms, immediate medical attention is crucial to reduce disability and death.

TABLE 56-3   Clinical Manifestations: Specific Cerebral Artery Involvement

Middle Cerebral Artery Involvement
Contralateral weakness (hemiparesis) or paralysis (hemiplegia)
Contralateral hemianesthesia; loss of proprioception, fine touch, localization
Dominant hemisphere: aphasia
Nondominant hemisphere: neglect of opposite side, anosognosia
Homonymous hemianopsia

Anterior Cerebral Artery Involvement
Occlusion of stem*
Occlusion distal to anterior communicating artery
- Contralateral sensory and motor deficits of foot and leg, greatest distally
- Contralateral weakness of proximal upper extremity
- Urinary incontinence (possibly unrecognized by patient)
- Sensory loss (discrimination, proprioception)
- Contralateral grasp and sucking reflexes may be present
- Apraxia
- Personality change: flat affect, loss of spontaneity, loss of interest in surroundings, distractibility, slowness in responding
- Possible cognitive impairment

Posterior Cerebral Artery and Vertebrobasilar Involvement†
Alert to comatose
Unilateral or bilateral sensory loss
Contralateral or bilateral weakness
Dysarthria
Dysphagia
Hoarseness
Ataxia
Horner syndrome: miosis, ptosis, decreased sweating
Vertigo
Unilateral hearing loss
Nausea, vomiting
Visual disturbances (blindness, homonymous hemianopsia, nystagmus, diplopia)

*There is usually no problem if the stem is occluded near the anterior communicating artery because perfusion from the opposite side is maintained.
†The site of occlusion, the origin of the basilar arteries, and the arrangement of the circle of Willis are involved in the type of deficit seen. This can occur from a thrombus or embolus.

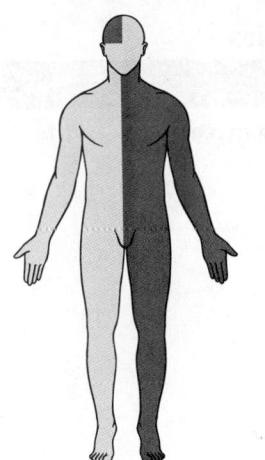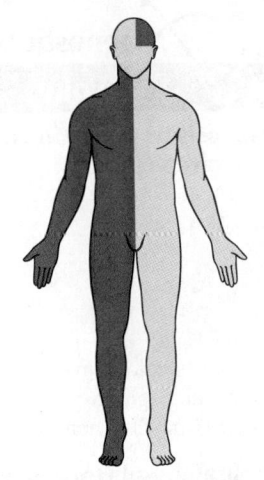

Right-brain damage (stroke on right side of the brain)	**Left-brain damage** (stroke on left side of the brain)
• Paralyzed left side: hemiplegia	• Paralyzed right side: hemiplegia
• Left-sided neglect	• Impaired speech/language aphasias
• Spatial-perceptual deficits	• Impaired right/left discrimination
• Tends to deny or minimize problems	• Slow performance, cautious
• Rapid performance, short attention span	• Aware of deficits: depression, anxiety
• Impulsive, safety problems	• Impaired comprehension related to language, math
• Impaired judgment	
• Impaired time concepts	

FIG. 56-6 Manifestations of right-brain and left-brain stroke.

Motor Function. Motor deficits are the most obvious effect of stroke. Motor deficits include impairment of (1) mobility, (2) respiratory function, (3) swallowing and speech, (4) gag reflex, and (5) self-care abilities. Symptoms are caused by the destruction of motor neurons in the pyramidal pathway (nerve fibers from the brain and passing through the spinal cord to the motor cells). The characteristic motor deficits include loss of skilled voluntary movement *(akinesia),* impairment of integration of movements, alterations in muscle tone, and alterations in reflexes. The initial *hyporeflexia* (depressed reflexes) progresses to *hyperreflexia* (hyperactive reflexes) for most patients.

Motor deficits after a stroke follow certain specific patterns. Because the pyramidal pathway crosses at the level of the medulla, a lesion on one side of the brain affects motor function on the opposite side of the brain (contralateral). The arms and legs of the affected side may be weakened or paralyzed to different degrees depending on which part of and to what extent the cerebral circulation was compromised. A stroke affecting the middle cerebral artery leads to a greater weakness in the upper extremity than the lower extremity. The affected shoulder tends to rotate internally, and the hip rotates externally. The affected foot is plantar flexed and inverted. An initial period of flaccidity may last from days to several weeks and is related to nerve damage. Spasticity of the muscles follows the flaccid stage and is related to interruption of upper motor neuron influence.

Communication. The left hemisphere is dominant for language skills in right-handed persons and in most left-handed per-

sons. Language disorders involve expression and comprehension of written and spoken words. The patient may experience **aphasia** (total loss of comprehension and use of language) when a stroke damages the dominant hemisphere of the brain. **Dysphasia** refers to difficulty related to the comprehension or use of language and is due to partial disruption or loss. Patterns of dysphasia may differ as the stroke affects different portions of the brain. Dysphasias can be classified as *nonfluent* (minimal speech activity with slow speech that requires obvious effort) or *fluent* (speech is present but contains little meaningful communication). Most dysphasias are mixed with impairment in both expression and understanding. A massive stroke may result in *global aphasia,* in which all communication and receptive function is lost.

Strokes affecting Wernicke's area of the brain exhibit symptoms of *receptive aphasia,* when neither the sounds of speech nor its meaning can be understood. This results in impairment of the patient's comprehension of both spoken and written language. Strokes affecting Broca's area of the brain cause *expressive aphasia* (difficulty in speaking and writing).

Many stroke patients also experience **dysarthria,** a disturbance in the muscular control of speech. Impairments may involve pronunciation, articulation, and phonation. Dysarthria does not affect the meaning of communication or the comprehension of language, but it does affect the mechanics of speech. Some patients experience a combination of aphasia and dysarthria.

Affect. Patients who have had a stroke may have difficulty controlling their emotions. Emotional responses may be exaggerated or unpredictable. Depression and feelings associated with changes in body image and loss of function can make this worse. Patients may also be frustrated by mobility and communication problems. An example of unpredictable affect is as follows. A reserved professional engineer has returned home from the hospital following a stroke. During meals with his family, he becomes frustrated and begins to cry because of the difficulty getting food into his mouth and chewing, something that he was able to do easily before his stroke.

Intellectual Function. Both memory and judgment may be impaired as a result of stroke. These impairments can occur with strokes affecting either side of the brain. A left-brain stroke is more likely to result in memory problems related to language. Patients with a left-brain stroke often are very cautious in making judgments. The patient with a right-brain stroke tends to be impulsive and to move quickly. An example of behavior with right-brain stroke is the patient who tries to rise quickly from the wheelchair without locking the wheels or raising the foot rests. The patient with a left-brain stroke would move slowly and cautiously from the wheelchair. Patients with either type of stroke may have difficulty making generalizations, which interferes with their ability to learn.

Spatial-Perceptual Alterations. A stroke on the right side of the brain is more likely to cause problems in spatial-perceptual orientation, although this can also occur with left-brain stroke. Spatial-perceptual problems may be divided into four categories. The first is related to the patient's incorrect perception of self and illness. This deficit follows damage to the parietal lobe. Patients may deny their illnesses or their own body parts. The second category concerns the patient's erroneous perception of self in space. The patient may neglect all input from the affected side. This may be worsened by *homonymous hemianopsia,* in which blindness occurs in the same half of the visual fields of both eyes. The patient also has difficulty with spatial orientation, such as judging distances. The third spatial-perceptual deficit is *agnosia*, the inability to recognize an object by sight, touch, or hearing. The fourth deficit is *apraxia*, the inability to carry out learned sequential movements on command. Patients may or may not be aware of their spatial-perceptual alterations.

Elimination. Fortunately, most problems with urinary and bowel elimination occur initially and are temporary. When a stroke affects one hemisphere of the brain, the prognosis for normal bladder function is excellent. At least partial sensation for bladder filling remains, and voluntary urination is present. Initially, the patient may experience frequency, urgency, and incontinence. Although motor control of the bowel is usually not a problem, patients are frequently constipated. Constipation is associated with immobility, weak abdominal muscles, dehydration, and diminished response to the defecation reflex. Urinary and bowel elimination problems may also be related to inability to express needs and to manage clothing.

Diagnostic Studies

When symptoms of a stroke occur, diagnostic studies are done to (1) confirm that it is a stroke and not another brain lesion, such as a subdural hematoma, and (2) identify the likely cause of the stroke (Table 56-4). Tests also guide decisions about therapy to prevent a secondary stroke. CT is the primary diagnostic test used after a stroke. CT can indicate the size and location of the lesion and differentiate between ischemic and hemorrhagic stroke. CT angiography (CTA) provides visualization of vasculature and can be performed at the same time as the CT scan. CTA allows detection of intracranial or extracranial occlusive disease. Serial CT scans may be used to assess the effectiveness of treatment and to evaluate recovery.

Magnetic resonance imaging (MRI) is used to determine the extent of brain injury. MRI has greater specificity compared with CT. Diffusion-weighted MRI is a more sensitive MRI that better delineates ischemic brain injury early after a stroke when CT and standard MRI may appear normal. Use of MRI may be restricted in patients with claustrophobia or with devices such as pacemakers that would be affected by the magnetic field. Magnetic resonance angiography (MRA) is a noninvasive method of assessing vascular occlusive disease in the head or neck, similar to CTA.

Other tests used to diagnose stroke and assess the extent of tissue damage include positron emission tomography (PET), magnetic resonance spectroscopy (MRS), xenon CT, single photon emission computed tomography (SPECT), and cerebral angiography. PET shows the metabolic activity of the brain and provides a depiction of the extent of tissue damage after a stroke. Less active or diseased tissue appears darker than healthy, active cells. MRS detects biochemical changes that may be present before physical changes are apparent. Its value in the clinical evaluation of stroke remains to be determined.

Angiography is the gold standard for imaging the carotid arteries. Angiography can identify cervical and cerebrovascular occlusion, atherosclerotic plaques, and malformation of vessels. Intraarterial digital subtraction angiography (DSA) reduces the dose of contrast material, uses smaller catheters, and shortens the length of the procedure compared with conventional angiography. DSA involves the injection of a contrast agent to visualize blood vessels in the neck and the large vessels of the circle of Willis. It is considered safer than cerebral angiography because

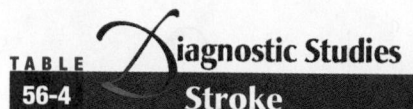

TABLE 56-4	Diagnostic Studies — Stroke
Diagnosis of Stroke, Including Extent of Involvement	CT, CTA MRI, MRA SPECT PET MRS Xenon CT Electroencephalogram Cerebral angiography Cerebrospinal fluid analysis*
Cerebral Blood Flow Measures	Cerebral angiography Digital subtraction angiography Doppler ultrasonography Transcranial Doppler Carotid duplex Carotid angiography
Cardiac Assessment	Electrocardiogram Chest x-ray Cardiac enzymes Echocardiography (transthoracic, transesophageal) Holter monitor (evaluation of arrhythmias)
Additional Studies	Complete blood count Platelets, prothrombin time, activated partial thromboplastin time Electrolytes, blood glucose Renal and hepatic studies Lipid profile Arterial blood gases (if hypoxia suspected)

*A lumbar puncture to obtain cerebrospinal fluid is avoided if increased intracranial pressure is suspected.

CT, Computed tomography; *CTA*, computed tomography angiography; *MRA*, magnetic resonance angiography; *MRI*, magnetic resonance imaging; *MRS*, magnetic resonance spectroscopy; *PET*, positron emission tomography; *SPECT*, single photon emission computed tomography.

less vascular manipulation is required. Risks of angiography include dislodging an embolus, vasospasm, inducing further hemorrhage, and allergic reaction to contrast media.

Transcranial Doppler (TCD) ultrasonography is a noninvasive study that measures the velocity of blood flow in the major cerebral arteries. TCD has been shown to be effective in detecting microemboli and vasospasm. Other neurodiagnostic tests such as skull x-rays, brain scan, lumbar puncture, and electroencephalogram (EEG) are currently used much less in the diagnosis of stroke. A skull x-ray result is usually normal after a stroke, but there may be a pineal gland shift with a massive infarction.

A lumbar puncture may be done to look for evidence of red blood cells in the cerebrospinal fluid if a subarachnoid hemorrhage is suspected but the CT does not show hemorrhage. A lumbar puncture is avoided if there are signs of increased ICP because of the danger of herniation of the brain downward leading to pressure on cardiac and respiratory centers in the brainstem and potentially death. An EEG may show low-voltage, slow-wave activity suggestive of ischemic infarction. If the stroke is due to a hemorrhage, the EEG may show high-voltage slow waves. If the suspected cause of the stroke includes emboli from the heart, diagnostic cardiac tests should be done (see Table 56-4).

Blood tests are also done to help identify conditions contributing to stroke and to guide treatment (see Table 56-4).

Collaborative Care

Prevention. Primary prevention is a priority for decreasing morbidity and mortality from stroke (Table 56-5). The goals of stroke prevention include health management for the well individual and education and management of modifiable risk factors to prevent a primary or secondary stroke. Health management focuses on (1) healthy diet, (2) weight control, (3) regular exercise, (4) no smoking, (5) limiting alcohol consumption, and (6) routine health assessments. Patients with known risk factors such as diabetes mellitus, hypertension, obesity, high serum lipids, or cardiac dysfunction require close management.

Drug therapy. Measures to prevent the development of a thrombus or embolus are used in patients at risk for stroke. Antiplatelet drugs are usually the chosen treatment to prevent further stroke in patients who have had a TIA related to atherosclerosis.[28] Aspirin is the most frequently used antiplatelet agent, commonly at a dose of 50 to 325 mg per day. Other drugs include ticlopidine (Ticlid), clopidogrel (Plavix), dipyridamole (Persantine), and combined dipyridamole and aspirin (Aggrenox). Oral anticoagulation using warfarin is the treatment of choice for individuals with atrial fibrillation who have had a TIA.[28]

Surgical therapy. Surgical interventions for the patient with TIAs from carotid disease include carotid endarterectomy, transluminal angioplasty, stenting, and extracranial-intracranial (EC-IC) bypass. In a carotid endarterectomy (CEA), the atheromatous lesion is removed from the carotid artery to improve blood flow[29] (Fig. 56-7).

Transluminal angioplasty is the insertion of a balloon to open a stenosed artery and improve blood flow. Stenting involves intravascular placement of a stent in an attempt to maintain patency of the artery. These procedures are still being evaluated as options to CEA.

EC-IC bypass involves anastomosing (surgically connecting) a branch of an extracranial artery to an intracranial artery (most commonly, superficial temporal to middle cerebral artery) beyond an area of obstruction with the goal of increasing cerebral perfusion. This procedure is generally reserved for those patients who do not benefit from other forms of therapy.[30] Further study is needed to determine the benefit of this therapy over medical therapy.

Acute Care. The goals for collaborative care during the acute phase are preserving life, preventing further brain damage, and reducing disability. Treatment differs according to the type of stroke and changes as the patient progresses from the acute to the rehabilitation phase.

TABLE 56-5	Collaborative Care
	Stroke

Diagnostic*
History and physical examination

Collaborative Therapy
Prevention
Control of hypertension
Control of diabetes mellitus
Treatment of underlying cardiac problem
Anticoagulation therapy for patients with atrial fibrillation
No smoking
Platelet inhibitors (e.g., aspirin)
Limiting alcohol intake
Surgical interventions for patients with aneurysms at risk of
   bleeding
Carotid endarterectomy
Stenting
Transluminal angioplasty
Extracranial-intracranial bypass
Acute Care
Maintenance of airway
Fluid therapy
Ischemic Stroke
Tissue plasminogen activator (tPA)
Anticoagulation
Ischemic and Hemorrhagic Stroke
Treatment of cerebral edema
Hemorrhagic Stroke
Surgical decompression if indicated
Subarachnoid Hemorrhage
Surgical obliteration (dependent on size and location of hemorrhage)
Embolic Stroke
Treatment of underlying cause

*Diagnostic studies are presented in Table 56-4.

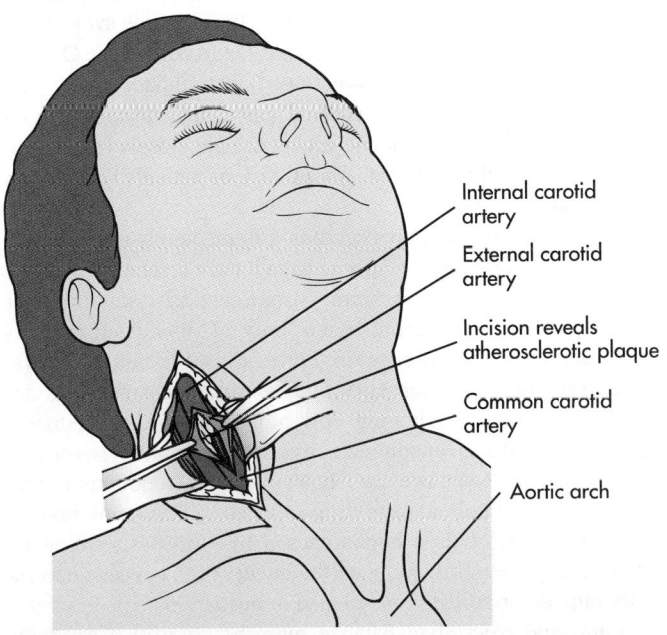

FIG. 56-7 Carotid endarterectomy. Atherosclerotic plaque in the internal carotid artery is removed to prevent impending cerebral infarction.

Internal carotid artery
External carotid artery
Incision reveals atherosclerotic plaque
Common carotid artery
Aortic arch

TABLE 56-6   Emergency Management   Stroke

ETIOLOGY	ASSESSMENT FINDINGS	INTERVENTIONS
• Sudden vascular compromise causing disruption of blood flow to the brain • Thrombosis • Trauma • Aneurysm • Embolism • Hemorrhage	• Altered level of consciousness • Weakness, numbness, or paralysis of portion of body • Speech or visual disturbances • Severe headache • Increased or decreased heart rate • Respiratory distress • Unequal pupils • Hypertension • Facial drooping on affected side • Difficulty swallowing • Seizures • Bladder or bowel incontinence • Nausea and vomiting • Vertigo	**Initial** • Ensure patent airway. • Remove dentures. • Perform pulse oximetry. • Maintain adequate oxygenation (SaO_2 >92%) with supplemental O_2, if necessary. • Establish IV access with normal saline. • Maintain BP according to guidelines (e.g., Advanced Cardiac Life Support).* • Remove clothing. • Obtain CT scan immediately. • Perform baseline laboratory tests, including blood glucose immediately, and treat if hypoglycemic. • Position head midline. • Elevate head of bed 30 degrees if no symptoms of shock or injury. • Institute seizure precautions. • Anticipate thrombolytic therapy for ischemic stroke. **Ongoing Monitoring** • Monitor vital signs and neurologic status, including level of consciousness (Glasgow Coma Scale), motor and sensory function, pupil size and reactivity, O_2 saturation, and cardiac rhythm. • Reassure patient and family.

BP, Blood pressure; *CT,* computed tomography; *IV,* intravenous.
*See Chapter 35.

Table 56-6 outlines the emergency management of the patient with a stroke. Acute care begins with managing the ABCs. Patients may have difficulty keeping an open and clear airway because of a decreased level of consciousness or decreased or absent gag and swallowing reflexes. Maintaining adequate oxygenation is important. Both hypoxia and hypercarbia are to be avoided because they can contribute to secondary neuronal injury. Oxygen administration, artificial airway insertion, intubation, and mechanical ventilation may be required. Baseline neurologic assessment is carried out, and patients are monitored closely for signs of increasing neurologic deficit. About 25% of patients will worsen in the first 24 to 48 hours.

Elevated blood pressure is common immediately after a stroke and may be a protective response to maintain cerebral perfusion. Immediately following ischemic stroke, use of drugs to lower blood pressure is recommended only if blood pressure is markedly increased (mean arterial pressure >130 mm Hg or systolic pressure >220 mm Hg). Oral antihypertensive drugs are generally preferred. Although low blood pressure immediately following stroke is uncommon, hypotension and hypovolemia should be corrected if present. Hypervolemic hemodilution using crystalloids and colloids and drug-induced hypertension may be used in patients with ischemia caused by vasospasm following subarachnoid hemorrhage once the aneurysm has been successfully clipped or coiled (coils placed in aneurysm sac).

Fluid and electrolyte balance must be controlled carefully. The goal generally is to keep the patient adequately hydrated to promote perfusion and decrease further brain injury. Overhydra-tion may compromise perfusion by increasing cerebral edema. Adequate fluid intake during acute care via oral, intravenous (IV), or tube feedings should be 1500 to 2000 ml per day. Urine output is monitored. If secretion of antidiuretic hormone (ADH) increases in response to the stroke, urine output decreases and fluid is retained. Low serum sodium (hyponatremia) may occur. IV solutions with glucose and water are avoided because they are hypotonic and may further increase cerebral edema and ICP. In addition, hyperglycemia may be associated with further brain damage and should be treated. In general, decisions regarding individualized fluid and electrolyte replacement therapy are based on the extent of intracranial edema, symptoms of increased ICP, central venous pressure levels, laboratory values for electrolytes, and intake and output.

Increased ICP is more likely to occur with hemorrhagic strokes but can occur with ischemic strokes. Increased ICP from cerebral edema usually peaks in 72 hours and may cause brain herniation. Management of increased ICP includes practices that improve venous drainage, such as elevating the head of the bed, maintaining head and neck in alignment, and avoiding hip flexion. Hyperthermia, which is seen commonly following stroke and may be associated with poorer outcome, is avoided. Increased temperature contributes to increased cerebral metabolism. Other measures include pain management, avoidance of hypervolemia, and management of constipation. Cerebrospinal fluid drainage may be used in some patients to reduce ICP. Diuretic drugs, such as mannitol (Osmitrol) and furosemide (Lasix), may be used to decrease cerebral edema. As a last resort in the management of ICP, a bone flap may be removed to allow for cerebral edema without increases in ICP. The bone flap is frozen and replaced later.[31]

Drug therapy. Recombinant tissue plasminogen activator (tPA) is used to reestablish blood flow through a blocked artery to prevent cell death in patients with the acute onset of ischemic stroke symptoms. Thrombolytic drugs, such as tPA, produce localized fibrinolysis by binding to the fibrin in the thrombi. The lytic action of tPA occurs as the plasminogen is converted to plasmin (fibrinolysin), whose enzymatic action digests fibrin and fibrinogen and thus lyses the clot. Because it is clot specific in its activation of the fibrinolytic system, tPA is less likely to cause hemorrhage compared with streptokinase or urokinase. (Thrombolytic therapy is discussed in Chapter 33.)

tPA must be administered within 3 hours of the onset of clinical signs of ischemic stroke. Therefore the single most important factor is timing. Patients are screened carefully before tPA can be given. Screening includes a CT or MRI scan to rule out hemorrhagic stroke, blood tests for coagulation disorders, and screening for recent history of gastrointestinal bleeding, stroke or head trauma within the past 3 months, or major surgery within 14 days. Thrombolytic therapy given within 3 hours of the onset of symptoms reduces disability, but at the expense of an increase in deaths within the first 7 to 10 days and an increase in intracranial hemorrhage.[32]

During infusion of the drug, the patient's vital signs and neurologic status are monitored closely to assess for improvement or for potential deterioration related to intracerebral hemorrhage. Control of blood pressure is critical during treatment and for 24 hours following. No anticoagulant or antiplatelet drugs are given for 24 hours after tPA treatment.

Patients with stroke caused by thrombi and emboli may also be treated with platelet inhibitors and anticoagulants (after the first 24 hours if treated with tPA) to prevent further clot formation. Common anticoagulants include heparin and warfarin (Coumadin, Panwarfin). Platelet inhibitors include aspirin, ticlopidine (Ticlid), clopidogrel (Plavix), and dipyridamole (Persantine). IV heparin or low-molecular-weight heparin may be given in the situation of rapidly evolving strokes or stroke caused by emboli traveling from the heart. IV heparin is administered via continuous infusion, and activated partial thromboplastin time is closely monitored.

Typically, heparin is replaced by oral warfarin for long-term administration. Warfarin dosage is regulated according to the international normalized ratio (INR), a standardized measure of prothrombin time that adjusts for assay variations. The therapeutic range for the INR is two to three times normal. Patients must be monitored closely for hemorrhage at other body sites while using anticoagulants and platelet inhibitors. A patient teaching guide for patients taking long-term warfarin is found in Table 37-14. Subcutaneous heparin may be administered for deep vein thrombosis prophylaxis.

Anticoagulants and platelet inhibitors are contraindicated for patients with hemorrhagic strokes. The calcium channel blocker nimodipine (Nimotop) is given to patients with subarachnoid hemorrhage to decrease the effects of vasospasm and minimize cerebral damage. Although nimodipine is a calcium channel blocker, its exact mechanism of action in reducing vasospasm is not known.[33]

Acetylsalicylic acid (aspirin) is also used to prevent platelet aggregation at the site of atherosclerotic plaque. Complications of aspirin include gastrointestinal bleeding with higher doses. Aspirin administration should be done cautiously if the patient has a history of peptic ulcer disease or is taking other anticoagulants.

Drug therapies to treat hyperthermia include aspirin or acetaminophen (Tylenol). A temperature elevation of even 1° C can increase brain metabolism by 10% and contribute to further brain damage. Cooling blankets may be used to cautiously lower temperature. The nurse must closely monitor the patient's temperature.[34]

Approximately 10% to 15% of patients who experience a stroke will have seizures, usually within 24 hours. An antiseizure drug, such as phenytoin (Dilantin), is given if a seizure occurs. The Stroke Council of the American Heart Association recommends uniform seizure prophylaxis in the acute period after intracerebral and subarachnoid hemorrhages.[35] In these patients, seizure activity may result in further neuronal injury and contribute to coma, although no clinical data support this recommendation. In other types of strokes, prophylactic use of antiseizure drugs is not recommended for patients who have not had a seizure.[35]

Surgical therapy. Surgical interventions for stroke include immediate evacuation of aneurysm-induced hematomas or cerebellar hematomas larger than 3 cm. Subarachnoid hemorrhage is usually caused by a ruptured aneurysm. Approximately 20% of patients will have multiple aneurysms. Treatment of an aneurysm involves clipping, wrapping, or coiling the aneurysm to prevent rebleeding (see Figs. 56-4 and 56-5). Treatment of arteriovenous malformation (AVM) is surgical resection and/or radiosurgery (i.e., gamma knife). Both may be preceded by interventional neuroradiology to embolize the blood vessels that supply the AVM.

Subarachnoid and intracerebral hemorrhage can involve bleeding into the ventricles of the brain. This situation produces hydro-

| TABLE 56-7 | Nursing Assessment Stroke |

Subjective Data
Important Health Information
Past health history: Hypertension; previous stroke, TIA, aneurysm, cardiac disease (including recent myocardial infarction), arrhythmias, congestive heart failure, valvular disease, infective endocarditis, hyperlipidemia, polycythemia, diabetes, gout, family history of hypertension, diabetes, stroke, or coronary artery disease
Medications: Use of oral contraceptives, use of and compliance with antihypertensive and anticoagulant agents
Functional Health Patterns
Health perception–health management: Positive family history; alcohol abuse, smoking
Nutritional-metabolic: Anorexia, nausea, vomiting; dysphagia, disturbances in taste and smell
Elimination: Change in bowel and bladder patterns
Activity-exercise: Loss of movement and sensation; syncope; weakness on one side; generalized weakness, easy fatigability
Cognitive-perceptual: Numbness, tingling of one side of the body; loss of memory; alteration in speech, language, problem-solving ability; pain; headache, possibly sudden and severe (hemorrhage); visual disturbances; denial of illness

Objective Data
General
Emotional lability, lethargy, apathy or combativeness, fever
Respiratory
Loss of cough reflex, labored or irregular respirations, tachypnea, rhonchi (aspiration), airway occlusion (tongue), apnea
Cardiovascular
Hypertension, tachycardia, carotid bruit
Gastrointestinal
Loss of gag reflex, bowel incontinence, decreased or absent bowel sounds, constipation
Urinary
Frequency, urgency, incontinence
Neurologic
Contralateral motor and sensory deficits, including weakness, paresis, paralysis, anesthesia; unequal pupils, hand grasps; akinesia, aphasia (expressive, receptive, global), dysarthria (slurred speech), agnosias, apraxia, visual deficits, perceptual or spatial disturbances, altered level of consciousness (drowsiness to deep coma) and Babinski sign, ↓ followed by ↑ deep tendon reflexes, flaccidity followed by spasticity, amnesia, ataxia, personality change, nuchal rigidity, seizures

Possible Findings
Positive CT, CTA, MRI, MRA, or other neuroimaging scans showing size, location, and type of lesion; positive Doppler ultrasonography and angiography indicating stenosis

CT, Computed tomography; *CTA,* computed tomography angiography; *MRA,* magnetic resonance angiography; *MRI,* magnetic resonance imaging; *TIA,* transient ischemic attack.

cephalus, which further damages brain tissue from increased ICP. Insertion of a ventriculostomy for cerebrospinal fluid drainage can result in dramatic improvement in these situations.

Rehabilitation Care. After the stroke has stabilized for 12 to 24 hours, collaborative care shifts from preserving life to lessening disability and attaining optimal function. The patient may be evaluated by a *physiatrist* (a physician who specializes in physical medicine and rehabilitation). It is important to remember that some aspects of rehabilitation actually begin in the acute care phase as soon as the patient is stabilized. Depending on the patient's status, other medical conditions, rehabilitation potential, and available resources, the patient may be transferred to a rehabilitation unit. Other options for rehabilitation include outpatient therapy and home care–based rehabilitation.

As part of the long-term collaborative care after a stroke, various members of the health care team may be involved in the effort to promote optimal function of the patient and family. The composition of the team depends on patient and family needs and rehabilitation facility resources.

NURSING MANAGEMENT STROKE

■ Nursing Assessment

Subjective and objective data that should be obtained from a person who has had a stroke are presented in Table 56-7. Primary assessment is focused on cardiac and respiratory status and neurologic assessment. If the patient is stable, the nursing history is obtained as follows: (1) description of the current illness with attention to initial symptoms, including onset and duration, nature (intermittent or continuous), and changes; (2) history of similar symptoms previously experienced; (3) current medications; (4) history of risk factors and other illnesses such as hypertension; and (5) family history of stroke or cardiovascular diseases. This information is gained through an interview of the patient, family members, significant others, or caregiver.

Secondary assessment should include a comprehensive neurologic examination of the patient. This includes (1) level of consciousness (Glasgow Coma Scale), (2) cognition, (3) motor abilities, (4) cranial nerve function, (5) sensation, (6) proprioception, (7) cerebellar function, and (8) deep tendon reflexes. Clear documentation of initial and ongoing neurologic examinations is essential to note changes in patient status.

■ Nursing Diagnoses

Nursing diagnoses for the person with a stroke may include, but are not limited to, those presented in NCP 56-1.

■ Planning

The patient, family, and nurse establish the goals of nursing care in a cooperative manner. Typical goals are that the patient will (1) maintain a stable or improved level of consciousness, (2) attain maximum physical functioning, (3) attain maximum self-care abilities and skills, (4) maintain stable body functions (e.g., bladder control), (5) maximize communication abilities, (6) maintain adequate nutrition, (7) avoid complications of stroke, and (8) maintain effective personal and family coping.

NURSING CARE PLAN 56-1

Patient with Stroke

NURSING DIAGNOSIS **Ineffective tissue perfusion (cerebral)** *related to* decreased cerebral blood flow secondary to thrombus, embolus, hemorrhage, or edema *as manifested by* ICP >15 mm Hg for 15 to 30 seconds or longer, decreasing Glasgow Coma Scale score, and altered respiratory pattern.

OUTCOMES–NOC

Tissue Perfusion: Cerebral (0406)
- Neurologic function _____
- Intracranial pressure WNL _____
- Unexplained anxiety not present _____
- Headache not present _____

_____

Outcome Scale
1 = Extremely compromised
2 = Substantially compromised
3 = Moderately compromised
4 = Mildly compromised
5 = Not compromised

INTERVENTIONS–NIC and *RATIONALES*

Cerebral Perfusion Promotion (2550)
- Assess neurologic status (ICP, LOC) at least hourly initially *to detect changes indicative of worsening or improving condition.*
- Monitor patient's ICP and neurologic response to activities *because ICP can increase with changes in positioning and movement.*
- Plan nursing care activities *to minimize increases in ICP.*
- Avoid neck flexion or extreme hip/knee flexion *to avoid obstruction of arterial and venous blood flow.*
- Monitor respiratory status *to assess changes in neurologic status.*

NURSING DIAGNOSIS **Ineffective airway clearance** *related to* inability to raise secretions *as manifested by* adventitious breath sounds, diminished breath sounds, and ineffective cough.

OUTCOMES–NOC

Respiratory Status: Airway Patency (0410)
- Moves sputum out of airway _____
- Free of adventitious breath sounds _____
- Choking not present _____

Outcome Scale
1 = Extremely compromised
2 = Substantially compromised
3 = Moderately compromised
4 = Mildly compromised
5 = Not compromised

INTERVENTIONS–NIC and *RATIONALES*

Cough Enhancement (3250)
- Assist patient to a sitting position with head slightly flexed, shoulders relaxed, and knees flexed *to provide optimal positioning for generating maximum intrathoracic pressure during cough.*
- Instruct patient to inhale deeply, bend forward slightly, and perform three or four huffs (against an open glottis) *to expel secretions.*
- Encourage use of incentive spirometry *to open collapsed alveoli, promote deep breathing, and prevent atelectasis.*

NURSING DIAGNOSIS **Impaired physical mobility** *related to* generalized weakness, muscle atrophy, or paralyzed extremities *as manifested by* decreased physical activity, limited range of motion, decreased muscle strength or control.

OUTCOMES–NOC

Mobility Level (0208)
- Balance performance _____
- Muscle movement _____
- Joint movement _____
- Ambulation: walking _____

_____

Outcome Scale
1 = Dependent, does not participate
2 = Requires assistive person and device
3 = Requires assistive person
4 = Independent with assistive device
5 = Completely independent

INTERVENTIONS–NIC and *RATIONALES*

Exercise Therapy: Muscle Control (0226)
- Assess and document range of motion, transfer abilities, and positioning ability *to determine extent of problem and plan appropriate interventions.*
- Determine patient's readiness to engage in activity or exercise protocol *to assess expected level of participation.*
- Maintain alignment with support pillows and footboard according to procedures; teach and assist family and patient with positioning techniques *to prevent contractures.*
- Encourage patient to practice exercises independently *to promote patient's sense of control.*
- Provide restful environment for patient after periods of exercise *to facilitate recuperation.*

ICP, Intracranial pressure; *LOC,* level of consciousness; *WNL,* within normal limits.

Continued

NURSING CARE PLAN 56-1

Patient with Stroke—cont'd

NURSING DIAGNOSIS **Impaired verbal communication** *related to* residual aphasia *as manifested by* refusal or inability to speak, word-finding problems, use of inappropriate words, inability to follow verbal directions.

OUTCOMES—NOC	INTERVENTIONS—NIC and *RATIONALES*
Communication: Expressive Ability (0903)	*Communication Enhancement: Speech Deficit (4976)*
▪ Use of spoken language: vocal _____ ▪ Use of written language _____ ▪ Use of sign language _____ ▪ Directs message appropriately _____ _____ **Outcome Scale** 1 = Extremely compromised 2 = Substantially compromised 3 = Moderately compromised 4 = Mildly compromised 5 = Not compromised	▪ Assess communication deficits and strengths *to determine type of communication problem and plan appropriate interventions.* ▪ Listen attentively *to convey the importance of patient's thoughts and to promote a positive environment for learning.* ▪ Provide positive reinforcement and praise *to build self-esteem and confidence.* ▪ Use short, simple questions that elicit "yes" and "no" answers; speak slowly and allow adequate time for response *to avoid overwhelming patient with verbal stimuli.* ▪ Provide verbal prompts and reminders (especially if patient is frustrated) *to assist patient to express self.*

NURSING DIAGNOSIS **Unilateral neglect** *related to* visual field cut and sensory loss on one side of body *as manifested by* consistent inattention to stimuli on affected side.

OUTCOMES—NOC	INTERVENTIONS—NIC and *RATIONALES*
Body Image (1200)	*Unilateral Neglect Management (2760)*
▪ Description of affected body part _____ ▪ Willingness to touch affected body part _____ ▪ Adjustment to changes in body function _____ ▪ Willingness to use strategies to enhance appearance and function _____ _____ **Outcome Scale** 1 = Never positive 2 = Rarely positive 3 = Sometimes positive 4 = Often positive 5 = Consistently positive	▪ Assess and document abnormal responses to three primary types of stimuli: sensory, visual, and auditory *to determine the presence of and degree to which unilateral neglect exists (i.e., inability to see objects on affected side, leaving food on a plate that corresponds to affected side, lack of sensation on affected side).* ▪ Teach patient to turn and look from left to right *to scan the entire environment.* ▪ Early in care, approach patient on unaffected side; place objects in patient's field of vision; give physical and verbal cues to aid in path finding *to compensate for visual field deficits.* ▪ Later in care, approach patient on affected side *to encourage patient to turn head.* ▪ Provide visual stimulation *to promote use of full range of visual capabilities.* ▪ Teach family and patient to stimulate paralyzed limbs using touch and warm and cold stimuli *to promote reintegration with the whole body.* ▪ Encourage patient to use cue cards and mirrors *as reminder to survey his/her whole body for position, cleanliness, and appropriate dress.*

NURSING DIAGNOSIS **Impaired urinary elimination** *related to* impaired impulse to void or inability to reach toilet or manage tasks of voiding *as manifested by* incontinence and flow of urine at unpredictable times.

OUTCOMES—NOC	INTERVENTIONS—NIC and *RATIONALES*
Urinary Continence (0502)	*Urinary Bladder Training (0570)*
▪ Recognizes urge to void _____ ▪ Responds in timely manner to urge _____ ▪ Maintains environment barrier free to independent toileting _____ ▪ Free of urine leakage between voidings _____ _____ **Outcome Scale** 1 = Never demonstrated 2 = Rarely demonstrated 3 = Sometimes demonstrated 4 = Often demonstrated 5 = Consistently demonstrated	▪ Keep a continence record for 3 days, specifically noting intake and output, *to establish voiding pattern and plan appropriate interventions.* ▪ Establish interval of initial toileting schedule based on voiding pattern *to initiate process of improving bladder functioning and increased muscle tone.* ▪ Toilet patient or remind patient to void at prescribed intervals *to assist patient in adapting to new toileting schedule.* ▪ Teach patient to consciously hold urine until the scheduled toileting time *to improve muscle tone.* ▪ Discuss daily record of continence with patient to provide reinforcement and *to allow time to ask questions, make comments, or share concerns.*

NURSING CARE PLAN 56-1

Patient with Stroke—cont'd

NURSING DIAGNOSIS   Impaired swallowing *related to* weakness or paralysis of affected muscles *as manifested by* drooling, difficulty in swallowing, choking.

OUTCOMES–NOC	INTERVENTIONS–NIC and *RATIONALES*
Swallowing Status (1010)	**Aspiration Precautions (3200)**
▪ Handles oral secretions _____	**Swallowing Therapy (1860)**
▪ Maintains food in mouth _____	▪ Assess patient *to determine ability to swallow and presence of gag reflex.*
▪ Choking, coughing, or gagging not present _____	▪ Assist patient to sit in an erect position (as close to 90-degree angle as possible) for feeding exercise *to provide optimal position for chewing and swallowing without aspirating.*
▪ Comfort with swallowing _____	▪ Teach patient to take small bites and place in unaffected side of mouth, keep chin down, and stroke throat *to stimulate swallowing.*
	▪ Assist to maintain sitting position for 30 minutes after completing meal *to prevent regurgitation of food.*
Outcome Scale	▪ Instruct caregiver on emergency measures for choking *to prevent complications in the home setting.*
1 = Extremely compromised	▪ After patient has eaten, check oral cavity for pocketed food and teach patient and family this technique *to prevent collection and putrefaction of food and resultant risk of infection.*
2 = Substantially compromised	▪ Give oral care after meals *to promote comfort and oral health.*
3 = Moderately compromised	▪ Monitor body weight *to determine adequacy of nutritional intake.*
4 = Mildly compromised	
5 = Not compromised	

NURSING DIAGNOSIS   Situational low self-esteem *related to* actual or perceived loss of function *as manifested by* refusal to touch or look at affected body parts, increasing dependence on others, refusal to participate in self-care.

OUTCOMES–NOC	INTERVENTIONS–NIC and *RATIONALES*
Self-Esteem (1205)	**Self-Esteem Enhancement (5400)**
▪ Maintenance of grooming/hygiene _____	▪ Encourage patient to verbalize feelings *to assess effect of stroke sequelae on self-esteem.*
▪ Acceptance of self-limitations _____	▪ Encourage patient to identify strengths *to facilitate patient's recognition of intrinsic value.*
▪ Open communications _____	▪ Establish achievable goals; explain all procedures and involve patient in planning goals; offer praise for every success and step of progress; involve patient as soon as possible in rehabilitation program *to promote sense of satisfaction, independence, and control and to reduce frustrations.*
▪ Description of self _____	▪ Monitor levels of self-esteem over time *to determine stressors or situations that trigger low self-esteem and to teach coping mechanisms.*
	Body Image Enhancement (5220)
Outcome Scale	▪ Monitor whether patient can look at the changed body part *to determine patient's level of acceptance with new image.*
1 = Never positive	▪ Help patient to determine the extent of actual changes in the body *to prevent misperceptions concerning new level of physiologic functioning.*
2 = Rarely positive	
3 = Sometimes positive	
4 = Often positive	
5 = Consistently positive	

▪ Nursing Implementation

Health Promotion. To reduce the incidence of stroke, the nurse should focus teaching efforts toward stroke prevention, particularly for persons with known risk factors (see Table 56-1). In any health care setting and for the population as a whole, nurses can play a major role in the promotion of a healthy lifestyle. An overall program to prevent events such as stroke includes recognizing that people are responsible to some degree for their own health and for the health of future generations.

Another very important aspect of health promotion is teaching patients and families about early symptoms associated with stroke or TIA and when to seek health care for symptoms (Table 56-8).

Acute Intervention

Respiratory system. During the acute phase following a stroke, management of the respiratory system is a nursing priority. Stroke patients are particularly vulnerable to respiratory problems. Advancing age and immobility increase the risk for atelectasis and pneumonia. Risk for aspiration pneumonia may be high because of impaired consciousness or dysphagia. Airway obstruction can occur because of problems with chewing and swallowing, food pocketing (food remaining in the buccal cavity of the mouth), and the tongue falling back. Some stroke patients, especially brainstem or hemorrhagic, may require endotracheal intubation and mechanical ventilation, initially and/or with in-

NURSING RESEARCH
Community Education Regarding Stroke

Citation Becker K et al: Community-based education improves stroke knowledge, *Cerebrovas Dis* 11:34, 2001.

Purpose To test the effectiveness of a community-based education campaign about stroke and the need to call 911.

Methods A pretest-posttest design was used with telephone interviews carried out before and after the community-based education campaign to assess stroke knowledge. The education campaign included public service announcements, television, newspaper, and public stroke screenings. Telephone interviews were completed for 547 individuals before and 511 individuals after the campaign.

Results and Conclusions Before the campaign, 45% of respondents knew that the brain was the organ injured in stroke. This increased to 50% following the campaign. On completion of the education campaign, respondents were 52% more likely to know a stroke risk factor and 35% more likely to know a stroke symptom. Overall, a severe knowledge deficit about stroke was identified, which was greatest among the elderly, the less educated, individuals with lower income, men, and Asian Americans.

Implications for Nursing Practice The general public's knowledge about stroke risk factors, symptoms, and treatment is lacking. This can contribute to greater mortality and morbidity from stroke. Further study is needed to develop strategies that result in translation of knowledge to changes in behavior. Particular efforts must be focused on high-risk groups and those with the greatest knowledge deficits. Nurses can have a key role in these efforts.

TABLE 56-8
Patient & Family Teaching Guide
Warning Signs of Stroke

If someone is having one or more of these signs, do not ignore them. Call 911 and get medical help immediately.
- Sudden weakness, paralysis, or numbness of the face, arm, or leg, especially on one side of the body
- Sudden dimness or loss of vision in one or both eyes
- Sudden loss of speech, confusion, or difficulty speaking or understanding speech
- Unexplained sudden dizziness, unsteadiness, loss of balance or coordination
- Sudden severe headache

creasing cerebral edema and/or ICP. Enteral tube feedings also place the patient at risk for aspiration pneumonia.

Nursing interventions to support adequate respiratory function are individualized to meet the needs of the patient. An oropharyngeal airway may be used in comatose patients to prevent the tongue from falling back and obstructing the airway and to provide access for suctioning. Alternately, a nasopharyngeal airway may be used to provide airway protection and access. When an artificial airway will be required for a prolonged time,

a tracheostomy may be performed. Nursing interventions include frequent assessment of airway patency and function, oxygenation, suctioning, patient mobility, positioning of the patient to prevent aspiration, and encouraging deep breathing. Patients who have an unclipped or uncoiled aneurysm may experience rebleeding and the possibility of further ICP increases with coughing exercises. Interventions related to maintenance of airway function are described in NCP 56-1.

Neurologic system. The patient's neurologic status must be monitored closely to detect changes suggesting extension of the stroke, increased ICP, vasospasm, or recovery from stroke symptoms. Neurologic assessment includes the Glasgow coma scale (a standardized assessment of level of consciousness), mental status, pupillary responses, and extremity movement and strength. (The Glasgow coma scale is shown in Table 55-5.) Vital signs are also closely monitored and documented. A decreasing level of consciousness may indicate increasing ICP. ICP and cerebral perfusion pressure may be monitored as well if the patient is in a critical care environment. Data from the nursing assessment are recorded on flow sheets to communicate evaluation of neurologic status to the interdisciplinary team.

Cardiovascular system. Nursing goals for the cardiovascular system are aimed at maintaining homeostasis. Many patients with stroke have decreased cardiac reserves from the secondary diagnoses of cardiac diseases. Cardiac efficiency may be further compromised by fluid retention, overhydration, dehydration, and blood pressure variations. Fluids are retained if there is increased production of ADH and aldosterone secondary to stress. Fluid retention plus overhydration can result in fluid overload. It can also increase cerebral edema and ICP. At the same time, dehydration can add to the morbidity and mortality associated with stroke, especially in the patient with vasospasm. IV therapy should be carefully regulated. The nurse should closely monitor intake and output. Central venous pressure, pulmonary artery pressure, or hemodynamic monitoring may be used as indicators of fluid balance or cardiac function in the critical care unit.

Nursing interventions include (1) monitoring vital signs frequently; (2) monitoring cardiac rhythms; (3) calculating intake and output, noting imbalances; (4) regulating IV infusions; (5) adjusting fluid intake to the individual needs of the patient; (6) monitoring lung sounds for crackles and rhonchi indicating pulmonary congestion; and (7) monitoring heart sounds for murmurs or for S_3 or S_4 heart sounds. Bedside monitors or telemetry may record cardiac rhythms. Hypertension is sometimes seen following a stroke as the body attempts to increase cerebral blood flow.

After a stroke, the patient is at risk for deep vein thrombosis, especially in the weak or paralyzed lower extremity. This is related to immobility, loss of venous tone, and decreased muscle pumping activity in the leg. The most effective prevention is to keep the patient moving. Active range-of-motion exercises should be taught if the patient has voluntary movement in the affected extremity. For the patient with hemiplegia, passive range-of-motion exercises should be done several times a day. Additional measures to prevent deep vein thrombosis include positioning to minimize the effects of dependent edema and the use of elastic compression gradient stockings or support hose. Intermittent pneumatic compression stockings may be ordered for bedridden patients. Deep vein thrombosis prophylaxis may include low-molecular-weight heparin (e.g., Lovenox). The nursing assessment for deep vein thrombosis includes measuring the calf and thigh daily, observing swelling of the lower extremities, noting unusual warmth of the leg, and asking the patient about pain in the calf.

Musculoskeletal system. The nursing goal for the musculoskeletal system is to maintain optimal function. This is accomplished by the prevention of joint contractures and muscular atrophy. In the acute phase, range-of-motion exercises and positioning are important nursing interventions. Passive range-of-motion exercise is begun on the first day of hospitalization. If the stroke is due to subarachnoid hemorrhage, the movement is limited to the extremities. The patient is taught to actively exercise as soon as possible. Muscle atrophy secondary to lack of innervation and activity can develop within 1 month following stroke.

The paralyzed or weak side needs special attention when the patient is positioned. Each joint should be positioned higher than the joint proximal to it to prevent dependent edema. Specific deformities on the weak or paralyzed side that may be present in patients with stroke include internal rotation of the shoulder; flexion contractures of the hand, wrist, and elbow; external rotation of the hip; and plantar flexion of the foot. Subluxation of the shoulder on the affected side is common. Careful positioning and moving of the affected arm may prevent the development of a painful shoulder condition. Immobilization of the affected upper extremity may precipitate a painful shoulder-hand syndrome.

Nursing interventions to optimize musculoskeletal function include (1) trochanter roll at the hip to prevent external rotation; (2) hand cones (not rolled washcloths) to prevent hand contractures; (3) arm supports with slings and lap boards to prevent shoulder displacement; (4) avoidance of pulling the patient by the arm to avoid shoulder displacement; (5) posterior leg splints, footboards or high-topped tennis shoes to prevent footdrop; and (6) hand splints to reduce spasticity. Use of a footboard for the patient with spasticity is controversial. Rather than preventing plantar flexion (footdrop), the sensory stimulation of a footboard against the bottom of the foot increases plantar flexion. Likewise, there is disagreement on whether hand splints facilitate or diminish spasticity. The decision regarding the use of footboards or hand splints is made on an individual patient basis.

Integumentary system. The skin of the patient with stroke is particularly susceptible to breakdown related to loss of sensation, decreased circulation, and immobility. This is compounded by patient age, poor nutrition, dehydration, edema, and incontinence. The nursing plan for prevention of skin breakdown includes (1) pressure relief by position changes, special mattresses, or wheelchair cushions; (2) good skin hygiene; (3) emollients applied to dry skin; and (4) early mobility. The ideal position change schedule is side-back-side with a maximum duration of 2 hours for any position. Nurses should position the patient on the weak or paralyzed side for only 30 minutes. If an area of redness develops and does not return to normal color within 15 minutes of pressure relief, the epidermis and dermis are damaged. The damaged area should not be massaged because this may cause additional damage. Control of pressure is the single most important factor in both the prevention and treatment of skin breakdown. Pillows can be used under lower extremities to reduce pressure on the heels. Vigilance and good nursing care are required to prevent pressure sores.

Gastrointestinal system. The stress of illness contributes to a catabolic state that can interfere with recovery. Neurologic, car-

diac, and respiratory problems are considered priorities in the acute phase of stroke. However, the nutritional needs of the patient require quick assessment and treatment. The patient may initially receive IV infusions to maintain fluid and electrolyte balance, as well as for administration of drugs. Patients with severe impairment may require enteral or parenteral nutrition support. Depending on the severity of the stroke, individual assessment and planning for nutrition are necessary.

The first oral feeding should be approached carefully because the gag reflex may be impaired. Before initiation of feeding, the gag reflex may be assessed by gently stimulating the back of the throat with a tongue blade. If a gag reflex is present, the patient will gag spontaneously. If it is absent, feeding should be deferred and exercises to stimulate swallowing should be started. The speech therapist or occupational therapist is usually responsible for designing this program. However, the nurse may be called on to develop the program in some clinical settings.

To assess swallowing ability, the nurse should elevate the head of the bed to an upright position (unless contraindicated) and give the patient a small amount of crushed ice or ice water to swallow. If the gag reflex is present and the patient is able to swallow safely, the nurse may proceed with feeding.

After careful assessment of swallowing, chewing, gag reflex, and pocketing, oral feedings can be initiated. Mouth care before feeding helps stimulate sensory awareness and salivation and can facilitate swallowing. The patient should remain in a high-Fowler's position, preferably in a chair with the head flexed forward for the feeding and for 30 minutes following. Various dietary items may be recommended by the speech therapist. Foods should be easy to swallow and provide enough texture, temperature (warm or cold), and flavor to stimulate a swallow reflex. Crushed ice can be used as a stimulant. The patient is instructed to swallow and then swallow again. Pureed foods are not usually the best choice because they are often bland and too smooth. Thin liquids are often difficult to swallow and may promote coughing. Milk products should be avoided because they tend to increase the viscosity of mucus and increase salivation. Food should be placed on the unaffected side of the mouth. The nurse should ensure an unrushed, nonstressful atmosphere. Feedings must be followed by scrupulous oral hygiene because food may collect on the affected side of the mouth.

The most common bowel problem for the patient who has experienced a stroke is constipation. Patients may be prophylactically placed on stool softeners and/or fiber (psyllium [Metamucil]). If the patient does not have a daily or every-other-day bowel movement, the patient should be checked for impaction. The patient who has liquid stools should also be checked for stool impaction. Depending on the patient's fluid balance status and swallowing ability, fluid intake should be 1800 to 2000 ml per day and fiber intake up to 25 g per day. Physical activity also promotes bowel function. Laxatives, suppositories, or additional stool softeners may be ordered if the patient does not respond to increased fluid and fiber. Similarly, enemas are used only if suppositories and digital stimulation are ineffective because they cause vagal stimulation and increase ICP.

Urinary system. In the acute stage of stroke, the primary urinary problem is poor bladder control, resulting in incontinence. Efforts should be made to promote normal bladder function and avoid the use of indwelling catheters. If an indwelling catheter must be used initially, it should be removed as soon as the patient is medically and neurologically stable. Long-term use of an indwelling catheter is associated with urinary tract infections and delayed bladder retraining. An intermittent catheterization program may be used for patients with urinary retention because of the lower incidence of urinary infections. An alternative to intermittent catheterizations is the external catheter for male patients with urinary incontinence. External catheters do not alleviate the problem of urine retention. Overdistention should be avoided.

A bladder retraining program consists of (1) adequate fluid intake with the majority given between 8 AM and 7 PM; (2) scheduled toileting every 2 hours using bedpan, commode, or bathroom; and (3) noting signs of restlessness, which may indicate the need for urination.

Communication. During the acute stage of stroke, the nurse's role in meeting the psychologic needs of the patient is primarily supportive. An alert patient is usually anxious because of lack of understanding about what has happened and because of difficulty with, or inability to, communicate. The patient is assessed both for the ability to speak and the ability to understand. The patient's response to simple questions can give the nurse a guideline for structuring explanations and instructions. If the patient cannot understand words, gestures may be used to support verbal cues. It is helpful to speak slowly and calmly, using simple words or sentences to enhance communication. The nurse must give the patient extra time to comprehend and respond to communication. The stroke patient with aphasia may easily be overwhelmed by verbal stimuli. (Guidelines for communicating with a patient who has aphasia are presented in Table 56-9.) Evaluation and treatment of language and communication deficits are often done by the speech pathologist once the patient has stabilized.

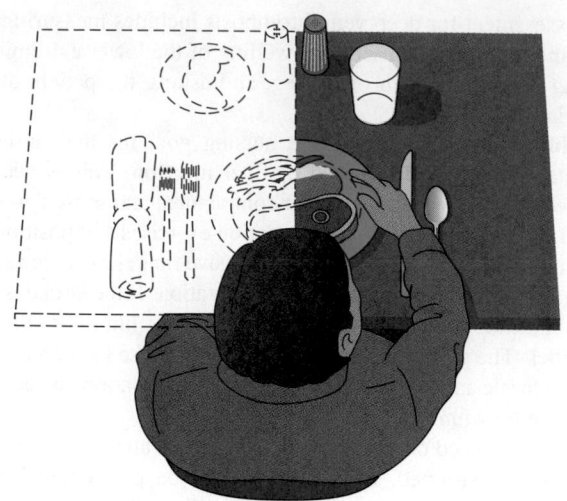

FIG. 56-8 Spatial and perceptual deficits in stroke. Perception of a patient with homonymous hemianopsia shows that food on the left side is not seen and thus is ignored.

Sensory-perceptual alterations. Homonymous hemianopsia (blindness in the same half of each visual field) is a common problem after a stroke (Fig. 56-8). Persistent disregard of objects in part of the visual field should alert the nurse to this possibility. Initially, the nurse helps the patient to compensate by arranging the environment within the patient's perceptual field, such as arranging the food tray so that all foods are on the right side or the left side to accommodate for field of vision (see Fig. 56-8). Later, the patient learns to compensate for the visual defect by consciously attending or scanning the neglected side. The weak or paralyzed extremities are carefully checked for adequacy of dressing, for hygiene, and for trauma.

In the clinical situation it is often difficult to distinguish between a visual field cut and a neglect syndrome. Both problems may occur with strokes affecting either the right or the left side of the brain. A person may be unfortunate enough to have both homonymous hemianopsia and a neglect syndrome, which increases the inattention to the weak or paralyzed side. A neglect syndrome results in decreased safety awareness and places the patient at high risk for injury. Immediately after the stroke, the nurse must anticipate potential safety hazards and provide protection from injury. Safety measures can include close observation of the patient, elevating side rails, lowering the height of the bed, and video monitors. The use of restraints and soft vests is avoided because this may agitate the patient.

Other visual problems may include *diplopia* (double vision), loss of the corneal reflex, and *ptosis* (drooping eyelid), especially if the area of stroke is in the vertebrobasilar distribution. Diplopia is often treated with an eye patch. If the corneal reflex is absent, the patient is at risk for corneal abrasion and should be observed closely and protected against eye injuries. Corneal abrasion can be prevented with artificial tears or gel to keep the eyes moist and an eye shield (especially at night). Ptosis is generally not treated because it usually does not inhibit vision.

Coping. A stroke is usually a sudden, extremely stressful event for the patient, family members, and significant others. A stroke is often a family disease, affecting the family emotionally, socially, and financially, as well as changing roles and responsibilities within the family. An older couple may perceive the

TABLE 56-9	Communication with a Patient with Aphasia

1. Decrease environmental stimuli that may be distracting and disrupting to communication efforts.
2. Treat the patient as an adult.
3. Present one thought or idea at a time.
4. Keep questions simple or ask questions that can be answered with "yes" or "no."
5. Let the person speak. Do not interrupt. Allow time for the individual to complete thoughts.
6. Make use of gestures or demonstration as an acceptable alternative form of communication. Encourage this by saying, "Show me . . ." or "Point to what you want."
7. Do not pretend to understand the person if you do not. Calmly say you do not understand and encourage the use of nonverbal communication, or ask the person to write out what he or she wants.
8. Speak with normal volume and tone.
9. Give the patient time to process information and generate a response before repeating a question or statement.
10. Allow body contact (e.g., the clasp of a hand, touching) as much as possible. Realize that touching may be the only way the patient can express feelings.
11. Organize the patient's day by preparing and following a schedule (the more familiar the routine, the easier it will be).
12. Do not push communication if the person is tired or upset. Aphasia worsens with fatigue and anxiety.

stroke as a very real threat to life and to accustomed lifestyle. Reactions to this threat vary considerably but may involve fear, apprehension, denial of the severity of stroke, depression, anger, and sorrow. During the acute phase of caring for the stroke patient and the family, nursing interventions designed to facilitate coping involve providing information and emotional support.

Explanations to the patient about what has happened and about diagnostic and therapeutic procedures should be clear and understandable. It is particularly challenging to keep the aphasic patient adequately informed. Tone, demeanor, and touch may also be used to convey support.

The patient's family should be given a careful, detailed explanation of what has happened to the patient. However, if the family is extremely anxious and upset during the acute phase, explanations may need to be repeated at a later time. Because family members usually have not had time to prepare for the illness, they may need assistance in arranging care for family members or pets and for transportation and finances. A social services referral is often helpful.

Ambulatory and Home Care. The patient is usually discharged from the acute care setting to home, an intermediate or long-term care facility, or a rehabilitation facility. Criteria for transfer to rehabilitation may include the patient's ability to participate in therapies for a minimum number of hours per day. Functional status scales such as the Barthel Index, Modified Rankin Scale, and Functional Independence Measure are used to evaluate the patient.[36] Ideally, discharge planning with the patient and family starts early in the hospitalization and promotes a smooth transition from one care setting to another. The interdisciplinary team provides the guidance for the appropriate care required after discharge. If the patient requires a short- or long-term health care facility, the team can make appropriate referrals that allow time for family selection and arrangement of care. A critical factor in discharge planning is the patient's level of independence in performing ADLs. If the patient is returning home, the team can make referrals for needed equipment and services in preparation for discharge.

Nurses have an excellent opportunity to prepare the patient and family for discharge through education, demonstration and return demonstration, practice, and evaluation of self-care skills before discharge. Total care is considered in discharge planning: medications, nutrition, mobility, exercises, hygiene, and toileting. Follow-up care is carefully planned to permit continuing nursing, physical, occupational, and speech therapy, as well as medical care. Community resources should be identified to provide recreational activities, group support, spiritual assistance, respite care, adult day care, and home assistance based on the individual patient's needs.

Rehabilitation is the process of maximizing the patient's capabilities and resources to promote optimal functioning related to physical, mental, and social well-being. The goals of rehabilitation are to prevent deformity and maintain and improve function. Regardless of the care setting, ongoing rehabilitation is essential to maximize the patient's abilities.

Rehabilitation requires a team approach so the patient and family can benefit from the combined, expert care of an interdisciplinary team. The team must communicate and coordinate care to achieve the patient's and family's goals. The nurse is in a good position to facilitate this process and is often key to successful rehabilitation efforts. The patient's and family's participation in

decision making during rehabilitation is essential to goal achievement after a stroke. The interdisciplinary team is composed of many members, including nurses, physicians, psychiatrist, physical therapist, occupational therapist, speech therapist, registered dietitian, respiratory therapist, vocational therapist, recreational therapist, social worker, psychologist, pharmacist, and chaplains. Physical therapy focuses on mobility, progressive ambulation, transfer techniques, and equipment needed for mobility. Occupational therapy emphasizes retraining for skills of daily living such as eating, dressing, hygiene, and cooking. Occupational therapists are also skilled in cognitive and perceptual evaluation and training. Speech therapy focuses on speech, communication, cognition, and eating abilities.

Many of the nursing interventions outlined in the nursing care plan for the patient with a stroke (see NCP 56-1) are initiated in the acute phase of care and continue throughout rehabilitation. Some of the interventions are independent nursing actions, whereas others involve the entire rehabilitation team.

The rehabilitation nurse assesses the patient and family with attention to (1) rehabilitation potential of the patient, (2) physical status of all body systems, (3) presence of complications caused by the stroke or other chronic conditions, (4) cognitive status of the patient, (5) family resources and support, and (6) expectations of the patient and family related to the rehabilitation program.

The goals for rehabilitation of the patient with stroke are mutually set by the patient, family, nurse, and other members of the rehabilitation team. The rehabilitation goals typically include the following:

- Learn techniques to self-monitor and maintain physical wellness
- Demonstrate self-care skills
- Exhibit problem-solving skills with self-care
- Avoid complications associated with stroke
- Establish and maintain a useful communication system
- Maintain nutritional and hydration status
- List community resources for equipment, supplies, and support
- Establish flexible role behaviors to promote family cohesiveness

Musculoskeletal function. The nurse initially emphasizes the musculoskeletal functions of eating, toileting, and walking for the rehabilitation of the patient. Initial assessment consists of determining the stage of recovery of muscle function. If the muscles are still flaccid several weeks after the stroke, the prognosis for regaining function is poor and the focus of care is on preventing additional loss. Most patients begin to show signs of spasticity with exaggerated reflexes within 48 hours following the stroke. Spasticity at this phase of stroke denotes progress toward recovery. As improvement continues, small voluntary movements of the hip or shoulder may be accompanied by involuntary movements in the rest of the extremity (synergy). The final stage of recovery occurs when the patient has voluntary control of isolated muscle groups.

Interventions for musculoskeletal system advance in a manner of progressive activity. Balance training is the initial step and begins with the patient sitting up in bed or dangling on the edge of the bed. The nurse evaluates tolerance by noting dizziness or syncope caused by vasomotor instability. The next step is transferring from bed to chair or wheelchair. The chair is placed beside the bed so that the patient can lead with the stronger arm and leg.

The patient sits on the side of the bed, stands, places the strong hand on the far wheelchair arm, and sits down. The nurse may either supervise the transfer or provide minimal assistance by guiding the patient's strong hand to the wheelchair arm, standing in front of the patient blocking the patient's knees with the nurse's knees to prevent knee buckling, and guiding the patient into a sitting position.

In some rehabilitation units the Bobath approach is used as an approach to mobility. The goal of this approach is to help the patient gain control over patterns of spasticity by inhibiting abnormal reflex patterns. Therapists and nurses use the Bobath approach to encourage normal muscle tone, normal movement, and promotion of bilateral function of the body. An example is to have the patient transfer into the wheelchair using the weak or paralyzed side and the stronger side to facilitate more bilateral functioning.

Another more recent approach to stroke rehabilitation is constraint-induced movement therapy (CIMT). CIMT encourages the patient to use the weakened extremity by restricting movement of the normal extremity. The ability of patients to comply with this approach is challenging and may limit its use.[37]

Supportive or assistive equipment, such as canes, walkers, and leg braces, may be needed on a short-term or long-term basis for mobility. The physical therapist usually selects the most appropriate supportive device(s) to meet individual needs and instructs the patient regarding use. The nurse should incorporate physical therapy activities into the patient's daily routine for additional practice and repetition of rehabilitation efforts.

Nutritional therapy. After the acute phase, a dietitian can assist in determining the appropriate daily caloric intake based on the patient's size, weight, and activity level. If the patient is unable to take in an adequate oral diet, a percutaneous gastrostomy (PEG) may be used for nutritional support if dysphagia persists. Most commercially prepared formulas provide about 1 calorie per milliliter. (Enteral feedings are described in Chapter 39.)

The nurse and speech therapist must assess the ability of the patient to swallow solids and fluids and adjust the diet appropriately. The dietitian plans the diet type, texture, calorie count, and fluids to meet the patient's nutritional needs. The occupational therapist and nurse must evaluate the patient's ability to feed himself or herself and recommend assistive devices to allow for independent eating. Nurses are involved in the daily planning, implementation, and evaluation of the nutritional status of the patient.

The inability to feed oneself can be frustrating and may result in malnutrition and dehydration. Interventions to promote self-feeding include using the unaffected upper extremity to eat; employing assistive devices such as rocker knives, plate guards, and nonslip pads for dishes (Fig. 56-9); removing unnecessary items from the tray or table, which can reduce spills; and providing a nondistracting environment to decrease sensory overload and distraction. The effectiveness of the dietary program is evaluated in terms of maintenance of weight, adequate hydration, and patient satisfaction.

Bowel function. A bowel management program is implemented for problems with bowel control, constipation, or incontinence. A high-fiber diet (see Table 41-9) and adequate fluid intake (2500 to 3000 ml) are usually recommended. Patients with

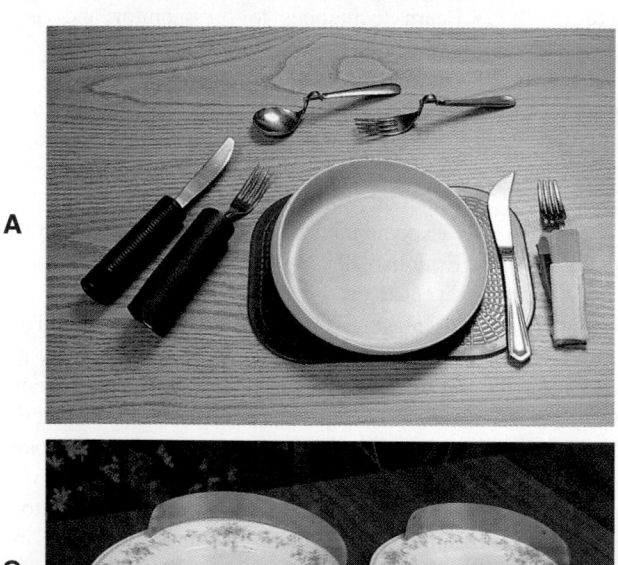
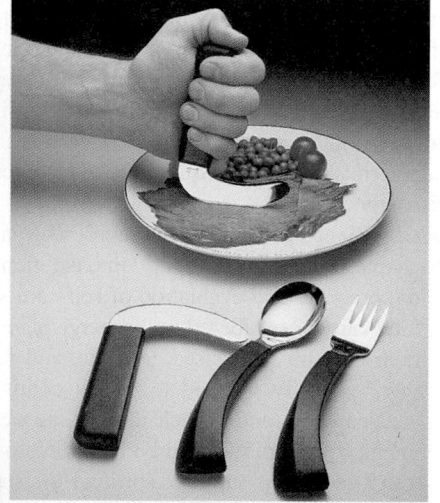
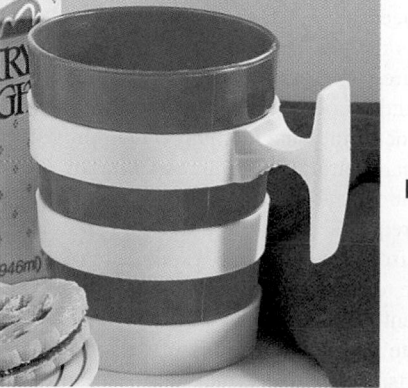

FIG. 56-9 Assistive devices for eating. **A,** The curved fork fits over the hand. The rounded plate helps keep food on the plate. Special grips and swivel handles are helpful for some persons. **B,** Knives with rounded blades are rocked back and forth to cut food. The person does not need a fork in one hand and a knife in the other. **C,** Plate guards help keep food on the plate. **D,** Cup with special handle.

stroke frequently have constipation, which responds to the following dietary management:

- Fluid intake of 2500 to 3000 ml daily unless contraindicated
- Prune juice (120 ml) or stewed prunes daily
- Cooked fruit three times daily
- Cooked vegetables three times daily
- Whole-grain cereal or bread three to five times daily

The bowel management program for incontinence consists of placing the patient on the bedpan or bedside commode or taking the patient to the bathroom at a regular time daily to reestablish bowel regularity. A good time for the bowel program is 30 minutes after breakfast because eating stimulates the gastrocolic reflex and peristalsis. The time can be adjusted for individual bowel habits and preferred timing. Sitting on the commode or toilet promotes bowel elimination through both gravity and increased abdominal pressure. Stool softeners or suppositories may be ordered if the bowel program is ineffective in reestablishing bowel regularity. A glycerin suppository can be inserted 15 to 30 minutes before evacuation time to stimulate the anorectal reflex. The bisacodyl (Dulcolax) suppository is a chemical stimulant to the bowel and is used when other measures are ineffective. Ideally the suppository use is for short-term management.

Bladder function. The nurse often assists the patient with urinary difficulties or incontinence that may follow a stroke. Often the patient with stroke has functional incontinence, which is associated with communication difficulties, mobility problems, and dressing or undressing difficulties. Nursing interventions focused on urinary continence include (1) assessment for bladder distention by palpation; (2) offering the bedpan, urinal, commode, or toilet every 2 hours during waking hours and every 3 to 4 hours at night; (3) focusing the patient on the need to urinate with direct command; (4) assistance with clothing and mobility; (5) scheduling the majority of fluid intake between 7 AM and 7 PM; and (6) encouraging the usual position for urinating (standing for men and sitting for women). Short-term interventions for urinary incontinence may include indwelling catheters, intermittent catheterization, external catheters for men, or incontinence briefs. These are not long-term solutions for urinary incontinence because complications such as urinary infections or skin irritation may occur. A coordinated program by the entire nursing staff is needed to achieve urinary continence.

Sensory-perceptual function. Patients who have had a stroke frequently have perceptual deficits. Patients with a stroke on the right side of the brain usually have difficulty in judging position, distance, and rate of movement. These patients are often impulsive and impatient and tend to deny problems related to strokes. They may fail to correlate spatial-perceptual problems with the inability to perform activities, such as guiding a wheelchair through the doorway. The patient with a right-brain stroke (left hemiplegia) is at higher risk for injury because of mobility difficulties. Directions for activities are best given verbally for comprehension. The task should be broken down to simple steps for ease of understanding. Environmental control such as removing clutter and obstacles, and good lighting, aids in concentration and safer mobility. One-sided neglect is common for people with right-brain stroke, so the nurse may assist or remind the patient to dress the weak or paralyzed side or shave the forgotten side of the face.

Patients with a left brain stroke (right hemiplegia) commonly are slower in organization and performance of tasks. They tend to have impaired spatial discrimination. These patients usually admit to deficits and have a fearful, anxious response to a stroke. Their behaviors are slow and cautious. Nonverbal cues and instructions are helpful for comprehension with patients who have had a left-brain stroke.

Affect. Patients who have had strokes often exhibit emotional responses that are not appropriate or typical for the situation. Patients may appear apathetic, depressed, fearful, anxious, weepy, frustrated, and angry. Some patients exhibit exaggerated mood swings, especially those with a stroke on the left side of the brain (right hemiplegia). The patient may be unable to control emotions and may suddenly burst into tears or laughter. This behavior is out of context and often is unrelated to the underlying emotional state of the patient. Nursing interventions for atypical emotional response are to (1) distract the patient who suddenly becomes emotional, (2) explain to the patient and family the reason for emotional outbursts, (3) maintain a calm environment, and (4) avoid shaming or scolding the patient during emotional outbursts.

Coping. The patient with a stroke may experience many losses, including sensory, intellectual, communicative, functional, role behavior, emotional, social, and vocational losses. The patient and family often go through the process of grief and mourning associated with the losses. Some patients experience long-term depression with symptoms such as anxiety, weight loss, loss of energy, poor appetite, and sleep disturbances. In addition, the time and energy required to perform previously simple tasks can result in anger and frustration.

The patient and family need help with coping with the losses associated with stroke. The nurse may assist the coping by (1) supporting communication between the patient and family; (2) discussing lifestyle changes resulting from stroke deficits; (3) discussing changing roles and responsibilities within the family; (4) being an active listener to allow the expression of fear, frustration, and anxiety; (5) including the family and patient in short- and long-term goal planning and patient care; and (6) supporting family conferences. Maladjusted dependence with inadequate coping occurs when the patient does not maintain optimal functioning for self-care, family responsibilities, decision making, or socialization. This situation can cause resentment from both the patient and family with a negative cycle of interpersonal dependency and control. Maladjusted independence occurs when the patient overestimates personal cognitive or physical capabilities and energy levels. These patients are at risk for injury.

Family members must cope with three aspects of the patient's behavior: (1) recognition of behavioral changes resulting from neurologic deficits that are not changeable, (2) responses to multiple losses both by the patient and the family, and (3) behaviors that may have been reinforced during the early stages of stroke as continued dependency. The patient and family may express feelings of guilt over not living healthy lifestyles or not seeking professional help sooner. Family therapy is a helpful adjunct to rehabilitation. The patient and family need support and reassurance. Open communication, information regarding the total effects of stroke, education regarding stroke treatment, and therapy are helpful. Stroke support groups within rehabilitation facilities and in the community are helpful in terms of mutual sharing, education, coping, and understanding.

Sexual function. A patient who has had a stroke may be concerned about the loss of sexual function. Many patients are comfortable talking about their anxieties and fears regarding sexual function if the nurse is comfortable and open to the topic. The nurse may initiate the topic with the patient and spouse or significant other. Common concerns of sexual activity involving the patient with a stroke are impotence and the occurrence of another stroke during sex. Nursing interventions for sexual activity include education on (1) optional positioning of partners, (2) timing for peak energy times, and (3) patient and partner counseling.

Communication. Speech, comprehension, and language deficits are the most difficult problems for the patient and family. Speech therapists can assess and formulate a plan of care to support communication. The nurse can be a role model for communication with the patient who has aphasia. Nursing interventions that support communication include (1) frequent, meaningful communication; (2) allowing time for the patient to comprehend and answer; (3) using simple, short sentences; (4) using visual cues; (5) structuring conversation so that it permits simple answers by the patient; and (6) praising the patient honestly for improvements with speech.

Community integration. Traditionally, successful community integration following stroke may be difficult for the patient because of persistent problems with cognition, coping, physical deficits, and emotional lability that interfere with functioning. Older patients who have had a stroke often have more severe deficits and frequently experience multiple health problems. Failure to continue the rehabilitation regimen at home may result in deterioration and further complications. Advances in health care have resulted in an increased survival rate for patients with extensive stroke damage. Successful community integration can be redefined by the patient, family, and interdisciplinary health team as successful mobility, achievement of ADLs, and quality of life with family and friends.

Community resources can be an asset to patients and their families. The National Stroke Association provides information, resources, referral services, and quarterly newsletters on stroke. The American Stroke Association, a division of the American Heart Association, has information regarding stroke, hypertension, diet, exercise, and assistive devices. This association sponsors self-help groups in many areas. The Easter Seal Society provides wheelchairs and other assistive devices for stroke patients.

Local groups can offer more daily assistance such as meals and transportation. These resources can be identified by nurse case managers, home health nurses, discharge planners, and clinical nurse specialists. (Resources are listed at the end of the chapter.)

■ Gerontologic Considerations: Stroke

Stroke is a significant cause of death and disability. The highest incidence of stroke occurs among older adults. Stroke can result in a profound disruption in the life of an older person. The magnitude of disability and changes in total function can leave patients wondering if they can ever return to their "old self," and loss of independence may be a major concern. The ability to perform ADLs may require many adaptive changes because of physical, emotional, perceptual, and cognitive deficits. Home management may be a particular challenge if the patient has an elderly spouse caretaker who also has health problems. There may be limited family members (including adult children) living in close proximity to provide help.

The rehabilitative phase and assisting the older patient to deal with the residual deficits of stroke, as well as aging, can provide a challenging nursing experience. Patients may become fearful and depressed because they think they may have another attack or die. The fear can become immobilizing and interfere with effective rehabilitation.

Changes may occur in the patient-spouse relationship. The dependency resulting from a stroke may be threatening. The spouse may also have chronic medical problems that affect the ability to take care of the stroke survivor. The patient may not want anyone other than the spouse to provide care, putting a significant burden on the spouse.

The nurse has the opportunity to assist the patient and family in the transition through acute hospitalization, rehabilitation, long-term care, and home care. The needs of the patient and family require ongoing nursing assessment and adaptation of interventions in response to changing needs to optimize quality of life for both the patient and family. ■

CRITICAL THINKING EXERCISES

Case Study
Stroke

Patient Profile. Suzanne, a 66-year-old white woman, awoke in the middle of the night and fell when she tried to get up and go to the bathroom. She fell because she was not able to control her left leg. Her husband took her to the hospital, where she was diagnosed with an acute ischemic stroke. Because she had awakened with symptoms, the actual time of onset was unknown and she was not a candidate for tPA.

Subjective Data
- Left arm and leg are weak and feel numb
- Feeling depressed and fearful
- Requires help with ADLs
- Concerned regarding having another stroke
- Says she has not taken her drugs for high cholesterol
- History of a brief episode of left-sided weakness and tingling of the face, arm, and hand 3 months earlier, which totally resolved and for which she did not seek treatment

Objective Data
- BP: 180/110
- Left-sided arm weakness (3/5) and leg weakness (4/5)
- Decreased sensation on the left side, particularly the hand
- Left homonymous hemianopsia
- Overweight
- Alert, oriented, and able to answer questions appropriately but mild slowness in responding

CRITICAL THINKING QUESTIONS
1. How does Suzanne's prior health history put her at risk for a stroke?
2. How can the nurse address Suzanne's concerns regarding having another stroke?
3. How can Suzanne and her family address activity issues such as driving after the stroke?
4. What strategies might the home health nurse use to help Suzanne and her family cope with her feeling depressed?

CRITICAL THINKING EXERCISES—cont'd

5. What lifestyle changes should Suzanne make to reduce the likelihood of another stroke?
6. How will homonymous hemianopsia affect Suzanne's hygiene, eating, driving, and community activities?
7. What factors should the nurse assess for related to outpatient rehabilitation for Suzanne?
8. Based on the assessment data provided, write one or more nursing diagnoses. Are there any collaborative problems?

Nursing Research Issues

1. Determine the effectiveness of weight loss and stop-smoking programs in reducing the incidence of stroke.
2. Examine the relationship between functional abilities and level of independence following a stroke.
3. Determine the effectiveness of nursing interventions to promote full-field visualization for patients with homonymous hemianopsia.
4. Examine the spouse-patient relationship and coping styles following a stroke.
5. Examine the impact of stroke on socialization, quality of life, and loneliness.

REVIEW QUESTIONS

The number of the question corresponds to the same-numbered objective at the beginning of the chapter.

1. Of the following patients, the nurse recognizes that the one with the highest risk for a stroke is
   a. an obese 45-year-old Native American.
   b. a 35-year-old Asian American woman who smokes.
   c. a 32-year-old white woman taking oral contraceptives.
   d. a 65-year-old African American man with hypertension.
2. The factor related to cerebral blood flow that most often determines the extent of cerebral damage from a stroke is the
   a. amount of cardiac output.
   b. oxygen content of the blood.
   c. degree of collateral circulation.
   d. level of carbon dioxide in the blood.
3. Information provided by the patient that would help differentiate a hemorrhagic stroke from a thrombotic stroke includes
   a. sensory disturbance.
   b. a history of hypertension.
   c. presence of motor weakness.
   d. sudden onset of severe headache.
4. A patient with right-sided hemiplegia and aphasia resulting from a stroke most likely has involvement of the
   a. brainstem.
   b. vertebral artery.
   c. left middle cerebral artery.
   d. right middle cerebral artery.
5. The nurse explains to the patient with a stroke who is scheduled for angiography that this test is used to determine the
   a. presence of increased ICP.
   b. site and size of the infarction.
   c. presence of blood in the cerebrospinal fluid.
   d. patency of the cerebral blood vessels.

6. A patient experiencing TIAs is scheduled for a carotid endarterectomy. The nurse explains that this procedure is done to
   a. decrease cerebral edema.
   b. reduce the brain damage that occurs during a stroke in evolution.
   c. prevent a stroke by removing atherosclerotic plaques blocking cerebral blood flow.
   d. provide a circulatory bypass around thrombotic plaques obstructing cranial circulation.
7. Nursing management of the patient with hemiplegia during the acute phase of a stroke includes
   a. restricting active movement.
   b. positioning each joint higher than the proximal joint.
   c. performing passive range of motion on all limbs every 4 hours.
   d. maintaining the patient in a recumbent, side-lying position.
8. Bladder training in a male patient who has urinary incontinence after a stroke includes
   a. limiting fluid intake.
   b. keeping a urinal in place at all times.
   c. assisting the patient to stand to void.
   d. catheterizing the patient every 4 hours.
9. The most common response of the stroke patient to the change in body image is
   a. denial.
   b. depression.
   c. disassociation.
   d. intellectualization.

REFERENCES

1. Goldstein et al: Primary prevention of ischemic stroke, *Circulation* 103:163, 2001.
2. Heart and Stroke Foundation of Canada (last updated Sept 19, 2001). General Info–Stroke Statistics. Available at *http://www.heartandstroke.ca/* (accessed Nov 21, 2001).
3. American Heart Association: *2001 Heart and stroke statistical update*, Dallas, 2002, American Heart Association.
4. Helgason CM, Wolf PA: American Heart Association prevention conference IV: prevention and rehabilitation of stroke, *Circulation* 96:701, 1997.
5. The Intercollegiate Working Party for Stroke: National clinical guidelines for stroke: a concise update, *Clin Med* 2:231, 2002.
6. Matchar DB et al: Improving the quality of anticoagulation of patients with atrial fibrillation in managed care organizations: results of the managing anticoagulation services trial, *Am J Med* 113:42, 2002.
7. Desbiens NA: Deciding on anticoagulating the oldest old with atrial fibrillation: insights from cost-effectiveness analysis, *J Am Geriatr Soc* 50:863, 2002.
8. Wolf PA et al: Probability of stroke: a risk profile from the Framingham Study, *Stroke* 22:3, 1991.
9. Kothari V et al: UKPDS 60: risk of stroke in type 2 diabetes estimated by the UK Prospective Diabetes Study risk engine, *Stroke* 33:1776, 2002.
10. Liao JK: Statins and ischemic stroke, *Atheroscler Suppl* 3:21, 2002.
11. Leys D et al: Stroke prevention: management of modifiable vascular risk factors, *J Neurol* 249:507, 2002.
12. Bolego C, Poli A, Paoletti R: Smoking and gender, *Cardiovasc Res* 53:568, 2002.
13. Tuhrim S: Management of stroke and transient ischemic attack, *Mt Sinai J Med* 69:121, 2002.
14. Sacco RL et al: The protective effect of moderate alcohol consumption on ischemic stroke, *JAMA* 281:1, 1999.
15. Rexrode KM et al: A prospective study of body mass index, weight change, and risk of stroke in women, *JAMA* 277:19, 1997.
16. Sacco RL et al: Leisure-time physical activity and ischemic stroke risk: the northern Manhattan stroke study, *Stroke* 29:2, 1998.
17. Petitti DB et al: Stroke and cocaine or amphetamine use, *Epidemiology* 9:6, 1998.
18. Neiman J, Haapaniemi HM, Hillbom M: Neurological complications of drug abuse: pathophysiological mechanisms, *Eur J Neurol* 6:595, 2000.
19. Gillum RF, Mussolino ME, Ingram DD: Physical activity and stroke incidence in women and men. The NHANES I epidemiologic follow-up study, *Am J Epidemiol* 143:9, 1996.
20. Heinemann et al: Thromboembolic stroke in young women: a European case-control study on oral contraceptives, *Contraception* 57:29, 1998.
21. Writing Group for the Women's Health Initiative Investigators: Risks and benefits of estrogen plus progestin in healthy postmenopausal women: principal results from the Women's Health Initiative randomized controlled trial, *JAMA* 288:321, 2002.
22. Hankey GJ et al: Inherited thrombophilia in ischemic stroke and its pathogenic subtypes, *Stroke* 32:1793, 2001.
23. Fisher M, Bogousslavsky J: *Current review of cerebrovascular disease*, ed 4, Philadelphia, 2001, Current Medicine.
24. Barnett HJM et al: *Stroke: pathophysiology, diagnosis, and management*, ed 3, New York, 1998, Churchill Livingstone.
25. Gilroy J: *Basic neurology*, New York, 2000, McGraw-Hill.
26. Broderick et al: Guidelines for the management of spontaneous intracerebral hemorrhage, *Stroke* 30:905, 1999.
27. Greener J, Langhorne P: Systematic reviews in rehabilitation for stroke: issues and approaches to addressing them, *Clin Rehabil* 16:69, 2002.
28. Coull BM et al: Anticoagulants and antiplatelets agents in acute ischemic stroke: report of the Joint Stroke Guideline Development Committee of the American Academy of Neurology and the American Stroke Association, *Stroke* 33:1934, 2002.
29. Bailes JE: Carotid endarterectomy, *Neurosurgery* 50:1290, 2002.
30. Nussbaum ES, Erickson DL: Extracranial-intracranial bypass for ischemic cerebrovascular disease refractory to maximal medical therapy, *Neurosurgery* 46:37, 2000.
31. Csokay A et al: Vascular tunnel creation to improve the efficacy of decompressive craniotomy in post-traumatic cerebral edema and ischemic stroke, *Neurosurgery* 57:126, 2002.
32. Wardlaw JM, del Zoppo G, Yamaguchi T: Thrombolysis for acute ischemic stroke, Cochrane Stroke Group, *Cochrane Database Syst Rev*, Issue 1, 2002.
33. Feigin VL et al: Calcium antagonists for aneurismal subarachnoid hemorrhage, *The Cochrane Library*, Issue 2, Oxford, 2002 Update Software.
34. Mitchell M: *Neuroscience nursing: a nursing diagnosis approach*, Baltimore, 2001, WB Saunders.
35. Broderick J et al: Guidelines for the management of spontaneous intracerebral hemorrhage: a statement for the healthcare professionals from a special writing group of the Stroke Council, American Heart Association, *Stroke* 30:905, 1999.
36. Pettersen R, Dahl T, Wyller TB: Prediction of long-term functional outcome after stroke rehabilitation, *Clin Rehabil* 16:149, 2002.
37. Page SJ et al: Stroke patients' and therapists' opinions of constraint-induced movement therapy, *Clin Rehabil* 16:55, 2002.

RESOURCES

American Association of Neuroscience Nurses (AANN)
4700 West Lake Avenue
Glenview, IL 60025
888-557-2266 or 847-375-4733
Fax: 847-375-6333
www.aann.org

American Stroke Association
National Center
7272 Greenville Avenue
Dallas, TX 75231
888-4-STROKE or 888-478-7653
www.strokeassociation.org

Association of Rehabilitation Nurses (ARN)
4700 West Lake Avenue
Glenview, IL 60025-1485
800-229-7530 or 847-375-4710
Fax: 877-734-9384
www.rehabnurse.org

Canadian Association of Neuroscience Nurses (CANN)
www.cann.ca

Heart and Stroke Foundation of Canada
222 Queen Street, Suite 1402
Ottawa, ON
K1P 5V9 Canada
613-569-4361
Fax: 613-569-3278
http://ww1.heartandstroke.ca

National Institute of Neurological Disorders and Stroke
NIH Neurological Institute
PO Box 5801
Bethesda, MD 20824
800-352-9424
www.ninds.nih.gov

National Stroke Association
9707 East Easter Lane
Englewood, CO 80112
800-STROKES (787-6537) or 303-649-9299
Fax: 303-649-1328
www.stroke.org

Society for Neuroscience
11 Dupont Circle NW, Suite 500
Washington, DC 20036
202-462-6688
Fax: 202-462-9740
www.sfn.org

Stroke Clubs International
805 12th Street
Galveston, TX 77550
409-762-1022
strokeclub@aol.com

For additional Internet resources, see the website for this book at *http://evolve.elsevier.com/Lewis/medsurg/*.

CHAPTER 57

NURSING MANAGEMENT
Chronic Neurologic Problems

Judith M. Ozuna

LEARNING OBJECTIVES

1. Compare and contrast tension-type, migraine, and cluster headaches in terms of etiology, clinical manifestations, collaborative care, and nursing management.
2. Describe the etiology, clinical manifestations, diagnostic studies, collaborative care, and nursing management of seizure disorder, multiple sclerosis, Parkinson's disease, and myasthenia gravis.
3. Describe the clinical manifestations and collaborative care of amyotrophic lateral sclerosis and Huntington's chorea.
4. Explain the potential impact of chronic neurologic disease on physical and psychologic well-being.
5. Outline the major goals of treatment for the patient with a chronic, progressive neurologic disease.

KEY TERMS

absence (petit mal) seizure, p. 1556
amyotrophic lateral sclerosis, p. 1577
atypical absence seizure, p. 1556
aura, p. 1550
cluster headaches, p. 1551
epilepsy, p. 1555
generalized seizures, p. 1556
headache, p. 1549
Huntington's disease, p. 1577

migraine headache, p. 1550
multiple sclerosis, p. 1563
myasthenia gravis, p. 1573
myasthenic crisis, p. 1574
Parkinson's disease, p. 1569
partial seizures, p. 1556
restless legs syndrome, p. 1576
seizure, p. 1555
status epilepticus, p. 1557
tension-type headache, p. 1549
tonic-clonic seizure, p. 1556

Headache

Headache is probably the most common type of pain experienced by humans. The majority of people have functional headaches, such as migraine or tension-type headaches; the remainder have organic headaches caused by intracranial or extracranial disease.

Not all tissues of the cranium are sensitive to pain. The pain-sensitive structures in the head include the venous sinuses, dura, cranial blood vessels, three divisions of the trigeminal nerve (CN V), facial nerve (CN VII), glossopharyngeal nerve (CN IX), vagus nerve (CN X), and first three cervical nerves. Thus headache pain can arise from both intracranial and extracranial sources.

Headaches are classified using the International Headache Society (IHS) diagnostic criteria based on the characteristics of the headache and the facial pain. The primary classifications include tension-type, migraine, and cluster headaches. Characteristics of these headaches are shown in Table 57-1. A patient may have more than one type of headache. The history and neurologic examination are diagnostic keys to determining the type of headache.

TENSION-TYPE HEADACHE

Tension-type headache, the most common type of headache, is characterized by a bilateral feeling of pressure around the head. Tension-type headache has been called muscle-contraction, tension, psychogenic, and rheumatic headache. Tension-type headaches are often subcategorized as acute or episodic and chronic.

Etiology and Pathophysiology

It was originally thought that tension-type headache was the result of sustained and painful contraction of the muscles of the scalp and the neck. Recent evidence, however, does not support this mechanism in all patients with tension-type headaches. It is likely that neurovascular factors similar to those involved in migraine headaches play a role in the development of tension-type headaches.

Clinical Manifestations

There is no *prodrome* (early manifestation of impending disease) in tension-type headache. The IHS classification system defines *tension-type headache* as involving at least two of the following characteristics: pressure or tightness sensation, mild to moderate severity, bilateral location, or worsening with physical activity. The headache does not involve nausea or vomiting but may involve sensitivity to light *(photophobia)* or sound *(phonophobia).* The headaches may occur intermittently for weeks, months, or even years. Many patients can have a combination of migraine and tension-type headaches, with features of both headaches occurring simultaneously. Patients with migraine headaches may experience tension-type headaches between migraine attacks.

Diagnostic Studies

Careful history taking is probably the most important diagnostic tool for tension-type headache. Electromyography (EMG) may be performed. This test may reveal sustained contraction of the neck, scalp, or facial muscles, but many patients may not show increased muscle tension with this test, even when the test

Reviewed by Mary S. Baird, RN, MN, CNRN, ARNP, Nurse Practitioner, Northwest Neuromuscular Association, Olympia, Wash.

TABLE 57-1	Comparison of Tension-Type, Migraine, and Cluster Headaches		
PATTERN	**TENSION-TYPE HEADACHE**	**MIGRAINE HEADACHE**	**CLUSTER HEADACHE**
Site	Bilateral, bandlike pressure at base of skull, in face, or in both	Unilateral (in 60%), may switch sides, commonly anterior	Unilateral, radiating up or down from one eye
Quality	Constant, squeezing tightness	Throbbing, synchronous with pulse	Severe, bone-crushing
Frequency	Cycles for several years	Periodic; cycles of several months to years	May have months or years between attacks; attacks occur in clusters: one to three times a day over a period of 4 to 8 weeks
Duration	Intermittent for months or years	Continuous for hours or days	30 to 90 minutes
Time and mode of onset	Not related to time	May be preceded by prodrome; onset after awakening; gets better with sleep	Nocturnal; commonly awakens patient from sleep
Associated symptoms	Palpable neck and shoulder muscles, stiff neck, tenderness	Nausea or vomiting, edema, irritability, sweating, photophobia, phonophobia, prodrome of sensory, motor, or psychic phenomena; family history (in 65%)	Vasomotor symptoms such as facial flushing or pallor, unilateral lacrimation, ptosis, and rhinitis

is done during the actual headache. Conversely, patients with diagnosed migraine headaches may show increased muscle tension on EMG. If tension-type headache is present during physical examination, increased resistance to passive movement of the head and tenderness of the head and neck may be present.

MIGRAINE HEADACHE

Migraine headache is a recurring headache characterized by unilateral or bilateral throbbing pain, a triggering event or factor, strong family history, and manifestations associated with neurologic and autonomic nervous system dysfunction. The onset of migraine usually occurs in childhood or adolescence. A family history of migraine can be found in 65% of patients with migraine. At some point in their lives, 7% to 9% of men and 16% to 25% of women will experience migraine headaches.[1]

Etiology and Pathophysiology

Although the exact cause of migraine headaches is not known, evidence suggests that neurologic, vascular, and chemical factors are involved.[2] The neurogenic model of migraine implies that a stimulus can trigger the trigeminovascular system (trigeminal nerve and its connections to meningeal blood vessels), producing inflammation of the blood vessels and vasodilation. This vasodilation ultimately results in headache. The neurotransmitter serotonin produces cerebrovascular dilation and stimulates afferent pain fiber activation, both of which are important in promoting migraine progression.

In addition to the headache itself, migraines can be preceded by prodrome and aura. The prodrome may precede the headache phase by several hours or several days. The **aura** (sensation of light or warmth) of migraine is associated with "spreading depression," a wave of *oligemia* (diminished cerebral blood flow) beginning in the occipital lobe and spreading forward in the brain at a rate of 2 to 3 mm per minute.

Migraine headaches, in many cases, have no known precipitating events. However, for other patients, the headache may be precipitated or triggered by stress, excitement, bright lights, menstruation, alcohol, or certain foods such as chocolate or cheese.

Clinical Manifestations

Migraines are subdivided by the IHS into those with aura (formerly called classic migraine) and those without aura (formerly called common migraine).

Migraine with aura is defined by IHS as involving at least three of the following: (1) reversible aura involves brain dysfunction; (2) aura symptoms develop gradually over more than 4 minutes, or two or more symptoms occur in succession; (3) no aura lasts more than 60 minutes; and (4) headache follows aura within 60 minutes. Migraine with aura occurs in only 10% of migraine headache episodes. The sharply defined aura may last for 10 to 30 minutes before the start of the headache and may include sensory dysfunction (e.g., visual field defects, tingling or burning sensations, paresthesias), motor dysfunction (e.g., weakness, paralysis), dizziness, confusion, and even loss of consciousness. The classic aura symptom is perception of flashing lights in one quadrant of the visual field, often termed *scintillating scotomata*. Migraine with aura usually peaks in 1 hour and may last several hours.

The IHS classification defines *migraine without aura* as involving at least two of the following characteristics: unilateral location, pulsating quality, moderate to severe intensity, worsening with activity, and at least one of either (1) nausea and vomiting or (2) photophobia and phonophobia. Migraine without aura is the most common type of migraine headache. The headache itself may last several hours or days.

Clinical manifestations that might occur in migraine with and without aura are generalized edema, irritability, pallor, nausea and vomiting, and sweating. In migraine with and without aura, the prodrome is not sharply defined. The prodrome can include psychic disturbances, gastrointestinal upset, and changes in fluid balance.

During the headache phase, some patients with migraine may tend to "hibernate"; that is, they seek shelter from noise, light, odors, people, and problems. The headache is described as a steady, throbbing pain that is synchronous with the pulse. However, the presentation of migraine is varied in its severity. Not all migraine headaches are disabling, and many patients who have migraine headaches do not seek health care treatment for them. Although the headache is usually unilateral, it may switch to the opposite side in another episode.

Diagnostic Studies

There are no specific laboratory or radiologic tests for migraine headache. The diagnosis of migraine headache is usually made from the history. The neurologic and other diagnostic examinations are often normal.

The IHS criteria are used as the clinical basis for migraine diagnosis. If atypical features are present, secondary headaches must be ruled out. Neuroimaging techniques (e.g., head computed tomography [CT], with or without contrast, and magnetic resonance imaging [MRI]) are not recommended for routine evaluation of headache unless abnormal findings are found on the neurologic examination.

CLUSTER HEADACHE

Cluster headaches are characterized by repeated headaches that can occur for weeks to months at a time, followed by periods of remission. It is one of the most severe forms of head pain. Cluster headache occurs less frequently than migraine (the cluster headache to migraine frequency is 1:10) and is more frequent in men than in women by a ratio of 8:1. The onset is usually between 20 and 50 years of age.

Etiology and Pathophysiology

Neither the cause nor the pathophysiologic mechanism of cluster headache is fully known. The vasodilation that occurs in the affected part of the face is extracranial. Similar to migraine headaches, the trigeminal nerve is implicated in the production of pain. Activation of this nerve causes release of substance P and other vasoactive substances that cause vasodilation, stimulation of afferent pain fibers, and neurogenic inflammation with extravasation (movement of fluid out of blood vessels). The periodicity (i.e., regularity in terms of timing) and autonomic symptoms of cluster headache indicate a dysfunction of the biologic clock mechanisms of the hypothalamus.[3] These headaches can also be triggered by alcohol ingestion.

Clinical Manifestations

The IHS classification defines *cluster headache* as involving severe unilateral orbital, supraorbital, or temporal pain and at least one of the following signs present on the pain side: conjunctival injection, lacrimation, nasal congestion, rhinorrhea, forehead and facial swelling, *miosis* (constricted pupil), *ptosis* (eyelid dropping), eyelid edema. The headache has an abrupt onset, usually without a prodrome. It peaks in 5 to 10 minutes and lasts 30 to 90 minutes. It is not uncommon for this type of headache to start at night, awakening the patient after a few hours of sleep. Headaches may recur several times a day over a period of several days, with each cluster lasting 2 to 3 months. It usually affects the upper face, the periorbital region, and the forehead on one side of the face and the head. The headache may not recur for months or years.

The patient may also exhibit conjunctivitis, increased lacrimation (tearing), and nasal congestion on the side of the headache.

Sweating may occur on the forehead of the affected side. A partial *Horner's syndrome* (miosis and ptosis on the affected side) may be seen. The headache is described as deep, steady, and penetrating but not throbbing.

Unlike the patient with migraine, who seeks isolation and quiet, the patient with a cluster headache paces the floor, cries out, and resents being touched. The patient with a cluster headache does not experience the systemic manifestations that accompany a migraine headache, such as nausea or vomiting. As with migraine headaches, there are usually no complications with cluster headaches.

Diagnostic Studies

The diagnosis of cluster headache is primarily based on the history. However, CT scan, MRI, or magnetic resonance angiography (MRA) may be performed to rule out an aneurysm, tumor, or infection.

OTHER TYPES OF HEADACHES

Although tension, migraine, and cluster headaches are by far the most common types of headaches, other types of headaches can also occur. These headaches may be the first symptom of a more serious illness. Headache can accompany subarachnoid hemorrhage; brain tumors; other intracranial masses; arteritis; vascular abnormalities; trigeminal neuralgia (tic douloureux); diseases of the eyes, nose, and teeth; and systemic illness (e.g., bacteremia, carbon monoxide poisoning, mountain sickness, polycythemia vera). The symptoms vary greatly. Because of the variety of causes of headache, clinical evaluation must be thorough. It should include an evaluation of personality, life adjustment, environment, and family situation, as well as a comprehensive evaluation of neurologic and physical status.

Collaborative Care for Headaches

If no systemic underlying disease is found, therapy is directed toward the functional type of headache. Table 57-2 outlines the general workup for a patient with headache to rule out any intracranial or extracranial disease. Table 57-3 summarizes the current therapies for prophylaxis and symptomatic relief of common

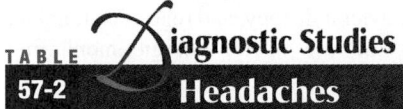

TABLE 57-2	Diagnostic Studies — Headaches

History and physical examination
Neurologic examination (often negative)
  Inspection for local infections
  Palpation for tenderness, bony swellings
  Auscultation for bruits over major arteries
Routine laboratory studies
  CBC
  Electrolytes
  Urinalysis
CT scan of sinuses
Special studies (e.g., CT scan, angiography, EMG, EEG, MRA, MRI)

CBC, Complete blood count; *CT,* computed tomography; *EEG,* electroencephalography; *EMG,* electromyography; *MRA,* magnetic resonance angiography; *MRI,* magnetic resonance imaging.

TABLE 57-3 Collaborative Care — Headaches

	TENSION-TYPE HEADACHE	MIGRAINE HEADACHE	CLUSTER HEADACHE
Diagnostic	History of neck and head tenderness, resistance to movement	History*	History
Collaborative Therapy			

Symptomatic	Nonnarcotic analgesics: aspirin, ibuprofen, acetaminophen
	Analgesic combinations: butalbital and aspirin (Fiorinal); butalbital and acetaminophen (Fioricet); dichloralphenazone, acetaminophen, and isometheptene (Midrin)
	Muscle relaxants
		Nonnarcotic analgesics:
		  aspirin, acetaminophen, ibuprofen
		Serotonin receptor agonists:
		  almotriptan (Axert)
		  eletriptan (Relpax)
		  frovatriptan (Frova)
		  naratriptan (Amerge)
		  rizatriptan (Maxalt)
		  sumatriptan (Imitrex)
		  zolmitriptan (Zomig)
		α-Adrenergic blockers:
		  ergotamine tartrate (Ergomar, DHE)
		Analgesic combination:
		  acetaminophen, dichloralphenazone, and isometheptene (Midrin)
		Corticosteroids:
		  dexamethasone (Decadron)
			α-Adrenergic blockers: ergotamine tartrate
			Vasoconstrictors
			Oxygen

Prophylactic	Tricyclic antidepressants:
	  doxepin (Sinequan)
	  amitriptyline (Elavil)
	β-Adrenergic blockers: propranolol (Inderal)
	Biofeedback
	Psychotherapy
	Muscle relaxation training
		β-Adrenergic blockers: propranolol (Inderal)
		Antidepressants: amitriptyline (Elavil)
		  imipramine (Tofranil)
		Calcium channel blockers: verapamil (Isoptin)
		Antiseizure: valproate (Depakene)
		Serotonin antagonist:† methysergide (Sansert)
		Biofeedback
		Relaxation therapy
		Cognitive-behavioral therapy
			α-Adrenergic blockers: ergotamine tartrate
			Serotonin antagonist:
			  methysergide (Sansert)
			Corticosteroids: prednisone
			Calcium channel blockers:
			  verapamil (Isoptin)
			Lithium
			Biofeedback

EMG, Electromyography.

*Magnetic resonance imaging (MRI) should be considered in nonacute headache patients with unexplained abnormal neurologic examination, atypical headache, headache features, or an additional risk factor, such as immune deficiency.

†Only for patients suffering from one or more severe headaches per week.

---

headaches. These therapies include drugs, meditation, yoga, biofeedback, cognitive-behavioral therapy, and relaxation training.

Biofeedback involves the use of physiologic monitoring equipment to give the patient information regarding muscle tension and peripheral blood flow (skin temperature of the fingers). The patient is trained to relax the muscles and raise the finger temperature and is given reinforcement (operant conditioning) in accomplishing these physiologic alterations.

Cognitive-behavioral therapy and relaxation therapy used alone or in conjunction with drug therapy may be beneficial to some patients. Acupuncture, acupressure, and hypnosis are also therapies that have worked well in some patients with headaches. These therapies are described further in Chapter 7. Treatments for tension-type headache include physical therapy (e.g., massage, hot packs, cervical collar), injection of local anesthetic into spastic muscles, and correction of faulty posture.

Drug Therapy

Tension-type headache. Drug treatment for tension-type headache usually involves a nonnarcotic analgesic (e.g., aspirin, acetaminophen) used alone or in combination with a sedative, muscle relaxant, tranquilizer, or codeine. However, many of these drugs have serious side effects. The patient should be cautioned about the long-term use of aspirin and aspirin-containing drugs because they can cause gastric bleeding and coagulation abnormalities in susceptible patients. Long-term use of Fiorinal should be avoided because in addition to aspirin it contains a barbiturate (butalbital), which may be habit forming. Drugs containing acetaminophen (Tylenol, Phenaphen, Midrin) can cause kidney damage with chronic use and liver damage when combined with alcohol.

Migraine headache. Drug treatment of the acute migraine attack is aimed at terminating or decreasing the symptoms of the attack. Many people with mild or moderate migraine can obtain relief with aspirin or acetaminophen. Ergotamine (Ergomar) is often used when simple analgesics do not relieve headache. Ergotamine inhibits the reuptake of norepinephrine into postganglionic nerve terminals of the sympathetic nervous system. This allows more norepinephrine to attach to α-adrenergic sites on smooth muscle in the artery wall, thereby causing prolonged vasoconstriction of cranial blood vessels. Ergotamine can be administered orally, sublingually, parenterally, rectally, or by inhalation. The usual dosage is 1 to 2 mg (oral or rectal) at the onset of the headache, followed by 2 mg within 1 hour. No more than 6 mg is given for any single attack. Dihydroergotamine mesylate is available as a nasal spray called Migranal.

Drugs that affect selected serotonin receptors, the "triptans," are aimed at treating the pathologic process of migraine. These drugs reduce neurogenic inflammation of the cerebral blood vessels and produce vasoconstriction. They include sumatriptan (Imitrex), naratriptan (Amerge), rizatriptan (Maxalt), almotriptan (Axert), frovatriptan (Frova), zolmitriptan (Zomig), and eletriptan (Relpax). Because these drugs cause constriction of coronary arteries, they are avoided in patients with heart disease. Triptans should be taken at the first symptom of migraine headache. Other drugs that may relieve migraine headache include butalbital with aspirin or acetaminophen (Fiorinal, Fioricet), isometheptene with acetaminophen and dichloralphenazone (Midrin, Migratine), and, in certain cases, narcotics.

A variety of drugs are used to reduce the frequency and severity of tension-type and migraine attacks. They are taken on a daily basis and are usually used when headaches occur more than twice a month. Preventive drugs for migraine headaches include β-adrenergic blockers (e.g., propranolol [Inderal], atenolol [Tenormin]), tricyclic antidepressants (e.g., amitriptyline [Elavil]), selective serotonin reuptake inhibitors (e.g., fluoxetine [Prozac]), calcium channel blockers (e.g., verapamil [Isoptin]), divalproex (Depakote), clonidine (Catapres), and thiazides. Another drug, methysergide (Sansert), competitively blocks serotonin receptors in the central and peripheral nervous systems. However, because of side effects, including retroperitoneal, pulmonary, and cardiac fibrosis, the patient taking methysergide requires regular follow-up. It is recommended that a patient taking methysergide have a break (drug holiday) every 4 to 6 months.

Cluster headache. Because cluster headaches occur suddenly, often at night, and are not long lasting, drug therapy is not as useful as it is for the other types of headaches. Prophylactic drugs may include verapamil, lithium, ergotamine, divalproex, or nonsteroidal antiinflammatory drugs (NSAIDs). Acute treatment of cluster headache is inhalation of 100% oxygen delivered at a rate of 7 to 9 L per minute for 15 to 20 minutes, which may relieve headache by causing vasoconstriction. It can be repeated after a 5 minute rest. However, a drawback to this treatment is that the patient must have continuous access to the oxygen supply. Sumatriptan is also effective in treating acute cluster headache. Methysergide may be used prophylactically when the cluster headache recurs at a known time.

Patients with frequent headaches may overuse analgesic drugs.[4] Such overuse can lead to chronic daily headache, also called *analgesic rebound headache* or drug-induced headache. Drugs known to cause this problem are acetaminophen, aspirin, NSAIDs (e.g., ibuprofen), butalbital, sumatriptan, and narcotics. Treatment involves abrupt withdrawal of the offending drug, except for opioids, which need to be tapered, and initiation of alternative drugs such as amitriptyline.

NURSING MANAGEMENT
HEADACHES

■ Nursing Assessment

Subjective and objective data that should be obtained from a patient with headache are presented in Table 57-4. Because the history provides the key to assessment of headache, it should include specific details of the headache itself, such as the location and type of pain, onset, frequency, duration, relation to events (emotional, psychologic, physical), and time of day of the occurrence. Information about previous illnesses, surgery, trauma, al-

TABLE 57-4	Nursing Assessment
	Headaches

Subjective Data

Important Health Information

Past health history: Seizures, cancer, recent fall or trauma, cranial infection, stroke; asthma or allergies; mental illness; relationship of headache to overwork, stress, menstruation, exercise, food, sexual activity, travel, bright lights, or noxious environmental stimuli

Medications: Use of hydralazine, bromides, nitroglycerin, ergotamine (withdrawal), nonsteroidal antiinflammatory drugs (in high daily doses), estrogen preparations, oral contraceptives, over-the-counter or prescription remedies

Surgery or other treatments: Craniotomy, sinus surgery, facial surgery

Functional Health Patterns

Health perception–health management: Positive family history; malaise

Nutritional-metabolic: Ingestion of alcohol, caffeine, cheese, chocolate, monosodium glutamate, aspartame, lunch meats (nitrites in cured meats), sausage, hot dogs, onions, avocados; anorexia, nausea, vomiting (migraine prodrome); unilateral lacrimation (cluster)

Activity-exercise: Vertigo, fatigue, weakness, paralysis, fainting

Sleep-rest: Insomnia

Cognitive-perceptual:

Migraine: aura; unilateral, severe, throbbing (possible switching of side) headache; visual disturbances; photophobia; phonophobia; dizziness; tingling or burning sensations

Cluster: unilateral and severe, nocturnal headache; nasal stuffiness

Tension-type: bilateral, bandlike, dull and persistent, base-of-skull headache, neck tenderness

Self-perception–self-concept: Depression

Coping–stress tolerance: Stress, anxiety, irritability, withdrawal

Objective Data

General

Anxiety, apprehension

Integumentary

Cluster: forehead diaphoresis, pallor, unilateral facial flushing with cheek edema, conjunctivitis

Migraine: generalized edema (prodrome), pallor, diaphoresis

Neurologic

Horner's syndrome, restlessness (cluster), hemiparesis (migraine)

Musculoskeletal

Resistance of head and neck movement, nuchal rigidity (meningeal, tension-type), palpable neck and shoulder muscles (tension-type)

Possible Findings

Possible evidence of disease, deformity, or infection on brain imaging (CT, MRI, MRA), cerebral angiogram, lumbar puncture, EEG, EMG; nonspecific brain imaging or laboratory tests

CT, Computed tomography; *EEG,* electroencephalography; *EMG,* electromyography; *MRA,* magnetic resonance angiography; *MRI,* magnetic resonance imaging.

lergies, family history, and response to medication should also be obtained. The nurse can suggest that the patient keep a diary of headache episodes with specific details. This type of record can be of great help in determining the type of headache and the precipitating events. If the patient has a history of migraine, tension-type, or cluster headaches, it is important to determine if the character, intensity, or location of the headache has changed. This may be an important clue as to the cause of the headache.

■ Nursing Diagnoses

Nursing diagnoses for the patient with headache may include, but are not limited to, those presented in NCP 57-1.

■ Planning

The overall goals are that the patient with a headache will (1) have reduced or no pain, (2) experience increased comfort and decreased anxiety, (3) demonstrate understanding of triggering events and treatment strategies, (4) use positive coping strategies to deal with chronic pain, and (5) experience increased quality of life and decreased disability.

■ Nursing Implementation

Patients with chronic headache present a great challenge to health care providers. Headaches may be related to an inability to cope with daily stresses. The most effective therapy may be to help patients examine their lifestyle, recognize stressful situations, and learn to cope with them more appropriately. Precipitating factors can be identified, and ways of avoiding them can be developed. Daily exercise, relaxation periods, and socializing can be encouraged because each can help decrease the recurrence of headache. The nurse can suggest alternative ways of handling the pain of headache through techniques such as relaxation, meditation, yoga, and self-hypnosis.

In addition to using analgesics and analgesic combination drugs for the symptomatic relief of headache, the patient should be encouraged to use relaxation techniques because they are effective in relieving tension-type and migraine headaches. The migraine sufferer often needs a quiet, dimly lit environment. Massage and moist hot packs to the neck and head can help a patient with tension-type headaches. The patient should learn about the drugs prescribed for prophylactic and symptomatic treatment of headache and should be able to describe the purpose, action, dosage, and side effects of the drug. To prevent accidental overdose, the patient should make a written note of each dose of drug or headache remedy.

For the patient whose headaches are triggered by food, dietary counseling may be provided. The patient is encouraged to eliminate foods that may provoke headaches, such as vinegar, chocolate, onions, alcohol (particularly red wine), excessive caffeine, cheese, fermented or marinated foods, monosodium glutamate,

NURSING CARE PLAN 57-1

Patient with Headache

EXPECTED PATIENT OUTCOMES	NURSING INTERVENTIONS and *RATIONALES*
NURSING DIAGNOSIS	**Acute pain** *related to* headache *as manifested by* complaint of steady, throbbing, or severe crushing pain.
▪ Reduced pain ▪ Satisfaction with pain relief	▪ Assess pain intensity, characteristics, location, and duration *to determine appropriate interventions*. ▪ Encourage patient to keep a pain log including associated or precipitating factors *to provide patient some control in identifying and controlling factors that may precipitate headaches*. ▪ Encourage patient to use alternative therapies such as massage, meditation, yoga, biofeedback, and relaxation techniques *to provide sense of control over pain*. ▪ Support patient's use of counseling or psychotherapy *to promote stress reduction*. ▪ Administer drugs as ordered *to reduce pain*.* ▪ Monitor patient following administration of pain medication *to assess drug efficacy and identify adverse drug effects*.
NURSING DIAGNOSIS	**Anxiety** *related to* lack of knowledge about headache's etiology and ways to treat it *as manifested by* ↑ heart rate, insomnia, feeling of helplessness.
▪ ↑ Psychologic comfort and ↓ anxiety ▪ Effective coping mechanisms to manage anxiety	▪ Assess level of anxiety *to determine appropriate interventions*. ▪ Encourage patient to verbalize concerns *because this reduces anxiety*. ▪ Explain possible etiology of patient's specific headache type *to reduce patient's fear of unknown*. ▪ Reinforce health care provider's explanation of diagnostic tests and treatment measures *to relieve concerns about cause and seriousness of headache*.
NURSING DIAGNOSIS	**Hopelessness** *related to* chronic pain, alteration of lifestyle, and ineffective treatment modalities *as manifested by* expressions of apathy and listlessness, lack of interest in doing usual activities.
▪ Expression of confidence in ability to function in spite of headaches	▪ Assess patient's degree of hopelessness *to enable appropriate planning*. ▪ Explore patient's self-treatment of pain and alterations in lifestyle *to make appropriate adjustments if necessary*. ▪ Promote verbalization of fears and concerns *to convey empathy and correct possible misconceptions*. ▪ Assist patient in identifying support systems that can be used *to bolster hopefulness*.

*See Table 57-3.

TABLE 57-5 Patient & Family Teaching Guide — Headaches

1. Keep a diary or calendar of headaches and possible precipitating events
2. Avoid factors that can trigger a headache:
   - Foods containing amines (cheese, chocolate), nitrites (meats such as hot dogs), vinegar, onions, monosodium glutamate
   - Fermented or marinated foods
   - Caffeine
   - Nicotine
   - Ice cream
   - Alcohol (particularly red wine)
   - Emotional stress
   - Fatigue
   - Drugs such as ergot-containing and monoamine oxidase inhibitors
3. Describe the purpose, action, dosage, and side effects of drugs taken
4. Be able to self-administer sumatriptan (Imitrex) subcutaneously if prescribed
5. Use stress-reduction techniques such as relaxation
6. Participate in regular exercise
7. Contact health care provider if the following occur:
   - Symptoms become more severe, last longer than usual, or are resistant to medication
   - Nausea and vomiting (if severe or not typical), change in vision, or fever occur with the headache
   - Problems with drugs

and aspartame. Active challenge and provocative testing with specific foods may be necessary to determine the specific causative agents. However, food triggers may change over time. Patients should avoid smoking and exposure to triggers such as strong perfumes, volatile solvents, and gasoline fumes. Cluster headache attacks may occur at high altitudes with low oxygen levels during air travel. Ergotamine, taken before the plane takes off, may decrease the likelihood of these attacks. A teaching guide for the patient with a headache is presented in Table 57-5.

■ Evaluation

Expected outcomes for the patient with headache are addressed in NCP 57-1.

Chronic Neurologic Disorders

SEIZURE DISORDERS AND EPILEPSY

Seizure is a paroxysmal, uncontrolled electrical discharge of neurons in the brain that interrupts normal function. Seizures are often symptoms of an underlying illness. They may accompany a variety of disorders, or they may occur spontaneously without any apparent cause. Seizures resulting from systemic and metabolic disturbances are not considered epilepsy if the seizures cease when the underlying problem is corrected. In the adult, metabolic disturbances that cause seizures include acidosis, electrolyte imbalances, hypoglycemia, hypoxia, alcohol and barbitu-

rate withdrawal, dehydration, and water intoxication. Extracranial disorders that can cause seizures are heart, lung, liver, or kidney diseases; systemic lupus erythematosus; diabetes mellitus; hypertension; and septicemia.

Epilepsy is a condition in which a person has spontaneously recurring seizures caused by a chronic underlying condition. The prevalence of epilepsy is 5 to 10 per 1000 persons.[5] It is higher in undeveloped countries. The incidence rates are high during the first year of life, decline through childhood and adolescence, plateau in middle age, and rise sharply again among the elderly.

Etiology and Pathophysiology

The most common causes of seizure disorder during the first 6 months of life are severe birth injury, congenital defects involving the central nervous system (CNS), infections, and inborn errors of metabolism. In patients between 2 and 20 years of age, the primary causative factors are birth injury, infection, trauma, and genetic factors. In individuals between 20 and 30 years of age, seizure disorder usually occurs as the result of structural lesions, such as trauma, brain tumors, or vascular disease. After 50 years of age the primary causes of seizure disorders are cerebrovascular lesions and metastatic brain tumors. Although many causes of seizure disorders have been identified, three fourths of all seizure disorder cases cannot be attributed to a specific cause and are considered *idiopathic*.

The role of heredity in the etiology of seizure disorders has been difficult to determine because of the problem of separating hereditary from environmental or acquired influences. In addition, some families carry a predisposition to seizure disorders in the form of an inherently low threshold to seizure-producing stimuli, such as trauma, disease, and high fever. Nevertheless, at least 40 seizure disorder syndromes have been linked to specific genetic defects.[6]

In recurring seizures (epilepsy) a group of abnormal neurons *(seizure focus)* seems to undergo spontaneous firing. This firing spreads by physiologic pathways to involve adjacent or distant areas of the brain. If this activity spreads to involve the whole brain, a generalized seizure occurs. The factor that causes this abnormal firing is not clear. Any stimulus that causes the cell membrane of the neuron to depolarize induces a tendency to spontaneous firing. Often the area of the brain from which the epileptic activity arises is found to have scar tissue *(gliosis)*. The scarring is thought to interfere with the normal chemical and structural environment of the brain neurons, making them more likely to fire abnormally.

Repetitive electrical discharges from an epileptic focus in experimental animals can produce long-lasting and possibly permanent changes in neuron excitability, both locally and in distant areas of the brain. This effect is called *kindling,* and it presents an interesting and important implication for epilepsy in humans: seizures can beget more seizures. Clinical experience indicates that the longer a patient goes without good seizure control, the lower the likelihood that the seizures will be controllable. Therefore a vigorous attempt must be made to control recurring seizures.

Clinical Manifestations

The specific clinical manifestations of a seizure are determined by the site of the electrical disturbance. The preferred method of classifying recurring seizures is the International Classification System[7] (Table 57-6). This system is based on the clinical and electroencephalographic manifestations of seizures. In this system, seizures are divided into two major classes: *general-*

TABLE 57-6 **International Classification of Seizure Disorders**

Generalized Seizures (Bilaterally Symmetric and without Local Onset)
Absence seizures, atypical absence seizures
Myoclonic seizures
Clonic seizures
Tonic seizures
Tonic-clonic seizures
Atonic seizures

Partial Seizures (Local Onset)
Simple partial seizures (no impairment of consciousness)
- With motor symptoms
- With somatosensory or special sensory symptoms
- With autonomic symptoms
- With psychic symptoms
Complex partial seizures (impairment of consciousness)
- Simple partial seizures with progression to impairment of consciousness
  With no other features
  With features of simple partial seizures
  With automatisms
- Impairment of consciousness at onset
  With no other features
  With features of simple partial seizures
  With automatisms

Unclassified Epileptic Seizures (Inadequate or Incomplete Data)

Modified from Commission on Classification and Terminology of the International League against Epilepsy: Proposal for revised clinical and electroencephalographic classification of epileptic seizures, *Epilepsia* 22:489, 1981.

---

ized and *partial.* Depending on the type, a seizure may progress through several phases, which include (1) the *prodromal* phase with signs or activity, which precede a seizure; (2) the *aural phase* with a sensory warning; (3) the *ictal phase* with full seizure; and (4) the *postictal phase,* which is the period of recovery after the seizure.

Generalized Seizures. **Generalized seizures** are characterized by bilateral synchronous epileptic discharges in the brain from the onset of the seizure. Because the entire brain is affected at the onset of the seizures, there is no warning or aura. In most cases, the patient loses consciousness for a few seconds to several minutes.

Tonic-clonic seizures. The most common generalized seizure is the generalized tonic-clonic, or grand mal, seizure. **Tonic-clonic seizure** is characterized by loss of consciousness and falling to the ground if the patient is upright, followed by stiffening of the body (tonic phase) for 10 to 20 seconds and subsequent jerking of the extremities (clonic phase) for another 30 to 40 seconds. Cyanosis, excessive salivation, tongue or cheek biting, and incontinence may accompany the seizure.

In the postictal phase the patient usually has muscle soreness, is very tired, and may sleep for several hours. Some patients may not feel normal for several hours or days after a seizure. The patient has no memory of the seizure.

Typical absence seizures. The **absence (petit mal) seizure** usually occurs only in children and rarely continues beyond ado-

lescence. This type of seizure may cease altogether as the child matures, or it may evolve into another type of seizure. The typical clinical manifestation is a brief staring spell that lasts only a few seconds, so it often occurs unnoticed. There may be an extremely brief loss of consciousness. When untreated, the seizures may occur up to 100 times a day.

The electroencephalogram (EEG) demonstrates a 3-Hz (cycles per second) spike-and-wave pattern that is unique to this type of seizure. Absence seizures can often be precipitated by hyperventilation and flashing lights.

Atypical absence seizures. Another type of generalized seizure is **atypical absence seizure,** which is characterized by a staring spell accompanied by other signs and symptoms, including brief warnings, peculiar behavior during the seizure, or confusion after the seizure. The EEG demonstrates atypical spike-and-wave patterns, usually greater or less than 3 Hz.

Other types of generalized seizures. Other generalized seizures are myoclonic and akinetic seizures. A *myoclonic seizure* is characterized by a sudden, excessive jerk of the body or extremities. The jerk may be forceful enough to hurl the person to the ground. These seizures are very brief and may occur in clusters.

The terms *akinetic* (arrest of movement), *atonic* (loss of tone), and *astatic* (loss of balance) have been used interchangeably to describe drop attacks or falling spells. This type of seizure involves either a tonic episode or a paroxysmal loss of muscle tone and begins suddenly with the person falling to the ground. Consciousness usually returns by the time the person hits the ground, and normal activity can be resumed immediately. Patients with this type of seizure are at a great risk of head injury and often have to wear protective helmets. A less severe akinetic seizure involves brief loss of muscle tone without falling.

Partial Seizures. **Partial seizures** are the other major class of seizures in the International Classification System. They are also referred to as partial focal seizures. Partial seizures begin in a specific region of the cortex, as indicated by the EEG and usually by the clinical manifestations. For example, if the discharging focus is located in the medial aspect of the postcentral gyrus, the patient may experience paresthesias and tingling or numbness in the leg on the side opposite the focus. If the discharging focus is located in the part of the brain that governs a particular function, sensory, motor, cognitive, or emotional manifestations may occur.

Partial seizures may be confined to one side of the brain and remain partial or focal in nature, or they may spread to involve the entire brain, culminating in a generalized tonic-clonic seizure. Any tonic-clonic seizure that is preceded by an aura or warning is a partial seizure that generalizes secondarily. Many tonic-clonic seizures that appear to be generalized from the outset may actually be secondary generalized seizures, but the preceding partial component may be so brief that it is undetected by the patient, by the observer, or even on the EEG. Unlike the primary generalized tonic-clonic seizure, the secondary generalized seizure may result in a transient residual neurologic deficit postictally. This is called *Todd's paralysis* (focal weakness), which resolves after varying lengths of time.

Partial seizures are further divided into (1) simple partial seizures (those with simple motor or sensory phenomena) and (2) complex partial seizures (those with complex symptoms). *Simple partial seizures* with elementary symptoms do not involve loss of consciousness and rarely last longer than 1 minute. They may involve motor, sensory, or autonomic phenomena or a combination of these. The terms *focal motor, focal sensory,* and *jacksonian* have been used to describe seizures of the simple partial type.

Complex partial seizures can involve a variety of behavioral, emotional, affective, and cognitive functions. The location of the discharging focus is usually in the temporal lobe, hence the term *temporal lobe seizure.* These seizures usually last longer than 1 minute and are frequently followed by a period of postictal confusion. Complex partial seizures are distinct from simple partial (focal motor, focal sensory) seizures in that they involve some alteration in consciousness. The sole manifestation of complex partial seizures may be clouding of consciousness or a confused state without any motor or sensory components. This type of attack is sometimes termed *temporal lobe absence.* There is rarely the complete loss of consciousness that is typical of the generalized absence attack, nor does the patient snap back to the preseizure state as does the patient who has had a generalized absence attack.

The most common complex partial seizure involves lip smacking and *automatisms* (repetitive movements that may not be appropriate). These are often called *psychomotor seizures.* The patient may continue an activity that was initiated before the seizure, such as counting out change or picking items from a grocery shelf, but after the seizure does not remember the activity performed during the seizure. Other automatisms are less organized, such as picking at clothing, fumbling with objects (real or imaginary), or simply walking away.

A variety of psychosensory symptoms may occur during a complex partial seizure, including distortions of visual or auditory sensations and vertigo. There may be alterations in memory, such as a feeling of having experienced an event before *(déjà vu),* or alterations in thought processes. Alterations in sexual functioning can vary from hyposexuality to hypersexuality. Many patients with temporal lobe seizures have decreased sexual drive or erectile dysfunction. However, some may experience sexual sensations during their seizures. This is because the abnormal electrical activity arises from the brain centers responsible for these sensations. Some experience increased sexual drive just after a seizure. In addition, some antiseizure drugs can cause a decrease in sexual drive because of sedation. Others can cause erectile dysfunction.

Complications

Physical. **Status epilepticus** is a state of continuous seizure activity or a condition in which seizures recur in rapid succession without return to consciousness between seizures. It is the most serious complication of epilepsy and is a neurologic emergency. Status epilepticus can involve any type of seizure. During repeated seizures the brain uses more energy than can be supplied. Neurons become exhausted and cease to function. Permanent brain damage may result. Tonic-clonic status epilepticus is the most dangerous because it can cause ventilatory insufficiency, hypoxemia, cardiac arrhythmias, hyperthermia, and systemic acidosis, all of which can be fatal.

Another complication of seizures is severe injury and even death from trauma suffered during a seizure. Patients who lose consciousness during a seizure are at greatest risk. Death can result from head injury incurred in a fall, from drowning in the bathtub, or from severe burns.

Psychosocial. Perhaps the most common complication of seizure disorders is the effect it has on a patient's lifestyle. Although attitudes have improved in recent years, epilepsy still carries a social stigma. It used to be associated with supernatural powers, possession by the devil, and insanity. Today the stigma probably exists because the characteristics of seizures are in direct conflict with modern societal values of self-control, conformity, and independence. The patient with epilepsy may experience discrimination in employment and educational opportunities. Transportation may be difficult because of legal sanctions against driving in most states and Canada. The patient may develop ineffective methods of coping.

Diagnostic Studies

The most useful diagnostic tools are accurate and comprehensive description of the seizures and the patient's health history (Table 57-7). The EEG is a useful diagnostic adjuvant to the history but only if it shows abnormalities. Abnormal findings help determine the type of seizure and help pinpoint the seizure focus. Unfortunately, only a small percentage of patients with seizure disorders have abnormal findings on the EEG the first time the test is done. EEGs may need to be repeated often, or continuous EEG monitoring may be needed to detect abnormalities. Abnormal discharges may not occur during the 30 to 40 minutes of sampling during EEG, and the test may never indicate an abnormality. It is not a definitive test because some patients who do not have seizure disorders have abnormal patterns on their EEGs, whereas many patients with seizure disorders have normal EEGs between

TABLE 57-7   Collaborative Care
Seizure Disorders and Epilepsy

Diagnostic

History and Physical Examination
Birth and development history
Significant illnesses and injuries
Family history
Febrile seizures
Comprehensive neurologic assessment

Seizure History
Precipitating factors
Antecedent events
Seizure description (including onset, duration, frequency, postictal state)

Diagnostic Studies
CBC, urinalysis, electrolytes, creatinine, fasting blood glucose
Lumbar puncture
CT, MRI, MRA, MRS, PET scan
Electroencephalography (EEG)

Collaborative Therapy
Antiseizure drugs (see Table 57-9)
Surgery (see Table 57-10)
Vagal nerve stimulation
Psychosocial counseling

CBC, Complete blood count; *CT,* computed tomography; *MRA,* magnetic resonance angiography; *MRI,* magnetic resonance imaging; *MRS,* magnetic resonance spectroscopy; *PET,* positron emission tomography.

seizures. Magnetoencephalography may be done in conjunction with the EEG. This test has greater sensitivity in detecting small magnetic fields generated by neuronal activity.

A complete blood count, serum chemistries, studies of liver and kidney function, and urinalysis should be done to rule out metabolic disorders. A CT or MRI scan should be done in any new-onset seizure to rule out a structural lesion. Cerebral angiography, single-photon emission computed tomography (SPECT), magnetic resonance spectroscopy (MRS), MRA, and positron emission tomography (PET) may be used in selected clinical situations.

Collaborative Care

Most seizures do not require professional emergency medical care because they are self-limiting and rarely cause bodily injury. However, if status epilepticus occurs, if significant bodily harm occurs, or if the event is a first-time seizure, medical care should be sought immediately. Table 57-8 summarizes emergency care of the patient with a generalized tonic-clonic seizure, the seizure most likely to warrant professional emergency medical care. The diagnostic studies and collaborative care of seizure disorders are summarized in Table 57-7.

Drug Therapy. Seizure disorders are treated primarily with antiseizure drugs (Table 57-9). Therapy is aimed at preventing seizures because cure is not possible. Drugs generally act by stabilizing nerve cell membranes and preventing spread of the epileptic discharge. In about 70% of the patients, seizure disorders are controlled by medication. The primary goal of antiseizure drug therapy is to obtain maximum seizure control with a minimum of toxic side effects. The principle of drug therapy is to begin with a single drug and increase the dosage until seizures are controlled or toxic side effects occur. Serum levels of the drug should be monitored if seizures continue to occur, if seizure fre-

TABLE 57-8 Emergency Management
Tonic-Clonic Seizures

ETIOLOGY	ASSESSMENT FINDINGS	INTERVENTIONS
Head Trauma Epidural hematoma Subdural hematoma Intracranial hematoma Cerebral contusion Traumatic birth injury **Drug-Related Processes** Overdose Withdrawal of alcohol, opioids, antiseizure drugs Ingestion, inhalation **Infectious Processes** Meningitis Septicemia Encephalitis **Intracranial Events** Brain tumor Subarachnoid hemorrhage Stroke Hypertensive crisis Increased ICP secondary to clogged shunt **Metabolic Imbalances** Fluid and electrolyte imbalance Hypoglycemia **Medical Disorders** Heart, liver, lung, or kidney disease Systemic lupus erythematosus **Other** Cardiac arrest Idiopathic Psychiatric disorders High fever	• Aura—peculiar sensations that precede seizure • Loss of consciousness • Bowel and bladder incontinence • Tachycardia • Diaphoresis • Warm skin • Pallor, flushing, or cyanosis • *Tonic phase:* continuous muscle contractions • *Hypertonic phase:* extreme muscular rigidity lasting 5 to 15 seconds • *Clonic phase:* rigidity and relaxation alternate in rapid succession • *Postictal phase:* lethargy, altered level of consciousness • Confusion and headache • Repeated tonic-clonic seizures for several minutes	**Initial** • Ensure patent airway. • Assist ventilations if patient does not breathe spontaneously after seizure. Anticipate need for intubation if gag reflex absent. • Suction as needed. • Stay with patient until seizure has passed. • Protect patient from injury during seizure. *Do not restrain.* Pad side rails. • Establish IV access. • Anticipate administration of phenobarbital, phenytoin (Dilantin), or benzodiazepines (diazepam [Valium], midazolam [Versed], lorazepam [Ativan]) to control seizures. • Remove or loosen tight clothing. **Ongoing Monitoring** • Monitor vital signs, level of consciousness, oxygen saturation, Glasgow coma scale, pupil size and reactivity. • Reassure and orient the patient after seizure. • Never force an airway between a patient's clenched teeth. • Give dextrose for hypoglycemia.

ICP, Intracranial pressure; *IV,* intravenous.

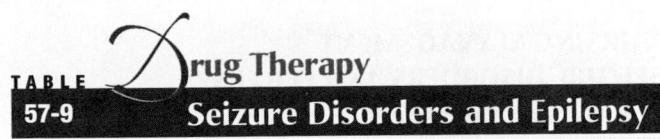

TABLE 57-9 Drug Therapy: Seizure Disorders and Epilepsy

Generalized Tonic-Clonic and Partial Seizures
carbamazepine (Tegretol)
divalproex (Depakote)
felbamate (Felbatol)
gabapentin (Neurontin)
lamotrigine (Lamictal)
levetiracetam (Keppra)
oxcarbazepine (Trileptal)
phenobarbital
phenytoin (Dilantin)
primidone (Mysoline)
tiagabine (Gabitril)
topiramate (Topamax)
valproic acid (Depakene)
zonisamide (Zonegran)

Absence, Akinetic, and Myoclonic Seizures
clonazepam (Klonopin)
divalproex (Depakote)
ethosuximide (Zarontin)
phenobarbital
valproic acid (Depakene)

Recently, many new drugs have become available, including gabapentin (Neurontin), lamotrigine (Lamictal), topiramate (Topamax), tiagabine (Gabitril), levetiracetam (Keppra), and zonisamide (Zonegran). These drugs are effective for partial seizures and for some of the primary generalized seizure disorders as well.

Felbamate (Felbatol) may be used to treat patients whose seizure disorders are refractory to other drugs. However, its use is limited because it can cause aplastic anemia and liver toxicity.

Treatment of status epilepticus requires initiation of a rapid-acting antiseizure drug that can be given intravenously. The drugs most commonly used are lorazepam (Ativan) and diazepam (Valium). Because these are short-acting drugs, they must be followed by administration of long-acting drugs such as phenytoin or phenobarbital.

Current drugs used in seizure management are shown in Table 57-9. Because many of these drugs (e.g., phenytoin, phenobarbital, ethosuximide, lamotrigine, topiramate) have a long half-life, they can be given in once- or twice-daily doses. This increases the patient's compliance with taking the drug by simplifying the drug regimen and avoiding the need to take it at work or school. Antiseizure drugs should not be discontinued abruptly because this can precipitate seizures.

Toxic side effects of antiseizure drugs involve the CNS and include diplopia, drowsiness, ataxia, and mental slowing. Neurologic assessment for dose-related toxicity involves testing the eyes for nystagmus, hand and gait coordination, cognitive functioning, and general alertness.

Idiosyncratic side effects involve organs outside the CNS, including the skin (rashes), gingiva (hyperplasia), bone marrow (blood dyscrasias), liver, and kidneys. Nurses should be knowledgeable about these side effects so that patients can be informed and proper treatment can be instituted. A common side effect of phenytoin is gingival hyperplasia (excessive growth of gingival tissue), especially in children and young adults. This can be limited by good dental hygiene, including regular toothbrushing and flossing. If gingival hyperplasia is extensive, the hyperplastic tissue may have to be surgically removed (gingivectomy), and phenytoin may have to be replaced by another antiseizure drug. Because phenytoin can also cause hirsutism in young people, other drugs are often used first.

Surgical Therapy. A significant number of patients whose epilepsy cannot be controlled with drug therapy are candidates for surgical intervention to remove the epileptic focus or prevent spread of epileptic activity in the brain (Table 57-10). The major types of surgery are removal of one lobe (usually the temporal

quency increases, or if drug compliance is questioned. The therapeutic range for each drug indicates the serum level above which most patients experience toxic side effects and below which most continue to have seizures. Therapeutic ranges are only guides for therapy. If the patient's seizures are well controlled with a subtherapeutic level, the drug dose need not be increased. Likewise, if a drug level is above the therapeutic range and the patient has good seizure control without toxic side effects, the drug dose need not be decreased. Many of the newer drugs do not require drug level monitoring because the therapeutic range is very large. If seizure control is not achieved with a single drug, the drug may be changed or a second drug may be added.

For many years the primary drugs for treatment of generalized tonic-clonic and partial seizures were phenytoin (Dilantin), carbamazepine (Tegretol), phenobarbital, and divalproex (Depakote). For treatment of absence, akinetic, and myoclonic seizures the drugs included ethosuximide (Zarontin), divalproex (Depakote), and clonazepam (Klonopin).

TABLE 57-10 Surgical Procedures for Seizure Disorders and Epilepsy

TYPE OF SEIZURE	SURGICAL PROCEDURE	RESULTS
Complex partial seizure of temporal lobe origin	Resectioning of epileptogenic tissue	Absence of seizures 5 yr postoperatively in 55%-70% of patients
Partial seizures of frontal lobe origin	Resectioning of epileptogenic tissue (if in resectable area)	Absence of seizures 5 yr postoperatively in 30%-50% of patients
Generalized seizures (Lennox-Gastaut syndrome or drop attacks)	Sectioning of corpus callosum	Persistence of seizures, less violent, less frequent, less disabling events
Intractable unilateral multifocal epilepsy associated with infantile hemiplegia	Hemispherectomy or callosotomy	Reduction in seizure frequency and type, improvement in behavior

lobe), removal of cortex, or separation of the two hemispheres (corpus callosotomy).[8]

The benefits of surgery include cessation or reduction in frequency of the seizures, but not all types of epilepsy benefit from surgery. An extensive preoperative evaluation is important, including continuous EEG monitoring and other specific tests to ensure precise localization of the focal point. Before surgery is performed, three requirements must be met: (1) the diagnosis of epilepsy must be confirmed; (2) there must have been an adequate trial with drug therapy without satisfactory results; and (3) the electroclinical syndrome (type of seizure disorder) must be defined.

Other Therapies. Another treatment for seizure disorders is vagal nerve stimulation. An electrode is surgically placed around the left vagus nerve in the neck. It is connected to a battery placed beneath the skin in the upper chest. The device is programmed to deliver intermittent electrical stimulation to the brain to reduce the frequency and intensity of seizures. The exact mechanism of action is unknown, although the stimulation may interrupt synchronization of epileptic brain-wave activity. This method is currently used in only a small number of patients.

Biofeedback to control seizures is aimed at teaching the patient to maintain a certain brain-wave frequency that is refractory to seizure activity. This method is still in the experimental stage.

NURSING MANAGEMENT
SEIZURE DISORDERS AND EPILEPSY

■ Nursing Assessment

Subjective and objective data that should be obtained from a patient with a seizure disorder are presented in Table 57-11. Data related to a specific seizure episode can be obtained from a witness.

■ Nursing Diagnoses

Nursing diagnoses for the patient with seizure disorders and epilepsy may include, but are not limited to, those presented in NCP 57-2.

■ Planning

The overall goals are that the patient with seizures will (1) be free from injury during a seizure, (2) have optimal mental and physical functioning while taking antiseizure drugs, and (3) have satisfactory psychosocial functioning.

■ Nursing Implementation

Health Promotion. Many cases of seizure disorders can be prevented by promotion of general safety measures, such as the wearing of helmets in situations involving risk of head injury. Improved perinatal, labor, and delivery care have reduced fetal

---

TABLE 57-11   Nursing Assessment
Seizure Disorders and Epilepsy

Subjective Data

Important Health Information

Past health history: Previous seizures, birth defects or injuries, anoxic episodes; CNS trauma, tumors, or infections; stroke; metabolic disorders, alcoholism; exposure to metals and carbon monoxide; hepatic or renal failure; fever; pregnancy, systemic lupus erythematosus

Medications: Compliance with antiseizure medications; barbiturate or alcohol withdrawal; use and overdose of cocaine, amphetamines, lidocaine, theophylline, penicillin, lithium, phenothiazines, tricyclic antidepressants, benzodiazepines

Functional Health Patterns

Health perception–health management: Positive family history

Cognitive-perceptual: Headaches, aura, mood or behavioral changes before seizure; mentation changes; abdominal pain, muscle pain (postictal)

Self-perception–self-concept: Anxiety, depression; loss of self-esteem, social isolation

Sexuality-reproductive: Decreased sexual drive, erectile dysfunction; increased sexual drive (postictal)

Objective Data

General

Precipitating factors, including severe metabolic acidosis or alkalosis, hyperkalemia, hypoglycemia, dehydration, or water intoxication

Integumentary

Bitten tongue, soft-tissue damage, cyanosis, diaphoresis (postictal)

Respiratory

Abnormal respiratory rate, rhythm, or depth; apnea (ictal); absent or abnormal breath sounds, possible airway occlusion

Cardiovascular

Hypertension, tachycardia or bradycardia (ictal)

Gastrointestinal

Bowel incontinence; excessive salivation

Urinary

Incontinence

Neurologic

Generalized

Tonic-clonic: Loss of consciousness, muscle tightening, then jerking; dilated pupils; hyperventilation, then apnea; postictal somnolence

Absence: Altered consciousness (5 to 30 seconds), minor facial motor activity

Partial

Simple: Aura; consciousness; focal sensory, motor, cognitive, or emotional phenomena (focal motor); unilateral "marching" motor seizure (jacksonian)

Complex: Altered consciousness with inappropriate behaviors, automatisms, amnesia of event

Musculoskeletal

Weakness, paralysis, ataxia (postictal)

Possible Findings

Positive toxicology screen or alcohol level; altered serum electrolytes, acidosis or alkalosis, very low blood glucose level, ↑ blood urea nitrogen or serum creatinine, liver function tests, ammonia; abnormal CT scan or MRI of head, abnormal findings from lumbar puncture; abnormal discharges on EEG

CNS, Central nervous system; *CT,* computed tomography; *EEG,* electroencephalogram; *MRI,* magnetic resonance imaging.

trauma and hypoxia and thereby have reduced brain damage leading to seizure disorders.

The patient with a seizure disorder should practice good general health habits (e.g., maintaining a proper diet, getting adequate rest, exercising). The patient should be helped to identify events or situations that precipitate the seizures and should be given suggestions for avoiding them or handling them better. Excessive alcohol intake, fatigue, and loss of sleep should be avoided, and the patient should be helped to handle stress constructively.

Acute Intervention. The nurse caring for a hospitalized patient with a seizure disorder or a patient who has had seizures as a result of metabolic factors involves several responsibilities, including observation and treatment of the seizure, education, and psychosocial intervention.

When a seizure occurs, the nurse should carefully observe and record details of the event because the diagnosis and subsequent treatment often rest solely on the seizure description. All aspects of the seizure should be noted. What events preceded the seizure? When did the seizure occur? How long did each phase (aural [if any], ictal, postictal) last? What occurred during each phase?

Both subjective data (usually the only type of data in the aural phase) and objective data are important. Objective data should

NURSING CARE PLAN 57-2

Patient with Seizure Disorder or Epilepsy

EXPECTED PATIENT OUTCOMES	NURSING INTERVENTIONS and *RATIONALES*
NURSING DIAGNOSIS	**Ineffective breathing pattern** *related to* neuromuscular impairment secondary to prolonged tonic phase of seizure or during postictal period *as manifested by* abnormal respiratory rate, rhythm, or depth.
• Appropriate rate, rhythm, and depth of respirations	• Loosen constricting clothing *to avoid restricting breathing.* • Assess breathing pattern, observing for labored respiration, tachypnea, bradypnea, dyspnea, and apnea *to determine presence and extent of problem and to initiate appropriate interventions.* • Provide manual ventilation or O_2 when necessary; be prepared to assist with endotracheal intubation *to maintain adequate oxygenation and prevent hypoxia.* • Insert oral airway (if indicated) only after seizure activity has ceased *to prevent mouth and teeth injury from forcing airway between clamped teeth.*
NURSING DIAGNOSIS	**Risk for injury** *related to* seizure activity and subsequent impaired physical mobility secondary to postictal weakness or paralysis.
• No injury • Verbalization of knowledge of potential for injury during seizure • Arrangement of environment to minimize risk for injury	• Assess for trauma to mouth, cheek, tongue, lips; abrasions, bruises; broken bones; burns *because these injuries may occur during seizure activity.* • Assess for weakness, paralysis of one side of body, ataxia, fatigue, lethargy *as potential postictal risks for injury to plan appropriate interventions.* • If patient anticipates a seizure may occur, assist to a safe location or position; use seizure precautions as appropriate; remove potentially harmful objects from surrounding area; gently guide arm or leg movements *to prevent injury during a seizure.* • Refrain from moving or restraining patient during a seizure *to prevent bone or soft tissue injury.* • Assist in determining whether operation of a motor vehicle or dangerous machinery is appropriate for patient *to assist patient in making the appropriate choice about driving.*
NURSING DIAGNOSIS	**Ineffective coping** *related to* perceived loss of control and denial of diagnosis *as manifested by* verbalizations about not having epilepsy, lack of truth-telling regarding seizure frequency, noncompliant behavior.
• Acceptance of disorder as evidenced by using the words *seizure disorder* or *epilepsy* to describe illness • Acknowledgment that a seizure has occurred	• Explore reasons for denial *to determine extent of problem and to plan appropriate interventions.* • Implement and individualize teaching plan about causes and mechanisms of seizures, effectiveness of drugs in controlling seizures, inaccuracy of myths about epilepsy, avoidance of precipitating factors, state law regarding driving, pros and cons of medical identification tags, moderation in drinking and eating, exposure to stress, and avoidance of hazardous activities *to promote effective coping by providing correct information.*
NURSING DIAGNOSIS	**Ineffective therapeutic regimen management** *related to* lack of knowledge about management of seizure disorder *as manifested by* verbalization of lack of knowledge, inaccurate perception of health status, noncompliance with prescribed health behavior.
• Therapeutic drug levels of antiseizure medication • Compliance with therapeutic regimen	• Provide teaching to patient and family about seizure activity and therapeutic management including diagnosis, treatment, lifestyle adjustments, and community resources *so that patient and family can make necessary lifestyle modifications to manage a chronic disease.*

include the exact onset of the seizure (which body part was affected first and how); the course and nature of the seizure activity (loss of consciousness, tongue biting, automatisms, stiffening, jerking, total lack of muscle tone); the body parts involved and their sequence of involvement; and the presence of autonomic signs, such as dilated pupils, excessive salivation, altered breathing, cyanosis, flushing, diaphoresis, or incontinence. Assessment of the postictal period should include a detailed description of the level of consciousness, vital signs, memory loss, muscle soreness, speech disorders (aphasia, dysarthria), weakness or paralysis, sleep period, and the duration of each sign or symptom.

During the seizure it is important to maintain a patent airway. This may involve supporting and protecting the head, turning the patient to the side, loosening constrictive clothing, or easing the patient to the floor, if seated. The patient should not be restrained, and no objects should be placed in the mouth. After the seizure the patient may require suctioning, and oxygen may be needed.

A seizure can be a frightening experience for the patient and for others who may witness it. The nurse should assess the level of their understanding and provide information about how and why the event occurred. This is an excellent opportunity for the nurse to dispel many common misconceptions about seizures.

Ambulatory and Home Care. Prevention of recurring seizures is the major goal in the treatment of epilepsy. Because many seizure disorders cannot be cured, drugs must be taken regularly and continuously, often for a lifetime. The nurse should ensure that the patient knows this, as well as the specifics of the drug regimen and what to do if a dose is missed. Usually the dose should be made up if the omission is remembered within 24 hours. The patient should be cautioned not to adjust drug doses without professional guidance because this can increase seizure frequency and even cause status epilepticus. The patient should be encouraged to report any medication side effects and to keep regular appointments with the health care provider.

Nurses play an important role in teaching the patient and the family. Guidelines for teaching are shown in Table 57-12. Nurses should teach family members and significant others the emergency management of tonic-clonic seizures (see Table 57-8). They should be reminded that it is not necessary to call an ambulance or send a person to the hospital after a single seizure unless the seizure is prolonged, another seizure immediately follows, or extensive injury has occurred.

Patients with a seizure disorder also experience concerns or fears related to recurrent seizures, incontinence, or loss of self-control. The nurse provides support for the patient through education and by helping to identify coping mechanisms.

Perhaps the greatest challenge that a seizure disorder presents to the patient is adjusting to the personal limitations imposed by the illness. Discrimination in employment is the most serious problem facing the person with a seizure disorder. For issues relating to job discrimination, patients can be referred to the State Human Rights Commission or the State Department of Vocational Rehabilitation.

A variety of other resources can be offered to the patient with a seizure disorder who has a specific problem. If the nurse believes that associating with others who have a seizure disorder would be beneficial, the patient can be referred to the local chapter of the Epilepsy Foundation (EF), a voluntary agency that offers a variety of services to patients with epilepsy. The

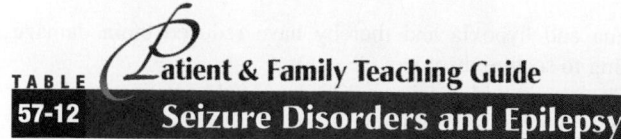

TABLE 57-12 **Patient & Family Teaching Guide**
Seizure Disorders and Epilepsy

The patient should be taught the following:
1. Drugs must be taken as prescribed. Any and all side effects of drugs should be reported to the health care provider. When necessary, blood drawings are done to ensure that therapeutic levels are maintained.
2. Use of nondrug techniques, such as relaxation therapy and biofeedback training, to potentially reduce the number of seizures.
3. Availability of resources in the community.
4. Need to wear a medical alert bracelet, necklace, and identification card.
5. Avoidance of excessive alcohol intake, fatigue, and loss of sleep.
6. Regular meals and snacks in between if feeling shaky, faint, or hungry.

Family members should be taught the following:
1. For first aid treatment of tonic-clonic seizure, it is not necessary to call an ambulance or send the patient to the hospital after a single seizure unless the seizure is prolonged, another seizure immediately follows, or extensive injury has occurred.
2. During an acute seizure, it is important to protect the patient from injury. This may involve supporting and protecting the head, turning the patient to the side, loosening constrictive clothing, and easing the patient to the floor, if seated.

patient who is an eligible veteran can be referred to a Department of Veterans Affairs medical center that provides comprehensive care.

The patient should be informed that medical alert bracelets, necklaces, and identification cards are available through the EF, local pharmacies, or companies specializing in identification devices (e.g., Medic Alert). However, the use of these medical identification tags is optional. Some patients have found them beneficial, but others have found them to be more a burden than a help because they prefer not to be identified as having a seizure disorder.

Social workers and welfare agencies can help with financial problems and living arrangements. State services for individuals with developmental disabilities include assistance with job training and placement for patients whose seizures are not well controlled. Sheltered housing and funding for special needs, such as medical and psychologic evaluation and transportation, are also offered. State agencies specializing in vocational rehabilitation services can offer vocational assessment, counseling, funding for training, and assistance with job placement. They can also offer financial assistance for transportation and medical costs that are necessary for vocational rehabilitation or job maintenance. If intensive psychologic counseling is needed, the nurse can refer the patient to a community mental health center.

The patient should be encouraged to learn more about epilepsy through self-education materials. The EF provides several information pamphlets and may facilitate support groups. Many agencies that offer services to epileptic patients, as well as local chapters of EF, have these available as teaching aids.

■ Evaluation

Expected outcomes for the patient with seizures are addressed in NCP 57-2.

MULTIPLE SCLEROSIS

Multiple sclerosis (MS) is a chronic, progressive, degenerative disorder of the CNS characterized by disseminated demyelination of nerve fibers of the brain and spinal cord. It is not known exactly how many people have MS. High prevalence rates (over 30 per 100,000) occur in northern Europe, northern United States, southern Canada, and southern Australia and New Zealand. Low prevalence rates (less than 5 per 100,000) occur in southern Europe, Japan, China, and South America. This difference may be related to climate or racial differences or both. MS is 5 times more prevalent in temperate climates (between 45 and 65 degrees of latitude), such as those found in the northern United States, Canada, and Europe, as compared with tropical regions.[9] MS is considered a disease of young to middle-age adults, with the onset usually being between 15 and 50 years of age. Women are affected more often than men.

Etiology and Pathophysiology

The cause of MS is unknown, although research findings suggest that MS is related to infectious (viral), immunologic, and genetic factors and is perpetuated as a result of intrinsic factors (e.g., faulty immunoregulation). The susceptibility to MS appears to be inherited. First-, second-, and third-degree relatives of patients with MS are at a slightly increased risk. Multiple genes confer susceptibility to MS.

The role of precipitating factors such as exposure to pathogenetic agents in the etiology of MS is controversial. It is possible that their association with MS is random and that there is no cause-and-effect relationship. Possible precipitating factors include infection, physical injury, emotional stress, excessive fatigue, pregnancy, and a poorer state of health.

MS is characterized by chronic inflammation, demyelination, and gliosis (scarring) in the CNS. The primary neuropathologic condition is an autoimmune disease orchestrated by autoreactive T cells (lymphocytes). This process may be initially triggered by a virus in genetically susceptible individuals. The activated T cells in the systemic circulation migrate to the CNS, causing blood-brain barrier disruption. This is likely the initial event in the development of MS. Subsequent antigen-antibody reaction within the CNS results in activation of the inflammatory response and through multiple effector mechanisms leads to demyelination of axons. The disease process consists of loss of myelin, disappearance of oligodendrocytes, and proliferation of astrocytes. These changes result in characteristic plaque formation, or sclerosis, with plaques scattered throughout multiple regions of the CNS.

Initially the myelin sheaths of the neurons in the brain and spinal cord are attacked (Fig. 57-1, *A* and *B*). Early in the disease the myelin sheath is damaged; but the nerve fiber is not affected, and nerve impulses are still transmitted (Fig. 57-1, *C*). At this point the patient may complain of a noticeable impairment of function (e.g., weakness). However, the myelin can regenerate, and the symptoms disappear, resulting in a remission.

In addition to myelin disruption, the axon also becomes involved (Fig. 57-1, *D*). Myelin is replaced by glial scar tissue, which forms hard, sclerotic plaques in multiple regions of the

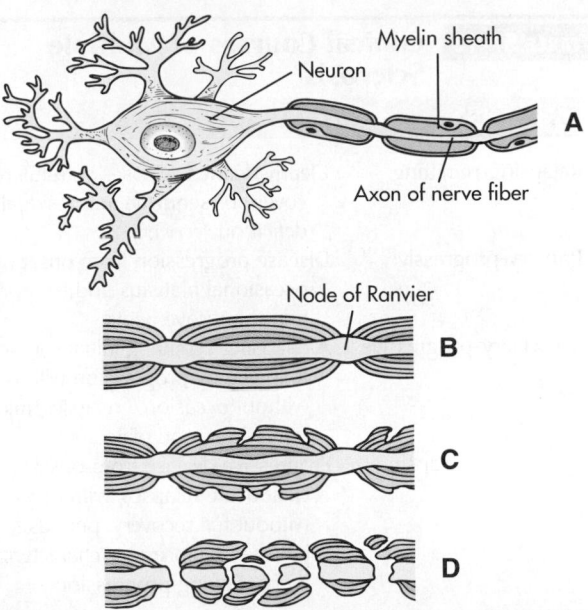

FIG. 57-1 Pathogenesis of multiple sclerosis. **A,** Normal nerve cell with myelin sheath. **B,** Normal axon. **C,** Myelin breakdown. **D,** Myelin totally disrupted; axon not functioning.

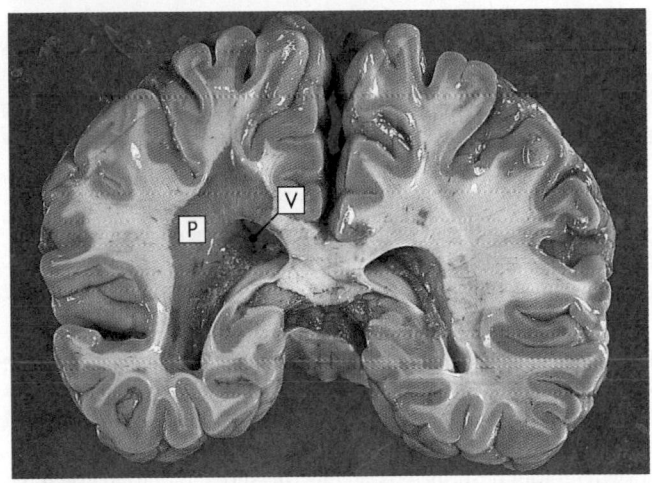

FIG. 57-2 Chronic multiple sclerosis. Demyelination plaque *(P)* at gray-white junction and adjacent partially remyelinated shadow plaque *(V)*.

CNS (Fig. 57-2). Without myelin, nerve impulses slow down, and with destruction of nerve axons, impulses are totally blocked, resulting in permanent loss of function. In many chronic lesions, demyelination continues with progressive loss of nerve function.

Clinical Manifestations

Because the onset is often insidious and gradual, with vague symptoms that occur intermittently over months or years, the disease may not be diagnosed until long after the onset of the first symptom. The disease process has a spotty distribution in the CNS, so the signs and symptoms vary over time. The disease is characterized by chronic, progressive deterioration in some persons and by remissions and exacerbations in others. With repeated exacerbations, however, progressive scarring of the myelin sheath occurs, and the overall trend is progressive deterioration in neurologic function.

TABLE 57-13 Clinical Courses of Multiple Sclerosis

CATEGORY	CHARACTERISTICS
Relapsing-remitting	Clearly defined relapses with full recovery or sequelae and residual deficit on recovery
Primary-progressive	Disease progression from onset with occasional plateaus and temporary minor improvements
Secondary-progressive	A relapsing-remitting initial course, followed by progression with or without occasional relapses, minor remissions, and plateaus
Progressive-relapsing	Progressive disease from onset, with clear acute relapses, with or without full recovery; periods between relapses are characterized by continuing progression

The clinical manifestations vary according to the areas of the CNS involved. Some patients have severe, long-lasting symptoms early in the course of the disease. Others may experience only occasional and mild symptoms for several years after onset. A classification scheme that identifies the various courses of MS has been developed[10] (Table 57-13).

Common signs and symptoms of MS include motor, sensory, cerebellar, and emotional problems. Motor symptoms include weakness or paralysis of the limbs, trunk, or head; diplopia; scanning speech; and spasticity of the muscles that are chronically affected. Patients with MS experience a variety of sensory abnormalities, including numbness and tingling and other paresthesias, patchy blindness (scotomas), blurred vision, vertigo, tinnitus, decreased hearing, and chronic neuropathic pain. Radicular (nerve root) pains may be present, particularly in the low thoracic and abdominal regions. Lhermitte's phenomenon is a transient sensory symptom described as an electric shock radiating down the spine or into the limbs with flexion of the neck. Cerebellar signs include nystagmus, ataxia, dysarthria, and dysphagia.

Bowel and bladder function can be affected if the sclerotic plaque is located in areas of the CNS that control elimination. Problems with defecation usually involve constipation rather than fecal incontinence. Urinary problems are variable. A common problem in MS patients is a spastic (uninhibited) bladder. This indicates a lesion above the second sacral nerve, which cuts off suprasegmental inhibiting influences on bladder contractility. As a result, the bladder has a small capacity for urine, and its contractions are unchecked. This is accompanied by urinary urgency and frequency and results in dribbling or incontinence. A flaccid (hypotonic) bladder indicates a lesion in the reflex arc governing bladder function. The bladder has a large capacity for urine because there is no sensation or desire to void, no pressure, and no pain. Generally, there is urinary retention, but urgency and frequency may also occur with this type of lesion. Another urinary problem is a combination of the previous two problems. Urinary problems cannot be adequately diagnosed and treated unless urodynamic studies are done.

Sexual dysfunction occurs in many persons with MS. Physiologic erectile dysfunction may result from spinal cord involvement in men. Women may experience decreased libido, difficulty with orgasmic response, painful intercourse, and decreased vaginal lubrication. Diminished sensation can prevent a normal sexual response in both sexes. The emotional effects of chronic illness and the loss of self-esteem also contribute to loss of sexual response.

MS has no apparent effect on the course of pregnancy, labor, delivery, or lactation. Some women with MS who become pregnant experience remission or an improvement in their symptoms during the gestation period. The hormonal changes associated with pregnancy appear to affect the immune system. However, during the postpartum period, women are at greater risk for exacerbation of the disease.[11]

Although intellectual functioning generally remains intact, emotional stability may be affected. Cognitive sequelae can produce significant disability for some patients with MS. Persons may experience anger, depression, or euphoria. Signs and symptoms of MS are aggravated or triggered by physical and emotional trauma, fatigue, and infection.

The average life expectancy after the onset of symptoms is more than 25 years. Death usually occurs because of infective complications (e.g., pneumonia) of immobility or because of an unrelated disease.

Diagnostic Studies

Because there is no definitive diagnostic test for MS, diagnosis is based primarily on history, clinical manifestations, and the presence of multiple lesions over time as measured by MRI (Table 57-14). Certain laboratory tests are currently used as adjuncts to the clinical examination. In some patients, cerebrospinal fluid (CSF) analysis may show an increase in oligo-

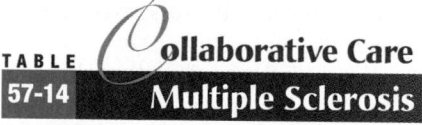

TABLE 57-14 Collaborative Care Multiple Sclerosis

Diagnostic
History and physical examination
CSF analysis
Evoked response testing (also called evoked potential testing, e.g., somatosensory evoked potential [SSEP], auditory evoked potential [AEP], visual evoked potential [VEP])
CT scan
MRI, MRS

Collaborative Therapy
*Drug Therapy**
Corticosteroids
Immunomodulators
Immunosuppressants
Cholinergics
Anticholinergics
Muscle relaxants
Surgical Therapy
Thalamotomy (unmanageable tremor)
Neurectomy, rhizotomy, cordotomy (unmanageable spasticity)

*See Table 57-15.
CSF, Cerebrospinal fluid; *CT*, computed tomography; *MRI*, magnetic resonance imaging; *MRS*, magnetic resonance spectroscopy.

clonal immunoglobulin G. The CSF also contains a high number of lymphocytes and monocytes. Evoked responses are often delayed in persons with MS because of decreased nerve conduction from the eye and the ear to the brain. MRI scan may be helpful because sclerotic plaques as small as 3 to 4 mm in diameter can be detected. Characteristic white-matter lesions scattered through the brain or spinal cord are evident on such a scan. MRS may also be used to evaluate patients with MS.

Collaborative Care

Drug Therapy. Because there is no cure for MS, collaborative care is aimed at treating the disease process and providing symptomatic relief (see Table 57-14). The disease process is treated with drugs (Table 57-15), and the symptoms are controlled with a variety of drugs and other forms of therapy.[12] Adrenocorticotropic hormone, methylprednisolone, and pred-

nisone are helpful in treating acute exacerbations of the disease, probably by reducing edema and acute inflammation at the site of demyelination. Although the dose and route of administration may vary, these drugs are used in patients with all types of MS. However, these drugs do not affect the ultimate outcome or degree of residual neurologic impairment from the exacerbation.

Immunosuppressive drugs, such as azathioprine (Imuran), methotrexate, and cyclophosphamide (Cytoxan), have been shown to produce some beneficial effects in patients with progressive-relapsing, secondary-progressive, and primary-progressive MS. However, the potential benefits of these drugs in patients with MS must be counterbalanced against the potentially serious side effects.

Immunomodulator drugs modify the disease process. Interferon β-1b (Betaseron) is used for ambulatory patients with relapsing-remitting MS. Interferon β-1a (Avonex) is similar to interferon β-1b in efficacy and is used in similar patient groups with

TABLE 57-15 Drug Therapy: Multiple Sclerosis

DRUG	SYMPTOMS RELIEVED	SIDE EFFECTS AND PRECAUTIONS	PATIENT TEACHING
Corticosteroids ACTH, prednisone, methylprednisolone	Exacerbations	Edema, mental changes (euphoria), weight gain, redistribution of body fat*; widespread effects on many metabolic processes; few adverse effects with use for less than 1 month at a time	• Restrict salt intake • Do not abruptly stop therapy • Know drug interactions
Immunomodulators β-interferon (Betaseron, Avonex, Rebif)	Exacerbations	Flulike symptoms, local skin reactions, depression; monitor CBC, blood chemistries, and liver function tests every 3 months	• Perform self-injection techniques • Report side effects
glatiramer acetate (Copaxone)	Exacerbations	Local skin reactions; chest pain, weakness; no laboratory monitoring required	• Perform self-injection techniques • Report side effects
Immunosuppressants mitoxantrone (Novantrone)	Exacerbations	Nausea, vomiting, diarrhea, mucositis, alopecia, hepatotoxicity, myelosuppression; cardiovascular disease; lifetime dose limit because of cardiotoxicity; monitor CBC and liver function every month	• Receive regular monitoring and follow-up • Consult health care provider before getting immunizations • Be aware that urine may turn a blue-green color initially • Maintain adequate fluid intake
Cholinergics bethanechol (Urecholine) neostigmine (Prostigmin)	Urinary retention (flaccid bladder)	Hypotension, diarrhea, diaphoresis, muscle weakness; history of cardiac dysfunction, hypotension, allergies, peptic ulcer disease, asthma	• Consult with health care provider before using other drugs, including over-the-counter drugs
Anticholinergics probanthine (Pro-Banthine) oxybutynin (Ditropan)	Urinary frequency† and urgency (spastic bladder)	Dry mouth, blurred vision, constipation, hypertension, flushing, urinary retention (too high of dose); contraindicated with history of glaucoma, prostatic hyperplasia, cardiac dysfunction, intestinal obstruction	• Consult health care provider before using other drugs, especially sleeping aids, antihistamines (possibly leading to potentiated effect)

*See Chapter 48 for effects of long-term corticosteroid therapy.
†Urodynamic studies must be done before initiation of therapy because patients with MS have multiple lesions and type of bladder dysfunction cannot be diagnosed from symptoms alone.
ACTH, Adrenocorticotropic hormone; *CBC,* complete blood count; *CNS,* central nervous system; *MAO,* monoamine oxidase.

Continued

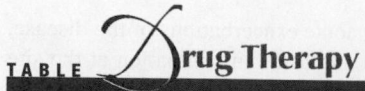

TABLE 57-15	Drug Therapy — Multiple Sclerosis—cont'd		
DRUG	**SYMPTOMS RELIEVED**	**SIDE EFFECTS AND PRECAUTIONS**	**PATIENT TEACHING**
Muscle Relaxants			
diazepam (Valium)	Spasticity	Drowsiness, ataxia, fatigue; contraindicated with history of narrow-angle glaucoma	• Avoid driving and similar activities because of CNS depressant effects • Be aware of addictive potential • Avoid long-term use • Avoid concomitant use of barbiturates, MAO inhibitors, antidepressants
baclofen (Lioresal)	Spasticity	Drowsiness, weakness; used cautiously with a history of hypersensitivity and renal damage; possible exacerbation of seizures in patients with seizure disorders	• Do not abruptly stop therapy (possibility of hallucinations) • Avoid driving and similar activities because of sedative effects • Avoid use of other CNS depressants • Take with food or milk
dantrolene (Dantrium)	Spasticity	Drowsiness, dizziness, malaise, fatigue, diarrhea; used cautiously in patients with a history of respiratory or cardiac dysfunction; risk of hepatotoxicity	• Avoid driving when drug is used • Avoid use with tranquilizers and alcohol (possibly causing photosensitivity) • Obtain baseline liver function tests
tizanidine (Zanaflex)	Spasticity	Drowsiness, dry mouth, fatigue, nausea; used cautiously in patients with history of hypersensitivity, liver or renal disease, hypotension, bradycardia	• Avoid driving when drug is used • Avoid use with tranquilizers and alcohol (possibly causing photosensitivity) • Eat small frequent meals to reduce nausea • Change position slowly when going from lying or sitting position to standing

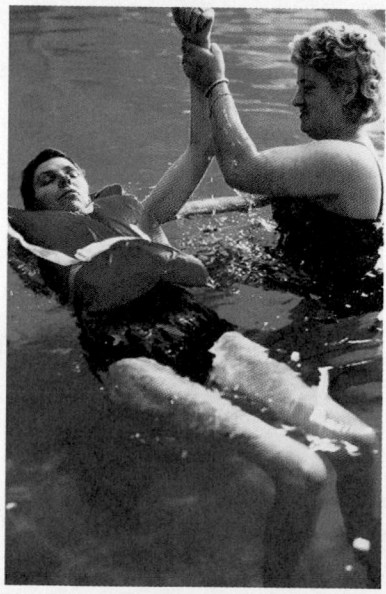

FIG. 57-3 Water therapy provides exercise and recreation for the patient with a chronic neurologic disease.

MS. It is given intramuscularly once a week. Interferon β-1a (Rebif) is administered subcutaneously 3 times weekly. Glatiramer acetate (Copaxone), formerly known as copolymer-1, is unrelated to interferon. It is given subcutaneously every day in patients with relapsing-remitting MS.[12] Natalizumab (Antegren), a recombinant monoclonal antibody to a leukocyte adhesion molecule, is a promising new therapy for MS. It works by inhibiting the migration of lymphocytes, thus decreasing the inflammatory process.

Mitoxantrone (Novantrone) is a new drug for the treatment of primary-progressive and progressive-relapsing MS. It is an immunosuppressant drug that reduces both B and T lymphocytes and impairs antigen presentation. It is given intravenously monthly. Unlike the other disease-modifying drugs, mitoxantrone has a lifetime dose limit because of cardiac toxicity. Therefore it cannot be used for more than 2 to 3 years.

Many other drugs are used to treat the symptoms of MS. Antispasmodics are used for spasticity. Amantadine (Symmetrel) and CNS stimulants (pemoline [Cylert], methylphenidate [Ritalin], and modafinil [Provigil]) are used for fatigue. Anticholinergics are used to treat bladder symptoms. Tricyclic antidepressants and antiseizure drugs are used for chronic pain syndromes.

Other Therapies. Spasticity is primarily treated with antispasmodic drugs. However, surgery (e.g., neurectomy, rhizotomy, cordotomy), dorsal-column electrical stimulation, or intrathecal baclofen (Lioresal) pump may be required. Tremors that become unmanageable with drugs are sometimes treated by thalamotomy or deep brain stimulation.

Neurologic dysfunction sometimes improves with physical therapy and speech therapy. Physical therapy is important in keeping the patient as functionally active as possible. The purpose of therapy is to relieve spasticity, increase coordination, and train the patient to substitute unaffected muscles for impaired ones. An especially beneficial type of physical therapy is water exercise (Fig. 57-3). Water gives buoyancy to the body and allows the patient to perform activities that would normally be impossible. In water, the patient experiences more control over the body.

Nutritional Therapy. Various nutritional measures have been used in the management of MS, including megavitamin therapy (cobalamin [vitamin B_{12}], vitamin C) and diets consisting of low-fat and gluten-free food and raw vegetables. These particular dietary measures have not come into widespread use because of lack of proof of their effectiveness.

A nutritious, well-balanced diet is essential. Although there is no standard prescribed diet, a high-protein diet with supplementary vitamins is often advocated. A diet high in roughage may help relieve the problem of constipation. Vitamins are merely supplemental and not curative.

NURSING MANAGEMENT
MULTIPLE SCLEROSIS

■ Nursing Assessment

Subjective and objective data that should be obtained from a patient with MS are presented in Table 57-16.

■ Nursing Diagnoses

Nursing diagnoses for the patient with MS may include, but are not limited to, those presented in NCP 57-3.

■ Planning

The overall goals are that the patient with MS will (1) maximize neuromuscular function, (2) maintain independence in activities of daily living for as long as possible, (3) optimize psychosocial well-being, (4) adjust to the illness, and (5) reduce factors that precipitate exacerbations.

■ Nursing Implementation

The patient with MS should be aware of triggers that may cause exacerbations or worsening of the disease. Exacerbations of MS are triggered by infection (especially upper respiratory and urinary tract infections), trauma, immunization, delivery after pregnancy, stress, and change in climate. Of these the best documented are upper respiratory infections, postpartum period, and head trauma.[13] Each person responds differently to these triggers. The nurse should help the patient identify particular triggers and develop ways to avoid them or minimize their effects.

The most common reasons for hospitalization of the patient with MS are for a diagnostic workup and treatment of an acute exacerbation. During the diagnostic phase the patient needs reassurance that even though there is a tentative diagnosis of MS, certain diagnostic studies must be done to rule out other neurologic disorders. The nurse should assist the patient in dealing with the anxiety caused by a diagnosis of a disabling illness. The patient with recently diagnosed MS may need assistance with the grieving process.

During an acute exacerbation the patient may be immobile and confined to bed. The focus of nursing intervention at this phase is to prevent major complications of immobility, such as respiratory and urinary tract infections and pressure ulcers.

Patient teaching should focus on building general resistance to illness, including avoiding fatigue, extremes of heat and cold, and exposure to infection. The last measure involves avoiding exposure to cold climates and to people who are sick, as well as

---

TABLE 57-16	Nursing Assessment
	Multiple Sclerosis

Subjective Data

Important Health Information

Past health history: Recent or past viral infections or vaccinations, other recent infections, residence in cold or temperate climates, recent physical or emotional stress, pregnancy, exposure to extremes of heat and cold

Medications: Use of and compliance in taking corticosteroids, immunomodulators, immunosuppressants, cholinergics, anticholinergics, antispasmodics

Functional Health Patterns

Health perception–health management: Positive family history; malaise

Nutritional-metabolic: Weight loss; difficulty in chewing, dysphagia

Elimination: Urinary frequency, urgency, dribbling or incontinence, retention; constipation

Activity-exercise: Generalized muscle weakness, muscle fatigue; tingling and numbness, ataxia (clumsiness)

Cognitive-perceptual: Eye, back, leg, joint pain; painful muscle spasms; vertigo; blurred or lost vision; diplopia; tinnitus

Sexuality-reproductive: Impotence, decreased libido

Coping-stress tolerance: Anger, depression, euphoria, social isolation

Objective Data

General

Apathy, inattentiveness

Integumentary

Pressure ulcers

Neurologic

Scanning speech, nystagmus, ataxia, tremor, spasticity, hyperreflexia, decreased hearing

Musculoskeletal

Muscular weakness, paresis, paralysis, spasms, foot dragging, dysarthria

Possible Findings

↓ T-suppressor cells, demyelinating lesions on MRI or MRS scans, increased IgG or oligoclonal banding in cerebrospinal fluid, delayed evoked potential

IgG, Immunoglobulin G; *MRI,* magnetic resonance imaging; *MRS,* magnetic resonance spectroscopy.

---

vigorous and early treatment of infection when it does occur. It is important to teach the patient to (1) achieve a good balance of exercise and rest, (2) eat nutritious and well-balanced meals, and (3) avoid the hazards of immobility (e.g., contractures, pressure ulcers). Patients should know their treatment regimens, the side effects of drugs and how to watch for them, and drug interactions with over-the-counter medications. The patient should consult a health care provider before taking nonprescription drugs.

Bladder control is a major problem for many patients with MS. Although anticholinergics may be beneficial for some patients to decrease spasticity, other patients may need to be taught self-catheterization (see Chapter 44). Bowel problems, particularly constipation, occur frequently in patients with MS. Increasing the dietary fiber intake may help some patients achieve regularity in bowel habits.

NURSING CARE PLAN 57-3

Patient with Multiple Sclerosis

EXPECTED PATIENT OUTCOMES	NURSING INTERVENTIONS and *RATIONALES*
NURSING DIAGNOSIS	**Impaired physical mobility** *related to* muscle weakness or paralysis and muscle spasticity *as manifested by* inability to ambulate, intermittent muscle spasms, pain associated with muscle spasms.
• Demonstration of use of adaptive devices • Maintenance of or increased strength of limbs • ↓ Muscle spasms	• Use assistive devices as indicated *to decrease fatigue and enhance independence, comfort, and safety.* • Do active range-of-motion exercises at least 2 times per day *to prevent contractures and minimize muscle atrophy.* • Encourage and assist with ambulation and transfer as indicated *to maintain mobility, promote independence, and provide for safety.* • Change position of patient (if bedridden) at least q2hr to prevent circulatory problems and pressure ulcers. • Perform stretching exercises every 6 to 8 hours *to relieve spasms and contracted muscles.*
NURSING DIAGNOSIS	**Dressing/grooming self-care deficit** *related to* muscle spasticity and neuromuscular deficits *as manifested by* inability to perform some or all activities of daily living (ADLs).
• Maximum level of functioning • ADL needs met by self or others	• Assess self-care problems *to plan appropriate interventions to meet care needs.* • Promote use of appropriate assistive devices *so that patient can maximally participate in self-care activities with minimum fatigue.* • Perform or assist with ADLs only as indicated *to promote patient's independence.*
NURSING DIAGNOSIS	**Risk for impaired skin integrity** *related to* immobility, sensorimotor deficits, and inadequate nutrition.
• Intact skin	• Assess skin for redness and breakdown *to monitor changes in skin integrity and make appropriate plan for interventions.* • Use circular massage of unreddened bony prominences with each turning *to improve circulation to these areas.* • Provide high-protein diet *to promote healthy skin resistant to breakdown.*
NURSING DIAGNOSIS	**Impaired urinary elimination pattern** *related to* sensorimotor deficits and/or inadequate fluid intake *as manifested by* posturination residual volume >50 ml, dribbling, bladder distention.
• Residual urine volume <50 ml • Maintenance of urinary continence	• Administer cholinergic drugs as ordered *to improve the muscle tone of bladder and facilitate bladder emptying.* • Follow intermittent catheterization protocol *to prevent distention or dribbling.* • Use Credé maneuver or reflex stimulation (manual stimulation) *as an alternative method of emptying bladder.* • Maintain fluid intake of 3000 ml per day *to dilute urine and reduce risk of urinary tract infection.* • Teach patient signs and symptoms of urinary tract infection *to ensure early identification and treatment.* • Initiate bladder training program *to help restore adequate bladder function.*
NURSING DIAGNOSIS	**Sexual dysfunction** *related to* neuromuscular deficits *as manifested by* impotence, verbalization of problem, decreased libido.
• Verbalization of satisfaction with expression of sexuality	• Initiate sexual counseling if indicated *because not all nurses have the education required for this type of counseling.* • Suggest alternative methods of achieving sexual gratification *because sexual intercourse may not be possible as a result of neuromuscular deficits.*
NURSING DIAGNOSIS	**Interrupted family processes** *related to* changing family roles, potential financial problems, and fluctuating physical condition *as manifested by* strained family relations, ineffective communication, verbalization of financial concerns.
• Open communication between family and patient • Able to seek outside assistance when indicated	• Facilitate open communication among patient and family *to promote better interpersonal relationships.* • Promote problem solving *to enable the family to handle the issues of long-term illness.* • Refer for family and financial counseling (if indicated) *to provide additional help in coping with a chronic debilitating disease.* • Educate family regarding fluctuating nature of disease *because lack of knowledge about MS affects ability to cope with the changes.*

NURSING RESEARCH
Health Promotion for Women with Multiple Sclerosis

Citation Shabas D, Weinreb H: Preventive health care in women with multiple sclerosis, *J Womens Health Gend Based Med* 9:389, 2000.

Purpose To evaluate the adequacy of preventive health care delivery (e.g., cancer and osteoporosis detection) in women with MS.

Methods 220 women with MS were surveyed regarding preventive medical practices.

Results and Conclusion Half of the women did not have regular medical preventive checkups; 25% did not have regular pelvic examinations; and 11% have not had a Pap smear within 3 to 5 years. Of women over 40 years old, 52% have not had yearly mammograms. Risk factors for osteoporosis included impaired mobility (53%), corticosteroid use (82%), and vitamin D deficiency as a result of sunlight avoidance. However, 85% have not had bone mineral density (BMD) testing, 50% are not taking calcium supplements, and 71% are not taking vitamin D. Among the postmenopausal women, 81% have never had BMD testing, 50% are not taking calcium supplements, and 70% are not receiving hormone replacement therapy. The benefits of preventive health care and prevention screening for cancer and osteoporosis should be stressed to women with MS.

Implications for Nursing Practice The presence of a chronic disabling condition affects the degree to which women engage in health promotion or disease prevention behaviors. Women with MS should be encouraged to seek regular medical checkups for disease prevention.

The patient with MS and the family must make many emotional adjustments because of the unpredictability of the disease, the need to change lifestyles, and the challenge of avoiding or decreasing precipitating factors. The National Multiple Sclerosis Society and its local chapters can offer a variety of services to meet the needs of patients with MS.

■ Evaluation

Expected outcomes for the patient with MS are addressed in NCP 57-3.

PARKINSON'S DISEASE

Parkinson's disease (PD) is a disease of the basal ganglia characterized by a slowing down in the initiation and execution of movement (bradykinesia), increased muscle tone (rigidity), tremor at rest, and impaired postural reflexes. It is the most common form of *parkinsonism* (a syndrome characterized by similar symptoms). Parkinson's disease is named after James Parkinson, who, in 1817, wrote a classic essay on "shaking palsy," a disease whose cause is still unknown.

Etiology and Pathophysiology

The prevalence of Parkinson's disease is about 160 per 100,000 and the incidence is about 20 per 100,000. The diagnosis of Parkinson's disease increases with age, with the peak onset in the sixth decade. Onset of Parkinson's disease before age 50 is more likely related to a genetic defect.[14] Parkinson's disease is more common in men by a ratio of 3:2.

There are many forms of parkinsonism other than Parkinson's disease. Encephalitis lethargica, or type A encephalitis, has been clearly associated with the onset of parkinsonism. However, the incidence of postencephalitic parkinsonism has dwindled since the 1920s, when there was a large outbreak of this infectious illness. Parkinsonism-like symptoms have occurred after intoxication with a variety of chemicals, including carbon monoxide and manganese (among copper miners) and the product of meperidine-analog synthesis, MPTP. Drug-induced parkinsonism can follow reserpine (Serpasil), methyldopa (Aldomet), lithium, haloperidol (Haldol), and phenothiazine (Thorazine) therapy. Parkinsonism can also be seen following the use of illicit drugs including amphetamine and methamphetamine. Other causes of parkinsonism include hydrocephalus, hypoxia, infections, stroke, tumor, and trauma.[15]

The pathologic process of Parkinson's disease involves degeneration of the dopamine-producing neurons in the substantia nigra of the midbrain (Figs. 57-4 through 57-6), which in turn disrupts the normal balance between dopamine (DA) and acetylcholine (ACh) in the basal ganglia. DA is a neurotransmitter essential for normal functioning of the extrapyramidal motor system, including control of posture, support, and voluntary motion. Symptoms of Parkinson's disease do not occur until 80% of neurons in the substantia nigra are lost.

Clinical Manifestations

The onset of Parkinson's disease is gradual and insidious, with a gradual progression and a prolonged course. It may involve only one side of the body initially. In the beginning stages, only a mild tremor, a slight limp, or a decreased arm swing may be evident. Later in the disease the patient may have a shuffling, propulsive gait with arms flexed and loss of postural reflexes. In some patients there may be a slight change in speech patterns. None of these alone is sufficient evidence for a diagnosis of the disease.

Tremor. *Tremor,* often the first sign, may be minimal initially, so the patient is the only one who notices it. This tremor can affect handwriting, causing it to trail off, particularly toward the ends of words. Parkinsonian tremor is more prominent at rest and is aggravated by emotional stress or increased concentration.

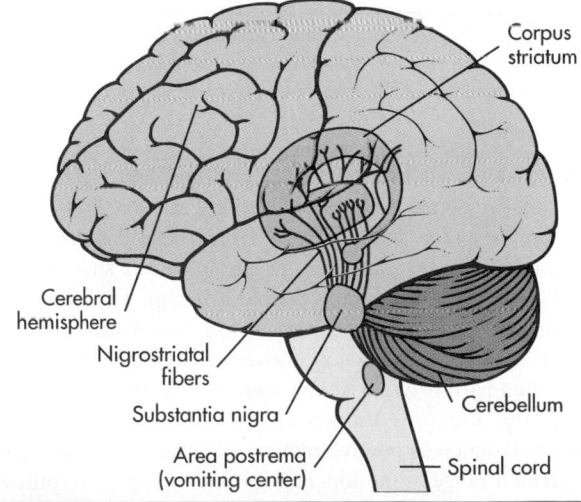

FIG. 57-4 Nigrostriatal disorders produce parkinsonism. Left-sided view of the human brain showing the substantia nigra and the corpus striatum (*shaded area*) lying deep within the cerebral hemisphere. Nerve fibers extend upward from the substantia nigra, divide into many branches, and carry dopamine to all regions of the corpus striatum.

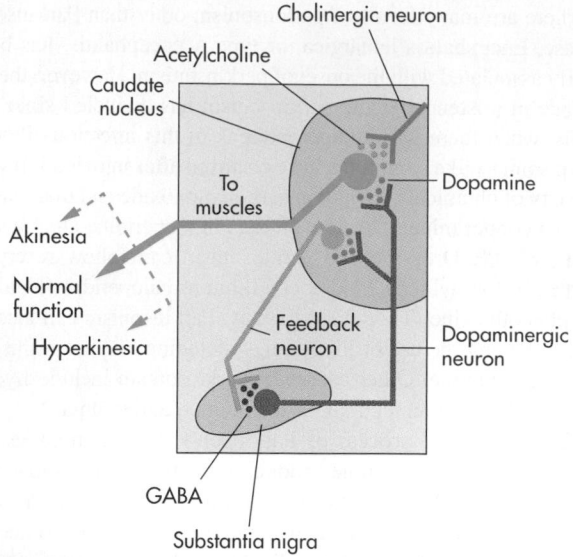

FIG. 57-5 Dopaminergic synaptic activity is mediated by dopamine. Cholinergic synaptic activity is mediated by acetylcholine. A balance between the two kinds of activity produces normal motor function. A relative excess of cholinergic activity produces akinesia and rigidity. A relative excess of dopaminergic activity produces involuntary movements. Neurons in the caudate nucleus contain γ-aminobutyric acid (GABA) and possibly control dopaminergic neurons in the substantia nigra through a feedback pathway.

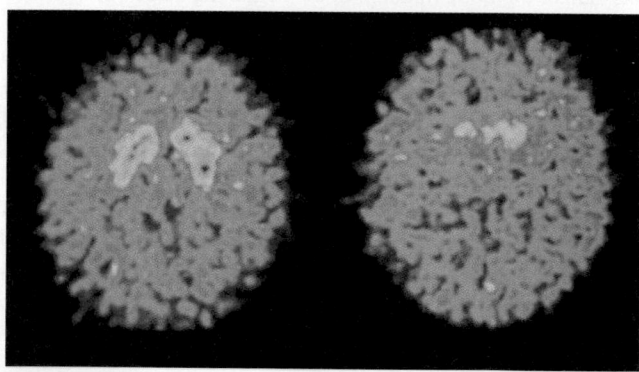

FIG. 57-6 Reduced fluorodopa in Parkinson's disease. Positron emission tomography (PET) scan showing reduced fluorodopa uptake in the basal ganglia *(right)* compared with a normal control *(left)*.

The hand tremor is described as "pill rolling" because the thumb and forefinger appear to move in a rotary fashion as if rolling a pill, coin, or other small object. Tremor can involve the diaphragm, tongue, lips, and jaw but rarely causes shaking of the head. Unfortunately, in many people a benign essential tremor has mistakenly been diagnosed as Parkinson's disease. Essential tremor occurs during voluntary movement, has a more rapid frequency than parkinsonian tremor, and is often familial.

Rigidity. *Rigidity,* the second sign of the triad, is the increased resistance to passive motion when the limbs are moved through their range of motion. Parkinsonian rigidity is typified by a jerky quality, as if there were intermittent catches in the movement of a cogwheel, when the joint is moved. This is termed *cogwheel rigidity.* The rigidity is caused by sustained muscle contraction and consequently elicits a complaint of muscle sore-

ness; feeling tired and achy; or pain in the head, upper body, spine, or legs. Another consequence of rigidity is slowness of movement because it inhibits the alternating of contraction and relaxation in opposing muscle groups (e.g., biceps and triceps).

Bradykinesia. *Bradykinesia* is particularly evident in the loss of automatic movements, which is secondary to the physical and chemical alteration of the basal ganglia and related structures in the extrapyramidal portion of the CNS. In the unaffected patient, automatic movements are involuntary and occur subconsciously. They include blinking of the eyelids, swinging of the arms while walking, swallowing of saliva, self-expression with facial and hand movements, and minor movement of postural adjustment. The patient with Parkinson's disease does not execute these movements, and there is a lack of spontaneous activity. This accounts for the stooped posture, masked facies (deadpan expression), drooling of saliva, and shuffling gait (festination) that are characteristic of a person with this disease. In addition, there is difficulty in initiating movement.

Complications

Many of the complications of Parkinson's disease are caused by the progressive deterioration and loss of spontaneity of movement. Swallowing may become very difficult (dysphagia) in severe cases, leading to malnutrition or aspiration. General debilitation may lead to pneumonia, urinary tract infections, and skin breakdown. Mobility is greatly decreased. The gait slows, and turning is especially difficult. The gait usually consists of rapid, short, shuffling ministeps. The posture is that of the "old man" image, with the head and trunk bent forward and the legs constantly flexed (Fig. 57-7). The lack of mobility may lead to constipation, ankle edema, and, more seriously, contractures.

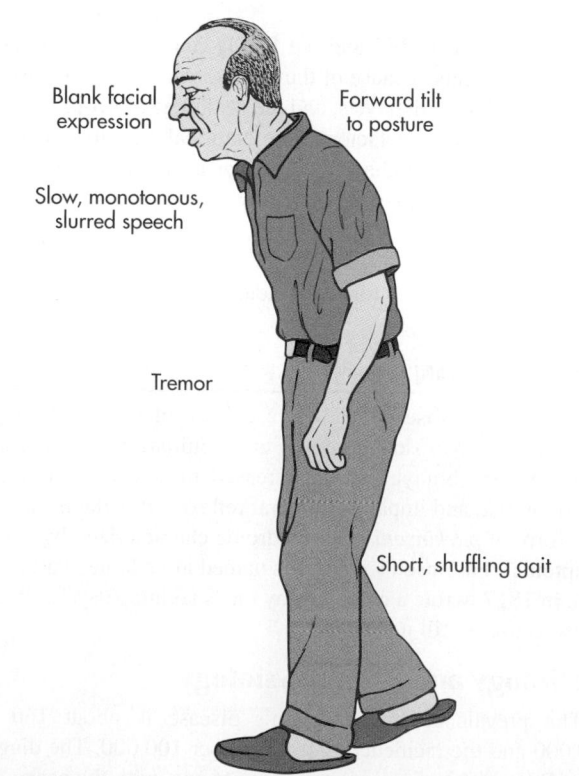

FIG. 57-7 Characteristic appearance of a patient with Parkinson's disease.

Orthostatic hypotension may occur in some patients and, along with loss of postural reflexes, may result in falls or other injury. Bothersome complications include seborrhea (increased oily secretion of the sebaceous glands of the skin), dandruff, excessive sweating, conjunctivitis, difficulty in reading, insomnia, incontinence, and depression.

Many of the apparent complications of Parkinson's disease are the result of side effects of drugs, particularly levodopa. These include *dyskinesias* (e.g., fidgeting movements of limbs), hallucinations, orthostatic hypotension, weakness, and akinesia (total immobility). These complications become apparent after prolonged levodopa (L-dopa) therapy.

Diagnostic Studies

Because there is no specific diagnostic test for Parkinson's disease, the diagnosis is based solely on the history and the clinical features. A firm diagnosis can be made only when at least two of the three characteristic signs of the classic triad are present: tremor, rigidity, and bradykinesia (slow or retarded movement). Dementia occurs in up to 40% of patients with Parkinson's disease.[16] The ultimate confirmation of Parkinson's disease is a positive response to antiparkinsonian drugs.

Collaborative Care

Because there is no cure for Parkinson's disease, collaborative management (Table 57-17) is aimed at relieving the symptoms.

Drug Therapy. Drug therapy for Parkinson's disease is aimed at correcting an imbalance of neurotransmitters within the CNS. Antiparkinsonian drugs either enhance the release or supply of DA (dopaminergic) or antagonize or block the effects of the overactive cholinergic neurons in the striatum (anticholinergic). Levodopa with carbidopa (Sinemet) is often the first drug to be used. Levodopa is a precursor of DA and can cross the blood-brain barrier. It is converted to DA in the basal ganglia. Sinemet is the preferred drug because it also contains carbidopa, an agent that inhibits the enzyme dopa-decarboxylase in the peripheral tissues. This enzyme breaks down levodopa before it reaches the brain. The net result of the combination of levodopa and carbidopa is that more levodopa reaches the brain, and therefore less drug is needed.

TABLE 57-17   Collaborative Care   Parkinson's Disease

Diagnostic
History and physical examination
Tremor
Rigidity
Bradykinesia
Positive response to antiparkinson drugs*
Rule out side effects of phenothiazines, reserpine, benzo-
    diazepines, haloperidol

Collaborative Therapy
Antiparkinson drugs*
Surgical destruction or deep brain stimulation of ventrolateral
    nucleus of the thalamus or posteroventral globus pallidus

*See Table 57-18.

Many patients are given Sinemet early in the disease course. However, some health care providers believe that after a few years of therapy, the effectiveness of Sinemet wears off, so they prefer to initiate therapy with a DA receptor agonist instead. These drugs include bromocriptine (Parlodel), pergolide (Permax), ropinirole (Requip), and pramipexole (Mirapex). These drugs directly stimulate DA receptors. When more moderate to severe symptoms are present, levodopa with carbidopa (Sinemet) is added to the drug regimen.

Anticholinergic drugs are also used to manage Parkinson's disease. These drugs act by decreasing the activity of acetylcholine, thus providing balance between cholinergic and dopaminergic actions. Antihistamines (e.g., diphenhydramine [Benadryl]) with anticholinergic properties or a β-adrenergic blocker (e.g., propranolol [Inderal]) are used to manage tremors. The antiviral agent amantadine (Symmetrel) is also an effective antiparkinsonian drug. Although its exact mechanism of action is not known, amantadine promotes the release of DA from neurons.

Selegiline (Eldepryl) is a monoamine oxidase (MAO) inhibitor that is sometimes used in combination with Sinemet. By inhibiting MAO, the degradative enzyme for DA, the levels of DA are increased. Entacapone (Comtan) and tolcapone (Tasmar) block the enzyme catechol-o-methyl transferase (COMT), which breaks down levodopa in the peripheral circulation, thus prolonging the effect of Sinemet. This helps to manage symptoms caused by "wearing off" of Sinemet before the next dose is due.

Table 57-18 summarizes the drugs commonly used in Parkinson's disease, the symptoms they relieve, and their common side effects. The use of only one drug is preferred because there are fewer side effects and the drug dosage is easier to adjust than when several drugs are used. However, as the disease progresses, combination therapy is often required. Excessive amounts of dopaminergic drugs can lead to *paradoxic intoxication* (aggravation rather than relief of symptoms).

Surgical Therapy. Surgical procedures are aimed at relieving symptoms of Parkinson's disease and are usually used in patients who are unresponsive to drug therapy or who have developed severe motor complications. Surgical procedures fall into three categories: ablation (destruction), deep brain stimulation (DBS), and transplantation. *Ablation surgery* involves stereotactic ablation of areas in the thalamus *(thalamotomy),* globus pallidus *(pallidotomy),* and subthalamic nucleus *(subthalamic nucleotomy).* Ablative procedures have been used for Parkinson's disease for over 50 years, but they have been replaced recently by DBS. DBS involves placing an electrode in either the thalamus, globus pallidus, or subthalamic nucleus and connecting it to a generator placed in the upper chest (like a pacemaker). The device is programmed to deliver a specific current to the targeted brain location. Unlike ablation procedures, DBS can be adjusted to control symptoms better and is reversible (the device can be removed). These ablative and DBS procedures work by reducing the increased neuronal activity produced by DA depletion.[17]

Transplantation of fetal neural tissue into the basal ganglia is designed to provide DA-producing cells in the brains of patients with Parkinson's disease. This form of therapy is still in the experimental stages.

Nutritional Therapy. Diet is of major importance to the patient with Parkinson's disease because malnutrition and constipation can be serious consequences of inadequate nutrition. Patients who have dysphagia and bradykinesia need appetizing

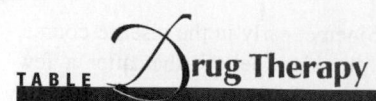

TABLE 57-18	Drug Therapy — Parkinson's Disease	
DRUG	**SYMPTOMS RELIEVED**	**SIDE EFFECTS AND PRECAUTIONS**
Dopaminergic		
levodopa (L-dopa)	Bradykinesia, tremor, rigidity	Nausea, dyskinesia, hypotension, palpitations, arrhythmias; agitation, hallucinations, confusion (in older patient); avoidance of vitamin pills and diet high in vitamin B_6 (reversal of effect of levodopa); contraindicated in narrow-angle glaucoma
levodopa-carbidopa (Sinemet)	Same as above	Less nausea but greater chance of dyskinesia, confusion, hallucinations; periodic check of BUN, AST, WBCs, Hct; contraindicated in melanoma, narrow-angle glaucoma, combination with MAO inhibitors, reserpine, methyldopa, guanethidine, antipsychotics
bromocriptine mesylate (Parlodel)	Same as above	Orthostatic hypotension, nausea, vomiting, toxic psychosis, limb edema, phlebitis, dizziness, headache, insomnia
pergolide (Permax)	Same as above	Same as above
pramipexole (Mirapex)	Same as above	
ropinirole (Requip)	Same as above	
amantadine (Symmetrel)	Rigidity, akinesia	Nervousness, insomnia, confusion, hallucinations, dry mouth, nausea, edema, orthostatic hypotension
Anticholinergic		
trihexyphenidyl (Artane)	Tremor	Dry mouth, blurred vision, constipation, delirium, anxiety, agitation, hallucinations; avoidance of drugs with similar actions, including over-the-counter drugs containing scopolamine or antihistamines (e.g., Sominex), antispasmodics (e.g., Donnatal, Bellergal), tricyclic antidepressants (e.g., imipramine [Tofranil], amitriptyline [Elavil])
cycrimine (Pagitane)		
procyclidine (Kemadrin)		
benztropine (Cogentin)		
biperiden (Akineton)		
Antihistamine		
diphenhydramine (Benadryl)	Tremor, rigidity	Sedation, same precautions as for anticholinergic drugs
orphenadrine (Disipal)		
chlorphenoxamine (Phenoxene)		
phenindamine (Thephorin)		
Monoamine Oxidase Inhibitor		
selegiline (Eldepryl, Carbex)	Bradykinesia, rigidity, tremor	Similar to dopaminergic drugs
Catechol-O-Methyl Transferase (COMT) Inhibitor		
entacapone (Comtan)	By blocking COMT, this drug slows down the breakdown of levodopa, thus prolonging the action of levodopa	Similar to dopaminergic drugs; works only when used in combination with Sinemet
tolcapone (Tasmar)		

AST, Aspartate aminotransferase; *BUN,* blood urea nitrogen; *Hct,* hematocrit; *MAO,* monoamine oxidase; *WBCs,* white blood cells.

foods that are easily chewed and swallowed. The diet should contain adequate roughage and fruit to avoid constipation. Food should be cut into bite-sized pieces before it is served, and it should be served on a warmed plate to preserve its appeal. Eating six small meals a day may be less exhausting than eating three large meals a day. Ample time should be planned for eating to avoid frustration and encourage independence. In addition, absorption of levodopa can be impaired by protein ingestion. Some patients are advised to limit their protein intake to the evening meal to avoid this problem.

NURSING MANAGEMENT
PARKINSON'S DISEASE

■ Nursing Assessment

Subjective and objective data that should be obtained from a patient with Parkinson's disease are presented in Table 57-19.

■ Nursing Diagnoses

Nursing diagnoses for the patient with Parkinson's disease may include, but are not limited to, those presented in NCP 57-4.

■ Planning

The overall goals are that the patient with Parkinson's disease will (1) maximize neurologic function, (2) maintain independence in activities of daily living for as long as possible, and (3) optimize psychosocial well-being.

■ Nursing Implementation

Promotion of physical exercise and a well-balanced diet are major concerns for nursing care. Exercise can limit the consequences of decreased mobility, such as muscle atrophy, contractures, and constipation. The American Parkinson Disease

TABLE 57-19	Nursing Assessment Parkinson's Disease

Subjective Data

Important Health Information

Past health history: CNS trauma, cerebrovascular disorders, exposure to metals and carbon monoxide, encephalitis

Medications: Use of major tranquilizers, especially haloperidol (Haldol), and phenothiazines, reserpine, methyldopa, amphetamines

Functional Health Patterns

Health perception–health management: Fatigue

Nutritional-metabolic: Excessive salivation, dysphagia; weight loss

Elimination: Constipation, incontinence; excessive sweating

Activity-exercise: Difficulty in initiating movements; frequent falls; loss of dexterity; micrographia (handwriting deterioration)

Sleep-rest: Insomnia

Cognitive-perceptual: Diffuse pain in head, shoulders, neck, back, legs, and hips; muscle soreness and cramping

Self-perception–self-concept: Depression; mood swings, hallucinations

Objective Data

General

Blank (masked) facies, slow and monotonous speech, infrequent blinking

Integumentary

Seborrhea, dandruff; ankle edema

Cardiovascular

Postural hypotension

Gastrointestinal

Drooling

Neurologic

Tremor at rest, first in hands (pill rolling), later in legs, arms, face, and tongue; aggravation of tremor with anxiety, absence in sleep; poor coordination; subtle dementia, impaired postural reflexes

Musculoskeletal

Cogwheel rigidity, dysarthria, bradykinesia, contractures, stooped posture, shuffling gait

Possible Findings

Lack of specific tests, diagnosis on basis of history and physical findings and ruling out of other diseases

CNS, Central nervous system.

Association (see Resources at the end of this chapter) publishes a series of booklets and videotapes that are helpful in terms of exercise that can be used by family members and health care professionals.

A physical therapist may be consulted to design a personal exercise program aimed at strengthening and stretching specific muscles. Overall muscle tone, as well as specific exercises to strengthen the muscles involved with speaking and swallowing, should be included. Although exercise will not halt the progress of the disease, it will enhance the patient's functional ability.

Because Parkinson's disease is a chronic degenerative disorder with no acute exacerbations, nurses should note that teaching and nursing care are directed toward maintenance of good health, encouragement of independence, and avoidance of complications such as contractures.

Problems secondary to bradykinesia can be alleviated by relatively simple measures. The following are helpful hints for patients who tend to "freeze" while walking: consciously think about stepping over imaginary or real lines on the floor, drop rice kernels and step over them, rock from side to side, lift the toes when stepping, take one step backward and two steps forward. The patient should be assessed for the possibility of levodopa overdose because it is a common cause of akinesia "freezing." A brief period of dyskinesia, usually *athetosis* (slow, writhing, continuous, and involuntary movement) of the neck, should alert the nurse to this possibility.

Getting out of a chair can be facilitated by using an upright chair with arms and placing the back legs on small (2-inch) blocks. Other aspects of the environment can be altered. Rugs and excess furniture can be removed to avoid stumbling. An ottoman can be used to elevate the legs and avoid dependent ankle edema. Clothing can be simplified by the use of slip-on shoes and Velcro hook-and-loop fasteners or zippers on clothing, instead of buttons and hooks. An elevated toilet seat can facilitate getting on and off the toilet. The nurse should work closely with the patient's family in exploring creative adaptations that allow maximum independence and self-care.

■ **Evaluation**

Expected outcomes for the patient with Parkinson's disease are addressed in NCP 57-4.

MYASTHENIA GRAVIS

Myasthenia gravis (MG) is an autoimmune disease of the neuromuscular junction characterized by the fluctuating weakness of certain skeletal muscle groups. The prevalence rate is 14 per 100,000 in the United States. MG can occur at any age but most commonly occurs between the ages of 10 and 65. The peak age at onset in women is 20 to 30 years. MG is three times more common in women, but at older ages both sexes are equally affected.[18]

Etiology and Pathophysiology

MG is caused by an autoimmune process in which antibodies attack acetylcholine (ACh) receptors, resulting in a decreased number of ACh receptor sites at the neuromuscular junction. This prevents ACh molecules from attaching and stimulating muscle contraction. Anti-ACh receptor antibodies are detectable in the serum of 85% to 90% of patients with generalized MG and in 50% to 60% of patients with ocular myasthenia.[18] Thymic tumors are found in about 15% of patients, and abnormal thymus tissue is found in most others.

Clinical Manifestations and Complications

The primary feature of MG is fluctuating weakness of skeletal muscle. Strength is usually restored after a period of rest. The muscles most often involved are those used for moving the eyes and eyelids, chewing, swallowing, speaking, and breathing. The muscles are generally the strongest in the morning and become exhausted with continued activity. Consequently, by the end of the day, muscle weakness is prominent.

In 90% of cases, the eyelid muscles or extraocular muscles are involved. Facial mobility and expression can be impaired. There may be difficulty in chewing and swallowing food. Speech is affected, and the voice often fades after a long conversation. The muscles of the trunk and limbs are less often affected. Of these, the proximal muscles of the neck, shoulder, and hip are more of-

NURSING CARE PLAN 57-4

Patient with Parkinson's Disease

EXPECTED PATIENT OUTCOMES	NURSING INTERVENTIONS and *RATIONALES*
NURSING DIAGNOSIS	**Impaired physical mobility** *related to* rigidity, bradykinesia, and akinesia *as manifested by* difficulty in initiation of purposeful movements.
• Safe ambulation • Maintenance of joint mobility	• Assist with ambulation *to assess degree of impairment and to prevent injury.* • Perform active range-of-motion (ROM) exercises to all extremities *to maintain joint ROM, prevent atrophy, and strengthen muscles.* • Consult physical therapist or occupational therapist for aids *to facilitate activities of daily living and safe ambulation.* • Teach techniques to assist with mobility by instructing patient to step over imaginary line, rock from side to side to initiate leg movements *because these are helpful in dealing with "freezing" (akinesia) while walking.*
NURSING DIAGNOSIS	**Impaired verbal communication** *related to* dysarthria and tremor or bradykinesia *as manifested by* decreased amount of communication, slow and slurred speech, inability to move facial muscles, decreased tongue mobility, and micrographia.
• Development of communication method to meet needs	• Allow sufficient time for communication *to reduce patient's frustration.* • Encourage deep breaths before speaking. • Consult speech therapist *to provide specialized guidance in care of the patient.* • Provide alternative communication methods such as picture books or flash cards *because muscle involvement has impaired writing and speaking ability.* • Massage patient's facial and neck muscles *to foster relaxation that can facilitate speech.*
NURSING DIAGNOSIS	**Imbalanced nutrition: less than body requirements** *related to* dysphagia *as manifested by* difficulty in swallowing and chewing, drooling, decreased gag reflex.
• Maintenance of satisfactory body weight	• Carefully monitor swallowing ability during drug administration and mealtime *to evaluate patient's level of impairment and minimize risk of aspiration.* • Provide soft-solid and thick-liquid diet *because these consistencies are more easily swallowed.* • Maintain patient in upright position for all meals *to reduce risk of aspiration.* • Consult speech therapist and dietitian *because they can provide specific plans to improve swallowing and intake.* • Have suction available *to remove pooled secretions and prevent choking and aspiration.*
NURSING DIAGNOSIS	**Deficient diversional activity** *related to* inability to perform usual recreational activities *as manifested by* boredom, lack of participation, restlessness, depression, hostility.
• Engagement in satisfying diversional activities • Expression of acceptance of diminished capabilities	• Assess patient's activity *to determine physical and emotional response to difficulties.* • Determine preferred diversional activities *so that individual needs are considered.* • Adapt difficult activities when possible *so that patient is able to continue performing activities.* • Initiate new activities within patient's capabilities *such as reading to replace activities patient can no longer perform.* • Encourage patient to discuss emotional response to decreasing capabilities *to provide opportunity to problem-solve and demonstrate a caring attitude.*

ten affected than the distal muscles. No other signs of neural disorder accompany MG; there is no sensory loss, reflexes are normal, and muscle atrophy is rare.

The course of this disease is highly variable. Some patients may have short-term remissions, others may stabilize, and others may have severe, progressive involvement. Restricted ocular myasthenia, usually seen only in men, has a good prognosis. Exacerbations of MG can be precipitated by emotional stress, pregnancy, menses, secondary illness, trauma, temperature extremes, and hypokalemia. Ingestion of drugs including aminoglycoside antibiotics, β-adrenergic blockers, procainamide, quinidine, and phenytoin can aggravate MG. Psychotropic drugs (e.g., lithium carbonate, phenothiazines, benzodiazepines, tricyclic antidepressants) have also been associated with worsening of myas-

thenia as have neuromuscular blocking agents (d-tubocurarine, pancuronium, succinylcholine [Anectine]).

Myasthenic crisis is an acute exacerbation of muscle weakness triggered by infection, surgery, emotional distress, or overdose of or inadequate drugs. The major complications of MG result from muscle weakness in areas that affect swallowing and breathing resulting in aspiration, respiratory insufficiency, and respiratory infection.

Diagnostic Studies

The diagnosis of MG can be made on the basis of history and physical examination. However, other tests may be used if the diagnosis is still in doubt. Blood tests show that antibodies to ACh receptors are found in 85% to 90% of patients with generalized MG.

EMG may show a decrementing response to repeated stimulation of the hand muscles, indicative of muscle fatigue. Use of drugs may also aid in the diagnosis. The Tensilon test in a patient with MG reveals improved muscle contractility after intravenous injection of the anticholinesterase agent edrophonium chloride (Tensilon). (Anticholinesterase blocks the enzyme acetylcholinesterase.) This test also aids in the diagnosis of cholinergic crisis (secondary to overdose of anticholinesterase drug). In this condition, Tensilon does not improve muscle weakness but may actually increase it. Atropine, a cholinergic antagonist, should be readily available to counteract Tensilon effects when it is used diagnostically.

Collaborative Care

Drug Therapy. Drug therapy for MG includes anticholinesterase drugs, alternate-day corticosteroids, and immunosuppressants (Table 57-20). Anticholinesterase drugs are aimed at enhancing function of the neuromuscular junction. Acetylcholinesterase is the enzyme that breaks down ACh in the synaptic cleft. Thus inhibition of this enzyme by an anticholinesterase inhibitor will prolong the action of ACh and facilitate transmission of impulses at the neuromuscular junction. Neostigmine (Prostigmin) and pyridostigmine (Mestinon) are the most successful drugs of this group in treating MG. Tailoring the dose to avoid a myasthenic or cholinergic crisis often presents a clinical challenge. Because of the autoimmune nature of the disorder, corticosteroids (specifically prednisone) are used to suppress the immune response. Drugs such as azathioprine (Imuran) and cyclophosphamide (Cytoxan) may also be used for immunosuppression.

Many drugs are contraindicated or must be used with caution in patients with MG. Classes of drug that should be cautiously evaluated before use include anesthetics, antiarrhythmics, antibiotics, quinine, antipsychotics, barbiturates and sedative-hypnotics, cathartics, diuretics, narcotics, muscle relaxants, thyroid preparations, and tranquilizers.

Surgical Therapy. Because the presence of the thymus gland in the patient with MG appears to enhance the production of ACh receptor antibodies, removal of the thymus gland results in improvement in a majority of patients. Thymectomy is indicated for almost all patients with thymoma, for patients with generalized MG between the ages of puberty and about 65 years, and for patients with purely ocular MG.[19]

Other Therapies. Plasmapheresis can yield a short-term improvement in symptoms and is indicated for patients in crisis or in preparation for surgery when corticosteroids must be avoided. (Plasmapheresis is discussed in Chapter 13.) Intravenous immunoglobulin G has been used with some success and is recommended as a second-line treatment for MG.[20]

NURSING MANAGEMENT
MYASTHENIA GRAVIS

■ Nursing Assessment

The nurse can assess the severity of MG by asking the patient about fatigability, what body parts are affected, and how severely they are affected. The patient's coping abilities and understanding of the disorder should also be assessed. Some patients become so fatigued that they are no longer able to work or even ambulate.

Objective data should include respiratory rate and depth, oxygen saturation, arterial blood gas analyses, pulmonary function tests, and evidence of respiratory distress in patients with acute myasthenic crisis. Muscle strength of all face and limb muscles should be assessed, as should swallowing, speech (volume and clarity), and cough and gag reflexes.

■ Nursing Diagnoses

Nursing diagnoses for the patient with MG may include, but are not limited to, the following:
- Ineffective breathing pattern *related to* intercostal muscle weakness
- Ineffective airway clearance *related to* intercostal muscle weakness and impaired cough and gag reflex
- Impaired verbal communication *related to* weakness of the larynx, lips, mouth, pharynx, and jaw
- Imbalanced nutrition: less than body requirements *related to* impaired swallowing
- Disturbed sensory perception (visual) *related to* ptosis, decreased eye movements, and disconjugate gaze
- Activity intolerance *related to* muscle weakness and fatigability
- Disturbed body image *related to* inability to maintain usual lifestyle and role responsibilities

■ Planning

The overall goals are that the patient with MG will (1) have a return of normal muscle endurance, (2) avoid complications, and (3) maintain a quality of life appropriate to disease course.

■ Nursing Implementation

The patient with MG who is admitted to the hospital usually has a respiratory tract infection or is in an acute myasthenic crisis. Nursing care is aimed at maintaining adequate ventilation, continuing drug therapy, and watching for side effects of therapy. The nurse must be able to distinguish cholinergic from myasthenic crisis (Table 57-21) because the causes and treatment of the two conditions differ greatly.

As with other chronic illnesses, care focuses on the neurologic deficits and their impact on daily living. A balanced diet with food that can be chewed and swallowed easily should be prescribed. Semisolid foods may be easier to eat than solids or

TABLE 57-20   Collaborative Care   Myasthenia Gravis

Diagnostic
History and physical examination
　Fatigability with prolonged upward gaze (2 to 3 minutes)
　Muscle weakness
EMG
Tensilon test
Acetylcholine receptor antibodies

Collaborative Therapy
Drugs
　Anticholinesterase agents
　Corticosteroids
　Immunosuppressive agents
Surgery (thymectomy)
Plasmapheresis

EMG, Electromyography.

TABLE 57-21   Comparison of Myasthenic Crisis and Cholinergic Crisis

	MYASTHENIC CRISIS	CHOLINERGIC CRISIS
Causes	Exacerbation of myasthenia following precipitating factors or failure to take drug as prescribed or drug dose too low	Overdose of anticholinesterase drugs resulting in increased ACh at the receptor sites, remission (spontaneous or after thymectomy)
Differential diagnosis	Improved strength after IV administration of anticholinesterase drugs; increased weakness of skeletal muscles manifesting as ptosis, bulbar signs (e.g., difficulty in swallowing, difficulty in articulating words), or dyspnea	Weakness within 1 hr after ingestion of anticholinesterase; increased weakness of skeletal muscles manifesting as ptosis, bulbar signs, dyspnea; effects on smooth muscle include pupillary miosis, salivation, diarrhea, nausea or vomiting, abdominal cramps, increased bronchial secretions, sweating, or lacrimation

ACh, Acetylcholine; *IV*, intravenous.

liquids. Scheduling doses of drugs so that peak action is reached at mealtime may make eating less difficult. Diversional activities that require little physical effort and match the interests of the patient should be arranged. Teaching should focus on the importance of following the medical regimen, potential adverse reactions to specific drugs, planning activities of daily living to avoid fatigue, the availability of community resources, and the complications of the disease and therapy (crisis conditions) and what to do about them. Contact with the Myasthenia Gravis Foundation or an MG support group may be helpful and should be explored.

■ **Evaluation**

The overall expected outcomes are that the patient with MG will

- maintain optimal muscle function
- be free from side effects of drugs
- not experience complications, in particular myasthenic or cholinergic crises, from the disease
- maintain a quality of life appropriate to the disease course

RESTLESS LEGS SYNDROME

Etiology and Pathophysiology

Restless legs syndrome (RLS) is characterized by unpleasant sensory (paresthesias) and motor abnormalities of one or both legs. Prevalence rates vary from 1% to 15%, although the numbers may be higher because the condition is underdiagnosed.[21] Although the exact cause of RLS is not known, probably more than half of all cases are transmitted in an autosomal dominant pattern.[21] RLS can be seen in metabolic abnormalities associated with iron deficiency, renal failure, polyneuropathy associated with diabetes mellitus, rheumatic disorders (e.g., rheumatoid arthritis), or pregnancy. However, the majority of cases are idiopathic.

Idiopathic RLS may be related to nervous system dysfunction. Although the exact cause remains to be determined, several theories include (1) an alteration in dopaminergic transmission in the basal ganglia, (2) axonal neuropathy, or (3) a brainstem disinhibition phenomenon resulting in motor and sensory disturbances.

Clinical Manifestations

The severity of RLS sensory symptoms ranges from infrequent minor discomfort (paresthesias including numbness, tingling, "pins and needles" sensation) to severe pain. Sensory symptoms often appear first and are manifested as an annoying and uncomfortable (but usually not painful) sensation in the legs. The sensation is often compared with the sensation of bugs creeping or crawling on the legs. The leg pain is localized within the calf muscles. Patients can also experience pain in the upper extremities and trunk. The discomfort occurs when the patient is sedentary and usually occurs in the evening or at night.

The pain at night can produce sleep disruptions and is often relieved by physical activity such as walking, stretching, rocking, or kicking. In the most severe cases, patients sleep only a few hours at night, resulting in daytime fatigue and disruption of the daily routine. The motor abnormalities associated with RLS consist of voluntary restlessness and stereotyped, periodic, involuntary movements. The involuntary movements usually occur during sleep. Symptoms are aggravated by fatigue. Over time, RLS advances to more frequent and more severe episodes.

Diagnostic Studies

RLS is a clinical diagnosis and is based in large part on the patient's history or the report of the bed partner related to nighttime activities. The International Restless Legs Study Group proposed four minimum diagnostic criteria.[22] They are (1) desire to move the limbs, (2) motor restlessness, (3) symptoms that are worse or exclusively present at rest with at least partial and temporary relief by activity, and (4) symptoms that are worse in the evening or night. Polysomnography studies during sleep may be performed for the patient with RLS to distinguish the problem from other clinical conditions (e.g., sleep apnea) that can disturb sleep. However, periodic leg movements in sleep are a common feature in RLS patients. The patient's history of diabetes mellitus and its management may provide information to determine whether paresthesias are caused by peripheral neuropathy or RLS.

NURSING *and* COLLABORATIVE MANAGEMENT RESTLESS LEGS SYNDROME

The goal of collaborative management is to reduce patient discomfort and distress and to improve sleep quality. When RLS is secondary to uremia or iron deficiency, correction of these conditions will decrease symptoms. Nonpharmacologic approaches to RLS management include establishing regular sleep habits, encouraging exercise, avoiding activities that cause symptoms, and eliminating aggravating factors such as alcohol, caffeine, and certain drugs (neuroleptics, lithium, antihistamines, and antidepressants).

If nonpharmacologic measures fail to provide symptom relief, drug therapy may be started. The main drugs used in RLS are dopaminergic agents, opioids, and benzodiazepines. Dopaminergic agents such as carbidopa-levodopa (Sinemet) and DA agonists (pergolide [Permax], bromocriptine [Parlodel], pramipexole [Mirapex]) are the drugs of choice in treating RLS. These agents are effective in managing sensory and motor symptoms. Dopaminergic agents have a number of side effects, including hypotension and gastric irritation.

Other agents that may be used include antiseizure drugs such as gabapentin (Neurontin), divalproex (Depakote), lamotrigine (Lamictal), and carbamazepine (Tegretol). Clonidine (Catapres) and propranolol (Inderal) are also effective in some patients. Opioids (e.g., oxycodone) are usually reserved for those patients with severe symptoms who fail to respond to other drug therapies. When used, opioids given in low doses have also been found to be effective in reducing the symptoms associated with RLS. The main side effect of opioids is constipation, so the patient may need to take a stool softener or laxative.

AMYOTROPHIC LATERAL SCLEROSIS

Amyotrophic lateral sclerosis (ALS) is a rare progressive neurologic disorder characterized by loss of motor neurons. ALS usually leads to death within 2 to 6 years after diagnosis. This disease became known as Lou Gehrig's disease when the famous baseball player was stricken with it in the early 1940s. The onset is usually between 40 and 70 years of age. ALS is more common in men than women by a ratio of 2:1.

For unknown reasons, motor neurons in the brainstem and spinal cord gradually degenerate in ALS (Fig. 57-8). Dead motor neurons cannot produce or transport vital signals to muscles. Consequently, electrical and chemical messages originating in the brain do not reach the muscles to activate them.

The typical symptoms are weakness of the upper extremities, dysarthria, and dysphagia. However, weakness may begin in the legs. Muscle wasting and fasciculations result from the denervation of the muscles and lack of stimulation and use. Death usually results from respiratory infection secondary to compromised respiratory function. Unfortunately, there is no cure for ALS. Riluzole (Rilutek) slows the progression of ALS.[23,24] This drug works to decrease the amount of glutamate (an excitatory neurotransmitter) in the brain. In clinical trials, riluzole has been shown to delay the need for tracheostomy and death by a few months.[25]

The illness trajectory for ALS is devastating because the patient remains cognitively intact while wasting away. The challenge of nursing care is to support the patient's cognitive and emotional functions by facilitating communication, reducing risk of aspiration, decreasing pain secondary to muscle weakness, decreasing risk of injury related to falls, providing diversional activities such as reading and human companionship, and helping the person and family with advance care planning and anticipatory grieving related to loss of motor function and ultimately death.

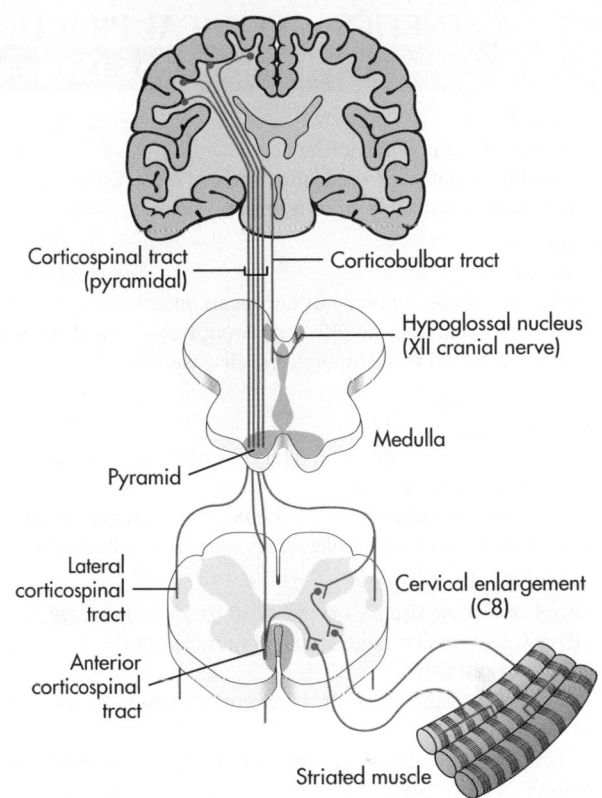

FIG. 57-8 Pathogenesis of amyotrophic lateral sclerosis. This disease is characterized by degeneration of the pyramidal tract and the motor cells in the anterior gray horns. In cases with corticobulbar involvement, the motor nuclei of cranial nerves V, VII, IX, X, XI, and XII also undergo degeneration.

HUNTINGTON'S DISEASE

Huntington's disease (HD) is a genetically transmitted, autosomal dominant disorder that affects both men and women of all races. The offspring of a person with this disease have a 50% risk of inheriting it (see Genetics in Clinical Practice box on p. 1578). The onset of HD is usually between 30 and 50 years of age. Often the diagnosis is made after the affected individual has had children. In the United States the incidence of HD is 1 in 10,000, and there are currently 30,000 Americans with HD.[26] Diagnosis in the past was based on family history and clinical symptoms. However, since the gene for HD has been discovered, one now can be tested for the presence of the gene. People who are asymptomatic but who have a positive family history of HD face the dilemma of whether or not to get tested. If the test is positive, the person will develop HD, but when and to what extent the disease develops cannot be determined.

Like Parkinson's disease, the pathologic process of HD involves the basal ganglia and the extrapyramidal motor system. However, instead of a deficiency of DA, HD involves a deficiency of the neurotransmitters ACh and γ-aminobutyric acid (GABA). The net effect is an excess of DA, which leads to symptoms that are the opposite of those of parkinsonism. The clinical manifestations are characterized by abnormal and excessive involuntary movements *(chorea).* These are writhing, twisting movements of the face, limbs, and body. The movements get

GENETICS in CLINICAL PRACTICE
Huntington's Disease

Genetic Basis
- Autosomal dominant disorder
- Caused by mutation of single gene located on chromosome 4
- Expression similar in homozygotes and heterozygotes

Incidence
- 1 in 10,000
- Higher incidence in people of European ancestry
- With each pregnancy an affected parent has a 50% chance of having a child with Huntington's disease (HD)

Genetic Testing
- DNA testing is available
- DNA testing can be done on fetal cells obtained by amniocentesis or chorionic biopsy
- Genetic testing can determine whether a person is a carrier
- No test is available to predict when symptoms will develop

Clinical Implications
- Onset of disease usually occurs at 30 to 50 years of age
- HD is a progressive, degenerative brain disorder
- No cure is available
- Drugs are available to control movements and behavioral problems
- Genetic counseling may be considered if there is a family history of HD

worse as the disease progresses. Facial movements involving speech, chewing, and swallowing are affected and may cause aspiration and malnutrition. The gait deteriorates, and ambulation eventually becomes impossible. Perhaps the most devastating deterioration is in mental functions, which include intellectual decline, emotional lability, and psychotic behavior. Death usually occurs 10 to 20 years after the onset of symptoms.

Because there is no cure, collaborative care is palliative. Antipsychotic (e.g., haloperidol [Haldol]), antidepressant (fluoxetine [Prozac], sertraline [Zoloft], nortriptyline [Aventyl]), and antichorea (clonazepam [Klonopin]) drugs are prescribed and have some benefit. However, they do not alter the course of the disease. Transplantation of fetal striatal neural tissues into the striatum (caudate and putamen) of the brain is an experimental treatment that may be effective.[26] HD presents a great challenge to health care professionals. The goal of nursing management is to provide the most comfortable environment possible for the patient and the family by maintaining physical safety, treating the physical symptoms, and providing emotional and psychologic support. Because of the choreic movements, caloric requirements are high. Patients may require as many as 4000 to 5000 calories per day to maintain body weight. As the disease progresses, meeting caloric needs becomes a greater challenge when the patient has difficulty swallowing and holding the head still. Depression and mental deterioration can also compromise nutritional intake.

CRITICAL THINKING EXERCISES

Case Study
Myasthenia Gravis

Patient Profile. Mr. D., a 58-year-old African American, was diagnosed with myasthenia gravis after an episode of double vision and drooping of the left eyelid years ago. He was offered thymectomy but refused it. He has been taking pyridostigmine (Mestinon) and prednisone since then and has had few symptoms until recently. While visiting his daughter, he developed severe weakness in his arms and legs and had breathing problems.

Subjective Data
- Reports difficulty "getting enough air"
- Tires easily
- Reports food "gets stuck in my throat" sometimes
- Reports trouble speaking clearly

Objective Data

Physical Examination
- Jaw muscle weakness
- Generalized weakness
- Tense and anxious
- Shallow respirations

Diagnostic Studies
- Chest CT scan shows large mediastinal mass, likely thymoma
- Pulmonary function tests show decreased expiratory effort

CRITICAL THINKING QUESTIONS
1. What is the pathogenesis of myasthenia gravis?
2. What is this exacerbation called?
3. What is the likely explanation for this exacerbation?
4. What teaching plan should be developed for Mr. D.?
5. What treatment would be appropriate for Mr. D.?
6. Write one or more appropriate nursing diagnoses based on the assessment data presented. Are there any collaborative problems?

Nursing Research Issues
1. What kinds of physical activity can enhance functioning and well-being in patients with multiple sclerosis and Parkinson's disease?
2. What are the most effective ways to assist patients with chronic neurologic problems to maintain a positive self-esteem?
3. What factors influence the quality of life for patients with epilepsy?
4. What can be done to promote self-efficacy in patients with chronic neurologic conditions?

REVIEW QUESTIONS

The number of the question corresponds to the same-numbered objective at the beginning of the chapter.

1. The nurse plans care for the patient with a migraine headache based on the knowledge that during a migraine the patient is most likely to
   a. withdraw from stimuli.
   b. act out with bizarre behavior.
   c. seek out the company of others.
   d. experience painful facial spasms and tearing.

2. The triad of symptoms the nurse would expect to find during assessment of the patient with Parkinson's disease is
   a. spasticity, diplopia, tremor.
   b. tremor, rigidity, bradykinesia.
   c. ataxia, drowsiness, dysarthria.
   d. diplopia, tremor, bradykinesia.

3. During assessment of the patient with ALS, the nurse would expect to find
   a. emotional lability.
   b. mental deterioration.
   c. muscle weakness and wasting.
   d. sensory loss in the extremities.

4. The emotional response of the patient with a chronic neurologic disease is often
   a. symptoms of intellectual deterioration.
   b. absent in patients with cognitive impairment.
   c. a result of physical disability and changes in body image.
   d. reduced in patients who have family members to care for them.

5. A major goal of treatment for the patient with a chronic, progressive neurologic disease is
   a. reversal of pathophysiologic features.
   b. total remission of the disease.
   c. continuation of usual lifestyle.
   d. adaptation by patient and family to the disease.

REFERENCES

1. Rasmussen BK, Stewart WF, Welch KMA: Epidemiology of migraine. In Olesen J, Tfelt-Hansen P, editors: *The headaches,* Philadelphia, 2000, Lippincott Williams & Wilkins.
2. Olesen J, Oadsby PJ: Synthesis of migraine mechanisms. In Olesen J, Tfelt-Hansen P, editors: *The headaches,* Philadelphia, 2000, Lippincott Williams & Wilkins.
3. Raskin N: Migraine and other headaches. In Rowland LP, editor: *Merritt's neurology,* Philadelphia, 2000, Lippincott Williams & Wilkins.
4. Zed P, Loewen P, Robinson G: Medication induced headache: overview and systematic review of therapeutic approaches, *Ann Pharmacother* 33:61, 1999.
5. Shorvon SD: *Handbook of epilepsy treatment,* London, 2000, Blackwell Science.
6. Prasad A et al: Recent advances in the genetics of epilepsy: insights from human and animal studies, *Epilepsia* 40:1329, 1999.
7. Commission on Classification and Terminology of the International League Against Epilepsy: Proposal for the revised clinical and electroencephalographic classification of epileptic seizures, *Epilepsia* 22:249, 1981.
8. Leppik IE: *Contemporary diagnosis and management of the patient with epilepsy,* Newton, Pa, 2000, Handbooks in Health Care.
9. Miller JR: Multiple sclerosis. In Rowland LP, editor: *Merritt's neurology,* Philadelphia, 2000, Lippincott Williams & Wilkins.
10. Lubin FD, Reingold SC: Defining the clinical course of multiple sclerosis, *Neurology* 46:907, 1996.
11. Confavreux C et al: Rates of pregnancy-related relapse in multiple sclerosis, *N Engl J Med* 339:285, 1998.
12. Polman CH, Uitdehaag BM: Drug treatment of multiple sclerosis, *BMJ* 321(7259):490, 2000.
13. Edwards S et al: Clinical relapses and disease activity on magnetic resonance imaging associated with viral upper respiratory infections in multiple sclerosis, *J Neurol Neurosurg Psychiatry* 64:736, 1998.
14. Fahn S, Przedborski S: Parkinsonism. In Rowland LP, editor: *Merritt's neurology,* Philadelphia, 2000, Lippincott Williams & Wilkins.
15. Waters CH: *Diagnosis and management of Parkinson's disease,* Caddo, Okla, 1998, Professional Communications Inc.
16. Glosser G: Neurobehavioral effects of movement disorders, *Neurol Clin* 19:535, 2001.
17. Ahlskog JE: Parkinson's disease: medical and surgical treatment, *Neurol Clin* 19:579, 2001.
18. Penn AS, Rowland LP: Myasthenia gravis. In Rowland LP, editor: *Merritt's neurology,* Philadelphia, 2000, Lippincott Williams & Wilkins.
19. Urschel JD, Grewal RP: Thymectomy for myasthenia gravis, *Postgrad Med J* 74:139, 1998.
20. Bril V et al: IGIV in neurology—evidence and recommendations, *Can J Neurol Sci* 26:139, 1999.
21. Tan E, Ondo W: Restless legs syndrome: clinical features and treatment, *Am J Med Sci* 319:397, 2000.
22. Walters AS: Toward a better definition of restless legs syndrome, *Mov Disord* 10:634, 1995.
23. Miller RG: New approaches to therapy of amyotrophic lateral sclerosis, *West J Med* 168:262, 1998.
24. Riviere M et al: An analysis of extended survival in patients with amyotrophic lateral sclerosis treated with riluzole, *Arch Neurol* 55:526, 1998.
25. Miller RG et al: Riluzole for amyotrophic lateral sclerosis (ALS)/motor neuron disease (MND) (Cochrane Review), *Cochrane Database Syst Rev* 2:CD001447, 2002.
26. Freeman TB et al: Transplanted fetal striatum in Huntington's disease: phenotypic development and lack of pathology, *Proc Natl Acad Sci* 97:13877, 2000.

RESOURCES

ALS Association (ALSA)
27001 Agoura Road, Suite 150
Calabasas Hills, CA 91301-5104
800-782-4747 or 818-880-9007
www.alsa.org

American Association of Neuroscience Nurses (AANN)
4700 West Lake Avenue
Glenview, IL 60025-1485
888-557-2266 or 847-375-4733
Fax: 847-375-6333
www.aann.org

American Council for Headache Education (ACHE)

19 Mantua Road
Mt. Royal, NJ 08061
857-423-0258
Fax: 856-423-0082
www.achenet.org

American Parkinson Disease Association

1250 Hylan Boulevard, Suite 4B
Staten Island, NY 10305-1946
800-223-2732 or 718-981-8001
Fax: 781-981-4399
www.apdaparkinson.com

Association of Rehabilitation Nurses (ARN)

4700 West Lake Avenue
Glenview, IL 60025-1485
800-229-7530 or 847-375-4710
Fax: 877-734-9384
www.rehabnurse.org

Epilepsy Foundation

4351 Garden City Drive
Landover, MD 20785-7223
800-332-1000 or 301-459-3700
www.efa.org

Huntington's Disease Society of America

158 West 29th Street, 7th Floor
New York, NY 10001-5300
800-345-HDSA
Fax: 212-239-3430
www.hdsa.org

Myasthenia Gravis Foundation of America

5841 Cedar Lake Road, Suite 204
Minneapolis, MN 55416
800-541-5454 or 952-545-9438
Fax: 952-545-6073
www.myasthenia.org

National Headache Foundation

428 West St. James Place, 2nd Floor
Chicago, IL 60614-2750
888-NHF-5552
www.headaches.org

National Institute of Neurological Disorders and Stroke

PO Box 5801
Bethesda, MD 20824
800-352-9424 or 301-468-5981
www.ninds.nih.gov

National Multiple Sclerosis Society

733 Third Avenue
New York, NY 10017
800-FIGHT-MS (344-4867)
www.nmss.org

Restless Legs Syndrome Foundation

819 Second Street SW
Rochester, MN 55902-2985
877-463-6757 or 507-287-6465
www.rls.org

For additional Internet resources, see the website for this book at
http://evolve.elsevier.com/Lewis/medsurg/.

CHAPTER 58

NURSING MANAGEMENT
Alzheimer's Disease and Dementia

Margaret McLean Heitkemper
Lissi Hansen
Sharon Mantik Lewis

LEARNING OBJECTIVES

1. Describe the etiology, pathophysiology, clinical manifestations, diagnostic studies, and collaborative management of delirium.
2. Define dementia and describe its impact on society.
3. Compare and contrast different etiologies of dementia.
4. Describe the clinical manifestations, diagnostic studies, and collaborative management of dementia.
5. Describe the clinical manifestations, diagnostic studies, and collaborative management of Alzheimer's disease.
6. Describe the nursing management of the patient with Alzheimer's disease.
7. Describe other neurodegenerative disorders associated with dementia, including Lewy body disease, Pick's disease, Creutzfeldt-Jakob disease, and normal-pressure hydrocephalus.

KEY TERMS

Alzheimer's disease, p. 1586
Creutzfeldt-Jakob disease, p. 1598
delirium, p. 1581
dementia, p. 1583
familial Alzheimer's disease, p. 1586
frontotemporal dementia, p. 1599
Lewy body disease, p. 1598

mild cognitive impairment, p. 1587
neuritic plaque, p. 1586
neurofibrillary tangles, p. 1586
normal pressure hydrocephalus, p. 1599
Pick's disease, p. 1599
vascular dementia, p. 1584

The three most common cognitive problems in adults are delirium (acute confusion), dementia, and depression. These problems often occur together. It is important to be able to identify the distinguishing characteristics because the treatment for each problem is very different.

DELIRIUM

Delirium, a state of temporary but acute mental confusion, is common in older adults who have a short-term illness such as lung or heart disease, infections, poor nutrition, drug interactions, and metabolic or hormone disorders. Approximately 10% to 40% of patients are delirious when admitted to the hospital, and another 25% to 60% develop delirium during hospitalization. It is also estimated that delirium will complicate the hospitalizations of more than 2.2 million persons each year. Patients who experience delirium are at greater risk for longer hospitalizations, further functional decline, and institutionalization.[1]

Reviewed by Catherine M. Harris, RNCS, PhD, Professor Emeritus, College of Nursing, University of New Mexico, Albuquerque, NM, and Senior Vice President, Dementia Care Design International, San Antonio, Tex.

Etiology and Pathophysiology

The pathophysiologic mechanism of delirium is poorly understood. Neuroimaging studies indicate that both cortical and subcortical structures (thalamus, basal ganglia, and pontine reticular formation) are involved.[1] The finding that subcortical structures are involved may explain the high risk of delirium in patients with Parkinson's disease. The neurotransmitter acetylcholine may be a critical factor in the development of delirium.[2] This is based in part on three observations: (1) anticholinergic drugs can precipitate delirium in older adults; (2) anticholinesterase agents (physostigmine [Antilirium]) can reverse delirium caused by anticholinergic drug use; and (3) other risk factors for delirium, such as hypoglycemia, hypoxia, and thiamine deficiency, decrease the central nervous system (CNS) production of acetylcholine.[3] Other neurotransmitters including γ-aminobutyric acid, norepinephrine, dopamine, and serotonin may also be involved in delirium but are less well studied.

Delirium associated with infection, inflammation, and cancer may be related to the action of specific cytokines such as interleukins and interferons.[4] In addition, patients treated with cytokine therapies (e.g., interferon for hepatitis C) can develop neuropsychiatric side effects including delirium.[5]

Clinically, delirium is rarely caused by a single factor. It is often the result of the interaction of the patient's underlying condition with a precipitating event. Delirium can occur following a relatively minor insult in a vulnerable patient. For example, the patient with underlying health problems such as congestive heart failure, cancer, cognitive impairment, or sensory limitations may develop delirium in response to a relatively minor change (e.g., use of a sleeping medication). In other nonvulnerable patients, it may take a combination of factors (e.g., anesthesia, major surgery, infection, prolonged sleep deprivation) to precipitate delirium.[1] Delirium can also be a symptom of a serious medical illness such as bacterial meningitis.

Understanding factors that can lead to delirium can help to determine effective interventions. Several factors identified as pre-

TABLE 58-1	**Factors That Can Precipitate Delirium**

- Absence of time and place cues (e.g., watch, clock)
- Change in environment
- Chronic illness (e.g., congestive heart failure)
- Dehydration
- Dementia
- Electrolyte imbalances (hyponatremia, hypercalcemia)
- Hospitalization (e.g., intensive care unit)
- Hypercarbia
- Hyperthermia
- Hypoglycemia
- Hypothermia
- Hypoxia
- Immobilization
- Infection
- Liver disease
- Medications (e.g., sedative-hypnotics, narcotics, benzodiazepines)
- Metabolic disorders
- Pain (untreated)
- Renal disease
- Sensory deprivation
- Sensory overload
- Stress
- Trauma

cipitating delirium are shown in Table 58-1. One of the most important risk factors for delirium is preexisting dementia. Many of the conditions that can precipitate delirium are more common in older patients. In addition, older patients have limited compensatory mechanisms to deal with physiologic insults such as hypoxia, hypoglycemia, and dehydration. Older adults are more susceptible to drug-induced delirium, in part because of their increased use of multiple drugs. Medications including sedative-hypnotics, narcotics (especially meperidine [Demerol]), benzodiazepines, and drugs with anticholinergic properties can cause or contribute to delirium, especially in older or vulnerable patients.

Clinical Manifestations

Patients with delirium can present with a variety of manifestations ranging from hypoactivity and lethargy to hyperactivity including agitation and hallucinations.[6] Patients can also have mixed delirium and manifest both hypoactive and hyperactive symptoms. In most patients delirium usually develops over a 2- to 3-day period. The early manifestations often include inability to concentrate, irritability, insomnia, loss of appetite, restlessness, and confusion. Later the manifestations may include agitation, misperception, misinterpretation, and hallucinations. Delirium is an acute problem.

Manifestations of delirium are sometimes confused with dementia and depression. Table 58-2 compares the features of delirium, dementia, and depression. A key distinction between delirium and dementia is that the person who exhibits sudden

TABLE 58-2	**Comparison of the Clinical Features of Delirium, Dementia, and Depression**		
FEATURE	DELIRIUM	DEMENTIA	DEPRESSION
Onset	Rapid, often at night	Usually insidious	Coincides with life changes; often abrupt
Course	Fluctuates, worse at night; lucid intervals	Long; symptoms progressive yet relatively stable over time	Diurnal effects, typically worse in the morning; situational fluctuations
Progression	Abrupt	Slow but even	Variable, rapid–slow but uneven
Duration	Hours to less than 1 month	Months to years	At least 2 weeks, but can be several months to years
Awareness	Reduced	Clear	Clear
Alertness	Fluctuates, lethargic or hypervigilant	Generally normal	Normal
Orientation	Fluctuates in severity, generally impaired	Progressive impairment	Selective disorientation resulting from impaired concentration and attention span, which may manifest as memory deficit
Thinking	Disorganized, distorted, fragmented; slow or accelerated incoherent speech	Difficulty with abstraction, thoughts impoverished, judgment impaired, words difficult to find	Intact but with apathy, fatigue; may not want to live; may be at risk for suicide
Perception	Distorted; illusions, delusions, and hallucinations	Misperceptions often present; delusions, illusions, and hallucinations	May deny depression
Psychomotor behavior	Variable; hypokinetic, hyperkinetic, or mixed	Apraxia	Variable; psychomotor retardation or agitation
Sleep–wake cycle	Disturbed, cycle reversed	Frequent awakenings	Disturbed, often early morning awakening
Mental status testing	Distracted from task; poor performance; improves when patient recovers	Frequent "near miss" answers, struggles with test, great effort to find an appropriate reply; consistently poor performances	Frequent "don't know" answers, little effort, frequently gives up, indifferent

cognitive impairment, disorientation, or clouded sensorium is more likely to have delirium rather than dementia.

Diagnostic Studies

A careful medical and psychologic history and physical examination are the first steps in the diagnosis of delirium. This includes careful attention to medications, both prescription and over-the-counter drug use. A variety of cognitive measures can be used, including the Mini-Mental State Examination (see Table 58-5 later in the chapter). The information may have to be obtained from a reliable informant if the patient is unable to provide the information. It is important to distinguish whether the delirium is part of an underlying problem of dementia.

Once delirium has been diagnosed, potential causes of the delirium are explored. These include careful review of the patient's health history and medication record. Laboratory tests include complete blood count, serum electrolytes, blood urea nitrogen and creatinine levels, electrocardiogram, urine analysis, liver function tests, thyroid function, and oxygen saturation level. Drug and alcohol levels may be obtained. If unexplained fever or nuchal rigidity is present and meningitis or encephalitis is suspected, a lumbar puncture may be performed. Cerebrospinal fluid (CSF) is examined for glucose and protein and the presence of bacteria. If the patient's history includes head injury, appropriate x-ray or scans may be ordered. In general, brain imaging studies, computed tomography (CT) or magnetic resonance imaging (MRI), are used only in those situations in which head injury is known or suspected.

NURSING and COLLABORATIVE MANAGEMENT
DELIRIUM

Preventing delirium in patients at risk for delirium is important. Patient groups at risk include those with neurologic disorders (e.g., stroke, dementia, CNS infection, Parkinson's disease), sensory impairment, and advanced age. Other risk factors include hospitalization in an intensive care unit, lack of a watch or calendar, and absence of reading glasses.[6,7] Untreated pain may also precipitate delirium.

Care of the patient with delirium is focused on eliminating precipitating factors. If it is drug-induced, medications are discontinued. It is important to keep in mind that delirium can also accompany drug and alcohol withdrawal. Depending on patient history, drug screening may be performed. Fluid and electrolyte imbalances and nutritional deficiencies (e.g., thiamine) are corrected if appropriate. If the problem is related to environmental conditions (e.g., overstimulating or understimulating environment), changes should be made. If delirium is secondary to infection, appropriate antibiotic therapy is started. Similarly, if delirium is secondary to chronic illness such as chronic kidney disease or congestive heart failure, treatment is focused on these conditions.

Care of the patient experiencing delirium includes protecting the patient from harm. Priority is given to creating a calm and safe environment. This may include encouraging family members to stay at the bedside, providing familiar objects, transferring the patient to a private room or one closer to the nurses' station, and planning for consistent staff care if possible. Reorientation and behavioral interventions should be used in all patients with delir-

ium. The patient is provided with reassurance and reorienting information as to place, time, and procedures. Clocks, calendars, and listing the patient's scheduled activities are also useful in reducing confusion. Environmental stimuli including noise and light levels may have to be reduced if possible.

Personal contact through touch and verbal communication can be important reorienting strategies. If the patient uses eyeglasses or a hearing aid, it should be made readily available because sensory deprivation can precipitate delirium. The use of restraints should be avoided. Other interventions, including relaxation techniques, music therapy, and massage, may also be appropriate for some patients with delirium.

Comprehensive, institutional-based programs focused on reducing risk factors for delirium (cognitive impairment, sleep deprivation, immobility, visual impairment, hearing impairment, and dehydration) have been shown to be effective in reducing overall episodes of delirium in hospitalized older patients.[8] An interdisciplinary team approach is needed to reduce polypharmacy, decrease pain, enhance nutritional intake, and reduce incontinence. The patient experiencing delirium is also at risk for the adverse consequences of immobility, including skin breakdown. Attention is given to increasing physical activity or providing range-of-motion exercises, when appropriate, and preventing skin breakdown.

The nurse should also focus on supporting the family and caregivers during episodes of delirium. Family members need to understand factors that may have precipitated the delirium, as well as the potential outcomes.

Drug Therapy. Drug therapy is reserved for those patients with severe agitation, especially in those patients whose agitation interferes with needed medical therapy (e.g., fluid replacement, intubation, dialysis). Agitation can put the patient at risk for falls and injury. Drug therapy is used cautiously because many of the drugs used to manage agitation have psychoactive properties.

Patients are often treated with low-dose antipsychotics (neuroleptics) such as haloperidol (Haldol). Haloperidol can be administered intravenously, intramuscularly, or orally and will produce sedation. In addition to sedation, other side effects include hypotension, extrapyramidal side effects including *tardive dyskinesia* (involuntary muscle movements of the face, trunk, and arms), *athetosis* (involuntary writhing movements of the limbs), muscle tone changes, and anticholinergic effects. Older patients receiving antipsychotic agents need to be carefully monitored. Newer antipsychotics including risperidone (Risperdal), olanzapine (Zyprexa), and quetiapine (Seroquel) can be used to manage agitated behavior in older adults. These drugs have fewer side effects compared with haloperidol.

Short-acting benzodiazepines (e.g., lorazepam [Ativan]) can be used to treat delirium associated with sedative and alcohol withdrawal or in conjunction with antipsychotics to reduce extrapyramidal side effects. However, these drugs may worsen delirium caused by other factors and must be used cautiously.

DEMENTIA

Dementia is a syndrome characterized by dysfunction or loss of memory, orientation, attention, language, and judgment and reasoning and by changes in behavior. Ultimately these problems result in alterations in the individual's ability to work, social and family responsibilities, and activities of daily living.

The World Health Organization has defined *dementia* as a syndrome caused by disease of the brain, usually of a chronic or progressive nature, in which there is disturbance of multiple cortical functions, calculation, learning capacity, language, and judgment. Impairments of cognitive function are commonly ac-

TABLE 58-3	Causes of Dementia
Neurodegenerative disorders	Alzheimer's disease
	Lewy body disease
	Frontal lobe dementia
	Frontal-temporal dementia (e.g., Pick's disease)
	Down syndrome
	Amyotrophic lateral sclerosis (ALS)
	Parkinson's disease
	Huntington's disease
Vascular diseases	Vascular (multiinfarct) dementia
	Cardiac disease producing emboli or decreased perfusion
	Binswanger's disease
	Subarachnoid hemorrhage*
	Chronic subdural hematoma*
Toxic or metabolic diseases	Alcoholism
	Thiamine (vitamin B₁) deficiency*
	Cobalamin (vitamin B₁₂) deficiency*
	Folate deficiency*
	Hyperthyroidism*
	Hypothyroidism*
	Hypoglycemia*
	Hypercalcemia*
Immunologic diseases or infections	Multiple sclerosis
	Chronic fatigue syndrome
	Infections (e.g., Creutzfeldt-Jakob disease)
	Acquired immunodeficiency syndrome (AIDS)
	Meningitis*
	Encephalitis *
	Neurosyphilis*
	Systemic lupus erythematosus*
Systemic diseases	Uremic encephalopathy*
	Dialysis dementia*
	Hepatic encephalopathy*
	Wilson's disease
Trauma	Head injury*
Cancer	Brain tumors (primary)*
	Metastatic tumors*
Ventricular disorders	Hydrocephalus*
Seizure disorders	Epilepsy
Drugs†	Diuretics
	digoxin
	Anticholinergics
	Narcotics
	Hypnotics
	Antihypertensives
	Antiparkinsonian drugs
	Antihistamines

*Potentially reversible.
†These are examples of drugs that may cause cognitive impairment that is potentially reversible.

companied and occasionally preceded by deterioration in emotional control, social behavior, and motivation.[9]

Dementia is a disorder that occurs most often in older adults. As the average life span of humans increases, the number of those affected with dementia is growing and is now a major international public health concern.[10] In the United States half of all patients in long-term care facilities have Alzheimer's disease (AD) or a related dementia. In Canada approximately 60,000 new cases of dementia are identified each year.[11]

Etiology and Pathophysiology

Causes of dementia are due to both treatable and nontreatable conditions (Table 58-3). The two most common causes of dementia are neurodegenerative conditions (e.g., AD) and vascular disorders. Neurodegenerative conditions account for 60% to 80% of all dementias. Advanced age and family history are important risk factors for dementia. Infectious conditions such as bacterial meningitis and viral encephalitis can result in both vascular and neurodegenerative changes that may ultimately result in dementia.

Dementia is sometimes caused by treatable conditions that are potentially reversible (see Table 58-3). Initially these conditions may be reversible. However, with prolonged exposure or disease, irreversible changes may occur.

Vascular causes are the second most common cause of dementia. **Vascular dementia,** also called multiinfarct dementia, is the loss of cognitive function resulting from ischemic, ischemic-hypoxic, or hemorrhagic brain lesions caused by cardiovascular disease. This type of dementia is the result of decreased blood supply from narrowing and blocking of arteries that supply the brain. Vascular dementia may be caused by a single stroke (infarct) or by multiple strokes.

A history of smoking, cardiac arrhythmias (e.g., atrial fibrillation), hypertension, hypercholesterolemia, diabetes mellitus, and coronary artery disease predispose to vascular dementia. Recently, high homocysteine levels have been associated with the development of dementia and AD.[12]

Clinical Manifestations

Depending on the cause of the dementia, the onset of symptoms may be insidious and gradual or somewhat more abrupt. Often dementia associated with neurologic degeneration is gradual and progressive over time. Causes of vascular dementia can result in more abrupt symptoms or symptoms that progress in a more stepwise pattern. However, it is difficult to distinguish the etiology of dementia (vascular versus neurodegenerative) based on symptom progression alone. An acute (days to weeks) or subacute (weeks to months) pattern of change may be indicative of an infectious or metabolic cause including encephalitis, meningitis, hypothyroidism, or drug-related dementia.

Clinical manifestations of dementia are classified as mild, moderate, and severe (Table 58-4). Regardless of the cause of dementia the initial symptoms are related to changes in cognitive functioning. Patients may have complaints of memory loss, mild disorientation, and/or trouble with words and numbers. Often it is a family member, in particular the spouse, who complains to the health care provider about the patient's declining memory. Almost all adults experience some changes with memory related to aging. Normal age-related memory decline

TABLE 58-4   Clinical Manifestations of Dementia

EARLY (MILD)	MIDDLE (MODERATE)	LATE (SEVERE)
• Forgetfulness beyond what is seen in a normal person • Short-term memory impairment, especially for new learning • Difficulty recognizing what numbers mean • Loss of initiative and interests • Decreased judgment • Geographic disorientation	• Impaired ability to recognize close family or friends • Agitation • Wandering, getting lost • Loss of remote memory • Confusion • Impaired comprehension • Forgets how to do simple tasks • Apraxia • Receptive aphasia • Expressive aphasia • Insomnia • Delusions • Illusions, hallucinations • Behavioral problems	• Little memory, unable to process new information • Cannot understand words • Difficulty eating, swallowing • Repetitious words or sounds • Unable to perform self-care activities • Immobility • Incontinence

is characterized as mild changes that do not impact on activities of daily living. In dementia the memory loss is initially for recent events with remote memories still intact. With time and progression of the dementia, memory loss includes both recent and remote memory and ultimately affects the ability to perform self care.

Diagnostic Studies

The diagnosis of dementia is focused on determining the cause (e.g., reversible versus nonreversible factors). An important first step is a thorough medical, neurologic, and psychologic history. A thorough physical examination is performed to rule out other potential medical conditions. Screening for cobalamin (vitamin B_{12}) deficiency and hypothyroidism are often performed. Based on patient history, testing for neurosyphilis (see Chapter 57) may be performed. The American Academy of Neurology recommends cognitive evaluation and ongoing clinical monitoring of persons with mild cognitive impairment because of their increased risk of developing dementia.[13]

Mental status testing is an important component for the patient evaluation. Patients with mild dementia may be able to compensate, making it difficult to evaluate cognitive function only through conversation. Cognitive testing is focused on evaluating memory, ability to calculate, language, visuospatial skills, and degree of alertness. The Mini-Mental State Examination (Table 58-5) is the most commonly used tool to assess cognitive functioning.

Depression is often mistaken for dementia in older adults, and, conversely, dementia for depression. Manifestations of depression (especially in the older adult) include sadness, difficulty thinking and concentrating, fatigue, apathy, feelings of despair, and inactivity. When the depression is severe, poor concentration and attention may occur, causing memory and functional impairment. When dementia and depression do occur together (which may be in as many as 40% of dementia cases), the intellectual deterioration may be more extreme. Depression, alone or in combination with dementia, is treatable. The challenge is to make an early assessment.

TABLE 58-5   Mini-Mental State Examination (MMSE)

MMSE SAMPLE ITEMS

Orientation to Time
"What is the date?"

Registration
"Listen carefully, I am going to say three words. You say them back after I stop. Ready? Here they are. . .
HOUSE (pause), CAR (pause), LAKE (pause). Now repeat those words back to me." (Repeat up to five times, but score only the first trial.)

Naming
"What is this?" (Point to a pencil or pen.)

Reading
"Please read this and do what it says." (Show examinee the words on the stimulus form.) CLOSE YOUR EYES

Diagnosis of dementia related to vascular causes is based on the presence of cognitive loss, the presence of vascular brain lesions demonstrated by neuroimaging techniques, and the exclusion of other causes of dementia (e.g., AD). The American Academy of Neurology guidelines include the use of structural neuroimaging with CT or MRI in the evaluation of patients with dementia.[14] Although both single photon emission computed tomography (SPECT) and positron emission tomography (PET) scanning techniques can be used to characterize CNS changes in dementia, these tools are not routinely used in the initial diagnosis of dementia. There are no genetic markers or CSF markers that are currently recommended for routine evaluation of patients with dementia.

NURSING *and* COLLABORATIVE MANAGEMENT
DEMENTIA

Collaborative and nursing management of the patient with dementia is similar to that described for AD (see later in this chapter). Vascular dementia can be prevented. Preventive measures include treatment of risk factors including hypertension, diabetes, smoking, hyperfibrinogenemia, hyperhomocysteinemia, orthostatic hypotension, and cardiac arrhythmias. (Stroke is discussed in Chapter 56.) Cholinesterase inhibitors (e.g., donepezil [Aricept]) that are used for patients with AD are also useful in patients with vascular dementia.

ALZHEIMER'S DISEASE

Alzheimer's disease (AD) is a chronic, progressive, degenerative disease of the brain. It is the most common form of dementia, accounting for approximately 60% to 80% of all cases of dementia. AD is named after Alois Alzheimer, a German physician who in 1906 described changes in the brain tissue of a 51-year-old woman who had died of an unusual mental illness.

Approximately 4 million Americans suffer from AD. It is estimated that 10% of people over age 65 and 50% of those over age 85 have AD. Worldwide it is estimated that more than 22 million individuals will have AD by 2025.[10] The course of the disease can span 5 to 20 years. The economic costs of AD in the United States range from approximately $19,000 annually for the care of the person with early disease to $37,000 annually for the person with late disease.[15] Nationally the annual costs of AD are estimated at $100 billion dollars. The burden on the individual, family, caregivers, and society as a whole is staggering.

The incidence of AD is approximately the same for all ethnic groups although the risk may be slightly higher in African Americans and Hispanic Americans. AD has been associated with lower socioeconomic status and education level and poor access to health care. Therefore additional research is needed to determine whether ethnic differences are related to genetic or environmental risk factors.[15] Women are more likely than men to develop AD primarily because they live longer. Individuals with Down syndrome are at high risk for AD. They may develop clinical signs around the age of 20, and by age 40, 95% of patients with Down syndrome will have evidence of AD based on autopsy findings.[15]

Etiology and Pathophysiology

The exact etiology of AD is unknown. Similar to other forms of dementia, age is the most important risk factor for developing AD. However, AD is not a normal part of aging. AD is a disease that destroys brain cells, which is not a normal part of aging. Only a small percentage of people younger than 60 years old will develop AD. When AD develops in someone less than the age of 60, it is referred to as *early onset AD*. AD that becomes evident in individuals after the age of 60 is called *late onset AD* (see the Genetics in Clinical Practice box on this page).

Persons in whom a clear pattern of inheritance within a family is established are said to have **familial Alzheimer's disease** (FAD). Others in whom no familial connection can be made are termed *sporadic*. FAD is associated with earlier onset (before 60 years of age) and more rapid disease course. In both FAD and sporadic AD, the pathogenesis of AD is similar.

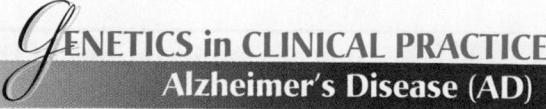

GENETICS in CLINICAL PRACTICE
Alzheimer's Disease (AD)

Genetic Basis
Early Onset (Familial) (<60 years old at onset)
- Autosomal dominant disorder
- Various mutations in the following genes:
  Amyloid precursor protein (APP) gene on chromosome 21
  Presenilin-1 (PSEN1) gene on chromosome 14
  Presenilin-2 (PSEN2) gene on chromosome 1

Late Onset (Sporadic) (>60 years old at onset)
- Genetically more complex than early onset form
- Presence of apolipoprotein E (ApoE)-4 gene on chromosome 19 increases the likelihood of developing AD
- If two ApoE-4 alleles are inherited, there is a higher risk of AD
- Presence of ApoE-2 allele is associated with a lower risk for AD

Incidence
Early Onset
- Rare form of AD accounting for less than 10% of cases
- 50% risk of disease for children of affected parents

Late Onset
- Many ApoE-4 positive people do not develop AD, and many ApoE-4 negative people do.

Genetic Testing
Early Onset
- Genetic screening for mutations on chromosomes 1, 14, and 21

Late Onset
- Blood test to identify presence of ApoE-4 gene
- No consensus on the clinical appropriateness of ApoE testing
- ApoE testing is mainly used for research

Clinical Implications
- AD is the most common cause of dementia.
- Overall the incidence of AD is three times higher among people with one affected parent than in those with no affected parents.
- Genetic testing and counseling for family members of patients with early onset AD may be appropriate.
- If person tests positive for ApoE-4, it does not mean that the person will develop AD.

The characteristic findings in AD are the presence of abnormal clumps (neuritic or senile plaques) and tangled bundles of fibers (neurofibrillary tangles) in the brain (Fig. 58-1). The **neuritic plaque** is a cluster of degenerating axonal and dendritic nerve terminals that contain amyloid-beta protein. **Neurofibrillary tangles** are seen in the cytoplasm of abnormal neurons in those areas of the brain (hippocampus, cerebral cortex) most affected by AD (Fig. 58-2). In the cerebral cortex they are found in those areas of brain associated with cognition, learning, sleep, and memory.

Genetic factors may play a critical role in how the brain processes the amyloid-beta protein.[15] Overproduction of amyloid-beta appears to be an important risk factor for AD. Amyloid-beta (A-beta) is part of a larger protein called amyloid precursor protein (APP) that is involved in cell membrane function and is produced by cells throughout the body. Large amounts of APP are

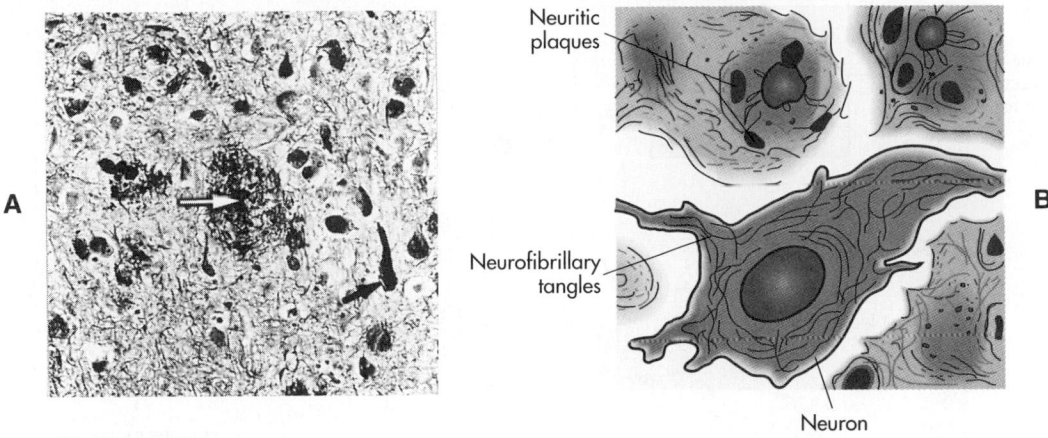

FIG. 58-1 Pathologic changes in Alzheimer's disease. **A,** Senile plaque with central amyloid core *(white arrow)* next to a neurofibrillary tangle *(black arrow)* on the histologic specimen from a brain autopsy. **B,** Schematic representation of neuritic plaque and neurofibrillary tangle.

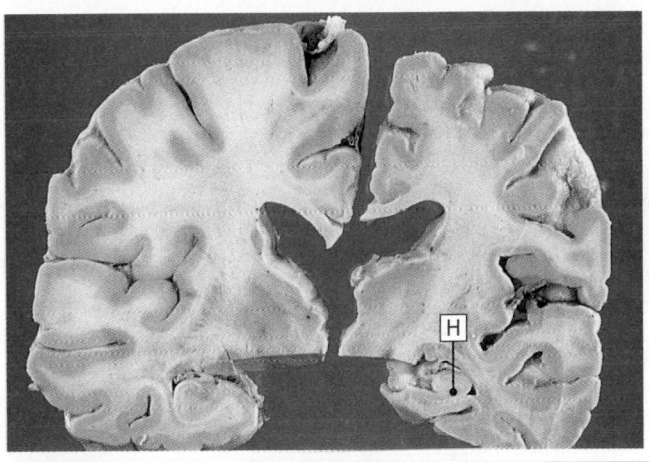

FIG. 58-2 Alzheimer's disease. This shows slices from two brains. On the left is a normal brain from a 70-year-old; on the right is the same region from a 70-year-old with Alzheimer's disease. The diseased brain is atrophic with loss of cortex and white matter, most marked in the hippocampal region *(H).*

produced in the brain. Neuritic plaques are composed of A-beta proteins. Abnormally high levels of A-beta are thought to produce cell damage either directly or through eliciting an inflammatory response and ultimately neuron death (Fig. 58-3, *A*).[16]

Understanding why neurons produce A-beta led researchers to examine the enzymes (and their genes) that are responsible for both the synthesis and processing of APP. In patients with early onset AD, three genes have been identified as important in the etiology of AD (see Genetics in Clinical Practice box on p. 1586). When the presenilin 1 and presenilin 2 genes are mutated, they cause brain cells to overproduce A-beta.

The first gene associated with AD was the epsilon (E) 4 allele of the apolipoprotein E (ApoE) gene on chromosome 19.[15] ApoE comes in several different forms or alleles, but three occur most commonly. People inherit one allele (ApoE-2, ApoE-3, ApoE-4) from each parent. ApoE may play a role in clearing amyloid

plaques. Mutations in this gene result in greater amyloid deposition. The presence of ApoE-4 increases the risk of a person developing late onset AD. However, the presence of the gene alone is not adequate to account for AD because many people with ApoE-4 do not develop AD.

An important part of the neurofibrillary tangle is a protein called tau. *Tau* proteins in the CNS are involved in providing support for intracellular structure through their support of microtubules. Tau proteins hold the microtubules together like railroad ties hold the railroad tracks together. In AD it appears that the tau protein is altered, and as a result, the microtubules twist together in a helical fashion (see Fig. 58-3, *B*). This ultimately forms the neurofibrillary tangles observed in the neurons of persons with AD.

The presence of neuritic plaques and neurofibrillary tangles appears to be related to neuronal death. However, whether they are directly toxic or predispose to cell injury via other mechanisms remains to be determined. For example, examination of autopsied brain tissue from AD patients shows evidence of inflammatory changes. These findings suggest that AD may involve an inflammatory process. This inflammatory response may be elicited by cell damage or death secondary to A-beta or neurofibrillary tangle formation.

Neuritic plaques and neurofibrillary tangles are not unique to patients with AD or dementia. They are also found in the brains of individuals without evidence of cognitive impairment. However, they are more plentiful in the brains of individuals with AD.

Cholinergic neurons are lost in people with AD, particularly in regions essential for memory and cognition. Other neurotransmitter systems, including serotonin and norepinephrine, also show losses over time in patients with AD. Such neurotransmitter changes are the basis of current drug therapies for AD.

Clinical Manifestations

Pathologic changes often precede clinical manifestations of dementia by anywhere from 5 to 20 years. **Mild cognitive impairment** refers to a state of cognition and functional ability between normal aging and early AD (Table 58-6). The Alzheimer's Association has developed a list of warning signs that include common

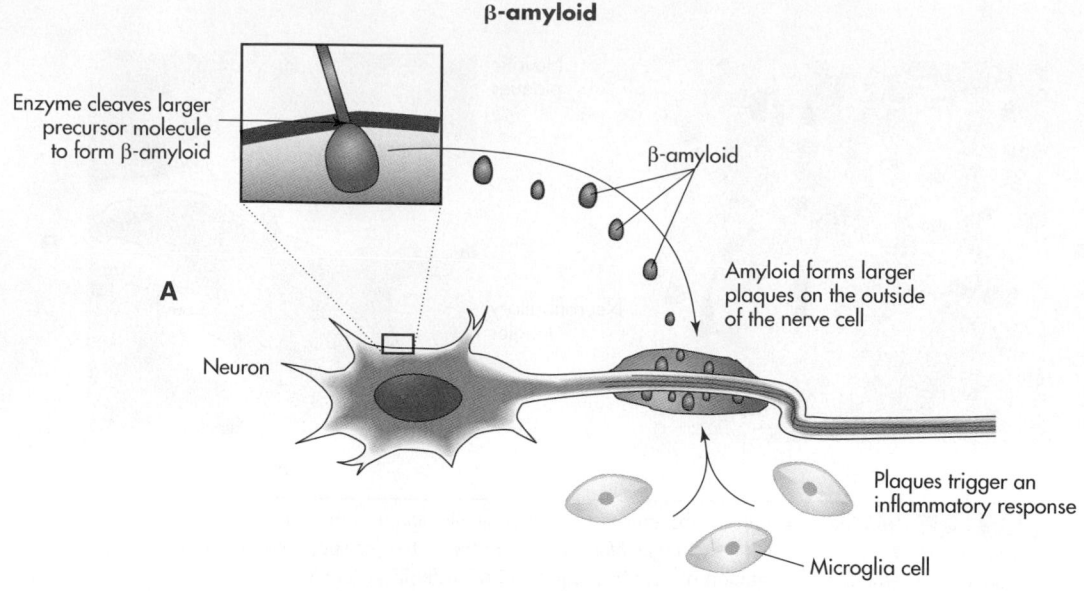

β-amyloid

Enzyme cleaves larger precursor molecule to form β-amyloid

β-amyloid

Amyloid forms larger plaques on the outside of the nerve cell

A

Neuron

Plaques trigger an inflammatory response

Microglia cell

Tau proteins

Normal   **Neurofibrillary tangle**

Tau proteins

Microtubules

Misshapen tau

B

Neuron

FIG. 58-3 Current etiologic theories for the development of Alzheimer's disease. **A,** Abnormal amounts of amyloid are cleaved and released into the circulation. The amyloid forms plaques that attach to the neuron. This stimulates an inflammatory response. **B,** Tau proteins provide structural support for the neuron microtubules. Chemical changes in the neuron produce structural changes in tau proteins. This results in twisting and tangling (neurofibrillary tangles).

manifestations of AD (Table 58-7). The manifestations of AD can be categorized similar to those for dementia as mild, moderate, and late (see Table 58-4). The rate of progression from mild to late is highly variable from individual to individual and ranges from 3 to 20 years. Some patients may have mild cognitive impairment for years, whereas others, especially those with early onset AD, may progress over a few years from mild to severe impairment.

An initial sign of AD is a subtle deterioration in memory. Inevitably this progresses to more profound memory loss that interferes with the patient's ability to function. As the disease progresses, manifestations are more easily noticed and become serious enough to cause people with AD or their family members to seek medical help. Recent events and new information cannot be recalled. Personal hygiene deteriorates, as does the ability to concentrate and maintain attention. Ongoing loss of neurons in

AD can cause a person to act in altered or unpredictable ways. Behavioral manifestations of AD (e.g., agitation) result from changes that take place within the brain. They are neither intentional nor controllable by the individual with the disease. Some patients develop psychotic manifestations (e.g., delusions, illusions, hallucinations).

With progression of AD, additional cognitive impairments are noted. These include *dysphasia* (difficulty comprehending language and oral communication), *apraxia* (inability to manipulate objects or perform purposeful acts), *visual agnosia* (inability to recognize objects by sight), and *dysgraphia* (difficulty communicating via writing). Eventually long-term memories cannot be recalled, and patients lose the ability to recognize family members and friends. Other problems include aggression and a tendency to wander.

TABLE 58-6   Mild Cognitive Impairment (MCI)

Description	• MCI refers to a state of cognition and functional ability between normal aging and early Alzheimer's disease (AD). • Individuals are memory impaired but otherwise functionally normal. • MCI may be considered a transitional state between aging and AD.
Characteristics	• Memory complaint • Abnormal memory for age • Intact activities of daily living • Normal general cognitive functioning • Not demented
Progression to AD	• More than 80% of patients with MCI develop AD within 10 years at a rate of 10% to 15% of patients per year.
Significance	• It is important to identify and treat patients with MCI. • Treatment strategies must be developed to stop or reverse the decline in cognitive function. • If treated appropriately, the progression to onset of AD may be delayed.

Later in the disease, the ability to communicate and to perform activities of daily living is lost. In the late or final stages of AD, the patient is unresponsive, incontinent, and requires total care.

Diagnostic Studies

The diagnosis of AD is primarily a diagnosis of exclusion. No single clinical test can be used to diagnose AD. In patients with cognitive impairment, there is increased emphasis on early and careful evaluation of the patient. As indicated earlier in this chapter, there are many conditions that can cause manifestations of dementia, some of which are treatable or "reversible" (see Table 58-3).

When all other possible conditions that can cause cognitive impairment have been ruled out, a clinical diagnosis of AD can be made. A comprehensive patient evaluation includes a complete health history, physical examination, neurologic and mental status assessments, and laboratory tests (Table 58-8). Brain imaging tests include CT or MRI. A CT or an MRI scan may show brain atrophy and enlarged ventricles in the later stages of the disease, although this finding occurs in other diseases and can also be seen in persons without cognitive impairment. Newer techniques include SPECT, magnetic resonance spectroscopy (MRS), and PET. These techniques allow for detection of changes early in the disease as well as monitoring of treatment response. Blood levels of ApoE-4 may be obtained (see Genetics in Clinical Practice box on p. 1586). Although neuroimaging, neuropsychologic testing, and examination of genetic markers may provide a diagnosis of possible or probable AD, a definitive diagnosis requires examination of brain tissue and the presence of neurofibrillary tangles and neuritic plaques at autopsy.

Neuropsychologic testing with tools such as the Mini-Mental State Examination (see Table 58-5) can help document the de-

TABLE 58-7   Patient & Family Teaching Guide
Early Warning Signs of Alzheimer's Disease

1. *Memory loss that affects job skills.* Frequent forgetfulness or unexplainable confusion at home or in the workplace may signal that something is wrong. This type of memory loss goes beyond forgetting an assignment, colleague's name, deadline, or phone number.
2. *Difficulty performing familiar tasks.* It is not abnormal for most people to become distracted and to forget something (e.g., leave something on the stove too long). People with Alzheimer's disease (AD) may cook a meal but then forget not only to serve it but also that they made it.
3. *Problems with language.* Most people have trouble with finding the "right" word from time to time. Persons with AD may forget simple words or substitute inappropriate words, making their speech difficult to understand.
4. *Disorientation to time and place.* While most individuals occasionally forget the day of the week or what they need from the store, people with AD can become lost on their own street, not knowing where they are, how they got there, or how to get back home.
5. *Poor or decreased judgment.* Many individuals from time to time may choose not to dress appropriately for the weather (e.g., not bringing a coat or sweater on a cold evening). A person with AD may dress inappropriately in more noticeable ways, such as wearing a bathrobe to the store or sweater on a hot day.
6. *Problems with abstract thinking.* For the person with AD this goes beyond challenges such as balancing a checkbook. The person with AD may have difficulty recognizing numbers or doing even basic calculations.
7. *Misplacing things.* For many individuals, temporarily misplacing keys, purses, or wallets is a normal albeit frustrating event. The person with AD may put items in inappropriate places (e.g., eating utensils in clothing drawers) but have no memory of how they got there.
8. *Changes in mood or behavior.* Most individuals experience mood changes. The person with AD tends to exhibit more rapid mood swings for no apparent reason.
9. *Changes in personality.* As most individuals age, they may demonstrate some change in personality (e.g., become less tolerant). The person with AD can change dramatically, either suddenly or over time. For example, someone who is generally easygoing may become angry, suspicious, or fearful.
10. *Loss of initiative.* The person with AD may become and remain uninterested and uninvolved in many or all of his or her usual pursuits.

Adapted from *Early warning signs,* Alzheimer's Association, Chicago, Ill.

gree of cognitive impairment. Neuropsychologic testing is important not only for diagnostic purposes but also to determine a baseline from which changes over time can be evaluated.

A urine test that measures isoprostanes (by-products of fat metabolism associated with free radicals) may provide a mechanism for assessing risk of AD in those with mild cognitive im-

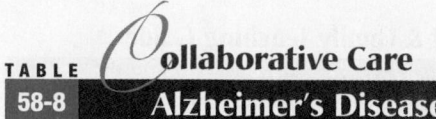

TABLE 58-8 Collaborative Care: Alzheimer's Disease

Diagnostic
History and physical examination, including psychologic evaluation
Neuropsychologic testing including Mini-Mental State Examination (see Table 58-5)
Brain imaging tests: CT, MRI, MRS, SPECT, PET
Complete blood count
Electrocardiogram
Serum glucose, creatinine, BUN
Serum levels of vitamins B_1, B_6, B_{12}
Thyroid function tests
Liver function tests
Screening for depression

Collaborative Therapy
Drug therapy for cognitive problems (see Table 58-9)
Drug therapy for behavioral problems (see Table 58-9)
Behavioral modification
Moderate exercise
Assistance with functional independence
Music, particularly with meals and bathing
Assistance and support for caregiver

BUN, Blood urea nitrogen; *CT*, computed tomography; *MRI*, magnetic resonance imaging; *MRS*, magnetic resonance spectroscopy; *PET*, positron emission tomography; *SPECT*, single photon emission computed tomography.

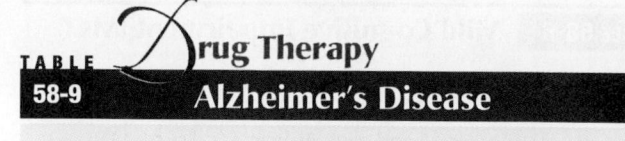

TABLE 58-9 Drug Therapy: Alzheimer's Disease

PROBLEM	DRUGS
Decreased memory and cognition	Cholinesterase inhibitors • donepezil (Aricept) • rivastigmine (Exelon) • galantamine (Reminyl)
Depression	Selective serotonin reuptake inhibitors (SSRIs) • sertraline (Zoloft) • fluvoxamine (Luvox) • citalopram (Celexa) • fluoxetine (Prozac) Tricyclic antidepressants • nortriptyline (Aventyl, Pamelor) • amitriptyline (Elavil) • imipramine (Tofranil) • doxepin (Sinequan) Atypical antidepressant • trazodone (Desyrel)
Behavioral problems (e.g., agitation, disinhibition)	Conventional antipsychotics (neuroleptics) • loxapine (Loxitane) • haloperidol (Haldol) Atypical antipsychotics (neuroleptics) • risperidone (Risperdal) • olanzapine (Zyprexa) • quetiapine (Seroquel) Benzodiazepines • lorazepam (Ativan) • temazepam (Restoril) • oxazepam (Serax)
Sleep disturbances	zolpidem (Ambien)

pairment.[17] However, widespread use of this marker is not currently available.

Collaborative Care

At this time there is no cure for AD. The collaborative management of AD is aimed at improving or controlling decline in cognition and controlling the undesirable manifestations that the patient may exhibit (see Table 58-8).

Drug Therapy. Drug therapy for AD is listed in Table 58-9. Cholinesterase inhibitors are used in the treatment of mild and moderate dementia.[18,19] They block cholinesterase, the enzyme responsible for the breakdown of acetylcholine in the synaptic cleft (Fig. 58-4). Cholinesterase inhibitors include donepezil (Aricept), rivastigmine (Exelon), and galantamine (Reminyl). These drugs have been shown to either improve or stabilize cognitive decline in some people with AD. As a result, they can enhance the patient's functional abilities. However, these drugs do not cure or reverse the progression of the disease. It is not known whether the long-term administration of these drugs will actually delay the progression of the neurologic damage.

Memantine (Ebixa) is a new drug for the treatment of the middle to late stages of AD. Memantine appears to protect the brain's nerve cells against excess amounts of glutamate, which is released in large amounts by cells damaged by AD. The attachment of glutamate to *N*-methyl-D-aspartate (NMDA) receptors permits calcium to flow freely into the cell, which in turn may lead to cell degeneration. Memantine may prevent this destructive sequence by adjusting the activity of glutamate.

Drug therapy is often used for the management of behavioral problems that occur in patients with AD. Conventional antipsychotic drugs (e.g., haloperidol [Haldol]) can be used to manage acute episodes of agitation, aggressive behavior, and psychosis.

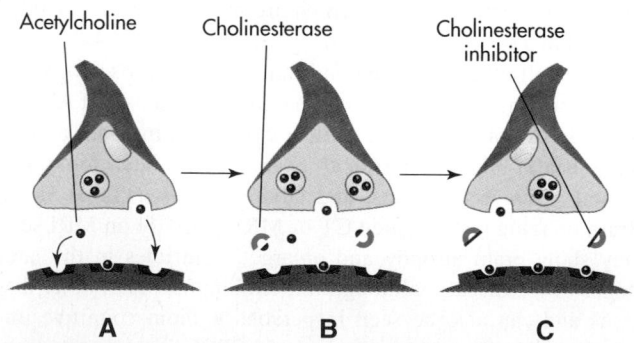

FIG. 58-4 Mechanism of action of cholinesterase inhibitors. Acetylcholine (A) is released from the nerve synapses and carries a message across the synapse. Cholinesterase (B) breaks down acetylcholine. Cholinesterase inhibitors (C) block cholinesterase, thus giving acetylcholine more time to transmit the message.

However, these antipsychotics are often associated with side effects including extrapyramidal symptoms and anticholinergic activity, especially in older adults. Therefore atypical antipsychotics are being used more commonly for behavioral management in AD. These include risperidone (Risperdal), olanzapine (Zyprexa), and quetiapine (Seroquel). They reduce aggression, improve behavior, and usually have fewer side effects.

Treating the depression that is often associated with AD may improve cognitive ability. Depression is often treated with selective serotonin reuptake inhibitors including fluoxetine (Prozac), sertraline (Zoloft), fluvoxamine (Luvox), and citalopram (Celexa). The antidepressant trazodone (Desyrel) may help with problems related to sleep. However, this agent may result in hypotension. Antiseizure drugs (neuroleptics) including valproic acid (Depakene) and carbamazepine (Tegretol) are also used to manage behavioral problems. These drugs tend to act as mood stabilizers.

There has been some debate about the ability of certain drugs, hormones, and herbs (e.g., ginkgo biloba) to prevent or treat AD. Early observational studies indicated that estrogen slowed the progression of AD in those who already had it. However, at this time estrogen is not recommended for the prevention or treatment of AD. Currently, several large studies are exploring the relationship between estrogen and AD. Ginkgo biloba (see the Complementary and Alternative Therapies box on this page) can be used in patients with AD. In Germany ginkgo is considered a form of treatment for AD patients.

Preliminary results from studies investigating the incidence and onset of AD in patients with arthritis who have taken nonsteroidal antiinflammatory drugs (NSAIDs) suggest that NSAIDs may have a protective effect. Although NSAIDs have been shown through epidemiologic studies to be associated with a reduced risk of AD, controlled clinical trials in patients with AD have not demonstrated a clear benefit.[19] When NSAIDs are used in older adults at high doses, there are concerns related to increased potential for upper gastrointestinal bleeding.

Antioxidants may prove to be helpful in slowing the progression of AD. Vitamin C, vitamin E, and selegiline (Eldepryl) are antioxidants and may prevent nerve cell damage by destroying toxic free radicals.[20] *Free radicals* are by-products of normal cell metabolism. Immune cells that are in the brain responding to chronic brain inflammation from AD may release free radicals. Studies of antioxidants and their potential role in prevention or slowing of AD are ongoing.

A number of ongoing clinical drug trials are attempting to find drugs that can limit or decrease the rate of disease progression, as well as manage the signs and symptoms of AD. These new agents will focus on enhancing communications between nerve cells, regulating defective cell processes (reducing A-beta deposition), protecting nerve cells from damage, and repairing nerve cells in the brain.[21]

COMPLEMENTARY & ALTERNATIVE THERAPIES
Ginkgo Biloba

Clinical Uses
Alzheimer's disease and dementia, depression, peripheral arterial vascular disease, tinnitus

Effects
Memory improvement. Increases blood flow to the brain and extremities. Is an antioxidant. Inhibits platelet aggregation.

Nursing Implications
Must be used with caution, or not at all, in people at risk for bleeding or taking anticoagulants. Needs 1 to 3 months to achieve full therapeutic effect. May be of some benefit in treating dementia. There is no evidence that ginkgo will cure or prevent dementia.

NURSING MANAGEMENT
ALZHEIMER'S DISEASE

■ Nursing Assessment

Subjective and objective data that should be obtained from a person with AD are presented in Table 58-10. Useful questions for the patient and informant are, "When did you first notice the memory loss?" and "How has the memory loss progressed since then?"

■ Nursing Diagnoses

Nursing diagnoses for AD may include, but are not limited to, those presented in the NCP 58-1.

■ Planning

The overall goals are that the patient with AD will (1) maintain functional ability for as long as possible, (2) be maintained in a safe environment with a minimum of injuries, (3) have personal care needs met, and (4) have dignity maintained. The over-

TABLE 58-10 Nursing Assessment Alzheimer's Disease

Subjective Data
Important Health Information
Past health history: Repeated head trauma, stroke, exposure to metals (e.g., mercury, aluminum), previous CNS infection, family history of dementia
Medications: Use of any drug to decrease symptoms (e.g., tranquilizers, hypnotics, antidepressants, antipsychotics)
Functional Health Patterns
Health perception–health management: Positive family history; emotional lability
Nutritional-metabolic: Anorexia, malnutrition, weight loss
Elimination: Incontinence
Activity-exercise: Poor personal hygiene; gait instability, weakness; inability to perform activities of daily living
Sleep-rest: Frequent nighttime awakening, daytime napping
Cognitive-perceptual: Forgetfulness, inability to cope with complex situations, difficulty with problem solving (early signs); depression, withdrawal, suicidal ideation (early)

Objective Data
General
Disheveled appearance, agitation
Neurologic
Early: Loss of recent memory; disorientation to date and time; flat affect; lack of spontaneity; impaired abstraction, cognition, and judgment
Middle: Agitation; impaired ability to recognize close family and friends; loss of remote memory; confusion, apraxia, agnosia, alexia (inability to understand written language); aphasia; inability to do simple tasks
Late: Inability to do self-care; incontinence; immobility; limb rigidity; flexor posturing
Possible Findings
Diagnosis by exclusion, cerebral cortical atrophy on CT scan, poor scores on mental status tests, hippocampal atrophy on MRI scan, abnormal changes on PET, SPECT, and MRS

CNS, Central nervous system; *MRI,* magnetic resonance imaging; *MRS,* magnetic resonance spectroscopy; *PET,* positron emission tomography; *SPECT,* single photon emission computed tomography.

all goals for the caregiver of a patient with AD are to (1) reduce caregiver stress, (2) maintain personal health, and (3) cope with the long-term effects of caregiving.

■ Nursing Implementation

Health Promotion. At this time there is no known method of reducing the risk of AD. Ongoing studies suggest that antioxidants may be beneficial. However, additional data are clearly needed. Because traumatic brain injury may be a risk factor for developing AD, the nurse should promote safety in physical activities and driving. Depression should be recognized and treated early. At this time genetic testing for AD is not performed on a regular basis.

Early recognition and treatment of AD are important. The nurse has a responsibility in terms of informing patients and their families regarding the early signs of AD. The warning signs of

NURSING CARE PLAN 58-1

Patient with Alzheimer's Disease

NURSING DIAGNOSIS **Disturbed thought processes** *related to* effects of dementia *as manifested by* loss of memory and other cognitive deficits.

OUTCOMES—NOC

Distorted Thought Control (1403)
- Behaviors indicate accurate interpretation of environment _____
- Asks for validation of reality _____
- Interacts with others appropriately _____

_____

Outcome Scale
1 = Never demonstrated
2 = Rarely demonstrated
3 = Sometimes demonstrated
4 = Often demonstrated
5 = Consistently demonstrated

INTERVENTIONS—NIC and *RATIONALES*

Dementia Management (6460)
- Include family members in planning, providing, and evaluating care to the extent desired *to plan appropriate and consistent interventions.*
- Determine physical, social, and psychologic history of patient, usual habits, and routines *to maintain familiar routines.*
- Prepare for interaction with eye contact and touch as appropriate *to provide respect and acceptance of the patient.*
- Give one simple direction at a time *to decrease potential for increasing confusion and frustration.*
- Use distraction, rather than confrontation, to manage behavior, *which will decrease anxiety.*
- Provide patient a general orientation to the season of the year by using appropriate cues such as calendars, pictures, and seasonal decorations *to promote memory and reduce confusion.*
- Refrain from arguing or contradicting the patient.

Cognitive Stimulation (4720)
- Stimulate memory by repeating patient's last expressed thought.
- Orient to time, place, and person *to promote memory and reduce confusion.*

NURSING DIAGNOSIS **Self-care deficit (bathing, dressing, toileting)** *related to* memory deficit and neuromuscular impairment *as manifested by* inability to independently and appropriately bathe, dress, or toilet.

OUTCOMES—NOC

Self-Care: Activities of Daily Living (0300)
- Dressing _____
- Bathing _____
- Toileting _____

_____

Outcome Scale
1 = Dependent, does not participate
2 = Requires assistive person and device
3 = Requires assistive person
4 = Independent with assistive device
5 = Completely independent

INTERVENTIONS—NIC and *RATIONALES*

Self-Care Assistance (1800)
- Monitor patient's ability for independent self-care *to plan appropriate interventions specific to patient's unique problems.*
- Use consistent repetition of daily health routines as a means of establishing them *because memory loss impairs patient's ability to plan and complete specific sequential activities.*
- Assist patient in accepting dependency *to ensure that all needs are met.*
- Teach family to encourage independence and to intervene only when the patient is unable to perform *to promote independence.*

Self-Care Assistance: Bathing/Hygiene (1801)
- Provide desired personal articles, such as bath soap and hairbrush, *to enhance memory and provide care.*
- Facilitate patient's bathing self as appropriate *to facilitate independence and provide appropriate help in hygiene.*

Self-Care Assistance: Dressing/Grooming (1802)
- Provide patient's clothes in accessible area *to facilitate dressing.*
- Be available for assistance in dressing as necessary *to facilitate independence and provide appropriate help in dressing.*

Self-Care Assistance: Toileting (1804)
- Assist patient to toilet at specified intervals *to promote regularity.*
- Facilitate toilet hygiene after completion of elimination *to prevent discomfort and skin breakdown.*

NURSING CARE PLAN 58-1

Patient with Alzheimer's Disease—cont'd

NURSING DIAGNOSIS   Risk for injury *related to* impaired judgment, possible gait instability, muscle weakness, and sensory/perceptual alteration.

OUTCOMES—NOC	INTERVENTIONS—NIC and *RATIONALES*
Safety Behavior: Fall Prevention (1909) • Correct use of assistive devices _____ • Use of restraints as needed _____ • Use of well-fitting tied shoes _____ • Use of vision-correcting devices _____ **Outcome Scale** 1 = Never demonstrated 2 = Rarely demonstrated 3 = Sometimes demonstrated 4 = Often demonstrated 5 = Consistently demonstrated	*Fall Prevention (6490)* • Identify cognitive or physical deficits of the patient that may increase potential of falling in a particular environment *to decrease or prevent occurrence of injury.* • Provide assistive devices, such as walker, *to steady gait and provide ambulation support.* • Ensure that patient wears shoes that fit properly, fasten securely, and have nonskid soles *to provide support during ambulation.* • Instruct patient to wear prescription glasses *to allow for proper vision.*

NURSING DIAGNOSIS   Ineffective coping *related to* depression in response to diagnosis of Alzheimer's disease *as manifested by* depression, withdrawal, fatigue, social isolation.

OUTCOMES—NOC	INTERVENTIONS—NIC and *RATIONALES*
Coping (1302) • Identifies effective coping patterns _____ • Uses effective coping strategies _____ **Outcome Scale** 1 = Never demonstrated 2 = Rarely demonstrated 3 = Sometimes demonstrated 4 = Often demonstrated 5 = Consistently demonstrated	*Coping Enhancement (5230)* • Appraise the impact of the patient's life situation on roles and relationships *to develop appropriate interventions.* • Encourage social and community activities *to provide pleasurable activities to relieve depression.* • Encourage the use of spiritual resources, if desired, *to allow familiarity and provide a sense of calming to the patient.* • Encourage the family to verbalize feelings about patient and increase communication *to foster mutual understanding among family members.* • Determine the risk of the patient inflicting self-harm *to identify possibility of violent behavior and initiate appropriate nursing plan.*

NURSING DIAGNOSIS   Ineffective therapeutic regimen management *related to* decreasing level of cognitive functioning and memory.

OUTCOMES—NOC	INTERVENTIONS—NIC and *RATIONALES*
Compliance Behavior (1601) • Performs activities of daily living as prescribed _____ • Reports following prescribed regimen _____ **Outcome Scale** 1 = Never demonstrated 2 = Rarely demonstrated 3 = Sometimes demonstrated 4 = Often demonstrated 5 = Consistently demonstrated	*Anticipatory Guidance (5210)* • Assist the patient to identify possible upcoming situations and the effects on the personal and family life *to establish possible outcomes and identify support systems.* • Provide information on realistic expectations related to the patient's behavior and lifestyle changes such as driving *to prepare for the future needs of daily living.* • Include the family and significant others as appropriate in planning *to ensure agreement of plans and to ensure patient's wishes are respected and health care needs are met.*

NURSING DIAGNOSIS   Wandering *related to* disease process *as evidenced by* getting lost numerous times a day and patient's statement of "I don't know where I am."

OUTCOMES—NOC	INTERVENTIONS—NIC and *RATIONALES*
Safety Behavior: Personal (1911) • Provision of secure environment _____ **Outcome Scale** 1 = Not adequate 2 = Slightly adequate 3 = Moderately adequate 4 = Substantially adequate 5 = Totally adequate	*Area Restriction (6420)* • Provide verbal reminders, as necessary, to remain in designated area *to reorient the patient.* *Surveillance: Safety (6654)* • Monitor environment for potential safety hazards *to prevent injury to patient.* • Monitor patient for alterations in physical or cognitive function that might lead to unsafe behavior *to assess any changes that may occur.* • Provide appropriate level of supervision/surveillance *to monitor patient and to allow for therapeutic actions.* • Provide appropriate activities *as diversion from restlessness associated with wandering.*

AD developed by the Alzheimer's Association are shown in Table 58-7.

Acute Intervention. The diagnosis of AD is traumatic for both the patient and the family. It is not unusual for the patient to respond with depression, denial, anxiety and fear, isolation, and feelings of loss. The nurse is in an important position to assess for depression and suicidal ideation. Antidepressant drugs and counseling may be appropriate interventions to assist the patient. Family members may also be in denial and may not seek medical attention early in the disease. The nurse must assess family members and their abilities to accept and cope with the diagnosis.

Although there is no current treatment for reversing AD, there is a need for ongoing monitoring of both the patient with AD and the patient's caregiver. An important nursing responsibility is to work collaboratively with the patient's caregiver to manage clinical manifestations effectively as they change over time. The nurse is often responsible for teaching the caregiver to perform the many tasks that are required to manage the patient's care. The nurse must consider both the patient with AD and the caregiver as patients with overlapping but unique problems. To aid in identifying the many problems of the caregiver, a nursing care plan for the caregiver of a person with AD is presented (NCP 58-2).

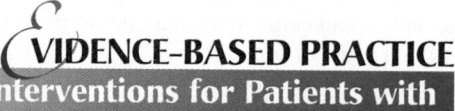

EVIDENCE-BASED PRACTICE
Interventions for Patients with Dementia and Their Caregivers

Clinical Problem

Do pharmacotherapy, educational, or other nonpharmacologic interventions improve outcomes in patients with dementia or for their caregivers?

Best Clinical Practice

- Cholinesterase inhibitors improve outcomes in some patients with Alzheimer's disease.
- Antipsychotics are effective in treating agitation, and antidepressants are effective in treating depression in patients with dementia.
- Educational interventions for family caregivers of patients with Alzheimer's disease improve caregiver and patient outcomes, thus delaying time to institutionalization of the patient.
- Nonpharmacologic interventions, such as behavior modification, are effective for patients with Alzheimer's disease.
- Educating staff in long-term care facilities about Alzheimer's disease minimizes the unnecessary use of antipsychotic drugs.
- Behavior modification, scheduled toileting, and prompted voiding reduce urinary incontinence in people with dementia.

Implications for Nursing Practice

- Effective management of patients with Alzheimer's disease requires a multifaceted approach including drugs specific for the disease, as well as for behavioral problems related to the disease.
- It is essential to consider the needs of the caregiver when planning care for the patient with dementia.

Reference for Evidence

Review: Pharmacologic and nonpharmacologic interventions improve outcomes in patients with dementia and for their caregivers, *ACP Journal Club* 135:94, 2001.

Patients with AD may be hospitalized for other health care problems. Patients with AD are subject to acute and other chronic illnesses and may require surgical interventions. Their inability to communicate symptoms of health problems places the responsibility for assessment and diagnosis on caregivers and health care professionals. Hospitalization of the patient with AD can be a traumatic event for both the patient and the caregiver and can precipitate a worsening of the disease or delirium. Patients with AD hospitalized in the acute care setting will need to be observed more closely because of concerns for safety, frequently oriented to place and time, and given reassurance. The use of the consistent nurses may be helpful in reducing anxiety or disruptive behavior.

Ambulatory and Home Care. Currently, family members and friends care for the majority of individuals who suffer from AD in their homes. Others with AD reside in various facilities, including long-term care and assisted living facilities. Care for these individuals requires further research to identify optimal methods for providing quality of life. A facility that is good for one person may not be suitable for another. Also, what is helpful for a person at one point in the disease process may be completely different from what is best when the disease progresses.

Patients with AD progress through the stages at variable rates. The nursing care needs of the patient with AD change as the disease progresses, emphasizing the need for regular assessment, monitoring, and support. Regardless of the setting, the severity of the problems and the amount of care required intensify over time. The specific manifestations of the disease will depend on the area of the brain involved. Nursing care is focused on decreasing clinical manifestations, preventing harm, and supporting the patient and caregiver through the disease process.

In the mild cognitive impairment phase, memory aids (e.g., calendars) may be beneficial. During this phase depression is likely to occur. Depression is related to the diagnosis of an incurable disorder, as well as the impact of the disease on activities of daily living (e.g., driving, socializing with friends, participating in hobbies or recreational activities). Drug therapy with cholinesterase inhibitors appears to be most effective during the early stages of AD. However, not all patients will show improvement. Drugs must be taken on a regular basis. Because memory is one of the key functions to be altered early in AD, drug compliance may be challenging.

Following the initial diagnosis, patients need to be aware that the progression of the disease is variable. Effective management of the disease can slow the progress of the disease and decrease the burden on the patient, caregiver, and family. However, decisions related to care should be made with the patient, family members, and the health care team early in the disease. The nurse has a role in advising the patient and the caregiver to initiate health care and advanced directives and decisions while the patient still has the capacity to do so. This can ease the burden for the caregiver as the disease progresses.

Adult day care is one of the options available to the person with AD. Although programs vary in size, structure, physical environment, and degree of experience of staff, the common goals of all day care programs are to provide respite for the family and a protective environment for the patient. During the early and middle stages of AD the person can still benefit from stimulating activities that encourage independence and decision making in a protective environment. Graded assistance, practice, and positive

NURSING CARE PLAN 58-2

Caregiver of the Patient with Alzheimer's Disease

EXPECTED PATIENT OUTCOMES	NURSING INTERVENTIONS and *RATIONALES*
NURSING DIAGNOSIS	**Caregiver role strain** *related to* grieving the family member's illness, change in role, and pressure from unrelieved caregiving *as manifested by* statements about stress and inadequate resources to provide care and worry about having to put the family member in a long-term care facility.
• Seeking of appropriate assistance by caregiver • Satisfactory care to the person with Alzheimer's disease	• Assess health status of caregiver *to determine if health planning is needed.* • Refer for medical evaluation when appropriate. • Discuss effects of caregiving with the caregiver *to determine status of caregiver and to enable open discussion of needs.* • Encourage visits and help from other family members *to provide support and relief to caregiver as needed.* • Acknowledge caregiver's fears of being unable to care for family member *to demonstrate empathy and awareness of this fear.* • Provide financial or social service referrals *to assist caregiver with planning for long-term care.* • Counsel and support caregiver if patient is placed in a long-term care facility to *allay guilt and reinforce services the patient now requires.*
NURSING DIAGNOSIS	**Social isolation** *related to* diminishing social relationships, behavioral problems of patient with Alzheimer's disease, and underdeveloped social support system *as manifested by* feelings of abandonment and uselessness, behavior changes, inability to make decisions or concentrate.
• Satisfactory contact with significant others or members of a support group	• Assess past social network and diversional activities *to determine size and scope of network and personal interests.* • Assess social support system of family and willingness and ability to participate in care *to develop care alternatives.* • Assist in planning respite care *to enable caregiver to continue with important activities and social contacts.* • Refer to social services *for realistic appraisal of financial resources for respite care and for linkage to community resources.* • Provide information regarding available support groups (e.g., Alzheimer's Association) *because these groups can meet socialization, recreational, and educational needs of caregiver.*
NURSING DIAGNOSIS	**Anxiety** *related to* uncertain outcome, perceived powerlessness, possible change in role functioning, behavioral problems of the person with Alzheimer's disease, and financial insecurity *as manifested by* apprehension, helplessness, fear, irritability, forgetfulness, inability to concentrate.
• Decreased anxiety • Sense of control of situation	• Assess past roles of patient with Alzheimer's disease and of caregiver *to determine extent of role changes required of caregiver.* • Document changes in role expectations and refer to community resources or provide instruction as needed; assess knowledge of behavioral management techniques and instruct as appropriate; assist caregiver in problem-solving techniques *to ensure that caregiver has skills to manage changing roles and patient status.* • Refer to appropriate agencies as indicated for complete list of community resources and possible sources of financial aid *to relieve anxiety related to financial insecurity.*
NURSING DIAGNOSIS	**Ineffective health maintenance** *related to* unrelieved caregiving responsibilities, fatigue, and chronic stress *as manifested by* failure to care for self.
• Optimal health • Appropriate health practices for age and sex	• Assess physical and emotional health status of caregiver *to determine if problem is present and to plan appropriate interventions.* • Collaborate with caregiver in planning interventions in major identified problem areas *to prevent further deterioration of health.* • Assist with planning of continued care of patient *so that caregiver's personal health needs can be pursued.* • Emphasize need for maintaining own health *to avoid increasing the complexity of the caregiving situation.*

EVIDENCE-BASED PRACTICE
Reality Orientation for Patients with Dementia

Clinical Problem

Is reality orientation effective as a therapy for elderly patients with dementia?

Best Clinical Practice

- Reality orientation (presentations of orientation information such as time, place, person) provides the person with dementia with a greater understanding of his or her surroundings, possibly resulting in an improved sense of control and self-esteem.
- Reality orientation has positive benefits on both cognition and behavior for patients with dementia.

Implications for Nursing Practice

- Nurses can use reality orientation in taking care of patients with dementia.
- Reality orientation can improve the quality of life of confused older adults.
- Continued reinforcement of reality orientation must be ongoing.

Reference for Evidence

Spector A et al: Reality orientation for dementia, *Cochrane Database Syst Rev*, issue 3, 2002.

---

reinforcement can help patients increase their functional independence.[20] The patient returns home tired, content, less frustrated, and ready to be with the family. The respite from the demands of care allows the caregiver to be more responsive to the patient's needs.

Although adult day care may delay the transition, the demands on the caregiver eventually exceed the resources, and the person with AD may be placed in a long-term care facility. Special units to care for persons with AD are becoming increasingly common in long-term care settings. The Alzheimer's unit is designed to be a safer environment for patients with AD. Although there are a variety of these units, many are characterized by spaces that allow the patient to walk freely on the unit yet are closed to prevent patients from wandering.

As the patient with AD progresses to the late stages (severe impairment) of AD, there is increased difficulty with the most basic functions, including walking and talking. Total care is required.

Specific problems relate to the care of the patient with AD across the phases of the disease. These problems are described in the following text.

Behavioral problems. Behavioral disturbances occur in about 90% of patients with AD. Behavioral problems can include repetitiveness (asking the same question repeatedly), delusions (false beliefs), illusions, hallucinations, agitation, aggression, altered sleeping patterns, and wandering. Many times these behaviors are unpredictable and challenge caregivers. Caregivers need to be aware that these behaviors are not intentional and are often difficult to control. Behavioral symptoms often lead to the placement of patients in institutional care settings.

Behaviors do not occur in a vacuum and are often in response to a precipitating factor (e.g., pain, frustration, temperature extremes, anxiety). Controlling the environment to reduce stimuli is the first step in behavior management. This includes identifying factors that can trigger behavior disruptions. Extremes in temperature, as well as excessive noise, may result in behavior change. The use of consistent routines may help to manage behavioral symptoms. Using touch and eye contact when communicating with the patient can have benefit in terms of orienting the patient.

Other strategies can be employed to deal with difficult behavior. These include redirection, distraction, and reassurance. For the patient who is restless or agitated, redirecting would involve having the patient perform activities such as sweeping, raking, or dusting. Examples of strategies to distract the agitated patient might include snacks, car rides, porch swing, rocker, favorite music or videotapes, looking at family photographs, or walking. Repetitive activities, songs, poems, music, massage, aromas, or a favorite object can be soothing to some patients. Reassuring involves letting the patient know that he or she will be protected from danger, harm, or embarrassment.

When nonpharmacologic therapies are ineffective or there is concern about self-injury, disruptive behavior may be treated by medications (see Table 58-9). However, many of these drugs have adverse side effects that can be distressing for the patient and caregiver. Thus the side effects of the drugs are weighed against the distress and potential safety concerns for the patient created by the behavior. As verbal skills decline, the caregiver and nurse may need to rely more on the patient's body language to anticipate care needs.

Safety. The person with AD is at risk for a number of problems related to personal safety. These include injury from falls, injury from ingesting dangerous substances, wandering, injury to others and self with sharp objects, fire or burns, and inability to respond to crisis situations.[22] These concerns require careful attention to the home environment to minimize risk, as well as the need for supervision. As the patient's cognitive function declines over time, the patient may have difficulty navigating physical spaces and interpreting environmental cues. Stairwells must be well lit. Handrails should be graspable with the end of rail shaped differently to alert the patient that it is the end of the stairway. Carpets should have their edges tacked down, and throw rugs should be removed. Polished floor surfaces and linoleum can predispose to falls. Extension cords should be removed because the patient may trip over them. In the bathroom, nonskid mats should be used in the tub or shower, and handrails should be installed in the bath and commode. The nurse can assist the caregiver to evaluate the home environment with safety in mind.

Wandering is a major concern for caregivers. Wandering may be due to loss of memory, side effects of drugs, an expression of a physical or emotional need, restlessness, curiosity, or stimuli that trigger memories of earlier routines.[23] Similar to other behaviors, the nurse should observe for factors or events that may precipitate wandering. For example, the patient may be sensitive to stress and tension in the environment. In such cases, wandering may reflect an attempt to leave the environment. AD patients who tend to wander can be registered with Safe Return, a federally supported program through the Alzheimer's Association. The Safe Return program includes identification products (e.g., wallet cards), a national photo/information database, a 24-hour toll-free emergency crisis line, local chapter support, and wandering behavior education and training for caregivers and families.[10]

Pain management. Because of difficulties with oral and written language associated with AD, patients may have difficulty expressing physical complaints, including pain. The nurse must rely on other clues, including the patient's behavior. Pain can result in alterations in the patient's behavior, such as increased vocalization, agitation, withdrawal, and changes in function. Similar to other patients, pain should be treated with drug therapies and the patient's response monitored.

Eating and swallowing difficulties. Loss of interest in food and decreased ability to feed self *(feeding apraxia),* as well as co morbid conditions, can result in significant nutritional deficiencies in the patient with AD. In long-term care facilities, inadequate assistance with feeding may further add to the problem.

Pureed foods, thickened liquids, and nutritional supplements can be used when chewing and swallowing become problematic for the patient. Patients may need to be reminded to chew their food and to swallow. Dietary restrictions such as a low-salt diet are eased to increase the patient's appetite. Patients need a quiet and unhurried environment for eating. Distractions at mealtimes, including the television, should be avoided. Low lighting, music, and simulated nature sounds may improve eating behaviors.[19] Easy-grip eating utensils and finger foods may allow the patient to self-feed. Liquids should be offered frequently.

When oral feeding is not possible, alternative routes may be explored. Nasogastric (NG) feeding may be used for short periods. However, for the long term the NG tube is uncomfortable and may add further to the patient's agitation. A percutaneous endoscopic gastrostomy (PEG) tube provides another option. Little long-term benefit including increased longevity or reduced complications has been noted in patients receiving PEG feedings.[24] In addition, patients with AD are particularly vulnerable to aspiration of feeding formula and tube dislodgment. The potential positive outcomes to be gained from nutritional therapies are considered in light of overall outcome goals and potential adverse effects of the specific therapy. Nutritional support therapies are described in Chapter 39.

Oral care. In the late stages of AD, the patient will be unable to perform oral self-care. With decreased tooth brushing and flossing, dental problems are likely to occur. Because of swallowing difficulties, patients may pocket food in the mouth, adding to the potential for tooth decay. Dental caries and tooth abscess can add to patient discomfort or pain and subsequently may increase agitation. The mouth should be inspected regularly and mouth care provided to those patients unable to do self-care.

Infection prevention. Urinary tract infection and pneumonia are the most common infections to occur in patients with AD. Such infections are ultimately the cause of death in many patients with AD. Because of feeding and swallowing problems, the patient with AD is at risk for aspiration pneumonia. Immobility can also predispose to pneumonia. Reduced fluid intake, prostate hyperplasia in men, poor hygiene, and urinary drainage devices (e.g., catheter) can predispose to bladder infection. Manifestations of infection including change in behavior, fever, cough (pneumonia), and pain on urination (bladder) are evaluated and appropriately treated.

Skin care. It is important to monitor the patient's skin over time. Rashes, areas of redness, and skin breakdown should be noted and treated as appropriate. In the late stages, incontinence along with immobility and undernutrition can place the patient at risk for skin breakdown. The skin should be kept dry and clean and the patient's position changed regularly to avoid areas of pressure over bony prominences.

Elimination problems. During the middle and late stages of AD, urinary and fecal incontinence become problems. If possible, habit or behavioral retraining of bladder and bowel function (e.g., scheduled toileting) may help decrease episodes of incontinence. Drug therapy including oxybutynin (Ditropan) may decrease bladder excitability and improve control. For women, estrogen cream may be helpful if atrophic vaginitis is present.

A variety of approaches may be used to help decrease problems with constipation. Constipation may be due to immobility, dietary intake (e.g., reduced fiber intake), and decreased fluid intake. Increasing dietary fiber, fiber supplements, and stool softeners are the first lines of management. The combination of aging, other health problems, and swallowing difficulties may increase the risk of complications associated with the use of mineral oil, stimulants, osmotic agents, and enemas. Management of constipation is discussed in Chapter 41.

Caregiver support. AD is a disease that disrupts all aspects of personal and family life. Persons caring for the person with AD spend significantly more time on caregiving tasks than do people caring for individuals with other illnesses.[15,22] Caregivers of patients with AD also exhibit more adverse consequences in terms of the impact on their employment, mental and physical health, family conflict, and caregiver strain. Caregivers with a history of depression may have greater difficulty in adjusting to the demands placed on them. Suggested caregiver needs based on disease stage are provided in Table 58-11.

As the disease progresses, the relationship of the caregiver to the patient changes. Family roles may be altered or reversed (e.g., son caring for father). A range of decisions must be made including when to tell the patient about the diagnosis, when to have the patient stop driving or doing activities that might be dangerous, when to ask for assistance, and when to place the patient with AD in adult day care or long-term care facility. With early onset AD, the adult is affected during his or her most productive years in terms of career and family. The consequences can be devastating for the individual and the family.

Sexual relations for couples are also seriously affected by AD. As the disease progresses, sexual interest may decline for both the patient and the partner. A number of reasons account for this, including caregiver fatigue, as well as memory impairment and episodes of incontinence in the patient with AD. It is also possible for the patient to become very sexually driven as the disease progresses and the patient becomes more uninhibited.

The nurse should work with the caregiver to determine stressors and strategies to reduce the burden of caregiving. For example, the nurse should ask which behaviors are most disruptive to family life and remember that this is likely to change over time as the disease progresses. Establishing what the caregiver views as most disruptive or distressful can help to establish priorities for care. Risk to the safety of the patient and caregiver is given high priority. It is also important to assess what the caregiver's expectations are regarding the patient's behavior. Are the expectations reasonable given the progression of the disease? Working with the caregiver to identify risk factors for complications including behavioral problems is an important responsibility of the nurse.

Caregivers, most of whom are women, may be older adults themselves. Caregiving stress or burden can have adverse outcomes for their health, especially for those who have chronic health problems. Adult children are often caregivers. The impact

TABLE 58-11   Family & Caregiver Teaching Guide
Alzheimer's Disease

Mild Stage

1. Confirm the diagnosis. Many treatable (and potentially reversible) conditions can mimic Alzheimer's disease (see Table 58-3).
2. Get the person to stop driving. Confusion and poor judgment can impair driving skills and potentially put others at risk.
3. Encourage activities such as visiting with friends and family, listening to music, participating in hobbies, and exercising.
4. Provide cues in the home, establish a routine, and determine specific location where essential items (e.g., glasses) need to be kept.
5. Do not correct misstatements or faulty memory.
6. Register with Safe Return, a program established by the Alzheimer's Association to locate individuals who may wander from their homes.
7. Make plans for the future in terms of care options, financial concerns, and personal preference for care.

Moderate Stage

1. Install door locks for patient safety.
2. Provide protective wear for urinary and fecal incontinence.
3. Ensure that the home has good lighting, install handrails in stairways and bathroom, and remove area rugs or ensure that they are tacked down.
4. Label drawers and faucets (hot and cold) to ensure safety.
5. Develop strategies such as distraction and diversion to cope with behavioral problems. Identify and reduce potential triggers (e.g., reduce stress, extremes in temperature) for disruptive behavior.
6. Provide memory triggers, such as pictures of family and friends.

Late Stage

1. Provide a regular schedule for toileting to reduce incontinence.
2. Provide care to meet needs, including oral care and skin care.
3. Monitor diet and fluid intake to ensure their adequacy.
4. Continue communication through talking and touching.
5. Consider placement in a long-term care facility when providing total care becomes too difficult.

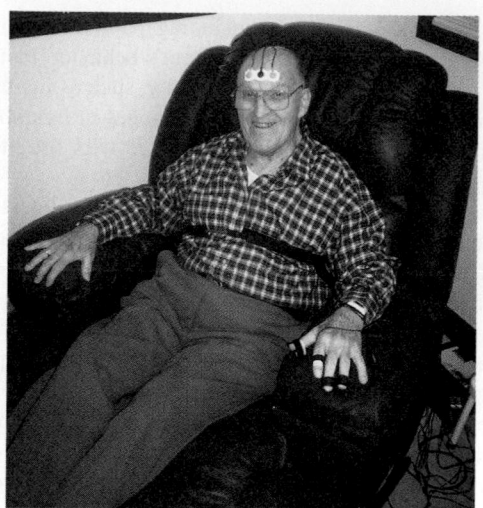

FIG. 58-5 Biofeedback can be used to teach relaxation techniques to caregivers.

■ Evaluation

Expected outcomes for the patient with AD are addressed in the NCP 58-1. Expected outcomes for the caregiver of a patient with AD are addressed in NCP 58-2.

OTHER NEURODEGENERATIVE DISEASES

Parkinson's disease and Huntington's disease are both neurodegenerative diseases (see Chapter 57). Both diseases are chronic, progressive, and incurable. Despite differences in the etiology and pathophysiology of these diseases, both are associated with the development of dementia in the later stages of disease.

Lewy body disease is a condition characterized by the presence of Lewy bodies (intraneural cytoplasmic inclusions) in the brainstem and cortex. The disease has features of both AD and Parkinson's disease. Patients with this form of dementia exhibit disabling mental impairment progressing to dementia, fluctuation in cognitive function, visual hallucinations, and features of Parkinson's disease, especially rigidity. The diagnostic criteria for Lewy body dementia is based on clinical signs and symptoms and confirmed at autopsy by histologic examination of brain tissue.

Creutzfeldt-Jakob disease (CJD) is a rare and fatal brain disorder thought to be caused by a prion protein. A *prion* is a small infectious pathogen containing protein but lacking nucleic acids. Worldwide, sporadic CJD affects one in a million individuals each year.

There are three types of CJD: sporadic CJD, hereditary CJD, and acquired CJD. A variant of CJD (vCJD) was first described in the mid-1980s. The source of this infection appeared to be beef used in baby food preparations obtained from animals contaminated with bovine spongiform encephalopathy, which is also called *mad cow disease.* Worldwide, approximately 110 cases of vCJD have been identified.[25]

The earliest symptom of the disease may be memory impairment and behavior changes. The disease progresses rapidly with mental deterioration, involuntary movements (muscle jerks), weakness in the limbs, blindness, and eventually coma. There is no diagnostic test for CJD. Only autopsy and examination of brain tissue can confirm the diagnosis. There is no treatment for CJD. Emphasis is on reducing the risk of acquiring CJD via food products.

of the caregiving role can be overwhelming for adult children caregivers. They may need to relocate their family or their parent(s), juggle employment and family responsibilities, face financial strain, and realize the "loss" of their own lives.

Support groups for caregivers and family members have been formed throughout the United States and other countries to provide an atmosphere of understanding and to give current information about the disease itself and related topics such as safety, legal, ethical, and financial issues. Nurses often receive personal and professional satisfaction in participating in such support groups. Other strategies related to stress management including relaxation and biofeedback training (Fig. 58-5) are discussed in Chapters 7 and 8.

The Alzheimer's Association has many educational and support systems available to help family caregivers. This organization can provide help in many different ways to caregivers.

Pick's disease, a type of **frontotemporal dementia,** is a rare brain disorder characterized by disturbances in behavior, sleep, personality, and eventually memory. The major distinguishing characteristic between these disorders and AD is marked symmetric lobar atrophy of the temporal and/or frontal lobes. The disease is relentless in its progression, which may ultimately include language impairment, erratic behavior, and dementia. Because of the strange behavior associated with Pick's disease and frontotemporal dementia, psychiatrists often see these patients first. There is no specific treatment. The diagnosis can be confirmed at autopsy.

Normal Pressure Hydrocephalus

Normal pressure hydrocephalus is an uncommon disorder characterized by an obstruction in the flow of CSF, which causes a buildup of this fluid in the brain. Symptoms of the condition include dementia, urinary incontinence, and difficulty in walking. Meningitis, encephalitis, or head injury may cause the condition. If diagnosed early in the disease, normal-pressure hydrocephalus is treatable by surgery in which a shunt is inserted to divert the fluid away from the brain.

CRITICAL THINKING EXERCISES

Case Study
Alzheimer's Disease
Patient Profile. Mr. Y., an 80-year-old African American man, was diagnosed with AD 3 years ago. Today his 78-year-old wife brings him to the emergency department because he wandered from his home, fell, and injured his left hip.

Subjective Data
- Can state his name
- Confused as to place and time
- Denies memory of wandering or falling
- Agitated, trying to get up
- Denies pain

Objective Data
Physical Examination
- Left leg shorter than right leg
- Tense and anxious

Diagnostic Studies
- X-ray of left hip indicates a fracture
- Mini-Mental State Examination shows cognitive impairment

CRITICAL THINKING QUESTIONS
1. What is the pathogenesis of AD?
2. What precipitating factors may have resulted in Mr. Y's fall?
3. What precautions need to be taken regarding the inpatient care of Mr. Y?
4. What teaching plan should be developed for Mr. Y and his wife?
5. Write one or more appropriate nursing diagnoses based on the assessment data presented. Are there any collaborative problems?

Nursing Research Issues
1. What nursing interventions can be used in long-term care facilities to reduce agitated behaviors in patients with dementia?
2. What specific factors can be used to rate a patient's risk of developing delirium while in the acute care facility?
3. What strategies can be used to reduce burden and enhance coping skills in caregivers of patients with AD?
4. Does early intervention in patients with AD reduce the progression of the disease?

REVIEW QUESTIONS

The number of the question corresponds to the same-numbered objective at the beginning of the chapter.

1. Which of the following patients is most at risk for developing delirium?
   a. A 50-year-old woman with cholecystitis
   b. A 19-year-old man with a fractured femur
   c. A 42-year-old woman having an elective hysterectomy
   d. A 78-year-old man admitted to the medical unit with complications related to congestive heart failure

2. Dementia is defined as a
   a. syndrome that results only in memory loss.
   b. disease associated with abrupt changes in behavior.
   c. disease that is always due to reduced blood flow to the brain.
   d. syndrome characterized by cognitive dysfunction and loss of memory.

3. Vascular dementia is associated with
   a. transient ischemic attacks.
   b. bacterial or viral infection of neuronal tissue.
   c. cognitive changes secondary to cerebral ischemia.
   d. abrupt changes in cognitive function that are irreversible.

4. The clinical diagnosis of dementia is based on
   a. brain biopsy.
   b. electroencephalogram.
   c. patient history and cognitive assessment.
   d. CT or MRS.

5. The early stage of AD is characterized by
   a. no noticeable change in behavior.
   b. memory problems and mild confusion.
   c. increased time spent sleeping or in bed.
   d. incontinence, agitation, and wandering behavior.

6. A major goal of treatment for the patient with AD is to
   a. maintain patient safety.
   b. maintain or increase body weight.
   c. return to a higher level of self-care.
   d. enhance functional ability over time.

7. Creutzfeldt-Jakob disease is characterized by
   a. remissions and exacerbations over many years.
   b. memory impairment, muscle jerks, and blindness.
   c. parkinsonian symptoms including muscle rigidity and tremors at rest.
   d. increased intracranial pressure secondary to decreased CSF drainage.

REFERENCES

1. Inouye SK: Assessment and management of delirium in hospitalized older patients, *Ann Long-Term Care* 8:53, 2000.
2. Burt T: Donepezil and related cholinesterase inhibitors as mood and behavioral controlling agents, *Curr Psychiatry Rep* 2:473, 2000.
3. Tune LE, Egeli S: Acetylcholine and delirium, *Dement Geriatr Cogn Disord* 10:342, 1999.
4. Broadhurst C, Wilson K: Immunology of delirium: new opportunities for treatment and research, *Br J Psychiatry* 179:288, 2001.
5. Hosoda S et al: Psychiatric symptoms related to interferon therapy for chronic hepatitis C: clinical features and prognosis, *Psychiatry Clin Neurosci* 54:565, 2000.
6. Henry M: Descending into delirium, *Am J Nurs* 102:49, 2002.
7. McCusker J et al: Environmental risk factors for delirium in hospitalized older people, *J Am Geriatr Soc* 49:1327, 2001.
8. Inouye SK et al: A multicomponent intervention to prevent delirium in hospitalized older patients, *N Engl J Med* 340:669, 1999.
9. Fleming KD, Adams AC, Petersen RC: Dementia: diagnosis and evaluation, *Mayo Clin Proc* 70:1093, 1995.
10. Alzheimer's Association: About Alzheimer's. Available at *www.alz.org/AboutAD/overview.htm* (accessed August 22, 2002).
11. The Canadian Study of Health and Aging Working Group: The incidence of dementia in Canada, *Neurology* 55:66, 2000.
12. Seshadri S et al: Plasma homocysteine as a risk factor for dementia and Alzheimer's disease, *N Engl J Med* 346:476, 2002.
13. Petersen RC et al: Practice parameter: early detection of dementia: mild cognitive impairment (an evidence-based review), *Neurology* 56:1133, 2001.
14. Knopman DS: Practice parameter: diagnosis of dementia (an evidence-based review), *Neurology* 56:1143, 2001.
15. National Institute on Aging, NIH: 2000 progress report on Alzheimer's disease, NIH Publication No. 00-4859. Available at *www.alzheimers.org/pubs/prog00.htm* (accessed August 22, 2002).
16. Sinha S: The role of beta-amyloid in Alzheimer's disease, *Med Clin North Am* 86:629, 2002.
17. Pratico D et al: Increase of brain oxidative stress in mild cognitive impairment: a possible predictor of Alzheimer disease, *Arch Neurol* 59:972, 2002.
18. Sramek JJ et al: Acetylcholinesterase inhibitors for the treatment of Alzheimer's disease, *Ann Long Term Care* 9:15, 2001.
19. Blais MA et al: The treatment and management of Alzheimer's disease, *Clin Geriatr* 9:58, 2001.
20. Doody RS: Practice parameter: management of dementia (an evidence-based review), *Neurology* 56:1154, 2001.
21. Bonner LT, Peskind ER: Pharmacologic treatments of dementia, *Med Clin North Am* 86:657, 2002.
22. Gitlin LN et al: A randomized, controlled trial of a home environmental intervention: effect on efficacy and upset in caregivers and on daily function of persons with dementia, *Gerontologist* 41:4, 2001.
23. Alzheimer's wandering, Mayo Clinic. Available at *www.mayohealth.org/mayo/9901/htm/wandering.htm* (accessed August 22, 2002).
24. Braun UK et al: Malnutrition in patients with severe dementia: is there a place for PEG tube feeding, *Ann Long Term Care* 9:47, 2001.
25. Taylor DM: Current perspectives on bovine spongiform encephalopathy and variant Creutzfeldt-Jakob disease, *Clin Microbiol Infect* 8:332, 2002.

RESOURCES

Administration on Aging (AoA)
330 Independence Avenue, SW
Washington, DC 20201
202-619-0724
www.aoa.dhhs.gov

Alzheimer's Association
919 North Michigan Avenue, Suite 1100
Chicago, IL 60611-1676
800-272-3900 or 312-335-8700
Fax: 312-335-1110
www.alz.org

Alzheimer's Disease Education and Referral Center
P.O. Box 8250
Silver Spring, MD 20907-8250
800-438-4380
www.alzheimers.org

American Association for Geriatric Psychiatry
7910 Woodmont Avenue, Suite 1050
Bethesda, MD 20814-3004
301-654-7850
Fax: 301-654-4137
www.aagponline.org

American Association of Retired Persons
601 E Street, NW
Washington, DC 20049
800-424-3410
www.aarp.org

National Alliance for Caregiving
4729 Montgomery Lane, Suite 642
Bethesda, MD 20814
www.caregiving.org

National Council on the Aging (NCOA)
409 Third Street SW, Suite 200
Washington, DC 20024
202-479-1200
Fax: 202-479-0735
www.ncoa.org

National Family Caregivers Association (NFCA)
10400 Connecticut Avenue, #500
Kensington, MD 20895-3944
800-896-3650
Fax: 301-942-2302
www.nfcacares.org

National Institute on Aging
Building 31, Room 5C27
31 Center Drive, MSC 2292
Bethesda, MD 20892
800-222-2225 or 301-496-1752
www.nia.nih.gov

National Institute of Mental Health (NIMH)
6001 Executive Boulevard
Room 8184, MSC 9663
Bethesda, MD 20892-9663
800-421-4211 or 301-443-4513
Fax: 301-443-4279
www.nimh.nih.gov

National Institute of Neurological Disorders and Strokes
NIH Neurological Institute
P.O. Box 5801
Bethesda, MD 20824
800-352-9424
www.ninds.nih.gov

National Mental Health Association
1021 Prince Street
2001 North Beauregard Street, 12th Floor
Alexandria, VA 22311
800-969-NMHA (6642) or 703-684-7722
Fax: 703-684-5968
www.nmha.org

For additional Internet resources, see the website for this book at *http://evolve.elsevier.com/Lewis/medsurg*.

CHAPTER 59

NURSING MANAGEMENT
Peripheral Nerve and Spinal Cord Problems

Catherine Warms

LEARNING OBJECTIVES

1. Explain the etiology, clinical manifestations, collaborative care, and nursing management of trigeminal neuralgia and Bell's palsy.
2. Explain the etiology, clinical manifestations, collaborative care, and nursing management of Guillain-Barré syndrome, botulism, tetanus, and neurosyphilis.
3. Describe the classification of spinal cord injuries and associated clinical manifestations.
4. Describe the clinical manifestations, collaborative care, and nursing management of spinal cord shock.

5. Correlate the clinical manifestations of spinal cord injury with the level of disruption and rehabilitation potential.
6. Describe the nursing management of the major physical and psychologic problems of the patient with a spinal cord injury.
7. Describe the effects of spinal cord injury on the older adult population.
8. Explain the types, clinical manifestations, collaborative care, and nursing management of spinal cord tumors.

KEY TERMS

anterior cord syndrome, p. 1612
autonomic dysreflexia, p. 1625
Bell's palsy, p. 1605
botulism, p. 1608
Brown-Séquard syndrome, p. 1612
central cord syndrome, p. 1612
Guillain-Barré syndrome, p. 1606
neurogenic bladder, p. 1626
neurogenic bowel, p. 1627

neurogenic shock, p. 1611
neurosyphilis, p. 1610
paraplegia, p. 1611
poikilothermism, p. 1614
posterior cord syndrome, p. 1612
spinal shock, p. 1611
tetanus, p. 1609
tetraplegia, p. 1610
trigeminal neuralgia, p. 1601

Cranial Nerve Disorders

Cranial nerve disorders are commonly classified as peripheral neuropathies. The 12 pairs of cranial nerves are considered the peripheral nerves of the brain. The disorders usually involve the motor or sensory (or both) branches of a single nerve (mononeuropathies). Causes of cranial nerve problems include tumors, trauma, infections, inflammatory processes, and idiopathic (unknown) causes. Two cranial nerve disorders are trigeminal neuralgia (tic douloureux) and acute peripheral facial paralysis (Bell's palsy).

TRIGEMINAL NEURALGIA

Etiology and Pathophysiology

Trigeminal neuralgia (tic douloureux) is a relatively uncommon cranial nerve disorder diagnosed in approximately 15,000 Americans each year. However, it is the most commonly diagnosed neuralgic condition. It is seen approximately twice as often in women as in men. The majority of cases (over 90%) are diagnosed

in individuals over the age of 40.[1] The trigeminal nerve is the fifth cranial nerve (CN V) and has both motor and sensory branches. In trigeminal neuralgia the sensory or afferent branches, primarily the maxillary and mandibular branches, are involved (Fig. 59-1).

The pathophysiology of trigeminal neuralgia is not fully understood. One theory is that compression of blood vessels, the superior cerebellar artery in particular, occurs, resulting in chronic irritation of the trigeminal nerve at the root entry zone. This irritation results in increased firing of the afferent or sensory fiber. Other factors that may result in neuralgia include herpesvirus infection, infection of teeth and jaw, and a brainstem infarct. The effectiveness of antiseizure drug therapy in reducing pain may be related to the ability of these drugs to stabilize the neuronal membrane and decrease paroxysmal afferent impulses of the nerve.[1]

Clinical Manifestations

The classic feature of trigeminal neuralgia is an abrupt onset of paroxysms of excruciating pain described as a burning, knifelike, or lightninglike shock in the lips, upper or lower gums, cheek, forehead, or side of the nose. Intense pain, twitching, grimacing, and frequent blinking and tearing of the eye occur during the acute attack (giving rise to the term tic). Some patients may experience facial sensory loss as well. The attacks are usually brief, lasting only seconds to 2 or 3 minutes, and are generally unilateral. Recurrences are unpredictable; they may occur several times a day or weeks or months apart. After the refractory (pain-free) period, a phenomenon known as clustering can occur. Clustering is characterized by a cycle of pain and refractoriness that continues for hours.

The painful episodes are usually initiated by a triggering mechanism of light cutaneous stimulation at a specific point (trigger zone) along the distribution of the nerve branches. Precipitating stimuli include chewing, teeth brushing, a hot or cold blast of air on the face, washing the face, yawning, or even talking. Touch and tickle seem to predominate as causative triggers rather than

---

Reviewed by Kathleen T. Lucke, RN, PhD, Assistant Professor, School of Nursing, University of Texas Health Science Center, San Antonio, Tex.

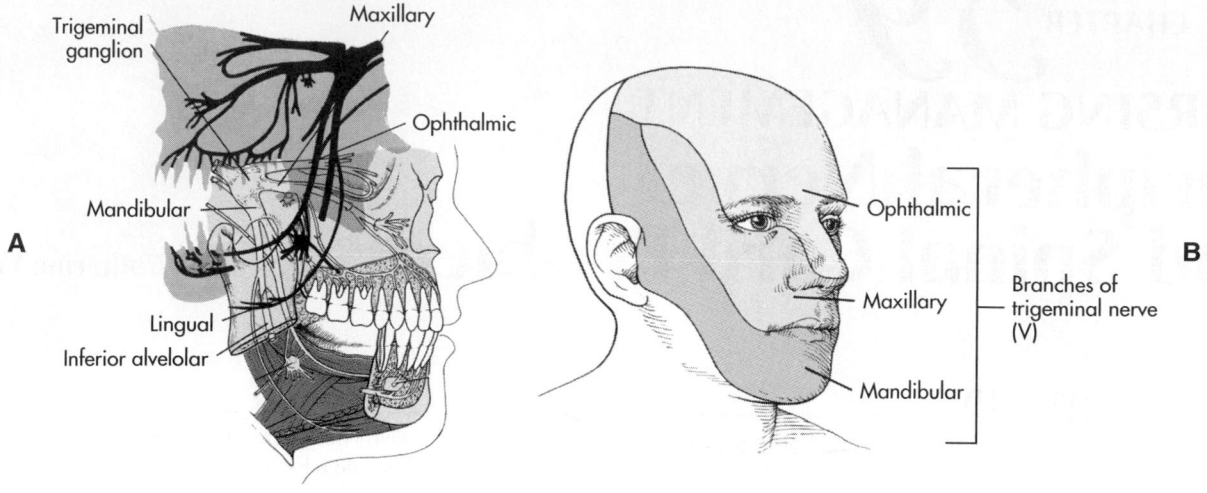

FIG. 59-1 **A,** Trigeminal (fifth cranial nerve and its three main divisions—the ophthalmic, maxillary, and mandibular nerves). **B,** Cutaneous innervation of the head.

pain or changes in temperature. As a result, the patient may eat improperly, neglect hygienic practices, wear a cloth over the face, and withdraw from interaction with other individuals. The patient may sleep excessively as a means of coping with the pain.

Although this condition is considered benign, the severity of the pain and the disruption of lifestyle can result in almost total physical and psychologic dysfunction or even suicide.

Diagnostic Studies

It is important to rule out other problems with similar manifestations, such as other forms of facial and cephalic neuralgias and pain arising from the sinuses, teeth, and jaws. In young adults with bilateral facial pain, a computed tomography (CT) scan is performed to rule out any lesions or vascular abnormalities, and a lumbar puncture and magnetic resonance imaging (MRI) are done to rule out multiple sclerosis. A complete neurologic assessment is done including audiologic evaluation, although results are usually normal. Additional tests used to rule out other pathologic conditions include electromyography (EMG), cerebrospinal fluid (CSF) analysis, arteriography, and myelography. Once the diagnosis is made, the goal of treatment is relief of pain either medically or surgically (Tables 59-1 and 59-2).

Collaborative Care

Drug Therapy. The majority of patients obtain adequate relief through antiseizure drugs such as carbamazepine (Tegretol), phenytoin (Dilantin), and valproate (Depakene). Carbamazepine is considered the first-line therapy for trigeminal neuralgia. By acting on sodium channels, carbamazepine and other antiseizure drugs lengthen the time needed for neuron repolarization, resulting in decreased neuron firing. Side effects of carbamazepine may include bone marrow suppression leading to blood abnormalities. Therefore routine complete blood cell (CBC) counts are required. Newer antiseizure drugs used in the management of trigeminal neuralgia include oxcarbazepine (Trileptal), gabapentin (Neurontin), lamotrigine (Lamictal), and topiramate (Topamax). These antiseizure drugs may prevent an acute attack or promote a remission of symptoms. Because drug therapy may not provide permanent pain relief, some patients may seek continued help by

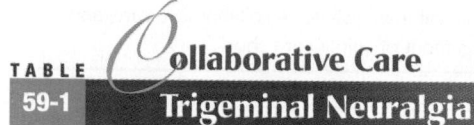

TABLE 59-1 **Collaborative Care**
Trigeminal Neuralgia

Diagnostic
History and physical examination
Audiologic evaluation
CT scan
MRI
EMG
CSF analysis
Arteriography
Posterior myelography

Collaborative Therapy
Drug therapy (e.g., phenytoin [Dilantin], carbamazepine [Tegretol], valproate [Depakene], oxcarbazepine [Trileptal], gabapentin [Neurontin], lamotrigine [Lamictal], topiramate [Topamax])
Local nerve blocking
Biofeedback
Surgical intervention (see Table 59-2)

CSF, Cerebrospinal fluid; *CT,* computed tomography; *EMG,* electromyography; *MRI,* magnetic resonance imaging.

numerous visits to otolaryngologists or from therapies such as acupuncture and megavitamins.

Conservative Therapy. Nerve blocking with local anesthetics is another treatment possibility. Local nerve blocking results in complete anesthesia of the area supplied by the injected branches. Relief of pain is temporary, lasting from 6 to 18 months. This treatment is usually tolerated well by older adults.

Biofeedback is another strategy that may be helpful for some patients. In addition to controlling the pain, the patient may experience a strong sense of personal control by mastering the technique and altering certain body functions. (Biofeedback is discussed in Chapter 7.)

Surgical Therapy. If a conservative approach including drug therapy is not effective, surgical therapy is available (see

TABLE 59-2	Surgical Interventions for Trigeminal Neuralgia	
PROCEDURE	**TECHNIQUE**	**BENEFIT**
Peripheral		
Glycerol rhizotomy (injection into one or more branches of the trigeminal nerve)	Chemical ablation	Total pain relief with sparing of touch and corneal reflex
Intracranial		
Percutaneous radiofrequency rhizotomy	Destruction of sensory fibers by low-voltage current	Total pain relief, sparing of touch and corneal reflex (increased risk for sensory changes)
Microvascular decompression (Jannetta procedure)	Lifting of artery pressing on nerve root in posterior fossa with wedge of sponge, leading to removal of pressure at nerve-root entry zone or removing the involved vessel	Pain relief without loss of sensation
Gamma knife radiosurgery	Technique that uses high doses of radiation focused on the trigeminal nerve root using stereotactic localization	Pain relief 1 day to 4 months post-treatment; noninvasive; no loss of sensation
Retrogasserian rhizotomy	Temporal craniotomy (sectioning of sensory root in middle cranial fossa)	Permanent anesthesia
Suboccipital craniotomy	Sectioning of sensory root of posterior fossa	Permanent anesthesia

Table 59-2). Glycerol rhizotomy is a percutaneous procedure. *Glycerol rhizotomy* consists of an injection of glycerol through the foramen ovale into the trigeminal cistern (Fig. 59-2). Glycerol rhizotomy is a more benign procedure with less sensory loss and fewer sensory aberrations than radiofrequency rhizotomy and with comparable or better pain relief. However, for some patients the pain will return over time.[2,3]

Percutaneous radiofrequency rhizotomy (electrocoagulation) and microvascular decompression afford the greatest relief of pain. *Percutaneous radiofrequency rhizotomy* consists of placing a needle into the trigeminal rootlets that are adjacent to the pons and destroying the area by means of a radiofrequency current. This can result in facial numbness (although some degree of sensation may be retained), corneal anesthesia, and trigeminal motor weakness. This procedure is easily performed with minimal risk to the patient and is based on the exchange of pain for numbness. The procedure is usually performed on an outpatient basis with few complications. It is tolerated well by older adults and avoids a major operative procedure in the high-risk patient.[2]

Microvascular decompression of the trigeminal nerve is another commonly used procedure for neuralgia. It is accomplished by displacing and repositioning blood vessels that appear to be compressing the nerve at the root entry zone where it exits the pons. This procedure relieves pain without residual sensory loss, but it is potentially dangerous, as is any surgery near the brainstem. Microvascular decompression has a long-term success rate equal to or superior to percutaneous procedures without the higher rate of permanent neurologic outcomes such as numbness. It is a safe procedure with an almost negligible mortality and low morbidity when performed in younger adults by a skilled surgeon.[2]

Gamma knife radiosurgery is another surgical treatment that is used for trigeminal neuralgia. Radiosurgery using the gamma knife provides precise radiation of the proximal trigeminal nerve identified on high-resolution imaging. This image-guided approach has been useful for both patients with persistent pain after other surgeries and as a primary surgical option.[3] Two other

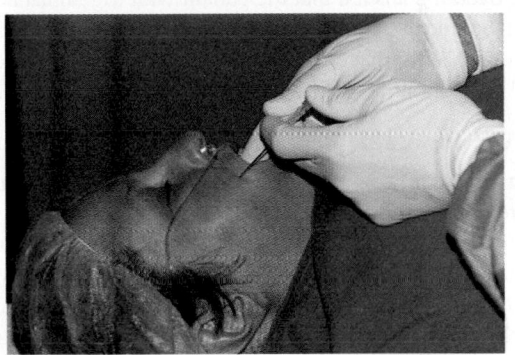
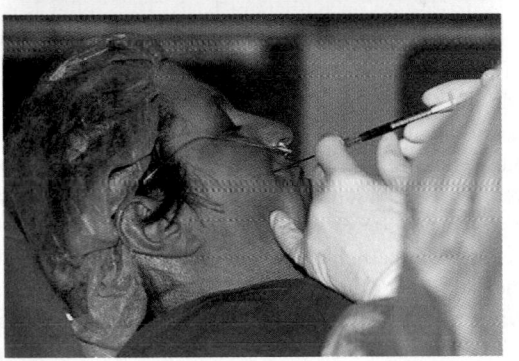

FIG. 59-2 A, Patient with trigeminal neuralgia having needle placed. B, Physician injecting glycerol.

intracranial procedures include the retrogasserian rhizotomy and suboccipital craniotomy (see Table 59-2).

NURSING MANAGEMENT
TRIGEMINAL NEURALGIA

■ Nursing Assessment

Assessment of the attacks, including the triggering factors, characteristics, frequency, and pain management techniques, helps the nurse plan for patient care. The nursing assessment should include the patient's nutritional status, hygiene (especially oral), and behavior (including withdrawal). Evaluation of the degree of pain and its effects on the patient's lifestyle, drug history, emotional state, and suicidal tendencies are other important factors.

■ Nursing Diagnoses

Nursing diagnoses for the patient with trigeminal neuralgia include, but are not limited to, the following:

- Acute pain *related to* inflammation or compression of the trigeminal nerve
- Imbalanced nutrition: less than body requirements *related to* fear of triggering pain by eating or chewing
- Anxiety *related to* uncertainty of timing and initiating event of pain and uncertainty regarding effectiveness of pain-relieving treatments
- Impaired oral mucous membrane *related to* unwillingness to practice oral hygiene measures secondary to potential for initiating pain
- Social isolation *related to* anxiety over pain attacks and desire to maintain nonstimulating environment

■ Planning

The overall goals are that the patient with trigeminal neuralgia will (1) be free of pain, (2) maintain adequate nutritional and oral hygiene status, (3) have minimal to no anxiety, and (4) return to normal or previous socialization and occupational activities.

■ Nursing Implementation

Health Promotion. Because the etiology of trigeminal neuralgia remains unknown, health promotion is directed at reducing recurrent episodes in those who have trigeminal neuralgia. Awareness and reduction of triggering events may be possible in some patients.

Acute Intervention. Patients with trigeminal neuralgia are treated primarily on an outpatient basis. Pain relief is primarily obtained by the administration of the recommended drug therapy. The nurse monitors the patient's response to therapy and notes any side effects. Strong narcotics such as morphine should be used cautiously because of the potential for addiction over time. Alternative pain relief measures, such as biofeedback, should be explored for the patient who is not a surgical candidate and whose pain is not controlled by other therapeutic measures. Careful assessment of pain, including history, pain relief, and drug dependency, can assist in selecting appropriate interventions.

Environmental management is essential during an acute period to lessen triggering stimuli. The room should be kept at an even, moderate temperature and free of drafts. A private room is preferred during an acute period. The nurse must use care to avoid touching the patient's face or jarring the bed. Many patients prefer to carry out their own care, fearing that someone else will inadvertently injure them.

The nurse must teach the patient about the importance of nutrition, hygiene, and oral care and convey understanding if previous oral neglect is apparent. The nurse should provide lukewarm water and soft cloths or cotton saturated with solutions not requiring rinsing for cleansing the face. A small, soft-bristled toothbrush or a warm mouthwash assists in promoting oral care. Hygiene activities are best carried out when analgesia is at its peak.

The patient will probably not engage in extensive conversation during the acute period. Alternative communication methods such as paper and pencil should be provided.

Food should be high in protein and calories and easy to chew. It should be served lukewarm and offered frequently. The diet should be individualized according to personal, cultural, and religious preferences. When oral intake is sharply reduced and the patient's nutritional status is compromised, a nasogastric tube can be inserted on the unaffected side for enteral feedings.

The nurse is responsible for instruction related to diagnostic studies to rule out other problems, such as multiple sclerosis, dental or sinus problems, and neoplasms, and for preoperative teaching if surgery is planned. The nurse may also need to reinforce the surgeon's instructions related to postoperative expectations; Appropriate teaching related to postoperative activities depends on the type of procedure planned (e.g., percutaneous, intracranial). The patient needs to know that he or she will be awake during local procedures so that he or she can cooperate when corneal and ciliary reflexes and facial sensations are checked. Patients are informed about the potential risk of postoperative facial numbness.

After the procedure the patient's pain is compared with the preoperative level. The corneal reflex, extraocular muscles, hearing, sensation, and facial nerve function are evaluated frequently (see Chapter 54). If there is impairment of the corneal reflex, special attention must be paid to eye protection. This includes the use of artificial tears or eye shields. General postoperative nursing care after a craniotomy is appropriate if intracranial surgery is performed. (Nursing care related to craniotomy is discussed in Chapter 55.) Diet and ambulation should be increased according to the patient's progress or specific orders.

After a radiofrequency percutaneous electrocoagulation procedure, an ice pack is applied to the jaw on the operative side for 3 to 5 hours. To avoid injuring the mouth, the patient should not chew on the operative side until sensation has returned.

Ambulatory and Home Care. Regular follow-up care should be planned. The patient needs instruction regarding the dosage and side effects of medications. Although relief of pain may be complete, the patient should be encouraged to keep environmental stimuli to a moderate level and to use stress reduction methods. The patient may have developed protective practices to prevent pain and may need counseling or psychiatric assistance in the readjustment, especially in reestablishing personal relationships. Herpes simplex infection (cold sores) can occur from manipulation of the gasserian ganglion. Treatment consists of antiviral agents such as acyclovir (Zovirax) (see Chapter 23).

Long-term management after surgical intervention depends on the residual effects of the type of procedure. If anesthesia is present or the corneal reflex is altered, the patient should be taught to (1) chew on the unaffected side; (2) avoid hot foods or beverages, which can burn the mucous membranes; (3) check the oral cavity after meals to remove food particles; (4) practice meticulous oral hygiene and continue with semiannual dental visits; (5) protect the face against extremes of temperature; (6) use an electric razor; and (7) wear a protective eye shield.

■ Evaluation

The expected outcomes are that the patient with trigeminal neuralgia will

- have decreased or relief from pain
- appear more comfortable and less anxious
- have normal facial sensation or expected paresthesias and anesthesias
- return to previous socialization and occupational activities

BELL'S PALSY

Etiology and Pathophysiology

Bell's palsy (peripheral facial paralysis, acute benign cranial polyneuritis) is a disorder characterized by a disruption of the motor branches of the facial nerve (CN VII) on one side of the face in the absence of any other disease such as a stroke. Bell's palsy is an acute, peripheral facial paresis of unknown cause. Each year approximately 20 per 100,000 individuals will be diagnosed with Bell's palsy. It can affect any age group, but it is more commonly seen in the 20- to 60-year-old age range. Despite its good prognosis, Bell's palsy leaves more than 8000 people a year in the United States with permanent, potentially disfiguring facial weakness.[4]

Although the exact etiology is not known, there is evidence that reactivated herpes simplex virus (HSV) may be involved in some cases. The reactivation of the HSV causes inflammation, edema, ischemia, and eventual demyelination of the nerve, creating pain and alterations in motor and sensory function.

Bell's palsy is considered benign with full recovery after 6 months in about 85% of patients, especially if treatment is instituted immediately. The remaining 15% of patients continue to be bothered by asymmetric movement of facial muscles.[4]

Clinical Manifestations

The onset of Bell's palsy is often accompanied by an outbreak of herpes vesicles in or around the ear. Patients may complain of pain around and behind the ear. In addition, manifestations may include fever, tinnitus, and hearing deficit. The paralysis of the motor branches of the facial nerve typically results in a flaccidity of the affected side of the face, with drooping of the mouth accompanied by drooling (Fig. 59-3). An inability to close the eyelid, with an upward movement of the eyeball when closure is attempted, is also evident. A widened *palpebral fissure* (the opening between the eyelids); flattening of the nasolabial fold; and inability to smile, frown, or whistle are also common. Unilateral loss of taste is common. Decreased muscle movement may alter chewing ability, and although some patients may experience a loss of tearing, many patients complain of excessive tearing. The muscle weakness causes the lower lid to turn out, allowing overflow of normal tear production. Pain may be present

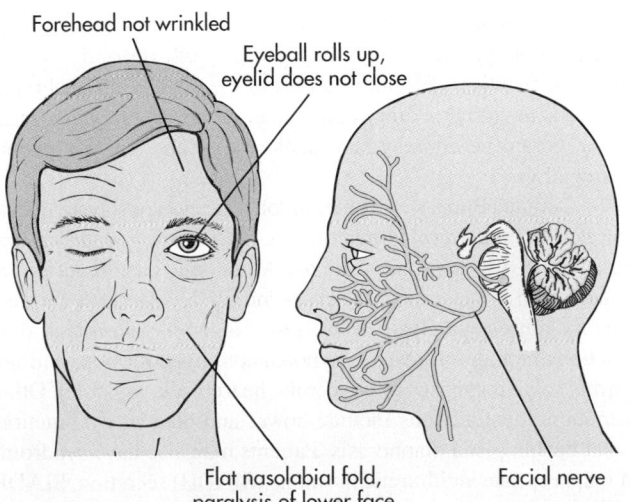

Forehead not wrinkled
Eyeball rolls up, eyelid does not close
Flat nasolabial fold, paralysis of lower face
Facial nerve

FIG. 59-3 Bell's palsy: facial characteristics.

behind the ear on the affected side, especially before the onset of paralysis.

Complications can include psychologic withdrawal because of changes in appearance, malnutrition, dehydration, mucous membrane trauma, corneal abrasions, muscle stretching, and facial spasms and contractures.

Diagnostic Studies

The diagnosis of Bell's palsy is one of exclusion. There is no definitive test. The diagnosis and prognosis are indicated by observation of the typical pattern of onset and signs and the testing of percutaneous nerve excitability by EMG.

Collaborative Care

Methods of treatment for Bell's palsy include moist heat, gentle massage, and electrical stimulation of the nerve and prescribed exercises. Stimulation may maintain muscle tone and prevent atrophy. Care is primarily focused on relief of symptoms, prevention of complications, and protection of the eye on the affected side.

Drug Therapy. Corticosteroids, especially prednisone, are started immediately, and the best results are obtained if corticosteroids are initiated before paralysis is complete.[4] When the patient improves to the point that the corticosteroids are no longer necessary, they should be tapered off over a 2-week period. Usually, the corticosteroid treatment decreases the edema and pain, but mild analgesics can be used if necessary. Because the HSV is implicated in approximately 70% of cases of Bell's palsy, treatment with acyclovir (Zovirax), alone or in conjunction with prednisone, is used.[4] Additional antiviral agents, including valacyclovir (Valtrex) and famciclovir (Famvir), have also been used in the management of Bell's palsy.

NURSING MANAGEMENT
BELL'S PALSY

■ Nursing Assessment

Early recognition of the possibility of Bell's palsy is important. Because HSV is a possible etiologic factor, any person who is prone to herpes simplex should be alerted to seek health care if pain occurs in or around the ear. Assessment of facial muscles for any signs of weakness should also be done. Careful recording of assessment data provides information related to the progress of the syndrome.

■ Nursing Diagnoses

The nursing diagnoses for the patient with Bell's palsy may include, but are not limited to, the following:
- Acute pain *related to* the inflammation of CN VII (facial nerve)
- Imbalanced nutrition: less than body requirements *related to* inability to chew secondary to muscle weakness
- Risk for injury (corneal abrasion) *related to* inability to blink
- Disturbed body image *related to* change in facial appearance secondary to facial muscle weakness

■ Planning

The overall goals are that the patient with Bell's palsy will (1) be pain free or have pain controlled, (2) maintain adequate nutritional status, (3) maintain appropriate oral hygiene, (4) not experience injury to the eye, (5) return to normal or previous perception of body image, and (6) be optimistic about disease outcome.

■ Nursing Implementation

The patient with Bell's palsy is treated on an outpatient basis. The following interventions are used throughout the course of the disease. Mild analgesics can relieve pain. Hot wet packs can reduce the discomfort of herpetic lesions, aid circulation, and relieve pain. The face should be protected from cold and drafts because trigeminal *hyperesthesia* (extreme sensitivity to pain or touch) may accompany the syndrome. Maintenance of good nutrition is important. The patient should be taught to chew on the unaffected side of the mouth to avoid trapping food and to enjoy the taste of food. Thorough oral hygiene must be carried out after each meal to prevent the development of parotitis, caries, and periodontal disease from accumulated residual food.

Dark glasses may be worn for protective and cosmetic reasons. Artificial tears (methylcellulose) should be instilled frequently during the day to prevent drying of the cornea. The eye should be inspected for the presence of eyelashes. Ointment and an impermeable eye shield can be used at night to retain moisture. In some patients, taping the lids closed at night may be necessary to provide protection. The patient is taught to report ocular pain, drainage, or discharge.

A facial sling may be helpful to support affected muscles, improve lip alignment, and facilitate eating. The facial sling is usually made and fitted by a physical or occupational therapist. Vigorous massage can break down tissues, but gentle upward massage has psychologic benefits even if physical effects other than the maintenance of circulation are questionable. When function begins to return, active facial exercises are performed several times a day.

The change in physical appearance as a result of Bell's palsy can be devastating. The patient must be reassured that a stroke did not occur and that chances for a full recovery are good. The patient's need for privacy should be respected, especially during meals, but the nurse's assistance in the patient's adjustment to the physical changes should not be delayed. Enlisting support from family and friends is important. It is important to share with the patient that most patients recover within about 6 weeks of the onset of symptoms.

■ Evaluation

The expected outcomes are that the patient with Bell's palsy will

- be free of pain
- not experience any complications
- maintain appropriate nutritional intake
- experience minimal side effects associated with corticosteroid treatment
- return to previous perception of body image

Polyneuropathies

GUILLAIN-BARRÉ SYNDROME

Etiology and Pathophysiology

Guillain-Barré syndrome (Landry-Guillain-Barré-Strohl syndrome, postinfectious polyneuropathy, ascending polyneuropathic paralysis) is an acute, rapidly progressing, and potentially fatal form of polyneuritis. It affects the peripheral nervous system and

results in loss of myelin (a segmental demyelination) and edema and inflammation of the affected nerves, causing a loss of neurotransmission to the periphery. The syndrome affects both genders equally and is more commonly seen in adults, although it is observed in all age groups. Worldwide the incidence has varied from 0.4 to 1.7 cases per 100,000 persons per year. Guillain-Barré syndrome has an estimated annual cost of 2 to 3 billion dollars in the United States. With adequate supportive care, 85% of these patients recover completely from this disorder.

The etiology of this disorder is unknown, but it is believed to be a cell-mediated immunologic reaction directed at the peripheral nerves. The syndrome is often preceded by immune system stimulation from a viral infection, trauma, surgery, viral immunizations, human immunodeficiency virus (HIV), or lymphoproliferative neoplasms. *Campylobacter jejuni* is the most recognized organism associated with Guillain-Barré syndrome.[5] *C. jejuni* gastroenteritis is thought to precede Guillain-Barré syndrome in approximately 30% of cases. Other potential pathogens include *Mycoplasma pneumoniae,* cytomegalovirus, Epstein-Barr virus, varicella-zoster virus, and vaccines (rabies, swine influenza). These stimuli are thought to cause an alteration in the immune system, resulting in sensitization of T lymphocytes to the patient's myelin and, ultimately, myelin damage. Demyelination occurs, and the transmission of nerve impulses is stopped or slowed down. The muscles innervated by the damaged peripheral nerves undergo denervation and atrophy. In the recovery phase, remyelination occurs slowly, and neurologic function returns in a proximal to distal pattern.

Clinical Manifestations

Guillain-Barré syndrome is a heterogeneous condition with symptoms ranging from mild to severe. Symptoms of Guillain-Barré syndrome usually develop 1 to 3 weeks after an upper respiratory or gastrointestinal (GI) infection. Weakness of the lower extremities (evolving more or less symmetrically) occurs over hours to days to weeks, usually peaking about the fourteenth day. Distal muscles are more severely affected. *Paresthesia* (numbness and tingling) is frequent, and paralysis usually follows in the extremities. *Hypotonia* (reduced muscle tone) and *areflexia* (lack of reflexes) are common, persistent symptoms. Objective sensory loss is variable, with deep sensitivity more affected than superficial sensations.

Miller Fisher syndrome is a clinical variant of Guillain-Barré syndrome, accounting for 5% to 10% of cases. It is characterized by a triad of symptoms including ataxia, areflexia, and *ophthalmoplegia* (paralysis of motor nerves of the eye).[6] Other subtypes include acute inflammatory demyelinating polyneuropathy, acute motor axonal neuropathy, and acute motor and sensory axonal neuropathy.

In Guillain-Barré syndrome, autonomic nervous system dysfunction results from alterations in both the sympathetic and parasympathetic nervous systems. Autonomic disturbances are usually seen in patients with severe muscle involvement and respiratory muscle paralysis. The most dangerous autonomic dysfunctions include orthostatic hypotension, hypertension, and abnormal vagal responses (bradycardia, heart block, asystole). Other autonomic dysfunctions include bowel and bladder dysfunction, facial flushing, and diaphoresis. Patients may also have syndrome of inappropriate antidiuretic hormone (SIADH) secretion. SIADH is discussed in Chapter 48. Progression of Guillain-Barré syndrome to include the lower brainstem involves the facial, abducens, oculomotor, hypoglossal, trigeminal, and vagus nerves (CNs VII, VI, III, XII, V, and X, respectively). This involvement manifests itself through facial weakness, extraocular eye movement difficulties, dysphagia, and paresthesia of the face.

Pain is a common symptom in the patient with Guillain-Barré syndrome. The pain can be categorized as paresthesias, muscular aches and cramps, and hyperesthesias. Pain appears to be worse at night. Narcotics may be indicated for those experiencing severe pain. Pain may lead to a decrease in appetite and may interfere with sleep.

Complications. The most serious complication of this syndrome is respiratory failure, which occurs as the paralysis progresses to the nerves that innervate the thoracic area. Constant monitoring of the respiratory system by checking respiratory rate, depth, forced vital capacity, and negative inspiratory force provides information about the need for immediate intervention including intubation and mechanical ventilation. Respiratory or urinary tract infections (UTIs) may occur. Fever is generally the first sign of infection, and treatment is directed at the infecting organism. Immobility from the paralysis can cause problems such as paralytic ileus, muscle atrophy, deep vein thrombosis, pulmonary emboli, skin breakdown, orthostatic hypotension, and nutritional deficiencies.

Diagnostic Studies

Diagnosis is based primarily on the patient's history and clinical signs. CSF is normal or has a low protein content initially, but after 7 to 10 days it shows an elevated protein level to 700 mg/dl (7 g/L) (normal protein is 15 to 45 mg/dl [0.15 to 0.45 g/L]) with a normal cell count. Results of EMG and nerve conduction studies are markedly abnormal (reduced nerve conduction velocity) in the affected extremities.

Collaborative Care

Management is aimed at supportive care, particularly ventilatory support, during the acute phase. Plasma exchange is used in the first 2 weeks of Guillain-Barré syndrome. In patients with severe disease who are treated within 2 weeks of onset, there is a distinct reduction in the length of hospital stay, length of time on ventilator, and time required to resume walking. Intravenous (IV) administration of high-dose immunoglobulin (Sandoglobulin) has also shown to be as effective as plasma exchange and has the advantage of immediate availability and greater safety. However, patients receiving high-dose immunoglobulin need to be well hydrated and have adequate renal function. (Plasmapheresis is discussed in Chapter 13.) After 3 weeks of disease onset, plasma exchange and immunoglobulin therapies have little value. Corticosteroids appear to have little effect on the prognosis or duration of the disease.[7]

Nutritional Therapy. Nutritional intake is compromised in the patient with Guillain-Barré syndrome. During the acute phase, the patient may experience difficulty swallowing because of cranial nerve involvement. Mild dysphagia can be managed by placing the patient in an upright position and flexing the head forward during feeding. For more severe dysphagia, tube feedings may be required. Patients who experience paralytic ileus or intestinal obstruction may require total parenteral nutrition. Later in the course of the disease, motor paralysis or weakness continues to affect the ability to self-feed. The patient's nutritional status, including body weight, serum albumin levels, and calorie counts, must be evaluated at regular intervals.

NURSING MANAGEMENT
GUILLAIN-BARRÉ SYNDROME

■ Nursing Assessment

Assessment of the patient is the most important aspect of nursing care during the acute phase. The nurse must monitor the ascending paralysis; assess respiratory function; monitor arterial blood gases (ABGs); and assess the gag, corneal, and swallowing reflexes during the routine assessment. Reflexes are usually decreased or absent.

Monitoring blood pressure and cardiac rate and rhythm is also important during the acute phase because transient cardiac arrhythmias have been reported. Autonomic dysfunction is common and usually takes the form of bradycardia and arrhythmias. Orthostatic hypotension secondary to muscle atony may occur in severe cases. Vasopressor agents and volume expanders may be needed to treat the low blood pressure. However, the presence of SIADH may require fluid restriction.

■ Nursing Diagnoses

Nursing diagnoses for the patient with Guillain-Barré syndrome may include, but are not limited to, the following:
- Impaired spontaneous ventilation *related to* progression of disease process resulting in respiratory muscle paralysis
- Risk for aspiration *related to* dysphagia
- Acute pain *related to* paresthesias, muscle aches and cramps, and hyperesthesias
- Impaired verbal communication *related to* intubation or paralysis of the muscles of speech
- Fear *related to* uncertain outcome and seriousness of the disease
- Self-care deficits *related to* inability to use muscles to accomplish activities of daily living (ADLs)

■ Planning

The overall goals are that the patient with Guillain-Barré syndrome will (1) maintain adequate ventilation, (2) be free from aspiration, (3) be pain free or have pain controlled, (4) maintain an acceptable method of communication, (5) maintain adequate nutritional intake, and (6) return to usual physical functioning.

■ Nursing Implementation

The objective of therapy is to support body systems until the patient recovers. Respiratory failure and infection are serious threats. Monitoring the vital capacity and ABGs is essential. If the vital capacity drops to less than 800 ml (15 ml/kg or two thirds of the patient's normal vital capacity) or the ABGs deteriorate, endotracheal intubation or tracheostomy may be done so that the patient can be mechanically ventilated (see Chapter 66). Meticulous suctioning technique is needed to prevent infection whether the patient has an endotracheal tube or tracheostomy. Thorough bronchial hygiene and chest physiotherapy help clear secretions and prevent respiratory deterioration. If fever develops, sputum cultures should be obtained to identify the pathogen. Appropriate antibiotic therapy is then initiated.

A communication system must be established with the use of the patient's available abilities. This is extremely difficult if the disease progresses to involvement of the cranial nerves. At the peak of a severe episode the patient may be incapable of communicating. The nurse must explain all procedures before doing them and reassure the patient that muscle function will return.

Urinary retention is common for a few days. Intermittent catheterization is preferred to an indwelling catheter to avoid UTIs. However, for the acutely ill patient receiving a large volume of fluids (>2.5 L/day), indwelling catheterization may be safer to reduce overdistention of a temporarily flaccid bladder and to prevent vesicoureteral reflux. Physical therapy is indicated early to help prevent problems related to immobility. Passive range-of-motion exercises and attention to body position help maintain function and prevent contractures. Patients who develop facial paralysis must receive meticulous eye care to avoid corneal irritation or damage (exposure keratitis). Artificial tears should be instilled frequently during the day to prevent drying of the cornea. The eyes should be inspected for the presence of eyelashes. Ointment and an impermeable eye shield can be used at night to retain moisture.

Nutritional needs must be met in spite of possible problems associated with delayed gastric emptying, paralytic ileus, and potential for aspiration if the gag reflex is lost. In addition to checking for the gag reflex, nurses should note drooling and other difficulties with secretions, which may be more indicative of an inadequate gag reflex. Initially, tube feedings or parenteral nutrition may be used to ensure adequate caloric intake. Because of delayed gastric emptying, residual volumes of the feedings should be assessed at regular intervals or before feedings (see Chapter 39). Fluid and electrolyte therapy must be monitored carefully to prevent electrolyte imbalances. A bowel program should be initiated because constipation is a common problem related to diet changes, immobility, and decreased GI motility.

Throughout the course of the illness, the nurse needs to provide support and encouragement to the family and patient. Because residual problems and relapses are uncommon except in the chronic form of the disease, complete recovery can be anticipated although it is generally a slow process that takes months or years if axonal degeneration occurs.

■ Evaluation

The expected outcomes are that the patient with Guillain-Barré syndrome will
- return to usual level of physical functioning
- be free from pain and discomfort
- maintain nutritional status

BOTULISM

Etiology and Pathophysiology

Botulism is the most serious type of food poisoning. It is caused by GI absorption of the neurotoxin produced by *Clostridium botulinum*. This organism is found in the soil, and the spores are difficult to destroy. It can grow in any food contaminated with the spores. Improper home canning of foods is often the cause. In 1999, there were 174 cases of botulism reported to the Centers for Disease Control.[8] It is thought that the neurotoxin destroys or inhibits the neurotransmission of acetylcholine at the myoneural junction, resulting in disturbed muscle innervation.

Clinical Manifestations

Symptoms are usually nausea, vomiting, and abdominal cramps, generally within 6 to 48 hours after consumption of the contaminated food. Neurologic manifestations develop rapidly over 2 to 4 days. They include difficulty in convergence of the eyes, photophobia, ptosis, paralysis of extraocular muscles, blurred vision, diplopia, dry mouth, sore throat, and difficulty in swallowing. Other manifestations include paralytic ileus, mild muscle weakness, seizures, and respiratory symptoms that can rapidly deteriorate to respiratory arrest and/or cardiac arrest. The course of the disease depends on the amount of toxin absorbed from the gut. If only a small amount is absorbed, symptoms are mild and recovery is complete. When large amounts are absorbed, death usually occurs in 4 to 8 days from circulatory failure, respiratory paralysis, or development of pulmonary complications.[8]

Because botulism is a reportable disease, local, state, and federal health agencies, particularly the Centers for Disease Control and Prevention (CDC) in Atlanta, must be notified. Botulism can also be contracted through nasal inhalation, as well as oral ingestion. It has been highlighted as a potential bioterrorism agent and is discussed further in Chapter 67.

Diagnostic Studies and Collaborative Care

Blood and CSF are obtained for studies to rule out other diseases. In the patient with botulism the blood and CSF results are normal.

Drug Therapy. The initial treatment of botulism is IV administration of botulinum antitoxin. Before administration of the antitoxin, an intradermal test dose for sensitivity to horse serum is given. If there are no reactions, the test dose is followed by daily doses of 50,000 units of botulism antitoxin until improvement begins.

The GI tract is purged by laxatives, high colonic enemas, and gastric lavage to decrease the absorption of the toxin. Activated charcoal is most effective if administered within 1 hour of ingestion.

NURSING MANAGEMENT
BOTULISM

■ Nursing Implementation

Primary prevention is the goal of nursing management through educating consumers to be alert to situations that may result in botulism. Particular attention should be given to foods with a low acid content, which support germination and the production of botulin, a deadly poison. These foods include fish, vichyssoise, and peppers. All varieties of spores are destroyed by boiling for 10 minutes or maintaining a temperature of 176° F (80° C) for 30 minutes. Specific suggestions related to the preparation, storage, and use of food include the following:
- In home canning, the equipment manufacturer's directions should be followed. Only fresh fruits and vegetables (with all questionable spots removed) should be used. All containers and utensils must be cleansed, and the seal on the can or jar must be airtight. Canned foods should be stored properly in a cool, dry place.
- A can with a swollen end should never be used; the swelling may be caused by gases from *C. botulinum*.
- If the food is forcefully expelled when a container is opened, it should be discarded immediately and the contents should not be tasted.

- If the contents of a can look or smell bad after opening, the can should be discarded without tasting the contents. Materials may be flushed down the toilet or disposed of in the garbage disposal if a large amount of water is used.

Nursing care during the acute illness is similar to that for Guillain-Barré syndrome. Supportive nursing interventions include rest, activities to maintain respiratory function, adequate nutrition, and prevention of loss of muscle mass. Because the recovery process is slow, the patient may develop problems related to a feeling of helplessness, boredom, and low morale.

TETANUS

Etiology and Pathophysiology

Tetanus (lockjaw) is an extremely severe polyradiculitis and polyneuritis affecting spinal and cranial nerves. It results from the effects of a potent neurotoxin released by the anaerobic bacillus *Clostridium tetani*. The toxin interferes with the function of the reflex arc by blocking inhibitory transmitters at the presynaptic sites in the spinal cord and brainstem. The spores of the bacillus are present in soil, garden mold, and manure. Thus *Clostridium tetani* enters the body through a traumatic or suppurative wound that provides an appropriate low-oxygen environment for the organisms to mature and produce toxin. Other possible sources include dental infection, injections of heroin, human and animal bites, frostbite, compound fractures, and gunshot wounds. The incubation period is usually 7 days but can range from 3 to 21 days, with symptoms frequently appearing after the original wound is healed. In general, the longer the incubation period, the milder the illness and the better the prognosis.

Worldwide the number of cases per year is estimated to be 1 million. In the United States about 100 to 200 cases occur each year and are due to infection of puncture wounds of the extremities by nails or splinters or IV drug use.[9] Of the reported cases the majority of patients are over the age of 59 years. However, the number of individuals under the age of 40 with tetanus is increasing, most likely related to IV drug use. Mortality rates vary according to age, with infants and persons over 50 years of age most seriously affected. Overall mortality rates are declining and are at about 10% in the United States.

Clinical Manifestations

Manifestations of generalized tetanus include a feeling of stiffness in the jaw *(trismus)* or neck, slight fever, and other symptoms of general infection. Generalized tonic spasms occur because of the lack of reciprocal innervation. As the disease progresses, the neck muscles, back, abdomen, and extremities become progressively rigid. In severe forms, continuous tonic convulsions may occur with *opisthotonos* (extreme arching of the back and retraction of the head). Laryngeal and respiratory spasms cause apnea and anoxia. Additional effects are manifested by overstimulation of the sympathetic nervous system, including profuse diaphoresis, labile hypertension, episodic tachycardia, hyperthermia, and arrhythmias. The slightest noise, jarring motion, or bright light can set off the seizure. These seizures are agonizingly painful. Mortality is almost 100% in the severe form. Death is usually attributable to asphyxia or heart failure, the result of constantly recurring spasms. Residual injury, such as vertebral fracture, muscle contracture, and brain damage secondary to hypoxia, may be long-term consequences.

Collaborative Care

Serum electrolytes, CBC count, albumin, clotting factors, glucose, and ABGs are monitored. Cardiac function is monitored by electrocardiogram and auscultation. As increasing numbers of nerve cells become involved, their inhibitory control over muscle activity decreases and symptoms develop.

Drug Therapy. The management of tetanus includes administration of tetanus toxoid booster (Td) and tetanus immune globulin (TIG) before the onset of symptoms to neutralize circulating toxins (see Table 67-6). Control of spasms is essential and is managed by deep sedation, usually with diazepam (Valium), barbiturates, or chlorpromazine (Thorazine). Chlorpromazine is also helpful in reducing hyperthermia. A 10-day course of penicillin is recommended to inhibit further growth of the organism.

Because of laryngospasm, a tracheostomy is usually performed early and the patient is maintained on mechanical ventilation. If sedation does not control seizures, skeletal muscle–paralyzing drugs such as D-tubocurarine (Curare) are used. Pain is relieved by means of codeine or meperidine, often with the addition of promethazine (Phenergan). Any recognized wound should be debrided or an abscess drained. Antibiotics may be given to prevent secondary infections.

Nutrition is maintained through parenteral nutrition or nasogastric feeding. The mortality rate associated with tetanus is declining. However, for those who recover there is a long convalescence that includes extensive physical therapy.

NURSING MANAGEMENT
TETANUS

■ Nursing Implementation

Health teaching is aimed at ensuring tetanus prophylaxis, which is the most important factor influencing the incidence of this disease. Tetanus prevention and immunization protocols are summarized in Table 67-6. The patient should be taught that immediate, thorough cleansing of all wounds with soap and water is important in the prevention of tetanus. If an open wound occurs and the patient has not been immunized within 10 years, the health care provider should be contacted so that a tetanus booster can be given.

If equine tetanus antitoxin is to be used, the patient should be tested for sensitivity. Administration of equine antitoxin is not recommended if sensitivity occurs; anaphylactic shock is potentially life threatening, and desensitization is ineffective. The side effects of routine administration of the antitoxin are mild and include a sore arm, swelling at the site, and itching. Serious side effects rarely occur. Routine administration of a booster shot to an adequately immunized patient can cause arm swelling and lymphadenopathy.

Every patient should receive a written record of immunizations and be encouraged to complete the active immunization schedule. The patient's immunization history should be accurately recorded to protect the patient and health care providers.

The acute nursing management of the patient with tetanus is aimed at supportive care based on the treatment of clinical manifestations. The patient should be placed in a quiet, darkened room that is insulated against noise. Judicious sedation should be given. Nursing care should be administered with the utmost caution to avoid triggering spasms. For example, the nurse should avoid unnecessary touching, use firm touching when necessary, avoid the use of linens to cover the patient, and maintain a slightly higher than normal ambient temperature. Nursing care related to tracheostomy and mechanical ventilation is given as appropriate. An indwelling urinary catheter may be used to prevent bladder distention and urinary reflux in the presence of spasms in the muscles of the pelvic floor. Attention is also given to skin care. The patient needs emotional support during the acute phase because the fear of death is real. The family also needs support and education.

NEUROSYPHILIS

Neurosyphilis (tertiary syphilis) is an infection of any part of the nervous system by the organism *Treponema pallidum*. It is the result of untreated or inadequately treated syphilis (see Chapter 51). The organism can invade the central nervous system within a few months of the original infection. Except for causing some changes in the CSF, including increased white blood cells (WBCs) and protein and positive serologic reaction, the organism lies dormant for years. Untreated neurosyphilis, although not contagious, can be fatal. Penicillin therapy is effective for syphilitic meningitis, but the neurologic deficits remain.

Late neurosyphilis results from degenerative changes in the spinal cord (tabes dorsalis) and brainstem (general paresis). *Tabes dorsalis* (progressive locomotor ataxia) is characterized by vague, sharp pains in the legs; ataxia; "slapping" gait; loss of proprioception and deep tendon reflexes; and zones of hyperesthesia. *Charcot's joints,* which are characterized by enlargement, bone destruction, and hypermobility, also occur as a result of joint effusion and edema. Other manifestations of neurosyphilis include seizures and vision and hearing problems.

Neurologic symptoms associated with neurosyphilis are numerous and many times nonspecific.[10] Neurosyphilis is a differential diagnosis for patients with neurologic and psychiatric symptoms. *Dementia paralytica* is an ongoing spirochetal meningoencephalitis that causes a general dissolution of mental and physical capabilities. It may mimic a number of major or minor psychoses. Management includes treatment with penicillin, symptomatic care, and protection from physical injury.

Spinal Cord Problems

SPINAL CORD TRAUMA

Before World War II, the life expectancy for the person with a spinal cord injury ranged from months to 10 years from the onset of injury. The leading causes of death were renal failure and sepsis. Today, with improved treatment strategies (specifically, intermittent catheterization), even the very young patient with a spinal cord injury can anticipate a long life. The prognosis for life is generally only about 5 years less than for persons of the same age without spinal cord injury. The cause of premature death in the patient with **tetraplegia** (paralysis of both arms and legs), which was formerly called quadriplegia, is usually related to compromised respiratory function.

The potential for disruption of individual growth and development, altered family dynamics, economic loss in terms of absence from work, and the high cost of rehabilitation and long-term health care make spinal cord trauma a major problem. According to estimates from the Centers for Diseases Control

and Prevention (CDC), 11,000 Americans suffer spinal cord injuries each year.[11] The number of persons with spinal cord injuries living in the United States at any one time ranges from 183,000 to 230,000. The cost of spinal cord injury care can be high. The average cost of care for a person with a high cervical injury is $572,178 in the first year and $102,491 in each subsequent year.[12] Although many people with spinal cord injuries can care for themselves independently, those with the highest level of injury may require round-the-clock care at home or in a long-term care facility. Today almost 90% of patients with spinal cord injury are discharged from the hospital to home or another non-institutionalized residence.[12] The remaining 10% are discharged to nursing homes, chronic care facilities, or group homes.

Etiology and Pathophysiology

The segment of the population with the greatest risk for spinal cord injury is young adult men between the ages of 16 and 30 years. Eighty percent of people with spinal cord injury are male, and the most common age at injury is 19.

Causes of spinal cord injury include many types of trauma. Motor vehicle crashes account for 39%; violence, 25%; falls, 22%; sports injuries, 7%; and other miscellaneous causes, 7% of spinal cord injuries.[12] In large urban areas, gunshot wounds have recently surpassed falls as the second most common cause of spinal cord injuries.

There has also been an increase in the number of older adults with spinal cord injuries. People who were at least 61 years of age when injured increased from 4.7% of patients with spinal cord injury in the 1970s to 10% currently. Besides having greater mortality, older adults with traumatic injuries experience more complications than younger ones, and they are hospitalized longer. This trend toward older age at time of injury explains the overall increase in mean age of people with spinal cord injury from 28 years in the 1970s to 35.3 years at this time.[12]

Initial Injury. Spinal cord injury can be due to cord compression by bone displacement, interruption of blood supply to the cord, or traction resulting from pulling on the cord. The spinal cord is wrapped in tough layers of dura and is rarely torn or transected by direct trauma. Penetrating trauma, such as gunshot and stab wounds, can result in tearing and transection. The initial mechanical disruption of axons as a result of stretch or laceration is referred to as the *primary injury. Secondary injury* refers to the ongoing, progressive damage that occurs after the initial injury.[13]

There are several theories on what causes this ongoing damage at the molecular and cellular levels. These include free radical formation, uncontrolled calcium influx, ischemia, and lipid peroxidation. At the molecular level, *apoptosis* (cell death) occurs and may continue sometimes for weeks or months after the initial injury. Thus the complete cord damage (previously thought to be transection) in severe trauma is related to autodestruction of the cord. This is confirmed by observations that shortly after the injury, petechial hemorrhages are noted in the central gray matter of the cord. Hemorrhagic areas in the center of the spinal cord appear within 1 hour, and by 4 hours there may be infarction in the gray matter.[13] This ongoing destructive process makes it critical that the initial care and management of the patient with a spinal cord injury limit further activation of these processes.

Fig. 59-4 illustrates the cascade of events causing secondary injury following traumatic spinal cord injury. The resulting hyp-

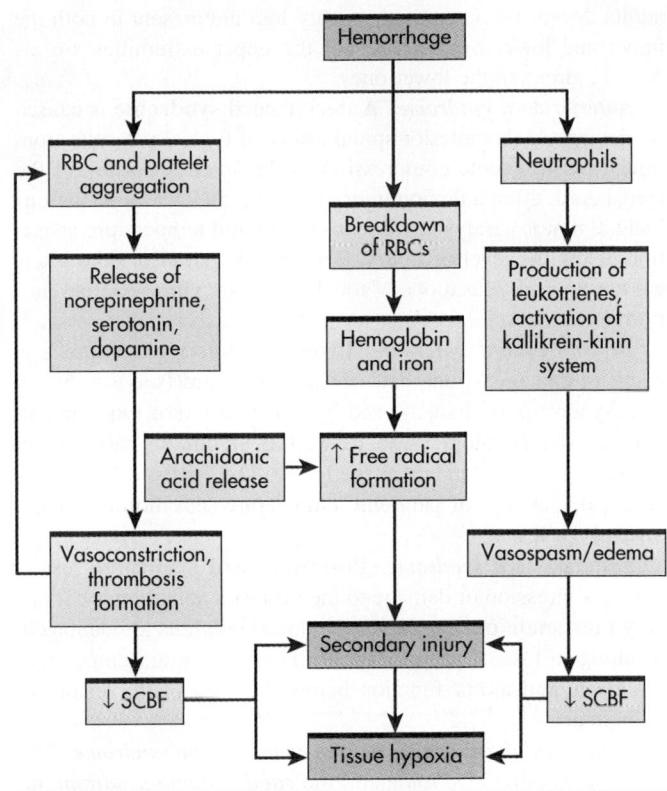

FIG. 59-4 Cascade of metabolic and cellular events that leads to spinal cord ischemia and hypoxia of secondary injury. *SCBF,* Spinal cord blood flow. (Redrawn from Marciano FF et al: *BNI Quarterly* 11:6, 1995.)

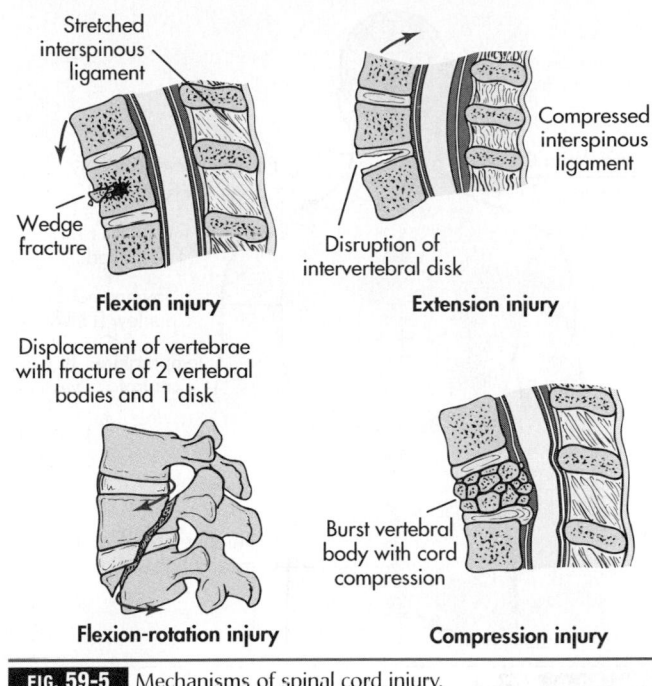

FIG. 59-5 Mechanisms of spinal cord injury.

oxia reduces the oxygen tension below the level that meets the metabolic needs of the spinal cord. Lactate metabolites and an increase in vasoactive substances including norepinephrine, serotonin, and dopamine are noted. At high levels, these vasoactive substances cause vasospasms and hypoxia, leading to subsequent necrosis. Unfortunately, the spinal cord has minimal ability to adapt to vasospasm.

By 24 hours or less, permanent damage may occur because of the development of edema. Edema secondary to the inflammatory response is particularly harmful because of lack of space for tissue expansion. Therefore resultant compression of the cord and extension of edema above and below the injury increase the ischemic damage.

The extent of the neurologic damage caused by a spinal cord injury results from primary injury damage (actual physical disruption of axons) and secondary injury damage (ischemia, hypoxia, microhemorrhage, and edema).[13] Because secondary injury processes occur over time, the extent of injury and prognosis for recovery are most accurately determined at 72 hours or more after injury.[14]

Spinal and neurogenic shock. About 50% of people with acute spinal cord injury experience a temporary neurologic syndrome known as **spinal shock** that is characterized by decreased reflexes, loss of sensation, and flaccid paralysis below the level of the injury.[15] This syndrome lasts days to months and may mask postinjury neurologic function. Active rehabilitation may begin in the presence of spinal shock. **Neurogenic shock,** in contrast, is due to the loss of vasomotor tone caused by injury and is char-

acterized by hypotension, bradycardia, and warm, dry extremities. Loss of sympathetic innervation causes peripheral vasodilation, venous pooling, and a decreased cardiac output. These effects are generally associated with a cervical or high thoracic injury.

Classification of Spinal Cord Injury. Spinal cord injuries are classified by the mechanism of injury, skeletal and neurologic level of injury, and completeness or degree of injury.

Mechanisms of injury. The major mechanisms of injury are flexion, hyperextension, flexion-rotation, extension rotation, and compression (Fig. 59-5). The flexion-rotation injury is the most unstable of all injuries because the ligamentous structures that stabilize the spine are torn. This injury is most often implicated in severe neurologic deficits.

Level of injury. *Skeletal level* of injury is the vertebral level where there is the most damage to vertebral bones and ligaments. *Neurologic level* is the lowest segment of the spinal cord with normal sensory and motor function on both sides of the body. The level of injury may be cervical, thoracic, or lumbar. Cervical and lumbar injuries are most common because these levels are associated with the greatest flexibility and movement. If the cervical cord is involved, paralysis of all four extremities occurs, resulting in tetraplegia. However, even with a cervical injury the arms are rarely completely paralyzed. If the thoracic or lumbar cord is damaged, the result is **paraplegia** (paralysis and loss of sensation in the legs). Fig. 59-6 shows affected structures and functions at different levels of cord injury.

Degree of injury. The degree of spinal cord involvement may be either complete or incomplete (partial). *Complete cord involvement* results in total loss of sensory and motor function below the level of the lesion (injury). *Incomplete cord involvement* results in a mixed loss of voluntary motor activity and sensation and leaves some tracts intact. The degree of sensory and motor

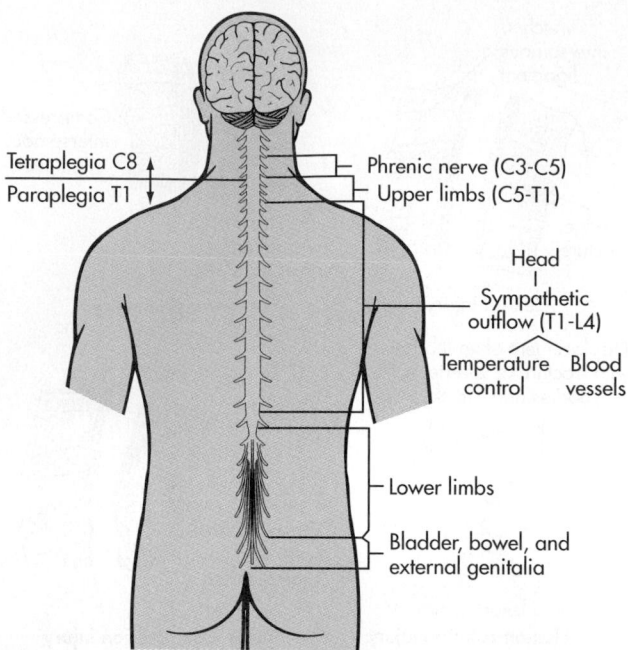

FIG. 59-6 Symptoms, degree of paralysis, and potential for rehabilitation depend on the level of the lesion.

loss varies depending on the level of the lesion and reflects the specific nerve tracts damaged and those spared. Six syndromes are associated with incomplete lesions: central cord syndrome, anterior cord syndrome, Brown-Séquard syndrome, posterior cord syndrome, cauda equina syndrome, and conus medullaris syndrome.

Central cord syndrome. Damage to the central spinal cord is termed **central cord syndrome** (Fig. 59-7). It occurs most commonly in the cervical cord region and is more common in older adults. Motor weakness and sensory loss are present in both the upper and lower extremities, but the upper extremities are affected more than the lower ones.

Anterior cord syndrome. **Anterior cord syndrome** is caused by damage to the anterior spinal artery. It typically results from injury causing acute compression of the anterior portion of the spinal cord, often a flexion injury (see Fig. 59-7). Manifestations include motor paralysis and loss of pain and temperature sensation below the level of injury. Because the posterior cord tracts are not injured, sensations of touch, position, vibration, and motion remain intact.

Brown-Séquard syndrome. **Brown-Séquard syndrome** is a result of damage to one half of the spinal cord (see Fig. 59-7). This syndrome is characterized by a loss of motor function and position and vibratory sense, as well as vasomotor paralysis on the same side *(ipsilateral)* as the lesion. The opposite *(contralateral)* side has loss of pain and temperature sensation below the level of the lesion.

Posterior cord syndrome. **Posterior cord syndrome** results from compression or damage to the posterior spinal artery. It is a very rare condition. Generally the dorsal columns are damaged, resulting in loss of proprioception. However, pain, temperature sensation, and motor function below the level of the lesion remain intact.

Conus medullaris syndrome and cauda equina syndrome. The *conus medullaris syndrome* and the *cauda equina syndrome* result from damage to the very lowest portion of the spinal cord *(conus)* and the lumbar and sacral nerve roots *(cauda equina)*. Injury to these areas produces flaccid paralysis of the lower limbs and areflexic (flaccid) bladder and bowel.

American Spinal Injury Association (ASIA) Impairment scale. The ASIA Impairment scale is commonly used for classifying the severity of impairment resulting from spinal cord injury. It combines assessments of motor and sensory function to determine neurologic level and completeness of injury (Figs. 59-8 and 59-9).[16] This scale is useful for recording changes in neurologic status and identifying appropriate functional goals for rehabilitation.[14]

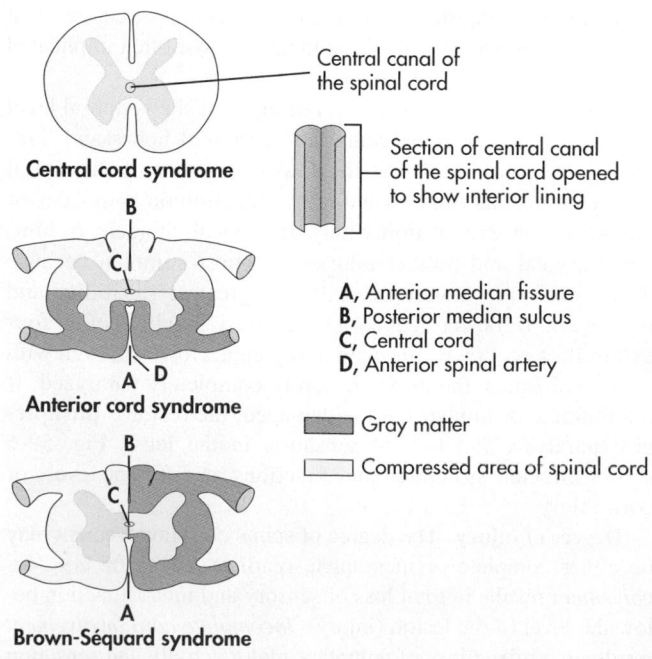

FIG. 59-7 Syndromes associated with incomplete cord lesions.

American Spinal Injury Association (ASIA) Impairment Scale

☐ **A = Complete:** No motor or sensory function is preserved in the sacral segments S4-S5.

☐ **B = Incomplete:** Sensory but not motor function is preserved below the neurologic level and includes the sacral segments S4-S5.

☐ **C = Incomplete:** Motor function is preserved below the neurologic level, and more than half of key muscles below the neurologic level have a muscle grade less than 3.

☐ **D = Incomplete:** Motor function is preserved below the neurologic level, and at least half of key muscles below the neurologic level have a muscle grade of 3 or more.

☐ **E = Normal:** Motor and sensory function are normal.

FIG. 59-8 The American Spinal Injury Association Impairment scale.

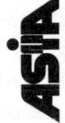

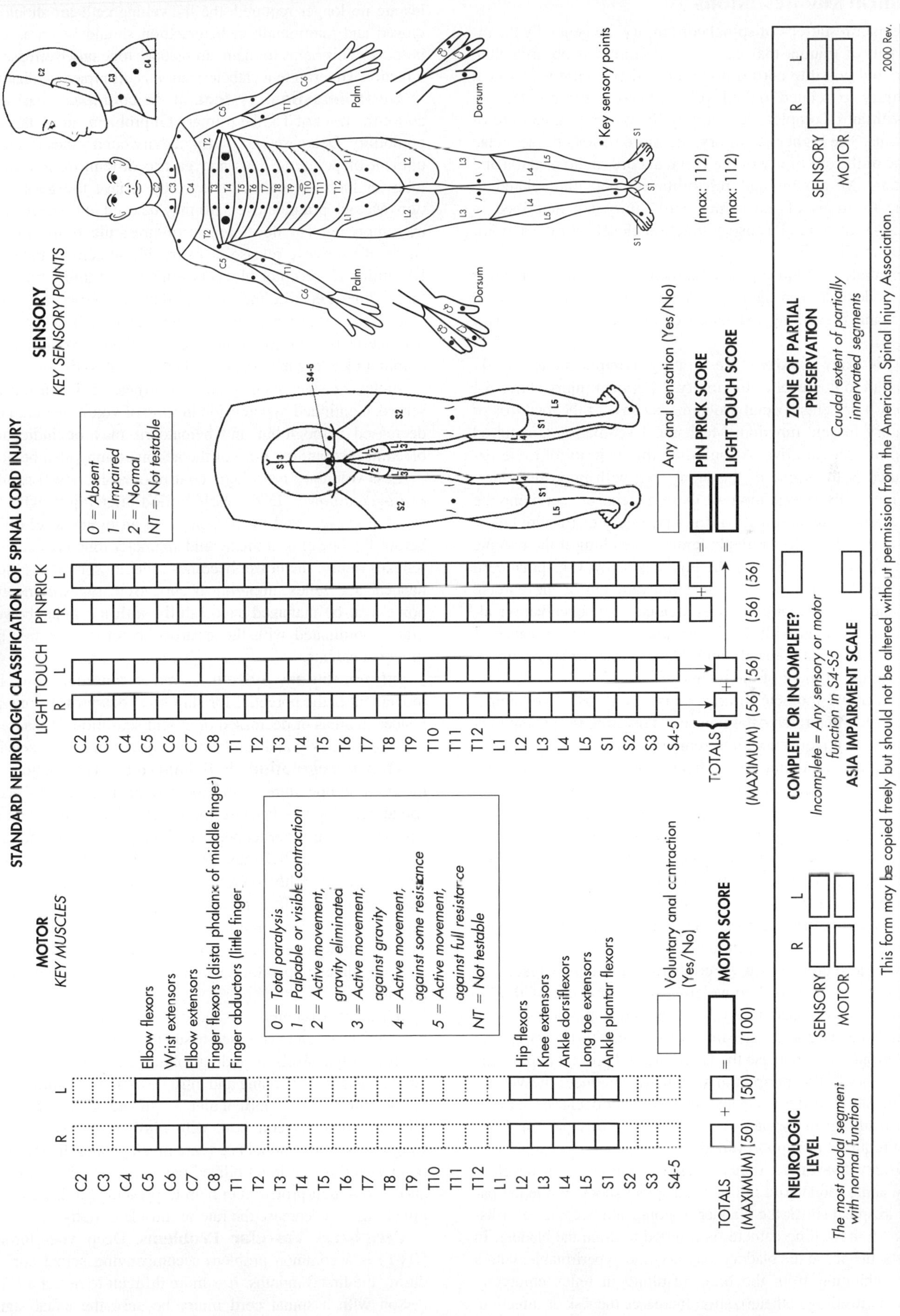

STANDARD NEUROLOGIC CLASSIFICATION OF SPINAL CORD INJURY

MOTOR
KEY MUSCLES

C2
C3
C4
C5   Elbow flexors
C6   Wrist extensors
C7   Elbow extensors
C8   Finger flexors (distal phalanx of middle finger)
T1   Finger abductors (little finger)
T2
T3
T4
T5
T6
T7
T8
T9
T10
T11
T12
L1
L2   Hip flexors
L3   Knee extensors
L4   Ankle dorsiflexors
L5   Long toe extensors
S1   Ankle plantar flexors
S2
S3
S4-5

0 = Total paralysis
1 = Palpable or visible contraction
2 = Active movement, gravity eliminated
3 = Active movement, against gravity
4 = Active movement, against some resistance
5 = Active movement, against full resistance
NT = Not testable

Voluntary anal contraction (Yes/No)

MOTOR SCORE

TOTALS [ ] + [ ] = [ ] (100)
(MAXIMUM) (50) (50)

SENSORY
KEY SENSORY POINTS

• Key sensory points

Palm
Dorsum

Palm
Dorsum

0 = Absent
1 = Impaired
2 = Normal
NT = Not testable

S4-5
S2
L5
S1
L4
L3
L2
S3

Any anal sensation (Yes/No) [ ]

PIN PRICK SCORE [ ] (max: 112)
LIGHT TOUCH SCORE [ ] (max: 112)

LIGHT TOUCH   PINPRICK
R   L   R   L

C2
C3
C4
C5
C6
C7
C8
T1
T2
T3
T4
T5
T6
T7
T8
T9
T10
T11
T12
L1
L2
L3
L4
L5
S1
S2
S3
S4-5

TOTALS { [ ] + [ ]   [ ] + [ ] }
        (MAXIMUM) (56) (56) (56) (56)
        = [ ] = [ ]

COMPLETE OR INCOMPLETE?
Incomplete = Any sensory or motor function in S4-S5   [ ]

ASIA IMPAIRMENT SCALE [ ]

	R	L
SENSORY	[ ]	[ ]
MOTOR	[ ]	[ ]

NEUROLOGIC LEVEL
The most caudal segment with normal function

ZONE OF PARTIAL PRESERVATION
Caudal extent of partially innervated segments

	R	L
SENSORY	[ ]	[ ]
MOTOR	[ ]	[ ]

2000 Rev.

This form may be copied freely but should not be altered without permission from the American Spinal Injury Association.

FIG. 59-9   Standard neurologic classification of spinal cord injury.

Clinical Manifestations

The manifestations of spinal cord injury are generally the direct result of trauma that causes cord compression, ischemia, edema, and possible cord transection. Manifestations of spinal cord injury are related to the level and degree of injury. The patient with an incomplete lesion may demonstrate a mixture of symptoms. The higher the injury, the more serious the sequelae because of the proximity of the cervical cord to the medulla and brainstem. Movement and rehabilitation potential related to specific locations of the spinal cord injury are described in Table 59-3. In general, sensory function closely parallels motor function at all levels.

Immediate postinjury problems include maintaining a patent airway, adequate ventilation, and adequate circulating blood volume and preventing extension of cord damage (secondary damage).

Respiratory System. Respiratory complications closely correspond to the level of the injury.[15] Cervical injury above the level of C4 presents special problems because of the total loss of respiratory muscle function. Mechanical ventilation is required to keep the patient alive. At one time the majority of these patients died at the scene of the injury, but with improved emergency medical services, more of these patients are surviving the initial events of their spinal cord injury. Injury or fracture below the level of C4 results in diaphragmatic breathing if the phrenic nerve is functioning. Even if the injury is below C4, spinal cord edema and hemorrhage can affect the function of the phrenic nerve and cause respiratory insufficiency. Hypoventilation almost always occurs with diaphragmatic respirations because of the decrease in vital capacity and tidal volume, which occurs as a result of impairment of the intercostal muscles.

Cervical and thoracic injuries cause paralysis of abdominal muscles and often intercostal muscles. Therefore the patient cannot cough effectively enough to remove secretions, leading to atelectasis and pneumonia. An artificial airway provides direct access for pathogens, making bronchial hygiene and chest physiotherapy extremely important to reduce infection. Neurogenic pulmonary edema may occur secondary to a dramatic increase in sympathetic nervous system activity at the time of injury, which shunts blood to the lungs. In addition, pulmonary edema may occur in response to fluid overload.

Cardiovascular System. Any cord injury above the level of T6 greatly decreases the influence of the sympathetic nervous system. Bradycardia occurs. Peripheral vasodilation results in hypotension. A relative hypovolemia exists because of the increase in venous capacitance. Cardiac monitoring is necessary. In marked bradycardia (heart rate <40 beats/min), appropriate drugs (atropine) to increase the heart rate and prevent hypoxemia are necessary.[15] The peripheral vasodilation reduces the venous return of blood to the heart and subsequently decreases cardiac output, resulting in hypotension. IV fluids or vasopressor drugs may be required to support blood pressure.

Urinary System. Urinary retention is a common development in acute spinal cord injuries and spinal shock. While the patient is in spinal shock the bladder is atonic and becomes overdistended. An indwelling catheter is inserted to drain the bladder. In the postacute phase the bladder may become hyperirritable, with a loss of inhibition from the brain resulting in reflex emptying. Chronic indwelling catheterization increases the risk of infection.

Once the patient is medically stable and large quantities of IV fluids are no longer required, the indwelling catheter should be removed and intermittent catheterization should begin as early as possible. This helps to maintain bladder tone and decrease risk of infection. (Intermittent catheterization is discussed in Chapter 44.)

Gastrointestinal System. If the cord injury has occurred above the level of T5, the primary GI problems are related to hypomotility. Decreased GI motor activity contributes to the development of paralytic ileus and gastric distention. A nasogastric tube for intermittent suctioning may relieve the gastric distention. Metoclopramide (Reglan) may be used to treat delayed gastric emptying. The development of stress ulcers is common because of excessive release of hydrochloric acid in the stomach. Histamine H_2-receptor blockers, such as ranitidine (Zantac) and famotidine (Pepcid), and proton pump inhibitors (e.g., omeprazole [Prilosec] or lansoprazole [Prevacid]) are frequently used to prevent the occurrence of ulcers during the initial phase. Intraabdominal bleeding may occur and is difficult to diagnose because no subjective signs such as pain, tenderness, and guarding are observed. Continued hypotension in spite of vigorous treatment and decreased hemoglobin and hematocrit may be indications of bleeding. Expanding girth of the abdomen may also be noted.

Less voluntary neurologic control over the bowel results in a *neurogenic bowel*. In the early period after injury when spinal shock is present and for patients with an injury level of T12 or below, the bowel is areflexic and sphincter tone is decreased. As reflexes return, the bowel becomes reflexic, sphincter tone is enhanced, and reflex emptying occurs. Both types of neurogenic bowel can be managed successfully with a regular bowel program coordinated with the gastrocolic reflex to minimize untimely accidents.

Integumentary System. A major consequence of lack of movement is the potential for skin breakdown over bony prominences in areas of decreased or absent sensation. Pressure ulcers can occur quickly and can lead to major infection or sepsis.

Thermoregulation. **Poikilothermism** is the adjustment of the body temperature to the room temperature. This occurs in spinal cord injuries because the interruption of the sympathetic nervous system prevents peripheral temperature sensations from reaching the hypothalamus. With spinal cord disruption there is also decreased ability to sweat or shiver below the level of the lesion, which also affects the ability to regulate body temperature. The degree of poikilothermism depends on the level of injury. Those with high cervical injuries have a greater loss of the ability to regulate temperature than do those with thoracic or lumbar injuries.

Metabolic Needs. Nasogastric suctioning may lead to metabolic alkalosis, and decreased tissue perfusion may lead to acidosis. Electrolyte levels, including sodium and potassium, can be altered by gastric suctioning and must be monitored until suctioning is discontinued and a normal diet is resumed. Loss of body weight (10% or more) is common, with nitrogen excretion mirroring weight loss.[15] Nutritional needs are much greater than what would be expected for an immobilized person. A positive nitrogen balance and a high-protein diet help to prevent skin breakdown and infections and decrease the rate of muscle atrophy.

Peripheral Vascular Problems. Deep vein thrombosis (DVT) is a common problem accompanying spinal cord injury during the first 3 months. It is more difficult to detect a DVT in a person with a spinal cord injury because the usual signs and symptoms, such as pain, tenderness, and a positive Homans' sign, will not be present.[17] Pulmonary embolism is one of the leading causes of death in patients with spinal cord injury. Techniques for assessment of DVT include Doppler examination, impedance plethysmography, and measurement of leg and thigh girth.

Diagnostic Studies

Once the patient is immobilized, diagnostic studies can be done. Complete spine films are performed to assess for vertebral fracture. X-rays including visualization of C1 through T1 are

TABLE 59-3   Functional Level of Spinal Cord Injury and Rehabilitation Potential

LEVEL OF INJURY	MOVEMENT REMAINING	REHABILITATION POTENTIAL
Tetraplegia		
C1-C3 Often fatal injury, vagus nerve domination of heart, respiration, blood vessels, and all organs below injury	Movement in neck and above, loss of innervation to diaphragm, absence of independent respiratory function	Ability to drive electric wheelchair equipped with portable ventilator by using chin control or mouth stick, headrest to stabilize head; computer use with mouth stick, head wand, or noise control; 24-hour attendant care, able to instruct others
C4 Vagus nerve domination of heart, respirations, and all vessels and organs below injury	Sensation and movement in neck and above; may be able to breathe without a ventilator	Same as C1-C3
C5 Vagus nerve domination of heart, respirations, and all vessels and organs below injury	Full neck, partial shoulder, back, biceps; gross elbow, inability to roll over or use hands; decreased respiratory reserve	Ability to drive electric wheelchair with mobile hand supports; indoor mobility in manual wheelchair; able to feed self with setup and adaptive equipment; attendant care 10 hours per day
C6 Vagus nerve domination of heart, respirations, and all vessels and organs below injury	Shoulder and upper back abduction and rotation at shoulder, full biceps to elbow flexion, wrist extension, weak grasp of thumb, decreased respiratory reserve	Ability to assist with transfer and perform some self-care; feed self with hand devices; push wheelchair on smooth, flat surface; drive adapted van from wheelchair; independent computer use with adaptive equipment; attendant care 6 hours per day
C7-C8 Vagus nerve domination of heart, respirations, and all vessels and organs below injury	All triceps to elbow extension, finger extensors and flexors, good grasp with some decreased strength, decreased respiratory reserve	Ability to transfer self to wheelchair; roll over and sit up in bed; push self on most surfaces; perform most self-care; independent use of wheelchair; ability to drive car with powered hand controls (in some patients); attendant care 0 to 6 hours per day
Paraplegia		
T1-T6 Sympathetic innervation to heart, vagus nerve domination of all vessels and organs below injury	Full innervation of upper extremities, back, essential intrinsic muscles of hand; full strength and dexterity of grasp; decreased trunk stability, decreased respiratory reserve	Full independence in self-care and in wheelchair; ability to drive car with hand controls (in most patients); independent standing in standing frame
T6-T12 Vagus nerve domination only of leg vessels, GI and genitourinary organs	Full, stable thoracic muscles and upper back; functional intercostals, resulting in increased respiratory reserve	Full independent use of wheelchair; ability to stand erect with full leg brace, ambulate on crutches with swing (although gait difficult); inability to climb stairs
L1-L2 Vagus nerve domination of leg vessels	Varying control of legs and pelvis, instability of lower back	Good sitting balance; full use of wheelchair; ambulation with long leg braces
L3-L4 Partial vagus nerve domination of leg vessels, GI and genitourinary organs	Quadriceps and hip flexors, absence of hamstring function, flail ankles	Completely independent ambulation with short leg braces and canes; inability to stand for long periods

GI, Gastrointestinal.

done to document the presence of vertebral injury. A CT scan may be used to assess the stability of the injury, location and degree of bony injury, soft and neural tissue changes, and degree of spinal canal compromise.[17] MRI is used in cases in which there is unexplained neurologic deficit or worsening of neurologic status. A comprehensive neurologic examination is performed along with assessment of head, chest, and abdomen for additional injuries or trauma. Patients with cervical injuries who demonstrate altered mental status may also need vertebral angiography to rule out vertebral artery damage.

Collaborative Care

The initial goals for the patient with a spinal cord injury are to sustain life and prevent further cord damage. Table 59-4 outlines the emergency management of the patient with a spinal cord injury. Systemic and neurogenic shock must be treated to maintain blood pressure. For injury at the cervical level, all body systems must be maintained until the full extent of the damage can be evaluated.

Collaborative care during the acute phase for a patient with a cervical injury is described in Table 59-5. The systemic support required by the patient is less intense for spinal cord injuries of the thoracic and lumbar vertebrae. Respiratory compromise is not as severe, and bradycardia is not a problem. Specific problems are treated symptomatically. After stabilization at the accident scene, the person is transferred to a medical facility. A thorough assessment is done to specifically evaluate the degree of deficit and to establish the level and degree of injury. A history is obtained, with emphasis on how the accident occurred and the extent of injury as perceived by the patient immediately after the accident. Assessment involves testing muscle groups rather than individual muscles. Muscle groups should be tested with and against gravity, alone and against resistance, and on both sides of the body. Spontaneous movement should be noted. The patient should be asked to move legs and then hands, spread fingers, extend wrists, and shrug shoulders. After assessment of motor status, a sensory examination including touch and pain as tested by pinprick should be carried out, starting at the toes and working upward. If time and conditions permit, position sense and vibration can also be assessed.

The types of accidents that cause spinal cord trauma may also result in brain injury. The patient should therefore be assessed for history of unconsciousness, signs of concussion, and increased intracranial pressure (see Chapter 55). In addition, a careful assessment for musculoskeletal injuries and trauma to internal organs should be performed. Because there are no muscle, bone, or visceral sensations, the only clue to internal trauma with hemorrhage may be a rapidly falling hematocrit level. Urinary output is examined for hematuria, which is also indicative of internal injuries.

The patient must be moved in alignment as a unit or moved "as a log" during transfers and when repositioning to prevent further injury. Respiratory, cardiac, urinary, and GI functions should be monitored closely. The patient may go directly to surgery following initial immobilization and stabilization or to the intensive care unit (ICU) for monitoring and management.

Nonoperative Stabilization. Nonoperative treatments are focused on stabilization of the injured spinal segment and decompression, either through traction or realignment. Stabilization methods eliminate damaging motion at the injury site. They

---

TABLE 59-4   Emergency Management
Spinal Cord Injury

ETIOLOGY	ASSESSMENT FINDINGS	INTERVENTIONS
Blunt • Compression, flexion, extension, or rotational injuries to spinal column • Motor vehicle accidents • Pedestrian accidents • Falls • Diving **Penetrating** • Stretched, torn, crushed, or lacerated spinal cord • Gunshot • Stab wounds	• Pain, tenderness, deformities, or muscle spasms adjacent to vertebral column • Numbness, paresthesias • Alterations in sensation: temperature, light touch, deep pressure, proprioception • Weakness or heaviness in limbs • Weakness, paralysis, or flaccidity of muscles • Spinal shock • Cuts; bruises; open wounds over head, face, neck, or back • Neurogenic shock: hypotension; bradycardia; dry, flushed skin • Bowel and bladder incontinence • Urinary retention • Difficulty breathing • Priapism • Diminished rectal sphincter tone	**Initial** • Ensure patent airway. • Stabilize cervical spine. • Administer oxygen via nasal cannula or nonrebreather mask. • Establish IV access with two large-bore catheters to infuse normal saline or lactated Ringer's solution as appropriate. • Assess for other injuries. • Control external bleeding. • Obtain cervical spine radiographs or CT scan. • Prepare for stabilization with cranial tongs and traction. • Administer high-dose methylprednisolone. **Ongoing Monitoring** • Monitor vital signs, level of consciousness, oxygen saturation, cardiac rhythm, urine output. • Keep warm. • Monitor for urinary retention, hypertension. • Anticipate need for intubation if gag reflex absent.

CT, Computed tomography; *IV*, intravenous.

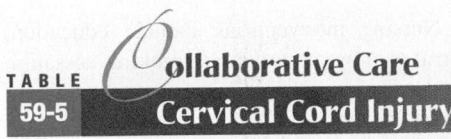

TABLE 59-5	Collaborative Care
	Cervical Cord Injury

Diagnostic
History and physical examination including complete neurologic examination
ABGs
Serial bedside PFTs
Electrolytes, glucose, hemoglobin, and hematocrit levels
Urinalysis
Anteroposterior, lateral, and odontoid spinal x-ray studies
CT scan, MRI
X-ray of vertebral spine
Myelography
EMG to measure evoked potentials
Venous duplex studies

Collaborative Therapy

Acute Care
Immobilization of vertebral column by skeletal traction
Maintenance of heart rate (e.g., atropine) and blood pressure (e.g., dopamine [Intropin])
Methylprednisolone high-dose therapy
Insertion of nasogastric tube and attachment to suction
Intubation (if indicated by ABGs and PFT)
O_2 by high humidity mask
Indwelling urinary catheter
Administration of IV fluids
Stress ulcer prophylaxis
Deep vein thrombosis prophylaxis
Bowel and bladder training

Rehabilitation and Home Care
Physical therapy
Range-of-motion exercises
Mobility training
Muscle strengthening
Occupational therapy (splints, activities of daily living training)
Bowel and bladder training
Autonomic dysreflexia prevention
Pressure ulcer prevention
Recreation therapy

ABGs, Arterial blood gases; CT, computed tomography; EMG, electromyography; MRI, magnetic resonance imaging; PFTs, pulmonary function tests.

are intended to prevent secondary spinal cord damage caused by repeated contusion or compression.[15]

Surgical Therapy. The decision to perform surgery on a patient with a spinal cord injury often depends on the preference of a particular physician. When cord compression is certain or the neurologic disorder progresses, benefit may be seen following immediate surgery. Surgery stabilizes the spinal column. There is some evidence to suggest that early cord decompression results in reduced secondary injury to the spinal cord and therefore improved outcomes.[18] Other criteria used in the decision for early surgery include (1) evidence of cord compression, (2) progressive neurologic deficit, (3) compound fracture of the vertebrae, (4) bony fragments (may dislodge and penetrate the cord), and (5) penetrating wounds of the spinal cord or surrounding structures.

The more common surgical procedures include decompression laminectomy by anterior cervical and thoracic approaches with fusion, posterior laminectomy with the use of acrylic wire mesh and fusion, and insertion of stabilizing rods (e.g., Harrington rods for the correction and stabilization of thoracic deformities). (Specific surgical and nursing interventions for these techniques are discussed in Chapter 61.)

Drug Therapy. The National Acute Spinal Cord Injury Study II (NASCIS II, 1990) and NASCIS III (1997) showed that methylprednisolone (MP), when administered early and in a large dose, resulted in greater recovery of neurologic function.[19-21] MP (Solu-Medrol) is effective if given within 8 hours of injury. When the loading dose of 30 mg/kg is given within 3 hours of injury, this is followed by 24 hours of 5.4 mg/kg IV MP drip (see Evidence-Based Practice box). If this loading dose is given between 3 and 8 hours postinjury, the IV drip is maintained for 48 hours. Patients do not benefit from MP if it is given more than 8 hours postinjury or the injury is penetrating. MP, a blocker of lipid peroxidation by-products, improves blood flow and reduces edema in the spinal cord. MP produces a number of effects that may account for the overall improvement noted in the spinal cord–injured patient, including reduction of posttraumatic spinal cord ischemia, improvement of energy balance, restoration of extracellular calcium, improvement of nerve impulse conduction, and repression of the release of free fatty acids from spinal cord tissues. Side effects of MP include immunosuppression, increased frequency of upper GI bleeding, and increased risk of infection.[19] Although MP treatment is currently considered to be the standard of care, controversy exists over whether the benefits outweigh the risks.

The NASCIS III also determined tirilazad mesylate (Freedox), a potent lipid peroxidation inhibitor, administered for 48 hours postinjury provided motor recovery rates equivalent to MP. There was an indication of fewer adverse effects in comparison with 48-hour treatment with MP. GM-1 ganglioside (Sygen), which enhances neuronal conductance and may pre-

Evidence-Based Practice
Drug Therapy for Spinal Cord Injury

Clinical Problem
Does pharmacologic treatment in the early hours following an acute spinal cord injury reduce the extent of permanent paralysis during the rest of the patient's life?

Best Clinical Practice
High-dose methylprednisolone therapy is the only pharmacologic therapy shown to be effective in reducing the extent of permanent paralysis when it is administered within 8 hours of injury.
High-dose methylprednisolone has been accepted as standard therapy in many countries.

Implications for Nursing Practice
- Assess involved systems before and periodically throughout the course of high-dose methylprednisolone therapy.
- Risk for infections and gastrointestinal bleeding is increased when this therapy is administered.

Reference for Evidence
Bracken MB: Pharmacological interventions for acute spinal cord injury, Cochrane Injuries Group, *Cochrane Database Syst Rev*, Issue 1, 2002.

vent postischemic neuronal damage, has also demonstrated safety and efficacy in early clinical trials.[18] Other neuroprotective drugs are being tested, and more treatment options may be available soon.

Vasopressor agents such as dopamine (Intropin) are employed in the acute phase as adjuvants to treatment. These agents are used to maintain the mean arterial pressure at a level greater than 80 to 90 mm Hg so that perfusion to the spinal cord is improved.

Pharmacologic properties and drug metabolism are altered in spinal cord injury. Therefore drug interactions may occur. The differences in drug metabolism correlate with level and completeness of injury, with greater change apparent in people with cervical injury than in those with injury of lower spinal levels.[22]

Pharmacologic agents are used to treat specific autonomic dysfunctions such as GI hypoactivity, bradycardia, orthostatic hypotension, inadequate emptying of the bladder, and autonomic dysreflexia. The nurse must know the intended effects of such agents, observe responses, and provide specific interventions when adverse reactions are seen.

NURSING MANAGEMENT
SPINAL CORD TRAUMA

■ Nursing Assessment

Subjective and objective data that should be obtained from a patient with a recent spinal cord injury are presented in Table 59-6.

■ Nursing Diagnoses

Nursing diagnoses for the patient with a spinal cord injury depend on the severity of the injury and the level of dysfunction. The nursing diagnoses for a patient with a spinal cord injury may include, but are not limited to, those presented in NCP 59-1. The care plan presented is for a patient with a complete cervical cord injury.

■ Planning

The overall goals are that the patient with a spinal cord injury will (1) maintain optimal level of neurologic functioning; (2) have minimal or no complications of immobility; (3) learn new skills, gain new knowledge, and acquire new behaviors to be able to care for self or successfully direct others to do so; and (4) return to home and the community at an optimal level of functioning.

■ Nursing Implementation

Health Promotion. Nursing interventions for injury prevention include identification of risk populations, counseling, and education. Support of local legislation related to seat belt use in cars, helmets for motorcyclists and bicyclists, child safety seats, and tougher penalties for drunk-driving offenses is a professional responsibility.

Roles of nursing in health promotion as it applies to spinal cord injury include injury prevention, counseling and education of people with spinal cord injury regarding health behaviors (e.g., smoking, substance abuse, diet, exercise), and ensuring that ongoing health care after hospital discharge includes appropriate general health screening and health promotion, as well as spinal cord injury care.

After injury, health-promoting behaviors can have a significant impact on the health and well-being of the individual with spinal cord injury. Nursing interventions include education, counseling, and referral to programs such as smoking cessation classes, recreation and exercise programs, or alcohol treatment programs. Outpatient health care requires that screening and prevention programs be accessible to people with spinal cord injury. Nurses in these settings should facilitate wheelchair-accessible

---

TABLE 59-6	Nursing Assessment Spinal Cord Injury

Subjective Data
Important Health Information
Past health history: Motor vehicle accident, sports injury, industrial accident, gunshot or stabbing injury, falls
Functional Health Patterns
Health perception–health management: Use of alcohol or recreational drugs; risk-taking behaviors
Activity-exercise: Loss of strength, movement, and sensation below level of injury; dyspnea, inability to breathe adequately ("air hunger")
Cognitive-perceptual: Presence of tenderness, pain at or above level of injury; numbness, tingling, burning, twitching of extremities
Coping–stress tolerance: Fear, denial, anger, depression

Objective Data
General
Poikilothermism (unable to regulate body heat)
Integumentary
Warm, dry, flushed extremities below level of injury (neurogenic shock)
Respiratory
Lesions at C1 to C3: apnea, inability to cough; lesions at C4: poor cough, diaphragmatic breathing, hypoventilation; lesions at C5 to T6: decreased respiratory reserve
Cardiovascular
Lesions above T5: bradycardia, hypotension, postural hypotension, absence of vasomotor tone
Gastrointestinal
↓ or absent bowel sounds (paralytic ileus in lesions above T5), abdominal distention, constipation, fecal incontinence, fecal impaction
Urinary
Retention (for lesions between T1 and L2); flaccid bladder (acute stages); spasticity with reflex bladder emptying (later stages)
Reproductive
Priapism, loss of sexual function
Neurologic
Complete: Flaccid paralysis and anesthesia below level of injury resulting in tetraplegia (for lesions above C8) or paraplegia (for lesions below C8), hyperactive deep tendon reflexes, bilaterally positive Babinski test (after resolution of spinal shock)
Incomplete: Mixed loss of voluntary motor activity and sensation
Musculoskeletal
Muscle atony (in flaccid state), contractures (in spastic state)
Possible Findings
Location of level and type of bony involvement on spinal x-ray: lesion, edema, compression on CT scan and MRI; positive finding on myelogram

CT, Computed tomography; *MRI,* magnetic resonance imaging.

examination rooms, adjustable height examination tables, and scheduling that allows extra time if needed.

Acute Intervention. High cervical injury caused by flexion-rotation is the most complex spinal cord injury and is discussed in this section. Interventions for this type of injury can be modified for patients with less severe problems.

Immobilization. Proper immobilization of the neck involves the maintenance of a neutral or slight extension position. Sandbags, hard cervical collars, and backboards can be used to stabilize the neck to prevent lateral rotation of the cervical spine. The body should always be correctly aligned, and turning should be performed so that the patient is moved as a unit (e.g., logrolling)

NURSING CARE PLAN 59-1

Patient with a Spinal Cord Injury*

EXPECTED PATIENT OUTCOMES	NURSING INTERVENTIONS and *RATIONALES*
NURSING DIAGNOSIS	**Impaired gas exchange** *related to* diaphragmatic fatigue or paralysis and retained secretions *as manifested by* decreased PaO_2 content, increased $PaCO_2$ concentration, fatigue, diminished breath sounds.
• ABGs and PFT within normal limits • Normal chest x-ray • Clear lungs on auscultation • Absence of respiratory distress	• Maintain a patent airway *to prevent respiratory arrest.* • Assess all respiratory parameters initially and at least q2hr *to determine extent of problem and plan appropriate interventions.* • Monitor ABGs and PFT *to determine oxygenation and ventilation status.* • Provide aggressive pulmonary toilet, including chest physical therapy and assisted coughing (see Chapter 66, Fig. 66-6) q4hr *to facilitate the raising of secretions.* • Assess strength of cough at least q4hr *to determine adequacy for raising secretions.* • Suction as necessary *to remove accumulated secretions.*
NURSING DIAGNOSIS	**Decreased cardiac output** *related to* venous pooling of blood, bradycardia, and immobility *as manifested by* hypotension, restlessness, oliguria, decreased pulmonary artery pressures.
• Adequate cardiac output • Stable blood pressure and pulse • Absence of arrhythmias • No complications such as venous thrombosis or pulmonary emboli	• Monitor blood pressure and pulse at least q2hr initially; monitor cardiac rhythm *as indicators of cardiac status.* • Mobilize gradually *to prevent orthostatic hypotension.* • Administer dopamine (Intropin) or other vasopressor agents *to maintain mean blood pressure >80 mm Hg.* • Apply pneumatic compression devices to calves and/or compression gradient stockings *to prevent venous pooling and thromboemboli.* • Perform range-of-motion to all extremities at least q8hr *to cause muscle contractions, which aid in venous return.*
NURSING DIAGNOSIS	**Impaired skin integrity** *related to* immobility and poor tissue perfusion *as manifested by* reddened skin over bony prominences and pin and tong sites.
• Intact skin • No pressure ulcers	• Inspect all skin areas, especially over bony prominences, at least q2hr; observe area around pins or tongs for signs of breakdown or infection *so that interventions can be initiated promptly if a problem develops.* • Turn patient at least q2hr; use kinetic treatment table (see Fig. 66-11) or other specialty care devices as needed *to prevent development of pressure areas.* • Ensure adequate nutritional intake *to maintain healthy skin resistant to breakdown.* • Wash and dry patient's skin thoroughly *to prevent moisture from predisposing to skin breakdown.* • Teach patient and family to inspect bony prominences *to detect reddened areas* and ways to prevent pressure ulcers (Table 12-25).
NURSING DIAGNOSIS	**Constipation** *related to* neurogenic bowel, inadequate fluid intake, diet low in roughage, and immobility *as manifested by* lack of bowel movement for more than 2 days, decreased bowel sounds, palpable impaction, hard stool or stool incontinence.
• Established bowel program • Bowel movement at least every other day	• Auscultate bowel sounds at least q4hr; monitor abdominal distention *to determine if peristalsis is present.* • Begin bowel program as soon as bowel sounds return and include suppository every other day and stool softeners *to establish a bowel routine as quickly as possible.* • Teach patient and family the bowel program *to ensure continuity of the program.* • Ensure appropriate food and fluid intake *because bulk, fiber, and fluid are necessary to the success of a bowel program.*

*This care plan is suitable for a patient with a high cervical injury caused by flexion-rotation. It can be modified for patients with less severe problems.
ABGs, Arterial blood gases; *PFT,* pulmonary function test.

Continued

NURSING CARE PLAN 59-1

Patient with a Spinal Cord Injury—cont'd

EXPECTED PATIENT OUTCOMES	NURSING INTERVENTIONS and *RATIONALES*
NURSING DIAGNOSIS	**Impaired urinary elimination** *related to* spinal injury and limited fluid intake *as manifested by* lack of urine output, bladder distention, involuntary emptying of bladder (after spinal shock).
▪ No urinary retention or infection ▪ Able to perform self-catheterization to empty bladder or able to void with adequate emptying	▪ Palpate bladder *because loss of autonomic and reflex control of bladder and sphincter can cause distention.* ▪ Insert indwelling catheter during acute phase *to ensure continuous flow of urine to prevent reflux of urine into the kidneys.* ▪ Begin intermittent catheterization program when appropriate; teach patient and family intermittent catheterization using a clean technique *to avoid long-term use of indwelling catheter with high potential for infection.* ▪ Maintain accurate intake and output records *to evaluate fluid balance.* ▪ Encourage fluids (2 to 4 L/day) *to maintain high volume of dilute urine,* which aids in preventing infection with indwelling catheter. ▪ Encourage fluids (2 L/day) divided into 200 to 250 ml every 2 to 3 hours while awake *to maintain regular bladder volumes (<500 ml) during intermittent catheterization.* ▪ Monitor bladder volumes regularly using bladder ultrasound for patients who are regaining ability to void *to assess adequacy of emptying and to prevent bladder overdistention.* ▪ Monitor blood urea nitrogen and creatinine levels, urine cultures, and WBC count *to monitor kidney function and presence of infection.*
NURSING DIAGNOSIS	**Impaired physical mobility** *related to* spinal cord injury, vertebral column instability, or forced immobilization by traction *as manifested by* inability to move purposefully, limited muscle strength, impaired perception of position or presence of body parts.
▪ No complications of immobility	▪ Assess motor and sensory function at least q4hr initially *to promptly detect deterioration of neurologic status.* ▪ Promote good pulmonary function *because pulmonary complications are a common sequelae of immobility.* ▪ Use specialty bed or turn patient q1-2hr *to prevent prolonged pressure, which can lead to pressure ulcers.* ▪ Perform full range-of-motion to all extremities several times a day *to promote circulation and prevent contractures.* ▪ Use splints and foot boards as appropriate *to prevent contractures and promote functional positioning.*
NURSING DIAGNOSIS	**Risk for autonomic dysreflexia** *related to* reflex stimulation of sympathetic nervous system after spinal shock resolves.
▪ No occurrence of dysreflexia ▪ Receive immediate and appropriate nursing or medical interventions if dysreflexia occurs	▪ Assess for hypertension, bradycardia, severe headache, sweating, blurred vision, flushed feeling, nasal congestion *as signs of dysreflexia.* ▪ Reduce or eliminate noxious stimuli such as fecal impaction, urinary retention, tactile stimulation, and skin lesions by appropriate interventions *to prevent occurrence of dysreflexia.* ▪ If dysreflexia occurs, check for elevated blood pressure and administer antihypertensive medication as ordered; check for and correct possible sources of irritation such as a distended bladder or bowel; elevate head of bed immediately *to reduce blood pressure by allowing blood to pool in the lower extremities.* ▪ If nursing interventions do not reverse symptoms, notify physician *so that immediate medical interventions can be initiated to prevent a life-threatening situation from developing.* ▪ Teach patient and family to recognize and treat dysreflexia *to reverse occurrence and prevent occurrence of status epilepticus, stroke, and possible death.*

NURSING CARE PLAN 59-1

Patient with a Spinal Cord Injury—cont'd

EXPECTED PATIENT OUTCOMES	NURSING INTERVENTIONS and *RATIONALES*
NURSING DIAGNOSIS	**Imbalanced nutrition: less than body requirements** *related to* increased metabolic demand, gastrointestinal hypomotility, and inability to eat independently *as manifested by* weight loss >10% of admission weight, decreased serum albumin or protein.
• Weight loss <10% • Normal values for serum protein and albumin	• Assess weight on admission *to provide baseline for comparison over time.* • Ensure enteral feedings are given as ordered during acute phase *so that nutrient intake is not interrupted.* • When patient is eating, encourage high-protein, high-carbohydrate, high-calorie diet with high bulk *to counteract the severe catabolism that occurs with spinal cord injury.* • Keep a calorie count and weigh patient at least weekly *to evaluate nutritional plan and continue or revise as necessary.*
NURSING DIAGNOSIS	**Risk for ineffective coping** *related to* loss of control over bodily functions and altered lifestyle secondary to paralysis.
• Verbalization of ability to cope with effects of spinal cord injury	• Assess for prolonged use of inappropriate defense mechanisms, inability to accept current status, refusal to use available support services *to determine presence of risk factors for ineffective coping.* • Offer support and acceptance of feelings; assist patient with problem solving *to bolster patient's confidence in ability to cope.* • Foster decision making regarding care *to increase feelings of control.* • Encourage use of support systems *to discuss concerns.* • Provide information *because knowledge of expectations can help patient cope with the future.* • Teach patient healthy coping behaviors such as relaxation techniques to *prevent patient from practicing ineffective behaviors such as smoking, drinking, or angry outbursts.*
NURSING DIAGNOSIS	**Disturbed body image** *related to* paralysis *as manifested by* expression of anger or other negative feelings, refusal to discuss changes in function, participate in social contacts, or look at body.
• Expression of feelings about self • Work through feelings to facilitate adaptation	• Encourage discussion of feelings *to aid patient in venting and clarifying feelings.* • Allow patient to grieve *because spinal cord injury results in a real loss, which requires adjustment through grieving.* • Encourage social interaction *to foster sense of returning normalcy to life.* • Assist family members in supporting patient *to enhance patient's sense of worth and value as a person.* • Make referral for counseling as needed.
NURSING DIAGNOSIS	**Interrupted family processes** *related to* change in function of ill family member *as manifested by* poor communication patterns among family members, use of ineffective coping techniques (e.g., shouting, blaming), inability of family members to meet needs of patient.
• Family will maximize individual and collective strengths and meet patient's needs	• Assess family dynamics related to roles and responsibilities *to determine problematic areas and strengths.* • Encourage open communication among family members regarding long-term planning to meet patient's needs, including financial aspects *so that ideas and concerns of all involved family members are considered.* • Assist family members to understand patient's feelings *to strengthen patient's feeling of worth and support.* • Assist family members to develop an action plan to meet patient's needs *to reduce sense of frustration and helplessness.* • Coordinate an organized team approach *to help the patient and family cope with the complex changes.*

NURSING RESEARCH
Interventions to Enhance Quality of Life Following Spinal Cord Injury

Citation
Phillips VL et al: Telehealth: reaching out to newly injured spinal cord patients, *Public Health Rep* 116:94, 2001.

Purpose
To describe health-related outcomes of a randomized trial of telehealth interventions that were designed to reduce secondary problems among spinal cord injury (SCI) patients with mobility impairment.

Methods
Patients were recruited during their stay in a rehabilitation unit. Patients were randomly assigned to receive a video-based intervention for 9 weeks, a telephone-based intervention for 9 weeks, or standard follow-up care. Measurements included days of hospitalization, depressive symptoms, and health-related quality of life. Measures were obtained immediately after the intervention and at 1 year.

Results and Conclusions
Quality of life did not differ significantly among the three groups at the end of the 9-week intervention. However, at 1 year, patients in the video and telephone intervention group had higher self-reported quality of life scores compared with the standard care group. In addition, at 1 year, mean annual hospital days were lower for the two intervention groups than for the standard care group. In-home telephone or video-based interventions did improve health-related outcomes for newly injured SCI patients.

Implications for Nursing Practice
Optimizing patient quality of life after a SCI remains a challenge. It is important to test interventions delivered in the rehabilitation unit and the home for their long-term effectiveness in reducing health problems and hospitalization, as well as improving quality of life.

to prevent movement of the spine. For cervical injuries, skeletal traction is usually provided by Crutchfield (Fig. 59-10), Vinke, or Gardner-Wells tongs or other types of skull tongs. Traction is provided by a rope that is extended from the center of the tongs over a pulley and has weights attached at the end. Traction must

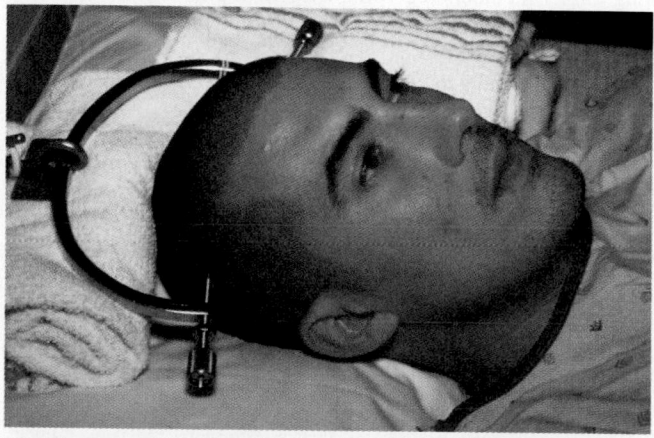

FIG. 59-10   Cervical traction is attached to tongs inserted in the skull.

be maintained at all times. One disadvantage of skull tongs is that the skull pins can be displaced. If this occurs, the head should be held in a neutral or extended position and help should be summoned. Sandbags can be positioned to stabilize the head while the physician reinserts the tongs.

Infection at the sites of tong insertion is another potential problem. Preventive care includes cleansing the sites twice a day with normal saline solution and applying an antibiotic ointment, which acts as a mechanical barrier to the entrance of bacteria. The preventive care of insertion sites may vary depending on individual hospital standards of care.

Special beds are often used in the management of the patient with a spinal cord injury (see Fig. 66-11). Kinetic therapy uses a continual side-to-side slow rotation 62 degrees laterally with the patient in constant motion. The bed allows a frequency of turns greater than 200 times per day. The bed is used to decrease the likelihood of pressure sores and cardiopulmonary complications. However, in some patients the turning can induce motion sickness and fear of falling out of bed when turned to the extremes. (Motion sickness is unlikely when automatic rather than manual turning is used.)

Depending on the type of injury and therapeutic interventions, the tongs and traction may be removed 1 to 4 weeks after injury. In a stable injury for which surgery is not done, halo traction may be applied. The removal of traction and application of a collar brace or halo traction device allow the patient to be more mobile and to begin active rehabilitation. After cervical fusion or other stabilization surgery, a Philadelphia collar or sternal-occipital-mandibular immobilizer brace is worn until the fusion becomes solid (Fig. 59-11).[13] The halo apparatus applies cervical traction by means of a jacketlike arrangement that allows greater mobility and wheelchair activity than other traction systems (Fig. 59-12). Patients with thoracic or lumbar spine injuries are immobilized with a custom thoracolumbar orthosis ("body jacket"), which controls spinal flexion, extension, and rotation, or with a Jewett brace, which restricts forward flexion.

Immobilization of the neck of the patient with a spinal cord injury prevents further injury, but the effects of immobility are profound. Meticulous skin care is critical because decreased sensation and circulation make the patient particularly susceptible to skin breakdown. Patients should be removed from backboards as soon as possible, and cervical collars should be properly fitted or replaced with other forms of immobilization to prevent coccygeal and occipital area skin breakdown. It is important that areas under the halo vest or jacket or under braces or orthoses be inspected to assess skin condition.

Respiratory dysfunction. During the first 48 hours after injury, spinal cord edema may increase the level of dysfunction and respiratory distress may occur. If the injury is at or above C3, or if the patient is exhausted from labored breathing or ABGs deteriorate (indicating inadequate oxygenation or ventilation), endotracheal intubation or tracheostomy and mechanical ventilation should be initiated. Respiratory arrest is a possibility that requires careful monitoring of the respiratory system and prompt action, should it occur. Pneumonia and atelectasis are potential problems because of reduced vital capacity and the loss of intercostal and abdominal muscle function, resulting in diaphragmatic breathing, pooled secretions, and an ineffective cough.[23] The older adult has a more difficult time responding to hypoxia and hypercapnia and is extremely intolerant of hypoxia caused by lack of reserve. Therefore aggressive chest physiotherapy, ad-

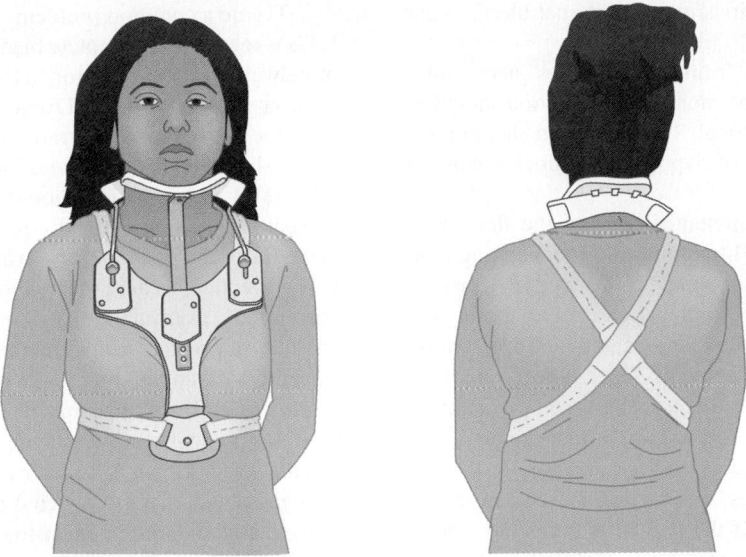

FIG. 59-11 Sternal-occipital-mandibular immobilizer (SOMI) brace.

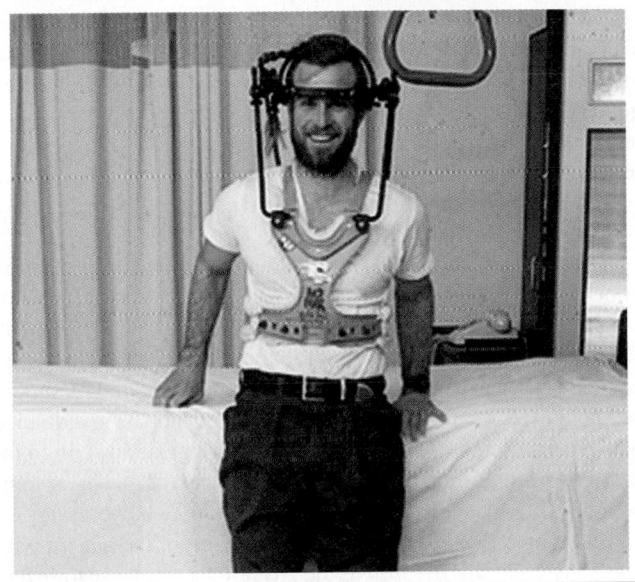

FIG. 59-12 Halo vest, Ace manufacturing design. Note the rigid shoulder straps and encompassing vest. Various vest sizes are available prefabricated. The halo ring, superstructure, and vest are MRI-compatible.

equate oxygenation, and proper pain management are essential to maximize respiratory function and gas exchange. Other problems include nasal stuffiness and bronchospasms.

The nurse needs to regularly assess (1) breath sounds, (2) ABGs, (3) tidal volume, (4) vital capacity, (5) skin color, (6) breathing patterns (especially the use of accessory muscles), (7) subjective comments about the ability to breathe, and (8) the amount and color of sputum. A PaO_2 (partial pressure of oxygen in arterial blood) above 60 mm Hg and a $PaCO_2$ (partial pressure of carbon dioxide in arterial blood) below 45 mm Hg are acceptable values in a patient with uncomplicated tetraplegia. A patient who is unable to count to 10 out loud without taking a breath needs immediate attention.

In addition to monitoring, the nurse can intervene in maintaining ventilation. Oxygen is administered until ABGs stabilize.

Chest physiotherapy and assisted coughing facilitate the raising of secretions. Assisted coughing simulates the action of the ineffective abdominal muscles during the expiratory phase of a cough. The nurse places the heels of both hands just below the xiphoid process and exerts firm upward pressure to the area timed with the patient's efforts to cough (see Fig. 66-6). Tracheal suctioning should be performed if crackles or rhonchi are present. Incentive spirometry is an additional technique that can be used to improve the patient's respiratory status.

Cardiovascular instability. Because of unopposed vagal response, the heart rate is slowed, often to below 60 beats per minute. Any increase in vagal stimulation such as turning or suctioning can result in cardiac arrest. Loss of sympathetic tone in peripheral vessels results in chronic low blood pressure with potential postural hypotension. Lack of muscle tone to aid venous return can result in sluggish blood flow and predispose the patient to DVT.

Vital signs should be assessed frequently. If bradycardia is symptomatic, an anticholinergic drug such as atropine is administered. A temporary pacemaker may be inserted in some instances. Hypotension is managed with a vasopressor agent, such as dopamine (Intropin) or norepinephrine, and fluid replacement.

In the older adult, the prevalence of cardiovascular disease must be considered. The cardiovascular system becomes less able to handle the stress of traumatic injury because heart contractions weaken, and cardiac output is reduced. Maximum heart rate is also reduced.

Compression gradient stockings can be used to prevent thromboemboli and to promote venous return. The stockings must be removed every 8 hours for skin care. The use of pneumatic compression devices for the calves is advocated, and they must be applied as soon as possible after admission and maintained throughout the hospitalization. Venous duplex studies may be performed before applying compression devices. The nurse should also perform range-of-motion exercises and stretching regularly. The thighs and calves of the legs should be assessed every shift for signs of DVT.

Prophylactic use of heparin or low-molecular-weight heparin (e.g., enoxaparin [Lovenox]) may be used to prevent DVT unless contraindicated. Contraindications include internal bleeding and recent surgery.

If blood loss has occurred from other injuries, hemoglobin and hematocrit levels should be monitored and blood should be administered according to protocol. The nurse also should monitor the patient for indications of hypovolemic shock secondary to hemorrhage.

Fluid and nutritional maintenance. During the first 48 to 72 hours after the injury the GI tract may stop functioning (paralytic ileus) and a nasogastric tube must be inserted. Because the patient cannot have oral intake, fluid and electrolyte needs must be carefully monitored. Specific solutions and additives are ordered based on individual requirements. Once bowel sounds are present or flatus is passed, oral food and fluids can gradually be introduced. Because of severe catabolism, a high-protein, high-calorie diet is necessary for energy and tissue repair. In patients with high cervical cord injuries, swallowing must be evaluated before starting oral feedings. If the patient is unable to resume eating, total parenteral nutrition may be started to provide nutritional support.

Some patients experience anorexia, which can be due to psychologic depression, boredom with institutional food, or discomfort at being fed (often by a hurried nurse). Some patients have a normally small appetite. Occasionally, refusal to eat is used as a means of maintaining control over the environment because of diminished or absent body control. If the patient is not eating adequately, the cause should be thoroughly assessed. On the basis of this assessment, a contract may be made with the patient using mutual goal setting regarding the diet. This gives the patient increased control of the situation and often results in improved nutritional intake. General measures such as providing a pleasant eating environment, allowing adequate time to eat (including any self-feeding the patient can achieve), encouraging the family to bring in special foods, and planning social rewards for eating may be useful. A calorie count should be kept, and the patient's daily weight recorded as a means of evaluating progress. If feasible, the patient should participate in recording calorie intake. Increased dietary fiber should be included to promote bowel function. The nurse should avoid allowing the patient's nutritional intake to become a basis for a power struggle.

Bladder and bowel management. Immediately after injury, urine is retained because of the loss of autonomic and reflex control of the bladder and sphincter. Because there is no sensation of fullness, overdistention of the bladder can result in reflux into the kidney with eventual renal failure. Bladder overdistention may even result in rupture of the bladder. Consequently, an indwelling catheter is usually inserted as soon as possible after injury. Its patency must be ensured by frequent inspection and irrigation if necessary. In some institutions a physician's order is required for this procedure. Strict aseptic technique for catheter care is essential to avoid introducing infection.

After the patient is stabilized, the best means of managing long-term urinary function is assessed. Usually the patient is started on an intermittent catheterization program. Intermittent catheterization has been shown to reduce UTIs when compared with an indwelling catheter, and it is the safest method of bladder management for protecting the kidneys.[23] The patient is often maintained on a fluid restriction of 1800 to 2000 ml per day to facilitate a bladder training program. Urinary output is monitored closely.

UTIs are a common problem. The best method for preventing UTIs is regular and complete bladder drainage. During the period of indwelling catheterization, a large fluid intake is required. The catheter should be checked frequently to prevent kinking and ensure free flow of urine. During intermittent catheterization, fluid intake should be moderate and regular (200 to 300 ml every 2 to 3 hours). Catheterization should be done every 3 to 4 hours to prevent bacterial overgrowth resulting from urinary stasis. Cranberry juice and/or cranberry extract tablets may be helpful for UTI prevention because there is some evidence that they may prevent bacteria from adhering to the bladder wall. Ascorbic acid and a urinary antiseptic, such as methenamine hippurate (Hiprex), are sometimes given although their use in preventing UTIs remains controversial. If the appearance or odor of the urine is suspicious or if the patient develops symptoms of a UTI (chills, fever, malaise), a specimen is sent for culture.

Age-related changes in renal function should be considered. The older adult is more likely to develop renal calculi, and older men may have prostatic hyperplasia, which may interfere with urinary flow and complicate urinary management.

Constipation is generally a problem during spinal shock because no voluntary or involuntary (reflex) evacuation of the bowels occurs. A bowel program should be started during acute care. This consists of choosing a rectal stimulant (suppository or mini-enema) to be inserted daily at a regular time of day followed by gentle digital stimulation or manual evacuation done by the nurse until evacuation is complete. Initially the program may be done in bed in the side-lying position, but as soon as the patient has resumed sitting, it should be done in the upright position on a padded bedside commode chair.[24]

Temperature control. Because there is no vasoconstriction, piloerection, or heat loss through perspiration below the level of injury, temperature control is largely external to the patient. Therefore the nurse must monitor the environment closely to maintain an appropriate temperature. Body temperature should be monitored regularly. The patient should not be overloaded with covers or unduly exposed (such as during bathing). If an infection with high fever develops, more extensive means of temperature control, such as a cooling blanket, may be necessary.

Stress ulcers. Stress ulcers are a problem for the patient with a spinal cord injury because of the physiologic response to severe trauma, psychologic stress, and high-dose corticosteroids. Peak incidence of stress ulcers is 6 to 14 days after injury. Stool and gastric contents are tested daily for blood, and the hematocrit is observed for a slow drop. When corticosteroids are given, they should be accompanied by antacids or food. Histamine H_2-receptor blockers, such as ranitidine (Zantac) and famotidine (Pepcid), or proton pump inhibitors, such as omeprazole (Prilosec), may be given prophylactically to decrease the secretion of hydrochloric acid.

Sensory deprivation. The nurse must compensate for the patient's absent sensations to prevent sensory deprivation. This is done by stimulating the patient above the level of injury. Conversation, music, strong aromas, and interesting flavors should be a part of the nursing care plan. Prism glasses are provided so that the patient can read and watch television. Every effort should be made to prevent the patient from withdrawing from the environment.

Patients with spinal cord injury often report altered sensorium and vivid dreams during the acute phase of their treatment. Whether this is due to drugs used to manage pain and anxiety is not known. Patients may also experience disrupted sleep patterns as a result of the hospital environment or posttraumatic stress disorder.

Reflexes. Once spinal cord shock is resolved, the return of reflexes may complicate rehabilitation. Lacking control from the higher brain centers, reflexes are often hyperactive and produce exaggerated responses. Penile erections can occur from a variety of stimuli, causing embarrassment and discomfort. Spasms ranging from mild twitches to convulsive movements below the level of the lesion may also occur. This reflex activity may be interpreted by the patient or family as a return of function, and the nurse must tactfully explain the reason for the activity. The patient may be informed of the positive use of these reflexes in sexual, bowel, and bladder retraining. Spasms may be controlled with the use of antispasmodic drugs. Most commonly prescribed are baclofen (Lioresal), dantrolene (Dantrium), and tizanidine (Zanaflex). Botulism toxin injections may also be given to treat severe spasticity.[25]

Autonomic dysreflexia. The return of reflexes after the resolution of spinal shock means that patients with an injury level at T6 or higher may develop autonomic dysreflexia. **Autonomic dysreflexia** is a massive uncompensated cardiovascular reaction mediated by the sympathetic nervous system. It occurs in response to visceral stimulation once spinal shock is resolved in patients with spinal cord lesions above T7. The condition is a life-threatening situation that requires immediate resolution. If resolution does not occur, this condition can lead to status epilepticus, stroke, myocardial infarction, and even death.

The most common precipitating cause is a distended bladder or rectum, although any sensory stimulation may cause autonomic dysreflexia. Contraction of the bladder or rectum, stimulation of the skin, or stimulation of the pain receptors may also cause autonomic dysreflexia. Manifestations include hypertension (up to 300 mm Hg systolic), blurred vision, throbbing headache, marked diaphoresis above the level of the lesion, bradycardia (30 to 40 beats per minute), *piloerection* (erection of body hair) as a result of pilomotor spasm, flushing of the skin above the level of the lesion, blurred vision or spots in the visual fields, nasal congestion, anxiety, and nausea. It is important to measure blood pressure when a patient with a spinal cord injury complains of a headache.[26]

The pathology of autonomic dysreflexia involves the stimulation of sensory receptors below the level of the cord lesion. The intact autonomic nervous system below the level of the lesion responds to the stimulation with a reflex arteriolar vasoconstriction that increases blood pressure. Baroreceptors in the carotid sinus and the aorta sense the hypertension and stimulate the parasympathetic system. This results in a decrease in heart rate, but the visceral and peripheral vessels do not dilate because efferent impulses cannot pass through the cord lesion.

Nursing interventions in this serious emergency are elevation of the head of the bed 45 degrees or sitting the patient upright, notification of the physician, and assessment to determine the cause. The most common cause is bladder irritation. Immediate catheterization to relieve bladder distention may be necessary. Lidocaine jelly should be instilled in the urethra before catheterization. If a catheter is already in place, it should be checked for kinks or folds. If plugged, small-volume irrigation should be performed slowly and gently to open a plugged catheter, or a new catheter may be inserted. Stool impaction can also result in auto-

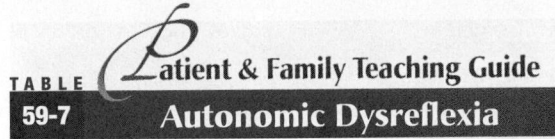

TABLE 59-7	**Patient & Family Teaching Guide** **Autonomic Dysreflexia**

Patient and family members must know the signs and symptoms of autonomic dysreflexia so that timely intervention can occur. These include the following:
- Sudden onset of acute headache
- Elevation in blood pressure and/or reduction in pulse rate
- Flushed face and upper chest (above the level of the lesion) and pale extremities (below the level of the lesion)
- Sweating above the level of the lesion
- Nasal congestion
- Feeling of apprehension

Immediate interventions include the following:
- Raise the person to a sitting position.
- Remove the stimulus (fecal impaction, kinked urinary catheter).
- Call the health care provider if above actions do not relieve the signs and symptoms.

Efforts to decrease the likelihood of autonomic dysreflexia include the following:
- Maintain regular bowel function.
- If manual rectal stimulation is used, local anesthetics may reduce stimulation of autonomic dysreflexia.
- Monitor urine output.
- Wear a medical alert bracelet indicating a history of autonomic dysreflexia.

nomic dysreflexia. A digital rectal examination should be performed only after application of an anesthetic ointment to decrease rectal stimulation and to prevent an increase of symptoms. The nurse should remove all skin stimuli, such as constrictive clothing and tight shoes. Blood pressure should be monitored frequently during the episode. If symptoms persist after the source has been relieved, an α-adrenergic blocker or an arteriolar vasodilator (e.g., nifedipine [Procardia]) is administered. Careful monitoring must continue until the vital signs stabilize.

The patient and family should be taught the causes and symptoms of autonomic dysreflexia (Table 59-7). They must understand the life-threatening nature of this dysfunction and must know how to relieve the cause.

Rehabilitation and Home Care. The physiologic and psychologic rehabilitation of the person with spinal cord injury is complex and involved. With physical and psychologic care and intensive and specialized rehabilitation, the patient with a spinal cord injury learns to function at the highest level of wellness. It is recommended that all patients with a new spinal cord injury receive comprehensive inpatient rehabilitation in a rehabilitation unit or center that specializes in spinal cord rehabilitation.

Many of the problems identified in the acute period become chronic and continue throughout life. Rehabilitation focuses on refined retraining of physiologic processes and extensive patient and family teaching about how to manage the physiologic and life changes resulting from injury (Fig. 59-13).

Rehabilitation is a multidisciplinary endeavor carried out through a team approach. Team members include rehabilitation nurses, physicians, physical therapists, occupational therapists, speech therapists, vocational counselors, psychologists, thera-

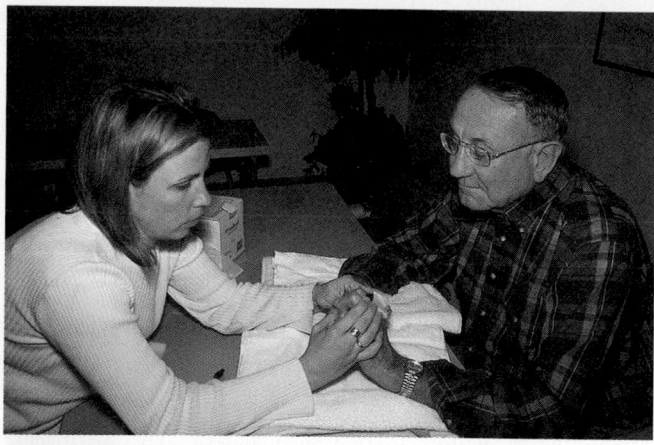

FIG. 59-13 Patient participating in occupational therapy.

who are not ventilator dependent should be taught assisted coughing and regular use of incentive spirometry or deep breathing exercises.

Neurogenic bladder. A **neurogenic bladder** is any type of bladder dysfunction related to abnormal or absent bladder innervation. After spinal cord shock resolves, depending on the completeness of the spinal cord injury, patients usually have some degree of neurogenic bladder. Normal voiding requires nervous system coordination of urethral and pelvic floor relaxation with simultaneous contraction of the detrusor muscle.[27] Depending on the lesion, a neurogenic bladder may have no reflex detrusor contractions (areflexic, flaccid), may have hyperactive reflex detrusor contractions (hyperreflexic, spastic), or may have lack of coordination between detrusor contraction and urethral relaxation (dyssynergia). Common problems with a neurogenic bladder include urgency, frequency, incontinence, inability to void, and high bladder pressures resulting in reflux of urine into the kidneys.

Neurogenic bladder can be classified according to reflex detrusor activity, intravesical filling pressure, and continence function. Types of neurogenic bladder are outlined in Table 59-8. Diagnostic and collaborative care of neurogenic bladder is described in Table 59-9. The patient with a spinal cord injury and a neurogenic bladder requires a comprehensive program to manage bladder function.

After the patient's overall condition is stable and there is evidence of neurologic reflexes, urodynamic testing, an IV pyelogram, and a urine culture are done. The method used for urinary drainage depends on the type of neurogenic bladder dysfunction, the preference of the patient, and availability of a family caregiver, the physician, and the nursing staff. Numerous drainage methods are possible, including bladder reflex retraining if partial voiding control remains, indwelling catheter, intermittent catheterization, and external catheter (condom catheter). Surgical options including sphincterectomy, implantation of a functional electrical stimulation device, and urinary diversion.

Many factors are considered when selecting a bladder management strategy. These include upper extremity function, caregiver burden, and lifestyle choices. The type of bladder dysfunction also defines treatment goals and management options. A

peutic recreation specialists, prosthetists, orthotists, and dietitians. Rehabilitation care is organized around the individual patient's goals and needs. During rehabilitation, patients are expected to be involved in therapies and learn self-care for several hours each day. Such intensive work at a time when the patient is dealing with the sudden change in health and functional status can be very stressful. Progress may be slow, and frequent encouragement may be required. The rehabilitation nurse has a pivotal role in providing encouragement, specialized nursing care, patient and family teaching, and helping to coordinate the efforts of the rehabilitation team.

Respiratory rehabilitation. The patient with high cervical spinal cord injury may have greatly increased mobility with phrenic nerve stimulators or electronic diaphragmatic pacemakers. These devices are not appropriate for all ventilator-dependent patients but may be helpful for those with an intact phrenic nerve. Today, ventilators are also reasonably portable, and ventilator-dependent tetraplegic patients can be mobile and somewhat independent. Patients and family members should be taught all aspects of home ventilator care, and referrals should be made to appropriate community agencies. Patients with cervical level injuries

TABLE 59-8   Types of Neurogenic Bladder

TYPE	CHARACTERISTICS	CAUSES	CLINICAL MANIFESTATIONS
Reflexic (spastic, uninhibited, upper motor neuron)	No inhibitions influence time and place of voiding; bladder empties in response to stretching of bladder wall	Corticospinal tract lesion; observed in spinal cord injury, stroke, multiple sclerosis, brain tumor, brain trauma	Incontinence, frequency, urgency; voiding is unpredictable and incomplete
Areflexic (autonomous, flaccid, lower motor neuron)	Bladder acts as if there were paralysis of all motor functions, fills without emptying	Lower motor neuron lesion caused by trauma involving S2-S4; lesions of cauda equina, pelvic nerves	If sensory function intact, feels bladder distention and hesitancy; no control of micturition, resulting in overdistention of bladder and overflow incontinence
Sensory	Lack of sensation of need to urinate	Damage to sensory limb of bladder spinal reflex arc; seen in multiple sclerosis, diabetes mellitus	Poor bladder sensation, infrequent voiding, large residual volume

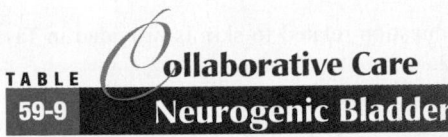

TABLE 59-9 Collaborative Care
Neurogenic Bladder

Diagnostic
History and physical examination including neurologic examination
Urodynamic testing
IV pyelogram
Urine culture

Collaborative Therapy
Drug therapy
Suppress bladder contractions (anticholinergics)
Relaxation of urethral sphincter (α-adrenergic blockers)
Suppress pelvic floor spasticity (baclofen [Lioresal])
Fluid intake of 1800 to 2000 ml/day
Urine drainage
Voluntary or reflex voiding
Intermittent catheterization
Indwelling catheter
Surgery
Sphincterotomy
Electrical stimulation
Urinary diversion

IV, Intravenous.

reflexic bladder with detrusor and sphincter dyssynergia requires interventions to provide low-pressure storage, low-pressure voiding, and adequate emptying. Anticholinergic drugs (oxybutynin [Ditropan], tolterodine [Detrol]) may be used to suppress bladder contraction. α-Adrenergic blockers (e.g., terazosin [Hytrin], doxazosin [Cardura]) may be used to decrease outflow resistance at the bladder neck, and antispasmodic drugs (e.g., baclofen [Lioresal] may be used to decrease spasticity of pelvic floor muscles.

Drainage options include intermittent catheterization, external catheter, or indwelling catheter. A reflexic bladder with detrusor hyperreflexia may be treated with anticholinergic drugs, intravesical capsaicin, or botulinum A toxin. An areflexic bladder is usually managed with intermittent catheterization or indwelling catheter.

The long-term use of an indwelling catheter should be carefully evaluated because of the associated high incidence of UTI, fistula formation, and diverticula. However, there may be patients for whom this is the best option. Adequate fluid intake and patency of the catheter should be ensured. The frequency of routine catheter changes ranges from 1 week to 1 month, depending on the type of catheter used and agency policy.

Intermittent catheterization is the most commonly recommended method of bladder management (see Chapter 44). Nursing assessment is important in selecting the time interval between catheterizations. Initially, catheterization is done every 4 hours. Bladder volume can be assessed before catheterization using the portable bladder ultrasound machine. If less than 200 ml of urine is measured, the time interval may be extended. If 500 ml or more of urine is measured, the time interval is shortened. An overdistended bladder can cause ischemia of the bladder wall, which may predispose tissues to bacterial invasion and infection. Patients often experience diuresis at a regular time during a 24-hour period. The number of intermittent catheterizations per day is usually five or six.

Urinary diversion surgery may be necessary if the patient has repeated UTIs with renal involvement or repeated stones or if therapeutic intervention has been unsuccessful (see Chapter 44). Surgical treatment of neurogenic bladder includes bladder neck revision (sphincterotomy), bladder augmentation (augmentation cystoplasty), penile prosthesis, artificial sphincter, perineal ureterostomy, cystotomy, vesicotomy, and anterior urethral transplantation.

No matter which bladder management strategy is selected, the nurse must teach the patient and the family or caregivers about how to accomplish successful self-management. Management techniques, how to obtain necessary supplies, care of supplies and equipment, and when to seek health care must be taught. Resources and referrals for supplies and ongoing care must be arranged.

Neurogenic bowel. Careful management of bowel evacuation is necessary in the patient with a spinal cord injury because voluntary control of this function may be lost as a result of a condition called **neurogenic bowel.** The usual measures for preventing constipation include a high-fiber diet and adequate fluid intake (see Table 41-9). Patient and family teaching guidelines related to bowel management are presented in Table 59-10. However, these measures by themselves may not be adequate to stimulate evacuation. In addition, suppositories (bisacodyl [Dulcolax] or glycerin) or small-volume enemas and digital stimulation by the nurse or patient may be necessary. In the patient with an upper motor neuron lesion, digital stimulation is necessary to relax the external sphincter to promote defecation. A stool softener such as docusate sodium (Colace) can be used to regulate stool consistency. Oral stimulant laxatives should be used only if absolutely necessary for a day or two and not on a regular basis.

Valsalva maneuver and manual stimulation are useful in patients with lower motor neuron lesions. The Valsalva maneuver requires intact abdominal muscles, so it is used in those patients with injuries below T12. In general, a bowel movement every other day is considered adequate. However, preinjury patterns should be considered. Incontinence can result from too much stool softener or a fecal impaction.

Careful recording of bowel movements, including amount, time, and consistency, is important to the overall success of the program. Timing of defecation may also be an important factor. If bowel evacuation is planned for 30 to 60 minutes following the first meal of the day, this may enhance success by taking advantage of the gastrocolic reflex induced by eating. Again, patient and family education is required to promote successful independent bowel management.

Neurogenic skin. Prevention of pressure ulcers and other types of injury to insensitive skin are essential for every patient with spinal cord injury. Nurses in rehabilitation are responsible for teaching these skills and providing information about daily skin care. A comprehensive visual and tactile examination of the skin should be done twice daily with special attention given to areas over bony prominences. The areas most vulnerable to breakdown include the ischia, trochanters, heels, and the sacrum. Careful positioning and repositioning should be done initially every 2 hours with gradual increases in the times between turns if there is no redness over bony prominences at the time of turning. Pressure-relieving cushions must be used in wheelchairs, and special

TABLE 59-10 Patient & Family Teaching Guide
Bowel Management after Spinal Cord Injury

The following are teaching guidelines for a patient with a spinal cord injury:

1. Optimal nutritional intake includes:
   Three well-balanced meals each day
   Two servings from the milk group
   Two or more servings from the meat group, including beef, pork, poultry, eggs, fish
   Four or more servings from the vegetable and fruit groups
   Four or more servings from the bread and cereal group
2. Fiber intake should be approximately 20 to 30 g per day. The amount of fiber eaten should be increased gradually over 1 to 2 weeks.
3. Three quarts of fluid per day should be consumed unless contraindicated. Water or fruit juices should be used, and caffeinated beverages such as coffee, tea, and cola should be avoided. Fluid softens hard stools; caffeine stimulates fluid loss through urination.
4. Foods that produce gas (e.g., beans) or upper GI upset (spicy foods) should be avoided.
5. *Timing*: A regular schedule for bowel evacuation should be established. A good time is 30 minutes after the first meal of the day.
6. *Position*: If possible, an upright position with feet flat on the floor or on a stepstool enhances bowel evacuation. Staying on the toilet, commode, or bedpan for longer than 20 to 30 minutes may cause skin breakdown. Based on stability, someone may need to stay with the patient.
7. *Activity*: Exercise is important for bowel function. In addition to improving muscle tone, it also increases GI transit time and increases appetite. Muscles should be exercised. This includes stretching, range-of-motion, position changing, and functional movement.
8. *Drug treatment*: Suppositories may be necessary to stimulate a bowel movement. Manual stimulation of the rectum may also be helpful in initiating defecation. Stool softeners should be used as needed to regulate stool consistency. Oral laxatives should be used only if necessary.

GI, Gastrointestinal.

mattresses may also be needed. Movement during turns and transfers should be done carefully to avoid stretching and folding of soft tissues (shear), as well as friction or abrasion.[27]

Nutritional status should be assessed regularly. Both body weight loss and weight gain can contribute to skin breakdown. Adequate intake of protein is essential for skin health. Measurement of prealbumin, total protein, and albumin can help identify inadequate protein intake. The importance of nutrition to skin health should be stressed to the patient and family.

Protection of the skin also requires avoidance of thermal injury. Burns can be caused by hot food or liquids, bath or shower water that is too warm, radiators, heating pads, and uninsulated plumbing. Thermal injury also can result from extreme cold (frostbite). Injuries may not be noticed until severe damage is done. Anticipatory guidance about potential risks is essential.

Patient and family education related to skin is provided in Tables 59-11 and 59-12.

Sexuality. Knowledge of the level and completeness of injury is needed to understand the male patient's potential for orgasm, erection, and fertility and the patient's capacity for sexual satisfaction (Table 59-13). Sexuality is an important issue regardless of the patient's age or gender. To provide accurate and sensitive counseling and education about sexuality, the nurse must have an awareness and an acceptance of personal sexuality, as well as knowledge of human sexual responses. When discussing sexual potential, the nurse should use scientific terminology rather than slang whenever possible.

Reflex sexual function capability is possible if the patient has an upper motor neuron lesion. The presence of tone in the external rectal sphincter indicates an upper motor lesion. The absence of external rectal sphincter tone, bulbocavernosus reflex, or both indicates that the patient has lower motor neuron involvement and may be capable of psychogenic erection but not reflex erection. If ejaculation occurs, it may be retrograde into the bladder.

The type of lesion determines the physical sexual response. Men with upper motor neuron lesions may have reflexogenic erections that are produced by reflex activity or external stimuli or that occur spontaneously. These spontaneous erections are often short lived and uncontrolled and cannot be maintained or summoned at the time of coitus. Orgasm and ejaculation are usually not possible for men with a complete upper motor neuron lesion.

Most patients with a complete lower motor neuron lesion are unable to have either psychogenic or reflexogenic erections. Patients with incomplete lower motor neuron lesions have the highest possibility of successful psychogenic erection with ejaculation, and up to 10% of these patients are fertile.

Treatments for erectile dysfunction include drugs, vacuum devices, and surgical procedures. Sildenafil (Viagra) has become the treatment of choice since several studies have documented its effectiveness in men with spinal cord injury. Penile injection of vasoactive substances (papaverine, prostaglandin E) is another

TABLE 59-11 Patient & Family Teaching Guide
Skin Care for Patient with Spinal Cord Injury

Skin breakdown is a potential problem after spinal cord injury. The following measures are used to decrease this possibility:
Change Position Frequently
- If in a wheelchair, lift self up and shift weight every 15 to 30 minutes.
- If in bed, a regular turning schedule (at least every 2 hours) that includes sides, back, and abdomen is encouraged to change position.
- Use special mattresses and wheelchair cushions.
- Use pillows to protect bony prominences when in bed.
Monitor Skin Condition
- Inspect skin frequently for areas of redness, swelling, and breakdown.
- Keep fingernails trimmed to avoid scratches and abrasions.
- If a wound develops, follow standard wound care management procedures.

medical treatment. Risks include *priapism* (prolonged penile erection) and scarring, so these substances are often considered only after failure of sildenafil. Vacuum suction devices use negative pressure to encourage blood flow into the penis. Erection is maintained by a constriction band placed at the base of the penis.

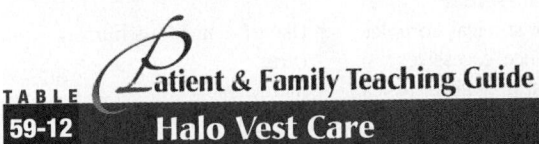

TABLE	*P*atient & Family Teaching Guide
59-12	**Halo Vest Care**

The following are teaching guidelines for a patient with a halo vest:

1. Inspect the pins on the halo traction ring. Report to health care provider if pins are loose or if there are signs of infection including redness, tenderness, swelling, or drainage at the insertion sites.
2. Clean around pin sites carefully with hydrogen peroxide on a cotton swab. Repeat the procedure using water.
3. Use alcohol swabs to cleanse pin sites of any drainage.
4. Apply antibiotic ointment as prescribed.
5. To provide skin care, have the patient lie down on a bed with his or her head resting on a pillow to reduce pressure on the brace. Loosen one side of the vest. Gently wash the skin under the vest with soap and water, rinse it, and then dry it thoroughly. At the same time, check the skin for pressure points, redness, swelling, bruising, or chafing. Close the open side and repeat the procedure on the opposite side.
6. If the vest becomes wet or damp, it can be carefully dried with a blow dryer.
7. An assistive device (e.g., cane, walker) may be used to provide greater balance. Flat shoes should be worn.
8. Turn the entire body, not just the head and neck, when trying to view sideways.
9. In case of an emergency, keep a set of wrenches close to the halo vest at all times.
10. Mark the vest strap such that consistent buckling and fit can be maintained.
11. Avoid grabbing bars or vest to assist patient.
12. Keep sheepskin pad under vest. Change and wash at least weekly.
13. If perspiration or itching is a problem, a cotton T-shirt can be worn under sheepskin. The T-shirt can be modified with Velcro seam closure on one side.

The main surgical option is implantation of a penile prosthesis.[28] (Erectile dysfunction is discussed in Chapter 53.)

Male fertility is affected by spinal cord injury causing poor sperm quality and ejaculatory dysfunction. Recent advances in methods of retrieving sperm (penile vibratory stimulation and electroejaculation) combined with ovulation induction and intrauterine insemination of the female partner have changed the prognosis for men with spinal cord injury to father children from unlikely to a reasonable possibility of successful outcomes.[29]

The effect of spinal cord injury on female sexual response is less clear. Lubrication is similar to erections in males, with reflex and psychogenic components. Women with upper motor neuron injuries may retain the capacity for reflex lubrication, whereas psychogenic lubrication depends on the completeness of injury. Orgasm is reported by about 50% of women with spinal cord injury.[29]

The woman of childbearing age with a spinal cord injury usually remains fertile. The injury does not affect the ability to become pregnant or to deliver normally through the birth canal. Menses may cease for as long as 6 months. If sexual activity is resumed, protection against an unplanned pregnancy is necessary. A normal pregnancy may be complicated by UTIs, anemia, and autonomic dysreflexia. Because uterine contractions are not felt, a precipitous delivery is always a danger.

Sexual rehabilitation for both men and women should begin informally after the acute phase of the injury has passed. Questions such as, "Have you had an erection since your accident?" and "Have your menstrual periods continued since the accident?" are nonthreatening ways to introduce the topic of sexual functioning. The male patient may pose a question such as, "Can I ever be a man again?"

Open discussion with the patient is essential. This important aspect of rehabilitation should be handled by someone specially trained in sexual counseling. A nurse or other rehabilitation professional with such expertise works with the patient and partner to provide support with the emphasis on open communication. The nurse's educational role requires respect for every couple's personal standards of religious and cultural beliefs. Alternative methods of obtaining sexual satisfaction such as oral-genital sex (cunnilingus and fellatio) may be suggested. Explicit films (e.g., *Touching*) may also be used. This film demonstrates the sexual activities of a patient with paraplegia and a nondisabled partner. Graphics should be used cautiously because they may be too lim-

TABLE 59-13	Potential for Sexual Function in Men with Spinal Cord Injury		
ERECTION	**EJACULATION**		**ORGASM**
Upper Motor Neuron			
Complete			
Frequent (92%), reflexogenic only	Rare (4%)		Rare
Incomplete			
Most frequent (99%) including reflexogenic (80%) and psychogenic (19%)	Less frequent (32%), after reflexogenic erection (74%), after psychogenic erection (26%)		Present (if ejaculation occurs)
Lower Motor Neuron			
Complete			
Infrequent (26%)	Infrequent (18%)		Present (if ejaculation occurs)
Incomplete			
Psychogenic and reflexogenic	Frequent (70%), after psychogenic and reflexogenic erections		Present (if ejaculation occurs)

iting or focus too much on the mechanics of sex rather than on the relationship.

Sexual activities may require more planning and be less spontaneous than before the injury. For example, an attendant may have to undress the patient and remove equipment. A relaxed atmosphere with music and perfume creates an attractive environment. Ample time for caressing, fondling, and kissing is essential. The partners should be encouraged to explore each other's erogenous areas, such as the lips, neck, and ears, which can arouse psychogenic erection or orgasm. Few demands should be made initially.

Care should be taken not to dislodge an indwelling catheter during sexual activity. If an external catheter is used, it should be removed before sexual activity and the patient should refrain from fluids. The bowel program should include evacuation the morning of sexual activity. The partner should be informed that an accident is always possible. The woman may need a water-soluble lubricant to supplement diminished vaginal secretions and facilitate vaginal penetration.

Grief and depression. Patients with spinal cord injuries may feel an overwhelming sense of loss. They may temporarily lose control over everyday life activities and must depend on others for ADLs and for life-sustaining measures. Patients may believe that they are useless and burdens to their families. At a stage when independence is often of the greatest importance, they may be totally dependent on others.

The patient's response and recovery differ in some important aspects from those experiencing loss from amputation or terminal illness. First, regression can and does occur at different stages. Working through grief is a difficult, lifelong process with which the patient needs support and encouragement. With recent advances in rehabilitation, it is usual for the patient to be independent physically and discharged from the rehabilitation center before completion of the grief process. The goal of recovery is related more to adjustment than to acceptance. Adjustment implies the ability to go on with living with certain limitations. Although the patient who is cooperative and accepting is easier to treat, the nurse should expect a wide fluctuation of emotions from a patient with a spinal cord injury. Depression may not be a component of the recovery process. Societal norms allow depression after severe loss and almost impose it on those confronted with death or radical lifestyle changes. However, every patient may not experience depression.

The nurse's role in grief work is to allow mourning as a component of the rehabilitation process. Table 59-14 summarizes the mourning process and appropriate nursing interventions. Maintaining hope is an important strategy during the grieving process and should not be interpreted as denial. During the shock and denial stage the nurse reassures the patient and stresses the expertise of the entire health care team. During the anger stage, the nurse assists the patient in achievement of control over the environment, particularly by allowing the patient's input into the plan of care. The nurse should not respond to anger or manipulation or become involved in a power struggle with the patient. As self-care abilities increase, the patient's independence increases.

The patient's family also requires counseling to avoid promoting dependency in the patient through guilt or misplaced sympathy. The family is also experiencing an intense grieving process. A support group of family members and friends of patients with

TABLE 59-14 Mourning Process and Nursing Interventions in Spinal Cord Injury

PATIENT BEHAVIOR	NURSING INTERVENTION
Shock and Denial Struggle for survival, complete dependence, excessive sleep, withdrawal, fantasies, unrealistic expectations	• Use of meticulous nursing care. • Be honest. • Use simple diagrams to explain injury. • Encourage patient to begin road to recovery. • Establish agreement to use and improve all current abilities while not denying the possibility of future improvement.
Anger Refusal to discuss paralysis, decreased self-esteem, manipulation, hostile and abusive language	• Coordinate care with patient and encourage self-care. • Support family members; prevent alleviation of guilt by supporting dependency. • Use humor liberally. • Allow patient outbursts. • Do not allow fixation on injury.
Depression Sadness, pessimism, anorexia, nightmares, insomnia, agitation, psychomotor retardation, "blues," suicidal preoccupation, refusal to participate in any self-care activities	• Encourage family involvement and resources. • Plan graded steps in rehabilitation to give success with minimal opportunity for frustration. • Give cheerful and willing assistance with activities of daily living. • Avoid sympathy. • Use firm kindness.
Adjustment Planning for future, active participation in therapy, finding of personal meaning in experience and continuation of growth, return to premorbid personality	• Remember that patients have individual personalities. • Balance support systems to encourage independence. • Set goals with patient input. • Emphasize potentials.

spinal cord injury can help increase family members' knowledge and participation in the grieving process, physical difficulties, rehabilitation plan, and the meaning of the disability in society.

During the stage of depression, the nurse must be patient and persistent and maintain a sense of humor. Sympathy is not helpful. The patient should be treated in an adult manner and be involved in decision making about care, but the nurse must insist that the care be performed. A primary nurse relationship is helpful. Staff planning and sessions in which staff members can express their feelings are helpful in providing consistency of care. To achieve the stage of adjustment, the patient needs continual support throughout the rehabilitation process in the forms of acceptance, affection, and caring. The nurse must be attentive when the patient needs to talk and sensitive to needs at the various stages of the grief process.

Although the stage of depression during the grief process usually lasts days to weeks, there are some individuals who may become clinically depressed and require treatment for depression. Evaluation by a psychiatric nurse or psychiatrist is recommended. Treatment may include drugs and psychotherapy.[30]

■ Evaluation

Expected outcomes for the patient with a spinal cord injury are presented in NCP 59-1 on p. 1619.

■ Gerontologic Considerations: Spinal Cord Injury

The demographics of patients living with spinal cord injury are changing. The fact that persons with spinal cord injury now have longer life spans has contributed to the increasing number of older adults living with spinal cord injury. Aging is also associated with an increased likelihood of other chronic illnesses that may have a serious impact on the older adult with a spinal cord injury. As patients with spinal cord injury age, both individual aging changes and duration since injury impact functional ability. For example, bowel and bladder dysfunction can increase with duration and severity of spinal cord injury. Musculoskeletal repetitive trauma injuries are more common.

Health promotion and screening are important for the older patient with a spinal cord injury. Daily skin inspections, UTI prevention measures, and monthly breast exams for women and regular prostate cancer screening for men are recommended. Cardiovascular disease is the most common cause of morbidity and mortality among spinal cord–injured persons. The lack of sensation including angina in those with high level injuries may mask acute myocardial ischemia. Altered autonomic nervous system function and decreases in physical activity can place the patient at risk for cardiovascular problems including hypertension.[31]

At the same time, because of increased work and recreational activities of older adults, more older adults are experiencing spinal cord injury. Health promotion to decrease injury risk includes fall prevention strategies (e.g., using a stepstool or a grab bar to reach high shelves, handrails on stairs). Rehabilitation for the older person who has undergone a spinal cord injury may likely take longer because of other preexisting conditions and poorer health status at the time of the initial injury. ■

SPINAL CORD TUMORS

Etiology and Pathophysiology

Tumors that affect the spinal cord account for 0.5% to 1% of all neoplasms. These tumors are classified as primary (arising from some component of cord, dura, nerves, or vessels) or secondary (from primary growths in the breast, thyroid, lung, kidney, and other sites). Spinal cord tumors are further classified as extradural (outside the spinal cord), intradural extramedullary (within the dura but outside the actual spinal cord), and intradural intramedullary (within the spinal cord itself). These latter tumors are usually astrocytomas or ependy-

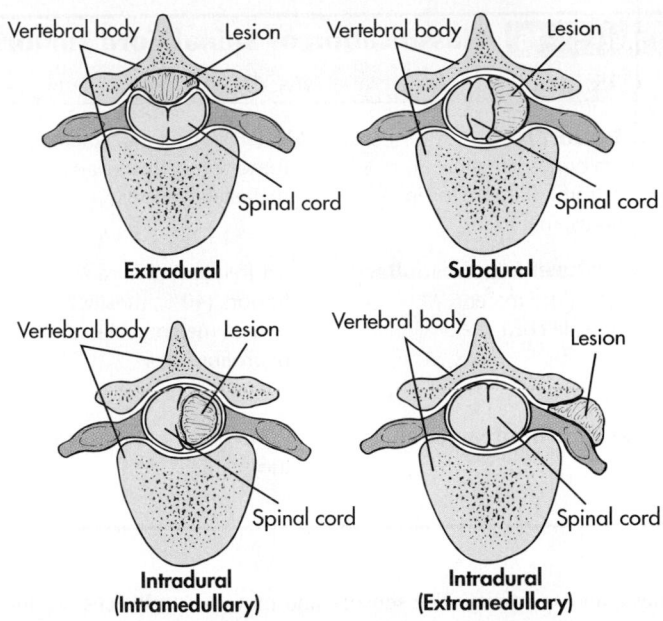

FIG. 59-14 Types of spinal cord tumors.

momas (Fig. 59-14, Table 59-15). Approximately 90% of all spinal tumors are extradural. Extradural tumors are usually metastatic and most often arise in the vertebral bodies. These metastatic lesions can invade intradurally and compress the spinal cord. Spinal intradural-extramedullary tumors account for two thirds of all intraspinal neoplasms and are mainly represented by meningiomas and schwannomas.

Because many of these tumors are slow growing, their symptoms stem from the mechanical effects of slow compression and irritation of nerve roots, displacement of the cord, or gradual obstruction of the vascular supply. The slowness of growth does not cause autodestruction (secondary injury) as in traumatic lesions. Therefore complete functional restoration may be possible when the tumor is removed, except with the intradural-intramedullary tumors.

Most metastatic tumors are extradural lesions. Tumors that commonly metastasize to the spinal epidural space are those that spread to bone, such as carcinomas of the breast, lung, prostate, and kidney.

Clinical Manifestations

Both sensory and motor problems may result with the location and extent of the tumor determining the severity and distribution of the problem. The most common early symptom of a spinal cord tumor outside the cord is pain in the back with radicular pain simulating intercostal neuralgia, angina, or herpes zoster. The location of the pain depends on the level of compression. The pain worsens with activity, coughing, straining, and lying down. Sensory disruption is later manifested by coldness, numbness, and tingling in an extremity or in several extremities, slowly progressing upward until it reaches the level of the lesion. Impaired sensation of pain, temperature, and light touch precedes a deficit in vibration and position sense that may progress to complete anesthesia. Motor weakness accompanies the sensory disturbances and consists of slowly increasing clumsiness, weak-

TABLE 59-15   Classification of Spinal Cord Tumors

TYPE	INCIDENCE	TREATMENT	PROGNOSIS
Extradural From bones of spine, in extradural space, or in paraspinal tissue	20%–50% of all intraspinal tumors, mostly malignant metastatic lesions	Relief of cord pressure by surgical laminectomy, radiation, chemotherapy, or combination approach	Poor
Intradural Extramedullary Within dura mater outside cord	Most frequent of intradural tumors (40%), mostly benign meningiomas and neurofibromas	Complete surgical removal of tumor (if possible), partial removal followed by radiation	Usually very good if lack of damage to cord from compression
Intradural Intramedullary	Least frequent of intradural tumors (5%–10%)	Partial surgical removal, radiation therapy (resulting in only temporary improvement)	Very poor

ness, and spasticity. The sensory and motor disturbances are ipsilateral to the lesion. Bladder disturbances are marked by urgency with difficulty in starting the flow and progressing to retention with overflow incontinence.

Manifestations of intradural spinal tumor develop as progressive damage to the long spinal tracts, producing paralysis, sensory loss, and bladder dysfunction. Pain can be severe as a result of compression of spinal roots or vertebrae.

NURSING *and* COLLABORATIVE MANAGEMENT SPINAL CORD TUMORS

Extradural tumors are seen early on routine spinal x-rays, whereas intradural and intramedullary tumors require MRI or CT scans for detection. CSF analysis may reveal tumor cells. The cord is decompressed after removal of the tumor by a laminectomy. More than 85% of primary neoplasms are benign and can be completely resected; 90% of patients recover without residual problems.

Compression of the spinal cord is an emergency. Relief of the ischemia related to the compression is the goal of therapy. Corticosteroids are generally prescribed immediately to relieve tumor-

related edema. Dexamethasone (Decadron) is usually used, often in large doses.

Treatment for nearly all spinal cord tumors is surgical removal. The exception is the metastatic tumor that is sensitive to radiation and that has caused only minimal neurologic deficits in the patient. In general, tumors of the extradural or intradural-extramedullary group can be completely removed surgically. Intramedullary tumors offer a less favorable prognosis; however, exploration and removal are usually attempted.

Radiation therapy after the operation is fairly effective. Maximum permissible tissue dose is given over 6 to 8 weeks. Chemotherapy has also been used in conjunction with radiation therapy.

Relief of pain and return of function are the ultimate goals of treatment. Nurses must be aware of the neurologic status of the patient before and after treatment. Ensuring that the patient receives pain medication as needed is an important nursing responsibility. Depending on the amount of neurologic dysfunction exhibited, the patient may need to be cared for as though recovering from a spinal cord injury. Rehabilitation of patients with spinal cord tumors is similar to spinal cord injury rehabilitation.[32]

CRITICAL THINKING EXERCISES

Case Study
Spinal Cord Injury

Patient Profile. Samuel D., a 25-year-old white man, is admitted to the emergency department with the diagnosis of a cervical spinal cord injury. Samuel was swimming at a neighbor's backyard pool. He dove into the shallow end, striking his head on the bottom of the pool. His friends noticed that he did not resurface. They rescued him and brought him to the side of the pool. They maintained neck immobilization until the rescue crews arrived.

Subjective Data
- Is awake and alert
- Has complaints of neck pain
- Is anxious and asking why he cannot move his legs
- Is asking to see his family

Objective Data
Physical Examination
- Weak biceps movement
- No triceps movement
- Gross elbow movement present
- Decreased sensation from the shoulders down
- No bladder or bowel control
- BP: 90/56; pulse: 56; respirations: 32 and labored

Diagnostic Studies
- X-rays revealed C5 fracture dislocation

Collaborative Care
- Placed in tongs and traction in the emergency department
- Started on methylprednisolone in the emergency department
- Admitted to ICU

CRITICAL THINKING EXERCISES—cont'd

CRITICAL THINKING QUESTIONS

1. What nursing activities would be a priority on Samuel D.'s arrival in the ICU?
2. What physiologic problems are causing Samuel D. to have hypotension and bradycardia?
3. What would the first line of treatment be for Samuel D.'s hypotension and bradycardia?
4. What signs and symptoms would indicate respiratory distress and what physiologic problem would cause respiratory distress in Samuel D.'s injury state?
5. What can the nurse do to decrease Samuel D.'s anxiety?
6. Based on the assessment data provided, write one or more nursing diagnoses. Are there any collaborative problems?

Nursing Research Issues

1. What is the best method of education in the prevention of spinal cord injuries?
2. What type of support or education is best for the families of patients with spinal cord injuries to help them cope with their situation?
3. What nursing interventions enhance self-care in the patient with a spinal cord injury?
4. What is the best method of preventing UTIs in the spinal cord injured patient?
5. What is the relationship between the functional ability of spinal cord injury and quality of life?

REVIEW QUESTIONS

The number of the question corresponds to the same-numbered objective at the beginning of the chapter.

1. During assessment of the patient with trigeminal neuralgia, the nurse should
   a. inspect all aspects of the mouth and teeth.
   b. lightly palpate the affected side of the face for edema.
   c. test for temperature and sensation perception on the face.
   d. ask the patient to describe factors that initiate an episode.
2. During routine assessment of a patient with Guillain-Barré syndrome, the nurse finds the patient to be short of breath. The patient's respiratory distress is caused by
   a. elevated protein levels in the CSF.
   b. immobility resulting from ascending paralysis.
   c. degeneration of motor neurons in the brainstem and spinal cord.
   d. paralysis ascending to the nerves that stimulate the thoracic area.
3. A patient is admitted to the ICU with a C7 spinal cord injury and diagnosed with Brown-Séquard syndrome. On physical examination, the nurse would most likely find
   a. upper extremity weakness only.
   b. complete motor and sensory loss below C7.
   c. loss of position sense and vibration in both lower extremities.
   d. ipsilateral motor loss and contralateral sensory loss below C7.
4. A patient is admitted to the hospital with a spinal cord injury following an automobile accident. The nurse recognizes that the pathophysiology of secondary spinal cord injury involves
   a. initial infarction of the white matter of the cord.
   b. mechanical transection of the cord by the trauma.
   c. necrotic destruction of the cord from hemorrhage and edema.
   d. release of epinephrine leading to massive vasodilation of spinal cord vessels.

5. A rehabilitation goal for the patient with an injury at the C5 level includes
   a. feeding self with hand devices.
   b. driving an electric wheelchair.
   c. assisting with transfer activities.
   d. controlling bowel and bladder functions.
6. A patient with a C7 spinal cord injury undergoing rehabilitation tells the nurse he must have the flu because he has a bad headache and nausea. The initial action of the nurse is to
   a. call the physician.
   b. check the patient's temperature.
   c. take the patient's blood pressure.
   d. elevate the head of the bed to 90 degrees.
7. For a 65-year-old female patient who has lived with a T1 spinal cord injury for 20 years, the nurse would emphasize the following health teaching information:
   a. A mammogram is needed every year.
   b. Bladder function tends to improve with age.
   c. Heart disease is not common in persons with spinal cord injury.
   d. As a person ages, the need to change body position is less important.
8. The most common early symptom of a spinal cord tumor is
   a. urinary incontinence.
   b. back pain that worsens with activity.
   c. paralysis below the level of involvement.
   d. impaired sensation of pain, temperature, and light touch.

REFERENCES

1. Rozen TD: Antiepileptic drugs in the management of cluster headache and trigeminal neuralgia, *Headache* 41:S25, 2001.
2. Peiper DR, Dickerson J, Hassenbusch SJ: Percutaneous retrogasserian glycerol rhizolysis for treatment of chronic intractable cluster headaches: long-term results, *Neurosurgery* 46:363, 2000.
3. Tronnier VM et al: Treatment of idiopathic trigeminal neuralgia: comparison of long-term outcome after radiofrequency rhizotomy and microvascular decompression, *Neurosurgery* 48:1261, 2001.
4. Grogan PM, Gronseth GS: Practice parameter: steroids, acyclovir, and surgery for Bell's palsy (an evidence-based review), *Neurology* 56:830, 2001.
5. Nachamkin I: Chronic effects of *Campylobacter* infection, *Microbes Infect* 4:399, 2002.
6. Willison HJ, O'Hanlon GM: The immunopathogenesis of Miller Fisher syndrome, *J Neuroimmunol* 100:3, 1999.
7. Hughes RA, van det Meche FG: Corticosteroids for treating Guillain-Barre syndrome, *Cochrane Database Syst Rev* 2:CD001446, 2000.
8. Centers for Disease Control and Prevention: Botulism. Available at *http://www.cdc.gov/nip/publications/pink/botulism* (accessed July 29, 2002).
9. Centers for Disease Control and Prevention: Tetanus. Available at *http://www.cdc.gov/nip/publications/pink/tetanus* (accessed July 29, 2002).
10. Hutto B: Syphilis in clinical psychiatry: a review, *Psychosomatics* 42:453, 2001.
11. Centers for Disease Control and Prevention: What you should know about spinal cord injuries. Available at *http://www.cdc.gov/safeusa/home/sci.htm* (accessed June 12, 2002).
12. Spinal cord injury facts and figures, May 2001. Available at *http://www.spinalcord.uab.edu* (accessed June 12, 2002).
13. Atrice MB et al: Traumatic spinal cord injury. In Umphred DA, editor: *Neurological rehabilitation*, ed 4, St Louis, 2001, Mosby.
14. Kirshblum SC, O'Connor KC: Levels of spinal cord injury and predictors of neurologic recovery, *Phys Med Rehabil Clin N Am* 11:1, 2000.
15. Nockels RP: Nonoperative management of acute spinal cord injury, *Spine* 26:531, 2001.
16. American Spinal Injury Association/International Medical Society of Paraplegic (ASIA/IMSOP): *International standards for neurological functional classification of spinal cord injury patients* (revised). Chicago, 2002, American Spinal Injury Association.
17. Kim V, Spandorfer J: Epidemiology of venous thromboembolic disease, *Emerg Med Clin North Am* 19:839, 2001.
18. Papadopoulos SM et al: Immediate spinal cord decompression for cervical spinal cord injury: feasibility and outcome, *J Trauma* 52:323, 2002.
19. Dumont RJ et al: Acute spinal cord injury, part II: contemporary pharmacotherapy. *Clin Neuropharmacol* 24:265, 2001.
20. Bracken MB, Holford TR: Neurological and functional status 1 year after acute spinal cord injury: estimates of functional recovery in National Acute Spinal Cord Injury Study II from results modeled in National Acute Spinal Cord Injury Study III, *J Neurosurg* 96:259, 2002.
21. Bracken MB: Steroids for acute spinal cord injury (Cochrane Review), *Cochrane Database Syst Rev* 3:CD001046, 2002.
22. Segal JL, Pathak MS: Optimal drug therapy and therapeutic drug monitoring after spinal cord injury: a population-specific approach, *Am J Ther* 8:451, 2001.
23. Ball PA: Critical care of spinal cord injury, *Spine* 26:S27, 2001.
24. Consortium for spinal cord medicine: neurogenic bowel management in adults with spinal cord injury, Clinical Practice Guidelines. Washington DC, 1998, Paralyzed Veterans of America.
25. Burchiel KJ, Hsu FPK: Pain and spasticity after spinal cord injury, *Spine* 26: S146, 2001.
26. Consortium for spinal cord medicine: Acute management of autonomic dysreflexia: individuals with spinal cord injury presenting to health-care facilities, *J Spinal Cord Med* 25:S67, 2002.
27. Consortium for spinal cord medicine: pressure ulcer prevention and treatment following spinal cord injury: a clinical practice guideline for health-care professionals, *J Spinal Cord Med* 24:S40, 2001.
28. Burns AS, Rivas DA, Dilunno JF: The management of neurogenic bladder and sexual dysfunction after spinal cord injury, *Spine* 26:S129, 2001.
29. Benevento BT, Sipski ML: Neurogenic bladder, neurogenic bowel, and sexual dysfunction in people with spinal cord injury, *Phys Ther* 82:601, 2001.
30. Consortium for spinal cord medicine: *Depression following spinal cord injury: a clinical practice guideline for primary care physicians,* Washington DC, 1998, Paralyzed Veterans of America.
31. Groah SL et al: Spinal cord injury medicine. 5. Preserving wellness and independence of the aging patient with spinal cord injury: a primary care approach for the rehabilitation medicine specialist, *Arch Phys Med Rehabil* 83:S82, 2002.
32. Kirshblum S et al: Rehabilitation of persons with central nervous system tumors, *Cancer* 92:1029, 2001.

RESOURCES

American Association of Spinal Cord Injury Nurses (AASCIN)
75-20 Astoria Boulevard
Jackson Heights, NY 11370-1177
718-803-3782
Fax: 718-803-0414
www.aascin.org

American Paraplegia Society
75-20 Astoria Boulevard
Jackson Heights, NY 11370
718-803-3782
Fax: 718-803-0414
www.apssci.org

Canadian Paraplegic Association
1101 prom. Prince of Wales Drive, Suite 230
Ottawa, ON
K2C 3W7 Canada
800-720-4933 or 613-723-1033
Fax: 613-723-1060
www.canparaplegic.org

Christopher Reeve Paralysis Foundation
500 Morris Avenue
Springfield, NJ 07081
800-225-0292 or 973-379-2690
Fax: 973-912-9433
www.christopherreeve.org

Guillain-Barré Syndrome Foundation International
P.O. Box 262
Wynnewood, PA 19096
610-667-0131
Fax: 610-667-7036
www.guillain-barre.com

National Institute of Neurological Disorders and Stroke (NINDS)
National Institutes of Health Neurological Institute
P.O. Box 5801
Bethesda, MD 20824
800-352-9424
www.ninds.nih.gov

National Rehabilitation Information Center (NARIC)
4200 Forbes Boulevard, Suite 202
Lanham, MD 20706
800-346-2742 or 301-459-5900
www.naric.com

National Spinal Cord Injury Association
6701 Democracy Boulevard, Suite 300-9
Bethesda, MD 20817
800-962-9629 or 301-588-6959
Fax: 301-588-9414
www.spinalcord.org

Paralyzed Veterans of America
801 18th Street NW
Washington, DC 20006-3517
800-424-8200
www.pva.org

Spinal Cord Society
19051 County Highway 1
Fergus Falls, MN 56537-7609
218-739-5252 or 739-5261
Fax: 218-739-5262
http://members.aol.com/scsweb

For additional Internet resources, see the website for this book at *http://www.evolve.elsevier.com/Lewis/medsurg.*

CHAPTER 60

NURSING ASSESSMENT
Musculoskeletal System

Dottie Roberts

LEARNING OBJECTIVES

1. Describe the gross anatomic and microscopic composition of bone.
2. Explain the classification system of joints and movements at synovial joints.
3. Describe the types and structure of muscle tissue.
4. Describe the functions of cartilage, muscles, ligaments, tendons, fascia, and bursae.
5. Describe age-related changes in the musculoskeletal system and differences in assessment findings.
6. Identify the significant subjective and objective data related to the musculoskeletal system that should be obtained from a patient.
7. Describe the appropriate techniques used in the physical assessment of the musculoskeletal system.
8. Differentiate normal from abnormal findings of a physical assessment of the musculoskeletal system.
9. Describe the purpose, significance of results, and nursing responsibilities related to diagnostic studies of the musculoskeletal system.

KEY TERMS

abduction (Table 60-3), p. 1643	flexion (Table 60-3), p. 1643
adduction (Table 60-3), p. 1643	isometric contractions, p. 1638
ankylosis (Table 60-6), p. 1644	isotonic contractions, p. 1638
arthrocentesis, p. 1648	kyphosis, (Table 60-6), p. 1644
arthroscopy, p. 1648	lordosis, (Table 60-6), p. 1644
atrophy (Table 60-6), p. 1644	motor end plate, p. 1638
contracture (Table 60-6), p. 1644	neuromuscular junction, p. 1638
crepitation (Table 60-6), p. 1644	scoliosis, p. 1644
extension (Table 60-3), p. 1643	x-ray, p. 1644

The unique structures of the musculoskeletal system allow human beings to complete complex movements in their interactions with the environment. The dexterity of the upper extremities enables an individual to perform complicated technical tasks, while stronger lower extremities allow mobility for varied activities. The musculoskeletal system is composed of voluntary muscle and five types of connective tissue: bones, cartilage, ligaments, tendons, and fascia.[1]

Resilient bone and cartilage absorb energy from any impact, minimizing the risk of injury to other body structures. However, this characteristic ability makes the musculoskeletal system itself particularly vulnerable to injury from external forces. Any damage to bone and related soft tissues can cause functional disruption for an individual. Deformity, alteration in body image, alteration in mobility, pain, or permanent disability may result from musculoskeletal injury.

STRUCTURES AND FUNCTIONS OF THE MUSCULOSKELETAL SYSTEM

Bone

Function. The main functions of bone are support, protection of internal organs, voluntary movement, blood cell production, and mineral storage.[2] Bones provide the supporting frame-

work that keeps the body from collapsing and also allow the body to bear weight. Bones also protect underlying vital organs and tissues. For example, the skull encloses the brain, the vertebrae surround the spinal cord, and the rib cage contains the lungs and heart. Bones serve as a point of attachment for muscles, which are connected to bones by tendons. Bones act as a lever for muscles, and movement occurs as a result of muscle contractions applied to these levers. Bones contain hematopoietic tissue for the production of red and white blood cells. Bones also serve as a site for storage of inorganic minerals such as calcium and phosphorus.

Bone was previously considered to be a static, inert substance. In reality, it is a dynamic tissue that continually changes form and composition. It contains both organic material (collagen) and inorganic material (calcium, phosphate). The internal and external growth and remodeling of bone are ongoing processes. Bone is classified according to structure as *cortical* (compact and dense) or *cancellous* (spongy).

Microscopic Structure. Cylinder-shaped structural units (*haversian* systems) fit closely together in compact bone, creating a dense bone structure (Fig. 60-1, *A*). Within the systems, the haversian canals run parallel to the bone's long axis and contain the blood vessels that travel to the bone's interior from the periosteum. Surrounding the haversian canals are concentric rings known as *lamellae*, which characterize mature bone. Smaller canals (*canaliculi*) extend from the haversian canals to the *lacunae*, where mature bone cells are embedded. Cancellous bone lacks the organized structure of cortical (compact) bone. The lamellae are not arranged in concentric rings but rather along the lines of maximum stress placed on the bone. Networks of bone tissue are filled with red or yellow marrow, and blood reaches the bone cells by passing through spaces in the marrow.

The three types of bone cells are osteoblasts, osteocytes, and osteoclasts. *Osteoblasts* synthesize organic bone matrix (collagen) and are the basic bone-forming cells. *Osteocytes* are the mature bone cells. *Osteoclasts* participate in bone remodeling by assisting in the breakdown of bone tissue. *Bone remodeling* is the removal of old bone by osteoclasts (*resorption*) and the deposi-

Reviewed by Helen L. Lamothe, RN, BSN, PHN, ONC, Nurse Consultant, Office Practice, Golden, Colo.

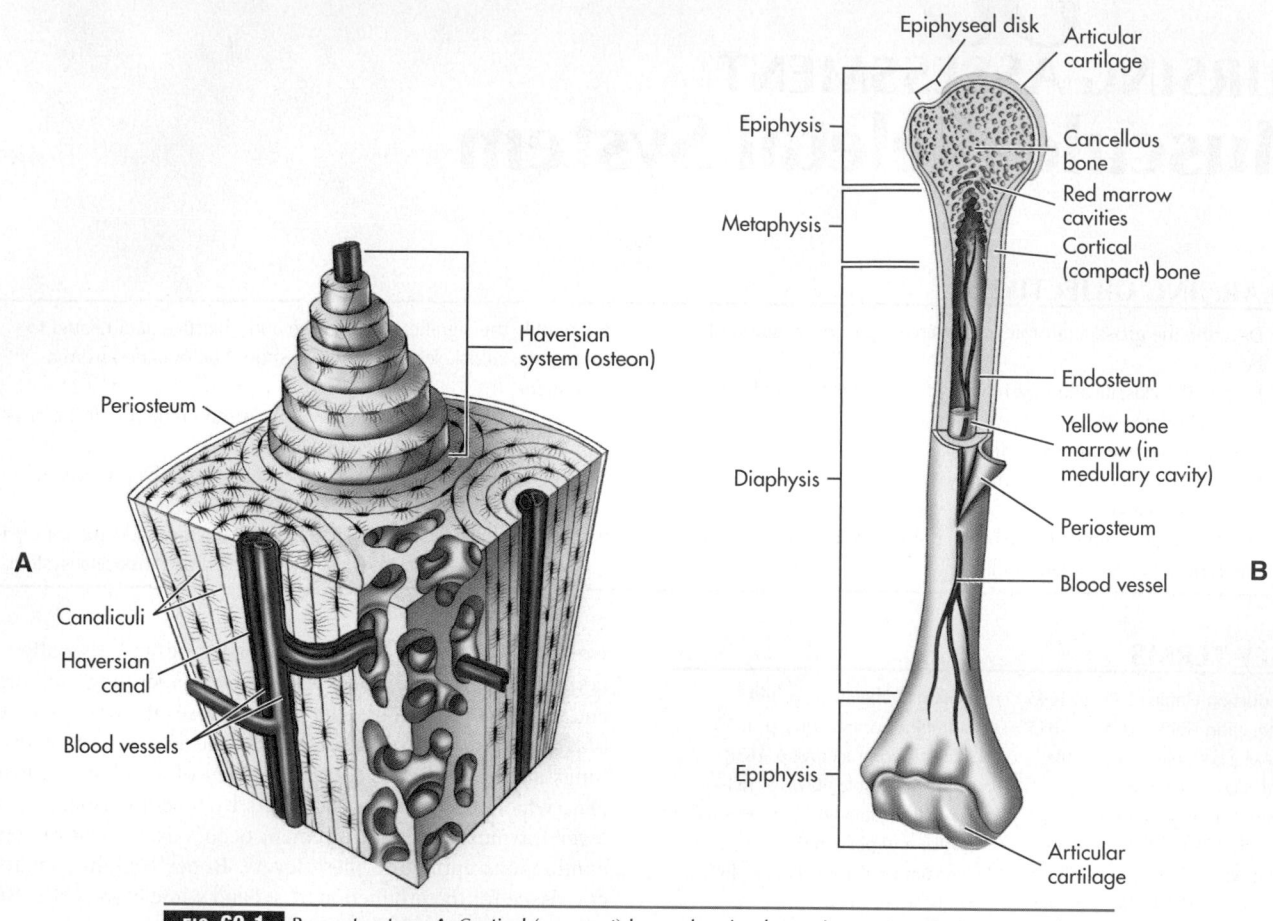

FIG. 60-1 Bone structure. **A**, Cortical (compact) bone showing haversian system. **B**, Anatomy of a long bone (humerus).

tion of new bone by osteoblasts (*ossification*). The inner layer of bone is primarily made up of osteoblasts with a few osteoclasts.

Gross Structure. The anatomic structure of bone is best represented by a typical long bone such as the humerus (see Fig. 60-1, *B*). Each long bone consists of the epiphysis, the diaphysis, and the metaphysis. The *epiphysis,* the widened area found at each end of a long bone, is composed primarily of cancellous bone. The wide epiphysis allows for greater weight distribution and provides stability for the joint. The epiphysis is also the location of muscle attachment. Articular cartilage covers the ends of the epiphysis to provide a smooth surface for joint movement. The *diaphysis* is the main shaft of the bone. It provides structural support and is composed of compact bone. The tubular structure of the diaphysis allows it to more easily withstand bending and twisting forces. The *metaphysis* is the flared area between the epiphysis and the diaphysis. Like the epiphysis, it is composed of cancellous bone. The *epiphyseal plate,* or growth zone, is the cartilaginous area between the epiphysis and metaphysis. It actively produces bone to allow longitudinal growth in children. Injury to the epiphyseal plate in a growing child can lead to a shorter extremity that can cause significant functional problems. In the adult, the metaphysis and epiphysis become joined as this plate hardens to mature bone.

The *periosteum* is composed of fibrous connective tissue that covers the bone. Tiny blood vessels penetrate the periosteum to provide nutrition to underlying bone. Musculotendinous fibers anchor to the outer layer of the periosteum. The inner layer of the periosteum is attached to the bone by bundles of collagen. No periosteum exists on the articular surfaces of long bones. These bone ends are covered by articular cartilage.

The medullary (marrow) cavity is in the center of the diaphysis and contains either red or yellow bone marrow.[3] In the growing child, red bone marrow is actively involved in hematopoiesis. In the adult, the medullary cavity of long bones contains yellow bone marrow, which is mainly adipose tissue. Yellow marrow will only be involved in hematopoiesis in times of great blood cell need. Blood cell production in the adult normally occurs in the red bone marrow of the skull, ribs, sternum, pelvis, vertebrae, and the shoulders.

Types. The skeleton consists of 206 bones, which are classified according to shape as long, short, flat, or irregular.

Long bones are characterized by a central shaft (diaphysis) and two widened ends (epiphyses) (Fig. 60-2). Examples include the femur, humerus, and radius. Short bones are composed of cancellous bone covered by a thin layer of compact bone. Examples include the carpals in the hand and the tarsals in the foot.

Flat bones have two layers of compact bone separated by a layer of cancellous bone. Examples include the ribs, skull, scapula, and sternum. The spaces in the cancellous bone contain

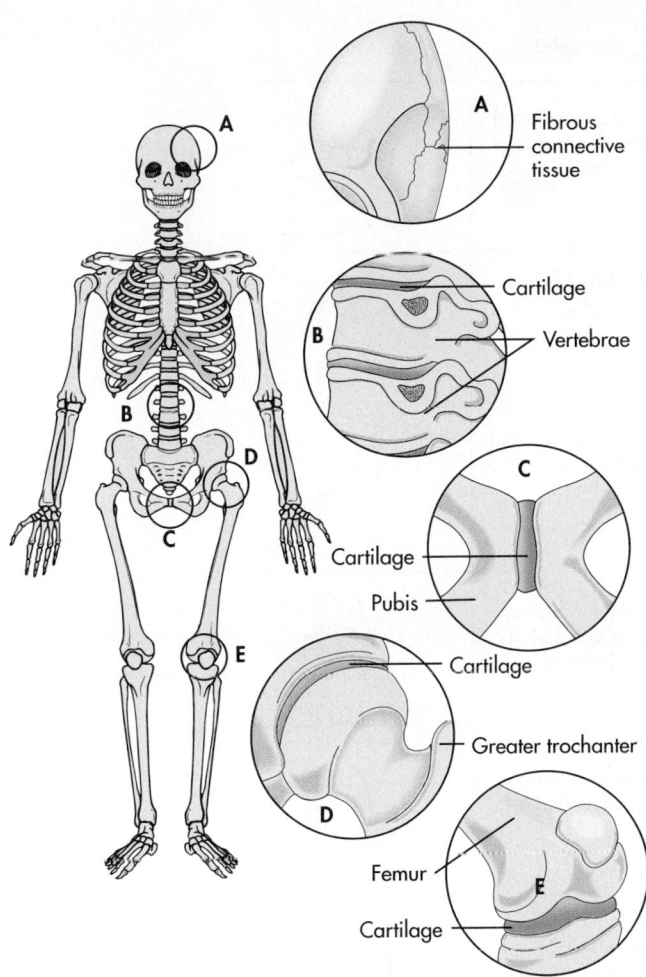

FIG. 60-2 | Classification of joints. A to C, Synarthrotic (immovable) and amphiarthrotic (slightly movable) joints. D and E, Diarthrodial (freely movable) joints.

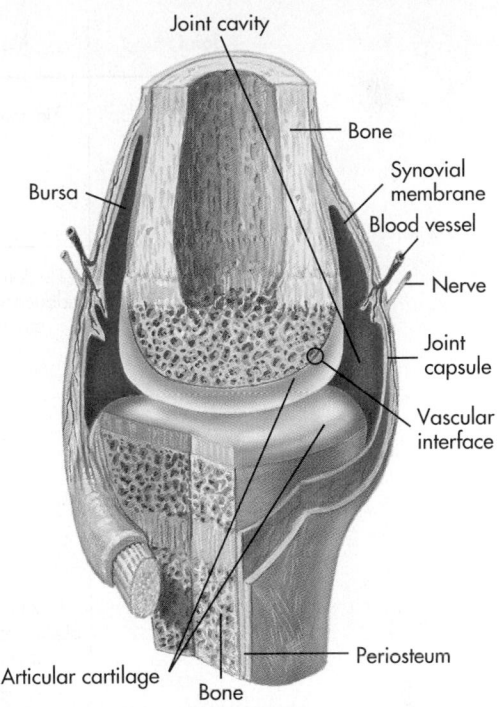

FIG. 60-3 | Structure of synovial joint.

bone marrow. Irregular bones appear in a variety of shapes and sizes. Examples include the vertebrae, sacrum, and mandible.

Joints

A *joint* (articulation) is a place where the ends of two bones are in proximity and move in relation to each other. Joints are classified according to the degree of movement that they allow (see Fig. 60-2).

The most common joint is the freely movable *diarthrodial* (synovial) type. Each joint is enclosed in a capsule of fibrous connective tissue, which joins the two bones together to form a cavity (Fig. 60-3). The capsule is lined by a synovial membrane, which secretes a thick synovial fluid to lubricate the joint and reduce friction. The end of each bone is covered with articular (hyaline) cartilage. Supporting structures (e.g., ligaments, tendons) reinforce the joint capsule and provide limits to joint movement.[4] Types of diarthrodial joints are shown in Fig. 60-4.

Cartilage

Cartilage is a rigid connective tissue that serves as a support for soft tissue and provides the articular surface for joint movement. It protects underlying tissues. The cartilage in the epiphyseal plate is also involved in the growth of long bones before

physical maturity is reached. Because articular cartilage is relatively avascular, it must receive nourishment by the diffusion of material from the synovial fluid. The lack of a direct blood supply contributes to the slow metabolism of cartilage cells and explains why cartilage tissue heals slowly.

The three types of cartilage tissue are hyaline, elastic, and fibrous. *Hyaline cartilage,* the most common, contains a moderate amount of collagen fibers. It is found in the trachea, bronchi, nose, epiphyseal plate, and articular surfaces of bones. *Elastic cartilage,* which contains both collagen and elastic fibers, is more flexible than hyaline cartilage. It is found in the ear, epiglottis, and larynx. Fibrous cartilage (fibrocartilage) consists mostly of collagen fibers and is a tough tissue that often functions as a shock absorber. It is found between the vertebral disks and also forms a protective cushion between the bones of the pelvic girdle, knee, and shoulder.

Muscle

Types. The three types of muscle tissue are *cardiac* (striated, involuntary), *smooth* (nonstriated, involuntary), and *skeletal* (striated, voluntary) muscle. Cardiac muscle is found in the heart. Its spontaneous contractions propel blood through the circulatory system. Smooth muscle occurs in the walls of hollow structures such as airways, arteries, gastrointestinal (GI) tract, urinary bladder, and uterus. Smooth muscle contraction is modulated by neuronal and hormonal influences. Skeletal muscle, which requires neuronal stimulation for contraction, accounts for about half of a human being's body weight. It is the focus of the following discussion.

Structure. The structural unit of muscle is the muscle cell or muscle fiber, which is highly specialized for contraction. Skeletal muscle fibers are long, multinucleated cylinders that contain many mitochondria to support their high metabolic activity. Mus-

Joint	Movement	Examples	Illustration
Hinge joint	Flexion, extension	Elbow joint (shown), interphalangeal joints, knee joint	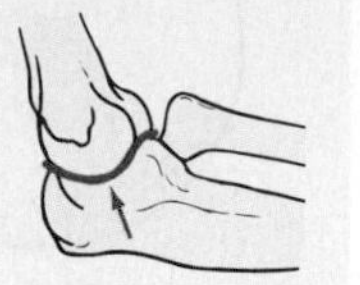
Ball and socket (spheroidal)	Flexion, extension; adduction, abduction; circumduction	Shoulder (shown), hip	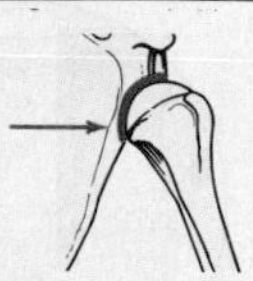
Pivot (rotary)	Rotation	Atlas-axis, proximal radioulnar joint (shown)	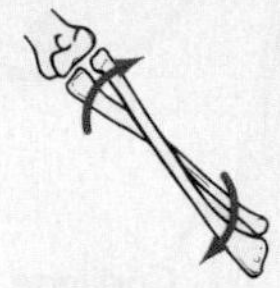
Condyloid	Flexion, extension; abduction, adduction; circumduction	Wrist joint (between radial and carpals) (shown)	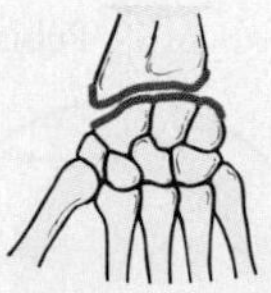
Saddle	Flexion, extension; abduction, adduction; circumduction, thumb-finger opposition	Carpometacarpal joint of thumb	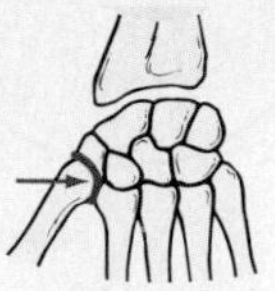
Gliding	One surface moves over another surface	Between tarsal bones, sacroiliac joint, between articular processes of vertebrae, between carpal bones (shown)	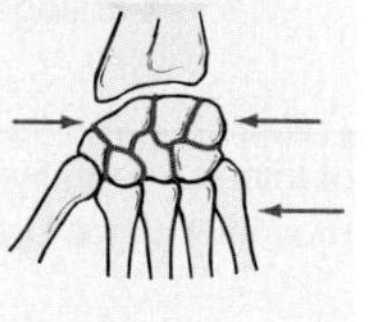

FIG. 60-4 Types of diarthrodial (synovial) joints.

cle fibers are composed of myofibrils, which in turn are made up of contractile filaments.

The *sarcomere* is the contractile unit of the myofibrils.[5] Each sarcomere consists of myosin (thick) filaments and actin (thin) filaments. The arrangement of the thin and thick filaments accounts for the characteristic banding of muscle when it is seen under a microscope. Muscle contraction occurs as thick and thin filaments slide past each other, causing the sarcomeres to shorten.

Contractions. Skeletal muscle contractions allow posture maintenance, movement, and facial expressions. **Isometric contractions** increase the tension within a muscle but do not produce movement. Repeated isometric contractions make muscles grow larger and stronger. **Isotonic contractions** shorten a muscle to produce movement. Most contractions are a combination of tension generation (isometric) and shortening (isotonic). Muscular *atrophy* (decrease in size) occurs with the absence of contraction that results from immobility, whereas increased muscular activity leads to *hypertrophy* (increase in size).

Skeletal muscle fibers are divided into two groups based on the type of activity they demonstrate. Slow-twitch muscle fibers support prolonged muscle activity such as marathon running. Because they also support the body against gravity, they assist in posture maintenance. Fast-twitch muscle fibers are used for rapid muscle contraction required for activities such as blinking the eye, jumping, or sprinting.

Neuromuscular Junction. Skeletal muscle fibers require a nerve impulse to contract. A nerve fiber and the skeletal muscle fibers it stimulates are called a **motor end plate.** The junction between the axon of the nerve cell and the adjacent muscle cell is called the *myoneural* or **neuromuscular junction** (Fig. 60-5).

Acetylcholine is released from the motor end plate of the neuron and diffuses across the neuromuscular junction to bind with receptors on the muscle fiber. In response to this stimulation, the sarcoplasmic reticulum releases calcium ions into the cytoplasm. The presence of calcium triggers the contraction in the myofibrils.

Energy Source. The direct energy source for muscle fiber contractions is adenosine triphosphate (ATP). ATP is synthesized by cellular oxidative metabolism in numerous mitochondria located close to the myofibrils. It is rapidly depleted through conversion to adenosine diphosphate (ADP) and must be rephos-

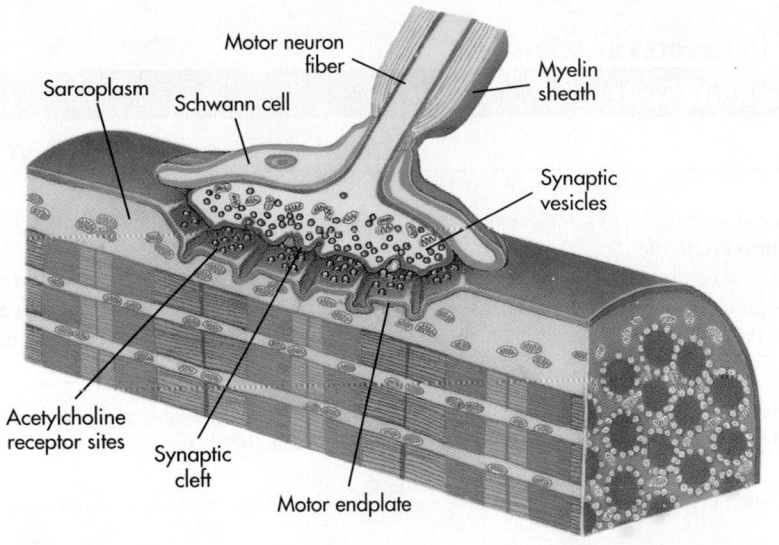

FIG. 60-5 Neuromuscular junction.

phorylated. Phosphocreatine provides a rapid source for the resynthesis of ATP, but it is in turn converted to creatine and must be recharged. Glycolysis can serve as a source of ATP when the oxygen supply is inadequate for the metabolic needs of the muscle tissue. Glucose is broken down to pyruvic acid, which can be further converted to lactic acid to make more oxygen available. An accumulation of lactic acid in tissues leads to fatigue and pain.

Ligaments and Tendons

Ligaments and tendons are both composed of dense, fibrous connective tissue that contains bundles of closely packed collagen fibers arranged in the same plane for additional strength. Tendons attach muscles to bones as an extension of the muscle sheath that adheres to the periosteum. Ligaments connect bones to bones (e.g., tibia to femur at knee joint). They have a higher elastic content than tendons.[6] Ligaments provide stability while permitting controlled movement at the joint.

Ligaments and tendons have a relatively poor blood supply, usually making tissue repair a slow process after injury. For example, the stretching or tearing of ligaments that occurs with a sprain may require a long time to mend.

Fascia

Fascia refers to layers of connective tissue with intermeshed fibers that can withstand limited stretching. Superficial fascia lies immediately under the skin. Deep fascia is a dense, fibrous tissue that surrounds the muscle bundles, nerves, and blood vessels. It also encloses individual muscles, allowing them to act independently and to glide over each other during contraction. In addition, fascia provides strength to muscle tissues.

Bursae

Bursae are small sacs of connective tissue lined with synovial membrane and containing synovial fluid. They are typically located at bony prominences or joints to relieve pressure and prevent friction between moving parts. For example, bursae are found between the patella and the skin (prepatellar bursa), between the olecranon process of the elbow and the skin (olecranon bursa), between the head of the humerus and the acromion process of the scapula (subacromial bursa), and between the greater trochanter of the proximal femur and the skin (trochanteric bursa). *Bursitis* is an inflammation of a bursa sac.

■ Gerontologic Considerations: Effects of Aging on the Musculoskeletal System

Many of the functional problems experienced by the aging adult are related to changes of the musculoskeletal system. Although some changes begin in early adulthood, obvious signs of musculoskeletal impairment may not appear until later adult years. Alterations may affect the older adult's ability to complete self-care tasks and pursue other customary activities. Effects of musculoskeletal changes may range from mild discomfort and decreased ability to perform activities of daily living to severe, chronic pain and immobility. The risk for falls also increases in the older adult.

The bone remodeling process is altered in the aging adult. Increased bone resorption and decreased bone formation cause a loss of bone density, contributing to development of osteopenia and osteoporosis (see Chapter 62). Muscle mass and strength also decrease with aging. Almost 30% of muscle mass is lost by the eighth decade of life.[7] A loss of motor neurons can cause additional problems with skeletal muscle movement. Tendons and ligaments become less flexible, and movement becomes more rigid. Joints in the aging adult are also more likely to be affected by osteoarthritis (see Chapter 63).

In addition to the usual musculoskeletal assessment with a particular emphasis on exercise practices, the nurse should determine the impact of age-related changes of the musculoskeletal system on the functional status of the older patient. Functional limitations that are accepted by older adults as a normal part of aging can often be halted or reversed with appropriate preventive strategies (see Chapter 61, Table 61-1).

Diseases such as osteoarthritis and osteoporosis are not the normal consequences of growing old. The nurse should carefully differentiate between expected changes and the effects of disease in the aging adult. Symptoms of disease can be treated in many

TABLE 60-1 *Gerontologic* Differences in Assessment — Musculoskeletal System

CHANGES	DIFFERENCES IN ASSESSMENT FINDINGS
Muscle	
Decreased number and diameter of muscle cells, replacement of muscle cells by fibrous connective tissue	Decreased muscle strength and bulk, abdominal protrusion, flabby muscle
Loss of elasticity in ligaments and cartilage	Decreased fine motor dexterity, decreased agility
Reduced ability to store glycogen; decreased ability to release glycogen as quick energy during stress	Slowed reaction times and reflexes as a result of slowing of impulse conduction along motor units; earlier fatigue with activity
Joints	
Increased risk for cartilage disruption that contributes to direct contact between bone ends and overgrowth of bone around joint margins	Joint stiffness, possible crepitation on movement; pain with motion and/or weight bearing
Loss of water from disks between vertebrae, narrowing of intervertebral spaces	Loss of height from disk compression; posture change
Bone	
Decrease in bone density	Loss of height from vertebral compression, back pain; deformity such as dowager's hump (kyphosis) caused by vertebral compression

cases, helping the older adult to return to a higher functional level. Age-related changes in the musculoskeletal system and differences in assessment findings are presented in Table 60-1. ■

ASSESSMENT OF THE MUSCULOSKELETAL SYSTEM

Correct diagnosis of any complaint depends on a complete patient history and thorough physical examination. Musculoskeletal assessment can focus on a specific body part, or it can be done as part of a general physical examination or as an examination in itself. The nurse uses the patient's complaint as a guide in selecting all or part of the components of the musculoskeletal history and physical examination. For example, accidents may result in multisystem trauma. Because serious or life-threatening injuries do not usually involve the musculoskeletal system, critical information about the patient's condition is obtained to support immediate treatment, and a complete assessment of the musculoskeletal system may be deferred.

The most common symptoms of musculoskeletal impairment include pain, weakness, deformity, limitation of movement, stiffness, and joint crepitation.[8] Information should also be sought about changes in sensation or in the size of a muscle.

Subjective Data

Important Health Information. Appropriate questions to ask during a musculoskeletal assessment are included in Table 60-2.

Past health history. Because certain illnesses are known to affect the musculoskeletal system either directly or indirectly, the nurse should carefully question the patient about past medical problems. These include tuberculosis, poliomyelitis, diabetes mellitus, parathyroid problems, hemophilia, rickets, scurvy, soft tissue infection, and neuromuscular disabilities. In addition, past or developing musculoskeletal problems can affect the patient's overall health. Trauma to the musculoskeletal system is a common reason for seeking medical evaluation. Questions should also

focus on symptoms of arthritic and connective tissue diseases (e.g., gout, psoriatic arthritis, systemic lupus erythematosus), osteomalacia, osteomyelitis, and fungal infection of the bones or joints. The patient should also be asked about possible sources of a secondary bacterial infection, such as the ears, tonsils, teeth, sinuses, or genitourinary tract. These infections can enter the bones, resulting in osteomyelitis. A detailed account of the course and treatment of any of these problems should be obtained.

Medications. The nurse should carefully question the patient regarding prescription and over-the-counter drugs and herbal products and nutritional supplements (see Complementary and Alternative Therapies box on p. 34). Detailed information should be obtained about each treatment, including its name, the dose and frequency, length of time it was taken, its effects, and any possible side effects. Specific inquiry should be made about skeletal muscle relaxants, opioids, nonsteroidal antiinflammatory drugs, and systemic and topical corticosteroids. The patient who has taken antiinflammatory drugs should be questioned about GI distress or signs of bleeding.

In addition to drugs taken for treatment of a musculoskeletal problem, the patient should be questioned about drugs that can have detrimental effects on this system. These drugs and their potential side effects include antiseizure drugs (osteomalacia), phenothiazines (gait disturbances), corticosteroids (avascular necrosis, decreased bone and muscle mass), and potassium-depleting diuretics (muscle cramps and weakness). Women should be questioned about their menstrual history. Episodes of amenorrhea can contribute to early development of osteoporosis. Questions about the use of hormone replacement therapy and calcium and vitamin D supplements are important for postmenopausal women.

Surgery or other treatments. Information should be obtained about past hospitalizations from a musculoskeletal problem. The nurse should carefully document the reason for hospitalization, the date and duration, and the treatment. Details of emergency treatment for musculoskeletal injuries should also be sought. Specific information should also be obtained regarding any sur-

TABLE	*H*ealth History
60-2	Musculoskeletal System

Health Perception–Health Management Pattern
- Describe your usual daily activities.
- Do you experience any difficulties performing these activities?* Describe what you do if you experience difficulty in dressing, preparing meals and feeding yourself, performing basic hygiene, or maintaining your home.
- Do you use any mechanical assistive devices?*
- Do you have to lift heavy objects? Describe any specialized equipment you use or wear when you work or exercise that helps protect you from injury.
- What other safety precautions do you take?
- Do you take any drugs or herbal products to manage your musculoskeletal problem? If so, what is the name of the drug(s) and what are the expected effects?
- When did you have your last tetanus and polio immunizations? When were you last tested for tuberculosis?

Nutritional-Metabolic Pattern
- Give a 24-hour diet recall.
- What dietary supplements do you take? (Ask specifically about calcium, vitamin D supplements, and herbal products.)
- What is your weight? Describe any recent weight loss or gain. Were your musculoskeletal symptoms affected by the change in your weight?*

Elimination Pattern
- Does your musculoskeletal problem make it difficult for you to reach the toilet in time?*
- Do you need any assistive devices or equipment to achieve satisfactory toileting?*
- Do you experience constipation related to decreased mobility or to drugs taken for your musculoskeletal problem?*

Activity-Exercise Pattern
- Do you require assistance in completing your usual daily activities because of a musculoskeletal problem?*
- Describe your usual exercise pattern. Do you experience musculoskeletal symptoms before, during, or after exercising?*

- Are you able to move all your joints comfortably through full range of motion? Describe any limitations in mobility.
- Do you use any prosthetic or orthotic devices?*

Sleep-Rest Pattern
- Do you experience any difficulty sleeping because of a musculoskeletal problem?* Do you require frequent position changes at night?*
- Do you wake up at night because of musculoskeletal pain?*

Cognitive-Perceptual Pattern
- Describe any musculoskeletal pain you experience. How do you manage your pain? (Ask specifically about adjunctive therapies such as heat and cold or alternative therapies such as acupuncture.)

Self-Perception–Self-Concept Pattern
- Describe how changes in your musculoskeletal system (posture, walking, muscle strength) and decreased ability to do certain things have affected how you feel about yourself. How have these changes affected your lifestyle?

Role-Relationship Pattern
- Do you live alone?
- Describe how family members or others assist you with your musculoskeletal problem.
- Describe the effect of your musculoskeletal problem on your work and on your social relationships.

Sexuality-Reproductive Pattern
- Describe any sexual concerns related to your musculoskeletal problem.

Coping-Stress Tolerance Pattern
- Describe how you deal with problems such as pain or immobility that have resulted from your musculoskeletal problem.

Value-Belief Pattern
- Describe any cultural practices or religious beliefs that may influence the treatment of your musculoskeletal problem.

*If yes, describe.

gical procedure and the postoperative course. If the patient experienced a period of prolonged immobilization, the development of osteoporosis and muscle atrophy should be considered.

Functional Health Patterns. The use of functional health patterns assists the nurse in organizing the data and formulating diagnoses based on information collected about the musculoskeletal system. Table 60-2 summarizes specific questions to ask in relation to functional health patterns.

Health perception–health management pattern. The nurse should ask about the patient's health practices related to the musculoskeletal system, such as maintenance of a normal body weight, avoidance of excessive stress on muscles and joints, and the use of proper body mechanics when lifting objects.[9]

The patient should be specifically questioned about tetanus and polio immunizations. The most current date and reaction to a tuberculin skin test should also be obtained.

Food or contact allergies have little direct relation to musculoskeletal problems, but the general malaise often associated with allergic reactions may manifest in musculoskeletal stiffness

and lethargy. Allergic reactions to drugs used to treat musculoskeletal problems can be significant if they interfere with therapy. An alternative treatment may have to be used if the reaction is severe.

The patient who is a good historian can recount numerous minor and major injuries of the musculoskeletal system. Information should be recorded chronologically and should include the following:

1. Mechanism of the injury (e.g., twist, crush, stretch)
2. Circumstances related to the injury
3. Diagnostic evaluations
4. Methods of treatment
5. Duration of treatment
6. Current status related to the injury
7. Need for assistive devices
8. Interference with activities of daily living

A family history should be obtained related to rheumatoid arthritis, sickle cell disease, osteoarthritis, gout, osteoporosis, and scoliosis because these problems have a familial predisposition.

Safety practices can affect the patient's predisposition for certain injuries and illnesses. Therefore the nurse should ask the patient about safety practices as they relate to work environment, recreation, and exercise. For example, if the patient is a computer programmer, the nurse should ask about ergonomic adaptations in the office that decrease the risk of carpal tunnel syndrome or low back pain. Identification of problems in this area will direct the plan for patient teaching.

Nutritional-metabolic pattern. The patient's description of a typical day's diet provides clues to areas of nutritional concern that can affect the musculoskeletal system. Adequate amounts of vitamins C and D, calcium, and protein are essential for a healthy, intact musculoskeletal system. Abnormal nutritional patterns can predispose individuals to problems such as osteomalacia and osteoporosis. In addition, maintenance of normal weight is an important nutritional goal. Obesity places additional stress on weight-bearing joints such as the knees, hips, and spine, and it predisposes individuals to ligamentous instability.

Elimination pattern. Questions about the patient's mobility may reveal difficulty with ambulating to the toilet. The patient should be asked if an assistive device such as an elevated toilet seat or a grab bar is necessary to accomplish toileting. Decreased mobility secondary to a musculoskeletal problem can lead to constipation. In addition, musculoskeletal problems can contribute to bowel or bladder incontinence.

Activity-exercise pattern. The nurse should obtain a detailed account of the type, duration, and frequency of exercise and recreational activities. Daily, weekend, and seasonal patterns should be compared because occasional or sporadic exercise can be more problematic than regular exercise. Many musculoskeletal problems can affect the patient's activity-exercise pattern. The nurse should question the patient about limitations of movement, pain, weakness, clumsiness, crepitus, or any change in the bones or joints that interferes with daily activities.

Extremes of activity related to occupation can also affect the musculoskeletal system. A sedentary occupation can negatively impact muscle flexibility and strength. Jobs that require extreme effort through heavy lifting or pushing can lead to damage of joints and supporting structures. The nurse should specifically question the patient about work-related injuries to the musculoskeletal system, including treatment and time lost from work.

Sleep-rest pattern. The discomfort caused by musculoskeletal disorders can interfere with a normal sleep pattern. The patient should be questioned about possible alterations in sleep patterns. If the patient describes sleep interference related to a musculoskeletal problem, the nurse should inquire further about the type of bedding and pillows used, sleeping partner, and sleeping positions.

Cognitive-perceptual pattern. Any pain experienced by the patient as a result of a musculoskeletal problem should be fully explored and documented. To provide a baseline for later reassessment, the patient should be asked to describe the intensity of the pain on a scale from 1 to 10 (0 = no pain, 10 = most severe pain imaginable). Reassessments over time will assist in determining the effectiveness of any treatment plan. The patient should also be questioned about measures used at home for pain management and about related problems such as joint swelling or muscle weakness. (Pain is discussed in Chapter 9.)

Self-perception–self-concept pattern. Many chronic musculoskeletal problems lead to deformities that can have a serious negative impact on the patient's body image and sense of personal worth. The nurse should address the patient's feelings about each of these changes.

Role-relationship pattern. Impaired mobility and chronic pain from musculoskeletal problems can negatively affect the patient's ability to perform in roles of spouse, parent, or employee. The ability to pursue and maintain meaningful social and personal relationships can also be affected by musculoskeletal problems. The nurse should carefully question the patient about role performance and relationships.

If the patient lives alone, the current musculoskeletal problem and its rehabilitation may make it difficult or impossible to continue this arrangement. The degree of assistance available from family, friends, and organized caregivers should be determined.

Sexuality-reproductive pattern. The pain of musculoskeletal problems can greatly affect the patient's ability to obtain sexual satisfaction. The nurse should sensitively explore this area, helping the patient feel comfortable in discussing any sexual problems related to pain, movement, and positioning.

Coping–stress tolerance pattern. Mobility limitations and pain, whether acute or chronic, are serious potential stressors that challenge the patient's coping resources. The nurse must recognize the potential for ineffective coping in the patient and family or significant other. Additional questioning will help determine if a musculoskeletal problem is causing coping difficulties.

Objective Data

Physical Examination. Examination involves observation, palpation, motion, and muscular assessment.[10] Although a general overview will be conducted, data obtained in a careful health history will guide the nurse in choosing areas on which to concentrate the local examination. Specific measurements may be taken as indicated by the local examination.

Inspection. Inspection begins during the nurse's initial contact with the patient. The patient's use of an assistive device such as a walker or cane should be noted. The nurse also observes general body build, muscle configuration, and symmetry of joint movement. If the patient is able to move independently, the nurse should assess posture and gait by watching the patient walk, stand, and sit. Musculoskeletal and neurologic problems can result in changes from a normal gait.

A systematic inspection is performed starting at the head and neck and proceeding to the upper extremities, the lower extremities, and the trunk. A specific order is not required, but the regular use of a systematic approach is important to avoid missing important aspects of the examination. The skin is inspected for general color, scars, or other overt signs of previous injury or surgery. The nurse notes any swelling, deformity, nodules or masses, and discrepancies in limb length or muscle size. The patient's opposite body part is used for comparison when an abnormality is suspected.

Palpation. Any area that has aroused concern because of a subjective complaint or appears abnormal on inspection should be carefully palpated. As with inspection, palpation usually proceeds cephalopedally (head to toe) to examine the neck, shoulders, elbows, wrists, hands, back, hips, knees, ankles, and feet. Both superficial and deep palpation are usually performed consecutively.

The nurse's hands should be warm to prevent muscle spasm, which can interfere with identification of essential landmarks or soft tissue structures. Palpation of both muscles and joints allows for evaluation of skin temperature, local tenderness, swelling, and crepitation. The nurse must establish the relationship of adjacent structures and evaluate the general contour, abnormal prominences, and local landmarks.

Motion. When assessing the patient's joint mobility, the nurse must carefully evaluate both passive and active range of joint motion. Measurements should be similar for both active and passive range of motion. *Active range of motion* means the patient takes his or her own joints through all movements without assistance. *Passive range of motion* occurs when someone else moves the patient's joints without his or her participation. The nurse should be cautious in performing passive range of motion because of the risk of injury to underlying structures. Manipulation must cease immediately if pain or resistance is encountered. If deficits in active or passive range of motion are noted, the nurse must also assess functional range of motion to determine if performance of activities of daily living has been affected by joint changes. This is done by asking the patient if activities such as eating and bathing must be performed with assistance or cannot be done at all.

Range of motion is most accurately assessed with a goniometer, which measures the angle of the joint (Fig. 60-6). Specific degrees of range of motion of all joints are usually not measured unless a musculoskeletal problem has been identified. A less exact but valuable assessment method is to compare the range of motion of one extremity with the range of motion on the opposite side. The most common movements that occur at the synovial joints are described in Table 60-3.

Muscle-strength testing. The nurse grades the strength of individual muscles or groups of muscles during contraction (Table 60-4). The patient should be instructed to apply resistance to the force exerted by the nurse. For example, the examiner tries to pull the bent arm down while the patient tries to raise it. Muscle strength should also be compared with the strength of the opposite extremity. Subtle variations in muscle strength may be noted when comparing the patient's dominant side with the nondominant side.

Measurement. When length discrepancies or subjective problems are noted, the nurse will often obtain limb length and circumferential muscle mass measurements. For example, leg length should be measured when gait disorders are observed. The affected limb is measured between two bony prominences and compared with the similar measurement of the opposite extremity. Muscle mass is measured circumferentially at the largest area of the muscle. When recording measurements, the

TABLE 60-3 Movement at Synovial Joints

MOVEMENT	DESCRIPTION
Abduction	Movement of part away from midline of body
Adduction	Movement of part toward midline of body
Circumduction	Combination of flexion, extension, abduction, and adduction resulting in circular motion of a body part
Eversion	Turning of sole outward away from midline of body
Extension	Straightening of joint that increases angle between two bones
External rotation	Movement along longitudinal axis away from midline of body
Flexion	Bending of joint as a result of muscle contraction that results in decreased angle between two bones
Hyperextension	Extension in which angle exceeds 180 degrees
Internal rotation	Movement along longitudinal axis toward midline of body
Inversion	Turning of sole inward toward midline of body
Pronation	Turning of palm downward
Supination	Turning of palm upward

TABLE 60-4 Muscle Strength Scale

0	No detection of muscular contraction
1	A barely detectable flicker or trace of contraction with observation or palpation
2	Active movement of body part with elimination of gravity
3	Active movement against gravity only and not against resistance
4	Active movement against gravity and some resistance
5	Active movement against full resistance without evident fatigue (normal muscle strength)

TABLE 60-5 Normal Physical Assessment of the Musculoskeletal System

Full range of motion of all joints without pain or laxity
No joint swelling, deformity, or crepitation
Normal spinal curvatures
No tenderness on palpation of spine
No muscle atrophy or asymmetry
Muscle strength of 5

nurse should document the exact location at which the measurements were obtained (e.g., the quadriceps muscle is measured 15 cm above the patella). This informs the next examiner of the exact area to be measured and ensures consistency during reassessment.

Other. Assessment of reflexes is discussed in Chapter 54. Table 60-5 is an example of how to record a normal physical assessment of the musculoskeletal system. Common abnormal as-

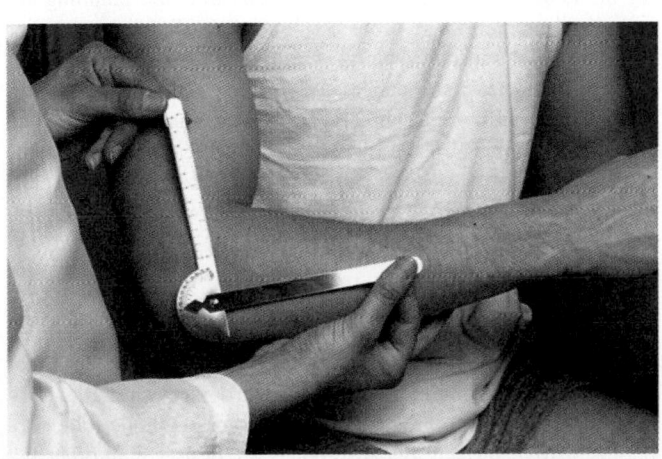

FIG. 60-6 Measurement of joint motion with a goniometer.

TABLE 60-6 Common Assessment Abnormalities
Musculoskeletal System

FINDING	DESCRIPTION	POSSIBLE ETIOLOGY AND SIGNIFICANCE
Ankylosis	Scarring within a joint leading to stiffness or fixation	Chronic joint inflammation
Atrophy	Wasting of muscle, characterized by decreased circumference and flabby appearance leading to decreased function and tone	Muscle denervation, contracture, prolonged disuse as a result of immobilization
Contracture	Resistance of movement of muscle or joint as a result of fibrosis of supporting soft tissues	Shortening of muscle or ligaments, tightness of soft tissue, incorrect positioning of immobilized extremity
Crepitation (crepitus)	Crackling sound or grating sensation as a result of friction or broken bone or cartilage bits in joint	Fracture, dislocation, chronic inflammation, osteoarthritis
Effusion	Fluid in joint possibly with swelling and pain	Trauma, especially to knees; inflammation
Ganglion	Small fluid-filled synovial cyst usually on dorsal surface of wrist or foot	Degeneration of connective tissue close to tendons and joints leading to formation of small cysts
Hypertrophy	Increase in size of muscle as a result of enlargement of existing cells	Exercise or other increased stimulation, increased androgens
Kyphosis (dowager's hump)	Anteroposterior or forward bending of thoracic spine with convexity of curve in posterior direction	Poor posture, tuberculosis, arthritis, osteoporosis, growth disturbance of vertebral epiphyses
Lordosis	Lumbar spinal deformity resulting in anteroposterior curvature with concavity in posterior direction	Secondary to other spinal deformities, muscular dystrophy, obesity, flexion contracture of hip, congenital dislocation of hip
Pes planus	Flatfoot	Congenital condition, muscle paralysis, mild cerebral palsy, early muscular dystrophy
Scoliosis	Deformity resulting in lateral curvature of thoracic spine (see Fig. 60-7)	Idiopathic or congenital condition, fracture or dislocation, osteomalacia
Subluxation	Partial dislocation of joint	Instability of joint capsule and supporting ligaments (e.g., from trauma, arthritis)
Valgus (bow legs)	Angulation of bone away from midline	Alteration in gait, pain, arthritis
Varus (knock-knees)	Angulation of bone toward midline	Alteration in gait, pain, arthritis

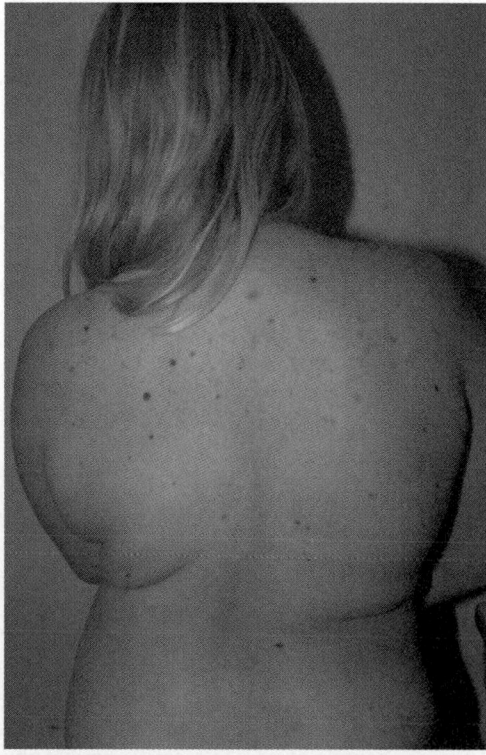

FIG. 60-7 Scoliosis in a standing erect posture.

sessment findings of the musculoskeletal system are presented in Table 60-6. **Scoliosis** is a lateral S-shaped curvature of the thoracic and lumbar spine.[9] Unequal shoulder and scapula height is usually noted (Fig. 60-7). If the deformity is greater than 45 degrees, lung and cardiac function is generally impaired.

DIAGNOSTIC STUDIES OF THE MUSCULOSKELETAL SYSTEM

Diagnostic studies provide important objective data that aid the nurse in monitoring the patient's condition and planning appropriate interventions. Table 60-7 contains diagnostic studies common to the musculoskeletal system. Use of studies such as x-rays and magnetic resonance imaging (MRI) has greatly improved orthopedic care, but diagnostic imaging has resulted in approximately 50% of the increase in health care costs over the last decade.[11] Tests must be carefully chosen to enhance or clarify information gained from the patient's history and physical examination.

X-ray

The **x-ray,** or roentgenogram, is the most common diagnostic study used to assess musculoskeletal problems and to monitor the effectiveness of treatment. A standard x-ray is a film produced by the action of x-rays emitted from a cathode tube on a photosensitive surface. Because bones are denser than other tissues, x-rays do not penetrate them. Dense areas show as white on

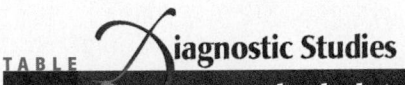

TABLE 60-7

Diagnostic Studies
Musculoskeletal System

STUDY	DESCRIPTION AND PURPOSE	NURSING RESPONSIBILITY
Radiologic Studies		
• Standard x-ray	An x-ray is taken to determine density of bone. Study evaluates structural or functional changes of bones and joints. In anteroposterior view, x-ray beam passes from front to back, allowing one-dimensional view; lateral position provides two-dimensional view.	Avoid excessive exposure of patient and self. Before procedure, remove any radiopaque objects that can interfere with results. Explain procedure to patient. Verify patient is not pregnant.
• Arthrogram	Study involves injection of contrast medium or air into joint cavity, which permits visualization of joint structures. Joint movement is followed with series of x-rays.	Assess patient for possible allergy to contrast medium. Explain procedure.
• Diskogram	An x-ray of cervical or lumbar intervertebral disk is done after injection of contrast dye into nucleus pulposus. Study permits visualization of intervertebral disk abnormalities.	Same as for arthrogram.
• Sinogram	An x-ray is taken after injection of contrast dye into sinus tract (deep draining wound). Study visualizes course of sinus and tissues involved.	Same as for arthrogram.
• Computed tomography (CT) scan	An x-ray beam is used with a computer to provide a three-dimensional picture. It is used to identify soft tissue abnormalities, bony abnormalities, and various musculoskeletal trauma.	Inform patient that procedure is painless. Inform patient of importance of remaining still during procedure.
• Magnetic resonance imaging (MRI)	Radio waves and magnetic field are used to view soft tissue. Study is especially useful in the diagnosis of avascular necrosis, disk disease, tumors, osteomyelitis, ligament tears, and cartilage tears. Patient is placed inside scanning chamber. Gadolinium may be injected into a vein to enhance visualization of the structures. Open MRI does not require the patient to be placed inside a chamber.	Inform patient that procedure is painless. Be aware that it is contraindicated in patient with aneurysm clips, metallic implants, pacemakers, electronic devices, hearing aids, shrapnel, and extreme obesity. Ensure that patient has no metal on clothing (e.g., snaps, zippers, jewelry, credit cards). Inform patient of importance of remaining still throughout examination. Inform patients who are claustrophobic that they may experience symptoms during examination. Administer antianxiety agent if indicated and ordered. Open MRI may be indicated for obese patient or patient with large chest and abdominal girth or severe claustrophobia. Open MRI may not be available at all facilities.
Bone Mineral Density (BMD) Measurements		
• Dual energy x-ray absorptiometry (DEXA)	Technique measures bone mass of spine, femur, forearm, and total body. Allows assessment of bone density with minimal radiation exposure; used to diagnose metabolic bone disease and to monitor changes in bone density with treatment.	Inform patient that procedure is painless.
• Quantitative ultrasound (QUS)	Evaluates density, elasticity, and strength of patella and calcaneus using ultrasound rather than radiation.	Inform patient that procedure is painless.
Radioisotope Studies		
• Bone scan	Technique involves injection of radioisotope (usually sodium pertechnetate) that is taken up by bone. Radiation detector (Geiger counter) scans entire body (front and back), and recording is made on paper. Degree of uptake is related to blood flow to bone. Increased uptake is seen in osteomyelitis, osteoporosis, primary and metastatic malignant lesions of bone, and certain fractures. Decreased uptake is seen in areas of avascular necrosis.	Explain that technician gives a calculated dose of radioisotope 2 hr before procedure. Ensure that bladder is emptied before scan. Inform patient that procedure requires 1 hr while patient lies supine and that no pain or harm will result from isotopes. Explain that no follow-up scans are required. Increase fluids after the examination.

Continued

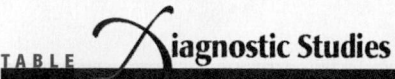

TABLE
60-7
Diagnostic Studies
Musculoskeletal System—cont'd

STUDY	DESCRIPTION AND PURPOSE	NURSING RESPONSIBILITY
Endoscopy		
• Arthroscopy	Study involves insertion of arthroscope into joint (usually knee) for visualization of structure and contents. It can be used for exploratory surgery (removal of loose bodies and biopsy) and for diagnosis of abnormalities of meniscus, articular cartilage, ligaments, or joint capsule. Other structures that can be visualized through the arthroscope include the shoulder, elbow, wrist, jaw, hip, and ankle.	Inform patient that procedure is performed in operating room with strict asepsis and that either local or general anesthesia is used. After procedure, cover wound with sterile dressing.
Mineral Metabolism		
• Alkaline phosphatase	This enzyme, produced by osteoblasts of bone, is needed for mineralization of organic bone matrix. Elevated levels are found in healing fractures, bone cancers, osteoporosis, osteomalacia, and Paget's disease. *Normal:* 20 to 90 U/L (0.3 to 2.7 mmol/L).	Obtain blood samples by venipuncture. Observe venipuncture site for bleeding or hematoma formation. Inform patient that procedure does not require fasting.
• Calcium	Bone is primary organ for calcium storage. Calcium provides bone with rigid consistency. Decreased serum level is found in osteomalacia, renal disease, and hypoparathyroidism; increased level is found in hyperparathyroidism, some bone tumors. *Normal:* 9 to 11 mg/dl (2.3 to 2.7 mmol/L).	Same as above.
• Phosphorus	Amount present is indirectly related to calcium metabolism. Decreased level is found in osteomalacia; increased level is found in chronic renal disease, healing fractures, osteolytic metastatic tumor. *Normal:* 2.8 to 4.5 mg/dl (0.9 to 1.5 mmol/L).	Same as above.
Serologic Studies		
• Rheumatoid factor (RF)	Study assesses presence of autoantibody (rheumatoid factor) in serum. Factor is not specific for rheumatoid arthritis and is seen in other connective tissue diseases, as well as in a small percentage of normal population. *Normal:* negative or titer <1:20.	Same as above.
• Erythrocyte sedimentation rate (ESR)	Study is nonspecific index of inflammation. Study measures rapidity with which red blood cells settle out of unclotted blood in 1 hr. Results are influenced by physiologic factors, as well as diseases. Elevated levels are seen with any inflammatory process (especially rheumatoid arthritis, rheumatic fever, osteomyelitis, and respiratory infections). *Normal:* <20 mm/hr. Some gender variation.	Same as above.
• Antinuclear antibody (ANA)	Study assesses presence of antibodies capable of destroying nucleus of body's tissue cells. Finding is positive in 95% of patients with systemic lupus erythematosus and may also be positive in individuals with systemic sclerosis (scleroderma) or rheumatoid arthritis and in a small percentage of normal population.	Same as above.
• Anti-DNA antibody	Study detects serum antibodies that react with DNA. It is the most specific test for systemic lupus erythematosus.	Same as above.
• Complement	Complement, a normal body protein, is essential to both immune and inflammatory reactions. Complement components used up in these reactions are depleted. Complement depletions may be found in patients with rheumatoid arthritis or systemic lupus erythematosus.	Same as above.

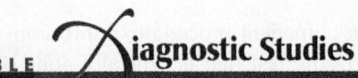

TABLE
60-7

Diagnostic Studies
Musculoskeletal System—cont'd

STUDY	DESCRIPTION AND PURPOSE	NURSING RESPONSIBILITY
Serologic Studies—cont'd		
• Uric acid	End product of purine metabolism is normally excreted in urine. Although not specific, levels are usually elevated in gout. *Normal:* men, 4.5 to 6.5 mg/dl (268 to 387 μmol/L); women, 2.5 to 5.5 mg/dl (149 to 327 μmol/L).	Obtain blood samples by venipuncture. Observe venipuncture site for bleeding or hematoma formation. Inform patient that procedure does not require fasting.
• C-reactive protein (CRP)	Study is used to diagnose inflammatory diseases, infections, and active widespread malignancy. CRP is synthesized by the liver and is present in large amounts in serum 18 to 24 hr after onset of tissue damage. *Normal:* negative.	Same as above.
• Human leukocyte antigen (HLA)-B27	Antigen present in disorders such as ankylosing spondylitis and rheumatoid arthritis.	Same as above.
Muscle Enzymes		
• Creatine kinase (CK)	Highest concentration is found in skeletal muscle. Increased values are found in progressive muscular dystrophy, polymyositis, and traumatic injuries. *Normal:* men, 5 to 55 U/L (0.1 to 0.9 μkat/L); women, 5 to 35 U/L (0.01 to 7.5 U/L (16.7-125 μkat/L).	Same as above.
• Aldolase	Study is useful in monitoring muscular dystrophy and dermatomyositis. *Normal:* 1 to 7.5 U/L (16.7 to 125 μkat/L).	Same as above.
Invasive Procedures		
• Arthrocentesis	Incision or puncture of joint capsule is done to obtain samples of synovial fluid from within joint cavity or to remove excess fluid. Local anesthesia and aseptic preparation are used before needle is inserted into joint and fluid aspirated. Study is useful in diagnosis of joint inflammation, infection, and subtle fractures.	Inform patient that procedure is usually done at bedside or in examination room. Send samples of synovial fluid to laboratory for examination (if indicated). After procedure apply compression dressing. Observe for leakage of blood or fluid on dressing.
• Electromyogram (EMG)	Study evaluates electrical potential associated with skeletal muscle contraction. Small-gauge needles are inserted into certain muscles. Needle probes are attached to leads that feed information to EMG machine. Recordings of electrical activity of muscle are traced on audiotransmitter, as well as on oscilloscope and recording paper. Study is useful in providing information related to lower motor neuron dysfunction and primary muscle disease.	Inform patient that procedure is usually done in electromyogram laboratory while patient lies supine on special table. Keep patient awake to cooperate with voluntary movement. Inform patient that procedure involves some discomfort from needle insertion. Avoid administration of stimulants including caffeine and sedatives 24 hr before procedure.
Miscellaneous		
• Thermography	Technique uses infrared detector, which measures degree of heat radiating from skin surface. Study is useful in investigation of cause of inflamed joint and in following up patient's response to antiinflammatory drug therapy.	Inform patient that procedure is painless and noninvasive.
• Plethysmography	Study records variations in volume and pressure of blood passing through tissues. Test is nonspecific.	Inform patient that procedure is painless and noninvasive.
• Somatosensory evoked potential (SSEP)	Study evaluates evoked potential of muscle contractions. Electrodes are placed on skin and provide recordings of electrical activity of muscle. Study is useful in identifying subtle dysfunction of lower motor neuron and primary muscle disease. SSEP measures nerve conduction along pathways not accessible by EMG. Transcutaneous or percutaneous electrodes are applied to the skin and help identify neuropathy and myopathy.	Inform patient that procedure is similar to EMG but does not involve needles. Electrodes are applied to the skin.

the standard x-ray. X-rays provide information about bone deformity, joint congruity, bone density, and calcification in soft tissue. Fracture diagnosis and management are the primary indications for x-ray, but it is also useful in the evaluation of hereditary, developmental, infectious, inflammatory, neoplastic, metabolic, and degenerative disorders.

The anteroposterior and lateral views are the most commonly used standard x-ray perspectives. Additional views in combination with other studies can aid in differential diagnosis.

Magnetic Resonance Imaging

MRI is a diagnostic study that shows the hydrogen density of tissues within the body. The body is composed primarily of hydrogen, and hydrogen possesses magnetic properties that make it appropriate as the basis for MRI. In MRI, radio waves and magnetic fields are used to construct soft tissue and bone images. The study is particularly advantageous in identifying soft tissue disorders, including cartilage or ligament tears and herniated disks, but it can also be helpful in diagnosing bone disorders such as avascular necrosis, tumors, and multiple myeloma.

Arthroscopy

A small fiberoptic tube called an arthroscope is used to directly examine the interior of a joint cavity in a procedure known as **arthroscopy.** Arthroscopy is performed under sterile conditions. After anesthesia has been administered, a large-bore needle is inserted into the joint, and the joint is distended with fluid or air (Fig. 60-8). When the arthroscope is inserted, the surgeon is able to perform extensive, accurate visualization of the joint cavity. Photographs or videotapes can be made through the scope, and a biopsy of the synovium or cartilage can be obtained. Torn tissue can be repaired through arthroscopic surgery, eliminating the need for a larger incision and greatly decreasing the recovery time.

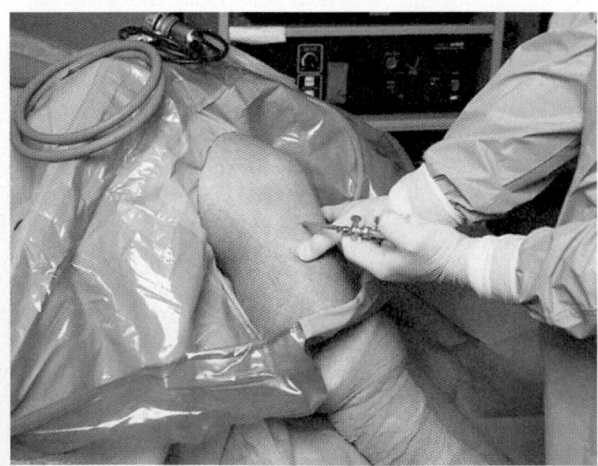

FIG. 60-8 Arthroscopy of a knee.

Typically performed as an outpatient procedure, arthroscopy is a highly cost-effective diagnostic test that is typically done on an ambulatory basis.

Arthrocentesis and Synovial Fluid Analysis

An **arthrocentesis** or joint aspiration is usually performed for a synovial fluid analysis. It may also be used to instill medications for the patient with septic arthritis or to remove fluid from joints to relieve pain. After the skin has been cleaned, a local anesthetic is instilled. An 18-gauge or larger needle is inserted into the joint, and fluid is withdrawn. The appropriate sterile container should be readily available to receive the aspirated fluid, which must be transported immediately to the laboratory. The fluid will be examined grossly for volume, color, clarity, viscosity, and mucin clot formation. Normal synovial fluid is transparent and colorless or straw-colored. It should be scant in amount and of low viscosity. Fluid from an infected joint may be purulent and thick or gray and thin. In gout the fluid may be whitish yellow. Blood may be aspirated if there is hemarthrosis because of injury or a bleeding disorder. The mucin clot test indicates the character of the protein portion of the synovial fluid. Normally a white, ropelike mucin clot is formed. In the presence of an inflammatory process, the clot breaks apart easily and fragments. The fluid is examined grossly for floating fat globules, which indicate bone injury.

The fluid is examined microscopically for cell count and identification. The normal white blood cell (WBC) count is less than 200 cells/μl, with fewer than 25% neutrophils and no bacteria. Infection would be suspected if the cell count reveals more than 25,000 WBC/μl and more than 25% polymorphonuclear cells. Protein content is elevated, and glucose is considerably decreased in septic arthritis. Presence of uric acid crystals suggests a diagnosis of gout. A Gram stain and culture may also be done of the aspirated fluid.

Muscle Enzymes

Muscle enzymes are released from injured or dead muscle cells. Determinations of muscle enzyme values are used to distinguish between muscle weakness that is due to nerve innervation problems and dystrophic disease of the muscle itself. The level of enzymes reflects the progress of the disorder and the effectiveness of treatment. Creatine kinase is a reliable measure of muscle damage.

Serologic Studies

Approximately 80% of people with rheumatoid arthritis and related diseases have an autoantibody known as rheumatoid factor (RF) in their serum. RF is an autoantibody directed against the immunoglobulin IgG. RF titers are higher during periods of increased disease activity. Elevated erythrocyte sedimentation rate and C-reactive protein are nonspecific indicators of active inflammation.

REVIEW QUESTIONS

The number of the question corresponds to the same-numbered objective at the beginning of the chapter.

1. The bone cells that function in the breakdown of bone tissue (resorption) are called
   a. osteoids.
   b. osteocytes.
   c. osteoclasts.
   d. osteoblasts.

2. While performing passive range of motion for a patient, the nurse puts a hinge joint through the movements of
   a. rotation.
   b. flexion and extension.
   c. flexion, extension, abduction, and adduction.
   d. flexion, extension, abduction, adduction, and circumduction.

3. The nurse teaches a patient with a leg immobilized in traction to prevent muscle atrophy in the affected leg by performing
   a. twitch contractions.
   b. tetanic contractions.
   c. isotonic contractions.
   d. isometric contractions.

4. A patient with bursitis of the shoulder asks the nurse what the bursa does. The nurse's response is based on the knowledge that bursae
   a. connect bone to bone.
   b. separate muscle from muscle.
   c. lubricate joints with synovial fluid.
   d. relieve friction between moving parts.

5. The decreased agility found during assessment of the older adult is caused by the age-related change of
   a. decrease in bone mass.
   b. erosion of articular cartilage.
   c. loss of elasticity in ligaments and cartilage.
   d. decrease in number and diameter of muscle cells.

6. While obtaining subjective assessment data related to the musculoskeletal system, it is particularly important for the nurse to ask about family history in the patient with
   a. osteomyelitis.
   b. osteomalacia.
   c. low back pain.
   d. rheumatoid arthritis.

7. When grading muscle strength, the nurse records a score of 2, indicating
   a. active movement against gravity.
   b. a barely detectable flicker of contraction.
   c. active movement with elimination of gravity.
   d. active movement against full resistance without evident fatigue.

8. A normal assessment finding of the musculoskeletal system is
   a. muscle strength of 4.
   b. a lateral curvature of the spine.
   c. angulation of bone toward midline.
   d. simultaneous occurrence of stance and swing phase of gait.

9. A patient is scheduled for an electromyogram. The nurse explains that this diagnostic test involves
   a. placement of thin needles into the muscles.
   b. placement of electrodes on the skin to record electrical activity of muscles.
   c. measurement of the heat of muscle contractions radiating from the skin surface.
   d. administration of a calculated dose of radioisotope 2 hours before the procedure.

REFERENCES

1. Maher AB, Salmond SW, Pellino TA, editors: *Orthopaedic nursing,* ed 3, Philadelphia, 2002, WB Saunders.
2. National Association of Orthopaedic Nurses: *An introduction to orthopaedic nursing,* ed 2, Pitman NJ, 1998, NAON.
3. Thibodeau GA, Patton KT: *The human body in health and disease,* ed 3, St Louis, 2002, Mosby.
4. Schoen DC: *Core curriculum for orthopaedic nursing,* ed 4, Pitman NJ, 2001, NAON.
5. McCance KL, Huether SE, editors: *Pathophysiology: the biologic basis for disease in adults and children,* ed 4, St Louis, 2002, Mosby.
6. Herlihy B, Maebius NK: *The human body in health and illness,* ed 2, Philadelphia, 2003, WB Saunders.
7. Ebersole P, Hess P, editors: *Toward healthy aging,* ed 5, St Louis, 1998, Mosby.

8. Swartz MH: *Textbook of physical diagnosis,* ed 4, Philadelphia, 2002, WB Saunders.
9. Jarvis C: *Physical examination and health assessment,* ed 4, Philadelphia, 2004, WB Saunders.
10. Brinker MR, Miller MD: *Fundamentals of orthopaedics,* Philadelphia, 1999, WB Saunders.
11. Galen B: Diagnostic imaging: an overview, *Prim Care Pract* 3:5, 1999.

RESOURCES

Resources for this chapter are listed after Chapter 61 on page 1691, Chapter 62 on page 1714, and Chapter 63 on page 1755.

CHAPTER 61

NURSING MANAGEMENT
Musculoskeletal Trauma and Orthopedic Surgery

Cathleen E. Kunkler

LEARNING OBJECTIVES

1. Explain the etiology, pathophysiology, clinical manifestations, and collaborative care of soft tissue injuries, including strains, sprains, dislocations, subluxations, bursitis, repetitive strain injury, carpal tunnel syndrome, rotator cuff injury, meniscus injury, and muscle spasms.
2. Describe the sequential events involved in fracture healing.
3. Differentiate among closed reduction, cast immobilization, open reduction, and traction regarding purpose, complications, and nursing management.
4. Describe the neurovascular assessment of an injured extremity.

5. Explain common complications associated with fracture injury and fracture healing.
6. Describe the collaborative care and nursing management of patients with specific fractures.
7. Describe the indications for and the collaborative care and nursing management of the patient with an amputation.
8. Describe the types of joint replacement surgery associated with arthritis and connective tissue diseases.
9. Identify the preoperative and postoperative management of the patient having joint replacement surgery.

KEY TERMS

arthroplasty, p. 1685	osteotomy, p. 1685
bursitis, p. 1656	phantom limb sensation, p. 1682
carpal tunnel syndrome, p. 1654	repetitive strain injury, p. 1653
compartment syndrome, p. 1671	sprain, p. 1650
debridement, p. 1685	strain, p. 1651
dislocation, p. 1652	subluxation, p. 1652
fat embolism syndrome, p. 1672	synovectomy, p. 1685
fracture, p. 1657	traction, p. 1664

The most common cause of musculoskeletal problems is injury from a traumatic event resulting in fracture, dislocations, and associated soft tissue injuries. Although most of these injuries are not fatal, the cost in terms of pain, disability, medical expense, and lost wages is enormous. For all ages, accidents are exceeded only by heart disease, cancer, and strokes as a cause of death. Accidents are the leading cause of death in children and young adults.

The nurse has an important role in educating the public about the basic principles of safety and accident prevention. The morbidity associated with accidents can be significantly reduced if people are aware of environmental hazards, use existing safety equipment, and apply safety and traffic rules. In the industrial setting, the nurse should teach employees and employers about the use of proper safety equipment and avoidance of hazardous working situations.

In the home environment, falls account for many musculoskeletal injuries. Preventive education should be directed toward the importance of wearing shoes with functional soles and

heels, avoidance of wet or slippery surfaces, careful placement of throw rugs, and removal of obstacles from the pathway of high-risk individuals such as persons with gait instability or visual or cognitive impairment. Ways to prevent common musculoskeletal problems in the older adult are listed in Table 61-1.

SOFT TISSUE INJURIES

Soft tissue injuries include sprains, strains, dislocations, and subluxation. These common injuries are usually caused by trauma. The increase in the number of people who have committed themselves to a regular fitness program or participating in sports has contributed to the increased incidence of soft tissue injuries. Common sports-related injuries are summarized in Table 61-2. Most sport injuries result from direct trauma, contusion, or indirect stretch injury.[1]

SPRAINS AND STRAINS

Sprains and strains are the two most common types of injury affecting the musculoskeletal system. These injuries are usually associated with abnormal stretching or twisting forces that may occur during vigorous activities. These injuries tend to occur around joints.

A **sprain** is an injury to ligamentous structures surrounding a joint, usually caused by a wrenching or twisting motion. A sprain is classified according to the amount of ligament fibers torn. A first-degree (mild) sprain involves tears of only a few fibers resulting in mild tenderness and slight swelling. A second-degree (moderate) sprain is partial disruption of the involved tissue with more swelling and tenderness. A third-degree (severe) sprain is a complete tearing of the ligament. A gap in the muscle may be apparent or palpated through the skin if the muscle is torn. Because these areas are rich in nerve endings, the injury can be extremely painful. The most common areas of sprains occur in the ankle and wrist.

Reviewed by Sharon G. Childs, RN, MS, CRNP-CS, ONC, CEN, Adult Nurse Practitioner, Orthopedic Clinical Specialist, Concentra Medical Center, Baltimore, Md.

A **strain** is an excessive stretching of a muscle and its facial sheath. It often also involves the tendon. Strains may also be classified as first-degree (mild or slightly pulled muscle), second-degree (moderate or moderately pulled muscle), and third-degree (severely pulled muscles).[2] The clinical manifestations of sprains and strains are similar and include pain, edema, decrease in function, and bruising. Pain aggravated by continued use is common.

Edema develops in the injured area because of tiny hemorrhages within the disrupted tissues and the ensuing inflammatory response. Usually the patient will recount a history of traumatic injury, possibly of a twisting nature, or recent exercise activity.

Minor sprains and strains are usually self-limiting, with full function returning within 3 to 6 weeks. A severe sprain can result in an *avulsion fracture*, in which the ligament pulls loose a fragment of bone. Alternatively, the joint structure may become unstable and result in subluxation or dislocation. At the time of injury, *hemarthrosis* (bleeding into a joint space or cavity) or disruption of the synovial lining may occur. An acute strain may involve partial or complete rupture of a muscle. Third-degree strains occasionally require surgical suturing of the muscle and surrounding fascia.

X-rays of the affected part are usually taken to rule out a fracture or widening of the joint structure. Surgical repair may be necessary if the injury is significant enough to produce severe disruption of ligamentous or muscle structures, fracture, or dislocation.

TABLE 61-1   Patient & Family Teaching Guide
Prevention of Musculoskeletal Problems in the Older Adult

1. Use ramps in buildings and at street corners instead of steps to prevent falls.
2. Eliminate scatter rugs in the home.
3. Treat pain and discomfort from osteoarthritis.
   - Rest in reclining position to decrease discomfort.
   - Use plain or enteric-coated aspirin or nonsteroidal antiinflammatory drugs to decrease inflammation of joints and reduce pain.
4. Use a walker or cane to help with walking to prevent falls.
5. Eat the amount and kind of foods to prevent excess weight gain because obesity adds stress to joints, which may predispose to osteoarthritis.
6. Get regular and frequent exercise.
   - Activities of daily living provide range-of-motion exercises.
   - Hobbies (e.g., jigsaw puzzles, needlework, model building) exercise finger joints and prevent stiffness.
   - Some weight-bearing exercise daily (e.g., walking) is essential and should be done two or three times daily.
7. Use shoes with good support to provide for safety and promote comfort.
8. Gradually initiate activities to promote optimal coordination. Rise slowly to a standing position to prevent dizziness, falls, and fractures.

NURSING MANAGEMENT
SPRAINS AND STRAINS

■ **Nursing Implementation**

Health Promotion. Stretching and warm-up exercises before vigorous activity significantly reduce sprains and strains. Preconditioning exercise protects an inherently weak joint because slow stretching is tolerated better by tissues than is quick stretching. Warm-up exercises "prelengthen" potentially strained tissues by avoiding the quick stretch often encountered in sports. Warm-up exercises also increase the temperature of muscle, which increases cell metabolism and nerve impulse transmission. The increased metabolism contributes to better oxygenation of muscle fiber during work. Stretching is also thought to improve kinesthetic awareness, thus lessening the chance of uncoordinated movement.

The use of elastic support bandages or adhesive tape wrapping before beginning a vigorous activity is thought to reduce the

TABLE 61-2   Common Sports-Related Injuries

INJURY	DEFINITION	TREATMENT
Impingement syndrome	Entrapment of soft tissue structures under coracoacromial arch of the shoulder	NSAIDs; rest until symptoms decrease and then gradual ROM and strengthening exercises
Rotator cuff tear	Tear within muscle or ligaments of shoulder	If minor tear, rest, NSAIDs, and gradual mobilization with ROM and strengthening exercises If major tear, surgical repair
Shin splints	Inflammation along tibial shaft from tearing away of tendons caused by improper shoes, overuse, or running on hard pavement	Rest, ice, NSAIDs, proper shoes; gradual increase in activity; if pain persists, x-ray should be done to rule out stress fracture of tibia
Tendinitis	Inflammation of tendon in upper or lower extremity as a result of overuse or incorrect use	Rest, ice, NSAIDs; gradual return to sport activity; protective brace (orthosis) may be necessary if symptoms recur
Ligament injury	Tearing or stretching of ligament; usually occurs as a result of direct blow; characterized by sudden pain, swelling, and instability	Rest, ice, NSAIDs; protection of affected extremity by use of brace; if symptoms persist, surgical repair may be necessary
Meniscal injury	Injury to fibrocartilage of the knee characterized by popping, clicking, or tearing sensation, swelling	Rest, ice, NSAIDs; gradual return to regular activities; if symptoms persist, surgical arthroscopy to diagnose and repair meniscal injury may be necessary

NSAIDs, Nonsteroidal antiinflammatory drugs; *ROM,* range of motion.

occurrence of sprains. However, some health care providers do not support preventive wrapping or taping because it may predispose the athlete to injury.

Acute Intervention. If an injury occurs, the immediate care focuses on (1) rest and limitation of movement, (2) application of ice to the injured area, (3) compression of the involved extremity, (4) elevation of the extremity, and (5) analgesia as necessary (Table 61-3). RICE (rest, ice, compression, elevation) has been found to be effective for most injuries of the musculoskeletal system.[3] Movement should be limited and the extremity rested as soon as pain is felt. Unless the injury is severe, prolonged rest is usually not necessary. Cold *(cryotherapy)* in several forms can be used to produce hypothermia to the involved part. Physiologic changes that occur in soft tissue as a result of the use of cold include vasoconstriction and reduction in the transmission of nerve impulses. These changes result in analgesia and anesthesia, reduction of muscle spasm without changes in muscular strength or endurance, reduction of local edema and inflammation, and reduction of local metabolic requirements. Few unwanted side effects accompany the use of cold to treat a soft tissue injury. Cold is most useful when applied immediately after the injury has occurred. Ice applications should not exceed 20 to 30 minutes per application, allowing a "warm-up" time of 10 to 15 minutes between applications.

Compression also helps limit swelling, which, if left uncontrolled, could lengthen healing time. An elastic compression bandage can be wrapped around the injured part. The bandage is too tight if numbness is felt in the area or there is cramping or additional pain or swelling beyond the edge of the bandage. The bandage can be left in place for 30 minutes and then removed for 15 minutes.

The injured part should be elevated above the heart level to help mobilize excess fluid from the area and impede further edema. The injured part should be elevated even during sleep. Mild analgesics such as nonsteroidal antiinflammatory drugs (NSAIDs) may be necessary to manage patient discomfort. The cyclooxygenase-2 (COX-2) inhibitors (celecoxib [Celebrex],

rofecoxib [Vioxx]) may be given to patients if gastrointestinal problems are a concern.[4]

After the acute phase (usually lasting 24 to 48 hours), warm, moist heat can be applied to the affected part to reduce swelling and provide comfort. Heat applications should not exceed 20 to 30 minutes, allowing a "cool-down" time between applications. NSAIDs may be recommended to decrease edema and pain. The patient is encouraged to use the limb, provided that the joint is protected by means of casting, bracing, taping, or splinting. Movement of the joint maintains nutrition to the cartilage, and muscle contraction improves circulation and resolution of the contusion.

Ambulatory and Home Care. With the exception of treatment in the emergency department following the injury, sprains and strains are treated in the outpatient setting. The patient should be instructed in the use of ice and elevation for 24 to 48 hours after the injury to reduce edema. The use of mild analgesics to promote comfort should be encouraged. Use of an elastic wrap may provide additional support during activity. To prevent reinjury, the patient should learn proper measures of prevention.

The physical therapist may help provide pain relief by means of specialized techniques such as ultrasound. The therapist may also teach the patient exercises to perform for flexibility and to strengthen shortened muscles. Referral to a sports medicine clinic may be appropriate to aid the patient in learning stretching and warm-up exercises to prevent future injury.

DISLOCATION AND SUBLUXATION

A **dislocation** is a severe injury of the ligamentous structures that surround a joint. Dislocation results in the complete displacement or separation of the articular surfaces of the joint. A **subluxation** is a partial or incomplete displacement of the joint surface. The clinical manifestations of a subluxation are similar to those of a dislocation but are less severe. Treatment of subluxation is similar to that of a dislocation, but subluxation may require less healing time.

Dislocations characteristically result from overwhelming forces transmitted to the joint that cause a disruption of the soft

TABLE 61-3   *Emergency Management*

Acute Soft Tissue Injury

ETIOLOGY	ASSESSMENT FINDINGS	INTERVENTIONS
Falls	• Edema	**Initial**
Direct blows	• Ecchymosis	• Ensure airway, breathing, and circulation.
Crush injury	• Pain, tenderness	• Assess neurovascular status of involved limb.
Motor vehicle collisions	• Decreased sensation with severe edema	• Elevate involved limb.
Sports injuries	• Decreased pulse, coolness, and capillary refill	• Apply compression bandage unless dislocation present.
	• Decreased movement	• Apply ice packs to affected area.
	• Pallor	• Immobilize affected extremity in the position found.
	• Shortening or rotation of extremity	• Anticipate x-rays of injured extremity.
	• Inability to bear weight when lower extremity involved	• Give analgesia as necessary.
		• Administer tetanus prophylaxis if skin integrity broken.
	• Decreased function with upper-extremity involvement	**Ongoing Monitoring**
	• Muscle spasms	• Monitor for changes in neurovascular status.
		• Eliminate weight bearing when lower extremity involved.
		• Anticipate compartment pressure monitoring if neurovascular status changes.

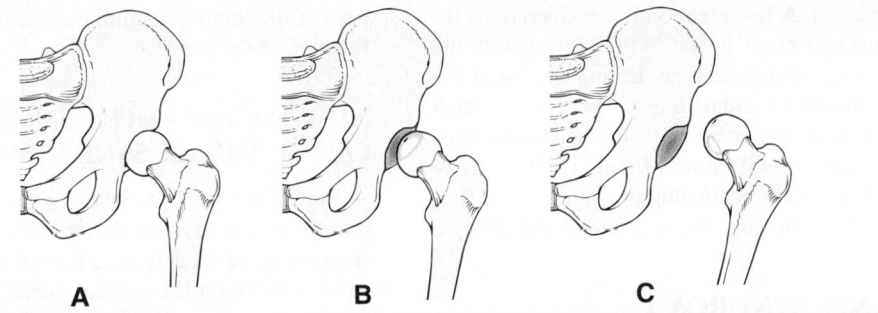

FIG. 61-1 Soft tissue injury of the hip. A, Normal. B, Subluxation (partial dislocation). C, Dislocation.

tissues surrounding the joint. The joints most frequently dislocated in the upper extremity include the thumb, elbow, and shoulder. In the lower extremity, the hip is vulnerable to dislocation occurring as a result of severe trauma, often associated with motor vehicle accidents (Fig. 61-1). The patella may dislocate because of instability of the tendons, ligaments, and muscles surrounding the knee or a severe twisting blow. Dislocations may also be the result of a congenital anomaly or of a pathologic origin.

The most obvious clinical manifestation of a dislocation is asymmetry of the musculoskeletal contour. For example, if a hip is dislocated, the limb is shorter on the affected side. Additional manifestations include local pain, tenderness, loss of function of the injured part, and swelling of the soft tissues in the region of the joint. The major complications of a dislocated joint are open joint injuries, intraarticular fractures, fracture dislocation, *avascular necrosis* (bone cell death as a result of inadequate blood supply), and damage to adjacent neurovascular tissue. Neurovascular assessment is critical.

X-ray studies are performed to determine the extent of shifting of the involved structures. The joint may also be aspirated to determine the presence of blood (hemarthrosis) or fat cells. Fat cells in the aspirate indicate a probable intraarticular fracture.

NURSING *and* COLLABORATIVE MANAGEMENT DISLOCATION

A dislocation requires prompt attention, especially the knee joint. A dislocation is considered an orthopedic emergency.[5] The longer the joint remains unreduced, the greater the possibility of avascular necrosis. The hip joint is particularly susceptible to avascular necrosis. The first goal of management is to realign the dislocated portion of the joint in its original anatomic position. This can be accomplished by a closed reduction, which may be performed under local or general anesthesia or intravenous (IV) conscious sedation. Anesthesia is often necessary to produce muscle relaxation so that the bones can be manipulated. In some situations, surgical open reduction may be necessary. After reduction, the extremity is usually immobilized by taping or using a sling to allow the torn ligaments and capsular tissue time to heal.

Nursing management of subluxation or dislocation is directed toward relief of pain and support and protection of the injured joint. After the joint has been reduced and immobilized, motion is usually restricted. A carefully regulated rehabilitation program can prevent the formation of contractures. Gentle range of motion (ROM) may be started if the joint is stable and the affected joint is well supported. The patient should not stretch the joint beyond its limits because the torn capsule and ligament heal in a

shortened position with fibrous scar tissue that is not as strong as the original tissue. An exercise program slowly and methodically restores the joint to its original ROM without causing another dislocation. The patient should gradually return to normal activities.

A patient who has dislocated a joint may be at greater risk for repeated dislocations because the joint has been weakened by shortened ligaments and scar tissue. Activity restrictions of the affected joint may be imposed to decrease the risk of repeatedly dislocating the joint.

REPETITIVE STRAIN INJURY

Repetitive strain injury (RSI) is a cumulative trauma disorder resulting from prolonged, forceful, or awkward movements. RSI is also reported as repetitive trauma disorder, nontraumatic musculoskeletal injury, overuse syndrome (sports medicine), regional musculoskeletal disorder, work-related disorder, and "nintendinitis" (Nintendo games).[6] Repeated movements strain tendons, ligaments, and muscles, causing tiny tears that become inflamed. If the tissues are not given time to heal properly, scarring can occur. Blood vessels of the arms and hands may become constricted, depriving tissues of vital nutrients and causing an accumulation of factors such as lactic acid. Without intervention, tendons and muscles can deteriorate and nerves can become hypersensitive. At this point even the slightest movement can cause pain.

In addition to the repetitive movements, other factors related to RSI include poor posture and positioning, poor work space ergonomics, a badly designed keyboard, and lifting of heavy workloads without sufficient muscle rest. The result may cause chronic dysfunction to the muscles, tendons, and nerves of the neck, shoulder, forearm, and hand. Symptoms of RSI include pain, weakness, numbness, or impairment of motor function. Persons most often affected by RSI include musicians, dancers, electricians, butchers, keyboard operators, cashiers, grocery clerks, packers, postal workers, poultry processors, and vibratory tool workers.

RSI is becoming a serious public health problem for youth. More young people are employed an average of 15 to 20 hours per week; many work in the fast food industry where the equipment has been designed for adult workers. Farm laborers, competitive athletes, and poorly trained athletes may develop RSI. Swimming, overhead throwing (e.g., baseball), weight lifting, gymnastics, dancing, tennis, skiing, soccer (kicking sports), and horseback riding require repetitive motion, and overtraining compounds the effects.

RSI can be prevented through education, ergonomics (consideration of the interaction of humans and their work environment), and appropriate job design. A few ergonomic considerations include keeping the hips and knees flexed to 90 degrees with the feet flat, keeping the wrist straight to type, having the top of the monitor even with the forehead, and taking at least hourly stretch breaks. Once diagnosed, the treatment of RSI consists of identifying precipitating activity, modification of equipment or activity, pain management including heat/cold application, NSAIDs, rest, physical therapy for strengthening exercises, and lifestyle changes.

CARPAL TUNNEL SYNDROME

Carpal tunnel syndrome (CTS) is a condition caused by compression of the median nerve beneath the transverse carpal ligament within the narrow confines of the carpal tunnel located in the wrist (Fig. 61-2). CTS is the most common compression neuropathy. This condition often is due to pressure from trauma or edema caused by inflammation of a tendon (tenosynovitis), neoplasm, rheumatoid synovial disease, or soft tissue masses such as ganglia. Symptoms of CTS are often seen during the premenstrual period, pregnancy, and menopause, in diabetes mellitus and thyroid dysfunction, or in conditions with increased fluid retention.[7] This syndrome is associated with occupations that require continuous wrist movement (e.g., butchers, dentists, seamstresses, machine operators, musicians, hair stylists, secretaries, painters, carpenters, computer operators, bowlers, knitters, guitarists).

The clinical manifestations of CTS are weakness (especially of the thumb), burning pain (causalagia) and numbness, or impaired sensation in the distribution of the median nerve and clumsiness in performing fine hand movements. Numbness and tingling may be present that awaken the patient at night. Holding the wrist in acute flexion for 60 seconds will produce tingling and numbness over the distribution of the median nerve, the palmar surface of the thumb, the index finger, the middle finger, and part of the ring finger. This is known as a positive *Phalen's sign.* Tapping gently over the area of the inflamed median nerve may reproduce the paresthesia. This is known as a positive *Tinel's sign.* In late stages there is atrophy of the thenar muscles around the base of the thumb, resulting in recurrent pain and eventual dysfunction of the hand.

NURSING *and* COLLABORATIVE MANAGEMENT CARPAL TUNNEL SYNDROME

Prevention of CTS involves educating employees and employers to identify risk factors. Adaptive devices such as wrist splints may be worn to hold the wrist in slight dorsiflexion to relieve pressure on the median nerve. Special keyboard pads that help prevent repetitive pressure on the median nerve are available for computer operators to help prevent or reduce CTS by decreasing tension on the carpal tunnel. Other ergonomic changes include workstation modifications, change in body positions, and frequent breaks.

Collaborative care of the patient with CTS is directed toward relieving the underlying cause of the nerve compression. The early symptoms associated with CTS can usually be relieved by stopping the aggravating movement and by placing the hand and wrist at rest by immobilizing them in a hand splint. If the cause is inflammation, injection of a corticosteroid drug directly into the carpal tunnel may provide short-term (up to 6 months) relief. The patient's sensation may be impaired during this time. Therefore the patient should be instructed to avoid hazards such as extreme heat because of the risk of thermal injury. The patient may be required to consider occupational changes because of discomfort and sensory and functional changes.

If the problem continues, the median nerve may have to be surgically decompressed by longitudinal division of the transverse carpal ligament under regional anesthesia (see Fig. 61-2). This surgery is done on an outpatient basis. After surgery, the neurovascular status of the hand should be evaluated before discharge, and the patient should be instructed in the appropriate assessments to perform at home. Endoscopic carpal tunnel release is a surgical procedure in which the decompression is performed through a small incision puncture site with the patient under local anesthesia. Modified open carpal tunnel release procedure is another alternative surgical intervention.

ROTATOR CUFF INJURY

The rotator cuff is a complex of four muscles in the shoulder: supraspinatus, infraspinatus, teres minor, and subscapularis. These muscles act to stabilize the humeral head in the glenoid fossa while assisting with the ROM of the shoulder joint and rotation of the humerus. Degenerative changes of the rotator cuff are associated with normal aging.

A tear in the rotator cuff may occur as a gradual, degenerative process resulting from aging, poor posture, repetitive stress (especially overhead arm motions), or use of an arm to break a fall. The rotator cuff will rupture as a result of sudden adduction forces applied to the cuff while the arm is held in abduction. In sports, repetitive overhead motions, such as in swimming, racquet sports (tennis, racquetball), and baseball (especially pitching), are often activities that initiate injury. A fall to an outstretched hand or a blow to the upper arm, heavy lifting, or repetitive work motions are also causative factors.[8]

Patients with a rotator cuff injury will complain of shoulder pain and inability to initiate or maintain abduction of the arm or shoulder. The weakness and decreased ROM accompany a positive Neer's test and Hawkin's test, which both will yield a positive

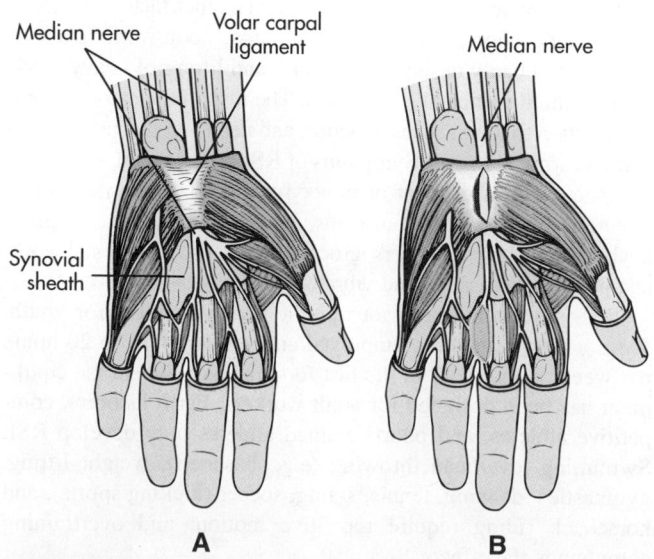

FIG. 61-2 A, Wrist structures involved in carpal tunnel syndrome. B, Decompression of median nerve.

Median nerve
Volar carpal ligament
Median nerve
Synovial sheath
A   B

response to pain. An x-ray alone is usually not beneficial in the diagnosis of a rotator cuff injury. A tear can be confirmed by arthrogram or magnetic resonance imaging (MRI).[9] The Simple Shoulder Test is also diagnostic in evaluating rotator cuff function. In this test patients are evaluated in their ability to place the arm comfortably at the side, ability to sleep with the arm at their side, ability to tuck in a shirt or blouse behind, place hand behind head, place a coin on a shelf, place a pound on a shelf, place 8 lb on a shelf, carry 20 lb, toss underhand, throw overhand, wash the opposite shoulder, and perform their usual work.[10]

The goal of treatment emphasizes maintaining passive ROM and the return of abduction strength. The patient may be treated conservatively with rest, ice and heat, NSAIDs, periodic corticosteroid injections into the joint, and physical therapy. If the patient does not respond to conservative treatment or if a complete tear is present, a surgical repair may be necessary. Surgical repair may be done through the arthroscope. If an extensive tear is present, acromioplasty (surgical removal of part of the acromion to relieve compression of rotator cuff during movement) may be necessary. An immobilization device such as a sling or, more commonly, a shoulder immobilizer may be used immediately after surgery. However, the shoulder should not be immobilized for too long a period because frozen shoulder or arthrofibrosis may occur. Pendulum exercises and physical therapy begin the first postoperative day.

MENISCUS INJURY

The meniscus is the fibrocartilage in the knee and other joints. Meniscus injuries are closely associated with ligament sprains commonly occurring in athletes engaged in sports such as basketball, rugby, football, soccer, and hockey. These activities produce rotational stress when the knee is in varying degrees of flexion and the foot is planted or fixed. A blow to the knee can cause the meniscus to be sheared between the femoral condyles and the tibial plateau, resulting in a torn meniscus. (The knee joint is shown in Fig. 61-3.) Occupations that require persons to work in a squatting or kneeling position may be at higher risk for meniscus injuries.

Meniscus injuries alone do not usually cause chronic edema because cartilage is avascular and aneural. However, a torn meniscus may be suspected when local tenderness or pain is reported. Pain is elicited by abduction or adduction of the leg at the knee. The usual clinical picture is a feeling by the patient that the knee is unstable and a report that the knee may "click, lock, and give away."[11] Quadriceps atrophy is evident if the injury has been present for some time. Traumatic arthritis may occur from repeated meniscal injury and chronic inflammation.

An arthrogram, arthroscopy, or both can diagnose knee problems. MRI is beneficial in confirming the diagnosis before arthroscopy is used. MRI has eliminated the use of an arthrogram as a diagnostic tool in many cases. Surgery may be indicated for a torn meniscus. Degree of knee pain and dysfunction, occupation, sport activities, and age may affect the patient's decision to have or postpone surgery.

NURSING and COLLABORATIVE MANAGEMENT
MENISCUS INJURY

Because meniscal injuries are commonly caused by sports-related activity, athletes should be taught to do warm-up activities. Proper stretching may make the patient less prone to meniscal injury when a fall or twisting occurs. Examination of the acutely injured knee should occur within 24 hours of injury. Initial care of this type of injury involves application of ice, immobilization, and partial weight bearing with crutches. Most meniscal injuries are treated in an outpatient setting. The patient should be allowed to ambulate as tolerated. Crutches may be necessary. Use of a knee brace or immobilizer during the first few days after the injury protects the knee and offers some pain relief.

After acute pain has decreased, gradual increases in flexion and muscle strengthening may assist the patient to full functioning. Physical therapy is generally recommended to help the patient to strengthen the quadricep muscles before returning to sport activities. Surgical repair or excision of part of the menis-

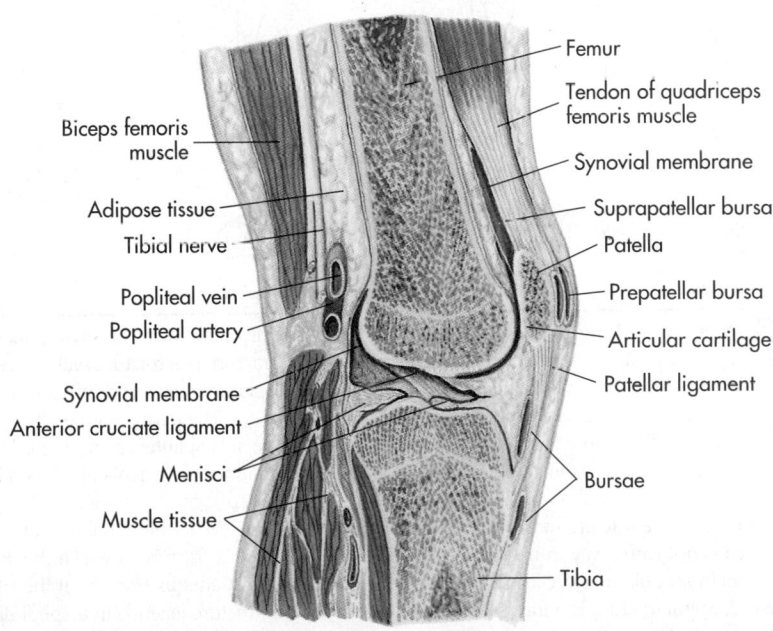

FIG. 61-3 Sagittal section through knee joint.

Labels (left side, top to bottom): Biceps femoris muscle; Adipose tissue; Tibial nerve; Popliteal vein; Popliteal artery; Synovial membrane; Anterior cruciate ligament; Menisci; Muscle tissue

Labels (right side, top to bottom): Femur; Tendon of quadriceps femoris muscle; Synovial membrane; Suprapatellar bursa; Patella; Prepatellar bursa; Articular cartilage; Patellar ligament; Bursae; Tibia

cus (meniscectomy) may be necessary. Often this can be done by arthroscopy. Pain relief may include NSAIDs, tramadol (Ultram), or a mild combination of drugs such as acetaminophen with hydrocodone. Rehabilitation starts soon after surgery, including ROM and quadricep and hamstring strengthening exercises. When the patient's strength is back to its preinjury level, normal activities may be resumed.

BURSITIS

Bursae are closed sacs that are lined with synovial membrane and contain a small amount of synovial fluid. They are located at sites of friction, such as between tendons and bones and near the joints. **Bursitis** (inflammation of the bursa) results from repeated or excessive trauma or friction, gout, rheumatoid arthritis, or infection. The primary clinical manifestations of bursitis are warmth, pain, swelling, and limited ROM in the affected part. Sites at which bursitis commonly occurs include the hand, knee, greater trochanter of the hip, shoulder, and elbow. Repetitive kneeling (carpet layers, coal miners, and gardeners), jogging in worn-out shoes, and prolonged sitting with crossed legs are common precipitators of injury.[12]

Attempts are made to determine and correct the cause of the bursitis. Rest is often the only treatment needed. Icing the area will decrease pain and may reduce inflammation. The affected part may be immobilized in a compression dressing or plaster splint. NSAIDs may be used to reduce inflammation and pain.[13] Aspiration of the bursal fluid (dark, bloody, cloudy) and injection of a corticosteroid may be necessary. If the bursal wall has become thickened and continues to interfere with normal joint function, surgical excision (bursectomy) may be necessary. For example, subacromial bursal thickening causes pain and loss of ROM on abduction of the shoulder. Septic bursae usually require surgical incision and drainage.

MUSCLE SPASMS

Local muscle spasms are a common condition often associated with sports and excessive everyday activities. Injury to a muscle results in inflammation and edema, which irritates nerve endings, resulting in muscle spasm. The spasms produce additional pain, creating a repetitive cycle. The clinical manifestations of muscle spasm include pain; palpable, tense, firm muscle mass; diminished ROM if a joint is involved; and limitation of daily or occupational activities.

A careful history and physical examination should be performed to rule out central nervous system (CNS) problems. Muscle spasms may be managed with drug therapy, physical therapy, or both. Drugs used for treatment of local muscle spasms include mild analgesics, NSAIDs, and skeletal muscle relaxants. A physical therapy program might include the use of heat or ice, supervised exercise, massage, hydrotherapy, local heat-producing ap-

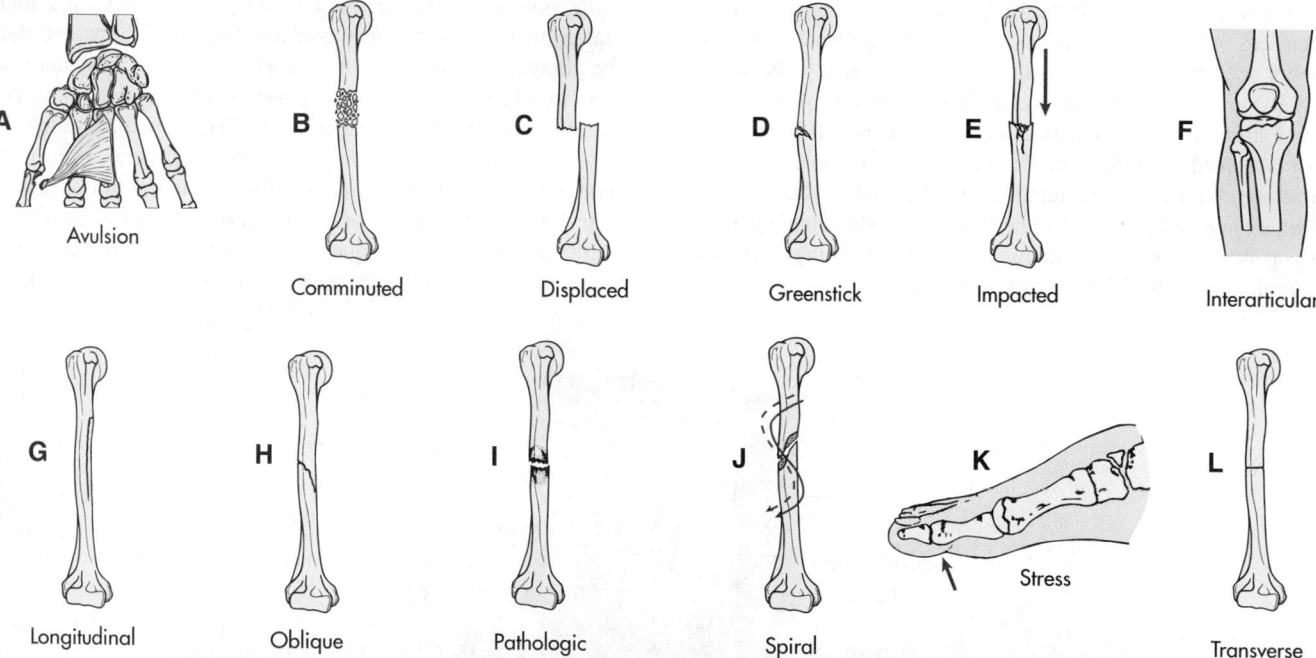

FIG. 61-4 Types of fractures. **A,** Avulsion is a fracture of bone resulting from the strong pulling effect of tendons or ligaments at the bone attachment. **B,** Comminuted fracture is a fracture with more than two fragments. The smaller fragments appear to be floating. **C,** Displaced (overriding) fracture involves a displaced fracture fragment that is overriding the other bone fragment. The periosteum is disrupted on both sides. **D,** Greenstick fracture is an incomplete fracture with one side splintered and the other side bent. **E,** Impacted fracture is a comminuted fracture in which more than two fragments are driven into each other. **F,** Interarticular fracture is a fracture extending to the articular surface of the bone. **G,** Longitudinal fracture is an incomplete fracture in which the fracture line runs along the longitudinal axis of the bone. The periosteum is not torn away from the bone. **H,** Oblique fracture is a fracture in which the line of the fracture extends in an oblique direction. **I,** Pathologic fracture is a spontaneous fracture at the site of a bone disease. **J,** Spiral fracture is a fracture in which the line of the fracture extends in a spiral direction along the shaft of the bone. **K,** Stress fracture is a fracture that occurs in normal or abnormal bone that is subject to repeated stress, such as from jogging or running. **L,** Transverse fracture is a fracture in which the line of the fracture extends across the bone shaft at a right angle to the longitudinal axis.

plications (oil of wintergreen), ultrasound (deep heat), manipulation, and bracing.

Fractures

Classification

A **fracture** is a disruption or break in the continuity of the structure of bone. Traumatic injuries account for the majority of fractures, although some fractures are secondary to a disease process (pathologic fractures). Fractures are described and classified according to (1) type (Fig. 61-4); (2) communication or noncommunication with the external environment (Fig. 61-5); and (3) anatomic location of fracture on the involved bone (Fig. 61-6) as well as the appearance, position, and alignment of the fragments; and classic names.[14]

Fractures are also described as stable or unstable. A *stable fracture* occurs when a piece of the periosteum is intact across the fracture and either external or internal fixation has rendered the fragments stationary. Stable fractures are usually transverse, spiral, or greenstick. An *unstable fracture* is grossly displaced during injury and is a site of poor fixation. Unstable fractures are usually comminuted or oblique.

A fracture can also be classified as closed (simple) or open. An *open fracture* (formerly called compound fracture) involves communication of the fracture through the skin with the external environment.

Clinical Manifestations

The patient's history indicates a mechanism of injury associated with numerous signs and symptoms, including immediate localized pain, decreased function, and inability to bear weight or use the affected part (Table 61-4). The patient guards and protects the extremity against movement. The fracture may not be accompanied by obvious bone deformity. If a fracture is suspected, the extremity is immobilized in the position in which it is found. Unnecessary movement increases soft-tissue damage and may convert a closed fracture to an open fracture or create further injury to adjacent neurovascular structures.

Fracture Healing

It is important to understand the principles of fracture healing (Fig. 61-7) to provide appropriate therapeutic interventions. Bone goes through a remarkable reparative process of self-healing (termed *union*) that occurs in the following stages:

1. *Fracture hematoma.* When a fracture occurs, bleeding and edema create a hematoma, which surrounds the ends of the fragments. The hematoma is extravasated blood that changes from a liquid to a semisolid clot. This occurs in the initial 72 hours after injury.

2. *Granulation tissue.* During this stage, active phagocytosis absorbs the products of local necrosis. The hematoma converts to granulation tissue. Granulation tissue (consisting of new blood vessels, fibroblasts, and osteoblasts) produces the basis for new bone substance called *osteoid* during days 3 to 14 postinjury.

3. *Callus formation.* As minerals (calcium, phosphorus, and magnesium and new bone matrix) are deposited in the osteoid, an unorganized network of bone is formed that is woven about the fracture parts. *Callus* is primarily composed of cartilage, osteoblasts, calcium, and phosphorus. It usually begins to appear by the end of the second week after injury. Evidence of callus formation can be verified by x-ray.

4. *Ossification.* Ossification of the callus occurs from 3 weeks to 6 months after the fracture and continues until the fracture has healed. Callus ossification is sufficient to prevent movement at the fracture site when the bones are gently stressed. However, the fracture is still evident on x-ray. During this stage of clinical union the patient can be converted from skeletal traction to a cast, or the cast can be removed to allow limited mobility.

5. *Consolidation.* As callus continues to develop, the distance between bone fragments diminishes and eventually closes. This stage is called consolidation, and ossification continues. It can be equated with radiologic union.

6. *Remodeling.* Excess bone tissue is reabsorbed in the final stage of bone healing, and union is completed. Gradual return of the injured bone to its preinjury structural strength and shape occurs. Bone remodels in response to physical stress.[14] Initially, stress is provided through exercise. Weight bearing is gradually introduced. New bone is deposited in sites subjected to stress and resorbed at areas where there is little stress. Radiologic union occurs when there is x-ray evidence of complete bony union. This phase can occur up to a year following injury.

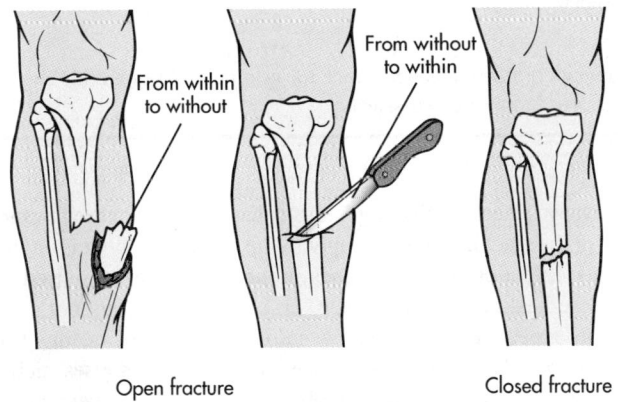

Open fracture   Closed fracture

FIG. 61-5 Fracture classification according to communication.

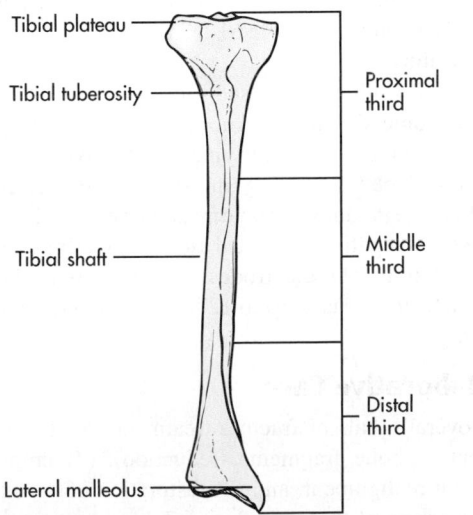

Tibial plateau
Tibial tuberosity
Proximal third
Tibial shaft
Middle third
Distal third
Lateral malleolus

FIG. 61-6 Fracture classification according to location.

TABLE 61-4   Clinical Manifestations of Fracture

MANIFESTATION	SIGNIFICANCE
Edema and Swelling Disruption of soft tissues or bleeding into surrounding tissues	Unchecked edema in closed space can occlude circulation and damage nerves (i.e., there is a risk of compartment syndrome).
Pain and Tenderness Muscle spasm as a result of involuntary reflex action of muscle, direct tissue trauma, increased pressure on sensory nerve, movement of fracture parts	Pain and tenderness encourage splinting of fracture with reduction in motion of injured area.
Muscle Spasm Protective response to injury and fracture	Muscle spasms may displace nondisplaced fracture or prevent it from reducing spontaneously.
Deformity Abnormal position of bone as result of original forces of injury and action of muscles pulling fragment into abnormal position; seen as a loss of normal bony contours	Deformity is cardinal sign of fracture; if uncorrected, it may result in problems with bony union and restoration of function of injured part.
Ecchymosis Discoloration of skin as a result of extravasation of blood in subcutaneous tissues	Ecchymosis may appear immediately after injury and may appear distal to injury. The nurse should reassure patient that process is normal.
Loss of Function Disruption of bone, preventing functional use	Fracture must be managed properly to ensure restoration of function.
Crepitation Grating or crunching together of bony fragments, producing palpable or audible crunching sensation	Crepitation may increase chance for nonunion if bone ends are allowed to move excessively.

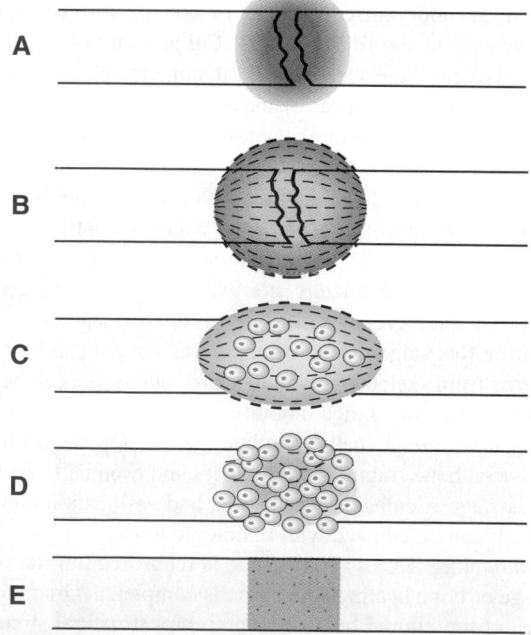

FIG. 61-7 Bone healing (schematic representation). **A,** Bleeding at broken ends of the bone with subsequent hematoma formation. **B,** Organization of hematoma into fibrous network. **C,** Invasion of osteoblasts, lengthening of collagen strands, and deposition of calcium. **D,** Callus formation: new bone is built up as osteoclasts destroy dead bone. **E,** Remodeling is accomplished as excess callus is reabsorbed and trabecular bone is laid down.

Many factors, such as age, initial displacement of the fracture, site of the fracture, blood supply to the area, immobilization, implants, infection, and hormones influence the time required for fracture healing to be complete. Fracture healing may not occur in the expected time *(delayed union)* or may not occur at all *(nonunion)*. The ossification process is arrested by causes such as inadequate reduction and immobilization, excess movement, infection, poor nutrition, and systemic disease. Healing time for fractures increases with age. For example, an uncomplicated midshaft fracture of the femur heals in 3 weeks in a newborn and in 20 weeks in an adult. Table 61-5 summarizes complications of fracture healing.

Electrical stimulation is used successfully to stimulate bone healing in some situations of nonunion or delayed union. The electric current acts by modifying cell behavior causing bone remodeling. The underlying mechanism for electrically induced bone remodeling remains unknown. It is thought to be related to negative electrical fields attracting positive ions such as calcium. The electrodes are placed over the patient's skin or cast and are used 10 to 12 hours each day, usually while sleeping.

Collaborative Care

The overall goals of fracture treatment are (1) anatomic realignment of bone fragments (reduction), (2) immobilization to maintain realignment, and (3) restoration of normal or near-normal function of the injured part. Table 61-6 summarizes the collaborative care of fractures.

TABLE 61-5	Complications of Fracture Healing
PROBLEM	**DESCRIPTION**
Delayed union	Fracture healing progresses more slowly than expected; healing eventually occurs.
Nonunion	Fracture fails to heal properly despite treatment, resulting in fibrous union or pseudarthrosis.
Malunion	Fracture heals in expected time but in unsatisfactory position, possibly resulting in deformity or dysfunction.
Angulation	Fracture heals in abnormal position in relation to midline of structure (type of malunion).
Pseudarthrosis	Type of nonunion occurring at fracture site in which false joint is formed on shaft of long bones. It is a fracture site that failed to fuse. Each bone end is covered with fibrous scar tissue.
Refracture	New fracture occurs at original fracture site.
Myositis ossificans	Condition occurring in response to muscle hemorrhage caused by trauma. Hematoma ossifies.

TABLE 61-6	Collaborative Care: Fractures

Diagnostic
History and physical examination
X-ray examination
CT scan, MRI

Collaborative Therapy
Fracture Reduction
Manipulation
Closed reduction
Traction devices
  Skin traction
  Skeletal traction
Open reduction
Fracture Immobilization
Casting
Traction
External fixation
Internal fixation
Open Fractures
Surgical debridement and irrigation
Tetanus immunization
Prophylactic antibiotic therapy
Immobilization

CT, Computed tomography; *MRI*, magnetic resonance imaging.

Fracture Reduction

Closed reduction. *Closed reduction* is a nonsurgical, manual realignment of bone fragments to their previous anatomic position. Traction and countertraction are manually applied to the bone fragments to restore position, length, and alignment. Closed reduction is usually performed with the patient under local or general anesthesia. After reduction, the injured part is immobilized by traction, casting, external fixation, splints, or orthoses (braces) to maintain alignment until healing occurs.

Open reduction. *Open reduction* is the correction of bone alignment through a surgical incision. It often includes internal fixation of the fracture with the use of wire, screws, pins, plates, intramedullary rods, or nails. The type and location of the fracture, age of patient, and concurrent disease, as well as the result of attempted closed reduction by means of traction, may influence the decision to use open reduction. The chief disadvantages of this form of treatment are the possibility of infection and the complications associated with anesthesia.

If open reduction with internal fixation (ORIF) is used for intraarticular fractures (involving joint surfaces), early initiation of ROM of the joint is indicated. Machines that provide continuous passive motion (CPM) to various joints are now available. Use of such machines can result in prevention of intraarticular adhesions, faster reconstruction of the subchondral (beneath cartilage) bone plate, more rapid healing of the articular cartilage, and possibly decreased incidence of later posttraumatic arthritis. ORIF facilitates early ambulation, which decreases the risk of complications related to prolonged immobility, and promotes fracture healing with gradually increasing increments of stress.

Traction. Traction devices apply a pulling force on the fractured extremity to attain realignment while countertraction pulls in the opposite direction. The two most common types of traction are skin traction and skeletal traction. *Skin traction* is generally used for short-term treatment (48 to 72 hours) until skeletal traction or surgery is possible. Tape, boots, or splints are applied directly to the skin to maintain alignment, assist in reduction, and

help diminish muscle spasms in the injured extremity. The traction weights are usually limited to 5 to 10 lb (2.3 to 4.5 kg). *Skeletal traction*, generally in place for longer periods, is used to align injured bones and joints or to treat joint contractures and congenital hip dysplasia. It provides a long-term pull that keeps the injured bones and joints aligned. To establish skeletal traction, the physician inserts a pin or wire into the bone, either partially or completely, to align and immobilize the injured body part. Weight for skeletal traction ranges from 5 to 45 lb (2.3 to 20.4 kg).

When traction is used to treat fractures, the forces are usually exerted on the distal fragment to obtain alignment with the proximal fragment. Several types of traction are used for this purpose (Table 61-7). Fracture alignment depends on the correct positioning and alignment of the patient while the traction forces remain constant. For extremity traction to be effective, forces must be pulling in the opposite direction (countertraction) to prevent the patient from sliding to the end or side of the bed. Countertraction is commonly supplied by the patient's body weight or may be augmented by elevating the end of the bed. It is imperative that the nurse maintain the traction constantly and not interrupt the weight applied to the traction.

Fracture Immobilization

Casts. A cast is a temporary circumferential immobilization device. Casting is a common treatment following closed reduction. It allows the patient to perform many normal activities of daily living while providing sufficient immobilization to ensure stability. Cast materials are natural (plaster of paris), synthetic, fiberglass free, latex-free polymer, or a hybrid of materials.[15]

After immersion in water, plaster of paris is wrapped and molded around the affected part. It is composed of anhydrous calcium sulfate embedded in gauze roll. The strength of the cast

TABLE 61-7 Common Types of Traction

TYPE	INDICATIONS	NURSING IMPLICATIONS
Skin Buck's 	Used for many conditions affecting hip, femur, knee, or back. It is generally used for temporary immobilization and stabilization of fractured hips or fractures of the femoral shaft. It can be unilateral or bilateral. May also be used to correct knee and hip joint contractures.	All assessments should be at least q4hr. Assess for altered neurovascular status caused by original injury or the application of the bandages used in Buck's traction. Especially note decreased peripheral vascular flow and peroneal nerve deficit by assessing for ability to dorsiflex toes and foot, and for changes in sensation in the first webspace between the great and second toes. Pressure from the elastic wrap may result in pressure necrosis, especially over bony prominences and areas prone to pressure (anterior tibial border, fibular head, both malleoli, Achilles tendon, calcaneus, and dorsum of the foot). In addition, assess for an allergic reaction to the adhesive material, rotation of the extremity, and constant traction and countertraction forces.
Russell's 	Used for fractures of femur or hip.	Same as above. An additional area prone to pressure necrosis is the area over the hamstring tendons in the popliteal space.
Bryant's 	Used for fractures of the femur, fractures in small children, and stabilization of hip joints in children under 2 yr or 30 lb (14 kg) in weight.	Be aware that with traction in place, buttocks should just clear the mattress. Check for undue pressure over the outer head and neck of fibula, dorsum of foot, Achilles tendon, scapulae, and shoulders. Check that bandages or boot has not slipped. Be aware that these are usually removed for skin care and assessment q4hr.
Pelvic belt (or girdle) 	Used for sciatica, muscle spasms (low back), and minor fractures of the lower spine.	Check for security of the pelvic belt. Check frequently for skin irritation over iliac crests and in the intergluteal fold. Use measures to prevent skin breakdown. Check and adjust pelvic belt straps so that they are unrestricted and equal in length. Secure the straps with adhesive tape. Use a footboard to prevent footdrop. Maintain the correct angle of pull of the traction. Be aware that the physician orders the type of countertraction.
Pelvic sling traction	Used for pelvic fractures to provide compression for a separated pelvic girdle.	The sling should keep the pelvis just above the surface of the bed. Assess for pressure necrosis and skin irritation q4hr; especially assess for pressure over the iliac crests, intergluteal fold, and greater trochanters. Monitor for soiling of the sling and change as needed; use a fracture bedpan for toileting. Limit use of trapeze because it will reduce compressive force from the sling. Use alternating air pressure mattress or other pressure-dispersing devices; provide frequent back care.

TABLE 61-7	Common Types of Traction—cont'd	
TYPE	**INDICATIONS**	**NURSING IMPLICATIONS**
Skin—cont'd **Head halter** 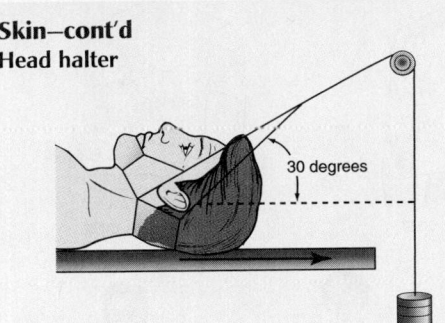	Used for soft tissue disorders and degenerative disk disease of the cervical spine. It is not commonly used for unstable fractures of the cervical spine.	Assess for alignment with trunk, areas of local pressure over the ears and mandibular joints and under the chin and occipital area, and pain or dysfunction in the temporomandibular joint. Patients may be permitted to remove traction for meals; if not, provide a liquid or mechanical soft diet to reduce temporomandibular joint pain. Because this traction is commonly used in the home, ensure patients can demonstrate safe and effective setup, application, and use of the traction before discharge.
Skeletal **Overhead arm (90 degrees-90 degrees)** 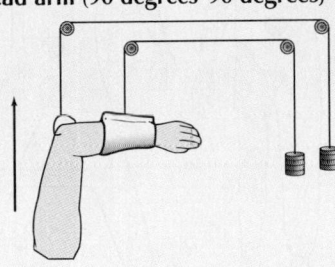	Commonly used for immobilization of fractures and dislocations of the upper arm and shoulder.	Be aware that the shoulder and elbow joint are maintained at 90-degree angles. Assess for pressure necrosis beneath the sling, especially over bony prominences. Assess distal neurovascular status; because of exposure, skin temperature may be cool and thus not indicative of decreased perfusion. Perform assessments q4hr. Inspect the pin site and perform pin site care according to protocol.
Lateral arm 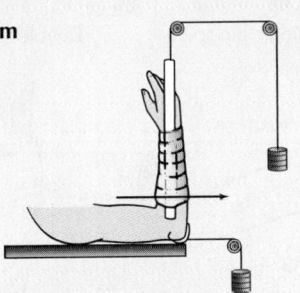	Commonly used in immobilization of fractures and dislocations of the upper arm and shoulder.	Inspect the pin site and perform pin site care according to protocol. Assess neurovascular status.
Balanced suspension traction 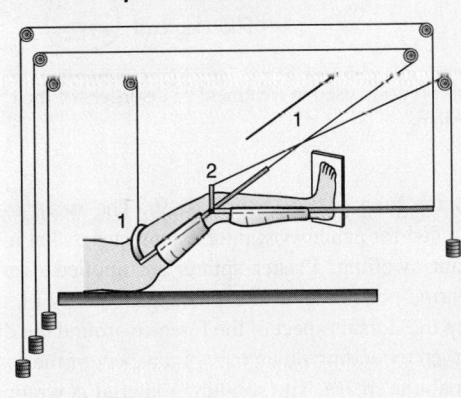	Used for injury or fracture of the femoral shaft of the femur, acetabulum, hip, tibia, or any combination of these.	Be aware that this traction uses half-ring Thomas splint (1) and Pearson attachment (2) and that suspension of the extremity and direct skeletal traction are applied. This allows raising of the buttocks off the bed for bedpan use and skin care without altering the line of traction. Maintain countertraction (e.g., position patient high in bed so that feet do not press on foot of bed; do not elevate the head of the bed >25 degrees if it causes continual movement toward foot of the bed). Encourage self-help in patient's performance of activities of daily living, movement in bed with help of trapeze, and flexion and extension of affected foot to prevent footdrop. Assess for pressure necrosis in areas contacted by the traction, especially the greater trochanter, ischial tuberosity, hamstring tendons, fibular head, and both malleoli. Assess distal neurovascular status q4hr. Inspect the pin site and perform pin site care according to protocol.

is determined by the number of layers of plaster bandage and the technique of application. As the cast dries a thermochemical reaction occurs in which the calcium sulfate recrystallizes and hardens. The patient may experience increased warmth about the fracture site. Increased edema as a result of the improved circulation may occur as a result of heat produced by the drying cast. After the cast is completely dry, it is strong and firm and can withstand stresses. The plaster hardens within 15 minutes, so the patient may move around without difficulty. However, it is not strong enough for weight bearing until about 24 to 72 hours.

A fresh cast should never be covered with a blanket because air cannot circulate and heat builds up in the cast. During the drying period the cast should not be subjected to any wetness, soiling, or abnormal stresses that can cause weakening or a break in the cast. It should be carefully handled by the palms of the hands rather than with the fingertips to avoid indentations that will dry and become potential pressure areas. Once the cast is thoroughly dry, the edges may need to be petaled to avoid skin irritation from rough edges and to prevent plaster of paris debris from falling into the cast and causing irritation or pressure necrosis (Fig. 61-8).

Synthetic casting materials (thermolabile plastic, thermoplastic resins, polyurethane, and fiberglass) are molded to fit the torso or extremity after being activated by submersion in cool or tepid water. Casts made of synthetic materials are frequently used because they are lightweight and relatively waterproof and support immediate mobilization.

Types of casts. Immobilization of an acute fracture or soft tissue injury of the upper extremity is often accomplished by use of (1) the sugar-tong splint, (2) the posterior splint, (3) the short

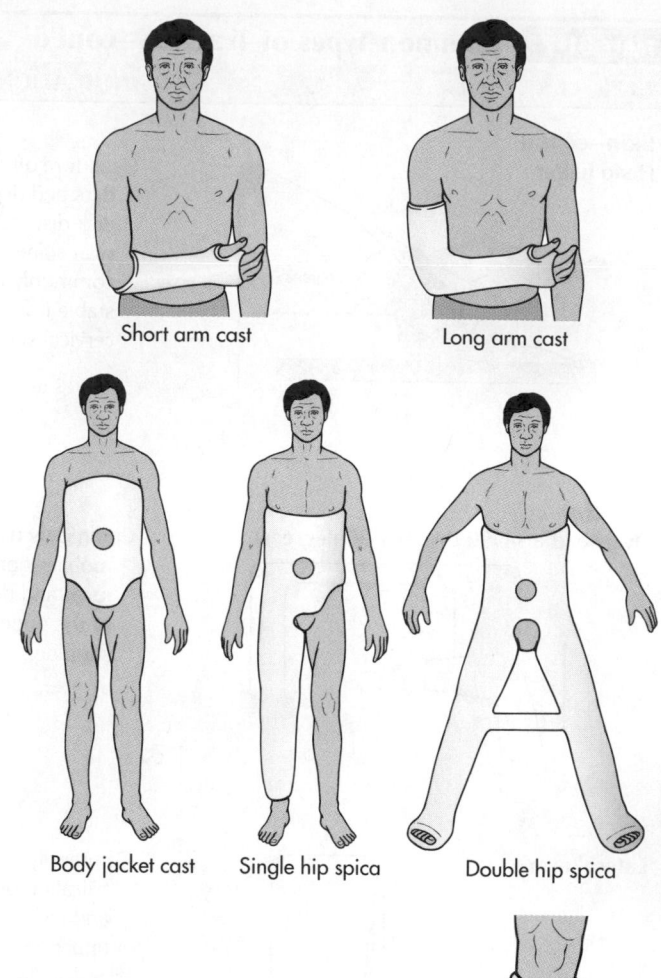

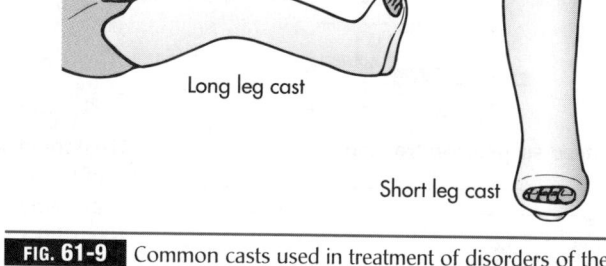

FIG. 61-9 Common casts used in treatment of disorders of the musculoskeletal system.

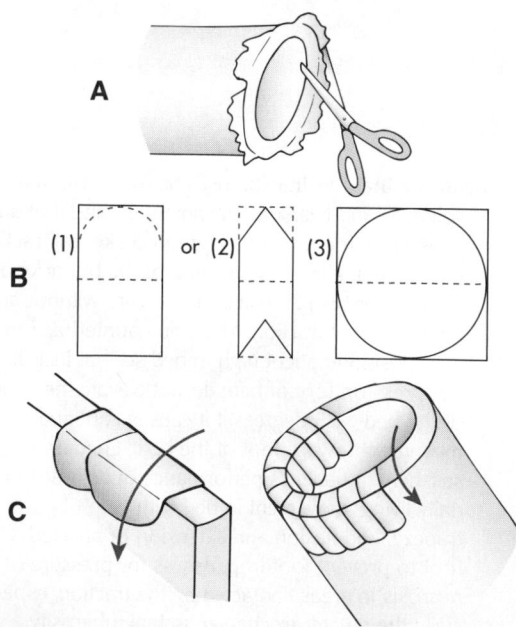

FIG. 61-8 Petaling edges of cast with waterproof adhesive strips. **A,** Cast must be thoroughly dry. The nurse trims the excess sheet wadding and stretches the stockinette over the cast edge (when possible). **B,** Several strips (petals) of waterproof adhesive tape (2-inch-wide strips for wide areas and 1-inch-wide strips for small areas, each 1 inch long) are made in advance. **C,** Uncut end of the tape is placed beneath the cast edge. Each succeeding petal overlaps the previous one by one-half inch, ensuring a smooth cast edge.

arm cast, and (4) the long arm cast (Fig. 61-9). The *sugar-tong splint* is typically used for acute wrist injuries or injuries that may result in significant swelling. Plaster splints are applied over a well-padded forearm, beginning at the phalangeal joints of the hand, extending up the dorsal aspect of the forearm around the distal humerus, and then extending down the volar aspect of the forearm to the distal palmar crease. The splinting material is wrapped with either elastic bandage or bias stockinette. The major advantage of the sugar-tong cast and posterior splint is avoidance of the circumferential effects of a nonelastic cylinder cast. The sugar-tong posterior splints accommodate for swelling in the fractured extremity that occurs postinjury.

The *short arm cast* is often used for the treatment of stable wrist or metacarpal fractures. An aluminum finger splint can be fabricated into the short arm cast for concurrent treatment of phalangeal injuries. The short arm cast is a circular cast extending from the distal palmar area to the proximal forearm. This cast provides wrist immobilization and permits unrestricted elbow motion.

The *long arm cast* is commonly used for stable forearm or elbow fractures and unstable wrist fractures. It is similar to the short arm cast but extends to the proximal humerus, restricting motion in the wrist and elbow. Nursing measures should be directed toward supporting the extremity and reducing the effects of edema by maintaining extremity elevation with a sling. However, when a hanging arm cast is used for a proximal humerus fracture, elevation or a supportive sling are contraindicated because hanging provides traction and promotes fracture healing.

When a sling is used, the nurse must ensure that the axillary area is well padded to prevent skin maceration associated with direct skin-to-skin contact. Placement of the sling should not put undue pressure on the posterior neck. Movement of the fingers (unless contraindicated) should be encouraged to enhance the pumping action of vascular and soft tissue structures to decrease edema. The nurse should also encourage the patient to actively move nonimmobilized joints of the upper extremity to prevent stiffness and contractures.

The *body jacket cast* is often used for immobilization and support for stable spine injuries of the thoracic or lumbar spine. This cast is applied around the chest and abdomen and extends from above the nipple line to the pubis. After application of the cast, the nurse must assess the patient for the development of *cast syndrome*. This condition occurs if the body cast is applied too tightly and the cast compresses the superior mesenteric artery against the duodenum. The patient generally complains of abdominal pain, abdominal pressure, nausea, and vomiting. The abdomen should be assessed for decreased bowel sounds (a window may be left over the umbilicus). Treatment includes gastric decompression with a nasogastric (NG) tube and suction. The cast may need to be removed or split. Nursing assessment also includes observation of respiratory status, bowel and bladder function, and areas of pressure over the bony prominences, especially the iliac crest. During the time required for the cast to dry, the nurse should reposition the patient every 2 to 3 hours to promote even cast drying and to relieve pressure and discomfort.

The *hip spica cast* is used for treatment of femoral fractures. The purpose of the hip spica cast is to immobilize the affected extremity and the trunk securely. It includes two casts joined together: (1) the body jacket cast and (2) the long leg cast. The location of the femoral fracture will determine whether the thigh of the unaffected extremity will have to be immobilized to restrict rotation of the pelvis and possible hip motion on the side of the femur fracture. The hip spica cast extends from above the nipple line to the base of the foot (single spica) and may include the opposite extremity up to an area above the knee (spica and a half) or both extremities (double spica).

The nurse should assess the patient with a hip spica cast for the same problems that are associated with the body jacket cast. During the initial drying stage the patient should not be placed in the prone position because the cast may break. The patient should be slightly turned from side to side and supported with pillows. When the patient is repositioned, the support bar joining the thighs must never be used to assist in moving because the bar can break and cause cast disruption. After the cast has dried, the nurse (with assistance) can turn the patient to the prone position and provide pillow support under the chest and immobilized ex-

tremity. Skin care around the cast edges (petaling) and the areas not encompassed by plaster is important to prevent any pressure sores. The nurse should instruct the patient in the positioning activities required to get on and off the bedpan. A fracture bedpan may be used to provide comfort and ease the movement of getting on and off the bedpan. After the hip spica cast has dried sufficiently, the patient may be instructed in ambulation techniques by the physical therapist.

Injuries to the lower extremity. Injuries to the lower extremity are often immobilized by a long leg cast, short leg cast, cylinder cast, or a Jones dressing. The usual indications for applying a long leg cast are an unstable ankle fracture, soft tissue injuries, a fractured tibia, and knee injuries. The cast usually extends from the base of the toes to the groin and gluteal crease. The short leg cast can be used for a variety of conditions but is primarily used for stable ankle and foot injuries. A cylinder cast is used for knee injuries or fractures. The cast extends from the groin to the malleoli of the ankle. A Jones dressing is composed of bulky padding materials (absorption dressing and sheet wadding), splints, and an elastic wrap or bias-cut stockinette. The Jones dressing, like the sugar-tong splint, is used for knee fractures or surgery when there is a risk of significant edema. After the application of a lower-extremity cast or dressing, the extremity should be elevated with pillows above the heart level for the first 24 hours. After the initial phase, the casted extremity should not be placed in a dependent position because of the possibility of excessive edema.

Initially, no weight can be put on the injured extremity. Later, a walking heel or cast shoe may be added to the cast if the patient is allowed to bear weight and walk on the affected leg. Following cast application, the nurse should observe for signs of pressure, especially in the regions of the heel, anterior tibial border, fibular head, and malleoli.

External fixation. An external fixator is a metallic device composed of metal pins that are inserted into the bone and attached to external rods to stabilize the fracture while it heals. It can be used to apply traction or to compress fracture fragments and to immobilize reduced fragments when the use of a cast or other traction is not appropriate. The external device holds fracture fragments in place much like surgically implanted internal devices do. The external fixator is attached directly to the bones by percutaneous transfixing pins or wires (Fig. 61-10). External fixation is indicated in simple fractures (either open or closed), complex fractures with extensive soft tissue damage, correction of bony defects (congenital), pseudoarthrosis, and nonunion or malunion and for limb lengthening.

External fixation has many advantages over other fracture management strategies and is often employed to salvage complex mangled extremity fractures that otherwise might be amputated at the time of injury. Because the use of an external device is a long-term process, assessment for pin loosening and infection is critical. Infection signaled by exudate, redness, tenderness, and pain may require removal of the device. Meticulous pin care must be taught to the patient and the support person. Although each physician has a protocol for pin care cleaning, half-strength hydrogen peroxide with normal saline is often used.

Internal fixation. Internal fixation devices (pins, plates, intramedullary rods and screws) are surgically inserted at the time of realignment. Biologically inert metal devices such as stainless steel, Vitallium, or titanium are used to realign and maintain bony

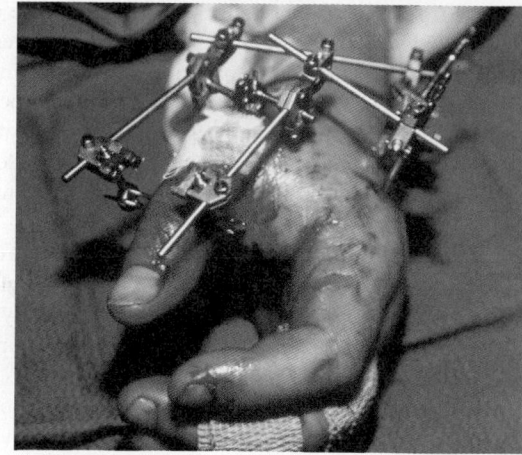

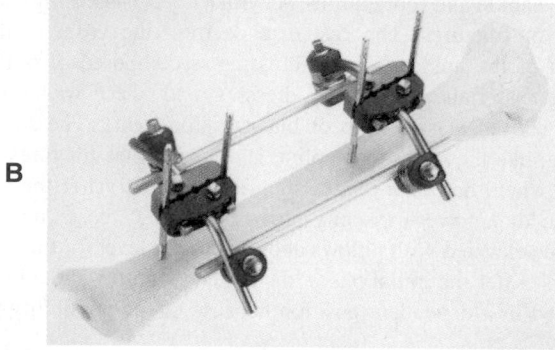

FIG. 61-10 External fixators. **A,** Mini–Hoffman system in use on hand. **B,** Hoffman II on the tibia (standard system).

fragments. Proper alignment is evaluated by x-ray studies at regular intervals.

Traction. **Traction** is the application of a pulling force to an injured or diseased part of the body or an extremity while countertraction pulls in the opposite direction. The purpose of any traction is to (1) prevent or reduce muscle spasm, (2) immobilize a joint or part of the body, (3) reduce a fracture or dislocation, and (4) treat a joint pathologic condition.[16] Traction is also indicated to (1) provide immobilization to prevent soft tissue damage (2) reduce muscle spasm associated with low back pain or cervical whiplash, (3) expand a joint space during arthroscopic procedures, and (4) expand a joint space before major joint reconstruction. A continuous pulling force can be applied directly to bone with wires and pins (skeletal traction) or can be applied indirectly by weights that are attached to the skin with slings, belts, adhesive straps, or boots (skin traction).

Skin traction is usually applied directly to the extremity by adhesive material that is wrapped circumferentially with a bandage or slings, belts, or a special splint that is attached to a rope with a weight. Skin traction for extremities is applied for a short time and usually consists of not more than 7 to 10 lb (3.2 to 4.5 kg) of traction weight because of skin intolerance to pressure. Pelvic or cervical skin traction may require heavier weights applied intermittently.

Skeletal traction is usually indicated when the traction forces are expected to exceed 10 lb (4.5 kg) or when traction will be used for a long time. Use of too much weight to maintain traction can result in delayed union or nonunion. The major disadvan-

tages of skeletal traction are infection in the area of bone where the skeletal pin has been inserted and the consequences of prolonged immobility necessitated by skeletal traction.

Drug Therapy. Patients with fractures often experience varying degrees of pain associated with muscle spasms. These spasms are caused by involuntary reflexes that result from edema following muscle injury. Muscle relaxants, such as carisoprodol (Soma), cyclobenzaprine (Flexeril), or methocarbamol (Robaxin), may be prescribed for relief of pain associated with muscle spasms.

Common side effects associated with muscle relaxants are drowsiness, lassitude, headache, weakness, fatigue, blurred vision, ataxia, and gastrointestinal upset. Hypersensitivity reactions may include skin rash or pruritus. Ingestion of large doses of muscle relaxants may cause hypotension, tachycardia, or respiratory depression. The possible habituating effects associated with long-term use and the potential for abuse must be carefully considered.

Some physicians do not advocate the use of muscle relaxants for relief of muscle spasms. Their rationale is that the reflex spasm will continue as long as the precipitating pain persists. If the pain is controlled by use of appropriate analgesia, the muscle spasms will cease.

In an open fracture the threat of tetanus occurring can be reduced with tetanus-diphtheria toxoid or immunoglobulin for the patient who has not been previously immunized. A bone-penetrating antibiotic (such as a cephalosporin) is used prophylactically.

Nutritional Therapy. Proper nutrition is an essential component of the reparative process in injured tissue. An adequate energy source is needed to promote muscle strength and tone, build endurance, and enhance ambulation and gait-training skills. The patient's dietary requirements must include ample protein (e.g., 1 g per kilogram of body weight), vitamins (especially D, B, and C), and calcium to ensure optimal soft tissue and bone healing. Low serum protein levels and vitamin C deficiencies interfere with tissue healing. Immobility and callus formation increase calcium needs. Three well-balanced meals a day will usually provide the necessary nutrients. The well-balanced meal should be supplemented by a fluid intake of 2000 to 3000 ml per day to promote optimal bladder and bowel function. Adequate fluid and a high-fiber diet with fruits and vegetables will prevent constipation. If immobilized in a body jacket or hip spica bandage, the patient should be instructed to eat six small meals so as not to overeat and thus avoid abdominal pressure and cramping.

NURSING MANAGEMENT FRACTURES

■ Nursing Assessment

A brief history of the accident, mechanism of injury, and the position in which the victim was found can be obtained from the patient or witnesses. As soon as possible, the patient should be transported to an emergency department where a thorough assessment and treatment can be initiated (Table 61-8). Subjective and objective data that should be obtained from an individual with a fracture are presented in Table 61-9.

Special emphasis must be focused on the region distal to the site of injury. Clinical findings must be documented before fracture treatment is initiated to avoid doubts about whether a prob-

TABLE 61-8 Emergency Management — Fractured Extremity

ETIOLOGY	ASSESSMENT FINDINGS	INTERVENTIONS

Blunt
Motor vehicle collision
Pedestrian event
Falls
Direct blows
Forced flexion or
  hyperextension
Twisting forces
 	
Penetrating
Gunshot
Blast
 	
Other
Pathologic conditions
Violent muscle
  contractions (seizures)
Crush injury
	• Deformity (loss of normal bony contours)
	  or unnatural position of affected limb
	• Edema and ecchymosis
	• Muscle spasm
	• Tenderness and pain
	• Loss of function
	• Numbness, tingling, loss of distal pulses
	• Grating (crepitus)
	• Open wound over injured site, exposure
	  of bone
		Initial
		• Treat life-threatening injuries first.
		• Ensure airway, breathing, and circulation.
		• Control external bleeding with direct pressure or sterile
		  pressure dressing.
		• Splint joints above and below fracture site.
		• Check neurovascular status distal to injury before and
		  after splinting.
		• Elevate injured limb if possible.
		• Do *not* attempt to straighten fractured or dislocated
		  joints.
		• Do *not* manipulate protruding bone ends.
		• Apply ice packs to affected area.
		• Obtain x-rays of affected limb.
		• Administer tetanus prophylaxis if skin integrity is violated.
		• Mark location of pulses to facilitate repeat assessment.
		• Splint fracture site, including joints above and below fracture site.
		
		Ongoing Monitoring
		• Monitor vital signs, level of consciousness, oxygen saturation, peripheral pulses, and pain.
		• Monitor for compartment syndrome characterized by excessive pain, pain with passive stretch, pallor, paresthesia, paralysis, pulselessness.
		• Monitor for fat embolism (dyspnea, chest pain).

TABLE 61-9 Nursing Assessment — Fracture

Subjective Data

Important Health Information

Past health history: Traumatic injury; long-term repetitive forces (stress fracture); bone or systemic diseases, prolonged immobility (pathologic fracture), osteopenia, osteoporosis

Medications: Use of corticosteroids (pathologic fractures); analgesics

Surgery or other treatments: First aid treatment of fracture

Functional Health Patterns

Health perception–health management: Estrogen replacement therapy, calcium supplementation

Activity-exercise: Loss of motion or weakness of affected part; muscle spasms

Cognitive-perceptual: Sudden and severe pain in affected area; numbness, tingling, loss of sensation distal to injury; chronic pain that increases with activity (stress fracture)

Objective Data

General

Apprehension, guarding of injured site

Integumentary

Skin lacerations, pallor and cool skin or bluish and warm skin distal to injury; ecchymosis, hematoma, edema at site of fracture

Cardiovascular

Reduced or absent pulse distal to injury, ↓ skin temperature, delayed capillary refill

Neurologic

Paresthesias, ↓ or absent sensation, hypersensation

Musculoskeletal

Restricted or lost function of affected part, local bony deformities, abnormal angulation, shortening, rotation, crepitation; muscle weakness

Possible Findings

Localization and extent of fractures on x-ray, bone scans, tomograms, CT scan, or MRI

CT, Computed tomography; *MRI,* magnetic resonance imaging.

lem discovered later was missed during the original examination or was caused by the treatment.

Neurovascular Assessment. Musculoskeletal injuries have the potential of causing changes in the neurovascular system. The original trauma, application of a cast or constrictive dressing, poor positioning, and the physiologic response to the injury can cause nerve or vascular damage, usually distal to the injury. A thorough neurovascular assessment consists of a peripheral vascular assessment (color, temperature, capillary refill, peripheral pulses, and edema) and a peripheral neurologic assessment (sensation, motor

NURSING CARE PLAN 61-1

Patient with a Fracture

EXPECTED PATIENT OUTCOMES	NURSING INTERVENTIONS and *RATIONALES*
NURSING DIAGNOSIS	**Risk for peripheral neurovascular dysfunction** *related to* nerve compression.
▪ Has normal neurovascular examination	▪ Assess for signs and symptoms of peripheral neurovascular dysfunction such as pain in affected extremity that is unrelieved by drugs, paresthesias, pain on passive movement, weakness, cool temperature, pallor, diminished pulses *to ensure early recognition and intervention.* ▪ Elevate extremity above heart level *to reduce edema by promoting venous return.* (Note: If compartment syndrome is suspected, elevate extremity no higher than heart level.) ▪ Apply ice compresses as ordered *to reduce edema and provide comfort.* (Note: If compartment syndrome is suspected, remove ice because it may decrease tissue perfusion.) ▪ Notify physician immediately if patient complains of increasing pain that is unrelieved by drugs *because this may indicate neurovascular impairment, which can result in significant injury if unrelieved.* ▪ Teach patient the signs of peripheral neurovascular dysfunction *to enable her or his participation in care.*
NURSING DIAGNOSIS	**Acute pain** *related to* edema, movement of bone fragments, and muscle spasms *as manifested by* pain descriptors, guarding, crying.
▪ Tolerable or no pain ▪ Satisfaction with plan for pain relief	▪ Gently and correctly position fractured extremity *to minimize pain and prevent bone displacement.* ▪ Use a pain scale *to assess pain and evaluate effectiveness of interventions.* ▪ Give patient analgesics and/or muscle relaxants as indicated *to relieve pain and promote muscle relaxation.* ▪ Elevate, apply ice (if prescribed), and support affected extremity *to reduce edema and promote comfort.* ▪ Be alert for pain that is not diminished after analgesic is administered *because this may indicate an impending compartment syndrome.*
NURSING DIAGNOSIS	**Risk for infection** *related to* disruption of skin integrity and presence of environmental pathogens secondary to open fracture, external fixation pins, surgical incision.
▪ No evidence of wound infection ▪ Temperature in normal range ▪ WBC count in normal range	▪ Assess fracture or pin insertion points for blistering, tenting discoloration, and drainage as indicators of infection. ▪ Use aseptic technique when providing pin or wound care or when performing dressing change *to prevent cross-contamination and possible introduction of infection.* ▪ Obtain culture of wound if infection is suspected *to identify infective organism.* ▪ Administer antibiotics as ordered *to provide prophylaxis or treatment of diagnosed infection.* ▪ Monitor temperature q2hr *because fever may indicate infection.* ▪ Monitor WBC count *because elevation may indicate infection.*
NURSING DIAGNOSIS	**Risk for impaired skin integrity** *related to* immobility and presence of cast.
▪ No evidence of skin breakdown	▪ Examine potential pressure areas q4hr *to assess condition of skin.* ▪ Petal cast edges *to prevent skin abrasion or cast crumbs from falling beneath the cast.* ▪ Assess exposed skin areas of traction sites for signs of infection or irritation *because improper positioning of traction devices can cause localized pressure necrosis.* ▪ Instruct patient not to insert items (e.g., hangers, forks) into cast to scratch *because these may cause tissue injury.* ▪ Instruct patient to report areas of warmth, pain, burning, or moisture beneath the cast; foul odor from cast ends; or areas of new or increasing drainage on cast surfaces.
NURSING DIAGNOSIS	**Impaired physical mobility** *related to* ineffective use of crutches *as manifested by* inability to move about independently.
▪ Crutches correctly used to move about as needed	▪ Teach gait-training principles to patient (non–weight-bearing gait status unless otherwise ordered by physician); sit with feet over edge of bed, stand with no weight on affected extremity, measure and adjust crutches *to promote mobility according to patient's abilities.* ▪ Ensure gait is compatible with weight-bearing status *to prevent malalignment.* ▪ Work with physical therapist regarding exercise and gait-training *to reinforce plan and to provide unified approach to patient.*

Patient with a Fracture—cont'd

EXPECTED PATIENT OUTCOMES	NURSING INTERVENTIONS and *RATIONALES*
NURSING DIAGNOSIS	**Ineffective therapeutic regimen management** *related to* lack of knowledge regarding muscle atrophy, exercise program, and cast care *as manifested by* questioning of long-term effect of casting and cast care, activity restrictions.
• Minimal loss of muscle bulk of affected extremity • Verbalization of confidence in ability to follow the prescribed discharge plan	• Instruct patient on home care measures related to exercise, cast care, and prevention of complications *so that patient can carry out prescribed discharge plan.* • Explain factors that contribute to atrophy; emphasize relationship of inactivity to muscle atrophy *so that patient will exercise involved extremity to maximum allowed and will not be alarmed at appearance of extremity when cast is removed.* • Provide written instructions of prescribed exercise plan.

function, and pain).[17] Throughout the neurovascular assessment, both extremities are compared to obtain an accurate assessment.

An extremity's color (pink, pale, cyanotic) and temperature (hot, warm, cool, cold) in the area of the affected extremity are assessed. Cyanosis or a cool/cold extremity below the injury could indicate arterial insufficiency. A warm, bluish extremity could indicate poor venous return. Capillary refill (blanching of the nailbed) is next assessed. The standard for a compressed nailbed to return to its original color is within 3 seconds. Accurate documentation and ongoing assessment of capillary refill are the cornerstones of nursing care for the individual with a musculoskeletal injury.

Pulses on both the unaffected and injured extremity are compared to identify differences in rate or quality. Pulses are described as strong, diminished, audible by Doppler, or absent. A diminished or absent pulse distal to the injury can indicate vascular insufficiency. However, some adults do not have specific pulses, including an absent dorsalis pedis (17% of all ethnic groups) and an absent posterior tibial (9% of African Americans).[18] Peripheral edema is also assessed, and pitting edema may be present with severe injury.

Sensation and motor innervation in the upper extremity are assessed by evaluating the ulnar, median, and radial nerves. Neurovascular status can be assessed by abduction and adduction of the fingers, opposition of the fingers, and supination and pronation of the hand. In the lower extremity, dorsiflexion and plantar flexion assess motor function of the peroneal and tibial nerves. Sensory innervation is evaluated for the peroneal nerve on the dorsal part of the foot between the web space of the great and second toes. Tibial nerve assessment is performed by stroking the volar part (sole) of the foot. Ipsilateral evaluation is critical. Paresthesia (abnormal sensation [e.g., numbness, tingling]), decreased sensation, hypersensation, partial or full loss of sensation [paresis/paralysis] may be reported by the patient. Reduced motion or strength in an injured extremity alerts the nurse to potential limb-threatening complications or disability.

Pain is the final element of the neurovascular assessment. The nurse must carefully assess the location, quality, and intensity of the pain. Current nursing practice is to evaluate the patient's level of pain on a scale of 1 to 10.[17] Pain unrelieved by drugs and out of proportion to the injury is an indication of compartment syndrome or complex regional pain syndrome.[19]

Patients should be instructed to report any changes in their neurovascular status. Patients must verbalize and demonstrate a thorough understanding of all elements before discharge from the emergency department or outpatient setting.

■ Nursing Diagnoses

Nursing diagnoses for the patient with a fracture may include, but are not limited to, those presented in NCP 61-1.

■ Planning

The overall goals are that the patient with a fracture will (1) have physiologic healing with no associated complications, (2) obtain satisfactory pain relief, and (3) achieve maximal rehabilitation potential.

■ Nursing Implementation

Health Promotion. The public should be taught to take appropriate safety precautions to prevent injuries while at home, at work, when driving, or when participating in sports. Nurses should be vocal advocates for personal actions known to reduce injuries such as regular use of seat belts, driving within posted speed limits, stretching before exercise, use of protective athletic equipment (helmets and knee, wrist, and elbow pads), and not combining drinking and driving.

Older adults should be encouraged to participate in moderate exercise to aid in the maintenance of muscle strength and balance. To reduce falls, their living environment should be examined to rule out the use of scatter rugs, to ensure adequate footwear and lighting, and to clear paths to bathrooms for nighttime use. The nurse should also stress the importance of adequate calcium and vitamin D intake.

Acute Intervention. Patients with fractures may be treated in an emergency department or a physician's office and released to home care, or they may require hospitalization for varying amounts of time. Specific nursing measures depend on the type of treatment used and the setting in which patients are placed.

Preoperative management. If surgical intervention is required to treat the fracture, patients will need preoperative preparation. In addition to the usual preoperative nursing measures (see Chapter 17), the nurse should inform patients of the type of immobilization device that will be used and the expected activity limitations. Patients must be assured that their needs will be met by the nursing staff until they can again meet their own needs. Assurance that pain medication will be available, if needed, is often beneficial.

Proper skin preparation is an important part of preoperative preparation. The protocol for skin preparation varies among agencies and may be the responsibility of the nurse. The aim of skin preparation is to clean the skin and remove debris and hair to reduce the possibility of infection. Careful attention to this preoperative treatment can influence the postoperative course.

Postoperative management. In general, postoperative nursing care and management are directed toward monitoring vital signs and applying the general principles of postoperative nursing care (see Chapter 19). Frequent neurovascular assessments of the affected extremity are necessary to detect changes. Any limitations of movement or activity related to turning, positioning, and extremity support should be monitored closely. Pain and discomfort can be minimized through proper alignment and positioning. Dressings or casts should be carefully observed for any overt signs of bleeding or drainage. A significant increase in size of the drainage area should be reported. If a wound drainage system is in place, the patency of the system and the volume of drainage should be regularly assessed. Whenever the contents of a drainage system are measured or emptied, the nurse should use sterile technique to avoid contamination. Additional nursing responsibilities depend on the type of immobilization used. A blood salvage and reinfusion system that allows for recovery and

reinfusion of the patient's own blood may be used. The blood is retrieved from a joint space or cavity, and the patient receives this blood in the form of an autotransfusion. (Autotransfusion is discussed in Chapter 30.)

Other measures. Patients with musculoskeletal injury often have reduced mobility as a result of the fracture. The nurse must plan care to prevent the many complications associated with limited mobility. Constipation can be prevented by activity and maintenance of a high fluid intake (more than 2500 ml per day) and a diet high in bulk and roughage (fresh fruit and vegetables). If these measures are not effective in maintaining the patient's normal bowel pattern, stool softeners, laxatives, or suppositories may be necessary. Maintaining a regular time for elimination aids in promoting regularity.

Renal calculi can develop as a result of bone demineralization. The resulting hypercalcemia causes a rise in urine pH and stone formation resulting from the precipitation of calcium. Unless contraindicated, a fluid intake of 2500 ml per day is recommended. Cranberry juice or ascorbic acid (500 mg per day) may be recommended to acidify the urine and prevent calcium precipitation. (Renal calculi are discussed in Chapter 44.)

Rapid deconditioning of the cardiopulmonary system can occur as a result of prolonged bed rest, resulting in orthostatic hypotension and decreased lung capacity. Unless contraindicated, these effects can be diminished by permitting the patient to sit on the side of the bed, allowing the patient's lower limbs to dangle over the bedside and the patient to perform standing transfers. When the patient is allowed to increase activity, careful evaluation should be made to assess for orthostatic hypotension. Patients must also be assessed for the risk of deep vein thrombosis (DVT) and pulmonary emboli.

Traction. The nurse is responsible for patient comfort and safety while traction is used and for ensuring proper functioning of the traction equipment. The equipment should be regularly examined for frayed ropes, loose knots, ropes out of the groove of the pulley, pulley clamps not fastened firmly to the bed frame, and weights not hanging freely.

When slings are used with traction, the nurse should inspect the skin area that is exposed in and near the sling regularly. Pressure over a bony prominence or a wrinkled area may cause pressure necrosis and can impair blood flow, causing injury to the peripheral neurovascular structures. Skeletal traction pin sites must be observed for signs of infection. Pin site care varies but usually includes regular removal of exudate with half-strength hydrogen peroxide, rinsing pin sites with sterile saline, and drying of the area with sterile gauze.[20]

External rotation of the hip can occur when skin traction is used on the lower extremity. The nurse can correct this position by placing a pillow, sandbag, or rolled-up draw sheet along the greater trochanteric region of the femur. When traction is used, the nurse should ensure that the patient's body is always correctly aligned. Generally, the patient should be in the center of the bed in a supine position. Incorrect alignment can result in increased pain, nonunion, or malunion.

To offset some of the problems associated with prolonged immobility, the nurse should discuss specific patient activity with the health care provider. If exercise is permitted, the nurse should encourage participation by the patient in a simple exercise regimen within activity restrictions. Activities that the patient should participate in include frequent position changes, ROM exercises of unaffected joints, deep breathing exercises, isometric exercises, and use of the trapeze bar (if permitted) to raise oneself off the bed for linen changes and use of the bedpan. These activities should be performed several times each day.

Active exercises that move uninvolved joints through the ROM are the preferred activity, if allowed. Frequent exercise of the trunk and extremities is an excellent stimulus to deep breathing. Active, resistive exercise (isotonic) of uninvolved extremities helps reduce deconditioning from prolonged immobility.

Ambulatory and Home Care

Cast care. Because many fractures are casted in an outpatient setting, the patient often requires only a short hospitalization or none at all. Regardless of the type of material of which it is made, a cast can interfere with circulation and nerve function from being applied too tightly or because of excessive edema after application. Thus frequent neurovascular assessments of the immobilized extremity are critical. The patient must be taught about signs of cast complications so that they can be reported promptly. Elevation of the extremity above the level of the heart to promote venous return and applications of ice to control or prevent edema are measures frequently used during the initial phase. The nurse should instruct the patient to exercise joints above and below the cast. Pulling out cast padding and scratching or placing foreign objects inside the cast is forbidden because it predisposes the patient to skin breakdown and infection.

Patient teaching is an important nursing responsibility to prevent complications. In addition to specific instructions for cast care and recognition of complications, the nurse should encourage the patient to contact the clinic or care provider should questions arise. Table 61-10 summarizes patient and family instructions for cast care. The nurse should validate the patient's and family's understanding of these instructions before discharge from the outpatient setting, emergency department, or hospital. A follow-up phone contact is appropriate, and home care nursing visits are warranted, especially with body or spica casts.

Cast removal is done in the outpatient setting. Patients often fear being cut by the oscillating blade of the cast saw, and the nurse should reassure the patient. More importantly, the nurse should educate the patient as to the possible alteration in the appearance of the skin, which has been beneath the cast. Anxiety will also be present related to weight bearing and continued follow-up care.

Psychosocial problems. Short-term rehabilitative goals are directed toward the transition from dependence to independence in performing simple activities of daily living and preservation or increasing strength and endurance. Long-term rehabilitative goals are aimed at preventing problems associated with musculoskeletal injury (Table 61-11). An important part of nursing care during the rehabilitative phase is assisting the patient to adjust to any problems caused by the injury (e.g., separation from family, financial impact of medical care, loss of income from inability to work, potential for lifetime disability). The nurse must exhibit gentleness, support, and encouragement and should actively listen to the patient's and family's fears.

Ambulation. The nurse must know the overall goals of physical therapy in relation to the patient's abilities, needs, and tolerance. Mobility training and instruction in the use of assistive aids constitute major areas of responsibility of the physical therapist. The patient with lower extremity dysfunction is usually started in mobility training when able to sit in bed and dan-

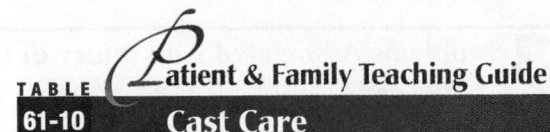

TABLE 61-10 — **Patient & Family Teaching Guide**

Cast Care

Do Not
1. Get plaster cast wet
2. Remove any padding
3. Insert any foreign object inside cast
4. Bear weight on new cast for 48 hr (not all casts are made for weight bearing; check with health care provider when unsure)
5. Cover cast with plastic for prolonged periods

Do
1. Apply ice directly over fracture site for first 24 hr (avoid getting cast wet by keeping ice in plastic bag and protecting cast with cloth)
2. Check with health care provider before getting fiberglass cast wet
3. Dry cast thoroughly after exposure to water
   - Blot dry with towel
   - Use hair dryer on low setting until cast is thoroughly dry
4. Elevate extremity above level of heart for first 48 hr
5. Move joints above and below cast regularly
6. Report signs of possible problems to health care provider
   - Increasing pain
   - Swelling associated with pain and discoloration of toes or fingers
   - Pain during movement
   - Burning or tingling under cast
   - Sores or foul odor under the cast
7. Keep appointment to have fracture and cast checked

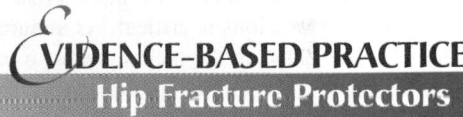

EVIDENCE-BASED PRACTICE
Hip Fracture Protectors

Clinical Problem
Do hip protectors reduce the risk of sustaining a fracture in a fall involving the hip in older adults?

Best Clinical Practice
- Hip protectors appear to reduce the risk of hip fracture within a selected population at high risk of sustaining a hip fracture.
- Generalization of the results is unknown beyond high-risk populations.
- User acceptability of the protectors remains a problem because of discomfort and practicality.

Implications for Nursing Practice
- Falls can be prevented in older persons.
- Older adults and their families need to be informed that hip protectors are available.
- The most effective interventions to prevent hip fractures are multifaceted (see Table 61-1) and targeted to individuals in high-risk categories.

References for Evidence
EBM Reviews: Falls can be prevented in older persons, but interventions should be multifaceted and targeted, *ACP Journal Club* 134:100, May/June 2001.

Parker MJ, Gillespie LD, Gillespie WJ: Hip protectors for preventing hip fractures in the elderly, Cochrane Musculoskeletal Injuries Group, *Cochrane Database Syst Rev*, Issue 3, 2002.

TABLE 61-11   Problems Associated with Injury of the Musculoskeletal System

PROBLEM	DESCRIPTION	NURSING CONSIDERATIONS
Muscle atrophy	Decreased muscle mass normally occurs as a result of disuse following prolonged immobilization.	An isometric muscle–strengthening exercise regimen within the confines of the immobilization device assists in reducing the amount of atrophy. Muscle atrophy interferes with and prolongs the rehabilitation process.
Contracture	Abnormal condition of joint characterized by flexion and fixation. Caused by atrophy and shortening of muscle fibers or by loss of normal elasticity of skin over a joint.	Can be prevented by frequent position change, correct body alignment, and active–passive range-of-motion exercises several times a day. Intervention requires gradual and progressive stretching of the muscles or ligaments in the region of the joint.
Footdrop	Plantar-flexed position of the foot (footdrop) occurs when the Achilles tendon in the ankle shortens because it has been allowed to assume an unsupported position.	Nursing management of the patient with long-term injuries must include preventive measures by supporting the foot in a neutral position. Once footdrop has developed, ambulation and gait training may be significantly hindered.
Pain	Frequently associated with fractures, edema, and muscle spasm; pain varies in intensity from mild to severe and is usually described as aching, dull, burning, throbbing, sharp, or deep.	Causes of pain include incorrect positioning and alignment of the extremity, incorrect support of the extremity, sudden movement of the extremity, and immobilization device that is applied too tightly or in an incorrect position, constrictive dressings, and motion occurring at the fracture site. Causes of pain should be determined so that corrective nursing action can be taken.
Muscle spasms	Caused by involuntary muscle contraction after fracture and may last as long as several weeks. Pain associated with muscle spasms is often intense and can last from several seconds to several minutes.	Nursing measures to reduce the intensity of the muscle spasms are similar to the corrective actions for pain control. Muscle spasms should not be massaged. Thermotherapy, especially heat, may reduce muscle spasm.

gle the feet over the side. This activity should be done two or three times for 10 to 15 minutes, with the nurse assisting as necessary. Collaboration of the nurse and physical therapist to coordinate pain management and thus increase patient participation at therapy sessions is critical. As endurance increases, the patient is instructed in the techniques of transferring from bed to chair. Progressive ambulation is usually started with parallel bars and progresses to ambulatory assistive devices. When the patient begins to ambulate, the nurse must know the weight bearing allowed for the affected extremity and the correct technique if the patient is using an assistive device. There are different degrees of weight-bearing ambulation: (1) non–weight-bearing (no weight borne) ambulation, (2) touch-down/toe-touch weight-bearing ambulation (contact with floor but no weight borne), (3) partial–weight-bearing ambulation (25% to 50% of patient's weight borne), (4) weight-bearing as tolerated (dictated by patient's pain and tolerance), and (5) full–weight-bearing ambulation (no limitations).[15]

Assistive devices. Devices for ambulation range from a cane, which can relieve up to 40% of the weight normally borne by a lower limb, to a walker or crutches, which may allow for complete non–weight-bearing ambulation. The decision about which device is appropriate for a patient involves weighing the need for maximum stability and safety versus maneuverability, which is required in small spaces such as bathrooms and buses. The decision is made more easily by discussing with patients the requirements of their lifestyles and determining the device with which each patient feels most secure and independent.

The technique for using assistive devices varies. The involved limb is usually advanced at the same time or immediately after the advance of the device. The uninvolved limb is advanced last.

In almost all cases, canes are held in the hand opposite the involved extremity.

The common gait patterns with assistive devices are the two-point gait, the four-point gait, the swing-to gait, and the swing-through gait:

- *Two-point gait.* Crutch on one side advances simultaneously with the opposite foot; this gait is also used with cane ambulation.
- *Four-point gait.* A slower version of the two-point gait, each "point" is advanced separately.
- *Swing-to gait.* Both crutches are advanced together, followed by the lifting of both lower limbs to the same place; this gait is also used with walkers.
- *Swing-through gait.* This gait is similar to the swing-to gait, but the patient swings body past the crutches. An alternate four-point sweep-through gait for patients with concurrent visual and neuromuscular disability provides exploration of upcoming terrain by the crutches before they are placed in the traditional position.[21]

A transfer belt should be placed around the patient's waist to provide stability during the learning stages. The nurse should discourage the patient from reaching for furniture or relying on another person for support. When there is inadequate upper limb strength or poorly fitted crutches, the patient bears weight at the axilla rather than at the hands, endangering the neurovascular bundle that passes across the axilla. If verbal coaching does not correct the problem, the patient should be instructed in another form of ambulation until strength is adequate (e.g., platform crutches, walker).

Patients who must ambulate without weight bearing require sufficient upper limb strength to lift their own weight at each step. Because the muscles of the shoulder girdle are not accustomed to this work, they require vigorous and diligent training in preparation for this task. Push-ups, pull-ups using the overhead trapeze bar, and lifting weights develop the triceps and biceps. Straight-leg raises and quadriceps-setting exercises strengthen the quadriceps.

Counseling and referrals. During the rehabilitative process the patient's family assumes an important role in the provision and follow-through of long-term care plans. The family must be instructed in the techniques of strength and endurance exercises, assistance with mobility training, and promoting activities that enhance the quality of daily living. Sexual counseling should be included in discharge planning. Unless nurses have specific preparation for sexual health counseling, they should remember that wrong answers may be more harmful than no answers. For referral purposes, nurses must know whether weight-bearing status will affect sexual activity and whether any immobilization or support devices are necessary.

Patients also need to be evaluated for posttraumatic stress disorder. This is especially important if significant injury to others or fatalities were associated with the patient's injuries.

■ Evaluation

The expected outcomes for a patient with a fracture are presented in NCP 61-1.

COMPLICATIONS OF FRACTURES

The majority of fractures heal without complications. If death occurs after a fracture, it is usually the result of damage to underlying organs and vascular structures or from complications of the fracture or immobility. Complications of fractures may be either direct or indirect. Direct complications include problems with bone infection, bone union, and avascular necrosis. Indirect complications of fractures are associated with blood vessel and nerve damage resulting in conditions such as compartment syndrome, venous thrombosis, fat embolism, and traumatic or hypovolemic shock.[18] Although most musculoskeletal injuries are not life threatening, open fractures or fractures accompanied by severe blood loss and fractures that damage vital organs (such as the lung, heart, or bladder) are medical emergencies requiring immediate attention.

Infection

Open fractures and soft tissue injuries have a high incidence of infection. An open fracture usually results from the impact of severe external forces. Massive or blunt soft tissue injury often has more serious consequences than the fracture. Devitalized and contaminated tissue is an ideal medium for many common pathogens, including gas-forming (anaerobic) bacilli. Treatment of infections is costly in terms of extended nursing and medical care, time for treatment, and loss of patient income. Osteomyelitis can become chronic (see Chapter 62).

Collaborative Care. Open fractures require aggressive surgical debridement. The wound is initially cleansed by jet pulsed lavage in the operating room. Gross contaminants are irrigated and mechanically removed. Contused, contaminated, and devitalized tissue such as muscle, subcutaneous fat, skin, and fragments of bone are surgically excised (debridement). The extent of the soft tissue damage determines whether the wound will be closed at the time of surgery, whether closed suction drainage

may be necessary, and whether skin grafting will be needed. Depending on the location and extent of the fracture, reduction may be maintained by external fixation or traction. During surgery the open wound may be irrigated with antibiotic solution. Antibiotic impregnated beads may also be placed in the surgical site. During the postoperative phase the patient will have antibiotics administered intravenously for 3 to 7 days. Antibiotics, in conjunction with aggressive surgical management, have greatly reduced the occurrence of infection.

Compartment Syndrome

Compartment syndrome is a condition in which elevated intracompartmental pressure within a confined myofascial compartment compromises the neurovascular function of tissues within that space.[22] Compartment syndrome causes capillary perfusion to be reduced below a level necessary for tissue viability and is classified as acute, chronic/exertional, or crush. Thirty-eight compartments are located in the upper and lower extremities. Two basic etiologies create compartment syndrome, including (1) decreased compartment size resulting from restrictive dressings, splints, casts, excessive traction, or premature closure of fascia and (2) increased compartment content related to bleeding, edema, chemical response to snakebite, or IV infiltration. Depending on the patient's age and body mass index, the expected range of intracompartmental readings is 0 to 8 mm Hg. Readings of 30 to 40 mm Hg indicate compartment syndrome.

Edema is a physiologic response to soft tissue injury in the general region of trauma and may elevate the compartment pressure. This can create sufficient pressure to obstruct circulation and cause venous occlusion, which increases edema. Eventually arterial flow is compromised, resulting in inadequate arterial circulation (ischemia) to the extremity. As ischemia continues, muscle and nerve cells are destroyed over time, and fibrotic tissue replaces the healthy tissue. Contracture, disability, and loss of function can occur. Delay in diagnosis and treatment can result in irreversible muscle and nerve ischemia, resulting in a functionally useless or severely impaired extremity.

Compartment syndrome is associated with fractures, extensive soft tissue damage, crush injury, reperfusion syndrome, severe burns, venomous snakebite, or following knee or leg surgery. Prolonged pressure on a muscle compartment may occur when someone is trapped under a heavy object or a person's limb is trapped beneath the body because of an obtunded state such as drug or alcohol overdose. It has even been known to occur as a result of massive infiltration of IV fluids. Exertional compartment syndrome may occur after intensive exercise. The upper arm and lower leg are the most common sites of compartment syndrome. Fractures of the distal humerus and proximal tibia are the most common fractures associated with compartment syndrome. In the upper extremity this condition is referred to as Volkmann's ischemic contracture (Fig. 61-11) and in the lower extremity as anterior tibial compartment syndrome, although the underlying pathophysiologic mechanism is similar.

Clinical Manifestations. Early recognition and treatment of compartment syndrome are essential to avoid permanent damage to muscles and nerves.[23] Ischemia can occur within 4 to 12 hours after onset. Regular neurovascular assessments should be performed on all patients with fractures, but especially those with injury of the distal humerus or proximal tibia or soft tissue disruption in these areas. Compartment syndrome may occur initially

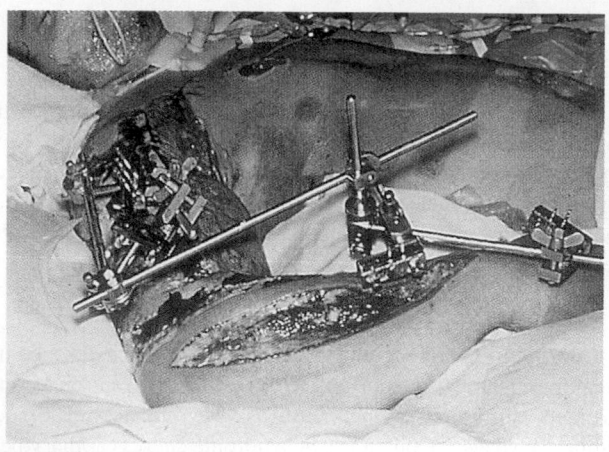

FIG. 61-11 Volkmann's ischemic contracture of the forearm following acute compartment syndrome secondary to a supracondylar fracture of the humerus. Note the incision line of an unsuccessful fasciotomy.

from the physiologic response of the body or may be delayed for several days from the original insult/injury.

The six *P*s are characteristic of an impending compartment syndrome: (1) *paresthesia* (numbness and tingling); (2) *pain* distal to the injury that is not relieved by narcotic analgesics and pain on passive stretch of muscle (positive Homans' sign in lower extremity) traveling through the compartment; (3) *pressure* of the compartment rises; (4) *pallor,* coolness, and loss of normal color of the extremity; (5) *paralysis* or loss of function; and (6) *pulselessness* or diminished/absent peripheral pulses. The patient may present with one or all of the six *P*s. Absence of a peripheral pulse is an ominous late sign that indicates severe disturbance of circulation.[24] Ongoing neurovascular assessment by the nurse must be accurately documented. The health care provider should be notified immediately of the patient's changing condition.

Because of the possibility of muscle damage, urine output must be assessed. Myoglobin, released from damaged muscle cells, can be trapped in renal tubules because of its high molecular weight. Large amounts of myoglobinemia may result in acute tubular necrosis, which precipitates acute renal failure. Common signs of myoglobinuria are (1) dark reddish brown urine and (2) clinical manifestations associated with acute renal failure (see Chapter 45).

Collaborative Care. Prompt, accurate diagnosis of compartment syndrome is critical. Prevention or early recognition is the key. Elevation of the extremity may raise venous pressure and slow arterial perfusion, thus the extremity should not be elevated above heart level. Similarly, the application of cold compresses may result in vasoconstriction and exacerbate compartment syndrome. Elevation and ice should not be used in patients with suspected compartment syndrome. It may also be necessary to remove or loosen the bandage and bivalve the cast. A reduction in traction weight may also decrease external circumferential pressures.

Surgical decompression (e.g., fasciotomy) of the involved compartment may be necessary.[25] The fasciotomy site is left open for several days to ensure adequate soft tissue decompression. Infection resulting from delayed wound closure is a potential problem following a fasciotomy. Severe compartment syndrome may require amputation to decrease myoglobinemia or to replace a functionally useless extremity with a prosthesis.

Venous Thrombosis

The veins of the lower extremities and pelvis are highly susceptible to thrombus formation after fracture, especially hip fracture. Precipitating factors are venous stasis caused by incorrectly applied casts or traction, local pressure on a vein, or immobility. Venous stasis is aggravated by inactivity of the muscles that normally assist in the pumping action of venous blood returning to the extremities. In addition to wearing compression gradient stockings (antiembolism hose) and using sequential compression devices, the patient should be instructed to move (dorsiflex/plantarflex) the fingers or toes of the affected extremity against resistance and to perform ROM exercises on the unaffected lower extremities.

Because of the high risk of venous thrombosis in the patient with limited mobility, prophylactic anticoagulant drugs such as aspirin, warfarin, or heparin may be ordered.[26] Low-molecular-weight heparin (LMWH) (e.g., enoxaparin [Lovenox]) is frequently used to prevent venous thrombosis. Because LMWH has a predictable dose response, monitoring of prothrombin time is not necessary. A new class of antithrombotic drugs (e.g., fondaparinux [Arixtra]) works by inhibiting factor Xa, a key blood-clotting component. (Assessment and management of venous thrombosis are discussed in Chapter 37.)

Fat Embolism Syndrome

Fat embolism syndrome (FES) is characterized by the presence of fat globules in tissues and organs after a traumatic skeletal injury.[27] FES is a contributory factor in many deaths associated with fractures. The fractures that most often cause FES are those of the long bones, ribs, tibia, and pelvis. FES has also been known to occur following total joint replacement, spinal fusion, liposuction, crush injuries, and bone marrow transplantation. Two theories related to the origin of fat emboli exist: the mechanical theory and the biochemical theory. The mechanical theory suggests that fat is released from the marrow of injured bone. It is driven out by an increase in intramedullary pressure and enters the circulation through draining veins traveling to pulmonary capillaries, where it lodges. Some fat droplets traverse the capillary bed to enter systemic circulation and embolize to other organs such as the brain. The biochemical theory postulates that catecholamines released at the time of trauma mobilize free fatty acids from the adipose tissue, causing loss of chylomicron emulsion stability. The chylomicrons form large fat globules that eventually lodge in the lungs. This is possibly due to some biochemical change initiated by injury. The tissues of the lungs, brain, heart, kidneys, and skin are most often affected.

Clinical Manifestations. Early recognition of FES is crucial in preventing a potentially lethal course. Initial manifestations usually occur 24 to 48 hours after injury. Severe forms have occurred within hours of injury. The fat globules transported to the lungs cause a hemorrhagic interstitial pneumonitis that produces signs and symptoms of acute respiratory distress syndrome (ARDS), such as chest pain, tachypnea, cyanosis, dyspnea, apprehension, tachycardia, and decreased partial pressure of arterial oxygen (PaO_2). All of these symptoms are caused by poor oxygen exchange. Because they are frequently the presenting symptoms, changes in the mental status as a result of hypoxemia are important to recognize. Memory loss, restlessness, confusion, elevated temperature, and headache prompt further investigation so that CNS involvement is not mistaken for alcohol withdrawal or acute head injury. The continued change in level of consciousness and petechiae located around the neck, anterior chest wall, axilla, buccal membrane, and conjunctiva of the eye help distinguish fat emboli from other problems. Petechiae result from intravascular thromboses caused by decreased oxygenation.

The clinical course of a fat embolus may be rapid and acute. Frequently the patient expresses a feeling of impending disaster. In a short time, skin color changes from pallor to cyanosis, and the patient may become comatose. No specific laboratory examinations are available to aid in the diagnosis. However, certain diagnostic abnormalities may be present. These include fat cells in the blood, urine, or sputum; a decrease of the PaO_2 to less than 60 mm Hg; ST segment changes on electrocardiogram; a decrease in the platelet count and hematocrit levels; and a prolonged prothrombin time resulting from hemorrhaging into the lungs. A chest x-ray may reveal areas of pulmonary infiltrate or multiple areas of consolidation. This is sometimes referred to as the white-out effect.

Collaborative Care. Treatment for fat embolism is directed at prevention. Careful immobilization of a long bone fracture is probably the most important factor in the prevention of fat embolism. Management of FES is essentially symptom related and supportive, and fluid resuscitation is given to prevent hypovolemic shock, correction of acidosis, and replacement of blood loss. Coughing and deep breathing should be encouraged. The patient should be repositioned as little as possible before fracture immobilization or stabilization because of the danger of dislodging more fat droplets into the general circulation. Use of corticosteroids to prevent or treat fat embolism is controversial. Oxygen is administered to treat hypoxia. Intubation or intermittent positive pressure breathing may be considered if a satisfactory PaO_2 cannot be obtained with supplemental oxygen alone. Some patients may develop pulmonary edema, ARDS, or both, leading to an increased mortality rate. Most survive FES with few sequelae.

Types of Fractures

COLLES' FRACTURE

A *Colles' fracture* is a fracture of the distal radius and is one of the most common fractures in adults. The styloid process of the ulna may be involved as well. The injury usually occurs when the patient attempts to break a fall with an outstretched hand. This type of fracture most often occurs in women over age 50 whose bones are osteoporotic. The clinical manifestations of Colles' fracture are pain in the immediate area of injury, pronounced swelling, and dorsal displacement of the distal fragment (dinner-fork deformity). This may appear as an obvious deformity on the wrist. The major complication associated with a Colles' fracture is vascular insufficiency as a result of edema.

A Colles' fracture is usually managed by closed manipulation of the fracture and immobilization by either a splint or a cast or, if displaced, by external fixation.[28] The elbow must be immobilized to prevent wrist supination and pronation. Nursing management should include measures to prevent or reduce edema and frequent neurovascular assessments. Support and protection of the extremity should be provided, along with encouragement of active movement of the thumb and fingers. This type of movement helps reduce edema and increases venous return. The patient should be instructed to perform active movements of the shoulder to prevent stiffness or contracture.

FRACTURE OF THE HUMERUS

Fractures involving the shaft of the humerus are a common injury among young and middle-aged adults. The prominent clinical manifestations are an obvious displacement of the humerus shaft, shortened extremity, abnormal mobility, and pain (Fig. 61-12). The major complications associated with fracture of the humerus are radial nerve injury and vascular injury to the brachial artery as a result of laceration, transection, or muscle spasm.

The treatment for a fracture of the humerus depends on the location and displacement of the fracture. Nonoperative treatment may include a hanging arm cast, a shoulder immobilizer, or the sling and swathe, which is a type of immobilization that prevents glenohumeral movement. The swathe encircles the trunk and

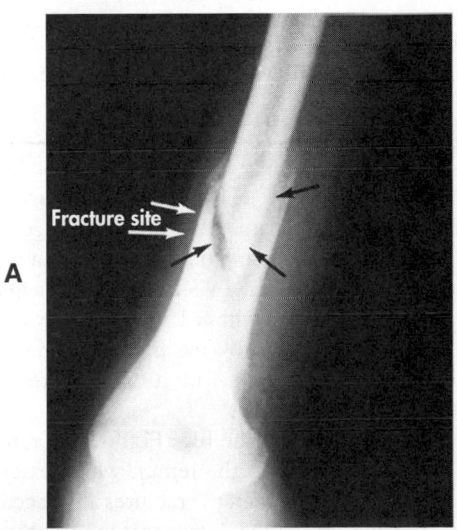
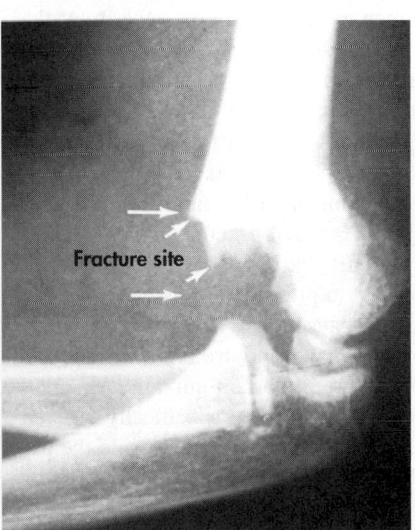

FIG. 61-12 A, Supracondylar fracture of the humerus. This type of injury results in the formation of a large hematoma. B, Fracture of distal shaft of humerus.

humerus as an additional binder. It is often used for surgical repairs and shoulder dislocation.

When these devices are used, the head of the bed should be elevated to assist gravity in reducing the fracture. The arm should be allowed to hang freely when the patient is sitting and standing. Nursing care should include measures to protect the axilla and prevent skin maceration by placing lightly powdered absorbable dressing pads in the axilla and changing them twice daily or as needed. Skin or skeletal traction may be used for purposes of reduction and immobilization.

During the rehabilitative phase an exercise program geared toward improving strength and motion of the injured extremity is extremely important. This should include assisted motion of the hand and fingers. The shoulder can also be exercised if the fracture is stable. This helps to prevent stiffness secondary to frozen shoulder or arthrofibrosis.

FRACTURE OF THE PELVIS

Pelvic fractures range from benign to life threatening depending on the mechanism of injury and associated vascular insult. High-speed vehicular or motorcycle accidents or skiing accidents can result in open book (anterior-posterior compression) fractures resulting in hemorrhagic life-threatening situations. An *open book fracture* is sustained when the external force pulls the pelvis apart, such as when struck or crushed from the front. A *closed book* (lateral compression) fracture is sustained from lateral force impact, whereas a vertical shear injury is the result of a fall. Although only a small percentage of all fractures are pelvic fractures, this type of injury is associated with the highest mortality rate.[29] Preoccupation with associated injuries at the time of a traumatic event may result in an oversight of pelvic injuries. Pelvic fractures may cause serious intraabdominal injury such as paralytic ileus, hemorrhage, and laceration of the urethra, bladder, or colon. Patients may survive the initial pelvic injury, only to die from sepsis, FES, or DVT complications.

Physical examination demonstrates local swelling, tenderness, deformity, unusual pelvic movement, and ecchymosis on the abdomen. The neurovascular status of the lower extremities and manifestations of associated injuries should be assessed. Pelvic fractures are diagnosed by x-ray study.

Treatment of a pelvic fracture depends on the severity of the injury. Stable, nondisplaced fractures such as those sustained in a fall require limited intervention and early mobilization. Bed rest for stable pelvic fractures is maintained from a few days to 6 weeks. More complex fractures may be treated with pelvic sling traction, skeletal traction, hip spica casts, external fixation, open reduction, or a combination of these methods. Open reduction and internal fixation of a pelvic fracture may be necessary if the fracture is displaced.[30] Extreme care in handling or moving the patient is important to prevent serious injury from a displaced fracture fragment. Because a pelvic fracture can damage other organs, assessment of bowel and urinary tract function and distal neurovascular status are important nursing measures.

The patient should be turned only when specifically ordered by the health care provider. Back care is provided while the patient is raised from the bed either by independent use of the trapeze or with adequate assistance. Weight bearing on the affected side should be avoided until healing is complete. If the pelvic fracture is nondisplaced, the patient is usually allowed to

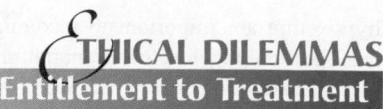

ETHICAL DILEMMAS
Entitlement to Treatment

Situation

A 35-year-old tourist from Germany had a hanggliding accident while touring the United States. He was taken to the regional trauma center for treatment of internal injuries, loss of blood, and severe pelvic fractures. He has become septic, is now in renal failure, and has acute respiratory distress syndrome. He has no health insurance. Despite a poor chance of survival, his wife and parents want all possible measures to be taken.

Important Points for Consideration

- Federal law requires hospitals receiving federal funds through Medicare and Medicaid, under the Emergency Medical Treatment and Labor Act (EMTALA, part of the Consolidated Omnibus Reconciliation Act [COBRA]), to provide emergency evaluation and treatment to stabilize patients. They are under no obligation to continue treatment and may transfer the patient to another facility.
- In addition, the Hill-Burton Act requires states to provide sufficient hospitals to provide necessary services for those unable to pay.
- Neither health care providers nor hospitals are required to provide medically futile care, that is, care that provides no benefit to the patient.
- Discussions with the family must take place to clarify the goals of treatment (i.e., recovery, survival, continued biologic existence, nonabandonment of the patient). There is no legal or ethical obligation to continue medical treatment when the treatment goals cannot be met.
- This man intentionally participated in a potentially dangerous activity although he had no health insurance coverage.

Critical Thinking Questions

1. How can the nurse facilitate discussions with the family regarding their goals for this patient?
2. What are your feelings about continuing treatment for this man?

ambulate using a walker or crutches to distribute the weight bearing between the upper and lower extremities.

FRACTURE OF THE HIP

Hip fractures are common in older adults. More than 200,000 hip fractures occur annually, and by age 80, one in five women will fracture a hip.[31] In adults over age 65, hip fracture occurs more frequently in women than in men because of osteoporosis. It is estimated that 14% to 36% of patients who experience a hip fracture will die within 1 year of injury because of medical complications caused by the fracture or resulting immobility. Only half of older adults with a hip fracture are able to return home and be independent.[32]

A fracture of the hip (Fig. 61-13) refers to a fracture of the proximal third of the femur, which extends up to 5 cm below the lesser trochanter. Fractures that occur within the hip joint capsule are called *intracapsular fractures*. Intracapsular fractures (femoral neck) are further identified by a name derived

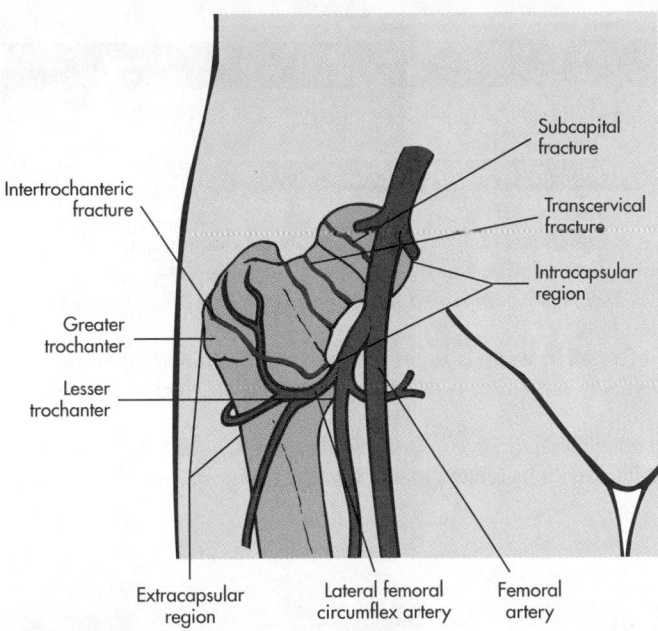

FIG. 61-13   Femur with location of various types of fracture.

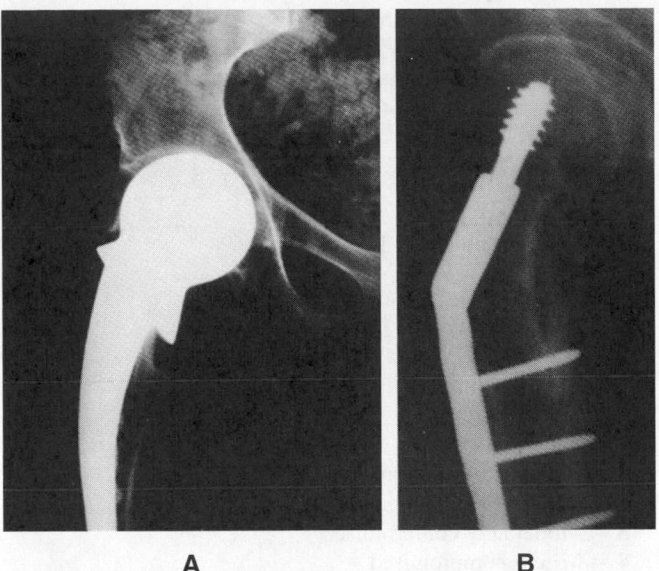

FIG. 61-14   Types of internal fixation for a hip fracture. A, Femoral head endoprosthesis. B, Type of hip compression screw with side plate.

from specific locations: (1) capital (fracture of the head of the femur), (2) subcapital (fractures just below the head of the femur), and (3) transcervical (fractures of the neck of the femur). These fractures are often associated with osteoporosis and minor trauma. *Extracapsular fractures* occur outside the joint capsule and are termed (1) *intertrochanteric* if they occur in a region between the greater and lesser trochanter or (2) *subtrochanteric* if they occur in the region below the lesser trochanter. Extracapsular fractures are usually caused by severe direct trauma or a fall.

Clinical Manifestations

The clinical manifestations of hip fractures are external rotation, muscle spasm, shortening of the affected extremity, and severe pain and tenderness in the region of the fracture site. Displaced femoral neck fractures cause serious disruption of the blood supply to the femoral head, which can result in avascular necrosis.

Collaborative Care

Surgical repair is the preferred method of managing intracapsular and extracapsular hip fractures. Surgical treatment permits early mobilization of the patient and decreases the risk of major complications. Initially the affected extremity may be temporarily immobilized by Buck's traction until the patient's physical condition is stabilized and surgery can be performed. Buck's traction relieves painful muscle spasms and is used for 24 to 48 hours maximum.

Intracapsular (femoral neck) fractures are usually repaired with the use of an endoprosthesis to replace the femoral head (hemiarthroplasty) (Fig. 61-14, *A*). Extracapsular fractures are repaired using fixed nail plates, sliding nail plates, intramedullary devices, and replacement prostheses (Fig. 61-14, *B*). The principles of patient care for these procedures are similar.

NURSING MANAGEMENT
HIP FRACTURE

■ Nursing Implementation

Preoperative Management. Because older adults are most prone to hip fractures, chronic health problems must often be considered when planning treatment. Diabetes mellitus, hypertension, cardiac decompensation, pulmonary disease, and arthritis are chronic problems that may complicate clinical status. Surgery may be delayed for a brief time until the patient's general health is stabilized.

Before surgery, severe muscle spasms can increase pain. Spasms are managed by appropriate analgesics or muscle relaxants, comfortable positioning unless contraindicated, and properly adjusted traction.

Careful preoperative patient teaching can affect future mobility.[33] Often this is done in the emergency department because quick surgical intervention is the standard of care today. Many patients will not have an overnight preoperative period in which to receive instructions, or the patient may not have the cognitive abilities to retain this important patient education. When possible, the patient can be taught the method and frequency for exercising the unaffected leg and both arms. The patient should also be encouraged to use the overhead trapeze bar and the opposite side rail to assist in changing positions. A physical therapist can begin to teach out-of-bed and chair transfers. The family must also be informed about the patient's weight-bearing status after surgery. Plans for discharge begin as the patient enters the hospital because the length of stay postoperatively will be only a few days.

Postoperative Management. The initial postoperative management of a patient following open reduction with internal fixation (ORIF) of a hip fracture is similar to that for any older surgical patient. The nurse must monitor vital signs, intake, and

NURSING CARE PLAN 61-2

Patient with a Hip Fracture

NURSING DIAGNOSIS   **Risk for peripheral neurovascular dysfunction** *related to* vascular insufficiency and nerve compression secondary to edema.

OUTCOMES—NOC	INTERVENTIONS—NIC and *RATIONALES*
Tissue Perfusion: Peripheral (0407)	*Circulatory Precautions (4070)*
▪ Peripheral edema not present _____	▪ Perform a comprehensive appraisal of peripheral circulation (e.g., peripheral pulses, edema, capillary refill, color, temperature of extremity) *to assess for diminished tissue perfusion and plan appropriate intervention.*
▪ Localized extremity pain not present _____	
▪ Distal peripheral pulses strong _____	
▪ Capillary refill brisk _____	
▪ Sensation level normal _____	▪ Prevent infection in wounds *to prevent further edema and inflammation, which may contribute further to vascular insufficiency and nerve compression.*
▪ Extremity temperature warm _____	
_____	
Outcome Scale	▪ Maintain adequate hydration *to prevent increased blood viscosity.*
1 = Extremely compromised	▪ For other interventions related to this nursing diagnosis, see NCP 61-1.
2 = Substantially compromised	
3 = Moderately compromised	
4 = Mildly compromised	
5 = Not compromised	

NURSING DIAGNOSIS   **Acute pain** *related to* tissue trauma, disruption of skin integrity and edema secondary to hip fracture *as manifested by* reluctance to move, guarding of affected area, persistent score of >8 on 10-point pain scale, and facial grimacing.

OUTCOMES—NOC	INTERVENTIONS—NIC and *RATIONALES*
Pain Control (1605)	*Pain Management (1400)*
▪ Recognizes pain onset _____	▪ Align and position extremity and patient correctly *to reduce pressure on nerves and tissue.*
▪ Uses nonanalgesic pain relief measures _____	
▪ Uses analgesics appropriately _____	▪ Encourage patient to monitor own pain and to intervene appropriately *to increase patient's control over pain management.*
▪ Reports pain controlled _____	
_____	▪ Implement the use of patient-controlled analgesia (PCA) *to give patient control.*
Outcome Scale	
1 = Never demonstrated	▪ Administer medication before an activity *to increase participation in mobility exercises, which will ultimately decrease healing time.*
2 = Rarely demonstrated	
3 = Sometimes demonstrated	▪ Evaluate the effectiveness of the pain control measures used through ongoing assessment of the pain experience *so that pain relief is in accordance with the healing process.*
4 = Often demonstrated	
5 = Consistently demonstrated	

NURSING DIAGNOSIS   **Risk for impaired skin integrity** *related to* immobility and shearing forces.

OUTCOMES—NOC	INTERVENTIONS—NIC and *RATIONALES*
Tissue Integrity (1101)	*Pressure Management (3500)*
▪ Skin intactness _____	▪ Elevate injured extremity *to increase venous return and decrease edema.*
▪ Tissue perfusion _____	
▪ Sensation in expected range (IER) _____	▪ Monitor patient's nutritional status *to ensure adequate intake to facilitate bone and wound healing.*
▪ Tissue lesion free _____	
_____	▪ Monitor for sources of pressure and friction to relieve *pressure and friction in a timely manner.*
Outcome Scale	
1 = Extremely compromised	▪ Monitor skin for areas of redness or breakdown using Braden scale (see Table 12-21) *to assess for signs and symptoms of skin breakdown.*
2 = Substantially compromised	
3 = Moderately compromised	
4 = Mildly compromised	▪ Monitor patient's mobility and activity *to assess for changes in range of motion in affected limb.*
5 = Not compromised	

output; supervise respiratory activities, such as deep breathing and coughing; administer pain medication cautiously; and observe the dressing and incision for signs of bleeding and infection. Specific nursing interventions for the patient with a fracture of the hip are described in NCP 61-2.

In the early postoperative period there is a potential for neurovascular impairment. The nurse assesses the patient's extrem-

ity for (1) color, (2) temperature, (3) capillary refill, (4) distal pulses, (5) edema, (6) sensation, (7) motor function, and (8) pain. Edema is alleviated by elevation of the leg whenever the patient is in a chair. The pain resulting from poor alignment of the affected extremity can be reduced by keeping pillows (or an abductor splint) between the knees when the patient is turning to either side. Sandbags and pillows are also used to prevent external

NURSING CARE PLAN 61-2

Patient with a Hip Fracture—cont'd

NURSING DIAGNOSIS   **Impaired physical mobility** *related to* decreased muscle strength, pain, presence of immobilization device *as manifested by* inability to purposefully move, limited joint ROM, inability to bear weight.

OUTCOMES—NOC	INTERVENTIONS—NIC and *RATIONALES*
Ambulation: Walking (0200) ▪ Bears weight _____ ▪ Walks at slow pace _____ ▪ Walks with effective gait ___ *Mobility Level (0208)* ▪ Body positioning performance ___ ▪ Joint movement ___ ▪ Ambulation: Walking_____ _____ **Outcome Scale** 1 = Dependent, does not participate 2 = Requires assistive person and device 3 = Requires assistive person 4 = Independent with assistive device 5 = Completely independent	*Exercise Therapy: Joint Mobility (0740)* *Exercise Therapy: Ambulation (0221)* ▪ Get patient out of bed and into chair, usually within 24 to 48 hours after surgery *to reduce the complications associated with immobility.* ▪ Instruct and assist patient with transfer from bed to chair to *prevent accidental falling and improper movements.* ▪ Collaborate with physical therapist in developing and implementing an exercise program to *maximize patient's progress in rehabilitation.* ▪ Provide written instructions for exercises for patient to refer to as needed. ▪ Provide positive reinforcement for performing exercises *to enhance motivation.* ▪ Encourage family to get involved with exercises *so that they can provide continuity of care.*

rotation. If an endoprosthesis was placed, the patient is at risk for hip dislocation. Hip precautions must be demonstrated and explained to the patient.

The physical therapist usually supervises active-assistance exercises for the affected extremity and ambulation when the surgeon permits it. Ambulation usually begins on the first or second postoperative day. The nurse in collaboration with the physical therapist monitors the patient's ambulation status for proper crutch walking or use of the walker. For the patient to be discharged home, the patient must be able to safely demonstrate use of crutches or a walker, the ability to transfer into and from a chair and bed, and the ability to ascend and descend stairs.

Complications associated with femoral neck fracture include nonunion, avascular necrosis, dislocation, and degenerative arthritis. As a result of an intertrochanteric fracture, the affected leg may be shortened. A cane or built-up shoe may be required for safe ambulation.

If the hip fracture has been treated by insertion of a femoral head prosthesis, measures to prevent dislocation must always be used (Table 61-12). The patient and family must be fully aware of positions and activities that predispose the patient to dislocation (greater than 90 degrees of flexion, adduction, or internal rotation). Many daily activities may reproduce these positions, including putting on shoes and socks, crossing the legs or feet while seated, assuming the side-lying position incorrectly, standing up or sitting down while the body is flexed relative to the chair, and sitting on low seats, especially low toilet seats. Until the soft tissue surrounding the hip has healed sufficiently to stabilize the prosthesis, these activities must be avoided, usually for at least 6 weeks. Sudden severe pain, a lump in the buttock, limb shortening, and external rotation indicate prosthesis dislocation. This requires a closed reduction with conscious sedation or open reduction to realign the femoral head in the acetabulum.

In addition to teaching the patient and family how to prevent prosthesis dislocation, the nurse should (1) place a large pillow between the patient's legs when turning, (2) keep leg abductor splints on the patient except when bathing, (3) avoid extreme hip flexion, and (4) avoid turning the patient on the affected side until approved by the surgeon.

If the hip fracture is treated by pinning, dislocation precautions are not necessary. The patient is out of bed on the first postoperative day. Weight bearing on the involved extremity varies. Weight bearing of especially fragile fractures may be restricted until x-ray examination indicates adequate healing, usually 6 to 12 weeks.

The nurse assists both the patient and the family in adjusting to the restrictions and dependence imposed by the hip fracture. Depression can easily occur, but creative nursing care and awareness of the problem can do much to prevent it. The patient and family may need to be informed about community referral services that can assist in the postdischarge rehabilitation phase. Hospitalization averages 4 days. Patients frequently require care in a subacute unit, at a skilled nursing facility, or in a rehabilitation facility for a few weeks before returning home. Regular follow-up care after discharge including home health nursing should be arranged.

■ Evaluation

The expected outcomes for the patient with fracture of the hip are presented in NCP 61-2.

■ Gerontologic Considerations: Hip Fracture

Factors that contribute to the occurrence of a hip fracture in older adults include a propensity to fall, inability to correct a postural imbalance, orientation of the fall, inadequacy of local tissue shock absorbers (e.g., fat, muscle bulk), and underlying skeletal strength. Several factors have been identified in older persons that increase their risk of falling. These include gait and balance problems, decreased vision and hearing, decreased reflexes, orthostatic hypotension, and medication use. Leading hazards of

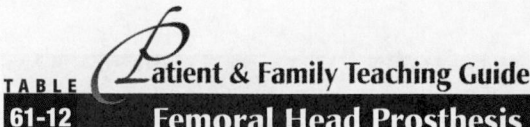

TABLE 61-12 Patient & Family Teaching Guide — Femoral Head Prosthesis

Do Not

- Force hip into greater than 90 degrees of flexion*
- Force hip into adduction
- Force hip into internal rotation
- Cross legs
- Put on own shoes or stockings until 8 wk after surgery without adaptive device (e.g., long-handled shoehorn or stocking-helper)
- Sit on chairs without arms to aid rising to a standing position*

Do

- Use toilet elevator on toilet seat*
- Place chair inside shower or tub and remain seated while washing
- Use pillow between legs for first 8 wk after surgery when lying on "good" side or when supine*
- Keep hip in neutral, straight position when sitting, walking, or lying*
- Notify surgeon if severe pain, deformity, or loss of function occurs*
- Inform dentist of presence of prosthesis before dental work so that prophylactic antibiotics can be given

*These precautions may also apply after a hip pinning.

falls are loose rugs and slippery or uneven surfaces. Many falls are associated with getting in or out of a chair or bed. Falls to the side, the most common type in the frail elderly, are more likely to result in a hip fracture than a forward fall.

Two important factors influencing the amount of force imposed on the hip are the presence of energy-absorbing soft tissue over the greater trochanter and the state of leg muscle contraction at the time of the fall. Because many elderly persons have poor muscle tone, these are important factors in the severity of a fall. Finally, elderly women often have osteoporosis and accompanying low bone density, which increases the risk of hip fracture.[34]

Targeted interventions to reduce hip fractures in the elderly include a variety of strategies. Calcium and vitamin D supplementation, estrogen replacement, and drug therapy have been shown to decrease bone loss or increase bone density and decrease the likelihood of fracture. (Osteoporosis is discussed in Chapter 62.) Nurses must be vigilant in planning interventions for the elderly that are known to reduce the incidence of hip fracture. ■

FEMORAL SHAFT FRACTURE

Femoral shaft fracture is a common injury occurring particularly in young adults. Severe direct force is required to produce this injury because the femur can bend slightly before actual fracture occurs. The force exerted to cause the fracture often causes damage to the adjacent soft tissue structures. These injuries may be more serious than the bone injury. Displacement of the fracture fragments often results in open fracture and increased soft tissue damage. This can result in considerable blood loss (1 to 1.5 L).

The clinical manifestations of a fracture of the femoral shaft are usually obvious. They include marked deformity and angulation, shortening of the extremity, inability to move either the hip

or knee, and pain. The common complications associated with fracture of the femoral shaft include fat embolism, nerve and vascular injury, and problems associated with bone union, open fracture, and soft tissue damage.

Initial management is directed toward stabilization of the patient and immobilization of the fracture. Treatment may consist of skeletal traction via a femoral or tibial pin and balanced suspension traction for 8 to 12 weeks. The nurse must encourage the patient to perform exercises and ROM activities for the uninvolved extremities and joints to discourage deconditioning. The physician determines when active exercise can be instituted on the affected extremity. When there is sufficient clinical evidence of bone union, a hip spica or long leg cast may be applied. Use of prolonged traction is uncommon as the current standard of care.

ORIF has become the preferred method to manage a femoral fracture. It is carried out with an intramedullary rod, compression plate, and screws or side plate with an intercondylar nail. Internal fixation is often the preferred treatment because it reduces hospital stay and the complications associated with prolonged bed rest. Other indications for internal fixation are failure to obtain satisfactory reduction by nonsurgical methods and multiple associated injuries. In some instances the surgically repaired femur may be supported by suspension traction for 3 to 4 days to prevent excessive movement of the extremity and to control rotation; non–weight-bearing gait training is then begun. Fractures associated with extensive soft tissue injury may be treated with external fixation.

Promotion and maintenance of strength in the affected extremity usually include gluteal and quadricep isometric exercises. It is important to ensure performance of ROM and strengthening exercises for all uninvolved extremities in preparation for ambulation. The patient may be immobilized in a hip spica cast and gradually progress to an articulating cast brace or may be allowed to begin non–weight-bearing activities with an ambulatory assistive device. Full weight bearing is usually restricted until there is x-ray evidence of union of the fracture fragments.

FRACTURE OF THE TIBIA

Although the tibia is vulnerable to injury because it lacks anterior muscle covering, strong force is required to produce a fractured tibia. As a result, soft tissue damage, devascularization, and open fracture are frequent. Other complications associated with tibial fractures are compartment syndrome, fat embolism, problems associated with bony union, and possible infection associated with open fracture. Amputation may be required if adequate muscle and tissue coverage is not achieved following muscle and flap grafts.

The recommended management for closed tibial fracture is closed reduction followed by immobilization in a long leg cast. ORIF with intramedullary rods or compression plate or external fixation is indicated for complex fractures and those with extensive soft tissue damage. With either method of reduction, emphasis is placed on maintaining the strength of the quadriceps.

The neurovascular status of the affected extremity must be assessed at least every 2 hours during the first 48 hours. Patients are instructed to perform active ROM exercises with all uninvolved extremities, as well as exercises for the upper extremities, to build the strength required for crutch walking. When the physician has determined that the patient is ready for gait training, the patient is instructed in the principles of crutch walking. The patient may be on non–weight-bearing status for 6 to 12 weeks depending on healing. Patients with external fixation must be taught pin care and dressing changes if extensive tissue has been debrided. Home nursing visits can be initiated to augment outpatient appointments and monitor the patient's progress.

STABLE VERTEBRAL FRACTURES

Stable fractures of the vertebral column are usually caused by motor vehicle accidents, falls, diving, or athletic injuries. A stable fracture is one in which the fracture or the fragment is not likely to move or cause spinal cord damage. This type of injury is frequently confined to the anterior element (vertebral body) of the spinal column in the lumbar region, and involves the cervical and thoracic regions less frequently. The vertebral bodies are usually protected from displacement by the intact spinal ligaments.

Most patients with spinal fractures have stable fractures and experience only brief periods of disability. However, if the ligamentous structures are significantly disrupted, dislocation of the vertebral structures may occur, resulting in instability and injury to the spinal cord (unstable fracture). These injuries generally require surgery. The most serious complication of vertebral fractures is fracture displacement, which can cause damage to the spinal cord (see Chapter 59). Although stable vertebral fractures are not associated with abnormal spinal cord pathologic conditions, all spinal injuries should initially be considered unstable and potentially serious until diagnostic tests are done and the physician determines that the fracture is stable.

The most common injury to the vertebral body is the compression type of fracture caused by excessive vertical loading, such as a severe fall on the buttocks or injury resulting from sudden flexion that forces the spine beyond its normal ROM. The patient usually complains of pain and tenderness in the affected region of the spine. Compression fractures are associated with a "gibbous" deformity (flexion angulation of several vertebrae). This deformity may be noted during the physical examination. In patients with osteoporosis, several vertebral levels may be involved as evidenced by a "dowager's hump" (abnormal backward curvature of thoracic spine). The cervical spine may also be involved. Bowel and bladder dysfunction may be an indication of an interruption of the autonomic nervous system or injury to the spinal cord.

The overall goal in management of stable fractures of a vertebral body is to keep the spine in good alignment until union has been accomplished. Many nursing interventions are aimed at assessing for the possibility of spinal cord trauma. Vital signs and bowel and bladder function should be evaluated regularly, as should the motor and sensory status of the peripheral nerves distal to the injured region. Any deterioration in the patient's neurovascular status should be promptly reported.

Treatment includes support, heat, and traction. The patient is usually placed in a standard hospital bed with firm support from the mattress or a bed board. The aim is to support the spinal column, relax muscles, and release any compression on nerve roots. Heat and traction may be used to relieve muscle spasms resulting from the fracture. Traction may also be used to reduce and immobilize fracture fragments. A trapeze is not usually allowed because its use disrupts spinal alignment. Both an upright position and turning of the torso are prohibited. When turning, the patient should be taught to keep the spine straight by turning shoulders and pelvis together. Nursing assistance is necessary for the patient to learn how to turn in this "logrolling" fashion.[35] Several days after the initial injury, the physician may apply a specially constructed orthotic device (e.g., Milwaukee, Jewett, or Taylor brace), a jacket cast, or a removable corset if there is no evidence of neurologic deficit.

If the fracture is in the cervical spine, a cervical collar may be worn by the patient. Some cervical fractures are immobilized by use of a halo vest (see Fig. 59-12). This consists of a plastic jacket or cast fitted about the chest and attached to a halo that is held in place by skeletal pins inserted into the cranium. These devices immobilize the spine in the fracture area but allow patient mobility. The patient is discharged after (1) regaining ambulation skills, (2) learning care of the cast or orthotic device, and (3) learning how to cope with interferences in safety and security imposed by injury and treatment.

FACIAL FRACTURES

Any bone of the face can be fractured as a result of trauma. Fractures can occur as a result of collision with another person or object, fighting, or blunt trauma. The primary concern after facial injury is to establish and maintain a patent airway and to provide adequate ventilation by removal of foreign material and blood. Suctioning may be necessary. An artificial airway (tracheostomy) may be needed if a patent airway cannot be maintained. Hemorrhage is controlled by pressure packing. Cervical spine injuries are common. All patients with facial injuries should be treated as though they have a cervical injury until proven otherwise by examination and imaging studies (e.g., x-ray). Table 61-13 describes the clinical manifestations of common facial fractures.

Concurrent soft tissue injury often makes assessment of a facial injury difficult. Oral and facial examinations should be performed after the patient has been stabilized and any life-threatening situations have been treated. Careful assessment is made of the ocular muscles and cranial nerve involvement. An x-ray documents the extent of the injury. Computed tomography (CT) imaging helps differentiate between bone and soft tissue and gives a more specific view of the fracture.

Injury to the eye must be suspected when a facial injury occurs, particularly if the injury is near the orbit. If a global rupture is suspected, the examination is stopped and a protective shield is placed over the eye until examined by the ophthalmologist. Signs

TABLE 61-13	Clinical Manifestations of Facial Fractures	
FRACTURE	**CLINICAL MANIFESTATION**
Frontal bone	Rapid edema that may mask underlying fractures
Periorbital	Possible frontal sinus involvement, entrapment of ocular muscles
Nasal	Displacement of nasal bones, epistaxis
Zygomatic arch	Depression of zygomatic arch
Maxilla	Segmental motion of maxilla
Mandible	Tooth fractures, bleeding, limited motion of mandible

of global rupture include brown tissue (iris or ciliary body) on the surface of the globe or penetrating through a laceration with an eccentric or teardrop-shaped pupil.[36] Specific treatment of a facial fracture depends on the site and extent of the fracture and the associated soft tissue injury. Immobilization or surgical stabilization may be necessary.

The patient who sustains a facial fracture requires sensitive nursing care because alteration in appearance after the trauma may be drastic. Edema and discoloration subside with time, but concurrent soft tissue injuries may result in permanent scarring. Attention to maintenance of a patent airway and adequate nutrition are ongoing concerns of the nurse throughout the recovery period. Suction should always be available to maintain a patent airway for these patients.

Mandible Fracture

A fracture of the mandible may result from trauma to the face or jaws. Maxillary fractures may also occur, but they are less common than mandibular fractures. The fracture may be simple, with no bone displacement, or it may involve loss of tissue and bone. The fracture may require immediate and sometimes long-term treatment to ensure survival and restore satisfactory appearance and function. Mandibular fracture may also be therapeutically performed to correct an underlying malocclusion problem that cannot be corrected by orthodontic procedures alone. In these conditions, the mandible is resected during surgery and manipulated forward or backward depending on the occlusion problem. For this patient, the procedure is performed on an elective basis.

Surgery consists of immobilization, usually by wiring the jaws (intermaxillary fixation). Internal fixation may be accomplished with screws and plates. In a simple fracture with no loss of teeth, the lower jaw is wired to the upper jaw. First, wires are placed around the teeth; then cross-wires or rubber bands are used to hold the lower jaw tight against the upper jaw (Fig. 61-15). Arch bars may be placed on the maxillary and mandibular arches of the teeth. Vertical wires are placed between the arch bars holding the jaws together. When teeth are missing or if there is bone displacement, other forms of fixation such as metal arch bars in the mouth or insertion of a pin in the bone may be used. The immobilization is usually necessary for only 4 to 6 weeks because the fractures heal rapidly.

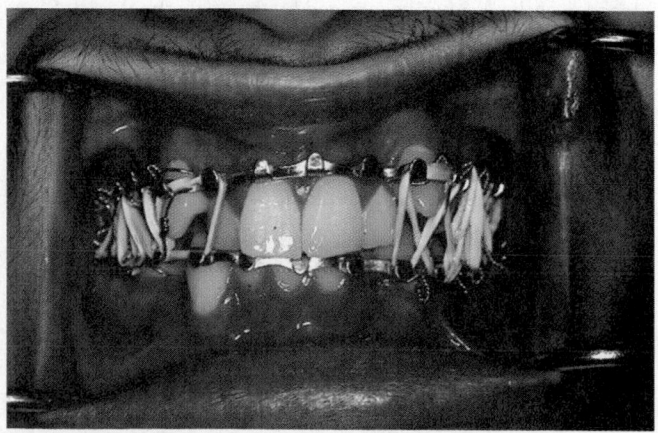

FIG. 61-15 Intermaxillary fixation.

NURSING MANAGEMENT
MANDIBULAR FRACTURE

■ Nursing Implementation

Preoperative Management. The patient should be told preoperatively about the surgical procedure, including what it involves, how the face will look, and alterations the surgery will cause. The patient must be reassured about the ability to breathe normally, speak, and swallow liquids. Usually hospitalization is brief unless there are other injuries or problems.

Postoperative Management. Postoperative care should focus on a patent airway, oral hygiene, communication, and adequate nutrition. Two major potential problems in the immediate postoperative period are airway obstruction and aspiration of vomitus. Because the patient cannot open the jaws, measures to ensure an airway are essential. The nurse must observe for signs of respiratory distress. The patient should be placed on the side with the head slightly elevated immediately after surgery. A wire cutter or scissors (for rubber bands) must be taped to the head of the bed and sent with the patient on all appointments and examinations away from the bedside. These may be used to cut the wires or elastic bands in case of an emergency. The wires should be cut only as a last resort. Once the patient is awake the wires should be cut only in case of cardiac or respiratory arrest.

The physician should explain, by using a picture, the appropriate wire or wires to cut, and this should be included in the care plan. In some cases, cutting the wires may cause the entire facial and upper jaw structure to collapse and worsen the problem. A tracheostomy tray or an endotracheal tray should always be available.

If the patient begins to vomit or choke, the nurse should try to clear the mouth and airway. Suctioning may be necessary and may be done by the nasopharyngeal or oral route, depending on the extent of injury and the type of repair. An NG tube may be used for decompression to remove fluids and gas from the stomach to help prevent aspiration. It also helps prevent vomiting. Antiemetics may also be used. The NG tube can later be used as a feeding tube. The nurse should teach the patient to clear secretions and vomitus.

Oral hygiene is an important part of the nursing care. The mouth should be rinsed frequently, particularly after meals and snacks, to remove food debris. Warm normal saline solution, water, or alkaline mouthwashes may be used. A soft rubber catheter or a Water-Pik is effective for a thorough oral cleansing. The nurse should inspect the mouth several times a day to see that it is clean. A flashlight is necessary, and a tongue depressor is used to retract the cheeks. The lips and corners of the mouth should be kept moist.

Communication may be a problem, particularly in the early postoperative period. An effective way of communication must be established preoperatively (e.g., use of picture board, pad and pencil, small chalkboard). Usually the patient can speak well enough to be understood, especially after the first few postoperative days.

Ingestion of sufficient nutrients poses a challenge because the diet must be liquid. The patient easily tires of sucking through a straw or laboriously using a spoon. The diet must be planned to include adequate calories, protein, and fluids. Liquid protein supplements may be helpful for improving the nutritional status. The nurse works with the dietitian and the patient to ensure adequate nutrition. The low-bulk, high-carbohydrate diet and the intake of air through the straw create a problem with constipation and flatus. Ambulation, prune juice, and bulk-forming laxatives may help relieve these problems.

The patient is usually discharged with the wires in place. The nurse should allow the patient to verbalize feelings about the altered appearance. Discharge teaching should include oral care, techniques of handling secretions, diet, and how and when to use wire cutters.

AMPUTATION

During the past 20 years, major advances have been made in surgical amputation techniques, prosthetic design, and rehabilitation programs. These advances are enabling amputees to return to productive and satisfying social roles. There are an estimated 400,000 amputees in the United States, with an annual increase of 20,000. The middle and older age-groups have the highest incidence of amputation because of the effects of peripheral vascular disease, atherosclerosis, and vascular changes related to diabetes mellitus.

Clinical Indications

The clinical indications for an amputation depend on the underlying disease or trauma. Amputation is required more often in persons engaged in hazardous occupations, with a greater incidence in men. Common indications for amputation include circulatory impairment resulting from a peripheral vascular disorder, traumatic and thermal injuries, malignant tumors, uncontrolled or widespread infection of the extremity (e.g., gas gangrene, osteomyelitis), and congenital disorders. These conditions may manifest as loss of sensation, inadequate circulation, pallor, and local or systemic manifestations of infection. Although pain is often present, it is not usually the primary reason for an amputation. The underlying problem dictates whether the amputation is performed as elective or emergency surgery. Consideration must also be given to the patient's ability to successfully use a prosthetic device.

Diagnostic Studies

The types of diagnostic studies performed depend on the underlying problem that makes the amputation necessary (Table 61-14). An elevated white blood cell (WBC) count may indicate infection. Vascular studies such as arteriography and venography provide information about the circulatory status of the extremity.

Collaborative Care

The potential for revascularization surgery rather than amputation can be assessed on the basis of vascular studies. If amputation is to be considered "elective," the patient's general health is carefully assessed. Chronic illnesses and infection are monitored closely. The patient and family should be helped to understand the need for the amputation and be assured that rehabilitation can result in an active, useful life. If the amputation is done on an emergency basis as a result of trauma, the management is physically and emotionally more complicated.

The goal of amputation surgery is to preserve extremity length and function while removing all infected, pathologic, or ischemic tissue. This improves the possibility of good prosthetic, cosmetic, and functional satisfaction. (Levels of amputation of upper and lower extremities are illustrated in Fig. 61-16.) The type of amputation depends on the reason for the surgery. A

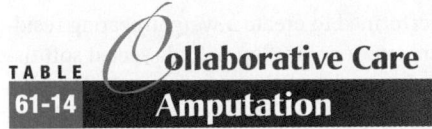

TABLE 61-14	Collaborative Care Amputation

Diagnostic
History and physical examination
    Physical appearance of soft tissues
    Skin temperature
    Sensory function
    Presence of peripheral pulses
Arteriography
Thermography
Plethysmography
Transcutaneous ultrasonic Doppler recordings

Collaborative Therapy
Medical
Appropriate management of underlying disease
Stabilization of trauma victim
Surgical
Appropriate type of amputation, leaving as long a residual
    limb as possible
Residual limb management
    Immediate prosthetic fitting
    Delayed prosthetic fitting
Rehabilitation
Coordination of prosthesis-fitting and gait-training activities
Coordination of muscle-strengthening and physical therapy
    regimens

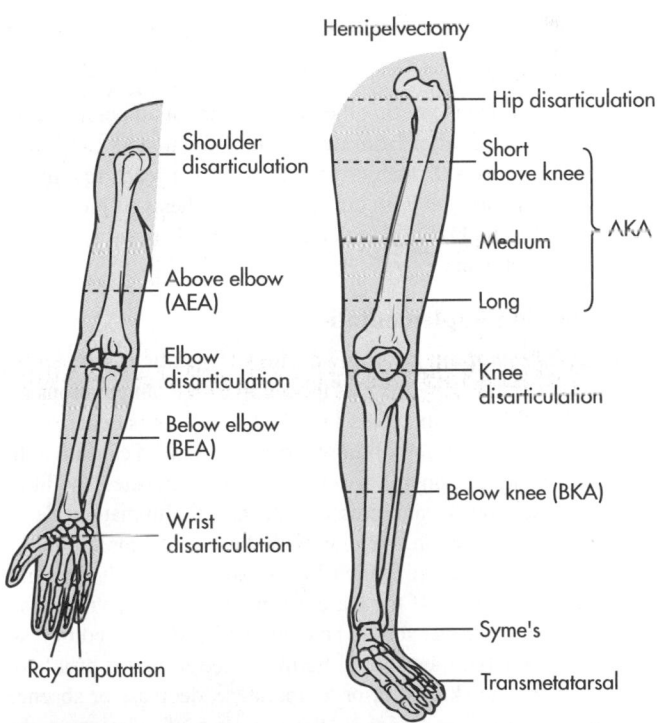

FIG. 61-16 Location and description of amputation sites of the upper and lower extremities. *AKA*, Above the knee amputation.

closed amputation is performed to create a weight-bearing residual limb (or stump). An anterior skin flap with dissected soft tissue padding covers the bony part of the residual limb. The skin flap is sutured posteriorly so that it will not be positioned in a weight-bearing area. Special care is necessary to prevent the accumulation of drainage, which can produce pressure and harbor infection. Disarticulation is an amputation performed through a joint. A Syme's amputation is a form of disarticulation at the ankle. An open amputation leaves a surface on the residual limb that is not covered with skin. This type of surgery is generally indicated for control of actual or potential infection. The wound is usually closed later by a second surgical procedure or closed by skin traction surrounding the residual limb. This type of amputation is often called a "guillotine amputation."

NURSING MANAGEMENT AMPUTATION

■ Nursing Assessment

Preexisting illnesses must be adequately assessed because most amputations are performed as a result of vascular problems. Assessment of the vascular and neurologic status is an important part of this assessment process (see Chapters 31 and 54).

■ Nursing Diagnoses

Nursing diagnoses for the patient with an amputation may include, but are not limited to, the following:

- Disturbed body image *related to* amputation and impaired mobility
- Impaired skin integrity *related to* immobility and improperly fitted prosthesis
- Chronic pain *related to* phantom limb sensation
- Impaired physical mobility *related to* amputation of lower limb

■ Planning

The overall goals are that the patient with an amputation will (1) have adequate relief from treatment of the underlying health problem, (2) have satisfactory pain control, (3) reach maximum rehabilitation potential with the use of a prosthesis (if indicated), (4) cope with the body image changes, and (5) make satisfying lifestyle adjustments.

■ Nursing Implementation

Health Promotion. Most lower-limb amputations result from peripheral vascular disease, and most upper-limb amputations result from severe trauma. This knowledge directs patient education related to prevention of amputation. Control of causative illnesses such as peripheral vascular disease, diabetes mellitus, chronic osteomyelitis, and pressure ulcers can eliminate or delay the need for amputation. Patients with these problems should be taught to carefully examine their lower extremities daily for signs of potential problems. If the patient cannot assume this responsibility, a family member should be instructed in the procedure. Patients and their families should be instructed to report problems such as change in skin color or temperature, decrease or absence of sensation, tingling, pain, or the presence of a lesion to the health care provider.

Instruction in proper safety precautions in recreation and in the performance of hazardous work is an important nursing responsibility, especially for occupational health nurses. Limb mutilation and subsequent amputation are serious consequences of trauma that can be avoided through such instruction.

Acute Intervention. The nurse must recognize the tremendous psychologic and social implications of an amputation for the patient. The disruption in body image caused by an amputation often causes a patient to go through psychologic stages similar to the grieving process. Allowing the patient to go through a grieving process or period of depression and recognizing it as a normal consequence may do much to aid the patient's acceptance of the amputation. The patient's family must also be helped to work through the process to arrive at a realistic and positive attitude about the future. The reasons for an amputation and the rehabilitation potential depend on age, diagnosis, occupation, personality, resources, and support systems.

Preoperative management. Before surgery, the nurse should reinforce information that the patient and family have received about the reasons for the amputation, the proposed prosthesis, and the mobility training program. In addition to the usual preoperative instructions, the patient undergoing an amputation has special education needs. To meet these needs, the nurse must know the level of amputation, the type of postsurgical dressing to be applied, and the type of prosthesis planned. The patient should receive instruction in the performance of upper-extremity exercises such as push-ups in bed or the wheelchair to promote arm strength. This instruction is essential for later crutch walking and gait training. General postoperative nursing care should be discussed, including positioning, support, and residual limb care. If a compression bandage is to be used after surgery the patient should be instructed about its purpose and how it will be applied. If an immediate prosthesis is planned, the general ambulation program should be discussed.

The patient should be warned that she or he may feel as though the amputated limb is still present after surgery. This phenomenon, termed **phantom limb sensation,** occurs in 80% of amputees and may cause patients grave concern unless they are forewarned. If pain was present in the affected limb preoperatively, the patient may also experience phantom limb pain postoperatively. The patient may have feelings of coldness and heaviness, cramping, shooting, burning, or crushing pain. Often, the patient may be extremely anxious about this pain because the patient knows the limb is gone but still feels pain in it. As recovery and ambulation progress, phantom limb sensation and pain usually subside, although the pain can become chronic.[37]

Postoperative management. General postoperative care for the patient who has had an amputation depends largely on the patient's general state of health, the reason for the amputation, and the patient's age. Nursing care must be individualized on the basis of these factors. For example, an older adult patient needs particularly careful monitoring of respiratory status. A victim of a motor vehicle accident may need careful neurologic monitoring. Individuals who undergo amputation as a result of a traumatic injury need to be monitored for posttraumatic stress disorder because they had no time to prepare or perhaps even participate in the decision to have a limb amputated.

Prevention and detection of complications are important nursing responsibilities during the postoperative period. Careful monitoring of the patient's vital signs and dressing can alert the nurse to hemorrhage in the operative area. Careful attention to sterile technique during dressing changes reduces the potential for wound infection and subsequent interruption of rehabilitation.

If an immediate postoperative prosthesis has been applied, the nurse must monitor vital signs carefully because the surgical site is heavily covered and may not be visible. A surgical tourniquet must always be available for emergency use. If hemorrhage occurs, the surgeon should be notified immediately, and efforts to control the hemorrhage should begin at once.

The orthopedic surgeon will decide the type of prosthetic fitting that will be used after surgery. An immediate prosthetic fitting, often called the immediate postsurgical fitting or the immediate postoperative fitting, is done in the operating room after the amputation. A rigid, castlike bandage is applied around the closed residual limb with a prosthetic pylon and an ankle-foot assembly. While the patient is still anesthetized, the prosthetic pylon and ankle-foot assembly are aligned and adjusted to provide a smooth gait and to avoid excessive pressure on the residual limb area. A strap is placed on the proximal anterior surface of the rigid plaster bandage and attached to a waistband to prevent slippage. The main advantages of this device are reduction of edema and the psychologic benefit of early ambulation. A disadvantage is the inability to directly visualize the surgical site.

The delayed prosthetic fitting may be the best choice for certain patients. Patients who have had amputations above the knee or below the elbow, older adults, debilitated individuals, and those with infection usually have delayed prosthetic fittings (Fig. 61-17). The appropriate time for use of a prosthesis depends on satisfactory healing of the residual limb, as well as on the general condition of the patient. A temporary prosthesis may be used for partial weight bearing once the sutures are removed. Barring any problems, patients can bear full weight on permanent prostheses by approximately 3 months after amputation.

Not all patients are candidates for a prosthesis. It is important that the surgeon discuss ambulation possibilities frankly with the patient and family. The seriously ill or debilitated patient may not have the energy required to use a prosthesis. Mobility with a wheelchair may be the most realistic goal for this type of patient.

Collaborative care also includes the direction and coordination of the rehabilitation program for the amputee. Success depends on the physical and emotional health of the patient. Chronic illness and debilitation complicate aggressive rehabilitation efforts. Both physical and occupational therapy must be an integral component of the patient's overall plan of care.

Flexion contractures may delay the rehabilitation process. The most common and debilitating contracture is hip flexion. Hip adduction contracture is rare. Patients should avoid sitting in a chair for more than 1 hour with hips flexed or having pillows under the surgical extremity to prevent flexion contractures. Unless specifically contraindicated, patients should lie on their abdomen for 30 minutes three to four times each day and position the hip in extension while prone.

Proper residual limb bandaging fosters shaping and molding for eventual prosthesis fitting (Fig. 61-18). The physician usually orders a compression bandage to be applied immediately after surgery to support the soft tissues, reduce edema, hasten healing, minimize pain, and promote residual limb shrinkage and maturation. This bandage may be an elastic roll applied to the residual limb or a residual limb shrinker, which is an elastic stocking that fits tightly over the residual limb and lower trunk area.[38]

The compression bandage is initially worn at all times except during physical therapy and bathing. The bandage is taken off and reapplied several times daily, and care is taken so that it is applied snugly but not so tight as to interfere with circulation. Shrinker bandages should be washed and changed daily. It is recommended that the patient have two residual limb shrinker bandages so that one can be worn while the other is being washed. After healing has occurred, the residual limb is bandaged only when the patient is not wearing the prosthesis. The patient should

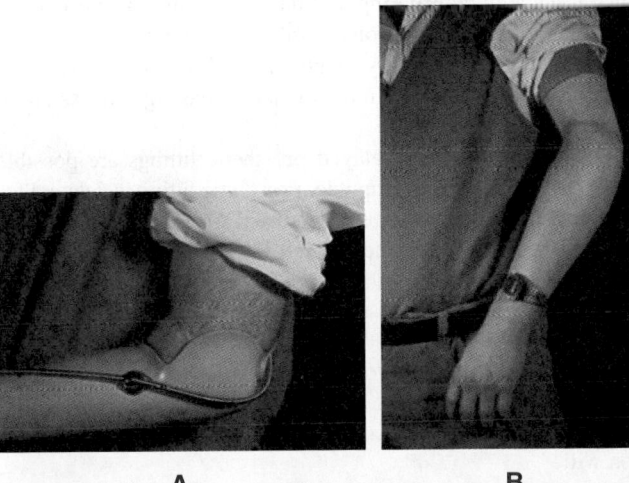

FIG. 61-17 Two types of prosthesis. A, Traditional fiberglass. B, New materials and techniques have made possible fabrication of prosthetic sockets that are light, soft, flexible, and secure.

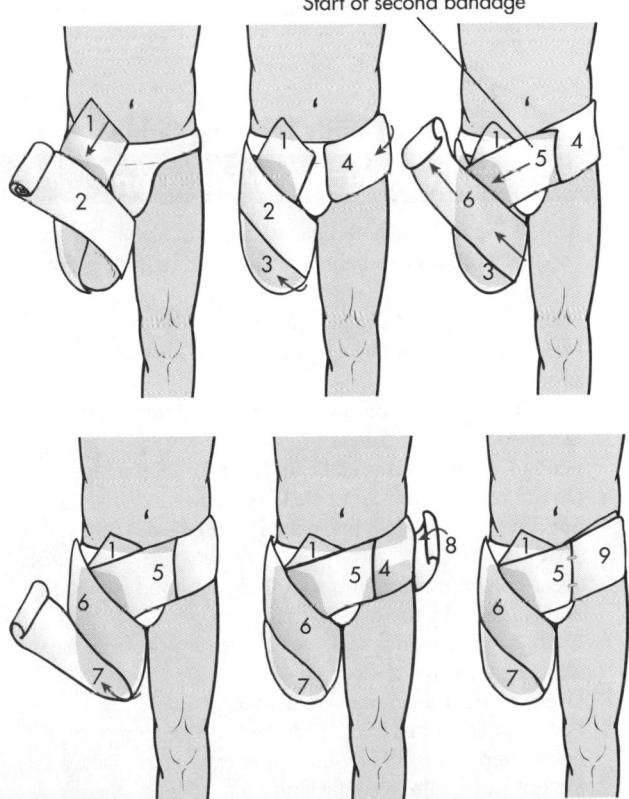

Start of second bandage

FIG. 61-18 Bandaging for the above-the-knee amputation residual limb. Figure-of-eight style covers progressive areas of the residual limb. Two elastic wraps are required.

be instructed to avoid dangling the residual limb over the bedside to minimize edema formation.

As the patient's overall condition improves, the nurse begins instruction in the principles and techniques of transferring from bed to chair and back. Active exercises and conditioning are essential in developing ambulation skills. The exercise regimen is normally started under the supervision of the physician and the physical therapist. The nurse must have a clear understanding of the exercise regimen to reinforce it and ensure that the exercises are performed correctly. Active ROM exercises of all joints should be started as soon after surgery as the patient's pain level and medical status permit. In preparation for mobility, the patient should increase triceps and shoulder strength and lower limb support and learn balance of the altered body. The loss of the weight of a limb requires adaptation of the patient's proprioceptive mechanisms to prevent falls and frustration.

Crutch walking is started as soon as patients are physically able. If they have had immediate postsurgical fitting, orders related to weight bearing must be carefully followed to avoid disruption of the skin flap and delay of the healing process. Initial periods of ambulation should not exceed 5 minutes to prevent dependent edema.

Before discharge, the patient and family need careful instruction related to residual limb care, ambulation, prevention of contractures, recognition of complications, exercise, and follow-up care. Table 61-15 outlines patient and family teaching following an amputation.

Ambulatory and Home Care. When the healing has occurred satisfactorily and the residual limb is well molded, the patient is ready for fitting a prosthesis. Walking with a below-the-knee prosthesis requires 40% additional energy, and an above-the-

knee prosthesis requires 60% more energy. Matching a patient with a suitable prosthesis involves many factors, including age, general health, intelligence, motivation, occupation, and finances. After the physician makes the recommendation, the patient is referred to a prosthetist, who initially makes a mold of the residual limb and measures landmarks for the fabrication of the prosthesis. The molded residual limb socket allows the residual limb to fit snugly into the prosthesis.[39] The residual limb is covered with a residual limb stocking to ensure good fit and prevent skin breakdown. The residual limb may continue to shrink, causing a loose fit, in which case a new socket has to be fabricated. The patient may need to have the prosthesis adjusted to prevent rubbing and friction between the residual limb and the socket. Excessive movement of a loose prosthesis can cause severe skin irritation and breakdown.

The prosthesis is fitted by the prosthetist, who may also train the amputee to use it. It is important for the nurse to be familiar with the training program to encourage and assist the patient. Most often this learning occurs after the patient has been discharged from the inpatient setting. Learning to use a prosthesis is frustrating, and the patient may easily become discouraged. The nurse must continually offer support until the patient is able to manage alone.

Artificial limbs become an integral part of the patient's body image. Proper care ensures their long life and useful functioning. The patient should be instructed to clean the prosthesis socket daily with a mild soap and rinse thoroughly to remove irritants. The leather and metal parts of the prosthesis should not get wet. The patient should be encouraged to have regular maintenance of the prosthesis. Consideration of the condition of the shoe is also necessary. A badly worn shoe alters the gait and may cause damage to the prosthesis.

Referral to a community health nurse can foster optimal physical and emotional adjustment. The family should be instructed on ambulation and transfer techniques and proper residual limb care.

Special Considerations in Upper-Limb Amputation. The emotional implications of an upper-limb amputation are often more devastating than those for lower-limb amputation. The enforced dependency brought about by one-handedness is both frustrating and humiliating to many patients. Because most upper-extremity amputations result from trauma, the patient has not had the opportunity to adjust psychologically to an amputation or to participate in the decision-making process about amputation.

Both immediate and delayed prosthetic fittings are possible for the below-the-elbow amputee. Prosthetic fitting is delayed for the above-the-elbow amputee. The usual functional prosthesis is the arm and hook. A cosmetic hand is available but has limited functional value. As with the lower-limb prosthesis, patient motivation and endurance are major factors contributing to a satisfactory outcome.

■ **Evaluation**

The expected outcomes are that the patient with an amputation will

- accept changed body image and integrate changes into lifestyle
- have no evidence of skin breakdown
- have reduction or absence of pain
- become mobile within limitations imposed by amputation

TABLE 61-15

Patient & Family Teaching Guide
Following an Amputation

1. Inspect the residual limb daily for signs of skin irritation, especially redness and abrasion. Pay particular attention to areas prone to pressure.
2. Discontinue use of the prosthesis if an irritation develops. Have the area checked before resuming use of the prosthesis.
3. Wash residual limb thoroughly each night with warm water and a bacteriostatic soap. Rinse thoroughly and dry gently. Expose the residual limb to air for 20 minutes.
4. Do not use any substance such as lotions, alcohol, powders, or oil unless prescribed by the health care provider.
5. Wear only a residual limb sock that is in good condition and supplied by the prosthetist.
6. Change residual limb sock daily. Launder in a mild soap, squeeze, and lay flat to dry.
7. Use prescribed pain management techniques.
8. Perform ROM to all joints daily. Perform general strengthening exercises including the upper extremities daily.
9. Do not elevate the residual limb on a pillow.
10. Lay prone with hip extension for 30 minutes three to four times daily.

ROM, Range of motion.

■ Gerontologic Considerations: Amputation

If a lower-limb amputation has been performed on an older adult, the patient's previous ability to ambulate may affect the extent of recovery. Use of a prosthesis requires a significant amount of energy for ambulation. Older adults whose general health is weakened by disorders such as cardiac or pulmonary problems may not be candidates for prosthesis use. This patient's ability to ambulate will be limited. If possible, this should be discussed with the patient and family before surgery so that realistic expectations can be set. ■

Common Joint Surgical Procedures

Surgery plays an important role in the treatment and rehabilitation of patients with various forms of arthritis, conditions related to trauma, and other painful conditions resulting in functional disability. Joint replacement surgery is the most common orthopedic operation performed on older adults. Significant advances in the field of reconstructive surgery have resulted in improvements in prosthetic design, materials, and surgical techniques that provide significant relief of pain and deformity and improve function and joint motion for patients with arthritis.

Indications for Joint Surgery

Surgery is aimed at relieving pain, improving joint motion, correcting deformity and malalignment, reducing vertical loads and shear stresses, and removing intraarticular causes of erosion. Debilitating joint pain is one of the primary reasons for arthroplasty. In addition to the effects of chronic pain on the physical and emotional well-being of the patient, any movement of the painful joint is often avoided. If this decreased functional ability is not corrected, contraction with permanent limitation of motion often occurs. Limitation of motion at any joint can be demonstrated on physical examination and by joint-space narrowing on radiologic examination.

There may also be a slow loss of cartilage in affected joints, which may be related to loss of motion. Synovitis can cause tendon damage, resulting in rupture or subluxation of the joint and subsequent loss of function. Continuing disease activity may cause loss of cartilage and bony surface and result in mechanical barriers to movement requiring surgical intervention.

Additional indications for hip or knee arthroplasty include failed prior procedures, sepsis, tumors, Paget's disease, congenital hip dysplasia, severe varus or valgus deformity, and spondyloarthropathies.[40]

TYPES OF JOINT SURGERIES

Synovectomy

Synovectomy (removal of synovial membrane) is used as a prophylactic measure and as a palliative treatment of rheumatoid arthritis (RA). Removal of synovial membrane, thought to be the location of the basic pathologic changes in joint destruction, helps prevent further progression of joint damage. A synovectomy is best performed early in the disease process to prevent serious destruction of joint surfaces. Removal of the thickened synovium prevents extension of the inflammatory process into the adjacent cartilage, ligaments, and tendons.

It is impossible to surgically remove all the synovium in a joint. The underlying disease process is still present and will again affect the regenerating synovium. However, the disease appears to be milder after synovectomy, and definite improvement in pain, weight bearing, and ROM can be expected. Common sites for this surgery include the elbow, wrist, and fingers. Synovectomy in the knee is done less frequently because knee joint replacement techniques are usually used.

Osteotomy

An **osteotomy** is performed by removing or adding a wedge or slice of bone to change its alignment and shift weight bearing, thereby correcting deformity and relieving pain. Cervical osteotomy may be used to correct deformity in some patients with ankylosing spondylitis. A halo and body jacket are worn until fusion occurs (3 or 4 months). Subtrochanteric or femoral osteotomy may provide some relief of pain and improve motion in selected patients with hip osteoarthritis. Osteotomy has proven ineffective in patients with inflammatory joint disease. Osteotomy of the knee provides relief of pain in selected patients, but advanced joint destruction is usually corrected by joint replacement surgery. The postoperative care is similar to the treatment of an internal fixation of a fracture at a comparable site (see p. 1668). The osteotomy is usually fixed by internal wires, screws and plates, bone grafts, or an external fixator.

Debridement

Debridement is the removal of degenerative debris such as loose bodies, osteophytes, joint debris, and degenerated menisci from a joint. This procedure is usually performed on the knee or the shoulder using a fiberoptic arthroscope. The procedure is usually done on an outpatient basis. A compression dressing is applied postoperatively. Weight bearing is permitted following knee arthroscopy. Patient education includes monitoring for signs of infection, managing pain, and restricting excessive activity for 24 to 48 hours.

Arthroplasty

Arthroplasty is the reconstruction or replacement of a joint. This surgical procedure is performed to relieve pain, improve or maintain ROM, and correct deformity. The most common uses of arthroplasty are for patients with osteoarthritis (OA), RA, avascular necrosis, congenital deformities or dislocations, and other systemic problems. There are several types of arthroplasty, including replacement of part of a joint (hemiarthroplasty), surgical reshaping of the bones of the joints, and total joint replacement. Replacement arthroplasty is available for the elbow, shoulder, phalangeal joint of the finger, hip, knee, ankle, and foot.[41]

Hip Arthroplasty. Total hip arthroplasty (THA) has provided significant relief of pain and improvement of function for patients with OA and RA. Implants are often "cemented" in place with polymethylmethacrylate, which bonds to the bone. With time, a significant number of femoral components loosen and require revision surgery. Because of this risk, cemented THAs are recommended for less active, older adults with compromised bone strength. Younger individuals receive "cementless" arthroplasties in an effort to prolong the lifetime of the prosthesis. Cementless THAs provide long-term implant stability by facilitating biologic ingrowth of new bone tissue into the porous surface

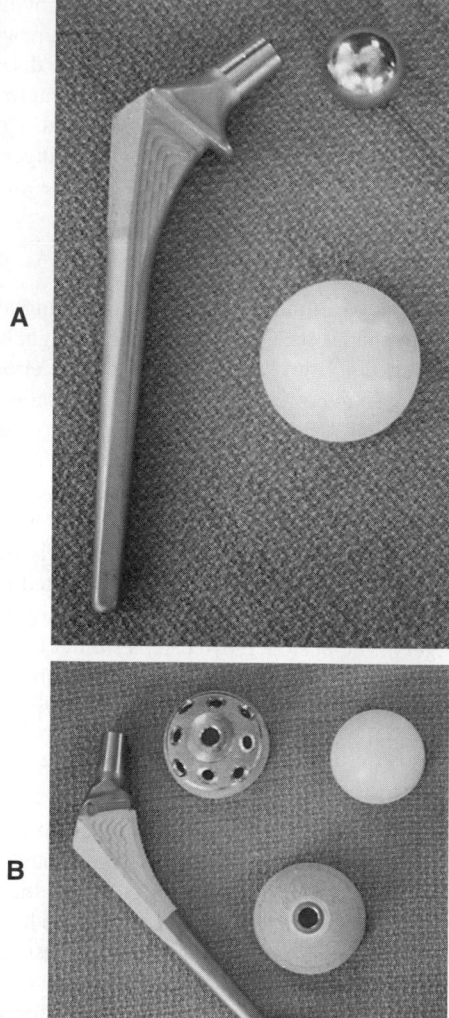

FIG. 61-19 Total hip replacements. **A,** Coated cemented components. **B,** Porous cementless components.

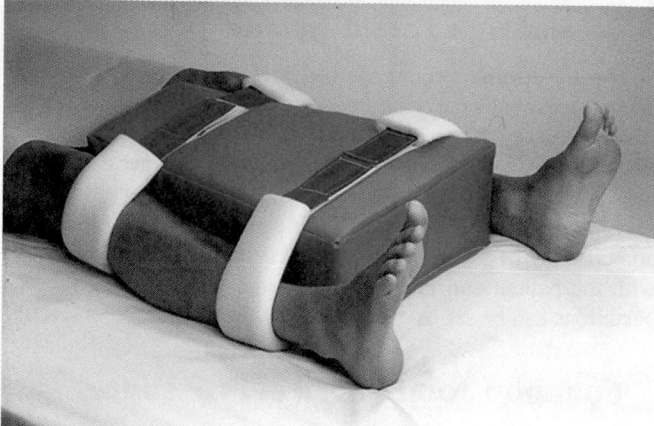

FIG. 61-20 Maintaining postoperative abduction following total hip replacement.

coating of the prosthesis. A patient with a high activity potential and a life expectancy of 25 years or more is an excellent candidate for a cementless prosthesis. Total hip replacements are shown in Fig. 61-19.

In both types of arthroplasties, extremes of internal rotation, adduction, and 90-degree flexion of the hip must be avoided for 4 to 6 weeks postoperatively. A foam abduction pillow is sometimes placed between the legs to prevent dislocation of the new joint (Fig. 61-20). Following surgery, patients must not allow their hips to be lower than their knees, and elevated toilet seats and chair alterations at home are necessary. Tub baths and driving a car are not allowed for 4 to 6 weeks. An occupational therapist may teach the patient to use assistive devices, such as reach bars ("reachers") to avoid bending over to pick something off the floor, long-handled shoehorns, or sock pullers. The knees must be kept apart; the patient must never cross the legs or twist to reach behind. Physical therapy is initiated the first postoperative day with ambulation and weight bearing with a walker for patients with a cemented prosthesis and weight bearing on the operative side for those with an uncemented prosthesis.

Exercises are designed to restore strength and muscle tone in the hip muscles essential to improved function and ROM. These include quadriceps setting, gluteal muscle setting, leg raises in supine and prone positions, and abduction exercises (swinging the leg out but never crossing midline) from supine and standing positions. The patient will continue these for many months after discharge, and the family should be well acquainted with the exercise program to offer encouragement at home.

Home care considerations include ongoing assessment of pain management, monitoring for infection, and prevention of DVT. Not all patients will qualify for home nursing visits. The incision may be closed with metal staples, which are removed at the surgeon's office. Because of the high risk for DVT, prothrombin times will be drawn weekly and anticoagulation adjusted accordingly if warfarin is used. Enoxaparin (Lovenox), a LMWH, is administered subcutaneously and can be given at home by the patient or family member. An advantage of enoxaparin is that it does not require monitoring of the patient's coagulation status. The patient should be instructed to use prophylactic antibiotics before dental appointments or procedures that might put the patient at risk for bacteremia.

A physical therapist will assess ROM, ambulation, and compliance with the exercise regimen. The patient will gradually increase the number of repetitions of exercises, add weights to ankles, swim, and may eventually use a stationary bicycle to tone quadriceps and improve cardiovascular fitness. High-impact exercises and sports, such as jogging and tennis, may loosen the implant and should be avoided. The elderly adult may require rehabilitation at a subacute or extended care facility until able to function independently.[42]

Knee Arthroplasty. Unremitting pain and instability as a result of severe destructive deterioration of the knee joint is the main indication for total knee arthroplasty (TKA). The presence of osteoporosis may necessitate bone grafting to augment defects and to correct bone deficiencies. Either part or all of the knee joint may be replaced with a metal and plastic prosthetic device. A compression dressing is used to immobilize the knee in extension immediately after the operation. This is removed before discharge and may be replaced with a knee immobilizer or posterior plastic shell, which maintains extension during ambulation and at rest for about 4 weeks.

Great emphasis is placed on postoperative exercising, and dislocation is not typical with TKA. Isometric quadriceps setting begins the first day after surgery. The patient progresses to straight-leg raises and gentle ROM to increase muscle strength and obtain 90-degree knee flexion. Active flexion exercises through the use of a CPM machine postoperatively promotes joint mobility.[43] Full weight bearing is begun before discharge. An active home exercise program involves progressive ROM, muscle strengthening, and stationary bicycle exercising.

Finger Joint Arthroplasty. A silicone rubber arthroplastic device is used to help restore function in the fingers of the patient with RA. The goal of hand surgery is primarily to restore function related to grasp, pinch, stability, and strength rather than to correct cosmetic deformity. The metacarpophalangeal and proximal interphalangeal joints take longer to heal.[44] Ulnar deviation is often present, which results in severe functional limitations of the hand. Before surgery the patient is instructed in hand exercises, including flexion, extension, abduction, and adduction of the fingers. Postoperatively, the hand is kept elevated with a bulky dressing in place. Neurovascular assessment is conducted postoperatively, and the nurse assesses for signs of infection. The success of the surgery depends largely on the postoperative treatment plan, which is often carried out under the direction of an occupational therapist. Once the dressing is removed, a guided splinting program is initiated. The patient is discharged with splints to use while sleeping and hand exercises to perform for 10 to 12 weeks at least three to four times a day. The patient is also instructed to avoid lifting heavy objects.

Elbow and Shoulder Arthroplasty. Although available, total replacement of elbow and shoulder joints is not as common as other forms of arthroplasty. Shoulder replacements are used in patients with severe pain because of RA, OA, avascular necrosis, or an old trauma. The shoulder replacement is usually considered if the patient has adequate surrounding muscle strength and bone stock. If joint replacement is necessary for both elbow and shoulder, the elbow is usually done first because a severely painful elbow interferes with the shoulder rehabilitation program.

Significant pain relief has been achieved following arthroplasty, with 90% of patients having no pain at rest or minimal pain with activity. Functional improvements have resulted in better hygiene and increased ability to perform activities of daily living in most patients. Rehabilitation is longer and more difficult than with other joint surgeries.

Ankle Arthroplasty. Total ankle arthroplasty (TAA) is indicated for RA, OA, and avascular necrosis. Ankle fusion is often selected over arthroplasty because the result is more durable. However, the patient is left with a stiff foot and the inability to change heel height. TAA is advantageous because a more normal gait pattern can be achieved. Postoperatively, the patient may not weight-bear for 6 weeks, must elevate the extremity to reduce and prevent edema, be extremely careful to prevent postoperative infection, and maintain immobilization as directed by the physician. Although the use of TAA is not widespread, it is becoming a viable alternative to fusion for the treatment of severe ankle arthritis in selected patients.

Arthrodesis

Arthrodesis is the surgical fusion of a joint. This procedure is indicated only if articular surfaces are too severely damaged or infected to allow joint replacement or for reconstructive surgery failures. Arthrodesis relieves pain and provides a stable but immobile joint. The fusion is usually accomplished by removal of the articular hyaline cartilage and the addition of bone grafts across the joint surface. The affected joint must be immobilized until bone healing has occurred. Common areas of fusion are the wrist, ankle, cervical spine, lumbar spine, and the metatarsophalangeal joint of the great toe.

Complications of Joint Surgery

Infection is a serious complication of joint surgery, particularly joint replacement surgery. The most common causative organisms are gram-positive aerobic streptococci and staphylococci. Infection almost always leads to pain and loosening of the prosthesis, generally requiring extensive surgery. Efforts to reduce the incidence of infection include the use of specially designed hypersterile operating rooms with laminar airflow and prophylactic antibiotic administration.

DVT is another potentially serious complication after joint surgeries, particularly those involving the lower extremities. Prophylactic measures such as aspirin, warfarin, low-molecular-weight heparin (LMWH), and pneumatic compression of the legs are usually instituted. Patients may be followed postoperatively with venous Doppler ultrasound to detect DVT, the source of most pulmonary emboli. FES may also occur after total hip arthroplasty.

Collaborative Care

Preoperative Management. As surgical techniques and care improve, more patients with chronic diseases such as RA are being considered as surgical candidates. Over 250,000 persons annually undergo total joint arthroplasty. The primary goal of preoperative assessment is to identify risk factors associated with postoperative complications so that nursing strategies can be implemented to promote optimal positive outcomes. A careful history will include previous medical diagnosis and complications such as diabetes and thrombophlebitis, pain tolerance and management preferences, current functional status and expectations following surgery, and level of social support and home care needs after discharge. The patient should be free from evidence of infection and acute joint inflammation.

If lower-extremity surgery is planned, upper-extremity muscle strength and joint function are assessed to determine the type of assistive devices needed postoperatively for ambulation and activities of daily living. Preoperative teaching informs the patient and family of the expected hospital course and postoperative management at home. In addition, it prepares them to maximize the usefulness and longevity of the prosthesis. Research has shown that preoperative education alone is not sufficient to ensure successful joint replacement; the patient must have a sense of self-efficacy for an optimal outcome to be achieved.[45] Patients also need to realize that recovery is "not going to happen overnight." Both patients and their families or significant others need to speak with individuals who have had a total joint arthroplasty to better understand the reality of dealing with a joint replacement.

Postoperative Management. Postoperatively, neurovascular assessment is performed to assess nerve function and circulatory status. Anticoagulation therapy, analgesia, and parenteral antibiotics are administered. In general, the affected joint is exercised, and ambulation is encouraged as early as possible to prevent complications of immobility. Specific protocols vary ac-

NURSING CARE PLAN 61-3

Patient with Joint Replacement Surgery

EXPECTED PATIENT OUTCOMES	NURSING INTERVENTIONS and *RATIONALES*
NURSING DIAGNOSIS	**Impaired physical mobility** *related to* pain, stiffness, and surgical procedure *as manifested by* difficulty in ambulating, inability to participate in physical rehabilitation, guarded movement.
• Functional ROM of joint	• Assess effect of surgery on patient's mobility *to plan appropriate interventions*. • Maintain proper positioning *to prevent dislocation or other complications*. • Begin exercise program as directed *to minimize mobility impairment and stiffness*. • Collaborate with physical and occupational therapist *to increase patient compliance and promote continuity of exercise*. • Give pain medication before exercise *to decrease discomfort from exercise and increase patient participation*.
NURSING DIAGNOSIS	**Self-care deficit** *related to* restrictions imposed by joint surgery, pain, weakness *as manifested by* inability to perform part or all activities of daily living.
• Activities of daily living (ADLs) met satisfactorily by patient or caregivers	• Assess patient's ability to perform ADLs *to plan appropriate assistance*. • Work with physical therapy and patient in learning to use assistive devices *to ensure independence*. • Assure patient that self-care abilities will be resumed with time *to decrease anxiety over dependency*. • Teach family how to assist with care.
NURSING DIAGNOSIS	**Risk for peripheral neurovascular dysfunction** *related to* edema and dislocated prosthesis.
• Palpable peripheral pulses • Warm extremities	• Assess nerve and circulatory status q1hr for first 24 hours, then every 2 to 4 hours *to determine if problem is present so that treatment can be initiated promptly*. • Notify surgeon immediately if abnormalities are noted *so that interventions are started without delay*. • Initiate measures such as cold packs and elevation of affected part *to minimize edema*. • Carry out measures to prevent dislocation *because this can be a cause of neurovascular dysfunction*. • Teach patient to report signs of neurovascular dysfunction such as paresthesia, coldness, pallor, excessive pain, swelling of affected extremity or body area *so that treatment is not delayed*.
NURSING DIAGNOSIS	**Ineffective therapeutic regimen management** *related to* lack of knowledge of follow-up care *as manifested by* expression of concern with ability to care for self after discharge, frequent questioning about follow-up care, lack of plan for follow-up care.
• Confidence in ability to manage self-care after discharge and to make necessary lifestyle changes	• Instruct patient on usual follow-up protocol, including activity limitations, drugs, follow-up visits, signs of infection, dislocation *to prepare patient for self-care and decision making*. • Assist patient to identify activities that require modification *so that appropriate changes can be made*. • Initiate a nurse referral *to monitor the long-term exercise program at home*.

COLLABORATIVE PROBLEM

NURSING GOALS	NURSING INTERVENTIONS AND *RATIONALES*
POTENTIAL COMPLICATION	**Deep vein thrombophlebitis** *related to* surgery and immobilization.
• Monitor and report signs of thrombosis • Carry out appropriate medical and nursing interventions	• Monitor for redness, swelling, and tenderness or pain of the extremity *to recognize and report signs of thrombophlebitis*. • Apply elastic compression stockings and instruct patient to perform isotonic exercises such as quadriceps setting, ankle rolling, and pushing on footboard *to promote circulation and prevent clot formation*. • Provide adequate parenteral and oral fluids *to prevent dehydration and thrombus formation*. • Instruct the patient in the importance of home exercise *to prevent venous stasis*. • Instruct the patient and caregivers in the proper administration and follow-up of anticoagulation drug therapy (e.g., low-molecular-weight heparin, warfarin) *to prevent side effects* (see Table 37-4).

cording to patient, type of prosthesis, and surgeon preference. Pain management postoperatively may use epidural analgesia, patient-controlled analgesia, IV injections, and oral narcotics or NSAIDs.[46]

The hospital stay after arthroplasty is 3 to 5 days depending on the patient's course and need for physical therapy. Physical therapy and ambulation enhance mobility, build muscle strength, and reduce the risk of thrombus formation. If the patient is taking warfarin, therapy starts on the day of surgery and continues for 3 weeks with a prothrombin time done on a regular basis. For those taking LMWH (e.g., enoxaparin), therapy starts 24 to 36 hours after surgery and continues for 2 weeks postoperatively. Daily monitoring of the patient's coagulation status is not necessary with LMWH. The decision to use warfarin or LMWH depends on many factors, including the patient's age and overall state of health.

NURSING MANAGEMENT
JOINT SURGERY

The nursing management of the patient undergoing joint surgery begins with preoperative teaching and realistic goal setting. It is important that the patient understands and accepts the limitations of the proposed surgery and realizes that it will not remove the underlying disease process. Postoperative procedures such as turning, deep breathing, use of bedpan and bedside com-

mode, and use of abductor pillows should be explained and opportunities for practice provided. The patient should be reassured that pain relief will be available. Patient-controlled analgesia can be helpful. A preoperative visit from a physical therapist allows practice of postoperative exercises and measurement for crutches or other assistive devices.

Discharge planning begins immediately. The duration of the hospital stay and the expected postoperative events should be discussed because the patient and family must prepare ahead. The home environment must be assessed for safety (e.g., presence of scatter rugs and electrical cords) and accessibility. Are the bathroom and bedroom on the first floor? Are door frames wide enough to accommodate a walker? Social support must also be assessed. Is a friend or family member available to assist the patient in the home? Will the patient require homemaker or meal services? The elderly patient may need the rehabilitation services of a subacute or extended care facility for a few weeks postoperatively to progressively develop independent living skills. Specific nursing interventions related to joint surgery are summarized in NCP 61-3.

Patient teaching includes instructions on reporting complications, including infection (e.g., fever, increased pain, drainage) and dislocation of the prosthesis (e.g., pain, loss of function, shortening or malalignment of an extremity). The home care nurse acts as the liaison between the patient and the surgeon, monitoring for postoperative complications, assessing comfort and ROM, and facilitating improvements in functional performance.

CRITICAL THINKING EXERCISES

Case Study
Lower Extremity Fracture
Patient Profile. Brad Hamil, a 32-year-old white construction worker, was admitted into the emergency department. A load of lumber fell from the forklift and crushed his legs. His legs were crushed for approximately 30 minutes before the weight could be relieved. He has a bone protruding from his left femur and his right leg is mangled. It appears he sustained an open fracture with massive internal bleeding into the left thigh muscle and lower extremity.

Subjective Data
- Complains of severe, excruciating pain involving both legs
- Complains of thirst and dizziness

Objective Data
Physical Examination
- Blood pressure: 90/60
- Diaphoretic and pale skin
- Pain not relieved by narcotic analgesic
- Moderately profuse bleeding from left femur wound
- Popliteal and posterior tibial pulses absent in both legs by Doppler auscultation
- Compartment pressures: left femur, 68 mm Hg; left proximal tibial region, 52 mm Hg

Diagnostic Studies
- X-rays of his left leg revealed an open comminuted, oblique fracture of the left femur and fractures of the proximal tibia, distal tibia, and fibula. No fractures are present in his right leg.
- Hematocrit 25%; hemoglobin 13 g/dl; WBC 15,000/μl (15×10^9/L); urine negative for myoglobin; chemistry panel within expected ranges

Collaborative Care
- Surgical reduction and fixation of fractures
- cefazolin (Ancef) 1 g intravenously every 8 hours
- Intake and output for 48 hours postoperatively
- morphine sulfate per patient-controlled analgesia pump

CRITICAL THINKING QUESTIONS
1. How do the pathophysiologic features of Brad's fracture predispose him to compartment syndrome?
2. What other complications of severe musculoskeletal trauma is Brad at high risk for developing?
3. What are the preoperative and postoperative priorities of nursing care for Brad?
4. What nursing interventions might help Brad cope with his long-term rehabilitation?
5. Based on the data presented, write one or more appropriate nursing diagnoses. Are there any collaborative problems?

Nursing Research Issues
1. What body image and self-concept issues does a patient who has undergone an amputation experience?
2. Are casual and weekend athletes using proper protective gear to prevent injury?
3. What is the most effective technique of providing pin care for a patient in skeletal traction?
4. Do nurses recognize the signs and symptoms of deep vein thrombosis and fat embolism syndrome?
5. What home health nursing interventions are most effective for increasing mobility in the patient recovering from a hip fracture?

REVIEW QUESTIONS

The number of the question corresponds to the same-numbered objective at the beginning of the chapter.

1. The nurse suspects an ankle sprain when a patient at the urgent care center
   a. is hit by another soccer player on the field.
   b. has ankle pain after running a 10-mile race.
   c. drops a 10-lb weight on his lower leg at the health club.
   d. has a twisting injury while running bases during a baseball game.

2. The nurse explains to a patient with a distal tibial fracture returning for a 3-week checkup that healing is indicated by
   a. callus formation.
   b. complete union of bone.
   c. presence of granulation tissue.
   d. formation of a hematoma at the fracture site.

3. A patient with a comminuted fracture of the femur is to have an open reduction with internal fixation (ORIF) of the fracture. The nurse explains that ORIF is indicated when
   a. a cast would be too large to provide normal mobility.
   b. the patient is able to tolerate long-term immobilization.
   c. adequate alignment cannot be obtained by other methods.
   d. the patient cannot tolerate the discomfort of a closed reduction.

4. An indication of a neurovascular problem noted during assessment of the patient with a fracture is
   a. exaggeration of extremity movement.
   b. petechiae on the head and upper thorax.
   c. decreased sensation distal to the fracture site.
   d. purulent drainage at the site of an open fracture.

5. A patient with a stable, closed fracture of the humerus caused by trauma to the arm has a temporary splint with bulky padding applied with an elastic bandage. The nurse suspects compartment syndrome and notifies the physician when the patient experiences
   a. pain at the fracture site.
   b. increasing edema of the limb.
   c. muscle spasms of the lower arm.
   d. pain when the nurse passively extends the fingers.

6. A patient with symphysis pubis and pelvic rami fractures should be monitored for
   a. sudden thirst.
   b. changes in urinary output.
   c. a palpable lump in the buttock.
   d. sudden decrease in blood pressure.

7. During the postoperative period, the patient with an above-the-knee amputation should be instructed that the residual limb should not be routinely elevated because
   a. this position reduces the development of phantom pain.
   b. the flexed position can promote hip flexion contracture.
   c. this position promotes clot formation at the incision site and thigh.
   d. unnecessary movement of the extremity can cause wound dehiscence.

8. A patient with rheumatoid arthritis is scheduled for an arthroplasty. The nurse explains that the purpose of this procedure is to
   a. fuse a joint and reduce pain.
   b. prevent further joint damage.
   c. assess the extent of joint damage.
   d. replace the joint and improve function.

9. The nurse teaches a patient recovering from a total hip replacement that it is important to avoid
   a. sleeping on the abdomen.
   b. sitting with the legs crossed.
   c. abduction exercises of the affected leg.
   d. bearing weight on the affected leg for 6 weeks.

REFERENCES

1. Schoen D: *Adult orthopaedic nursing,* Philadelphia, 2000, Lippincott.
2. Maher A: Trauma. In Schoen D, editor: *Core curriculum for orthopaedic nursing,* ed 4, Pitman, NJ, 2001, Jannetti.
3. Childs S: Nursing care for hand and wrist problems. In Schoen D, editor: *Core curriculum for orthopaedic nursing,* ed 4, Pitman, NJ, 2001, Jannetti.
4. Barry M: Ankle sprains, *AJN* 101:38, 2001.
5. Perron A, Brady W, Sing R: Orthopedic pitfalls in the ED: vascular injury associated with knee dislocation, *Am J Emerg Med* 19:583, 2001.
6. Bagwell-Crum C: The shoulder. In Schoen D, editor: *Core curriculum for orthopedic nursing,* ed 4, Pitman, NJ, 2001, Jannetti.
7. Ferry S et al: Carpal tunnel syndrome: a nested case-control study of risk factors in women, *Am J Epidemiol* 151:6, 2000.
8. Litaker D et al: Returning to the bedside: using the history and physical examination to identify rotator cuff tears, *J Am Geriatr Soc* 48:2, 2000.
9. Skinner H et al: Identifying structural hip and knee problems, *Postgrad Med* 106:7, 1999.
10. Breuninger C et al: *Diseases,* ed 3, Springhouse, Pa, 2001, Springhouse Corporation.
11. Kunkler C: Fractures. In Maher AB, Salmond SW, Pellino TA, editors: *Orthopaedic nursing,* ed 3, St Louis, 2002, Mosby.
12. Ruda S: Fracture biomechanics and healing. In Williamson V, editor: *Management of lower extremity fractures,* Pitman, NJ, 1998, Jannetti.
13. Sanchez Y, Bush T: Bursitis and tendonitis: injection therapy basics, *J Musculoskeletal Med* 19:21, 2002.
14. Kunkler C: Therapeutic modalities. In Schoen D, editor: *Core curriculum for orthopaedic nursing,* ed 4, Pitman, NJ, 2001, Jannetti.
15. Ceccio C: Key concepts in the care of patients in traction. In Schoenly L, editor: *An introduction to orthopaedic nursing,* ed 2, Pitman, NJ, 1999, Jannetti.
16. Kunkler C: Neurovascular assessment. In Schoenly L, editor: *An introduction to orthopaedic nursing,* ed 2, Pitman, NJ, 1999, Jannetti.
17. Kunkler C: Care of the casted lower extremity. In Williamson V, editor: *Management of lower extremity fractures,* Pitman, NJ, 1998, Jannetti.

18. Childs S, Holmes S: *Guidelines for orthopaedic nursing: adult trauma,* National Association of Orthopaedic Nurses, 1998, Jannetti.
19. Astifidia R: Reflex sympathetic dystrophy complex regional pain syndrome of the upper extremity. In Childs S, editor: *The upper extremity: traumatic injuries and conditions,* Pitman, NJ, 1999, Jannetti.
20. McKenzie L: In search of a standard for pin care, *Orthop Nurs* 18:73, 1999.
21. Pellino T et al: Complications of orthopaedic disorders and orthopaedic surgery. In Maher AB, Salmond SW, Pellino TA, editors: *Orthopaedic nursing,* ed 3, St Louis, 2002, Mosby.
22. Harvey C: Compartment syndrome: when it is least expected, *Orthop Nur* 20:3, 2001.
23. Perrin A, Brady W, Keats T: Orthopedic pitfalls in the ED: acute compartment syndrome, *Am J Emerg Med* 19:413, 2001.
24. Ross D: Complications of lower extremity trauma. In Williamson V, editor: *Management of lower extremity fractures,* Pitman, NJ, 1998, Jannetti.
25. Tumbarello C: Acute extremity compartment syndrome, *J Trauma Nurs* 7:30, 2000.
26. Crowther C: *Primary orthopedic care,* St Louis, 1999, Mosby.
27. Choi H: Management of post-traumatic fat embolism in the emergency department, *Aust Emerg Nurs J* 2:10, 1999.
28. Newport M: Colles fracture: managing a common upper extremity injury, *J Musculoskeletal Med* 17:292, 2000.
29. Rose D, Rowen D: AANA Journal Course I: update for nurse anesthetists: perioperative considerations in major orthopedic trauma: pelvic and long bone fractures, *AANA J* 70:131, 2002.
30. Korovessis P et al: Medium and long-term results of open reduction and internal fixation for unstable pelvic ring fractures, *Orthopedics* 23:1165, 2000.
31. Yarnold B: Hip fracture, *AJN* 99:36, 1999.
32. Gallagher B et al: A fall prevention program for the home environment, *Home Care Provid* 6:157, 2001.
33. Richmind J, Zuckerman J, Koval K: Geriatric hip fractures, *J Musculosketal Med* 17:626, 2000.
34. Kamel H et al: Hormone replacement therapy and fractures in older adults, *J Am Geriatr Soc* 49:179, 2001.
35. Groeneveld A et al: Logrolling: establishing consistent practice, *Orthop Nurs* 20:2, 2001.
36. Beers M, Berkow R, editors: Eye injuries. In *Merck manual of diagnosis and therapy,* ed 17 [electronic version], Whitehouse Station, NJ, 1999, Merck and Co.
37. Dillingham T et al: Use and satisfaction with prosthetic devices among persons with trauma related amputations: a long-term outcome study, *Am J Phys Rehabil* 80:563, 2001.
38. Bryant G: Stump care, *AJN* 101:2, 2001.
39. Kapp S: Transfemoral socket design and suspension options, *Phys Med Rehabil Clin North Am* 11:569, 2000.
40. Roberts D: Degenerative disorders. In Maher AB, Salmond SW, Pellino TA, editors: *Orthopaedic nursing,* ed 3, St Louis, 2002, Mosby.
*41. Kelly M et al: Total joint arthroplasty: a comparison of post-acute settings on patient functional outcomes, *Orthop Nurs* 18:5, 1999.
*42. Ridge R et al: The relationship between multidisciplinary discharge outcomes and functional status after total hip replacement, *Orthop Nurs* 19:1, 2000.
43. O'Driscoll S, Giori N: Continuous passive motion (CPM): theory and principles of clinical application, *J Rehabil Res Dev* 37:179, 2000.
44. Childs S: Finger injury, *Lippincotts Prim Care Pract* 3:397, 1999.
*45. Moon LB et al: Relationships among self-efficacy, outcome expectancy, and postoperative behaviors in total joint replacement patients, *Orthop Nurs* 19:2, 2000.
46. Curtiss C: JCAHO: meeting the standards for pain management, *Orthop Nurs* 20:2, 2001.

*Nursing research–based reference.

RESOURCES

American Academy of Orthopedic Surgeons (AAOS)
6300 North River Road
Rosemont, IL 60018-4262
800-346-AAOS or 847-823-7186
Fax: 847-823-8125
www.aaos.org

American College of Sports Medicine (ACSM)
P.O. Box 1440
401 West Michigan Street
Indianapolis, IN 46202
317-637-9200
Fax: 317-634-7817
www.acsm.org

Amputees in Motion
P.O. Box 2703
Escondido, CA 92033
619-454-9300

National Amputation Foundation
38-40 Church Street
Malverne, NY 11565
516-887-3600
Fax: 516-887-3667
www.nationalamputation.org

National Arthritis/Musculoskeletal and Skin Diseases Information Clearinghouse
9000 Rockville Pike
Bethesda, MD 20892-2350
800-283-7800
www.nih.gov/niams

National Association of Orthopaedic Nurses, Inc. (NAON)
East Holly Avenue, Box 56
Pitman, NJ 08071-0056
800-289-NAON (6266) or 856-256-2310
Fax: 856-589-7463
www.orthonurse.org

National Easter Seal Society
230 West Monroe Street, Suite 1800
Chicago, IL 60606
800-221-6827 or 312-726-6200
Fax: 312-726-1494
www.easter-seals.org

Older Women's League
666 11th Street NW, Suite 700
Washington, DC 20001
800-825-3695 or 202-783-6686
Fax: 202-638-2356
www.owl-national.org

For additional Internet resources, see the website for this book at *http://www.evolve.elsevier.com/Lewis/medsurg.*

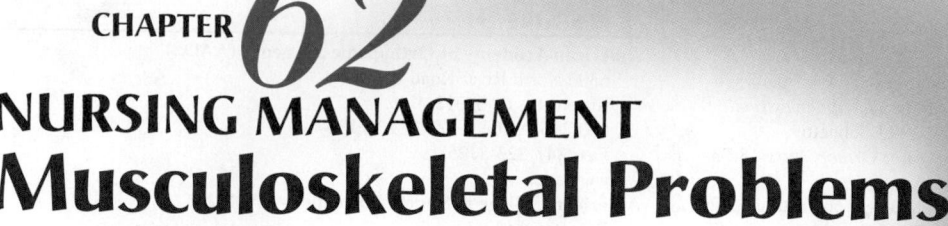

CHAPTER 62

NURSING MANAGEMENT
Musculoskeletal Problems

Cathleen E. Kunkler

LEARNING OBJECTIVES

1. Describe the pathophysiology, clinical manifestations, collaborative care, and nursing management of osteomyelitis.
2. Describe the types, pathophysiology, clinical manifestations, and collaborative care of bone cancer.
3. Differentiate between the causes and characteristics of acute and chronic low back pain.
4. Describe the conservative and surgical therapy of herniated intervertebral disk.

5. Describe the postoperative nursing management of a patient who has undergone spinal surgery.
6. Explain the etiology and nursing management of common foot disorders.
7. Describe the etiology, pathophysiology, clinical manifestations, and collaborative and nursing management of osteomalacia, osteoporosis, and Paget's disease.

KEY TERMS

Ewing's sarcoma, p. 1697
herniated intervertebral disk, p. 1702
low back pain, p. 1699
multiple myeloma, p. 1696
muscular dystrophy, p. 1698

osteoclastoma, p. 1696
osteogenic sarcoma, p. 1696
osteomalacia, p. 1707
osteomyelitis, p. 1692
osteoporosis, p. 1708
Paget's disease, p. 1711

OSTEOMYELITIS

Etiology and Pathophysiology

Osteomyelitis is a severe infection of the bone, bone marrow, and surrounding soft tissue. The most common infecting microorganism is *Staphylococcus aureus*. A variety of microorganisms can cause osteomyelitis, including *Escherichia coli, Salmonella, Neisseria gonorrhoeae, Staphylococcus epidermidis,* and *Pseudomonas aeruginosa*[1,2] (Table 62-1). Aerobic gram-negative bacteria alone or mixed with gram-positive organisms are often found. The widespread use of antibiotics in conjunction with surgical treatment has significantly reduced the mortality rate and complications associated with osteomyelitis.

The infecting microorganisms can invade by indirect or direct entry. The *indirect entry (hematogenous)* of microorganisms in osteomyelitis most frequently affects growing bone in boys less than 12 years old, and is associated with their higher incidence of blunt trauma. The most common sites of indirect entry in children are the distal femur, proximal tibia, humerus, and radius.[3] Adults with vascular insufficiency disorders (e.g., diabetes mellitus) and genitourinary and respiratory infections are at higher risk for a primary infection to spread via the blood to the bone. The pelvis and vertebrae, which are vascular-rich sites of bone, are the most common sites of infection.

Direct entry osteomyelitis can occur at any age when there is an open wound (e.g., penetrating wounds, fractures) and microorganisms gain entry to the body. Osteomyelitis may also occur in the presence of a foreign body such as an implant or an orthopedic prosthetic device (e.g., plate, total joint prosthesis). After gaining entrance to the bone by way of the blood, the microorganisms then lodge in an area of bone in which circulation slows, usually the metaphysis. The microorganisms grow, resulting in an increase in pressure because of the nonexpanding nature of most bone. This increasing pressure eventually leads to ischemia and vascular compromise of the periosteum. Eventually the infection passes through the bone cortex and marrow cavity, ultimately resulting in cortical devascularization and necrosis. Once ischemia occurs, the bone dies. The area of devitalized bone eventually separates from the surrounding living bone, forming *sequestra*. The part of the periosteum that continues to have a blood supply forms new bone called *involucrum* (Fig. 62-1).

TABLE 62-1	Causative Organisms in Osteomyelitis
ORGANISM	**POSSIBLE PREDISPOSING PROBLEM**
Staphylococcus aureus	Pressure ulcer, penetrating wound, open fracture, orthopedic surgery, abscessed tooth, vascular insufficiency disorders (e.g., diabetes, atherosclerosis)
Staphylococcus epidermidis	Indwelling prosthetic devices (e.g., joint replacements, fractured fixation devices)
Escherichia coli	Urinary tract infection
Mycobacterium tuberculosis	Tuberculosis
Neisseria gonorrhoeae	Gonorrhea
Pseudomonas	Puncture wounds, intravenous drug use
Salmonella	Sickle cell disease
Fungi, mycobacteria	Immunocompromised host

Reviewed by Brenda Elliff, RN, MPA, ONC, CCM, LNCC, Nurse Consultant, Elliff Legal and Medical Services, Coeur d'Alene, Idaho.

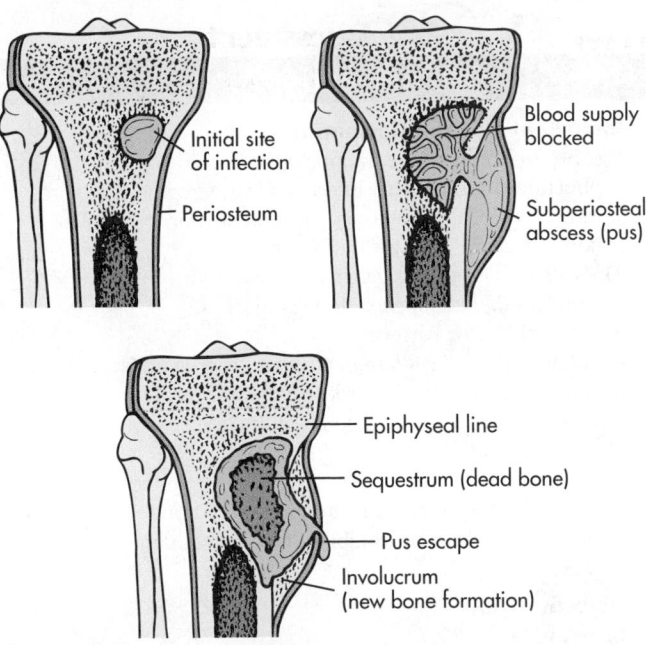

FIG. 62-1 Development of osteomyelitis infection with involucrum and sequestrum.

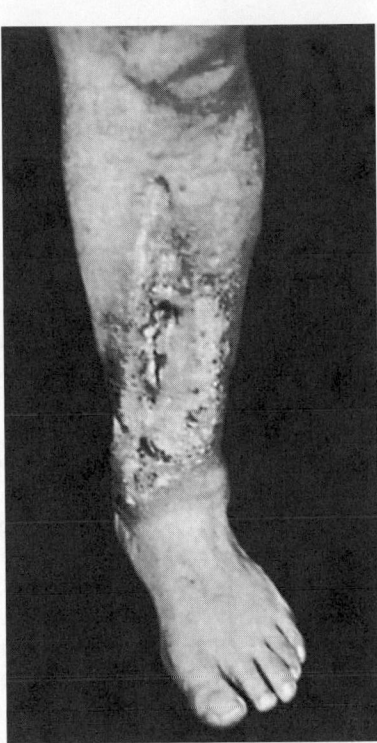

FIG. 62-2 Chronic osteomyelitis of the tibia. Marked skin scarring and draining sinuses are evident.

Once formed, a sequestrum continues to be an infected island of bone, surrounded by pus and difficult to reach by blood-borne antibiotics or white blood cells (WBCs). Sequestrum may enlarge and serve as a site for microorganisms that spread to other sites, including the lungs and brain. The sequestrum can move out of the bone and into the soft tissue. Once outside the bone, the sequestrum may revascularize and then undergo removal by normal immune processes. Another possibility is that the sequestrum can be surgically removed through debridement of the necrotic bone. If the necrotic sequestrum is not resolved naturally or surgically, it may develop a sinus tract, resulting in a chronic, purulent cutaneous drainage (Fig. 62-2).

Chronic osteomyelitis is either a continuous, persistent problem (a result of inadequate acute treatment) or a process of exacerbations and remission. Over time, granulation tissue turns to scar tissue. This avascular scar tissue provides an ideal site for continued microorganism growth and is impenetrable to antibiotics.

Clinical Manifestations

Acute osteomyelitis refers to the initial infection or an infection of less than 1 month in duration. The clinical manifestations of acute osteomyelitis are both systemic and local. Systemic manifestations include fever, night sweats, chills, restlessness, nausea, and malaise. Local manifestations include constant bone pain that is unrelieved by rest and worsens with activity; swelling, tenderness, and warmth at the infection site; and restricted movement of the affected part. Later signs include drainage from sinus tracts to the skin and/or the fracture site.

Chronic osteomyelitis refers to a bone infection that persists for longer than 1 month or an infection that has failed to respond to the initial course of antibiotic therapy. Systemic signs may be diminished, with local signs of infection more common, including constant bone pain and swelling, tenderness, and warmth at the infection site.

Diagnostic Studies

A bone or soft tissue biopsy is the definitive way to determine the causative microorganism. The patient's blood and/or wound cultures are frequently positive for the presence of microorganisms. An elevated WBC and erythrocyte sedimentation rate (ESR) may also be found. Radiologic signs suggestive of osteomyelitis usually do not appear until 10 days to weeks after the appearance of clinical symptoms, by which time the disease will have progressed. Radionuclide bone scans (gallium and indium) are helpful in diagnosis and are usually positive in the area of infection. Magnetic resonance imaging (MRI) and computed tomography (CT) scans may be used to help identify the extent of the infection including soft tissue involvement.[4]

Collaborative Care

Vigorous and prolonged intravenous (IV) antibiotic therapy is the treatment of choice for acute osteomyelitis, as long as bone ischemia has not yet occurred. Cultures or a bone biopsy should be done if possible before drug therapy is initiated. If antibiotic therapy is delayed, surgical debridement and decompression are often necessary.

Treatment for osteomyelitis previously involved an extended hospital stay for IV antibiotic treatment. Today patients are often discharged to home care with IV antibiotics delivered via a central venous catheter or peripherally inserted central catheter. IV antibiotic therapy may initially be started in the hospital and continued in the home for 4 to 6 weeks or as long as 3 to 6 months. A variety of antibiotics may be prescribed depending on the microorganism. These drugs include penicillin, nafcillin (Nafcil), neomycin, cephalexin (Keflex), cefazolin (Ancef), cefoxitin (Mefoxin), gentamicin (Garamycin), and tobramycin (Nebcin).

In adults with chronic osteomyelitis, oral therapy with a fluoroquinolone (ciprofloxacin [Cipro]) for 6 to 8 weeks may be prescribed instead of IV antibiotics. Oral antibiotic therapy may also be given after acute IV therapy is complete to ensure resolution of the infection. The patient's response to drug therapy is monitored through bone scans and ESR tests.

Surgical treatment for chronic osteomyelitis includes removal of the poorly vascularized tissue and dead bone and the extended use of antibiotics.[5] Antibiotic-impregnated polymethylmethacrylate bead chains may also be implanted at this time to aid in combating the infection.[6] After debridement of the devitalized and infected tissue, the wound may be closed, and a suction irrigation system is inserted. Intermittent or constant irrigation of the affected bone with antibiotics may also be initiated. Protection of the limb or surgical site with casts or braces is frequently done.

Hyperbaric oxygen therapy of 100% oxygen may be administered in chronic osteomyelitis. This therapy is thought to promote antibiotic activity and stimulate circulation and healing in the infected tissue. Orthopedic prosthetic devices (if a source of chronic infection) may have to be removed. Myocutaneous flaps or skin and bone grafting may be necessary if destruction is extensive. Amputation of the extremity may then be necessary to preserve life and improve the quality of life.

Long-term and mostly rare complications of osteomyelitis include septicemia, septic arthritis, pathologic fractures, squamous cell carcinoma, and amyloidosis.

NURSING MANAGEMENT
OSTEOMYELITIS

■ Nursing Assessment

Subjective and objective data that should be obtained from an individual with osteomyelitis are presented in Table 62-2.

■ Nursing Diagnoses

Nursing diagnoses for the patient with osteomyelitis may include, but are not limited to, those presented in NCP 62-1.

■ Planning

The overall goals are that the patient with osteomyelitis will (1) have satisfactory pain and fever control, (2) not experience any complications associated with osteomyelitis, (3) cooperate with the treatment plan, and (4) maintain a positive outlook on the outcome of the disease.

■ Nursing Implementation

Health Promotion. The control of infections already in the body (e.g., urinary, respiratory tract) is important in preventing osteomyelitis. Adults who are immunocompromised, have orthopedic prosthetic devices, and/or have vascular insufficiencies are especially susceptible. These patients should be instructed regarding the local and systemic manifestations of osteomyelitis. Families should also be aware of their role in monitoring the patient's health. Symptoms of bone pain, fever, swelling, and restricted limb movement should be reported immediately to the health care provider.

Acute Intervention. Some immobilization of the affected limb (e.g., splint, traction) is usually indicated to decrease pain. The involved limb should be handled carefully to avoid excessive manipulation, which increases pain and may cause pathologic

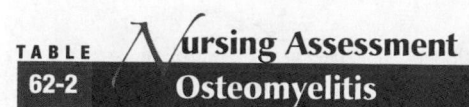

TABLE 62-2	Nursing Assessment Osteomyelitis

Important Health Information
Past health history: Bone trauma, open fracture, open or puncture wounds, other infections (e.g., streptococcal sore throat, bacterial pneumonia, sinusitis, skin or tooth infection, chronic urinary tract infection)
Medications: Use of analgesics or antibiotics
Surgery or other treatments: Bone surgery

Functional Health Patterns
Health perception–health management: IV drug abuse; malaise
Nutritional-metabolic: Anorexia, weight loss; chills
Activity-exercise: Weakness, paralysis, muscle spasms around affected bone
Cognitive-perceptual: Local tenderness over affected area, increase in pain with movement of affected bone
Coping–stress tolerance: Irritability, withdrawal, dependency, anger

Objective Data
General
Restlessness; high, spiking temperature; night sweats
Integumentary
Diaphoresis; erythema, warmth, edema at infected bone
Musculoskeletal
Restricted movement; wound drainage; spontaneous fractures
Possible Findings
Leukocytosis, positive blood and/or wound cultures, ↑ erythrocyte sedimentation rate; presence of sequestrum and involucrum on x-rays, radionuclide bone scans, CT, and MRI

CT, Computed tomography; *IV,* intravenous; *MRI,* magnetic resonance imaging.

fracture. An important nursing responsibility is to assess the patient's pain. Minor to severe pain may be experienced with muscle spasms. Nonsteroidal antiinflammatory drugs (NSAIDs), narcotic analgesics, and muscle relaxants may be prescribed to provide patient comfort. Nonpharmacologic (e.g., guided imagery, hypnosis) approaches to pain should be encouraged by the nurse (see Chapters 7 and 9).

Dressings are used to absorb the exudate from draining wounds and to debride devitalized tissue from the wound site when removed. Types of dressings used include dry, sterile dressings; dressings saturated in saline or antibiotic solution; and wet-to-dry dressings. Soiled dressings should be handled carefully to prevent cross-contamination of the wound or spread of the infection to other patients. When the dressing is changed, sterile technique is essential.

The patient is frequently on bed rest in the early stages of the acute infection. Good body alignment and frequent position changes prevent complications associated with immobility and promote comfort. Flexion contracture, especially of the hip or knee, is a common sequela of osteomyelitis of the lower extremity because the patient frequently positions the affected extremity in a flexed position to promote comfort. The contracture may then progress to a deformity. Footdrop can develop quickly in the lower extremity if the foot is not correctly supported by a splint. The patient should be instructed to avoid any activities such as exercise or heat application that increase circulation and serve as

NURSING CARE PLAN 62-1

Patient with Osteomyelitis

EXPECTED PATIENT OUTCOMES	NURSING INTERVENTIONS and *RATIONALES*
NURSING DIAGNOSIS	**Acute pain** *related to* inflammatory process secondary to infection *as manifested by* guarding, moaning, crying, restlessness, altered muscle tone, decreased activity, rated pain as >4 on a 10-point rating scale.
• Decrease in or absence of pain • Satisfaction with pain relief	• Assess location and severity of pain and previous pain-relieving measures *to plan appropriate interventions.* • Use a pain scale *to assess pain and evaluate effectiveness of interventions.* • Give analgesics as indicated *to relieve pain.* • Instruct patient to request analgesia *before pain becomes severe.* • Use gentle handling and support when moving extremity *to reduce pain and prevent pathologic fractures.* • Use the prescribed immobilization device and maintain patient's body in correct alignment and positioning *to prevent unusual position or muscle stretching from increasing pain.* • Restrict ambulation or teach patient to use assistive device (e.g., crutches) *to prevent pathologic fracture, pain, and increased stress on bone.* • Elevate extremity *to reduce swelling and provide comfort.* • Instruct patient in nonpharmacologic methods of pain control such as distraction, relaxation breathing, guided imagery *to reduce the need for analgesics.*
NURSING DIAGNOSIS	**Impaired physical mobility** *related to* pain, immobilization devices, and weight-bearing limitations *as manifested by* inability or unwillingness to move.
• Consistent increase in mobility and range of motion with minimal pain or discomfort	• Assist patient as needed *to reduce patient's frustration with impaired mobility and prevent injury.* • Explain the rationale for immobilization *to foster the patient's cooperation.* • Increase mobility as ordered and tolerated *to maintain muscle function and strength.* • Provide assistive devices (e.g., pick-up stick, long-handled shoehorn, stocking helpers) *to increase independence in activities of daily living.*
NURSING DIAGNOSIS	**Ineffective therapeutic regimen management** *related to* lack of knowledge regarding long-term management of osteomyelitis *as manifested by* verbalization of concern and uncertainty about procedures and skills needed for home care.
• Verbalization of confidence in self or caregiver's ability to carry out home management routine	• Provide information and instruction regarding wound care, aseptic technique, and dressing disposal *to reduce risk of cross-contamination and encourage wound healing.* • Review drug regimen including schedule, name, dosage, purpose, and side effects *because long-term antibiotic therapy is required.* • Stress importance of proper diet, rest, follow-up, and physical rehabilitation *to facilitate wound healing and reduce risk of chronic osteomyelitis.* • Provide written instructions about the preceding information along with a phone number to call with any questions.

stimuli to the spread of infection. Uninvolved joints and muscles should continue to be exercised.

The patient should also be taught the potential adverse and toxic reactions associated with prolonged and high-dose antibiotic therapy. These reactions include hearing deficit, fluid retention, and neurotoxicity, which can occur with the aminoglycosides (e.g., tobramycin, neomycin), and jaundice, colitis, and photosensitivity from the extended use of the cephalosporins (e.g., cefazolin). Peak and trough blood levels of most antibiotics must be carefully monitored throughout the course of therapy to avoid these adverse effects. Lengthy antibiotic therapy can also result in an overgrowth of *Candida albicans* in the genitourinary and oral cavities, especially in immunosuppressed and older patients. The nurse should instruct the patient to report any whitish, yellow, curdlike lesions to the health care provider.

The patient and family are often frightened and discouraged because of the serious nature of the disease, uncertainty of the outcome, and the lengthy cost and course of treatment. Continued psychologic and emotional support is an integral part of nursing management.

Ambulatory and Home Care. With the introduction of various intermittent venous access devices, IV antibiotics can be administered to the patient in a long-term care or home setting. If at home, the patient and family must be instructed on the proper care and management of the venous access device. They must also be taught how to administer the antibiotic when scheduled and the need for follow-up laboratory testing. The importance of continuing to take antibiotics after the symptoms have subsided should be stressed. Periodic home nursing visits provide the family with support, which helps to reduce anxiety. If there is an open wound, dressing changes are often necessary. The patient and family may require supplies and instruction in the technique. Family members also need to understand that the infection is not contagious.

If the osteomyelitis becomes chronic, patients need physical and psychologic support for a prolonged period. They may become suspicious and hostile toward the health care providers when treatment plans do not result in a cure. Well-informed patients are better able to participate in decisions and cooperate in treatment plans.

■ Evaluation

The expected outcomes for the patient with osteomyelitis are presented in NCP 62-1.

Bone Cancer

Primary malignant bone neoplasms are rare in adults. In 2002, 2400 new cases of bone cancer occurred in the United States with an estimated 1300 deaths.[7] Primary neoplasms occur most often during childhood through young adulthood. They are characterized by their rapid metastasis and bone destruction.

MULTIPLE MYELOMA

In adults, multiple myeloma (plasma cell myeloma) is the most frequently occurring primary tumor arising in bone. **Multiple myeloma** is a malignant neoplasm of plasma cells causing widespread infiltration and destruction of bone marrow and cortex, which produces osteolytic lesions throughout the skeletal system. The most commonly involved bones are those with active marrow, such as the axial skeleton, sternum, ribs, spine, clavicles, skull, pelvis, and long bones. Recurrent infection, anorexia, fatigue, weight loss, back pain, anemia, thrombocytopenia, and bleeding tendencies are common presenting manifestations. The diagnosis of multiple myeloma is confirmed by bone marrow biopsy and x-rays indicating lytic lesions.

Patients with multiple myeloma generally have a poor prognosis because by the time a diagnosis has been confirmed, the disease has usually invaded the axial skeleton. Chemotherapeutic treatment of multiple myeloma is directed toward suppressing plasma cell growth and includes melphalan (Alkeran), vincristine (Oncovin), or doxorubicin (Adriamycin).[8] Corticosteroid therapy is commonly used in conjunction with chemotherapy drugs. Radiation therapy may be helpful in reducing pain. Early aggressive cell therapy with autologous stem cell transplantation may prolong survival. Myeloma in the spinal cord may require decompression. (Multiple myeloma is discussed in further detail in Chapter 30).

OSTEOGENIC SARCOMA

Osteogenic sarcoma (osteosarcoma) is a primary neoplasm of bone that is extremely malignant and is characterized by rapid growth and metastasis. It usually occurs in the metaphyseal region of the long bones of the extremities, particularly in the regions of the distal femur, proximal tibia, and proximal humerus, as well as the pelvis (Fig. 62-3). Osteogenic sarcoma is the most common malignant bone tumor affecting children and young adults; the highest incidence is in males in the 10- to 25-year-old age-group. Secondary osteosarcoma is known to occur in adults over age 60 and is most commonly associated with Paget's disease.

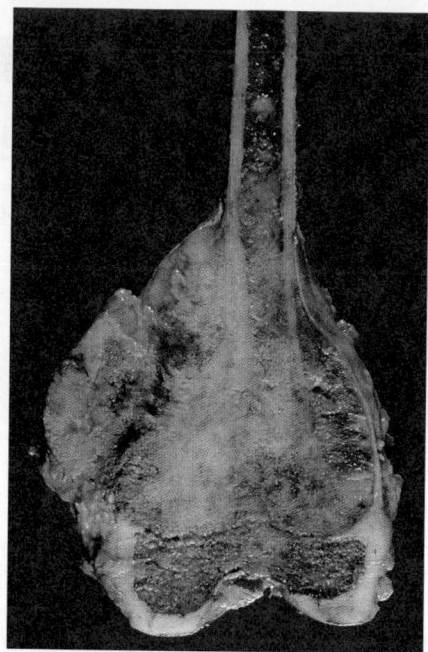

FIG. 62-3 Osteogenic sarcoma in the femur. Bone cortex has been destroyed.

Clinical manifestations of osteogenic sarcoma are usually associated with a gradual onset of pain and swelling, especially around the knee. A minor injury does not cause the neoplasm but may bring the preexisting condition to medical attention. The neoplasm grows rapidly and can restrict joint motion if the tumor is close to a joint structure. The diagnosis is confirmed from biopsied tissue specimens; elevation of serum alkaline phosphatase and calcium levels; and findings on x-ray, CT or positron emission tomogram (PET) scans, and MRI. Metastasis is present in 10% to 20% of individuals on diagnosis, with the lung being the most frequent site.

Major advances continue to be made in the treatment of osteosarcoma. Preoperative (neoadjuvant) chemotherapy is used to decrease tumor size. As a result, limb-salvage procedures, including a wide surgical resection of the tumor, are being used more often. Limb-salvage procedures are considered when there is a clear 6- to 7-cm margin surrounding the lesion. Limb salvage is contraindicated if there is major neurovascular involvement, pathologic fracture, infection, skeletal immaturity, or extensive muscle involvement.[9] Quality-of-life considerations also factor in the decision of limb salvage compared with amputation. Current use of adjunct chemotherapy following amputation has increased the projected 5-year survival rate to 60%.[10] Chemotherapeutic agents include methotrexate, doxorubicin (Adriamycin), cisplatin (Platinol), cyclophosphamide (Cytoxan), bleomycin (Blenoxane), dactinomycin (Cosmegen), and ifosfamide (Ifex).

OSTEOCLASTOMA

Osteoclastoma *(giant cell tumor)* is a destructive tumor that arises in the cancellous ends of long bones in young adults. Most (98%) of these variant giant cell tumors are benign, but they can be locally aggressive and spread to the lungs. Giant cell tumors most commonly occur in females between the ages of 20 and 35. Common tumor sites are in the distal ends of the femur, tibia, and radius.[11] Clinical manifestations are usually swelling, local pain,

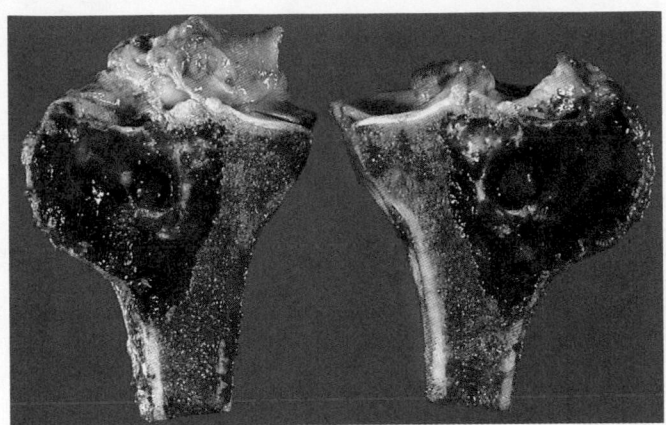

FIG. 62-4 Osteoclastoma (giant cell tumor) in a long bone.

and some disturbances in joint function. X-ray evidence of giant cell tumor is variable but usually reveals local areas of bone destruction and eventual expansion of the bone ends (Fig. 62-4).

Biopsy is used to establish the diagnosis. After diagnosis, surgical curettage of the tumor is usually done, followed by bone grafting. Cryosurgery aids to preserve joint motion and reduce the need for amputation. Complications from cryosurgery include future pathologic fracture and delayed union. After treatment there is a greater than 50% chance of recurrence. Recurrent giant cell tumors may have to be treated with amputation.

EWING'S SARCOMA

Ewing's sarcoma is one of the most common primary malignant neoplasms of bone and soft tissue. It occurs more often in males during periods of rapid bone growth (5 to 15 years of age). This neoplasm is characterized by rapid growth within the medullary cavity of long bone, especially the femur, humerus, pelvis, and tibia. Metastasis occurs early, and the most frequent site is the lungs. Common manifestations are progressive local pain, swelling, palpable soft tissue mass, noticeable increase in size of the affected part, fever, and leukocytosis. Initially, x-rays, CT, and MRI show periosteal bone destruction. Bone biopsy confirms the diagnosis. Treatment usually involves radiation therapy and wide surgical resection of the tumor or amputation. Multidrug chemotherapy has improved survival rates. Chemotherapeutic agents commonly used are cyclophosphamide (Cytoxan), vincristine (Oncovin), ifosfamide (Ifex), doxorubicin (Adriamycin), etoposide (VePesid), and dactinomycin (Cosmegen). These drugs are also used in treating metastatic Ewing's sarcoma.[12] Surgical resection of the tumor has helped decrease the rate of recurrence. The use of radiation, surgical resection, and chemotherapy has increased the 5-year survival rate to 60%.[13]

METASTATIC BONE DISEASE

The most common type of malignant bone tumor occurs as a result of metastasis from a primary tumor. Common sites for the primary tumor include the breast, prostate, gastrointestinal tract, lungs, kidney, ovary, and thyroid.[14] Metastatic cancer cells travel to other sites from the primary tumor via the lymph and blood. The metastatic bone lesion is commonly found in the vertebrae, pelvis, femur, humerus, or ribs. Pathologic fractures at the site of metastasis are common because of weakening of the involved bone.

Once a primary lesion has been identified, radionuclide bone scans are often done to detect the presence of metastatic lesions before they are visible on x-ray. It is important to note that metastatic bone lesions may occur at any time (even years later) following diagnosis and treatment of the primary tumor. Metastasis to the bone should be suspected in any patient who has local bone pain and a past history of cancer. Treatment may be palliative and consists of pain management and radiation. Surgical stabilization of the fracture may be indicated if there is a fracture or pending fracture. Prognosis depends on the extent of metastasis and location.

NURSING MANAGEMENT
BONE CANCER

■ Nursing Assessment

The patient with bone cancer should be assessed for the location and severity of pain. Weakness caused by anemia and decreased mobility may also be noted. Swelling at the involved site and decreased joint function, depending on the tumor site, should also be monitored.

■ Nursing Diagnoses

Nursing diagnoses for the patient with bone cancer may include, but are not limited to, the following:
- Acute pain *related to* the disease process or inadequate pain medication or comfort measures
- Impaired physical mobility *related to* disease process, pain, weakness, and debility
- Disturbed body image *related to* possible amputation, deformity, swelling, and effects of chemotherapy
- Anticipatory grieving *related to* poor prognosis of the disease
- Risk for injury *related to* disease process, possible pathologic fracture, or inadequate handling or positioning of affected body part
- Impaired home maintenance *related to* lack of knowledge about care needed at home or how to perform the necessary skills

■ Planning

The overall goals are that the patient with bone cancer will (1) have satisfactory pain relief; (2) maintain preferred activities as long as possible; (3) demonstrate acceptance of body image changes resulting from chemotherapy, radiation, and surgery; (4) e free from injury; and (5) verbalize a realistic idea of disease progression and prognosis.

■ Nursing Implementation

Health Promotion. The nurse should teach the public to recognize the warning signs of bone cancer, including swelling, bone pain of unexplained origin, limitation of joint function, and changes in skin temperature. As with all forms of cancer, health promotion should stress the importance of periodic screening and health examinations.

Acute Intervention. Nursing care of the patient with a malignant bone neoplasm does not differ significantly from the care given to the patient with a malignant disease of any other body system (see Chapter 15). However, special attention is required to reduce the complications associated with prolonged bed rest and to prevent falls and pathologic fractures. Careful handling and support of the affected extremity and logrolling for those on bed rest is important to prevent pathologic fractures.[15] The patient is often reluctant to participate in therapeutic activities because of weakness from the disease and treatment and fear of pain. Regular rest periods should be provided between activities.

Ambulatory and Home Care. The nurse must be able to assist the patient and family in accepting the guarded prognosis associated with bone neoplasms. Inability to accomplish age-specific developmental tasks can increase the frustrations with this condition. General principles related to cancer nursing are applicable (see Chapter 15). Special attention is necessary for the problems of pain and disability, chemotherapy, and specific surgery such as spinal cord decompression or amputation.

■ Evaluation

The expected outcomes are that the patient with bone cancer will

- have minimal to no pain
- have no falls
- have no pathologic fractures
- accept changes in body image
- retain dignity and active participation in treatment decisions
- have maximal functional ability

Muscular Dystrophy

Muscular dystrophy (MD) is a group of genetically transmitted diseases characterized by progressive symmetric wasting of skeletal muscle without evidence of neurologic involvement. In all forms of MD an insidious loss of strength occurs with increasing disability and deformity. The types of MD differ in the groups of muscles affected, age of onset, rate of progression, and mode of genetic inheritance.[16] Types of MD are presented in Table 62-3.

Duchenne and Becker MD are sex-linked recessive disorders usually seen only in males. In these disorders there is a genetic mutation of the dystrophin gene. Dystrophin in normal muscle cells helps to attach skeletal muscle fibers to the basement membrane. Abnormalities in dystrophin can lead to defects in the plasma membrane of muscle fiber with subsequent muscle fiber degeneration.

Diagnostic studies for MD include muscle serum enzymes (especially creatine kinase), electromyogram (EMG) testing, muscle fiber biopsy, electrocardiogram abnormalities reflective of cardiomyopathy, and genetic pedigree (see Chapter 13). Mus-

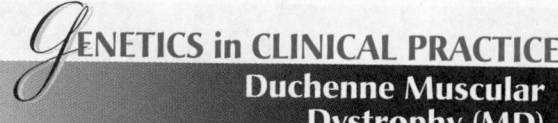

GENETICS in CLINICAL PRACTICE
Duchenne Muscular Dystrophy (MD)

Genetic Basis
- Sex-linked recessive disorder

Incidence
- About 30 in 100,000 males

Genetic Testing
- DNA testing for mutation in dystrophin gene

Clinical Implications
- Duchenne MD is present at birth but does not usually become clinically apparent until at least age 3.
- Very few individuals with the disease live to adulthood.
- Genetic testing and counseling should be considered in individuals with a family history of Duchenne MD.
- Because there are many types of MD with different genetic bases, establishing the type of MD is important to determine treatment and possible genetic counseling recommendations.

cle biopsy confirms the diagnosis with classic findings of fat and connective tissue deposits, degeneration and necrosis of muscle fibers, and a deficiency of the muscle protein dystrophin.[17]

Presently, no definitive therapy is available to stop the progressive wasting of MD. Corticosteroid therapy may significantly halt the disease progression for up to 3 years. The goal of treatment is to preserve mobility and independence through exercise, physical therapy, and orthopedic appliances. The nurse should encourage communication among family members (and parents) to cope with the emotional and physical strains of MD. An emphasis should be placed on teaching the patient and family range-of-motion exercises, nutrition, and signs of progression. Genetic testing and counseling may be recommended for individuals with a family history of MD.

Nursing care should focus on keeping the patient active as long as possible. Prolonged bed rest should be avoided because immobility can lead to further muscle wasting. As the disease progresses, the focus will shift to teaching the patient to limit sedentary periods when skin integrity or respiratory complications could develop. Ongoing medical and nursing care will be required throughout the individual's lifetime.

TABLE 62-3 Types of Muscular Dystrophy		
TYPE	**GENETIC BASIS**	**CLINICAL MANIFESTATIONS**
Duchenne (pseudohypertrophic)	X-linked Mutation of dystrophin gene	Onset before age 5; progressive weakness of pelvic and shoulder muscles; unable to walk after age 12; cardiomyopathy; respiratory failure in second or third decade; mental impairment
Becker (benign pseudohypertrophic)	X-linked Mutation of dystrophin gene	Onset between 5 and 15 years; slower course of pelvic and shoulder muscle wasting than Duchenne; cardiomyopathy; respiratory failure; may survive into fourth or fifth decade
Landouzy-Dejerine (facioscapulohumeral)	Autosomal dominant deletion of chromosome 4q35	Onset before age 20; slowly progressive weakness of face, shoulder muscles, and foot dorsiflexion; deafness
Erb (limb-girdle)	Autosomal recessive or autosomal dominant	Onset ranges from early childhood to early adulthood; slow progressive weakness of shoulder and hip muscles

Low Back Pain

Etiology and Pathophysiology

Low back pain is common and has probably affected about 80% of adults in the United States at least once during their lifetime. Backache is second only to headache as the most common pain complaint.[18] Low back pain in persons under age 45 is responsible for more lost working hours than any other medical condition and represents one of the nation's most costly health problems.[19] Low back pain is a common problem because the lumbar region (1) bears most of the weight of the body, (2) is the most flexible region of the spinal column, (3) contains nerve roots that are vulnerable to injury or disease, and (4) has an inherently poor biomechanical structure.

Several risk factors are associated with low back pain, including lack of muscle tone and excess body weight, poor posture, cigarette smoking, and stress. Jobs that require repetitive heavy lifting, vibration (such as a jackhammer operator), and prolonged periods of sitting are also associated with low back pain.

Low back pain is most often due to a musculoskeletal problem. The causes of low back pain of musculoskeletal origin include (1) acute lumbosacral strain, (2) instability of lumbosacral bony mechanism, (3) osteoarthritis of the lumbosacral vertebrae, (4) intervertebral disk degeneration, and (5) herniation of the intervertebral disk. Of these, the most common cause is mechanical strain of paravertebral muscles. Herniation of the nucleus pulposus is another common cause of low back pain. Other causes include metabolic, circulatory, gynecologic, urologic, or psychologic problems.

ACUTE LOW BACK PAIN

Acute low back pain lasts 4 weeks or less. Acute low back pain is usually associated with some type of activity that causes undue stress (often hyperflexion) on the tissues of the lower back. Often symptoms do not appear at the time of injury but develop later because of a gradual increase in paravertebral muscle spasms. Few definitive diagnostic abnormalities are present with paravertebral muscle strain. One test is the straight-leg raise, which may produce pain in the lumbar area without radiation along the sciatic nerve. MRI and CT scans are generally not done unless trauma or systemic disease (e.g., cancer, spinal infection) is suspected.

Collaborative Care

If the acute muscle spasms and accompanying pain are not severe and debilitating, the patient may be treated on an outpatient basis with a combination of the following: (1) analgesics, such as NSAIDs; (2) muscle relaxants (e.g., cyclobenzaprine [Flexeril]); (3) massage and back manipulation; and (4) the daytime use of a corset. Severe pain may require a brief course of narcotic analgesics. A corset prevents rotation, flexion, and extension of the lower back.

A brief period (1 to 2 days) of rest at home may be necessary for some persons, whereas others do better with a continuation of regular activities.[18] The effectiveness of invasive treatments, such as epidural corticosteroid injections and implanted devices that deliver pain medication, remains controversial.[20] All patients during this time should avoid activities that aggravate the pain, including lifting, bending, twisting, and prolonged sitting. Most cases spontaneously improve within 2 weeks.

NURSING MANAGEMENT
ACUTE LOW BACK PAIN

■ Nursing Assessment

Subjective and objective data that should be obtained from the patient with low back pain are summarized in Table 62-4.

■ Nursing Diagnoses

Nursing diagnoses for the patient with low back pain may include, but are not limited to, those presented in NCP 62-2.

■ Planning

The overall goals are that the patient with low back pain will (1) have satisfactory pain relief, (2) avoid constipation secondary to medication and immobility, (3) learn back-sparing practices, and (4) return to previous level of activity within prescribed restrictions.

TABLE 62-4	Nursing Assessment Low Back Pain

Subjective Data
Important Health Information
Past health history: Acute or chronic lumbosacral strain, osteoarthritis, degenerative disk disease, obesity
Medications: Use of analgesics, muscle relaxants, nonsteroidal antiinflammatory drugs, corticosteroids, over-the-counter remedies including herbal products and nutritional supplements
Surgery or other treatments: Previous back surgery, epidural corticosteroid injections
Functional Health Patterns
Health perception–health management: Smoking, lack of exercise
Nutritional-metabolic: Obesity
Activity-exercise: Poor posture, muscle spasms; activity intolerance
Elimination: Constipation
Sleep-rest: Interrupted sleep
Cognitive-perceptual: Pain in back, buttocks, or leg associated with walking, turning, straining, coughing, leg raising; numbness or tingling of legs, feet, toes
Role-relationship: Occupation requiring heavy lifting, vibrations, or extended driving

Objective Data
General
Guarded movement
Neurologic
Depressed or absent Achilles tendon reflex; positive straight-leg raise test
Musculoskeletal
Tense, tight paravertebral muscles on palpation, decreased range of motion of spine
Possible Findings
Localization of site of lesion or disorder on myelogram, CT scan, or MRI; determination of nerve irritation on electromyography

CT, Computed tomography; *MRI,* magnetic resonance imaging.

NURSING CARE PLAN 62-2

Patient with Low Back Pain

ACUTE MANAGEMENT

EXPECTED PATIENT OUTCOMES	NURSING INTERVENTIONS and *RATIONALES*
NURSING DIAGNOSIS	**Acute pain** *related to* herniated nucleus pulposus, muscle spasms, and ineffective comfort measures *as manifested by* verbalization of back pain on movement, guarded movements, palpable muscle spasm, decreased physical activity, rating pain as >4 on a 10-point pain scale.
▪ Reduction or absence of pain and muscle spasms ▪ Expression of satisfaction with pain relief (rates pain as <4 on pain scale of 10)	▪ Assess location, severity, and characteristics of pain *to plan appropriate interventions.* ▪ Use a pain scale and evaluate pain relief interventions *to assess pain and treatment measures.* ▪ Enforce decreased activity *to reduce paravertebral muscle spasms and resulting pain.* ▪ Keep head of bed elevated 20 degrees and knee of bed flexed *to promote comfort by reducing stress on lower back muscles.* ▪ Apply moist heat or ice to lower back *to reduce pain and muscle spasm.* ▪ Administer analgesics, nonsteroidal antiinflammatory drugs, and/or muscle relaxants as ordered; document effect *to promote comfort and evaluate effectiveness.*
NURSING DIAGNOSIS	**Impaired physical mobility** *related to* pain *as manifested by* limited active joint range of motion (ROM), movement restrictions, muscle spasms.
▪ Unrestricted gait ▪ Ambulation within normal limits ▪ Resumption of previous level of mobility ▪ Performance of prescribed exercises	▪ Have patient perform ROM and muscle-strengthening exercises daily *to strengthen the supporting muscles and maintain all joints in normal ROM.* ▪ Start ambulation program and progress with assistance *to promote gradual and progressive return to previous mobility level.* ▪ Avoid having patient bend, sit, or lift *to prevent back strain and increased pain.* ▪ Provide written instructions that describe each exercise and activity and a phone number to call with any questions.

CHRONIC MANAGEMENT

NURSING DIAGNOSIS	**Chronic pain** *related to* progression of problem *as manifested by* verbal report or evidence of pain longer than 6 months in duration.
▪ Development of effective methods of managing pain ▪ Expression of satisfaction with pain control measures	▪ Assess variety and effectiveness of pain management techniques *to determine extent of problem and develop appropriate interventions.* ▪ Use a pain scale *to assess pain and to evaluate pain control interventions.* ▪ Instruct patient and family about home care and alternative methods of pain control, including use of heat, transcutaneous electrical nerve stimulation *to provide information about supplementary methods of pain management.* ▪ Assist in identifying activities that exacerbate pain *to make adjustments so that pain is reduced.*
NURSING DIAGNOSIS	**Ineffective coping** *related to* effects of chronic pain *as manifested by* verbalization of inability to cope, irritability, tension, inability to meet role expectations, altered participation in social events, ineffective or inappropriate use of defense mechanisms.
▪ Return to previous levels of work and lifestyle or successfully adapt to lifestyle changes	▪ Explain factors that may contribute to development of maladaptive coping behavior *to communicate information and a caring attitude.* ▪ Discuss how to develop therapeutic coping skills that enhance self-esteem and social interaction *to foster effective coping behaviors and adjustment to chronic pain.*
NURSING DIAGNOSIS	**Ineffective therapeutic regimen management** *related to* lack of knowledge regarding posture, exercises, body mechanics, and weight reduction *as manifested by* lack of necessary knowledge to participate in treatment plan, inadequate understanding, or inaccurate follow-through of previous instructions.
▪ Use of proper body mechanics at all times ▪ Maintenance of weight within normal limits ▪ Maintenance of activity and ambulation appropriate to age and state of health	▪ Assess body mechanics *to identify incorrect techniques and intervene appropriately.* ▪ Instruct patient on proper body mechanics and use of firm mattress or bed board *to reduce risk of reinjury, provide back support, and maintain proper body alignment.* ▪ Assess for decreasing muscle strength *to identify complications and modify care plan.* ▪ Refer to physical therapist for low back exercises *to develop abdominal and paravertebral muscle strength to provide increased support.* ▪ Encourage activity and ambulation within limitations *to maintain physical mobility.* ▪ Teach about weight reduction and/or refer to dietitian if indicated *because increased abdominal weight puts strain on low back.*

■ Nursing Implementation

Health Promotion. The nurse is a significant role model and teacher for patients with low back problems. As a role model, the nurse should use proper body mechanics at all times. This should be a primary consideration when teaching patients and health care providers transfer and turning techniques. The nurse should assess the patient's use of body mechanics and offer advice when activities that could produce back strain are used (Table 62-5).

Some health care providers refer patients with back pain to a program called "Back School." It is a formal program usually taught by health professionals such as physicians, nurses, and physical therapists. It is designed to teach the patient how to minimize back pain and avoid repeat episodes of low back pain. Tips for prevention of back injury are listed in Table 62-5. Exercises to strengthen the back are presented in Table 62-6.

Patients are also advised to maintain appropriate body weight. Excess body weight places extra stress on the lower back and weakens the abdominal muscles that support the lower back.

The position assumed while sleeping is also important in preventing low back pain. Sleeping in a prone position should be avoided because it produces excessive lumbar lordosis, placing excessive stress on the lower back. A firm mattress is recommended. The patient should sleep in either a supine or side-lying position with the knees and hips flexed to prevent unnecessary pressure on support muscles, ligamentous structures, and lumbosacral joints. Patients should be educated about the necessity

to avoid or cease smoking. Nicotine has been shown to decrease circulation to the vertebral disks, and a causal relationship exists between smoking and some types of low back pain.[21]

Acute Intervention. The primary nursing responsibilities in acute low back pain are to assist the patient to maintain activity limitations, promote comfort, and educate the patient about the health problem and appropriate exercises. Other nursing interventions are summarized in NCP 62-2. Use of analgesics, NSAIDs, thermotherapy (ice and heat), and muscle relaxants to promote comfort is incorporated into the plan of care.

Muscle stretching and strengthening exercises may be part of the management plan. Although the actual exercises are often taught by the physical therapist, it is the nurse's responsibility to ensure that the patient understands the type and frequency of exercise prescribed, as well as the rationale for the program.

Ambulatory and Home Care. The goal of management is to make an episode of acute low back pain an isolated incident. If the lumbosacral mechanism is unstable, repeated episodes can be anticipated. The lumbosacral spine may be unable to meet the demands placed on it without strain because of factors such as obesity, poor posture, poor muscular support, advancing age, or local trauma. Intervention is aimed at strengthening the supporting muscles by exercise. The use of a corset limits extremes of movement. In addition, weight reduction decreases the mechanical demands on the lower back.

Persistent use of poor body mechanics may result in repeated episodes of low back pain. If the strain is work related, occupa-

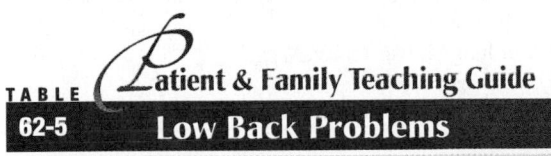

TABLE 62-5   Patient & Family Teaching Guide — Low Back Problems

Do Not
- Lean forward without bending knees
- Lift anything above level of elbows
- Stand in one position for prolonged time
- Sleep on abdomen or on back or side with legs out straight
- Exercise without consulting health care provider if having severe pain
- Exceed prescribed amount and type of exercises without consulting health care provider

Do
- Prevent lower back from straining forward by placing a foot on a step or stool during prolonged standing
- Sleep in a side-lying position with knees and hips bent
- Sleep on back with a lift under knees and legs or on back with 10-inch-high pillow under knees to flex hips and knees
- Sit in a chair with knees higher than hips and support arms on chair or knees
- Exercise 15 min in the morning and 15 min in the evening regularly; begin exercises with a 2- or 3-min warm-up period by moving arms and legs, by alternately relaxing and tightening muscles; exercise slowly with smooth movements as directed by a physical therapist
- Avoid chilling during and after exercising
- Maintain appropriate body weight
- Use local heat and cold application
- Use a lumbar roll or pillow for sitting

EVIDENCE-BASED PRACTICE — Nonspecific Low Back Pain

Clinical Problem
Are back schools and/or massage effective for patients with nonspecific low back pain?

Best Clinical Practice
- Evidence exists that back schools have better short-term effects than other treatments for chronic low back pain.
- Evidence exists that back schools in an occupational setting are more effective than placebo or wait-list control groups.
- Insufficient evidence exists to recommend massage as a stand-alone treatment for nonspecific low back pain.

Implications for Nursing Practice
- Back schools usually involve information-giving interventions where patients are taught about anatomy and function of the back, mechanical strain, and posture. Isometric exercises for abdominal muscles and physical activity programs are also taught.
- Back schools may be effective for patients with recurrent and chronic low back pain, especially in occupational settings. Little is known about the cost-effectiveness of back schools.
- Additional high-quality controlled trials are needed to evaluate the effects of massage for nonspecific low back pain.

References for Evidence
Furlan AD et al: Massage for low back pain, Cochrane Back Review Group, *Cochrane Database Syst Rev*, issue 1, 2002.
Tulder MW et al: Back schools for non-specific low back pain, Cochrane Back Review Group, *Cochrane Database Syst Rev*, issue 1, 2002.

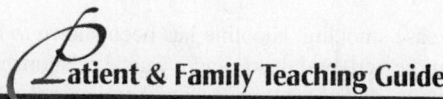

TABLE
62-6 **Patient & Family Teaching Guide**

Back Exercises

Knee-to-chest lift (to stretch hip, buttocks, lower back muscles)

- Lie on back on the floor with knees bent and feet flat on floor.
- Draw both knees up to chest.
- Place both hands around knees and pull them firmly against chest. Hold for 30 seconds.
- Lower legs and return to starting position.
- Repeat 5-10 times.

Simple leg lift

- Lie flat on back on floor with left knee bent and left foot flat on floor.
- Raise right leg as high as comfortably possible.
- Hold for 5 counts.
- Slowly return leg to floor.
- Bend right knee and put right foot flat on floor.
- Raise left leg and hold for 5 counts.
- Repeat 5-10 times for each leg.

Double leg lift

- Lie flat on back.
- Slowly lift legs until feet are 12 inches from the floor.
- Keep legs straight and hold this position for 10 counts.
- Lower legs to floor.
- Repeat 5 times.

Pelvic tilt

- Lie flat on back on floor with knees bent and feet flat on the floor.
- Firmly tighten your buttock muscles.
- Hold for 5 counts.
- Relax buttocks.
- Repeat 5-10 times.
- Be sure to keep lower back flat against floor.

Half sit-ups (to strengthen abdominal muscles)

- Lie flat on floor on back with knees bent, feet flat on floor, and hands on chest.
- Slowly raise head and neck to top of chest.
- Reach both hands forward and place them on knees.
- Hold for 5 counts.
- Return to starting position.
- Repeat 5-10 times.

Elbow props (to extend lower back)

- Lie face down with your arms beside your body and your head turned to one side.
- Stay in this position for 2-5 minutes, making sure that you relax completely.
- Remain face down and prop yourself on your elbows.
- Hold this position for 2-3 minutes.
- Return to starting position and relax for 1 minute.
- Repeat 5-10 times.

Hip tilts

- Lie flat on back with knees bent.
- Slowly bend legs and hips to one side as far as possible.
- Bend to other side.
- Repeat 5 times.

Toe touches

- Stand straight and relaxed.
- Lower head and body and try to touch floor with fingertips.
- Keep knees straight.
- Do not jerk or lunge toward floor.
- Bend only as far as you can.
- Repeat 5 times.

From Canobbio MM: *Mosby's handbook of patient teaching,* ed 2, St Louis, 2000, Mosby.

tional counseling may be necessary. The frustration, pain, and disability imposed on the patient with low back pain require emotional support and understanding care by the nurse.

■ Evaluation

The expected outcomes for the patient with low back pain are presented in NCP 62-2.

CHRONIC LOW BACK PAIN

Chronic back pain lasts more than 3 months or is a repeated incapacitating episode. The causes of chronic low back pain include degenerative disk disease, lack of physical exercise, prior injury, obesity, structural and postural abnormalities, and systemic disease. Osteoarthritis (OA) of the lumbar spine is found in patients over 50, whereas chronic back pain in younger patients with OA usually involves the thoracic or lumbar spine.[2] Periods of inactivity, particularly on awakening or after long periods of sitting, increase the discomfort.

Treatment regimens are much the same as acute low back pain: a reduction in the pain associated with daily activities, a formal back pain program, and ongoing medical care. Cold, damp weather aggravates the back pain but can be relieved with rest and local heat application. Relief of pain and stiffness by the use of mild analgesics, such as NSAIDs, is integral to the daily comfort of the individual with chronic low back pain. Weight reduction, sufficient rest periods, local heat or cold application, and exercise and activity throughout the day help to keep the muscles and joints mobilized.

Surgery may be indicated in patients with severe chronic low back pain who do not respond to conservative care and/or have continued neurologic deficits.[22] (Surgery for low back pain is discussed on p. 1704.)

HERNIATED INTERVERTEBRAL DISK

Etiology and Pathophysiology

An intervertebral disk is interposed between the adjacent surfaces of vertebral bodies from the cervical axis to the sacrum. An acute **herniated intervertebral disk** (slipped disk) can be the result of natural degeneration with age or repeated stress and trauma to the spine. The nucleus pulposus (gelatinous center of the disk) may rupture to cause acute injury and back pain. The most common sites of rupture are the lumbosacral disks, specifically L4-5 and L5-S1. Disk herniation may also occur at C5-6 and C6-7.

COMPLEMENTARY & ALTERNATIVE THERAPIES
Acupuncture

Acupuncture is a traditional Chinese medical practice of inserting very fine needles into the skin to stimulate specific anatomic points in the body (called acupoints) for therapeutic purposes. Used to regulate the flow of Qi (life force or energy), the acupuncture needles unblock the obstruction of Qi through the meridians (see Chapter 7).

Clinical Uses
Lower back pain and other types of pain. Postoperative and chemotherapy-associated nausea and vomiting. Addiction, stroke rehabilitation, menstrual cramps, fibromyalgia, and myofascial pain. Table 7-2 on p. 98 lists other conditions that may benefit from acupuncture.

Effects
Release of endorphins, activation of the hypothalamus and pituitary gland, and alterations in the levels of neurotransmitters.

Nursing Implications
Acupuncture is considered a safe therapy when (1) the practitioner has been appropriately trained and (2) the practitioner uses sterilized or disposable needles. Acupuncture should be used with caution with those who have a history of seizures; are carriers of hepatitis B or have chronic hepatitis C; or have human immunodeficiency viral infection, bleeding disorders, thrombocytopenia, or skin infections.

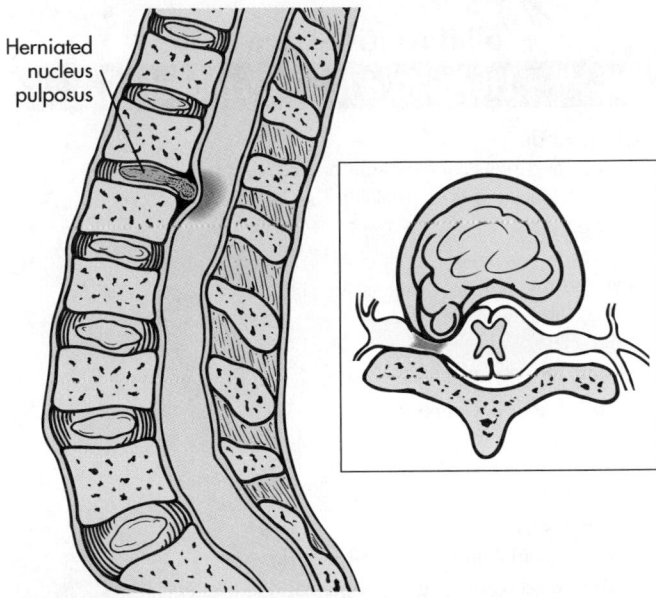

FIG. 62-5 Compression of spinal cord caused by herniation of nucleus pulposus into spinal cord. *Inset,* Pressure on nerves as they leave the spinal canal.

Structural degeneration of the intervertebral disk is a result of degenerative disk disease. The degeneration results in intervertebral narrowing and a lessening of the efficiency of the intervertebral disks in acting as shock absorbers. As stress on the degenerated disk continues and eventually exceeds the strength of the disk, herniation of the intervertebral disk may result. Compression of the nerve roots and cord may then occur (Fig. 62-5).

Clinical Manifestations

The most common feature of a lumbar herniated disk is low back pain, radiating down the buttock and below the knee, along the distribution of the sciatic nerve *(radiculopathy).* (Specific manifestations based on the level of lumbar disk herniation are summarized in Table 62-7.) The straight-leg raise test may be positive, indicating nerve root irritation. Back or leg pain may be reproduced by raising the leg and flexing the foot at 90 degrees. Low back pain from other causes may not be accompanied by leg pain. Reflexes may be depressed or absent, depending on the spinal nerve root involved. Paresthesia or muscle weakness in the legs, feet, or toes may be reported by the patient. Multiple nerve root (cauda equina) compression may be manifested as bowel and bladder incontinence or impotence.

Diagnostic Studies

X-rays are done to note any structural defects. A myelogram, MRI, or CT scan is helpful in localizing the site of herniation. An epidural venogram or diskogram may be necessary if other methods of diagnosis are unsuccessful. An EMG of the extremities can be performed to determine the severity of nerve irritation caused by herniation or to rule out other pathologic conditions such as peripheral neuropathy.

Collaborative Care

The patient with a suspected disk herniation is usually managed first with conservative therapy (Table 62-8). This includes limitation of extremes of spinal movement (brace, corset, or belt), local heat or ice, ultrasound and massage, traction, and

TABLE 62-7	Neurologic Assessment of Herniated Intervertebral Disk*				
INTERVERTEBRAL LEVEL	**SUBJECTIVE PAIN**	**AFFECTED REFLEX**	**MOTOR FUNCTION**	**SENSATION**
L3-L4	Back to buttocks to posterior thigh to inner calf	Patellar	Quadriceps, anterior tibialis	Inner aspect of lower leg, anterior part of thigh
L4-L5	Back to buttocks to dorsum of foot and big toe	None	Anterior tibialis, extensor hallucis longus, gluteus medius	Dorsum of foot and big toe
L5-S1	Back to buttocks to sole of foot and heel	Achilles	Gastrocnemius, hamstring, gluteus maximus	Heel and lateral foot

*A disk herniation can involve pressure on more than one nerve root.

TABLE 62-8	Collaborative Care
	Herniated Intervertebral Disk

Diagnostic

History and physical examination with emphasis on neuro-
logic deficits and straight-leg raising
CT scan
MRI
Myelogram
Diskogram
EMG
Somatosensory evoked potential

Collaborative Therapy

Conservative
Restricted activity
Medication
   Analgesics
   Nonsteroidal antiinflammatory drugs
   Muscle relaxants (e.g., cyclobenzaprine [Flexeril])
Local ice or heat
Physical therapy
Surgical
Laminectomy with or without spinal fusion
Diskectomy
Percutaneous laser diskectomy
Spinal fusion with or without instrumentation

CT, Computed tomography; *EMG,* electromyogram; *MRI,* magnetic resonance imaging.

transcutaneous electrical nerve stimulation. Drug therapy includes NSAIDs, short-term narcotic opioids, and muscle relaxants. Conservative treatment can result in a healing over of the herniated area with a concomitant decrease in pain. Once the symptoms subside, back strengthening exercises are begun twice a day and are encouraged for a lifetime. The patient should be taught the principles of good body mechanics. Extremes of flexion and torsion are strongly discouraged.

Most patients with a herniated disk recover with a conservative treatment plan. However, if conservative treatment is unsuccessful, *radiculopathy* (nerve root pain) becomes progressively worse, or loss of bowel or bladder control (cauda equina) is documented, surgery may then be indicated.

Surgical Therapy. Surgery for disk disease is generally indicated when diagnostic tests point out a herniation not responding to conservative treatment, consistent pain, and/or a persistent neurologic deficit.[23]

The traditional and most common procedure for lumbar disk disease is a *laminectomy.* It involves the surgical excision of part of the posterior arch of the vertebra (referred to as the lamina) to gain access to part or all of the protruding disk to remove it.

A *diskectomy* is another common type of surgical procedure that may be performed to decompress the nerve root. Microsurgical diskectomy is a version of the standard diskectomy in which the surgeon uses a microscope to allow better visualization of the disk and disk space during surgery to aid in the removal of the herniated portion.

A *percutaneous laser diskectomy* is an outpatient surgical procedure using a tube that is passed through the retroperitoneal soft tissues to the lateral border of the disk with local anesthesia and the aid of fluoroscopy. A laser is then used on the herniated portion of the disk. Small stab wounds are used, and minimal blood loss occurs during the procedure. The procedure is effective and safe and has been shown to decrease rehabilitation time.[24]

A *spinal fusion* may be performed if an unstable bony mechanism is present. The spine is stabilized by creating an ankylosis (fusion) of contiguous vertebrae with a bone graft from the patient's fibula or iliac crest or from a donated cadaver bone. Metal fixation with rods, plates, or screws may be implanted at the time of spinal surgery to provide more stability and decrease vertebral motion. A posterior lumbar interbody fusion may be performed in patients to provide extra support for bone grafting or a prosthetic device. A new device, the InFuse Bone Graft/LT-CAGE, is being used to eliminate the need to use bone from the patient in grafting. The device contains genetically engineered protein that stimulates the body to grow new bone at the spinal fusion site.[25]

NURSING MANAGEMENT
SPINAL SURGERY

Postoperative nursing interventions focus on maintaining proper alignment of the spine at all times until healing has occurred. Flat bed rest may be maintained for 1 to 2 days depending on the extent of surgery. Log rolling patients when turning is essential to maintain proper body alignment. Pillows can be used under the thighs of each leg when supine and between the legs when in the side-lying positions to provide comfort and ensure alignment. The patient often fears turning or any movement that increases pain by straining the surgical area. The nurse must offer reassurance to the patient that the proper technique is being used to maintain body alignment. Sufficient staff should be available to move the patient without undue pain or strain on staff members or the patient.

Postoperatively, most patients will require narcotic opioids such as morphine intravenously for 24 to 48 hours. Patient-controlled analgesia allows for optimal analgesic levels and is the preferred method of continued pain management during this time. Once fluids are being taken, the patient may be switched to oral drugs such as acetaminophen with codeine, hydrocodone (Vicodin), or oxycodone (Percocet). Diazepam (Valium) may be prescribed for muscle relaxation. The nurse should monitor pain management and its effectiveness for at least 3 weeks after the surgery.

Because the spinal canal may be entered during surgery, there is potential for cerebrospinal fluid (CSF) leakage. Severe headache or leakage of CSF on the dressing should be reported immediately. CSF appears as clear or slightly yellow drainage on the dressing. It has a high glucose concentration and will be positive for glucose when a dipstick test is done. The amount and characteristics of drainage should be noted.

Frequent monitoring of peripheral neurologic signs of the extremities is a routine postoperative nursing responsibility after spinal surgery. Movement of the arms and legs and assessment of sensation should be unchanged when compared with the preoperative status. Table 62-9 summarizes a lumbar laminectomy assessment appropriate for the patient who has undergone back

TABLE 62-9	Postoperative Assessment Following Lumbar Surgery

Sensation*

Assess sensation of extremities for paresthesia in all appropriate dermatomes.

Movement*

Assess ability to move all extremities.

Muscle Strength*

Assess for any weakness of the extremities.

Wound

Assess dressing for drainage and note amount, color, characteristics.

Pain

Document location of the pain.

Ask patient to rate the pain on a scale of 1 to 10, with
  1 being no pain and 10 being worst pain.

Evaluate pain after analgesia has been administered.

*Postoperative findings should be compared with preoperative assessments. It is not unusual for the patient to continue to experience these symptoms after surgery. Symptoms gradually decrease over several months.

surgery. These assessments are repeated every 2 to 4 hours during the first 48 hours after surgery, and findings are compared with the preoperative assessment. Paresthesias, such as numbness and tingling, may not be relieved immediately after surgery. Any new muscle weakness or paresthesias should be documented and reported to the surgeon immediately.

Paralytic ileus and interference with bowel function may occur for several days and may manifest as nausea, abdominal distention, and constipation. The nurse should assess whether the patient is passing flatus, has bowel sounds in all quadrants, and has a flat, soft abdomen. Stool softeners (e.g., docusate [Colace]) may aid in relieving and preventing constipation.

Adequate bladder emptying may be altered because of activity restrictions, narcotics, or anesthesia. If allowed by the surgeon, men should be encouraged to dangle or stand to urinate. Patients should use the commode or ambulate to the bathroom when allowed to promote adequate emptying of the bladder. The nurse should ensure that privacy is maintained. It is necessary to clarify whether the patient can be allowed up to the bathroom without the corset or brace. Intermittent catheterization or an indwelling catheter may be necessary for patients who have difficulty urinating.

Loss of sphincter tone or bladder tone may indicate nerve damage. Incontinence or difficulty evacuating the bowel or bladder must be monitored closely and reported to the surgeon.

Activity prescriptions vary with surgeons, but the patient who has had spinal surgery usually ambulates early in the postoperative period. It is a nursing responsibility to know the specific orders related to activity for any patient.

In addition to the nursing care appropriate for a patient who has had a laminectomy, there are other nursing responsibilities if the patient has also had a spinal fusion. Because a bone graft is usually involved, the postoperative healing time is prolonged compared with that of a laminectomy. Immobilization over an extended time may

be necessary. A rigid orthosis (thoracic-lumbar-sacral orthosis or chairback brace) is often used during the period of immobilization. Some surgeons require that the patient be taught to put it on and take it off by log rolling in bed, whereas others allow their patients to apply the brace in a sitting or standing position. The nurse should verify the preferred method before initiating this activity. The extended immobilization required by a spinal fusion carries with it all the potential problems related to immobility.

In addition to the primary surgical site, the donor site for the bone graft must be regularly assessed. The posterior iliac crest is the most commonly used donor site, although the fibula may also be used. The donor site usually causes greater postoperative pain than the fused area. The donor site is bandaged with a pressure dressing to prevent excessive bleeding. If the donor site is the fibula, neurovascular assessments of the extremity are a postoperative nursing responsibility.

As the bone graft heals, the patient must adjust to the permanent immobility at the graft or fusion site. Instruction in proper body mechanics is essential and should be evaluated during the hospital stay.

The patient should be instructed to avoid sitting or standing for prolonged periods. Activities that should be encouraged include walking, lying down, and shifting weight from one foot to the other when standing. The patient should learn to mentally think through an activity before starting any potentially injurious task such as bending, lifting, or stooping. Any twisting movement of the spine is contraindicated. The thighs and knees, rather than the back, should be used to absorb the shock of activity and movement. A firm mattress or bed board is essential.

NECK PAIN

Cervical neck sprains and strains occur from hyperflexion and hyperextension injury. Patients have symptoms of stiffness and neck pain and possible pain radiating into the arm and hand. Pain may also radiate into the head, anterior chest, thoracic spine region, and shoulders. Cervical nerve root compression from degenerative disk disease or herniation may be indicated by weakness or paresthesia of the arm and hand. Diagnosing the cause of neck pain is done by history, physical examination, x-ray, MRI, CT scan, and myelogram. An EMG of the upper extremities is done to diagnose cervical radiculopathy.

Nonoperative treatment options for neck pain include head support via cervical collars, heat applications, massage, physical therapy, ultrasound, and NSAIDs. Surgical intervention on the cervical spine is similar to that performed on the lower back, including a diskectomy, laminectomy, and spinal fusion. If surgery is done on the cervical spine, the nurse must be alert for symptoms of spinal cord edema such as respiratory distress and a worsening neurologic status of the upper extremities. After surgery, the patient's neck is immobilized in either a soft or hard cervical collar.

FOOT DISORDERS

The foot is the platform that provides support for the weight of the body and absorbs considerable shock in ambulation. It is a complicated structure composed of bony structures, muscles, tendons, and ligaments. It can be affected by (1) congenital conditions, (2) structural weakness, (3) traumatic injuries, and (4) systemic conditions such as diabetes mellitus and rheumatoid arthritis. Abnormalities of the foot affect over 80 million persons in the United States. Much of the pain, deformity, and disability associated with foot disorders can be directly attributed to or accentuated by improperly fitting shoes, which cause crowding and angulation of the toes and inhibition of the normal movement of

foot muscles. The purposes of footwear are to (1) provide support, foot stability, protection, shock absorption, and a foundation for orthoses; (2) increase friction with the walking surface; and (3) treat foot abnormalities. (Table 62-10 summarizes common foot disorders.) One of the most common forefoot disorders

TABLE 62-10 Common Foot Disorders

DISORDER	DESCRIPTION	TREATMENT
Forefoot		
Hallux valgus (bunion)	Painful deformity of great toe consisting of lateral angulation of great toe toward second toe, bony enlargement of medial side of first metatarsal head, and formation of bursa or callus over bony enlargement (see Fig. 62-6)	Conservative treatment includes wearing shoes with wide forefoot or "bunion pocket" and use of bunion pads to relieve pressure on bursal sac. Surgical treatment is removal of bursal sac and bony enlargement and correction of lateral angulation of great toe; may include temporary or permanent internal fixation.
Hallux rigidus	Painful stiffness of first metatarsophalangeal joint caused by osteoarthritis or local trauma	Conservative treatment includes intraarticular corticosteroids and passive manual stretching of first metatarsophalangeal joint. A shoe with a stiff sole decreases pain in the joint during walking. Surgical treatment is joint fusion or arthroplasty with silicone rubber implant.
Hammertoe	Deformity of second through fifth toes, including dorsiflexion of metatarsophalangeal joint, plantar flexion of proximal interphalangeal joint, and callus on dorsum of proximal interphalangeal joint and end of involved toe; complaints related to hammertoe include burning on bottom of foot and pain and difficulty in walking when wearing shoes	Conservative treatment consists of passive manual stretching of proximal interphalangeal joint and use of metatarsal arch support. Surgical correction consists of resection of base of middle phalanx and head of proximal phalanx and bringing raw bone ends together. Kirschner wire maintains straight position.
Morton's neuroma (Morton's toe or plantar neuroma)	Neuroma in web space between third and fourth metatarsal heads, causing sharp, sudden attacks of pain and burning sensations	Surgical excision is the usual treatment.
Midfoot		
Pes planus (flatfoot)	Loss of metatarsal arch causing pain in foot or leg	Symptoms are relieved by use of resilient longitudinal arch supports. Surgical treatment consists of triple arthrodesis or fusion of subtalar joint.
Pes cavus	Elevation of longitudinal arch of foot resulting from contracture of plantar fascia or bony deformity of arch	Treatment is manipulation and casting (in patients <6 yr of age); surgical correction is necessary if it interferes with ambulation (in patients >6 yr of age).
Hindfoot		
Painful heels	Complaint of heel pain with weight bearing; common cause of plantar bursitis or calcaneal spur in adult	Corticosteroids are injected locally into inflamed bursa and sponge rubber heel cushion is used; surgical excision of bursa or spur is performed.
Local Problems		
Corn	Localized thickening of skin caused by continual pressure over bony prominences, especially metatarsal head, frequently causing localized pain	Corn is softened with warm water or preparations containing salicylic acid and trimmed with razor blade or scalpel. Pressure on bony prominences caused by shoes is relieved.
Soft corn	Painful lesion caused by bony prominence of one toe pressing against adjacent toe; usual location in web space between toes; softness caused by secretions keeping web space relatively moist	Pain is relieved by placing cotton between toes to separate them. Surgical treatment is excision of projecting bone spur (if present).
Callus	Similar formation to corn but covering of wider area and usual location on weight-bearing part of foot	Same as for corn.
Plantar wart	Painful papillomatous growth caused by virus that may occur on any part of skin on sole of foot	Excision with electrocoagulation or surgical removal is done; ultrasound may also be used.

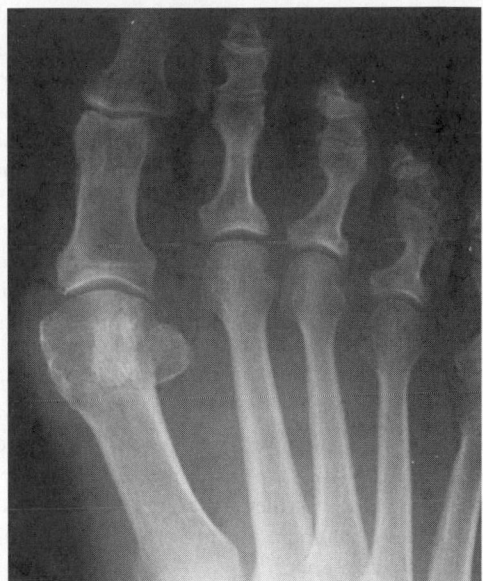

FIG. 62-6 Hallux valgus, with bunion of the great toe.

is a bunion (Fig. 62-6). A lateral deviation of the great toe, termed *hallux valgus*, occurs with a bunion.[26]

NURSING MANAGEMENT
FOOT DISORDERS

■ Nursing Implementation

Health Promotion. Well-constructed and properly fitted shoes are essential for healthy, pain-free feet. Fashion styles, especially for women, often influence selection of footwear instead of considerations of comfort and support. Patient teaching should stress the importance of having a shoe that conforms to the foot rather than to current fashion trends. The shoe must be long enough and wide enough to prevent crowding of the toes and forcing of the great toe into a position of hallux valgus. At the metatarsal head, the width of the shoe should be sufficient to allow free movement of the foot muscles and permit bending of the toes. The shank (narrow part of sole under the instep) of the shoe should be rigid enough to give optimal support. The height of the heel should be realistic in relation to the purpose for which the shoe is worn. Ideally, the heel of the shoe should not rise more than 1 inch higher than the forefoot support.

Acute Intervention. Many foot problems require referral to a podiatrist. Depending on the problem, conservative therapy is usually tried first (Table 62-10). These therapies include NSAIDs, shock-wave therapy, icing, physical therapy, alterations in foot wear, stretching, warm soaks, ultrasound, and corticosteroid injections. If these methods do not offer relief, surgery may then be recommended.

When surgery is performed, the foot is usually immobilized by a bulky dressing, short leg cast, slipper (plaster) cast, or a platform "shoe" that fits over the dressing and has a rigid sole (known as a bunion boot). The foot should be elevated with the heel off the bed to help reduce discomfort and prevent edema. The neurovascular status should be assessed frequently during the immediate postoperative period. Depending on the type of surgery, pins or wires may extend through the toes, or a protec-

tive splint that extends over the end of the foot may be in place. Care must be taken not to jar these devices and cause pain. The devices may interfere with or preclude assessment for movement. The nurse should be aware that sensation may be difficult to evaluate because postoperative pain can interfere with the patient's ability to differentiate pain caused by the surgical procedure from pain resulting from nerve pressure or circulatory impairment.

The type and extent of surgery determine the degree of ambulation allowed. Crutches or canes may be necessary. The patient may experience pain or a throbbing sensation when starting ambulation. The nurse should reinforce instructions given by the physical therapist and ensure that the patient does not develop a faulty gait pattern such as walking on the heels in an attempt to avoid excessive pain or pressure. The nurse must reinforce the importance of walking with an erect posture and with proper weight distribution. Dysfunction of gait or continued pain should be reported to the physician. The nurse should instruct the patient on the importance of frequent rest periods with the foot elevated.

Ambulatory and Home Care. Foot care should include daily hygienic care and the wearing of clean stockings. Stockings should be long enough to avoid wrinkling and the development of pressure areas. Trimming toenails straight across helps prevent ingrown toenails and reduces the possibility of infection. Persons with impaired circulation or diabetes mellitus require detailed instruction to prevent serious complications associated with blisters, pressure areas, and infections. (See Table 47-21 for guidelines for foot care.)

■ Gerontologic Considerations: Foot Problems

The older adult is prone to developing foot problems because of poor circulation, atherosclerosis, and decreased sensation in the lower extremities. This is especially a problem for older patients with diabetes mellitus. A patient may develop an open wound but not feel it because of altered sensation. This may be the result of peripheral vascular disease or diabetic neuropathy. Older adults should be instructed to inspect their feet daily and report any open wounds or breaks in the skin to their physician. If left untreated, wounds may become infected, lead to osteomyelitis, and require surgical debridement. If the infection becomes widespread, lower limb amputation may be necessary.[27] ■

Metabolic Bone Diseases

Normal bone metabolism is affected by hormones, nutrition, and hereditary factors. When there is dysfunction in any of these factors, a generalized reduction in bone mass and strength may result. Metabolic bone diseases include osteomalacia, osteoporosis, and Paget's disease.

OSTEOMALACIA

Osteomalacia is a rare condition of adult bone associated with vitamin D deficiency, resulting in decalcification and softening of bone. This disease is the same as rickets in children except that the epiphyseal growth plates are closed in the adult. Vitamin D with its complex actions and method of synthesis is required for the absorption of calcium from the intestine. Insufficient vitamin D intake can interfere with the normal mineralization of bone, causing failure or insufficient calcification of bone, which results in bone softening. Etiologic factors in the development of osteomalacia include lack of exposure to ultraviolet rays (which is needed for vitamin D synthesis), gastrointestinal malabsorption, extensive burns, chronic diarrhea, pregnancy, kidney disease, and drugs such as phenytoin (Dilantin).

The most common clinical feature of osteomalacia is persistent skeletal pain, especially during weight bearing. Other clinical manifestations include low back and bone pain; progressive muscular weakness, especially in the pelvic girdle; weight loss; and progressive deformities of the spine (kyphosis) or extremities. Fractures are common and demonstrate delayed healing when they occur. Mineralization may take 2 to 3 months as opposed to the normal 6 to 10 days.[28]

Laboratory findings commonly associated with osteomalacia are decreased serum calcium or phosphorus levels, decreased 25-hydroxyvitamin D, and elevated serum alkaline phosphatase. X-rays may demonstrate the effects of generalized bone demineralization, especially loss of calcium in the bones of the pelvis and the presence of associated bone deformity. Looser's transformation zones (ribbons of decalcification in bone found on x-ray) are diagnostic of osteomalacia. However, significant osteomalacia may exist without demonstrable x-ray changes.

Collaborative care of osteomalacia is directed toward correction of the vitamin D deficiency. Vitamin D_3 (cholecalciferol) and vitamin D_2 (ergocalciferol) can be supplemented, and the patient often shows a dramatic response. Calcium salts or phosphorus supplements may also be prescribed. Dietary ingestion of eggs, low-fat milk, fish, and vegetables is encouraged. Exposure to sunlight (and ultraviolet rays) is also valuable, along with weight-bearing exercise.

OSTEOPOROSIS

Osteoporosis, or porous bone (fragile bone disease), is a chronic, progressive metabolic bone disease characterized by low bone mass and structural deterioration of bone tissue, leading to increased bone fragility (Fig. 62-7). At least 28 million persons in the United States have some degree of osteoporosis, and with the projected increase in life expectancy, this number is expected to grow. One in two women and one in eight men over the age of 50 will sustain an osteoporosis-related fracture during their lifetime. In the United States, the total cost of osteoporosis in terms of medical care, nursing home fees, and loss of income is estimated to exceed $13 billion. Osteoporosis is known as the "silent thief" because it slowly and insidiously over many years robs the skeleton of its banked resources. Bones can eventually become so fragile that they cannot withstand normal mechanical stress.[29]

Osteoporosis is 8 times more common in women than in men for several reasons: (1) women tend to have lower calcium intake than men throughout their lives (men between 15 and 50 years of age consume twice as much calcium as women); (2) women have less bone mass because of their generally smaller frame; (3) bone resorption begins at an earlier age in women and is accelerated at menopause; (4) pregnancy and breastfeeding deplete a woman's skeletal reserve unless calcium intake is adequate; and (5) longevity increases the likelihood of osteoporosis, and women live longer than men. Although osteoporosis is more common in women than men, it is important to realize that men can also develop osteoporosis.[30]

Etiology and Pathophysiology

Risk factors for osteoporosis are female gender, increasing age, family history of osteoporosis, white (European descent) or Asian race, small stature, early menopause, anorexia, oophorectomy, sedentary lifestyle, and insufficient dietary calcium. In-

CULTURAL & ETHNIC CONSIDERATIONS
Osteoporosis

- White and Asian American women have a higher incidence of osteoporosis than African American women.
- African American women have 10% more bone mass than non–African American women.
- Hispanic women have a lower incidence of osteoporosis than white women.
- Postmenopausal women are at the highest risk for osteoporosis regardless of ethnic group.

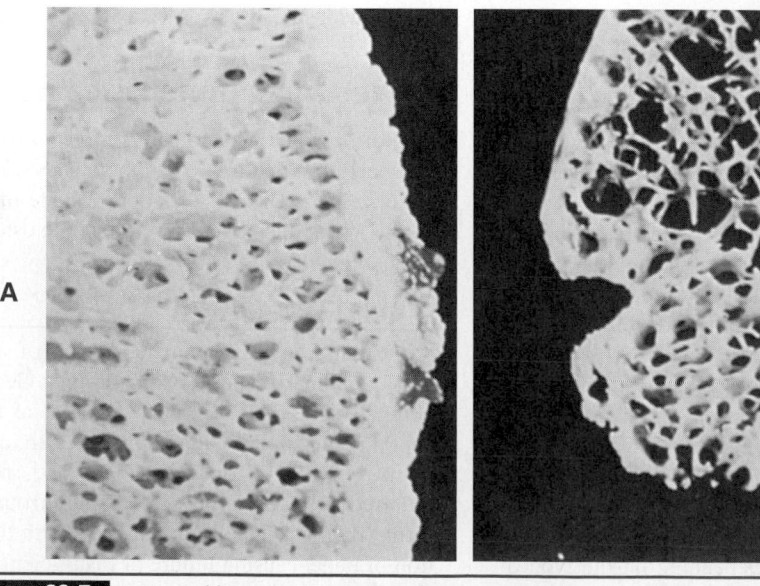

FIG. 62-7   A, Normal bone. B, Osteoporotic bone.

TABLE 62-11	Risk Factors for Osteoporosis

- Female gender
- Thin, small framed
- Family history of osteoporosis
- Diet low in calcium
- White or Asian ethnicity
- Excessive use of alcohol
- Cigarette smoking
- Inactive lifestyle
- Long-term use of corticosteroids, thyroid replacements, or antiseizure medications
- Postmenopausal, including early or surgically induced menopause
- History of anorexia nervosa or bulimia, chronic liver disease, or malabsorption

From National Osteoporosis Foundation: *Position paper: current perspectives on diagnosis, prevention, and treatment of osteoporosis,* Washington, DC, 1998, The Foundation.

creased risk is associated with cigarette smoking and alcoholism, and decreased risk is associated with regular weight-bearing exercise and fluoride and vitamin D ingestion.[31] Risk factors for osteoporosis are listed in Table 62-11. Low testosterone levels is a major risk factor in men.[30]

Peak bone mass (maximum bone tissue) is mainly achieved before age 20. It is determined by a combination of four major factors: hereditary, nutrition, exercise, and hormone function. Heredity may be responsible for up to 70% of a person's peak bone mass. Bone loss from midlife (age 35 to 40 years) onward is inevitable, but the rate of loss varies. At menopause, women experience rapid bone loss when the decline in estrogen production is the sharpest. This rate of loss then slows, and eventually matches the rate of bone lost by men 65 to 70 years old.

Bone is continually being deposited by osteoblasts and resorbed by osteoclasts, a process called remodeling. Normally the rates of bone deposition and resorption are equal to each other so that the total bone mass remains constant. In osteoporosis, bone resorption exceeds bone deposition. Although resorption affects the entire skeletal system, osteoporosis occurs most commonly in the bones of the spine, hips, and wrists. Over time, wedging and fractures of the vertebrae produce gradual loss of height and a humped back known as *"dowager's hump,"* or *kyphosis.* The usual first signs are back pain or spontaneous fractures.[32] The loss of bone substance causes the bone to become mechanically weakened and prone to either spontaneous fractures or fractures from minimal trauma.

Specific diseases associated with osteoporosis include intestinal malabsorption, kidney disease, rheumatoid arthritis, hyperthyroidism, advanced alcoholism, cirrhosis of the liver, hypogonadism, and diabetes mellitus.

Many drugs can interfere with bone metabolism, including corticosteroids, antiseizure drugs (e.g., valproate [Depakote], phenytoin [Dilantin]), aluminum-containing antacids, heparin, certain cancer treatments, and excessive thyroid hormones. At the time a drug is prescribed, the patient should be informed of this possible side effect.[33] Long-term corticosteroid use is a major contributor to osteoporosis. When a corticosteroid is taken, there is a disproportionate loss of bone resulting from the inhibition of new bone formation.

Clinical Manifestations

Osteoporosis is often called the "silent disease" because bone loss occurs without symptoms. People may not know they have osteoporosis until their bones become so weak that a sudden strain, bump, or fall causes a hip, vertebral, or wrist fracture. Collapsed vertebrae may initially be manifested as back pain, loss of height, or spinal deformities such as kyphosis or severely stooped posture.

Diagnostic Studies

Osteoporosis often goes unnoticed because it cannot be detected by conventional x-ray until more than 25% to 40% of calcium in the bone is lost. Serum calcium, phosphorus, and alkaline phosphatase levels usually are normal, although alkaline phosphatase may be elevated after a fracture. Bone mineral density (BMD) measurements are typically used to measure the bone density. BMD assesses the mass of bone per unit volume, or how tightly the bone is packed. (BMD measurements are presented in Table 60-7.) Quantitative ultrasound measures bone density with sound waves in the heel, kneecap, or shin.[34] One of the most common BMD studies is dual-energy x-ray absorptiometry (DEXA), which measures bone density in the spine, hips, and forearm (the most common sites of fractures resulting from osteoporosis). DEXA studies are also useful to evaluate changes in bone density over time and to assess the effectiveness of treatment. Bone biopsy is effective to differentiate the diagnosis of osteoporosis from osteomalacia.

NURSING *and* COLLABORATIVE MANAGEMENT OSTEOPOROSIS

Collaborative care of osteoporosis focuses on proper nutrition, calcium supplementation, exercise, prevention of fractures, and drugs (Table 62-12). Prevention and treatment of osteoporosis focuses on adequate calcium intake (1000 mg per day in pre-

TABLE 62-12	Collaborative Care Osteoporosis

Diagnostic
History and physical examination
Serum calcium, phosphorus, and alkaline phosphatase levels
Bone mineral densitometry
Dual energy x-ray absorptiometry (DEXA)
Quantitative ultrasound

Collaborative Therapy
Calcium supplements (see Table 62-14)
Diet high in calcium (see Table 62-13)
Vitamin D supplements
Exercise program
Estrogen replacement therapy
Bisphosphonates
    etidronate (Didronel)
    alendronate (Fosamax)
    raloxifene (Evista)
calcitonin (Calcimar)

menopausal women and postmenopausal women taking estrogen and 1500 mg per day in postmenopausal women who are not receiving supplemental estrogen). If dietary intake of calcium is inadequate, supplemental calcium should be taken.[35] Foods that are high in calcium content include whole and skim milk, yogurt, turnip greens, cottage cheese, ice cream, sardines, and spinach

TABLE 62-13   Nutritional Therapy — Sources of Calcium

FOOD	CALCIUM (MG)
1 cup milk	
Buttermilk	285
Chocolate	284
Whole	291
Low-fat	300
Skim	302
Half and half	254
Evaporated, canned	657
Egg nog	330
1 oz cheese	
American	174
Blue	150
Brie	52
Camembert	110
Cheddar	130
Cottage	130
Mozzarella	207
Parmesan	390
Swiss	272
8 oz yogurt	415
1 cup ice cream	176
Soft serve	272
3 oz seafood	
Salmon	167
Sardines with bones	372
Shrimp	98
Oysters	113
1 med stalk cooked broccoli	158
1 cup cooked spinach	200
1 cup cooked mustard greens	193
1 cup turnip greens	252
1 cup cooked collard greens with stems	289
1 cup bok choy	250
1 cup kale	206
Bonus Sources	
1 cup almonds	304
1 cup hazelnuts	240
1 tbs blackstrap molasses	137
Poor Sources	
Egg	28
1 cup cabbage	44
1 oz cream cheese	23
3 oz beef, pork, poultry	10
Apple, banana	10
½ grapefruit	20
1 med potato	14
1 med carrot	14
¼ head lettuce	27

TABLE 62-14   Elemental Calcium Content of Various Oral Calcium Preparations

CALCIUM PREPARATION	ELEMENTAL CALCIUM CONTENT
Calcium carbonate (Tums 500)	500 mg/tablet
Calcium carbonate + 5 μg vitamin D_2 (Os-Cal 250)	250 mg/tablet
Calcium gluconate	40 mg/500 mg
Calcium carbonate	400 mg/g
Calcium lactate	80 mg/600 mg
Calcium citrate	40 mg/300 mg

(Table 62-13). The amount of elemental calcium varies in different calcium preparations (Table 62-14). Calcium supplementation inhibits age-related bone loss; however, no new bone is formed.

Vitamin D is important in calcium absorption and function and may have a role in bone formation. Most people get enough vitamin D from the diet or naturally through synthesis in the skin from exposure to sunlight. However, supplemental vitamin D (400 to 800 IU) may be recommended for older adults, those who are homebound, and those who get minimal sun exposure.

Moderate amounts of exercise are important to build up and maintain bone mass. Exercise also increases muscle strength, coordination, and balance. The best exercises are weight-bearing exercises that force an individual to work against gravity. These exercises include walking, hiking, weight training, stair climbing, tennis, and dancing. Walking is preferred to high-impact aerobics or running, both of which may put too much stress on the bones of patients with osteoporosis. Walking 30 minutes, three times a week, is recommended.

Cigarette smoking and excess alcohol intake are risk factors for osteoporosis. Regular consumption of 2 to 3 ounces of alcohol a day may increase the degree of osteoporosis, even in young men and women. Patients should be instructed to quit smoking and cut down on alcohol intake to decrease the likelihood of losing bone mass.

Although loss of bone cannot be significantly reversed, further loss can be prevented if the patient follows a regimen of calcium and vitamin D supplementation, exercise, estrogen replacement, and alendronate (Fosamax) or raloxifene (Evista), if indicated. Efforts should be made to keep patients with osteoporosis ambulatory to prevent further loss of bone substance as a result of immobility. Treatment also involves protecting areas of potential pathologic fractures; for example, a corset can be used to prevent vertebral collapse.

■ **Drug Therapy**

Estrogen replacement therapy after menopause is used to prevent osteoporosis. Although the exact mechanism for the protective function of estrogen is not known, it is believed that estrogen inhibits osteoclast activity, leading to decreased bone resorption and preventing both cortical and trabecular bone loss. Estrogen replacement therapy is most effective when combined with calcium (see Table 62-14). The greatest benefit of estrogen is probably in the first 10 years after menopause. Transdermal estrogen treatment has been shown to be effective in the treatment of postmenopausal

EVIDENCE-BASED PRACTICE
Osteoporosis

Clinical Problem

In postmenopausal women with osteoporosis, what is the effectiveness of parathyroid hormone (PTH) in decreasing fracture rates and increasing bone mineral density (BMD)?

Best Clinical Practice

- In postmenopausal women with osteoporosis, PTH decreases the development of new fractures and increases BMD.

Implications for Nursing Practice

- PTH stimulates the growth of new bone
- PTH therapy offers a different approach from other osteoporosis treatments currently available.
- Serum calcium levels and bone density should be periodically assessed during therapy with PTH.

Reference for Evidence

EBM Reviews: Parathyroid hormone decreased fracture rates and increased bone mineral density in postmenopausal women, *ACP Journal Club* 135:95, November/December 2001.

women with established osteoporosis. (See Chapter 52 for further discussion of estrogen replacement therapy.)

Calcitonin is secreted by the thyroid gland and inhibits osteoclastic bone resorption by directly interacting with active osteoclasts. Calcitonin (Calcimar) is available in intramuscular, subcutaneous, and intranasal forms. The nasal form is easy to administer, and patients should be taught to alternate nostrils daily. Nasal dryness and irritation are the most frequent side effects. Administration of the intramuscular or subcutaneous form of the drug at night has been shown to decrease the side effects of nausea and facial flushing. Nausea does not occur with the nasal spray. When calcitonin is used, calcium supplementation is necessary to prevent secondary hyperparathyroidism.[36]

Bisphosphonates inhibit osteoclast-mediated bone resorption, thereby increasing BMD and total bone mass. This group of drugs includes etidronate (Didronel), alendronate (Fosamax), pamidronate (Aredia), risedronate (Actonel), clodronate (Bonefos), and tiludronate (Skelid). Common side effects are anorexia, weight loss, and gastritis. The most commonly used bisphosphonate drug in treating osteoporosis is alendronate. Patients should be instructed on the proper administration of alendronate to aid in its absorption.[36] It should be taken after rising in the morning with a full glass of water. The patient should not eat or drink anything for 30 minutes after taking it. The patient should also be instructed not to lie down after taking the drug. These precautions have shown to decrease gastrointestinal side effects (especially esophageal irritation) and increase absorption. Alendronate is available as a once-per-week oral tablet.

Another type of drug used in treating osteoporosis is selective estrogen receptor modulators, such as raloxifene (Evista). These drugs mimic the effect of estrogen on bone by reducing bone resorption without stimulating the tissues of the breast or uterus. Raloxifene in postmenopausal women significantly increases BMD.[37] The most commonly reported side effects are leg cramps and hot flashes.

Teriparatide (Forteo) is used for the treatment of osteoporosis in men and postmenopausal women who are at high risk for having a fracture. Teriparatide is a portion of human parathyroid hormone (PTH) and works by increasing the action of osteoblasts. Teriparatide is the first drug approved for the treatment of osteoporosis that stimulates new bone formation. Most drugs used to treat osteoporosis prevent further bone loss. Teriparatide is administered by subcutaneous injection once a day.

Medical management of patients receiving corticosteroids includes prescribing the lowest possible dose of the drug, as well as calcium and vitamin D supplementation. If osteopenia is evident on bone densitometry, treatment with bisphosphonate agents, such as alendronate (Fosamax), should be considered.

PAGET'S DISEASE

Paget's disease *(osteitis deformans)* is a skeletal bone disorder in which there is excessive bone resorption followed by replacement of normal marrow by vascular, fibrous connective tissue. The new bone is larger, disorganized, and structurally weaker. The regions of the skeleton commonly affected are the pelvis, long bones, spine, ribs, sternum, and cranium. The etiology of Paget's disease is unknown, although a viral cause has been proposed.[38] Up to 40% of all patients with Paget's disease have at least one relative with the disorder. Men are affected 2:1 over women, and Paget's disease is rarely seen in persons under 40 years of age.

In milder forms of Paget's disease, patients may remain free of symptoms, and the disease may be discovered incidentally on x-ray or serum chemistry. The initial clinical manifestations are usually insidious development of bone pain (which may progress to severe intractable pain), complaints of fatigue, and progressive development of a waddling gait. Patients may complain that they are becoming shorter or that their heads are becoming larger. Headaches, dementia, visual deficits, and loss of hearing can result with an enlarged, thickened skull. Increased bone volume in the spine can cause spinal cord or nerve root compression. Pathologic fracture is the most common complication of Paget's disease and may be the first indication of the disease. Other complications include malignant osteosarcoma, fibrosarcoma, and osteoclastoma (giant cell) tumors.

Serum alkaline phosphatase levels are markedly elevated (indicating high bone turnover) in advanced forms of the disease. X-rays may demonstrate that the normal contour of the affected bone is curved and the bone cortex is thickened and irregular, especially the weight-bearing bones and cranium. Bone scans using a radiolabeled biphosphate demonstrate increased uptake in the skeletal areas affected.

Collaborative care of Paget's disease is usually limited to symptomatic and supportive care and correction of secondary deformities by either surgical intervention or braces. Bone resorption, relief of acute symptoms, and lowering the serum alkaline phosphatase levels may be significantly influenced by the administration of calcitonin (Cibacalcin), which inhibits osteoclastic activity. Response to calcitonin therapy is not permanent and often stops when therapy is discontinued. Bisphosphonate drugs including risedronate (Actonel), etidronate (Didronel), pamidronate (Aredia), tiludronate (Skelid), and alendronate (Fosamax) are also used to retard bone resorption.[39] Calcium and vitamin D are often given to decrease hypocalcemia, a common side effect with these drugs. Drug effectiveness may be monitored by serum alkaline phosphatase levels. Salmon calcitonin (Calcimar) is recommended for patients who cannot tolerate bisphosphonate drugs.

Pain is usually managed by NSAIDs (acetaminophen), and the COX-2 inhibitor drugs (e.g., celecoxib [Celebrex]). Orthopedic surgery for fractures, hip and knee replacements, and knee re-alignment may be necessary.

A firm mattress should be used to provide back support and to relieve pain. The patient may be required to wear a corset or light brace to relieve back pain and provide support when in the up-right position. The patient should be proficient in the correct ap-plication of such devices and know how to regularly examine ar-eas of the skin for friction damage. Activities such as lifting and twisting should be discouraged. Physical therapy may increase muscle strength. Good body mechanics are essential. A properly balanced nutritional program is important in the management of metabolic disorders of bone, especially pertaining to vitamin D, calcium, and protein, which are necessary to ensure the avail-ability of the components for bone formation. Prevention mea-sures such as patient education, use of an assistive device, and environmental changes should be actively pursued to prevent falls and subsequent fractures.

■ Gerontologic Considerations: Metabolic Bone Diseases

Osteoporosis and Paget's disease are common in older adults. Patients should be instructed in proper nutritional man-agement to prevent further bone loss such as that occurring from osteoporosis.

Because metabolic bone disorders increase the possibility of pathologic fractures, the nurse must use extreme caution when the patient is turned or moved. It is important to keep the patient as ac-tive as possible to retard demineralization of bone resulting from dis-use or extended immobilization. A supervised exercise program is an essential part of the treatment program. If the patient's condition permits, ambulation without causing fatigue must be encouraged. ■

CRITICAL THINKING EXERCISES

Case Study
Osteoporosis

Patient Profile. Rose Tan is a 56-year-old Asian American li-brarian who had a total hysterectomy and salpingo-oophorectomy for removal of a benign ovarian cyst 4 years ago.

Subjective Data
- Experiences chronic, mild lumbar pain and tenderness that radiates to her right hip and the lateral thigh
- Regular walking offers some relief
- Had a stress fracture in wrist 6 months ago
- Reports no noticeable loss of height
- Has maternal history of osteoporosis
- Has been taking corticosteroids for past 6 years for Addison's disease
- Drinks socially—two alcoholic beverages per day
- Dislikes dairy products

Objective Data
- 5 feet 6 inches tall, 116 lb

Diagnostic Studies
- Bone mass/density tests show decreased bone mineral density at spine and hip
- Laboratory tests reveal normal serum calcium, phosphorus, and alkaline phosphatase levels

Collaborative Care
- Premarin 0.625 mg PO daily
- Alendronate (Fosamax) 70 mg once/wk
- Calcium supplements 1200 mg PO daily
- High-calcium diet
- Reduce alcohol intake
- Maintain regular exercise program

CRITICAL THINKING QUESTIONS

1. What risk factors made Rose prone to develop osteoporosis?
2. Why does regular exercise help Rose's symptoms?
3. What is the purpose of prescribing estrogen replacement for Rose?
4. What teaching should the nurse provide to Rose regard-ing alendronate?
5. How might the nurse assist Rose in increasing her intake of calcium?
6. Based on the assessment data presented, write one or more nursing diagnoses. Are there any collaborative problems?

Nursing Research Issues

1. What factors are important for the nurse to address in helping an adolescent female increase her calcium intake?
2. What are the differences in pain management in the ado-lescent patient with Ewing's sarcoma compared with the adult patient with osteosarcoma?
3. How does patient teaching regarding back care and exer-cise affect the long-tern outcomes for chronic low back pain?
4. What are the risks of postoperative complications on laminectomy patients who are hospitalized versus those who have same-day procedures?
5. How can nurses best influence the footwear purchase of urban and rural young adult women related to heel height and toe box configuration?

REVIEW QUESTIONS

The number of the question corresponds to the same-numbered objective at the beginning of the chapter.

1. A patient with osteomyelitis is treated with surgical debridement followed by continuous irrigation of the affected bone with antibiotics. In responding to the patient who asks why oral or IV antibiotics cannot be used alone, the nurse explains that
   a. the irrigation is necessary to wash out dead tissue and pus from the infected area.
   b. the ischemia and bone death associated with osteomyelitis are frequently impenetrable to most blood-borne antibiotics.
   c. there are no effective oral or IV antibiotics to treat *S. aureus,* the most common cause of osteomyelitis.
   d. an irrigation can penetrate involucrum created by the infection and prevent bacterial spreading to other tissue.

2. A patient with an osteogenic sarcoma of the left femur has a nursing diagnosis of risk for injury (pathologic fracture) related to bone tissue changes. The nursing management of this patient is primarily directed toward
   a. preventing pain.
   b. relieving edema.
   c. increasing physical mobility.
   d. supporting and positioning the leg.

3. In identifying people at risk for back injuries, the nurse recognizes that the person at greatest risk for low back pain is a(n)
   a. long-distance truck driver.
   b. 62-year-old widow who walks daily.
   c. aerobics instructor who weighs 100 lb.
   d. 25-year-old nurse who works in a newborn nursery.

4. The primary nursing responsibility in caring for a patient with acute low back pain associated with severe pain and muscle spasms is
   a. teaching exercises such as straight-leg raises to decrease pain.
   b. positioning the patient on the abdomen with the legs extended.
   c. providing pain medication to promote exercise and ambulation.
   d. assisting the patient to maintain activity restrictions with a gradual increase in activity.

5. In caring for the patient after a spinal fusion, the nurse recognizes that interventions for this surgery differ from a simple laminectomy in that
   a. body alignment is maintained by the fusion procedure.
   b. earlier ambulation is permitted because the spine is more stabilized.
   c. the donor site for the bone graft may be more painful than the spinal incision.
   d. teaching regarding body mechanics and prevention of future back injuries is not as critical.

6. Before discharge from the same-day surgery unit, the nurse instructs the patient who has had a surgical correction of bilateral hallux valgus to
   a. rest frequently with the feet elevated.
   b. soak the feet in warm water several times a day.
   c. walk primarily on the heels to relieve pressure on the toes.
   d. expect the feet to be numb for several days postoperatively.

7. The nurse advises the patient with early osteoporosis to
   a. lose weight.
   b. stop smoking.
   c. eat a high-protein diet.
   d. start swimming for exercise.

REFERENCES

1. Breuninger C, Wittig P, editors: *Disease,* ed 3, Springhouse, Pa, 2001, Springhouse.
2. Schoen D: *Adult orthopaedic nursing,* Philadelphia, 2000, JB Lippincott.
3. Darville T, Jacobs R: Acute osteomyelitis in children: intervening for early control, *J Musculoskeletal Med* 16:49, 1999.
4. Tehranzadeh J et al: Imaging of osteomyelitis in the mature skeleton, *Radiol Clin North Am* 39:223, 2001.
5. DiPasquale D: Chronic osteomyelitis in adults: aggressive management required, *J Musculoskeletal Med* 17:250, 2000.
6. Roeder B et al: Antibiotic beads in the treatment of diabetic pedal osteomyelitis, *J Foot Ankle Surgery* 39:124, 2000.
7. Jemal A et al: Cancer statistics 2002, *CA Cancer J Clinicians* 52:23, 2002.
8. Barrick M, Mitchell S: Multiple myeloma, *AJN* 11(suppl):4, 2001.
9. Bridge J et al: Sarcomas of bone. In Abcloff M, Lichter A, Niederhuber J, editors: *Clinical oncology,* ed 2, New York, 2000, Livingstone.
10. Kelley C, Thomas R: Osteogenic sarcoma. In Miaskowski C, Buchsel P, editors: *Oncology nursing: assessment and clinical care,* St Louis, 1999, Mosby.
11. Haynes K: Tumors of the musculoskeletal system. In Schoen, D. editor: *Core curriculum for orthopaedic nursing,* ed 4, Pitman, NJ, 2001, Jannetti.
12. Pinkerton C et al: Treatment strategies for metastatic Ewing's sarcoma, *Eur J Cancer* 37:1338, 2001.
13. Ruyman F, Grovas A: Progress in the diagnosis and treatment of rhabdomyosarcoma and related soft tissue sarcomas, *Cancer Invest* 18:223, 2000.
14. Coleman R et al: Bone metastases. In Abeloff M, Lichter A, Niederhuber J, editors: *Clinical oncology,* ed 2, New York, 2000, Livingstone.
15. Hayes K: Neoplasms of the musculoskeletal system. In Maher AB, Salmond SW, Pellino TA, editors: *Orthopaedic nursing,* ed 3, Philadelphia, 2002, WB Saunders.
16. Mason K: Pediatric and congenital disorders. In Schoen D, editor: *Core curriculum for orthopaedic nursing,* ed 4, Pitman, NJ, 2001, Jannetti.
17. Alexander M: Congenital and developmental disorders. In Maher AB, Salmond SW, Pellino TA, editors: *Orthopedic nursing,* ed 3, Philadelphia, 2002, WB Saunders.
18. Deyo R, Weinstein J: Low back pain, *N Engl J Med* 344:363, 2001.
19. Andersson G: Epidemiologic features of chronic low back pain, *Lancet* 354:581, 1999.
20. Katz J: Controlling pain: getting the low down on back pain, *Nursing 2001* 31:24, 2001.
21. Stein R: An overview of the lumbar spine. In *An introduction to orthopaedic nursing,* ed 2, Pitman, NJ, 1999, Jannetti.
22. Dawson E, Bernbeck J: The surgical management of low back pain, *Phys Med Rehabil Clin North Am* 9:489, 1999.
23. Hellmann D, Stone J: Arthritis and musculoskeletal disorders. In Tierney L et al, editors: *Current medical diagnosis and treatment 2001,* ed 40, New York, 2001, Lange/McGraw-Hill.

24. Choy D: Percutaneous laser disc decompression: twelve years' experience with 752 procedures in 518 patients, *J Clin Laser Surg* 16:325, 1998.

25. Food and Drug Administration: FDA approves first device to utilize genetically engineered protein to treat degenerative disc disease. FDA Talk Paper [on-line]. Available at *www.fda.gov/bbs/topics* (accessed Aug 8, 2002).

26. Chou L: Disorders of the metatarsophalangeal joint: diagnosis of great-toe pain, *Physician Sportsmed* 28:32, 2000.

27. Findlow A et al: The management of diabetic foot ulcers, *Diabetic Foot* 4:112, 2001.

28. Pacala J: Osteoporosis and osteomalacia, *Clin Geriat* 8:13, 2000.

29. Turner L et al: Osteoporosis diagnosis and fracture, *Orthop Nurs* 18:5, 1999.

30. Tsitouras P et al: Equal time for the older male, *Annals Long-Term Care* 9:15, 2001.

31. Curry L, Hogstel M: Osteoporosis, *AJN* 102:26, 2002.

32. Burke S: Boning up on osteoporosis, *Nursing* 31:36, 2001.

33. Field-Munves E: Evidence-based decisions for the treatment of osteoporosis, *Annals Long-Term Care* 9:3, 2001.

34. Overdorf J et al: Osteoporosis: there's so much we can do, *RN* 64:30, 2001.

35. Taft L et al: Osteoporosis: a disease management opportunity, *Orthop Nurs* 19:2, 2000.

36. Capriotti T: Pharmacologic prevention and treatment of osteoporosis in women, *Med Surg Nurs* 9:2, 2000.

37. McCoy PW: Pharmacologic management of osteoporosis, *Topics Geriatr Rehabil* 17:38, 2001.

38. Helfrich MH et al: A negative search for a paramyxoviral etiology of Paget's disease of bone: molecular, immunological, and ultrastructural studies in UK patients, *J Bone Miner Res* 15:2315, 2000.

39. Vasikaran S: Biphosphates: an overview with special reference to alendronate, *Ann Clin Biochem* 38:608, 2001.

RESOURCES

American Academy of Orthopedic Surgeons (AAOS)
6300 North River Road
Rosemont, IL 60018-4262
800-346-AAOS or 847-823-7186
Fax: 847-823-8125
www.aaos.org

American Cancer Society
1599 Clifton Road, NE
Atlanta, GA 30329-4251
800-ACS-2345
www.cancer.org

American College of Foot and Ankle Surgeons
515 Busse Highway
Park Ridge, IL 60068
847-292-2237 or 800-421-2237
www.acfas.org

American College of Sports Medicine
P.O. Box 1440
401 W Michigan Street
Indianapolis, IN 46202
317-637-9200
Fax: 317-634-7817
www.acsm.org

American Orthopedic Foot and Ankle Society
2517 Eastlake Avenue East
Seattle, WA 98102
206-223-1120
Fax: 206-223-1178
www.aofas.org

American Podiatric Medical Association
9312 Old Georgetown Road
Bethesda, MD 20814
800-ASK-APMA or 301-571-9200
Fax: 301-530-2752
www.apma.org

Calcium Information Center
Oregon Health Sciences University
1221 SW Yamwill, Suite 303
Portland, OR 97205
800-321-2681

Cancer Survivors Network
800-333-HOPE (4673)
www.acscsn.org

Muscular Dystrophy Association
National Headquarters
3300 East Sunrise Drive
Tucson, AZ 85718
800-572-1717
www.mdausa.org

National Arthritis and Musculoskeletal and Skin Diseases
Information Clearinghouse, National Institutes of Health
1 AMS Circle
Bethesda, MD 20892-3675
877-22-NIAMS or 301-495-4484
Fax: 301-718-6366
www.nih.gov/niams

National Association of Orthopaedic Nurses (NAON)
Box 56
Pitman, NJ 08071
856-256-2310
Fax: 856-589-7463
http://naon.inurse.com

National Easter Seal Society
230 West Monroe Street, Suite 1800
Chicago, IL 60606
800-221-6827 or 312-726-6200
Fax: 312-726-1494
www.easter-seals.org

National Institutes of Health, Osteoporosis, and Related Bone Diseases—National Resource Center
1232 22nd Street NW
Washington, DC 20037-1292
800-624-BONE or 202-223-0644
Fax: 202-293-2356
www.osteo.org

National Osteoporosis Foundation
1232 22nd Street NW
Washington, DC 20037-1292
800-223-9994 or 202-223-2226
www.nof.org

Older Women's League
666 Eleventh Street SW, Suite 700
Washington, DC 20001
800-TAKE-OWL or 202-783-6686
Fax: 202-638-2356
www.owl-national.org

Osteoporosis Society of Canada
33 Laird Drive
Toronto, ON
M4G 3S9 Canada
416-696-2663
Fax: 416-696-2673
www.osteoporosis.ca

The Paget Foundation for Paget's Disease of Bone and Related Disorders
120 Wall Street, Suite 1602
New York, NY 10005-4001
800-23-PAGET or 212-509-5335
Fax: 212-509-8492
www.paget.org

For additional Internet resources, see the website for this book at *http://www.evolve.elsevier.com/Lewis/medsurg/*.

CHAPTER *63*
NURSING MANAGEMENT
Arthritis and Connective Tissue Diseases

Dottie Roberts

LEARNING OBJECTIVES

1. Compare and contrast the sequence of events leading to joint destruction in osteoarthritis and rheumatoid arthritis.
2. Describe the clinical manifestations, collaborative care, and nursing management of osteoarthritis and rheumatoid arthritis.
3. Compare and contrast the pathophysiology, clinical manifestations, collaborative care, and nursing management of ankylosing spondylitis, psoriatic arthritis, and Reiter syndrome.
4. Describe the pathophysiology, clinical manifestations, and collaborative care of septic arthritis, Lyme disease, and gout.
5. Describe the pathophysiology, clinical manifestations, collaborative care, and nursing management of systemic lupus erythematosus, polymyositis, dermatomyositis, and Sjögren syndrome.
6. Describe the drug therapy and related nursing management associated with arthritis and connective tissue diseases.
7. Compare and contrast the possible etiologies, clinical manifestations, and collaborative and nursing management of myofascial pain syndrome, fibromyalgia syndrome, and chronic fatigue syndrome.

KEY TERMS

ankylosing spondylitis, p. 1734
chronic fatigue syndrome, p. 1751
CREST syndrome, p. 1745
dermatomyositis, p. 1746
fibromyalgia syndrome, p. 1749
gout, p. 1737
Lyme disease, p. 1736
myofascial pain syndrome, p. 1748
osteoarthritis, p. 1715

polymyositis, p. 1746
Raynaud's phenomenon, p. 1745
Reiter syndrome, p. 1735
rheumatoid arthritis, p. 1724
septic arthritis, p. 1735
Sjögren syndrome, p. 1748
spondyloarthropathies, p. 1733
systemic lupus erythematosus, p. 1739
systemic sclerosis, p. 1744

OSTEOARTHRITIS

Osteoarthritis (OA), the most common form of joint (articular) disease in North America, is a slowly progressive noninflammatory disorder of the diarthrodial (synovial) joints. Previously identified as *degenerative joint disease*, it is now known to involve the formation of new joint tissue in response to cartilage destruction.[1]

Although OA is no longer considered to be a normal part of the aging process, growing older continues to be the most consistently identified risk factor for disease development.[2] Cartilage destruction can actually begin between ages 20 and 30, and more than 90% of adults are affected by age 40. Few patients experience symptoms until after age 60, but as many as 60% of those over 65 years of age have symptomatic disease. Before the age of 50, men are more often affected than women. However, the incidence of OA after age 50 is twice as great in women as in men.[3]

Etiology and Pathophysiology

OA may occur as an idiopathic (formerly primary) or secondary disorder.[4] The cause of idiopathic OA is unknown. Secondary OA, on the other hand, is caused by a known event or condition that directly damages cartilage or causes joint instability (Table 63-1).

TABLE 63-1	Causes of Secondary Osteoarthritis	
CAUSE	**EFFECTS ON JOINT CARTILAGE**
Trauma	Dislocations or fractures may lead to avascular necrosis or uneven stress on cartilage.
Mechanical stress	Repetitive physical activities (e.g., sports activities) cause cartilage deterioration.
Inflammation	Release of enzymes in response to local inflammation can affect cartilage integrity.
Joint instability	Damage to supporting structures causes instability, placing uneven stress on articular cartilage.
Neurologic disorders	Pain and loss of reflexes from neurologic disorders, such as diabetic neuropathy, and Charcot joint cause abnormal movements that contribute to cartilage deterioration.
Skeletal deformities	Congenital or acquired conditions such as Legg-Calvé-Perthes disease or dislocated hip contribute to cartilage deterioration.
Hematologic/endocrine disorders	Chronic hemarthrosis (e.g., hemophilia) can contribute to cartilage deterioration.
Use of selected drugs	Drugs such as indomethacin (Indocin), colchicine, and corticosteroids can stimulate collagen-digesting enzymes in joint synovium.

Reviewed by Sharon G. Childs, RN, MS, CRNP-CS, ONC, CEN, Adult Nurse Practitioner, Orthopedic Clinical Specialist, Concentra Medical Center, Baltimore, Md.

Researchers have been unable to identify a single cause for OA, but a number of factors have been linked to disease development. The increased incidence of OA in aging women is believed to be due to estrogen reduction at menopause. Genetic factors also appear to play a significant role in the occurrence of OA. Modifiable risk factors have been identified, including obesity, which contributes to knee OA. Regular moderate exercise, which also helps with weight control, has been shown to decrease the likelihood of disease development and progression. On the other hand, strenuous exercise through activities such as football and soccer has been linked to an increased risk of OA.

OA results from cartilage damage that triggers a metabolic response at the level of the chondrocytes (Fig. 63-1). Progression of OA causes the normally smooth, white, translucent articular cartilage to become dull, yellow, and granular. Affected cartilage gradually becomes softer, less elastic, and less able to resist wear with heavy use. The body's attempts at cartilage repair cannot keep up with the destruction that is occurring. Continued changes in the collagen structure of the cartilage lead to fissuring, fibrillation, and erosion of the articular surfaces. As the central cartilage becomes thinner, cartilage and bony growth (osteophytes) increase at the joint margins. The resulting incongruity in joint surfaces creates an uneven distribution of stress across the joint and contributes to a reduction in motion.

While inflammation is not characteristic of OA, a secondary synovitis may result when phagocytic cells try to rid the joint of small pieces of cartilage torn from the joint surface. These inflammatory changes contribute to the early pain and stiffness of OA. The pain of later disease results from contact between exposed bony joint surfaces after the articular cartilage has completely deteriorated.

Clinical Manifestations

Systemic. Systemic manifestations, such as fatigue or fever, are not present in OA. Organ involvement is also absent, marking an important distinction between OA and inflammatory joint disorders such as rheumatoid arthritis.

Joints. Manifestations of OA range from mild discomfort to significant disability. Joint pain is the predominant symptom of OA and the typical reason that the patient seeks medical attention. Pain generally worsens with joint use. In the early stages of OA, joint pain is relieved by rest. In advanced disease, however, the patient may complain of pain with rest or experience sleep disruptions caused by increasing joint discomfort. Pain may also become worse as barometric pressures fall before inclement weather. As OA progresses, increasing pain can contribute significantly to disability and loss of function. The pain of OA may be referred to the groin, buttock, or medial side of the thigh or

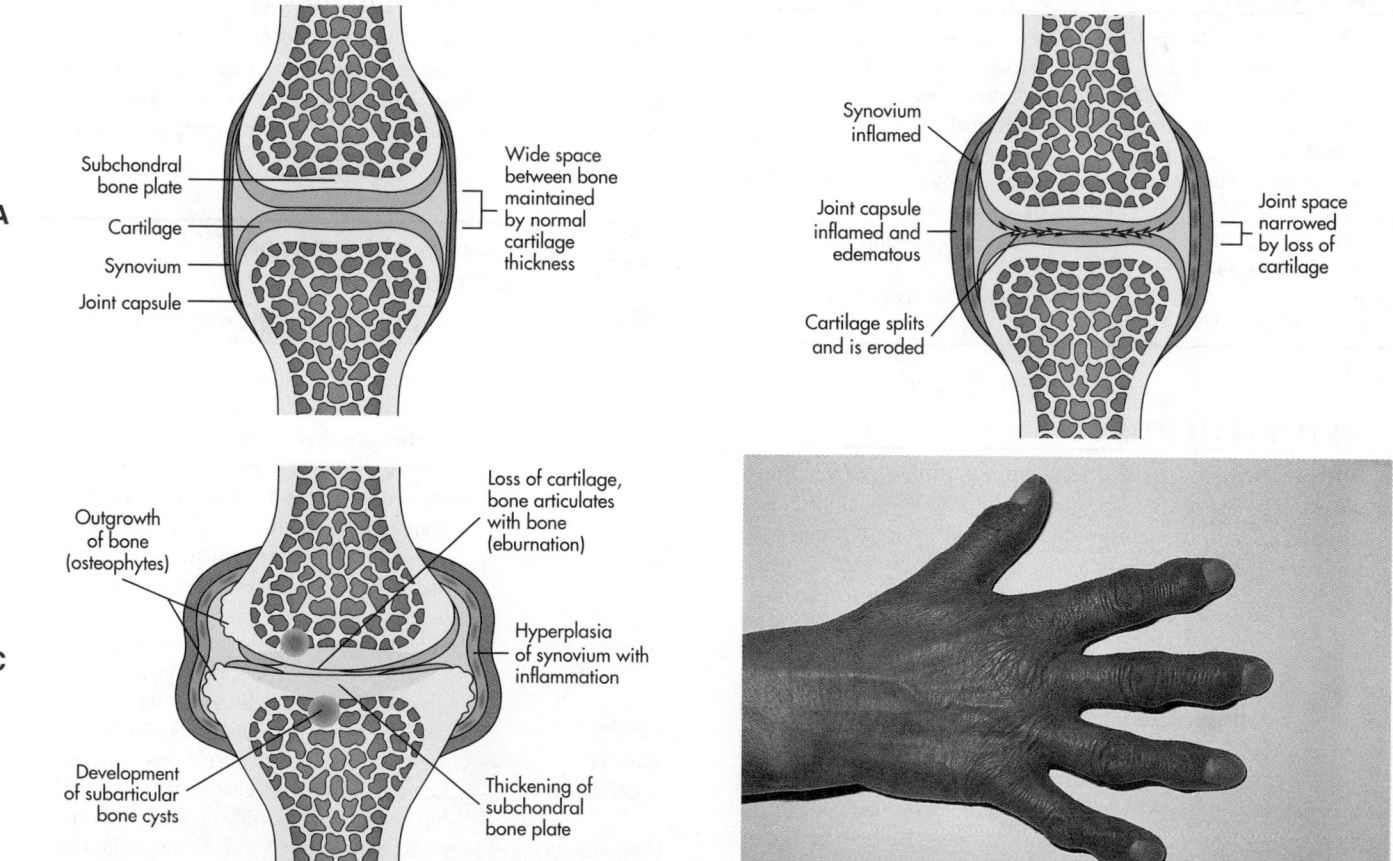

FIG. 63-1 Pathologic changes in osteoarthritis. **A,** Normal synovial joint. **B,** Early change in osteoarthritis is destruction of articular cartilage and narrowing of the joint space on x-ray. There is inflammation and thickening of the joint capsule and synovium. **C,** With time, there is thickening of subarticular bone caused by constant friction of the two bone surfaces, leading to a highly polished bony articular surface. Osteophytes form around the periphery of the joint by irregular outgrowths of bone. **D,** In osteoarthritis of the hands, osteophytes on the interphalangeal joints of the fingers are termed Heberden's nodes and appear as small nodules.

knee. Sitting down becomes difficult, as does rising from a chair when the hips are lower than the knees. As OA develops in the intervertebral (apophyseal) joints of the spine, localized pain and stiffness are common.

Unlike pain, which is typically provoked by activity, joint stiffness occurs after periods of rest or static position. Early morning stiffness is common but generally resolves within 30 minutes, a factor distinguishing OA from inflammatory arthritic disorders. Overactivity can cause a mild joint effusion that temporarily increases stiffness. *Crepitation,* a grating sensation caused by loose particles of cartilage in the joint cavity, can also contribute to stiffness. Crepitation indicates the loss of cartilage integrity and is present in more than 90% of patients with knee OA.

OA usually affect joints asymmetrically. The most commonly involved joints are the distal interphalangeal (DIP) and proximal interphalangeal (PIP) joints of the fingers, the carpometacarpal joint of the thumb, weight-bearing joints (hips, knees), the metatarsophalangeal (MTP) joint of the foot, and the cervical and lower lumbar vertebrae (Fig. 63-2).

Deformity. Deformity or instability associated with OA is specific to the involved joint. For example, *Heberden's nodes* occur on the DIP joints as an indication of osteophyte formation and loss of joint space (see Fig. 63-1). They can appear in the OA patient as early as age 40 and tend to be seen in family members. *Bouchard's nodes* on the PIP joints indicate similar disease involvement. Heberden's and Bouchard's nodes are often red, swollen, and tender. Although these bony enlargements do not usually cause significant loss of function, the patient may be distressed by the visible disfigurement.

Knee OA often leads to joint malalignment as a result of cartilage loss in the medial compartment. The patient has a characteristic bow-legged appearance and may develop an altered gait in response to the obvious deformity. In advanced hip OA, one of the patient's legs may become shorter from a loss of joint space.

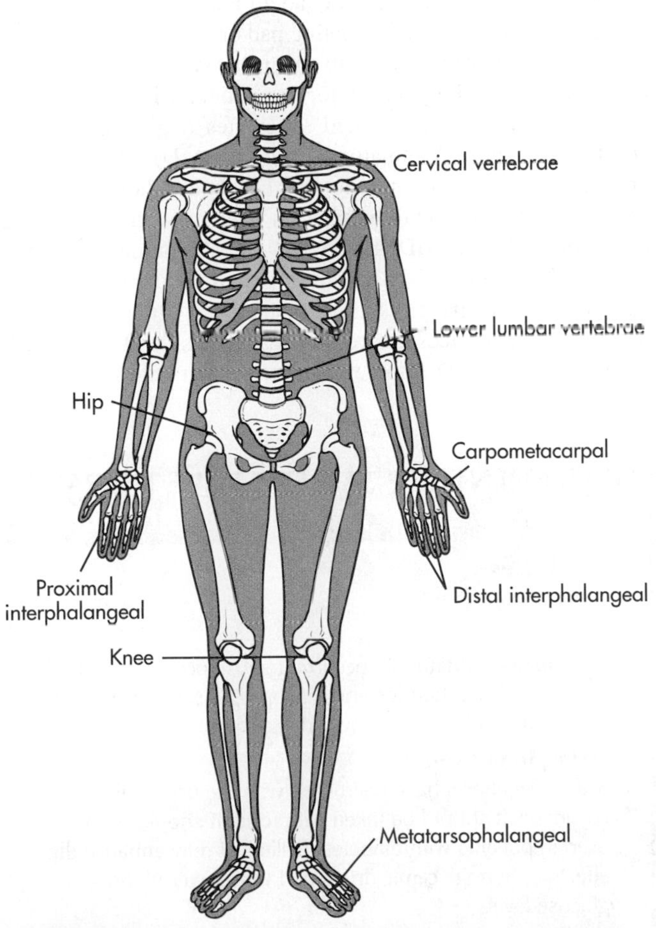

Diagnostic Studies

A bone scan, computed tomography scan, or magnetic resonance imaging may be useful in early OA because of the sensitivity of these tests to joint changes. X-rays are helpful in confirming disease and monitoring the effectiveness of treatment. As OA progresses, x-rays typically show joint space narrowing, bony sclerosis, and osteophyte formation. However, these changes do not always correlate with the degree of pain experienced by the patient. Despite significant radiologic indications of disease, the patient may be relatively free of symptoms. Conversely, another patient may have severe pain with only minimal x-ray changes.

No laboratory abnormalities are a specific diagnostic indicator of OA. The erythrocyte sedimentation rate (ESR) is normal except in instances of acute synovitis, when minimal elevations may be noted. Other routine blood tests (e.g., complete blood count [CBC], renal and liver function tests) are useful only in screening for related conditions or for establishing baseline values before the initiation of therapy. Synovial fluid analysis allows differentiation between OA and other forms of inflammatory arthritis. In the presence of OA, the fluid remains clear yellow with little or no sign of inflammation.

Collaborative Care

Because there is no cure for OA, collaborative care focuses on managing pain and inflammation, preventing disability, and maintaining and improving joint function (Table 63-2). Nonpharmacologic interventions are the foundation for OA management and

FIG. 63-2 Joints most frequently involved in osteoarthritis.

TABLE 63-2	Collaborative Care Osteoarthritis
Diagnostic	
History and physical examination	
Radiologic studies of involved joints	
Synovial fluid analysis	
Collaborative Therapy	
Nutritional counseling	
Rest and joint protection, use of assistive devices	
Therapeutic exercise	
Heat and cold	
Complementary and alternative therapies	
Herbal products	
Movement therapies	
Nutritional supplements	
Drug therapy*	
Acetaminophen	
Nonsteroidal antiinflammatory drugs	
Intraarticular hyaluronic acid	
Reconstructive surgery	

*See Table 63-3.

should be maintained throughout the patient's treatment period. Drug therapy serves as an adjunct to nonpharmacologic treatments. Symptoms of disease are often managed conservatively for many years, but the patient's loss of joint function, unrelieved pain, and diminished ability to independently perform self-care may prompt a recommendation for surgery. Reconstructive surgical procedures are discussed in Chapter 61. In general, arthroscopic surgery for debridement is usually not recommended for OA. However, arthroscopic surgery to repair cartilage or ligament tears or remove bone bits or cartilage is effective.[5]

Rest and Joint Protection. The OA patient must understand the importance of a balance of rest and activity. The affected joint should be rested during any periods of acute inflammation and maintained in a functional position with splints or braces if necessary. However, immobilization should not exceed 1 week because of the risk of joint stiffness with inactivity. The patient may need to modify his or her usual activities to decrease stress on affected joints. For example, the patient with knee OA should avoid prolonged periods of standing, kneeling, or squatting. Using an assistive device such as a cane, walker, or crutches can also help decrease stress on arthritic joints.

Heat and Cold Applications. Applications of heat and cold may help reduce complaints of pain and stiffness. Although ice is not used as often as heat in the treatment of OA, it can be appropriate if the patient experiences acute inflammation. Heat therapy is especially helpful for stiffness, including hot packs, whirlpool baths, ultrasound, and paraffin wax baths.

Nutritional Therapy and Exercise. If the patient is overweight, a weight-reduction program is a critical part of the total treatment plan. The nurse should help the patient evaluate the current diet to make appropriate changes. (Chapter 39 discusses ways to assist the patient in attaining and maintaining a healthy body weight.) Because the load on the joints and the degree of joint mobilization are essential to the preservation of articular cartilage integrity, the American College of Rheumatology has identified exercise as a fundamental part of OA management.[5] Aerobic conditioning and specific programs for muscle strengthening have led to a modest reduction in pain and disability for some patients with knee OA.

Complementary and Alternative Therapies. Complementary and alternative therapies for symptom management of arthritis have become increasingly popular with patients who have failed to find relief through traditional medical care. Acupuncture, for example, has been found to be a safe and effective method for arthritis pain management[6] (see the Evidence-Based Practice box below). Other therapies include the use of yoga, massage, guided imagery, and therapeutic touch (see Chapter 7). In particular, the use of nutritional supplements such as glucosamine and chondroitin sulfate for relieving arthritis pain and improving joint mobility have shown promising results[7] (see the Complementary and Alternative Therapies box below).

Drug Therapy. Drug therapy is based on the severity of the patient's symptoms (Table 63-3). The patient with mild-to-moderate joint pain may receive relief from acetaminophen (Tylenol). The patient may receive up to 1000 mg every 6 hours, with the daily dose not to exceed 4 g. A topical agent such as capsaicin cream may also be beneficial, either alone or in conjunction with acetaminophen. Capsaicin comes from cayenne red pepper. It blocks pain by locally interfering with substance P, which is responsible for the transmission of pain impulses. The cream can be applied to affected joints four times daily. A concentrated product is available by prescription, but creams of 0.025% to 0.075% capsaicin are sold over the counter (OTC). The patient should be told that a local burning sensation may accompany initial use. The cream should not be used with an external heat source such as a heating pad or hot water bottle.

For the patient who fails to obtain adequate pain management with acetaminophen or for the patient with moderate to severe OA pain, nonacetylated salicylates (e.g., aspirin) or a nonsteroidal antiinflammatory drug (NSAID) may provide greater relief. Ibuprofen (Motrin) has been shown to offer greater relief than acetaminophen in patients with severe knee pain from OA.[8] NSAID therapy is typically initiated in low-dose OTC strengths (200 mg up to four times daily), with the dose increased as patient symptoms indicate. If the patient is at risk for or experiences gastrointestinal (GI) side effects with a conventional NSAID, supplemental treatment with a protective

EVIDENCE-BASED PRACTICE
Acupuncture for Osteoarthritis

Clinical Problem

Is acupuncture effective in relieving pain related to osteoarthritis?

Best Clinical Practice

- Acupuncture is becoming a common therapeutic modality for pain relief.
- Acupuncture is more effective for symptomatic treatment of osteoarthritis of the hip than advice and exercise.

Implications of Nursing Practice

- The nurse should become knowledgeable about acupuncture and what problems can be treated with it. (Acupuncture is discussed in Chapter 7.)
- In addition to teaching patients with osteoarthritis about exercise, diet, and other measures to manage osteoarthritis (see Table 63-4), the nurse should inform the patient about acupuncture as a potential treatment modality.

Reference for Evidence

Haslam R: A comparison of acupuncture with advice and exercises on the symptomatic treatment of osteoarthritis of the hip—a randomized controlled trial, *Acupunct Med* 9:19, 2001.

COMPLEMENTARY & ALTERNATIVE THERAPIES
Glucosamine

Clinical Uses

Osteoarthritis

Effects

Glucosamine is a naturally occurring substance that is found in mucopolysaccharides and mucoproteins. It may have a role in the synthesis of new cartilage.

Nursing Implications

Few adverse effects have been seen with the use of glucosamine. It should be taken with food. It should not be used in patients with diabetes mellitus. It may enhance the effects of hypoglycemic drugs and thus lower blood glucose levels.

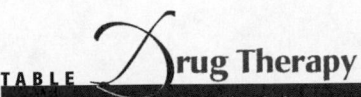

TABLE 63-3 Drug Therapy

Arthritis and Connective Tissue Disorders

DRUG	MECHANISM OF ACTION	SIDE EFFECTS	NURSING CONSIDERATIONS
Salicylates aspirin, salsalate (Disalcid, Asaphen) choline salicylate (Arthropan) choline magnesium trisalicylate (Trilisate)	Antiinflammatory Analgesic Antipyretic Act by inhibiting synthesis of prostaglandins	GI irritation (dyspepsia, nausea, ulcer, hemorrhage) Prolonged bleeding time Exacerbation of asthma (aspirin-sensitive asthma) Tinnitus, dizziness with repeated large doses	Administer drug with food, milk, antacids as prescribed, or full glass of water; may use enteric-coated aspirin. Report signs of bleeding (e.g., tarry stools, bruising, petechiae, nosebleeds).
Nonsteroidal Antiinflammatory Drugs ibuprofen (Motrin, Advil, Novoprofen) naproxen (Naprosyn, Anaprox, Aleve, Rhodiaprox, Synflex) ketoprofen (Orudis, Actron, Orafen) piroxicam (Feldene, Fexicam, Novopirocam) indomethacin (Indocin, Indocid) sulindac (Clinoril, Apo-Sulin, Novo-Sundac) tolmetin (Tolectin) diclofenac (Voltaren, Diclo SR) meclofenamate (Meclomen) oxaprozin (Daypro) meloxicam (Mobic) celecoxib (Celebrex) rofecoxib (Vioxx) valdecoxib (Bextra)	Antiinflammatory Analgesic Antipyretic Act by inhibiting synthesis of prostaglandins	GI irritation (dyspepsia, nausea, ulcer, hemorrhage) Prolonged bleeding time Headache, tinnitus Rash Acute renal insufficiency and other renal medullary changes Exacerbation of asthma (cross-reactivity with aspirin)	Administer drug with food, milk, or antacids as prescribed. Report signs of bleeding (e.g., tarry stools, bruising, petechiae, nosebleeds), edema, skin rashes, persistent headaches, visual disturbances. Monitor BP for elevations related to fluid retention. Needs to be used regularly for maximal effect.
Nonopioid Analgesics acetaminophen (Tylenol, Abenol) capsaicin cream (Zostrix)	Analgesic Antipyretic Topical analgesic Depletes substance P from nerve endings, interrupting pain signals to the brain	Rash, urticaria Hepatotoxicity (especially in presence of alcohol abuse) Leukopenia Localized burning sensation, erythema	Advise patient that concomitant use of alcohol may cause liver damage. Teach patient not to exceed recommended dosage. Must be used regularly over time for maximal effect. Aloe vera cream may moderate burning sensation. Advise patient not to use cream with external heat source (heating pad) because of risk of burns. Available in OTC and prescriptive strengths.
tramadol (Ultram)	Analgesic Centrally acting, binds to opioid receptors	GI irritation (dyspepsia, nausea, ulcer, hemorrhage) Dizziness, headache Somnolence Pruritus	Not recommended with concomitant MAO inhibitors or CNS depressants. May potentiate seizure risk with MAO inhibitors or neuroleptics. Advise patient to make position changes slowly because orthostatic hypotension may occur.

BP, Blood pressure; *CNS,* central nervous system; *GI,* gastrointestinal; *MAO,* monoamine oxidase; *OTC,* over-the-counter.

Continued

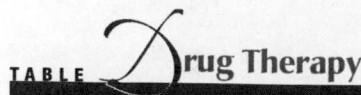

TABLE
63-3

Drug Therapy
Arthritis and Connective Tissue Disorders—cont'd

DRUG	MECHANISM OF ACTION	SIDE EFFECTS	NURSING CONSIDERATIONS
Opioid Analgesics			
propoxyphene with acetaminophen or aspirin (Darvocet, Darvon, Darvon-N) codeine with acetaminophen or aspirin (Tylenol #3 or #4, Empirin #3 or #4) hydrocodone (Hycodan, Robidone); with acetaminophen or aspirin (Lortab, Vicodin, Lortab ASA) oxycodone (OxyContin); with acetaminophen or aspirin (Percodan, Percocet, Tylox, Supeudol)	Analgesic	GI irritation (dyspepsia, nausea/vomiting, constipation) Dizziness, headache, orthostatic hypotension Sedation, respiratory depression	Advise patient regarding potential for constipation; encourage fluids and fiber if not contraindicated. Administer with antiemetic if nausea occurs. Report signs of bleeding with aspirin-containing products. Monitor CBC and liver function tests. Teach patient and family to report any CNS or respiratory changes.
Corticosteroids **Intraarticular Injections**			
methylprednisolone acetate (Depo-Medrol) triamcinolone (Aristospan)	Antiinflammatory Analgesic Act by inhibiting synthesis and/or release of mediators of inflammation	Local osteoporosis, tendon rupture, neuropathic arthropathy from frequent injection Dermal/subdermal changes leading to depression at injection site Possibility of local infection	Use strict aseptic technique for joint fluid aspiration or corticosteroid injection. Inform patient that joint may feel worse immediately after injection. Inform patient that improvement lasts weeks to months after injection. Advise patient to avoid overusing affected joint after injection.
Systemic			
hydrocortisone sodium succinate (Solu-Cortef) methylprednisolone sodium succinate (Solu-Medrol) dexamethasone (Decadron) prednisone triamcinolone (Aristocort, Triaderm)		Cushing syndrome (including fluid retention), GI irritation, osteoporosis, insomnia, hypertension, steroid psychosis, diabetes mellitus, acne, menstrual irregularities, hirsutism, risk of antibiotic-resistant infection, bruising	Use only in life-threatening exacerbation or when symptoms persist after treatment with less potent antiinflammatory drugs. Administer for limited time only, tapering dose slowly. Be aware that exacerbation of symptoms occurs with abrupt withdrawal of drug. Monitor BP, weight, CBC, and potassium level. Limit sodium intake. Report signs of infection. Instruct patient to report corticosteroid use to surgeon or dentist to avoid postoperative adrenal insufficiency.
Disease-Modifying Antirheumatic Drugs (DMARDs)			
methotrexate (Rheumatrex)	Antimetabolite Antirheumatic Inhibits DNA, RNA, protein synthesis	Hepatotoxicity occurs more often with frequent small doses than with large intermittent doses. Smaller dose and different administration schedule for RA make it less likely that patient will develop symptoms related to drug's antineoplastic activity (e.g., GI and skin toxicity, bone marrow depression, nephropathy).	Monitor CBC and hepatic and renal function. Advise patient to report signs of anemia (fatigue, weakness). Keep patient well hydrated. Teratogenic potential cautions against use for children or women of childbearing age. Inform patient that contraception should be used during and 3 mo after treatment.

CBC, Complete blood count.

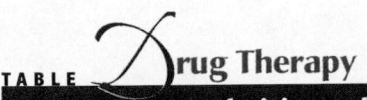

TABLE 63-3 Drug Therapy — Arthritis and Connective Tissue Disorders—cont'd

DRUG	MECHANISM OF ACTION	SIDE EFFECTS	NURSING CONSIDERATIONS
Disease-Modifying Antirheumatic Drugs (DMARDs)			
sulfasalazine (Azulfidine, Salazopyrin)	Sulfonamide Antiinflammatory Blocks prostaglandin synthesis	GI effects (anorexia, nausea/vomiting) Bleeding, bruising, jaundice Headache Rash, urticaria, pruritus	Advise patient that drug may cause orange-yellow discoloration of urine or skin. Space doses evenly around the clock, taking drug after food with 8 oz water. Treatment may be continued even after symptoms are relieved. Monitor CBC.
leflunomide (Arava)	Antiinflammatory Antirheumatic Immunomodulatory agent that inhibits proliferation of lymphocytes	Nausea, diarrhea Respiratory tract infection Alopecia Rash	Evaluate for relief of pain, swelling, stiffness; increase in joint mobility. Advise patient that medication can be taken without regard to food. Advise patient that improvement may take >8 wk.
penicillamine	Antiinflammatory Exact mechanism of action in RA unknown but may decrease cell-mediated immune response	GI irritation (nausea/vomiting, anorexia, diarrhea), reduced/altered taste Rash Proteinuria, hematuria Iron deficiency (especially in menstruating women)	Monitor WBC, platelets, urinalysis. Advise patient to take medication 1 hr before or 2 hr after meals or at least 1 hr from any other drug, food, or milk. Advise women of childbearing age to avoid pregnancy.
Gold Compounds			
Parenteral (gold sodium thiomalate [Myochrysine], aurothioglucose [Solganal]) Oral (auranofin [Ridaura])	Alters immune responses, suppressing synovitis of active RA Antirheumatic	Decreased hemoglobin, leukopenia, thrombycytopenia Proteinuria, hematuria Stomatitis	Rule out pregnancy before beginning treatment. Monitor CBC, urinalysis, and hepatic and renal function. Advise patient that therapeutic response may not occur for 3 to 6 mo. Advise patient to immediately report pruritus, rash, sore mouth, indigestion, or metallic taste.
Antimalarials			
hydroxychloroquine (Plaquenil)	Antirheumatic action unknown but may suppress formation of antigens	Ocular toxicity (retinopathy) may progress even after drug is discontinued Ototoxicity Peripheral neuritis, neuromyopathy, hypotension, electrocardiogram changes with prolonged therapy	Monitor CBC and hepatic function. Advise patient that therapeutic response may not occur for up to 6 mo. Advise patient to immediately report visual difficulties, muscular weakness, and decreased hearing/tinnitus.
Immunosuppressants			
azathioprine (Imuran) cyclophosphamide (Cytoxan)	Inhibits DNA, RNA, protein synthesis	GI irritation (nausea/vomiting; anorexia with large doses) Rash	Evaluate for relief of pain, swelling, stiffness; increase in joint mobility. Advise patient to immediately report unusual bleeding or bruising. Advise patient that therapeutic response may take up to 12 wk. Advise women of childbearing age to avoid pregnancy.

RA, Rheumatoid arthritis.

Continued

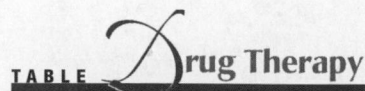

TABLE
63-3

Drug Therapy
Arthritis and Connective Tissue Disorders—cont'd

DRUG	MECHANISM OF ACTION	SIDE EFFECTS	NURSING CONSIDERATIONS
Biologic Therapy			
etanercept (Enbrel)	Binds TNF, blocking its interaction with cell surface receptors to decrease inflammatory and immune responses	Injection site reaction including erythema, pain, itching, swelling Abdominal pain, vomiting Dizziness, headache Rhinitis, pharyngitis, cough	Evaluate for relief of pain, swelling, stiffness; increase in joint mobility. Advise patient that injection site reaction generally occurs in first month of treatment and decreases with continued therapy. Advise patient to not receive live vaccines during treatment.
infliximab (Remicade) adalimumab (Humira)	Monoclonal antibody that binds to TNF; reduces infiltration of inflammatory cells	Abdominal pain, nausea/vomiting Dizziness, headache Rhinitis, cough, sinusitis, pharyngitis	Evaluate for relief of pain, swelling, stiffness; increase in joint mobility.
anakinra (Kineret)	Blocks the action of interleukin-1, thus decreases the inflammatory response	Injection site reaction Leukopenia, headache Abdominal pain, rash	Evaluate for relief of pain, swelling, stiffness; increase in joint mobility. Advise patient that injection site reaction generally occurs in first month of treatment and decreases with continued therapy. Evaluate renal function. Monitor for infection. Do not take drug with other biologic therapy.
Antibiotics			
minocycline (Minocin) (antirheumatic use needs additional validation in clinical studies)	Antirheumatic effect possibly related to immunomodulatory/antiinflammatory properties	GI effects (nausea/vomiting, diarrhea, stomach cramps) Dizziness Photosensitivity (severe)	May be reasonable alternative for patient with mild disease but probably not appropriate in severe destructive disease.

TNF, Tumor necrosis factor.

agent such as misoprostol (Cytotec) may be indicated. Arthrotec, a combination of misoprostol and the NSAID diclofenac (Voltaren), is also available.

Because traditional NSAIDs block the production of prostaglandins from arachidonic acid by inhibiting the production of cyclooxygenase-1 (COX-1) and cyclooxygenase-2 (COX-2) (see Fig. 12-7), the risk for GI erosion and bleeding is increased. Traditional NSAIDs affect platelet aggregation, leading to a prolonged bleeding time. Concerns have also been raised regarding the possible negative effects of long-term NSAID treatment on cartilage metabolism, particularly in older patients who may already have diminished cartilage integrity. As an alternative to traditional NSAIDs, treatment with the newer, selective COX-2 inhibitors may be considered, including celecoxib (Celebrex), valdecoxib (Bextra), and rofecoxib (Vioxx). These drugs inhibit production of COX-2 without affecting COX-1, an enzyme that primarily protects the stomach lining. Research continues to focus on the potential side effects of these drugs.[9]

When given in equivalent antiinflammatory dosages, all NSAIDs are considered comparable in efficacy but vary widely in cost. Individual responses to the NSAIDs are also variable. Aspirin is no longer a common treatment, and it should not be used in combination with NSAIDs because both inhibit platelet function and prolong bleeding time.

Intraarticular injections of corticosteroids may be appropriate for the elderly patient with local inflammation and effusion. Four or more injections without relief should suggest the need for additional intervention. Systemic use of corticosteroids is not indicated and can actually accelerate the disease process.

Another treatment for OA is hyaluronic acid (HA). HA contributes to both the viscosity and elasticity of synovial fluid, and its degradation can result in joint damage. Intraarticular HA injections have been shown to be safe and effective in treating the pain and functional impairment of knee OA.[10] Synthetic and naturally occurring HA derivatives (Orthovisc, Synvisc, Artz, and Hyalgan) are administered in three weekly injections. Although the exact mechanism of action is unknown, these compounds appear to have antiinflammatory benefits and a short-term lubricant effect. In addition, an analgesic effect may occur through the direct buffering effect of HA on synovial nerve endings.

NURSING MANAGEMENT
OSTEOARTHRITIS

■ Nursing Assessment

The nurse should carefully assess and document the type, location, severity, frequency, and duration of the patient's joint pain and stiffness. The patient should also be questioned about the extent to which these symptoms affect his or her ability to perform activities of daily living. Pain-relieving practices should be noted, and the patient should be questioned about the duration and success of treatment for each intervention. Physical examination of the affected joint or joints includes assessment of tenderness, swelling, limitation of movement, and crepitation. An involved joint should be compared with the contralateral joint if it is not affected.

■ Nursing Diagnoses

Nursing diagnoses for the patient with OA may include, but are not limited to, the following:

- Acute and chronic pain *related to* physical activity and lack of knowledge of pain self-management techniques
- Disturbed sleep pattern *related to* pain
- Impaired physical mobility *related to* weakness, stiffness, or pain on ambulation
- Self-care deficits *related to* joint deformity and pain with activity
- Imbalanced nutrition: more than body requirements *related to* intake in excess of energy output
- Chronic low self-esteem *related to* changing physical appearance and social and work roles

■ Planning

The overall goals are that the patient with OA will (1) maintain or improve joint function through a balance of rest and activity, (2) use joint protection measures (Table 63-4) to improve activity tolerance, (3) achieve independence in self-care and maintain optimal role function, and (4) use pharmacologic and nonpharmacologic strategies to manage pain satisfactorily.

■ Nursing Implementation

Health Promotion. Prevention of primary OA is not possible. However, community education should focus on the elimination of modifiable risk factors through weight loss and the reduction of occupational and recreational hazards. Athletic instruction and physical fitness programs should include safety measures that protect and reduce trauma to the joint structures. Congenital conditions, such as Legg-Calvé-Perthes disease, that are known to predispose a patient to the development of OA should be treated promptly.

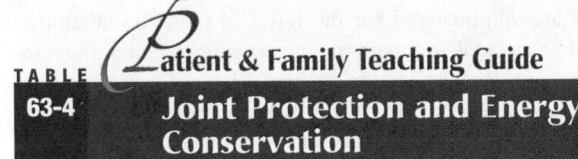

TABLE 63-4

Patient & Family Teaching Guide
Joint Protection and Energy Conservation

- Lose or maintain weight.
- Use assistive devices, if indicated.
- Avoid forceful repetitive movements.
- Avoid positions of joint deviation and stress.
- Use good posture and proper body mechanics.
- Seek assistance with necessary tasks that may cause pain.
- Develop organizing and pacing techniques for routine tasks.
- Modify home and work environment to create less stressful ways to perform tasks.

Acute Intervention. The person with OA most often complains of pain, stiffness, limitation of function, and the frustration of coping with these physical difficulties on a daily basis. The older adult may believe that OA is an inevitable part of the aging process and that nothing can be done to ease the discomfort and related disability.

The OA patient is usually treated on an outpatient basis, often by an interdisciplinary team of health care providers that includes a rheumatologist, a nurse, an occupational therapist, and a physical therapist. Health assessment questionnaires are often used to pinpoint areas of difficulty for the patient with arthritis. Questionnaires are updated at regular intervals to document disease and treatment progression. Treatment goals can be developed based on data from the questionnaires and the physical examination, with specific interventions to target identified problems. The patient is usually hospitalized only if joint surgery is planned (see Chapter 61).

EVIDENCE-BASED PRACTICE
Exercise in Osteoarthritis of the Knee

Clinical Problem
How effective is physical therapy and exercise in patients with osteoarthritis of the knee?

Best Clinical Practice
- In patients with osteoarthritis of the knee, physical therapy and exercise decrease pain and stiffness and increase function and ability to walk.

Implications for Nursing Practice
- Assessment of patients with osteoarthritis should include careful documentation of the nature, location, severity, and frequency of joint pain and stiffness.
- Overall goals for the patient with osteoarthritis of the knee are to balance rest and exercise and use joint protection measures.

Reference for Evidence
EMB Reviews: Manual physical therapy and exercise improve function in osteoarthritis of the knee, *ACP Journal Club* 133:57, 2000.

Drugs are administered for the relief of pain and inflammation. Nonpharmacologic pain management strategies may include massage, the application of heat (thermal packs) or cold (ice packs), relaxation, and guided imagery. Splints may be prescribed to rest and stabilize painful or inflamed joints. Once an acute flare has subsided, a physical therapist can provide valuable assistance in planning an exercise program. Therapists may often recommend Tai Chi as a low-impact form of exercise. Tai Chi can be performed by patients of all ages and may be done in a wheelchair. The nurse should emphasize the importance of warming up before practice to prevent stretch injuries.

Patient and family teaching related to OA is an important nursing responsibility in any care setting and is the foundation of successful disease management. Teaching should include information about the nature and treatment of the disease, pain management, correct posture and body mechanics, correct use of assistive devices such as a cane or walker, principles of joint protection and energy conservation (see Table 63-4), nutritional choices and weight management, stress management, and a therapeutic exercise program. The patient should be assured that OA is a localized disease and that severe deforming arthritis is not the usual course. The patient can also gain support and understanding of the disease process through community resources such as the Arthritis Foundation's Self-Help Course.

Ambulatory and Home Care. Chronic pain and a loss of function of the affected joints continue to be a primary concern. Home management goals must be individualized to meet the patient's needs, and family members or significant others should be included in goal setting and teaching. Home and work environment modification is essential for patient safety.[11] Measures include removing scatter rugs, providing rails at the stairs and bathtub, using night-lights, and wearing well-fitting supportive shoes. Assistive devices such as canes, walkers, elevated toilet seats, and grab bars also reduce the load on the joint and promote safety. The nurse should urge the patient to continue all prescribed pharmacologic and nonpharmacologic therapies at home and also be open to the discussion of new approaches to symptom management.

Sexual counseling may help the patient and significant other to enjoy physical closeness by introducing the idea of alternate positions and timing for intercourse. Discussion also increases awareness of each partner's needs. The nurse should encourage the patient to take analgesics or a warm bath to decrease joint stiffness before sexual activity.

■ Evaluation

The expected outcomes are that the patient with OA will
- experience adequate amounts of rest and activity
- achieve satisfactory pain management
- maintain joint flexibility and muscle strength through joint protection and therapeutic exercise
- verbalize acceptance of OA as a chronic disease, collaborating with health care providers in disease management

RHEUMATOID ARTHRITIS

Rheumatoid arthritis (RA) is a chronic, systemic disease characterized by inflammation of connective tissue in the diarthrodial (synovial) joints, typically with periods of remission and exacerbation. RA is frequently accompanied by extraarticular manifestations.

RA occurs globally, affecting all ethnic groups. It can occur at any time of life, but the incidence increases with age, peaking between the fourth and sixth decades. Women are affected by RA two to three times more frequently than men.[12] Smoking appears to be linked to both disease development and severity.[13]

Etiology and Pathophysiology

The cause of RA is unknown. Despite past theories, no infectious agent has been cultured from blood and synovial tissue or fluid with enough reproducibility to suggest an infectious cause for the disease. An autoimmune etiology is currently the most widely accepted.

1. *Autoimmunity.* The autoimmune theory suggests that changes associated with RA begin when a susceptible host experiences an initial immune response to an antigen. The antigen, which is probably not the same in all patients, triggers the formation of an abnormal immunoglobulin G (IgG). RA is characterized by the presence of autoantibodies against this abnormal IgG. The autoantibodies are known as *rheumatoid factor* (RF), and they combine with IgG to form immune complexes that initially deposit on synovial membranes or superficial articular cartilage in the joints. Immune complex formation leads to the activation of complement, and an inflammatory response results. (Complement activation is discussed in Chapter 12, and immune complex formation is discussed in Chapter 13.) Neutrophils are attracted to the site of inflammation, where they release proteolytic enzymes that can damage articular cartilage and cause the synovial lining to thicken (Fig. 63-3). Other inflammatory cells include T helper (CD4) cells, which are the primary orchestrators of cell-mediated immune responses. Activated CD4 cells stimulate monocytes, macrophages, and synovial fibroblasts to secrete the proinflammatory cytokines interleukin-1 (IL-1), interleukin-6 (IL-6), and tumor necrosis factor (TNF). These cytokines are the primary factors that drive the inflammatory response in RA.

Joint changes from chronic inflammation begin when the hypertrophied synovial membrane invades the surrounding cartilage, ligaments, tendons, and joint capsule. *Pannus* (highly vascular granulation tissue) forms within the joint. It eventually covers and erodes the entire surface of the articular cartilage. The production of inflammatory cytokines at the pannus-cartilage junction further contributes to cartilage destruction. The pannus also scars and shortens supporting structures such as

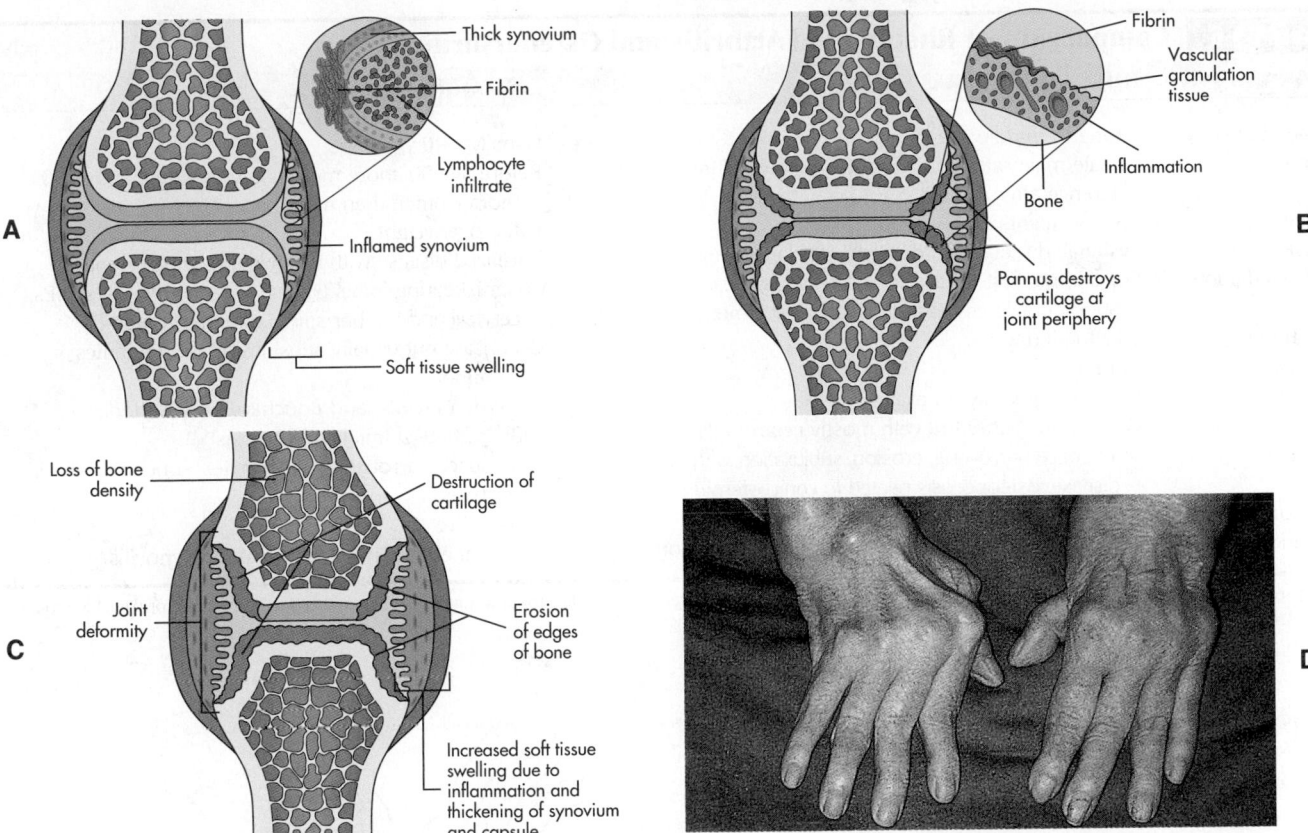

FIG. 63-3 Rheumatoid arthritis. **A,** Early pathologic change in rheumatoid arthritis is rheumatoid synovitis. The synovium is inflamed. There is a great increase in lymphocytes. **B,** With time, there is articular cartilage destruction; vascular granulation tissue grows across the surface of the cartilage (pannus) from the edges of the joint, and the articular surface shows loss of cartilage beneath the extending pannus, most marked at the joint margins. **C,** Inflammatory pannus causes focal destruction of bone. At the edges of the joint there is osteolytic destruction of bone, responsible for erosions seen on x-rays. This phase is associated with joint deformity. **D,** Characteristic deformity and soft tissue swelling associated with long-standing rheumatoid disease of the hands.

tendons and ligaments, ultimately causing joint laxity, subluxation, and contracture.

2. *Genetic factors.* Genetic predisposition appears to be important in the development of RA. For example, a higher occurrence of the disease has been noted in identical rather than fraternal twins. The strongest evidence for a familial influence is the increased occurrence of a human leukocyte antigen (HLA) known as HLA-DR4 in white RA patients. Other HLA variants have also been identified in patients from other ethnic groups. (HLA is discussed in Chapter 13.)

The pathogenesis of RA is more clearly understood than its etiology. If unarrested, the disease progresses through four stages, which are identified in Table 63-5.

Clinical Manifestations

Joints. The onset of RA is typically insidious. Nonspecific manifestations such as fatigue, anorexia, weight loss, and generalized stiffness may precede the onset of arthritic complaints. The stiffness becomes more localized in the following weeks to months. Some patients report a history of a precipitating stressful event such as infection, work stress, physical exertion, childbirth, surgery, or emotional upset. However, research has been unable to correlate such events directly with the onset of RA.

TABLE 63-5   Anatomic Stages of Rheumatoid Arthritis

Stage I—Early
No destructive changes on x-ray, possible x-ray evidence of osteoporosis

Stage II—Moderate
X-ray evidence of osteoporosis, with or without slight bone or cartilage destruction, no joint deformities (although possibly limited joint mobility), adjacent muscle atrophy, possible presence of extraarticular soft tissue lesions (e.g., nodules, tenovaginitis)

Stage III—Severe
X-ray evidence of cartilage and bone destruction in addition to osteoporosis; joint deformity, such as subluxation, ulnar deviation, or hyperextension, without fibrous or bony ankylosis; extensive muscle atrophy; possible presence of extraarticular soft tissue lesions (e.g., nodules, tenosynovitis)

Stage IV—Terminal
Fibrous or bony ankylosis, criteria of stage III

Data from Kirwan JR: Using the Larsen Index to assess radiographic progression in rheumatoid arthritis, *J Rheumatology* 27:264, 2000.

TABLE 63-6	Comparison of Rheumatoid Arthritis and Osteoarthritis	
PARAMETER	**RHEUMATOID ARTHRITIS**	**OSTEOARTHRITIS**
Age at onset	Young to middle age	Usually >40 yr of age
Gender	Female/male ratio is 2:1 or 3:1; less marked gender difference after age 60	Before age 50, more men than women; after age 50, more women than men
Weight	Lost or maintained weight	Often overweight
Disease	Systemic disease with exacerbations and remissions	Localized disease with variable, progressive course
Affected joints	Small joints first (PIPs, MCPs, MTPs), wrists, elbows, shoulders, knees; usually bilateral, symmetric	Weight-bearing joints (knees, hips), MCPs, DIPs, PIPs, cervical and lumbar spine; often asymmetric
Stiffness	1 hr to all day	On arising but usually subsides after 30 minutes
Effusions	Common	Uncommon
Nodules	Present, especially on extensor surfaces	Heberden's (DIPs) and Bouchard's (PIPs) nodes
Synovial fluid	WBC count >2000/μl with mostly neutrophils	WBC <2000/μl (mild leukocytosis)
X-rays	Joint space narrowing, erosion, subluxation with advanced disease; osteoporosis related to corticosteroid use	Joint space narrowing, osteophytes, subchondral cysts, sclerosis
Laboratory findings	RF positive in 80% of patients Elevated ESR, CRP indicative of active inflammation	RF negative Transient elevation in ESR related to synovitis

CRP, C-reactive protein; *DIP*, distal interphalangeal; *ESR*, erythrocyte sedimentation rate; *MCP*, metacarpophalangeal; *MTP*, metatarsophalangeal; *PIP*, proximal interphalangeal; *RF*, rheumatoid factor.

Specific articular involvement is manifested clinically by pain, stiffness, limitation of motion, and signs of inflammation (e.g., heat, swelling, tenderness).[14] Joint symptoms occur symmetrically and frequently affect the small joints of the hands (PIP and metacarpophalangeal) and feet (MTP). Larger peripheral joints such as the wrists, elbows, shoulders, knees, hips, ankles, and jaw may also be involved. The cervical spine may be affected, but the axial spine is generally spared. Table 63-6 compares the manifestations of RA and OA.

The patient characteristically experiences joint stiffness after periods of inactivity. Morning stiffness may last from 60 minutes to several hours or more, depending on disease activity. Metacarpal and PIP joints are typically swollen. In early disease, the fingers may become spindle shaped from synovial hypertrophy and thickening of the joint capsule (see Fig. 63-3). Joints become tender, painful, and warm to the touch. Joint pain increases with motion, varies in intensity, and may not be proportional to the degree of inflammation. Tenosynovitis frequently affects the extensor and flexor tendons around the wrists, producing manifestations of carpal tunnel syndrome and making it difficult for the patient to grasp objects.

As disease activity progresses, inflammation and fibrosis of the joint capsule and supporting structures may lead to deformity and disability. Atrophy of muscles and destruction of tendons around the joint cause one articular surface to slip past the other (*subluxation*). Typical distortions of the hand include ulnar drift ("zig zag deformity"), swan-neck, and boutonnière deformities (Fig. 63-4). Metatarsal-head subluxation and hallux valgus (bunion) in the feet may cause pain and walking disability.

Extraarticular Manifestations. RA can affect nearly every system in the body. Extraarticular manifestations of RA are depicted in Fig. 63-5. The three most common are rheumatoid nodules, Sjögren syndrome, and Felty syndrome.

Rheumatoid nodules develop in up to 25% of all patients with RA. Those affected with nodules usually have high titers of RF. Rheumatoid nodules appear subcutaneously as firm, nontender, granuloma-type masses and are usually over the extensor sur-

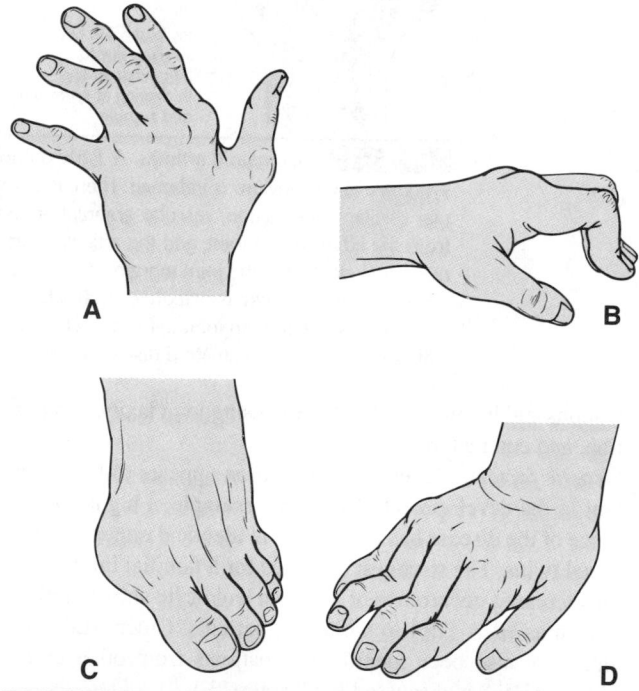

FIG. 63-4 Typical deformities of rheumatoid arthritis. **A,** Ulnar drift. **B,** Boutonnière deformity. **C,** Hallux valgus. **D,** Swan-neck deformity.

faces of joints such as fingers and elbows. Nodules at the base of the spine and back of the head are common in older adults. Nodules develop insidiously and can persist or regress spontaneously. They are usually not removed because of the high probability of recurrence, but they can easily break down or become infected. Nodules may also appear on the sclera or lungs; these indicate active disease and a poorer prognosis.

Sjögren syndrome is seen in 10% to 15% of patients with RA. Sjögren syndrome can occur as a disease by itself or in conjunction with other arthritic disorders such as RA and systemic lupus

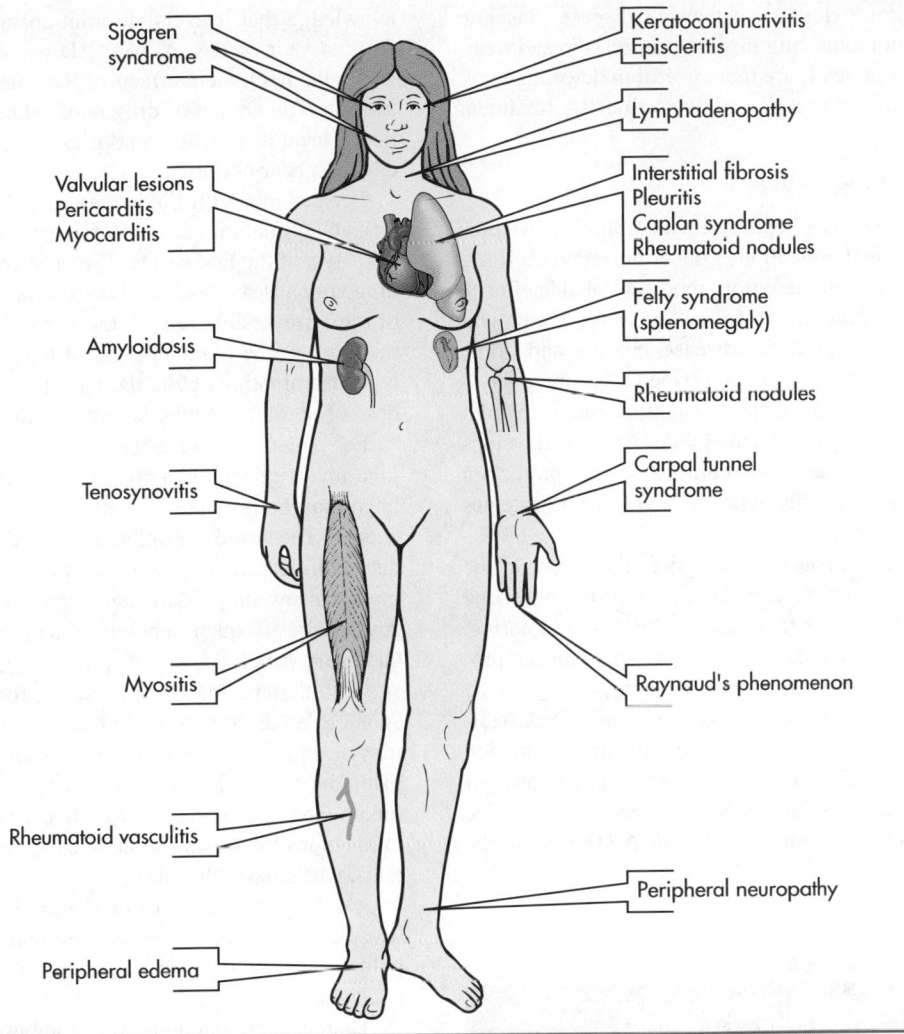

FIG. 63-5 Extraarticular manifestations of rheumatoid arthritis.

Labels (clockwise from top left): Sjögren syndrome; Keratoconjunctivitis; Episcleritis; Lymphadenopathy; Interstitial fibrosis; Pleuritis; Caplan syndrome; Rheumatoid nodules; Felty syndrome (splenomegaly); Rheumatoid nodules; Carpal tunnel syndrome; Raynaud's phenomenon; Peripheral neuropathy; Peripheral edema; Rheumatoid vasculitis; Myositis; Tenosynovitis; Amyloidosis; Valvular lesions; Pericarditis; Myocarditis

erythematosus (SLE). Affected patients have diminished lacrimal and salivary gland secretion, leading to complaints of burning, gritty, itchy eyes. They experience decreased tearing and photosensitivity (see p. 1748).

Felty syndrome occurs most commonly in patients with severe, nodule-forming RA. It is characterized by inflammatory eye disorders, splenomegaly, lymphadenopathy, pulmonary disease, and blood dyscrasias (anemia, thrombocytopenia, granulocytopenia).

Complications

Without treatment, joint destruction begins as early as the first year of the disease. Flexion contractures and hand deformities cause diminished grasp strength and affect the patient's ability to perform self-care tasks. Nodular myositis and muscle fiber degeneration can lead to pain similar to that of vascular insufficiency. Cataract development and loss of vision can result from scleral nodules. Complications can also result from rheumatoid nodules. On the skin, these nodules can ulcerate, similar to pressure sores. Nodules on the vocal cords lead to progressive hoarseness, and nodules in the vertebral bodies can cause bone destruction. In later disease, cardiopulmonary effects are not uncommon. These may include pleurisy, pleural effusion, peri-

carditis, pericardial effusion, and cardiomyopathy. Carpal tunnel syndrome results from neuromuscular involvement.

Diagnostic Studies

An accurate diagnosis is essential to the initiation of appropriate treatment and the prevention of unnecessary disability. A diagnosis is often made based on history and physical findings, but some laboratory tests are useful for confirmation and to monitor disease progression (Table 63-6). Positive RF occurs in approximately 80% of patients, and titers rise during active disease. ESR and C-reactive protein (CRP) are general indicators of active inflammation. Antinuclear antibody (ANA) titers are also seen in some RA patients.

Synovial fluid analysis in early disease often shows a straw-colored fluid with many fibrin flecks. The white blood cell (WBC) count of synovial fluid is elevated (up to $25,000/\mu l$). Inflammatory changes in the synovium can be confirmed by tissue biopsy.

X-rays are not specifically diagnostic of RA. They may be inconclusive during early stages of the disease, revealing only soft tissue swelling and possible bone demineralization. In later disease, narrowing of the joint space, destruction of articular cartilage, erosion, subluxation, and deformity are seen. Malalignment and ankylosis are often evident in advanced disease. Baseline films may be useful in monitoring disease progression and treatment effectiveness. Bone scans are more useful in detecting early joint changes and confirming a diagnosis so that RA treatment can be initiated.

Collaborative Care

Care of the patient with RA begins with a comprehensive program of drug therapy and education. Education regarding drug therapy includes correct administration, reporting of side effects, and frequent medical and laboratory follow-up visits. The patient and family are educated about the disease process and home management strategies. NSAIDs are prescribed to promote physical comfort. Physical therapy helps the patient maintain joint motion and muscle strength. Occupational therapy develops upper-extremity function and encourages joint protection through the use of splints or other assistive devices and strategies for activity pacing.

An individualized treatment plan considers the nature of the disease activity, joint function, age, gender, family and social roles, and response to previous treatment (Table 63-7). A caring, long-term relationship with an arthritis health care team can promote the patient's self-esteem and positive coping.

Drug Therapy. Drugs remain the cornerstone of RA treatment (see Table 63-3). Instead of maintaining the patient on high doses of aspirin or NSAIDs until x-rays show clear evidence of the disease, health care providers now aggressively prescribe disease-modifying antirheumatic drugs (DMARDs) with the

knowledge that irreversible joint changes can occur as early as the first year of RA. A DMARD is a drug with the potential to lessen the permanent effects of RA, such as joint erosion and deformity. The choice of drug is based on disease activity, the patient's level of function, and lifestyle considerations, such as the desire to bear children.

For patients with mild disease, hydroxychloroquine (Plaquenil), an antimalarial drug, is often prescribed initially. It is one of the safest of the DMARDs. The most common side effects of this drug are nausea, abdominal discomfort, and rash. The possibility of rare, irreversible retinal degeneration caused by deposition of this drug in the pigment layer of the retina requires ophthalmologic examination before therapy and at 6-month intervals. A low dose of prednisone may be given with hydroxychloroquine.

For patients with moderate to severe disease with symmetric joint involvement and a positive RF, a more aggressive drug regimen may be initiated. Usually methotrexate is the first drug of choice. The rapid antiinflammatory effect of methotrexate reduces clinical symptoms in days to weeks. Side effects include bone marrow suppression and hepatotoxicity. Methotrexate therapy requires frequent laboratory monitoring, including CBC and chemistry panel.

Gold therapy may be considered for patients who do not respond to methotrexate. Gold has an antiinflammatory action and may decrease phagocytosis and lysosomal activity.[15] It is usually given in a weekly injection for 5 months, then biweekly or monthly to sustain the clinical effects. Gold therapy often causes minor side effects, such as skin rashes, mouth sores, and GI problems, particularly diarrhea.

Azathioprine (Imuran) or D-penicillamine (Cuprimine) may be used if the patient does not respond to either methotrexate or gold therapy. Azathioprine and penicillamine may cause mild pancytopenia.

There is increased interest in combination therapy to treat RA. Possible combinations include methotrexate plus sulfasalazine (Azulfidine) and hydroxychloroquine plus sulfasalazine. Multiple agents may provide a synergistic effect and more adequately control symptoms.[16]

The newer-generation NSAIDs, COX-2 inhibitors, are effective in RA, as well as OA. These include celecoxib (Celebrex), rofecoxib (Vioxx), and valdecoxib (Bextra) (see Table 63-3).

Biologic therapy using TNF inhibitors is a new class of drugs used to slow disease progression in RA.[17] These drugs include etanercept (Enbrel), infliximab (Remicade), adalimumab (Humira), and anakinra (Kineret). These drugs can be used to treat patients with moderate to severe disease who have not responded to DMARDs.

Etanercept is a biologically engineered copy (using recombinant DNA technology) of the TNF cell receptor. This soluble TNF receptor binds to TNF in circulation before TNF can bind to the cell surface receptor. By inhibiting binding of TNF, etanercept inhibits the inflammatory response. This drug is given two times per week as a subcutaneous injection.

Infliximab and adalimumab are monoclonal antibodies against TNF. They bind to TNF, thus preventing it from binding to TNF receptors on cells. Infliximab is given IV on a weekly basis. Adalimumab is given subcutaneously every other week.

Anakinra (Kineret) is a recombinant version of IL-1 receptor antagonist (IL-1Ra). It blocks the biologic activity of IL-1 by competitively inhibiting IL-1 binding to the IL-1 receptor. It is given as

---

TABLE 63-7   Collaborative Care
Rheumatoid Arthritis

Diagnostic
History and physical examination
Laboratory studies
    Complete blood cell count (CBC)
    Erythrocyte sedimentation rate (ESR)
    Rheumatoid factor (RF)
    Antinuclear antibody (ANA)
    C-reactive protein (CRP)
Radiologic studies of involved joints
Synovial fluid analysis

Collaborative Therapy
Nutritional counseling
Therapeutic exercise
Rest and joint protection, use of assistive devices
Heat and cold
Complementary and alternative therapies
    Herbal products
    Movement therapies
Drug therapy*
    Disease-modifying antirheumatic drugs (DMARDs)
    Intraarticular or systemic corticosteroids
Biologic therapy
Orthopedic surgery
    Implants
    Arthroplasty

*See Table 63-3.

a subcutaneous injection. Anakinra is used to reduce the pain and swelling associated with moderate to severe RA.[18] Side effects are minor, including redness and swelling at the injection site. It can be used in combination with DMARDs but not with TNF inhibitors. Concurrent use of these agents can cause serious infection and neutropenia.

Corticosteroid therapy can be used to aid in symptom control. Intraarticular injections may temporarily relieve the pain and inflammation associated with disease flare-ups. Long-term use of oral corticosteroids should not be a mainstay of RA treatment because of the risk of osteoporosis and avascular necrosis. However, low-dose prednisone may be used for a limited time in select patients to decrease disease activity until a DMARD effect is seen.

Various NSAIDs and salicylates continue to be included in the drug regimen to treat arthritis pain and inflammation. Aspirin is often used in high dosages of 4 to 6 g per day (10 to 18 tablets). Because enteric-coated aspirin is absorbed in the small intestine, it can be prescribed in higher doses than regular tablets. The ability to obtain serum salicylate levels is helpful in developing and evaluating individualized treatment plans.

NSAIDs have antiinflammatory, analgesic, and antipyretic properties. Although many NSAIDs are potent inhibitors of inflammation, they do not appear to alter the natural history of RA. Some relief may be noted within days of the start of treatment with NSAIDs, but full effectiveness may take 2 to 3 weeks. NSAIDs may be used when the patient cannot tolerate high doses of aspirin. Those antiinflammatory drugs that are taken only once or twice a day may improve the patient's ability to follow the treatment regimen (see Table 63-3).

Antibiotics may be used in treatment of RA. The antirheumatic effect of minocycline (Minocin) may be due to its immunomodulatory and antiinflammatory properties. The drug is usually given for mild cases because of its only moderate effect on the disease. Dosage is typically 200 mg daily.

Apheresis. A blood filtration device used in apheresis called the Prosorba column is now being used to treat severe RA in patients who are not responding to other treatments. RF is removed from the patient's blood as it passes through the column. Patients are treated once a week for 12 weeks. Limited data have shown a decrease in RA signs and symptoms in most patients treated.[19] (Apheresis is discussed in Chapter 13.)

Nutritional Therapy. Although there is no special diet for RA, balanced nutrition is important. Fatigue, pain, depression, limited endurance, and mobility deficits often accompany RA and may cause a loss of appetite or interfere with the patient's ability to shop for and prepare food. Weight loss may result. The occupational therapist may help the patient to modify the home environment and to use assistive devices to make food preparation easier.

Corticosteroid therapy or immobility secondary to pain may result in unwanted weight gain. A sensible weight loss program consisting of balanced nutrition and exercise reduces stress on arthritic joints. Corticosteroids also increase the appetite, resulting in a higher caloric intake. In addition, the patient may become distressed as signs and symptoms of Cushing syndrome, including moon face and the redistribution of fatty tissue to the trunk, change one's physical appearance. The patient must be encouraged to continue a balanced diet and not to alter the corticosteroid dose or stop therapy abruptly. Weight slowly adjusts to normal several months after cessation of therapy.

NURSING MANAGEMENT
RHEUMATOID ARTHRITIS

■ Nursing Assessment

Subjective and objective data that should be obtained from the patient with RA are presented in Table 63-8.

■ Nursing Diagnoses

Nursing diagnoses for the patient with RA may include, but are not limited to, those presented in NCP 63-1.

TABLE 63-8	Nursing Assessment Rheumatoid Arthritis

Subjective Data

Important Health Information

Past health history: Recent infections; presence of precipitating factors such as emotional upset, infections, overwork, childbirth, surgery; pattern of remissions and exacerbations

Medications: Use of aspirin, NSAIDs, corticosteroids, DMARDs

Surgery or other treatments: Any joint surgery

Health Patterns

Health perception–health management: Positive family history for rheumatoid arthritis, malaise, ability to participate in therapeutic regimen

Nutritional-metabolic: Anorexia, weight loss; dry mucous membranes of mouth and pharynx

Activity-exercise: Stiffness and joint swelling, muscle weakness, difficulty walking, fatigue

Cognitive-perceptual: Paresthesias of hands and feet; numbness, tingling, loss of sensation; symmetric joint pain and aching that increases with motion or stress on joint

Objective Data

General

Lymphadenopathy, fever

Integumentary

Keratoconjunctivitis; subcutaneous rheumatoid nodules on forearm, elbows; skin ulcers; shiny, taut skin over involved joints; peripheral edema

Cardiovascular

Symmetric pallor and cyanosis of fingers (Raynaud's phenomenon); distant heart sounds, murmurs, arrhythmias

Respiratory

Chronic bronchitis, tuberculosis, histoplasmosis, fibrosing alveolitis

Gastrointestinal

Splenomegaly (Felty syndrome)

Musculoskeletal

Symmetric joint involvement with swelling, erythema, heat, tenderness, and deformities; enlargement of proximal phalangeal and metacarpophalangeal joints; limitation of joint movement; muscle contractures, muscle atrophy

Possible Findings

Positive rheumatoid factor, ↑ ESR, anemia; ↑ WBC in synovial fluid; evidence of joint space narrowing, and bony erosion and deformity on x-ray (osteoporosis with advanced disease)

DMARDs, Disease-modifying antirheumatic drugs; *ESR,* erythrocyte sedimentation rate; *NSAIDs,* nonsteroidal antiinflammatory drugs; *WBC,* white blood cells.

■ Planning

The overall goals are that patient with RA will (1) have satisfactory pain relief, (2) have minimal loss of functional ability of the affected joints, (3) participate in planning and carrying out the therapeutic regimen, (4) maintain a positive self-image, and (5) perform self-care to the maximum amount possible.

■ Nursing Implementation

Health Promotion. Prevention of RA is not possible at this time. However, community education programs should focus on symptom recognition to promote early diagnosis and treatment of RA. The Arthritis Foundation offers many publications, classes, and support activities (see the Resources at end of this chapter).

Acute Intervention. The primary goals in the management of RA are reduction of inflammation, management of pain, maintenance of joint function, and prevention or correction of joint deformity. Goals may be met through a comprehensive program of drug therapy, rest, joint protection, heat and cold applications, exercise, and patient and family teaching. The nurse is an integral member of the health team, working closely with the health care provider, physical and occupational therapists, and social worker to restore function and to help the patient make appropriate lifestyle adjustments to chronic illness.

NURSING CARE PLAN 63-1

Patient with Rheumatoid Arthritis

NURSING DIAGNOSIS   **Chronic pain** *related to* joint inflammation, overuse of joint, and ineffective pain and/or comfort measures *as manifested by* communication of pain descriptors, guarding behavior, and limited joint function; hot, swollen, painful joints.

OUTCOMES–NOC	INTERVENTIONS–NIC and *RATIONALES*
Pain Control (1605) ▪ Recognizes causal factors _____ ▪ Uses preventive measures _____ ▪ Uses nonanalgesic relief measures _____ ▪ Uses analgesics appropriately _____ **Outcome Scale** 1 = Never demonstrated 2 = Rarely demonstrated 3 = Sometimes demonstrated 4 = Often demonstrated 5 = Consistently demonstrated *Comfort Level (2100)* ▪ Expressed satisfaction with pain control _____ ▪ Reported satisfaction with symptom control _____ **Outcome Scale** 1 = None 2 = Limited 3 = Moderate 4 = Substantial 5 = Extensive	*Pain Management (1400)* ▪ Perform a comprehensive pain assessment to include location, characteristics, onset/duration, frequency, quality, intensity or severity of pain, and precipitating factors *to establish a pattern and baseline assessment and to plan appropriate interventions.* ▪ Evaluate with the patient, family, and the health care team the effectiveness of past pain control measures that have been used *to assess what has helped and not helped in the past.* ▪ Reduce or eliminate factors that precipitate or increase the pain experience such as fear, fatigue, and lack of knowledge *to minimize negative stimuli that may increase pain.* ▪ Teach the use of nonpharmacologic techniques, such as relaxation, distraction, warm applications and massage, before pain occurs or increases *to promote muscle relaxation and decrease tension.* ▪ Provide the patient with optimal pain relief with prescribed analgesics as appropriate *to help decrease pain and inflammation.*

NURSING DIAGNOSIS   **Impaired physical mobility** *related to* joint pain, stiffness, and deformity *as manifested by* limitation of joint motion, strength, and endurance; inability to perform routine activities of daily living.

OUTCOMES–NOC	INTERVENTIONS–NIC and *RATIONALES*
Mobility Level (0208) ▪ Joint movement _____ ▪ Body positioning performance _____ **Outcome Scale** 1 = Dependent, does not participate 2 = Requires assistive person and device 3 = Requires assistive device 4 = Independent with assistive device 5 = Completely independent	*Exercise Therapy: Joint Mobility (0224)* ▪ Determine limitations of joint movement and effect on function *to establish baseline for plan of care.* ▪ Collaborate with physical therapy in developing and executing an exercise program *to maintain and improve joint function.* ▪ Explain to patient and family the purpose and plan for joint exercises *to provide information and support for the patient.* ▪ Apply moist heat to affected joints (e.g., hot packs, warm shower) *to relieve stiffness and increase mobility.* ▪ Instruct patient on correct application of resting splints, selection of properly fitting footwear, maintenance of proper posture and body alignment, and selection and use of assistive devices *to prevent or limit joint deformity.*

NURSING CARE PLAN 63-1

Patient with Rheumatoid Arthritis—cont'd

NURSING DIAGNOSIS   **Disturbed body image** *related to* chronic disease activity, long-term treatment, deformities, stiffness, and inability to perform usual activities *as manifested by* social withdrawal, flat affect, altered self-concept, and reduced sexual interest.

OUTCOMES–NOC

Psychosocial Adjustment: Life Changes (1305)
- Maintenance of self-esteem _____
- Expressions of productivity _____
- Expressions of feeling socially engaged _____

Outcome Scale
1 = None
2 = Limited
3 = Moderate
4 = Substantial
5 = Extensive

INTERVENTIONS–NIC and *RATIONALES*

Body Image Enhancement (5220)
- Identify the significance of the patient's culture, religion, race, sex, and age on body image *to determine extent of problems and plan appropriate interventions.*
- Assist patient to discuss changes caused by illness *to identify problems and plan appropriate interventions.*
- Assist patient to separate physical appearance from feelings of personal worth *so that a positive body image is fostered in spite of physical manifestations.*
- Facilitate contact with individuals with similar changes in body image *to promote sharing and socialization for patient.*

Sexual Counseling (5248)
- Provide referral/consultation with other members of the health care team, such as a sex therapist, *because sexual problems and concerns can have a serious impact on body image.*
- Include the spouse/sexual partner in the counseling as much as possible *to encourage communication.*

NURSING DIAGNOSIS   **Ineffective therapeutic regimen management** *related to* complexity of chronic health problem, pain, and fatigue *as manifested by* questioning management plan, self-doubt about ability to manage disease, ability to perform activities for only short periods.

OUTCOMES–NOC

Participation: Health Care Decisions (1606)
- Seeks information _____
- Demonstrates self-direction in decision making _____
- States intent to act on decision _____
- Seeks services to meet desired outcomes _____

Outcome Scale
1 = Never demonstrated
2 = Rarely demonstrated
3 = Sometimes demonstrated
4 = Often demonstrated
5 = Consistently demonstrated

INTERVENTIONS–NIC and *RATIONALES*

Anticipatory Guidance (5210)
- Assess patient's knowledge of disease *to plan appropriate interventions.*
- Determine the patient's usual method of problem solving *to identify where interventions should focus.*
- Provide information on realistic expectations related to the patient's behavior and illness *to ensure correct understanding of disease management.*
- Refer the patient to community agencies, such as Meals on Wheels or the Arthritis Foundation, as appropriate *to allow the patient to meet desired outcomes.*
- Include the family/significant others in disease management *to increase their sense of control and to increase patient's sense of support.*
- Discuss patient's problems of pain and fatigue *because these are major deterrents to successful disease management and must be addressed.*

NURSING DIAGNOSIS   **Self-care deficit (total)** *related to* disease progression, weakness, and contracture *as manifested by* inability to perform activities of daily living.

OUTCOMES–NOC

Self-Care: Activities of Daily Living (ADL) (0300)
- Eating _____
- Dressing _____
- Toileting _____
- Bathing _____
- Grooming _____

Outcome Scale
1 = Dependent, does not participate
2 = Requires assistive person and device
3 = Requires assistive person
4 = Independent with assistive device
5 = Completely independent

INTERVENTIONS–NIC and *RATIONALES*

Self-Care Assistance (1800)
- Monitor patient's ability for independent self-care *to plan appropriate interventions.*
- Monitor patient's need for adaptive devices for personal hygiene, dressing, grooming, toileting, and eating *to compensate for contractures and weakness so that patient can perform as many self-care activities as possible.*
- Establish a routine for self-care activities with rest periods *to foster maximum independence with minimal fatigue.*
- Assist patient in accepting dependency needs *to ensure all needs are met.*
- Teach family to encourage independence and to intervene only when the patient is unable to perform *to promote independence.*

The newly diagnosed RA patient is usually treated on an outpatient basis, although hospitalization may be necessary for patients with extraarticular complications or advancing disease requiring reconstructive surgery for disabling deformities. Nursing intervention begins with a careful physical assessment (e.g., joint pain, swelling, range of motion [ROM], and general health status). The nurse must also evaluate psychosocial needs (e.g., family support, sexual satisfaction, emotional stress, financial constraints, vocation and career limitations) and environmental concerns (e.g., transportation, home or work modifications). After problem identification, a carefully planned program for rehabilitation and education can be coordinated by the nurse for the interdisciplinary health care team.

Suppression of inflammation is most effectively achieved through the administration of NSAIDs and DMARDs. Careful attention to timing is critical to sustain a therapeutic drug level and reduce early morning stiffness. The nurse should discuss the action and side effects of each prescribed drug and the importance of necessary laboratory monitoring. Many patients with RA will take several different drugs, and the nurse must make the drug regimen as understandable as possible.

Nonpharmacologic relief of pain may include the use of therapeutic heat and cold, rest, relaxation techniques, joint protection (see Tables 63-4 and 63-9), biofeedback (see Chapter 7), transcutaneous electrical nerve stimulation (see Chapter 9), and hypnosis. Assessment for individual differences and preference allows the nurse to help the patient and family choose therapies that promote optimal comfort within the parameters of their lifestyle.

Lightweight splints may be prescribed to rest an inflamed joint and prevent deformity from muscle spasms and contractures. The occupational therapist may help to identify additional self-help devices that can assist in activities of daily living. Splints should be removed at regular intervals to give skin care and perform ROM exercises. After assessment has been completed and supportive care has been given, the splints should be reapplied as prescribed.

Morning care and procedures should be planned around the patient's morning stiffness. Sitting or standing in a warm shower, sitting in a tub with warm towels around the shoulders, or simply soaking the hands in a basin of warm water may help relieve joint stiffness and allow the patient to more comfortably perform activities of daily living. Careful skin care should be offered, particularly if the patient is confined to bed.

Ambulatory and Home Care

Rest. Alternating scheduled rest periods with activity throughout the day helps relieve fatigue and pain. The amount of rest needed varies according to the severity of the disease and the patient's limitations. The patient should rest before becoming exhausted. Total bed rest is rarely necessary and should be avoided to prevent stiffness and immobility. However, even a patient with mild disease may require daytime rest in addition to 8 to 10 hours of sleep at night. The nurse should help the patient identify ways to modify daily activities to avoid overexertion that can lead to fatigue and an exacerbation of disease activity. For example, the patient may tolerate meal preparation more easily if the patient sits on a high stool in front of the sink. The nurse should assist the patient to pace activities and set priorities on the basis of realistic goals.

Good body alignment while resting can be maintained through use of a firm mattress or bed board. Positions of extension should be encouraged, and positions of flexion should be avoided. Splints and casts may be helpful in maintaining proper alignment and promoting rest, especially when joint inflammation is present. Lying prone for half an hour twice daily is also recommended. Pillows should never be placed under the knees. A small, flat pillow may be used under the head and shoulders.

Joint protection. Protecting joints from stress is important. The nurse can help the patient to identify ways to modify tasks to put less stress on joints during routine activities (see Table 63-9). Energy conservation requires careful planning. The emphasis is on work simplification techniques. Work should be done in short periods with scheduled rest breaks to avoid fatigue (pacing). Work should be spread throughout the week rather than attempted at one time (e.g., all cleaning should not be done on the weekend). Activities should be carefully organized to avoid going up and down stairs repeatedly. Carts should be used to carry supplies, or materials that are used often can be stored in a convenient, easily reached area. Time-saving joint protective devices (e.g., electric can opener) should be used whenever possible. Tasks can also be delegated to other family members.

Patient independence may be increased by occupational therapy training with assistive devices that help simplify tasks, such as built-up utensils, buttonhooks, modified drawer handles, lightweight plastic dishes, and raised toilet seats.[20] Wearing shoes with Velcro fasteners and clothing with buttons or a zipper down the front instead of the back makes dressing easier. A cane or a walker offers support and relief of pain when walking. A platform-wheeled walker further minimizes strain on the small joints of the hands and wrists. The Arthritis Foundation offers many programs to assist people and is an excellent resource for additional suggestions related to self-care.

TABLE 63-9   Patient & Family Teaching Guide

Protection of Small Joints

1. Maintain joint in neutral position to minimize deformity.
   - Press water from a sponge instead of wringing.
2. Use strongest joint available for any task.
   - When rising from chair, push with palms rather than fingers.
   - Carry laundry basket in both arms rather than with fingers.
3. Distribute weight over many joints instead of stressing a few.
   - Slide objects instead of lifting them.
   - Hold packages close to body for support.
4. Change positions frequently.
   - Do not hold book or grip steering wheel for long periods without resting.
   - Avoid grasping pencil or cutting vegetables with knife for extended periods.
5. Avoid repetitive movements.
   - Do not knit for long periods.
   - Rest between rooms when vacuuming.
6. Modify chores to avoid stress on joints.
   - Avoid heavy tasks.
   - Sit on stool instead of standing during meal preparation.

Heat and cold therapy and exercise. Heat and cold applications can help relieve stiffness, pain, and muscle spasm. Application of ice is especially beneficial during periods of disease exacerbation, whereas moist heat appears to offer better relief of chronic stiffness. The treatment modality should be selected according to disease severity, ease of application, and cost. Superficial heat sources such as heating pads, moist hot packs, paraffin baths, whirlpool baths, and warm baths or showers can relieve stiffness to allow participation in therapeutic exercises. Plastic bags of frozen vegetables (peas or corn), which can easily mold around the shoulder, wrists, or knees, are an easy home treatment. The patient can also use ice cubes or small paper cups of frozen water to massage proximally or distally to a painful joint. Heat and cold can be used as often as desired; however, the heat application should not exceed 20 minutes at one time, and the cold application should not exceed 10 to 15 minutes at one time. The nurse should alert the patient to the possibility of a burn, especially if a heat-producing cream (e.g., capsaicin) is used together with another external heat device.

Individualized exercise is an integral part of the treatment plan.[21] A therapeutic exercise program is usually developed by a physical therapist and includes exercises to improve flexibility, strength, and endurance. The nurse should reinforce program participation and ensure that the exercises are being done correctly. Inadequate joint movement can result in progressive joint immobility and muscle weakness, and overaggressive exercise can result in increased pain, inflammation, and joint damage.

Gentle ROM exercises are usually done daily to keep the joints functional. The patient should have the opportunity to practice the exercises with supervision. The nurse should emphasize that usual daily activities do not provide adequate exercise to maintain joint motion. Careful adherence to the prescribed exercise program should be a prime goal of the teaching program. Aquatic exercises in warm water (78° to 86° F [25° to 30° C]) allow easier joint movement because of the buoyancy of the water. At the same time, although movement seems easier, water provides two-way resistance that makes muscles work harder than they would on land. Aerobic conditioning programs have been shown to improve the physical fitness levels of patients with arthritis. During acute inflammation, exercise should be limited to one or two repetitions.

Psychologic support. Self-management and adherence to an individualized home treatment program can only be accomplished if the patient has a thorough understanding of RA, the nature and course of the disease, and the goals of therapy. In addition, the patient's value system and perception of the disease must be considered. The patient is constantly threatened by problems of limited function and fatigue, loss of self-esteem, altered body image, and fear of disability and deformity. Alterations in sexuality should be discussed. Chronic pain or loss of function may make the patient vulnerable to unproven or even dangerous remedies through the claims of false advertising. The nurse can help the patient recognize fears and concerns that are faced by all people who live with chronic illness.

Evaluation of the family support system is important. Financial planning may be necessary.[22] Community resources such as a home care nurse, homemaker services, and vocational rehabilitation may be considered. Self-help groups are beneficial for some patients.

▪ Gerontologic Considerations: Arthritis

The prevalence of arthritis in older adults is high, and the disease is accompanied by problems unique to this age group. The most problematic areas related to rheumatic disease in older adults include the following:

1. The high incidence of OA expected in older adults often keeps the health care provider from considering the presence of other types of arthritis.
2. Age alone causes changes in serologic profiles, making interpretation of laboratory values such as RF and ESR more difficult.
3. Polypharmacy in the older adult can result in iatrogenic arthritis.
4. Nonorganic musculoskeletal pain syndromes and weakness may be related to depressive reactions and physical inactivity.
5. Diseases such as SLE, which commonly occurs in younger adults, can develop in a milder form in older adults.

Aging brings many physical and metabolic changes that may increase the older patient's sensitivity to both the therapeutic and toxic effects of some drugs. The use of NSAIDs with a shorter half-life may require more frequent dosing but may also produce fewer side effects in the older patient with altered drug metabolism. The older adult who takes NSAIDs has an increased risk for side effects, particularly GI bleeding and renal toxicity. The common occurrence of polypharmacy makes the use of additional drugs in RA treatment particularly problematic in the older adult because of the increased likelihood of untoward drug interactions. The frequency of taking drugs and the complexity of the drug regimen should be simplified as much as possible to increase compliance in the older adult, particularly for the patient without regular assistance.

A major concern of treatment in the older patient relates to the use of corticosteroid therapy. Corticosteroid-induced osteopenia adds to the problem of age-related and inactivity-related loss of bone density and can increase the occurrence of pathologic fractures, especially compression fractures of vertebrae. Corticosteroid-induced myopathy can be minimized or prevented by an age-appropriate exercise program. Although important for all age-groups, an adequate support system for the older adult is a critical factor in the ability to follow a treatment regimen that includes nutritional planning, exercise, general health maintenance, and appropriate pharmacotherapy. ▪

Spondyloarthropathies

The **spondyloarthropathies** are a group of interrelated multisystem inflammatory disorders that affect the spine, peripheral joints, and periarticular structures. These disorders are all negative for RF, thus they are often referred to as seronegative arthropathies. Inheritance of HLA-B27 is strongly associated with occurrence of these diseases. Both genetic and environmental factors play a role in the development of this group of diseases, which includes ankylosing spondylitis, psoriatic arthritis, and Reiter syndrome. (HLAs and their relationship to autoimmune diseases are discussed in Chapter 13.) The spondyloarthropathies share clinical and laboratory characteristics that make it difficult to distinguish among them in early disease. According to the European Spondyloarthropathy Study Group criteria, a diagnosis is made when inflammatory spinal pain or asymmetric synovitis is accompanied by one or more of the following: (1) episodes of alternating buttock pain; (2) radiographic evidence of sacroiliitis; (3) heel enthesopathy (e.g., plantar fasciitis, Achilles tendinitis); (4) positive family history of spondyloarthropathy in first-degree relative; (5) current psoriasis or documented history of psoriasis; (6) current chronic inflammatory bowel disease or documented history of disease; and (7) urethritis, cervicitis, or acute diarrhea that occurred within the month preceding onset of arthritic symptoms.[23]

ANKYLOSING SPONDYLITIS

Ankylosing spondylitis (AS) is a chronic inflammatory disease that primarily affects the axial skeleton, including the sacroiliac joints, intervertebral disk spaces, and costovertebral articulations. The HLA-B27 antigen is found in approximately 90% of whites and 50% of African Americans with AS. Although the usual age of onset is 15 to 35 years of age, the highest incidence of the disease is in persons 25 to 34 years of age. Men are three to four times more likely to develop AS than women.[24] The disease may go undetected in women because of a milder course.

Etiology and Pathophysiology

The cause of AS is unknown. Genetic predisposition appears to play an important role in the disease pathogenesis, but the precise mechanisms are unknown. Aseptic synovial inflammation in joints and adjacent tissue causes the formation of granulation tissue (pannus) and the development of dense fibrous scars that lead to fusion of articular tissues. Extraarticular inflammation can affect the eyes, lungs, heart, kidneys, and peripheral nervous system.

GENETICS in CLINICAL PRACTICE
Ankylosing Spondylitis

Genetic Basis
- Inheritance of HLA-B27 antigen

Incidence
- More than 90% of white patients with ankylosing spondylitis (AS) have HLA-B27 antigen.
- Only 2% of people with HLA-B27 have clinically detectable disease.
- AS is three times more common in men than women.
- It occurs more often in whites.
- It affects 7 in 100,000 people.

Genetic Testing
- HLA testing for B27

Clinical Implications
- AS usually occurs in the second and third decades of life.
- AS has a strong association with inflammatory bowel disease (IBD).
- About 50% to 70% of patients with both AS and IBD are HLA-27 positive.
- It is a systemic disease often affecting the eyes and heart.
- Genetic and environmental factors play a role in pathogenesis of disease.

Clinical Manifestations and Complications

AS is characterized by symmetric sacroiliitis and progressive inflammatory arthritis of the axial skeleton. Symptoms of inflammatory spine pain are the first clues to a diagnosis of AS. The patient typically complains of low back pain, stiffness, and limitation of motion that is worse during the night and in the morning but improves with mild activity. In women, early symptoms of disease may present as pain and stiffness in the neck rather than the lower back. General symptoms such as fever, fatigue, anorexia, and weight loss are rarely present. Iritis is the most common nonskeletal symptom. It can appear as an initial presentation of the disease years before arthritic symptoms develop. AS patients may also experience chest pain that mimics the pain of angina or pleurisy.[25]

Severe postural abnormalities and deformity can lead to significant disability for the patient with AS. Impaired spinal ROM and fixed kyphosis contribute to altered visual function, raising concerns about safe ambulation. Aortic insufficiency and pulmonary fibrosis are frequent complications. Cauda equina syndrome can also result, contributing to lower-extremity weakness and bladder dysfunction. In addition, the patient is at risk for spinal fracture because of osteoporosis.

Diagnostic Studies

X-rays are essential for the diagnosis of AS. Spinal views are seldom useful in initial diagnosis. Instead, pelvic x-rays demonstrate characteristic changes of sacroiliitis that range from subtle erosion to completely fused joints in which joint spaces have been obliterated. Changes on later spinal films include the appearance of "bamboo spine," which is due to calcifications (syndesmophytes) that bridge from one vertebra to another. Laboratory testing is not specific, but an elevated ESR and mild anemia may be seen. HLA-B27 testing is often done, but because the antigen can occur in unaffected individuals, it is of little diagnostic value. The test can be used to exclude the disease if negative.[25]

Collaborative Care

Prevention of AS is not possible. However, families with other diagnosed HLA-B27–positive rheumatic diseases should be alert to signs of low back pain for early identification and treatment of AS.

Care of the AS patient is aimed at maintaining maximal skeletal mobility while decreasing pain and inflammation. Heat applications can help in the relief of local symptoms. NSAIDs and salicylates are commonly prescribed. Intractable pain may respond to DMARDs including sulfasalazine (Azulfidine) or methotrexate. The use of infliximab (Remicade), which is also used in the treatment of RA, shows promise for treating AS.[26]

Once pain and stiffness are managed, exercise is essential. Postural control is important to minimize spinal deformity. The exercise regimen should include back, neck, and chest stretches. Hydrotherapy has also been shown to decrease pain and facilitate spinal extension. Surgery may be indicated for severe deformity and mobility impairment. Spinal osteotomy and total joint replacement are the most commonly performed procedures (see Chapter 61).

NURSING MANAGEMENT
ANKYLOSING SPONDYLITIS

The key nursing responsibility for the patient with AS is education about the disease and principles of therapy. The home management program should include regular exercise and attention to posture, local moist heat applications, and knowledgeable use of drugs.

Baseline ROM assessment by the nurse should include chest expansion (using breathing exercises). Smoking cessation should be encouraged to decrease the risk for lung complications in those with reduced chest expansion. Ongoing physical therapy should include gentle, graded stretching and strengthening exercises to preserve ROM and improve thoracolumbar flexion and extension. Excessive physical exertion during periods of active flare-up of the disease should be discouraged. Proper positioning at rest is essential. The mattress should be firm, and the patient should sleep on the back with a flat pillow, avoiding positions that encourage flexion deformity. Postural training emphasizes avoiding spinal flexion (e.g., leaning over a desk); heavy lifting; and prolonged walking, standing, or sitting. Sports that facilitate natural stretching, such as swimming and racquet games, should be encouraged. Family counseling and vocational rehabilitation are important.

PSORIATIC ARTHRITIS

Psoriasis is a common benign, inflammatory skin disorder that appears to have a genetic predisposition (see Chapter 23). Approximately 10% of the 3 million people with psoriasis develop psoriatic arthritis (PsA). PsA is now recognized as a progressive inflammatory disease that can cause significant disability. The exact cause of PsA is unknown, but a combination of immune, genetic, and environmental factors is suspected.[27] PsA can occur in five forms:

- Arthritis involving primarily the small joints of the hands and feet
- Asymmetric arthritis involving joints of the extremities
- Symmetric polyarthritis resembling RA
- Arthritis of the sacroiliac joints and spine (psoriatic spondylitis)
- Arthritis mutilans, a rare but very deforming and destructive disease[28]

On x-ray, the cartilage loss and erosion resemble that of RA. Advanced cases of PsA often reveal widened joint spaces, and a "pencil in cup" deformity is common at the DIP joints.[29] Elevated ESR, mild anemia, and elevated blood uric acid levels can be seen in some patients; gout must be excluded. Treatment includes splinting, joint protection, and physical therapy. Although intramuscular gold therapy has been used with some success in the treatment of PsA, methotrexate continues to be one of the most effective agents for both cutaneous and articular manifestations. Sulfasalazine (Azulfidine) has been successfully used in treating PsA.

REITER SYNDROME

Reiter syndrome *(reactive arthritis)* more commonly occurs in young men and is associated with a symptom complex that includes urethritis or cervicitis, conjunctivitis, and mucocutaneous lesions.[30] Although the exact etiology is unknown, Reiter syndrome appears to occur after a genitourinary infection or gas-

troenteritis. *Chlamydia trachomatis* is most often implicated in sexually transmitted Reiter syndrome. Men and women appear to have equal risk for developing dysenteric Reiter syndrome, which typically occurs within days or weeks after infection with *Shigella, Salmonella, Campylobacter,* or *Yersinia.*[31] Most affected individuals have inherited HLA-B27.

Urethritis develops within 1 to 2 weeks after sexual contact or dysentery. Low-grade fever, conjunctivitis, and arthritis may occur over the next several weeks. The arthritis of Reiter syndrome tends to be asymmetric, frequently involving the large joints of the lower extremities and the toes. Lower back pain may occur with severe disease. Mucocutaneous lesions commonly occur as small, painless, superficial ulcerations on the tongue, oral mucosa, and glans penis. Soft tissue manifestations commonly include enthesopathies such as Achilles tendinitis or plantar fasciitis. Few laboratory abnormalities occur, although the ESR may be elevated.

Prognosis is favorable, with most patients recovering after 2 to 16 weeks. Because Reiter syndrome is often associated with *C. trachomatis* infection, treatment of patients and their sexual partners with tetracycline (Doxycycline) 100 mg twice daily for up to 3 months is widely recommended. Conjunctivitis and lesions require no treatment, but topical ophthalmic corticosteroids are typically prescribed for treatment of iritis. Physical therapy may be helpful during disease recovery.

Joints heal completely, and many patients have complete remission with full joint function. Up to 50% may develop chronic or recurring disease, which can result in major disability. X-ray changes in chronic disease closely resemble those of AS. Treatment of chronic Reiter syndrome is symptomatic.

SEPTIC ARTHRITIS

Septic arthritis (infectious or bacterial arthritis) is an invasion of the joint cavity with microorganisms. Bacteria can travel through the bloodstream from another site of active infection, resulting in hematogenous seeding of the joint. Organisms can also be introduced directly through trauma or surgical incision. Any bacteria can cause the infection. In the immunocompromised patient, even nonpathogenic bacteria can be responsible for development of septic arthritis. *Staphylococcus aureus* is the most common causative organism. *Streptococcus hemolyticus* is also seen. *Neisseria gonorrhoeae* is the most common cause in sexually active young adults. Septic arthritis occurs twice as often as does osteomyelitis.[32] Factors that increase the risk of infection include diseases where there is decreased host resistance, such as leukemia and diabetes mellitus; treatment with corticosteroids or immunosuppressive drugs; and debilitating chronic illness.

Large joints such as the knee and hip are most frequently involved. Inflammation of the joint cavity causes severe pain, erythema, and swelling. Because infection has often spread from a primary site elsewhere in the body, fever or shaking chills often accompany articular manifestations. Precise diagnosis is made by aspiration of the joint (arthrocentesis) and culture of the synovial fluid. Blood cultures for aerobic and anaerobic organisms should also be obtained.

Septic arthritis is a medical emergency that requires prompt diagnosis and treatment to prevent joint destruction. Based on identification of the causative organism, parenteral antibiotics are prescribed and administered until there are no clinical signs of active synovitis or inflammation in the joint fluid. Infections may respond to treatment within 2 weeks or may take as long as 4 to 8 weeks, depending on the causative organism. Open surgical drainage may be required. If diagnosis and treatment are delayed, destruction of articular cartilage can occur, followed by loss of joint function. Chronic infection can develop. Septic arthritis of the hip can also contribute to development of avascular necrosis.

Nursing intervention includes assessment and monitoring of joint inflammation, pain, and fever. Immobilization of affected joints to control pain can be achieved by use of resting splints or traction. Gentle ROM exercises should be performed on a regular schedule. Strict aseptic technique should be used during assistance with joint aspiration procedures. The nurse should explain the need for antibiotics and the importance of their continued use until the infection is resolved. Support should be offered to the patient who requires arthrocentesis or operative drainage.

LYME DISEASE

Lyme disease is a spirochetal infection caused by *Borrelia burgdorferi* and transmitted by the bite of an infected deer tick.[33] It was first identified in 1975 in Lyme, Connecticut, after an unusual clustering of arthritis in children and is now the most common vector-borne disease in the United States. The tick typically feeds on mice, dogs, cats, cows, horses, deer, and humans. Wild animals do not exhibit the illness, but clinical Lyme disease does occur in domestic animals. Person-to-person transmission does not occur. The peak season for human infection is during the summer months. Most U.S. cases occur in three endemic areas: along the northeastern coast from Maryland to Massachusetts; in the midwestern states of Wisconsin and Minnesota; and along the northwestern coast of northern California and Oregon. The reported incidence of Lyme disease has doubled in the last 10 years to 16,700 cases annually.[34]

Lyme disease is often called the "great imitator" because its symptoms can mimic other diseases such as multiple sclerosis, mononucleosis, and meningitis. The most characteristic clinical symptom of early localized disease is erythema migrans (EM), a skin lesion that occurs at the site of the tick bite within 2 to 30 days after exposure (Fig. 63-6). The lesion begins as a red macule or papule that slowly expands to form a large round lesion with a bright red border and central clearing. The EM lesion is often accompanied by acute viral-like symptoms, such as fever, chills, headache, stiff neck, fatigue, swollen lymph nodes, and migratory joint and muscle pain.

If not treated, symptoms of Lyme disease can progress within several weeks or months to include nervous system problems such as severe headaches, temporary facial paralysis (e.g., Bell's palsy), or poor motor coordination. In late disease, which can occur from months to years after the initial infection, arthritis pain and swelling may occur in a few large joints. Arthritic symptoms are often temporary, but about 10% of people with Lyme disease will develop chronic Lyme arthritis if untreated. Neurologic disorders can also occur at this stage, including one condition known as tertiary neuroborreliosis that results in confusion and forgetfulness.

A diagnosis of Lyme disease is often based on clinical manifestations, in particular, the EM lesion, and a history of exposure in an endemic area. Routine laboratory tests play only a minor

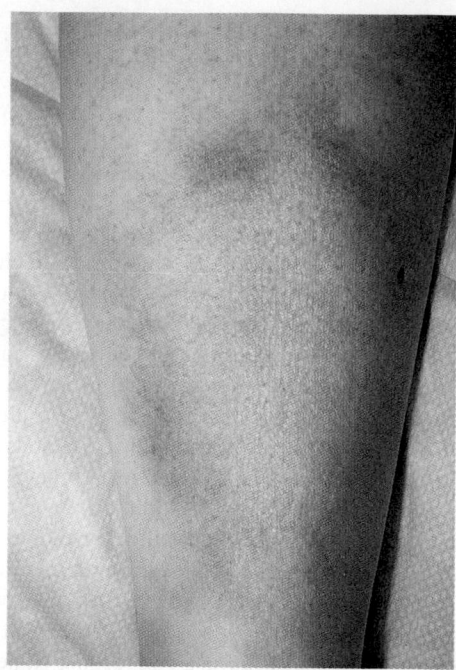

FIG. 63-6   Erythema migrans. Early skin lesion in Lyme disease.

role in diagnosis. CBC and ESR results are usually normal. Lyme serology tests for antibodies are not usually positive initially because it takes many weeks to get clinical detectable levels of circulating antibodies.[34] Cerebrospinal fluid should be examined in individuals with neurologic involvement.

Active lesions can be treated with antibiotic therapy. Oral doxycycline (Vibramycin) or amoxicillin is often effective in early stage infection and in prevention of later stages of the disease. Doxycycline has also proven to be very effective in preventing Lyme disease when given within 3 days after the bite of a deer tick. Short-term therapy of 2 to 3 weeks is usually effective for solitary EM, but long-standing infection may require extended parenteral antibiotic therapy. Intravenous ceftriaxone (Rocephin) is prescribed for cardiac or neurologic abnormalities. LYMErix, a vaccine, is given optimally in three doses over a 2-month period and is 76% effective against the disease.[35] The vaccine is recommended for individuals whose occupations or recreational activities place them at risk for *B. burgdorferi* exposure. However, the manufacturer recently discontinued the commercial availability of the vaccine. New vaccines are currently being investigated. Patient and family teaching for the prevention of Lyme disease in endemic areas is outlined in Table 63-10.

HUMAN IMMUNODEFICIENCY VIRUS–ASSOCIATED RHEUMATIC DISEASE

A group of inflammatory musculoskeletal disorders develop in the course of human immunodeficiency virus (HIV) infection.[36] The cause of these disorders in HIV-infected persons is not clearly known. However, it appears that an autoimmune process and an inflammatory response are occurring at the same time in the patient who is immunosuppressed.[37] Up to 70% of HIV-infected patients may develop a rheumatic disease. Rheumatic diseases associated with HLA-B27 appear to be more severe in HIV-infected patients. Conditions typically associated with HIV

TABLE 63-10 Patient & Family Teaching Guide
Prevention of Lyme Disease (Endemic Areas)

- Avoid walking through tall grasses and low brush.
- Mow grass and remove brush along paths, and around buildings and campsites.
- Move woodpiles and bird feeders away from house.
- Wear long pants or nylon tights of tightly woven, light-colored fabric so that ticks can be easily seen.
- Tuck pants into boots or long socks, tuck long-sleeved shirts into pants, and wear closed shoes when hiking.
- Check often for ticks crawling from legs to open skin.
- Thoroughly inspect and wash clothes.
- Spray insect repellant containing DEET on skin or permethrin on clothes, especially on lower extremities.
- Have pets wear tick collars, inspect them often, and do not allow them on furniture or beds.
- Remove attached ticks with tweezers (not fingers). Grasp tick's mouth parts as close to skin as possible and gently pull straight out. Do not twist or jerk.
- Dispose of tick in alcohol or flush down toilet. Do not crush with fingers.
- Wash bitten area with soap and water and apply antiseptic. Wash hands.
- See a doctor immediately if flulike symptoms or "bull's-eye" rash appears within a 2 to 30 days after removal of tick.

DEET, N,N-diethyl-M-toluamide.

TABLE 63-11 Conditions That Can Cause Hyperuricemia

Acidosis or ketosis
Alcoholism
Atherosclerosis
Chemotherapeutic drugs
Diabetes mellitus
Drug-induced renal impairment
Hyperlipidemia
Hypertension
Malignant disease
Myeloproliferative disorders
Obesity or starvation
Renal disease
Sickle cell anemia
Use of certain common drugs (salicylates, diuretics)

infection include SLE, Reiter syndrome, PsA, Sjögren syndrome, polymyositis, and vasculitis. The knees and ankles are generally the most affected joints. Most patients improve with conventional arthritis treatments such as NSAIDs, but patients with Reiter syndrome or PsA may not respond as well and develop progressive deformities. As with other patients, appropriate physical therapy is recommended.

GOUT

Gout is caused by an increase in uric acid production, underexcretion of uric acid by the kidneys, or increased intake of foods containing purines, which are metabolized to uric acid by the body. Characteristic deposits of monosodium urate crystals occur in articular, periarticular, and subcutaneous tissues. Joint involvement includes recurrent attacks of acute arthritis.

Gout may be classified as primary or secondary.[38] In *primary gout,* a hereditary error of purine metabolism leads to the overproduction or retention of uric acid. *Secondary gout* may be related to another acquired disorder (Table 63-11) or may be the result of drugs known to inhibit uric acid excretion. Secondary gout may also be caused by drugs that increase the rate of cell death, such as the chemotherapeutic agents used in treating leukemia. Primary gout, which accounts for 90% of cases, occurs predominantly in middle-aged men, with almost no incidence in premenopausal women. Hyperuricemia may also develop in patients taking thiazide diuretics, postmenopausal women, and in organ transplant recipients who are receiving immunosuppressive agents.

Etiology and Pathophysiology

Uric acid is the major end product of purine catabolism and is primarily excreted by the kidneys. Hyperuricemia may be the result of increased purine synthesis, decreased renal excretion, or both. A high dietary intake of purine alone has relatively little effect on uric acid levels. Hyperuricemia may result from prolonged fasting or excessive alcohol drinking because of the increased production of keto acids, which then inhibit uric acid excretion.

Clinical Manifestations and Complications

In the acute phase, gouty arthritis may occur in one or more joints but usually less than four. Affected joints may appear dusky or cyanotic and are extremely tender. Inflammation of the great toe *(podagra)* is the most common initial problem. Other affected joints may include the midtarsal area of the foot, ankle, knee, and wrist. Olecranon bursae may also be involved. Acute gouty arthritis is usually precipitated by events such as trauma, surgery, alcohol ingestion, or systemic infection. Onset of symptoms is typically rapid, with swelling and pain peaking within several hours, often accompanied by low-grade fever. Individual attacks usually subside, treated or untreated, in 2 to 10 days. The affected joint returns entirely to normal, and patients are often free of symptoms between attacks.

Chronic gout is characterized by multiple joint involvement and visible deposits of sodium urate crystals called *tophi.* These are typically noted in the synovium, subchondral bone, olecranon bursae, and vertebrae; along tendons; and in the skin and cartilage (Fig. 63-7). Tophi are rarely present at the time of the initial attack and are generally noted only many years after the onset of disease.

The severity of gouty arthritis is variable. The clinical course may consist of infrequent mild attacks or multiple severe episodes associated with a slowly progressive disability. In general, the higher the serum uric acid level, the earlier the appearance of tophi and the greater the tendency toward more frequent, severe episodes of acute gout. Chronic inflammation may result in joint deformity, and cartilage destruction may predispose the joint to secondary OA. Large and unsightly tophaceous deposits

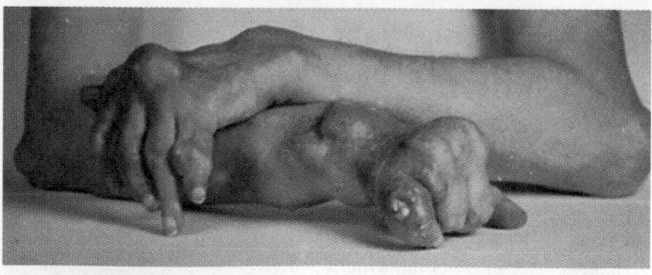

FIG. 63-7 Tophaceous gout.

may perforate overlying skin, producing draining sinuses that often become secondarily infected. Excessive uric acid excretion may lead to kidney or urinary tract stone formation. Pyelonephritis associated with intrarenal sodium urate deposits and obstruction may contribute to renal disease.

Diagnostic Studies

Serum uric acid levels are almost always elevated to 8 mg/dl. However, hyperuricemia is not specifically diagnostic of gout because increased levels may be related to a variety of drugs or may exist as a totally asymptomatic abnormality in the general population. Specimens for 24-hour urine uric acid levels may be obtained to determine if the disease is caused by undersecretion or overproduction of uric acid. Synovial fluid aspiration is a potentially controversial part of patient evaluation because an accurate diagnosis of gout is possible in 80% of patients based on clinical symptoms alone. However, aspiration may have therapeutic value by decompressing a swollen joint capsule. Joint aspiration is also the only reliable method to distinguish gout from septic arthritis and pseudogout. Affected fluid characteristically contains needlelike crystals of sodium urate.

Collaborative Care

Goals for care of the patient with gout (Table 63-12) include termination of an acute attack through use of an antiinflammatory agent such as colchicine, with NSAIDs prescribed adjunctively for pain management. Future attacks are prevented by a maintenance dose of allopurinol (Zyloprim) in combination with weight reduction, as needed, and possible avoidance of alcohol and food high in purine (red and organ meats). Treatment is also aimed at preventing the formation of uric acid kidney stones and the development of associated conditions such as hypertriglyceridemia and hypertension.

Drug Therapy. Acute gouty arthritis is treated with colchicine and NSAIDs. Colchicine has known antiinflammatory effects but no analgesic properties, so an NSAID is added to the treatment regimen primarily for pain management. Oral administration of colchicine generally produces dramatic pain relief within 24 to 48 hours. Colchicine also has diagnostic merit in that a good response to treatment gives further evidence for the diagnosis of gout. As another possible therapy, intraarticular injection of corticosteroids can be helpful in monoarthritic gout. Systemic corticosteroids may be used only if routine therapies are contraindicated or ineffective. Adrenocorticotropic hormone (ACTH) may also be used for treating acute gout.[39]

For many years the standard therapy for hyperuricemia caused by urate underexcretion has been uricosuric drugs such as

TABLE 63-12	*Collaborative Care* Gout

Diagnostic
History and physical examination
Family history of gout
Presence of monosodium urate monohydrate crystals in synovial fluid
Elevated serum uric acid levels
Elevated 24 hr urine for uric acid levels

Collaborative Therapy
Joint immobilization
Local application of heat or cold
Joint aspiration and intraarticular corticosteroids
Drug therapy
   Nonsteroidal antiinflammatory drugs
   colchicine
   probenecid (Benemid)
   allopurinol (Zyloprim)
Dietary avoidance of food/fluids with high purine content (e.g., anchovies, liver, wine/beer)

probenecid (Benemid), which inhibit renal tubular reabsorption of urates. However, this class of drugs is ineffective when creatinine clearance is reduced, as can occur in patients over the age of 60. Aspirin inactivates the effect of uricosurics, resulting in urate retention, and should be avoided while patients are taking uricosuric drugs. Acetaminophen can be used safely if analgesia is required.

Adequate urine volume with normal renal function (2 to 3 L per day) must be maintained to prevent precipitation of uric acid in the renal tubules. Allopurinol (Zyloprim), which blocks the production of uric acid, is particularly useful in patients with uric acid stones or renal impairment in whom uricosuric drugs may be ineffective or dangerous. For patients who cannot tolerate allopurinol because of minor reactions, oxypurinol can be prescribed. Oxypurinol is the active metabolite of allopurinol. The angiotensin II receptor antagonist losartan (Cozaar) may be especially useful for treatment of elderly patients with both gout and hypertension. Losartan given 50 mg daily will promote urate diuresis and may normalize serum urate levels. Combination therapy with losartan and allopurinol may also be given. Regardless of which drugs are prescribed, serum uric acid levels must be checked regularly to monitor treatment effectiveness.

Nutritional Therapy. Traditional dietary restrictions include limiting the use of alcohol and the consumption of foods high in purine (see Table 44-12). However, drugs can often control gout without necessitating these changes. Obese patients should be instructed in a carefully planned weight-reduction program.

NURSING MANAGEMENT
GOUT

Nursing intervention for the patient with acute gouty arthritis includes supportive care of the inflamed joints. Special care is taken to avoid causing pain to an inflamed joint by careless handling. Bed rest may be appropriate, with affected joints properly immobilized. Involvement of a lower extremity may require use of a cradle or foot board to protect the painful area from the weight of bed clothes. The limitation of motion and degree of pain should be assessed, and treatment effectiveness should be documented.

The nurse should help the patient and the family to understand that hyperuricemia and gouty arthritis are chronic problems that can be controlled with careful adherence to a treatment program. Thorough explanations should be given concerning the importance of drug therapy and the need for periodic determination of serum uric acid levels. The patient should be able to demonstrate knowledge of precipitating factors that may cause an attack, including excessive caloric intake or overindulgence in purine-containing foods and alcohol; starvation (fasting); drug use (e.g., aspirin, diuretics); and major medical events (e.g., surgery, myocardial infarction).

SYSTEMIC LUPUS ERYTHEMATOSUS

Systemic lupus erythematosus (SLE) is a chronic multisystem inflammatory disease associated with abnormalities of the immune system. It typically affects the skin, joints, and serous membranes (pleura, pericardium), along with the renal, hematologic, and neurologic systems. The overall incidence of SLE in the United States is 2 to 8 per 100,000. Most cases of SLE occur in women in their childbearing years.[40] African Americans, Asian Americans, and Native Americans are approximately three times more likely to develop SLE than whites. SLE is characterized by variability within and among persons, and its chronic unpredictable course is marked by alternating periods of exacerbations and remissions.

Etiology and Pathophysiology

The etiology of SLE is unknown.[41] Based on the high prevalence of SLE among family members, a genetic influence has long been suspected. Multiple susceptibility genes from the HLA complex show associations with SLE. Hormones are also known to play a role in the etiology of SLE. Onset or exacerbation of disease symptoms sometimes occurs after the onset of menarche, with the use of oral contraceptives, and during and after pregnancy. The disease tends to worsen in the immediate postpartum period.

Environmental factors are believed to contribute to the occurrence of SLE, with sun exposure and burns as the most significant environmental triggers. Infectious agents could serve as a stimulus for immune hyperactivity. SLE may also be precipitated or aggravated by certain drugs such as procainamide (Pronestyl), hydralazine (Apresoline), and a number of antiseizure drugs.

SLE is a disorder of immunoregulation. Autoimmune reactions are directed against constituents of the cell nucleus, particularly DNA. The overaggressive antibody response is related to B and T cell hyperactivity.[42] When autoantibodies bind to their specific antigens, complement activation occurs, and immune complexes are deposited in the basement membranes of capillaries in the kidneys, heart, skin, brain, and joints. The specific manifestations of SLE depend on which cell types or organs are involved.

Clinical Manifestations and Complications

SLE is extremely variable in its severity, ranging from a relatively mild disorder to a rapidly progressive one affecting many organ systems (Fig. 63-8). No characteristic pattern occurs in the progressive organ involvement of SLE. Theoretically, any organ can be affected by an accumulation of circulating immune complexes. The most commonly affected tissues are the skin and muscle, the lining of the lungs, the heart, nervous tissue, and the kidneys. Generalized complaints such as fever, weight loss, arthralgia, and excessive fatigue may precede an exacerbation of disease activity.

Dermatologic Manifestations. Cutaneous vascular lesions can appear in any location but are most likely to develop in sun-exposed areas. Severe skin reactions can occur in persons who are photosensitive. The classic butterfly rash over the cheeks and bridge of the nose occurs in 50% of patients with SLE (Fig. 63-9). A small number of patients have persistent lesions, photosensitivity, and mild systemic disease in a syndrome referred to as *subacute cutaneous lupus.*

Ulcers of the oral or nasopharyngeal membranes occur in up to one third of patients with SLE. Transient diffuse or patchy hair loss (alopecia) is also common, with or without underlying scalp lesions. The hair may grow back during remission, but hair loss may be permanent over lesions. The scalp becomes dry, scaly, and atrophied.

Musculoskeletal Problems. Polyarthralgia with morning stiffness is often the patient's first complaint and may precede the onset of multisystem disease by many years. Arthritis occurs in more than 90% of patients with SLE. Diffuse swelling is accompanied by joint and muscle pain, and some stiffness may be experienced. Lupus-related arthritis is generally nonerosive, but it may cause deformities such as swan-neck appearance of the fingers (see Fig. 63-4), ulnar deviation, and subluxation with hyperlaxity of the joints.

Cardiopulmonary Problems. Tachypnea and cough in patients with SLE are suggestive of restrictive lung disease. Pleurisy with or without pleural effusion is also possible. Cardiac involvement may include arrhythmias resulting from fibrosis of the sinoatrial and atrioventricular nodes. This occurrence is an ominous sign of advanced disease, contributing significantly to the morbidity and mortality seen in SLE. Clinical factors such as hypertension and hypercholesterolemia require aggressive therapy and careful monitoring. SLE accelerates coronary artery disease (CAD), and the risk of developing CAD also increases.[43]

Renal Problems. Lupus nephritis (LN) occurs in about 50% of patients within 1 year of diagnosis with SLE. Manifestations of LN vary from mild proteinuria to rapid, progressive glomerulonephritis. Nearly all patients with SLE show renal histologic abnormalities in renal biopsy studies or autopsy results.

The primary goal in treating LN is to slow the progression of nephropathy and preserve renal function by managing the underlying disease. The importance of obtaining a renal biopsy is controversial, but findings can help to guide treatment, which typically includes corticosteroids, cytotoxic agents (cyclophosphamide [Cytoxan]), and immunosuppressive agents (azathioprine [Imuran], cyclosporine [Sandimmune]). Cyclophosphamide is the most effective cytotoxic therapy, but azathioprine is considered to be less toxic. Oral prednisone or pulsed intravenous methylprednisolone may also be used as an intervention for LN, especially in the initial treatment period when cytotoxic agents have not had time to take effect.

Nervous System Problems. Along with renal involvement, neurologic effects are the most prevalent in SLE. Generalized or focal seizures are the most common manifestation in-

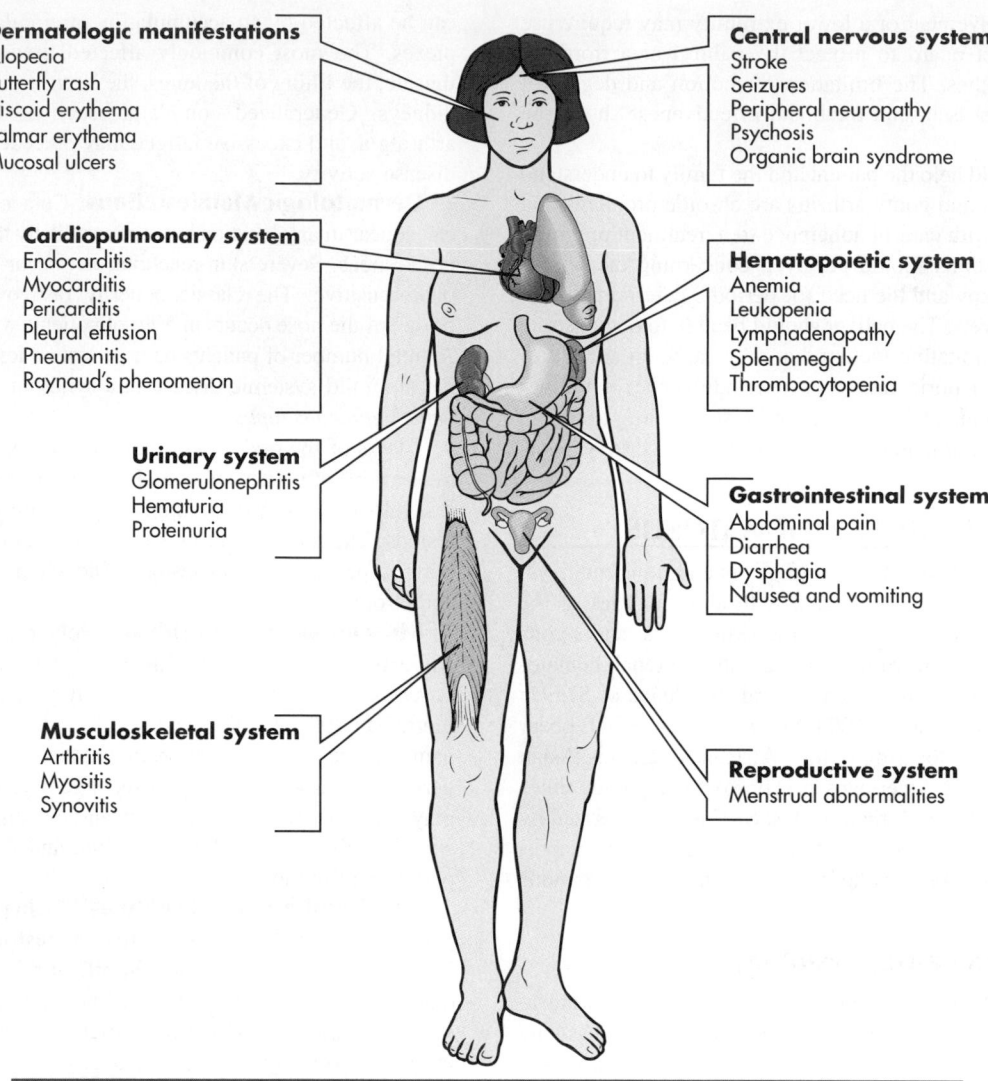

Dermatologic manifestations
Alopecia
Butterfly rash
Discoid erythema
Palmar erythema
Mucosal ulcers

Cardiopulmonary system
Endocarditis
Myocarditis
Pericarditis
Pleural effusion
Pneumonitis
Raynaud's phenomenon

Urinary system
Glomerulonephritis
Hematuria
Proteinuria

Musculoskeletal system
Arthritis
Myositis
Synovitis

Central nervous system
Stroke
Seizures
Peripheral neuropathy
Psychosis
Organic brain syndrome

Hematopoietic system
Anemia
Leukopenia
Lymphadenopathy
Splenomegaly
Thrombocytopenia

Gastrointestinal system
Abdominal pain
Diarrhea
Dysphagia
Nausea and vomiting

Reproductive system
Menstrual abnormalities

FIG. 63-8   Multisystem involvement in systemic lupus erythematosus.

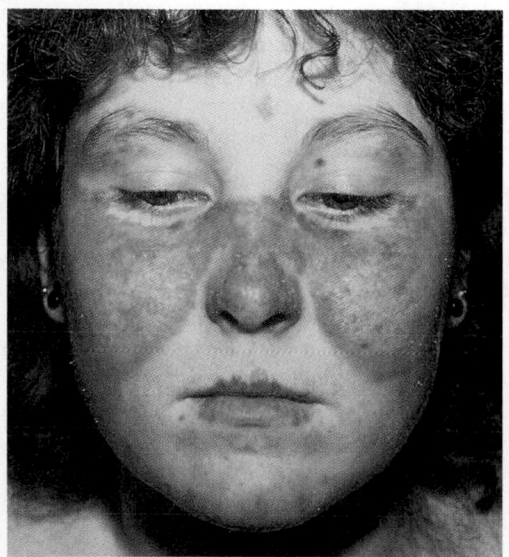

FIG. 63-9   Butterfly rash of systemic lupus erythematosus.

volving the central nervous system (CNS), and occur in as many as 15% of patients with SLE by the time of diagnosis. Seizures are generally controlled by corticosteroids or antiseizure drugs. Peripheral neuropathy can also occur, leading to sensory and motor deficits.

Organic brain syndrome, recognized as a CNS manifestation of SLE, may result from the deposition of immune complexes within brain tissue. It is characterized by disordered thought processes, disorientation, memory deficits, and psychiatric symptoms such as severe depression and psychosis. Recovery from organic brain disease is expected, although some residual impairment may result. Occasionally a stroke or aseptic meningitis may be attributable to SLE. It is difficult to differentiate neuropsychiatric SLE from non-SLE neurologic problems.

Hematologic Problems. The formation of antibodies against blood cells, such as erythrocytes, leukocytes, thrombocytes, and coagulation factors, is also a common feature of SLE. Anemia, mild leukopenia, and thrombocytopenia are often present in SLE. Some patients develop a tendency toward coagulopathy involving either excessive bleeding or blood clot development. A manifestation of antiphospholipid antibody syndrome is a common cause of hypercoagulability in SLE patients, many of whom benefit from high-intensity treatment with warfarin sodium (Coumadin).

Infection. Patients with SLE appear to have increased susceptibility to infections, possibly related to defects in their ability to phagocytize invading bacteria, deficiencies in production of antibodies, and the immunosuppressive effect of many antiinflammatory drugs. Infection is a major cause of death, with pneumonia being the most common infection. Fever should be considered serious because it may indicate an underlying infectious process rather than lupus activity alone. Vaccinations are generally safe for patients with SLE. The exception is avoidance of live-virus vaccines with patients who are being treated with corticosteroids or cytotoxic agents.

Diagnostic Studies

The diagnosis of SLE is based on the presence of distinct criteria revealed through patient history, physical examination, and laboratory findings (Table 63-13). No specific test is diagnostic for SLE, but a variety of abnormalities may be present in the blood. SLE is characterized by the presence of ANA. Other antibodies include anti-DNA, antineuronal, anticoagulant, anti-WBC, anti–red blood cell (RBC), antiplatelet, and anti–basement membrane. The tests that are most specific for SLE include the anti–double-stranded DNA and the anti-Smith (Sm). High levels of anti-DNA are rarely found in any condition other than SLE, and anti-Sm seems to be found almost exclusively in SLE. The lupus erythematosus (LE) cell prep test is a nonspecific test for SLE and is positive in other rheumatic diseases. ESR and CRP levels are not diagnostic of SLE but may be used to monitor disease activity.

Collaborative Care

A major challenge in treatment of SLE is to manage the active phase of the disease while preventing complications of treatments that cause long-term tissue damage. An improving prognosis of SLE may be the result of earlier diagnosis, prompt recognition of serious organ involvement, and better therapeutic regimens. Survival is influenced by several factors, including age, race, gender, socioeconomic status, accompanying morbid conditions, and severity of disease.

Drug Therapy. NSAIDs continue to be an important intervention, especially for patients with mild polyarthralgias or polyarthritis. Because prolonged therapy is likely, careful patient monitoring must include the potential for GI effects from NSAID use. Antimalarial agents such as hydroxychloroquine (Plaquenil) are also often used to treat polyarthritis. Retinopathy can develop with use of these agents, but it generally reverses when they are discontinued. If the patient cannot tolerate an antimalarial agent, an antileprosy drug such as dapsone may be used.

Corticosteroid exposure should be limited, but tapering doses of intravenous methylprednisolone may be useful in controlling severe exacerbations of polyarthritis. Steroid-sparing drugs such as methotrexate can serve as an alternate treatment and are prescribed in combination with folic acid to decrease minor side effects. However, high doses of corticosteroids may be especially appropriate for the patient with very severe cutaneous SLE. Immunosuppressive drugs such as azathioprine (Imuran) and cyclophosphamide (Cytoxan) may be prescribed to reduce the need for long-term corticosteroid therapy. Close monitoring is necessary to minimize drug toxicity and side effects.[44]

Disease management is most appropriately monitored by serial anti-DNA titers (Table 63-14). Simpler and less costly tests such as ESR or CRP may also help in monitoring treatment effectiveness.

TABLE 63-13   Criteria for Diagnosis of Systemic Lupus Erythematosus*

Malar rash
Discoid rash
Photosensitivity
Oral ulcers
Arthritis: nonerosive, involvement of two or more joints characterized by tenderness, swelling, and effusion
Serositis: pleuritis or pericarditis
Renal disorder: persistent proteinuria or cellular casts in urine
Neurologic disorder: seizures or psychosis
Hematologic disorder: hemolytic anemia, leukopenia, lymphopenia, or thrombocytopenia
Immunologic disorder: positive LE preparation; anti-DNA antibody or antibody to Sm nuclear antigen; or false-positive serologic tests for syphilis
Antinuclear antibodies

Data from American College of Rheumatology [on-line]. Available at *www. rheumatology.org/research/classification/sle/html.*
*A person is classified as having SLE if four or more of the criteria are present, serially or simultaneously, during any interval of observation. Revised criteria by a subcommittee of the American College of Rheumatology are used for the purpose of *classification* in population surveys, *not* for the diagnosis of individual patients.
Sm, Smith.

TABLE 63-14   Collaborative Care — Systemic Lupus Erythematosus

Diagnostic
History and physical examination
Antibodies
    Anti-DNA antibody
    Anti-Sm antibody
    Antinuclear antibody (ANA)
Complete blood cell count
LE cell prep
Urinalysis
X-ray of affected joints
Chest x-ray
ECG to determine extraarticular involvement

Collaborative Therapy
NSAIDs
Steroid-sparing drugs (e.g., methotrexate)
Antimalarials (e.g., hydroxychloroquine [Plaquenil])
Corticosteroids for exacerbations and severe disease
Immunosuppressive drugs
    cyclophosphamide (Cytoxan)
    azathioprine (Imuran)

LE, Lupus erythematosus; *NSAIDs,* nonsteroidal antiinflammatory drugs; *Sm antibody,* Smith antibody.

Patient teaching related to prescribed drugs must include their indications for use, proper administration, and possible side effects (see Chapter 48). The patient should understand that abrupt cessation may precipitate exacerbation of disease activity.

NURSING MANAGEMENT
SYSTEMIC LUPUS ERYTHEMATOSUS

■ Nursing Assessment

As in the majority of rheumatic diseases, the chronic and unpredictable nature of SLE presents many challenges to the patient and family. The physical, psychologic, and sociocultural problems associated with the long-term management of SLE require the varied approaches and skills of the multidisciplinary health care team.

Subjective and objective data that should be obtained from the patient with SLE are presented in Table 63-15. In particular, the extent to which pain and fatigue influence activities of daily living must be evaluated. A developmental approach focuses on age-appropriate education and counseling on issues such as personal relationships, family planning, occupational responsibilities, and recreational activities.

■ Nursing Diagnoses

Nursing diagnoses for the patient with SLE may include, but are not limited to, those presented in NCP 63-2.

■ Planning

As overall disease management goals, the patient with SLE will (1) have satisfactory pain relief, (2) comply with therapeutic regimen to achieve maximum symptom management, (3) demonstrate awareness of and avoid activities that cause disease exacerbation, and (4) maintain optimal role function and a positive self-image.

■ Nursing Implementation

Health Promotion. Prevention of SLE is not possible at this time. However, education of health professionals and the community should promote a clear understanding of the disease and the need for earlier diagnosis and treatment.

Acute Intervention. During an exacerbation of SLE, the patient may become abruptly and dramatically ill. Nursing interventions include accurately recording the severity of symptoms and documenting the response to therapy. Fever pattern, joint inflammation, limitation of motion, location and degree of discomfort, and fatigability should be specifically assessed. The patient's weight and fluid intake and output should be monitored if corticosteroids are prescribed because of the fluid-retention effect of these drugs and the possibility of renal failure. Collection of 24-hour urine samples for protein and creatinine clearance may be ordered. The nurse should observe for signs of bleeding that result from drug therapy, such as pallor, skin bruising, petechiae, or tarry stools.

TABLE 63-15	Nursing Assessment: Systemic Lupus Erythematosus
Subjective Data	**Objective Data**
Important Health Information	**General**
Past health history: Exposure to ultraviolet radiation, drugs, chemicals, viral infections; physical or psychologic stress; states of increased estrogen activity, including early onset of menarche, pregnancy, and postpartum period; pattern of remissions and exacerbations	Fever, lymphadenopathy, periorbital edema
	Integumentary
	Alopecia; dry, scaly scalp; keratoconjunctivitis, malar "butterfly" rash, palmar or discoid erythema, urticaria, periungual erythema, purpura, or petechiae; leg ulcers
Medications: Use of oral contraceptives, procainamide (Pronestyl), hydralazine (Apresoline), isoniazid (INH), antiseizure drugs, antibiotics (possibly precipitating symptoms of SLE); corticosteroids, NSAIDs	**Respiratory**
	Pleural friction rub, decreased breath sounds
Functional Health Patterns	**Cardiovascular**
Health perception–health management: Family history of autoimmune disorders; frequent infections; malaise	Vasculitis; pericardial friction rub; hypertension, edema, arrhythmias, murmurs; bilateral, symmetric pallor and cyanosis of fingers (Raynaud's phenomenon)
Nutritional-metabolic: Weight loss, oral and nasal ulcers; nausea and vomiting; xerostomia (salivary gland dryness), dysphagia; photosensitivity with rash; frequent infections	**Gastrointestinal**
	Oral and pharyngeal ulcers; splenomegaly
Elimination: Decreased urine output; diarrhea or constipation	**Neurologic**
Activity-exercise: Morning stiffness; joint swelling and deformity; shortness of breath, dyspnea; excessive fatigue	Facial weakness, peripheral neuropathies, papilledema, dysarthria, confusion, hallucination, disorientation, psychosis, seizures, aphasia, hemiparesis
Sleep-rest: Insomnia	**Musculoskeletal**
Cognitive-perceptual: Visual disturbances; vertigo; headache; polyarthralgia; chest pain (pericardial, pleuritic); abdominal pain; joint pain; pain, throbbing, coldness of fingers with numbness and tingling	Myopathy, myositis, arthritis
	Urinary
	Proteinuria
Sexuality-reproductive: Amenorrhea, irregular menstrual periods	**Possible Findings**
Coping-stress tolerance: Depression, withdrawal	Presence of anti-DNA, Sm, and antinuclear antibodies; anemia, leukopenia, thrombocytopenia; ↑ erythrocyte sedimentation rate (ESR); positive LE cell prep; ↑ serum creatinine; microscopic hematuria, cellular casts in urine; pericarditis or pleural effusion evident on chest x-ray

ANA, Antinuclear antibody; *NSAIDs,* nonsteroidal antiinflammatory drugs.

NURSING CARE PLAN 63-2

Patient with Systemic Lupus Erythematosus

EXPECTED PATIENT OUTCOMES	NURSING INTERVENTIONS and *RATIONALES*
NURSING DIAGNOSIS	**Fatigue** *related to* disease process *as manifested by* lack of energy, inability to maintain usual routine.
• Completion of priority activities • Pacing of activities • Verbalization of having more energy	• Analyze energy level patterns *to plan daily activities.* • Assist patient to prioritize activities *to establish preferred daily routine.* • Teach energy conservation techniques, such as sitting at kitchen sink, enlisting aid of others *to accomplish as much as possible with minimum energy expended.* * • Include family in planning *to increase patient's support and family's understanding of disease and related problems.* • Teach techniques such as meditation and yoga *to provide patient with stress-reducing strategies.* • Encourage patient to rest regularly and as needed *to temporarily reverse effect of fatigue.*
NURSING DIAGNOSIS	**Acute pain** *related to* disease process and inadequate comfort measures *as manifested by* complaints of joint pain, lack of relief from pain-relieving measures; reduction of activity to avoid exacerbating pain.
• Expression of satisfaction with pain relief measures • Performance of activities of daily living without pain	• Assess pain location and severity *to plan appropriate interventions.* • Administer analgesia as ordered and monitor effect, teach joint protection measures; apply heat or cold as determined *to relieve pain.* • Use nonpharmacologic pain interventions such as relaxation and imagery *to replace or supplement analgesics.*
NURSING DIAGNOSIS	**Impaired skin integrity** *related to* photosensitivity, skin rash, and alopecia *as manifested by* rash anywhere on body, butterfly rash on face, hair loss, areas of ulceration on fingertips, complaints of urticaria and photosensitivity.
• Limitation of direct exposure to sun and use of sunscreens • No open skin lesions • Strategies to cope with alopecia	• Assess and monitor location and progression of rash *to plan appropriate interventions.* • Administer drugs and apply ointments as ordered *to control skin manifestations.* • Keep skin clean and dry *to avoid secondary infections.* • Discuss need to limit direct sun exposure and use of sunscreens and sun protective clothing when outdoors *because sun exacerbates manifestations.*
NURSING DIAGNOSIS	**Activity intolerance** *related to* arthralgia, weakness, and fatigue *as manifested by* inability or unwillingness to ambulate or engage in physical activity, abnormal response to activity (e.g., increased pulse, respiratory rate).
• Expression of satisfaction with activity pattern • Pacing of activities to match level of tolerance	• Teach patient to pace activities and allow periods of rest between activities *to promote recuperation and to foster maximum participation in activities.* • Encourage patient to assist in setting activity schedule *to allow patient a sense of control and foster cooperation with the plan.* • Provide rest during exacerbation *to conserve energy for vital activities.* • Encourage use of assistive devices *to minimize energy expenditure.*
NURSING DIAGNOSIS	**Ineffective therapeutic regimen management** *related to* lack of knowledge of long-term management of disease *as manifested by* questions about SLE or incorrect answers to questions by patient or family, use of unproven remedies.
• Expression of confidence in ability to manage SLE over time and in home environment	• Teach patient about disease process, including chronic management *to increase probability of successful long-term management.* • Include family in teaching *to provide support during exacerbation and increase their sense of involvement.* • Discuss need to wear medical alert bracelet *to alert health care providers in time of emergency.* • Teach patient to report signs and symptoms of complications of disease such as fever, edema, decreased urine output, chest pain, and dyspnea *to ensure early intervention.* • Inform patient of availability of assistance from Lupus Foundation and Arthritis Foundation *to provide additional sources of information and support.*

*See Tables 63-4 and 63-9.

Careful assessment of neurologic status includes observation for visual disturbances, headaches, personality changes, seizures, and forgetfulness. Psychosis may indicate CNS disease or may be the effect of corticosteroid therapy. Irritation of the nerves of the extremities (peripheral neuropathy) may produce numbness, tingling, and weakness of the hands and feet.

The nurse must explain the nature of the disease, modes of therapy, and all diagnostic procedures. Emotional support for the patient and family is essential.

Ambulatory and Home Care. Nursing interventions must emphasize health teaching and the importance of patient cooperation for successful home management. The patient must understand that even perfect adherence to the treatment plan is not a guarantee against exacerbation because the course of the disease is unpredictable. However, a variety of factors may increase disease activity, such as fatigue, sun exposure, emotional stress, infection, drugs, and surgery. Nursing interventions should be directed toward assisting the patient and family to eliminate or minimize exposure to precipitating factors (Table 63-16).

Lupus and pregnancy. Because SLE is most common in women of childbearing age, treatment during pregnancy must be considered. The women's primary physician (or rheumatologist) and obstetrician should thoroughly discuss with the woman her desire to become pregnant. Infertility may have already resulted from renal involvement and the use of high-dose corticosteroid therapy. The SLE patient should understand that spontaneous abortion, stillbirth, and intrauterine growth retardation are common problems with pregnancy. They occur because of deposits of immune complexes in the placenta and because of inflammatory responses in the placental blood vessels. Renal, cardiovascular, pulmonary, and central nervous systems may be especially affected during pregnancy. Women who already demonstrate serious SLE involvement in these systems should be counseled against pregnancy. For the best outcome, pregnancy should be planned at a point when the disease activity is minimal. Exacerbation is common during the postpartum period. Therapeutic abortion offers the same risk of postdelivery exacerbation as carrying the fetus to term.

Neonatal lupus erythematosus (NLE) may occur in infants born of women with SLE. A risk for congenital heart block is correlated with high antibody titers.[45] A characteristic skin rash is seen in more than 30% of the cases of NLE.

Psychosocial issues. The patient with SLE confronts many psychosocial issues.[46] Disease onset may be vague, and SLE may be undiagnosed for long periods. Supportive therapies may become as important as medical treatment. The nurse should counsel the patient and family that SLE has a good prognosis for the majority of persons. Families are anxious about hereditary aspects and want to know whether their children will also have SLE. Many couples require pregnancy and sexual counseling. Individuals making decisions about marriage and careers worry about how SLE will interfere with their plans. The nurse may have to educate teachers, employers, and coworkers.

The obvious physical effects of skin rashes, discoid lesions, and alopecia may cause social isolation for the patient with SLE, affecting the individual's self-esteem and body image. However, pain and fatigue are cited most frequently as interfering with quality of life. Friends and relatives are confused by the patient's complaints of transient joint pain and overwhelming fatigue. Pacing techniques and relaxation therapy can help the patient remain involved in day-to-day activities. The nurse should stress the importance of planning both recreational and occupational activities. Young adults find sun restrictions and physical limitations particularly difficult to follow. Nursing interventions should assist the patient in developing and accomplishing reasonable goals for improving or maintaining mobility, energy levels, and self-esteem.

■ **Evaluation**

The expected outcomes for the patient with SLE are presented in NCP 63-2.

SYSTEMIC SCLEROSIS

Systemic sclerosis (SS), or *scleroderma,* is a disorder of connective tissue characterized by fibrotic, degenerative, and occasionally inflammatory changes in the skin, blood vessels, synovium, skeletal muscle, and internal organs. Skin thickening and tightening are the cardinal features.[47] The disease course of SS is variable. A localized or limited form of the disease, which is more common in children, is characterized by fewer symptoms mostly on the skin or in the muscles. Rarely does this localized sclerosis develop into systemic disease.[48]

SS affects women four times more often than men. SS has been reported in all ethnic groups but is more common in African Americans than whites. Although symptoms may begin at any time, the usual age at onset is between 30 and 50 years. Overall incidence increases with age. SS affects approximately 300,000 people in the United States.

Etiology and Pathophysiology

The exact cause of SS remains unknown. Immunologic dysfunction and vascular abnormalities are believed to play a role in development of widespread systemic disease. Other risk factors associated with skin thickening include environmental occupational exposure to coal, plastics, and silica dust. Collagen, the protein that gives normal skin its strength and elasticity, is overproduced (Fig. 63-10). Disruption of the cell is followed by platelet aggregation and fibrosis. Proliferation of collagen dis-

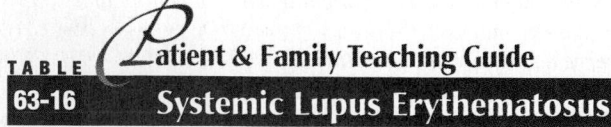

TABLE 63-16 ***Patient & Family Teaching Guide*** **Systemic Lupus Erythematosus**

Teaching related to the disease and appropriate management should include:
1. Disease process
2. Names of drugs, actions, side effects, dosage, administration
3. Pain management strategies
4. Energy conservation and pacing techniques
5. Therapeutic exercise, use of heat therapy (for arthralgia)
6. Avoidance of physical and emotional stress
7. Avoidance of exposure to individuals with infection
8. Avoidance of drying soaps, powders, household chemicals
9. Use of sunscreen protection (at least SPF 15), with minimal sun exposure from 11 AM to 3 PM
10. Regular medical and laboratory follow-up
11. Marital and pregnancy counseling as needed
12. Community resources and health care agencies

SPF, Sun protection factor.

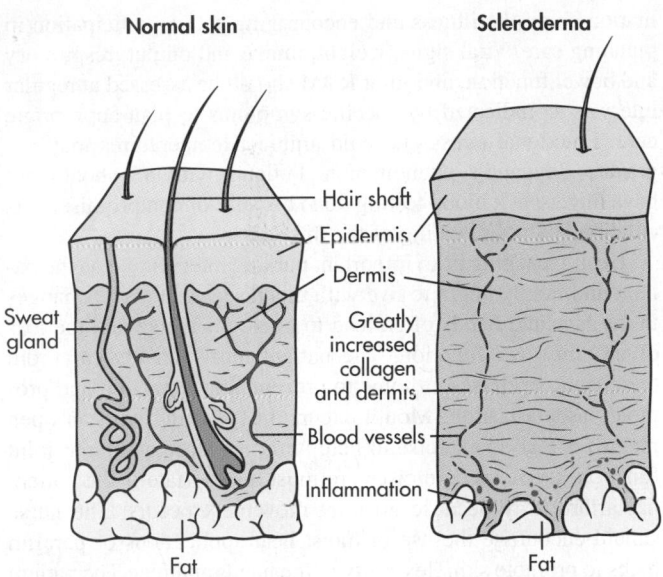

FIG. 63-10 Scleroderma skin changes.

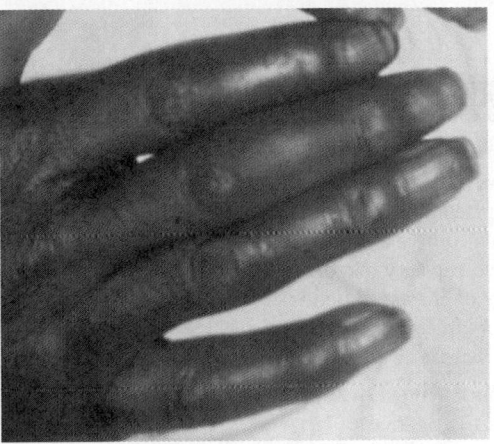

FIG. 63-11 Hand of a patient with systemic sclerosis showing sclerodactyly.

rupts the normal functioning of internal organs, such as the lungs, kidney, heart, and GI tract.

Clinical Manifestations

Manifestations of SS range from a diffuse cutaneous thickening with rapidly progressive and fatal visceral involvement to a more benign variant called CREST syndrome. **CREST syndrome** is characterized by the following five symptoms[49]:

Calcinosis—painful deposits of calcium in the skin

Raynaud's phenomenon—abnormal blood flow in response to cold or stress (Raynaud's phenomenon is explained in Chapter 37.)

Esophageal dysfunction—difficulty with swallowing caused by internal scarring

Sclerodactyly—tightening of the skin on the fingers and toes

Telangiectasia—red spots on the hands, forearms, palms, face and lips

Raynaud's Phenomenon. Raynaud's phenomenon (paroxysmal vasospasm of the digits) is the most common initial complaint in CREST syndrome. Patients have diminished blood flow to the fingers and toes on exposure to cold (blanching or white phase), followed by cyanosis as hemoglobin releases oxygen to the tissues (blue phase) and then erythema during rewarming (red phase). The color changes are often accompanied by numbness and tingling. Raynaud's phenomenon may precede the onset of systemic disease by months, years, or even decades.

Skin and Joint Changes. Symmetric painless swelling or thickening of the skin of the fingers and hands may progress to diffuse scleroderma of the trunk. In CREST syndrome, skin thickening is generally limited to the fingers and face. The skin loses elasticity and becomes taut and shiny, producing the typical expressionless facies with tightly pursed lips. Skin changes in the face may also contribute to reduced ROM in the temporomandibular joint. The hands may be affected by *sclerodactyly* in which the fingers are in a semiflexed position, with tightened skin to the wrist (Fig. 63-11). Reduced peripheral joint function may occur as an early symptom of polyarthritis.

Internal Organ Involvement. Esophageal fibrosis causes dysphagia and frequent reflux of gastric acid. If swallowing becomes difficult, the patient often decreases food intake and loses weight. GI effects include constipation resulting from colonic hypomotility and diarrhea caused by malabsorption from bacterial overgrowth.

Lung involvement includes pleural thickening, pulmonary fibrosis, and pulmonary function abnormalities. The patient develops a cough and dyspnea.

Primary heart disease consists of pericarditis, pericardial effusion, and cardiac arrhythmias. Myocardial fibrosis resulting in congestive heart failure occurs most frequently in patients with diffuse SS.

Renal disease is a major cause of death in SS. Malignant hypertension associated with rapidly progressive and irreversible renal insufficiency is often present. Recent improvements in dialysis, bilateral nephrectomy in patients with uncontrollable hypertension, and kidney transplantation have offered some hope to patients with renal failure.

Diagnostic Studies

Laboratory findings are relatively normal. Blood studies may reveal a mildly elevated ESR and mild hemolytic anemia as a result of RBC damage from diseased small vessels. The scleroderma antibody SCL-70 is found in about 35% of patients with systemic disease, and serum RF is found in 30% of affected patients. An anticentromere antibody is seen in many patients with CREST syndrome. If renal involvement is present, urinalysis may show proteinuria, microscopic hematuria, and casts. X-ray evidence of subcutaneous calcification, distal esophageal hypomotility, or bilateral pulmonary fibrosis is diagnostic of SS. Pulmonary function studies reveal decreased vital capacity and lung compliance.

Collaborative Care

The collaborative care of SS (Table 63-17) offers no specific treatment with long-term effects. Care is directed toward attempts to prevent or treat secondary complications of involved organs. Various drugs such as antiinflammatory agents, D-penicillamine (Cuprimine), minocycline (Minocin), and colchicine have been used with varying degrees of success.

TABLE 63-17	Collaborative Care Systemic Sclerosis

Diagnostic
History and physical examination
Antinuclear antibody titers
Anticentromere antibody
Nailbed capillary microscopy
X-rays of chest and hands
Skin or visceral biopsy
Urinalysis (proteinuria, hematuria, casts)

Collaborative Therapy
Vasoactive agents
Calcium channel blockers (diltiazem [Cardizem])
reserpine (Serpasil)
Nonsteroidal antiinflammatory drugs
penicillamine (Cuprimine)
Corticosteroids
Physical therapy

Physical therapy helps maintain joint mobility and preserve muscle strength. Occupational therapy assists the patient in maintaining functional abilities. Gastroesophageal reflux disease (GERD) may be treated by antacids and periodic dilation of the esophagus. (GERD is discussed in Chapter 40.)

Drug Therapy. No specific drugs or combination of drugs has been proven effective for the treatment of SS. Treatment is directed at symptoms and the prevention of complications. Vasoactive agents are often prescribed in early disease, and calcium channel blockers (nifedipine [Adalat, Procardia] and diltiazem [Cardizem]) are now a common treatment choice for Raynaud's phenomenon. Reserpine (Serpasil), an adrenergic blocking agent, increases blood flow to the fingers.

Corticosteroids are generally reserved for patients with significant joint or muscle involvement or severe skin disease with ulcerations. D-penicillamine increases the solubility of dermal collagen and may cause thinning of the skin. However, it is not accepted as a treatment option by all health care providers because of its possible toxic side effects, including myasthenia gravis and blood and liver dyscrasias. Topical agents may provide some relief from joint pain. Capsaicin cream may be useful not only as a local analgesic but also as a vasodilator. Other therapies are prescribed to address specific systemic problems, such as tetracycline for diarrhea caused by bacterial overgrowth, an H_2 histamine receptor blocker (e.g., cimetidine [Tagamet]) and proton pump inhibitor (e.g., omeprazole [Prilosec]) for esophageal symptoms, and an antihypertensive agent (e.g., captopril [Capoten], propranolol [Inderal], methyldopa [Aldomet]) for hypertension with renal involvement.

NURSING MANAGEMENT
SYSTEMIC SCLEROSIS

Because prevention is not possible, nursing intervention often begins during a hospitalization for diagnostic purposes. Diagnostic studies should be thoroughly explained. The nurse can help the patient resolve feelings of helplessness by providing information about the illness and encouraging active participation in planning care. Vital signs, weight, intake and output, respiratory and bowel function, and joint ROM should be assessed at regular intervals as indicated by specific symptoms to plan appropriate care. Emotional stress and cold ambient temperatures may aggravate Raynaud's phenomenon. Patients with SS should not have finger-stick blood testing done because of compromised circulation and poor healing of the fingers.

Health teaching is an important nursing intervention as the patient and family begin to live with this disease. Obvious changes in the face and hands often lead to poor self-image and the loss of mobility and function. The patient must actively carry out therapeutic exercises at home to prevent skin retraction and promote vascularization. Mouth excursion (yawning with an open mouth) is a good exercise to help with temporomandibular joint function. Isometric exercises are most appropriate if the patient has arthropathy because no joint movement occurs. The nurse should encourage the use of moist heat applications or paraffin baths to promote skin flexibility in the hands and feet. The patient should use assistive devices as appropriate and organize activities to preserve strength and reduce disability.

Hands and feet should be protected from cold exposure and possible burns or cuts that might heal slowly. Smoking should be avoided because of its vasoconstricting effect. Signs of infection should be promptly reported. Lotions may help alleviate skin dryness and cracking, but they must be rubbed in for an unusually long time because of the thickness of the skin.

Dysphagia may be reduced by eating small, frequent meals; chewing carefully and slowly; and drinking fluids. Heartburn may be minimized by using antacids 45 to 60 minutes after each meal and by sitting upright for at least 2 hours after eating. Using additional pillows or raising the head of the bed on blocks may help reduce nocturnal gastroesophageal reflux.

Job modifications are often necessary because stair climbing, typing, writing, and cold exposure may pose particular problems. The patient may become socially withdrawn as skin tightening alters the appearance of the face and hands. Dining out may become a socially embarrassing event because the patient's small mouth, difficulty swallowing, and reflux make eating less enjoyable. Some individuals with SS wear gloves to protect fingertip ulcers and to provide extra warmth. Sensitive areas on fingertips resulting from ulcers or calcinosis may require padded utensils or special assistive devices to reduce discomfort. Daily oral hygiene must be emphasized, or neglect may lead to increased tooth and gingival problems. The patient needs a dentist who is familiar with SS and can deal with a small oral aperture. Psychologic support reduces stress and may positively influence peripheral motor response. Biofeedback training and relaxation techniques can reduce tension, improve sleeping habits, and raise the temperature of the fingers and toes.

Sexual dysfunction resulting from body changes, pain, muscular weakness, limited mobility, decreased self-esteem, erectile dysfunction, and decreased vaginal secretions may require sensitive counseling by the nurse. Specific suggestions based on individual patient assessment should be offered.

POLYMYOSITIS AND DERMATOMYOSITIS

Polymyositis (PM) and **dermatomyositis** (DM) are diffuse, idiopathic, inflammatory myopathies of striated muscle, producing bilateral weakness usually most severe in the proximal or limb-girdle muscles. These disorders, which are relatively rare, occur twice as often in women as in men. In a bimodal distribution, children ages 5 to 14 years and adults ages 45 to 65 years are most often affected by PM and DM.[50] Some cases of DM are associated with concurrent malignant disease.[51]

Etiology and Pathophysiology

The exact cause of PM and DM is unknown. Theories include an infectious agent, neoplasms, drugs or vaccinations, and stress. Because disease severity is not well correlated with altered immune complexes, it is unclear if the complexes occur as primary or secondary phenomena. Because cytotoxic T cells and macrophages have been found near the damaged muscle fibers of PM, the disease is believed to be caused by cell-mediated injury.

Clinical Manifestations and Complications

Muscular. Over several months, the patient experiences weight loss and increasing fatigue. Gradually developing weakness of the muscles leads to difficulty in performing routine activities. The most commonly affected muscles are those of the shoulders, legs, arms, and pelvic girdle. The patient may have difficulty rising from a chair or bathtub, climbing stairs, combing the hair, or reaching into a high cupboard. Neck muscles may become so weak that the patient is unable to raise the head from the pillow. Muscle discomfort or tenderness is uncommon. Muscle examination reveals an inability to move against resistance or even gravity. Weak pharyngeal muscles may produce dysphagia and dysphonia (nasal or hoarse voice).

Dermal. Skin changes include the classic violet-colored, cyanotic, or erythematous symmetric rash (heliotrope) with edema around the eyelids. Reddened, smooth, or scaly patches appear at the PIP joints (Gottron's sign) and can be confused with psoriasis or seborrheic dermatitis. Violet-colored or erythematous papules and small plaques can also develop on the knuckles (Gottron's papules).[52] On the back and on the extensor surfaces of the forearms, an erythematous scaling rash may develop (poikiloderma). Hyperemia and telangiectasias are often present at the nailbeds. Calcium nodules (calcinosis cutis), which can develop throughout the skin, are especially common in long-standing DM.

Other Manifestations. Joint redness, pain, and inflammation often occur and contribute to limitations in joint ROM. Contractures and muscle atrophy may occur with advanced disease. Weakened pharyngeal muscles can lead to a poor cough effort, difficulty swallowing, and increased risk for aspiration pneumonia. "Cotton-wool" patches can occur in the retina. Childhood DM appears to have a more progressive, crippling course.

Diagnostic Studies

Diagnosis of PM or DM is confirmed after excluding other neuromuscular diseases. The most important laboratory finding is an elevation of the enzyme creatine kinase (CK). Increased levels of CK indicate muscle damage. Because test results change with disease activity, serum CK levels can also be valuable in determining the patient's response to treatment. Elevation of ESR is also expected with active disease. An electromyogram suggestive of PM will show bizarre high-frequency discharges and spontaneous fibrillation, with positive spikes at rest. Muscle biopsy reveals necrosis, degeneration, regeneration, and fibrosis. Complete pulmonary function testing is necessary to determine the extent of lung involvement.

Collaborative Care

PM and DM are initially treated with high-dose corticosteroids. Improvement is generally achieved if corticosteroid therapy is promptly instituted, and the dosage can typically be reduced as improvement is noted. Relapses are common. If corticosteroids prove ineffective or lead to myopathy, immunosuppressive drugs may be administered (methotrexate, azathioprine [Imuran] or cyclophosphamide [Cytoxan]) using oral or intermittent intravenous dosing. Topical corticosteroids may also be prescribed to treat the skin rash.

Physical therapy can be helpful and should be tailored to the activity of the disease. Massage and passive movement are appropriate during active disease. More aggressive exercises should be reserved for periods when disease activity is minimal, as evidenced by low serum enzyme levels.

A careful search for possible malignant lesions should be undertaken for the patient more than 40 years of age.[53] If malignant disease is found, it should be treated appropriately. Complete remission of DM may occur if the malignant lesion is removed.

NURSING MANAGEMENT
POLYMYOSITIS AND DERMATOMYOSITIS

Prevention is not possible. However, improved ability to discriminate PM from other muscular disorders may favorably influence prognosis by more rapid diagnosis and institution of therapy.

Nursing interventions should include a thorough explanation of the nature of the disease, the prescribed therapies, all diagnostic tests, and the importance of regular medical care. Assessment of muscular weakness and limitation of motion should be performed. It is important for the patient to understand that the benefits of therapy are often delayed. For example, weakness may increase during the first few weeks of corticosteroid therapy. The nurse should maintain the patient on bed rest and assist the patient with activities of daily living when extreme weakness is present. Special attention is paid to patient safety. To prevent aspiration, the patient should be encouraged to rest before meals, maintain an upright position when eating, and choose a diet of easily swallowed foods. Use of assistive devices should be encouraged as a fall prevention strategy.

The nurse should assist the patient to organize activities and use pacing techniques to conserve energy. Daily ROM exercises are encouraged to prevent contractures. When active inflammation is not evident, muscle-strengthening (repetitive) exercises may be started. Home care will be necessary during the acute phase of PM because profound muscle weakness renders the patient unable to carry out activities of daily living. Homemaker services, visiting nurses, and family caregivers are needed to assist the patient in routine hygiene, meal preparation and eating, and ambulation.

OVERLAPPING FORMS OF CONNECTIVE TISSUE DISEASE

Patients having a combination of clinical features of several rheumatic diseases are described as having *overlapping* or *mixed connective tissue disease*. Although this combination was originally believed to be a distinct clinical disorder, follow-up revealed an evolution primarily from SLE or SS. This early undifferentiated or transitional form of connective tissue disease has a typical serologic pattern, including high titers of a speckled pattern of ANA, high levels of antibody to ribonuclease-sensitive extractable nuclear antibody, and autoantibodies to ribonucleoprotein.

SJÖGREN SYNDROME

Sjögren syndrome is an autoimmune disease that targets moisture-producing glands, leading to the common symptoms of *xerostomia* (dry mouth) and keratoconjunctivitis *sicca* (dry eyes). The nose, throat, airways, and skin can also become dry. The disease can affect other glands as well, including those in the stomach, pancreas, and intestines (extraglandular involvement). The disease is usually diagnosed in women over age 40.[54]

In primary Sjögren syndrome, symptoms can be traced to problems with the lacrimal and salivary glands. The patient with primary disease is likely to have antibodies against the cytoplasmic antigens SS-A and SS-B, as well as ANA. The patient with secondary Sjögren syndrome typically has had another autoimmune disease (e.g., RA, SLE) before Sjögren develops.

Sjögren syndrome appears to be caused by genetic and environmental factors. Several genes seem to be involved. One gene predisposes whites to the disease, whereas other genes are linked to the disease in people of Japanese, Chinese, and African American heritage. The trigger may be a viral or bacterial infection that adversely stimulates the immune system. In Sjögren syndrome, lymphocytes attack and damage the lacrimal and salivary glands.

Dry eyes and dry mouth are the main symptoms. Decreased tearing leads to a "gritty" sensation in the eyes, burning, blurred vision, and photosensitivity. Dry mouth produces buccal membrane fissures, altered sense of taste, dysphagia, and increased frequency of mouth infections or dental caries. Dry skin and rashes, joint and muscle pain, and thyroid problems may also be present. Other exocrine glands can be affected. For example, vaginal dryness may lead to dyspareunia (painful intercourse). Autoimmune thyroid disorders are common with Sjögren syndrome, including Graves' disease or Hashimoto's thyroiditis. Histologic study reveals lymphocyte infiltration of salivary and lacrimal glands. The disease may become more generalized and involve the lymph nodes, bone marrow, and visceral organs (pseudolymphoma). Lymphoma develops in about 5% of patients with Sjögren syndrome.

Ophthalmologic examination (Schirmer test), salivary flow rates, and lower lip biopsy of minor salivary glands confirm the diagnosis.[55] The treatment is symptomatic, including (1) instillation of artificial tears as often as necessary to maintain adequate hydration and lubrication, (2) surgical punctual occlusion, and (3) increased fluids with meals. Dental hygiene is important. Pilocarpine (Salagen) and cevimeline (Evoxac) can be used to treat symptoms of dry mouth.[56] Increased humidity at home may reduce respiratory infections. Vaginal lubrication with a water-soluble product such as K-Y jelly may increase comfort during intercourse. Corticosteroids and immunosuppressive drugs are indicated for treatment of pseudolymphoma.

Soft Tissue Rheumatic Syndromes

Myofascial pain syndrome, fibromyalgia syndrome (FMS), and chronic fatigue syndrome (CFS) are three soft tissue disease syndromes that have many commonalities and may be related.

Ongoing research continues to explore links among these three syndromes. A multidisciplinary team approach consisting of a rheumatologist, nurse, mental health professional, and physical therapist may be especially helpful for patients with these syndromes whose disease course may be chronic.

MYOFASCIAL PAIN SYNDROME

Myofascial pain syndrome is characterized by musculoskeletal pain and tenderness in one anatomic region of the body. The pain has been shown to originate in anterior and posterior trigger points that have resulted from muscle trauma and/or chronically strained muscles (e.g., desk or computer work). Regions of pain are often within the taut bands and fascia of skeletal muscles. When activated by pressure, trigger points are thought to activate a characteristic pattern of pain. The incidence and the age groups and gender that are most affected are not known.

Patients complain of the pain as deep and aching accompanied by a sensation of burning, stinging, and stiffness.[57] The muscles frequently involved are located in the chest, neck, lower back, and shoulders. Referred pain from these muscle groups can also travel to the buttock, hand, and the head, causing severe headaches. Additional systemic manifestations have not been reported.

A test used to diagnose myofascial pain syndrome is the palpation of trigger points. On physical examination of the patient, palpation reveals induration and frequently a muscle twitch in the area of a trigger point. Once a trigger point is palpated, pain is then referred to a region often at some distance away.[58] These findings have also been noted to occur in normal healthy persons and in persons with FMS. Similarities in myofascial pain syndrome with FMS have led to the suggestion that myofascial pain may be a form of or evolve into FMS. A comparison of the two syndromes is shown in Table 63-18.

The active management of myofascial pain can often result in relief of the patient's pain. Positive results have been seen by locally injecting the trigger points with a local anesthetic (e.g., 1% lidocaine), passive muscle stretching and manipulation, and spraying the trigger point with a cold agent such as ethyl chloride. Massage, acupuncture, biofeedback, and ultrasound therapy have also shown to benefit some patients.

Patient and family teaching is an important nursing responsibility. Instruction should focus on the prevention of muscle tension in work and leisure activities. Good posture and resting and sleeping positions should also be reviewed. Most patients with

TABLE 63-18 Comparison of Fibromyalgia and Myofascial Pain Syndromes

VARIABLE	FIBROMYALGIA	MYOFASCIAL PAIN
Location		Regional
Examination		Trigger points
Response to local therapy		Curative
Gender		Equal or unknown
Systemic features		Unknown

From McCance KL, Huether SE: *Pathophysiology: the biologic basis for disease in adults and children,* ed 4, St Louis, 2002, Mosby.

myofascial pain syndrome are able to lead a normal and active lifestyle.

FIBROMYALGIA SYNDROME

Fibromyalgia syndrome (FMS) is a chronic disorder characterized by widespread, nonarticular musculoskeletal pain and fatigue with multiple tender points. People with FMS also typically experience nonrestorative sleep, morning stiffness, irritable bowel syndrome, and anxiety. The former name for this disorder, fibrositis, implied inflammation of the muscles and soft tissues. However, FMS is now known to be nondegenerative, nonprogressive, and noninflammatory.

Fibromyalgia is a commonly diagnosed musculoskeletal disorder and a major cause of disability. FMS affects over 6 million Americans, typically occurring in women 20 to 55 years old.[59,60] FMS and CFS share many commonalities (Table 63-19).

Etiology and Pathophysiology

Research continues to focus on identifying the underlying causes and pathophysiologic mechanisms of FMS. Currently multiple theories exist regarding the etiology of FMS. One possible factor may involve the CNS. Neurotransmitters in the CNS including serotonin, substance P, and norepinephrine are at abnormal levels in patients with FMS.[61] These neurotransmitters regulate mood, sleep, and pain perception. Sleep disturbances, depression, and widespread soft tissue pain are common in FMS.

A hyperfunctioning of the hypothalamic-pituitary-adrenal (HPA) axis, which plays a major role in the stress response, may also exist. Changes in the HPA axis can negatively affect a person's physical and mental state. An increase in cortisol levels, with a concomitant decrease in ACTH levels, has been noted in persons with FMS.[62,63] These findings can be linked to depression

and a decreased response to stress. It is not known if depression is a cause or an effect of the disease.

A dysfunction in the autonomic nervous system may cause changes in the vascular system leading to orthostatic hypotension and decreased heart rate variability. A recent viral illness or Lyme disease may serve as an infectious trigger in susceptible persons. A noted decrease in growth hormone may be responsible for the muscle pain.

Clinical Manifestations and Complications

Clinical manifestations of FMS overlap with those of CFS.[64] The patient complains of a widespread burning pain that worsens and improves through the course of a day. It is often difficult for the patient to discriminate if pain occurs in the muscles, joints, or soft tissues. Head or facial pain often results from stiff or painful neck and shoulder muscles. It can accompany temporomandibular joint dysfunction, which affects an estimated one third of FMS patients. Nonrestorative sleep and resulting fatigue are typical. Physical examination characteristically reveals point tenderness at 11 or more of 18 identified sites[65] (Fig. 63-12). Patients with FMS are sensitive to painful stimuli throughout the body and not merely at the identified tender sites. In addition, point tenderness can vary from day to day. On some occasions, the FMS patient may respond to fewer than 11 tender points; at other times, palpation of all sites may elicit pain.

Cognitive effects range from difficulty concentrating to memory lapses and a feeling of being overwhelmed when dealing with multiple tasks. Many individuals report migraine headaches. Depression and anxiety often occur and may require drugs. Numbness or tingling in the hands or feet (paresthesia) often accompanies FMS. Restless legs syndrome is also typical, with the patient describing an irresistible urge to move the legs when at rest or lying down.

Irritable bowel syndrome with manifestations of digestive disturbances, abdominal pain, and bloating is common. FMS patients may also experience difficulty swallowing, perhaps because of abnormalities in esophageal smooth muscle function. Increased frequency of urination and urinary urgency, in the absence of a bladder infection, are typical complaints. Women with FMS may experience more difficult menstruation, with a worsening of disease symptoms during this time.

Diagnostic Studies

A definitive diagnosis of FMS is often difficult to establish. Laboratory results in most cases serve to rule out other suspected disorders based on the patient's history and physical examination. Occasionally a low ANA titer is seen, but it is not considered diagnostic. Muscle biopsy may reveal a nonspecific moth-eaten appearance or fiber atrophy. The American College of Rheumatology classifies an individual as having FMS if two criteria are met: (1) pain is experienced in 11 of the 18 tender points on palpation (see Fig. 63-12) and (2) a history of widespread pain is noted for at least 3 months. Widespread pain is defined as occurring on both sides of the body and above and below the waist. Up to 70% all patients with FMS will also meet the criteria for a diagnosis of CFS.[61]

Collaborative Care

The treatment of FMS is symptomatic and requires a high level of patient motivation. The nurse can play a key role in teaching the patient to be an active participant in the therapeutic

TABLE 63-19	Commonalities Between Fibromyalgia Syndrome and Chronic Fatigue Syndrome
Occurrence	Previously healthy, young, and middle-aged women
Etiology (theories)	Infectious trigger, dysfunction in HPA axis, alteration in CNS
Clinical manifestations	Malaise and fatigue, cognitive dysfunction, headaches, sleep disturbances, depression, anxiety, fever, generalized musculoskeletal pain
Course of disease	Variable-intensity of symptoms fluctuate over time
Diagnosis	No definitive laboratory tests or joint and muscle examinations, mainly a diagnosis of exclusion
Collaborative care	Treatment is symptomatic and may include antidepressant drugs such as amitriptyline (Elavil) and fluoxetine (Prozac). Other measures are heat, massage, regular stretching, biofeedback, stress management, and relaxation training. Patient and family teaching is essential.

CNS, Central nervous system; *HPA,* hypothalamic-pituitary-adrenal.

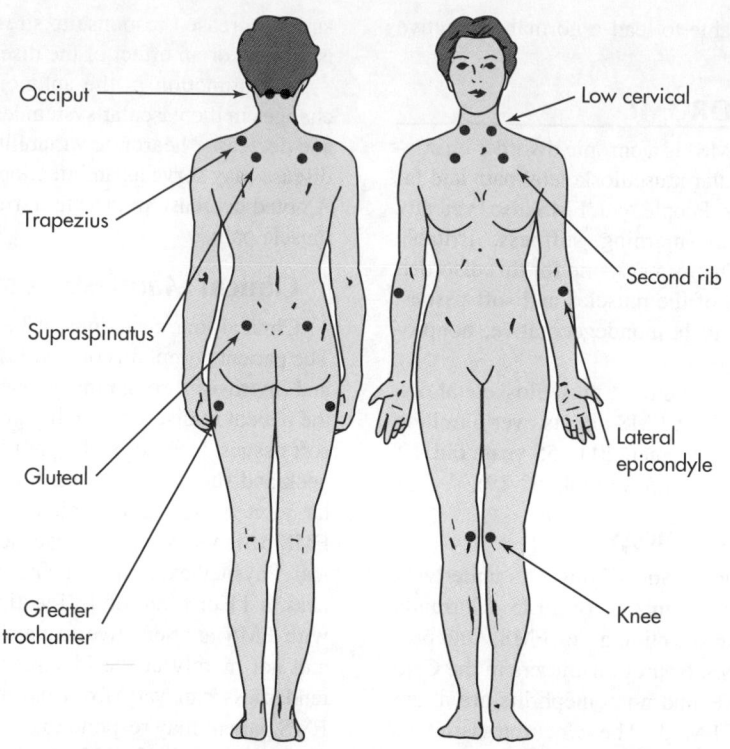

Occiput

Trapezius

Supraspinatus

Gluteal

Greater
trochanter

Low cervical

Second rib

Lateral
epicondyle

Knee

FIG. 63-12 Tender points in fibromyalgia syndrome.

regimen. Pain, aching, and tenderness can be helped by rest. Analgesics such as acetaminophen (Tylenol), and NSAIDs (e.g., tramadol [Ultram]) are effective for some patients. Stress, fatigue, and sleep disturbances can be helped by taking a low-dose tricyclic antidepressant such as amitriptyline (Elavil), which has undergone extensive clinical testing for use in the treatment of FMS (see the Evidence-Based Practice box). The skeletal muscle relaxant cyclobenzaprine (Flexeril) is also commonly used to treat sleep disturbances. Both drugs have sedative effects that can help in improving nighttime rest for the patient with FMS. If amitriptyline is not well tolerated, other similar drugs can be sub-

stituted (e.g., doxepin [Sinequan], imipramine [Tofranil], or trazodone [Desyrel]). Selective serotonin reuptake inhibitor (SSRI) antidepressants (e.g., sertraline [Zoloft] or paroxetine [Paxil]) tend to be reserved for FMS patients who also have depression. SSRIs are often prescribed at low doses during the day and sometimes combined with a tricyclic antidepressant at bedtime.

Benzodiazepines (e.g., diazepam [Valium], alprazolam [Xanax], clonazepam [Klonopin]) are often prescribed with low doses of ibuprofen (Motrin, Advil) to treat anxiety, as well as the muscle spasms that affect many FMS patients. The drug zolpidem tartrate (Ambien) is sometimes prescribed for short-term intervention in patients with severe sleep disturbances.

EVIDENCE-BASED PRACTICE
Antidepressants for Fibromyalgia

Clinical Problem
Are antidepressants effective in the treatment of fibromyalgia?

Best Clinical Practice
- Antidepressants improve overall symptoms related to fibromyalgia.
- Antidepressants improve individual symptoms of fatigue, sleep, and pain in patients with fibromyalgia.

Implications for Nursing Practice
- Fibromyalgia can be a devastating disease and significantly affect quality of life.
- Patients with fibromyalgia should be offered antidepressants as a form of treatment to decrease their symptoms.

Reference for Evidence
EMB Reviews: Antidepressants improve symptoms of fibromyalgia, *ACP Journal Club* 134:85, 2001.

NURSING MANAGEMENT
FIBROMYALGIA SYNDROME

Because of the chronic nature of FMS and the necessity of maintaining an ongoing rehabilitation program, the patient with FMS needs consistent support from the nurse and other members of the health care team. Massage is often combined with ultrasound or the application of alternating heat and cold packs to soothe tense, sore muscles and increase blood circulation. Gentle stretching can be performed by a physical therapist or practiced by the FMS patient at home to relieve muscle tension and spasm. Yoga and Tai Chi are often appropriate choices. Low-impact aerobic exercise such as walking can help prevent muscle atrophy. A cardinal rule for the FMS patient is to start slowly and build up exercise tolerance in increments.[66]

Dietitians often urge FMS patients to limit their consumption of sugar, caffeine, and alcohol because these substances have been shown to be muscle irritants. Vitamin and mineral supplements may be appropriate to combat stress, correct deficiencies, and support the immune system. However, unproven "miracle diets" or supplements should be carefully investigated by the FMS patient and discussed with the health care provider before using them. The patient should understand that some foods and supplements may cause serious or even dangerous side effects when mixed with certain drugs.

Pain and the related symptoms of FMS can cause significant stress. There is also some indication that FMS patients simply do not process stress well. Effective relaxation strategies include biofeedback, guided imagery, and autogenic training. Patients need to receive initial training for these interventions, but they can then continue to practice in their own homes. Psychologic counseling (individual or group) may also prove beneficial for the FMS patient.

CHRONIC FATIGUE SYNDROME

Chronic fatigue syndrome (CFS), also called chronic fatigue and immune dysfunction syndrome, is a disorder characterized by debilitating fatigue and a variety of associated complaints. Immune abnormalities are also frequently present. CFS is three times more common in women than in men. Its onset typically occurs between the ages of 25 and 45. The prevalence of CFS is difficult to determine. It is estimated that 500,000 people in the United States have a CFS-like condition.[67] CFS is a poorly understood condition and can have a devastating impact on the lives of patients and their families. CFS and FMS share some common features (see Table 63-19).

Etiology and Pathophysiology

Despite numerous attempts to determine the etiology and pathology of CFS, the precise mechanisms remain unknown. However, there are many theories about the cause of CFS.[68] It was once thought that CFS was postinfectious and followed a viral infection. Several microorganisms have been investigated as etiologic agents, including herpesviruses (e.g., Epstein Barr [EBV], cytomegalovirus [CMV]), retroviruses, enteroviruses, *Candida albicans,* and mycoplasma. Antibody titers to many infectious agents are elevated in patients with CFS. However, studies have shown no causal relationships between these specific viral agents and CFS. It is known that viruses can precipitate the syndrome. In addition, EBV and CMV infections may contribute to the fatigue and exhaustion experienced in CFS.

Abnormal immune function appears to be a central event in CFS. These abnormalities include decreased immunoglobulin production, reduced NK cell activity, altered cytokine production, decreased lymphocyte proliferation, altered CD4/CD8 ratio, and an increased percentage of activated T cells. If the mechanism of CFS involves a continuing immune response to an initial viral infection, the symptoms may be due in part to the production of cytokines. These immune mediators can cause muscle and CNS manifestations, including fatigue. However, immune alterations do not occur in all patients.

Dysfunctioning of the HPA axis may exist, causing neuroendocrine regulation alterations.[69,70] Changes in the HPA axis can alter the immune system, cause a decrease in energy, and affect mood states in patients with CFS. Because of the activation of the HPA axis, there is a reduced production of corticotropin-releasing hormone in the hypothalamus. Serum cortisol levels are low, and ACTH levels are correspondingly high.

Alterations in the CNS are thought to play a role in CFS. Patients often manifest cognitive deficits including problems with memory, attention, and concentration. A disturbance in the regulation of blood pressure and pulse is commonly found in patients with CFS.

Because mild to moderate depression occurs in many of these patients, it has been proposed that CFS is a psychiatric disorder. However, it is difficult to determine if depression is a cause or an effect of debilitating chronic fatigue.

Clinical Manifestations

It is often difficult to distinguish between CFS and FMS because many clinical features are similar (see Table 63-19). In about half of the cases, CFS develops insidiously, or the patient may have intermittent episodes that gradually become chronic. Incapacitating fatigue is the most common symptom of CFS and is the problem that causes the patient to seek health care. Associated symptoms (Table 63-20) may fluctuate in intensity over time. In other situations, CFS arises suddenly in a previously active, healthy individual. An unremarkable flulike illness or other acute stress is often identified as a triggering event.

The patient may become angry and frustrated with the inability of health care providers to diagnose a problem. The disorder may have a major impact on work and family responsibilities. Some individuals may even need help with activities of daily living.

Diagnostic Studies

Physical examination and diagnostic studies can be used to rule out other possible causes of the patient's symptoms. No laboratory test can diagnose CFS or measure its severity. The Centers for Disease Control and Prevention have developed diagnostic criteria based on the patient's symptoms (see Table 63-20). In general, it remains a diagnosis of exclusion.[71]

TABLE 63-20 Diagnostic Criteria for Chronic Fatigue Syndrome*

Major Criteria
- Unexplained, persistent, or relapsing chronic fatigue is of new and definite onset (not lifelong).
- Fatigue is not due to ongoing exertion.
- Fatigue is not substantially alleviated by rest.
- Fatigue results in substantial reduction in occupational, educational, social, or personal activities.

Minor Criteria
- Substantial impairment in short-term memory or concentration
- Sore throat
- Tender cervical or axillary lymph nodes
- Muscle pain
- Multijoint pain without joint swelling or tenderness
- Headaches of a new type, pattern, or severity
- Unrefreshing sleep
- Postexertional malaise lasting more than 24 hours

Adapted from Fukuda K et al (International Chronic Fatigue Syndrome Study Group): The chronic fatigue syndrome: a comprehensive approach to its definition and study, *Ann Intern Med* 121:953, 1994.
*For a diagnosis to be made, the patient must fulfill all the major criteria, plus four or more of the minor criteria. Each minor criterion must have persisted or recurred during 6 or more consecutive months of illness and must not have predated the fatigue. These criteria were prepared by the Centers for Disease Control and Prevention, National Institutes of Health, and International Chronic Fatigue Syndrome Study Group.

NURSING and COLLABORATIVE MANAGEMENT CHRONIC FATIGUE SYNDROME

Because there is no definitive treatment for CFS, supportive management is essential. The patient should be informed about what is known about the disease, and all complaints should be taken seriously. NSAIDs can be used to treat headaches, muscle and joint aches, and fever. Because many patients with CFS also have allergies and sinusitis, antihistamines and decongestants can be used to treat allergic symptoms. Tricyclic antidepressants (e.g., doxepin [Sinequan], amitriptyline [Elavil]) and SSRIs (e.g., fluoxetine [Prozac], paroxetine [Paxil]) can improve mood and sleep problems. Clonazepam (Klonopin) can also be used to treat sleep disturbances and panic disorders. The use of low-dose hydrocortisone is being studied to decrease fatigue and disability.

Total rest is not advised because it can potentiate the self-image of being an invalid. On the other hand, strenuous exertion can exacerbate the exhaustion. Therefore it is important to plan a carefully graduated exercise program. A well-balanced diet including fiber and fresh dark-colored fruits and vegetables for antioxidant action is essential in treatment. Behavioral therapy may be used to promote a positive outlook, as well as improve overall disability, fatigue, and other symptoms.[72,73]

One of the major problems facing many CFS patients is financial instability. When the illness strikes, they cannot work or must decrease the amount of time working. Loss of a job often leads to loss of medical insurance. Obtaining disability benefits can be frustrating because of the difficulty of establishing a diagnosis of CFS.

CFS does not appear to progress. Although most patients recover or at least gradually improve over time, some never show substantial improvement. Recovery is more common in individuals with a sudden onset of CFS. Patients with CFS suffer from substantial occupational and psychosocial impairments and loss, including the social pressure and isolation from being characterized as lazy or "crazy."

CRITICAL THINKING EXERCISES

Case Study
Systemic Lupus Erythematosus

Patient Profile. Grace Anderson, a 30-year-old married African American woman, is seen at the rheumatology clinic following a recent vacation to Hawaii.

Subjective Data
- Works in a flower shop
- Complains of joint pain, photosensitivity, fatigue, and a facial rash
- Is 4 months pregnant
- Has Raynaud's phenomenon when she works in the refrigerator room stocking flowers
- Fears something is horribly wrong with her
- Is afraid to take drugs because of pregnancy

Objective Data

Physical Examination
- Malar rash
- Swelling of third and fourth metacarpophalangeal joints of both hands
- Dry, scaly scalp
- Pain on motion of both wrists, shoulders, and knees with no obvious swelling

Diagnostic Studies
- WBC count 4000/μl (4 × 10^9/L)
- Platelets 100,000/μl (150 × 10^9/L)
- Complement (C3) 60 mg/dl (0.6 g/L)
- Positive ANA and Sm antibodies

Collaborative Care
- Diagnosed with SLE
- Started on prednisone 10 mg daily

CRITICAL THINKING QUESTIONS

1. How might the nurse explain the pathophysiology of SLE to Grace?
2. How might the vacation have influenced the symptoms that she is currently experiencing?
3. What are some home and work modifications that the nurse can suggest to Grace that will reduce her symptoms?
4. Discuss the types of prenatal and postpartum considerations essential in caring for Grace.
5. What other sources of information regarding SLE might the nurse suggest to Grace and her family?
6. Based on the assessment data presented, write one or more nursing diagnoses. Are there any collaborative problems?

Nursing Research Issues

1. What is the relationship between social support systems and quality of life for people with rheumatoid arthritis?
2. What are the needs of the family when the patient is diagnosed with SLE?
3. Are gender and age of the patient related to use of alternative therapies with arthritic pain?
4. What are effective measures that the nurse can institute to improve patient compliance with arthritis home management programs?
5. Does regular well-tolerated exercise by a patient with arthritis or connective tissue disease improve quality of life?

REVIEW QUESTIONS

The number of the question corresponds to the same-numbered objective at the beginning of the chapter.

1. In assessing the joints of a patient with rheumatoid arthritis, the nurse understands that the joints are damaged by
   a. the development of Heberden's nodes in the joint capsule.
   b. the deterioration of cartilage by the enzyme hyaluronidase.
   c. invasion of pannus into the joint capsule and subchondral bone.
   d. bony ankylosis following inflammation of the joints in HLA-B27–positive individuals.

2. Assessment data noted by the nurse in the patient with osteoarthritis commonly include
   a. elevated ESR.
   b. evening but no morning stiffness.
   c. progressive joint pain with activity.
   d. symmetric swelling of metacarpophalangeal joints.

3. An important nursing intervention in caring for the patient with ankylosing spondylitis is to teach the patient
   a. thoracic stretching and ROM exercises to prevent deformity.
   b. to sleep on the side with the legs flexed and supported with pillows.
   c. to prevent enteric and venereal infections that precipitate recurring attacks.
   d. that continuous therapeutic blood levels of NSAIDs can limit the progression of the disease.

4. When teaching the patient with gout, the nurse should instruct the patient to
   a. avoid foods high in fat and calories.
   b. drink plenty of fluids on a daily basis.
   c. apply ice packs to decrease joint pain.
   d. have CBC and WBC levels monitored regularly.

5. In teaching a patient with SLE about the disorder, the nurse uses the knowledge that the pathophysiology of SLE includes
   a. production of autoantibodies directed against constituents of cellular DNA.
   b. an autoimmune reaction resulting in degeneration, necrosis, and fibrosis of muscle fibers.
   c. deposition in tissues of immune complexes formed from IgG autoantibodies reacting with IgG.
   d. chronic inflammation and cytokine activity, which results in synovial proliferation and cartilage and bone damage.

6. The nurse planning teaching for the patient with rheumatoid arthritis who is receiving multiple drug therapy includes information related to the need to
   a. use aspirin only on an as-needed basis for pain relief.
   b. use birth control during and 3 months following gold therapy.
   c. have frequent laboratory monitoring while taking methotrexate.
   d. stop taking any corticosteroids as soon as symptoms are relieved.

7. In teaching a patient with fibromyalgia (FMS) about this disorder, the nurse understands that
   a. more men than women are affected.
   b. trigger points are a definitive diagnostic test.
   c. many symptoms are similar to chronic fatigue syndrome.
   d. FMS is characterized by progression of worsening inflammation.

REFERENCES

1. Roberts D: Arthritis and connective tissue disorders. In Schoen D, editor: *NAON core curriculum for orthopaedic nursing,* ed 4, Pitman, NJ, 2001, Jannetti.
2. Ling SM, Bathon JM: Osteoarthritis in older adults, *Am Geriatr Soc* 46:215-225, 1998.
3. Kee CC: Osteoarthritis: manageable scourge of aging, *Nurs Clin North Am* 35:1, 2000.
4. Roberts D: Degenerative disease. In Maher AB, Salmond SW, Pellino TA, editors: *Orthopaedic nursing,* ed 3, Philadelphia, 2002, Saunders.
5. Moseley JB et al: A controlled trial of arthroscopic surgery for osteoarthritis of the knee, *N Engl J Med* 347:81, 2002.
6. Horstman J: *The Arthritis Foundation's guide to alternative therapies,* Atlanta, 1999, Arthritis Foundation.
7. University of California, Berkeley: *Wellness Letter* 17:8, 2001, School of Public Health. Available at *www.WellnessLetter.com.*
8. Altman RD, IAP Study Group: Ibuprofen, acetaminophen and placebo in osteoarthritis of the knee: a six-day double-blind study, *Arthritis Rheum* 42:S9, 1999.
9. Food and Drug Administration: Labeling Changes for Celebrex [online]. Available at *www.fda.gov/bbs/topics/answers/2002* (accessed June 7, 2002).
10. Goorman SD et al: Functional outcome in knee osteoarthritis after treatment with Hylan G-F 20: A prospective study, *Arch Phys Med Rehab* 81:2000.
11. Mann W et al: Changes in health, functional and psychosocial status and coping strategies of home based older persons with arthritis over three years, *Occup Therapy Research* 19:126, 1999.
12. McDonald PA: Autoimmune and inflammatory disorders. In Maher AB, Salmond SW, Pellino TA, editors: *Orthopaedic nursing,* ed 3, Philadelphia, 2002, Saunders.

13. Dunkin MA, Morgan P: AT research spotlight: smoking linked to RA, *Arthritis Today* 15:3, 2001.

14. Wilson S, Giddens J: *Health assessment for nursing practice*, ed 2, St. Louis, 2001, Mosby.

15. Edmunds M, Mayhew M, editors: *Pharmacology for the primary care provider*, St Louis, 2000, Mosby.

16. O'Dell et al: Treatment of rheumatoid arthritis with methotrexate and hydroxychloroquine, methotrexate and sulfasalazine, or a combination of the three medications: results of a two-year, randomized, double-blind, placebo-controlled trial, *Arthritis Rheum* 46:1164, 2002.

17. Kassimos D et al: Biological response modifiers in rheumatoid arthritis, *Lancet* 359:352, 2002.

18. Dayer J, Bresnihan B: Targeting interleukin-1 in the treatment of rheumatoid arthritis, *Arthritis Rheum* 43:1001, 2000.

19. Food and Drug Administration: Prosorba column, summary of safety and effectiveness data [on-line]. Available at *www.fda.gov/cdrh* (accessed June 17, 2002).

20. Eckloff S, Thorntin B: Prescribing assistive devices for patients with rheumatoid arthritis: careful selection of equipment helps patients perform daily functions, *J Musculoskeletal Med* 19:27, 2002.

21. Westby M: A health professional's guide to exercise prescription for people with arthritis: a review of aerobic fitness activities, *Arthritis Care Res* 45:50, 2001.

22. Escalante A, Del Rincon I: The disablement process in rheumatoid arthritis, *Arthritis Care Res* 47:333, 2002.

23. Glaser V: Recognizing the spondyloarthropathies, Patient Care [on-line]. Available at *http://pc.pdr.net/pc/content/journals/p/data/1999/p4a/p4a/183.html* (accessed 1999).

24. Harvard Medical School, Boston: *Harvard Health Letter Special Report-Arthritis*, 1999, Health Publications Group, Boston, Mass.

25. Spondylitis Association of America: What is AS? [on-line]. Available at *www.spondylitis.org* (accessed 2002).

26. Stone M et al: Clinical and imaging correlates of response to treatment with infliximab in patients with ankylosing spondylitis, *J Rheumatology* 28:1605, 2001.

27. American College of Rheumatology: Psoriatic arthritis [on-line]. Available at *www.rheumatology.org/patients/factsheet/psoriati.html* (accessed 2002).

28. Danning C: Psoriatic arthritis: diagnosis and management of a diverse disease, *J Musculoskeletal Med* 17:169, 2000.

29. Psoriatic arthritis. *Wheeless' textbook of orthopaedics* [on-line]. Available at *www.medmedia.com/oa4/62.htm* (accessed 2002).

30. The Merck manual: Reiter's syndrome [on-line]. Available at *www.merck.com/pubs/mmanual/section5/chapter51/51b.htm* (accessed 2002).

31. Stone M, Inman R: Recognizing and managing reaction arthritis: the physician must search for the inciting event, *J Musculoskeletal Med* 19:37, 2002.

32. Zorn KE: Infections. In Schoen D, editor: *NAON core curriculum for orthopaedic nursing*, ed 4, Pitman, NJ, 2001, National Association of Orthopaedic Nurses.

33. Centers for Disease Control and Prevention: CDC Lyme disease home page [on-line]. Available at *www.cdc.gov/ncidod/diseases* (accessed June 10, 2002).

34. Centers for Disease Control and Prevention: Lyme disease-United States 2000, *MMWR* 51:29, 2002.

35. Eppes S: Lyme disease: current therapies and prevention, *Infect Med* 18:388, 2001.

36. American College of Rheumatology: HIV-associated rheumatic disease syndromes [on-line]. Available at *www.rheumatology.org/patients/factsheet/hiv.html* (accessed 2002).

37. Dequeker J (International League of Associations for Rheumatology): HIV infection and arthritis [on-line]. Available at *www.rheuma21st.com/archives/cutting_dequeker-hiv.html* (accessed 2001).

38. Crowther C: *Primary orthopedic care*, St Louis, 1999, Mosby.

39. Terkeltaub R: Pathogenesis and treatment of crystal-induced inflammation. In Koopman W, editor: *Arthritis and allied conditions*, ed 14, Philadelphia, 2001, JB Lippincott.

40. Kammer G et al: Abnormal T cell signal transduction in systemic lupus erythematosus, *Arthritis Rheum* 46:1139, 2002.

41. Centers for Disease Control and Prevention: Trends in deaths from systemic lupus erythematosus-United States 1979-1998, *MMWR* 51:371, 2002.

42. Lipsky P: Systemic lupus erythematosus: an autoimmune disease of B cell hyperactivity, *Nat Immunol* 2:764, 2002.

43. Maddison P et al: The rate and pattern of organ damage in late onset systemic lupus erythematosus, *J Rheumatoid* 29:913, 2002.

44. Godfrey T, Ryan P: Systemic lupus erythematosus: current management, *Med J Aust* 175:125, 2001.

45. Salomonsson S et al: A serologic marker for fetal risk of congenital heart block, *Arthritis Rheum* 46:1223, 2002.

46. Dobkin P et al: Psychosocial contributors to mental and physical health in patients with systemic lupus erythematosus, *Arthritis Care Res* 11:23, 1998.

47. Sabir S, Werth V: Cutaneous manifestation of sclerosing conditions, *J Musculoskeletal Med* 17:207, 2000.

48. Scleroderma Foundation: Scleroderma fact sheet [on-line]. Available at *www.scleroderma.org/fact.html* (accessed 2002).

49. Scleroderma Research Foundation: Scleroderma facts [on-line]. Available at *www.srfcure.org* (accessed 2002).

50. O'Rourke K: Myopathies in the elderly, *Rheum Dis Clin North Am* 26:647, 2000.

51. Paget S: Atypical rheumatic diseases, *Postgrad Med* 111:71, 2002.

52. Brown C, Marschall S: Connective tissue update: focus on dermatomyositis, *Consultant* 39:2876, 1999.

53. Yazici Y, Kagen L: The association of malignancy with myositis, *Curr Opin Rheum* 12:498, 2000.

54. National Institute of Arthritis and Musculoskeletal and Skin Disease: Questions and answers about Sjögren's syndrome [on-line]. Available at *www.niams.nih.gov/topics/sjogrens/index.htm* (accessed 2001).

55. Manthorpe R: How should we interpret the lower lip biopsy findings in patients investigated for Sjögren's syndrome? [on-line] Available at *www3.interscience.wiley.com/* (accessed April 5, 2002).

56. Hashimi I: The management of Sjögren's syndrome in dental practice, *J Am Dental Assoc* 132:1409, 2001.

57. Sheon R: Overview of soft-tissue rheumatic diseases [on-line]. Available at *www.uptodateonline.com* (accessed July 1, 2002).

58. Graff-Radford SB: Regional myofascial pain syndrome and headache: principles of diagnosis and treatment, *Curr Pain Headache Rep* 5:376, 2001.

59. Leslie M: Fibromyalgia syndrome: a comprehensive approach to identification and management, *Clin Excellence Nurse Pract* 3:165, 1999.

60. American College of Rheumatology: Criteria for classification of fibromyalgia [on-line]. Available at *www.nfra.net* (accessed July 23, 2002).

61. Goldenberg D: Pathogenesis and treatment of fibromyalgia [on-line]. Available at *www.uptodateonline.com* (accessed July 1, 2002).

62. Deuschle M et al: Effects of major depression, aging and gender upon calculated diurnal free plasma cortisol concentrations: a re-evaluation study, *Stress* 2:21, 1998.

63. Adler G et al: Reduced hypothalamic-pituitary and sympathoadrenal responses to hypoglycemia in women with fibromyalgia syndrome, *Am J Med* 106:534, 1999.

64. Goldenberg D: Differential diagnosis of fibromyalgia [on-line]. Available at *www.uptodateonline.com* (accessed July 1, 2002).

65. Russell I: Fibromyalgia syndrome: formulating a strategy for relief, *J Musculoskeletal Med* 15:4, 1998.

66. Coward B: Fibromyalgia, *AJN* 99:42, 1999.

67. Centers for Disease Control and Prevention: Chronic fatigue syndrome-demographics [on-line]. Available at *www.cdc.gov.ncidod.diseases* (accessed July 20, 2002).

68. Straus SE: Chronic fatigue syndrome. In Braunwald E et al, editors: *Harrison's principles of internal medicine*, ed 5, New York, 2001, McGraw-Hill.

69. Buskila D, Press J: Neuroendocrine mechanisms in fibromyalgia-chronic fatigue, *Best Pract Res Clin Rheumatol* 15:747, 2001.

70. Parker AJ, Wessely S, Cleare AJ: The neuroendocrinology of chronic fatigue syndrome and fibromyalgia, *Psychol Med* 31:1331, 2001.

71. Craig T, Kakumanu S: Chronic fatigue syndrome: evaluation and treatment, *Am Fam Physician* 65:6, 2002.

72. Kinsella P: Review: behavioural interventions show the most promise for chronic fatigue syndrome, *Evid Based Nurs* 5:46, 2002.

73. Smith RC: Review: behavioral interventions show the most promise for the chronic fatigue syndrome, *ACP J Club* 136:61, 2002.

RESOURCES

American Association for Chronic Fatigue Syndrome
515 Minor Avenue, Suite 8
Seattle, WA 98104
206-781-3544
Fax: 206-749-9052
www.aacfs.org

American College of Rheumatology
1800 Century Place, Suite 250
Atlanta, GA 30345
404-633-3777
Fax: 404-633-1870
www.rheumatology.org

Arthritis Foundation
P.O. Box 7669
Atlanta, GA 30309-0669
800-283-7800
www.arthritis.org

Lupus Foundation of America, Inc.
1300 Piccard Drive, Suite 200
Rockville, MD 20850-4303
800-558-0121 or 301-670-9292
Fax: 301-670-9486
www.lupus.org

National Fibromyalgia Research Association
P.O. Box 500
Salem, OR 97302
www.nfra.net

National Institute of Arthritis and Musculoskeletal and Skin Diseases Information Clearinghouse, National Institutes of Health
1 AMS Circle
Bethesda, MD 20892-3675
877-22-NIAMS (226-4267) or 301-495-4484
Fax: 301-718-6366
www.niams.nih.gov

National Institute of Neurological Disorders and Stroke
NIH Neurological Institute
P.O. Box 5801
Bethesda, MD 20824
800-352-9424
www.ninds.nih.gov

National Organization for Rare Disorders (NORD)
55 Kenosia Avenue
P.O. Box 1968
Danbury, CT 06813-1968
800-999-6673 or 203-744-0100
Fax: 203-798-2291
www.rarediseases.org

National Psoriasis Foundation
6600 SW 92nd Avenue, Suite 300
Portland, OR 97223-7195
800-723-9166 or 503-244-7404
Fax: 503-245-0626
www.psoriasis.org

Scleroderma Foundation
12 Kent Way, Suite 101
Byfield, MA 01922
978-463-5843
Info line: 800-722-HOPE (4673)
Fax: 978-463-5809
www.scleroderma.org

Scleroderma Research Foundation
2320 Bath Street, Suite 315
Santa Barbara, CA 93105
800-441-CURE or 805-563-9133
www.srfcure.org

Spondylitis Association of America
14827 Ventura Boulevard, # 222
Sherman Oaks, CA 91403
800-777-8189 or 818-981-1616
www.spondylitis.org

For additional Internet resources, see the website for this book at *http://www.evolve.elsevier.com/Lewis/medsurg.*

Nursing Care in Specialized Settings

SECTION OUTLINE

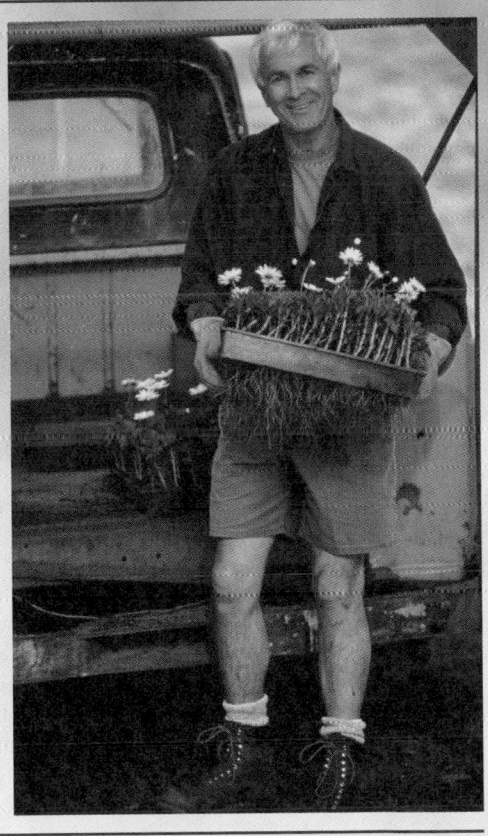

CHAPTER 64
NURSING MANAGEMENT
Critical Care Environment

Linda Bucher

LEARNING OBJECTIVES

1. Differentiate the certification roles of the critical care nurse: CCRN, CCNS, and ACNP.
2. Select appropriate nursing interventions to manage common problems and needs of critically ill patients.
3. Develop effective strategies to manage issues related to the families of critically ill patients.
4. Discuss the principles of hemodynamic monitoring and related collaborative care of critically ill patients.
5. Describe the purpose, indications, and function of circulatory assist devices and related collaborative care.
6. Select appropriate nursing interventions to manage the care of an intubated patient.
7. Differentiate the indications for and modes of mechanical ventilation.
8. Describe the principles of mechanical ventilation and related collaborative care of critically ill patients.

KEY TERMS

assist-control ventilation, p. 1783
bag-valve-mask, p. 1777
circulatory assist devices, p. 1772
closed-suction technique, p. 1778
continuous positive airway pressure, p. 1785
controlled mandatory ventilation, p. 1783
endotracheal intubation, p. 1776
extubation, p. 1780
hemodynamic monitoring, p. 1762
high-frequency ventilation, p. 1785
impedance cardiography, p. 1770
intraaortic balloon pump, p. 1772
mechanical ventilation, p. 1781

negative pressure ventilation, p. 1781
open-suction technique, p. 1778
partial liquid ventilation, p. 1785
phlebostatic axis, p. 1764
positive end-expiratory pressure, p. 1785
positive pressure ventilation, p. 1781
pressure support ventilation, p. 1784
pressure ventilators, p. 1782
synchronized intermittent mandatory ventilation, p. 1783
ventricular assist device, p. 1775
volume ventilators, p. 1782
weaning, p. 1788

CRITICAL CARE NURSING

Critical Care Units

Critical care units (CCUs) or intensive care units (ICUs) are designed to meet the special needs of acutely and critically ill patients. Florence Nightingale forwarded the concept of clustering the most acutely ill patients as far back as the 1800s.[1] During poliomyelitis and tuberculosis pandemics in the middle of the twentieth century, special units were established, equipped with technical equipment to manage the airway and ventilate the patient, and staffed by specialized care providers. Finally, lessons learned from World War II and the Korean War solidified the concepts of triage and specialty nursing units, and by the late 1950s, these concepts were being incorporated into hospital systems.[2]

Reviewed by Elisabeth G. Bradley, RN, APN, CCRN, Cardiac Clinical Nurse Specialist, Christiana Care Health Systems, Newark, Del.; and Michelle Kelly, RN, BSc, MN, Faculty of Nursing, Midwifery, and Health, University of Technology, Sydney, New South Wales, Australia.

In the 1960s technologic developments allowed for more accessible monitoring of the electrocardiogram (ECG), arterial and central venous pressures, and arterial blood gases (ABGs). Coronary care units were developed for patients with acute myocardial infarction. In these units patients were continually monitored for cardiac arrhythmias. Nurses followed protocols to aggressively manage arrhythmias. By the 1970s the ICU was a standard unit in most general hospitals worldwide. Since that time, technical advances have continued at a rapid pace, bringing improved monitoring capabilities and new strategies to manage life-threatening problems.

The term *critical care nursing* is often used interchangeably with the term *intensive care nursing*, but it is not exclusively restricted to that specialty area. The critical care nurse is responsible for assessing life-threatening conditions, instituting appropriate interventions, and evaluating the outcomes of the interventions. The biotechnology available in the ICU is extensive and continually evolving. The capability exists to continuously monitor ECG, blood pressure, oxygenation saturation, ventilation, intracranial pressure, and temperature. More advanced monitoring devices allow for the measurement of cardiac index, stroke volume, ejection fraction, end-tidal carbon dioxide (CO_2), and tissue oxygen consumption. (See Table 64-1 for common abbreviations used in critical care nursing.) Patients may be receiving continual support from mechanical ventilators, intraaortic balloon pumps, or dialysis machines. A typical CCU is illustrated in Fig. 64-1.

Critical Care Nurse

The critical care nurse cares for patients and the families of patients with acute and unstable physiologic problems in an environment equipped for technically advanced methods of assessing and managing patient problems. The American Association of Critical Care Nurses (AACN) defines critical care nursing as that specialty dealing with human responses to life-threatening problems. Critical care nursing requires in-depth knowledge of anatomy, physiology, pathophysiology, pharmacology, and advanced assessment skills, as well as the ability to use advanced biotechnology. The critical care nurse provides ongoing assessment and early recognition and management of complications

TABLE 64-1	Abbreviations Commonly Used in the Intensive Care Unit	
ABBREVIATION	**TERM**	
CI	Cardiac index	
CO	Cardiac output	
CVP	Central venous pressure	
FIO$_2$	Fraction of inspired oxygen	
IABP	Intraaortic balloon pump	
MAP	Mean arterial pressure	
PA	Pulmonary artery	
PAS, PAD	PA systolic (pressure), PA diastolic (pressure)	
PAWP	Pulmonary artery wedge pressure	
PVR	Pulmonary vascular resistance	
SpO$_2$	Percent oxygen saturation of hemoglobin measured by pulse oximetry	
SvO$_2$	Percent oxygen saturation of hemoglobin in mixed venous blood (e.g., in the PA)	
SVI	Stroke volume index	
SV	Stroke volume	
SVR	Systemic vascular resistance	
VAD	Ventricular assist device	

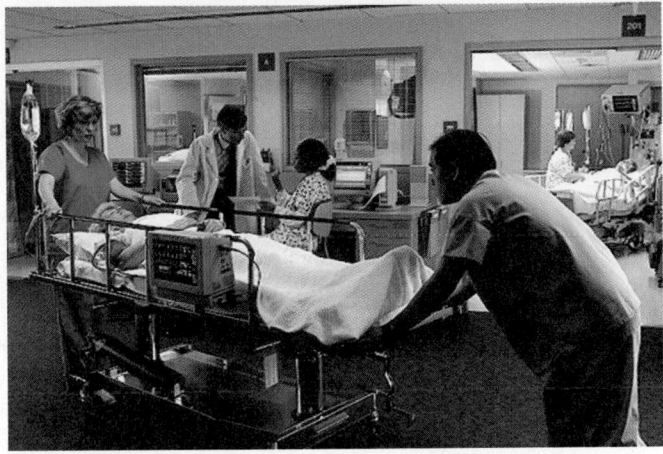

FIG. 64-1 Typical intensive care unit.

problems and disease-related symptoms, prescribes treatments, and coordinates care during transitions in settings. The ACNP may practice independently (e.g., providing comprehensive care to the chronically critically ill) or collaboratively (e.g., providing symptom management in conjunction with physicians). Certification as an ACNP is available through the AACN Certification Corporation and the American Nurses Credentialing Center. Prescriptive authority regulations for advanced practice nurses vary by state.

while fostering healing and recovery. Appropriate actions by an astute nurse can prevent many complications. The nurse must also be able to provide psychologic support to the patient and the family. To be effective, the critical care nurse must be able to communicate and collaborate effectively with all health team providers (e.g., physician, dietitian, respiratory therapist, occupational therapist).

Nursing practice in the ICU often follows a primary care model with the patient cared for by a limited group of nurses who become thoroughly familiar with the patient's condition and the needs of the patient and the family. The ICU nurse spends most working hours near the patient's bedside. Specialization in ICU nursing usually requires formal, in-service education combined with a preceptored clinical orientation.

The AACN Certification Corporation offers critical care certification (CCRN) in adult, pediatric, and neonatal critical care nursing. The designation requires registered nurse licensure, practice experience in critical care nursing, and successful completion of a written test. Continued critical care practice and retesting or continuing education is required for recertification. CCRN certification validates knowledge of critical care nursing; it is not the same as advanced practice.

Advanced practice critical care nurses have a graduate (master's or doctorate) degree. These nurses are employed in a variety of roles: patient and staff educators, consultants, administrators, researchers, or expert practitioners. The advanced practice critical care nurse who is a clinical nurse specialist (CNS) typically functions in one or more of these roles. Certification for the CNS in acute and critical care (CCNS) is available through the AACN Certification Corporation. Another advanced practice role is the acute care nurse practitioner (ACNP). This advanced practice nurse provides comprehensive care to select critically ill patients and their families. The ACNP conducts comprehensive assessments, orders and interprets diagnostic tests, manages health

Critical Care Patient

A patient is generally admitted to the ICU for one of three reasons. First, the patient may be physiologically unstable, requiring advanced and sophisticated clinical judgments by the nurse or physician. Second, the patient may be at risk for serious complications and require frequent and often invasive assessments. Third, the patient may require intensive and complicated nursing support related to the use of intravenous polypharmacy (e.g., neuromuscular blockade, thrombolytics, drugs requiring titration) and advanced biotechnology (e.g., ventricular assist devices, mechanical ventilation, intracranial pressure monitoring, continuous renal replacement therapy, hemodynamic monitoring).

ICU patients can be clustered by disease condition (e.g., neurology, pulmonary) or age-group (e.g., neonatal, pediatrics). ICU patients are sometimes clustered by acuity (e.g., acute and unstable versus technology dependent but stable). Patients commonly treated in the ICU include those with respiratory distress, myocardial ischemia or infarction, or acute neurologic impairment or those receiving care after cardiac surgery or major organ transplantation. The care of the critically injured patient is provided in trauma and burn ICUs. The patient with a medical emergency (e.g., sepsis, diabetic ketoacidosis, drug overdoses, or poisonings or thyroid, adrenal, or hematologic crises) is often treated in a medical ICU. The patient with multiple comorbidities may be monitored in the ICU while receiving care for unrelated conditions. The patient who is not expected to recover from an illness is usually not admitted to an ICU. For example, the ICU should not be used to manage the patient in a persistent coma, nor should ICU care be used to prolong the natural process of death.

Despite the emphasis on caring for the patient who can survive, death is common in ICU patients. It is reported that 10% of patients admitted to ICUs will die, and another 20% may leave the ICU but will not survive to discharge. This suggests a need for caution and coordination of care when transferring patients from ICUs to general care units. In general, nonsurvivors were older, had preexisting health problems, and experienced longer ICU stays.[3,4]

Progressive care units (PCUs), also called high-dependency units or stepdown units, have been established as intermediate units between the ICU and the general care unit. Generally, patients in PCUs are at risk for serious complications, but their risk is lower than that of ICU patients. Examples of patients found in PCUs include patients scheduled for interventional cardiac procedures (e.g., stent placement, pacemaker implantation), awaiting heart transplant, receiving vasoactive intravenous drugs (e.g., diltiazem [Cardizem]), or being weaned from prolonged mechanical ventilation. Patients in these units can be monitored for cardiac rhythm, arterial blood pressure, oxygen saturation, and end-tidal CO_2.[5] The use of PCUs provides specialized nursing care for an at-risk patient population in a more cost-effective environment.

Common Problems of Critical Care Patients. The patient admitted to the ICU is at risk for numerous complications and special problems. Critically ill patients are usually immobile and at risk for skin problems (see Chapter 23). The use of multiple, invasive devices predisposes the patient to iatrogenic infections. Sepsis and multiple organ dysfunction syndrome (MODS) may follow (see Chapter 65). Adequate nourishment for the critically ill patient is paramount but frequently overlooked. Other special problems for ICU patients relate to anxiety, pain, impaired communication, sensory-perceptual problems, and sleep difficulties.

Nutrition. Patients are often admitted to ICUs with conditions that result in either hypermetabolic states (e.g., burns, trauma, sepsis) or catabolic states (e.g., acute renal failure). Other times, patients may be admitted in severely malnourished states, such as those that occur with wasting syndrome and chronic liver disease. In general, malnutrition has been linked to increases in mortality and morbidity. Determining who to feed, what to feed, when to feed, and how to feed (e.g., route of administration) are crucial questions that must be asked when caring for a critically ill patient.[6] The critical care nurse must collaborate with the physician and the dietitian to determine how best to meet the nutritional needs of ICU patients.

The primary goal of nutritional support is to prevent or correct nutritional deficiencies. This is usually accomplished by the provision of enteral nutrition (i.e., delivery of calories via the gastrointestinal [GI] tract) or parenteral nutrition (i.e., delivery of calories intravenously). Enteral nutrition is thought to preserve the structure and function of the gut mucosa and help to prevent translocation of gut bacteria, a major trigger of MODS (see Chapter 65).[5,6] In addition, enteral nutrition is associated with fewer complications and is less expensive when compared with parenteral nutrition.[6] (See Evidence-Based Practice box on nutritional support on this page.) (Enteral and parenteral nutrition are discussed in Chapter 39.)

Parenteral nutrition should be considered only when the enteral route is unsuccessful in providing adequate nutrition or contraindicated. Examples of these conditions are paralytic ileus, diffuse peritonitis, intestinal obstruction, pancreatitis, GI ischemia, intractable vomiting, and severe diarrhea.[6]

EVIDENCE-BASED PRACTICE
Nutritional Support in Critically Ill Patients

Clinical Problem
What is the relationship between nutritional support and outcomes for critical care patients?

Best Clinical Practice
- When nutrition support is indicated, enteral nutrition should be preferentially used over parenteral nutrition.
- Parenteral nutrition is not recommended for critically ill patients with an intact gastrointestinal tract.
- In adult surgical patients, the early use of enteral nutrition is associated with a reduction in complications and shorter hospital stay.
- Early use of enteral nutrition is recommended in critically ill surgical patients and should be considered for other critically ill patients.
- Further studies are needed to determine the optimal timing and composition of parenteral nutrition in patients not tolerating enteral nutrition.

Implications for Nursing Practice
- Nurses have a very important role in assessing the nutritional status of critically ill patients.
- Providing nutritional support should be a standard of practice for critically ill patients.

References for Evidence
Heyland DK: Nutritional support in the critically ill patient: a critical review of the evidence, *Database of Abstracts of Reviews of Effectiveness* 2:2002.
Heyland DK: Parenteral nutrition in the critically ill patient: more harm than good? *Proc Nutr Soc* 59:457, 2000.
Heyland DK: Enteral and parenteral nutrition in the seriously ill, hospitalized patient: a critical review of the evidence, *J Nutr Health Aging* 4:31, 2000.

Anxiety. It has been reported that as many as 70% to 80% of ICU patients experience some degree of anxiety.[7] The primary sources of anxiety for patients include the perceived or anticipated threat to physical health and the seemingly hostile environment. Many patients and families feel uncomfortable in the ICU environment with its complex equipment, high noise and light levels, isolation from family, and intense pace of activity. Pain and sleeplessness enhance anxiety as do immobilization, loss of control, and impaired communication.[7]

In one study of over 700 critical care nurses, 71% reported that assessing patients for anxiety was very important. The nurses also identified agitation, increased blood pressure, increased heart rate, patient verbalization of anxiety, and restlessness as the five most important clinical indicators of anxiety.[7] To help reduce anxiety, the nurse should encourage patients and families to express concerns, ask questions, and state their needs. The nurse should include the patient and family in all conversations and explain the purpose of equipment and procedures. The nurse should also structure the patient's surrounding environment in a way that may decrease anxiety. For example, family members can be encouraged to bring in photographs and personal items. Judicious use of antianxiety drugs (e.g., lorazepam [Ativan]) and complementary therapies (e.g., imagery, music, massage) may reduce the stress response that can be triggered by anxiety and should be considered.[8,9]

Pain. The control of pain in the ICU patient is paramount. It is reported that as many as 70% of ICU patients recount having moderate to severe unrelieved pain.[10] Inadequate pain control is often linked with agitation and anxiety and is known to contribute to the stress response. ICU patients at high risk for pain include patients (1) who have medical conditions that include ischemic, infectious, or inflammatory processes; (2) who are immobilized; (3) who have invasive monitoring devices; (4) and who are scheduled for any invasive or noninvasive procedures.[10]

For some critically ill patients, continuous intravenous sedation (e.g., propofol [Diprivan]) is a practical and effective strategy for pain control. However, patients receiving deep sedation are unresponsive, and this prevents the nurse and other health care providers from properly assessing the patient's neurologic status. To address this limitation, policies that include a daily, scheduled interruption of sedation have been developed. Daily, sedative interruption allows the patient to awaken and the health care provider to conduct a neurologic examination.[8] In one study, patients who had interrupted sedation were extubated faster and discharged sooner from the ICU than patients who did not have their sedation interrupted.[11] (Chapter 9 has more detailed information on pain management.)

Impaired communication. Inability to communicate can be a distressing problem for the patient who may be unable to speak because of the use of paralyzing drugs or an endotracheal tube. As part of any procedure the nurse should explain what will happen or is happening to the patient. When the patient cannot speak, the nurse should explore alternative methods of communication, including the use of devices such as picture boards, notepads, magic slates, or computer keyboards. When speaking with the patient, the nurse should look directly at the patient and use hand gestures when appropriate. For patients who do not speak English, the use of a medical interpreter is strongly recommended (see Chapter 2).

Nonverbal communication is important. High levels of procedure-related touch and decreased levels of affection-related or comfort-related touch characterize the ICU. Patients have different levels of tolerance for being touched, usually related to cultural background and personal history. It may be appropriate to provide comforting touch with ongoing evaluation of the patient's response. Often the ICU nurse encourages the family to touch and talk with the patient.

Sensory-perceptual problems. Acute and reversible sensory-perceptual changes are common in ICU patients. The combination of alterations in mentation (e.g., delusions, short attention span, loss of recent memory), psychomotor behavior (e.g., restlessness, lethargy), and sleep-wake cycle (e.g., daytime sleepiness, nighttime agitation) has been inappropriately labeled *ICU psychosis*. The patient experiencing these alterations is not psychotic but is suffering from delirium. It is estimated that the prevalence of delirium in ICU patients ranges from 15% to 40%.[12] Demographic factors predisposing the patient to delirium include advanced age, preexisting cerebral illnesses (e.g., dementia), and a history of drug or alcohol abuse. Environmental factors that can contribute to delirium include sleep deprivation, anxiety, sensory overload, and immobilization. Physical conditions such as hemodynamic instability, hypoxemia, electrolyte disturbances, and severe infections can precipitate delirium. Last, certain drugs (e.g., sedatives [benzodiazepines], furosemide [Lasix], antimicrobials [aminoglycosides]) have been associated with the development of delirium.[12] (Delirium is discussed in Chapter 58.)

The task of the ICU nurse is to identify all predisposing factors and attempt to improve the patient's mental clarity and cooperation with therapy. It is imperative that physiologic factors be addressed (e.g., correction of oxygenation, perfusion, and electrolyte problems). The use of clocks and calendars may help the patient remain oriented. If the patient demonstrates unsafe behavior, hyperactivity, insomnia, or delusions, symptoms may be managed pharmacologically with neuroleptic drugs (e.g., haloperidol [Haldol]).[12] In addition, the presence of family members may help reorient the patient and reduce agitation.

Sensory overload can also result in patient distress and anxiety. Environmental noise levels are particularly high in the ICU.[13,14] The nurse can limit noise and assist the patient in understanding noises that cannot be prevented. Conversation is a particularly stressful noise, especially when the discussion concerns the patient and is conducted in the presence of, but without participation from, the patient. The nurse can eliminate this source of stress by identifying suitable places for patient-related discussions and, whenever possible, by including the patient in the discussion. The nurse can also limit noise levels directly by muting phones, setting alarms appropriate to the patient's condition, and eliminating unnecessary alarms. For example, the nurse should silence the blood pressure alarms while manipulating invasive lines and then reactivate the alarms when the procedures are complete. Similarly, ventilator alarms should be transiently silenced during endotracheal suctioning. Overhead paging and other unnecessary noise should be limited in patient care areas.

Sleep problems. Nearly all ICU patients experience sleep disturbances. Patients may have difficulty falling asleep or have disrupted sleep because of noise, anxiety, pain, frequent monitoring, or treatment procedures.[14] Drugs such as sedatives and hypnotics may result in disturbed sleep patterns, including reductions in slow wave and rapid eye movement (REM) sleep.[15] Sleep disturbance is a significant stressor in the ICU, contributing to delirium and possibly affecting recovery. The ICU nurse can structure the environment to promote the patient's sleep-wake cycle. Strategies include clustering activities, scheduling rest periods, dimming lights at nighttime, opening curtains during the daytime, obtaining physiologic measurements without disrupting the patient, limiting noise, and providing comfort measures (e.g., massage, evening care).

Issues Related to Families

When someone becomes critically ill, care must be extended beyond the patient to the patient's family because they are intimately connected. Family members play a valuable role in the patient's recovery and should be considered members of the health care team. They can contribute to the patient's well-being by:

1. Providing a link to the patient's personal life (e.g., news of friends, family, and job)
2. Advising the patient in health care decisions or functioning as the decision maker when the patient cannot
3. Helping with activities of daily living (e.g., bathing, oral suctioning)
4. Providing positive, loving, and caring support

To be effective in caring for their loved one, family members need guidance and support from the nurse. The experience of having a friend or family member in the ICU is physically and emotionally difficult. Anxiety regarding the patient's condition and prognosis and concerns regarding the patient's pain and other discomforts are some of the issues families confront. They may question the quality of care that the patient is receiving. In addition, it is common for families to experience anxiety regarding the financial issues related to the provision of care in the recovery phase of the illness.

The family will typically be experiencing disruption of their daily routines to support the patient. They may be far from their own home and supportive friends and family members. Ultimately, families of the critically ill are considered in crisis, and family-centered care is imperative.[16,17] To provide family-centered care effectively, the nurse must be skilled in crisis intervention. The nurse should conduct a family assessment and intervene as necessary. Interventions can include active listening, reduction of anxiety, and support of those who become upset or angry.[17] The family's feelings should be acknowledged and accepted and their decisions supported. Other health team members, such as chaplains, social workers, and psychologists, may be helpful in assisting the family to adjust and should be consulted as necessary. The extent to which family-centered care is provided will, in turn, affect the patient's clinical course in the ICU.

The major needs of families of critically ill patients have been categorized as informational needs, reassurance needs, and convenience needs.[16] Lack of information is a major source of anxiety for the family. The nurse should assess the family's understanding of the patient's status, treatment plan, and prognosis and provide information as appropriate. The nurse should also provide information to the family when the patient's condition changes. It is recommended that a spokesperson for the family be identified so that information between the health care team and the family can be coordinated.

The family needs reassurance regarding the way in which the patient's care is managed and decisions are made. The family should have the opportunity to be involved in decision making. If the patient has an advance directive or living will, the family will need to see that the patient's wishes are understood and respected. When patients are incapable of making their own health care decisions, they may have designated a durable power of attorney, and this person should be involved in the patient's plan of care.[18] The family should also be invited to meet the health care team members, including physicians, dietitian, respiratory therapist, social worker, physical therapist, and chaplain. The nurse should evaluate the appropriateness of including family members in multidisciplinary care conferences. It helps family members to accept and cope with problems if they observe that health care providers are hopeful, caring, and competent; decisions are deliberate; and they have the opportunity to help shape the course of care.

Research has demonstrated that families of critically ill patients need the convenience of access to the patient and that limiting family visitation does not protect that patient from adverse physiologic consequences.[16] Rigid visitation policies in ICUs should be abolished, and a move toward less restrictive, individualized visiting policies is strongly recommended by the AACN.[17] This can be accomplished by assessing the patient's and family members' needs and preferences and incorporating these into the plan of care. The first time family members visit, it is important for the nurse to prepare them for the experience by briefly describing the patient's appearance and the physical environment (e.g., equipment, noise). It is helpful if the nurse can accompany the family members as they enter the room. They should be encouraged to participate in the patient's care if they desire. The nurse should observe the responses of both the patient and family. In some ICUs, visitation has been expanded to include the family pet visitation or animal-assisted therapy. The positive benefits of pet visitation (e.g., decreases in blood pressure and anxiety) far outweigh the risks (e.g., transmission of infection from pet to patient) and should be considered as part of the visitation policy.[16,19]

■ Culturally Competent Care: Critical Care Patients

Providing culturally competent care to critically ill patients and families is challenging. Often, the nurse is focused on meeting the physiologic needs of the patient and may not appreciate the influence of the patient's culture on the illness experience. Minimally, the cultural dimensions of the meaning of sickness and health, pain, dying and death, and grief should be explored when caring for critically ill patients and their families. (See Chapter 2 for discussions on cultural issues related to sickness, health, and pain.)

Cultural perspectives on dying and death are complex. Telling some patients that they are dying as a way of letting them prepare for death is considered an infringement on the role of the family.[20] Others view a discussion about advance directives as a legal device to deny care. One study of African American patients found that most would opt to extend life even at the expense of the quality of life.[20] Similarly, customs surrounding dying and death vary widely, from leaving a window open to allow the spirit of the deceased to leave to providing the final bath for the deceased.[21] The nurse caring for the dying patient must make every attempt to understand and accommodate the family's cultural traditions. The expressions of grief that follow the loss of a loved one are highly individualized and influenced by several variables. These include the relationship between the grieving person and the person lost, whether the loss is sudden or anticipated, the support systems available to the grieving person, past experiences with loss, and the person's religious and cultural beliefs.[21] It is of utmost importance that the critical care nurse proceeds cautiously when approaching patients facing death and their families. Asking patients, "What do you want to know?" and "Who do you want with you when discussing options?" is a good starting point.[20] (See Chapter 10 for additional information on end-of-life care.) ■

HEMODYNAMIC MONITORING

Hemodynamic monitoring refers to measurement of pressure, flow, and oxygenation within the cardiovascular system. Both invasive (internally placed devices) and noninvasive (external devices) hemodynamic measurements are made in the ICU. Values commonly measured include systemic and pulmonary arterial pressures, central venous pressure (CVP), pulmonary artery wedge pressure (PAWP), cardiac output/index, stroke volume/index, and oxygen saturation of the hemoglobin of arterial blood (SaO_2) and mixed venous blood (SvO_2). From these measurements the clinician calculates several values, including the resistance of the systemic and pulmonary arterial vasculature and oxygen content, delivery, and consumption. When these data are integrated with clinical assessment data, the nurse can derive a picture of the patient's hemodynamic status and the effect of therapy. It is important that all measures be made with attention to technical accuracy. False or inaccurate data are potentially misleading and thus dangerous.

Hemodynamic Terminology

Cardiac Output and Cardiac Index. *Cardiac output* (CO) is the volume of blood pumped by the heart in 1 minute. *Cardiac index* (CI) is the measurement of the CO adjusted for body size and it is a more precise measurement of the efficiency of the pumping action of the heart. Although minor beat-to-beat changes may occur, generally the left and right ventricles pump the same volume. The volume pumped with each heartbeat is the stroke volume (SV). Like CI, stroke volume index (SVI) is the measurement of SV adjusted for body size. CO and the forces opposing blood flow determine blood pressure, the force exerted by blood on the vessel wall. The opposition to blood flow offered by the vessels is called systemic vascular resistance (SVR) or pulmonary vascular resistance (PVR). Preload, afterload, and contractility (see Chapter 31) determine SV (and thus CO and blood pressure). Understanding these concepts and relationships is essential for the critical care nurse. In addition, the nurse must understand the effects of manipulation of each of these variables. The formulas and normal values for common hemodynamic parameters are given in Table 64-2.

Preload. *Preload* is the volume within a cardiac chamber at the end of diastole. Unfortunately, chamber volume measurements are difficult to obtain. Instead, various pressures are used to estimate volume. Left ventricular preload is called left ventricular end-diastolic pressure. PAWP, a measure of pulmonary capillary pressure, reflects left ventricular end-diastolic pressure under normal conditions (i.e., when there is no mitral valve pathologic condition, intracardiac defect, or arrhythmia). CVP, measured in the right atrium or in the vena cava close to the heart, is the right ventricular preload or right ventricular end-diastolic pressure when there is no tricuspid valve pathologic condition, intracardiac defect, or arrhythmia.

The effects of preload are explained by *Starling's law,* which states that the more a myocardial fiber is stretched during filling, the more it shortens during systole and the greater the force of the contraction. As preload increases, force generated in the following contraction increases, thus SV and CO increase. The greater the preload, the greater the myocardial (heart muscle) stretch and the greater the oxygen requirement of the myocardium. Hence, increases in CO via increased preload require increased delivery of oxygen to the myocardium. It should be remembered that the change in SV with preload comes about because of stretching of the heart muscle. However, the clinical measurement made is not a direct measurement of the muscle length; the measurement made is pressure at the time of the peak stretch (end diastole) (see Table 64-2). This pressure indirectly indicates the amount of stretch and the volume. This pressure is also important because it indicates pressure in the blood vessels of the lung or in the blood returning to the heart. Preload can be increased by fluid administration and decreased by diuresis.

Afterload. *Afterload* refers to the forces opposing ventricular ejection. These forces include systemic arterial pressure, the resistance offered by the aortic valve, and the mass and density of the blood to be moved. Clinically, although the measures fail to include all the components of afterload, SVR and arterial pressure are indices of left ventricular afterload. Similarly, PVR and pulmonary arterial pressure are indices of right ventricular after-

---

TABLE 64-2   Hemodynamic Parameters at Rest

INDICATORS	NORMAL RANGE
Preload	
Right atrial pressure (RAP) or central venous pressure (CVP)	2-8 mm Hg
Pulmonary artery wedge pressure (PAWP) or left atrial pressure (LAP)	6-12 mm Hg
Pulmonary artery diastolic pressure (PADP)	4-12 mm Hg
Afterload	
Pulmonary vascular resistance (PVR) = $\dfrac{(\text{Pulmonary artery mean pressure [PAMP]} - \text{PAWP}) \times 80}{\text{Cardiac output (CO)}}$	<250 dynes/sec/cm^{-5}
Pulmonary vascular resistance index (PVRI) = (PAMP − PAWP) × 80/Cardiac index (CI)	160-380 dynes/sec/cm^{-5}/m^2
Systemic vascular resistance (SVR) = (Mean arterial pressure [MAP] − CVP) × 80/CO	800-1200 dynes/sec/cm^{-5}
Systemic vascular resistance index (SVRI) = (MAP − CVP) × 80/CI	1970-2390 dynes/sec/cm^{-5}/m^2
Mean arterial pressure (MAP) = $\dfrac{\text{Systolic blood pressure} + 2(\text{Diastolic blood pressure})}{3^*}$	70-105 mm Hg
Pulmonary artery mean pressure (PAMP) = $\dfrac{\text{Pulmonary artery systolic pressure (PASP)} + 2\text{PADP}}{3^*}$	10-20 mm Hg
Other	
Stroke volume (SV) = CO/Heart rate	60-150 ml/beat
Stroke volume index (SVI) = CI/Heart rate	30-65 ml/beat/m^2
Heart rate (HR)	60-100 beats/min
CO = SV × HR	4-8 L/min
Cardiac index (CI) = CO/Body surface area (BSA)	2.2-4 L/min/m^2
Arterial hemoglobin oxygen saturation	95%-99%
Mixed venous hemoglobin oxygen saturation	60%-80%

*This formula is an approximation because it does not take into consideration the heart rate. The monitor looks at the area under the pressure curve, as well as the heart rate, to calculate MAP and PAMP.

load. Increased afterload often results in a decreased CO. CO can be restored by decreasing afterload (i.e., decreasing forces opposing contraction). When afterload is reduced, myocardial oxygen needs are decreased. Thus CO is increased, and myocardial oxygen requirements are decreased. Drug therapy directed at reducing afterload (e.g., milrinone [Primacor]) is often used in the management of heart failure (see Chapter 34).

Vascular Resistance. *Systemic vascular resistance* (SVR) is the resistance of the systemic vascular bed. *Pulmonary vascular resistance* (PVR) is the resistance of the pulmonary vascular bed. Both of these measures reflect afterload as described earlier and can be adjusted for body size (see Table 64-2).

Contractility. *Contractility* describes the strength of contraction. Contractility is said to increase when preload is not changed yet the heart contracts more forcefully. Epinephrine, norepinephrine, isoproterenol (Isuprel), dopamine, dobutamine, digitalis-like drugs, calcium, and milrinone (Primacor) increase contractility. These agents are termed *positive inotropes.* Contractility is diminished by *negative inotropes,* such as acidosis and certain drugs (e.g., barbiturates, alcohol, procainamide [Pronestyl], calcium channel blockers, β-adrenergic blockers). Increased contractility results in increased SV and increased myocardial oxygen requirements. There are no direct clinical measures of cardiac contractility. To indirectly determine contractility, the nurse measures the patient's preload (PAWP) and CO and graphs the results. If preload, heart rate, and afterload remain constant yet CO changes, contractility is altered. Contractility is diminished in the failing heart.

Principles of Invasive Pressure Monitoring

Invasive lines are commonly used in the ICU to measure systemic and pulmonary blood pressures. Components of a typical invasive arterial pressure monitoring system are illustrated in Fig. 64-2. Catheter, pressure tubing, flush system, and usually the transducer are disposable.

To accurately measure pressure, equipment must be referenced and zero balanced and dynamic response characteristics optimized. *Referencing* means positioning the transducer so that the zero reference point is at the level of the atria of the heart.[22] The stopcock nearest the transducer is usually the zero reference for the transducer. To place this level with the atria, the nurse uses an external landmark, the phlebostatic axis. To identify the **phlebostatic axis,** two imaginary lines are drawn with the patient supine (Fig. 64-3, *A*). The first line, a horizontal line, is drawn through the midchest, halfway between the outermost anterior and posterior surfaces. The second line, a vertical line, is drawn through the fourth intercostal space at the sternum. The phlebostatic axis is the intersection of the two imaginary lines. Once the phlebostatic axis is identified, it should be marked on the patient's chest with a permanent marker. The port of the stopcock nearest the transducer must be positioned level with the phlebostatic axis. It is recommended that the transducer be taped to the patient's chest at the phlebostatic axis or mounted on a bedside pole.[22]

Zeroing confirms that when pressure within the system is zero, the equipment reads zero. This is accomplished by opening the reference stopcock to room air and observing the monitor for a reading of zero. Most transducers in current use are disposable and have little zero drift. Zeroing the transducer is recommended during initial setup, immediately after insertion of the arterial

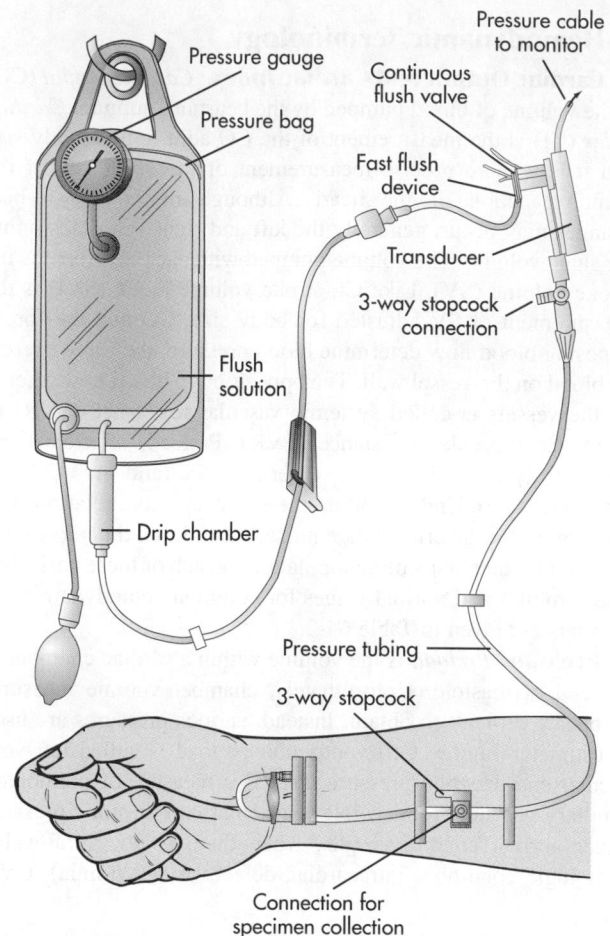

FIG. 64-2 Components of a pressure monitoring system. The cannula, shown entering the radial artery, is connected via pressure (nondistensible) tubing to the transducer. The transducer converts the pressure wave into an electronic signal. The transducer is wired to the electronic monitoring system, which amplifies, conditions, displays, and records the signal. Stopcocks are inserted into the line for specimen withdrawal and for referencing and zero-balancing procedures. A flush system, consisting of a pressurized bag of intravenous fluid, tubing, and a flush device, is inserted into the line. The flush system provides continuous slow (approximately 3 ml/hr) flushing and provides a mechanism for fast flushing of lines. All items except the electronic monitoring system are commonly disposable equipment.

line, when the transducer has been disconnected from the pressure cable or the pressure cable has been disconnected from the monitor, and when the accuracy of the measurements is questioned, and it should be done according to the manufacturer's guidelines.[22,23]

Optimizing dynamic response characteristics involves checking that the equipment reproduces without distortion a signal that changes rapidly. A *dynamic response test (square wave test)* is performed every 8 to 12 hours and when the system is opened to air or the accuracy of the measurements is questioned. It involves checking that the equipment reproduces a distortion-free signal (Fig. 64-4).[24]

Steps in obtaining blood pressure measurements with an invasive line are given in Table 64-3. Pressure measurements can be obtained from both digital and printed analog outputs, but accurate readings are best obtained from a printed pressure tracing

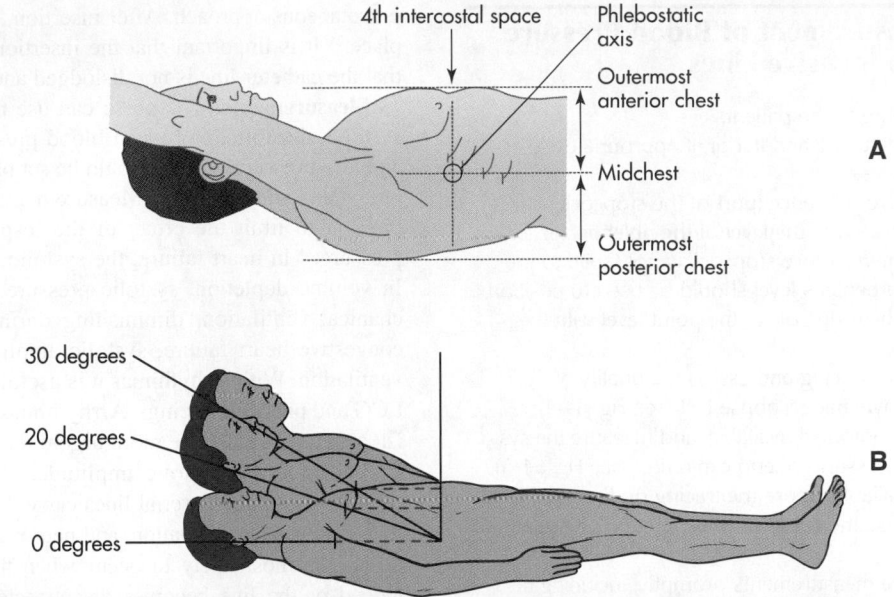

FIG. 64-3 Identification of phlebostatic axis. **A,** Phlebostatic axis is an external landmark used to identify the level of the atria in the supine patient. The phlebostatic axis is defined as the intersection of two imaginary lines: one drawn vertically through the fourth intercostal space at the sternum and another drawn horizontally through the midchest, halfway between the outermost anterior and outermost posterior points of the chest. **B,** As the backrest of the supine patient is elevated, the phlebostatic axis remains at the same anatomic location, becoming progressively elevated from the floor. The zero reference point must be repositioned with changes in backrest elevation to keep it at the phlebostatic level.

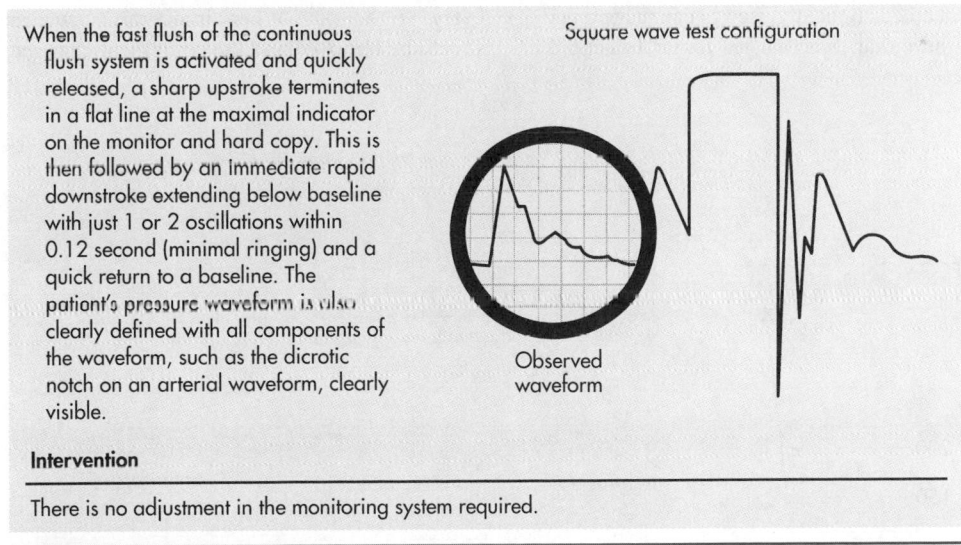

When the fast flush of the continuous flush system is activated and quickly released, a sharp upstroke terminates in a flat line at the maximal indicator on the monitor and hard copy. This is then followed by an immediate rapid downstroke extending below baseline with just 1 or 2 oscillations within 0.12 second (minimal ringing) and a quick return to a baseline. The patient's pressure waveform is also clearly defined with all components of the waveform, such as the dicrotic notch on an arterial waveform, clearly visible.

Square wave test configuration

Observed waveform

Intervention

There is no adjustment in the monitoring system required.

FIG. 64-4 Optimally damped system. Dynamic response test (square wave test) using the fast flush system: normal response.

at the end of expiration. Initial readings are made with the patient flat. Unless the patient's blood pressure is extremely sensitive to orthostatic changes, values at modest degrees of backrest elevation (up to 45 degrees) are generally equivalent to measurements with the patient flat. Studies have not demonstrated

the accuracy of readings obtained for patients in the lateral position.[22] It is not necessary to reposition the patient for each pressure reading. However, it is necessary to move the zero reference stopcock to keep it positioned at the phlebostatic axis (see Fig. 64-3, *B*).

TABLE 64-3   Measurement of Blood Pressure with Invasive Lines

1. Explain the procedure to the patient.
2. Position the patient supine and flat or, if appropriate, elevated up to 45 degrees.
3. Confirm that the zero reference (port of the stopcock nearest the transducer) is placed at the level of the phlebostatic axis (see Fig. 64-3). If the reference stopcock is not taped to the patient's chest, a carpenter's level should be used to position the stopcock on a bedside pole at the point level with the phlebostatic axis.
4. Observe the monitor tracing and assess the quality of the tracing. Perform a dynamic response test (see Fig. 64-4).
5. Obtain an analog printout, if available, and measure the systolic and diastolic pressures at end expiration (see Fig. 64-5). If no printout is available, freeze the tracing on the oscilloscope screen and use the cursor to measure the pressures at end expiration.
6. Record the pressure measurements promptly, including (if available) the printout marked to identify the points read.

Types of Invasive Pressure Monitoring

Arterial Blood Pressure. Continuous arterial pressure monitoring is indicated for patients in many situations, including acute hypertension and hypotension, respiratory failure, shock, neurologic injury, coronary interventional procedures, continuous infusion of vasoactive drugs (sodium nitroprusside [Nipride]), and frequent ABG sampling. A 20-gauge, 2-inch (5.1 cm) nontapered Teflon cannula-over-the needle is typically used to cannulate a peripheral artery, such as the radial, brachial, or femoral, using a percutaneous approach. After insertion, the catheter is sutured in place.[25] It is important that the insertion site be immobilized so that the catheter line is not dislodged and lines are not kinked.

Measurements. The nurse can use the arterial line to obtain systolic, diastolic, and mean blood pressures (Fig. 64-5). High- and low-pressure alarms should be set based on the patient's current status and activated. Measurements are obtained at end expiration to limit the effect of the respiratory cycle on arterial pressure.[24] In heart failure, the systolic upstroke may be slower. In volume depletion, systolic pressure varies greatly with mechanical ventilation, diminishing during inspiration. In severe congestive heart failure, systolic amplitude does not vary with ventilation. With arrhythmias it is useful to observe simultaneous ECG and pressure tracings. Arrhythmias that significantly diminish arterial pressure are more urgent than those that cause only a slight decrease in systolic amplitude.

Complications. Arterial lines carry the risk of hemorrhage, infection, thrombus formation, and neurovascular impairment. Hemorrhage is most likely to occur when the catheter becomes dislodged or the line becomes disconnected. To avoid this serious complication, the nurse uses Luer-Lok connections and always checks the arterial waveform and that the alarms are activated. If the pressure in the line falls (e.g., when the line is disconnected), the low-pressure alarm sounds immediately, allowing prompt correction of the problem. Pressure is always monitored when an arterial line is in place, even if the line was placed for ABG sampling.

Infection is a risk with any invasive line. The nurse should inspect the insertion site for local signs of inflammation and monitor the patient for signs of systemic infection. To limit the risk of contamination and catheter-related infection, the catheter site, pressure tubing, flush bag, and transducer should be changed every 96 hours.[24] When infection is suspected, the catheter should be removed and the equipment changed.

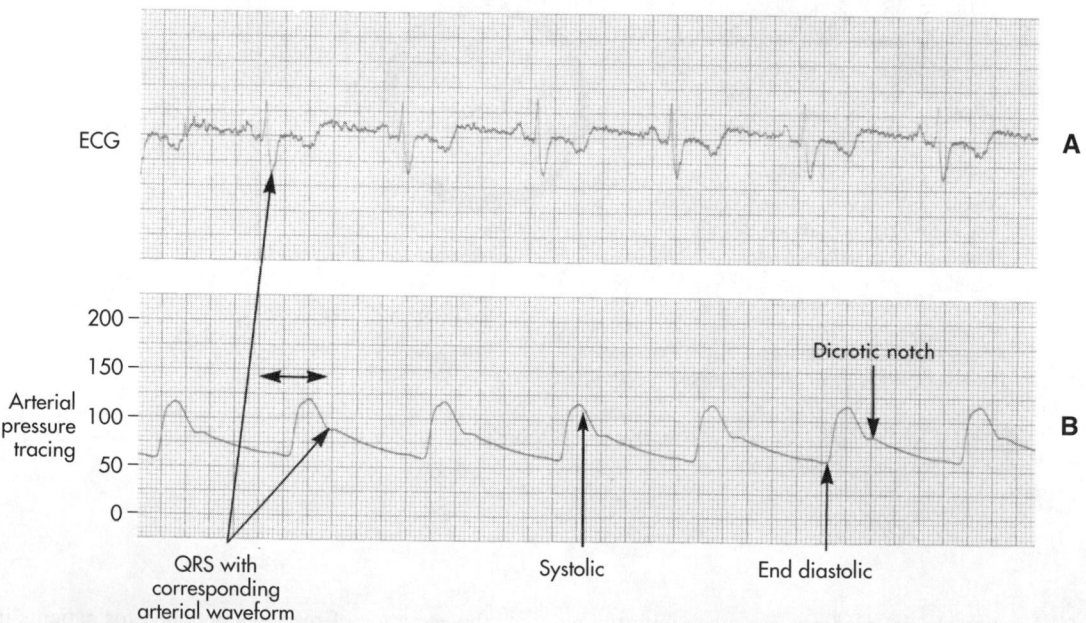

FIG. 64-5 **A,** Simultaneously recorded electrocardiogram (ECG) tracing and, **B,** systemic arterial pressure tracing. Systolic pressure is the peak pressure. The dicrotic notch indicates aortic valve closure. Diastolic pressure is the lowest value before contraction. Mean pressure is the average pressure over time calculated by the monitoring equipment.

Circulatory impairment can result from formation of a thrombus around the catheter, release of an embolus, spasm, or occlusion of the circulation by the catheter. Before inserting a line into the radial artery, an Allen test should be performed to confirm that ulnar circulation is sufficient to sustain the hand. In this test, pressure is applied to the radial and ulnar arteries simultaneously. The patient is instructed to open and close the hand repeatedly. The hand should blanch. The nurse then releases the pressure on the ulnar artery while compressing the radial artery. If pinkness fails to return within 6 seconds, the ulnar artery is insufficient, indicating that the radial artery should not be used for line insertion.

To help maintain line patency and limit thrombus formation, the nurse should assess the continuous flush irrigation system every 1 to 4 hours to determine that the pressure bag is inflated to 300 mm Hg, the flush bag contains fluid, and the system is delivering 1 to 3 ml per hour. It is recommended that a solution of heparinized saline (e.g., 1 to 4 U/ml) be used for the flush solution unless contraindicated.[24]

Once the catheter is inserted, the nurse should evaluate the neurovascular status distal to the arterial insertion site hourly. The limb with compromised arterial flow will appear cool and pale, with capillary refill greater than 3 seconds. There may be symptoms of neurologic impairment, such as tingling or paresthesia. Neurovascular impairment can result in loss of a limb and is an emergency.

Pulmonary Artery Flow-Directed Catheter. Pulmonary artery (PA) pressure monitoring is used to guide acute-phase management of patients with complicated cardiac, pulmonary, and intravascular volume problems (Table 64-4). PA diastolic (PAD) pressure and PAWP are sensitive indicators of fluid volume status and cardiac function. PAD pressure and PAWP are increased in fluid volume overload and heart failure. They are decreased with volume deficit. Fluid therapy based on PA pressure allows restoration of fluid balance while avoiding overcorrection of the problem. Monitoring PA pressures can allow precise therapeutic manipulation of preload, which allows CO to be maintained without placing the patient at risk for pulmonary edema.

A PA flow-directed catheter (e.g., Swan-Ganz) is used to measure PA pressures, including PAWP. The standard PA catheter is number 7.5 French, 43 inches (110 cm) long, with four or five lu-

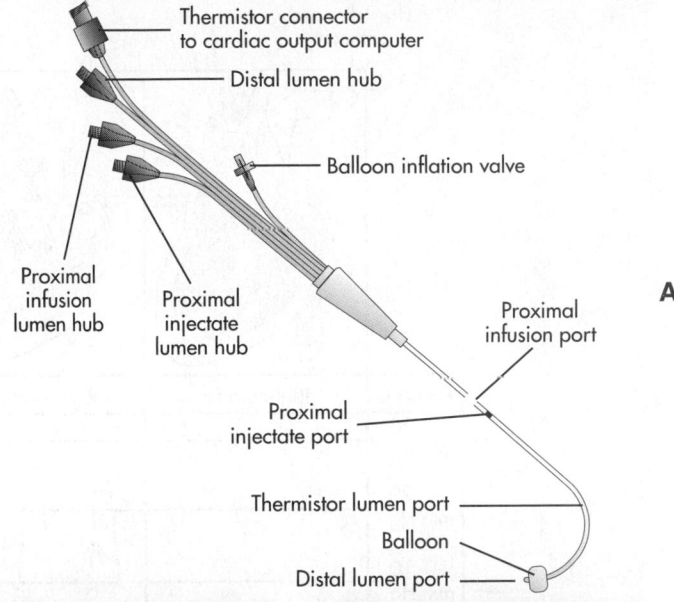

A

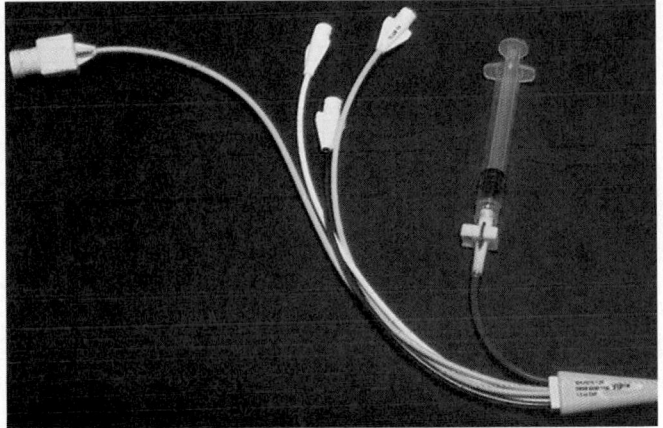

B

FIG. 64-6 Pulmonary artery (PA) catheter. **A,** Illustrated catheter has five lumens. When properly positioned, the distal lumen port is in the PA, and the proximal lumen ports are in the right atrium and right ventricle. The distal and one of the proximal ports are used to measure PA and central venous pressures, respectively. A balloon surrounds the catheter near the distal end. The balloon inflation valve is used to inflate the balloon with air to allow reading of the pulmonary artery wedge pressure. A thermistor located near the distal tip senses PA temperature and is used to measure thermodilution cardiac output when solution cooler than body temperature is injected into a proximal port. **B,** Photo of an actual catheter.

TABLE 64-4	Clinical Indications for Pulmonary Artery Catheterization

Acute respiratory distress syndrome
Acute respiratory failure in patients with chronic obstructive pulmonary disease
Cardiac tamponade
Complex fluid imbalance (e.g., trauma, burns, sepsis)
Evaluation of circulatory syndromes (e.g., heart failure, mitral valve regurgitation, intraventricular shunts)
Intraaortic balloon pump therapy
Myocardial infarction with complications (e.g., left ventricular failure, cardiogenic shock, ventricular septal rupture)
Perioperative fluid imbalance in high-risk patients (e.g., cardiac history)
Shock states (e.g., cardiogenic, septic, hypovolemic)
Vasoactive drug therapy support

mens (Fig. 64-6). When properly positioned, the distal lumen port (catheter tip) is within the PA (Fig. 64-7). This port is used to monitor PA pressures and withdraw mixed venous blood specimens (e.g., to evaluate oxygen saturation). A balloon connected to an external valve via the second lumen surrounds the distal lumen port. Balloon inflation has two purposes: (1) to allow moving blood to float the catheter forward and (2) to allow PAWP measurement. There will be one or two proximal lumens, with exit ports in the right atrium (if only one) or right atrium and right ventricle (if two). The right atrium port is used for measurement of CVP, injection of fluid for CO determination, and withdrawal of

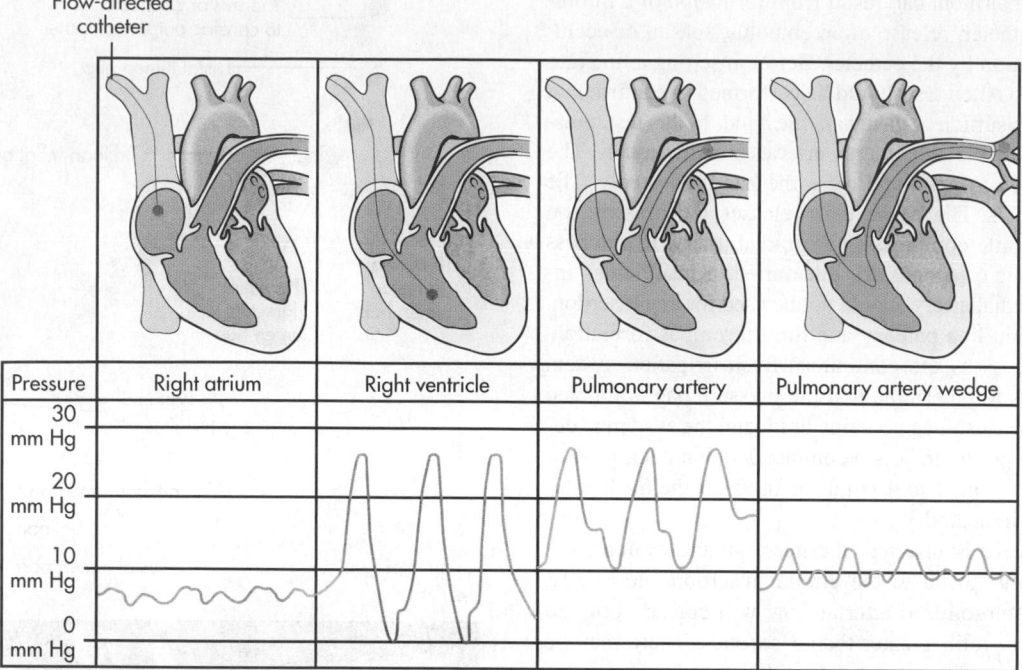

Flow-directed
catheter

Pressure	Right atrium	Right ventricle	Pulmonary artery	Pulmonary artery wedge

FIG. 64-7 Position of the pulmonary artery flow–directed catheter during progressive stages of insertion with corresponding pressure waveforms.

blood specimens. If a second proximal port is available, it is used for infusion of fluids and drugs or blood sampling. A thermistor lumen port located near the distal tip is wired to an external connector. This port is used for monitoring blood or core temperature and in the thermodilution method of measuring CO.

In addition to these relatively standard and common features of the PA flow-directed catheter, catheters with other features are available. One modification is the inclusion of an atrial electrode, useful in recording the atrial ECG or pacing the heart. Another common modification is inclusion of a fiberoptic sensor in the distal tip that detects mixed venous oxygen saturation. Another type of catheter provides continuous measurement of right ventricular volume and ejection fraction, while another catheter provides continuous CO monitoring.[26] The PA catheter sheath usually has a side port that serves as another intravenous line. Most catheters also have a plastic "sleeve" connected to the sheath, which permits manipulation of the catheter while maintaining sterility.

Pulmonary artery catheter insertion. Before PA catheter insertion, the nurse notes the patient's electrolyte, acid-base, oxygenation, and coagulation status. Imbalances such as hypokalemia, hypomagnesemia, hypoxemia, or acidosis can make the heart more irritable and increase the risk of ventricular arrhythmia during catheter insertion. Coagulopathy increases the risk of hemorrhage. The nurse prepares for the procedure by arranging the monitor, cables, and flush and infusion solutions. The system is zero referenced to the phlebostatic axis. The procedure is explained to the patient, and informed consent is obtained. The patient is positioned supine with the head of the bed flat.[27] The PA catheter is inserted through a sheath percutaneously into the internal jugular, subclavian, antecubital, or femoral vein using surgical asepsis. Venous cut-down is rarely required. The line is then advanced through the venous system to the right side of the heart.

Catheter insertion is guided by continuously observing the characteristic waveforms on the monitor as the catheter is advanced through the heart to the PA (see Fig. 64-7). When the tip reaches the right atrium, the balloon is inflated.[27] Inflation of the balloon should not exceed the balloon's capacity (usually 1 to 1.5 ml of air). The catheter is then floated through the tricuspid valve into the right ventricle and then through the pulmonic valve and into the PA. Once a typical PAWP tracing is observed, the balloon is deflated, and the PA waveform should return on the monitor. Following insertion, a chest x-ray is obtained to confirm the position. To maintain the catheter in its proper position, the catheter is then secured at its point of entry into the skin. The measurement at the exit point should be noted and recorded. An occlusive dressing is applied and changed according to unit protocol. It is necessary to monitor the ECG continuously during insertion because of the risk for arrhythmias, particularly when the catheter reaches the right ventricle.

Pulmonary artery pressure measurements. Systolic, diastolic, and mean pressures are routinely monitored. PA systolic is the peak pressure and PA diastolic is the lowest pressure point on the PA waveform. Mean PA pressure is the time-weighted average. Because PA ports are in the chest, intrathoracic pressures alter PA pressure. To produce accurate data, PA measurements are obtained at the end of expiration.[27,28]

The measurement of PAWP is obtained by slowly inflating the balloon with air (not to exceed balloon capacity) until the PA waveform changes to a PAWP waveform (Fig. 64-8). Before inflation the PA pressure tracing on the monitor looks like an arterial tracing, with a systolic peak, dicrotic notch, and then the diastolic low point. As the waveform becomes "wedged," the tracing changes shape and amplitude. Generally, the PAWP waveform is characterized by two small positive waves, the *a* and *v* waves. The *a wave* indicates atrial contraction, and it is followed by the

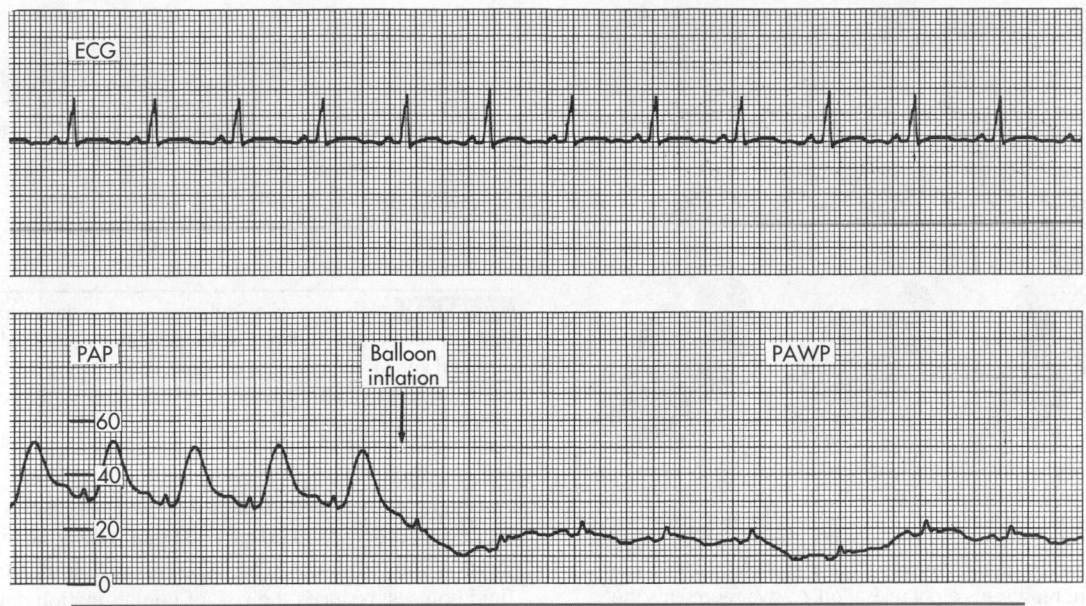

FIG. 64-8 Change in pulmonary artery pressure *(PAP)* waveform to pulmonary artery wedge pressure *(PAWP)* waveform with balloon inflation. The balloon is inflated while observing the bedside monitor for change in the waveform. Balloon inflation *(arrow)* in patient with a normal PAWP.

x descent, indicating atrial relaxation. At times, a *c wave* may be seen following the *a* wave and indicates closure of the mitral valve. The *v wave* is seen during the interval between the T and P waves of the ECG. The *v* wave indicates inflow into the left atrium when the mitral valve is closed and the ventricle is contracting. The *v* wave is followed by the *y descent*, indicating the emptying of the left atrium when the mitral valve opens and the ventricle fills.[28]

When measuring the PAWP, the balloon should be inflated for no more than four respiratory cycles or 8 to 15 seconds.[26,27] There

is danger of rupture of the PA if the catheter migrates distally into a smaller vessel or if the balloon is overinflated. This is suspected when less than 1 ml is needed to wedge the tracing or an "overwedge" tracing is obtained (Fig. 64-9). Readings should be acquired from an analog strip pressure recording, and the strip should be placed into the patient's record. If a printout of the tracing is not available, the readings can be taken from the monitor using the cursor.

Central venous or right atrial pressure measurement. CVP is a measurement of right ventricular preload. It can be measured

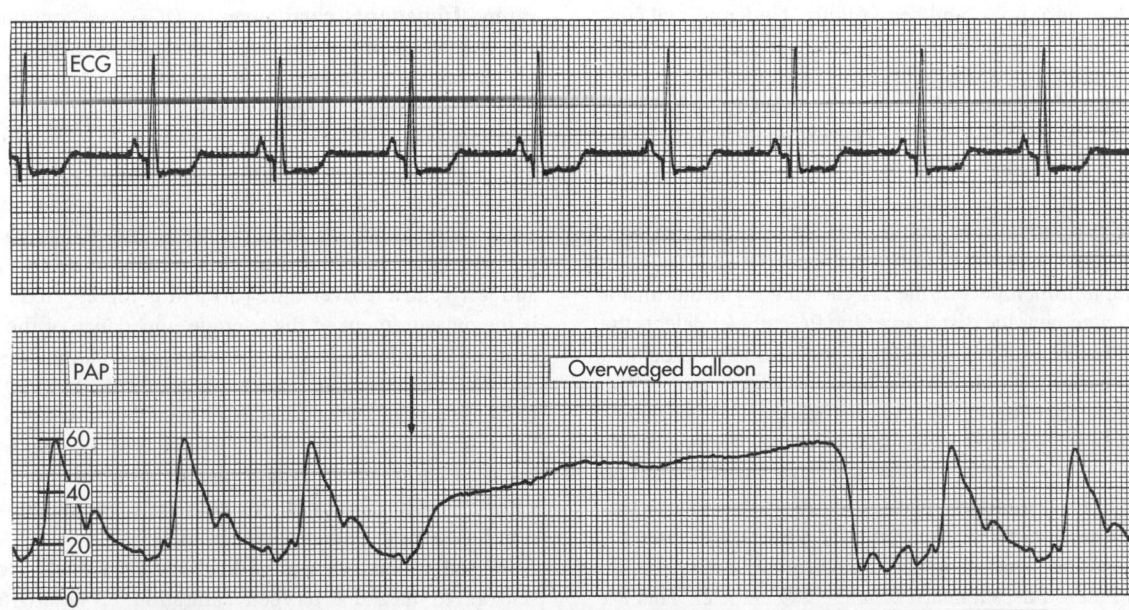

FIG. 64-9 Balloon inflation *(arrow)* in patient with elevated wedge pressure. Overwedging of balloon (balloon has been overinflated). The danger of overinflating the balloon is that the pulmonary artery *(PA)* vessel may rupture from the pressure of the balloon. *PAP,* Pulmonary artery pressure.

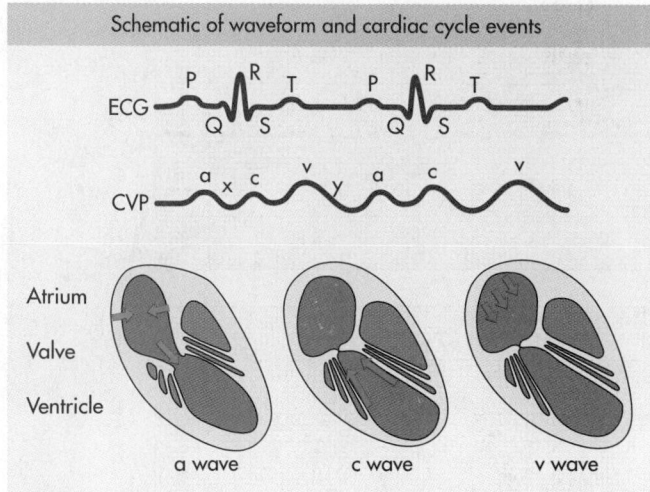

Schematic of waveform and cardiac cycle events

FIG. 64-10 Cardiac events that produce the central venous pressure (CVP) waveform with *a*, *c*, and *v* waves. *a* wave represents atrial contraction. *x* descent represents atrial relaxation. *c* wave represents the bulging of the closed tricuspid valve into the right atrium during ventricular systole. *v* wave represents atrial filling. *y* descent represents opening of the tricuspid valve and filling of the ventricle.

with a PA catheter using one of the proximal lumens or with a central venous catheter placed in the internal jugular or subclavian vein. CVP is measured as a mean pressure at the end of expiration. CVP waveforms (Fig. 64-10) are similar to PAWP waveforms. Although the PA diastolic pressure and PAWP are more sensitive indicators of fluid volume status, CVP also reflects fluid volume problems. An elevated CVP indicates right ventricular failure or volume overload. A low CVP indicates hypovolemia.

Invasive cardiac output measurement techniques. CO is frequently monitored in patients with hemodynamic instability. Normal resting CO is 4 to 8 L per minute and varies with body size. CI accounts for variations in body size and is normally 2.2 to 4 $L/min/m^2$. CO is decreased in conditions such as hypovolemia, cardiogenic shock, and heart failure. Under normal conditions, CO increases with exercise. Increases in CO at rest indicate a hyperdynamic state seen with fever or sepsis.

The PA catheter is commonly used to measure CO via the intermittent bolus *thermodilution* CO (TDCO) method or the *continuous* CO (CCO) method. With the TDCO method, a fixed volume (5 to 10 ml) of 5% dextrose solution (or saline, if contraindicated) of room temperature (or iced for patients with low or high COs) is injected rapidly (≤4 seconds) and smoothly into the proximal lumen port of the PA catheter.[29] The thermistor lumen port located near the distal tip of the PA catheter detects the drop in blood temperature. The CO is mathematically calculated from the area under the temperature curve by the computer. The larger the area under the curve, the smaller the CO, and, conversely, the smaller the area under the curve, the larger the CO (Fig. 64-11).[29] This procedure is repeated three times, with each measurement 1 to 2 minutes apart. Any CO measurement that does not have a normal curve is discarded. An average of three acceptable measurements is calculated to determine the CO.

The CCO method uses a heat-exchange CO catheter. This PA catheter contains a thermal filament that is located in the right atrium. This filament emits a pulsed signal every 30 to 60 seconds that allows for the mixing of blood with heat as it passes through the right ventricle. The thermistor lumen port detects the

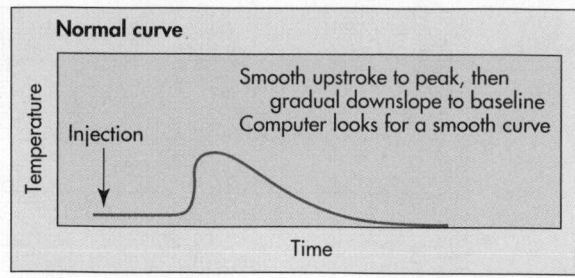

Normal curve

FIG. 64-11 Normal cardiac output curve. Cardiac output is calculated from the temperature change in the pulmonary artery when a fixed volume and known temperature of a solution is injected into the proximal port in the right atrium. The nurse should observe the curve during injection to make sure that it is smooth.

change in temperature. A bedside computer displays digital measurements every 30 to 60 seconds that reflect the average CO for the past 3 to 6 minutes. The CCO method eliminates the need for fluid boluses, reduces the risk of contamination, and permits ongoing evaluation (or trending) of the CO. Comparisons of the TDCO method with the CCO method have shown the CCO method to be reliable.[29]

SVR, SVR index (SVRI), SV, and SV index (SVI) can be calculated each time that CO is measured. The formulas for calculating these parameters are shown in Table 64-2. Increased SVR (>1200 $dynes/sec/cm^{-5}$) indicates vasoconstriction from shock, increased release or administration of epinephrine or norepinephrine, or left ventricular failure. A low SVR (<800 $dynes/sec/cm^{-5}$) indicates vasodilation, which may occur during sepsis, septic shock, or neurogenic shock or with drugs that reduce afterload. Changes in SV are rapidly becoming more important indicators of the pumping status of the heart. A high SV may be seen in bradycardia and exercise and with the use of positive inotropes (e.g., milrinone). Low SV is seen with tachyarrhythmias, extreme vasodilation, and cardiac tamponade.

Noninvasive hemodynamic monitoring: impedance cardiography. Impedance cardiography (ICG) is a continuous, noninvasive method of obtaining CO and assessing thoracic fluid status. Based on the concepts of impedance (the resistance to the flow of electrical current [Z]), ICG uses four sets of external electrodes to deliver a high-frequency, low-amplitude current that is similar to that used in apnea monitors.[30] Blood is an excellent conductor of electricity (lowers impedance), and pulsatile blood flow generates electrical impedance changes. ICG measures the change in impedance (dZ) in the ascending aorta and left ventricle over time (dt) and is represented as dZ/dt. Zo is the measurement of the average impedance of the fluid in the thorax. Impedance-based hemodynamic parameters (CO, SV, and SVR) can be calculated from Zo, dZ/dt, MAP, CVP, and the ECG. Some indications for ICG include early signs and symptoms of cardiac dysfunction, evaluation of cardiac or pulmonary cause of shortness of breath, justification for insertion of a PA catheter, evaluation of pharmacotherapy, and diagnosis of rejection following cardiac transplantation.[30]

Mixed venous oxygen saturation. PA catheters can include sensors to measure oxygen saturation of hemoglobin of PA blood. This value is the *mixed venous oxygen saturation* (SvO_2), and it is useful in determining the adequacy of tissue oxygenation. SvO_2 reflects the dynamic balance between oxygenation of the arterial blood, tissue perfusion, and tissue oxygen consump-

TABLE 64-5	Clinical Interpretation of SvO$_2$ Measurements	
SvO$_2$ MEASUREMENT	PHYSIOLOGIC BASIS FOR CHANGE IN SvO$_2$	CLINICAL DIAGNOSIS AND RATIONALE
High SvO$_2$ (80%-95%)	Increased oxygen supply Decreased oxygen demand	Patient receiving more oxygen than required by clinical condition Anesthesia, which causes sedation and decreased muscle movement Hypothermia, which lowers metabolic demand (e.g., with cardiopulmonary bypass) Sepsis caused by decreased ability of tissues to use oxygen at the cellular level False high positive because pulmonary artery catheter is wedged in a pulmonary capillary
Normal SvO$_2$ (60%-80%)	Normal oxygen supply and metabolic demand	Balanced oxygen supply and demand
Low SvO$_2$ (<60%)	Decreased oxygen supply caused by: Low hemoglobin Low arterial saturation (SaO$_2$) Low cardiac output Increased oxygen consumption (VO$_2$)	Anemia or bleeding with compromised cardiopulmonary system Hypoxemia resulting from decreased oxygen supply or lung disease Cardiogenic shock caused by left ventricular pump failure Metabolic demand exceeds oxygen supply in conditions and increases metabolic rate, including physiologic states such as shivering, seizures, and hyperthermia and nursing interventions such as obtaining bed scale weight and repositioning that increase muscle movement

From Urden LD, Stacy KM, Lough ME: *Thelan's critical care nursing: diagnosis and management*, ed 4, St Louis, 2002, Mosby.

tion (VO$_2$). SvO$_2$, when considered in conjunction with the arterial oxygen saturation, is useful in analyzing hemodynamic status and response to treatments or activities (Table 64-5). Normal SvO$_2$ at rest is 60% to 80%.

Sustained decreases and increases in SvO$_2$ must be analyzed carefully. Decreased SvO$_2$ may indicate decreased arterial oxygenation, low CO, low hemoglobin, or increased oxygen consumption. If the SvO$_2$ falls, the nurse determines which of these four factors has changed. The nurse observes for changes in arterial oxygenation by monitoring pulse oximetry or ABGs. By noting any changes in level of consciousness, strength and quality of peripheral pulses, urine output, and skin color and temperature, the nurse can grossly assess CO and tissue perfusion. If arterial oxygenation, CO, and hemoglobin are unchanged, a fall in SvO$_2$ indicates increased oxygen consumption, which could result from an increased metabolic rate, pain, movement, or fever. If oxygen consumption increases without a comparable increase in oxygen delivery, more oxygen is extracted from the blood, and SvO$_2$ will continue to fall.

Increased SvO$_2$ is also clinically significant and may indicate a clinical improvement (e.g., increased arterial oxygen saturation, improved perfusion, decreased metabolic rate) or problems (e.g., sepsis, ventricular septal defect). In sepsis, oxygen may not be extracted properly at the tissue level, resulting in increased mixed venous oxygen saturation.

Nursing interventions may be guided by changes in SvO$_2$. The nurse might note that the patient's heart rate increased moderately during repositioning but that the SvO$_2$ remained stable. In this case the nurse might conclude that the position change was tolerated. If the SvO$_2$ had dropped, this would be an indication to stop the activity until the SvO$_2$ returns to the previous level.

In many cases as activity or metabolism increases, heart rate and CO increase, and SvO$_2$ remains constant or varies slightly. However, it is not uncommon for critically ill patients to have

conditions that prevent substantial increases in CO. For example, this could occur in the patient with heart failure, shock, arrhythmias, or cardiac transplantation. In these cases, SvO$_2$ can provide a useful indicator of the balance between oxygen delivery and consumption.

Complications with PA catheters. Infection and sepsis are serious problems associated with PA catheters. Careful surgical asepsis for insertion and maintenance of the catheter and tubing line is mandatory to prevent infection. The skin is cleaned according to unit procedure, usually with an iodine preparation. The insertion site is covered with a sterile occlusive dressing. The nurse should monitor the patient for local and systemic signs of infection (e.g., redness and exudate at the insertion site, fever, increased white blood cell count). The PA catheter must be removed if there are local or systemic signs of infection. To reduce the risk of infection, the flush bag, pressure tubing, transducer, and stopcock should be changed every 72 hours, and the PA catheter should be removed once hemodynamic monitoring is no longer needed.[22]

Air embolus is another risk associated with PA catheters. Air embolus can be caused by injection of air into the lumen of a ruptured balloon or by balloon rupture. The nurse decreases the risk of air embolus by first aspirating to check for the absence or presence of blood and by injecting only the prescribed volume of air into the balloon before obtaining the PAWP. Catheters are also checked for balloon leak before insertion; defective catheters are not used. If the nurse aspirates blood from the balloon port or observes that injected air does not flow back into the syringe, the catheter should be so labeled and the physician notified. Air can also be introduced into the system if connections are not tight, and Luer-Lok connections should be used on all pressure lines. In addition, the low-pressure alarm is activated for all pressure lines to signal any substantial drop in the pressure. Any time the line needs to be disconnected to change the apparatus, the nurse closes the line to the patient via clamping or stopcocks.

The patient with a PA catheter is at risk for pulmonary infarction or PA rupture from the following causes: (1) the balloon may rupture, releasing fragments that could embolize; (2) prolonged balloon inflation may obstruct blood flow; (3) the catheter may advance into a wedge position, obstructing blood flow; and (4) a thrombus could form and embolize. To reduce the risk of pulmonary infarction and rupture, the balloon must never be inflated beyond the balloon's capacity (usually 1 to 1.5 ml of air). The balloon must not be left inflated for more than four breaths (except during insertion) or 15 seconds.[26,27] PA pressure waveforms are monitored continuously for evidence of catheter occlusion, dislocation, or spontaneous wedging. The pressure tracing will be blunted if the catheter starts to be occluded. The pressure tracing will appear wedged if the PA catheter advances and becomes spontaneously wedged. In each of these cases, the catheter must be immediately repositioned. To reduce the risk of thrombus and embolus formation, the PA catheter is continuously flushed with a slow infusion of heparinized (unless contraindicated) saline solution to prevent thrombus formation.[22]

Ventricular arrhythmias can occur during PA catheter insertion or removal or if the tip migrates back from the PA to the right ventricle and irritates the ventricular wall. In addition, the nurse may observe that the PA catheter cannot be wedged. In these situations, the catheter may need to be repositioned by the physician or a qualified nurse.

Noninvasive Arterial Oxygenation Monitoring. *Pulse oximetry* is a noninvasive and continuous method of determining arterial oxygenation (SpO_2), and monitoring SpO_2 may reduce the frequency of ABG sampling (see Chapter 25). SpO_2 is normally 95% to 100%. A common use for pulse oximetry is to evaluate the effectiveness of oxygen therapy. Decreased SpO_2 indicates inadequate oxygenation of the blood in the pulmonary capillaries. This may be corrected by increasing the fraction of inspired oxygen (FIO_2) and evaluating the patient's response. Similarly, the nurse uses SpO_2 to monitor how the patient tolerates decreases in FIO_2 and responds to changes in position and treatments. For example, the nurse might note that SpO_2 falls when the patient is positioned in a left lateral recumbent position. The nurse could then plan position changes that pose less risk for the patient.

Accurate SpO_2 measurements may be difficult to obtain on patients who are hypothermic, receiving intravenous vasopressor therapy (e.g., norepinephrine [Levophed]), or experiencing hypoperfusion (e.g., shock). Alternate locations for placement of the pulse oximetry probe may need to be considered (e.g., forehead, earlobe).

NURSING MANAGEMENT HEMODYNAMIC MONITORING

Assessment of hemodynamic status requires integration of data from many sources and comparison of the data over time. Thorough, basic nursing observations provide important clues about the patient's hemodynamic status. The nurse should begin by obtaining baseline data regarding the patient's general appearance, level of consciousness, skin color and temperature, vital signs, peripheral pulses, and urine output. Does the patient appear tired, weak, exhausted? There may be too little cardiac reserve to sustain even minimum activity. Pallor, cool skin, and diminished pulses may indicate decreased CO. Changes in mental clarity may reflect problems with cerebral perfusion or oxygenation. Monitoring urine output reflects the adequacy of perfusion to the kidneys. The patient with diminished perfusion to the GI tract may develop hypoactive or absent bowel sounds. If the patient is bleeding and developing shock, blood pressure might initially be relatively stable, yet the patient may become increasingly pale and cool from peripheral vasoconstriction. Conversely, the patient experiencing septic shock may remain warm and pink yet develops tachycardia and blood pressure instability. Although heart rates of 100 beats per minute are common among stressed, compromised, critically ill patients, sustained tachycardia greatly increases myocardial oxygen demand and may result in diminished CO.

The astute critical care nurse correlates observational data with data obtained from biotechnology (e.g., ECG; arterial, PA, PAWP pressures; SvO_2). Single hemodynamic values are rarely significant. The nurse must evaluate the whole clinical picture with the goals of recognizing early clues and intervening before problems escalate.

CIRCULATORY ASSIST DEVICES

Mechanical **circulatory assist devices** (CADs), such as the intraaortic balloon pump (IABP) and left ventricular assist device (VAD), are used to decrease cardiac work and improve organ perfusion in patients with heart failure when conventional drug therapy is no longer adequate. The type of device used depends on the extent and nature of the myocardial problem and the capabilities of the institution and staff. CADs provide interim support in three types of situations: (1) the left ventricle requires support while recovering from acute injury; (2) the heart requires surgical repair (e.g., a ruptured septum), but the patient must be stabilized; and (3) the heart has failed, and the patient is awaiting cardiac transplantation. All CADs decrease left ventricular workload, increase myocardial perfusion, and augment circulation. The most commonly used CAD is the IABP. Several types of VADs are available, and additional devices are under development.

Intraaortic Balloon Pump

The **intraaortic balloon pump** (IABP) provides temporary circulatory assistance to the compromised heart by reducing afterload (via reduction in systolic pressure) and augmenting the aortic diastolic pressure. Table 64-6 lists clinical conditions for which the IABP is used. The IABP consists of a sausage-shaped balloon, a pump that inflates and deflates the balloon, control devices for synchronizing the balloon inflation to the cardiac cycle, and fail-safe devices (Fig. 64-12). The balloon is inserted percutaneously or surgically, under strict aseptic technique, into the femoral artery, advanced toward the heart, and positioned in the descending thoracic aorta just below the left subclavian artery (Fig. 64-13). Following placement, the position is confirmed by x-ray. A pneumatic device cyclically fills the balloon with helium at the start of diastole (immediately after aortic valve closure) and deflates it just before systole. The ECG is the primary trigger used to initiate the deflation on the R wave (of the QRS) and inflation on the T wave, and the dicrotic notch of the arterial pressure tracing is used to refine timing (Fig. 64-14, *A*). IABP support is referred to as *counterpulsation* because the timing of balloon inflation is opposite to ventricular contraction. The IAPB assist ratio is 1:1 in the acute phase of treatment, that is, one IABP cycle of inflation and deflation for every heartbeat.[31]

TABLE 64-6   Indications and Contraindications for the Intraaortic Balloon Pump

Indications

Refractory unstable angina (when drugs have failed)
Short-term bridge to cardiac transplantation
Acute myocardial infarction with any of the following:*
  Ventricular aneurysm accompanied by ventricular arrhythmias
  Acute ventricular septal defect
  Acute mitral valve dysfunction
  Cardiogenic shock
  Recurrent chest pain with or without ventricular arrhythmias
Preoperative, intraoperative, and postoperative cardiac surgery
  (e.g., prophylaxis before surgery, failure to wean from cardiopulmonary bypass, left ventricular failure after cardiopulmonary bypass)
High-risk interventional cardiology procedures

Contraindications

Irreversible brain damage
Terminal or untreatable diseases of any major organ system
Abdominal aortic and thoracic aneurysms
Moderate to severe aortic insufficiency
Generalized peripheral vascular disease†

*Allows time for emergent angiography and corrective cardiac surgery to be performed.
†May inhibit placement of balloon and is considered a relative contraindication; sheathless insertion may be used.

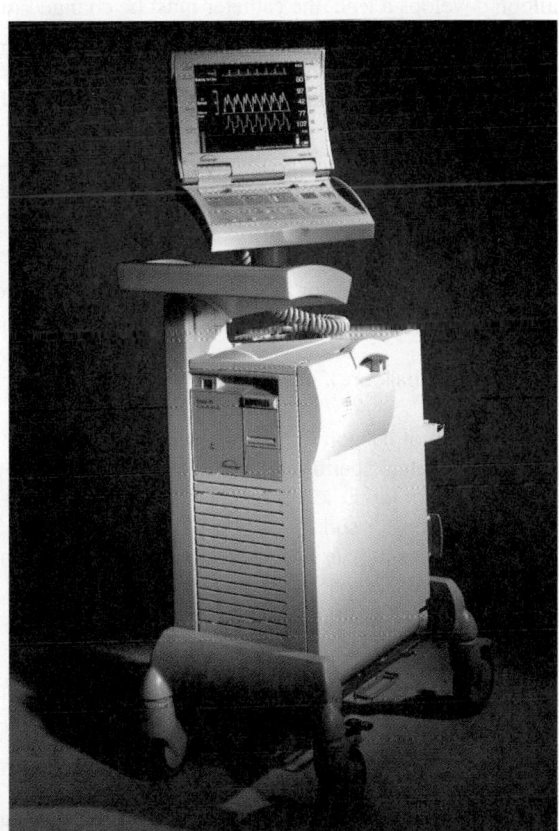

FIG. 64-12 Intraaortic balloon pump machine.

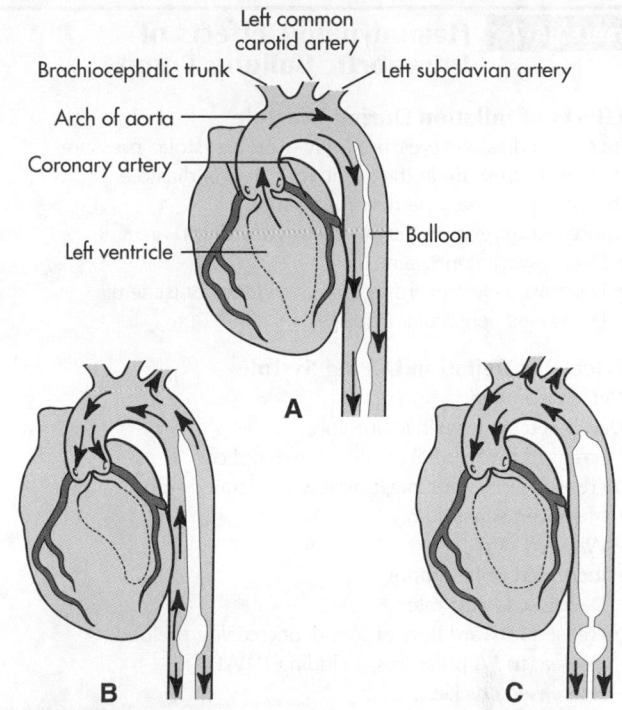

FIG. 64-13 Intraaortic balloon pump. A, During systole the balloon is deflated, which facilitates ejection of the blood into the periphery. B, In early diastole, the balloon begins to inflate. C, In late diastole, the balloon is totally inflated, which augments aortic pressure and increases the coronary perfusion pressure with the end result of increased coronary and cerebral blood flow.

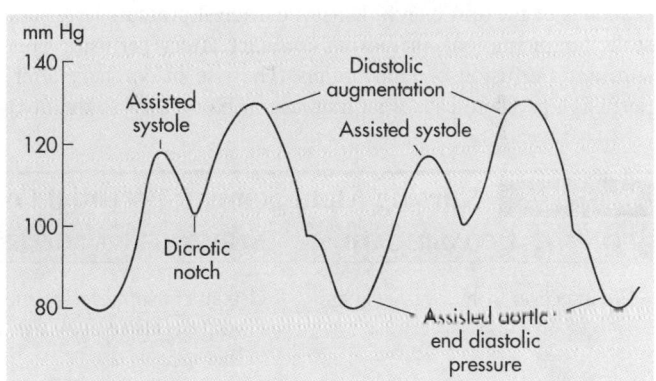

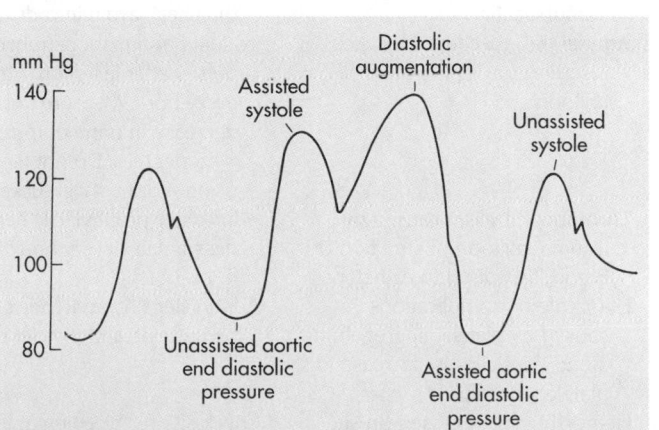

FIG. 64-14 A, Correct 1:1 intraaortic balloon pump frequency. B, Correct 1:2 intraaortic balloon pump frequency.

TABLE 64-7 Hemodynamic Effects of Intraaortic Balloon Pumps

Effects of Inflation During Diastole

Increased diastolic pressure (may exceed systolic pressure)
Increased pressure in the aortic root during diastole
Increased coronary perfusion pressure
Improved oxygen delivery to the myocardium
- Decreased angina pain
- Decreased electrocardiographic evidence of ischemia
- Decreased ventricular ectopy

Effects of Deflation During Systole

Decreased afterload
Decreased peak systolic pressure
Decreased myocardial oxygen consumption
Increased stroke volume, possibly associated with:
- Improved sensorium
- Warmed skin
- Increased urine output
- Decreased heart rate
Increased forward flow of blood, decreasing preload
- Decreased PA pressures, including PAWP
- Decreased crackles

PA, Pulmonary artery; PAWP, PA wedge pressure.

Effects of Counterpulsation. In late diastole when the balloon is totally inflated, blood is forcibly displaced distally to the extremities and proximally to the coronary arteries and main branches of the aortic arch. Diastolic arterial pressure rises (diastolic augmentation), increasing coronary artery perfusion pressure and perfusion of vital organs. The rise in coronary artery perfusion pressure causes an increase in blood flow to the myocardium. The balloon is rapidly deflated just before systole. The suddenly created vacuum causes aortic pressure to drop. With aortic resistance to left ventricular ejection reduced (reduced afterload), the left ventricle empties more easily and completely. As with other types of afterload reduction, the SV increases, yet the myocardial oxygen consumption decreases.[31] Hemodynamic effects of the IABP are summarized in Table 64-7.

Complications with Intraaortic Balloon Pumps. Complications are common with the IABP (Table 64-8). Vascular injuries such as dislodging of plaque, aortic dissection, and compromised distal circulation are common, occurring in 3% to 65% of cases. Thrombus and embolus formation add to the risk of circulatory compromise to the extremity. Peripheral nerve damage can occur, particularly when a cut-down is performed for insertion.[32,33] To reduce these risks, cardiovascular, neurovascular, and hemodynamic assessments are necessary every 15 to 60 minutes depending on the patient's status.[31] The action of the balloon pump can cause physical destruction of platelets, and thrombocytopenia is common. Coagulation profiles must be monitored, and the patient must be assessed for evidence of systemic bleeding. Displacement of the balloon can occlude the left subclavian, renal, or mesenteric arteries and can result in diminished or absent radial pulse, decreased urine output, and diminished or absent bowels sounds. Patients receiving IABP therapy are prone to infection, and local or systemic signs of infection necessitate catheter removal.[31]

Mechanical complications are rare but may occur. Improper timing of balloon inflation may cause increased afterload, decreased CO, myocardial ischemia, and increased myocardial oxygen use and must be immediately recognized by the nurse. If the balloon develops a leak, the catheter must be changed immediately to avoid a helium gas embolus. Signs of a leak include less effective augmentation, repeated alarms for gas loss, and blood backing up into the catheter. A malfunction of the balloon

TABLE 64-8 Nursing Management: Potential Complications of the Intraaortic Balloon Pump

POTENTIAL COMPLICATION	NURSING MANAGEMENT
Site infection from invasive lines	Use strict aseptic technique for insertion and dressing changes for all lines. Cover all insertion sites with occlusive dressings. Administer prescribed prophylactic antibiotic for entire course of therapy.
Pneumonia associated with immobilization	Reposition patient q2hr, being careful not to displace balloon. If patient requires physical therapy of the chest, avoid introducing an ECG artifact.
Arterial trauma caused by insertion or displacement of balloon	Evaluate and mark peripheral pulses before insertion of balloon to use as baseline for assessing pulses after insertion. After insertion of balloon, evaluate perfusion to both extremities at least every hour. Measure urine output at least every hour (occlusion of renal arteries causes severe decrease in urine output). Observe arterial waveforms for sudden changes. Keep head of bed <45 degrees. Do not flex cannulated leg at the hip. Immobilize cannulated leg to prevent flexion using a draw sheet tucked under the mattress, soft ankle restraint, or knee immobilizer.
Thromboembolism caused by trauma, balloon obstruction of blood flow distal to catheter	Administer prophylactic heparin if ordered. Evaluate pulses, urine output, and level of consciousness at least every hour. Check circulation, sensation, and movement in both legs at least every hour.
Hematologic complications caused by platelet aggregation along the balloon (decrease in platelets possible)	Administer Rheomacrodex (low-molecular-weight dextran) if ordered. Monitor coagulation profiles, hematocrit, and platelet count.
Hemorrhage from insertion site	Check site for bleeding at least every hour. Observe vital signs for hypovolemia with each vital sign check.

ECG, Electrocardiogram.

or console triggers fail-safe alarms and automatic shutdown of the unit.

The patient with an IABP is relatively immobile, limited to side-lying or supine positions with the head of the bed elevated less than 45 degrees.[31] The leg in which the catheter is inserted must not be flexed at the hip. The patient may be receiving ventilatory support and will likely have multiple invasive lines that increase the challenge of comfortable positioning. The patient may experience sleeplessness and anxiety. Adequate sedation, pain relief, skin care, and comfort measures are required.

IABP therapy is weaned as the patient improves; that is, circulatory support provided by the IABP is gradually reduced. Weaning involves reducing the IABP assist ratio from 1:1 to 1:2 and assessing the patient's response (see Fig. 64-14, *B*). If hemodynamic parameters remain stable, the ratio can be changed from 1:3 to 1:8 until the IABP catheter is removed. Even if the patient is stable without IABP, pumping is continued until the line is removed.[31] This reduces the risk of thrombus formation around the catheter. Frequent hemodynamic assessment continues to be required during the weaning phase.

Ventricular Assist Devices

The **ventricular assist device** (VAD) provides longer-term support for the failing heart (usually months) and allows more mobility than the IABP. VADs are inserted into the path of flowing blood to augment or replace the action of the ventricle. Some VADs are implanted (e.g., peritoneum), and others are positioned externally. A typical VAD would shunt the blood from the left atrium or ventricle to the device and then to the aorta (Fig. 64-15). Some VADs provide biventricular support.

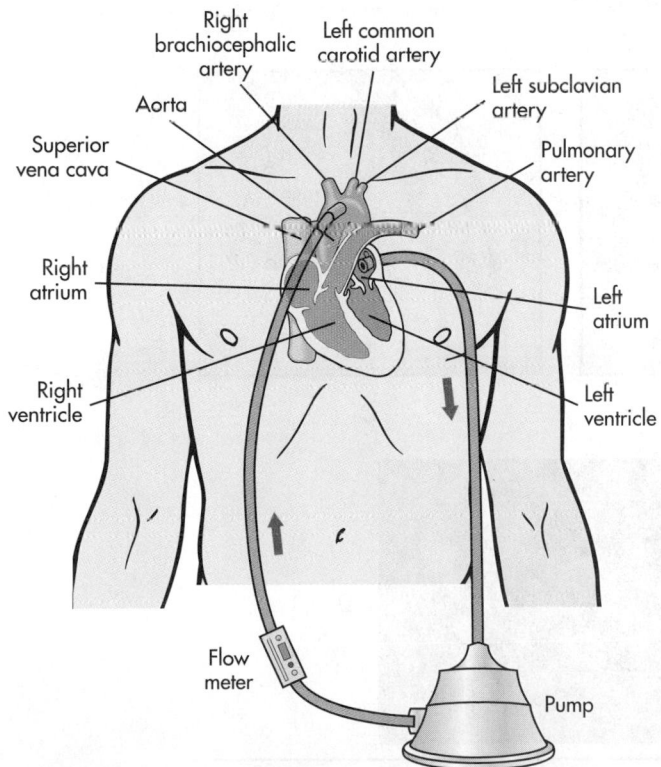

Failure to wean from cardiopulmonary bypass (CPB) after surgery has been the primary indicator for VAD support. Increasingly the VAD is used to support patients with ventricular failure caused by myocardial infarction and patients awaiting cardiac transplantation. A VAD is a temporary device with the capability to partially or totally support circulation until the heart recovers or a donor heart can be obtained. Cannula sites depend on the type of device used. For support of the right side of the heart, the right atrium and PA are cannulated. The left ventricular apex can be cannulated for left VADs. Direct cannulation of the atria and great vessels occurs in the operating room through a sternotomy.

Patient selection for VAD therapy is critical. Indications for VAD therapy include (1) extension of CPB for failure to wean or postcardiotomy cardiogenic shock, (2) bridge to recovery or cardiac transplantation, and (3) patients with New York Heart Association Classification IV (See Table 34-4) who have failed medical therapy. Relative contraindications for VAD therapy include (1) body surface area <1.3 m², (2) renal or liver failure unrelated to cardiac incident, and (3) untreatable metastatic cancer.[34]

Implantable Artificial Heart

Every year in the United States approximately 2000 patients receive donor hearts, yet the demand for these hearts far exceeds the supply. Research on mechanical CADs has led to the development of a fully implantable artificial heart that can sustain the body's circulatory system. This device is designed not only to extend life but also to provide a satisfactory quality of life for the thousands of patients with irreversible heart disease who never receive a donor heart. One major anticipated advantage of the artificial heart compared with heart transplantation is decreased costs for implantation and drug therapies. Patients will not require immunosuppression therapy, nor will they experience the inevitable, long-term effects of this therapy.[35]

NURSING MANAGEMENT
CIRCULATORY ASSIST DEVICES

The patient with an IABP requires highly skilled nursing care. Detailed cardiovascular assessment, including measurement of hemodynamic parameters (e.g., PA and arterial pressures, CO, CI, SVR, SV), cardiac and thoracic auscultation; and evaluation of the ECG (e.g., rate, rhythm), is performed frequently. Assessment of adequate tissue perfusion (e.g., skin color and temperature, mentation, peripheral pulses, urine output, bowel sounds) is also performed at regular intervals.[31] It is expected that with IABP therapy these parameters should improve.

Nursing care of the patient with a VAD is similar to that of the patient with an IABP. The patient is observed for bleeding, cardiac tamponade, ventricular failure, infection, arrhythmias, renal failure, hemolysis, and thromboembolism. Unlike the patient with an IABP, who must remain in bed with limited position change, the patient with VAD may be mobile and require an activity plan.[34] In some cases, patients with VADs may go home. Preparation for discharge is complex and requires in-depth teaching about the device. Patients must have a competent caregiver present at all times.

Ideally, patients with CADs will recover through ventricular improvement, heart transplantation, or artificial heart implantation. However, many patients die, or the decision to terminate the device is made and death follows. Both the patient and family require psychologic support. Nursing care should include the family as much as possible. Other members of the health care team, such as social workers or clergy, should be consulted as needed.

ARTIFICIAL AIRWAYS

The patient in the ICU often requires mechanical assistance to maintain airway patency. Inserting a tube into the trachea, bypassing upper airway and laryngeal structures, creates an artificial airway. The tube is placed into the trachea via the mouth or nose past the larynx (**endotracheal [ET] intubation**) or through a stoma in the neck (*tracheostomy*). ET intubation is more common in ICU patients. It can be performed quickly and safely at the bedside. Indications for ET intubation include (1) upper airway obstruction (e.g., secondary to trauma, tumor, bleeding), (2) high risk of aspiration, (3) ineffective clearance of secretions, and (4) respiratory distress.[36] ET tubes are illustrated in Fig. 64-16.

A *tracheotomy* is a surgical procedure that is performed when the need for an artificial airway is long term. There is ongoing debate regarding the timing of a tracheotomy in the patient with an ET tube. The situation varies with the patient, physician, and institution. Some institutions use ET intubation in patients for up to 6 weeks without harmful sequelae. Tracheostomy tubes and related nursing management are discussed in Chapter 26.

Endotracheal Tubes

In *oral intubation* the ET tube is passed through the mouth and vocal cords and into the trachea with the aid of a laryngoscope or bronchoscope. In nasal intubation, the ET tube is manipulated through the nose, nasopharynx, and vocal cords. Oral ET intubation is the procedure of choice for most emergencies because the airway can be secured rapidly. Compared with the nasal route, a larger-diameter tube can be used for oral intubation. With a larger-bore ET tube, work of breathing is reduced because there is less airway resistance. It is easier to remove secretions and perform fiberoptic bronchoscopy if needed.

There are disadvantages of oral ET intubation. It is difficult to place an oral tube if head and neck mobility are limited (e.g., suspected spinal cord injury). Teeth can be chipped or inadvertently dislodged during the procedure. Salivation is increased, and swallowing is difficult. Often a patient will obstruct the ET tube by biting down on it. A bite block or oropharyngeal airway can be used to avoid this. The ET tube and bite block (if used) should be secured (separately) to the face. Mouth care is a challenge. Finally, the larger tubes used in oral intubation are associated with laryngeal trauma and subglottic stenosis, particularly in smaller individuals.

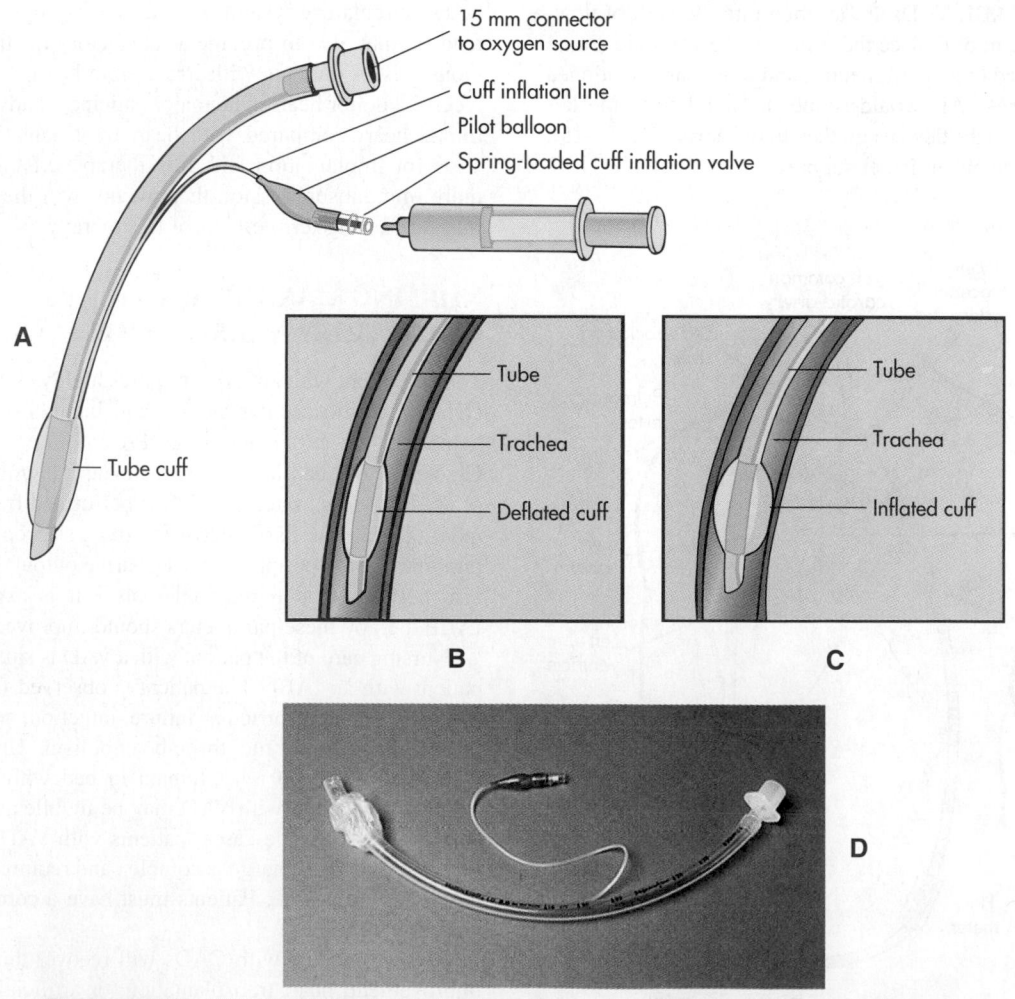

15 mm connector to oxygen source

Cuff inflation line

Pilot balloon

Spring-loaded cuff inflation valve

A

Tube cuff

B
Tube
Trachea
Deflated cuff

C
Tube
Trachea
Inflated cuff

D

FIG. 64-16 Endotracheal tube. **A,** Parts of an endotracheal tube. **B,** Tube in place with cuff deflated. **C,** Tube in place with the cuff inflated. **D,** Photo of tube before placement.

Nasal ET intubation is sometimes preferred because it is more stable than the oral tube and more difficult to dislodge. It is placed "blindly," that is, without visualizing the larynx, and is indicated when head and neck manipulation is risky. The nasal tube may be uncomfortable for some patients because it presses on the septum, whereas others may prefer it because there is no need for a bite block and mouth care is more easily accomplished. However, nasal ET tubes are more subject to kinking than oral tubes; the work of breathing is greater because the longer, narrower tube offers more airflow resistance; and suctioning and secretion removal are more difficult. Nasal tubes have been linked with increased incidence of sinus infections, which may be a source of sepsis.[37]

Endotracheal Intubation Procedure

Before the procedure, the patient and family should be told the reason for ET intubation, the steps that will occur in the procedure, and the patient's role in the procedure (if indicated). It is also important to explain that while intubated, the patient will not be able to speak, but that other means of communication will be provided, and that the patient's hands may be immobilized for safety purposes.[38]

All patients undergoing intubation and receiving mechanical ventilation need to have a self-inflating **bag-valve-mask** (BVM) device (e.g., *Ambu bag*) attached to oxygen and suctioning equipment ready and available at the bedside. The BVM device should contain a reservoir to sequester oxygen so that oxygen concentrations of 90% to 95% can be delivered. The slower the bag is deflated and inflated, the higher the oxygen concentration that will be delivered. The nurse assembles and checks the equipment to be used, removes the patient's dentures and/or partial plates (for oral intubation), and administers drugs as ordered. Premedication varies, depending on the patient's level of consciousness (e.g., awake, obtunded) and the nature of the procedure (e.g., emergent, nonemergent). A sedative-hypnotic-amnesic (e.g., midazolam [Versed]) is used if the patient is agitated, disoriented, or combative. A rapid-onset narcotic such as fentanyl (Sublimaze) may be used to blunt the pain of laryngoscopy and intubation. A paralytic drug such as succinylcholine (Anectine) may be used to produce skeletal muscle paralysis. Atropine may be used to limit secretions. Pulse oximetry is used during the procedure to assess oxygenation.

For oral intubation, the patient is placed supine with the head extended and the neck flexed *("sniffing position")*. This position allows for visualization of the vocal cords by aligning the axes of the mouth, pharynx, and trachea.[38] For nasal intubation it may be helpful to have the patient extrude the tongue. Before intubation is attempted, the patient is preoxygenated using a self-inflating BVM device with 100% O_2 for 3 to 5 minutes. Each intubation attempt is limited to 30 seconds. If unsuccessful, the patient is ventilated between successive attempts using the BVM device with 100% O_2.[36,38]

Following intubation, the cuff is inflated, and the placement of the ET tube is confirmed while manually ventilating the patient with 100% O_2. A disposable CO_2 detector is placed between the BVM device and the ET tube and observed for a color change (indicating the presence of CO_2). The lung bases and apices are auscultated for bilateral breath sounds, and the chest is observed for symmetric chest wall movement. In addition, SpO_2 should be >95%.[36] If the evidence supports proper ET tube placement, the tube is connected to an O_2 source and secured in place per insti-

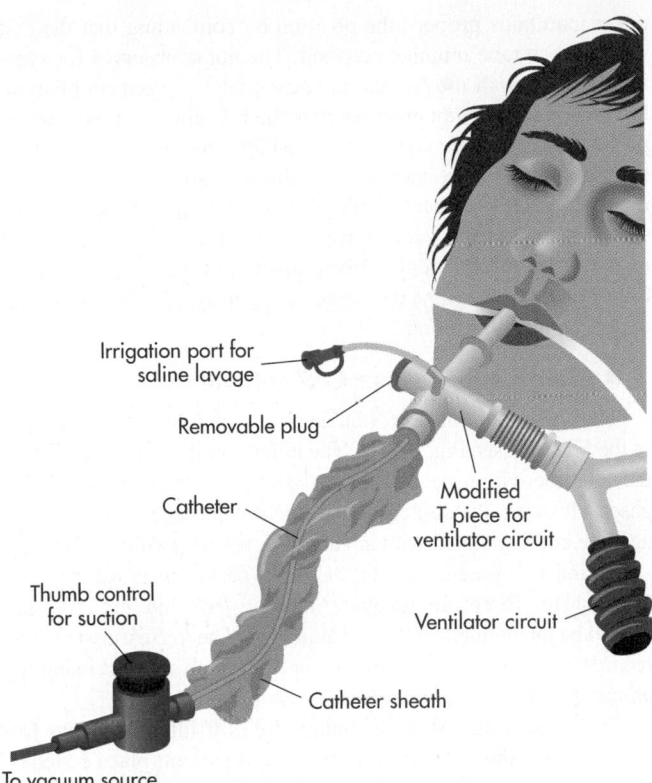

Irrigation port for saline lavage

Removable plug

Catheter

Thumb control for suction

To vacuum source

Modified T piece for ventilator circuit

Ventilator circuit

Catheter sheath

FIG. 64-17   Closed tracheal suction system.

tutional policy (Fig. 64-17). A bite block is inserted as needed. The ET tube and the pharynx should be suctioned as needed. A chest x-ray is immediately obtained to confirm tube placement (3 to 5 cm above the carina in the adult). This position allows the patient to move the neck without dislodging the tube or causing it to enter the right mainstem bronchus. Once proper positioning is confirmed with x-ray, the position of the tube at the teeth (usually 21 cm for women and 23 cm for men) or nose ("exit mark") is recorded and marked.[36] Excess tubing is cut to reduce dead space.

The ET tube is connected either to humidified air, O_2, or a mechanical ventilator. ABGs should be obtained 10 to 20 minutes after intubation to determine oxygenation and ventilation status. ABG values are reviewed and used to guide oxygenation and ventilation changes. Pulse oximetry provides useful continuous monitoring of arterial oxygenation.

NURSING MANAGEMENT ARTIFICIAL AIRWAY

Nursing responsibilities for the patient with an artificial airway include (1) maintaining correct tube placement, (2) maintaining proper cuff inflation, (3) monitoring oxygenation and ventilation, (4) maintaining tube patency, (5) assessing for complications, (6) providing oral care and maintaining skin integrity, and (7) fostering comfort and communication (see NCP 64-1 on p. 1790).

■ Maintaining Correct Tube Placement

The nurse must monitor the patient with an ET tube for proper placement at least every 2 to 4 hours.[38] If the tube is dislodged, it could terminate in the pharynx or enter the esophagus or the right mainstem bronchus (thus ventilating only the right lung). The nurse maintains proper tube position by confirming that the exit mark on the tube remains constant. The nurse observes for symmetric chest wall movement and auscultates to confirm bilateral breath sounds. It is an emergency if the ET tube is not positioned properly. The nurse stays with the patient, maintains the airway, supports ventilation, and secures the appropriate assistance to immediately reposition the tube. It may be necessary to ventilate the patient with a BVM device. If a malpositioned tube is not repositioned, no oxygen will be delivered to the lungs or the entire tidal volume will be delivered to one lung, placing the patient at risk for pneumothorax.

■ Maintaining Proper Cuff Inflation

The cuff is an inflatable, pliable sleeve encircling the outer wall of the ET tube (see Fig. 64-16). The inflated cuff stabilizes and seals the ET tube within the trachea and prevents escape of ventilating gases. However, the cuff can cause tracheal damage. To avoid damage, the cuff is inflated with air, and the pressure in the cuff is measured and monitored. Normal capillary perfusion is estimated at 30 mm Hg. To ensure adequate tracheal perfusion, cuff pressure should be maintained at 20 to 25 mm Hg.[38] The nurse measures and records cuff pressure after intubation and every 8 hours using the *minimal occluding volume (MOV) technique.*

The steps in the MOV technique for cuff inflation are as follows: (1) for the mechanically ventilated patient, place a stethoscope over the trachea and inflate the cuff to MOV by adding air until no air leak is heard at peak inspiratory pressure (end of ventilator inspiration); (2) for the spontaneously breathing patient, inflate until no sound is heard after a deep breath or after inhalation with an BVM; (3) use a manometer to verify that cuff pressure is between 20 and 25 mm Hg; and (4) record cuff pressure in the chart. If adequate cuff pressure cannot be maintained or larger volumes of air are needed to keep the cuff inflated, the cuff could be leaking or there could be tracheal dilation at the cuff site. In these situations the ET tube should be changed within 24 hours or sooner if the patient decompensates.

■ Monitoring Oxygenation and Ventilation

The patient with an ET tube is vigilantly monitored for adequate oxygenation by assessing clinical findings, ABGs, SpO_2, and SvO_2. The nurse must assess for clinical signs of hypoxemia such as confusion, anxiety, dusky skin, and arrhythmias. Periodic ABGs (specifically PaO_2) and continuous SpO_2 provide objective data regarding oxygenation. Lower values are expected in patients with obstructive pulmonary disease. PA catheters with SvO_2 capability can give an indirect indication about the patient's oxygenation status (see Table 64-5).

Indicators of ventilation include assessment of clinical findings, $PaCO_2$, and partial pressure of end-tidal CO_2 ($PETCO_2$). The patient's respirations should be assessed for rate and rhythm and use of accessory muscles. The patient who is hyperventilating will be breathing rapidly and deeply and may experience circumoral and peripheral numbness and tingling. The patient who is hypoventilating will be breathing shallowly or slowly and may appear dusky. $PaCO_2$ is the best indicator of alveolar hyperventilation (e.g., decreased $PaCO_2$, increased pH indicate respiratory alkalosis) or hypoventilation (e.g., increased $PaCO_2$, decreased pH indicate respiratory acidosis).

PETCO_2 monitoring is done by analyzing exhaled gas directly at the patient-ventilator circuit (*mainstream sampling*) or by transporting a sample of gas via a small-bore tubing to a bedside monitor (*sidestream sampling*).[39] Continuous $PETCO_2$ monitoring can be used to assess the patency of the airway and the presence of breathing. In addition, gradual changes in $PETCO_2$ values may accompany an increase in CO_2 production (e.g., sepsis, hypoventilation, neuromuscular blockade) or decrease in CO_2 production (e.g., hypothermia, decreased CO, metabolic acidosis). In patients with normal ventilation-to-perfusion ratios (see Chapter 66), $PETCO_2$ can be used as an estimate of $PaCO_2$, with $PETCO_2$ generally 1 to 5 mm Hg lower than $PaCO_2$. However, in patients with unusually large dead space or serious mismatch between ventilation and perfusion, $PETCO_2$ is not a reliable estimate of $PaCO_2$.[39]

■ Maintaining Tube Patency

The patient should be assessed routinely to determine a need for suctioning, but the patient should not receive suctioning routinely. Indications for suctioning include (1) visible secretions in the ET tube, (2) sudden onset of respiratory distress, (3) suspected aspiration of secretions, (4) increase in peak airway pressures, (5) auscultation of adventitious breath sounds over the trachea and/or bronchi, (6) increase in respiratory rate and/or sustained coughing, and (7) sudden or gradual decrease in PaO_2 and/or SpO_2.[39]

When the presence of secretions is confirmed, the nurse encourages the patient to cough to expel the secretions through the ET tube. If the patient cannot expel the secretions, suctioning is indicated. Two recommended suctioning methods, the **closed-suction technique** (CST) and the **open-suction technique** (OST), are described in Table 64-9. The CST uses a suction catheter that is enclosed in a plastic sleeve connected directly to the patient-ventilator circuit (see Fig. 64-17). With the CST, oxygenation and ventilation are maintained during suctioning and exposure to the patient's secretions is reduced. The CST should be considered for patients who require high levels of positive end-expiratory pressure (PEEP) (>10 cm H_2O) and/or FIO_2 (>80%), who have bloody pulmonary secretions and/or active tuberculosis, and who experience hemodynamic instability with the OST.[40]

Potential complications associated with suctioning include hypoxemia, bronchospasm, increased intracranial pressure, arrhythmias, mucosal damage, pulmonary bleeding, and infection.[40] The nurse must closely assess the patient before, during, and after the suctioning procedure. If the patient does not tolerate suctioning (e.g., decreased SpO_2, increased blood pressure, sustained coughing, development of arrhythmias), the procedure is halted, and the patient is manually ventilated with 100% oxygen or placed back on the ventilator until equilibration occurs and before another suction pass is attempted. Hypoxemia is prevented by hyperoxygenating the patient before and after each suctioning pass and limiting each suctioning pass to 10 seconds or less (see Table 64-9). There are only limited data that support the effectiveness of ventilator-delivered hyperoxygenation in increasing arterial oxygen levels over other methods.[40] If SvO_2 and/or SpO_2 are used, trends should be assessed throughout the suctioning procedure. Spontaneously breathing patients with chronic hypercapnia (e.g., patients with chronic obstructive pulmonary disease [COPD]) should be hyperoxygenated with FIO_2 ≤60%. Spontaneous respirations should be confirmed after the suctioning procedure to rule out oxygen-induced apnea.

TABLE 64-9   Suctioning Procedures for a Patient on a Mechanical Ventilator

General Measures

1. Gather all equipment.
2. Wash hands and don personal protective equipment.
3. Explain procedure and anticipated sensations to patient.
4. Monitor patient's cardiopulmonary status (e.g., vital signs, SpO_2, SvO_2, ECG, level of consciousness) before, during, and after the procedure.
5. Turn on suction and set vacuum to 100 to 120 mm Hg.
6. Pause ventilator alarms.

Open-Suction Technique

1. Open sterile catheter package using the inside of the package as a sterile field. Note: Suction catheter should be no wider than half the diameter of the ET tube (e.g., for a 7-mm ET tube, select a 10-French suction catheter).
2. Fill the sterile solution container with sterile normal saline or water.
3. Don sterile gloves.
4. Pick up sterile suction catheter with dominant hand. Using nondominant hand, secure the connecting tube (to suction) to the suction catheter.
5. Check equipment for proper functioning by suctioning a small volume of sterile saline solution from the container. (Go to Step 7.)

Closed-Suction Technique

6. Connect the suction tubing to the closed suction port.
7. Hyperoxygenate the patient for 30 seconds using one of the following methods:
    - Activate the suction hyperoxygenation setting on the ventilator using nondominant hand.
    - Increase FIO_2 to 100%. For patients with chronic hypercapnia who are breathing spontaneously, use FIO_2 of ≤60%.

Note: FIO_2 must be returned to baseline level at the completion of the procedure.
- Disconnect the ventilator tubing from the ET tube and manually ventilate the patient with 100% O_2 using a BVM device. Administer 5 to 6 breaths over 30 seconds. Note: Use of a second person to deliver the manual breaths will significantly increase the tidal volume delivered.

8. With suction off, gently and quickly insert the catheter using the dominant hand. When resistance is met, pull back 1 to 2 cm.
9. Apply continuous or intermittent suction using the nondominant thumb. Rotate the catheter between the dominant thumb and forefinger and withdraw the catheter over 10 seconds or less.
10. Hyperoxygenate for 30 seconds as described in Step 7.
11. If secretions remain and the patient has tolerated the procedure, two to three suction passes may be performed as described in Steps 8 and 9. Note: Rinse the suction catheter with sterile saline solution between suctioning passes as needed.
12. Reconnect patient to ventilator (open-suction technique).
13. At the completion of ET tube suctioning, rinse the catheter and connecting tubing with the sterile saline solution.
14. Suction nasal and/or oral pharynx. Note: A separate catheter must be used for this step when using the closed-suction technique.
15. Discard the suction catheter and rinse the connecting tubing with the sterile saline solution (open-suction technique).
16. Reset FIO_2 (if necessary) and ventilator alarms.
17. Reassess patient for signs of effective suctioning.

Adapted from Chulay M: Endotracheal or tracheostomy tube suctioning. In Lynn-McHale DJ, Carlson KK, editors: *AACN procedure manual for critical care*, ed 4, Philadelphia, 2001, WB Saunders.
BVM, Bag-valve-mask; *ECG*, electrocardiogram; *ET*, endotracheal.

Causes of arrhythmias during suctioning include hypoxemia resulting in myocardial hypoxia; vagal stimulation caused by tracheal irritation; and sympathetic nervous system stimulation caused by anxiety, discomfort, or pain. Arrhythmias include tachycardia, bradycardia, premature beats, and asystole. Suctioning should be halted if any new arrhythmias develop. Excessive suctioning should be avoided in patients with severe hypoxemia or bradycardia.

Tracheal mucosal damage may occur because of excessive suction pressures, overly vigorous catheter insertion, and the characteristics of the suction catheter itself. The presence of blood streaks or tissue shreds in aspirated secretions indicates that mucosal damage has occurred. Mucosal damage increases the risk of infection and bleeding.[40] Trauma to the mucosa can be prevented by following the steps described in Table 64-9.

Secretions may be thick and difficult to suction because of inadequate hydration, inadequate humidification, infection, or inaccessibility of the left mainstem bronchus or lower airways. Adequately hydrating the patient (e.g., oral or intravenous fluids) and providing supplemental humidification of inspired gases may assist in thinning secretions. Instillation of normal saline into the ET tube, a common practice thought to facilitate the removal of secre-

tions with suctioning, is to be discouraged. It is not effective and may cause decreases in arterial oxygenation. If infection is the cause of thick secretions, the patient should be given appropriate antibiotics. Postural drainage, percussion, and turning the patient every 2 hours may help move secretions into larger airways.[40]

■ Providing Oral Care and Maintaining Skin Integrity

When an oral ET tube is in place, the patient's mouth is always open, and the lips and mouth should be moistened with saline or water swabs to prevent mucosal drying. Oral care, including cleaning of teeth, tongue, and gums, should be performed every 2 to 4 hours and as needed to provide comfort and to prevent injury to the gums and plaque accumulation. If excessive nasal or oral secretions are noted, naso-oropharyngeal suctioning should be performed.

Meticulous care is required to prevent skin breakdown on the face, lips, tongue, and/or nares as a result of pressure from the ET tube and/or bite block or from the method used to secure the ET tube to the patient's face. The ET tube should be retaped or secured every 24 hours and as needed.[37] If the patient is nasally intubated, the nurse should remove the old tape or ties and clean the

FIG. 64-18 Methods for securing adhesive tape. Example of protocol for securing endotracheal tube using adhesive tape:

1. Clean the patient's skin with mild soap and water.
2. Remove oil from the skin with alcohol and allow to dry.
3. Apply a skin adhesive product to enhance tape adherence. (When tape is removed, an adhesive remover will be necessary.)
4. Place a hydrocolloid membrane over the cheeks to protect friable skin.
5. Secure with adhesive tape as shown here..

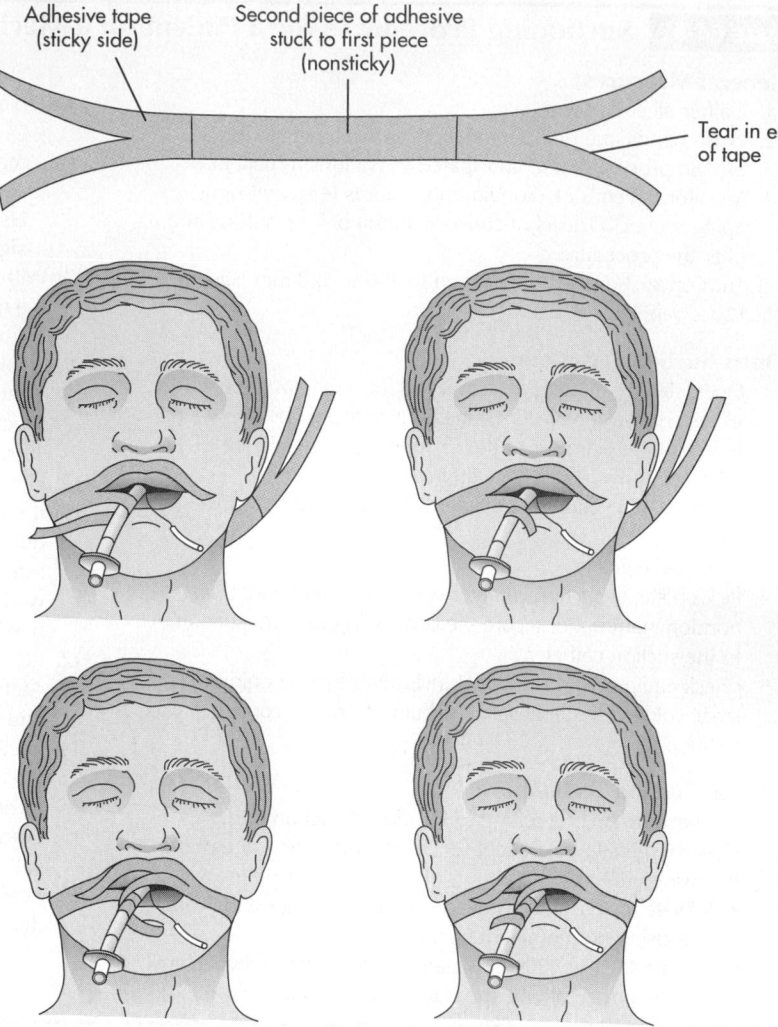

skin around the ET tube with saline-soaked gauze or cotton swabs. If the patient is orally intubated, the nurse should remove the bite block (if present) and the old tape or ties. Oral hygiene should be provided, and the ET tube should be repositioned to the opposite side of the mouth. The nurse replaces the bite block (if appropriate) and reconfirms proper cuff inflation and tube placement.[37] The ET tube is resecured per institutional policy (Fig. 64-18). If a manufactured tube holder is used, the straps can be loosened, the area under the straps massaged, and the straps reapplied. If the patient is anxious or uncooperative, it is recommended that two caregivers perform the repositioning procedure to prevent accidental dislodgment. The patient should be monitored for any signs of respiratory distress throughout the procedure.

■ Fostering Comfort and Communication

Patients have reported that intubation is a major stressor in the ICU.[41] The intubated patient may experience anxiety because of the inability to communicate and not knowing what to expect. Communicating with the intubated patient can be a frustrating experience for the patient, family, and the nurse. To communicate more effectively, the nurse should employ a variety of methods (see earlier section, Common Problems of Critically Care Patients).

The physical discomfort associated with ET intubation and mechanical ventilation often necessitates sedating the patient or administering an analgesic until the ET tube is no longer required. The patient may require morphine, lorazepam (Ativan),

or other sedatives to blunt the anxiety and discomfort related to intubation. The nurse should evaluate the effectiveness of the drugs used to achieve an acceptable level of patient comfort. In addition, the nurse should consider initiating alternative therapies (e.g., music therapy) to complement drug therapy.[9]

Complications of Endotracheal Intubation

Two major complications of ET intubation are inadvertent extubation and aspiration. Inadvertent (unplanned) **extubation** (removal of the ET tube from the trachea) can be a catastrophic event and usually complicates the patient's recovery. Usually the inadvertent extubation is obvious (the patient is holding the ET tube). Other times, the tip of ET tube is in the hypopharynx or esophagus and the extubation is not so obvious. Signs of inadvertent extubation may include patient vocalization, activation of the low-pressure ventilator alarm, diminished or absent breath sounds, respiratory distress, and gastric distention.[42] The nurse is responsible for preventing inadvertent extubation by immobilizing the patient's hands through the use of soft wrist restraints (per institutional policy) and/or sedation. The nurse should reinforce the purpose of the restraints to the patient and family. In one study of elderly ICU patients, being intubated and not being able to breathe were more distressing and memorable than being restrained.[41]

Should an accidental extubation occur, the nurse should stay with the patient. Interventions are directed at maintaining the patient's airway, supporting ventilation (usually by manually ventilating the patient with 100% oxygen), and securing the appropriate assistance to immediately reintubate the patient (if necessary).

Aspiration is a potential hazard for the patient with an ET tube. The ET tube passes through the epiglottis, splinting it in an open position. Thus the intubated patient cannot protect the airway from aspiration. The cuff cannot totally prevent the trickle of oral or gastric secretions into the trachea. Furthermore, secretions accumulate above the cuff. When the cuff is deflated, those secretions move into the lungs. Oral intubation increases salivation, yet swallowing is difficult, so the mouth must be suctioned frequently. The posterior pharynx should always be suctioned before cuff deflation. This may be performed with a Yankauer (tonsil-tip) suction catheter by the patient. Other contributing factors to aspiration include improper cuff inflation and tracheoesophageal fistula. The patient with an ET tube is at risk for aspiration of gastric contents. Even when the cuff is properly inflated, the nurse must take precautions to avoid emesis, which can lead to aspiration. Frequently, a nasogastric (NG) tube is inserted and connected to low, intermittent suction when a patient is intubated. If the patient is receiving enteral feedings through an NG tube, the head of the bed should be elevated.

MECHANICAL VENTILATION

Mechanical ventilation is the process by which room air or oxygen-enriched air is moved into and out of the lungs mechanically. Mechanical ventilation is not curative. It is a means of supporting patients until they recover the ability to breathe independently or a decision is made to withdraw ventilatory support. Indications for mechanical ventilation are listed in Table 64-10.

Patients with chronic pulmonary disease and their families should be given the opportunity to decide the issue of mechanical ventilation before terminal respiratory disease develops. Other patients with chronic illnesses should also be encouraged to discuss the subject. It is much easier for the health care team, patient, and family to decide not to institute ventilatory support initially than it is to remove the support once it has been initiated. The decision to use mechanical ventilation must be made carefully, respecting the informed wishes of the patient and family.

Types of Mechanical Ventilation

The two major types of mechanical ventilation are negative pressure and positive pressure ventilation.

Negative Pressure Ventilation. **Negative pressure ventilation** involves the use of chambers that encase the chest or body and surround it with intermittent subatmospheric or negative pressure. Intermittent negative pressure around the chest wall causes the chest to be pulled outward. This reduces intrathoracic pressure. Air rushes in via the upper airway, which is outside the sealed chamber. Expiration is passive; the machine cycles off, allowing chest retraction. This type of ventilation is similar to normal ventilation in that decreased intrathoracic pressures produce inspiration and expiration is passive. An artificial airway is not required.

New developments in negative pressure ventilation enable both control and assist-control ventilation modes. Lightweight, portable negative pressure ventilators are used in the home for patients with neuromuscular diseases, central nervous system disorders, diseases and injuries of the spinal cord, and severe COPD (Fig. 64-19). Negative pressure ventilators are not used extensively for acutely ill patients.

Positive Pressure Ventilation. **Positive pressure ventilation** (PPV) is the primary method used with acutely ill patients (Figs. 64-20 and 64-21). During inspiration the ventilator pushes

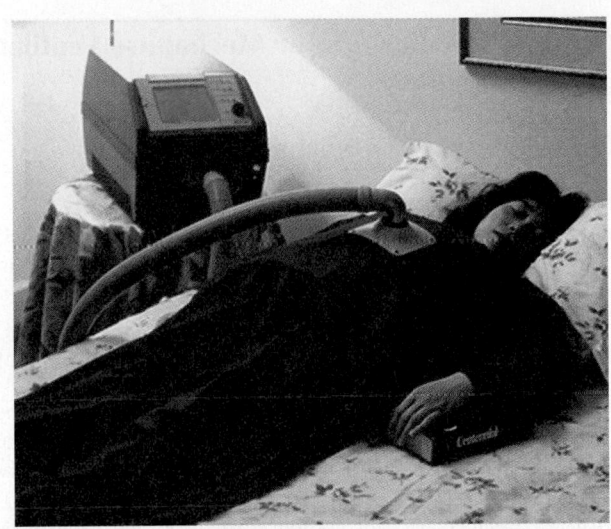
FIG. 64-19 Negative pressure ventilator.

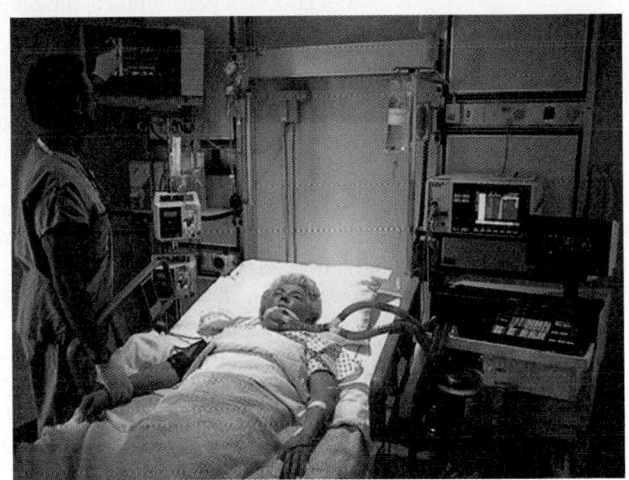
FIG. 64-20 Patient receiving mechanical ventilation.

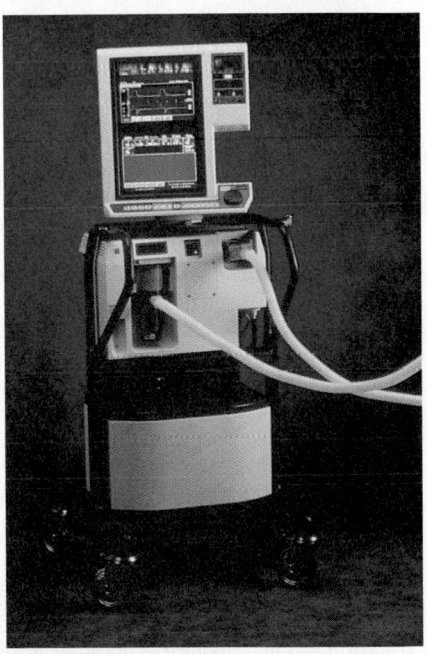
FIG. 64-21 Typical positive pressure ventilator.

TABLE 64-10   Indicators for Mechanical Ventilation and Weaning

MEASUREMENT	SIGNIFICANCE	NORMAL VALUES*	MECHANICAL VENTILATION INDICATED*	WEANING FEASIBLE*
Tests of Ventilatory Reserve or Mechanical Ability				
Spontaneous tidal volume (SV$_T$)	Amount of air exchanged during normal breathing at rest; measure of muscle endurance	7-9 ml/kg	<5 ml/kg	≥5 ml/kg
Spontaneous respiratory rate (fx)		12-20	<10 or >35	12-20
Vital capacity (VC)	Maximal inspiration and then measurement of air during maximal forced expiration; measure of respiratory muscle endurance or reserve or both; requires patient cooperation	65-75 ml/kg	<10-15 ml/kg	≥15 ml/kg
Positive expiratory pressure (PEP) or force (PEF)	After complete occlusion of expiratory valve, pressure manometer attached to airway or mouth for 10-20 seconds while positive expiratory efforts of patient noted; measure of expiratory muscle strength and ability to cough; requires patient cooperation	60-85 cm H_2O	<30 cm H_2O	≥30 cm H_2O
Maximal inspiratory pressure (MIP) or negative inspiratory pressure (NIP)	After complete occlusion of inspiratory valve, pressure manometer attached to airway or mouth for 10-20 seconds while negative inspiratory efforts of patient noted; measure of inspiratory muscle strength; measurement is effort independent (patient does not have to actively cooperate); most reliable of the weaning criteria	−75 to −100 cm H_2O	>−20 cm H_2O	≤−20 cm H_2O
Forced expiratory volume in 1 sec (FEV$_1$)	Volume of air measured in first second of exhalation of forced vital capacity maneuver; used in patients with COPD to determine degree of obstruction	50-60 ml/kg	<10 ml/kg	>16 ml/kg
Resting minute ventilation	Multiplication of tidal volume by respiratory rate for 1 min, general indication of patient's total ventilation	5-10 L/min	>10 L/min	≤10 L/min
Dead space to tidal volume ratio (V$_D$/V$_T$)	Estimation from V$_T$; accurate calculation requiring PaCO$_2$ and partial pressure of CO$_2$ in mixed expired gas; measurement of portion of V$_T$ that does not participate in gas exchange; indication of lungs' efficiency in removing CO_2	0.25-0.40	>0.6	<0.6
PaCO$_2$	Indication of lungs' efficiency in removing CO_2 and reflection of body's acid-base status	35-45 mm Hg	>55 mm Hg (acute)	<45 mm Hg
Tests of Oxygenation Capability				
FIO$_2$	Fraction (percent) of inspired O$_2$ needed to maintain adequate PaO$_2$	21% (room air)	>50%	≤50%
PaO$_2$/FIO$_2$	Provision of evidence of lung's ability to oxygenate arterial blood; couples PO$_2$ with amount of oxygen given	350-400	<200	>300

*These parameters are only guidelines and must be related to the individual patient's status (e.g., patients with severe COPD may have a normal PaCO$_2$ of 60 mm Hg and values lower than normal for FEV$_1$).
COPD, Chronic obstructive pulmonary disease.

air into the lungs under positive pressure. Unlike spontaneous ventilation, intrathoracic pressure is raised during lung inflation rather than lowered. Expiration occurs passively as in normal expiration. Positive pressure ventilators are categorized into volume and pressure ventilators.

Volume ventilators. With **volume ventilators,** a predetermined tidal volume (V$_T$) is delivered with each inspiration, and

the amount of pressure needed to deliver the breath varies based on the compliance and resistance factors of the patient-ventilator system. Consequently, the V$_T$ is consistent from breath to breath, but airway pressures will vary.[42,43]

Pressure ventilators. With **pressure ventilators,** the peak inspiratory pressure is predetermined, and the V$_T$ delivered to the patient varies based on the selected pressure and the compliance and resistance factors of the patient-ventilator system.[42,43] With this understanding, careful attention must be given to the V_T to prevent unplanned hyperventilation or hypoventilation. For example, when the patient breathes out of synchrony with the ventilator, the pressure limit may be reached quickly, and the volume of gas delivered may be small. Initially, pressure ventilation was used only in stable patients being weaned from the ventilator. Today, pressure ventilation is frequently selected to treat critically ill patients.[42]

Settings of Mechanical Ventilators

Mechanical ventilator settings regulate the rate, depth, and other characteristics of ventilation (Table 64-11). Settings are based on the patient's status (ABGs, body weight, level of consciousness, muscle strength). The ventilator is tuned as finely as possible to match the patient's ventilatory pattern. Settings are evaluated and adjusted frequently until the patient achieves optimal ventilation. Some settings serve as a fail-safe mechanism, alerting staff to problems with ventilation. It is important that the nurse ensure and document that all ventilator alarms are on at all times. Alarms sense potentially dangerous situations such as mechanical malfunction, apnea, or patient asynchrony with the ventilator. On many ventilators the alarms can be temporarily suspended or silenced for up to 2 minutes for suctioning or testing. After that period of time, the alarm system automatically becomes functional again.

Modes of Volume Ventilation

The variable methods by which the patient and the ventilator interact to deliver effective ventilation are called modes. The *ventilator mode* selected is based on how much work of breathing (WOB) the patient ought to or can perform and is determined by the patient's ventilatory status, respiratory drive, and ABGs. Generally, ventilator modes are controlled or assisted. With controlled ventilatory support, the ventilator does all of the work of breathing, and with assisted ventilatory support, the ventilator and the patient share the work of breathing.[43] Modes are further categorized as volume modes and pressure modes. For the past 25 years, volume modes such as controlled mandatory ventilation (CMV), assist-control ventilation (ACV), and synchronized intermittent mandatory ventilation (SIMV) have been used to treat critically ill patients. Over the last decade, pressure modes such as pressure support ventilation (PSV) and pressure-controlled inverse ratio ventilation (PC-IRV) have become more widespread.[43] These modes are described in Table 64-12.

Controlled Mandatory Ventilation. With **controlled mandatory ventilation** (CMV), breaths are delivered at a set rate per minute and V_T, which are independent of the patient's ventilatory efforts. Although CMV is used infrequently, it is used when the patient has no drive to breathe (e.g., the anesthetized patient) or is unable to breathe spontaneously (e.g., the paralyzed patient). The patient performs no WOB in this mode and cannot adjust respirations to changing demands.

Assist-Control Mechanical Ventilation. With **assist-control ventilation** (ACV), the ventilator delivers a preset V_T at a preset frequency, and when the patient initiates a spontaneous breath, a full V_T is delivered. The ventilator senses a decrease in intrathoracic pressure and then delivers the preset V_T. The patient can breathe faster than the preset rate but not slower. This mode has the advantage of allowing the patient some control over ventilation while providing some assistance. ACV is used in patients with a variety of conditions, including neuromuscular disorders (e.g., Guillain-Barré syndrome), pulmonary edema, and acute respiratory failure. The patient with ACV mode has the potential for hypoventilation and hyperventilation. The spontaneously breathing patient can easily be overventilated, resulting in hyperventilation. If the volume or minimum rate is set low and the patient is apneic or weak, the patient will be hypoventilated. Thus these patients require vigilant assessment and monitoring of ventilatory status, including respiratory rate, ABGs, SpO_2, and SvO_2. It is important that the amount of negative pressure required to initiate a breath is appropriate to the patient's condition. For example, if it is too difficult to initiate a breath, the WOB is increased and the patient may tire.

Synchronized Intermittent Mandatory Ventilation. With **synchronized intermittent mandatory ventilation** (SIMV), the ventilator delivers a preset V_T at a preset frequency in synchrony with the patient's spontaneous breathing. Between ventilator-delivered breaths, the patient is able to breathe spon-

---

TABLE 64-11   Settings of Mechanical Ventilation

PARAMETER	DESCRIPTION
Respiratory rate (f)	Number of breaths the ventilator delivers per minute; usual setting is 4-20 breaths/min
Tidal volume (V_T)	Volume of gas delivered to patient during each ventilator breath; usual volume is 5-15 ml/kg
Oxygen concentration (FIO_2)	Fraction of inspired oxygen delivered to patient; may be set between 21% (essentially room air) and 100%; usually adjusted to maintain PaO_2 level >60 mm Hg or SaO_2 level >90%
I:E ratio	Duration of inspiration (I) to duration of expiration (E); usual setting is 1:2 to 1:1.5 unless IRV is desired
Flow rate	Speed with which the V_T is delivered; usual setting is 40-100 L/min
Sensitivity/trigger	Determines the amount of effort the patient must generate to initiate a ventilator breath; it may be set for pressure triggering or flow triggering; usual setting for a pressure trigger is 0.5-1.5 cm H_2O below baseline pressure and for a flow trigger is 1-3 L/min below baseline flow
Pressure limit	Regulates the maximal pressure the ventilator can generate to deliver the V_T; when the pressure is reached, the ventilator terminates the breath and spills the undelivered volume into the atmosphere; usual setting is 10-20 cm H_2O above peak inspiratory pressure

From Urden LD, Stacy KM, Lough ME: *Thelan's critical care nursing: diagnosis and management,* ed 4, St Louis, 2002, Mosby.
IRV, Inverse ratio ventilation.

TABLE 64-12 Modes of Mechanical Ventilation

Volume Modes

Control Ventilation (CV) or Controlled Mandatory Ventilation (CMV)

With this mode, the ventilator provides all of the patient's minute ventilation. The clinician sets the rate, V_T, inspiratory time, and positive end-expiratory pressure (PEEP). Generally, this term is used to describe those situations in which the patient is chemically relaxed or is paralyzed from a spinal cord or neuromuscular disease and is therefore unable to initiate spontaneous breaths. The ventilator mode setting may be set on CMV, assist-control (AC), or synchronized intermittent mandatory ventilation (SIMV) because all these options provide volume breaths at the clinician-selected rate.

Assist-Control (AC) or Assisted Mandatory Ventilation (AMV)

This option requires that a rate, V_T, inspiratory time, and PEEP be set for the patient. The ventilator sensitivity is also set, and when the patient initiates a spontaneous breath, a full volume breath is delivered.

Intermittent Mandatory Ventilation (IMV) and Synchronized Intermittent Mandatory Ventilation (SIMV)

This mode requires that rate, V_T, inspiratory time, sensitivity, and PEEP are set by the clinician. In between "mandatory breaths," patients can spontaneously breathe at their own rates and V_T. With SIMV, the ventilator synchronizes the mandatory breaths with the patient's own inspirations.

Pressure Modes

Pressure Support Ventilation (PSV)

This mode provides an augmented inspiration to a spontaneously breathing patient. The clinician selects an inspiratory pressure level, PEEP, and sensitivity. When the patient initiates a breath, a high flow of gas is delivered to the preselected pressure level and pressure is maintained throughout inspiration. The patient determines the parameters of V_T, rate, and inspiratory time.

Pressure-Controlled Inverse Ratio Ventilation (PC-IRV)

This mode combines pressure-limited ventilation with an inverse ratio of inspiration to expiration. The clinician selects the pressure level, rate, inspiratory time (1:1, 2:1, 3:1, 4:1), and the PEEP level. With the prolonged inspiratory times, auto-PEEP may result. The auto-PEEP may be a desirable outcome of the inverse ratios. Some clinicians use PC without IRV. Conventional inspiratory times are used and rate, pressure level, and PEEP are selected.

Positive End-Expiratory Pressure (PEEP) and Continuous Positive Airway Pressure (CPAP)

PEEP

This ventilatory option creates positive pressure at end exhalation. PEEP restores functional residual capacity (FRC). The term PEEP is used when end-expiratory pressure is provided during ventilator positive pressure breaths.

Continuous Positive Airway Pressure (CPAP)

Similar to PEEP, CPAP restores functional residual capacity. However, this pressure is continuous during spontaneous breathing; no positive pressure breaths are present.

From Burns SM: Ventilatory management: volume and pressure modes. In Lynn-McHale DJ, Carlson KK, editors: *AACN procedure manual for critical care,* ed 4, Philadelphia, 2001, WB Saunders.

taneously through the ventilator circuit. Thus the patient receives the preset FIO_2 concentration during the spontaneous breaths but self-regulates the rate and depth of those breaths. This mode of ventilation differs from ACV, in which all breaths are of the same preset volume. SIMV is the most common mode of ventilatory support. It is used during continuous ventilation and during weaning from the ventilator. Potential benefits of SIMV include improved patient-ventilator synchrony (the patient "fights" the ventilator less), lower mean airway pressure, and prevention of muscle atrophy as the patient takes on more of the WOB.[43]

SIMV has advantages over other modes with respect to cardiovascular effects. Spontaneous inspiration decreases intrathoracic pressure, reduces mean intrathoracic pressure, and enhances venous blood return to the heart. Thus the patient with an extracellular fluid volume deficit is better able to maintain CO. Because of the lower mean intrathoracic pressure, higher levels of PEEP may be used with SIMV than with other modes of volume ventilation.

There are disadvantages with SIMV. If spontaneous breathing decreases when the preset rate is low, ventilation might not be adequately supported. Low-rate SIMV should be used only in patients with regular, spontaneous breathing. Weaning with SIMV demands close monitoring and may take longer because the rate of breathing is gradually reduced. Patients being weaned with SIMV may become fatigued, especially during the night.

Pressure Support Ventilation. With **pressure support ventilation** (PSV), positive pressure is applied to the airway only during inspiration and is used in conjunction with the patient's spontaneous respirations. A preset level of positive airway pressure is selected so that the gas flow rate is greater than the patient's inspiratory flow rate. As the patient initiates a breath, the machine senses the spontaneous effort and supplies a rapid flow of gas at the initiation of the breath and variable flow throughout the breath. With PSV the patient determines inspiratory length, V_T, and respiratory rate.[42,43] V_T depends on the pressure level and airway compliance. PSV is used with continuous ventilation and is especially helpful in combination with SIMV during weaning. PSV is not used as a sole ventilatory support during acute respiratory failure because of the risk of hypoventilation. Advantages to PSV include increased patient comfort, decreased WOB (because inspiratory efforts are augmented), decreased oxygen consumption (because inspiratory work is reduced), and increased endurance conditioning (because the patient is exercising respiratory muscles).[42,43]

Pressure-Controlled Inverse Ratio Ventilation. *Pressure-controlled inverse ratio ventilation* (PC-IRV) combines pressure-limited ventilation with an inverse ratio of inspiration (I) to expiration (E). The I/E ratio is the ratio of duration of inspiration (I) to the duration of expiration (E). This value is normally <1. With IRV the I/E ratio approaches 1. With IRV a prolonged positive pressure is applied, increasing inspiratory time. IRV progressively expands collapsed alveoli. The short expiratory time has a PEEP-like effect, preventing alveolar collapse. Because IRV imposes a nonphysiologic breathing pattern, the patient requires sedation or paralysis. IRV is indicated for patients with acute respiratory distress syndrome (ARDS) who continue to have refractory hypoxemia despite high levels of PEEP. Not all patients with poor oxygenation respond to IRV.

Other Ventilatory Maneuvers

Positive End-Expiratory Pressure. **Positive end-expiratory pressure** (PEEP) is a ventilatory maneuver in which positive pressure is applied to the airway during exhalation. Normally during exhalation, airway pressure drops to zero, and exhalation occurs passively. With PEEP, exhalation remains passive, but pressure falls to a preset level greater than zero, often 3 to 20 cm H_2O. With PEEP, lung volume during expiration and between breaths is greater than normal. Thus PEEP increases functional residual capacity (FRC), and this often improves oxygenation. The mechanisms by which PEEP increases FRC and oxygenation include increased aeration of patent alveoli, aeration of previously collapsed alveoli, and prevention of alveolar collapse throughout the respiratory cycle.[43]

PEEP is prescribed in increments of 2 to 5 cm H_2O and is titrated to the point that oxygenation improves without compromising hemodynamics.[43] This is termed best or optimal PEEP. Often 5 cm H_2O PEEP (referred to as *physiologic PEEP*) is used prophylactically to replace the glottic mechanism, help maintain a normal FRC, and prevent alveolar collapse. PEEP of 5 cm H_2O is also used for patients with a history of alveolar collapse during weaning. PEEP has demonstrated improvements in gas exchange, vital capacity, and inspiratory force when used during weaning.

In general, the major purpose of PEEP is to maintain or improve oxygenation while limiting risk of oxygen toxicity. FIO_2 can often be reduced when PEEP is used. PEEP is thought to be useful in pulmonary edema, providing a counterpressure opposing fluid extravasation. PEEP is indicated in lungs with diffuse disease, severe hypoxemia unresponsive to FIO_2 >50%, and loss of compliance or stiffness. The classic indication for PEEP therapy is ARDS (see Chapter 66). PEEP is generally contraindicated or used with extreme caution in patients with highly compliant lungs (e.g., COPD), unilateral or nonuniform disease, hypovolemia, and low CO. In these situations the adverse effects of PEEP may outweigh any benefits.

Continuous Positive Airway Pressure. **Continuous positive airway pressure** (CPAP) restores FRC and is similar to PEEP. However, the pressure in CPAP is delivered continuously during spontaneous breathing, thus preventing the patient's airway pressure from falling to zero. For example, if CPAP is 5 cm H_2O, airway pressure during expiration is 5 cm H_2O. During inspiration, 1 to 2 cm H_2O of negative pressure is generated, thus reducing airway pressure to 3 or 4 cm H_2O. The patient receiving SIMV with PEEP receives CPAP when breathing spontaneously. CPAP is commonly used in the treatment of obstructive sleep apnea. CPAP can be administered by a tight-fitting mask or an ET or tracheal tube. CPAP increases work of breathing because the patient must forcibly exhale against the CPAP and so must be used with caution in patients with myocardial compromise.

High-Frequency Ventilation. **High-frequency ventilation** (HFV) involves delivery of a small tidal volume (usually 1 to 5 ml per kg of body weight) at rapid respiratory rates (100 to 300 breaths per minute) in an effort to recruit and maintain lung volume and reduce intrapulmonary shunting (see Chapter 66). One benefit of HFV may be the ability to support gas exchange while minimizing the risk of barotrauma. HFV has been widely accepted in neonatal and pediatric ICUs, but its use in adults is still considered investigational and limited to patients with ARDS.[44]

There are three types of HFV. *High-frequency jet ventilation (HFJV)* delivers humidified gas from a high pressure source through a small-bore cannula positioned in the airway. With HFJV, precise V_T is difficult to predict and is a function of numerous variables. *High-frequency percussive ventilation (HFPV)* attempts to combine the positive effects of both HFV and conventional mechanical ventilation. A piston mechanism positioned at the end of the ET tube is driven by a high-pressure gas supply at a rate of 200 to 900 beats per minute. These high-frequency beats are superimposed on a conventional pressure-controlled ventilator mode.[44] *High-frequency oscillatory ventilation (HFOV)* uses a diaphragm or a piston in the ventilator to generate vibrations (or oscillations) of subphysiologic volumes of gas. HFOV can produce respiratory frequencies in excess of 3000 breaths per minute.[44] Patients receiving HFV must be paralyzed to suppress spontaneous respiration. In addition, patients must receive concurrent sedation and analgesia as necessary adjuncts when inducing paralysis (see Chapter 66).

Partial Liquid Ventilation. Currently, clinical trials are investigating the use of perflubron (LiquiVent) in **partial liquid ventilation** (PLV) for patients with ARDS. Perflubron is an inert, biocompatible, clear, odorless liquid derived from organic compounds that has an affinity for both oxygen and carbon dioxide and surfactant-like qualities.[45] Perflubron is trickled down a specially designed ET tube through a side port into the lungs of a mechanically ventilated patient. The amount used is usually equivalent to a patient's FRC. Perflubron evaporates quickly and must be replaced to maintain a constant level during the therapy (usually 3 to 5 days). Patients receiving PLV need close observation. Frequent assessment of vital signs, ABGs, and continuous SpO_2 and SvO_2 monitoring are required before, during, and after PLV. PLV has demonstrated few detrimental effects on hemodynamics and may evolve as an important adjunct in the management of ARDS.[45]

Complications of Positive Pressure Ventilation

Although mechanical ventilation may be essential to maintain ventilation and oxygenation, it can cause adverse effects. It is often difficult to distinguish complications of mechanical ventilation from the underlying disease.

Cardiovascular System. PPV can affect circulation because of the transmission of increased mean airway pressure to the thoracic cavity. With increased intrathoracic pressure, thoracic vessels are compressed. This results in decreased venous return to the heart, decreased left ventricular end-diastolic volume (preload), decreased CO, and hypotension. Mean airway pressure is further increased if titrating PEEP to improve oxygenation.

If the lungs are noncompliant (as in ARDS), airway pressures are not as easily transmitted to the heart and blood vessels. Thus effects of PPV on CO are reduced. Conversely, with compliant lungs (e.g., emphysema), there is increased danger of transmission of high airway pressures and negative effects on hemodynamics.

Compromise of venous return by PPV is exaggerated by hypovolemia (e.g., hemorrhage, multiple trauma) and decreased venous tone (e.g., sepsis, spinal shock). Restoration and maintenance of the circulating blood volume are important in minimizing cardiovascular complications.

Pulmonary System

Barotrauma. As lung inflation pressures increase, risk of *barotrauma* increases. Patients with compliant lungs (e.g., COPD) are at greater risk for barotrauma because the increased airway pressure readily distends the lungs and may rupture alveoli or emphysematous blebs. Patients with stiff lungs (e.g., ARDS) who are given high inspiratory pressures and high levels of PEEP and patients with suppurative lung abscesses resulting from necrotizing organisms (e.g., staphylococci) are also susceptible to barotrauma.

Air can escape into the pleural space from alveoli or interstitium, accumulate, and become trapped. Pleural pressure increases and collapses the lung, causing pneumothorax. (Clinical manifestations of pneumothorax are discussed in Chapter 27.) The lung receives air during inspiration but cannot expel it during expiration. Respiratory bronchioles are larger on inspiration than expiration. They may close on expiration, and air becomes trapped. With PPV, a simple pneumothorax can become a life-threatening tension pneumothorax. With tension pneumothorax, the mediastinum and contralateral lung are compressed, compromising CO. Immediate treatment of the pneumothorax is required.

Pneumomediastinum usually begins with rupture of alveoli into the lung interstitium; progressive air movement then occurs into the mediastinum and subcutaneous neck tissue. This is commonly followed by pneumothorax. Occurrence of new, unexplained subcutaneous emphysema is an indication for immediate chest x-ray. Pneumomediastinum and subcutaneous emphysema in the neck may be too small to be detected radiographically or clinically before the development of a pneumothorax.

Volu-pressure trauma. The concept of *volu-pressure trauma* in PPV relates to the lung injury that occurs when large tidal volumes are used to ventilate noncompliant lungs (e.g., ARDS). Volu-pressure trauma results in alveolar fractures and movement of fluids and proteins into the alveolar spaces. To limit this complication, it is recommended that smaller tidal volumes or pressure ventilation be used in patients with stiff lungs. A recent development in ventilator technology is a *volume-assured pressure mode.* This mode combines the advantages of pressure ventilation while ensuring a preset tidal volume on a breath-to-breath basis.[42]

Alveolar hypoventilation. *Hypoventilation* can be caused by inappropriate ventilator settings, leakage of air from the ventilator tubing or around the ET tube or tracheostomy cuff, lung secretions or obstruction, and low ventilation/perfusion ratio. Low V_T or respiratory rate decreases minute ventilation, causing hypoventilation. A leaking cuff or tubing that is not secured may cause air leakage, lowering the delivered V_T. Too low a SIMV rate in a patient who is unable to produce adequate spontaneous respirations causes hypoventilation, respiratory acidosis, and additional problems related to acidosis such as cardiac arrhythmias. Excess lung secretions can cause hypoventilation. Turning the patient every 1 to 2 hours, providing chest physical therapy to lung areas with increased secretions, encouraging deep breathing and coughing, and suctioning as needed can alleviate this. Atelectasis may develop. Increasing the V_T, adding small increments of PEEP, and adding a preset number of sighs to the ventilator settings lessen the likelihood of atelectasis.

Alveolar hyperventilation. Respiratory alkalosis can occur if the respiratory rate or V_T is set too high (*mechanical overventilation*) or if the patient receiving assisted ventilation is *hyperventilating.* It is easy to overventilate a patient on PPV. Particularly at risk are patients with chronic alveolar hypoventilation and CO_2 retention (e.g., patients with COPD). The patient with COPD may have a chronic $PaCO_2$ elevation (acidosis) and compensatory bicarbonate retention by the kidneys. When the patient is ventilated, the patient's "normal baseline" rather than the standard normal values should be the therapeutic goal. If the COPD patient is returned to a standard normal $PaCO_2$, the patient will develop alkalosis because of the retained bicarbonate. Such a patient could move from compensated respiratory acidosis to serious metabolic alkalosis. The presence of alkalosis makes weaning from the ventilator difficult. Alkalosis, especially if the onset is abrupt, can have additional serious consequences, including hypokalemia, hypocalcemia, and arrhythmias. Neuromuscular irritability, seizures, coma, and death can occur. Usually the patient with COPD who is supported on the ventilator does better with a short inspiratory and longer expiratory time.

If hyperventilation is spontaneous, it is important to determine the cause and treat it. Causes might include hypoxemia, pain, fear, anxiety, or compensation for metabolic acidosis. Patients who fight the ventilator or breathe out of synchrony may be anxious or in pain. If the patient is anxious and fearful, sitting with the patient and verbally coaching the patient to breathe with the ventilator may help. If these measures fail, manually ventilating the patient slowly with 100% oxygen source may slow breathing enough to bring it in synchrony with the ventilator.

Ventilator-associated pneumonia. The risk for iatrogenic pneumonia is highest in patients requiring PPV because the ET or tracheostomy tube bypasses normal upper airway defenses. In addition, poor nutritional state, immobility, and the underlying disease process (e.g., immunosuppression, organ failure) make the patient more prone to infection. The prevalence of *ventilator-associated pneumonia (VAP)* has been reported to range from 5.6 to 21.1 cases per 1000 ventilator days. In addition, patients who develop VAP have significantly longer hospital stays and higher mortality rates than those who do not develop VAP.[46]

In patients receiving prolonged PPV, sputum cultures often grow gram-negative bacteria such as *Pseudomonas, Serratia,* and *Klebsiella.* These are abundant in the hospital environment and the patient's GI tract. Organisms can spread in a number of ways, including contaminated respiratory equipment, inadequate hand washing, adverse environmental factors such as poor room ventilation and high traffic flow, and decreased patient ability to cough and clear secretions. Colonization of the oropharynx tract by gram-negative organisms is a predisposing factor in the development of gram-negative pneumonia.

Clinical evidence suggesting VAP includes fever, elevated white blood cell count, purulent sputum, odorous sputum, crackles or rhonchi on auscultation, and pulmonary infiltrates noted on chest x-ray. The patient is treated with antibiotics after appropriate cultures are taken by tracheal suctioning or bronchoscopy and when infection is evident.

Infection can be minimized by using strict aseptic technique while suctioning or handling the artificial airway (see earlier section, Nursing Management: Artificial Airway on p. 1777). Frequent hand washing is imperative. The nurse should wear latex or other impermeable gloves when in contact with the patient or equipment and change gloves between activities (e.g., bathing the patient, administering an intravenous drug). Finally, condensation that collects in the ventilator tubing should be drained away from the patient as it collects.

Sodium and Water Imbalance. Progressive fluid retention often occurs after 48 to 72 hours of PPV. PPV, especially with PEEP, is associated with decreased urinary output and increased sodium retention. Fluid balance changes may be due to decreased CO, which in turn results in diminished renal perfusion. Consequently, renin release is stimulated with subsequent production of angiotensin and aldosterone (Fig. 43-4). This results in sodium and water retention. It is also possible that pressure changes within the thorax are associated with decreased release of atrial natriuretic peptide, also causing sodium retention. Mild water retention is also associated with PPV. There is less insensible water loss via the airway because ventilated delivered gases are humidified with body temperature water. In addition, as a part of the stress response, release of antidiuretic hormone and cortisol may be increased, contributing to sodium and water retention.

Neurologic System. In patients with head injury, PPV, especially with PEEP, can impair cerebral blood flow. This is related to increased intrathoracic positive pressure impeding venous drainage from the head, as evidenced by jugular venous distention. As a result of the impaired venous return and increase in cerebral volume, the patient may exhibit increases in intracranial pressure. Elevating the head of the bed and keeping the patient's head in alignment may decrease the deleterious effects of PPV on intracranial pressure.

Gastrointestinal System. Patients receiving PPV are often stressed because of serious illness, immobility, and discomforts associated with the ventilator. Thus the ventilated patient is at risk for developing stress ulcers and GI bleeding. Patients with a preexisting ulcer or those receiving corticosteroid therapy are at an especially increased risk. Any kind of circulatory compromise, including reduction of CO caused by PPV, may contribute to ischemia of the gastric and intestinal mucosa and possibly increase the risk of translocation of GI bacteria.[6]

Prophylactic administration of histamine H_2-receptor blockers (e.g., ranitidine [Zantac]) or proton pump inhibitors (e.g., omeprazole [Prilosec]) decrease gastric acidity and diminish the risk of stress ulcer and hemorrhage. Target gastric pH is >5. Specially designed feeding tubes with a pH-sensitive probe allow for the measurement of gastric pH. Other methods of assessment include checking the pH of gastric aspirates.

Gastric and bowel dilation may occur as a result of gas accumulation in the GI tract from swallowed air. The irritation of an artificial airway may cause excessive air swallowing and subsequent gastric dilation. Gastric or bowel dilation may put pressure on the vena cava, decrease CO, and prohibit adequate diaphragmatic excursion during spontaneous breathing. Elevation of the diaphragm as a result of paralytic ileus or bowel dilation leads to compression of the lower lobes of the lungs, which may cause atelectasis and compromise respiratory function. Decompression of the stomach can be accomplished by the insertion of an NG tube.

Immobility, sedation, circulatory impairment, decreased oral intake, use of opioid pain medications, and stress contribute to decreased peristalsis. The patient's inability to exhale against a closed glottis may make defecation difficult. As a result, the ventilated patient could be predisposed to constipation. With the early use of enteral nutrition, constipation is usually not a problem.

Musculoskeletal System. Maintenance of muscle strength and prevention of the problems associated with immobility are important. Exercise tolerance is enhanced by adequate analgesia and adequate nutrition. Progressive ambulation of patients receiving long-term PPV can be attained without interruption of mechanical ventilation. The ventilator can be pushed around the room, or the patient can be manually ventilated with a BVM device while ambulating. Passive and active exercises, consisting of movements to maintain muscle tone in the upper and lower extremities, should be done in bed. Simple maneuvers such as leg lifts, knee bends, quadriceps setting, or arm circles are appropriate. Prevention of contractures, pressure ulcers, footdrop, and external rotation of the hip and legs by proper positioning is important.

Psychosocial Needs. The patient receiving mechanical ventilation may experience physical and emotional stress. In addition to the problems related to critical care patients discussed at the beginning of this chapter, the patient supported by a mechanical ventilator is unable to speak, eat, move, or breathe normally. Tubes and machines may cause pain, fear, and anxiety. Ordinary activities of daily living such as eating, elimination, and coughing are extremely complicated.

In studying the psychosocial needs of ICU patients, one researcher discovered that feeling safe was an overpowering need of ICU patients. In addition, four related needs were the need to know (information), the need to regain control, the need to hope, and the need to trust. Patients reported that when these needs were met, they felt safe.[47] The nurse should work to strengthen the various factors that affect feeling safe. Communication must be creative in the case of the intubated patient and information must be forthright. Patients should be involved in decision making as much as possible. The nurse should encourage hope and build trusting relationships with the patient and family.[47]

Patients receiving PPV usually require some type of sedation (e.g., propofol [Diprivan]) and/or analgesia (e.g., fentanyl) to facilitate optimal ventilation. Before initiating sedation and/or analgesia in the mechanically ventilated patient who is agitated or anxious, it is important to assess for the cause of distress. Common problems that can result in patient agitation or anxiety include PPV, nutritional deficits, pain, hypoxemia, hypercapnia, drugs, and environmental stressors (e.g., sleep deprivation).[48]

At times the decision is made to paralyze the patient with a neuromuscular blocking agent (e.g., pancuronium [Pavulon]) to provide more effective synchrony with the ventilator and increased oxygenation. If the patient is paralyzed, the nurse should remember that the patient can hear, see, smell, think, and feel. Intravenous sedation and analgesia must always be administered concurrently when the patient is paralyzed. Many patients have few memories of their time in the ICU, whereas others remember vivid details.[47] Although appearing to be asleep, sedated, or paralyzed, patients may be aware of their surroundings and should always be addressed as though awake and alert.

Machine Disconnection or Malfunction. Mechanical ventilators may become disconnected or malfunction. When turned on and operative, alarms alert the nurse to problems. Most deaths from accidental ventilator disconnection occur while the alarm is turned off, and most accidental disconnections in critical care settings are discovered by low-pressure alarm activation. The most frequent site for disconnection is between the tracheal tube and the adapter. Connections should be pushed together and then twisted to secure more tightly. The nurse should ascertain that alarms are set at all times and should chart that this is the case. Alarms can be paused (not inactivated) during suctioning or removal from the ventilator.

Ventilator malfunction may also occur and may be related to several factors. Although most institutions have emergency generators in the event of a power failure, the nurse should always consider the possibility that power may fail and have a plan for manually ventilating all the patients who are dependent on a ventilator. If, at any time, the nurse determines that the ventilator is malfunctioning (e.g., failure of oxygen supply), the patient should be disconnected from the machine and manually ventilated with 100% oxygen until the ventilator is fixed or replaced.

Nutritional Therapy: Patient Receiving Positive Pressure Ventilation

PPV and the hypermetabolism associated with critical illness can contribute to inadequate nutrition. Presence of an ET tube eliminates the normal route for eating. Although patients who are nasotracheally intubated may be allowed liquid and semiliquid feedings orally, it is difficult to ingest sufficient calories, protein, and fat. A patient with a tracheostomy can eat normally once the stoma has healed. When a tracheostomy tube is present, the patient should tilt the head slightly forward to facilitate swallowing and to prevent aspiration. Often, soft foods (e.g., puddings, ice cream) are more easily swallowed than liquids.

Patients likely to be without food for 3 to 5 days should have a nutritional program initiated. Inadequate nutrition makes the patient receiving prolonged mechanical ventilation more prone to poor oxygen transport secondary to anemia and to poor tolerance of minimal exercise. Poor nutrition and the disuse of respiratory muscles contribute to decreased respiratory muscle strength. In addition, the hypermetabolism associated with critical illness, trauma, and surgery and the presence of anxiety, pain, and increased WOB greatly increase caloric expenditure. Serum protein levels (e.g., albumin, prealbumin, transferrin, total protein) are usually decreased. Inadequate nutrition can delay weaning, decrease resistance to infection, and decrease the speed of recovery.[49] Enteral feeding via a small-bore feeding tube is the preferred method to meet caloric needs of ventilated patients (see Chapter 39 for discussion of enteral feeding).

A concern regarding the nutritional support of patients receiving PPV is the carbohydrate content of the diet. Metabolism of carbohydrates can contribute to an increase in serum CO_2 levels. The resulting CO_2 load results in a higher required minute ventilation. This, in turn, can cause an increase in WOB. Limiting carbohydrate content in the diet may lower CO_2 production. Preparations such as Pulmocare, which are high in protein and fat but low in carbohydrate content, may be beneficial to ventilated patients. The dietitian can provide useful consultation for the ventilated patient.

Weaning from Positive Pressure Ventilation and Extubation

The process of reducing ventilator support and resuming spontaneous ventilation is termed **weaning.** The weaning process differs for patients requiring short-term ventilation (≤ 3 days) versus long-term ventilation (>3 days). Patients requiring short-term ventilation (e.g., after cardiac surgery) will experience a linear weaning process. Patients likely to require prolonged PPV (e.g., patients with COPD who develop respiratory failure) will most likely experience a weaning process that consists of peaks and valleys.[50] Conceptually, preparation for weaning should begin when PPV is initiated and should involve a team approach (e.g., nurse, physician, patient, family, respiratory therapist, dietitian, physical therapist).[51]

Weaning can be viewed as consisting of three phases: the *preweaning phase,* the *weaning process,* and the *outcome phase.* The preweaning or assessment phase determines the patient's ability to breathe spontaneously. Assessment in this phase depends on a combination of respiratory (see Table 64-10) and nonrespiratory factors. Standard respiratory weaning criteria assess muscle strength (negative inspiratory pressure [NIP] and positive expiratory pressure [PEP]) and endurance (spontaneous tidal volume [SV_T] and vital capacity [VC]).[50,52] In addition, the patient's lungs should be reasonably clear on auscultation and chest x-ray. Nonrespiratory factors include the assessment of the patient's neurologic status, hemodynamics, fluid and electrolytes/acid-base balance, nutrition, and hemoglobin.[51] It is important to have an alert, well-rested, and well-informed patient relatively free from pain who can cooperate with the weaning plan. This does not mean complete withdrawal from sedatives or analgesics. Instead, drugs should be titrated to achieve comfort without causing excessive drowsiness.

A variety of weaning modes is available, and no single method is superior. All methods can be delivered with the patient remaining connected to the ventilator circuit. The patient receiving SIMV can have the ventilator breaths gradually reduced as the patient's ventilatory status permits. CPAP or PSV can be added to SIMV. Another method involves PSV, CPAP, or both delivered without SIMV. PSV is thought to provide gentle, slow respiratory muscle conditioning and may be especially beneficial for patients who are deconditioned or have cardiac problems. Some patients may be weaned by simply providing humidified oxygen (T-piece or flow-by method).[50]

Weaning is usually carried out during the day, with the patient ventilated at night. Regardless of the weaning mode selected, all team members should be familiar with the weaning plan. For example, a weaning plan using CPAP might involve placing the patient on CPAP at 0 cm H_2O for up to 2 hours (as tolerated). CPAP trials may be scheduled twice a day, with the second trial scheduled 6 hours after the first. Extubation is considered once the patient can tolerate 2 hours of CPAP.[50] Regardless of the method used, it is important to permit the patient's respiratory muscles to rest between weaning trials. Once the respiratory muscles become fatigued, they may require 12 to 24 hours to recover.

The patient being weaned and the family should be provided continuing psychologic support. The weaning process should be explained, and the patient and family informed of progress. The patient should be placed in a sitting or semirecumbent position and made comfortable. Baseline vital signs and respiratory parameters are measured (V_T, NIP, PEP, VC, SpO_2). During the weaning trial, the patient must be monitored closely for noninvasive criteria that may signal intolerance and result in cessation of the trial (e.g., tachypnea, dyspnea, tachycardia, arrhythmias, sustained desaturation [SpO_2 <91%], hypertension or hypotension, agitation, diaphoresis, anxiety, sustained V_T <5 ml/kg, changes in level of consciousness).[50] Documentation of the patient's tolerance throughout the weaning process is important and should include statements regarding the patient and family's perceptions.

The weaning outcome phase refers to the period when weaning stops and the patient is extubated or weaning is stopped because no further progress is being made. The patient who is ready for *extubation* (tube removal) should receive hyperoxygenation and suctioning (e.g., oropharynx, ET tube). The patient should be instructed to take a deep breath, and at the peak of inspiration, the cuff should be deflated and the tube removed in one motion.[53] After removal, the patient should be encouraged to deep breathe and cough, and the pharynx should be suctioned as needed. Supplemental oxygen should be applied and naso-oral care provided. The nurse must carefully monitor the patient's vital signs, respiratory status, and oxygenation immediately following extubation, within 1 hour, and per institutional policy.[53] If the patient cannot tolerate extubation, immediate reintubation may be necessary.

Home Mechanical Ventilation

Mechanical ventilators are no longer limited to the ICU but are now a part of home care.[54] In some instances, terminally ill, ventilated patients may be discharged to hospice.[55] In either case, the emphasis on controlling hospital health care costs has increased the early discharge of patients and the need to provide highly technical care such as mechanical ventilation in home settings.[56] The success of home mechanical ventilation will depend, in part, on careful predischarge assessment and planning.

Both negative pressure and positive pressure ventilators can be used in the home. Negative pressure ventilators are often the ventilator of choice because they do not require an artificial airway and are less complicated to use. Several types of small, portable (battery-powered) positive pressure ventilators are available and can be attached to a wheelchair or placed on a bedside table. Settings and alarms on these ventilators are similar to the standard ventilators used in ICUs.[56]

Home mechanical ventilation has advantages and disadvantages. Having the patient in the home eliminates the strain that the hospital setting may impose on family dynamics. The feeling of helplessness by family members when they first hear about the necessity for long-term mechanical ventilation is frequently countered by the ability of the family to participate fully in the patient's care in the home setting. At home the patient may be able to participate more in activities of daily living around a more individualized schedule and, because of the smaller size of the home ventilator, be more mobile.[54] Another advantage of home

mechanical ventilation is the reduction in the patient's risk of nosocomial infection.

Disadvantages of home mechanical ventilation include problems related to reimbursement, equipment, caregiver stress, and the complex needs of these patients. Ventilated patients are usually dependent, requiring extensive nursing care, at least initially. Disposable products may be nonreimbursable. Financial resources must be carefully assessed when arranging home mechanical ventilation, and a consultation with a social worker should be initiated. Another disadvantage of home mechanical ventilation is its potential impact on the family. Family members may seem enthusiastic about caring for their loved one in the home but may be motivated by numerous, complex factors. They may lack understanding of the potential sacrifices they may have to make financially and in personal time and commitment. Families should be encouraged to consider respite care to periodically relieve caregiver stress and strain.[56]

NURSING MANAGEMENT MECHANICAL VENTILATION

Nursing management of the patient receiving mechanical ventilation is presented in NCP 64-1.

OTHER CRITICAL CARE CONTENT

Table 64-13 lists additional critical care content presented in other chapters of this book.

TABLE 64-13 Cross-References to Other Critical Care Content

TOPIC	DISCUSSED IN CHAPTER
Acute congestive heart failure	34
Acute respiratory distress syndrome	66
Acute respiratory failure	66
Advanced cardiac life support	35
Burns	24
Cardiac arrhythmias	35
Cardiac pacemakers	35
Cardiac surgery	34
Cardiopulmonary resuscitation	35
Emergencies	67
Enteral nutrition	39
Head injury, including ICP monitoring	55
Myocardial infarction	33
Multiple organ dysfunction syndrome	65
Oxygen delivery	28
Pulmonary edema	34
Renal dialysis, including renal replacement therapy	45
Shock	65
Systemic inflammatory response syndrome	65
Total parenteral nutrition	39
Tracheostomy	26
Trauma	67

ICP, Intracranial pressure.

NURSING CARE PLAN 64-1

Patient Receiving Mechanical Ventilation

EXPECTED PATIENT OUTCOMES	NURSING INTERVENTIONS and *RATIONALES*

NURSING DIAGNOSIS | **Risk for injury** *related to* artificial airway, possible machine malfunction, accidental disconnection or extubation, inability to breathe unassisted, asynchrony with ventilator, and settings ineffective in maintaining adequate oxygenation.

- ABGs within normal range for patient
- Early detection of signs and symptoms of ↓ PaO_2 and ↑ $PaCO_2$
- Synchronous breathing with ventilator
- Early detection, correction, or prevention of complications associated with mechanical malfunction or disconnection
- Properly placed and patent artificial airway with appropriate cuff pressure

- Monitor for risk factors such as hypoxemia, hypercapnia, tachycardia, tachypnea, ↑ BP, agitation, confusion, pain, lethargy, cyanosis; respiratory pattern asynchronous with machine's pattern of ventilation; machine malfunction or disconnection *to determine presence of risk factors and plan for appropriate intervention.*
- Begin mechanical ventilation slowly (especially in patients with COPD); lower $PaCO_2$ only to patient's baseline level *to prevent alkalosis, especially in patient with compensated respiratory acidosis.*
- Assess patient for possible causes of hyperventilation such as retained secretions, hypoxemia, pain, fear, and anxiety *in order to treat appropriately.*
- Check ventilator settings (FIO_2, respiratory rate, V_T, O_2 flow rate, PEEP, airway pressure, thermistor temperature, and I:E ratio) *to determine if appropriate to clinical situation.*
- Keep BVM device connected to O_2 source at bedside *for use in case of an emergency.*
- If patient is fighting ventilation, slowly bag for three to six breaths and verbally coach patient to breathe *to help synchronize patient with ventilator.*
- If asynchrony persists, consider chemical paralysis and sedation and analgesia *to facilitate effective ventilation.*
- Turn all alarms on; pause, but do not turn off alarms during suctioning and disconnections *to prevent unnoticed ventilator malfunction.*
- Respond immediately to all alarms *because potentially dangerous situations of mechanical malfunction, accidental disconnection or extubation, or patient asynchrony with the ventilator may be present.*
- Check ET tube for proper placement and cuff for proper pressure and/or leaks *to prevent loss of ventilation gas and aspiration of oral secretions and to avoid inadvertent dislodgment of the ET tube.*
- Monitor ventilator tubing q1-2hr for condensed water and drain *to prevent aspiration of accumulated fluid.*
- Immobilize patient's hands with soft wrist restraints if needed *to prevent inadvertent extubation by the patient.*
- Use bite block or oral airway *to keep patient from biting and obstructing the ET tube opening.*

NURSING DIAGNOSIS | **Decreased cardiac output** *related to* impeded venous return by PPV *as manifested by* ↓ BP, ↓ SV and PAWP, ↑ heart rate, decreased urine output, presence of arrhythmias, mental confusion.

- BP and CO within normal range or patient's normal baseline
- Adequate urinary output

- Monitor vital signs and level of consciousness q1-4hr *to track trends.*
- Observe and monitor for clinical manifestations of ↓ CO *to identify decreased venous return to the heart, decreased left ventricular end-diastolic volume, and lowered BP.*
- Monitor hemodynamic parameters, especially when >10 cm H_2O of PEEP is used *to anticipate need for plasma expanders, vasopressors, and intravenous fluids as ordered because hemodynamic complications of decreased venous return induced by PPV are exaggerated by hypovolemia.*

NURSING DIAGNOSIS | **Ineffective airway clearance** *related to* presence of artificial airway, problems with positioning, accumulation of secretions, and immobility *as manifested by* presence of abnormal breath sounds, absent cough, presence of thick or copious secretions.

- Normal breath sounds
- Thin and easily removed secretions

- Change patient's position q2hr and perform postural drainage, vibration, and percussion maneuvers when indicated *to prevent pooling of secretions in the lungs.*
- Have patient cough and, if feasible, deep breathe q2hr *to remove secretions and to prevent hypoventilation.*
- Suction oropharynx q1-2hr and as needed *to remove pooled secretions.*
- Perform tracheobronchial suctioning *to remove retained secretions and improve oxygenation* (see Table 64-9).
- Assess breath sounds and other respiratory parameters (e.g., SpO_2, SvO_2, V_T, respiratory rate) q2-4hr *to monitor trends and effectiveness of interventions.*
- Assess for adequate systemic hydration and provide supplemental humidification of ventilator-delivered gases *because these will assist with the thinning of secretions.*

V_T, Tidal volume.

NURSING CARE PLAN 64-1

Patient Receiving Mechanical Ventilation—cont'd

EXPECTED PATIENT OUTCOMES	NURSING INTERVENTIONS and *RATIONALES*
NURSING DIAGNOSIS	**Impaired physical mobility** *related to* restricted movement *as manifested by* inability to perform active range-of-motion exercises, inability to get out of bed.
• Normal range of motion of joints • Absence of contractures, footdrop, pressure ulcer	• Perform active and passive range-of-motion exercises (e.g., leg lifts, knee bends, quadriceps setting, arm circles) *to maintain patient's joint and muscle functioning and improve circulation.* • Position patient properly *to prevent contractures and other musculoskeletal complications (e.g., external rotation of hips).* • Use footboard, high-top sneakers, and frequent foot flexion *to prevent foot drop.* • Change patient's position q2hr and assess skin *to maintain skin integrity and prevent the development of pressure ulcers.* • Get patient out of bed unless contraindicated *to improve circulation and oxygenation and facilitate exercises.* • Provide progressive ambulation for patients receiving long-term ventilation *to prevent complications of immobility.*
NURSING DIAGNOSIS	**Anxiety** *related to* clinical condition, pain, inability to communicate, and fear of death, suffocation, choking, and ICU environment *as manifested by* expression of feelings of anxiety, anxious appearance, agitation, rigid body posture.
• Effective communication of needs • Absent or manageable anxiety level	• Give simple, honest explanations regarding care and progress *to foster a realistic understanding of activities and to help patient make informed decisions and feel safe.* • When possible, allow patient to make decisions regarding all aspects of care *to help patient regain and maintain a sense of control.* • Provide patient with an appropriate means of communication (e.g., alphabet board) *to reduce anxiety associated with inability to speak and to provide means for patient to communicate anxieties.* • Provide for diversion (e.g., music therapy, pet therapy, occupational therapy) as desired and tolerated by the patient *to relieve anxiety.* • Keep call bell accessible to patient *to enable patient to call for assistance.* • Refer to psychiatric clinical nurse specialist, psychiatrist, and/or hospital chaplain when appropriate *to offer additional counseling and support.* • Be available to family; offer support and help *to lessen their anxiety and increase their cooperation.* • Administer and evaluate effectiveness of antianxiety medications and/or analgesics *to chemically manage patient's anxiety and/or pain.*
NURSING DIAGNOSIS	**Dysfunctional ventilatory weaning response** *related to* too-rapid pacing of weaning plan, insufficient knowledge of the weaning plan, and anxiety *as manifested by* restlessness, tachypnea, dyspnea, cyanosis, pallor, fatigue, ↑ or ↓ BP, use of accessory muscles, tachycardia, oxygen desaturation.
• Achievement of progressive weaning goals • Communication of increased comfort during weaning • Less tired from WOB • Remain extubated	• Assess respiratory parameters (e.g., negative inspiratory pressure, positive expiratory pressure, spontaneous tidal volume and vital capacity) *to determine patient's weaning ability.* • Explain the weaning process so that patient understands what is expected *to decrease anxiety and facilitate cooperation.* • Jointly negotiate progressive weaning goals *to provide patient a level of control in establishing the plan.* • Adopt a weaning pace that will ensure success and minimize setbacks *to maintain patient confidence.* • Monitor patient's tolerance during weaning trials (e.g., SpO_2, respirations, ECG, level of consciousness, ABGs) *to evaluate patient's weaning progress.* • Monitor for respiratory distress and place patient back on ventilator if observed *to ensure adequate ventilation.* • If the weaning process is discontinued, explain rationale and revised plan to patient *to minimize frustration and disappointment and enhance cooperation.*

Continued

NURSING CARE PLAN 64-1

Patient Receiving Mechanical Ventilation—cont'd

EXPECTED PATIENT OUTCOMES	NURSING INTERVENTIONS and *RATIONALES*
NURSING DIAGNOSIS	**Risk for infection** *related to* exposure to pathogens and loss of normal protective barrier to infection.
• No evidence of infection • Negative sputum cultures	• Monitor for global signs of infection: change in color, quantity, odor, and viscosity of sputum; difficulty in suctioning secretions; increase in cough; fever; chills; diaphoresis; abnormal breath sounds (e.g., crackles, wheezing); tachycardia; deterioration of ABGs; flushing of skin; elevated white blood cell count; evidence of infiltrate or atelectasis on chest x-ray; positive sputum cultures *to determine if infection is present or developing.* • Obtain sputum culture and order sensitivity test if secretions become purulent or tenacious, change color, or become odorous and/or obtain blood cultures if patient develops fever *to diagnose infectious agent.* • Keep head of bed elevated (especially if receiving enteral nutrition) *to prevent aspiration.* • Keep ventilator tubing cleared of condensed water *to eliminate source of infection.* • Use sterile technique with suctioning (see Table 64-9) *to reduce the risk of infection.* • Administer antiinfectives as ordered and monitor effectiveness (e.g., decrease in secretions, decrease in fever) *to determine efficacy of the drugs.*
NURSING DIAGNOSIS	**Imbalanced nutrition: less than body requirements** *related to* inability to take in adequate nourishment orally and increased caloric demands secondary to clinical condition and need for PPV *as manifested by* loss of 10% of body weight.*

COLLABORATIVE PROBLEMS

NURSING GOALS	NURSING INTERVENTIONS and *RATIONALES*
POTENTIAL COMPLICATION	**Barotrauma, volu-pressure trauma** *related to* PPV.
• Monitor for signs of pneumothorax, pneumo-mediastinum, subcutaneous emphysema • Monitor for changes in breath sounds • Report positive findings • Carry out appropriate emergency interventions as needed	• Record level of peak inspiratory pressure *to establish baseline data to evaluate changes in lung compliance.* • Observe for sudden increase (by 5 cm H_2O or more) in peak inspiratory pressure, sudden patient agitation or coughing, frequent activation of high-pressure alarm, decrease in compliance, palpable subcutaneous emphysema over neck and anterior chest areas, deterioration in ABGs and BP, decrease or absence of breath sounds, hyperresonance on percussion; pneumothorax on chest x-ray *to detect consequences of barotrauma.* • Determine minimal tidal volume needed for adequate ventilation *to limit risk of volu-pressure trauma.* • Ventilate with a BVM with 100% O_2 *to reduce airway pressures until a chest tube can be inserted.* • Notify physician and set up for chest tube insertion immediately *because pneumothorax can convert to a life-threatening tension pneumothorax.* • Check and record ventilator settings q2hr *to maintain accuracy.*
POTENTIAL COMPLICATION	**Gastric distention** *related to* improper ET tube placement, GI bleeding, or ileus.
• Perform abdominal assessment q4hr • Report deviations from expected findings	• Assess for abdominal distention, tympany, and bowel sounds and measure abdominal girth *to detect signs of bowel dilation and/or ileus.* • Test stools and gastric drainage for occult blood *because the patient is at risk of developing stress ulcers and GI bleeding.* • Check for gastric air on chest x-ray *to confirm or eliminate suspicions.* • Administer H_2-receptor blocker, proton pump inhibitor, and tube feedings as ordered *to reduce the occurrence of GI bleeding and to decrease the acidity of gastric secretions.* • If abdominal distention is present, elevate head of bed *to allow for optimal diaphragmatic excursion.* • Obtain order and place NG tube or, if present, confirm patency by irrigating *to relieve gastric tension.* • Confirm correct position of NG tube *to prevent aspiration and the accumulation of GI fluids.*

*Interventions for this nursing diagnosis are presented in the nursing care plan for the patient with acute respiratory failure (NCP 66-1) on pp. 1832-1833.

CRITICAL THINKING EXERCISES

Case Study
Critical Care and Mechanical Ventilation

Patient Profile. An older man was found lying on the street by the police. He had no identification on him. He was unconscious on admission and remains unconscious. He has an ET tube in place and is receiving mechanical ventilation. He weighs 198 lb. An arterial line was placed for blood pressure monitoring. The nurses in the ICU call him Mr. R.

Subjective Data
None; patient is unresponsive to painful stimuli

Objective Data
Physical Examination
- Arterial blood pressure is 100/75; heart rate is 120 (uncontrolled atrial fibrillation); temperature is 102° F (38.8° C); SpO_2 is 98%
- Purulent secretions from ET tube
- Breath sounds: rhonchi bilaterally, decreased breath sounds on the right

Diagnostic Studies
- Chest x-ray reveals right lower lung consolidation
- ABGs: pH, 7.48; PaO_2, 94 mm Hg; $PaCO_2$, 30 mm Hg; HCO_3, 34 mEq/L

Collaborative Care
- Positive pressure ventilation settings: assist-control mode at 16 breaths per minute; tidal volume, 900 ml; FIO_2, 60%
- Enteral nutrition at 25 ml/hr via small-bore feeding tube
- Indwelling urinary catheter to bedside drainage
- Change position every 2 hours
- Perform chest physical therapy every 2 to 4 hours
- gentamycin (Garamycin) 80 mg IV q8hr
- ceftriaxone (Rocephin) 1 g IV q12hr
- D_5NS with KCl 20 mEq/L at 100 ml/hr

CRITICAL THINKING QUESTIONS

1. Identify two reasons for intubating and providing mechanical ventilation for Mr. R.
2. What do Mr. R.'s ABGs indicate, and which ventilator setting(s) should be changed?
3. What is his PaO_2/FIO_2 ratio, and what does it signify?
4. Mr. R.'s blood pressure drops to 80 mm Hg, and he remains in atrial fibrillation with a ventricular rate of 138. A PA catheter is inserted for hemodynamic monitoring. What would be the purpose of hemodynamic monitoring in this patient? Identify two major nursing considerations for a patient with a PA catheter.
5. Mr. R.'s initial PAWP is 14 mm Hg, CI is 2 L/min/m², and SVRI is 2667 dynes/sec/cm⁻⁵/m². How would you interpret these values? What medical interventions might be considered?
6. Mr. R.'s pulmonary condition deteriorates. PaO_2 drops to 70 mm Hg, and SpO_2 is 89%. PEEP is added to the ventilator settings. What implications does this have for Mr. R. given his hemodynamic status?
7. Based on the data presented, identify two priority nursing diagnoses. Are there any collaborative problems?
8. After 6 days, Mr. R. remains unresponsive and is developing renal failure. The physician believes the situation is hopeless and wishes to discuss termination of life support. What approach should the nurse take in locating Mr. R.'s next of kin?
9. Based on the assessment data provided, write one or more nursing diagnoses. Are there any collaborative problems?

Nursing Research Issues

1. Are hemodynamic parameters obtained when patients are in a lateral (side-lying) position accurate?
2. How can communication be best facilitated in the mechanically ventilated patient?
3. What interventions can reduce the incidence of ventilator-associated pneumonia?
4. How can pet therapy be initiated safely and effectively in a critical care unit?

REVIEW QUESTIONS

The number of the question corresponds to the same-numbered objective at the beginning of the chapter.

1. Certification in critical care nursing by the American Association of Critical Care Nurses indicates that a nurse
   a. has earned a master's degree in the field of providing advanced critical care nursing.
   b. is an advanced practice nurse in the care of acutely ill patients.
   c. may practice independently to provide symptom management for the critically ill.
   d. has practiced in critical care and successfully completed a test of critical care knowledge.

2. An appropriate nursing intervention for the patient with delirium in the ICU is to
   a. use tranquilizers to establish normal sleep patterns.
   b. identify the factors contributing to the patient's confusion and irritability.
   c. silence all alarms, overhead paging, and conversations around the patient.
   d. sedate the patient with psychotropic drugs to protect the patient from harmful behaviors.

Continued

REVIEW QUESTIONS—cont'd

3. The critical care nurse recognizes that an ideal plan for family involvement includes
   a. a family member at the bedside at all times.
   b. allowing family at the bedside at preset, brief intervals.
   c. an individually devised plan with family involved with care and comfort measures.
   d. restriction of visiting in the ICU because the environment is overwhelming to visitors.

4. To establish hemodynamic monitoring for a patient, the nurse zeros the
   a. cardiac output monitoring system to the level of the left ventricle.
   b. pressure monitoring system to the level of the catheter tip located in the patient.
   c. pressure monitoring system to the level of the atrium, identified as the midaxillary line.
   d. pressure monitoring system to the level of the atrium, identified as the phlebostatic axis.

5. The hemodynamic changes the nurse expects to find after successful initiation of an intraaortic balloon pump in a patient in cardiogenic shock include
   a. decreased PAWP and increased CO.
   b. decreased SVR and decreased SV.
   c. increased diastolic BP and decreased systolic BP.
   d. decreased CVP and increased right atrial pressure.

6. The nursing management of a patient with an artificial airway includes
   a. routine suctioning of the tube at least every 2 hours.
   b. observing for cardiac arrhythmias during suctioning.
   c. maintaining ET tube cuff pressure at 30 cm H_2O.
   d. preventing tube dislodgment by limiting mouth care to lubrication of the lips.

7. The purpose of adding PEEP to positive pressure ventilation is to
   a. increase functional residual capacity and improve oxygenation.
   b. increase FIO_2 in an attempt to wean the patient and avoid oxygen toxicity.
   c. determine if the patient is able to be weaned and avoid the risk of pneumomediastinum.
   d. determine if the patient is in synchrony with the ventilator or needs to be paralyzed.

8. The nurse monitors the patient with positive pressure mechanical ventilation for
   a. paralytic ileus because pressure on the abdominal contents affects bowel motility.
   b. diuresis and sodium depletion because of increased release of atrial natriuretic peptide.
   c. signs of cardiovascular insufficiency because pressure in the chest impedes venous return.
   d. respiratory acidosis in a patient with COPD because of alveolar hyperventilation and increased PaO_2 levels.

REFERENCES

1. Nightingale F: *Notes on hospitals,* ed 3, London, 1863, Longman, Roberts, & Green.
*2. Lynaugh JE, Fairman J: *Critical care nursing: a history,* Philadelphia, 1998, University of Pennsylvania Press.
3. Goldhill DR, Summer A: Outcome of intensive care patients in a group of British intensive care units, *Crit Care Med* 26:1337, 1998.
4. Miller PA, Forbes S, Boyle DK: End-of-life care in the intensive care unit: a challenge for nurses, *Am J Crit Care* 10:230, 2001.
5. Bucher L, Melander S: Critical care across the health care continuum. In Bucher L, Melander S, editors: *Critical care nursing,* Philadelphia, 1999, Saunders.
6. Trujillo EB, Robinson MK, Jacobs DO: Feeding critically ill patients: current concepts, *Crit Care Nurse* 21:60, 2001.
*7. Frazier SK et al: Critical care nurses' assessment of patients' anxiety: reliance on physiological and behavioral parameters, *Am J Crit Care* 11:57, 2002.
8. White SK et al: A renaissance in critical care nursing: technological advances and sedation strategies, *Crit Care Nurse* 21(suppl):1, 2001.
*9. Keegan L: Alternative and complementary modalities for managing stress and anxiety in acute and critical care. In Chulay M, Molter NC, editors: *Protocols for practice: creating a healing environment,* Aliso Viejo, Calif, 1998, AACN.
*10. Stanik-Hutt J: Pain management in the acutely ill. In Chulay M, Molter NC, editors: *Protocols for practice: creating a healing environment,* Aliso Viejo, Calif, 1998, AACN.
*11. Kress JP et al: Daily interruption of sedative infusions in critically ill patients undergoing mechanical ventilation, *N Engl J Med* 342:1471, 2000.
12. Roberts BL: Managing delirium in adult intensive care patients, *Crit Care Nurse* 21:48, 2001.

13. Kahn DM et al: Identification and modification of environmental noise in an ICU setting, *Chest* 114:535, 1998.
*14. Richards KC et al: Promoting sleep in acute and critical care. In Chulay M, Molter NC, editors: *Protocols for practice: creating a healing environment,* Aliso Viejo, Calif, 1998, AACN.
15. Grozinger M et al: Effects of lorazepam on the automatic online evaluation of sleep EEG data in healthy volunteers, *Pharmacopsychiatry* 31:55, 1998.
16. Doherty MH et al: Impact of critical illness on the patient and family. In Bucher L, Melander S, editors: *Critical care nursing,* Philadelphia, 1999, WB Saunders.
*17. Titler MG: Family visitation and partnership in the critical care unit. In Chulay M, Molter NC, editors: *Protocols for practice: creating a healing environment,* Aliso Viejo, Calif, 1997, AACN.
18. Green ML: Legal and ethical issues in critical care nursing. In Bucher L, Melander S, editors: *Critical care nursing,* Philadelphia, 1999, WB Saunders.
*19. Titler MG, Drahozal R: Family pet visiting, animal-assisted activities, and animal-assisted therapy in critical care. In Chulay M, Molter NC, editors: *Protocols for practice: creating a healing environment,* Aliso Viejo, Calif, 1997, AACN.
20. Mitty EL: Ethnicity and end-of-life decision-making, *Reflec Nurs Leadersh* 27:28-31, 2001.
21. Germain C: Cultural issues in critical care nursing. In Bucher L, Melander S, editors: *Critical care nursing,* Philadelphia, 1999, WB Saunders.
*22. Arnone M: Single and multiple pressure transducer system. In Lynn-McHale DJ, Carlson KK, editors: *AACN procedure manual for critical care,* ed 4, Philadelphia, 2001, WB Saunders.
*23. Imperial-Perez F, McRae M: Arterial pressure monitoring. In Chulay M, Gawlinski A, editors: *Protocols for practice: hemodynamic monitoring,* Aliso Viejo, Calif, 1998, AACN.

*Nursing research–based reference.

*24. Shaffer RB: Arterial catheter insertion (assist), care, and removal. In Lynn-McHale DJ, Carlson KK, editors: *AACN procedure manual for critical care,* ed 4, Philadelphia, 2001, WB Saunders.

*25. Becker DE: Arterial catheter insertion (perform). In Lynn-McHale DJ, Carlson KK, editors: *AACN procedure manual for critical care,* ed 4, Philadelphia, 2001, WB Saunders.

*26. Keckeisen M: Pulmonary artery pressure monitoring. In Chulay M, Gawlinski A, editors: *Protocols for practice: hemodynamic monitoring,* Aliso Viejo, Calif, 1998, AACN.

*27. Lynn-McHale DJ, Preuss T: Pulmonary artery catheter insertion (assist) and pressure monitoring. In Lynn-McHale DJ, Carlson KK, editors: *AACN procedure manual for critical care,* ed 4, Philadelphia, 2001, WB Saunders.

28. Bridges EJ: Monitoring pulmonary artery pressures: just the facts, *Crit Care Nurse* 20:59, 2000.

*29. Gould KA, Hartigan C, Keane SF: Cardiac output measurement techniques (invasive). In Lynn-McHale DJ, Carlson KK, editors: *AACN procedure manual for critical care,* ed 4, Philadelphia, 2001, WB Saunders.

*30. Von Rueden KT: Noninvasive hemodynamic monitoring: impedance cardiography. In Lynn-McHale DJ, Carlson KK, editors: *AACN procedure manual for critical care,* ed 4, Philadelphia, 2001, WB Saunders.

*31. Lynn-McHale DJ: Intra-aortic balloon pump management. In Lynn-McHale DJ, Carlson KK, editors: *AACN procedure manual for critical care,* ed 4, Philadelphia, 2001, WB Saunders.

32. Davidson J et al: Intra-aortic balloon pump: indications and complications, *J Natl Med Assoc* 90:137, 1998.

33. Busch T et al: Vascular complications related to intraaortic balloon counterpulsation: an analysis of ten years experience, *Thorac Cardiovasc Surg* 45:55, 1997.

*34. Ruess LA: Ventricular assist devices. In Lynn-McHale DJ, Carlson KK, editors: *AACN procedure manual for critical care,* ed 4, Philadelphia, 2001, Saunders.

35. Berger EE: Abiomed: AbioCor frequently asked questions. AbioCor clinical trial information. Available at *www.abiomed.com/abiocor/faq.html* (accessed Feb 26, 2002).

*36. Goodrich C: Performing endotracheal intubation. In Lynn-McHale DJ, Carlson KK, editors: *AACN procedure manual for critical care,* ed 4, Philadelphia, 2001, WB Saunders.

*37. Deutsch JM: Endotracheal tube care. In Lynn-McHale DJ, Carlson KK, editors: *AACN procedure manual for critical care,* ed 4, Philadelphia, 2001, WB Saunders.

*38. Deutsch JM: Assisting with endotracheal intubation. In Lynn-McHale DJ, Carlson KK, editors: *AACN procedure manual for critical care,* ed 4, Philadelphia, 2001, WB Saunders.

*39. Good VS: Continuous end tidal carbon dioxide monitoring. In Lynn-McHale DJ, Carlson KK, editors: *AACN procedure manual for critical care,* ed 4, Philadelphia, 2001, WB Saunders.

*40. Chulay M: Endotracheal or tracheostomy tube suctioning. In Lynn-McHale DJ, Carlson KK, editors: *AACN procedure manual for critical care,* ed 4, Philadelphia, 2001, WB Saunders.

*41. Minnick A, Leipzig RM, Johnson ME: Elderly patients' reports of physical restraint experiences in intensive care units, *Am J Crit Care* 10:168, 2001.

*42. Burns SM: Ventilatory management—volume and pressure modes. In Lynn-McHale DJ, Carlson KK, editors: *AACN procedure manual for critical care,* ed 4, Philadelphia, 2001, WB Saunders.

*43. Pierce LNB: Traditional and nontraditional modes of mechanical ventilation. In Chulay M, Burns SM, editors: *Protocols for practice: care of the mechanically ventilated patient,* Aliso Viejo, Calif, 1998, AACN.

44. Hynes-Gay P, MacDonald R: Using high-frequency oscillatory ventilation to treat adults with acute respiratory distress syndrome, *Crit Care Nurse* 21:38, 2001.

45. Schlicher ML: Using liquid ventilation to treat patients with acute respiratory distress syndrome: a guide to a breath of fresh liquid, *Crit Care Nurse* 21:55, 2001.

*46. Byers JF, Sole ML: Analysis of factors related to the development of ventilator-associated pneumonia: use of existing databases, *Am J Crit Care* 9:344, 2000.

*47. Hupcey JE: Feeling safe: the psychosocial needs of ICU patients, *J Nurs Scholarsh* 32:361, 2000.

48. Arbour R: Sedation and pain management in critically ill adults, *Crit Care Nurse* 21:39, 2000.

*49. Stamps DC: Enteral nutrition. In Lynn-McHale DJ, Carlson KK, editors: *AACN procedure manual for critical care,* ed 4, Philadelphia, 2001, WB Saunders.

*50. Burns SM: Weaning procedure. In Lynn-McHale DJ, Carlson KK, editors: *AACN procedure manual for critical care,* ed 4, Philadelphia, 2001, WB Saunders.

51. Henneman EA: Liberating patients from mechanical ventilation—a team approach, *Crit Care Nurse* 21:25, 2001.

*52. Burns SM: Standard weaning criteria: negative inspiratory pressure, positive expiratory pressure, spontaneous tidal volume, and vital capacity. In Lynn-McHale DJ, Carlson KK, editors: *AACN procedure manual for critical care,* ed 4, Philadelphia, 2001, WB Saunders.

*53. Greenlee KK: Performing extubation and decannulation. In Lynn-McHale DJ, Carlson KK, editors: *AACN procedure manual for critical care,* ed 4, Philadelphia, 2001, WB Saunders.

*54. Glass CA: Home care management of ventilator-assisted patients. In Chulay M, Burns SM, editors: *Protocols for practice: care of the mechanically ventilated patient,* Aliso Viejo, Calif, 1998, AACN.

55. Creechan T: Combining mechanical ventilation with hospice care in the home: death with dignity, *Crit Care Nurse* 20:49, 2000.

56. McNeal GJ: *AACN guide to acute care procedures in the home,* Philadelphia, 2000, Lippincott.

RESOURCES

American Association of Critical Care Nurses (AACN)
101 Columbia
Aliso Viejo, CA 92656-4109
800-899-2226 or 949-362-2000
Fax: 949-362-2020
www.aacn.org

Australian College of Critical Care Nurses
P.O. Box 219
South Carlton
Victoria, Australia 3053
www.acccn.com.au

Canadian Association of Critical Care Nurses (CACCN)
P.O. Box 25322
London, ON N6C 6B1
519-649-5284
Fax: 519-649-1458
www.caccn.ca

Society of Critical Care Medicine (SCCM)
701 Lee Street, Suite 200
Des Plaines, IL 60016
847-827-6869
Fax: 847-827-6886
www.sccm.org

For additional Internet resources, see the website for this book at *http://evolve.elsevier.com/Lewis/medsurg/.*

CHAPTER 65

NURSING MANAGEMENT
Shock and Multiple Organ Dysfunction Syndrome

JoAnne K. Phillips

LEARNING OBJECTIVES

1. Define *shock.*
2. Differentiate the two major classifications of shock: low blood flow and maldistribution of blood flow.
3. Describe the pathophysiology and clinical manifestations of shock.
4. Compare and contrast the effects of sepsis, systemic inflammatory response syndrome, shock, and multiple organ dysfunction syndrome on the major body systems.
5. Compare the collaborative care, drug therapy, and nursing management of patients with different types of shock.
6. Describe the nursing management of a patient experiencing multiple organ dysfunction syndrome.

KEY TERMS

absolute hypovolemia, p. 1798	relative hypovolemia, p. 1798
anaphylactic shock, p. 1802	sepsis, p. 1802
cardiogenic shock, p. 1796	septic shock, p. 1802
hypovolemic shock, p. 1798	shock, p. 1796
multiple organ dysfunction syndrome, p. 1819	systemic inflammatory response syndrome, p. 1818
neurogenic shock, p. 1801	

Shock, systemic inflammatory response syndrome (SIRS), and multiple organ dysfunction syndrome (MODS) are serious and interrelated problems. Fig. 65-1 shows the relationship among shock, SIRS, and MODS. Shock is a complex process that often leads to the development of SIRS and MODS. This chapter provides an overview of shock, SIRS, and MODS.

SHOCK

Shock is a syndrome characterized by decreased tissue perfusion and impaired cellular metabolism. This results in an imbalance between the supply of and demand for oxygen and nutrients. The exchange of oxygen and nutrients at the cellular level is essential to life. When a cell experiences a state of hypoperfusion, the demand for oxygen and nutrients exceeds the supply.

Classification of Shock

Although the cause and initial presentation of various types of shock differ, the physiologic responses of the cell to hypoperfusion are similar. In addition, the management strategies for each type of shock vary widely. For the purposes of discussion, shock will be classified as *low blood flow* (cardiogenic and hypovolemic shock) or *maldistribution of blood flow* (septic, anaphylactic, and neurogenic shock)[1,2] (Table 65-1).

Reviewed by Joseph J. Napolitano, RN, MPH, MSN, APRN, Program Officer, Dorothy Rider Pool Health Care Trust, Allentown, Pa.

Low Blood Flow Shock

Cardiogenic shock. **Cardiogenic shock** occurs when either systolic or diastolic dysfunction of the myocardium results in compromised cardiac output. The heart's inability to pump the blood forward is classified as *systolic dysfunction.* Systolic dysfunction primarily affects the left ventricle, because systolic pressure and tension are greater on the left side of the heart. When systolic dysfunction affects the right side of the heart, blood flow through the pulmonary circulation is compromised. Precipitating causes of systolic dysfunction include myocardial infarction (MI), cardiomyopathies, severe systemic or pulmonary hypertension, blunt cardiac injury, and myocardial depression from sepsis. From 5% to 10% of patients who experience an acute MI will develop cardiogenic shock, most within 48 hours of the initial insult.[3]

Diastolic dysfunction is an impaired ability of the right or left ventricle to fill during diastole. Decreased filling of the ventricle will result in decreased stroke volume (amount of blood ejected from the heart with each contraction).

Fig. 65-2 describes the pathophysiology of cardiogenic shock. Whether the initiating event is an MI, a structural problem (e.g., valvular abnormality, papillary muscle dysfunction, acute ventricular septal defect), or arrhythmias, the physiologic responses are similar. The patient experiences impaired tissue perfusion and impaired cellular metabolism as a result of cardiogenic shock.[4]

The early clinical presentation of a patient with cardiogenic shock is similar to that of a patient with acute heart failure (see Chapter 34). The patient will have tachycardia, hypotension, and a narrowed pulse pressure. An increase in systemic vascular resistance (SVR) increases the workload of the heart, thus increasing the myocardial oxygen consumption.[5] The heart's inability to pump blood forward will result in a low cardiac index (less than 2.1 L/min/m²). On examination, the patient will be tachypneic and pulmonary congestion will be evident by the presence of crackles. The hemodynamic profile will demonstrate an increase in the pulmonary artery wedge pressure (PAWP) and pulmonary

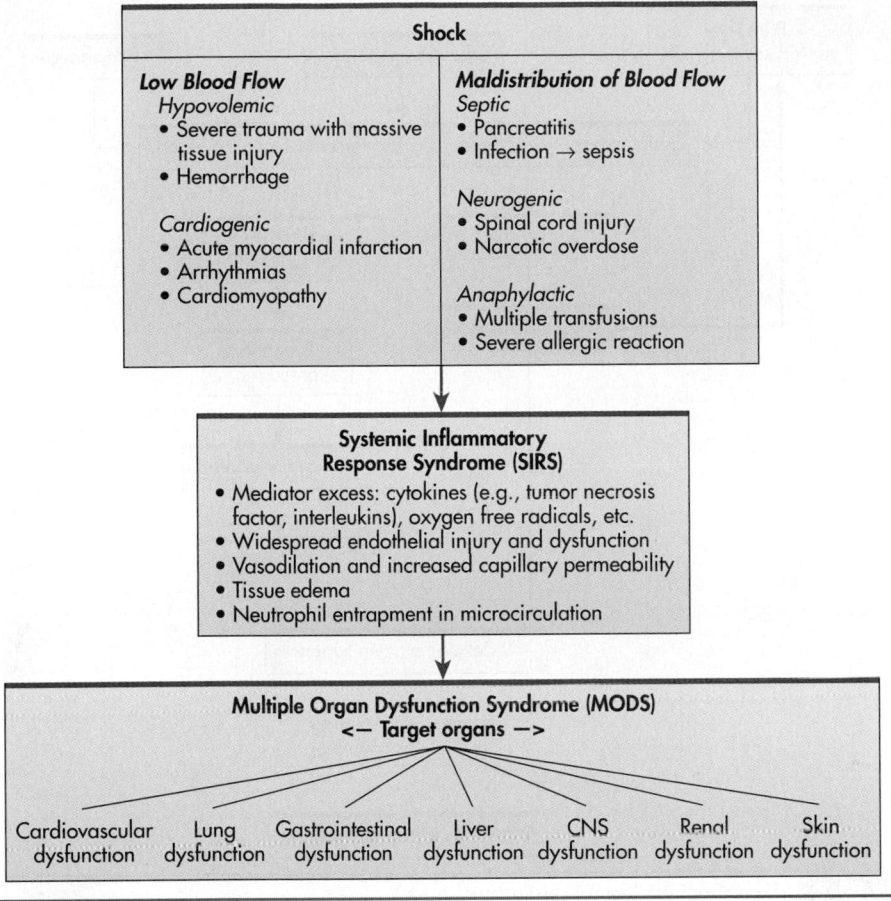

FIG. 65-1 Relationship of shock, systemic inflammatory response syndrome, and multiple organ dysfunction syndrome. *CNS,* Central nervous system.

TABLE 65-1	**Classification and Precipitating Factors of Shock**

LOW BLOOD FLOW	MALDISTRIBUTION OF BLOOD FLOW
Cardiogenic Shock • Systolic dysfunction: inability of the heart to pump blood forward (e.g., myocardial infarction, cardiomyopathy) • Diastolic dysfunction: inability of the heart to fill during diastole (e.g., cardiac tamponade) • Arrhythmias (e.g., bradycardia, tachycardia) • Structural factors: valvular abnormality (e.g., stenosis or regurgitation), papillary muscle dysfunction, acute ventricular septal defect **Hypovolemic Shock** **Absolute hypovolemia** • Loss of whole blood (e.g., hemorrhage from trauma, surgery, GI bleeding) • Loss of plasma (e.g., burn injuries) • Loss of other body fluids (e.g., vomiting, diarrhea, excessive diuresis, diaphoresis, diabetes insipidus, diabetes mellitus) **Relative hypovolemia** • Pooling of blood or fluids (e.g., ascites, peritonitis, bowel obstruction) • Internal bleeding (e.g., fracture of long bones, ruptured spleen, hemothorax, severe pancreatitis) • Massive vasodilation (e.g., sepsis)	**Neurogenic Shock** • Hemodynamic consequence of injury and/or disease to the spinal cord at or above T5 • Spinal anesthesia • Vasomotor center depression (e.g., severe pain, drugs, hypoglycemia, injury) **Septic Shock** • Infection (e.g., urinary tract, respiratory tract, invasive procedure, indwelling lines and catheters) • At risk patients: older adults, patients with chronic diseases (e.g., diabetes mellitus, chronic renal failure, congestive heart failure), patients receiving immunosuppressive therapy or who are malnourished or debilitated • Gram-negative bacteria most common; also gram-positive bacteria, viruses, fungi, and parasites **Anaphylactic Shock** • Contrast media, blood/blood products, drugs, insect bites, anesthetic agents, food/food additives, vaccines, environmental agents, latex

GI, Gastrointestinal.

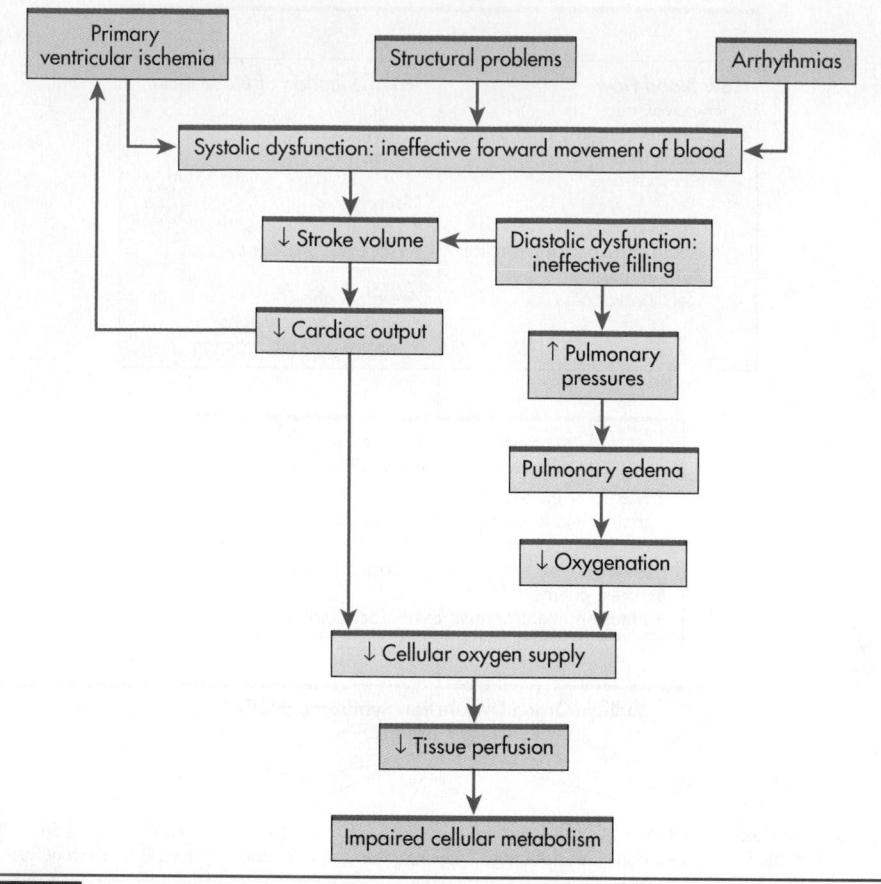

FIG. 65-2 The pathophysiology of cardiogenic shock.

TABLE 65-2 Effects of Shock, Systemic Inflammatory Response Syndrome, and Multiple Organ Dysfunction Syndrome on Hemodynamic Parameters

TYPE	HR	PULSE PRESSURE	BP	SVR	PVR	CVP	PAP	PAWP	CO	SvO$_2$
Cardiogenic shock	↑	↓	↓	↑	↑	≈↑	↑	↑	↓	↓
Hypovolemic shock	↑	↓	↓	↑	↑	↓	↓	↓	↓	↓
Anaphylactic shock	↑	↓	↓	↓	≈↑	↓	↓	↓	↓	↓
Neurogenic shock	↓	↓	↓	↓	≈	↓	↓	↓	↓	↓
Septic shock	↑	↓	↓	↓	≈↑	↓	↑≈↓	↓	↑	↑≈↓
SIRS	↑	≈	≈	↓	≈↑	↓	↑≈↓	↓	↑	↑≈↓
MODS	↑	≈	≈	↓	↑	↓	↑≈↓	↓≈↑	↓	↑

NOTE: Hemodynamic effects in some illnesses are highly variable. The hemodynamic findings in MODS depend on the system failing.
KEY: ↓, decrease; ↑, increase; ≈, no change.
BP, Blood pressure; *CO*, cardiac output; *CVP*, central venous pressure; *HR*, heart rate; *MODS*, multiple organ dysfunction syndrome; *PAP*, pulmonary artery pressure; *PAWP*, pulmonary artery wedge pressure; *PVR*, pulmonary vascular resistance; *SIRS*, systemic inflammatory response syndrome; *SvO$_2$*, mixed venous oxygen saturation; *SVR*, systemic vascular resistance.

vascular resistance (Table 65-2). Signs of peripheral hypoperfusion (e.g., cyanosis, pallor, cool and clammy skin, decreased capillary refill time) will be apparent. Decreased renal blood flow will result in sodium and water retention and decreased urine output. Anxiety and delirium may develop as cerebral perfusion is impaired. Studies that may be helpful in diagnosing cardiogenic shock include laboratory studies (e.g., cardiac enzymes, troponin levels) (Table 65-3), electrocardiogram (ECG), chest x-ray, and echocardiogram. The overall clinical presentation of a patient with cardiogenic shock is presented in Table 65-4.

Hypovolemic shock. The second type of low blood flow shock is hypovolemic shock. **Hypovolemic shock** occurs when there is a loss of intravascular fluid volume. In hypovolemic shock, the volume is inadequate to fill the vascular space. The volume loss may be either an absolute or relative volume loss. **Absolute hypovolemia** results when fluid is lost through hemorrhage, gastrointestinal (GI) loss (e.g., vomiting, diarrhea), fistula drainage, diabetes insipidus, or diuresis. In **relative hypovolemia,** fluid volume moves out of the vascular space into extravascular space (e.g., interstitial or intracavitary space). This type of

TABLE
65-3
Diagnostic Studies
Laboratory Abnormalities in Shock

LABORATORY STUDY	FINDING	SIGNIFICANCE OF FINDING
Blood		
Red blood cell count, hematocrit, hemoglobin	Normal	▪ Remains within normal limits in shock because of relative hypovolemia and pump failure and in hemorrhagic shock before fluid restoration
	Decreased	▪ Decreases in hemorrhagic shock after fluid resuscitation when fluids other than blood are used
	Increased	▪ Increases in nonhemorrhagic shock due to actual hypovolemia because fluid lost does not contain erythrocytes
DIC screen		
Fibrin split products (FSP)	Increased	▪ Acute DIC can develop within hours to days after an initial assault on the body (e.g., shock)
Fibrinogen level	Decreased	
Platelet count	Decreased	
PTT and PT	Prolonged	
Thrombin time	Increased	
D–Dimer	Increased	
Creatine kinase	Increased	▪ Increases in trauma, myocardial infarction in response to cellular damage and/or hypoxia
Troponin	Increased	▪ Increases in myocardial infarction
BUN	Increased	▪ Indicates impaired kidney function due to hypoperfusion as a result of severe vasoconstriction or occurs secondary to catabolism of cells (e.g., trauma, infection)
Creatinine	Increased	▪ Indicates impaired kidney function due to hypoperfusion as a result of severe vasoconstriction; is more sensitive indicator of renal function than BUN
Glucose	Increased	▪ Found in early shock because of release of liver glycogen stores in response to sympathetic nervous system stimulation and cortisol; insulin insensitivity develops
	Decreased	▪ Occurs because of depleted glycogen stores with hepatocellular dysfunction possible as shock progresses
Serum electrolytes		
Sodium	Increased	▪ Found in early shock because of increased secretion of aldosterone, causing renal retention of sodium
	Decreased	▪ May occur iatrogenically when excess hypotonic fluid is administered after fluid loss
Potassium	Increased	▪ Results when cellular death liberates intracellular potassium; also occurs in acute renal failure and in the presence of acidosis
	Decreased	▪ Found in early shock because of increased secretion of aldosterone, causing renal excretion of potassium
Arterial blood gases	Respiratory alkalosis	▪ Found in early shock secondary to hyperventilation
	Metabolic acidosis	▪ Occurs later in shock when organic acids, such as lactic acid, accumulate in blood from anaerobic metabolism
Base deficit	>−6	▪ Indicates acid production secondary to hypoxia
Blood cultures	Growth of organisms	▪ May grow organisms in patients who are in septic shock
Lactate	Increased	▪ Usually increases once significant hypoperfusion and impaired oxygen utilization at the cellular level have occurred; by-product of anaerobic metabolism
Liver enzymes (ALT, AST, GGT)	Increased	▪ Elevations indicate liver cell destruction in progressive stage of shock
Urine		
Specific gravity	Increased	▪ Occurs secondary to the action of ADH
	Fixed at 1.010	▪ Occurs in renal failure

ADH, Antidiuretic hormone; *ALT,* alanine aminotransferase; *AST,* aspartate aminotransferase; *BUN,* blood urea nitrogen; *DIC,* disseminated intravascular coagulation; *GGT,* gamma–glutamyl transferase; *PT,* prothrombin time; *PTT,* partial thromboplastin time.

TABLE 65-4   Clinical Presentation of the Major Types of Shock

	CARDIOGENIC SHOCK	HYPOVOLEMIC SHOCK	NEUROGENIC SHOCK	ANAPHYLACTIC SHOCK	SEPTIC SHOCK
Cardiovascular (see Table 65-2 for hemodynamic profile)	↓ Capillary refill time ↑ MVO$_2$ Cardiac index <2.1 L/min/m^2 PAWP >20 mm Hg Chest pain may or may not be present	↓ Preload ↓ Stroke volume ↓ Capillary refill time	↓/↑ Temperature	Chest pain Third spacing of fluid	**Early** ↓/↑ Temperature ↑ HR ↓ SVR, ↑ CO ↓ BP Biventricular dilation: ↓ ejection fraction ↑ SvO$_2$ **Late** ↓/↑ Temperature ↓ CO/↑ SVR ↓ SvO$_2$
Pulmonary	Tachypnea Cyanosis Crackles Rhonchi	Tachypnea → bradypnea (late)	Dysfunction related to level of injury	Swelling of lips and tongue Shortness of breath Edema of larynx and epiglottis Wheezing Rhinitis Stridor	Hyperventilation Respiratory alkalosis → respiratory acidosis Hypoxemia Respiratory failure ARDS Pulmonary hypertension Crackles ↓ Urine output
Renal	↑ Na$^+$ and H$_2$O retention ↓ Renal blood flow ↓ Urine output	↓ Urine output			
Skin	Pallor Cool, clammy	Pallor Cool, clammy	↓ Skin perfusion Cool or warm Dry	Flushing Pruritus Urticaria Angioedema	**Early** Warm and flushed **Late** Cool and mottled
Neurologic	↓ Cerebral perfusion: anxiety, confusion, agitation	Anxiety Confusion Agitation	Flaccid paralysis below the level of the lesion Loss of reflex activity, bowel and bladder function	Anxiety Feeling of impending doom Confusion ↓ LOC Metallic taste	**Early** Alteration in mental status Agitation **Late** Coma
Gastrointestinal	↓ Bowel sounds Nausea/vomiting	Absent bowel sounds		Cramping Abdominal pain Nausea Vomiting Diarrhea	GI bleeding Paralytic ileus
Diagnostic findings (also see Table 65-3)	↑ Cardiac markers ↑ Blood glucose ↑ BUN ECG (e.g., arrhythmias) Echocardiogram (e.g., left ventricular dysfunction) Chest x-ray (e.g., pulmonary infiltrates)	↓ Hematocrit ↑ Lactate ↑ Urine specific gravity Changes in electrolytes		Sudden onset History of allergies Exposure to contrast media	↑/↓ WBC ↓ Platelets ↑ Lactate ↑ Urine specific gravity ↓ Urine Na$^+$ Positive blood cultures

BP, Blood pressure; *BUN*, blood urea nitrogen; *ECG*, electrocardiogram; *GI*, gastrointestinal; *LOC*, level of consciousness; *MVO$_2$*, myocardial oxygen consumption; *PAWP*, pulmonary artery wedge pressure; *SvO$_2$*, mixed venous oxygen saturation; *SVR*, systemic vascular resistance; *WBC*, white blood cell.

fluid shift is called *third spacing*. One example of relative volume loss is leakage of fluid from the vascular space to the interstitial space from increased capillary permeability, as seen in sepsis. Other examples include sequestration of fluid into the colon from a bowel obstruction, loss of blood volume into a fracture site (e.g., pelvic fracture), burns (Chapter 24), and ascites (see Table 65-1).

In hypovolemic shock, the size of the vascular compartment remains unchanged while the volume of blood or plasma decreases. Whether the loss of intravascular volume is absolute or relative, the physiologic consequences are similar. A reduction in intravascular volume results in a decreased venous return to the heart, decreased preload, decreased stroke volume, and decreased cardiac output (see Table 65-2). A cascade of events results in decreased tissue perfusion and impaired cellular metabolism, the hallmarks of shock (Fig. 65-3).

The patient's response to acute volume loss is dependent on a number of factors, including extent of injury or insult, age, and general state of health (see Table 65-4). An overall assessment of physiologic reserve may indicate the patient's ability to compensate. A healthy young adult can compensate for a sudden loss of up to 15% of the total blood volume (or approximately 750 ml out of the average 5 L total blood volume in a 70 kg person).[6] Further loss of volume (15% to 30%) will result in a sympathetic nervous system (SNS)–mediated response. This response results in an increase in heart rate, cardiac output, and respiratory rate and depth. The stroke volume and PAWP are decreased because of the decreased circulating blood volume. The patient may appear anxious and urine output will begin to decrease. If hypovolemia is corrected at this time, tissue dysfunction is generally reversible. If volume loss is greater than 30%, blood volume must be replaced aggressively with blood or blood products, as the compensatory mechanisms become overwhelmed. Loss of more than 40% of the total blood volume is characterized by loss of autoregulation in the microcirculation and results in irreversible tissue destruction.[7,8] Laboratory studies that may be done include measurements of serial hemoglobin and hematocrit levels, urine specific gravity, serum electrolytes, and lactic acid (see Table 65-3).

Maldistribution of Blood Flow Shock

Neurogenic shock. Neurogenic shock is a hemodynamic phenomenon that occurs after a spinal cord injury at the fifth thoracic (T5) vertebra or above.[9] The injury results in a massive vasodilation without compensation as a consequence of the loss of SNS vasoconstrictor tone. This massive vasodilation leads to a pooling of blood in the blood vessels. The most important clinical manifestations are hypotension (from the massive vasodilation) and bradycardia. The unopposed activation of the parasympathetic nervous system leads to bradycardia.

The patient in neurogenic shock also characteristically has hypothalamic dysfunction, which may result in temperature dysregulation. The patient will often have *poikilothermia* (taking on the temperature of the environment), which, combined with massive vasodilation, promotes heat loss, often resulting in hypothermia. With poikilothermia, the skin could be cool or warm depending on the ambient temperature. In either case, the skin will usually be dry. Initially, the skin will be warm due to the massive dilation without compensation. As the heat dissipates, the skin loses heat and the patient is at risk for hypothermia.

The pathophysiology of neurogenic shock is described in Fig. 65-4. Hypoperfusion associated with neurogenic shock also results in impaired tissue perfusion. Onset of neurogenic shock

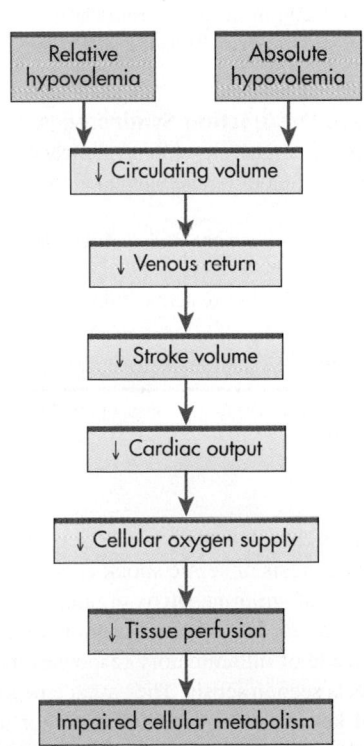

FIG. 65-3 The pathophysiology of hypovolemic shock.

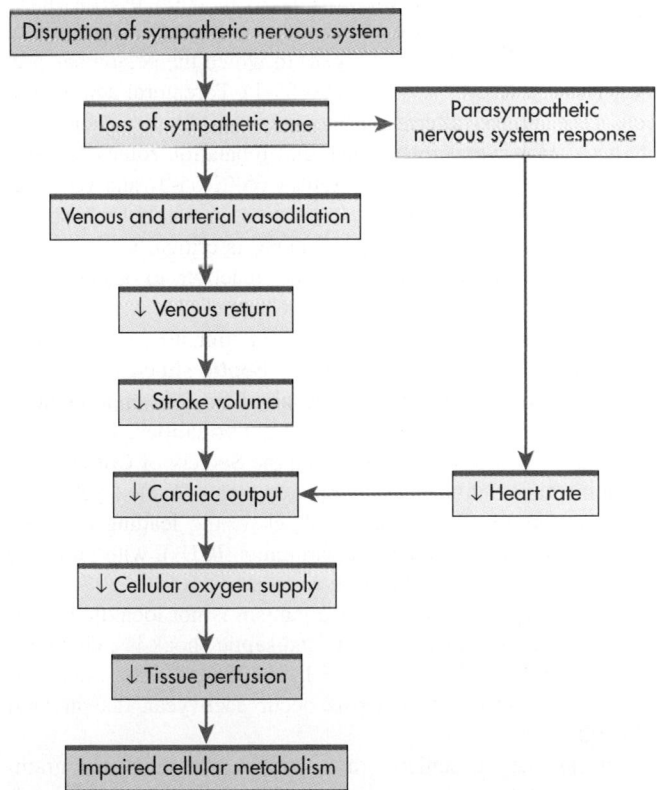

FIG. 65-4 The pathophysiology of neurogenic shock.

can begin as soon as 30 minutes after the injury, and may last from days to weeks following spinal cord injury.

Table 65-1 lists the causes of neurogenic shock. In addition to spinal cord injury, spinal anesthesia can also block transmission of impulses from the SNS. Depression of the vasomotor center of the medulla as a result of drugs (e.g., benzodiazepines, narcotics) can also result in decreased vasoconstrictor tone of the peripheral blood vessels, resulting in neurogenic shock. Tables 65-2, 65-3, and 65-4 further describe the clinical presentation of a patient with neurogenic shock.

Although spinal shock and neurogenic shock often occur in the same patient, they are not the same disorder. *Spinal shock* is a phenomenon that is present after an acute spinal cord injury (see Chapter 59). The patient with spinal shock will experience the absence of all voluntary and reflex neurologic activity below the level of the injury.[9]

Anaphylactic shock. **Anaphylactic shock** is an acute and life-threatening hypersensitivity (allergic) reaction to a sensitizing substance (e.g., drug, chemical, vaccine, food, or insect venom). It is an immediate reaction that causes massive vasodilation, release of vasoactive mediators, and an increase in capillary permeability. As capillary permeability increases, fluid leaks from the vascular space into the interstitial space. Anaphylactic shock can lead to respiratory distress, as a result of laryngeal edema or severe bronchospasm, and circulatory failure, as a result of massive vasodilation.[10] The patient experiences a sudden onset of symptoms, including hypotension, chest pain, swelling of the lips and tongue, wheezing, and stridor. Skin changes include flushing, pruritus, urticaria, and angioedema. In addition, the patient may feel an impending sense of doom and become very anxious and confused.

A patient can develop a severe allergic reaction, possibly leading to anaphylactic shock, after contact, inhalation, ingestion, or injection with an antigen (allergen) to which the person has previously been sensitized (see Table 65-1). Parenteral administration of the antigen (allergen) is the route most likely to cause anaphylaxis. However, oral, topical, and inhalation routes can also cause anaphylactic reactions. Tables 65-2, 65-3, and 65-4 describe the clinical presentation of a patient in anaphylactic shock. Quick and decisive action by the nurse is critical to preventing the progression of an anaphylactic reaction to anaphylactic shock. (Anaphylaxis is discussed in Chapter 13.)

Septic shock. **Sepsis** is a systemic inflammatory response to a documented or suspected infection.[11] **Septic shock** is the presence of sepsis with hypotension despite fluid resuscitation along with the presence of tissue perfusion abnormalities. The American College of Chest Physicians and the Society of Critical Care Medicine have defined a continuum of sepsis (Table 65-5).

Sepsis progressing to septic shock is the leading cause of death in noncoronary intensive care units (ICUs), with mortality rates as high as 40% to 60%. In as many as 10% to 30% of patients with sepsis, the causative organism is not identified. Thus managing the patient with sepsis and septic shock is a challenge for the entire health care team.[12] In the United States, approximately 750,000 cases of sepsis occur each year, and at least 225,000 are fatal.

The primary organisms that cause septic shock are gramnegative and gram-positive bacteria. The morbidity and mortality rates from infections with gram-negative organisms are greater than those from gram-positive organisms.[12] Parasites,

---

TABLE 65-5	Definitions of Sepsis, Severe Sepsis, Septic Shock, and Multiple Organ Dysfunction Syndrome*

Infection
- Disease caused by an invasion of the body by pathogenic organisms

Bacteremia
- Presence of viable bacteria in the blood; demonstrated by positive blood cultures

Systemic Inflammatory Response Syndrome (SIRS)
- Systemic inflammatory response to a variety of insults, including infection, ischemia, infarct, injury; manifested by two or more of the following:
  1. Temperature >100.4° F (38° C) or <97.0° F (36° C)
  2. Heart rate >90 beats/min
  3. Respiratory rate >20 breaths/min or $PaCO_2$ <32 mm Hg
  4. White blood cell count >12,000 cells/μl or <4000 cells/μl or >10% immature neutrophils (bands)

Sepsis
- A systemic inflammatory response to a documented or suspected infection

Severe Sepsis
- Sepsis associated with organ dysfunction, hypoperfusion, or hypotension

Septic Shock
- Sepsis with hypotension despite adequate fluid resuscitation along with the presence of tissue perfusion abnormalities (e.g., lactic acidosis, oliguria, alteration in mental status)

Hypotension
- A systolic BP of <90 mm Hg or a reduction of >40 mm Hg from baseline and in which BP is not adequate for normal perfusion

Multiple Organ Dysfunction Syndrome (MODS)
- Failure of more than one organ in an acutely ill patient such that homeostasis cannot be maintained without intervention

Primary MODS
- Occurs early and results from well-defined illness or injury

Secondary MODS
- Results from uncontrolled systemic inflammation with resultant organ dysfunction
- Develops latently after several insults

*These definitions are from the American College of Chest Physicians and Society of Critical Care Medicine.
BP, Blood pressure.

---

fungi, and viruses can also lead to the development of septic shock. The pathogenesis of septic shock is complex (Fig. 65-5).

The cell walls of gram-negative organisms contain a substance called *endotoxin.* The release of endotoxin into circulation stimulates a cascade of inflammatory responses that produce the detrimental effects seen in sepsis. The cascade begins with the release of several key mediators, including tumor necrosis factor (TNF) and interleukin 1 (IL-1). These mediators stimulate the release of other inflammatory mediators, such as platelet activating factor, thromboxanes, leukotrienes, prostaglandins, and inter-

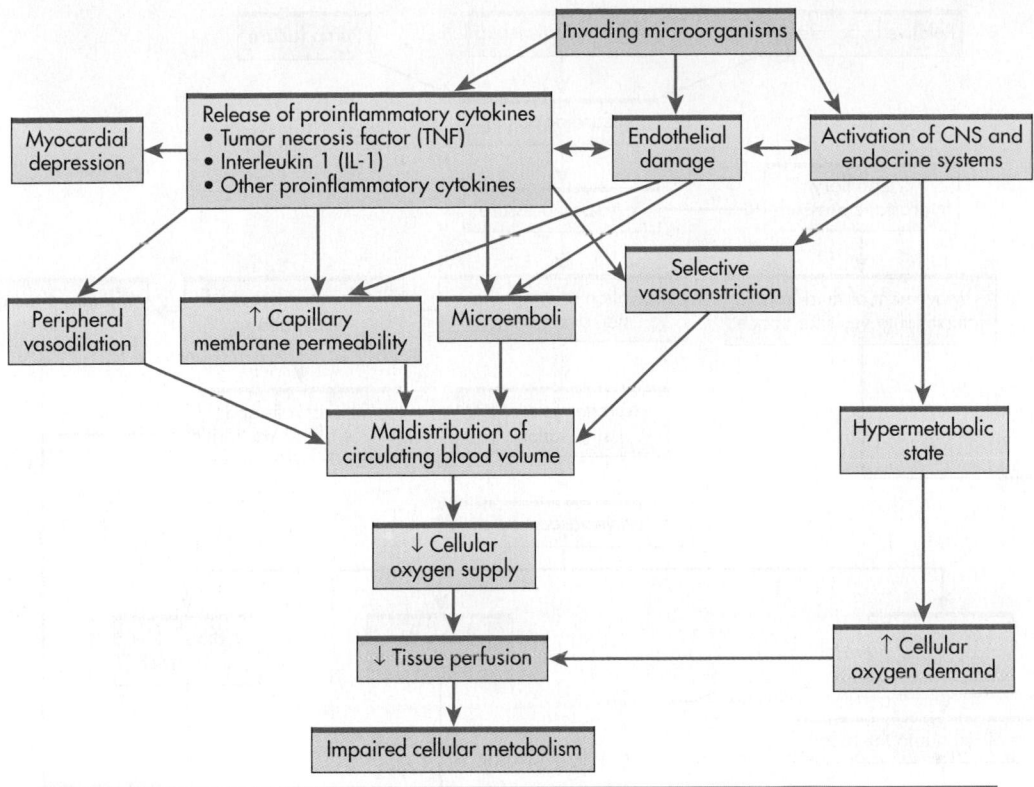

FIG. 65-5   The pathophysiology of septic shock. *CNS,* Central nervous system.

leukin 6 (IL-6) and interleukin 8 (IL-8).[13] (See Chapters 12 and 13 for discussion of the inflammatory response.) The combined effects of the mediators result in damage to the endothelium, vasodilation, increased capillary permeability, and neutrophil and platelet aggregation and adhesion to the endothelium.

In septic shock there is an increase in coagulation and inflammation and a decrease in fibrinolysis. The release of platelet activating factor results in the formation of microthrombi and obstruction of the microvasculature.

The clinical presentation of sepsis includes decreased SVR with a compensatory increase in cardiac output, hypotension, tachypnea, and temperature dysregulation (high or low). Tables 65-2 and 65-4 further delineate the clinical presentation of a patient with septic shock.

The combination of TNF and IL-1 is thought to have a role in sepsis-induced myocardial dysfunction. The ejection fraction is decreased for the first few days after the initial insult. Because of a decreased ejection fraction, the ventricles will dilate in order to maintain the stroke volume. The ejection fraction typically improves and the ventricular dilation resolves over 7 to 10 days. Persistence of a high cardiac output and a low SVR beyond 24 hours is an ominous finding and is often associated with an increased development of hypotension and MODS. Coronary perfusion and myocardial oxygen metabolism are normal in septic shock.[13]

In addition to the cardiovascular dysfunction that accompanies sepsis, respiratory failure is common. The patient will initially hyperventilate as a compensatory mechanism, resulting in respiratory alkalosis. Once the patient can no longer compensate, respiratory acidosis will develop. Respiratory failure will develop in 85% of patients with sepsis, and 40% will develop acute respiratory distress syndrome (ARDS). Other clinical signs of septic shock include decreased urine output, alteration in neuro-

logic status, and GI dysfunction, such as GI bleeding and paralytic ileus (see Table 65-4).

Stages of Shock

In addition to understanding the underlying pathogenesis of the type of shock the patient is experiencing, monitoring and management are also guided by knowing where the patient is on the shock "continuum." This continuum begins with the initial stage of shock, followed by the compensatory and progressive stages. If tissue perfusion is not restored, and the progression of the shock is not halted, the patient will deteriorate to the refractory (final) stage of shock, from which recovery is unlikely. Although there are no clear cut divisions between the stages, they provide a framework for discussing shock.

Initial Stage. The *initial stage* of shock may not be clinically apparent. The patient will have no outward signs of decreased tissue perfusion despite the fact that the body begins to respond to the imbalance of oxygen supply and demand at the cellular level. Metabolism changes from aerobic to anaerobic, and as a result, lactic acid, which is harmful to cells, begins to accumulate as a waste product. The lactic acid must be removed by the blood and broken down by the liver. This process also requires oxygen, which is unavailable at the cellular level in shock.[14]

Compensatory Stage. The next stage of shock is the *compensatory stage*. In this stage, the body activates several compensatory mechanisms in an attempt to overcome the increasing consequences of anaerobic metabolism and to maintain homeostasis (Fig. 65-6). There are neural, hormonal, and biochemical compensatory mechanisms. The patient's clinical presentation begins to reflect the body's responses to the imbalance in oxygen supply and demand (Table 65-6).

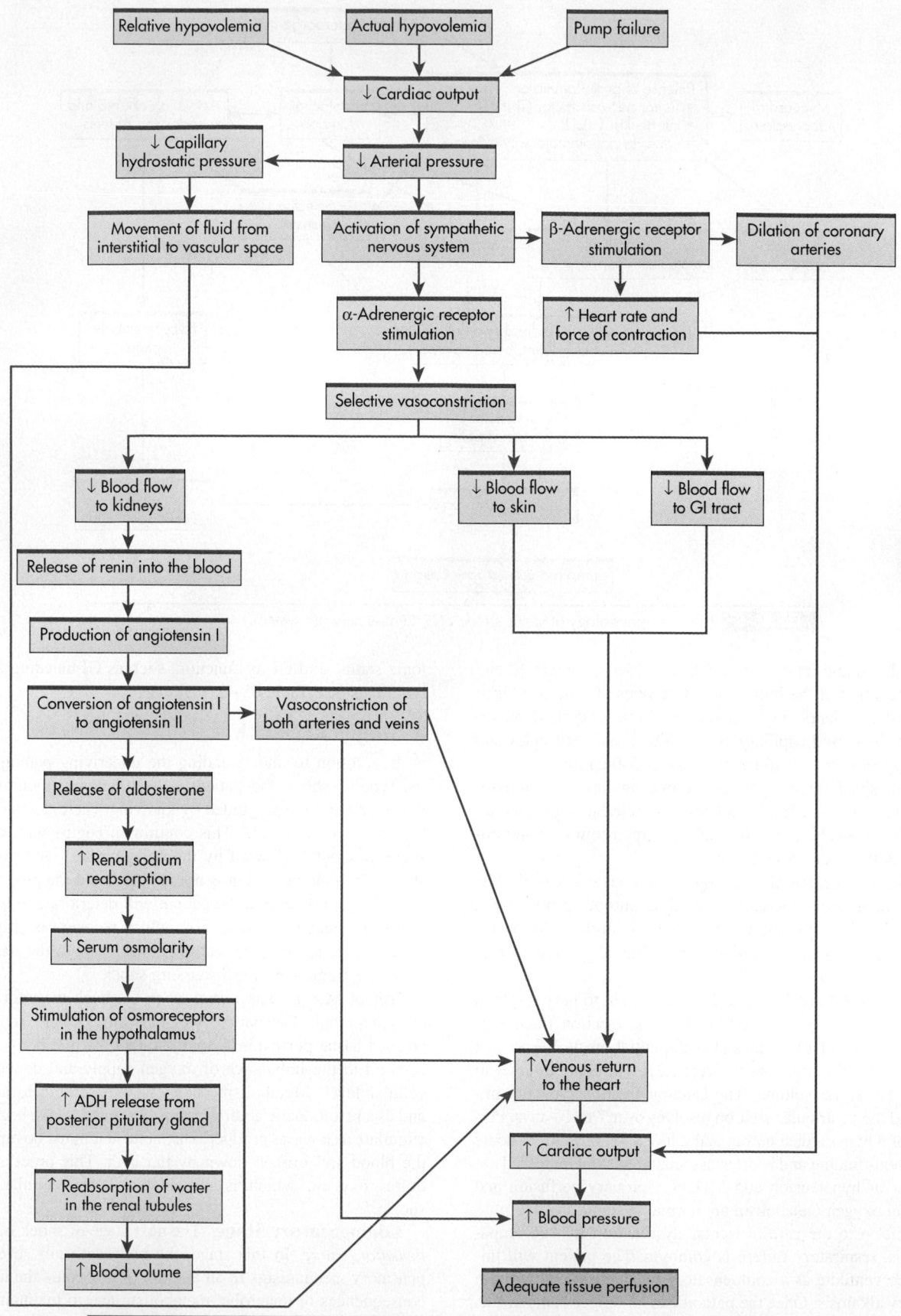

FIG. 65-6 Compensated stage: reversible stage during which compensatory mechanisms are effective and homeostasis is maintained.

TABLE 65-6	Clinical Manifestations of the Stages of Shock		
SYSTEM	**COMPENSATORY STAGE**	**PROGRESSIVE STAGE**	**REFRACTORY STAGE**
Neurologic	Oriented to person, place, time Restless, agitated, apprehensive Change in level of consciousness	↓ Cerebral perfusion pressure ↓ Cerebral blood flow Listless or agitated ↓ Responsiveness to stimuli	Unresponsive Areflexia (loss of reflexes) Pupils unreactive and dilated
Cardiovascular	Sympathetic nervous system response: Release of epinephrine/norepinephrine, which promotes vasoconstriction ↑ MVO_2 ↑ Contractility ↑ HR Coronary artery dilation BP adequate to perfuse vital organs (heart, brain)	Loss of autoregulation in microcirculation ↑ Capillary permeability → systemic interstitial edema ↓ Cardiac output → ↓ BP and ↑ HR MAP <60 mm Hg (or 40 mm Hg drop in BP from baseline) ↓ Coronary perfusion → • Arrhythmias • Myocardial ischemia • Myocardial infarction • Myocardial dysfunction → impaired cardiac output ↓ Peripheral perfusion → ischemia of distal extremities, diminished pulses, ↓ Capillary refill	Profound hypotension ↓ Cardiac output Bradycardia; irregular rhythm ↓ BP inadequate to perfuse vital organs
Respiratory	↓ Blood flow to the lungs • ↑ Physiologic dead space • ↑ Ventilation-perfusion mismatch • Hyperventilation • ↑ Minute ventilation (VE)	Noncardiogenic pulmonary edema (ARDS) • ↑ Capillary permeability • Pulmonary vasoconstriction • Pulmonary interstitial edema • Alveolar edema • Diffuse infiltrates • ↑ Respiratory rate • ↓ Compliance Moist crackles	Severe refractory hypoxemia Respiratory failure
Gastrointestinal	↓ Blood supply Hypoactive bowel sounds	Vasoconstriction and ↓ perfusion → ischemic gut (e.g., stomach, small and large intestines, gall bladder, pancreas) • Erosive ulcers • GI bleeding • Translocation of GI bacteria • Impaired absorption of nutrients	Ischemic gut
Renal	↓ Renal blood flow ↑ Renin resulting in release of angiotensin (vasoconstrictor) ↑ Aldosterone resulting in Na^+ and H_2O reabsorption ↑ Antidiuretic hormone resulting in H_2O reabsorption	Renal tubules become ischemic → acute tubular necrosis ↓ Urine output ↑ BUN/creatinine ratio ↑ Urine sodium ↓ Urine osmolarity and specific gravity ↓ Urine potassium Metabolic acidosis	Anuria
Hepatic		Failure to metabolize drugs and waste products Jaundice (decreased clearance of bilirubin) ↑ NH_3 and lactate	Metabolic changes from accumulation of waste products (e.g., NH_3, lactate, CO_2)
Hematologic		DIC • Thrombin clots in microcirculation • Consumption of clots in microcirculation	DIC
Temperature	Normal or abnormal	Hypothermia Sepsis: hypothermia or hyperthermia	Hypothermia
Skin	Pale and cool Warm and flushed (early stage of septic shock)	Cold and clammy	Mottled, cyanotic
Key Laboratory Findings	↑ Blood glucose ↑ pH ↓ PaO_2 ↓ $PaCO_2$	↑ Liver enzymes: ALT, AST, GGT ↑ Bleeding times Thrombocytopenia	↓ Blood glucose ↑ NH_3, lactate, and K^+ Metabolic acidosis

ALT, Alanine aminotransferase; *ARDS,* acute respiratory distress syndrome; *AST,* aspartate aminotransferase; *BUN,* Blood urea nitrogen; *DIC,* disseminated intravascular coagulation; *GGT,* gamma-glutamyl transferase; *GI,* gastrointestinal; *HR,* heart rate; *MAP,* mean arterial pressure; *MVO₂,* myocardial oxygen consumption.

One of the first clinical signs of shock may be a fall in BP, which occurs as a result of a decrease in cardiac output. The baroreceptors in the carotid and aortic bodies immediately respond by activating the SNS. The SNS stimulates vasoconstriction and the release of epinephrine and norepinephrine, both of which are potent vasoconstrictors. Blood flow to the most essential (vital) organs, the heart and the brain, is maintained, while blood flow to the nonvital organs, such as the kidneys, GI tract, skin, and lungs, is diverted or shunted.

Decreased blood flow to the kidneys activates the renin-angiotensin system. Renin is released, which activates angiotensinogen to produce angiotensin I, which is then converted to angiotensin II (see Chapter 43, Fig. 43-4). Angiotensin II is a potent vasoconstrictor, which causes both arterial and venous vasoconstriction. The net result is an increase in venous return to the heart and an increase in blood pressure. Angiotensin II also stimulates the adrenal cortex to release aldosterone, which results in sodium that water reabsorption and potassium excretion by the kidneys. The increase in sodium reabsorption raises the serum osmolality and stimulates the release of antidiuretic hormone (ADH) from the posterior pituitary gland. ADH works by increasing water reabsorption by the kidneys, thus further increasing blood volume. The increase in total circulating volume results in an increase in cardiac output and BP.

The shunting of blood from other organ systems also results in clinically important changes. The decrease in blood flow to the GI tract results in impaired motility and a slowing of peristalsis, thus increasing the risk for the development of a paralytic ileus. Decreased blood flow to the skin results in the patient feeling cool and clammy. The exception is the patient in early septic shock who will feel warm and flushed.

Shunting blood away from the lungs has an important clinical effect in the patient in shock. Decreased blood flow to the lungs increases the patient's physiologic dead space. *Physiologic dead space* is the anatomic dead space (the amount of air that will not reach gas-exchanging units) plus any inspired air that cannot participate in gas exchange. The clinical result of an increase in dead space ventilation is a ventilation-perfusion mismatch. There will be areas of the lungs participating in ventilation that will not be perfused because of the decreased blood flow to the lungs. Arterial oxygen levels will decrease, and the patient will have a compensatory increase in the rate and depth of respirations.[14]

The myocardium responds to the SNS stimulation and the increase in oxygen demand by increasing the heart rate and contractility. However, increased contractility also increases myocardial oxygen consumption (MVO_2). The coronary arteries dilate in an attempt to meet the increased oxygen demands of the myocardium.

A multisystem response to decreasing tissue perfusion is initiated in the compensatory stage of shock. At this stage, the body is able to compensate for the changes in tissue perfusion, whatever the cause. If the perfusion deficit (the cause of the shock) is corrected, the patient will recover with little or no residual sequelae. If the perfusion deficit is not corrected and the body is unable to compensate, the patient enters the progressive stage of shock.

Progressive Stage. The *progressive stage* of shock begins as compensatory mechanisms fail (Fig. 65-7). In this stage of shock, aggressive interventions are necessary to prevent the de-

velopment of MODS. The hallmarks of this stage of shock are decreased cellular perfusion and altered capillary permeability. The altered capillary permeability allows leakage of fluid and protein out of the vascular space into the surrounding interstitial space. In addition to the decrease in circulating volume, there is an increase in systemic interstitial edema. The patient may have *anasarca,* or diffuse profound edema. Fluid leakage from the vascular space affects the solid organs (e.g., liver, spleen, GI tract, lungs), as well as the peripheral tissues.

The pulmonary system is often the first system to display signs of critical dysfunction. During the compensatory stage, blood flow to the lungs is already reduced. In response to the decreased blood flow and the SNS stimulation, the pulmonary arterioles constrict, resulting in increased pulmonary artery pressure. As the pressure within the pulmonary vasculature increases, blood flow to the pulmonary capillaries decreases, and ventilation-perfusion mismatch worsens. Another key response in the lungs is the movement of fluid from the pulmonary vasculature into the interstitium. As capillary permeability increases, the movement of fluid from the pulmonary vasculature to the interstitium results in interstitial edema, bronchoconstriction, and a decrease in functional residual capacity. With further increases in capillary permeability the fluid moves to the alveoli, with resultant alveolar edema and a decrease in surfactant production. The combined effects of pulmonary vasoconstriction and bronchoconstriction are impaired gas exchange, decreased compliance, and worsening ventilation-perfusion mismatch. Clinically, the patient has tachypnea, crackles, and an overall increased work of breathing.

The cardiovascular system is profoundly affected in the progressive stage of shock. Cardiac output begins to fall, with a resultant decrease in BP and peripheral perfusion, including a decrease in coronary artery perfusion. Capillary permeability continues to increase, enhancing the movement of fluid from the vascular space into the interstitial space. Sustained hypoperfusion results in weak peripheral pulses, and ischemia of the distal extremities eventually occurs. Myocardial dysfunction from decreased perfusion results in arrhythmias, myocardial ischemia, and potentially MI. The end result is a complete deterioration of the cardiovascular system.

The effect of prolonged hypoperfusion on the kidneys is renal tubular ischemia. The resulting acute tubular necrosis (ATN) may lead to the development of acute renal failure, which can be worsened by nephrotoxic drugs, including certain antibiotics, anesthetics, and diuretics (see Chapter 45). Renal function is markedly impaired during the progressive stage of shock. The patient will have a decreased urine output and an elevated blood urea nitrogen (BUN) and serum creatinine. Metabolic acidosis occurs from an inability to excrete acids and reabsorb bicarbonate.

The GI system is also affected by prolonged decreased tissue perfusion. As the blood supply to the GI tract is decreased, the normally protective mucosal barrier becomes ischemic. This ischemia predisposes the patient to erosive ulcers and GI bleeding and increases the risk for translocation of bacteria from the GI tract to the blood. The decreased perfusion also leads to a decreased ability to absorb nutrients from the GI system.[13]

Other systems are also affected by the sustained hypoperfusion in the progressive stage of shock. The loss of the functional ability of the liver leads to a failure of the liver to metabolize drugs and waste products such as ammonia and lactate. Jaundice results from an accumulation of bilirubin. As the liver cells die,

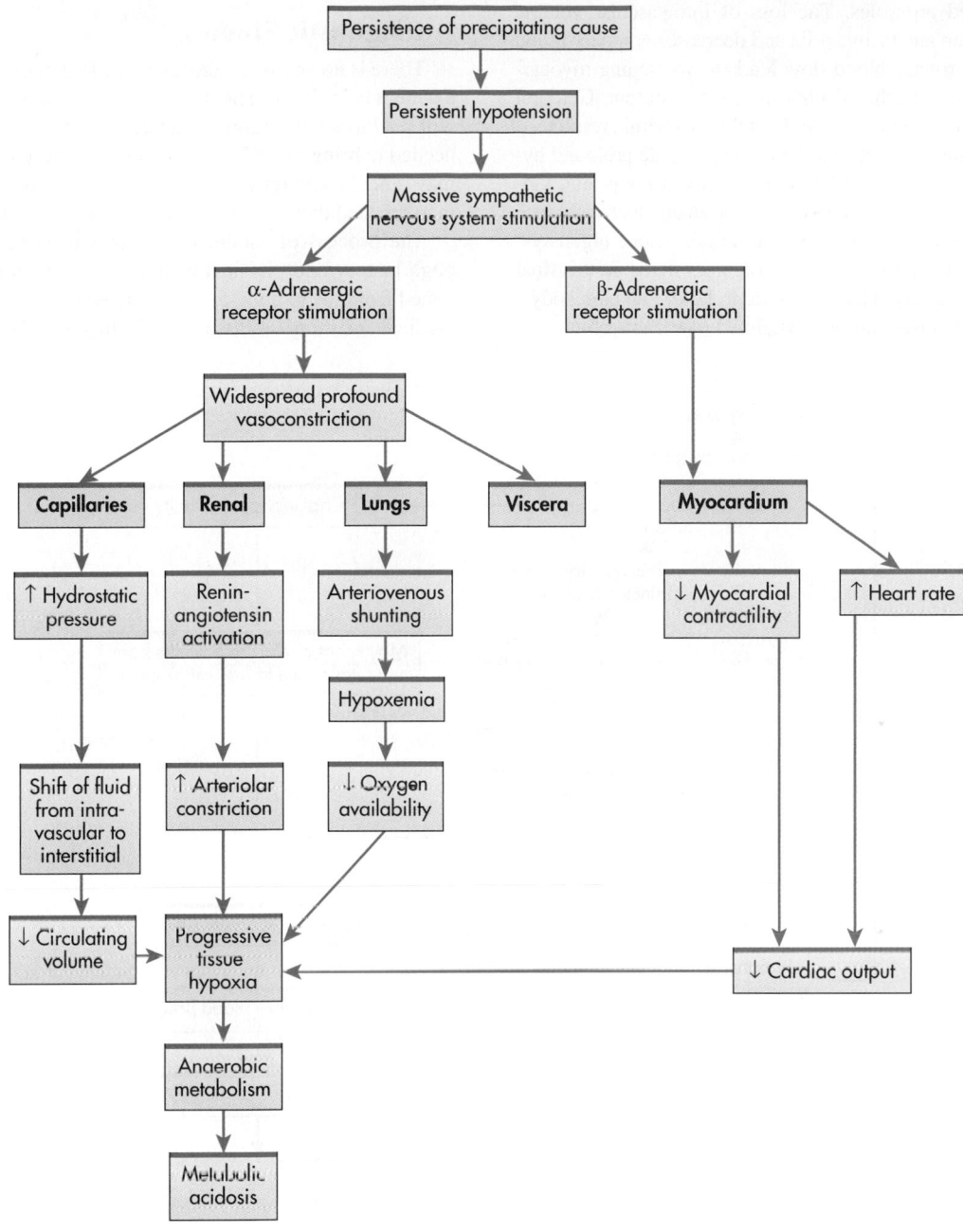

FIG. 65-7 Progressive stage: compensatory mechanisms are becoming ineffective and fail to maintain perfusion to vital organs.

enzymes become elevated, in particular alanine aminotransferase (ALT), aspartate aminotransferase (AST), and γ-glutamyl transferase (GGT). The liver also loses its ability to function as an immune organ. The bacteria that have translocated from the GI system are unable to be scavenged by the Kupffer cells. Instead, they are released into the bloodstream, thus increasing the possibility of the development of bacteremia.

Dysfunction of the hematologic system adds to the complexity of the clinical picture. The patient is at risk for the development of disseminated intravascular coagulation (DIC). In DIC, there is a consumption of the platelets and clotting factors with secondary fibrinolysis. This results in clinically significant bleeding from many orifices, including, but not limited to, the

GI tract, lungs, and puncture sites (see Chapter 30). Altered laboratory values in DIC include decreased platelets, prolonged prothrombin time, prolonged partial thromboplastin time, decreased fibrinogen, and increased fibrin split products (see Tables 65-3 and 65-6).

Refractory Stage. In the final stage of shock, the *refractory stage,* decreased perfusion from peripheral vasoconstriction and decreased cardiac output exacerbate anaerobic metabolism (Fig. 65-8). The accumulation of lactic acid contributes to an increased capillary permeability and dilation of the capillaries. Increased capillary permeability allows fluid and plasma proteins to leave the vascular space and move to the interstitial space. Blood pools in the capillary beds secondary to the constricted venules and dilated arterioles. The loss of intravascular volume worsens hypotension and tachycardia and decreases coronary blood flow. Decreased coronary blood flow leads to worsening myocardial depression and a further decline in cardiac output. Cerebral blood flow cannot be maintained, and cerebral ischemia results.

The patient in this stage of shock will demonstrate profound hypotension and hypoxemia. The failure of the liver, lungs, and kidneys will result in an accumulation of waste products, such as lactate, urea, ammonia, and carbon dioxide. The failure of one organ system will have an effect on several other organ systems. In this final stage, recovery is unlikely. The organs are in failure and the body's compensatory mechanisms are overwhelmed (see Table 65-6).

Diagnostic Studies

There is no single diagnostic study to determine whether or not a patient is in shock. The decreased tissue perfusion seen in shock will lead to an elevation of lactate and a base deficit (the amount needed to bring the pH back to normal). These laboratory changes may reflect an increase in anaerobic metabolism. Table 65-3 summarizes the laboratory findings that may be seen in shock.

The process of establishing a diagnosis begins with a thorough history and physical examination. The history may be obtained from the patient, family, or friends. Obtaining the patient's medical and surgical history, and a history of recent events (e.g.,

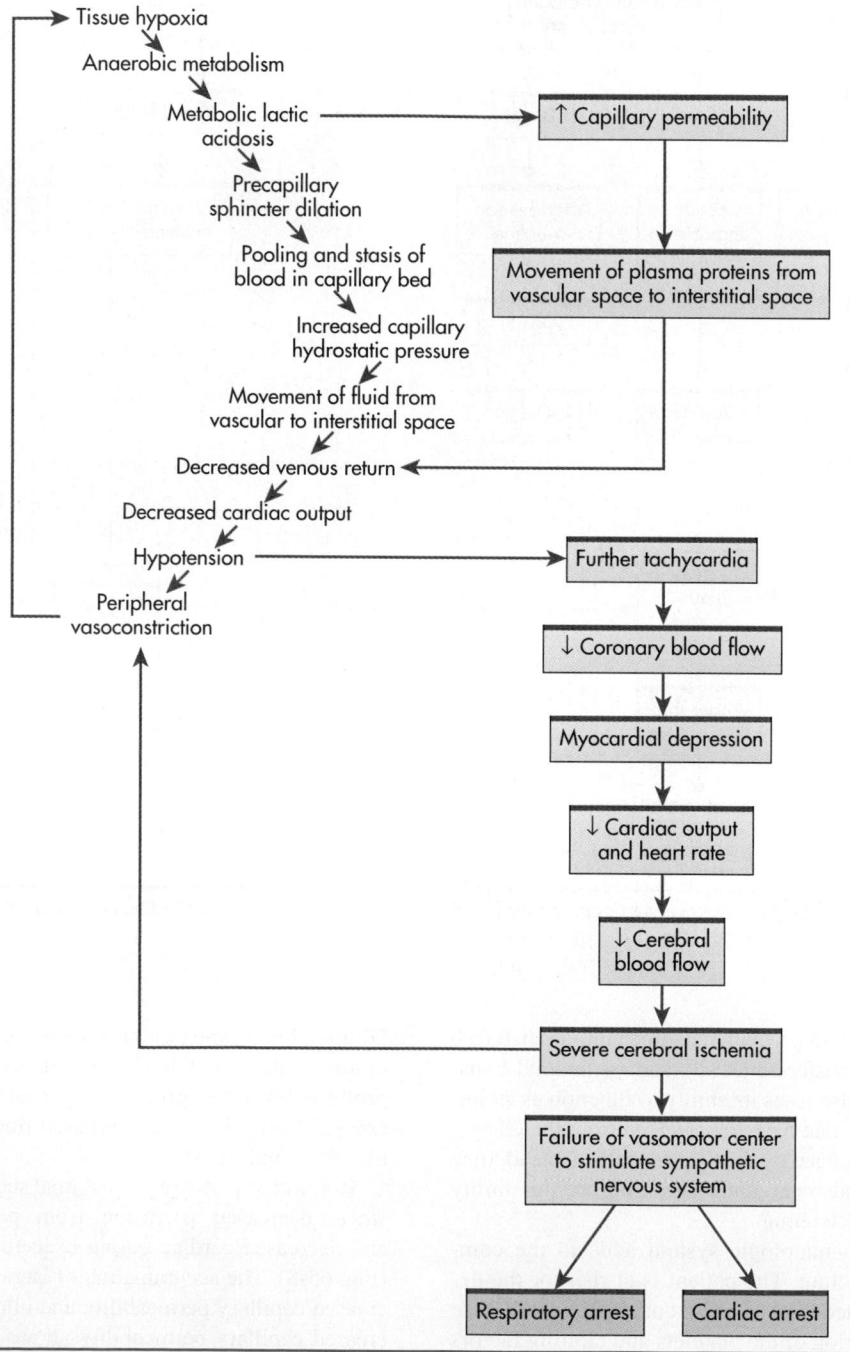

FIG. 65-8 Irreversible or refractory stage: compensatory mechanisms are not functioning or are totally ineffective, leading to multiple organ dysfunction syndrome.

upper respiratory tract infection, surgery, chest pain), will provide valuable data. Important diagnostic studies include a 12-lead ECG, continuous cardiac monitoring, chest x-ray, hemodynamic monitoring (e.g., arterial pressure monitoring, pulmonary artery pressure monitoring), and continuous pulse oximetry (see Chapter 64).

Collaborative Care: General Measures

Critical factors in the successful management of a patient experiencing shock relate to the early recognition and treatment of the shock state. Prompt intervention in the early stages of shock (initial and compensatory stages) may prevent the decline to the progressive or refractory stage. Successful management of the patient in shock includes the following:

1. Identification of patients at risk for the development of shock
2. Integration of the patient's history, physical examination, and clinical findings to establish a diagnosis
3. Interventions to control or eliminate the cause of the decreased perfusion
4. Protection of target and distal organs from dysfunction
5. Provision of multisystem supportive care

Table 65-7 provides an overview of the initial assessment findings and interventions for the emergency care of patients in shock. General management strategies for a patient in shock begin with ensuring that the patient has a patent airway. Once the airway is established, either with a natural airway or an endotracheal tube, oxygen delivery must be optimized. Mechanical ventilation may be necessary to support the delivery of oxygen to maintain an arterial oxygen saturation of 90% or greater (PaO_2 >60 mm Hg) to avoid hypoxemia (see Chapter 64). The mean arterial pressure and circulating blood volume are optimized with fluid replacement and drug therapy.

Oxygen and Ventilation. Oxygen delivery is dependent on cardiac output (CO), available hemoglobin, and arterial oxygen saturation (SaO_2). Methods to optimize oxygen delivery are directed at increasing supply and decreasing demand. Supply can be increased by (1) optimizing the CO with drug therapy or fluid replacement, (2) increasing the hemoglobin by the transfusion of blood or packed red blood cells (RBCs), and/or (3) increasing the arterial oxygen saturation with supplemental oxygen and mechanical ventilation.

Care must be planned so as not to disrupt the balance of oxygen supply and demand. The nurse must evaluate interventions that increase the patient's oxygen demand and appropriately space those interventions so that the patient's supply and demand balance is not disrupted. The use of a pulmonary artery (PA) catheter that includes a sensor to measure the mixed venous oxygen saturation (SvO_2) may be useful in determining the adequacy of tissue oxygenation. SvO_2 reflects the dynamic balance between oxygenation of the arterial blood, tissue perfusion, and tissue oxygen consumption. SvO_2, when considered in conjunction with the arterial oxygen saturation, is useful in analyzing the patient's hemodynamic status and response to treatments or activities (see Chapter 64).

TABLE 65-7 *Emergency Management*
Shock

ETIOLOGY*	ASSESSMENT FINDINGS	INTERVENTIONS
Surgical • Postoperative bleeding • Ruptured organ/vessel • Gastrointestinal bleeding • Aortic dissection • Vaginal bleeding • Ruptured ectopic pregnancy or ovarian cyst **Medical** • Myocardial infarction • Dehydration • Addisonian crisis • Diabetes insipidus • Sepsis • Diabetes mellitus • Pulmonary embolus **Trauma** • Ruptured or lacerated vessel or organ (e.g., spleen) • Fractures • Multisystem or multiorgan injury	• Decreased level of consciousness • Restlessness • Anxiety • Weakness • Rapid, weak, thready pulses • Arrhythmias • Hypotension • Narrowed pulse pressure • Cool, clammy skin (warm skin in early stage of septic shock) • Tachypnea, dyspnea, or shallow, irregular respirations • Decreased O_2 saturation • Extreme thirst • Nausea and vomiting • Chills • Feeling of impending doom • Pallor • Cyanosis • Obvious hemorrhage or injury • Temperature dysregulation	**Initial** • Establish and maintain patent airway. • Administer high-flow oxygen (100%) by non-rebreather mask or bag-valve mask. • Anticipate need for intubation. • Stabilize cervical spine as appropriate. • Establish IV access with two large-bore catheters (14-16 gauge) and begin fluid resuscitation with crystalloids (e.g., normal saline solution, lactated Ringer's solution). • Control any external bleeding with direct pressure or pressure dressing. • Assess for life-threatening injuries (e.g., cardiac tamponade, liver laceration, tension pneumothorax). • Consider vasopressor therapy only after hypovolemia has been corrected. • Insert an indwelling bladder catheter and nasogastric tube. • Treat arrhythmias. **Ongoing Monitoring** • Vital signs, including pulse oximetry, peripheral pulses, capillary refill • Level of consciousness • Cardiac rhythm • Urine output

*See Table 65-1 for additional etiologies of shock.

Fluid Replacement. Except for cardiogenic shock, all other classifications of shock involve decreased circulating blood volume. The cornerstone of therapy for septic, hypovolemic, neurogenic, and anaphylactic shock is volume expansion with the administration of the appropriate fluid. Before beginning fluid resuscitation, two large-bore (e.g., 14 to 16 gauge) IV catheters must be inserted, preferably into the antecubital veins.

Both crystalloids (e.g., normal saline solution) and colloids (e.g., albumin) have a role in fluid resuscitation (Table 65-8). The choice of fluid for resuscitation remains controversial. Currently, it is generally accepted that isotonic crystalloids, such as normal saline, are used in the initial resuscitation of shock, even though approximately two thirds of the crystalloid volume will diffuse out of the vascular space and into the interstitial space. Lactated Ringer's solution should be used cautiously in all shock situations because the failing liver cannot convert lactate to bicarbonate, thus increasing the serum lactate levels. Colloids are effective volume expanders because the size of their molecules keeps them in the vascular space for a longer period of time. Despite this fact, no definitive studies demonstrate that using colloids for resuscitation improves patient outcomes.[15]

The choice of fluid for resuscitation must also be based on the type and volume of fluid lost and the patient's clinical status. If the patient does not respond to 2 L of crystalloids, blood administration and central venous monitoring may be instituted. Serial blood pressures with an automatic BP cuff or an indwelling arterial catheter can be used to monitor the patient's status. An indwelling bladder catheter will also assist in monitoring the patient's fluid status.

When large amounts of fluid replacement are required, the patient must be protected against complications. Two major complications are hypothermia and coagulopathy. The patient can be protected from hypothermia by warming both crystalloid and colloid solutions used during massive fluid resuscitation. If the patient is receiving large volumes of packed RBCs, it is important to remember that they do not contain clotting factors. Therefore clotting factors will need to be replaced. Generally, 1 to 2 U of fresh frozen plasma are administered for every 5 U of packed RBCs.[16]

If the patient does not respond to volume replacement, a PA catheter may be considered to assist in evaluating the status of the intravascular volume. A PA catheter allows the measurement and/or computation of cardiac output (CO), preload, afterload, and SvO_2. If the patient has persistent hypotension after adequate volume resuscitation, a vasopressor agent, such as dopamine (Intropin), may be added. The goal for resuscitation remains the restoration of tissue perfusion. Thus decisions on which vasopressor or inotrope to use should be based on the physiologic goal. Although BP helps determine whether the patient's CO is adequate, an assessment of end-organ perfusion (e.g., urine output, neurologic function, peripheral pulses) provides more relevant information.

Drug Therapy. The primary goal of drug therapy for shock is the correction of decreased tissue perfusion. Medications used to improve perfusion in shock are administered intravenously via an infusion pump and often via a central venous line. One of the key reasons for administration of these medications via a central line is that many of the medications that have vasoconstrictor properties may have deleterious effects if administered peripherally and the drug extravasates (Table 65-9).[17]

TABLE 65-8	Fluid Therapy in Shock		
FLUID TYPE	**MECHANISM OF ACTION**	**TYPE OF SHOCK**	**NURSING IMPLICATIONS**
Crystalloids **Isotonic** • 0.9% NaCl (NSS) • Lactated Ringer's (LR)	Fluid primarily remains in the intravascular space, increasing intravascular volume	Used for initial volume replacement in most types of shock	Monitor patient closely for circulatory overload. LR should not be used in patients with liver failure.
Blood/Blood Products • Whole blood/packed red blood cells	Replaces blood loss, increases oxygen-carrying capability	All types of shock if hemoglobin is <12 g/dl (120 g/L) or if the patient does not respond to crystalloids	Same precautions as any blood administration (see Chapter 30).
Colloids • Hetastarch (Hespan)	Made from starch and acts as volume expander; is at least as effective as albumin; can exert osmotic effect for up to 36 hours	All types of shock	May be 50% less costly than albumin. Use cautiously in patients with congestive heart failure, renal failure, or bleeding disorders (due to anticoagulant effect).
• Human serum albumin (5%, 25%), plasma protein fraction (5% albumin in 500 ml NSS)	Can increase plasma colloid osmotic pressure; rapid volume expansion	All types of shock except cardiogenic	Monitor for circulatory overload. Mild side effects of chills, fever, and urticaria may develop. More expensive than other colloids.
• dextran dextran 40 dextran 70	Hyperosmotic glucose polymer; has similar degrees of volume expansion with dextran 40 and dextran 70; longer duration of action with dextran 70	Limited use because of side effects including reducing platelet adhesion, diluting clotting factors	Increases risk of bleeding. Important to monitor patient for allergic reactions and acute renal failure.

NSS, Normal saline solution.

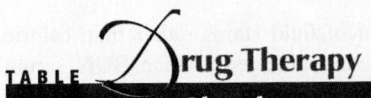

TABLE
65-9

Drug Therapy
Shock

DRUG*	MECHANISM OF ACTION	HEMODYNAMIC EFFECTS	TYPE OF SHOCK	NURSING IMPLICATIONS
dobutamine (Dobutrex)	↑ Myocardial contractility ↓ Ventricular filling pressures	↓ SVR/PAWP ↑ CO/stroke volume/ CVP ↑↓ HR	Used in cardiogenic shock with severe systolic dysfunction Used in septic shock with normal CO that is not meeting ↑ metabolic demands	Correct hypovolemia. Do not administer in same line with NaHCO₃. Administration via central line recommended. Monitor HR. Monitor for arrhythmias.
dopamine (Intropin)	Precursor to epinephrine and norepinephrine Hemodynamic effects from release of norepinephrine Positive inotropic effects: ↑ Myocardial contractility ↑ Automaticity ↑ Atrioventricular conduction Low doses: ↑ blood flow to renal, mesenteric, and cerebral circulation High doses: can cause progressive vasoconstriction	↑ HR ↑ CO ↑ BP	Cardiogenic shock: ↑ Mean arterial pressure ↑ HR ↑ MVO₂	Correct hypovolemia. Administer via central line. Do not administer with NaHCO₃. Monitor for peripheral vasoconstriction at moderate to high doses. Monitor for tachyarrhythmias.
epinephrine (Adrenalin)	Low doses: β-adrenergic agonist (cardiac stimulation, bronchial dilation, peripheral vasodilation) High doses: α-adrenergic agonist (peripheral vasoconstriction)	↑ HR/contractility/ CO ↓ SVR ↑ Stroke volume ↑ Systolic/↓ diastolic BP, widened pulse pressure ↑ CVP/PAWP	Cardiogenic shock combined with afterload reduction Anaphylactic shock Cardiac arrest, pulseless ventricular tachycardia, ventricular fibrillation, asystole	Correct hypovolemia if appropriate. Monitor for HR >110. Monitor for dyspnea, pulmonary edema. Monitor for chest pain, arrhythmias secondary to ↑ MVO₂. Monitor for renal failure secondary to ischemia.
norepinephrine (Levophed)	β₁-adrenergic agonist (cardiac stimulation) α-adrenergic agonist (peripheral vasoconstriction) Renal/splanchnic vasoconstriction	↑ BP, MAP ↑ CVP/PAWP ↑ SVR ↑↓ CO	Cardiogenic shock after myocardial infarction Septic shock: works by increasing vascular tone	Used for hypotension unresponsive to adequate fluid resuscitation. Administer via a central line (infiltration leads to tissue sloughing). Monitor for arrhythmias secondary to ↑ MVO₂ requirements.
phenylephrine (Neo-Synephrine)	α-adrenergic agonist Vasoconstriction: renal, mesenteric, splanchnic, cutaneous, and pulmonary vessels	↑ HR ↑ BP ↑ SVR ↑↓ CO	Neurogenic shock	Monitor for reflex bradycardia, headache, restlessness. Monitor for renal failure secondary to ↓ renal blood flow. Infiltration leads to tissue sloughing.
nitroglycerin (Tridil)	Venodilation Dilates coronary arteries ↓ Preload ↓ MVO₂	↓ SVR ↓ BP ↓ CVP/PAWP ↓↑ CO	Cardiogenic shock	Monitor for postural hypotension; reflex tachycardia. Use glass bottles for storage.
sodium nitroprusside (Nipride)	Arterial and venous vasodilation ↓ Preload/afterload	↓ BP ↓ CO	Cardiogenic shock with ↑ SVR	Continuously monitor BP. Protect solution from light; wrap infusion bottle with opaque covering. Administer with D₅W only. Monitor for cyanide toxicity (e.g., tinnitus, hyperreflexia, confusion, seizures).

*Consult individual facility's guidelines, pharmacist, pharmacology references, and drug manufacturer's administration materials for additional information and exact dosing.
BP, Blood pressure; *CO*, cardiac output; *CVP*, central venous pressure; *HR*, heart rate; *MVO₂*, myocardial oxygen consumption; *PAWP*, pulmonary artery wedge pressure; *SVR*, systemic vascular resistance.

Sympathomimetic drugs. Many of the drugs used in the treatment of shock have an effect on the SNS. Drugs that mimic the action of the SNS are termed *sympathomimetic*. The effects of these drugs are mediated through their binding to α-adrenergic or β-adrenergic receptors. The various drugs differ in their relative α-adrenergic and β-adrenergic effects. (See Chapter 32, Table 32-1, for a discussion of adrenergic receptors.)

Many of the sympathomimetic drugs cause peripheral vasoconstriction and are referred to as vasopressor drugs (e.g., epinephrine [Adrenalin], norepinephrine [Levophed]). At high doses these vasopressor drugs have the potential to cause severe peripheral vasoconstriction and further jeopardize tissue perfusion, either directly or indirectly. The increased SVR increases the workload of the heart and can be detrimental to a patient in cardiogenic shock by causing further myocardial damage. Use of vasopressor drugs is generally reserved for patients who have been unresponsive to other therapies. Adequate volume replacement must be administered before the use of any vasopressor because peripheral vasoconstrictor effects in patients with low blood volume will cause further reduction in tissue perfusion.

The goals of vasopressor therapy are to achieve and maintain a mean arterial pressure (MAP) of at least 60 mm Hg. The nurse must continuously monitor end-organ perfusion (e.g., urine output, neurologic function) to ensure that the BP is providing adequate perfusion.

Vasodilator drugs. Some patients in shock show evidence of excessive vasoconstriction and poor tissue perfusion in spite of volume replacement and normal or even high systemic BP. This is especially true of patients in cardiogenic shock. Although generalized sympathetic vasoconstriction is a useful compensatory mechanism for maintaining systemic pressure, excessive constriction can reduce tissue blood flow and increase the workload of the heart. The rationale for using vasodilator therapy for a patient in shock is to break the deleterious cycle in which widespread vasoconstriction causes a decrease in CO and BP, resulting in further sympathetic-induced vasoconstriction.

The goal of vasodilator therapy, as in vasopressor therapy, is to maintain MAP at 60 mm Hg or greater. It is also important to closely monitor PA pressures along with MAP so that fluid administration can be increased or the dose of the vasodilator decreased if a serious fall in BP occurs. The vasodilator agent most often used for the patient in cardiogenic shock is nitroglycerin (Tridil). Vasodilation may be enhanced with nitroprusside (Nipride) in noncardiogenic shock.

Nutritional Therapy. Protein-calorie malnutrition is one of the primary manifestations of hypermetabolism in shock. Nutrition is vital to decreasing morbidity. Some type of nutrition should be implemented within the first 24 hours. Generally, parenteral feeding is used only if enteral feedings have failed, are contraindicated, or fail to meet the patient's caloric requirements. (Total parenteral nutrition and enteral tube feedings are discussed in Chapter 39.) The patient is started on continuous drip of very small amounts of enteral feedings. Early enteral feedings are thought to enhance perfusion of the GI tract and prevent translocation of gut bacteria.

A patient in shock should be weighed daily on the same scale at the same time of day. If the patient experiences a significant weight loss, dehydration should be ruled out before additional calories are provided parenterally. Large weight gains are common because of third spacing of fluids. Therefore daily weights may function as an indicator of fluid status rather than caloric needs and balance. Serum protein, nitrogen balance, BUN, serum glucose, and serum electrolytes are all used to assess nutritional status.

Collaborative Care: Specific Measures

Cardiogenic Shock. For a patient in cardiogenic shock, the overall goal is to restore blood flow to the myocardium by restoring the balance between oxygen supply and demand. Definitive measures to restore blood flow include thrombolytic therapy, angioplasty with stenting, and emergency revascularization (see Chapter 33). Cardiac catheterization should be performed as soon as possible after the initial insult. Coronary angioplasty with or without stenting may be performed during the cardiac catheterization. Until these interventions can be performed, the heart must be supported to optimize stroke volume and CO in an effort to facilitate optimal perfusion (Tables 65-9 and 65-10).

Hemodynamic management of a patient in cardiogenic shock is geared toward reducing the workload of the heart through drug therapy or mechanical interventions. Drug selection is based on the clinical goal and a thorough understanding of the pharmacodynamics of each drug. Drugs can be used to decrease the workload of the heart by dilating coronary arteries (e.g., nitrates), reducing preload (e.g., diuretics), reducing afterload (e.g., angiotensin-converting enzyme [ACE] inhibitors), and reducing heart rate and contractility (e.g., β-adrenergic blockers).

The patient may also benefit from a circulatory assist device such as an intraaortic balloon pump (IABP) or a ventricular assist device (VAD) (see Chapter 64). The IABP is a circulatory assist device that is inserted into the femoral artery and placed in the aorta just distal to the aortic arch. The goal of this intervention is to decrease the SVR and thus left ventricular workload. Another type of circulatory assist device, the VAD, may also be used on a temporary basis for the patient in cardiogenic shock and/or awaiting cardiac transplantation. Cardiac transplantation is an option for a small and select group of patients with cardiogenic shock.

Hypovolemic Shock. The underlying principles of managing patients with hypovolemic shock focus on stopping the loss of fluid and restoring the circulating volume. Table 65-8 delineates the different types of fluid used for volume resuscitation, the mechanisms of action, and specific nursing implications for each fluid type.

Septic Shock. Patients in septic shock require large amounts of fluid replacement, sometimes as much as 6 to 10 L of isotonic crystalloids and 2 to 4 L of colloids.[18] Predetermined end points of resuscitation are suggested in Table 65-10. To optimize and evaluate large-volume resuscitation, hemodynamic monitoring with a PA catheter and continuous BP monitoring with an arterial catheter may be necessary. The overall goal of fluid resuscitation is to restore perfusion. If that cannot be accomplished with intravenous fluids, vasopressor drug therapy may be added. Vasodilation and low cardiac index, or vasodilation alone, can cause low blood pressure in spite of adequate volume resuscitation. The addition of a vasopressor drug may increase BP but may also result in a decrease in stroke volume. An inotropic agent is often added to offset the decrease in stroke volume (see Table 65-9).

In an attempt to meet the increasing tissue demands coupled with a low SVR, the patient may demonstrate a high CO. If the

TABLE 65-10	Collaborative Care

Specific Measures for the Treatment of Shock

CARDIOGENIC SHOCK	HYPOVOLEMIC SHOCK	SEPTIC SHOCK	NEUROGENIC SHOCK	ANAPHYLACTIC SHOCK

• Improve O_2 delivery by ↓ demand
• Reestablish blood flow with thrombolytics, angioplasty, emergency revascularization
• ↑ O_2 supply by providing supplemental O_2
• Drug therapy:
  • Dilate coronary arteries (e.g., nitrates)
  • Improve contractility (e.g., inotropes)
  • Reduce preload (e.g., nitrates, morphine, diuretics, ACE inhibitors)
  • Reduce afterload (e.g., ACE inhibitors, phosphodiesterase inhibitors, β-adrenergic agonists, vasodilators)
  • Reduce heart rate (e.g., β-adrenergic blockers, calcium channel blockers)
  • Reduce contractility (e.g., β-adrenergic blockers [contraindicated with ↓ ejection fraction])
• Correct arrhythmias
• Circulatory assist devices: IABP, VAD
	• Optimize oxygenation
	• Correct the cause (e.g., stop bleeding, GI losses)
	• Volume replacement (e.g., blood/blood products, crystalloids, colloids)
	• Rapid fluid replacement with two large-bore (14-16 gauge) peripheral IVs
	• Use warmed fluids
	• Endpoints of resuscitation:
	  • CVP 15 mm Hg
	  • PAWP 10-12 mm Hg
	  • CI >3 L/min/m²
	  • Blood lactate <4 mmol/L
	  • Base deficit −3 to +3 mmol/L
		• Optimize oxygen delivery by ↑ supply/↓ demand
		• Fluid resuscitation
		• Optimize cardiac output:
		  • Volume
		  • Vasopressors
		  • Vasopressors and inotropes (e.g., dobutamine)
		• Vasopressors (↑ BP) (e.g., dopamine, norepinephrine, phenylephrine)
		• Correct acidosis
		• Obtain culture before beginning antibiotics
		• Antibiotics as ordered
			• Treat according to the cause (see Table 65-1)
			• Minimize spinal cord trauma with stabilization
			• Careful administration of fluids
			• Drug therapy:
			  • Dopamine for hypotension and bradycardia
			  • Administration of phenylephrine or norepinephrine to increase SVR
			• Monitor for hypothermia
				• Prevention via avoidance of known allergens
				• Premedication with history of prior sensitivity (e.g., contrast media)
				• Identify and remove offending cause
				• Maintain patent airway
				• Intubation/mechanical ventilation
				• Drug therapy:
				  • Epinephrine subcutaneous, IV, nebulized
				  • Bronchodilators: nebulized, IV
				  • Antihistamines
				  • Corticosteroids (if hypotension persists)
				• Fluid resuscitation with colloids

ACE, Angiotensin-converting enzyme; *BP*, blood pressure; *CI*, cardiac index; *CVP*, central venous pressure; *GI*, gastrointestinal; *IABP*, intraaortic balloon pump; *PAWP*, pulmonary artery wedge pressure; *VAD*, ventricular assist device.

patient is unable to achieve and maintain an adequate CO and has unmet tissue oxygen demands, the CO may need to be increased using drug therapy (e.g., dobutamine [Dobutrex]). The adequacy of the CO can be determined using the mixed venous oxygen saturation (SvO_2). The SvO_2 (normal, 60% to 80%) is a reflection of the balance between oxygen delivery and consumption (see Chapter 64). If the balance is maintained, the tissue demands will be met and CO will be adequate.

Septic shock is always associated with a documented or suspected infection (see Table 65-5), and antibiotics are an important component of therapy. Before beginning definitive treatment for the infection, the cause of the infection must first be identified. Cultures (e.g., blood, wound exudate, urine, stool, sputum) are obtained before antibiotics are started. Broad-spectrum antibiotics are given initially, followed by more specific antibiotics once the organism has been identified.

Mortality rates from septic shock remain high, and until recently research efforts had not helped to improve outcomes for patients with septic shock. Drotrecogin (Xigris), a recombinant form of activated protein C, has demonstrated promise in treating patients with severe sepsis. Activated protein C is a naturally occurring substance whose exact mechanism of action is unknown. It is thought to produce an antiinflammatory effect by inhibiting TNF production and limiting inflammation. Activated protein C is found in subnormal levels in patients with sepsis. Drotrecogin interrupts the body's response to severe sepsis, including bleeding, clotting abnormalities, and cardiovascular and renal failure. The use of drotrecogin has resulted in a significant decrease in mortality rate when it is used for patients with severe sepsis.[19] Bleeding is the most common serious adverse effect associated with its use.

Neurogenic Shock. The specific treatment of neurogenic shock is dependent on the cause. If the cause is spinal cord injury, general measures to promote spinal stability (e.g., spinal precautions, cervical stabilization with a collar) are initially used. Once the spine is stabilized, definitive treatment of the hypotension and bradycardia is essential to prevent further spinal cord damage. Hypotension, which occurs as a result of a loss of sympathetic tone, is associated with peripheral vasodilation and decreased venous return. If the venous return is not optimized by volume, the addition of an α-adrenergic agonist (e.g., phenylephrine [Neo-Synephrine]) may be indicated (see Table 65-9).

The patient with a spinal cord injury will also need to be monitored for hypothermia due to hypothalamic dysfunction (see Table 65-10). Although corticosteroids do not have an effect in neurogenic shock, methylprednisolone (Solu-Medrol) is used for patients with a spinal cord injury to prevent secondary spinal cord damage caused by the release of chemical mediators (see Chapter 59).

Anaphylactic Shock. The first strategy in managing patients at risk for anaphylactic shock is prevention. A thorough history is key in avoiding the risk factors for anaphylaxis (see Table 65-1). The clinical presentation of anaphylactic shock is dramatic, and immediate intervention is required. Epinephrine is the drug of choice to treat anaphylactic shock.[15] It causes peripheral vasoconstriction and bronchodilation and opposes the effect of histamine. Diphenhydramine (Benadryl) is administered to block the massive release of histamine from the allergic reaction.

Maintaining a patent airway is important, because the patient can quickly develop airway compromise from laryngeal edema or bronchoconstriction. Nebulized bronchodilators are highly effective. Aerosolized epinephrine can also be used to treat laryngeal edema. Endotracheal intubation or cricothyroidotomy may be necessary to secure and maintain a patent airway.

Hypotension results from leakage of fluid out of the intravascular space into the interstitial space as a result of increased vascular permeability and vasodilation. Aggressive fluid replacement, predominantly with colloids, is necessary. Intravenous corticosteroids may be helpful in anaphylactic shock if significant hypotension persists after 1 to 2 hours of aggressive therapy (see Tables 65-9 and 65-10).

NURSING MANAGEMENT
SHOCK

▪ Nursing Assessment

The role of the nurse is vital in caring for patients who are at risk for developing shock or are in a state of shock. The initial assessment should be geared toward the ABCs: airway, breathing, and circulation. Further assessment should focus on the assessment of tissue perfusion and includes evaluation of vital signs, peripheral pulses, level of consciousness, capillary refill, skin (e.g., temperature, color, moisture), and urine output. As shock progresses, the patient's skin will become cooler and mottled, urine output will decrease, and neurologic status will continue to deteriorate.

To understand the complexity of the patient's clinical status, the nurse must integrate all of the assessment data. As care is initiated (see Tables 65-7 and 65-10), it is essential for the nurse to obtain a brief history from the patient or other knowledgeable person. This information should include a description of the events leading to the shock condition, time of onset and duration of symptoms, and a health history (e.g., medications, allergies, date of last tetanus vaccination). In addition, details regarding any care that the patient received before hospitalization are also important.

▪ Nursing Diagnoses

Nursing diagnoses for the patient with shock may include, but are not limited to, those presented in NCP 65-1.

▪ Planning

The overall goals for caring for a patient in shock include (1) assurance of adequate tissue perfusion, (2) restoration of normal BP, (3) return/recovery of organ function, and (4) avoidance of complications from prolonged states of hypoperfusion.

▪ Nursing Implementation

Health Promotion. It is important for nurses to become involved in the prevention of shock. To prevent shock, the nurse needs to identify patients at risk. In general, patients who are older, those with debilitating illnesses, and those who are immunocompromised are at an increased risk. Any person who sustains surgical or accidental trauma is at high risk for shock resulting from hemorrhage, spinal cord injury, and other conditions (see Table 65-1). Any patient who is at risk for decreased oxygen delivery or tissue hypoxia is also at risk for the development of shock.

Planning is essential to help prevent shock after a susceptible individual has been identified. For example, a person with an acute MI, especially an anterior wall MI, is at risk for cardiogenic shock. The primary goal for the patient with an acute MI is to limit the size of the infarction. The infarct size can be limited by restoring coronary blood flow through thrombolytic therapy, percutaneous coronary intervention (PCI), or surgical revascularization. Rest, analgesics, sedation, and judicious use of paralytic agents (if the patient is intubated) can reduce the myocardial demand for oxygen. The nurse can modify the patient's environment to provide care at intervals that will not increase the patient's oxygen demand. For example, if the patient becomes anxious with bathing, that activity can be planned at a time so as not to interfere with x-rays or other activities that may also increase oxygen demand.

A person with a severe allergy to such substances as drugs, shellfish, and insect bites is at increased risk to develop anaphylactic shock. The risk of anaphylactic shock can be decreased if the patient is carefully questioned about allergies before administering a new drug (even if the patient has received this drug in the past) or before undergoing diagnostic procedures involving the use of contrast media. Patients with severe allergies should wear a Medic Alert tag and report their allergies to their health care providers. These patients should also be instructed about the availability of special kits that contain equipment and medication (e.g., epinephrine [EpiPen]) for the treatment of acute hypersensitivity reactions. If a patient's condition warrants receiving a medication to which he or she is at high risk for an allergic reaction (e.g., contrast media), the patient should receive a premedication such as diphenhydramine or methylprednisolone.

Careful monitoring of fluid balance can help to prevent hypovolemic shock. Ongoing monitoring of intake and output and daily weights are important. In addition, monitoring of the patient's clinical status is essential because trends in clinical findings are more meaningful than any single piece of clinical information.

All patients must be carefully monitored for the development of infection. Progression from an infection to sepsis and septic shock is dependent on the patient's host defense mechanisms. Pa-

NURSING CARE PLAN 65-1

Patient in Shock

EXPECTED PATIENT OUTCOMES	NURSING INTERVENTIONS and *RATIONALES*

NURSING DIAGNOSIS

Decreased cardiac output *related to* shock state *as manifested by* increased diastolic BP, decreased systolic BP; postural hypotension; tachycardia; weak, thready pulses; flat neck veins; low CVP and PAWP; thirst and dry mucous membranes; urinary output <0.5 ml/kg/hr; altered mentation; arrhythmias; tachypnea; hypoxemia; pallor or cyanosis; cool, clammy skin.

- Normal or baseline BP (for patient)
- HR 60-100 beats/min and regular
- Strong peripheral pulses
- Normal CVP (1-8 mm Hg) and PAWP (6-12 mm Hg)
- Warm, dry skin
- Urinary output >0.5 ml/kg/hr
- Normal mentation
- Respiratory rate >12 and <20 breaths/min
- SaO$_2$ ≥90%

- Monitor vital signs, CVP, pulmonary artery pressures every 15 min to 1 hr *to monitor patient's status and detect fluid deficits or excesses, and to assess patient's response to treatment.*
- Administer crystalloids, colloids, and/or blood *to restore blood and fluid volume to maintain perfusion of vital organs.*
- Titrate drug therapy (as indicated) to support BP *to maintain perfusion.*
- Record accurate intake and output; daily weights *to monitor fluid balance status.*
- Monitor laboratory and x-ray findings *to evaluate patient's response to treatment.*
- Keep patient at normal body temperature *to prevent an increase in metabolic need for O$_2$ and increased CO$_2$ production.*
- Administer oxygen *to keep SaO$_2$ ≥90%.*

NURSING DIAGNOSIS

Fear and anxiety *related to* severity of condition *as manifested by* verbalization of anxiety about condition and fear of death, or withdrawal with no communication; restlessness; sleeplessness; increase in heart and respiratory rate.

- Verbalization of anxieties and/or fears
- Verbalization of reduced anxiety and/or fear

- Acknowledge expressed fear and anxiety *to validate patient's feelings.*
- Demonstrate concern and respect for patient.
- Provide time to listen to patient and to draw out patient if withdrawn *to encourage verbalization and discussion of fears.*
- Seek out significant other's perception of situation *to enlist help.*
- Maintain calm and reassuring demeanor and environment *to reduce patient's anxieties and oxygen need.*
- Explain interventions, patient status, and equipment simply and honestly *to reduce patient's fear of the unknown and assist patient in making informed decisions.*

COLLABORATIVE PROBLEMS

NURSING GOALS	NURSING INTERVENTIONS and *RATIONALES*

POTENTIAL COMPLICATION

Organ ischemia/dysfunction *related to* decreased tissue perfusion.

Neurologic Ischemia/Dysfunction
- Monitor for signs of neurologic ischemia
- Report deviations from acceptable parameters
- Carry out medical and nursing interventions

- Perform neurologic assessment every hour, including assessment of changes in mentation or level of consciousness, *to provide information regarding status of cerebral blood flow.*
- Record and report any changes *to guide selection of appropriate interventions.*
- Closely observe and protect confused patient *to prevent injury.*
- Take measures to minimize noise *to control sensory input and allow for rest.*

Renal Ischemia/Dysfunction
- Monitor for signs of renal ischemia
- Report deviations from acceptable parameters
- Carry out medical and nursing interventions

- Monitor for urine output <0.5 ml/kg/hr, increase in urine specific gravity, elevation in serum BUN and creatinine, abnormal serum electrolytes, low urine sodium, protein and blood in urine, metabolic acidosis *to assess renal function.*
- Insert bladder catheter *to accurately measure urinary output.*
- Perform daily weights *to monitor fluid status and evaluate renal function.*
- Administer fluids and drug therapy as ordered and assess results *to maintain adequate renal perfusion.*
- Monitor signs and symptoms of fluid overload *to identify a possible complication of overtreatment.*

BP, Blood pressure; *BUN,* blood urea nitrogen; *CVP,* central venous pressure; *HR,* heart rate; *PAWP,* pulmonary artery wedge pressure.

Continued

NURSING CARE PLAN 65-1

Patient in Shock—cont'd

COLLABORATIVE PROBLEMS

NURSING GOALS	NURSING INTERVENTIONS and *RATIONALES*
POTENTIAL COMPLICATION—cont'd	**Organ ischemia/dysfunction** *related to* decreased tissue perfusion.

Gastrointestinal Ischemia/Dysfunction

- Monitor for signs of GI ischemia
- Report deviations from acceptable parameters
- Carry out medical and nursing interventions

- Monitor for presence of abdominal pain, distention, nausea, vomiting, anorexia, diarrhea, thirst; auscultate bowel sounds every 4 hr *to assess GI status.*
- Measure intake and output and daily weight *to determine fluid balance.*
- Initiate enteral or parenteral nutrition as soon as possible (if ordered) *to provide adequate calories to meet metabolic demands.*

Peripheral Vascular Ischemia/Dysfunction

- Monitor for signs of peripheral vascular ischemia
- Report deviations from acceptable parameters
- Carry out appropriate medical and nursing interventions

- Monitor for presence of cool, pale, or cyanotic extremities; diminished or absent peripheral pulses; pain, tingling, or numbness in extremities; necrotic or gangrenous extremities; poor capillary refill *as indicators of peripheral vascular ischemia.*
- Report any changes in peripheral perfusion *so treatment can be initiated promptly.*
- Initiate proper skin care measures *to maintain skin integrity and prevent pressure ulcers because they can develop quickly when immobility is combined with tissue ischemia.*
- Keep patient warm and dry *to promote comfort and prevent vasoconstriction.*

Respiratory Ischemia/Dysfunction

- Monitor for signs of respiratory distress
- Report deviations from acceptable parameters
- Carry out appropriate medical and nursing interventions

- Monitor for the following: altered respiratory rate and depth, dyspnea, use of accessory muscles, cyanosis, adventitious breath sounds, cough, abnormal chest x-ray *to assess for respiratory distress.*
- Initiate oxygen and maintain $SaO_2 \geq 90\%$ *to ensure adequate oxygenation.*
- Monitor ABGs *to evaluate gas exchange in the lungs and acid-base balance.*
- Auscultate and record breath sounds every 1-2 hr *to determine presence of crackles, wheezes, and decreased or unequal breath sounds as indicators of impaired respirations.*
- Assist patient to deep breathe *to open up alveoli and improve gas exchange.*
- Suction as needed *to remove secretions patient cannot remove independently.*
- Maintain patent airway and prepare for possible intubation and mechanical ventilation.

ABGs, Arterial blood gases; *GI,* gastrointestinal.

---

tients who are immunocompromised or immunosuppressed are at especially high risk to develop an opportunistic infection. Interventions to decrease the risk of infection for hospitalized patients include decreasing the number of indwelling catheters (e.g., central lines, indwelling urinary catheters), using aseptic technique during invasive procedures, and strict attention to hand washing. In addition, all equipment must be changed according to institutional policy, or thoroughly cleaned or discarded (if disposable) between patient use.

Acute Intervention. The role of the nurse in shock involves (1) monitoring the patient's ongoing physical and emotional status to detect subtle changes in the patient's condition, (2) planning and implementing nursing interventions and therapy, (3) evaluating the patient's response to therapy, (4) providing emotional support to the patient and family, and (5) collaborating with other members of the health team when warranted by the patient's condition (see NCP 65-1).

Neurologic status. Neurologic status, including orientation and level of consciousness, should be assessed at least every hour. The patient's neurologic status is the best indicator of cerebral blood flow. The nurse should be aware of the clinical manifestations that may indicate neurologic involvement, such as changes

in behavior, restlessness, hyperalertness, blurred vision, confusion, and paresthesias. The astute nurse must also be alert to any subtle changes in the neurologic status (e.g., mild agitation).

Attempts should be made to orient the patient to time, place, person, and events. If the patient is in an ICU, orientation to the environment is particularly important. Measures such as minimizing noise and light levels should be taken to control sensory input. A day-night cycle of activity and rest should be maintained as much as possible. Sensory overload and disruption of the patient's diurnal cycle may contribute to delirium.

Cardiovascular status. Much of the therapy for shock is based on information about the patient's cardiovascular status. If the patient is unstable, the heart rate, blood pressure (BP), central venous pressure (CVP), and PA pressures (if available) should be determined at least every 15 minutes. PAWP should be measured every 1 to 2 hours. (Hemodynamic monitoring is discussed in Chapter 64.) Once the patient is stable, the PAWP should be obtained only as often as needed to avoid complications associated with balloon inflation. If the pulmonary artery diastolic pressure and the PAWP correlate, the pulmonary artery diastolic pressure may be used to estimate the PAWP. The PAWP most accurately reflects left ventricular function, especially in the presence of lung problems (e.g., pulmonary embolism, chronic lung disease), when the PA pressure is often elevated. Monitoring trends in PA pressure and other hemodynamic parameters yields more important information than individual numbers. Integration of hemodynamic data with physical assessment data is essential in planning strategies to manage the patient with shock.

The patient's ECG should be continuously monitored to detect arrhythmias that may result from the cardiovascular and metabolic derangements associated with shock. Heart sounds should be assessed for the presence of an S_3 or S_4 sound or new murmurs. The presence of an S_3 sound in an adult usually indicates heart failure. The frequency of this monitoring is decreased as the patient's condition improves.

In addition to monitoring the patient's cardiovascular status, the nurse must administer the prescribed therapy that is designed to correct the dysfunctions of the cardiovascular system. The response to fluid and medication administration must be assessed at least every 15 minutes. Appropriate adjustments should be made as needed. Once tissue perfusion is restored, medications that are being used to support blood pressure and tissue perfusion are slowly weaned after the patient becomes stabilized.

Respiratory status. The respiratory status of the patient in shock must be frequently assessed to ensure adequate oxygenation, detect complications early, and provide data regarding the patient's acid-base status. The rate, depth, and rhythm of respirations are initially monitored every 15 to 30 minutes. Increased rate and depth provide information regarding the patient's attempts to correct metabolic acidosis. Breath sounds should be assessed every 4 hours for any changes, which may indicate fluid overload or accumulation of secretions.

Pulse oximetry is used to continuously monitor oxygen saturation. Pulse oximetry using a patient's finger or toe may not be accurate in an advanced shock state because of poor peripheral circulation. In this situation, the probe should be attached to the nose, ear, or forehead (according to the manufacturer's guidelines) to increase accuracy. Arterial blood gases (ABGs) provide definitive information on oxygenation status and acid-base balance. Initial interpretation of ABGs is often the nurse's responsibility. A PaO_2 below 60 mm Hg (in the absence of chronic lung disease) indicates the presence of hypoxemia and the need for the administration of higher oxygen concentrations or for a different mode of oxygen administration. A low $PaCO_2$ in the presence of a low pH and low bicarbonate level may indicate that the patient is hyperventilating in an attempt to compensate for the metabolic acidosis. A rising $PaCO_2$ in the presence of a persistently low pH and PaO_2 may indicate the need for intubation and mechanical ventilation.

Most patients in shock will be intubated and on mechanical ventilation. Maintaining a patent airway and monitoring for ventilator-related complications are critical. (Artificial airways and mechanical ventilation are discussed in Chapter 64.)

Renal status. Hourly measurements of urinary output are essential in assessment of the adequacy of renal perfusion. An indwelling bladder catheter is inserted to facilitate measurements. Urine output of less than 0.5 ml/kg per hour may indicate inadequate perfusion of the kidneys. BUN and serum creatinine values are additional indicators used to assess renal function. Serum creatinine is a better indicator of renal function because BUN levels can be influenced by the catabolic state of the patient.

Body temperature and skin changes. In the presence of an elevated or subnormal temperature, tympanic or pulmonary arterial temperatures should be obtained hourly. If normal, the temperature should be monitored only every 4 hours. The patient should be kept comfortably warm with the use of light covers and the control of environmental temperature. If the patient's temperature rises above 101.5° F (38.6° C) and the patient becomes uncomfortable or experiences cardiovascular compromise, the fever may be managed with nonsteroidal antiinflammatory drugs (NSAIDs) (e.g., ibuprofen), with acetaminophen, or by removing some of the patient's covers.

The patient's skin should be monitored for pallor, flushing, cyanosis, diaphoresis, or piloerection. In addition, the rapidity of capillary refill should be monitored as an indicator of peripheral perfusion.

Gastrointestinal status. Bowel sounds should be auscultated at least every 4 hours, and abdominal distention should be assessed. If a nasogastric tube is used, the drainage should be measured as part of the fluid output and tested for occult blood. If the patient has a bowel movement, the stool should be checked for occult blood.

Personal hygiene. Hygiene is especially important to the patient in shock because impaired tissue perfusion predisposes the patient to skin breakdown and infection. However, bathing and other nursing measures must be carried out judiciously because a patient in shock is experiencing problems with oxygen delivery to tissues. The nurse must use clinical judgment in determining priorities of care in order to limit the demands for increased oxygen.

Oral care for the patient in shock is essential because mucous membranes may become dry and fragile in the volume-depleted patient. In addition, the intubated patient usually has difficulty swallowing, resulting in pooled secretions in the mouth. A water-soluble lubricant applied to the lips prevents drying and cracking. Moist swabbing of the tongue and oral mucosa with saline solution or diluted mouthwash is also beneficial. Lemon glycerin swabs should not be used because they can cause further drying of the mucosa.

Passive range of motion should be performed three to four times per day to maintain joint mobility. The patient should be turned at least every 1 to 2 hours and positioned in good body alignment to help prevent pressure ulcers. Use of a pressure-relieving mattress or a specialty bed may also be needed. If possible, oxygen consumption (SvO_2) should be monitored during all nursing interventions to monitor the patient's tolerance to activity.

Emotional support and comfort. The effects of anxiety and fear in the face of a critical, life-threatening situation on the patient and family are frequently overlooked or underestimated. Anxiety, fear, and pain may aggravate respiratory distress and increase the release of catecholamines. When implementing care, the nurse should assess and monitor the patient's anxiety and pain. Medication to decrease anxiety and pain are common modes of therapy. Continuous infusions of a benzodiazepine (e.g., lorazepam [Ativan]), a narcotic (e.g., morphine), and occasionally a neuromuscular blocking agent (e.g., pancuronium [Pavulon]) are extremely helpful in decreasing anxiety, pain, and oxygen utilization.

The nurse should talk to the patient, even if the patient is intubated, sedated, and paralyzed or appears comatose. Hearing is often the last sense to be diminished, and even if the patient cannot respond, he or she may still be able to hear. If the intubated patient is capable of writing, a "magic slate" or a pencil and pa-

NURSING RESEARCH
Effects of Positioning Critically Ill Patients on Measures of Tissue Oxygenation

Citation

Banasik JL, Emerson RJ: Effect of lateral positions on tissue oxygenation in the critically ill, *Heart Lung* 30:269, 2001.

Purpose

To determine the effects of lateral positions on tissue oxygenation in adult critical care patients.

Methods

A prospective, quasi-experimental design was used. Critically ill patients (n = 12) who required hemodynamic monitoring, including arterial pressure monitoring, and who were mechanically ventilated were included in the study. All patients had impaired arterial oxygenation (PaO_2 ≤70 mm Hg) and/or cardiac index ≤2.0 L/min/m². Patients were passively turned to each of three positions (supine, 45 degrees right lateral, and 45 degrees left lateral) using a randomized positioning schedule. Data on dependent variables (heart rate, cardiac output, arterial and venous blood gases, oxygen consumption, arterial oxygen content, and serum lactate) were collected 15 minutes after each position change.

Results and Conclusions

Analysis of variance for repeated measures revealed no differences in the dependent variables among the various positions. These findings suggest that positioning patients who are hypoxemic and/or had low cardiac outputs does not further impair tissue oxygenation.

Implications for Nursing Practice

Repositioning critically ill patients to prevent or limit the complications of immobility is essential. Evidence exists that some patients with impaired oxygenation tolerate repositioning without any untoward effects. Nurses should continue to monitor patient responses (i.e., physiologic data) to position changes when caring for them.

per should be provided. Alphabet boards or signboards with common requests (e.g., turn, fan, lights) are also useful. The patient should also receive simple explanations of procedures before they are carried out, as well as information regarding the current plan of care and its rationale. If the patient asks questions about progress and prognosis, simple and honest answers should be given.

Many patients desire a visit from a priest, rabbi, or minister. One way to provide support is to offer to call a member of the clergy rather than wait for the patient or family to express a wish for spiritual counseling.

Family and significant others can have a therapeutic effect on the patient. To perform this role, they need to be supportive and comforting. Family and significant others (1) link the patient to the outside world, (2) facilitate decision making and advise the patient, (3) assist with activities of daily living, (4) act as liaisons to advise the health care team of the patient's wishes for care, and (5) provide safe, caring, familiar relationships for the patient.[20] The fam-

ily primarily needs to be kept informed of the patient's condition. If possible, the same nurses should continuously care for the patient to decrease anxiety, limit contradictory information, and increase trust. Should the prognosis become increasingly grave, the patient's family should be given support when making difficult decisions regarding continuation of life support. The nursing staff must support the family's decisions and facilitate realistic expectations and outcomes. It is important for the nurse to remember that compassionate understanding is as essential as scientific and technical expertise in the total care of a patient and family.

Family time with the patient should be facilitated, provided this time is perceived as comforting by the patient. The nurse should explain in simple terms the purpose of tubes and equipment surrounding the patient, and the family should be informed of what they may and may not touch. If possible, the patient's hands and arms can be kept outside the sheets to encourage therapeutic touch. If desired, the family may be encouraged to perform simple comfort measures. Privacy should be provided as much as possible, but the patient and family should be assured that assistance is readily available should it be required. The call bell should be in reach at all times.

Ambulatory and Home Care. Rehabilitation of the patient who has experienced critical illness necessitates correction of the precipitating cause and prevention or early treatment of complications. The nurse should continue to monitor the patient for indications of complications throughout the recovery period. Complications may include decreased range of motion, decreased physical endurance, chronic renal failure following acute tubular necrosis, and the development of fibrotic lung disease as a result of ARDS (see Chapters 45 and 66). Thus patients recovering from shock may require diverse services on discharge. These can include admission to transitional care units (e.g., for weaning), rehabilitation centers (inpatient or outpatient), or home health care agencies. The nurse should begin to anticipate and facilitate a safe transition from the hospital to home on admission.

■ Evaluation

Expected outcomes for the patient with shock are addressed in NCP 65-1.

SYSTEMIC INFLAMMATORY RESPONSE SYNDROME AND MULTIPLE ORGAN DYSFUNCTION SYNDROME

Etiology and Pathophysiology

Systemic inflammatory response syndrome (SIRS) is a systemic inflammatory response to a variety of insults, including infection, ischemia, infarct, and injury (see Table 65-5). SIRS is characterized by generalized inflammation in organs remote from the initial insult. Normally, the inflammatory process is contained within a confined environment.

A systemic inflammatory response can be triggered by many mechanisms (see Fig. 65-1). Examples include the following:
- Mechanical tissue trauma: burns, crush injuries, surgical procedures
- Abscess formation: intraabdominal, extremities
- Ischemic or necrotic tissue: pancreatitis, vascular disease, myocardial infarction
- Microbial invasion: bacteria, viruses, fungi, parasites

- Endotoxin release: gram-negative bacteria
- Global perfusion deficits: post–cardiac resuscitation
- Regional perfusion deficits: distal perfusion deficits

Multiple organ dysfunction syndrome (MODS) is the failure of more than one organ system in an acutely ill patient such that homeostasis cannot be maintained without intervention (see Table 65-5 and Fig. 65-1). MODS results from SIRS. These two entities represent a continuum, and transition from SIRS to MODS does not occur in a clear-cut manner.[21]

MODS can develop as a result of a primary injury (primary MODS) or a secondary injury (secondary MODS). Primary MODS occurs early and results from a well-defined illness or injury (e.g., pulmonary contusion, aspiration, inhalation injury). Secondary MODS results from uncontrolled systemic inflammation with resultant organ dysfunction. It develops latently, often after many insults.[22]

Organ and Metabolic Dysfunction. When the inflammatory response is not controlled, consequences occur. These include activation of inflammatory cells and release of mediators, direct damage to the endothelium, and hypermetabolism. Vasodilation becomes excessive and leads to decreased SVR and hypotension. In addition, there is also an increase in vascular permeability that allows mediators and protein to leak out of the endothelium and into the interstitial space. The white blood cells begin to phagocytize the foreign debris, and the coagulation cascade is activated (see Chapter 29). Organ perfusion may be compromised because of hypotension, decreased perfusion, microemboli, and redistributed or shunted blood flow.

The respiratory system is often the first system to show signs of dysfunction in SIRS and MODS. Inflammatory mediators have a direct effect on the pulmonary vasculature. The endothelial damage from the release of inflammatory mediators results in an increase in capillary permeability and facilitates movement of proteinaceous fluid from the pulmonary vasculature into the pulmonary interstitial spaces. The fluid then moves to the alveoli, causing alveolar edema. Type I pneumocytes (alveolar cells) are destroyed. Type II pneumocytes become dysfunctional, and there is a decrease in surfactant production. The alveoli collapse, creating an increase in *shunt* (blood flow to the lungs that does not participate in gas exchange) and a worsening of the ventilation perfusion mismatch. The end result is ARDS. Patients with ARDS require aggressive pulmonary management with mechanical ventilation. (See Chapter 66 for a complete discussion of ARDS.)

Cardiovascular changes include myocardial depression and massive vasodilation in response to increasing tissue demands. Vasodilation results in decreased SVR (decreased afterload) and decreased blood pressure. The baroreceptor reflex causes release of *inotropic* (increasing force of contraction) and *chronotropic* (increasing heart rate) factors that enhance cardiac output. To compensate for hypotension, CO increases by an increase in heart rate and stroke volume. Increases in capillary permeability cause a shift of albumin and fluid out of the vascular space, further diminishing venous return and thus preload. The patient becomes warm and tachycardic with a high CO and a low SVR. Other signs include poor capillary refill, skin mottling, increased CVP and PAWP, and arrhythmias. SvO$_2$ may be abnormally high because the patient is perfusing areas not consuming much oxy-

gen (e.g., skin, nonworking muscle) while other areas may have blood shunted away from them. Eventually, either perfusion of vital organs becomes insufficient or the cells are unable to use oxygen and their function is compromised. As MODS progresses, myocardial dysfunction worsens.[23] The effects of SIRS and MODS on hemodynamic parameters are summarized in Table 65-2.

Neurologic dysfunction commonly manifests as mental status changes with SIRS and MODS. Acute alteration in mental status can be an early sign of MODS. The patient may become confused and agitated, combative, disoriented, lethargic, or comatose. These changes may be due to hypoxemia, the direct effect of the inflammatory mediators, or impaired perfusion. Mediators may damage neuronal tissue directly or indirectly via capillary leakage and related tissue damage. This in turn may produce cerebral edema, resulting in increased intracranial pressure.[24]

Acute renal failure (ARF) is frequently seen in SIRS and MODS. ARF can be caused not only by hypoperfusion but also by the effects of the mediators. When there is decreased perfusion to the kidneys, the SNS and the renin-angiotensin system are activated. The stimulation of the renin-angiotensin system results in systemic vasoconstriction and aldosterone-mediated sodium and water reabsorption. Another risk factor for the development of ARF is the use of nephrotoxic drugs. Antibiotics commonly used to treat gram-negative bacteria, such as aminoglycosides, can also be nephrotoxic. Careful monitoring of drug levels is essential to avoid the nephrotoxic effects.

The GI tract also plays a key role in the development of MODS. In the early stages of SIRS and MODS, the highly vascular GI mucosa has blood shunted away, making it highly vulnerable to ischemic injury. Decreased perfusion leads to a breakdown of this normally protective mucosal barrier, thus increasing the risk for ulceration and GI bleeding. With the breakdown of the mucosal barrier of the gut, bacteria translocate from the GI tract into circulation, resulting in the development of bacteremia. Gastrointestinal motility is also decreased in critical illness, causing abdominal distention and paralytic ileus.

Metabolic changes are pronounced in SIRS and MODS. Both syndromes trigger a hypermetabolic response. Glycogen stores are rapidly converted to glucose (glycogenolysis). Once glycogen is depleted, amino acids are converted to glucose (gluconeogenesis), reducing protein stores. Fatty acids are mobilized for fuel. Catecholamines and glucocorticoids are released and result in hyperglycemia and insulin resistance. The net result is a catabolic state, and lean body mass (muscle) is lost.

The hypermetabolism that is associated with SIRS and MODS may last for several days and results in liver dysfunction. Liver dysfunction in MODS may exist long before clinical evidence is present. Protein synthesis is impaired. The liver is unable to synthesize albumin, one of the key proteins that has an essential role in maintaining plasma oncotic pressure. Consequently, plasma oncotic pressure is altered and fluid and protein leak from the vascular spaces to the interstitial space. Administration of albumin does not normalize oncotic pressure in these patients.

As the state of hypermetabolism persists, the patient is unable to convert lactate to glucose, and lactate accumulates (lactic acidosis). Despite increases in glycogenolysis and gluconeogenesis, eventually the liver is unable to maintain a glucose level and the patient becomes hypoglycemic.

TABLE 65-11   Multiple Organ Dysfunction Syndrome: Clinical Manifestations and Management

SYSTEM	CLINICAL MANIFESTATIONS OF ORGAN FAILURE	MANAGEMENT
Respiratory	Development of ARDS (see Chapter 66): • Severe dyspnea • PaO_2/FIO_2 ratio <200 • Bilateral fluffy infiltrates on chest x-ray • PAWP <18 mm Hg • Ventilation-perfusion ($\dot{V}/\dot{Q}$) mismatch • Pulmonary hypertension • Increased minute ventilation • Increased respiratory rate • Decreased compliance • Refractory hypoxemia	Prevention Optimize oxygen delivery/minimize oxygen consumption Mechanical ventilation (see Chapter 64) • Positive end-expiratory pressure • Pressure control inverse ratio ventilation • Permissive hypercapnia Positioning (e.g., continuous lateral rotation therapy, prone positioning)
Renal	Prerenal: renal hypoperfusion • BUN/creatinine ratio >20:1 • ↓ Urine Na^+ <20 mEq/L • ↑ Urine specific gravity >1.020 • ↑ Urine osmolality Intrarenal: acute tubular necrosis • BUN/creatinine ratio <10:1-15:1 • ↑ Urine Na^+ >20 mEq/L • ↓ Urine osmolality • Urine specific gravity (~1.010)	Diuretics • Loop diuretics (e.g., furosemide [Lasix]) • May need to increase dose due to ↓ glomerular filtration rate Dopamine (Intropin) • Enhances renal blood flow • Improves renal perfusion • Increases urine output (if volume resuscitated) • May work synergistically with diuretics Renal replacement therapy (see Chapter 45)
Hepatic	Bilirubin >2 mg/dl (34 μmol/L) ↑ Liver enzymes (ALT, AST, GGT) ↑ Serum NH_3 ↓ Serum albumin, prealbumin, transferrin Jaundice Hepatic encephalopathy	Maintain adequate tissue perfusion Provide nutritional support (e.g., enteral feedings) Judicious use of hepatically metabolized drugs
Gastrointestinal	Mucosal ischemia • ↓ Intramucosal pH • Gut "leakiness" → translocation of gut bacteria Hypoperfusion → ↓ peristalsis, paralytic ileus Mucosal ulceration on endoscopy GI bleeding	Stress ulcer prophylaxis • Antacids (e.g., Maalox) • Histamine H_2 receptor blockers (e.g., cimetidine [Tagamet]) • Proton pump inhibitors (e.g., omeprazole [Prilosec]) • Sucralfate (Carafate) Enteral feedings • Stimulate mucosal activity • Provide nutrients
Central Nervous	Acute change in neurologic status Fever Hepatic encephalopathy Seizures Confusion/disorientation Failure to wean/prolonged rehabilitation	Evaluate for hepatic/metabolic encephalopathy Optimize cerebral blood flow ↓ Cerebral oxygen requirements Prevent secondary tissue ischemia • Calcium channel blockers (reduce cerebral vasospasm) Prevent further compromise
Cardiovascular	Myocardial depression Biventricular failure Systolic/diastolic dysfunction ↑ HR/CO/SVR ↓ Stroke volume ↓ MAP ↓ Ejection fraction/contractility	Volume management • PA catheter for hemodynamic monitoring • ↑ preload via volume replacement • Maximize myocardial function • Maintain CO • Maintain MAP >60 mm Hg Vasopressors Balance O_2 supply and demand Continuous ECG monitoring Circulatory assist devices • Intraaortic balloon pump • Ventricular assist device

ALT, Alanine aminotransferase; *ARDS,* acute respiratory distress syndrome; *AST,* aspartate aminotransferase; *BUN,* blood urea nitrogen; *CO,* cardiac output; *ECG,* electrocardiogram; *GGT,* gamma-glutamyl transferase; *GI,* gastrointestinal; *MAP,* mean arterial pressure; *PA,* pulmonary artery; *PAWP,* pulmonary artery wedge pressure; *SVR,* systemic vascular resistance.

TABLE 65-11	Multiple Organ Dysfunction Syndrome: Clinical Manifestations and Management—cont'd	
SYSTEM	**CLINICAL MANIFESTATIONS OF ORGAN FAILURE**	**MANAGEMENT**
Hematologic	↑ Bleeding times, ↑ PT, ↑ PTT ↓ Platelet count (thrombocytopenia) ↑ Fibrin split products ↑ D-dimer test	Observe for bleeding from obvious and/or occult sites Replace factors being lost (e.g., platelets) Minimize traumatic interventions (e.g., intramuscular injections, multiple venipunctures)

PT, prothrombin time; *PTT*, partial thromboplastin time.

Failure of the coagulation system manifests as DIC. DIC results in simultaneous microvascular clotting and bleeding because of the depletion of clotting factors and platelets and excessive fibrinolysis. (DIC is discussed in Chapter 30.)

Electrolyte imbalances, which are common, are related to hormonal and metabolic changes and fluid shifts. These changes exacerbate mental status changes, neuromuscular dysfunction, and arrhythmias. The release of antidiuretic hormone and aldosterone results in sodium and water retention. Aldosterone increases urinary potassium loss, and catecholamines cause potassium to move into the cell, resulting in hypokalemia. Hypokalemia is associated with arrhythmias and muscle weakness. Metabolic acidosis results from impaired tissue perfusion, hypoxia, and a shift to anaerobic metabolism with a resultant increase in hydrogen ion production. Progressive renal dysfunction also contributes to metabolic acidosis. Hypocalcemia, hypomagnesemia, and hypophosphatemia are common.

Clinical Manifestations of SIRS and MODS

The defining manifestations of SIRS and MODS are delineated in Table 65-5. The clinical manifestations of MODS are presented in Table 65-11.

NURSING *and* COLLABORATIVE MANAGEMENT
SIRS AND MODS

The prognosis for the patient with MODS is poor, with estimated mortality rates at 90% to 95% when three or more organ systems fail.[24] Therefore the most important goal is to prevent the progression of SIRS to MODS. A critical component of the nursing role is vigilant assessment and ongoing monitoring to detect early signs of deterioration or organ dysfunction.

Collaborative care for patients with MODS focuses on (1) prevention and treatment of infection, (2) maintenance of tissue oxygenation, (3) nutritional and metabolic support, and (4) appropriate support of individual failing organs. Table 65-11 summarizes the management for patients with MODS.

■ Prevention and Treatment of Infection

Aggressive infection control strategies are essential to decrease the risk for nosocomial infections. Despite aggressive strategies, host dysfunction may lead to the development of an infection. Once an infection is suspected, interventions to control the source must be instituted. Appropriate cultures should be sent, and broad-spectrum antibiotic therapy should be initiated. Early, aggressive surgery is recommended to remove necrotic tissue (e.g., early debridement of burn tissue) that may provide a culture medium for microorganisms. Once a specific organism is identified, therapy should be modified. Aggressive pulmonary management, including early ambulation, can reduce the risk of infection. Strict asepsis can decrease infections related to intraarterial lines, endotracheal tubes, urinary catheters, IV lines, and other invasive devices or procedures.

■ Maintenance of Tissue Oxygenation

Hypoxemia frequently occurs in patients with SIRS or MODS. These patients have greater oxygen needs and decreased oxygen supply to the tissues. Interventions that decrease oxygen demand and increase oxygen delivery are essential. Sedation, mechanical ventilation, analgesia, paralysis, and rest may decrease oxygen demand and should be considered. Oxygen delivery may be increased by maintaining normal levels of hemoglobin (e.g., transfusion of packed RBCs) and PaO_2 (80 to 100 mm Hg), using positive end-expiratory pressure (PEEP), increasing preload or myocardial contractility to enhance cardiac output, or reducing afterload to increase cardiac output.

■ Nutritional and Metabolic Needs

Hypermetabolism in SIRS or MODS can result in profound weight loss, cachexia, and further organ failure. Protein-calorie malnutrition is one of the primary manifestations of hypermetabolism and MODS. Total energy expenditure is often increased 1.5 to 2.0 times the normal metabolic rate. Because of their relatively short half-life, plasma transferrin and prealbumin levels are monitored to assess hepatic protein synthesis.

The goal of nutritional support is to preserve organ function. Providing adequate nutrition decreases morbidity and mortality rates in patients with SIRS and MODS. The use of the enteral route is preferable to parenteral nutrition and may limit translocation of gut bacteria. If the enteral route cannot be used, parenteral nutrition should be initiated. (Enteral and parenteral nutrition are discussed in Chapter 39.)

■ Support of Failing Organs

Support of any failing organ is a primary goal of therapy. For example, the patient with ARDS requires aggressive oxygen therapy and mechanical ventilation (see Chapter 64). DIC should be treated appropriately (e.g., blood products) (see Chapter 30). Renal failure may require renal replacement therapy. Continuous renal replacement therapy is better tolerated than hemodialysis, especially in a patient with hemodynamic instability (see Chapter 45).

CRITICAL THINKING EXERCISES

Case Study
Shock

Patient Profile. Mr. S., a 25-year-old Korean American, was an unrestrained driver involved in a motor vehicle crash. He was found face down 15 feet from his car. There were no passengers. The windshield was broken and the car was found up against a tree. Mr. S. was found conscious and moaning. He was taken to the emergency department (ED).

Subjective Data
- States, "I can't breathe."
- Cries out when abdomen is palpated.

Objective Data
Physical Examination
- Cardiovascular: BP 84/70; apical pulse 120 but no radial or brachial pulses palpable; carotid pulse present but weak
- Lungs: respiratory rate 35/min; labored breathing with severe respiratory distress; asymmetric chest wall movement; absence of breath sounds on left side
- Abdomen: slightly distended and painful on palpation

Diagnostic Studies
- Chest x-ray: hemopneumothorax and rib fractures on left side
- Hematocrit: 28%

Collaborative Care
- In the ED, placement of chest tube, which drained bright red blood

Surgical Procedure
- Splenectomy
- Repair of torn thoracic artery

CRITICAL THINKING QUESTIONS
1. What type of shock was present in Mr. S.? What clinical manifestations did he display?
2. What were the causes of Mr. S.'s shock? What are other causes of this type of shock?
3. What are the initial nursing responsibilities for Mr. S.?
4. What continual nursing assessment parameters are essential for this patient?
5. Based on the assessment data presented, write one or more nursing diagnoses. Are there any collaborative problems?

Nursing Research Issues
1. What nursing measures can be implemented to conserve oxygen and decrease oxygen utilization in patients with shock or MODS?
2. Which patient positions maximize oxygenation and circulatory status in patients with different types of shock?
3. Is there a difference in the accuracy of the following BP monitoring devices used to detect BP changes in shock: invasive arterial monitoring versus noninvasive devices?

REVIEW QUESTIONS

The number of the question corresponds to the same-numbered objective at the beginning of the chapter.

1. Shock is best defined as
   a. cardiovascular collapse.
   b. loss of sympathetic tone.
   c. inadequate tissue perfusion.
   d. blood pressure less than 90 mm Hg systolic.

2. A patient has a spinal cord injury at T4. Vital signs include a falling blood pressure with bradycardia. The nurse recognizes that the patient is experiencing
   a. a relative hypervolemia.
   b. an absolute hypovolemia.
   c. neurogenic shock from low blood flow.
   d. neurogenic shock from a maldistribution of blood flow.

3. The effect that shock has on the body includes
   a. sympathetic nervous system activation that results in stimulation of adrenergic receptors.
   b. massive vasoconstriction in the heart and brain that causes stimulation of the renin-angiotensin system.
   c. heart rate that is usually slow and irregular in the compensatory stage because of parasympathetic nervous stimulation.
   d. decreased tissue perfusion that causes the cells to undergo aerobic metabolism, leading to the development of lactic acidosis.

4. A 78-year-old man has confusion and temperature of 104° F (40° C). He is a diabetic with purulent drainage from his right great toe. His hemodynamic findings are BP 84/40; heart rate 110; respiratory rate 42 and shallow; CO 8 L/min; and PAWP 4 mm Hg. This patient's symptoms are most likely indicative of
   a. sepsis.
   b. septic shock.
   c. multiple organ dysfunction syndrome.
   d. systemic inflammatory response syndrome.

5. Appropriate treatment modalities for the management of cardiogenic shock include
   a. dopamine to increase myocardial contractility.
   b. vasopressors to increase systemic vascular resistance.
   c. corticosteroids to stabilize the cell wall in the infarcted myocardium.
   d. plasma volume expanders such as albumin to decrease an elevated preload.

6. The most accurate assessment parameters for the nurse to use to determine adequate tissue perfusion in the patient with MODS are
   a. blood pressure, pulse, and respirations.
   b. breath sounds, blood pressure, and body temperature.
   c. pulse pressure, level of consciousness, and pupillary response.
   d. level of consciousness, urine output, and skin color and temperature.

REFERENCES

1. Rice V: *Shock, a clinical syndrome,* ed 2, Aliso Viejo, Calif, 1997, American Association of Critical Care Nurses.
2. Edwards S: Shock: types, classifications and explorations of their physiological effects, *Emergency Nurse* 9:29, 2001.
3. Silvestry FE, Herling IM: Cardiogenic shock and other pump failure states. In Lanken PE, Hanson CW, Manaker S, editors: *Intensive care manual,* Philadelphia, 2001, WB Saunders.
4. Prieto A, Eisenberg J, Thakur RK: Nonarrhythmic complications of acute myocardial infarction, *Emerg Med Clin North Am* 19:397, 2001.
5. Hand H: Myocardial infarction, part II, *Nursing Standard* 15:45, 2001.
6. Mower-Wade DM et al: Shock: do you know how to respond? *Nursing* 30:34, 2000.
7. DoNofrio D, Loh E: Cardiogenic pulmonary edema. In Lanken PE, Hanson CW, Manaker S, editors: *Intensive care manual,* Philadelphia, 2001, WB Saunders.
8. Schiller HJ, Anderson HL: Hemorrhagic shock and other low preload states. In Lanken PE, Hanson CW, Manaker S, editors: *Intensive care manual,* Philadelphia, 2001, WB Saunders.
9. Marcotte P, Freese A: Spinal injury. In Lanken PE, Hanson CW, Manaker S, editors: *Intensive care manual,* Philadelphia, 2001, WB Saunders.
10. Jurewicz MA: Anaphylaxis: when the body over reacts, *Nursing* 30:58, 2000.
11. Balk RA: Severe sepsis and septic shock: definitions, epidemiology, and clinical manifestations, *Crit Care Clin* 16:179, 2000.
12. Lent M, Hirshberg P, Margolis G: Systemic toxins: signs, symptoms and management of patients in septic shock, *JEMS* 26:54, 2001.
13. Manaker S: Septic shock and other low afterload states. In Lanken PE, Hanson CW, Manaker S, editors: *Intensive care manual,* Philadelphia, 2001, WB Saunders.
14. Collins T: Understanding shock, *Nursing Standard* 14:35, 2000.
15. McQuillan KA: Initial management of traumatic shock. In McQuillan K et al: *Trauma nursing from resuscitation through rehabilitation,* ed 3, Philadelphia, 2002, WB Saunders.
16. DeJong MJ, Karch AM: *Lippincott's critical care drug guide,* Philadelphia, 2000, Lippincott.
17. Jindal N, Hollenberg SM, Dellinger RP: Pharmacologic issues in the management of septic shock, *Crit Care Clin* 16:233, 2000.
*18. Hollenberg SM et al: Practice parameters for hemodynamic support of sepsis in adult patients in sepsis, *Crit Care Med* 27:639, 1999.
19. Bernard GR et al: Efficacy and safety to recombinant human activated protein C for sever sepsis, *N Engl J Med* 344:699, 2001.
*20. Eichhorn DJ et al: Family presence during invasive procedures and resuscitation: hearing the voice of the patient, *Am J Nurs* 101:48, 2001.
21. Cryer HG et al: Multiple organ failure: by the time you predict it, it's already there, *J Trauma* 46:597, 1999.
22. Evans TW, Smithies M: ABCs of intensive care: organ dysfunction, *Br J Med* 318:1606, 1999.
23. Marshall JC: Inflammation, coagulopathy, and the pathogenesis of multiple organ dysfunction syndrome, *Crit Care Med* 29:S99, 2001.
24. Johnson D, Mayers I: Multiple organ dysfunction syndrome: a narrative review, *Can J Anaesth* 48:502, 2001.

RESOURCES

Resources for this chapter are listed after Chapter 64 on page 1795 and Chapter 67 on page 1868.

*Nursing research–based reference.

CHAPTER 66
NURSING MANAGEMENT
Respiratory Failure and Acute Respiratory Distress Syndrome

Richard B. Arbour

LEARNING OBJECTIVES

1. Compare the pathophysiologic mechanisms that result in hypoxemic and hypercapnic respiratory failure.
2. Differentiate between early and late clinical manifestations of acute respiratory failure.
3. Describe the nursing and collaborative management of the patient with hypoxemic or hypercapnic respiratory failure.
4. Relate the pathophysiologic mechanisms that result in acute respiratory distress syndrome (ARDS) to the clinical manifestations.
5. Describe the nursing and collaborative management of the patient with ARDS.
6. Identify complications that may result from acute respiratory failure or ARDS and measures to prevent or reverse these complications.

KEY TERMS

acute respiratory distress syndrome, p. 1837
alveolar hypoventilation, p. 1827
diffusion limitation, p. 1827
hypercapnia, p. 1824
hypercapnic respiratory failure, p. 1825

hypoxemia, p. 1824
hypoxemic respiratory failure, p. 1824
hypoxia, p. 1829
refractory hypoxemia, p. 1839
shunt, p. 1827

ACUTE RESPIRATORY FAILURE

The major function of the respiratory system is gas exchange, which involves the transfer of oxygen (O_2) and carbon dioxide (CO_2) between the atmosphere and the blood (Fig. 66-1).[1] *Respiratory failure* results when one or both of these gas-exchanging functions are inadequate. For example, insufficient O_2 is transferred to the blood or inadequate CO_2 is removed from the lungs. Clinical states that interfere with adequate O_2 transfer result in **hypoxemia,** which is manifested by a decrease in arterial O_2 tension (PaO_2) and a decrease in arterial O_2 saturation (SaO_2). Insufficient CO_2 removal results in **hypercapnia,** which is manifested by an increase in arterial CO_2 tension ($PaCO_2$).[2] Arterial blood gases (ABGs) can be used to assess changes in pH, PaO_2, $PaCO_2$, and SaO_2, and pulse oximetry can be used to intermittently or continuously assess arterial oxygen saturation (SpO_2). Data should be interpreted within the context of the clinical assessment findings, as well as the patient's baseline. For example, an individual with chronic lung disease may have a baseline $PaCO_2$ higher than what is considered the "normal" range.

Respiratory failure is not a disease; it is a condition that occurs as a result of one or more diseases involving the lungs or other body systems (Tables 66-1 and 66-2). Respiratory failure can be classified as hypoxemic or hypercapnic (Fig. 66-2). Hypoxemic respiratory failure is also referred to as *oxygenation failure* because the primary problem is inadequate O_2 transfer between the alveoli and the pulmonary capillary bed.[2,3] Although no universal definition exists, **hypoxemic respiratory failure** is commonly defined as a PaO_2 of 60 mm Hg or less when the patient is receiving an inspired O_2 concentration of 60% or greater. This definition incorporates two important concepts: (1) the PaO_2 is at a level that indicates inadequate O_2 saturation of hemoglo-

Glossary of Abbreviations

Arterial Blood Monitoring

ABGs	Arterial blood gases
pH	Negative log of the free hydrogen ion [H$^+$]
PaO_2	Partial pressure of oxygen in arterial blood
$PaCO_2$	Partial pressure of carbon dioxide in arterial blood
SaO_2	Oxygen saturation in arterial blood measured by ABGs
SpO_2	Oxygen saturation in arterial blood measured by pulse oximetry

Oxygen and Lung Function Monitoring

FIO_2	Fraction of inspired oxygen concentration
FRC	Functional residual capacity (volume of air in lung at end of expiration)
PEEP	Positive end-expiratory pressure (pressure in lungs at end of expiration)
PEFR	Peak expiratory flow rate (maximum airflow during a forced expiration)
$\dot{V}/\dot{Q}$	Ventilation/perfusion ratio (relationship of ventilation to perfusion in the lungs)
V_E	Minute ventilation (product of tidal volume times respiratory rate)
V_T	Tidal volume (volume of air inspired with each breath)

Reviewed by John J. Gallagher, RN, MSN, CCNS, CCRN, CEN, RRT, Clinical Nurse Specialist for Critical Care, Crozer Chester Medical Center, Upland, Pa.

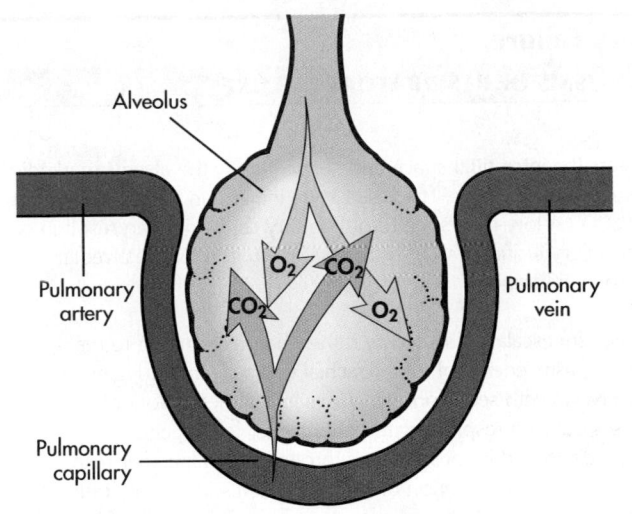

FIG. 66-1 Normal gas exchange unit in the lung.

TABLE 66-1	Types of Respiratory Failure and Common Causes
HYPOXEMIC RESPIRATORY FAILURE*	**HYPERCAPNIC RESPIRATORY FAILURE***
Respiratory System	**Respiratory System**
Acute respiratory distress syndrome	Asthma
Pneumonia	COPD
Toxic inhalation (smoke inhalation)	Cystic fibrosis
Hepatopulmonary syndrome (low-resistance flow state, $\dot{V}/\dot{Q}$ mismatch)	**Central Nervous System**
	Brainstem infarction
	Sedative and narcotic over-dose
Massive pulmonary embolism (e.g., thrombus emboli, fat emboli)	Spinal cord injury
	Severe head injury
Cardiac System	**Chest Wall**
Anatomic shunt (ventricular septal defect)	Thoracic trauma (e.g., flail chest)
	Kyphoscoliosis
Cardiogenic pulmonary edema	Pain
Shock (decreasing blood flow through pulmonary vasculature)	Massive obesity
	Neuromuscular System
	Myasthenia gravis
	Critical illness polyneuropathy
	Acute myopathy
	Toxic ingestion (tree tobacco)
	Amyotrophic lateral sclerosis
	Phrenic nerve injury
	Guillain-Barré syndrome
	Poliomyelitis
	Muscular dystrophy
	Multiple sclerosis

*This list is not all-inclusive.
COPD, Chronic obstructive pulmonary disease.

bin; and (2) this PaO$_2$ level exists despite administration of supplemental O$_2$ at a percentage (60%) that is about three times that in room air (21%). Disorders that interfere with O$_2$ transfer into the blood include pneumonia, pulmonary edema, pulmonary emboli, and alveolar injury related to inhalation of toxic gases (e.g., smoke inhalation). In addition, low-cardiac-output states (e.g., congestive heart failure, shock) can also cause hypoxemic respiratory failure.[1]

Hypercapnic respiratory failure is also referred to as *ventilatory failure* because the primary problem is insufficient CO$_2$ removal. **Hypercapnic respiratory failure** is commonly defined as a PaCO$_2$ above normal (greater than 45 mm Hg) in combination with acidemia (arterial pH less than 7.35). This definition incorporates three important concepts: (1) the PaCO$_2$ is higher than normal; (2) there is evidence of the body's inability to compensate for this increase (acidemia); and (3) the pH is at a level where a further decrease may lead to severe acid-base imbalance. (See Chapter 16 for a discussion of acid-base balance.) Disorders that compromise lung ventilation and subsequent CO$_2$ removal include drug overdoses with central nervous system (CNS) depressants, neuromuscular diseases (e.g., myasthenia gravis), and trauma or diseases involving the spinal cord and its role in lung ventilation. Many patients experience both hypoxemic and hypercapnic respiratory failure.

Etiology and Pathophysiology

Hypoxemic Respiratory Failure. Common diseases and conditions that cause hypoxemic respiratory failure are listed in Table 66-1. Four physiologic mechanisms may cause hypoxemia and subsequent hypoxemic respiratory failure: (1) mismatch between ventilation ($\dot{V}$) and perfusion ($\dot{Q}$), commonly referred to as $\dot{V}/\dot{Q}$ mismatch; (2) shunt; (3) diffusion limitation; and (4) hypoventilation. The most common causes are $\dot{V}/\dot{Q}$ mismatch and shunt.[1-3]

Ventilation-perfusion ($\dot{V}/\dot{Q}$) mismatch. In the normal lung, the volume of blood perfusing the lungs each minute (4 to 5 L) is approximately equal to the amount of fresh gas that reaches the alveoli each minute (4 to 5 L). In a perfectly matched system, each portion of the lung would receive about 1 ml of air for each 1 ml of blood flow. This match of ventilation and perfusion

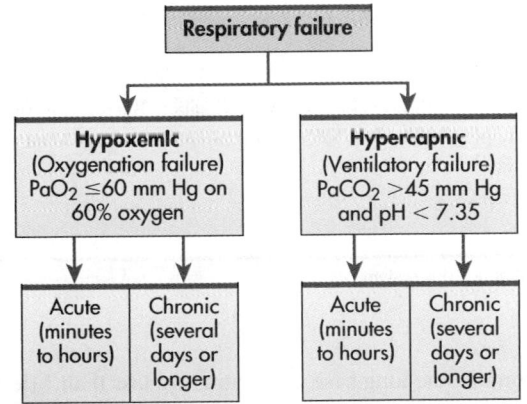

FIG. 66-2 Classification of respiratory failure.

would result in a $\dot{V}/\dot{Q}$ ratio of 1:1 (e.g., 1 ml of air per 1 ml of blood), which is expressed as $\dot{V}/\dot{Q} = 1$. Ventilation is ideally matched with perfusion.

Although this example implies that ventilation and perfusion are ideally matched in all areas of the lung, this situation does not normally exist. In reality, there is some regional mismatch. At the lung apex, $\dot{V}/\dot{Q}$ ratios are greater than 1 (more ventilation than

TABLE 66-2	Predisposing Factors for Acute Respiratory Failure
PREDISPOSING FACTORS	**MECHANISMS OF RESPIRATORY FAILURE**
Airways and Alveoli	
Acute respiratory distress syndrome *Direct lung injury:* aspiration; severe, disseminated pulmonary infection; near-drowning; toxic gas inhalation; or airway contusion *Indirect lung injury:* sepsis/septic shock, severe nonthoracic trauma, cardiopulmonary bypass	Fluid enters the interstitial space and subsequently the alveoli, markedly impairing gas exchange. The result is an initial ↓ in PaO_2 and later an ↑ in $PaCO_2$. A low-flow state to pulmonary capillaries can result in ischemic injury to lung tissues with loss of integrity of the alveolar-capillary membrane.
Asthma	Bronchospasm escalates in severity rather than responding to therapy. Bronchospasm, edema of the bronchial mucosa, and plugging of small airways with secretions greatly reduce airflow. Work of breathing increases, causing respiratory muscle fatigue. ↓ PaO_2 and ↑ $PaCO_2$.
Chronic obstructive pulmonary disease (COPD)	Alveoli are destroyed by protease-antiprotease imbalance or respiratory infection, or an exacerbation of COPD escalates in severity rather than responding to therapy. Secretions obstruct airflow. Work of breathing increases and causes respiratory muscle fatigue. ↓ PaO_2 and ↑ $PaCO_2$.
Cystic fibrosis	Abnormal Na^+ and Cl^- transport produces secretions that are viscous, poorly cleared, and therefore foci for infection. Over time the airways become clogged with copious, purulent, often greenish colored sputum. Secretions obstruct airflow. Repeated infections destroy alveoli. Work of breathing increases, causing respiratory muscle fatigue. ↓ PaO_2 and ↑ $PaCO_2$.
Central Nervous System	
Narcotic or other drug overdose with CNS depressant	Respirations slowed by drug effect. Insufficient CO_2 is excreted, resulting in ↑ $PaCO_2$.
Brainstem infarction, head injury	Medulla cannot alter respiratory rate in response to changes in $PaCO_2$.
Chest Wall	
Severe soft tissue injury, flail chest, rib fracture, pain	Prevent normal rib cage expansion resulting in inadequate gas exchange.
Kyphoscoliosis	Change in spinal configuration compresses the lungs and prevents normal expansion of the chest wall.
Massive obesity	Weight of the chest and abdominal contents prevents normal rib cage movement.
Neuromuscular Conditions	
Cervical cord injury, phrenic nerve injury	Neural control is lost, preventing use of the diaphragm, the major muscle of respiration. As a consequence, the patient inspires a smaller tidal volume, which predisposes to an ↑ in $PaCO_2$.
Amyotrophic lateral sclerosis (ALS), Guillain-Barré, muscular dystrophy, multiple sclerosis, poliomyelitis, myasthenia gravis	Respiratory muscle weakness or paralysis occurs, preventing normal CO_2 excretion. Dysfunction may be slowly progressive (muscular dystrophy, multiple sclerosis), progressive with no potential of recovery (ALS), rapid with good expectation of recovery (Guillain-Barré), or stable for extended periods of time (poliomyelitis, myasthenia gravis).

CNS, Central nervous system.

perfusion). At the lung base, $\dot{V}/\dot{Q}$ ratios are less than 1 (less ventilation than perfusion). Because changes at the lung apex balance changes at the base, the net effect is a close overall match (Fig. 66-3).

Many diseases and conditions alter overall $\dot{V}/\dot{Q}$ matching and thus cause $\dot{V}/\dot{Q}$ *mismatch* (Fig. 66-4). The most common are those in which increased secretions are present in the airways (e.g., chronic obstructive pulmonary disease [COPD]), alveoli (e.g., pneumonia), and when bronchospasm is present (e.g., asthma). $\dot{V}/\dot{Q}$ mismatch may also result from alveolar collapse (atelectasis) or as a result of pain. Unrelieved or inadequately relieved pain interferes with chest and abdominal wall movement,

compromising lung ventilation. Additionally, pain increases muscle and motor tension, producing generalized muscle rigidity; causes systemic vasoconstriction and activation of the stress response; and increases O_2 consumption and CO_2 production.[4,5] All of these conditions result in limited airflow (ventilation) to alveoli but have no effect on blood flow (perfusion) to the gas exchange units.[4] The consequence is $\dot{V}/\dot{Q}$ mismatch. A pulmonary embolus affects the perfusion portion of the $\dot{V}/\dot{Q}$ relationship. The embolus limits blood flow but has no effect on airflow to the alveoli, again causing $\dot{V}/\dot{Q}$ mismatch (see Fig. 66-4).

O_2 therapy is an appropriate first step to reverse hypoxemia caused by $\dot{V}/\dot{Q}$ mismatch because not all gas exchange units are

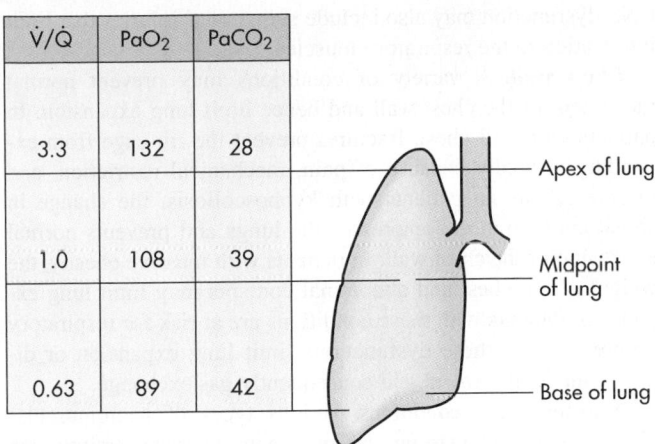

V̇/Q̇	PaO₂	PaCO₂
3.3	132	28
1.0	108	39
0.63	89	42

— Apex of lung

— Midpoint of lung

— Base of lung

FIG. 66-3 Regional $\dot{V}/\dot{Q}$ differences in the normal lung. At the lung apex, the $\dot{V}/\dot{Q}$ ratio is 3.3, at the midpoint 1.0, and at the base 0.63. This difference causes the PaO₂ to be higher at the apex of the lung and lower at the base. Values for PaCO₂ are the opposite (i.e., lower at the apex and higher at the base). Blood that exits the lung is a mixture of these values.

affected. O₂ therapy increases the PaO₂ in blood leaving normal gas exchange units, thus causing a higher than normal PaO₂. The well-oxygenated blood mixes with poorly oxygenated blood, raising the overall PaO₂ of blood leaving the lungs. Ultimately, the optimal approach to hypoxemia caused by a $\dot{V}/\dot{Q}$ mismatch is one directed at the cause.

Shunt. Shunt occurs when blood exits the heart without having participated in gas exchange. A shunt can be viewed as an extreme $\dot{V}/\dot{Q}$ mismatch (see Fig. 66-4). There are two types of shunt: anatomic and intrapulmonary. An *anatomic shunt* occurs when blood passes through an anatomic channel in the heart (e.g., a ventricular septal defect) and therefore does not pass through the lungs. An *intrapulmonary shunt* occurs when blood flows through the pulmonary capillaries without participating in gas exchange. Intrapulmonary shunt is seen in conditions in which the alveoli fill with fluid (e.g., acute respiratory distress syndrome [ARDS], pneumonia, pulmonary edema). O₂ therapy alone may be ineffective in increasing the PaO₂ if hypoxemia is due to shunt because (1) blood passes from the right to the left side of the heart without passing through the lungs (anatomic shunt); or (2) the alveoli are filled with fluid, which prevents gas exchange (intrapulmonary shunt). Patients with shunt are usually more hypoxemic than patients with $\dot{V}/\dot{Q}$ mismatch, and they may require mechanical ventilation and a high fraction of inspired oxygen (FIO₂) to improve gas exchange.

Diffusion limitation. Diffusion limitation occurs when gas exchange across the alveolar-capillary membrane is compromised by a process that thickens or destroys the membrane (Fig. 66-5). Diffusion limitation can also be worsened by conditions that affect the pulmonary vascular bed such as severe emphysema or recurrent pulmonary emboli. Some diseases cause the alveolar-capillary membrane to become thicker (fibrotic), which slows gas transport. These diseases include pulmonary fibrosis, interstitial lung disease, and ARDS. Diffusion limitation is more likely to cause hypoxemia during exercise than at rest. During exercise, blood moves more rapidly through the lungs. Because transit time is increased, red blood cells are in the lungs for a shorter time, de-

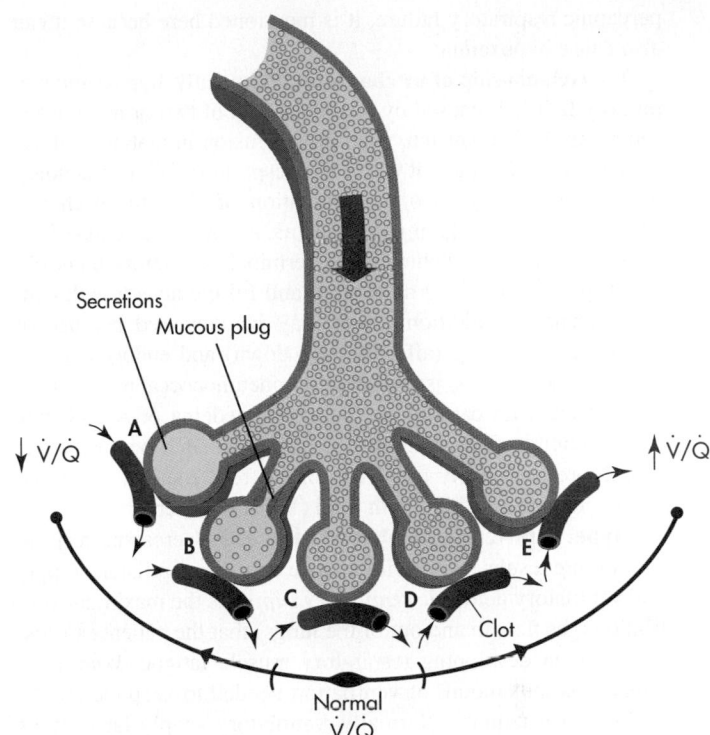

Secretions

Mucous plug

$\downarrow \dot{V}/\dot{Q}$ $\uparrow \dot{V}/\dot{Q}$

A   B   C   D   E

Clot

Normal
$\dot{V}/\dot{Q}$

FIG. 66-4 Range of ventilation to perfusion ($\dot{V}/\dot{Q}$) relationships. **A,** Absolute shunt, no ventilation due to fluid filling the alveoli. **B,** $\dot{V}/\dot{Q}$ mismatch, ventilation partially compromised by secretions in the airway. **C,** Normal lung unit. **D,** $\dot{V}/\dot{Q}$ mismatch, perfusion partially compromised by emboli obstructing blood flow. **E,** Dead space, no perfusion due to obstruction of the pulmonary capillary.

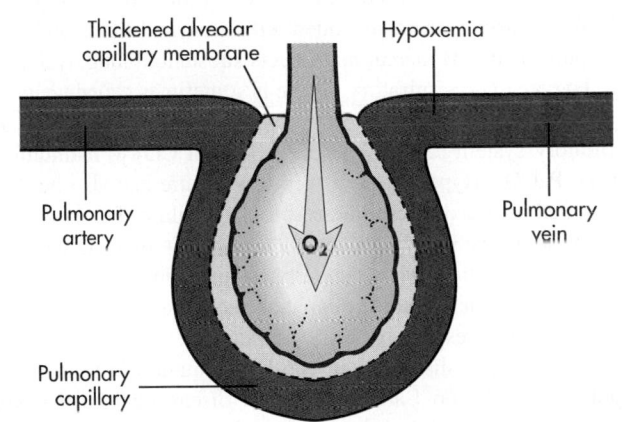

Thickened alveolar capillary membrane   Hypoxemia

Pulmonary artery   Pulmonary vein

O₂

Pulmonary capillary

FIG. 66-5 Diffusion limitation. Exchange of CO₂ and O₂ cannot occur because of the thickened alveolar–capillary membrane.

creasing the time for diffusion of O₂ across the alveolar-capillary membrane. The classical sign of diffusion limitation is hypoxemia that is present during exercise but not at rest.

Alveolar hypoventilation. Alveolar hypoventilation is a generalized decrease in ventilation that results in an increase in the PaCO₂ and a consequent decrease in PaO₂. Alveolar hypoventilation may be the result of restrictive lung disease, CNS disease, chest wall dysfunction, or neuromuscular disease. Although alveolar hypoventilation is primarily a mechanism of hypercapnic respiratory failure, it is mentioned here because it can also cause hypoxemia.

Interrelationship of mechanisms. Frequently, hypoxemic respiratory failure is caused by a combination of two or more of the following: $\dot{V}/\dot{Q}$ mismatch, shunting, diffusion limitation, and hypoventilation. The patient with acute respiratory failure secondary to pneumonia may have a combination of $\dot{V}/\dot{Q}$ mismatch and shunt because the inflammation, edema, and hypersecretion of exudate within the bronchioles and terminal respiratory units obstruct the airways ($\dot{V}/\dot{Q}$ mismatch) and fill the alveoli with exudate (shunt). In addition, shunt may be increased because of improper positioning (affected lung down) and endogenous vasodilator mediators as is the case with pneumococcal pneumonia.[6] The patient with cardiogenic pulmonary edema or ARDS may have a combination of shunt and $\dot{V}/\dot{Q}$ mismatch because some alveoli are completely filled with fluid from edema (shunt) and others are partially filled with fluid ($\dot{V}/\dot{Q}$ mismatch).

Hypercapnic Respiratory Failure. Hypercapnic respiratory failure results from an imbalance between ventilatory supply and ventilatory demand. *Ventilatory supply* is the maximum ventilation (gas flow in and out of the lungs) that the patient can sustain without developing respiratory muscle fatigue. *Ventilatory demand* is the amount of ventilation needed to keep the $PaCO_2$ within normal limits. Normally, ventilatory supply far exceeds ventilatory demand. As a consequence, individuals with normal lung function can engage in strenuous exercise, which greatly increases CO_2 production without an elevation in $PaCO_2$. Patients with preexisting lung disease such as severe emphysema do not have this advantage and cannot effectively increase lung ventilation in response to exercise or metabolic demands. However, considerable dysfunction is typically present before ventilatory demand exceeds ventilatory supply.

When ventilatory demand does exceed ventilatory supply, the $PaCO_2$ can no longer be sustained within normal limits and hypercapnia occurs. Hypercapnia reflects substantial lung dysfunction. Hypercapnic respiratory failure is sometimes called *ventilatory failure* because the primary problem is the inability of the respiratory system to ventilate out sufficient CO_2 to maintain a normal $PaCO_2$. Hypercapnic respiratory failure can also be differentiated as acute or chronic respiratory failure. For example, an episode of respiratory failure may represent an acute decompensation in a patient whose underlying lung function has deteriorated to the point that some degree of decompensation is always present (chronic respiratory insufficiency).

Many different diseases can cause a limitation in ventilatory supply (see Tables 66-1 and 66-2). These diseases can be grouped into four categories: (1) abnormalities of the airways and alveoli, (2) abnormalities of the CNS, (3) abnormalities of the chest wall, and (4) neuromuscular conditions.

Airways and alveoli. Patients with asthma, emphysema, chronic bronchitis, and cystic fibrosis are at high risk for hypercapnic respiratory failure because the underlying pathophysiology of these conditions results in airflow obstruction and air trapping.

Central nervous system. A variety of problems may suppress the drive to breathe. A common example is an overdose of a narcotic or other respiratory depressant drug. A brainstem infarction or severe head injury may also interfere with normal function of the respiratory center in the medulla. Patients with these conditions are at risk for respiratory failure because the medulla does not alter the respiratory rate in response to a change in $PaCO_2$.

CNS dysfunction may also include spinal cord injuries that limit innervation to the respiratory muscles.

Chest wall. A variety of conditions may prevent normal movement of the chest wall and hence limit lung expansion. In patients with flail chest, fractures prevent the rib cage from expanding normally because of pain, mechanical restriction, and muscle spasm. In patients with kyphoscoliosis, the change in spinal configuration compresses the lungs and prevents normal expansion of the chest wall. In patients with massive obesity, the weight of the chest and abdominal contents may limit lung expansion. Patients with these conditions are at risk for respiratory failure because these dysfunctions limit lung expansion or diaphragmatic movement and consequently gas exchange.

Neuromuscular conditions. Various types of neuromuscular diseases may result in respiratory muscle weakness or paralysis (see Table 66-1). For example, patients with Guillain-Barré syndrome, muscular dystrophy, or multiple sclerosis are at risk for respiratory failure because the respiratory muscles are weakened or paralyzed as a consequence of the underlying neuromuscular condition. Therefore they are unable to maintain normal $PaCO_2$ levels.

In summary, respiratory failure may occur in three of these categories (CNS, chest wall, neuromuscular conditions) despite the presence of normal lungs. Respiratory failure occurs because the medulla, chest wall, peripheral nerves, or respiratory muscles are not functioning normally. The patient may have no damage to lung tissue but may be unable to inspire a tidal volume sufficient to expel CO_2 from the lungs.

Tissue Oxygen Needs. It is important to remember that even though PaO_2 and $PaCO_2$ determine the definition of respiratory failure, the major threat of respiratory failure is the inability of the lungs to meet the oxygen demands of the tissues. This inability may occur as a result of inadequate tissue O_2 delivery or because the tissues are unable to use the O_2 delivered to them. It may also occur as a result of the stress response and dramatic increases in tissue oxygen consumption.[5] Tissue O_2 delivery is determined by the amount of O_2 carried in the hemoglobin, as well as cardiac output. Therefore respiratory failure places the patient at greater risk if there are coexisting cardiac problems or anemia. Failure of O_2 utilization most commonly occurs as a result of septic shock. In this situation, adequate O_2 may be delivered to the tissues, but an abnormally high amount of O_2 returns in the venous blood, indicating that it is not being extracted and used at the tissue level. (Shock is discussed in Chapter 65.)

Clinical Manifestations

Respiratory failure may develop suddenly (minutes or hours) or gradually (several days or longer). A sudden decrease in PaO_2 or a rapid rise in $PaCO_2$ implies a serious condition, which can rapidly become a life-threatening emergency. An example is the patient with asthma who develops severe bronchospasm and a marked decrease in airflow, resulting in respiratory arrest. A more gradual change in PaO_2 and $PaCO_2$ is better tolerated because compensation can occur. An example is the patient with COPD who develops a progressive increase in $PaCO_2$ over several days following the onset of a respiratory infection. Because the change occurred over several days, there is time for renal compensation (e.g., retention of bicarbonate), which will minimize the change in arterial pH. The patient has compensated respiratory acidosis.[3,7] (See Chapter 16 for a discussion of renal compensation for acid-base disorders.)

Manifestations of respiratory failure are related to the extent of change in PaO_2 or $PaCO_2$, the rapidity of change (acute versus chronic), and the ability to compensate to overcome this change. When the patient's compensatory mechanisms fail, respiratory failure occurs. Because clinical manifestations are variable, it is important to monitor trends in ABGs and/or pulse oximetry to evaluate the extent of change. These measurements cannot substitute for clinical assessment and should be interpreted within the context of clinical assessment findings. Frequently, the initial indication of respiratory failure is a change in the patient's mental status. Because the cerebral cortex is so sensitive to variations in oxygenation and acid-base balance, mental status changes will occur early and frequently before ABG results are obtained. Restlessness, confusion, agitation, and combative behavior suggest inadequate delivery of O_2 to the brain and should be fully investigated.

The nurse may detect manifestations of respiratory failure that are specific (arise from the respiratory system) or nonspecific (arise from other body systems) (Table 66-3). An understanding of the significance of these manifestations is critical to the ability to detect the onset of respiratory failure and effectiveness of treatment.

Tachycardia and mild hypertension can also be early signs of respiratory failure. Such changes may indicate an attempt by the heart to compensate for decreased O_2 delivery. A severe morning headache may suggest that hypercapnia may have occurred during the night, increasing cerebral blood flow by vasodilation and causing a morning headache. At night the respiratory rate is slower and the lungs of patients at risk for respiratory failure may remove less $PaCO_2$. Rapid, shallow breaths suggest that the tidal volume may be inadequate to remove CO_2 from the lungs. Cyanosis is an unreliable indicator of hypoxemia and is a late sign of respiratory failure because it does not occur until hypoxemia is severe ($PaO_2 \leq 45$ mm Hg).

Consequences of Hypoxemia and Hypoxia. *Hypoxemia* occurs when the amount of O_2 in arterial blood is less than the normal value (see Chapter 25 for normal values). **Hypoxia** occurs when the PaO_2 has fallen sufficiently to cause signs and symptoms of inadequate oxygenation (see Table 66-3). Hypoxemia can lead to hypoxia if not corrected. If hypoxia or hypoxemia is severe, the cells shift from aerobic to anaerobic metabolism. Anaerobic metabolism uses more fuel and produces less energy and is less efficient than aerobic metabolism. The waste product of anaerobic metabolism, lactic acid, is more difficult to remove from the body than CO_2 because lactic acid has to be buffered with sodium bicarbonate. When the body does not have adequate amounts of sodium bicarbonate to buffer the lactic acid produced by anaerobic metabolism, metabolic acidosis results and cell death may occur.

Hypoxia and metabolic acidosis have adverse effects on the vital organs, especially the heart and CNS. The heart tries to compensate for the decreased O_2 level in the blood by increasing the heart rate and cardiac output. As the PaO_2 decreases and acidosis increases, the heart muscle may become dysfunctional and cardiac output may decrease. In addition, angina and arrhythmias may occur. All of these consequences result in a further decrease in oxygen delivery. Permanent brain damage may occur because of O_2 deprivation. Renal function may also be impaired, and sodium retention, edema formation, acute tubular necrosis, and uremia may occur. Gastrointestinal (GI) system alterations include tissue ischemia, increased permeability of the intestinal wall, and possible translocation of bacteria from the GI tract into circulation.

Specific Clinical Manifestations. The patient in respiratory failure may have several clinical findings indicating distress. The patient may have a rapid, shallow breathing pattern or a respiratory rate that is slower than normal. Both changes predispose to insufficient CO_2 removal. The patient may increase the respiratory rate in an effort to blow off accumulated CO_2. This breathing pattern requires a substantial amount of work and predisposes to respiratory muscle fatigue. A change from a rapid rate to a slower rate in a patient in acute respiratory distress suggests extreme fatigue and the possibility of an impending respiratory arrest.

The position that the patient assumes is an indication of the effort associated with breathing. The patient may be able to lie

TABLE 66-3	Clinical Manifestations of Hypoxemia and Hypercapnia*	
SPECIFIC		**NONSPECIFIC**
Hypoxemia		
Respiratory		**Cerebral**
Dyspnea		Agitation
Tachypnea		Disorientation
Prolonged expiration (I:E = 1:3, 1:4)		Delirium
		Restless, combative behavior
Intercostal muscle retraction		Confusion
		$\downarrow$ Level of consciousness
Use of accessory muscles in respiration		Coma (late)
		Cardiac
$\downarrow$ SpO_2 (<80%)		Tachycardia
Paradoxic chest/abdominal wall movement with respiratory cycle (late)		Hypertension
		Skin cool, clammy, and diaphoretic
		Arrhythmias (late)
Cyanosis (late)		Hypotension (late)
		Other
		Fatigue
		Unable to speak without pausing to breathe
Hypercapnia		
Respiratory		**Cerebral**
Dyspnea		Morning headache
$\downarrow$ Respiratory rate or $\uparrow$ rapid rate with shallow respirations		Disorientation
		Progressive somnolence
		Coma (late)
$\downarrow$ Tidal volume		**Cardiac**
$\downarrow$ Minute ventilation		Arrhythmias
		Hypertension
		Tachycardia
		Bounding pulse
		Neuromuscular
		Muscle weakness
		$\downarrow$ Deep tendon reflexes
		Tremor, seizures (late)
		Other
		Pursed-lip breathing
		Use of tripod position

*List is not all-inclusive.

down (mild distress), be able to lie down but prefer to sit (moderate distress), or be unable to breathe unless sitting upright (severe distress). A common position is to sit with the arms propped on the overbed table. This position, called the tripod position, helps decrease the work of breathing because propping the arms increases the anterior-posterior diameter of the chest and changes pressure in the thorax. Pursed-lip breathing may be used. This strategy causes an increase in SaO_2 because it slows respirations, allows more time for expiration, and prevents the small bronchioles from collapsing, thus facilitating air exchange. (Pursed-lip breathing is discussed in Chapter 28.) Another assessment parameter is the number of pillows the patient requires to breathe comfortably when resting. This is termed *orthopnea* and may be documented as one-, two-, three-, or four-pillow orthopnea.

The person who is experiencing dyspnea is working hard to breathe and may be able to speak only a few words at a time between breaths. The ability of the patient to speak without pausing to breathe is an indication of the severity of dyspnea. The patient may speak in sentences (mild or no distress), phrases (moderate distress), or words (severe distress). The number of words is also a clue (e.g., how many words can the patient say without pausing to breathe?). The patient may have "two-word" or "three-word" dyspnea, signifying that only two or three words can be said before pausing to breathe. There may also be earlier onset of fatigue with walking. An additional assessment parameter is how far the patient is able to walk without stopping to rest.

There may be a change in the *inspiratory (I) to expiratory (E) (I:E) ratio*. Normally, the I:E ratio is 1:2, which means that expiration is twice as long as inspiration. In patients in respiratory distress, the ratio may increase to 1:3 or 1:4. This change signifies airflow obstruction and that more time is required to empty the lungs.

The nurse may observe *retraction* (inward movement) of the intercostal spaces or the supraclavicular area and use of the accessory muscles during inspiration or expiration. Use of the accessory muscles signifies moderate distress. Paradoxic breathing indicates severe distress. Normally, the thorax and abdomen move outward on inspiration and inward on exhalation. During *paradoxic breathing*, the abdomen and chest move in the opposite manner—outward during exhalation and inward during inspiration. Paradoxic breathing results from maximal use of the accessory muscles of respiration. The patient may also be diaphoretic from the work associated with breathing.

Auscultation should be performed in order to assess the patient's baseline breath sounds, as well as any changes from baseline. The nurse should note the presence and location of any adventitious breath sounds. Crackles and rhonchi may indicate pulmonary edema or emphysema. Absent or diminished breath sounds may indicate atelectasis or pleural effusion. The presence of bronchial breath sounds over the lung periphery often results from lung consolidation that is seen with pneumonia. A pleural friction rub may also be heard in the presence of pneumonia that has involved the pleura.

A thorough nursing assessment may result in early detection of manifestations associated with respiratory insufficiency, allowing therapy to be instituted before the patient experiences respiratory failure. Patients with end-stage (severe) chronic lung disease may have low PaO_2 values or elevated $PaCO_2$ levels and crackles as their "normal" baseline. It is especially important to monitor specific and nonspecific signs of respiratory failure in patients with COPD because a small change can cause significant decompensation (see Table 66-3). Any deterioration in mental status, such as agitation, combative behavior, confusion, or decreased level of consciousness, should be reported immediately because this change may indicate the onset of rapid deterioration in clinical status and the need for mechanical ventilation.

Diagnostic Studies

After physical assessment, the most common diagnostic study used to determine respiratory failure is ABG analysis. ABGs are used to determine the levels of $PaCO_2$, PaO_2, and pH. An indwelling catheter may be inserted into a peripheral artery for monitoring systemic blood pressure and obtaining blood for ABGs. Pulse oximetry is frequently used for monitoring oxygenation status, but tells little regarding lung ventilation. In respiratory failure, ABGs are necessary to obtain both oxygenation (PaO_2) and ventilation ($PaCO_2$) status, as well as information related to acid-base balance.

Other diagnostic studies that may be done include a chest x-ray, complete blood cell count, serum electrolytes, urinalysis, and electrocardiogram (ECG). Cultures of the sputum and blood are obtained as necessary to determine sources of possible infection. If pulmonary embolus is suspected, a ventilation/perfusion ($\dot{V}/\dot{Q}$) lung scan or pulmonary angiography may be done. Although not commonly done in acute situations, pulmonary function tests may be performed. For the patient in severe respiratory failure requiring endotracheal intubation, end-tidal CO_2 ($EtCO_2$) may be used to assess tube placement within the trachea immediately following intubation. $EtCO_2$ may also be used during ventilator management to assess trends in lung ventilation as determined by expired CO_2.

In severe respiratory failure, a pulmonary artery catheter may be inserted to measure heart pressures and cardiac output, as well as mixed venous oxygen saturation. This information is helpful in determining the adequacy of tissue perfusion and the patient's response to treatment measures. Pulmonary artery, pulmonary artery wedge, and left atrial pressures are monitored to determine whether the accumulation of fluid in the lungs is the result of cardiac or pulmonary problems. These parameters are also monitored to determine the response of the lung and heart to hypoxemia and the patient's response to therapy. Pulmonary arterial pressure monitoring can also provide feedback on the physiologic effects of mechanical ventilation on hemodynamic status. (Hemodynamic monitoring is discussed in detail in Chapter 64.)

NURSING *and* COLLABORATIVE MANAGEMENT
ACUTE RESPIRATORY FAILURE

Because many different problems cause respiratory failure, specific care of these patients varies. This section discusses general assessment and collaborative care measures that apply to patients with acute respiratory failure. In acute care settings there is often an overlap of function between nursing and other members of the health care team.

■ Nursing Assessment

Subjective and objective data that should be obtained from the patient with acute respiratory failure are presented in Table 66-4.

TABLE 66-4	Nursing Assessment
	Acute Respiratory Failure

Subjective Data

Important Health Information

Past health history: Chronic lung disease; potential occupational exposures to lung toxins; smoking (pack–years); previous hospitalizations related to lung disease; thoracic or spinal cord trauma; extreme obesity; altered consciousness; age (physiologic and chronologic); use/abuse of alcohol, other drugs

Medications: Use of oxygen, inhalers (bronchodilators), home nebulization, over-the-counter medications; immunosuppressant (corticosteroid) therapy, CNS depressants

Surgery or other treatments: Previous intubation and mechanical ventilation; recent thoracic or abdominal surgery

Functional Health Patterns

Health perception–health management: Exercise, self-care activities; immunizations (flu, pneumonia, hepatitis)

Nutritional-metabolic: Anorexia, bloatedness, heartburn; weight gain or loss; decreased appetite; diaphoresis, eating habits, vitamin/herbal supplements

Activity-exercise: Fatigue, dizziness; dyspnea at rest or with activity, wheezing, cough (productive or nonproductive); sputum (volume, color, viscosity); palpitations, swollen feet

Sleep-rest: Changes in sleep pattern

Cognitive-perceptual: Headache, chest pain or tightness

Coping–stress tolerance: Anxiety, depression

Objective Data

General

Restlessness, agitation

Integumentary

Pale, cool, clammy skin or warm flushed skin; peripheral and central cyanosis; peripheral dependent edema

Respiratory

Shallow, increased respiratory rate progressing to decreased rate; use of accessory muscles with evidence of retractions, altered I:E ratio; increased diaphragmatic excursion or asymmetric chest expansion; asynchronous respirations; tactile fremitus, crepitus, or deviated trachea on palpation; resonant, hyperresonant, or dull percussion note; absent, diminished, or adventitious breath sounds; bronchial or bronchovesicular sounds heard in other than normal location, inspiratory stridor, pleural friction rub

Cardiovascular

Tachycardia progressing to bradycardia, arrhythmias, extra heart sounds (S_3, S_4); bounding pulse; hypertension progressing to hypotension; pulsus paradoxus; jugular vein distention; pedal edema

Gastrointestinal

Abdominal distention with tympany; ascites, epigastric tenderness, hepatojugular reflex

Neurologic

Somnolence, confusion, slurred speech, restlessness, delirium, agitation, tremors, seizures, coma; asterixis, decreased deep tendon reflexes; papilledema

Possible Laboratory Findings

$\uparrow/\downarrow$ pH, $\uparrow/\downarrow$ $PaCO_2$, $\downarrow$ PaO_2, $\downarrow$ SaO_2, $\downarrow$ PEFR, $\downarrow$ tidal volume, $\downarrow$ forced vital capacity, $\downarrow$ minute ventilation, $\downarrow$ negative inspiratory force; altered values of serum electrolytes, hemoglobin, and hematocrit; abnormal findings on chest x-ray; abnormal pulmonary artery and pulmonary artery wedge pressures

CNS, Central nervous system; *I:E,* inspiratory:expiratory; *PEFR,* peak expiratory flow rate.

■ Nursing Diagnoses

Nursing diagnoses for the patient with acute respiratory failure include, but are not limited to, those presented in NCP 66-1.

■ Planning

The overall goals are that the patient in acute respiratory failure will have (1) ABG values within the patient's baseline, (2) breath sounds within the patient's baseline, (3) no dyspnea or breathing patterns within the patient's baseline, and (4) effective cough and ability to clear secretions.

■ Prevention

As part of the plan of care for any patient who may be at risk for respiratory failure, prevention and early recognition of respiratory distress is important. Prevention involves a thorough physical assessment and history to identify the patient at risk for respiratory failure and, then, the initiation of appropriate nursing interventions. For example, a patient at risk for respiratory failure should receive appropriate patient teaching regarding coughing, deep breathing, incentive spirometry, and ambulation as appropriate. Prevention of atelectasis, pneumonia, and complications of immobility, as well as optimizing hydration and nutrition, can po-

tentially decrease the risk of respiratory failure in the acutely or critically ill patient.

■ Respiratory Therapy

The major goals of care for acute respiratory failure include maintaining adequate oxygenation and ventilation. This goal is accomplished by collaboration among the nursing, medical, and respiratory care teams. The interventions used include O_2 therapy, mobilization of secretions, and positive pressure ventilation (Table 66-5).

Oxygen Therapy. The primary goal of O_2 therapy is to correct hypoxemia. If hypoxemia is secondary to $\dot{V}/\dot{Q}$ mismatch, supplemental O_2 administered at 1 to 3 L/min by nasal cannula or 24% to 32% by simple face mask or Venturi mask should improve the PaO_2 and SaO_2. Hypoxemia secondary to an intrapulmonary shunt is usually not responsive to high O_2 concentrations, and the patient will usually require positive pressure ventilation (PPV). PPV offers a means of providing O_2 therapy and humidification, decreasing the work of breathing, and reducing respiratory muscle fatigue. In addition, the positive pressure may assist in opening collapsed airways and decreasing shunt. PPV may be provided via an endotracheal tube (most frequently) or noninva-

NURSING CARE PLAN 66-1

Patient with Acute Respiratory Failure*

EXPECTED PATIENT OUTCOMES	NURSING INTERVENTIONS and *RATIONALES*
NURSING DIAGNOSIS	**Ineffective airway clearance** *related to* excessive secretions, ↓ level of consciousness, presence of an artificial airway, neuromuscular dysfunction, and pain *as manifested by* difficulty in expectorating sputum, presence of rhonchi or crackles, ineffective or absent cough.
▪ No abnormal breath sounds (e.g., rhonchi, crackles) ▪ Normal baseline breath sounds ▪ Presence of effective cough ▪ Effective expectoration of sputum	▪ Assess patient's ability to cough *to determine need for assistance in secretion removal.* ▪ Implement deep breathing/coughing exercises, assistive coughing strategies, and incentive spirometry *to promote secretion removal.* ▪ Position patient with head of bed elevated at least 45 degrees or in the tripod position *to promote maximal chest expansion and cough efforts.* ▪ Humidify O₂ if over 3 L/min *to prevent drying of the mucosa.* ▪ Perform tracheobronchial suctioning if cough is ineffective or if artificial airway is present *to remove secretions and improve oxygenation.* ▪ Perform chest physical therapy *to enhance removal of secretions.* ▪ Splint any abdominal or chest incision with pillow *to reduce pain and allow for improved inspiratory efforts.* ▪ Turn every 2 hours *to prevent stasis of secretions and promote optimal ventilation.* ▪ Ensure adequate fluid intake of 2-3 L/day *to liquefy secretions.* ▪ Administer prescribed routine and as needed bronchodilator and mucolytic medications *to promote better airflow and secretion removal.*
NURSING DIAGNOSIS	**Ineffective breathing pattern** *related to* neuromuscular impairment of respirations, pain, anxiety, ↓ level of consciousness, respiratory muscle fatigue, and bronchospasm *as manifested by* respiratory rate <12 or >24 breaths/min, altered I:E ratio, irregular breathing pattern, use of accessory muscles, asynchronous thoracoabdominal movement, wheezing, apnea.
▪ Respiratory rate, depth, and rhythm within normal limits for patient ▪ Synchronous thoraco-abdominal movement ▪ Use of accessory muscles appropriate for level of activity	▪ Monitor for ↑ or ↓ respiratory rate, periods of apnea, and ↓ inspiratory depth between chest and abdomen *to assess for presence of inability to sustain ventilation.* ▪ Position patient with head of bed elevated at least 45 degrees or in a tripod position *to promote diaphragmatic excursion.* ▪ Place oral or nasal airway and Ambu bag at the bedside *because airway support may be needed in the event of severely impaired ventilation or apnea.* ▪ Provide comfort measures (e.g., analgesics, positioning) *to reduce anxiety and promote patient cooperation.* ▪ Anticipate the need for possible application of NIPPV or intubation with mechanical ventilation *to maintain adequate oxygenation and ventilation.*
NURSING DIAGNOSIS	**Risk for imbalanced fluid volume** *related to* ↑ in peripheral or pulmonary fluid.
▪ Normal breath sounds ▪ ↓ or absent peripheral edema ▪ Normal pulmonary artery or pulmonary artery wedge pressures	▪ Assess for manifestations of fluid volume excess such as abnormal breath sounds (crackles), dyspnea, weight gain, jugular venous distention, peripheral or sacral edema *to identify if problem is present.* ▪ Monitor fluid status by intake and output measurements, daily weights, pulmonary artery or pulmonary artery wedge pressures, and central venous pressure *to monitor for changes in systemic fluid volume.* ▪ Restrict fluid intake and administer diuretics as ordered *to prevent or reduce fluid overload.*
NURSING DIAGNOSIS	**Anxiety** *related to* dyspnea, intubation, severity of illness, loss of personal control, and uncertain outcome *as manifested by* ↑ heart rate, respiratory rate, and blood pressure; agitation, restlessness; verbalization of anxiety.
▪ ↓ Anxiety ▪ Relaxed demeanor ▪ ↑ Sense of personal control ▪ Verbalization of positive attitude toward outcome	▪ Perform interventions in a calm, assured manner *to ↓ patient's anxiety.* ▪ Reassure patient of competence of caregivers *to encourage patient relaxation.* ▪ Answer questions simply and honestly *to provide patient with needed information for decision making.* ▪ Teach and demonstrate relaxation techniques of slow pursed-lip breathing, progressive relaxation, and guided imagery *to promote restoration of control over breathing.* ▪ Administer and evaluate patient's response to any prescribed antianxiety medication *to determine therapeutic efficacy.*

*The nursing care for the patient on mechanical ventilation is presented in NCP 64-1 and discussed in Chapter 64.
I:E, Inspiratory:expiratory; *NIPPV,* noninvasive positive pressure ventilation.

NURSING CARE PLAN 66-1

Patient with Acute Respiratory Failure—cont'd

EXPECTED PATIENT OUTCOMES	NURSING INTERVENTIONS and *RATIONALES*
NURSING DIAGNOSIS	**Impaired gas exchange** *related to* alveolar hypoventilation, intrapulmonary shunting, $\dot{V}/\dot{Q}$ mismatch, and diffusion impairment *as manifested by* hypoxemia or hypercapnia.
• PaO_2 and $PaCO_2$ within normal ranges for patient • Normal breath sounds	• Monitor for clinical manifestations of hypoxemia and hypercapnia *to detect systemic manifestations of* $\downarrow O_2$ *and* $\uparrow CO_2$. • Administer O_2 as ordered *to* $\uparrow PaO_2$ *and* SaO_2 *levels.* • Monitor ABGs for PaO_2 below 60 mm Hg, SaO_2 below 90%, and $PaCO_2$ above 50 mm Hg *to assess pulmonary gas exchange.* • Place the patient on continuous pulse oximetry *to assess for* $\uparrow$ *or* $\downarrow$ *in blood* O_2 *levels.* • Monitor apical-radial heart rate for irregular rhythm, tachycardia, bradycardia, and cardiac arrhythmias on the cardiac monitor *because hypoxemia may precipitate cardiac arrhythmias.* • Teach and encourage pursed-lip breathing *to improve gas exchange.* • Anticipate the need for ventilatory support *to improve oxygenation and ventilation status.* • Withhold sedative drugs unless discussed with physician *because they can depress respirations.*
NURSING DIAGNOSIS	**Imbalanced nutrition: less than body requirements** *related to* poor appetite, shortness of breath, presence of artificial airway, $\downarrow$ energy level, and $\uparrow$ caloric requirements *as manifested by* weight loss, weakness, muscle wasting, dehydration, poor muscle tone, poor skin integrity.
• Maintenance of weight or weight gain • Serum albumin and protein within normal ranges	• Provide high-protein, high-calorie, enteral or parenteral nutrition as ordered *to meet* $\uparrow$ *nutritional requirements.* • If able to take nutrition orally, provide six small meals per day *to* $\downarrow O_2$ *energy expenditure during digestion.* • Provide between-meal nutritional supplements *to maintain adequate caloric intake.* • Maintain the ordered O_2 delivery device during meals *to prevent shortness of breath and blood oxygen desaturation while eating.* • Monitor for signs of $\uparrow CO_2$ with parenteral nutrition *because carbohydrates may* $\uparrow CO_2$ *levels in patients with hypercapnia.*

sively by means of a tight-fitting mask.[8] (Mechanical ventilation is discussed in detail in Chapter 64.)

The type of O_2 delivery system chosen for the patient in acute respiratory failure should (1) be tolerated by the patient, because anxiety caused by feelings of claustrophobia related to the face mask or dyspnea may prompt the patient to remove the O_2 device; and (2) maintain PaO_2 at 55 to 60 mm Hg or more and SaO_2 at 90% or more at the lowest O_2 concentration possible. High O_2 concentrations replace the nitrogen gas normally present in the alveoli, causing instability and atelectasis. In intubated patients, exposure to 60% or greater O_2 for longer than 48 hours poses a significant risk for O_2 toxicity. In nonintubated patients, the risk is less clear. The effects of prolonged exposure to high levels of O_2 include increased pulmonary microvascular permeability, decreased surfactant production and surfactant inactivation, and fibrotic changes in the alveoli. (O_2 delivery devices are discussed in Chapter 28.)

Additional risks of O_2 therapy are specific to the patient with chronic hypercapnia such as the patient with COPD. Chronic hypercapnia may blunt the response of chemoreceptors in the medulla, a condition termed *CO_2 narcosis*. In this situation, respirations are stimulated by hypoxia. If the PaO_2 is suddenly

increased, the patient will no longer be hypoxemic, will have a decreased stimulus to breathe, and may experience a respiratory arrest. Patients with chronic hypercapnia should receive O_2 through a low-flow device such as a nasal cannula at 1 to 2 L/min or a Venturi mask at 24% to 28%. They should be closely monitored for changes in mental status and respiratory rate and ABG results until their PaO_2 level has reached their baseline normal value.

Mobilization of Secretions. Retained pulmonary secretions may cause or exacerbate acute respiratory failure by blocking movement of O_2 into the alveoli and pulmonary capillary blood and removal of CO_2 during the respiratory cycle. Secretions can be mobilized through effective coughing, adequate hydration and humidification, chest physical therapy, and tracheal suctioning.

Effective coughing and positioning. If secretions are obstructing the airway, the patient should be encouraged to cough. The patient with a neuromuscular weakness from a disease or exhaustion may not be able to generate sufficient airway pressures to produce an effective cough. *Augmented coughing (quad coughing)* may be of benefit to these patients. Augmented cough-

TABLE 66-5	Collaborative Care
	Acute Respiratory Failure

Diagnostic
History and physical examination
Arterial blood gases
Pulse oximetry
Chest x-ray
CBC
Serum electrolytes and urinalysis
ECG
Blood and sputum cultures (if indicated)
PAP, PAWP, LAP

Collaborative Therapy
Respiratory Therapy
O_2 therapy
Mobilization of secretions
• Effective coughing
• Incentive spirometry
• Hydration/humidification
• Chest physical therapy
• Airway suctioning
Positive pressure ventilation
• Noninvasive positive pressure ventilation
• Intubation with mechanical ventilation
Drug Therapy
Relief of bronchospasm (e.g., albuterol [Proventil])
Reduction of airway inflammation (corticosteroids)
Reduction of pulmonary congestion (e.g., furosemide [Lasix])
Treatment of pulmonary infections (e.g., antibiotics)
Reduction of severe anxiety and restlessness (e.g., lorazepam [Ativan])
Medical Supportive Therapy
Management of the underlying cause of respiratory failure
Maintenance of adequate cardiac output
Maintenance of adequate hemoglobin concentration
Nutritional Therapy
Parenteral nutrition support
Enteral nutrition support

CBC, Complete blood count; *ECG,* electrocardiogram; *LAP,* left atrial pressure; *PAP,* pulmonary artery pressure; *PAWP,* pulmonary artery wedge pressure.

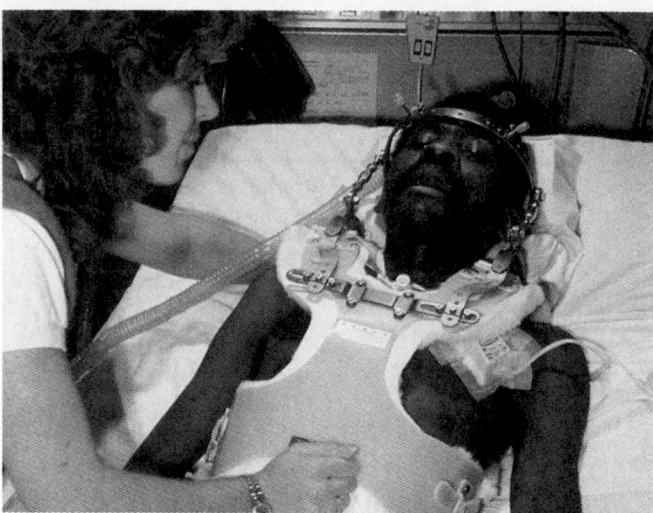

FIG. 66-6 Augmented cough. Augmented coughing is performed by placing the palm of the hand on the abdominal musculature below the xiphoid process. As the patient ends a deep inspiration and begins the expiration, the hand should be moved forcefully downward, increasing abdominal pressure, resulting in a forceful cough.

ing is performed by placing the palm of the hand or hands on the abdomen below the xiphoid process (Fig. 66-6). As the patient ends a deep inspiration and begins the expiration, the hands should be moved forcefully downward, increasing abdominal pressure and facilitating the cough. This measure helps increase expiratory flow and thereby facilitate secretion clearance.

Some patients may benefit from therapeutic cough techniques. *Huff coughing* is a series of coughs performed while saying the word "huff." This technique prevents the glottis from closing during the cough. Patients with COPD generate higher flow rates with a huff cough than is possible with a normal cough. The huff cough is effective in clearing only the central airways, but it may assist in moving secretions upward. The staged cough also assists secretion mobilization. To perform the *staged cough,* the patient sits in a chair, breathes three or four times in

and out through the mouth, and coughs while bending forward and pressing a pillow inward against the diaphragm.

Positioning the patient either by elevating the head of the bed at least 45 degrees or by using a reclining chair or chair bed may help maximize thoracic expansion, thereby decreasing dyspnea and improving secretion mobilization. A sitting position improves pulmonary function and assists in venous pooling in dependent body areas such as the lower extremities. When lungs are upright, ventilation and perfusion are best in the lung bases. Lateral or side-lying positioning may be used in patients with disease involving only one lung. This position, termed *down with the good lung,* allows for improved $\dot{V}/\dot{Q}$ matching in the affected lung. Pulmonary blood flow and ventilation are optimal in dependent lung areas. This positioning also allows for secretions to drain out of the affected lung to the point where they may be removed by suctioning. For example, in patients with a significant right middle lobe pneumonia, optimal positioning would be to place them on their left side to maximize ventilation and perfusion in the "good" lung and facilitate secretion removal from the affected lung (postural drainage). All patients should be side lying if there is any possibility that the tongue will obstruct the airway or that aspiration may occur. An oral or nasal airway should be kept at the bedside for use if necessary.

Hydration and humidification. Thick and viscous secretions are difficult to raise and should be thinned. Adequate fluid intake (2 to 3 L per day) is necessary to keep secretions thin and easy to expel. If the patient is unable to take sufficient fluids orally, intravenous (IV) hydration will be used. Thorough assessment of the patient's cardiac and renal status is paramount to determine whether he or she can tolerate the intravascular volume and avoid congestive heart failure (CHF) and pulmonary edema. Assessment for signs of fluid overload (e.g., crackles, dyspnea, and increased central venous pressure) at regular intervals is paramount. These considerations would also apply to the patient with renal dysfunction. An appropriate humidification device is an adjunct in secretion management. Aerosols of sterile normal saline, administered by a nebulizer, may be used to liquefy secretions. Oxygen may also be administered by aerosol mask to thin secretions and facilitate their removal. Aerosol therapy may induce bronchospasm and severe coughing, causing a decreased PaO_2. As such, frequent assessment of patient tolerance to therapy is paramount.[9] Mucolytic agents such as nebulized acetylcysteine (Mucomyst) mixed with a bronchodilator may be used to thin secretions but, as a side effect, may also cause airway erythema and bronchospasm. Therefore it is used only in special situations (e.g., during bronchoscopy to remove thick, copious secretions).

Chest physical therapy. Chest physical therapy is indicated in patients who produce more than 30 ml of sputum per day or have evidence of severe atelectasis or pulmonary infiltrates. If tolerated, postural drainage, percussion, and vibration to the affected lung segments may assist in moving secretions to the larger airways where they may be removed by coughing or suctioning. Because positioning may affect oxygenation, patients may not tolerate head-down or lateral positioning because of extreme dyspnea or hypoxemia caused by $\dot{V}/\dot{Q}$ mismatch. (Chest physical therapy is discussed in Chapter 28.)

Airway suctioning. If the patient is unable to expectorate secretions, nasopharyngeal, oropharyngeal, or nasotracheal suctioning (blind suctioning without a tracheal tube in place) is indicated. Suctioning through an artificial airway, such as endotracheal or tracheostomy tubes, may also be performed (see Chapters 26 and 64). A mini-tracheostomy (or mini-trach) may be used to suction patients who have difficulty mobilizing secretions and when blind suctioning is difficult or ineffective. The *mini-trach* is a 4 mm indwelling plastic cuffless cannula inserted through the cricothyroid membrane. It is used to instill sterile normal saline solution to elicit a cough and to perform suctioning using a size 10 or less French catheter. Contraindications for a mini-trach include an absent gag reflex, history of aspiration, and the need for long-term mechanical ventilation.

Positive Pressure Ventilation. If intensive measures fail to improve ventilation and oxygenation and the patient continues to exhibit manifestations of acute respiratory failure, ventilatory assistance may be initiated. Positive pressure ventilation (PPV) may be provided invasively through endotracheal or nasotracheal intubation or noninvasively through a nasal or face mask. Patients who require PPV are typically cared for in a critical care unit. (See Chapter 64 for a discussion of artificial airways and mechanical ventilation.)

Noninvasive positive pressure ventilation (NIPPV) may be used as a treatment for patients with acute or chronic respiratory failure. During NIPPV a mask is placed over the patient's nose or nose and mouth and the patient breathes spontaneously while PPV is delivered (Fig. 66-7). With NIPPV it is possible to decrease the work of breathing without the need for endotracheal intubation. Bilevel positive airway pressure (BiPAP ventilatory support system) is a form of NIPPV in which different positive pressure levels are set for inspiration and expiration (Fig. 66-7). Continuous positive airway pressure (CPAP) is another form of NIPPV in which a constant positive pressure is delivered to the airway during inspiration and expiration.[8,10]

NIPPV is most useful in managing chronic respiratory failure in patients with chest wall and neuromuscular disease (see

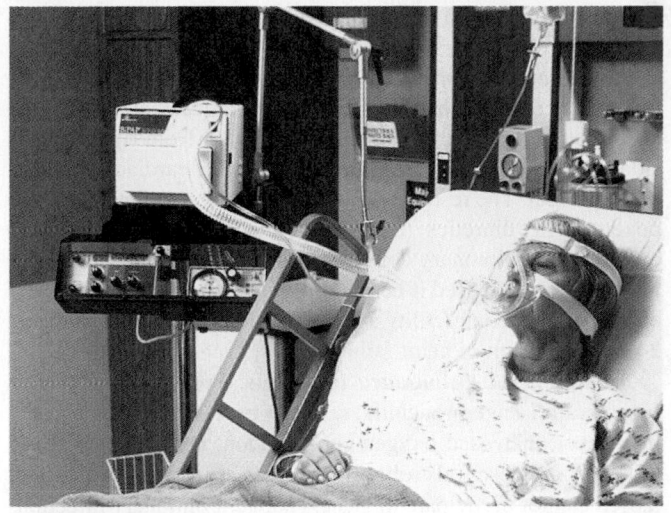

FIG. 66-7 Noninvasive bilevel positive pressure ventilation. A mask is placed over the nose or nose and mouth. Positive pressure from a mechanical ventilator assists the patient's breathing efforts, decreasing the work of breathing.

Table 66-1). NIPPV has been used in patients with hypoxemic respiratory failure (e.g., ARDS, cardiogenic pulmonary edema), but with less success. NIPPV may also be used for patients who refuse endotracheal intubation but still desire some palliative ventilatory support (e.g., patients with end-stage COPD). NIPPV is not appropriate for the patient who has absent respirations, excessive secretions, decreased level of consciousness, high O_2 requirements, facial trauma, or hemodynamic instability.[8,10-12]

■ Drug Therapy

Goals of drug therapy for patients in acute respiratory failure include relief of bronchospasm, reduction of airway inflammation and pulmonary congestion, treatment of pulmonary infection, and reduction of severe anxiety and restlessness.

Relief of Bronchospasm. Alveolar ventilation will be increased with relief of bronchospasm. Short-acting *bronchodilators,* such as metaproterenol (Alupent) and albuterol (Ventolin), are frequently administered to reverse bronchospasm using either a handheld nebulizer or a metered-dose inhaler with a spacer.[8] In acute bronchospasm these drugs may be given at 30- to 60-minute intervals until it can be determined that a response is occurring. If severe bronchospasm continues, IV aminophylline may be administered. The bronchodilator effects of all of these medications can sometimes cause a worsening of arterial hypoxemia by redistributing the inspired gas to areas of decreased perfusion. Administering the bronchodilator with an O_2-enriched gas mixture usually alleviates this effect.[1] (See Chapter 28 for nursing management related to bronchodilators.)

Reduction of Airway Inflammation. Corticosteroids (e.g., methylprednisolone [Solu-Medrol]) may be used in conjunction with bronchodilating agents when bronchospasm and inflammation are present. When administered intravenously, corticosteroids have an immediate onset of action. Inhaled corticosteroids are not used for acute respiratory failure, because they require 4 to 5 days before optimum therapeutic effects are seen.[13]

Reduction of Pulmonary Congestion. Pulmonary interstitial fluid can occur as a consequence of direct or indirect injury to the alveolar capillary membrane (e.g., ARDS) or from right- or left-sided heart failure, and therefore can be either cardiac or noncardiac in origin. The result is decreased alveolar ventilation and hypoxemia. IV diuretics (e.g., furosemide [Lasix]) are used to decrease the pulmonary congestion caused by heart failure. Digitalis may also be used if heart failure or atrial fibrillation is present to increase contractility and decrease heart rate. (See Chapter 34 for discussion of heart failure.)

Treatment of Pulmonary Infections. Pulmonary infections (pneumonia, acute bronchitis) result in excessive mucus production, fever, increased oxygen consumption, and inflamed, fluid-filled, or collapsed alveoli. Alveoli that are fluid filled or collapsed cannot participate in gas exchange. Pulmonary infections can either cause or exacerbate acute respiratory failure. IV antibiotics, such as vancomycin (Vancocin, Lyphocin) or ceftriaxone (Rocephin), are frequently administered to inhibit bacterial growth. Chest x-rays are performed to determine the location and extent of a suspected infectious process. Sputum cultures are used to determine the type of organisms causing the infection and their sensitivity to antimicrobial medications.

Reduction of Severe Anxiety, Pain, and Agitation. Anxiety, restlessness, and agitation result from cerebral hypoxia. In addition, fear caused by the inability to breathe and a sense of loss of control may exacerbate anxiety. Anxiety, pain, and agitation increase O_2 consumption, which may worsen the degree of hypoxemia. Anxiety, pain, and agitation also increase CO_2 production, affect ventilator management, and increase morbidity.[14,15] Several nursing strategies can assist the patient in reducing the level of anxiety and pain (see NCP 66-1).

Sedation and analgesia with drug therapy such as benzodiazepines (e.g., lorazepam [Ativan], midazolam [Versed]) and narcotics (e.g., morphine, fentanyl [Sublimaze]) may be used to decrease anxiety, agitation, and pain. Continued agitation will increase the patient's work of breathing, O_2 consumption, CO_2 production, and risk of injury (e.g., accidental extubation). When receiving any sedative or analgesic agent, patients must be monitored closely for cardiovascular and respiratory depression.[14,15] In the critical care setting, sedation and analgesia are commonly used for severely restless, anxious, and agitated patients who may be experiencing pain and are in acute respiratory failure.

Patients who breathe asynchronously with mechanical ventilation may also benefit from titration of ventilator flow rates and other settings, as well as addressing treatable causes of agitation such as hypoxemia, pain, or hypercapnia. Patients who remain asynchronous with mechanical ventilation may require neuromuscular blockade with agents such as vecuronium (Norcuron) or cisatracurium (Nimbex) to produce skeletal muscle relaxation and synchrony with mechanical ventilation. Neuromuscular blockade may also decrease the patient's risk of lung injury related to excessive inspiratory/intrathoracic pressures. In this way, the ventilator can then provide optimal respiratory support. Patients receiving neuromuscular blockade should receive sedation and analgesia to the point of unconsciousness for patient comfort, to eliminate patient awareness and to avoid the terrifying experience of being awake and in pain while paralyzed (see Nursing Research box).[14-16]

NURSING RESEARCH
Sedation Practices in Critical Care

Citation

Weinert CR, Chlan L, Gross C: Sedating critically ill patients: factors affecting nurses' delivery of sedative therapy, *Am J Crit Care* 10:156, 2001.

Purpose

To explore the beliefs and attitudes of nurses toward critical illness and sedation practices, and to identify processes that nurses use to assess patients' need for sedation.

Methods

A qualitative design was used to interview 34 experienced critical care nurses in focus group settings. All interviews were audiotaped and transcribed.

Results and Conclusions

Five themes were extracted from the data and validated by four of the study participants and two experienced critical care nurses who did not participate. It was discovered that patients' family members and the nurses' workload influence nurses' sedation practices. Conflicts with physicians were reported when sedation goals for the patient were not shared. Nurses believed that the goals of sedation were to provide for patient comfort, amnesia, and safety. Finally, nurses used a variety of patient cues to determine level of sedation and reported mixed feelings about the efficacy of sedation protocols.

Implications for Nursing Practice

Several nonpatient factors (e.g., social, personal) were reported to influence the sedation practices of nurses. Ideally, these factors should be limited. Sedation goals should reflect the individual patient's needs. The use of sedation protocols could achieve this directive and should be studied.

■ Medical Supportive Therapy

Therapeutic goals and interventions to maximize O_2 delivery and treat the underlying cause of the respiratory failure are essential to improving the patient's oxygenation and ventilation status. The primary goal is to treat the underlying cause of the respiratory failure. Other goals include maintaining an adequate cardiac output and hemoglobin concentration.

Treating the Underlying Cause. Interventions are directed toward reversing the disease process that resulted in the development of acute respiratory failure. Patients with hypoventilation can be diagnosed and treated rapidly. Patients with $\dot{V}/\dot{Q}$ mismatch, shunting, or diffusion limitation are managed differently depending on the underlying cause. In all patient situations, monitoring treatment effects, including trends in ABGs and changes in respiratory status, is a continuous process.

Maintaining Adequate Cardiac Output. Cardiac output reflects the blood flow reaching the tissues. Blood pressure is an important indicator of the adequacy of cardiac output. Usually a systolic blood pressure of at least 90 mm Hg is adequate to maintain perfusion to the vital organs. If the systolic blood pressure is at least 90 mm Hg, changes in mental status may be attributed to the level of O_2 and CO_2 rather than decreased cerebral perfusion. Decreased cardiac output is treated by administration of IV fluids, medications, or both. (See Chapter 65 for a discussion of drugs used to treat decreased cardiac output and shock.) Cardiac output may also be decreased by changes in intrathoracic or intrapulmonary pressures from positive pressure ventilation. Consequently, clinical indicators of adequate cardiac output and tissue perfusion should be monitored closely with initiation or titration of mechanical ventilation by mask or endotracheal intubation.

Maintaining Adequate Hemoglobin Concentration. Hemoglobin is the primary carrier when delivering O_2 to the tissues. If the patient is anemic, tissue O_2 delivery will be compromised. A hemoglobin concentration of 9 to 10 g/dl (90 to 100 g/L) or greater typically ensures adequate O_2 saturation of the hemoglobin. The patient should be monitored for sites of blood loss and transfused with packed red blood cells if an adequate hemoglobin concentration cannot be maintained.

■ Nutritional Therapy

Maintenance of protein and energy stores is especially important in patients who experience acute respiratory failure because nutritional depletion causes a loss of muscle mass, including the respiratory muscles, and may prolong recovery. During the acute manifestations of respiratory failure, the risk of aspiration typically prevents oral nutritional intake. Therefore enteral or parenteral nutrition may be administered. When the acute manifestations subside, the patient may resume oral intake as tolerated. A multitude of nutritional supplements are available for this patient population. A high-carbohydrate diet may need to be avoided in the patient who retains CO_2 because carbohydrates metabolize into CO_2 and increase the CO_2 load of the patient. However, research is currently being done in this area, and it remains controversial.

■ Evaluation

The expected outcomes for the patient with acute respiratory failure are presented in NCP 66-1.

■ Gerontologic Considerations
Respiratory Failure

The elderly population is the fastest growing age-group in North America, a trend that is increasingly reflected within the patient populations in acute care and critical care settings. Multiple factors contribute to an increased risk of respiratory failure in older adults. They are at higher risk of developing respiratory failure because of the reduction in ventilatory capacity that accompanies aging, especially if other risk factors are present. Physiologic aging of the lung may produce alveolar dilation, larger air spaces, and loss of surface area. Diminished elastic recoil within the airways, decreased chest wall compliance, and decreased respiratory muscle strength also occur. In older adults, the PaO_2 falls further and the $PaCO_2$ rises to a higher level before the respiratory system is stimulated to alter the rate and depth of breathing. This delayed response can contribute to the development of respiratory failure. In addition, a history of smoking is a risk factor. Lifelong smoking can accelerate age-related respiratory changes. Poor nutritional status and less available physiologic reserve in cardiovascular, respiratory, and autonomic nervous systems increase the risk of additional disease states such as pneumonia and cardiac disease

that may compromise respiratory function and precipitate respiratory failure.[17,18]

Assessment parameters must also be adjusted for age. For example, heart rate and blood pressure generally increase with age and related changes in the cardiovascular system. Therefore determination of the patient's baseline vital signs and using them as a basis for comparison of physical assessment findings is most appropriate in evaluating changes in cardiopulmonary function in the older adult. ■

ACUTE RESPIRATORY DISTRESS SYNDROME

Acute respiratory distress syndrome (ARDS) is a sudden and progressive form of acute respiratory failure in which the alveolar capillary membrane becomes damaged and more permeable to intravascular fluid (Fig. 66-8). The alveoli fill with fluid, resulting in severe dyspnea, hypoxemia refractory to supplemental O_2, reduced lung compliance, and diffuse pulmonary infiltrates.[19-22]

The incidence of ARDS in the United States is estimated at more than 150,000 cases annually. Despite supportive therapy, the mortality rate from ARDS is approximately 50%. Patients who have both gram-negative septic shock and ARDS have a mortality rate of 70% to 90%.[20]

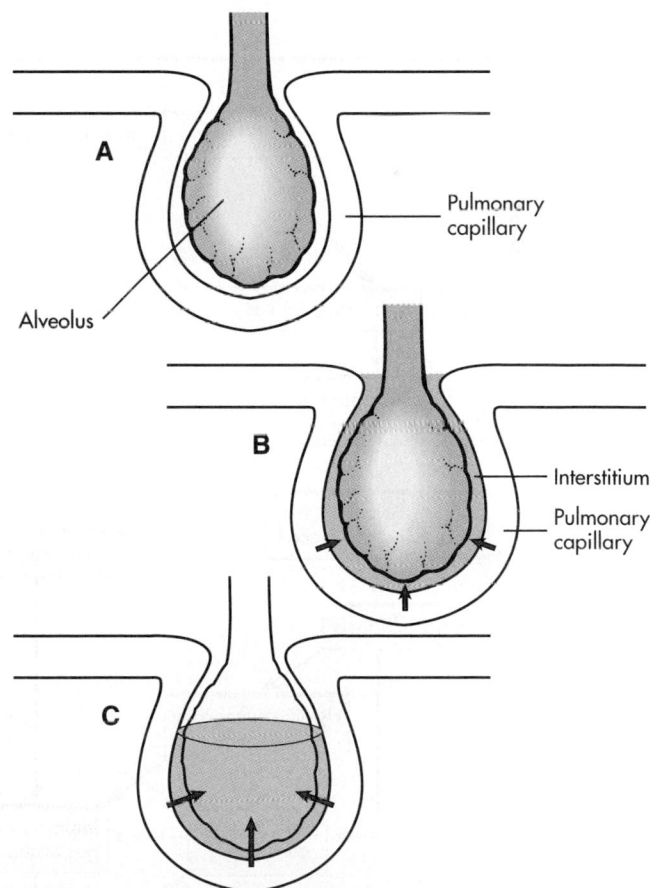

FIG. 66-8 Stages of edema formation in acute respiratory distress syndrome. **A,** Normal alveolus and pulmonary capillary. **B,** Interstitial edema occurs with increased flow of fluid into the interstitial space. **C,** Alveolar edema occurs when the fluid crosses the blood-gas barrier.

TABLE 66-6	Conditions Predisposing to Acute Respiratory Distress Syndrome

Direct Lung Injury

Common Causes
Aspiration of gastric contents or other substances
Viral/bacterial pneumonia

Less Common Causes
Chest trauma
Embolism: fat, air, amniotic fluid
Inhalation of toxic substances
Near-drowning
O_2 toxicity
Radiation pneumonitis

Indirect Lung Injury

Common Causes
Sepsis (especially gram–negative infection)
Severe massive trauma

Less Common Causes
Acute pancreatitis
Anaphylaxis
Cardiopulmonary bypass
Disseminated intravascular coagulation
Multiple blood transfusions
Narcotic drug overdose (e.g., heroin)
Nonpulmonary systemic diseases
Severe head injury
Shock states

Etiology and Pathophysiology

Table 66-6 lists conditions that predispose patients to the development of ARDS. The most common cause of ARDS is sepsis. Patients with multiple risk factors are three to four times more likely to develop ARDS.

Direct lung injury may cause ARDS (Fig. 66-9), or ARDS may develop as a consequence of the systemic inflammatory response syndrome (SIRS) (see Chapter 65, Fig. 65-1). SIRS may have an infectious or a noninfectious etiology and is characterized by widespread inflammation or clinical responses to inflammation following a variety of physiologic insults, including severe trauma, gut ischemia, lung injury, and sepsis.[22] ARDS may also develop as a consequence of multiple organ dysfunction syndrome (MODS). MODS results from organ system dysfunction that progressively increases in severity and ultimately results in multisystem organ failure. (SIRS and MODS are discussed in Chapter 65.)

An exact cause for the damage to the alveolar-capillary membrane is not known. However, the pathophysiologic changes of ARDS are thought to be due to stimulation of the inflammatory and immune systems, which causes an attraction of neutrophils to the pulmonary interstitium.[10] The neutrophils cause a release of biochemical, humoral, and cellular mediators (Table 66-7) that produce changes in the lung, including increased pulmonary capillary membrane permeability, destruction of elastin and collagen, formation of pulmonary microemboli, and pulmonary artery vasoconstriction (see Fig. 66-9).[20-22] (These mediators are discussed in Chapters 12 and 13.)

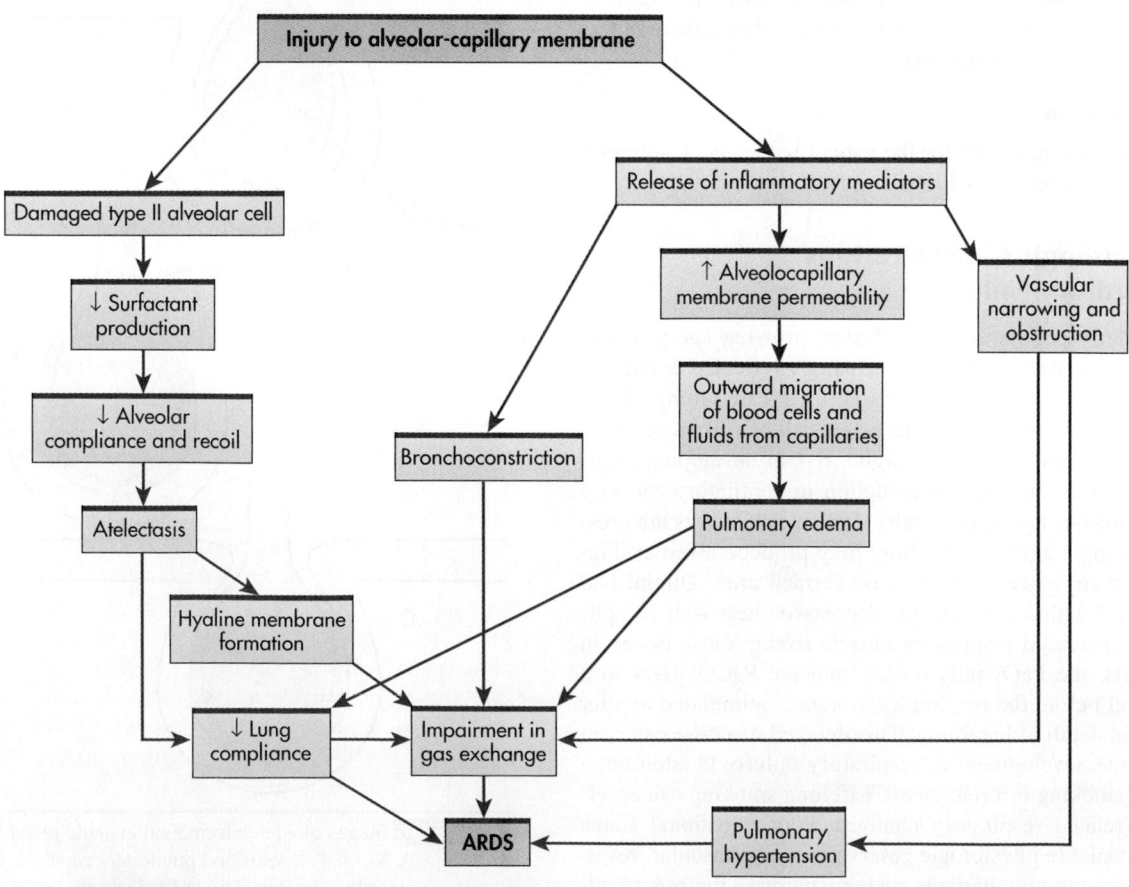

FIG. 66-9   Pathophysiology of acute respiratory distress syndrome (ARDS).

TABLE 66-7	Mediators of Acute Lung Injury

Complement component C5a
Neutrophil products, including proteases and O_2 radicals
Monocyte and macrophage products, including tumor necrosis factor, interleukin-1, and colony-stimulating factor
Arachidonic acid metabolites, including prostaglandins and leukotrienes
Coagulation products, including kallikreins, kinins, fibrin degradation products, and plasminogen-activating factor
Histamine
Serotonin
Endotoxin
Elastase
Collagenase

The pathophysiologic changes in ARDS are divided into three phases: (1) injury or exudative phase, (2) reparative or proliferative phase, and (3) fibrotic phase.

Injury or Exudative Phase. The *injury or exudative phase* occurs approximately 1 to 7 days (usually 24 to 48 hours) after the initial direct lung injury or host insult. Neutrophils adhere to the pulmonary microcirculation, causing damage to the vascular endothelium and increased capillary permeability. In the earliest phase of injury, there is engorgement of the peribronchial and perivascular interstitial space, which produces interstitial edema. Next, fluid from the interstitial space crosses the alveolar epithelium and enters the alveolar space. Intrapulmonary shunt develops because the alveoli fill with fluid, and blood passing through them cannot be oxygenated (see Figs. 66-4 and 66-8).

Alveolar type I and type II cells (which produce surfactant) are damaged by the changes caused by ARDS. This damage, in addition to further fluid and protein accumulation, results in surfactant dysfunction. The function of *surfactant* is to maintain alveolar stability by decreasing alveolar surface tension and preventing alveolar collapse. Decreased synthesis of surfactant and inactivation of existing surfactant cause the alveoli to become unstable and collapse (atelectasis). Widespread atelectasis further decreases lung compliance, compromises gas exchange, and contributes to hypoxemia.[21,22]

Also during this stage, hyaline membranes begin to line the alveoli. The hyaline membrane is composed of necrotic cells, protein, and fibrin and lies adjacent to the alveoli wall. These hyaline membranes are thought to result from the exudation of high-molecular-weight substances (particularly fibrinogen) in the edema fluid. Hyaline membranes contribute to the development of fibrosis and atelectasis, leading to a decrease in gas exchange capability and lung compliance.

The primary pathophysiologic changes that characterize the *injury or exudative phase* of ARDS are interstitial and alveolar edema (noncardiogenic pulmonary edema) and atelectasis.[23] Severe $\dot{V}/\dot{Q}$ mismatch and shunting of pulmonary capillary blood result in hypoxemia unresponsive to increasing concentrations of O_2 (termed **refractory hypoxemia**). Diffusion limitation, caused by hyaline membrane formation, further contributes to the severity of the hypoxemia. As the lungs become less compliant because of decreased surfactant, pulmonary edema, and atelectasis, the patient must generate higher airway pressures to inflate "stiff" lungs. Reduced lung compliance greatly increases the patient's work of breathing.

Hypoxemia and the stimulation of juxtacapillary receptors in the stiff lung parenchyma (J reflex) initially cause an increase in respiratory rate and decrease in tidal volume. This breathing pattern increases CO_2 removal, producing respiratory alkalosis. Cardiac output increases in response to hypoxemia, a compensatory effort to increase pulmonary blood flow. However, as atelectasis, pulmonary edema, and pulmonary shunt increase, compensation fails, and hypoventilation, decreased cardiac output, and decreased tissue O_2 perfusion eventually occur.

Reparative or Proliferative Phase. The *reparative or proliferative phase* of ARDS begins 1 to 2 weeks after the initial lung injury. During this phase, there is an influx of neutrophils, monocytes, and lymphocytes and fibroblast proliferation as part of the inflammatory response. The injured lung has an immense regenerative capacity after acute lung injury. The proliferative phase is complete when the diseased lung becomes characterized by dense, fibrous tissue. Increased pulmonary vascular resistance and pulmonary hypertension may occur in this stage because fibroblasts and inflammatory cells destroy the pulmonary vasculature. Lung compliance continues to decrease as a result of interstitial fibrosis. Hypoxemia worsens because of the thickened alveolar membrane, causing diffusion limitation and shunting. If the reparative phase persists, widespread fibrosis results. If the reparative phase is arrested, the lesions resolve.[19,21]

Fibrotic Phase. The *fibrotic phase* of ARDS occurs approximately 2 to 3 weeks after the initial lung injury. This phase is also called the *chronic or late phase* of ARDS. By this time, the lung is completely remodeled by sparsely collagenous and fibrous tissues. There is diffuse scarring and fibrosis, resulting in decreased lung compliance. In addition, the surface area for gas exchange is significantly reduced because the interstitium is fibrotic, and therefore hypoxemia continues. Pulmonary hypertension results from pulmonary vascular destruction and fibrosis.

Clinical Progression

Progression of ARDS varies among patients. Some persons survive the acute phase of lung injury; pulmonary edema resolves and complete recovery occurs in a few days. The chance for survival is poor in patients who enter the fibrotic (chronic or late) stage, which requires long-term mechanical ventilation. It is not known why injured lungs repair and recover in some patients, and in others ARDS progresses. Several factors seem to be important in determining the course of ARDS, including the nature of the initial injury, extent and severity of coexisting diseases, and pulmonary complications.[1,20,21]

Clinical Manifestations

The initial presentation of ARDS is often insidious. At the time of the initial injury, and for several hours to 1 to 2 days afterward, the patient may not experience respiratory symptoms, or the patient may exhibit only dyspnea, tachypnea, cough, and restlessness. Chest auscultation may be normal or reveal fine, scattered crackles. ABGs usually indicate mild hypoxemia and respiratory alkalosis caused by hyperventilation. Respiratory alkalosis results from hypoxemia and the stimulation of juxtacapillary receptors. The chest x-ray may be normal or exhibit evidence of minimal scattered interstitial infiltrates. Edema may not show on the x-ray until there is a 30% increase in fluid content in the lung.[20,21]

As ARDS progresses, symptoms worsen because of increased fluid accumulation and decreased lung compliance. Respiratory discomfort becomes evident as the work of breathing increases. Tachypnea and intercostal and suprasternal retractions may be present. Pulmonary function tests in ARDS reveal decreased compliance and decreased lung volumes, particularly a decreased functional residual capacity (FRC). Tachycardia, diaphoresis, changes in sensorium with decreased mentation, cyanosis, and pallor may be present. Chest auscultation usually reveals scattered to diffuse crackles and rhonchi. The chest x-ray demonstrates diffuse and extensive bilateral interstitial and alveolar infiltrates. A pulmonary artery catheter may be inserted. Pulmonary artery wedge pressure does not increase in ARDS because the cause is noncardiogenic (not related to cardiac function).

Hypoxemia and a PaO_2/FIO_2 ratio below 200 despite increased FIO_2 by mask, cannula, or endotracheal tube are hallmarks of ARDS. ABGs may initially demonstrate a normal or decreased $PaCO_2$ despite severe dyspnea and hypoxemia. Hypercapnia signifies that hypoventilation is occurring, and the patient is no longer able to maintain the level of ventilation needed to provide optimum gas exchange.

As ARDS progresses it is associated with profound respiratory distress requiring endotracheal intubation and positive pressure ventilation (PPV). The chest x-ray is often termed *whiteout* or *white lung,* because consolidation and coalescing infiltrates are widespread throughout the lungs, leaving few recognizable air spaces. Pleural effusions may also be present. Severe hypoxemia, hypercapnia, and metabolic acidosis, with symptoms of target organ or tissue hypoxia, may ensue if prompt therapy is not instituted.

In summary, no precise criteria define ARDS. ARDS is considered to be present if the patient has (1) refractory hypoxemia, (2) a chest x-ray with new bilateral interstitial or alveolar infiltrates, (3) a pulmonary artery wedge pressure of 18 mm Hg or less and no evidence of heart failure, and (4) a predisposing condition for ARDS within 48 hours of clinical manifestations (Table 66-8).

Complications

Complications may develop as a result of ARDS itself or its treatment. (Table 66-9 lists the common complications of ARDS.) The major cause of death in ARDS is MODS, often accompanied by sepsis. The vital organs most commonly involved are the kidneys, liver, and heart. The organ systems most often involved are the CNS, hematologic system, and gastrointestinal system.

Nosocomial Pneumonia. A frequent complication of ARDS is nosocomial pneumonia, occurring in as many as 68%

TABLE 66-8 Diagnostic Findings in Acute Respiratory Distress Syndrome

Refractory Hypoxemia
PaO_2 <50 mm Hg on FIO_2 >40% with PEEP >5 cm H_2O
PaO_2/FIO_2 ratio <200

Chest X-ray
New bilateral interstitial and alveolar infiltrates

Pulmonary Artery Wedge Pressure
≤18 mm Hg and no evidence of heart failure

Predisposing Condition
Identification of a predisposing condition for ARDS within 48 hours of clinical manifestations

ARDS, Acute respiratory distress syndrome; *PEEP,* positive end-expiratory pressure.

TABLE 66-9 Complications Associated with Acute Respiratory Distress Syndrome

Infection
Catheter-related infection
Nosocomial pneumonia
Sepsis (bacteremia)

Respiratory Complications
O_2 toxicity
Pulmonary barotrauma (e.g., pneumothorax, pneumomediastinum, subcutaneous emphysema)
Pulmonary emboli
Pulmonary fibrosis

Gastrointestinal Complications
Paralytic ileus
Pneumoperitoneum
Stress ulceration and hemorrhage

Renal Complications
Acute renal failure

Cardiac Complications
Arrhythmias
Decreased cardiac output

Hematologic Complications
Anemia
Disseminated intravascular coagulation
Thrombocytopenia

ET Intubation Complications
Laryngeal ulceration
Tracheal malacia
Tracheal stenosis
Tracheal ulceration

ET, Endotracheal tube.

of patients with ARDS. Risk factors include impaired host defenses, contaminated medical equipment, invasive monitoring devices, aspiration of gastrointestinal contents, and prolonged mechanical ventilation, as well as colonization of the respiratory tract. Strategies to prevent nosocomial pneumonia include infection control measures (e.g., strict hand washing and sterile technique during endotracheal suctioning) and elevating the head of the bed 45 degrees or more to prevent aspiration.[24] (See Chapter 27 for discussion of pneumonia.)

Barotrauma. *Barotrauma* may result from rupture of overdistended alveoli during mechanical ventilation. The high peak airway pressures that may be required in patients with ARDS predispose to this complication. Barotrauma results in the presence of alveolar air in locations where it is not usually found. This can lead to pulmonary interstitial emphysema, pneumothorax, subcutaneous emphysema, pneumoperitoneum, pneumomediastinum, and tension pneumothorax. (See Chapter 27 for discussion of pneumothorax.) To avoid barotrauma, the patient with ARDS is sometimes ventilated with smaller tidal volumes, resulting in higher $PaCO_2$. This method of mechanical ventilation is termed *permissive hypercapnia* because the $PaCO_2$ is allowed (permitted) to rise above normal limits.[9]

Volu-pressure Trauma. *Volu-pressure trauma* can occur in patients with ARDS when large tidal volumes are used to ventilate noncompliant lungs. Volu-pressure trauma results in alveolar fractures and movement of fluids and proteins into the alveolar spaces. To limit this complication, it is recommended that smaller tidal volumes or pressure ventilation be used in patients with ARDS (see Chapter 64).[25]

Stress Ulcers. Critically ill patients with acute respiratory failure are at high risk for stress ulcers. Bleeding from stress ulcers occurs in 30% of patients with ARDS who require PPV, a higher incidence than other causes of acute respiratory failure. Management strategies include correction of predisposing conditions such as hypotension, shock, and acidosis. Prophylactic management includes antiulcer agents (e.g., famotidine [Pepcid], omeprazole [Prilosec], sucralfate [Carafate]) and early initiation of enteral nutrition (see Chapters 39 and 64).

Renal Failure. Renal failure can occur from decreased renal tissue oxygenation as a result of hypotension, hypoxemia, or hypercapnia. Renal failure may also be caused by administration of nephrotoxic drugs (e.g., aminoglycosides), which are used to treat infections associated with ARDS.

NURSING and COLLABORATIVE MANAGEMENT ACUTE RESPIRATORY DISTRESS SYNDROME

The collaborative care for acute respiratory failure (see Table 66-5) is applicable to ARDS. The following section discusses additional collaborative care measures for the patient with ARDS (Table 66-10). Patients with ARDS are commonly cared for in critical care units. The nursing care plan for acute respiratory failure (see NCP 66-1) is applicable to patients with ARDS.

■ Nursing Assessment

Because ARDS causes acute respiratory failure, the subjective and objective data that should be obtained from a person with ARDS are the same as that for acute respiratory failure (see Table 66-4). Abnormal findings on physical examination are indications that ARDS has progressed beyond the initial stages.

■ Nursing Diagnoses

Nursing diagnoses for the patient with ARDS may include, but are not limited to, those described for acute respiratory failure (see NCP 66-1).

■ Planning

With appropriate therapy, the overall goals for the patient with ARDS are a PaO_2 of at least 60 mm Hg and adequate lung ventilation to maintain normal pH. The patient following recovery from ARDS will have (1) PaO_2 within normal limits for age or baseline values on room air (FIO_2 of 21%), (2) SaO_2 greater than 90%, (3) patent airway, and (4) clear lungs on auscultation.

TABLE 66-10 Collaborative Care Acute Respiratory Distress Syndrome

Diagnostic
See Table 66-8.

Collaborative Therapy

Respiratory Therapy
O_2 administration
Prone positioning
Lateral rotation therapy
Mechanical ventilation with PEEP

Supportive Therapy
Identification and treatment of underlying cause
Hemodynamic monitoring
Inotropic/vasopressor medications
   Dopamine (Intropin)
   Dobutamine (Dobutrex)
Diuretics
IV fluid administration

PEEP, Positive end-expiratory pressure.

■ Respiratory Therapy

Oxygen Administration. The primary goal of O_2 therapy is to correct hypoxemia. O_2 administered via a simple face mask or nasal cannula is usually inadequate to treat refractory hypoxemia that is associated with ARDS. Masks with high-flow systems that deliver higher O_2 concentrations are initially used to maximize O_2 delivery. Pulse oximetry (SpO_2) is continuously monitored to assess the effectiveness of O_2 therapy. The general standard for O_2 administration is to give the patient the lowest concentration that results in a PaO_2 of 60 mm Hg or greater. When the FIO_2 exceeds 60% for more than 48 hours, the risk for O_2 toxicity increases. Patients with ARDS commonly need intubation with mechanical ventilation because the PaO_2 cannot otherwise be maintained at acceptable levels.

Mechanical Ventilation. Endotracheal intubation and mechanical ventilation provide additional respiratory support. However, even with these interventions it may be necessary to maintain the FIO_2 at 60% or greater to maintain the PaO_2 at 60 mm Hg or greater. During mechanical ventilation, it is common to apply positive end-expiratory pressure (PEEP) at 5 cm H_2O to compensate for loss of glottic function caused by the presence of the endotracheal tube. In patients with ARDS, higher levels of PEEP (e.g., 10 to 20 cm H_2O) may be used. The mechanism of action of PEEP is related to its ability to increase FRC and recruit (open up) collapsed alveoli. PEEP is typically applied in 3 to 5 cm H_2O increments until oxygenation is adequate with FIO_2 of 60% or less. PEEP may improve $\dot{V}/\dot{Q}$ in respiratory units that collapse at low airway pressures, thus allowing the FIO_2 to be lowered.

However, PEEP is not a benign therapy. The additional intrathoracic and intrapulmonic pressures can compromise venous return to the right side of the heart, thereby decreasing preload, cardiac output, and blood pressure. PEEP can also cause hyperinflation of the alveoli, compression of the pulmonary capillary bed, a reduction in blood return to the left side of the heart, and a dramatic reduction in blood pressure. In addition, PEEP or excessive inspiratory pressures can result in barotrauma and volu-pressure trauma.[25]

If hypoxemic failure persists in spite of high levels of PEEP, alternative modes and therapies may be used. These include pressure support ventilation, pressure release ventilation, pressure control ventilation, inverse ratio ventilation, high-frequency ventilation, and permissive hypercapnia (low tidal volumes that allow $PaCO_2$ to increase slowly, maintaining normal pH and low airway pressures).[26,27] Additional information on mechanical ventilation and PEEP is provided in Chapter 64.

Extracorporeal membrane oxygenation (ECMO) and extracorporeal CO_2 removal ($ECCO_2R$) pass blood across a gas-exchanging membrane outside the body and then return oxygenated blood back to the body. $ECCO_2R$ with low-frequency PPV allows the lung to heal while the lung is not functional.[19,28]

Positioning Strategies. Some patients with ARDS demonstrate a marked improvement in PaO_2 when turned from the supine to prone position (e.g., PaO_2 70 mm Hg supine, PaO_2 90 mm Hg prone) with no change in inspired O_2 concentration (Fig. 66-10). The response may be sufficient to allow a reduction in inspired O_2 concentration or PEEP.

In the early phases of ARDS, fluid moves freely throughout the lung. Because of gravity, this fluid pools in dependent regions of the lung. As a consequence, some alveoli are fluid filled (dependent areas), whereas others are air filled (nondependent areas). In

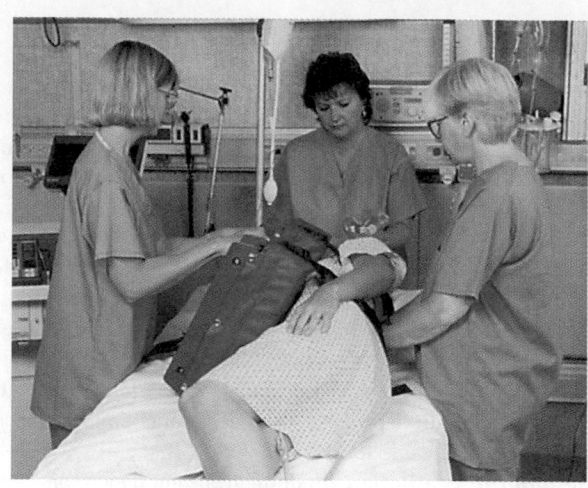
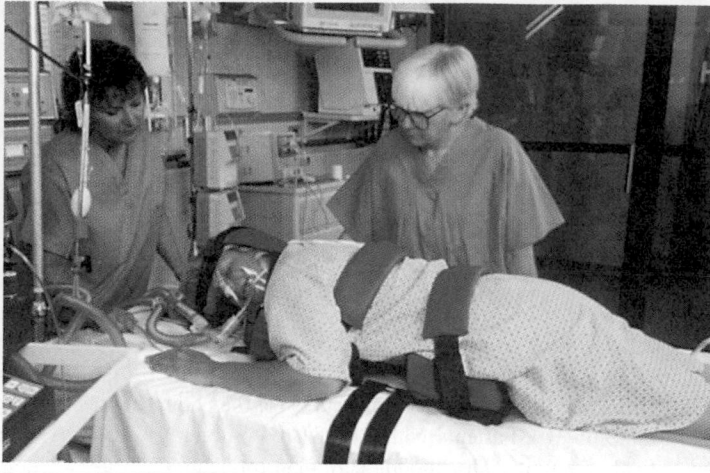

FIG. 66-10 A, Turning patient prone on Vollman Prone Positioner. B, Patient lying prone on Vollman Prone Positioner. (© 2001 Hill-Rom Services, Inc. REPRINTED WITH PERMISSION. ALL RIGHTS RESERVED.)

addition, when the patient is supine the heart and mediastinal contents place more pressure on the lungs than in the prone position, which changes pleural pressure and predisposes to atelectasis. If the patient is turned from supine to prone, air-filled, nonatelectic alveoli in the ventral (anterior) portion of the lung become dependent. Perfusion may be better matched to ventilation, causing less $\dot{V}/\dot{Q}$ mismatch. Not all patients respond to prone positioning with an increase in PaO_2, and there is no reliable way of predicting who will respond. Prone positioning is typically reserved for patients with refractory hypoxemia who do not respond to other strategies to increase PaO_2. When this positioning strategy is used, there must be a plan in place for immediate repositioning for cardiopulmonary resuscitation in the event of a cardiac arrest.[26,29-31]

Another positioning strategy that can be considered for patients with ARDS is lateral rotation therapy. The purpose of this therapy is to provide continuous, slow, side-to-side turning of the patient by rotating the actual bed frame (Fig. 66-11). The lateral movement of the bed is maintained for 18 of every 24 hours to simulate postural drainage and to help mobilize pulmonary secretions. In addition, the bed may also contain a vibrator pack that can provide chest physical therapy to further assist with secretion mobilization and removal. Baseline assessment of the patient's pulmonary status (e.g., respiratory rate and rhythm, breath sounds, ABGs, SpO_2) should be obtained before the initiation of the therapy and continued throughout the use of the therapy.[32]

■ Medical Supportive Therapy

Maintenance of Cardiac Output and Tissue Perfusion. Patients on PPV and PEEP frequently experience decreased cardiac output. One cause is decreased venous return, which results from the PEEP-induced increase in intrathoracic pressure. Cardiac output may also be decreased by impaired contractility and decreased preload. Continuous hemodynamic monitoring is essential to detect these changes and titrate therapy. An arterial catheter is inserted to permit continuous monitoring of blood pressure and sampling of blood for ABGs. A pulmonary artery catheter is normally inserted to allow monitoring of pulmonary artery pressure and pulmonary artery wedge pressures (which indicate the fluid status of the left side of the heart) and cardiac output. If the cardiac output falls, it may be necessary to administer

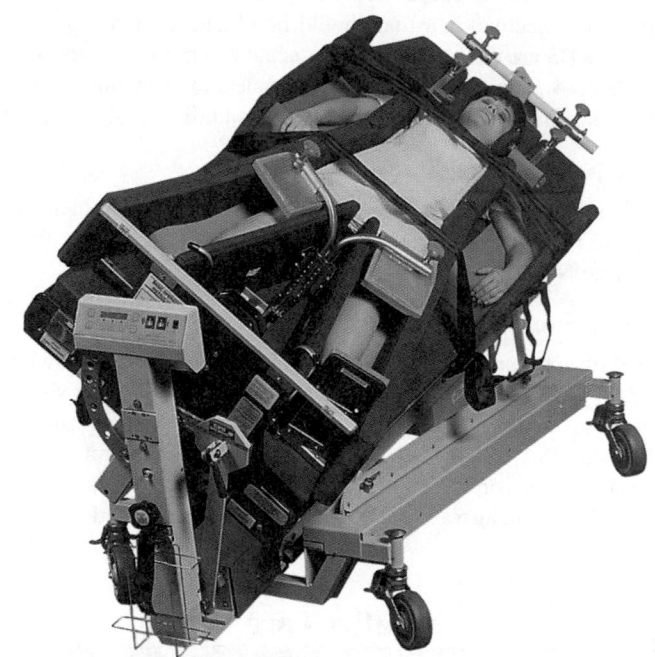

FIG. 66-11 Lateral rotation therapy bed.

crystalloid fluids or colloid solutions or to lower PEEP. Use of inotropic drugs such as dobutamine (Dobutrex) or dopamine (Intropin) may also be necessary. (See Chapter 64 for discussion of hemodynamic monitoring.)

The hemoglobin level is usually kept at levels of more than 9 to 10 g/dl (90 to 100 g/L) with an oxygen saturation of 90% or greater (when PaO_2 is more than 60 mm Hg). Packed red blood cells may be administered to increase hemoglobin and thus the O_2-carrying capacity of the blood.

Maintenance of Fluid Balance. Maintenance of fluid balance is challenging in the patient with ARDS. Increasing pulmonary capillary permeability results in fluid in the lungs and causes pulmonary edema. At the same time, the patient may be volume depleted and therefore prone to hypotension and decreased cardiac output from mechanical ventilation and PEEP.

Pulmonary artery wedge pressures, daily weights, and intake and output are monitored to assess the patient's fluid status. Controversy exists as to the benefits of fluid replacement with crystalloids versus colloids. Critics of colloid replacement believe that proteins in colloid fluid may leak into the pulmonary interstitium, exacerbating the movement of proteinaceous fluid into the alveoli. Advocates of colloid replacement believe that colloids help keep fluid from leaking into the alveoli. The pulmonary artery wedge pressure is kept as low as possible without impairing cardiac output in order to limit pulmonary edema. The patient is usually placed on mild fluid restriction, and diuretics are used as necessary.[33]

▪ Evaluation

The expected outcomes for the patient with ARDS are similar to those for a patient with acute respiratory failure and are presented in NCP 66-1.

SEVERE ACUTE RESPIRATORY SYNDROME

Severe acute respiratory syndrome (SARS) is a serious, acute respiratory infection caused by a coronavirus. The virus spreads by close contact between people. SARS is most likely spread via droplets in the air. It is possible that SARS may also be spread more broadly through the air or from touching objects that have become contaminated.

In general, SARS begins with a fever greater than 100.4° F (>38.0° C). Other manifestations may include headache, an overall feeling of discomfort, and muscle aches. Some people also experience mild respiratory symptoms. After 2 to 7 days, SARS patients may develop a dry cough and have trouble breathing.

Because the disease is severe, treatment needs to be started based on the symptoms and before the cause of the illness is confirmed. First, people who are suspected of having SARS should be placed in isolation to protect other patients and health care workers. Although there is no definitive treatment, antiviral medications (such as ribavirin), antibiotics, and corticosteroids may be used. Although antibiotics will not help with SARS (because it is believed to be caused by a virus), they may be used in cases where the person also has a bacterial infection.

About 80% to 90% of infected people start to recover after 6 to 7 days. However, 10% to 20% go on to develop very severe breathing problems and may need mechanical ventilation to breathe. The risk of death is higher for this group, and appears to be linked to the person's preexisting health conditions. People over age 40 are more likely to develop severe breathing problems.[34]

CRITICAL THINKING EXERCISES

Case Study
Acute Respiratory Distress Syndrome
Patient Profile. Mr. J. is a 55-year-old African American man who was admitted 72 hours ago to a general surgical unit after surgery for a bowel obstruction. The surgical procedure involved extensive abdominal surgery to repair a perforated colon, irrigate the abdominal cavity, and provide hemostasis. During surgery his systolic blood pressure dropped to 70 mm Hg. Seven units of packed red blood cells and 4 L of normal saline were administered intravenously to restore blood loss and circulating volume. He is receiving 60% O_2 through an aerosol face mask. He is being monitored with a cardiac monitor and pulse oximeter. He has a central intravenous catheter in place and is receiving 0.9% normal saline intravenously at 125 ml per hour. A urinary catheter is in place.

Subjective Data
- Complains of shortness of breath, inability to lie flat, and diffuse abdominal pain

Objective Data
Physical Assessment
- General: alert, well-nourished man who appears restless and anxious; head of bed elevated 45 degrees; skin cool with moderate diaphoresis.
- Respiratory: no accessory muscle use, retractions, or paradoxic breathing; respiratory rate 28 breaths/min; SpO_2 88%; fine crackles at lung bases.
- Cardiovascular: BP 100/60 mm Hg; cardiac monitor shows sinus tachycardia at 120 beats/min, with equal apical-radial pulse; temperature 101° F (38° C) orally.
- Gastrointestinal: surgical dressing dry and intact; sharp pain on palpation over incisional area.
- Urologic: urinary catheter draining concentrated urine, less than 30 ml per hour.

Diagnostic Findings
- ABG results: pH 7.35, PaO_2 59 mm Hg, $PaCO_2$ 27 mm Hg, bicarbonate 16 mEq/L, O_2 sat 89%.
- Chest x-ray shows new scattered interstitial infiltrates compatible with an ARDS pattern as interpreted by the radiologist.

CRITICAL THINKING QUESTIONS
1. How does the pathophysiology of ARDS predispose to the development of refractory hypoxemia?
2. What clinical manifestations does Mr. J. exhibit that support a diagnosis of ARDS?
3. What are the possible causes of ARDS in Mr. J.?
4. What are the possible complications that Mr. J. is at risk for developing secondary to ARDS?
5. What respiratory care interventions might be implemented to improve Mr. J's hypoxemia?
6. Based on the assessment data presented, write one or more appropriate nursing diagnoses.
7. Discuss any collaborative problems that might apply to this patient.

Nursing Research Issues
1. What should be the key components of an assessment tool to predict patients at risk for acute respiratory failure?
2. Compare the efficacy of prone positioning and continuous lateral rotation therapy in patients with ARDS.
3. What are the effects of a nurse-implemented sedation protocol for patients requiring mechanical ventilation on patient and family comfort and satisfaction with care?

REVIEW QUESTIONS

The number of the question corresponds to the same-numbered objective at the beginning of the chapter.

1. Hypercapnic respiratory failure can be caused by
   a. ARDS.
   b. asthma.
   c. pneumonia.
   d. pulmonary emboli.

2. An early sign of acute respiratory failure is
   a. coma.
   b. cyanosis.
   c. restlessness.
   d. paradoxic breathing.

3. The oxygen delivery system chosen for the patient in acute respiratory failure should
   a. always be a low-flow device, such as a nasal cannula.
   b. correct the PaO_2 to a normal level as quickly as possible.
   c. administer positive pressure ventilation to prevent CO_2 narcosis.
   d. maintain the PaO_2 at 60 mm Hg or greater at the lowest O_2 concentration possible.

4. The most common early clinical manifestations of ARDS that the nurse may observe are
   a. dyspnea and tachypnea.
   b. cyanosis and apprehension.
   c. hypotension and tachycardia.
   d. respiratory distress and frothy sputum.

5. Maintenance of fluid balance in the patient with ARDS involves
   a. hydration using colloids.
   b. administration of surfactant.
   c. mild fluid restriction and diuretics as necessary.
   d. keeping the hemoglobin at levels of 15 to 16 g/dl (150 to 160 g/L).

6. Which of the following interventions is designed to prevent or limit barotrauma in the patient with ARDS who is mechanically ventilated?
   a. increasing PEEP
   b. increasing the tidal volume
   c. use of permissive hypercapnia
   d. use of pressure support ventilation

REFERENCES

1. Murray JF et al, editors: *Textbook of respiratory medicine,* ed 3, New York, 2000, WB Saunders.
2. Grippi MA: Respiratory failure: an overview. In Fishman AP et al, editors: *Fishman's pulmonary diseases and disorders,* ed 3, New York, 1998, McGraw-Hill.
3. Hornick DB: An approach to the analysis of arterial blood gases and acid-base disorders. University of Iowa Health Care. Available at *www.int-med.uiowa.edu/education/abg.htm* (accessed Nov 13, 2001).
4. Desai PM: Pain management and pulmonary dysfunction, *Crit Care Clin* 15:151, 1999.
5. Epstein J, Breslow MJ: The stress response of critical illness, *Crit Care Clin* 15:17, 1999.
6. Light RB: Pulmonary pathophysiology of pneumococcal pneumonia, *Semin Respir Infect* 14:218, 1999.
7. Panettiere RA, Murray RK: Chronic obstructive pulmonary disease. In Foshman AP, editor: *Pulmonary diseases and disorders: companion handbook,* ed 3, New York, 1998, McGraw-Hill.
8. Mehta S, Hill NS: State of the art: noninvasive ventilation, *Am J Respir Crit Care Med* 163:540, 2001.
9. Vines DL, Shelledy DC, Peters J: Current respiratory care: oxygen therapy, oximetry, bronchial hygiene, *J Crit Illn* 15:507, 2000.
10. Moore MJ, Schmidt GA: Keys to effective noninvasive ventilation: initial steps, *J Crit Illn* 16:64, 2001.
11. Crawshaw L, Pennock BE: Noninvasive ventilatory support: who benefits. SpringNet-Nursing Community. Available at *www.springnet.com/criticalcare/noninvas.htm* (accessed Nov 13, 2001).
12. Hill NS, Meyer TJ: Lesson 3, volume 9: noninvasive positive pressure ventilation. Available at *www.chestnet.org/education/pccu/best/lesson03-09.html* (accessed Nov 13, 2001).
13. Que LG, Huang YCT: Pharmacological adjuncts during mechanical ventilation, *Semin Respir Crit Care Med* 21. Available at *http://respiratorycare.medscape.com/thieme/SRCCM/2000/v21.n03/r...pnt-rcm2103.02que.htm* (accessed Sept 9, 2001).
14. Lowson SM, Sawh S: Adjuncts to analgesia: sedation and neuromuscular blockade, *Crit Care Clin* 15:119, 1999.
15. Arbour R: Sedation and pain management in critically ill adults, *Crit Care Nurse* 20:39, 2000.
16. Arbour R: Mastering neuromuscular blockade, *DCCN* 19:4, 2000.
17. Janssens JP, Pache JC, Nicod LP: Physiological changes in respiratory function associated with aging, *Eur Respir J* 13:197, 1999.
18. Sue DS: Acute respiratory failure in the elderly patient, *Clin Geriatr* 8:37, 2000.
19. Zwischenberger JB: ARDS and mechanical ventilation, *J Respir Care Pract* 13:47, 2000.
20. Steinberg KS, Hudson LD: Acute lung injury and acute respiratory distress syndrome—the clinical syndrome, *Clin Chest Med* 21:401, 2000.
21. Soeren MH et al: Pathophysiology and implications for treatment of acute respiratory distress syndrome, *AACN Clin Issues* 11:179, 2000.
22. Davies P: Guarding your patient against ARDS, *Nursing* 32:36, 2002.
23. Urden LD, Stacy KM, Lough ME: *Thelan's critical care nursing: diagnosis and management,* ed 3, St Louis, 1998, Mosby.
24. Mayer J, Campbell D: ATS recommendations for treatment of adults with hospital-acquired pneumonia. Available at *www.medscape.com/SCP/IIM/1996/v13.n12/m1991.mayer/m1991.mayer.html* (accessed July 20, 2002).
*25. Burns SM: Ventilatory management—volume and pressure modes. In Lynn-McHale DJ, Carlson KK, editors: *AACN procedure manual for critical care,* ed 4, Philadelphia, 2001, WB Saunders.
26. Hirvela ER: Advances in the management of acute respiratory distress syndrome, *Arch Surg* 135:126, 2000.
27. Houston P: An approach to ventilation in acute respiratory distress syndrome, *Can J Surg* 43:263, 2000.
28. Bartlett RH: Extracorporeal life support in the management of severe respiratory failure, *Clin Chest Med* 21:555, 2000.
*29. Breilburg AN et al: Efficacy and safety of prone positioning for patients with acute respiratory distress syndrome, *J Adv Nurs* 32:922, 2000.
30. Ball C et al: Clinical guidelines for the use of the prone position in acute respiratory distress syndrome, *Intensive Crit Care Nurs* 17:94, 2001.
31. Marion BS: A turn for the better: "prone positioning" of patients with ARDS, *Am J Nurs* 101:26, 2001.
*32. Tomaselli NL, Goldberg MT, Wind S: Pressure-reducing devices: lateral rotation therapy. In Lynn-McHale DJ, Carlson KK, editors: *AACN procedure manual for critical care,* ed 4, Philadelphia, 2001, WB Saunders.
33. Sadikot RT, Christman JW: ARDS: what's new in management, *J Respir Dis* 20:499, 1999.
34. http://www.cdc.gov/ncidod/sars/

RESOURCES

Resources for this chapter are listed after Chapter 64 on page 1795.

*Nursing research–based references.

CHAPTER 67

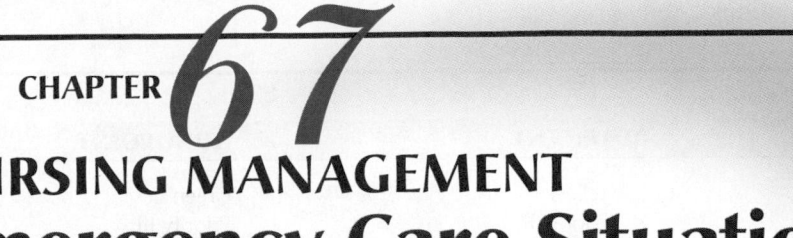

NURSING MANAGEMENT
Emergency Care Situations

Linda Bucher

LEARNING OBJECTIVES

1. Apply the sequential steps in the primary and secondary survey to a patient in an emergency situation.
2. Describe the pathophysiology, assessment, and collaborative care of select environmental emergencies, including hyperthermia, hypothermia, submersion injury, and animal bites.
3. Discuss the pathophysiology, assessment, and collaborative care of select toxicologic emergencies.
4. Differentiate between the various types and victims of violence.
5. Describe the difference between emergency and disaster preparedness from the perspective of the emergency department.
6. Identify the agents most likely to be used in a terrorist attack.

KEY TERMS

bioterrorism, p. 1862
disaster, p. 1866
domestic violence, p. 1862
emergency, p. 1866
frostbite, p. 1854
heat cramps, p. 1852
heat exhaustion, p. 1852
heat stroke, p. 1852
hypothermia, p. 1854
jaw-thrust maneuver, p. 1847

pneumatic antishock garment, p. 1848
primary survey, p. 1847
rapid-sequence intubation, p. 1847
secondary survey, p. 1848
submersion injury, p. 1856
triage, p. 1847
violence, p. 1862

Most patients with life-threatening or potentially life-threatening problems arrive at the hospital through the emergency department (ED). Many more patients report to the ED for less urgent conditions. Visits to the ED have increased significantly because of the lack of health insurance or a primary care provider, increased violence, and inability to access a health care provider.[1] Emergency nurses care for patients of all ages and with a variety of problems. However, some EDs specialize in certain patient populations or conditions, such as pediatric ED or trauma ED.

The Emergency Nurses Association (ENA) is the largest specialty nursing organization aimed at advancing emergency nursing practice. The ENA provides standards of care for nurses working in the ED, as well as a certification process that allows nurses to become a certified emergency nurse (CEN). This certification validates the knowledge that a nurse needs to provide competent care in emergency settings.[2]

Specific emergency management of patients with various medical, surgical, and traumatic emergencies is presented throughout this book where the disorders are discussed. Tables that highlight emergency management of specific problems are presented throughout the book. Table 67-1 lists each emergency management table by title, number, and page. This chapter focuses on ini-

tial assessment and management of the trauma patient and emergency conditions not addressed elsewhere in this book, including heat- and cold-related emergencies, submersion injuries, bites, stings, and poisonings. In addition, a brief overview of issues related to violence and emergency and disaster preparedness is presented.

TABLE 67-1 Emergency Management — Emergency Management Tables

TITLE	CHAPTER	PAGE
Abdominal trauma	41	1065
Acute abdominal pain	41	1061
Acute soft tissue injury	61	1652
Anaphylactic shock	13	251
Arrhythmias	35	867
Chemical burns	24	520
Chest pain	33	818
Chest trauma	27	619
Cocaine and amphetamine toxicity	11	182
Depressant drugs, overdose of	11	186
Diabetic ketoacidosis	47	1293
Electrical burns	24	521
Eye injury	21	445
Fractured extremity	61	1665
Head injury	55	1510
Hyperthermia	67	1853
Hypothermia	67	1855
Inhalation injury	24	521
Sexual assault	52	1413
Shock	65	1809
Spinal cord injury	59	1616
Stroke	56	1534
Submersion injuries	67	1857
Surface skin wound	23	495
Thermal burns	24	522
Thoracic injuries	27	620
Tonic-clonic seizures	57	1558

Reviewed by Linda Laskowski-Jones, RN, MS, CS, CCRN, CEN, Director of Trauma, Emergency, and Aeromedical Services, Christiana Care Health System, Newark, Del.

TABLE 67-2 Triage Acuity Systems

	EMERGENT	URGENT	NONURGENT
Colors	Red	Yellow	Green
Numbers	Priority I	Priority II	Priority III
Urgency	Life, limb, eye threatening; needs immediate attention	Needs treatment in 20 minutes to 2 hours	Can wait hours or days
Recommended reevaluation	Continuous	Every 30-60 min	Every 1-2 hr
Examples	Trauma, chest pain, cardiac arrest, severe respiratory distress, chemicals in the eyes, limb amputation, acute neurologic deficits	Fever >104° F (40° C), diastolic blood pressure >130 mm Hg, kidney stone, simple fracture, abdominal pain, asthma/no respiratory distress	Sprain, minor laceration, cold symptoms, rash, simple headache

TABLE 67-3 Primary Survey of an Emergency Patient

ASSESSMENT	INTERVENTIONS
Airway with Simultaneous Cervical Spine Stabilization and/or Immobilization	
• Clear and open airway • Assess for obstructed airway • Assess for respiratory distress • Check for loose teeth or foreign objects • Assess for bleeding, vomitus, or edema	• Suction • Jaw thrust • Nasal or oral airway, endotracheal tube, cricothyroidotomy • Cervical spine immobilization using collar, backboard, soft rolls; tape forehead
Breathing	

• Assess ventilation
  • Look for paradoxic movement of the chest wall during inspiration and expiration
  • Note use of accessory muscles or abdominal muscles
  • Listen for air being expired through nose and mouth
  • Feel for air being expelled
• Observe and count respiratory rate
• Note color of nail beds, mucous membranes, skin
• Auscultate lungs
• Assess for jugular venous distention and position of trachea
	• Ventilate with bag-valve-mask with 100% O_2
	• Prepare to intubate if respiratory arrest
	• Have suction available
	• Give supplemental O_2 via appropriate delivery system
	• If absent breath sounds, prepare for needle thoracostomy and chest tube insertion

Circulation	
• Check carotid or femoral pulse • Palpate pulse for quality and rate • Assess color, temperature, and moisture of skin • Check capillary refill • Assess for external bleeding • Auscultate blood pressure	• If absent pulse, initiate cardiopulmonary resuscitation and advanced life support measures • If shock symptoms or hypotensive, start two large-bore (14- to 16-gauge) IVs and initiate infusions of normal saline or lactated Ringer's solution • Administer blood products if ordered • Consider autotransfusion if isolated chest trauma • Consider use of a pneumatic antishock garment in the presence of pelvic fracture • Obtain blood samples for type and crossmatch • Control bleeding with direct pressure
Disability—Brief Neurologic Assessment	
• Assess level of consciousness by determining response to verbal and/or painful stimuli • Assess pupils for size, shape, equality, and response to light	• Periodically reassess level of consciousness • Consider hyperventilation if signs of brain herniation (e.g., motor posturing)

IVs, Intravenous lines.

CARE OF THE EMERGENCY PATIENT

Recognition of life-threatening illness or injury is one of the most important aspects of emergency care. Before a diagnosis can be made, recognition of dangerous clinical signs and symptoms with initiation of interventions to reverse or prevent a crisis is essential. This process begins with the first patient contact. The emergency nurse is usually confronted with multiple patients who have a variety of problems. Prompt identification of patients requiring immediate treatment and determination of appropriate treatment area are essential in a busy ED.[3]

A *triage system* identifies and categorizes patients so that the most critical are treated first. **Triage** is a French word meaning "to sort."[4] The process is based on the premise that patients who have a threat to life, vision, or limb should be treated before other patients. When patients call the ED with health-related questions, triage is conducted over the telephone.[5] The ED uses a system of words, color coding, or numbers for determining triage decisions (Table 67-2).

The emergency nurse must complete an initial assessment to determine the presence of actual or potential threats to life and then rapidly initiate interventions appropriate for the patient's condition.[6] A history is obtained simultaneously. A systematic approach to the initial patient assessment decreases the time required to identify potential threats and minimizes the risk of missing a life-threatening condition. Two systematic approaches, a primary survey and a secondary survey, were initially developed for use with the trauma patient, but these can be easily applied to assessment of any emergency patient.

Primary Survey

The **primary survey** (Table 67-3) focuses on airway, breathing, circulation, and disability and serves to identify life-threatening conditions so that appropriate interventions can be initiated. Life-threatening conditions related to airway, breathing, circulation, and disability (Table 67-4) may be identified at any point during the primary survey. When this occurs, interventions are started immediately and before proceeding to the next step of the survey.

A = Airway with Cervical Spine Stabilization and/or Immobilization. Nearly all immediate trauma deaths occur because of airway obstruction. Saliva, bloody secretions, vomitus, laryngeal trauma, facial trauma, fractures, and the tongue can obstruct the airway. Medical patients at risk for airway compromise include those who have seizures, near-drowning, anaphylaxis, foreign body obstruction, or cardiopulmonary arrest. If an airway is not maintained, obstruction of airflow occurs and hypoxia, acidosis, and death result.

Primary signs and symptoms in a patient with a compromised airway include dyspnea, inability to vocalize, presence of foreign body in the airway, and trauma to the face or neck. Airway maintenance should progress rapidly from the least to the most invasive method. Treatment includes opening the airway using the **jaw-thrust maneuver** (avoiding hyperextension of the neck) (Fig. 67-1), suctioning and/or removal of foreign body, insertion of a nasopharyngeal or oropharyngeal airway (will cause gag if patient is conscious), and endotracheal intubation. If unable to intubate because of airway obstruction, an emergency cricothyroidotomy or tracheotomy should be performed (see

TABLE 67-4	Causes of Life-Threatening Conditions Identified during the Primary Survey*

Airway
- Inhalation injury
- Obstruction, partial or complete, from foreign bodies, debris (e.g., vomitus), or the tongue
- Penetrating wounds and/or blunt trauma to the upper airway structures

Breathing
- Anaphylaxis
- Flail chest with pulmonary contusion
- Hemothorax
- Open pneumothorax
- Tension pneumothorax

Circulation
- Direct cardiac injury (e.g., myocardial infarction, trauma)
- Pericardial tamponade
- Shock (e.g., massive burns)
- Uncontrolled external hemorrhage

Disability
- Head injury
- Stroke

*List is not all-inclusive.

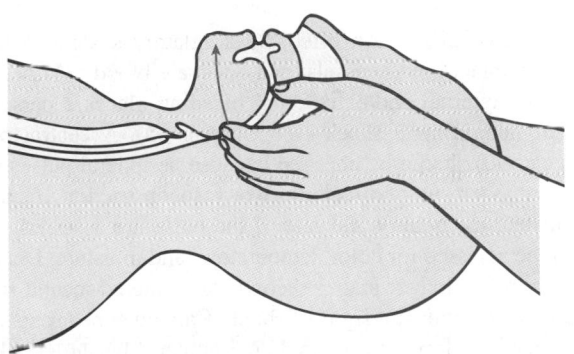

FIG. 67-1   Jaw-thrust maneuver is the only widely recommended procedure for use on an unconscious patient with possible neck or spinal injuries. The patient should be lying supine with the rescuer kneeling at the top of the head. The rescuer should carefully reach forward and gently place one hand on each side of the patient's chin at the lateral angles of the lower jaw. The patient's head should be stabilized with the rescuer's forearms, then the jaw pushed forward while pressure is applied with the index fingers.

Chapter 26). Patients should be ventilated with 100% oxygen using a bag-valve-mask (BVM) device before intubation or cricothyroidotomy.[7]

Rapid-sequence intubation is the preferred procedure for securing an unprotected airway in the ED. It involves the use of sedation (e.g., etomidate [Amidate]) and paralysis (e.g., succinylcholine [Anectine]) to facilitate intubation while minimizing the risk of aspiration and airway trauma.[8,9]

Any patient with significant upper torso injuries or face, head, or neck trauma should always be suspected of cervical spine trauma. The cervical spine must be stabilized (head maintained in a neutral position) and/or immobilized during assessment of the airway. At the scene of the injury, the cervical spine is immobilized with a rigid cervical collar or a cervical immobilization device (CID) (also known as "head blocks"), and towel rolls are taped to a backboard on either side of the head. Finally, the patient's forehead is taped to the backboard. Sandbags should not be used because the weight of the bags could move the head if the patient must be logrolled.

B = Breathing. Adequate airflow through the upper airway does not ensure adequate ventilation. Breathing alterations are caused by many conditions, including fractured ribs, pneumothorax, penetrating injury, allergic reactions, pulmonary emboli, and asthma attacks. Patients with these conditions may experience a variety of signs and symptoms, including dyspnea (e.g., due to pulmonary emboli), paradoxic or asymmetric chest wall movement (e.g., flail chest), decreased or absent breath sounds on the affected side (e.g., pneumothorax), visible wound to chest wall (e.g., penetrating injury), cyanosis (e.g., due to asthma), tachycardia, and hypotension.

Every critically injured or ill patient has an increased metabolic and oxygen demand and should have supplemental oxygen. High-flow oxygen (100%) via a non-rebreather mask should be administered and the patient's response monitored. Life-threatening conditions, such as tension pneumothorax and flail chest, can severely compromise ventilation. Interventions in these situations include BVM ventilation with 100% oxygen, intubation, and treatment of the underlying cause.

C = Circulation. An effective circulatory system includes the heart, intact blood vessels, and adequate blood volume. Uncontrolled internal and/or external bleeding places a person at risk for hemorrhagic shock (see Chapter 65). A central pulse (e.g., carotid) should be checked because peripheral pulses may be absent as a result of direct injury or vasoconstriction. If a pulse is palpated, the quality and rate of the pulse are assessed. Skin should be assessed for color, temperature, and moisture. Delayed capillary refill (longer than 3 seconds) and altered mental status are the most significant signs of shock. Care must be taken when evaluating capillary refill in cold environments because cold delays refill.

Intravenous (IV) lines are inserted into veins in the upper extremities unless contraindicated, such as in a massive fracture or an injury that affects limb circulation. Two large-bore (14- to 16-gauge) IV catheters should be inserted and aggressive fluid resuscitation initiated using lactated Ringer's solution or normal saline. Direct pressure with a sterile dressing should be applied to obvious bleeding sites. Blood samples are obtained for typing to determine ABO and Rh group. Type-specific packed red blood cells should be administered if needed. In an emergency (life-threatening) situation, uncrossmatched blood may be given if immediate transfusion is warranted.

The use of the **pneumatic antishock garment** (PASG) is a temporary strategy that can be considered for pelvic fracture bleeding with hypotension. The PASG is a three-chambered suit that is applied to the patient's legs and abdomen and is inflated with a foot pump. Physiologically, the PASG increases peripheral resistance in the patient's lower extremities, thus elevating blood pressure, and works to control pelvic fracture bleeding.[10]

D = Disability. A brief neurologic examination completes the primary survey. The degree of disability is measured by the patient's level of consciousness. Determining the patient's response to verbal and/or painful stimuli is one approach to assessing level of consciousness. A simple mnemonic to remember is AVPU: A = alert, V = responsive to voice, P = responsive to pain, and U = unresponsive. In addition, the Glasgow Coma Scale (GCS) is used to further assess the arousal aspect of the patient's consciousness (see Chapter 55). Finally, pupils should be also assessed for size, shape, equality, and response to light.

Secondary Survey

After each step of the primary survey is addressed and any lifesaving interventions are initiated, the secondary survey begins. The **secondary survey** is a brief, systematic process that is aimed at identifying *all* injuries (Table 67-5).

E = Exposure/Environmental Control. All trauma patients should have their clothes removed so that a thorough physical assessment can be performed. Once the patient is exposed, it is important to limit heat loss and prevent hypothermia by using warming blankets, overhead warmers, and warmed IV fluids.

F = Full Set of Vital Signs/Five Interventions/Facilitate Family Presence. A complete set of vital signs, including blood pressure, heart rate, respiratory rate, and temperature, should be obtained after the patient is exposed. Blood pressure should be obtained in both arms if the patient has sustained or is suspected of having sustained chest trauma.

At this point, it must be determined whether to proceed with the secondary survey or to perform additional interventions. The availability of other team members often influences this decision. For patients who have sustained significant trauma and/or have required lifesaving interventions during the primary survey, the following five interventions should be performed at this time.

First, the patient should be monitored by electrocardiogram (ECG) for heart rate and rhythm. Second, pulse oximetry should be initiated and oxygen saturation (SpO_2) monitored. Third, an indwelling catheter should be inserted to monitor urine output and to check for hematuria. An indwelling catheter should not be inserted if a urethral tear is suspected. Patients with pelvic injuries or blood at the meatus, and men with a high-riding prostate gland on digital rectal examination, are at risk for a urethral tear or transection. A urethrogram should be obtained before a catheter is inserted. Fourth, an orogastric or a nasogastric tube should be inserted to provide gastric decompression and emptying to reduce the risk of aspiration and to test the contents for blood. A nasogastric tube should not be placed in the nares in a patient suspected of having facial fractures or a basilar skull fracture because the tube could enter the brain through the cribriform plate; rather, it should be placed orally. Fifth, laboratory studies for typing and crossmatching, hematocrit, hemoglobin, blood urea nitrogen, creatinine, blood alcohol, toxicology screening, arterial blood gases, electrolytes, coagulation profile, liver enzymes, cardiac enzymes, and pregnancy should be facilitated.

Facilitating *family presence* (FP) completes this step of the secondary survey. Research supports the positive benefits of FP during invasive procedures (IPs) and cardiopulmonary resuscitation (CPR) to patients, families, and staff.[11,12] Patients reported that having family members present comforted them, served as an advocate for them, and helped to remind the health care team of their "personhood."[11] Family members who wished to be pre-

TABLE 67-5	Secondary Survey of an Emergency Patient	
PARAMETER	**ASSESSMENT**
Exposure and Environmental Control	Remove clothing for adequate examination. Keep patient warm with blankets, warmed IV fluids, overhead lights.
Full Set of Vital Signs	Obtain vital signs: temperature, heart rate, respiratory rate, blood pressure bilaterally.
Five Interventions	Heart rhythm, O_2 saturation, insertion of a urinary catheter (if not contraindicated), insertion of gastric tube, blood for laboratory studies.
Facilitate Family Presence	Determine family's desire to be present during invasive procedures or cardiopulmonary resuscitation.
Give Comfort Measures	Level of pain, anxiety.
History and Head-to-Toe Assessment	
History	Details of the incident/illness, mechanism and pattern of injury, length of time since incident occurred, injuries suspected, treatment provided and patient's response, level of consciousness. Allergies. Medication history. Past health history (e.g., preexisting medical conditions, last menstrual period). Last meal. Events/environment preceding illness or injury.
Head, neck, face	Note general appearance, including skin color. Examine face and scalp for lacerations, bone or soft tissue deformity, tenderness, bleeding, and foreign bodies. Examine eyes, ears, nose, and mouth for bleeding, foreign bodies, drainage, pain, deformity, ecchymosis, lacerations. Examine head for depressions of cranial or facial bones, contusions, hematomas, areas of softness, bony crepitus. Examine neck for stiffness, pain in cervical vertebrae, tracheal deviation, distended neck veins, bleeding, edema, difficulty swallowing, bruising, subcutaneous emphysema, bony crepitus.
Chest	Observe rate, depth, and effort of breathing, including chest wall movement. Palpate for bony crepitus, subcutaneous emphysema. Use of accessory muscles. Auscultate breath sounds. Obtain ECG. External signs of injury: petechiae, bleeding, cyanosis, bruises, abrasions, lacerations, old scars.
Abdomen and flanks	Symmetry of external abdominal wall and bony structures. External signs of injury: bruising, abrasions, lacerations, punctures. Assess for masses, guarding, femoral pulses. Type and location of pain, rigidity, or distention of abdomen. Assess bowel sounds.
Pelvis and perineum	Assess genitalia for blood at the meatus, priapism, ecchymosis, rectal bleeding, anal sphincter tone.
Extremities	Signs of external injury: deformity, ecchymosis, abrasions, lacerations, swelling. Pain. Movement and strength in arms and legs. Sensation in each limb. Color of skin. Presence and quality of peripheral pulses.
Inspect posterior surfaces	Logroll and inspect and palpate back for deformity, bleeding, lacerations, bruising.

ECG, Electrocardiogram; IV, intravenous.

sent during IPs and CPR viewed themselves as active participants in the care process. They also believed that they provided comfort to the patient and that it was their right to be with the patient.[12] Staff nurses reported that family members who participated in FP functioned as "patient helpers" (e.g., providing support) and "staff helpers" (e.g., acting as a translator) and reinforced that FP helped to convey the sense of the patient's personhood.[12] Should a family member request FP, it is essential that a member of the team explain care delivered and be available to answer questions.

G = Give Comfort Measures. Provision of comfort measures is of paramount importance when caring for patients in the ED. It has been reported that as many as 78% of all patients who come to the ED are in pain.[13] Pain management strategies should include a combination of pharmacologic (e.g., IV narcotics) and nonpharmacologic (e.g., imagery) measures.[14,15] Emergency nurses play a pivotal role in pain management because of their frequent contact with patients. However, emergency nurses have reported knowledge deficits regarding pain management principles (e.g., pharmacology; differentiating physical dependence, addiction, and tolerance).[13,14] General comfort measures such as verbal reassurance, listening, reducing stimuli (e.g., dimming lights), and developing a trusting relationship with the patient and family should be provided to all patients in the ED.

H = History and Head-to-Toe Assessment. The history of the incident, injury, or illness provides clues to the cause of the crisis and suggests specific assessment and intervention needs. The patient may be unable to give a history. However, family, friends, witnesses, and prehospital personnel can frequently provide important information. Prehospital information should focus on the mechanism and pattern of injury, injuries suspected, vital signs, and treatment initiated and patient responses.

Details of the incident are extremely important because the mechanism of injury and injury patterns can predict specific injuries. For example, a front-seat passenger with a seat belt may have a head injury from hitting the steering wheel; knee, femur, or hip fractures or dislocation from striking the dashboard; and an abdominal injury from the seat belt. If other victims were dead at the scene, the patient has a high chance of significant injury.

Patients who jump from buildings or bridges may have bilateral calcaneal (heel) fractures, bilateral wrist fractures, and lumbar spine compression fractures, and they may be at risk for aortic tears. Older patients who have climbed ladders and fallen may have had a stroke or myocardial infarction that led to the fall.

Prehospital personnel will often provide a detailed description of the patient's general condition, level of consciousness, and apparent injuries. An experienced ED team can complete a history within 5 minutes of the patient's arrival. If the patient is emergently ill, a thorough history is obtained from family or friends after the patient is taken to the treatment area. The history should include the following questions:

1. What is the chief complaint? What caused the patient to seek attention?
2. What are the patient's subjective complaints?
3. What is the patient's description of pain (e.g., location, duration, quality, character)?
4. What are witnesses' (if any) descriptions of the patient's behavior since the onset?
5. What is the patient's health care history? The mnemonic *AMPLE* assists the nurse in remembering to ask about the following:

   A   Allergies
   M   Medication history
   P   Past health history (e.g., preexisting medical conditions, previous hospitalizations/surgeries, smoking history, recent use of drugs/alcohol, tetanus immunization, last menstrual period)
   L   Last meal
   E   Events/environment preceding illness or injury

Head, neck, and face. The patient should be assessed for general appearance, skin color, and temperature. The eyes should be evaluated for extraocular movements. A disconjugate gaze is an indication of neurologic damage. "Raccoon eyes," or periorbital ecchymosis, is usually caused by a basilar skull fracture. The tympanic membranes and external canal are checked for blood and cerebrospinal fluid (see Chapter 55). Clear drainage from the ear or nose should not be stopped.

The airway is assessed for foreign bodies, bleeding, edema, and loose or missing teeth. Assess for difficulty swallowing, movement of the palate, and ability to open the mouth. The neck should be examined for bruising, edema, bleeding, or distended neck veins. The trachea is palpated and visualized to determine whether it is in the midline. A deviated trachea may signal a life-threatening tension pneumothorax. Subcutaneous emphysema may indicate laryngotracheal disruption. A stiff or painful cervical spine area may signify a fracture of a cervical vertebra. The cervical spine must be protected using a rigid collar and supine positioning. Patients must be logrolled when movement is necessary.

Chest. The chest is examined for paradoxic chest movements and large sucking chest wounds. The sternum, clavicles, and ribs are palpated for deformity and point tenderness. The chest is assessed for pain on palpation, respiratory distress, decreased breath sounds, distant heart sounds, and distended neck veins. In addition to tension pneumothorax and open pneumothorax, the patient should be evaluated for rib fractures, pulmonary contusion, blunt cardiac injury, and simple pneumothorax. A 12-lead ECG should be obtained, particularly on an older patient or a patient with suspected heart disease. The ECG should be done to detect arrhythmias and evidence of ischemia or infarction.

Abdomen and flanks. The abdomen and flanks are more difficult to assess. Frequent evaluation for subtle changes in the abdominal examination is essential. Motor vehicle collisions and assaults can cause blunt trauma. Penetrating trauma tends to injure specific organs. Decreased bowel sounds may indicate a temporary paralytic ileus. Bowel sounds in the chest may indicate a diaphragmatic rupture. The abdomen is percussed for distention (e.g., tympany [excessive air], dullness [excessive fluid]) and palpated for peritoneal irritation.

If intraabdominal hemorrhage is suspected, a diagnostic peritoneal lavage (DPL) may be performed to determine the presence of blood in the peritoneal space (hemoperitoneum). Before the procedure, a gastric tube and a bladder catheter must be inserted to decompress these organs and reduce the possibility of perforation. An alternative to DPL that is gaining support is an ultrasonography procedure called a *focused abdominal sonography for trauma* (FAST). This procedure is noninvasive and can be performed quickly.[10]

Pelvis and perineum. The pelvis is gently palpated. If pain is elicited, it may indicate a pelvic fracture. The genitalia are inspected for bleeding and obvious injuries. A rectal examination is performed to check for blood, a high-riding prostate gland, and loss of sphincter tone. Assess for bladder distention, hematuria, dysuria, or the inability to void.

Extremities. The upper and lower extremities are assessed. Injured extremities are splinted above and below the injury to decrease further soft tissue injury and pain. Grossly deformed, pulseless extremities should be realigned and splinted. Pulses are checked before and after movement or splinting of an extremity. A pulseless extremity represents a time-critical vascular or orthopedic emergency.

The extremities are palpated for point tenderness, crepitus, and abnormal movements. Injured extremities should be elevated and ice packs applied. Prophylactic antibiotics are administered for open fractures. Patients with fractures should receive IV analgesia.[14]

I = Inspect the Posterior Surfaces. The trauma patient should always be turned (using spinal precautions) to inspect the patient's posterior surfaces. The back is inspected for ecchymosis, abrasions, puncture wounds, cuts, and obvious deformities. The entire spine is palpated for misalignment, deformity, and pain.

Intervention and Evaluation

Once the secondary survey is complete, all findings are recorded. All patients should be evaluated to determine their need for tetanus prophylaxis. Information about the patient's past vaccination history and the condition of any wounds is needed in order to make an appropriate decision (Table 67-6).

Regardless of the patient's chief complaint, ongoing patient monitoring and evaluation of interventions are critical in an emergency situation. The nurse is responsible for providing appropriate interventions and assessing the patient's response. The evaluation of airway patency and the effectiveness of breathing will always assume highest priority. The nurse will monitor O_2 saturation and arterial blood gases (ABGs) to help determine the patient's progress in these areas. Level of consciousness, vital signs, quality of peripheral pulses, urine output, and skin temperature, color, and moisture provide key information about circulation and perfusion and are also monitored.

Depending on the patient's injuries and/or illness, the patient may be (1) transported for diagnostic tests such as a computed tomography (CT) scan, x-ray, or magnetic resonance imaging (MRI); (2) admitted to a general or intensive care unit; or (3) transferred to another facility. The emergency nurse is responsible for monitoring the patient during transport and notifying the team should the patient's condition change from baseline. Nurses accompanying critically ill patients on intrafacility or interfacility transports must be competent in advanced life support measures.

Death in the Emergency Department

Unfortunately, there are a number of emergency patients who do not benefit from the skill, expertise, and technology available in the ED. It is important for the emergency nurse to be able to deal with feelings about sudden death so that the nurse can help families and significant others begin the grieving process.[16]

The emergency nurse should recognize the importance of certain hospital rituals in preparing the bereaved to grieve, such as collecting the belongings, arranging for an autopsy, viewing the body, and making mortuary arrangements. The death must seem real so that the significant others can begin to grieve and accept the death. The emergency nurse plays a significant role in providing comfort to the surviving loved ones after a death in the ED.

Many patients who die in the ED could potentially be a candidate for non–heart beating donation (NHBD). Certain tissues and organs such as corneas, heart valves, bone, and kidneys can be harvested from patients after death. Approaching families about donation after an unexpected death is distressing to both the staff and the family. For many families, however, the act of donation may be the first positive step in the grieving process.[17] Organ procurement agencies (OPAs) are available to assist in the process of screening potential donors, counseling donor families, obtaining informed consent, and harvesting organs from patients who have died in the ED.

■ Gerontologic Considerations: Emergency Care

The proportion of the population over age 65 is growing, with most leading active lives. Regardless of a patient's age, aggressive interventions are warranted for all injuries or illnesses unless the patient is known to have a preexisting terminal illness, an extremely low probability of survival, or an advance directive indicating a different course of action.[18]

The elderly population is at high risk for injury due to many of the anatomic and physiologic changes that occur with aging (e.g., reduced visual acuity, limited neck rotation, slower gait, reduced reaction time). Of the injury-related admissions for people age 65 or older, approximately 52% are for fractures, with many of these resulting from falls. The three most common causes of falls in the elderly are generalized weakness, environmental hazards (e.g., loose mats, furniture), and orthostatic hypotension (e.g., side effect of medications).[18] When assessing a patient who has experienced a fall, it is important to determine whether the physical findings may have actually caused the fall or may be due to the fall itself. For example, a patient may exhibit acute confusion. The confusion may be due to an acute myocardial infarction that caused the patient to lose consciousness and fall, or the patient may have suffered a head injury as a result of a fall from tripping.

Knowledge of the concepts of aging will improve the care delivered to the elderly in the ED (see Chapter 5). Unfortunately, many older adults dismiss symptoms as simply "normal for their age." Any complaint by an older adult must be fully investigated. ■

Environmental Emergencies

Increased interest in outdoor activities such as running, hiking, cycling, skiing, sailing, and swimming has increased the number of environmental emergencies seen in the ED. Illness or injury may be caused by the activity, exposure to weather, or at-

TABLE 67-6	Prophylaxis against Tetanus in Wound Management				
	TYPE OF WOUND				
	TETANUS-PRONE WOUND		**NON–TETANUS-PRONE WOUND**		
HISTORY OF TETANUS TOXOID (DOSES)	**Td**	**TIG***		**Td**	**TIG**
Unknown to fewer than three	Yes	Yes		Yes	No
Three or more†	No‡	No		No§	No

*When TIG and Td are administered concurrently, separate sites and syringes must be used.
†If only three doses of fluid toxoid have been received, a fourth dose of toxoid, preferably absorbed toxoid, should be given.
‡Yes, if more than 5 years since last dose. More frequent boosters are not needed and can accentuate side effects.
§Yes, if more than 10 years since last dose.
Td, Tetanus-diphtheria toxoid absorbed (for adult use); TIG, tetanus immune globulin (human).

tack from various animals or humans. Specific environmental emergencies discussed in this section include heat-related emergencies, cold-related emergencies, submersion injuries, bites, and stings.

HEAT-RELATED EMERGENCIES

Brief exposure to intense heat or prolonged exposure to less intense heat leads to heat stress when thermoregulatory mechanisms such as sweating, vasodilation, and increased respirations cannot compensate for exposure to increased ambient temperatures.[19] Ambient temperature is a product of environmental temperature and humidity. Strenuous activities in hot or humid environments, clothing that interferes with perspiration, high fevers, and preexisting illnesses predispose individuals to heat stress (Table 67-7). Effects can be mild (heat rash and heat edema) or severe (heat exhaustion and heat stroke). The management of heat-related emergencies is summarized in Table 67-8.

Heat rash (miliaria or prickly heat) is a fine, red, papular rash that occurs on the torso, neck, and skinfolds. The rash occurs when sweat ducts are obstructed and become inflamed so that sweat excretion does not occur. The rash usually occurs in warm weather, but has also been reported in cold weather as a result of clothing.

Heat syncope is associated with prolonged standing and heat exposure. Manifestations include dizziness, orthostatic hypotension, and syncope. Inadequate vasomotor tone associated with aging places the elderly at greater risk for heat syncope.

Heat edema is characterized by swelling of the hands, feet, and ankles, usually in nonacclimatized individuals as a result of prolonged standing or sitting. Swelling usually resolves in days with rest, elevation, and support hose. Diuretics are not recommended because this condition is self-limiting and requires no additional treatment.

Heat Cramps

Heat cramps are severe cramps in large muscle groups fatigued by heavy work. Cramps are brief, intense, and tend to occur during rest after exercise or heavy labor. Nausea, tachycardia, pallor, weakness, and profuse diaphoresis are often present. The condition is seen most often in healthy, acclimated athletes with inadequate fluid intake. Cramps resolve rapidly with rest and oral or parenteral replacement of sodium and water. Elevation, gentle massage, and analgesia minimize pain associated with heat cramps. The patient should avoid strenuous activity for at least 12 hours after the development of heat cramps. Education should emphasize salt replacement during strenuous exercise in hot, humid environments. Commercially prepared electrolyte solutions (e.g., sports drinks) are recommended.

Heat Exhaustion

Prolonged exposure to heat over hours or days leads to **heat exhaustion,** a clinical syndrome characterized by fatigue, lightheadedness, nausea, vomiting, diarrhea, and feelings of impending doom (see Table 67-8). Tachypnea, hypotension, tachycardia, elevated body temperature, dilated pupils, mild confusion, ashen color, and profuse diaphoresis are also present. Hypotension and mild to severe temperature elevation (99.6° to 104° F [37.5° to 40° C]) are due to dehydration.[19] Heat exhaustion usually occurs in individuals engaged in strenuous activity in hot, humid weather, but it also occurs in sedentary individuals.

Treatment begins with placement of the patient in a cool area and removal of constrictive clothing. The patient is monitored for airway, breathing, and circulation (ABCs), including cardiac arrhythmias (due to electrolyte imbalances). Oral fluid and electrolyte replacement is initiated unless the patient is nauseated. Salt tablets are not recommended because of potential gastric irritation and hypernatremia. A 0.9% normal saline solution is initiated intravenously when oral solutions are not tolerated. An initial fluid bolus may be used to correct hypotension. However, fluid replacement should be correlated to clinical and laboratory parameters. A moist sheet placed over the patient decreases core temperature through evaporative heat loss. Hospital admission is considered for the elderly, the chronically ill, or those who do not improve within 3 to 4 hours.

Heat Stroke

Heat stroke, the most serious form of heat stress, results from failure of the central thermoregulatory mechanisms and is considered a medical emergency. Table 67-7 lists risk factors for

---

TABLE 67-7	**Risk Factors for Heat-Related Emergencies**

Age
Elderly
Infants

Environmental Conditions
High environmental temperature
High relative humidity
Low wind

Preexisting Illness
Cardiovascular disease
Cystic fibrosis
Diabetes
Obesity
Previous stroke or other central nervous system lesion
Skin disorders (e.g., large burn scars)

Prescription Drugs
Anticholinergics
Antihistamines
Antiparkinsonian drugs
Antispasmodics
β–Adrenergic blockers
Butyrophenones
Diuretics
Phenothiazines
Tricyclic antidepressants

Street Drugs
Amphetamines
Jimsonweed
Lysergic acid diethylamide (LSD)
Phencyclidine (PCP)

Alcohol

From Emergency Nurses Association, Newberry L, editor: *Sheehy's emergency nursing: principles and practice,* ed 5, St Louis, 2003, Mosby.

TABLE 67-8   Emergency Management

Hyperthermia

ETIOLOGY	ASSESSMENT FINDINGS	INTERVENTIONS
Environmental	**Heat Cramps**	**Initial**
• Lack of acclimatization	• Severe muscle contractions in exerted muscles	• Manage and maintain ABCs.
• Prolonged exposure to extreme temperatures	• Thirst	• Provide high-flow O_2 via non-rebreather mask or BVM.
• Physical exertion, especially during hot weather	**Heat Exhaustion**	• Establish IV access and begin fluid replacement for significant heat injury.
	• Pale, ashen	• Place patient in a cool environment.
Trauma	• Fatigue, weakness	• For patient with heat stroke, initiate rapid cooling measures: remove patient's clothing, place wet sheets over patient, and place in front of fan; immerse in ice water bath; administer cool IV fluids or lavage with cool fluids.
• Head injury	• Profuse sweating	
• Spinal cord injury	• Altered mental status (e.g., irritable)	
	• Hypotension	
Metabolic	• Tachycardia	
• Dehydration	• Weak, thready pulse	• Obtain ECG.
• Thyrotoxicosis	• Temperature >100° F (37.8° C) but <104° F (40° C)	• Obtain blood for electrolytes and CBC.
• Diabetes		• Insert urinary catheter.
Drugs	**Heat Stroke**	**Ongoing Monitoring**
• Phenothiazines	• Hot, dry skin	• Monitor ABCs, vital signs, level of consciousness.
• Tricyclic antidepressants	• Altered mental status (e.g., ranging from confusion to coma)	• Monitor cardiac rhythm, O_2 saturation, electrolytes, and urinary output.
• Diuretics	• Hypotension	• Monitor urine for development of myoglobinuria.
• Cocaine	• Tachycardia	• Monitor clotting studies for development of disseminated intravascular coagulation.
• Ethanol	• Weakness	
• Antihistamines	• Temperature >104° F (40° C)	
Other		
• Cardiovascular disease		
• CNS disorders		
• Alcoholism		

ABCs, Airway, breathing, circulation; *BVM,* bag-valve-mask; *CBC,* complete blood count; *CNS,* central nervous system; *ECG,* electrocardiogram; *IV,* intravenous.

---

heat-related emergencies, especially heat stroke. Increased sweating, vasodilation, and increased respiratory rate (the body's attempt to lower temperature) deplete fluids and electrolytes. Eventually, sweat glands stop functioning, so core temperature increases rapidly. The patient has core temperature greater than 104° F (40° C), altered mentation, absence of perspiration, and circulatory collapse. The skin is hot, dry, and ashen. Because the brain is extremely sensitive to thermal injuries, a range of neurologic symptoms occur, such as hallucinations, loss of muscle coordination, and combativeness. Cerebral edema and hemorrhage may occur as a result of direct thermal injury to the brain and decreased cerebral blood flow.

The development of heat stroke is directly related to the amount of time that the patient's body temperature remains elevated.[19] Prognosis is related to age, baseline health status, and length of exposure. Older adults and individuals with diabetes mellitus, chronic renal disease, cardiovascular disease, pulmonary disease, or other physiologic compromise are particularly vulnerable.

Collaborative Care. Treatment of heat stroke focuses on stabilizing the patient's ABCs and rapidly reducing the core temperature. Administration of 100% O_2 compensates for the patient's hypermetabolic state. Ventilation with a BVM or intubation and mechanical ventilation may be required. Fluid and electrolyte imbalances are corrected, and continuous cardiac monitoring for arrhythmias is initiated.

Various cooling methods are available, such as removal of clothing, covering with wet sheets, and placing the patient in front of a large fan (evaporative cooling); providing an ice water bath (conductive cooling); and administering cool fluids or lavaging with cool fluids.[20] Whatever method is selected, the nurse is responsible for closely monitoring the patient's temperature and controlling shivering. Shivering increases core temperature (due to the associated heat generated by muscle activity) and complicates cooling efforts. Chlorpromazine (Thorazine) IV is the drug of choice to suppress shivering. Aggressive temperature reduction should continue until core temperature reaches 102° F (38.9° C).[20] Antipyretics are not recommended.

The patient is also monitored for signs of *rhabdomyolysis* (a fatal disease characterized by breakdown of skeletal muscle). The muscle breakdown leads to myoglobinuria, which places the kidneys at risk for acute failure. Therefore urine should be carefully monitored for color, amount, pH, and myoglobin. Finally, clotting studies are performed to monitor the patient for signs of disseminated intravascular coagulation (DIC) (see Chapter 30).

Patient and family teaching focuses on how to avoid future problems. Essential information regarding proper hydration during hot weather and physical exercise is imperative. Patients should also be instructed on the early signs of and interventions for heat-related stress.

COLD-RELATED EMERGENCIES

Cold injuries may be localized (frostbite) or systemic (hypothermia). Contributing factors include age, duration of exposure, environmental temperature, homelessness, preexisting conditions (e.g., diabetes mellitus), medications that suppress shivering (narcotics, heroin, psychotropic agents, and antiemetics), and alcohol intoxication, which causes peripheral vasodilation, increases sensations of warmth, and depresses shivering. Smokers have an increased risk of cold-related injury as a result of the vasoconstrictive effects of nicotine.

Frostbite

Frostbite can be described as "true tissue freezing," which results in the formation of ice crystals in the tissues and cells. Peripheral vasoconstriction is the initial response to cold stress and results in a decrease in blood flow and vascular stasis. As cellular temperature decreases and ice crystals form in intracellular spaces, intracellular sodium and chloride increase, the cell membrane is destroyed, and organelles are damaged. These alterations result in edema. Depth of frostbite is the result of ambient temperature, length of exposure, type and condition (wet or dry) of clothing, and contact with metal surfaces. Other factors that affect severity include skin color (dark-skinned people are more prone to frostbite), lack of acclimatization, previous episodes, exhaustion, and poor peripheral vascular status.

Superficial frostbite involves skin and subcutaneous tissue, usually the ears, nose, fingers, and toes. The skin appearance will range from pale to blue to mottled, and the skin will feel crunchy and frozen. The patient may complain of tingling, numbness, or a burning sensation. Injured tissue is easily damaged, so the area should be handled carefully and never squeezed, massaged, or scrubbed. Clothing and jewelry should be removed because they may constrict the extremity and decrease circulation. The affected area should be immersed in a water bath (102° to 108° F) [38.9° to 42.2° C]).[21] Warm soaks may be used for the face. The patient often experiences a warm, stinging sensation as tissue thaws. Blisters form within a few hours (Fig. 67-2). The blisters should be debrided and a sterile dressing applied. Heavy blankets and clothing should be avoided because friction and weight can lead to sloughing of damaged tissue. Rewarming is extremely painful. Residual pain may last weeks or even years. Analgesia should be administered and tetanus prophylaxis should be given as appropriate (see Table 67-6). The patient should be evaluated for systemic hypothermia.

Deep frostbite involves muscle, bone, and tendon. The skin is white, hard, and insensitive to touch. The area has the appearance of deep thermal injury with mottling gradually progressing to gangrene (Fig. 67-3). The affected extremity is submersed in a circulating water bath (102° to 108° F [38.9° to 42.2° C]) until distal flush occurs. After rewarming, the extremity should be elevated to lessen edema.[21] Significant edema may begin within 3 hours, with blistering in 6 hours to days. Intravenous analgesia is always required in severe frostbite because of the pain associated with tissue thawing. Tetanus prophylaxis should be given (see Table 67-6), and the patient should be evaluated for systemic hypothermia. Amputation may be required if the injured area is untreated or treatment is unsuccessful. The patient may be admitted to the hospital for observation over 24 to 48 hours with bed rest, elevation of the injured part, and prophylactic antibiotics if the wound is at risk for infection.

Hypothermia

Hypothermia, defined as a core temperature less than 95° F (35° C), occurs when heat produced by the body cannot compensate for heat lost to the environment. From 55% to 60% of all body heat is lost as radiant energy, with the greatest loss from the head, thorax, and lungs (with each breath).[19] Wet clothing increases evaporative heat loss five times greater than normal; immersion in cold water increases heat loss by a factor of 25. Environmental exposure to freezing temperatures, cold winds, and wet, damp terrain in the presence of physical exhaustion, inadequate clothing, and/or inexperience predisposes individuals to hypothermia.[6] Near-drowning and water immersion are also associated with hypothermia.

The elderly are more prone to hypothermia resulting from decreased body fat, diminished energy reserves, decreased basal metabolic rate, decreased shivering response, decreased sensory perception, chronic medical conditions, and medications that alter body defenses. In addition, certain drugs, alcohol, and diabetes are considered risk factors for hypothermia.

Hypothermia mimics cerebral or metabolic disturbances causing ataxia, confusion, and withdrawal, so the patient may be misdiagnosed. Peripheral vasoconstriction is the body's first attempt to conserve heat. As cold temperatures persist, shivering and movement are the body's only mechanisms for producing heat. Death usually occurs when core temperature falls below 78° F (25.6° C).

Core temperature below 87° F (30.6° C) is severe and potentially life threatening. Assessment findings in hypothermia are variable and dependent on core temperature (Table 67-9). Patients with *mild hypothermia* (90° to 95° F [32.2° to 35° C]) have

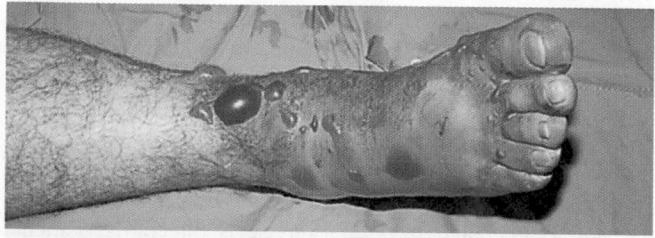

FIG. 67-2 Edema and blister formation 24 hours after frostbite injury occurring in an area covered by a tightly fitted boot.

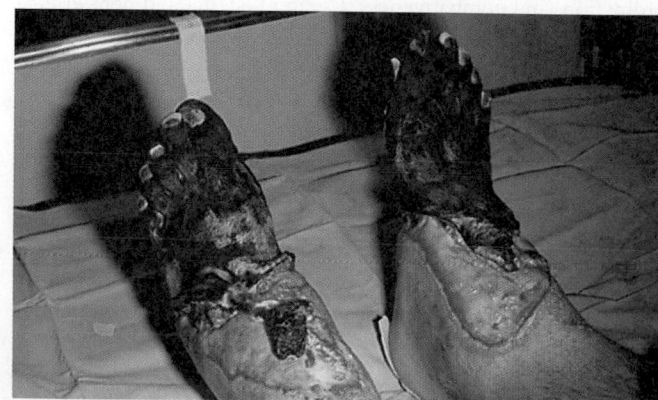

FIG. 67-3 Gangrenous necrosis 6 weeks after the frostbite injury shown in Fig. 67-2.

TABLE 67-9 Emergency Management — Hypothermia

ETIOLOGY	ASSESSMENT FINDINGS	INTERVENTIONS

Environmental
• Prolonged exposure to cold
• Prolonged submersion
• Inadequate clothing for environmental temperature
 	
Metabolic
• Hypoglycemia
• Hypothyroidism
 	
Iatrogenic
• Cold IV fluids
• Blood administration
• Inadequate warming or rewarming in the ED or surgery
• Administration of neuromuscular blocking agents
 	
Other
• Phenothiazines
• Barbiturates
• Alcohol
• Trauma
• Shock
	• Core body temperature:
	  Mild hypothermia: 90°-95° F (32.2°-35° C)
	  Moderate hypothermia: 87°-90° F (30.6°-32.2° C)
	  Profound hypothermia: <87° F (30.6° C)
	• Shivering (diminished or absent at core body temperature ≤ 92° F) (33.3° C)
	• Hypoventilation
	• Hypotension
	• Altered mental status (ranging from confusion to coma)
	• Areflexia (absence of reflexes)
	• Pale, cyanotic skin
	• Blue, white, or frozen extremities
	• Arrhythmias: bradycardia, atrial fibrillation, ventricular fibrillation, asystole
	• Fixed, dilated pupils
		Initial
		• Remove patient from cold environment.
		• Manage and maintain ABCs.
		• Provide high-flow O₂ via non-rebreather mask or BVM.
		• Anticipate intubation for diminished or absent gag reflex.
		• Rewarm patient:
		  Passive: remove wet clothing, apply dry clothing and warm blankets, administer warm fluids.
		  Active external: use body-to-body contact, apply heating devices (e.g., air-filled warming blankets) or radiant lights.
		  Active core warming: administer warmed IV fluids; heated, humidified O₂; peritoneal, gastric, or colonic lavage with warmed fluids.
		• Anticipate the need for hemodialysis or cardiopulmonary bypass.
		• Warm central trunk first in patients with profound hypothermia to avoid aftershock.
		• Establish IV access with two large-bore catheters for fluid resuscitation.
		• Assess for other injuries.
		• Keep patient's head covered with warm, dry towels, or stocking cap, to limit loss of heat.
		• Treat patient gently to avoid increased cardiac irritability.
		
		Ongoing Monitoring
		• Monitor ABCs, level of consciousness, temperature, vital signs.
		• Monitor O₂ saturation, cardiac rhythm.
		• Monitor electrolytes, glucose.

ABCs, Airway, breathing, circulation; *BVM,* bag-valve mask; *ED,* emergency department; *IV,* intravenous.

shivering, lethargy, confusion, rational to irrational behavior, and minor heart rate changes. Shivering disappears at temperatures less than 92° F (33.3° C). *Moderate hypothermia* (87° to 90° F [30.6° to 32.2° C]) causes rigidity, bradycardia, slowed respiratory rate, blood pressure obtainable only by Doppler, metabolic and respiratory acidosis, and hypovolemia.

As core temperature drops, basal metabolic rate decreases two or three times. The cold myocardium is extremely irritable, so any movement can precipitate ventricular fibrillation. Decreased renal blood flow decreases glomerular filtration rate, which impairs water reabsorption and leads to dehydration. The hematocrit increases as intravascular volume decreases. Cold blood becomes thick and acts as a thrombus, placing the patient at risk for stroke, myocardial infarction, pulmonary emboli, acute tubular necrosis, and renal failure. Decreased blood flow leads to lactic acid accumulation from anaerobic metabolism and subsequent metabolic acidosis.

Profound hypothermia (less than 87° F [30.6° C]) makes the person appear dead. Metabolic rate, heart rate, and respirations are so slow that they may be difficult to detect. Reflexes are absent and the pupils fixed and dilated. Profound bradycardia, asystole, or ventricular fibrillation may be present. Every effort is made to warm the patient to at least 90° F (32.2° C) before the

person is pronounced dead. The cause of death is usually refractory ventricular fibrillation.

Collaborative Care. Treatment of hypothermia focuses on managing and maintaining ABCs, rewarming the patient, correcting dehydration and acidosis, and treating cardiac arrhythmias (see Table 67-9). Passive or active external rewarming is used for mild hypothermia. *Passive external rewarming* involves moving the patient to a warm, dry place, removing damp clothing, and placing warm blankets on the patient. Gentle handling is essential to prevent stimulation of the cold myocardium. *Active external rewarming* involves body-to-body contact, fluid- or air-filled warming blankets, or radiant heat lamps. The patient should be closely monitored for marked vasodilation and hypotension during rewarming.

Active core rewarming is used for moderate to profound hypothermia and refers to heat applied directly to the core. Techniques include heated (105° to 115° F [40.6° to 46.1° C]), humidified oxygen; warmed intravenous fluids; and peritoneal, gastric, or colonic lavage with warmed fluids. Hemodialysis or cardiopulmonary bypass may also be considered in profound hypothermia.[19,20]

Core temperature should be carefully monitored during rewarming procedures. Warming places the patient at risk for *afterdrop,* a further drop in core temperature, which occurs when cold peripheral blood returns to the central circulation. Aftershock can produce hypotension and arrhythmias. Thus patients with moderate to profound hypothermia should have the core warmed before the extremities. Rewarming should be discontinued once the core temperature reaches 93° F (33.9° C).[19,21]

Patient teaching should focus on how to avoid future cold-related problems. Essential information includes dressing in layers for cold weather, covering the head, carrying high-carbohydrate foods for extra calories, and developing a plan for survival should an injury occur.

SUBMERSION INJURIES

Submersion injury results when a person becomes hypoxic due to submersion in a substance, usually water. Approximately 8000 deaths occur from submersion injuries annually in the United States. Forty percent of these victims are children under 5 years of age. The primary risk factors for submersion injury include inability to swim, use of alcohol or drugs, trauma, seizures, hypothermia, and stroke.

Drowning is death from suffocation after submersion in water or other fluid medium. *Near-drowning* is defined as survival from potential drowning. *Immersion syndrome* occurs with immersion in cold water, which leads to stimulation of the vagus nerve and potentially fatal arrhythmias (e.g., bradycardia).

Death from a submersion injury is caused by hypoxia secondary to aspiration and swallowing of fluid, usually water. Swallowed water may cause vomiting and additional aspiration. The majority of all drowning victims aspirate water into the pulmonary tree and develop pulmonary edema. Victims who do not aspirate fluid develop intense bronchospasm and airway obstruction, the cause of death in "dry drowning." Regardless of what fluid is aspirated into the pulmonary tree, the ultimate result is pulmonary edema. The osmotic gradient caused by aspirated fluid causes fluid imbalances in the body. Hypotonic fresh water is rapidly absorbed into the circulatory system through the alveoli. Fresh water may be contaminated with chlorine, mud, and algae, causing the breakdown of lung surfactant, fluid seepage, and pulmonary edema. Hypertonic salt water draws protein-rich fluid from the vascular space into the alveoli, impairing alveolar ventilation and resulting in hypoxia. Fig. 67-4 shows the pulmonary effects of saltwater and freshwater aspiration.

The body attempts to compensate for hypoxia by shunting blood to the lungs. This results in increased pulmonary pressures and deteriorating respiratory status. More and more blood is shunted through the alveoli. However, the blood is not adequately oxygenated, so the hypoxemia worsens. Anaerobic metabolism occurs, which leads to lactic acidosis.

The assessment findings of a patient with a submersion injury are listed in Table 67-10. Aggressive resuscitation efforts and the mammalian diving reflex improve survival of near-drowning victims even after submersion in cold water for long periods of time.[20,22] Cold water lowers the body's metabolic rate and oxygen demand. The mammalian diving reflex causes apnea, bradycardia, and peripheral vasoconstriction and further decreases metabolic rate. Blood flow is redistributed to the most vital organs (i.e., heart, lungs, and brain).

Collaborative Care

Treatment of submersion injuries focuses on correcting hypoxia, acid-base imbalances, and fluid imbalances; supporting basic physiologic functions; and rewarming when hypothermia is

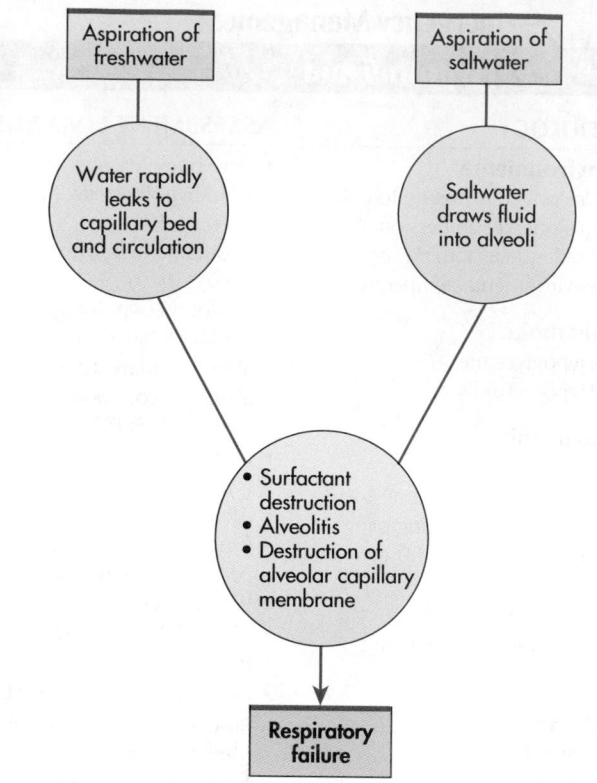

FIG. 67-4 Pulmonary effects of water aspiration.

present. Initial evaluation involves assessment of airway, cervical spine, breathing, and circulation. Other interventions are listed in Table 67-10.

Mechanical ventilation with positive end-expiratory pressure or continuous positive airway pressure may be used to improve gas exchange across the alveolar-capillary membrane when significant pulmonary edema is present. Ventilation and oxygenation are the primary techniques used to treat acidosis. Mannitol or furosemide (Lasix) may be given to decrease free water and treat cerebral edema.

Deterioration in neurologic status suggests cerebral edema, increased hypoxia, or profound acidosis. Near-drowning victims may also have head injuries that cause prolonged alterations in level of consciousness. All victims of near-drowning should be observed in a hospital for a minimum of 4 to 6 hours. Delayed pulmonary edema (also called *secondary drowning*), pneumonia, and cerebral edema have been reported in patients who were essentially free of symptoms immediately after the near-drowning episode but later developed problems.

Teaching should focus on water safety and minimizing the risks for drowning. Swimming pool gates should be locked; life jackets should be used on all water craft, including inner tubes and rafts; and water survival skills (i.e., swimming lessons) should be a priority. The dangers of combining alcohol and drugs with swimming and other water sports should be emphasized.[20]

BITES AND STINGS

Animals, spiders, and insects cause injury and even death by biting or stinging. Morbidity is a result of either direct tissue damage or lethal toxins. Direct tissue damage is a product of an-

TABLE 67-10	Emergency Management — Submersion Injuries	
ETIOLOGY	**ASSESSMENT FINDINGS**	**INTERVENTIONS**
• Inability to swim or exhaustion while swimming • Entrapment or entanglement with objects in water • Loss of ability to move secondary to trauma, stroke, hypothermia, acute myocardial infarction • Poor judgment due to alcohol or drugs • Seizure while in water	**Pulmonary** • Ineffective breathing • Dyspnea • Respiratory distress • Respiratory arrest • Crackles, rhonchi • Cough with pink-frothy sputum • Cyanosis **Cardiac** • Tachycardia • Bradycardia • Arrhythmia • Hypotension • Cardiac arrest **Other** • Panic • Exhaustion • Coma • Coexisting illness (e.g., acute MI) or injury (e.g., cervical spine injury) • Core temperature slightly elevated or below normal depending on water temperature and length of submersion	**Initial** • Manage and maintain ABCs. • Assume cervical spine injury in all drowning victims and stabilize and/or immobilize cervical spine. • Provide 100% O_2 via non-rebreather mask or BVM. • Anticipate need for intubation if gag reflex is absent. • Establish IV access with two large-bore catheters for fluid resuscitation and infuse warmed fluids if appropriate. • Assess for other injuries. • Remove wet clothing and cover with warm blankets. • Obtain temperature and begin rewarming if needed. • Obtain cervical spine and chest x-rays. • Insert gastric tube. **Ongoing Monitoring** • Monitor ABCs, vital signs, level of consciousness. • Monitor O_2 saturation, cardiac rhythm. • Monitor temperature and maintain normothermia. • Monitor for signs of acute respiratory failure.

ABCs, Airway, breathing, circulation; *BVM,* bag-valve mask; *IV,* intravenous; *MI,* myocardial infarction.

imal size, characteristics of the animal's teeth, and strength of the jaw. Tissue may be lacerated, crushed, or chewed while toxins released through teeth, fangs, stingers, spines, or tentacles have local or systemic effects. Death associated with animal bites is due to blood loss, allergic reactions, or lethal toxins. Injuries caused by insects, spiders, scorpions, ticks, snakes, dogs, cats, rodents, and humans are described below.

Hymenopteran Stings

The *Hymenoptera* family includes bees, yellow jackets, hornets, and wasps. Stings can cause mild discomfort or life-threatening anaphylaxis (see Chapters 13 and 65). Venom may be cytotoxic, hemolytic, allergenic, or vasoactive. Symptoms may begin immediately or be delayed up to 48 hours. Reactions are more severe with multiple stings. Most hymenopterans sting repeatedly. However, the honeybee stings only once, usually leaving the stinger in the skin so that release of venom continues. A scraping motion with a fingernail, knife, or needle is recommended for removing the stinger. Tweezers squeeze the stinger and may cause more venom release. However, the fastest method of removing the stinger is ultimately the best, so if tweezers are available, they can be used.

Manifestations vary from stinging, burning, swelling, and itching to edema, headache, fever, syncope, malaise, nausea, vomiting, wheezing, bronchospasm, laryngeal edema, and hypotension. Treatment depends on the severity of the reaction. Mild reactions are treated with elevation, cool compresses, antipruritic lotions, and oral antihistamines. Rings, watches, and restrictive clothing are removed. More severe reactions require intramuscular or intravenous antihistamines (diphenhydramine [Benadryl]), subcutaneous epinephrine, and corticosteroids. Allergic reactions and anaphylaxis are discussed in Chapter 13.

Spider Bites (Arachnid)

Although there are 20,000 species of venomous spiders in the world, only 50 species cause illness. Two venomous spiders found in the United States are the black widow spider and the brown recluse spider.[19] Their venom can cause a localized reaction or systemic anaphylaxis. Tarantulas appear more dangerous than they actually are because their bite causes only localized stinging and pain. Other types of spiders release venom when they bite and may cause allergic reactions in some individuals, but they are not considered poisonous.

Black Widow Spiders. Black widow spiders are the most feared of all spiders. The female's venom is especially poisonous to people. Both the female and male are black in color (Fig. 67-5). The female rarely leaves the web, biting defensively if disturbed. Black widow spiders are found among fallen branches, among firewood, and under objects of many kinds, including furniture, outhouse seats, and trash.

The black widow spider venom is neurotoxic. When bitten, the patient will feel a pinprick-like sensation and a tiny, red bite mark will appear. Approximately 15 to 60 minutes later, the patient will report severe pain that will increase over the next 12 to 48 hours. Systemic symptoms will develop 30 minutes after *envenomation* (the introduction of poisonous venoms into the body by a bite or a sting). These can include nausea, vomiting, abdominal cramping,

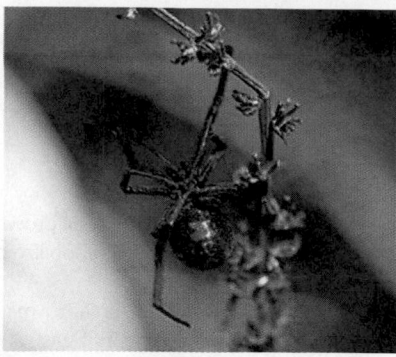

FIG. 67-5 Female black widow spider. The fully grown female is about 1.2 cm (0.5 in) long and is jet black, with an hourglass-shaped red mark on the underside of the abdomen. The female's sting is poisonous to humans. Males are only about half as long and usually have four pairs of red dots along the sides of the abdomen. Males are rarely seen and are harmless.

hypertension, dyspnea, paresthesias, and tachycardia. Symptoms usually peak 2 to 3 hours after onset; however, muscle spasms and hypertension can recur for 12 to 24 hours. Chest and abdominal pain, seizures, and shock can also occur. Bites on the lower body cause abdominal rigidity, whereas bites on the upper body lead to chest, back, and shoulder rigidity. A black widow spider bite is not prominent and can be easily missed. Patients not aware of the bite can be misdiagnosed, because symptoms mimic a perforated ulcer, appendicitis, pancreatitis, or other abdominal emergency.

Treatment includes cooling the area to slow the action of the neurotoxin. IV access should be established and oxygen administered as needed. The wound should be cleaned and tetanus prophylaxis given as appropriate. Muscle spasms are treated with calcium gluconate, methocarbamol (Robaxin), or diazepam (Valium). Severe pain may require narcotic analgesia. Although antivenin is rarely used, it can be used for severe reactions, young children, or adults with hypertension or cardiac disease.[19]

Brown Recluse Spiders. Brown recluse spiders are usually found in dark areas such as garages, closets, and boxes. The spider, common in the southeastern, south-central, and southwestern United States, is a light brown color with a characteristic dark brown fiddle shape that extends from the eyes down the back. The venom is cytotoxic, so local tissue effects can be dramatic. Initially, the bite is insignificant, with a local reaction beginning in 2 to 8 hours. A painful, purple purpura develops in a ring around the bite, and eventually may progress to a necrotic ulcerating wound by 7 to 14 days. The wound can extend deep into tissue and may persist for weeks. Occasionally, systemic manifestations of envenomation occur and can include fever, chills, joint pain, malaise, nausea, and vomiting.[19]

Treatment depends on severity of the reaction. Treatment is necessary when there is bleb or bulla formation, intense pain, and signs of rapidly progressive ischemia and necrosis. Initial interventions include cleansing the bite with mild antiseptic soap, providing cool compresses, and elevating the affected extremity. Analgesia, tetanus prophylaxis, antihistamines, corticosteroids, and antibiotics for prevention of secondary infection may also be required. Surgical debridement with grafting is necessary for some patients. Hyperbaric oxygen therapy may also be considered to enhance tissue healing. Dapsone (Avlosulfon), a polymorphonuclear leukocyte inhibitor, has been used for patients

with deep crater wounds. Patients with systemic manifestations are hospitalized and monitored for hemolysis, disseminated intravascular coagulation, and acute renal failure.

Tick Bites

Ticks are found in various parts of the United States, but they are most common in the Rocky Mountain region and the Northwest. Emergencies associated with tick bites include Rocky Mountain spotted fever, Lyme disease, and tick paralysis. Disease is caused by an infected tick or by the release of neurotoxin. Ticks release a neurotoxic venom as long as the tick head is attached to the body. Therefore removal of the attached tick is essential for effective treatment. Forceps may be used to safely remove the tick by grasping at the point of entry and pulling upward in a steady motion. Covering the tick with alcohol, mineral oil, petroleum jelly, or ether causes the tick to release from the skin. These methods work because the tick breathes through the skin in which it is embedded.

Rocky Mountain spotted fever caused by *Rickettsia rickettsii* has an incubation period of 2 to 14 days. A pink, macular rash appears on the palms, wrists, soles, feet, and ankles within 10 days of exposure. Other symptoms include fever, chills, malaise, myalgias, and headache. Treatment is antibiotic therapy.

Lyme disease is the most common arthropod-borne disease in the United States. Symptoms appear within 4 to 20 days of a bite from the *Ixodes* tick and result from exposure to the spirochete *Borrelia burgdorferi* that is found on the tick. The initial stage of this disease is characterized by nonspecific flulike symptoms (e.g., headache, stiff neck, fatigue) and a characteristic bull's-eye rash—an expanding circular area of redness of 5 cm diameter or more. Symptoms will disappear in 2 weeks if not treated. Monoarticular arthritis, meningitis, and neuropathies occur days or weeks after the initial symptoms. Chronic arthritis and myocarditis characterize the later stage of the disease, which can develop several months to 2 years after the initial skin lesion. Treatment includes antibiotic therapy; however, controversy exists over what the most effective regimen should be. (Lyme disease is discussed in Chapter 63.)

Tick paralysis occurs 5 to 7 days after exposure to the wood tick or dog tick. Classic symptoms are flaccid ascending paralysis, which develops over 1 to 2 days. Without tick removal, the patient dies as respiratory muscles become paralyzed. Tick removal leads to return of muscle movement, usually within 48 to 72 hours.

Snakebite

Only 375 of the 3000 species of snakes in the world are poisonous. Poisonous snakes indigenous to the United States are members of the Crotalidae and Elapidae family. Crotalidae, or pit vipers, include rattlesnakes, copperheads, and water moccasins. Coral snakes belong to the Elapidae family. Other poisonous snakes in the Elapidae family not indigenous to the United States are the highly venomous cobras, kraits, mambas, and sea snakes. Coral snakes do not exhibit the triangular head of pit vipers but are recognized by their bright colors. Coral snakes always have a blunt black snout and red, yellow, and black rings that completely encircle the body (Fig. 67-6). There is a yellow ring on both sides of every red ring. The beauty of this snake represents a true danger because small children may readily pick it up, thus providing an opportunity for a bite from this otherwise docile reptile. Other poisonous snakes in

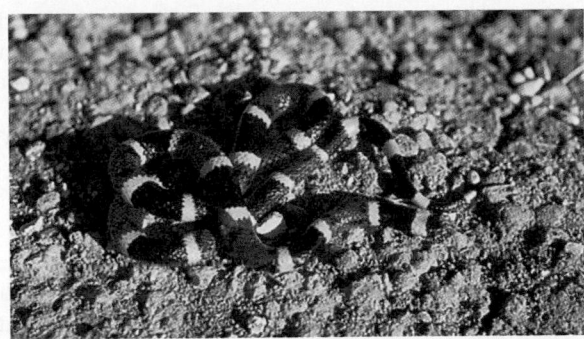

FIG. 67-6 Western coral snake. The venom from this snake is neurotoxic.

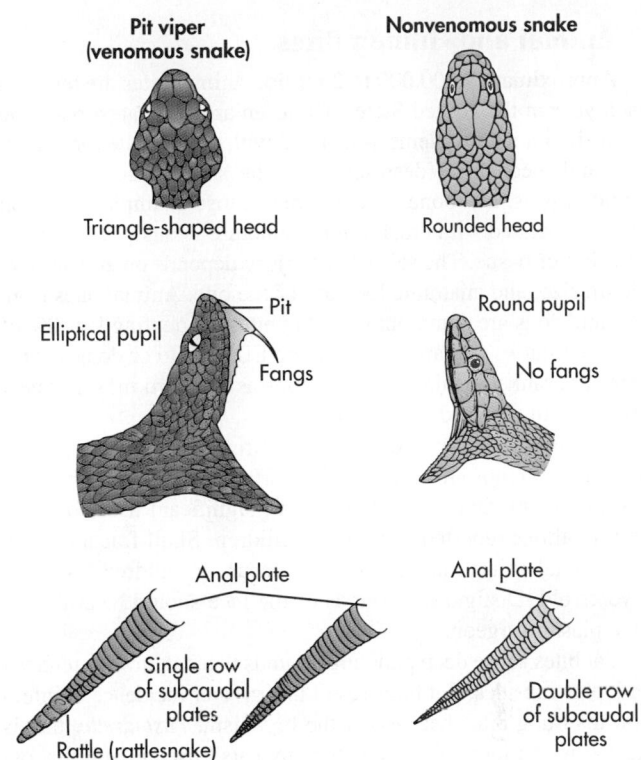

FIG. 67-7 Comparison of pit viper (a type of venomous snake) and nonvenomous snake.

the Elapidae family not indigenous to the United States are the cobra and the mamba. Fig. 67-7 highlights differences between the pit viper (a poisonous snake) and a nonpoisonous snake.

Venom from the pit viper is hemolytic, whereas coral snake venom is neurotoxic. Envenomation occurs in approximately 75% to 80% of all snakebites. If swelling does not occur within 30 minutes after the bite, envenomation is unlikely. Local reaction is characterized by one or two fang marks associated with pain, bruising, and edema within 36 hours of injury, petechiae, ecchymosis, and erythema. Loss of function and necrosis of the affected limb may occur 16 to 36 hours after the bite. Systemic reactions include nausea and vomiting, dizziness, tachycardia, muscle fasciculations, gastrointestinal bleeding, and respiratory problems. The patient may experience a metallic or rubber taste. Neurologic symptoms such as constricted pupils, drowsiness, weakness, fasciculations, muscle weakness, and seizures occur with neurotoxic venom. Life-threatening problems associated with systemic envenomation include severe hemorrhage, renal failure, and hypovolemic shock.

Treatment focuses on preventing the spread of venom. Rings, watches, and restrictive clothing should be removed, and then the affected limb should be immobilized at the level of the heart. Ice and tourniquets are not recommended. Incision of the wound is controversial. If done within 3 minutes of injury with the appropriate device (e.g., Sawyer extractor), 25% to 30% of the venom may be removed. Caffeine, alcohol, and smoking increase the spread of venom and should be avoided.

ED management includes vascular access with a large-bore (14- to 16-gauge) catheter and administration of crystalloids to maintain blood pressure. Diagnostic tests include complete blood count, urinalysis, coagulation studies, blood urea nitrogen, creatinine, creatine kinase, and electrolytes. Other measures include assessment of extremity swelling, usually through documentation of circumference every 30 to 60 minutes. Pain should be treated with acetaminophen. Aspirin and nonsteroidal antiinflammatory drugs should be avoided because they may exacerbate bleeding; narcotics may cause respiratory depression. Tetanus prophylaxis should be administered as needed (see Table 67-6). Secondary infection caused by microorganisms in the snake's mouth or other contaminants may require antibiotic therapy. Debridement or fasciotomy (see Chapter 24) is necessary in some patients. Antivenin (polyvalent Crotalidae antivenin ovine Fab [Cro-Fab]) therapy is used in mild to moderate reactions; the amount of antivenin required depends on the timing, type, and severity of envenomation (Table 67-11). Incomplete dosage is the most common cause of treatment failure.

TABLE 67-11	**Antivenin* Snakebite Treatment**	
ENVENOMATION	**SIGNS AND SYMPTOMS**	**NUMBER OF VIALS OF ANTIVENIN†**
None	Fang marks, no local swelling, hemorrhage, or paresthesia	No antivenin, tetanus prophylaxis, observation
Mild to moderate	*Mild:* Fang marks, local swelling of hands or feet, pain, no systemic reactions *Moderate:* Fang marks, progressive swelling beyond bite, mild systemic reaction (e.g., nausea, vomiting, paresthesias, hypotension)	*Initial dose:* 4-6 vials (3000-4500 mg) infused over 1 hour; infusion should be initiated slowly for the first 10 minutes to detect any allergic reactions; if initial control of symptoms is not achieved, dose may be repeated once *Additional regimen:* 2 vials every 6 hours for 18 hours

*Polyvalent Crotalidae antivenin ovine Fab (Cro-Fab).
†For Crotalidae envenomation (e.g., rattlesnakes, copperheads).

Animal and Human Bites

Approximately 500,000 to 2 million animal bites are reported each year in the United States. Children are at greatest risk. The most significant problems associated with animal bites are infection and mechanical destruction of the skin, muscle, tendons, blood vessels, and bone. The bite may cause a simple laceration or be associated with crush injury, puncture wound, or tearing or avulsion of tissue. The severity of injury depends on animal size, victim size, and anatomic location of the bite. Animal bites from cats and dogs are common, with dog bites accounting for 90% of the bite injuries that are treated in the ED.[19] Wild or domestic rodents are ranked behind cats and dogs as the third most frequent offenders in reported animal bites.

Dog bites usually occur on the extremities; however, facial bites are common in small children. Most victims own the dogs that bite them. Dog bites may involve significant tissue damage with fatalities reported, usually in children. Skull fractures with intracranial injury and death may occur in children less than 2 years old. Disfiguring wounds of the face should be evaluated by a plastic surgeon.

Cat bites cause deep puncture wounds that can involve tendons and joint capsules. Cat bites result in a greater incidence of infection than dog bites because of the organism, *Pasteurella,* that is carried in the mouths of most healthy cats.[19] Septic arthritis, osteomyelitis, and tenosynovitis have been reported in cat bites.

Humans bites also cause puncture wounds or lacerations and carry a high risk of infection from oral bacterial flora, most commonly *Staphylococcus aureus* and streptococci, and hepatitis virus. Hands, fingers, ears, nose, vagina, and penis are the most common sites of human bites and are frequently a result of violence or sexual activity. Boxer's fracture, fracture of the fifth metacarpal, is often associated with an open wound when the knuckles strike teeth. The human jaw has great crushing ability, causing laceration, puncture, crush injury, soft tissue tearing, and even amputation. More than 40 potential pathogens found in the human mouth account for an infection rate of approximately 50% in cases where victims did not seek medical intervention within 24 hours of injury.

Collaborative Care. Initial treatment for animal and human bites includes cleaning with copious irrigation, debridement, tetanus prophylaxis, and analgesics as needed. Prophylactic antibiotics are used for animal and human bites at risk for infection such as wounds over joints, those greater than 6 to 12 hours old, puncture wounds, and bites of the hand or foot. Individuals at greatest risk of infection are infants, older adults, immunosuppressed patients, alcoholics, diabetics, and people taking corticosteroids.

Puncture wounds are left open, whereas lacerations are loosely sutured. Wounds over joints are splinted. However, initial closure is reserved only for facial wounds. The patient is admitted for IV antibiotic therapy when an infection is present. There is an increased incidence of cellulitis, osteomyelitis, and septic arthritis in these patients. Human bites must be reported to the police in some states.

Consideration of rabies prophylaxis is an essential component in management of animal bites. A neurotoxic virus found in the saliva of some mammals causes rabies. If untreated, the condition is fatal in humans. Rabies exposure should be considered if an animal attack was not provoked, involved a wild animal, or involved a domestic animal not immunized against rabies. Rabies prophylaxis is always given when the animal cannot be found or a carnivorous wild animal causes the bite. An initial injection of rabies immune globulin (RIG) to provide passive immunity starts the prophylaxis regimen. This is followed by a series of five injections of human diploid cell vaccine (HDCV) on days 0, 3, 7, 14, and 28 to provide active immunity. Dosage is based on the patient's weight.

POISONINGS

A poison is any chemical that harms the body. In 2000, more than 2 million cases of human poison exposure were reported in the United States.[23] Poisonings can be accidental, occupational, recreational, or intentional. Natural or manufactured toxins can be ingested, inhaled, injected, splashed in the eye, or absorbed through the skin. Common poisons are reviewed in Table 67-12. Other poisonings related to the use of illegal drugs such as amphetamines, narcotics, and hallucinogens are discussed in Chapter 11. Poisoning may also be due to toxic plants or contaminated foods. (Food poisoning is discussed in Chapter 40.)

Severity of the poisoning depends on type, concentration, and route of exposure. Toxins can affect every tissue of the body, so symptoms can be seen in any body system. Specific management of toxins involves decreasing absorption, enhancing elimination, and implementation of toxin-specific interventions. The local poison control center is available 24 hours a day and should be consulted for the most current treatment protocols for specific poisons.

Options for decreasing absorption of poisons include emesis, gastric lavage, activated charcoal, dermal cleansing, and eye irrigation. Ipecac syrup (15 to 45 ml for adults) followed by 250 to 500 ml of water is used to induce emesis. This process is most effective if used within 30 minutes of ingestion. Use of ipecac has lost favor over the past decade for a variety of reasons. Onset of action is delayed and unpredictable, overall rate of drug return is low, and ipecac syrup is not effective with drugs that are rapidly absorbed, such as alcohol.[24] Ipecac is also potentially cardiotoxic if emesis does not occur or if a large dose is given. Other problems associated with induced emesis include fluid losses, electrolyte abnormalities, and acid-base disturbances secondary to protracted vomiting.

Gastric lavage involves oral insertion of a large-diameter (36 to 40 French) gastric tube for installation of copious amounts of saline. The head of the bed should be elevated or the patient placed on the side to prevent aspiration. Patients with an altered level of consciousness or diminished gag reflex are intubated before lavage. Lavage is contraindicated in patients who ingested caustic agents, coingested sharp objects, or ingested nontoxic substances.[25] Problems associated with lavage include epistaxis, esophageal perforation, and aspiration.

The most effective intervention for management of poisonings is administration of activated charcoal orally or via a gastric tube. Toxins adhere to charcoal and are excreted through the gastrointestinal (GI) tract rather than absorbed into the portal circulation. Adults receive 50 to 100 g of charcoal. Activated charcoal can absorb a number of poisons from the GI tract, but it does not absorb ethanol, alkali, iron, boric acid, lithium, methanol, or cyanide. For some toxins (e.g., phenobarbital) multiple-dose charcoal may be required.[25] Contraindications to charcoal administration are diminished bowel sounds, ileus, ingestion of a substance poorly absorbed by charcoal, or previous administration of N-acetylcysteine (NAC [Mucomyst]). Charcoal inactivates NAC, the antidote used for acetaminophen toxicity.

TABLE 67-12	Common Poisons	
POISON	**MANIFESTATIONS**	**TREATMENT**
• Acetaminophen (Tylenol)	*Phase 1:* within 24 hours of ingestion: malaise, diaphoresis, nausea and vomiting *Phase 2:* 24-28 hours: right upper quadrant pain, decreased urine output, diminished nausea, LFTs rise *Phase 3:* 72-96 hours: nausea and vomiting, malaise, jaundice, hypoglycemia, enlarged liver, possible coagulopathies, including DIC *Phase 4:* 7-8 days after ingestion: recovery, resolution of symptoms, LFTs return to normal	Activated charcoal, *N*-acetylcysteine (oral form may cause vomiting, IV form available on experimental basis).

• Acids and alkalis
  Acids: toilet bowel cleaners, antirust compounds
  Alkalis: drain cleaners, dishwashing detergents, ammonia
	Excess salivation, dysphagia, epigastric pain, pneumonitis; burns of mouth, esophagus, and stomach	Immediate dilution (water, milk), corticosteroids (for alkali burns), induced vomiting is contraindicated.

• Aspirin and aspirin-containing medications	Tachypnea, tachycardia, hyperthermia, seizures, pulmonary edema, occult bleeding/hemorrhage, metabolic acidosis	Gastric lavage, activated charcoal with or without cathartic, urine alkalinization, hemodialysis for severe acute ingestion, intubation and mechanical ventilation, supportive care.
• Bleaches	Irritation of lips, mouth, and eyes, superficial injury to esophagus; chemical pneumonia and pulmonary edema	Washing of exposed skin and eyes, dilution with water and milk, gastric lavage, prevention of vomiting and aspiration.
• Carbon monoxide	Dyspnea, headache, tachypnea, confusion, impaired judgment, cyanosis, respiratory depression	Removal from source, administration of 100% O_2 via non-rebreather mask, BVM, or intubation and mechanical ventilation; consider hyperbaric oxygen therapy.
• Cyanide	Almond odor to breath, headache, dizziness, nausea, confusion, hypertension, bradycardia followed by hypotension and tachycardia, tachypnea followed by bradypnea and respiratory arrest	Amyl nitrate (nasally), IV sodium nitrate, IV sodium thiosulfate, supportive care.
• Ethylene glycol	Sweet aromatic odor to breath, nausea and vomiting, slurred speech, ataxia, lethargy, respiratory depression	Gastric lavage, activated charcoal, supportive care.
• Iron	Vomiting (often bloody), diarrhea (often bloody), fever, hyperglycemia, lethargy, hypotension, seizures, coma	Gastric lavage, chelation therapy (deferoxamine [Desferal]).
• Nonsteroidal antiinflammatory drugs	Gastroenteritis, abdominal pain, drowsiness, nystagmus, hepatic and renal damage	Gastric lavage, activated charcoal, cathartics, supportive care.
• Tricyclic antidepressants (e.g., amitriptyline [Elavil])	In low doses: anticholinergic effects, agitation, hypertension, tachycardia; in high doses: central nervous system depression, arrhythmias, hypotension, respiratory depression	Multidose activated charcoal, gastric lavage, serum alkalinization with sodium bicarbonate, intubation and mechanical ventilation, supportive care; never induce vomiting.
• Alcohol, barbiturates, benzodiazepines, cocaine, hallucinogens, stimulants	See Chapter 11	See Chapter 11

LFTs, Liver function tests; *BVM,* bag-valve-mask; *DIC,* disseminated intravascular coagulation; *IV,* intravenous.

Skin and ocular decontamination involves removal of toxins from eyes and skin using copious amounts of water or saline. With the exception of mustard gas, most toxins can be safely removed with water or saline.[25] Water mixes with mustard gas and releases chlorine gas. As a general rule, dry substances should be brushed from the skin and clothing before water is used. Powdered lime should not be removed with water; it should just be brushed off. Personal protective equipment (gloves, gowns, goggles, and respirators) should be worn for decontamination to prevent secondary exposure. Decontamination procedures are usually done by those specially trained in hazardous material decontamination before the patient arrives at the hospital. Decontamination takes priority over all interventions except basic life support techniques.

Elimination of poisons is increased through administration of cathartics, whole-bowel irrigation, hemodialysis, hemoperfusion, urine alkalinization, chelating agents, and antidotes. Cathartics such as sorbitol, magnesium citrate, or magnesium sulfate are given together with activated charcoal to stimulate intestinal motility and increase elimination. Multiple doses of cathartics should be avoided because of potentially fatal electrolyte abnormalities. Whole bowel irrigation is controversial and involves administration of a nonabsorbable bowel evacuant solution (e.g., GoLYTELY). The solution is administered every 4 to 6 hours until stools are clear. This process can be effective for swallowed objects such as cocaine-filled balloons or condoms. There is a high risk of electrolyte imbalance due to fluid and electrolyte losses with this procedure.[25]

Hemodialysis and hemoperfusion are reserved for patients who develop severe acidosis from ingestion of toxic substances (e.g., aspirin). Other interventions include alkalinization and chelation therapy. Sodium bicarbonate administration raises the pH (greater than 7.5), which is particularly effective for phenobarbital and salicylate poisoning. Vitamin C may be added to IV fluids to enhance excretion of amphetamines and quinidine. Chelation therapy may be considered for heavy metal poisoning (e.g., edetate calcium disodium [EDTA] for lead poisoning). A limited number of true antidotes are available, and many of these agents are themselves toxic.[25]

Education for toxic emergencies focuses on how the poisoning occurred. Patients who experience poisoning because of a suicide attempt or related to substance abuse should be evaluated by a mental health counselor and then referred for alcohol or drug detoxification or scheduled for follow-up with a mental health professional. The Occupational Safety and Health Administration should evaluate all poisoning related to an occupational hazard.

VIOLENCE

Violence is the acting out of the emotions of fear or anger to cause harm to someone or something. It may be the result of organic disease (e.g., temporal lobe epilepsy), psychosis (e.g., schizophrenia), or antisocial behavior (e.g., homicide).[26] The patient cared for in the ED may be the victim of violence or the perpetrator of violence. Violence can take place in a variety of settings, including the home, workplace, and community.

Domestic violence is a pattern of coercive behavior in a relationship that involves fear, humiliation, intimidation, neglect, and/or intentional physical, emotional, financial, or sexual injury (see Chapter 52 for information on sexual assault). It is found in all professions, cultures, socioeconomic groups, ages, and genders. Although men can be victims of domestic violence, most victims are women, children, and the elderly. It has been estimated that 20% to 50% of women treated at EDs have been *battered* (assaulted) by spouses, significant others, or individuals known to them.[27,28]

ED nurses are well situated to conduct domestic violence screening, yet research indicates that this is not always done (see Nursing Research box). Barriers to conducting effective screening include limited privacy for screening, lack of time, and lack of knowledge about how to inquire about domestic violence. The development and implementation of specific policies, procedures, and staff education programs can improve the domestic violence screening practices of ED staff.[27-30] For any patient who is found to be a victim of abuse, appropriate interventions such as making referrals, providing emotional support, and informing victims about their options (e.g., safe house, legal rights) should be initiated.[27] See Resources at the end of this chapter for additional information on domestic violence.

NURSING RESEARCH
Caring for Battered Women in the Emergency Department

Citation
Yam M: Seen but not heard: battered women's perceptions of the emergency department (ED) experience, *J Emerg Nurs* 26:464, 2000.

Purpose
To describe the experiences of battered women seen in the ED.

Methods
A phenomenologic approach was used to allow women to express themselves in their own words. Five women were interviewed individually, and all interviews were audiotaped and transcribed.

Results and Conclusions
Five categories emerged from the data and were confirmed by an expert consultant in the phenomenologic method. The women reported a multitude of emotions during their visit (e.g., fear of their partner, loneliness, concern for children) and a belief that the ED staff does not understand abuse and may even blame the victim. The women did report a satisfaction with the care that they received for their physical injuries but dissatisfaction with how the issue of abuse was managed. All women found it difficult to discuss the abuse with the staff. Reasons for this difficulty included fear (of the abuser), embarrassment, and lack of resources and/or support. Finally, the women requested that caregivers display compassion and take time to talk to them privately about their injuries and options.

Implications for Nursing Practice
These findings provide important insights into the perceptions of abused women seen in the ED. The dissatisfaction reported by this sample is similar to findings from previous studies. Nurses need to evaluate their practice and care models that provide for the physical, emotional, and safety needs of victims of abuse. It is extremely important for nurses to focus on the emotional needs of women who have been abused.

AGENTS OF TERRORISM

The threat of terrorism has emerged as a growing concern. Terrorism involves overt actions such as the dispensing of disease pathogens (e.g., **bioterrorism**) or other agents (e.g., chemical, radiologic) as weapons for the expressed purpose of causing harm. Prompt recognition and identification of potential health hazards are essential in the preparedness of health care professionals.

Table 67-13 summarizes general information regarding biologic agents of terrorism. The pathogens most likely to be used in a bioterrorist attack are anthrax, smallpox, botulism, plague, tularemia, and hemorrhagic fever.

Among the agents considered likely to be biologic weapons, those that cause anthrax, plague, and tularemia could be treated effectively with commercially available antibiotics if sufficient supplies were available and the organisms were not resistant. Smallpox can be prevented or ameliorated by vaccination even when first given after exposure. Botulism can be treated with antitoxin. There is no established treatment for viruses that cause hemorrhagic fever.[31]

TABLE 67-13 Agents of Bioterrorism

PATHOGEN AND DESCRIPTION	CLINICAL MANIFESTATIONS	TRANSMISSIBILITY	TREATMENT
Anthrax *Bacillus anthracis* ***Inhalation*** • Bacterial spores multiply in the alveoli • Toxins cause hemorrhage and destruction of lung tissue • High mortality rate	• Incubation period: 1–2 days to 6 weeks • Abrupt onset • Dyspnea • Diaphoresis • Fever • Cough • Chest pain • Septicemia • Shock • Meningitis • Respiratory failure • Widened mediastinum (seen on chest x-ray) • Incubation period: up to 12 days	• No person-to-person spread • Found in nature and most commonly infects wild and domestic hoofed animals • Spread through direct contact with bacteria and its spores • Spores are dormant, encapsulated bacteria that become active when they enter a living host	• Antibiotics prevent systemic manifestations • Effective only if treated early • Ciprofloxacin (Cipro) is the treatment of choice • Penicillin • Doxycycline • Postexposure prophylaxis for 30 days (if vaccine available) or 60 days (if vaccine not available) • Vaccine has limited availability
Cutaneous • 95% of anthrax infections • Least lethal form • Spores enter skin through cuts or abrasions • Handling of contaminated animal skin products • Toxins destroy surrounding tissue	• Small papule resembles an insect bite • Advances to a depressed, black ulcer • Swollen lymph nodes in adjacent areas • Edema		
Gastrointestinal • Ingestion of contaminated, undercooked meat • Intestinal lesions in ileum or cecum • Acute inflammation of intestines	• Nausea • Vomiting • Anorexia • Hematemesis • Diarrhea • Abdominal pain • Ascites • Sepsis		
Smallpox Variola major and minor viruses • United States ended routine vaccination in 1971 • Global eradication declared in 1980	• Incubation period: 7–17 days • Sudden onset of symptoms • Fever • Headache • Myalgia • Lesions that progress from macules to papules to pustular vesicles • Malaise • Back pain	• Highly contagious • Direct person-to-person spread • Transmitted in air droplets • Transmitted by handling contaminated materials	• No known care • Cidofovir (Vistide) under testing • Isolation for containment • Vaccine available for those exposed • Vaccinia immune globulin (VIG) available
Botulism *Clostridium botulinum* • Spore-forming anaerobe • Found in soil • Seven different toxins • Lethal bacterial neurotoxin • Can die within 24 hours	• Incubation period: 12–72 hr • Abdominal cramps • Diarrhea • Nausea • Vomiting • Cranial nerve palsies (diplopia, dysarthria, dysphonia, dysphagia) • Skeletal muscle paralysis • Respiratory failure	• Spread through air or food • No person-to-person spread • Improperly canned foods • Contaminated wound	• Induce vomiting • Enemas • Antitoxin • Mechanical ventilation • Penicillin • No vaccine available • Toxin can be inactivated by heating food or drink to 85° C for at least 5 minutes

Continued

TABLE 67-13   Agents of Bioterrorism—cont'd

PATHOGEN AND DESCRIPTION	CLINICAL MANIFESTATIONS	TRANSMISSIBILITY	TREATMENT
Plague *Yersinia pestis* • Bacteria found in rodents and fleas ***Forms*** • Bubonic (most common) • Pneumonic • Septicemic (most deadly)	• Incubation period: 2–4 days • Hemoptysis • Cough • High fever • Chills • Myalgia • Headache • Respiratory failure • Lymph node swelling	• Direct person-to-person spread • Transmitted through flea bites • Ingestion of contaminated meat	• Antibiotics only effective if administered immediately • Drug of choice: streptomycin or gentamicin • Vaccine under development • Hospitalization • Isolation for containment
Tularemia *Francisella tularensis* • Bacterial infectious disease of animals • Mortality rate about 35% without treatment	• Incubation period: 3–10 days • Sudden onset • Fever • Swollen lymph nodes • Fatigue • Sore throat • Weight loss • Pneumonia • Pleural effusion • Ulcerated sore from tick bite	• No person-to-person spread • Aerosol or intradermal route • Spread by rabbits and ticks • Contaminated food, air, water	• Gentamicin treatment of choice • Streptomycin, doxycycline, and ciprofloxacin are alternatives • Vaccine in developmental stage
Hemorrhagic Fever • Caused by several viruses, including Marburg, Lassa, Junin, and Ebola • Ebola virus is life threatening	• Fever • Conjunctivitis • Headache • Malaise • Prostration • Hemorrhage of tissues and organs • Nausea • Vomiting • Hypotension • Organ failure	• Carried by rodents and mosquitoes • Direct person-to-person spread by body fluids • Virus can be aerosolized	• No intramuscular injections • No antiplatelet drugs • Isolation for containment • Ribavirin (Virazole) effective in some cases • No known treatment available

TABLE 67-14   Chemical Agents of Terrorism by Target Organ or Effect

NERVE	BLOOD	PULMONARY	BLISTER/VESICANTS
Sarin (isopropyl methylphosphanofluoridate) Tabun (ethyl *N,N*-dimethylphosphoramido–cyanidate) Soman (pinacolyl methyl phosphonofluoridate) GF (cyclohexylmethylphosphonofluoridate) VX (O-ethyl S-[2-diisopropylaminoethyl] methylphosphonothiolate)	Hydrogen cyanide Cyanogen chloride	Phosgene Chlorine Vinyl chloride	Nitrogen and sulfur mustards Lewisite (an aliphatic arsenic compound, 2-chlorovinyldichloroarsine) Phosgene oxime

Chemicals may also be used as agents of terrorism and are categorized according to their target organ or effect (Table 67-14).[32] For example, sarin is a highly toxic nerve gas that can cause death within minutes of exposure. It enters the body through the eyes and skin and acts by paralyzing the respiratory muscles. Phosgene is a colorless gas normally used in chemical manufacturing. If inhaled at high concentrations for a long enough period, it causes severe respiratory distress, pulmonary edema, and death. Mustard gas is yellow to brown in color and has a garlic-like odor. The gas irritates the eyes and causes skin burns and blisters. Protocols to treat victims of chemical exposure are varied and relate to the specific agent.[33]

Ionizing radiation, such as that from a nuclear bomb or damage to a nuclear reactor, represents another major agent of terrorism. Exposure to radiation may or may not include skin contamination with radioactive material. If external radioactive contaminants are present, decontamination procedures must be initiated. Acute radiation syndrome develops after a substantial exposure to radiation and follows a predictable pattern (Table 67-15).[34]

TABLE 67-15   Acute Radiation Syndrome

PHASE OF SYNDROME	FEATURE	WHOLE BODY RADIATION FROM EXTERNAL RADIATION OR INTERNAL ABSORPTION					
		SUBCLINICAL RANGE		SUBLETHAL RANGE		LETHAL RANGE	
		0-100 RAD	100-200 RAD	200-600 RAD	600-800 RAD	600-3000 RAD	>3000 RAD
Initial or prodromal	Nausea, vomiting	None	5%-50%	50%-100%	75%-100%	90%-100%	100%
	Time of onset		3-6 hr	2-4 hr	1-2 hr	<1 hr	<1 hr
	Duration		<24 hr	<24 hr	<48 hr	<48 hr	<48 hr
	Lymphocyte count/μl			<1000 at 24 hr	<500 at 24 hr		
	CNS function	No impairment	No impairment	Routine task performance; cognitive impairment for 6-20 hr	Simple and routine task performance; cognitive impairment for >24 hr	Progressive incapacitation occurs	Progressive incapacitation occurs
"Manifest illness" (obvious illness)	Signs and symptoms	None	Moderate leukopenia	Severe leukopenia, purpura, hemorrhage Pneumonia Hair loss after 300 rad	Severe leukopenia, purpura, hemorrhage	Diarrhea Fever Electrolyte disturbance	Convulsions, ataxia, tremor, lethargy
	Time of onset		>2 wk	2 days-2 wk	2 days-2 wk	2-3 days	2-3 days
	Critical period		None	4-6 wk	4-6 wk	5-14 days	1-48 hr
	Organ system	None		Hematopoietic and respiratory (mucosal) systems	Hematopoietic and respiratory (mucosal) systems	GI tract Mucosal systems	CNS
%	Hospitalization	0	<5%	90%	100%	100%	100%
	Fatality	0%	0%	0%-80%	90%-100%	90%-100%	90%-100%
	Time to death			3 wk-3 mo	3 wk-3 mo	1-2 wk	1-2 days

From Armed Forces Radiobiology Research Institute: *Pocket guide for responders to ionizing radiation terrorism.* Available at *www.afrri.usuhs.mil/www/outreach/pocketguide.htm* (accessed July 25, 2002).
CNS, Central nervous system; *GI,* gastrointestinal.

EMERGENCY AND DISASTER PREPAREDNESS

The term **emergency** usually refers to any extraordinary event (e.g., multivictim train crash) that requires a rapid and skilled response and that can be managed by a community's existing resources.[35] An *emergency* is differentiated from a *disaster* in that a **disaster** is a manmade (e.g., biologic warfare) or natural (e.g., hurricane) event that overwhelms a community's ability to respond with existing resources.[36] Disasters result in mass casualties (more than 100 victims), physical and emotional suffering, and permanent changes within a community. In addition, disasters require assistance from people and resources outside the affected community (Fig. 67-8).[35]

The ED nurse has an important role in emergency and disaster management. Knowledge of the agency's *emergency response plan*, including individual roles and responsibilities of the members of the response team, and participation in emergency/disaster preparedness drills are necessary. See Resources at the end of this chapter for additional information on emergency and disaster preparedness.

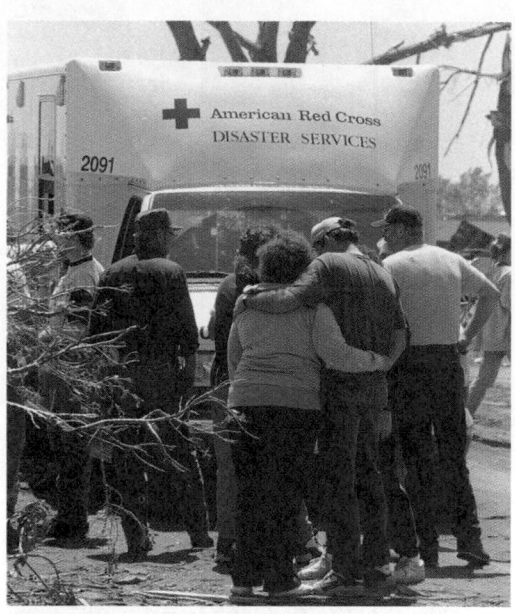

FIG. 67-8 American Red Cross.

CRITICAL THINKING EXERCISES

Case Study

Trauma

Patient Profile. A 20-year-old Hispanic female trauma patient is brought to the ED in an ambulance. She was the driver in a motor vehicle collision and was not wearing a seat belt. Two children in the car were pronounced dead at the scene. The paramedics stated that there was significant damage to the car on the driver's side.

Subjective Data
- Patient asks, "What happened? Where are the children?"
- Complains of shortness of breath and abdominal pain

Objective Data

Physical Examination
- 4 cm head laceration
- Badly deformed right lower leg with a pedal pulse by Doppler only
- Glasgow Coma Score = 14; unequal pupils
- Decreased breath sounds on left side of chest
- Asymmetric chest movement
- Vital signs: blood pressure 90/40, heart rate 130 beats/min, respiratory rate 36 breaths/min
- O_2 saturation 82%

CRITICAL THINKING QUESTIONS

1. What life-threatening injury does this patient probably have?
2. What is the priority of care?
3. What interventions are needed immediately?
4. What other interventions should the nurse consider?
5. Several family members have arrived in the ED, including the mother of one of the children who died. The second child who died was the patient's child. How should the nurse approach the family?
6. Based on assessment data presented, write one or more nursing diagnoses. Are there any collaborative problems?

Nursing Research Issues

1. Can the use of complementary therapies in the ED help patients manage pain?
2. What are the most effective teaching strategies for patients and their families following discharge from the ED?
3. Can the use of a screening tool for domestic violence increase the number of appropriate referrals?
4. What are the most effective strategies for helping family members in an ED setting?

REVIEW QUESTIONS

The number of the question corresponds to the same-numbered objective at the beginning of the chapter.

1. An elderly man arrives at the ED disoriented and breathing rapidly. He has hot, dry skin. The priority for treatment at this point is to
   a. assess his airway, breathing, and circulation.
   b. obtain a detailed medical history from his family.
   c. determine the kind of insurance he has before treating him.
   d. start oxygen administration and have the ED physician see him.

2. A patient has a core temperature of 90° F (32.2 °C). The most appropriate rewarming technique would be
   a. passive rewarming with body-to-body contact.
   b. active core rewarming using warmed IV fluids.
   c. passive rewarming using air-filled warming blankets.
   d. active external rewarming by submersing in a warm bath.

3. The most effective intervention in decreasing absorption of an ingested poison is
   a. ipecac syrup.
   b. milk dilution.
   c. gastric lavage.
   d. activated charcoal.

4. An elderly patient arrives in the ED with his son. The older man is in no apparent distress, although his clothes are soiled with urine and feces and he is tearful. The nurse should consider
   a. cancer.
   b. stroke.
   c. neglect.
   d. depression.

5. A chemical spill has occurred in a nearby industrial site. The first responders report that approximately 20 victims need to be transported to the ED after decontamination at the site. This is an example of
   a. an emergency.
   b. a natural disaster.
   c. a manmade disaster.
   d. an emergency response plan.

6. Which of the following biologic agents of bioterrorism has no effective treatment?
   a. anthrax
   b. botulism
   c. smallpox
   d. hemorrhagic fever

REFERENCES

*1. MacLean SL et al: The LUNAR project: a description of individuals who seek health care at emergency departments, *J Emerg Nurs* 25:269, 1999.

2. Emergency Nurses Association: ENA position statement on specialty certification in emergency nursing. Available at *www.ena.org/services/posistate/statements/Specialty/Certification.htm* (accessed Feb 20, 2002).

*3. Gerdtz MF, Bucknall TK: Triage nurses' clinical decision making: an observational study of urgency assessment, *J Adv Nurs* 35:550, 2001.

4. Rund DA, Rausch TS: *Triage,* St Louis, 1981, Mosby.

5. Rutenberg CD: Telephone triage, *Am J Nurs* 100:77, 2000.

6. Emergency Nurses Association, Newberry L, editor: *Sheehy's emergency nursing: principles and practice,* ed 5, St Louis, 2003, Mosby.

7. Jacobs BB, Hoyt KS, editors: *Trauma nursing core course,* ed 5, Des Plaines, Ill., 2000, Emergency Nurses Association.

*8. Li J et al: Complications of emergency intubation with and without paralysis, *Am J Emerg Med* 17:141, 1999.

*9. Sakles JC et al: Airway management in the emergency department: a one-year study of 610 tracheal intubations, *Ann Emerg Med* 33:325, 1998.

10. Laskowski-Jones L: Trauma. In Bucher L, Melander S, editors: *Critical care nursing,* Philadelphia, 1999, WB Saunders.

*11. Eichhorn DJ et al: Family presence during invasive procedures and resuscitation: hearing the voice of the patient, *Am J Nurs* 101:48, 2001.

*12. Meyers TA et al: Family presence during invasive procedures and resuscitation, *Am J Nurs* 100:32, 2000.

*13. Tanabe P, Buschmann M: Emergency nurses' knowledge of pain management principles, *J Emerg Nurs* 26:299, 2000.

*14. Kelly AM: A process approach to improving pain management in the emergency department: development and evaluation, *J Accid Emerg Med* 17:185, 1999.

*15. Tanabe P et al: The effect of standard care, ibuprofen, and music on pain relief and patient satisfaction in adults with musculoskeletal trauma, *J Emerg Nurs* 27:124, 2001.

*16. Socorro LL, Tolson D, Fleming V: Exploring Spanish emergency nurses' lived experience of the care provided for suddenly bereaved families, *J Adv Nurs* 35:562, 2001.

*17. Boulstridge HPM: Tissue donation after death in the accident and emergency department: an opportunity wasted? *J Accid Emerg Med* 16:117, 1999.

18. Linder JE, Fleming AW: Trauma in the elderly, *Clin Geriatr* 9:52, 2001.

19. Semonin-Holleran R: Environmental emergencies. In Jordan KS, editor: *Emergency nursing core curriculum,* ed 5, Philadelphia, 2000, WB Saunders.

20. Laskowski-Jones L: Responding to summer emergencies, *DCCN* 19:2, 2000.

21. Laskowski-Jones L: Responding to winter emergencies, *DCCN* 18:13, 1999.

22. DeBoer SL: Neurologic outcomes after near drowning, *Crit Care Nurse* 17:4, 1997.

*Nursing research–based reference.

23. Litovitz TL et al: 2000 Annual report of the American Association of Poison Control Centers toxic exposure surveillance system, *Am J Emerg Med* 19:337, 2001.

24. Emergency Nurses Association, Newberry L, editor: *Sheehy's emergency nursing: principles and practice,* ed 5, St Louis, 2003, Mosby.

25. McDeed-Breault C: Toxicological emergencies. In Jordan KS, editor: *Emergency nursing core curriculum,* ed 5, Philadelphia, 2000, WB Saunders.

26. Polli GE, Lazear SE: Mental health emergencies. In Jordan KS, editor: *Emergency nursing core curriculum,* ed 5, Philadelphia, 2000, WB Saunders.

*27. Ellis JM: Barriers to effective screening for domestic violence by registered nurses in the emergency department, *Crit Care Nurs Q* 22:27, 1999.

28. Emergency Nurses Association: ENA position statement on domestic violence. Available at *www.ena.org/services/posistate/data/domvio.htm* (accessed Feb 2, 2002).

*29. Brymer C et al: The effect of a geriatric education program on emergency nurses, *J Emerg Nurs* 27:27, 2001.

*30. Fulmer T et al: Elder neglect assessment in the emergency department, *J Emerg Nurs* 26:436, 2000.

31. On drugs and therapeutics, *Med Lett* 43:87, 2001.

32. Centers for Disease Control and Prevention: Biological and chemical terrorism: strategic plan for preparedness and response, October 2001. Available at *www.cdc.gov/mmwr/preview/mmwrhtml/rr4904a1.htm* (accessed July 23, 2002).

33. National Center for Environmental Health: Demilitarization of chemical weapons: emergency room procedures in chemical hazard emergencies—a job aid. Last reviewed May 4, 2002. Available at *www.cdc.gov/nceh/demil/articles/initialtreat.htm* (accessed July 23, 2002).

34. Armed Forces Radiobiology Research Institute: Pocket guide for responders to ionizing radiation terrorism. Last update June 25, 2002. Available at *www.afrri.usuhs.mil/www/outreach/pocketguide.htm* (accessed July 23, 2002).

35. Gebbie KM, Qureshi K: Emergency and disaster preparedness: core competencies for nurses, *Am J Nurs* 102:46, 2002.

36. Klein J: Disaster preparedness/disaster management. In Jordan KS, editor: *Emergency nursing core curriculum,* ed 5, Philadelphia, 2000, WB Saunders.

RESOURCES

American College of Emergency Physicians
1125 Executive Circle
Irving, TX 75038-2522
800-798-1822 or 972-550-0911
Fax: 972-580-2816
www.acep.org

American Nurses Association
Bioterrorism and Disaster Response Website
www.nursingworld.org/news/disaster

American Red Cross
P.O. Box 37243
Washington, DC 20013
800-HELP-NOW
www.redcross.org

American Trauma Society
8903 Presidential Parkway, Suite 512
Upper Marlboro, MD 20772
800-556-7890 or 301-420-4189
www.amtrauma.org

Association of Emergency Physicians (AEP)
127 Branchaw Boulevard
New Lenox, IL 60451
800-449-4237
Fax: 815-463-9230
www.aep.org

CDC Public Health Awareness and Response Website
Bioterrorism Preparedness and Response Planning
Centers for Disease Control and Prevention
Mailstop C-18
1600 Clifton Road
Atlanta, GA 30333
888-246-2675
www.bt.cdc.gov

Center for the Prevention of Sexual and Domestic Violence
2400 North 45th Street, #10
Seattle, WA 98103
206-634-1903
Fax: 206-634-0115
www.cpsdv.org

Emergency Nurses Association (ENA)
915 Lee Street
Des Plaines, IL 60016-6569
800-243-8362
www.ena.org

Federal Emergency Management Agency
500 C Street, SW
Washington, DC 20472
202-566-1600
www.fema.gov

National Coalition Against Domestic Violence
P.O. Box 18749
Denver, CO 80218
National Domestic Violence Hotline: 800-799-SAFE (7233)
303-839-1852
Fax: 303-831-9251
www.ncadv.org

National Domestic Violence Hotline
P.O. Box 16180
Austin, TX 78716
800-799-SAFE
Fax: 512-453-8541
www.ndvh.org

National Response Center
c/o United States Coast Guard (G-OPF)
2100 2nd Street, SW, Room 2611
Washington, DC 20593-0001
800-424-8802 or 202-267-2675
Fax: 202-267-2165
www.nrc.uscg.mil/index.htm

U.S. Department of Health and Human Services, Office of Emergency Preparedness
National Disaster Medical System
12300 Twinbrook Parkway, Suite 360
Rockville, MD 20857
301-443-1167 or 800-USA-NDMS
Fax: 301-443-5146 or 800-USA-KWIK
www.ndms.dhhs.gov/index.html

Wilderness Medicine Institute
National Outdoor Leadership School
284 Lincoln Street
Lander, WY 82520
307-332-7800
http://wmi.nols.edu

For additional Internet resources, see the website for this book at *http://evolve.elsevier.com/Lewis/medsurg/*.

APPENDIX 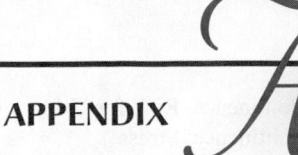 Nursing Diagnoses

ALPHABETICAL LISTING

Activity Intolerance
Activity Intolerance, Risk for
Adjustment, Impaired
Airway Clearance, Ineffective
Allergy Response, Latex
Allergy Response, Risk for Latex
Anxiety
Anxiety, Death
Aspiration, Risk for
Attachment, Risk for Impaired
    Parent/Infant/Child
Autonomic Dysreflexia
Autonomic Dysreflexia, Risk for
Body Image, Disturbed
Body Temperature, Risk for Imbalanced
Bowel Incontinence
Breastfeeding, Effective
Breastfeeding, Ineffective
Breastfeeding, Interrupted
Breathing Pattern, Ineffective
Cardiac Output, Decreased
Caregiver Role Strain
Caregiver Role Strain, Risk for
Communication, Impaired Verbal
Communication, Readiness for
    Enhanced
Conflict, Decisional
Conflict, Parental Role
Confusion, Acute
Confusion, Chronic
Constipation
Constipation, Perceived
Constipation, Risk for
Coping, Ineffective
Coping, Ineffective Community
Coping, Readiness for Enhanced
Coping, Readiness for Enhanced
    Community
Coping, Defensive
Coping, Compromised Family
Coping, Disabled Family
Coping, Readiness for Enhanced Family

Denial, Ineffective
Dentition, Impaired
Development, Risk for Delayed
Diarrhea
Disuse Syndrome, Risk for
Diversional Activity, Deficient
Energy Field, Disturbed
Environmental Interpretation Syndrome,
    Impaired
Failure to Thrive, Adult
Falls, Risk for
Family Processes, Dysfunctional:
    Alcoholism
Family Processes, Interrupted
Family Processes, Readiness for
    Enhanced
Fatigue
Fear
Fluid Balance, Readiness for Enhanced
Fluid Volume, Deficient
Fluid Volume, Excess
Fluid Volume, Risk for Deficient
Fluid Volume, Risk for Imbalanced
Gas Exchange, Impaired
Grieving, Anticipatory
Grieving, Dysfunctional
Growth and Development, Delayed
Growth, Risk for Disproportionate
Health Maintenance, Ineffective
Health-Seeking Behaviors
Home Maintenance, Impaired
Hopelessness
Hyperthermia
Hypothermia
Identity, Disturbed Personal
Incontinence, Functional Urinary
Incontinence, Reflex Urinary
Incontinence, Stress Urinary
Incontinence, Total Urinary
Incontinence, Urge Urinary
Incontinence, Risk for Urinary Urge
Infant Behavior, Disorganized
Infant Behavior, Risk for Disorganized
Infant Behavior, Readiness for
    Enhanced Organized
Infant Feeding Pattern, Ineffective
Infection, Risk for
Injury, Risk for
Injury, Risk for Perioperative-Positioning

Intracranial Adaptive Capacity,
    Decreased
Knowledge, Deficient
Knowledge, Readiness for Enhanced
Loneliness, Risk for
Memory, Impaired
Mobility, Impaired Bed
Mobility, Impaired Physical
Mobility, Impaired Wheelchair
Nausea
Neglect, Unilateral
Noncompliance
Nutrition, Imbalanced: Less than Body
    Requirements
Nutrition, Imbalanced: More than Body
    Requirements
Nutrition, Readiness for Enhanced
Nutrition, Risk for Imbalanced: More
    than Body Requirements
Oral Mucous Membrane, Impaired
Pain, Acute
Pain, Chronic
Parenting, Impaired
Parenting, Readiness for Enhanced
Parenting, Risk for Impaired
Peripheral Neurovascular Dysfunction,
    Risk for
Poisoning, Risk for
Post-Trauma Syndrome
Post-Trauma Syndrome, Risk for
Powerlessness
Powerlessness, Risk for
Protection, Ineffective
Rape-Trauma Syndrome
Rape-Trauma Syndrome: Compound
    Reaction
Rape-Trauma Syndrome: Silent Reaction
Relocation Stress Syndrome
Relocation Stress Syndrome, Risk for
Role Performance, Ineffective
Self-Care Deficit, Bathing/Hygiene
Self-Care Deficit, Dressing/Grooming
Self-Care Deficit, Feeding
Self-Care Deficit, Toileting
Self-Concept, Readiness for Enhanced
Self-Esteem, Chronic Low
Self-Esteem, Situational Low
Self-Esteem, Risk for Situational Low
Self-Mutilation

Modified from NANDA International (2002).
*NANDA Nursing Diagnoses: Definitions and
Classification 2003-2004*. Philadelphia: NANDA;
and Gordon M: *Manual of nursing diagnosis,*
ed 10, St. Louis, 2002, Mosby.

Self-Mutilation, Risk for
Sensory Perception, Disturbed
Sexual Dysfunction
Sexuality Patterns, Ineffective
Skin Integrity, Impaired
Skin Integrity, Risk for Impaired
Sleep Deprivation
Sleep Pattern, Disturbed
Sleep, Readiness for Enhanced
Social Interaction, Impaired
Social Isolation
Sorrow, Chronic
Spiritual Distress
Spiritual Distress, Risk for
Spiritual Well-Being, Readiness for
    Enhanced
Sudden Infant Death Syndrome, Risk for
Suffocation, Risk for
Suicide, Risk for
Surgical Recovery, Delayed
Swallowing, Impaired
Therapeutic Regimen Management,
    Effective
Therapeutic Regimen Management,
    Ineffective
Therapeutic Regimen Management,
    Ineffective Community
Therapeutic Regimen Management,
    Ineffective Family
Therapeutic Regimen Management,
    Readiness for Enhanced
Thermoregulation, Ineffective
Thought Processes, Disturbed
Tissue Integrity, Impaired
Tissue Perfusion, Ineffective
Transfer Ability, Impaired
Trauma, Risk for
Urinary Elimination, Impaired
Urinary Elimination, Readiness for
    Enhanced
Urinary Retention
Ventilation, Impaired Spontaneous
Ventilatory Weaning Response,
    Dysfunctional
Violence, Risk for Other-Directed
Violence, Risk for Self-Directed
Walking, Impaired
Wandering

GROUPED BY FUNCTIONAL HEALTH PATTERNS

Health Perception–Health Management Pattern

Energy Field, Disturbed
Falls, Risk for
Health Maintenance, Ineffective
Health-Seeking Behaviors
Infection, Risk for

Injury, Risk for
Injury, Risk for Perioperative-
    Positioning
Noncompliance
Poisoning, Risk for
Protection, Ineffective
Suffocation, Risk for
Therapeutic Regimen Management,
    Effective
Therapeutic Regimen Management,
    Ineffective
Therapeutic Regimen Management,
    Ineffective Family
Therapeutic Regimen Management,
    Ineffective Community
Therapeutic Regimen Management,
    Readiness for Enhanced
Trauma, Risk for

Nutritional-Metabolic Pattern

Allergy Response, Latex
Allergy Response, Risk for Latex
Aspiration, Risk for
Body Temperature, Risk for Imbalanced
Breastfeeding, Effective
Breastfeeding, Ineffective
Breastfeeding, Interrupted
Dentition, Impaired
Failure to Thrive, Adult
Fluid Volume, Deficient
Fluid Volume, Risk for Deficient
Fluid Volume, Excess
Fluid Volume, Risk for Imbalanced
Fluid Volume, Readiness for Enhanced
Hyperthermia
Hypothermia
Infant Feeding Pattern, Ineffective
Nausea
Nutrition, Imbalanced: Less than Body
    Requirements
Nutrition, Imbalanced: More than Body
    Requirements
Nutrition, Risk for Imbalanced: More
    than Body Requirements
Nutrition, Readiness for Enhanced
Oral Mucous Membrane, Impaired
Skin Integrity, Impaired
Skin Integrity, Risk for Impaired
Swallowing, Impaired
Thermoregulation, Ineffective
Tissue Integrity, Impaired

Elimination Pattern

Constipation
Constipation, Perceived
Constipation, Risk for
Diarrhea
Incontinence, Bowel
Incontinence, Functional Urinary
Incontinence, Reflex Urinary

Incontinence, Risk for Urinary Urge
Incontinence, Stress
Incontinence, Total
Incontinence, Urge
Urinary Elimination, Impaired
Urinary Elimination, Readiness for
    Enhanced
Urinary Retention

Activity-Exercise Pattern

Activity Intolerance
Activity Intolerance, Risk for
Airway Clearance, Ineffective
Autonomic Dysreflexia
Autonomic Dysreflexia, Risk for
Breathing Pattern, Ineffective
Cardiac Output, Decreased
Development, Risk for Delayed
Disuse Syndrome, Risk for
Diversional Activity, Deficient
Fatigue
Gas Exchange, Impaired
Growth and Development, Delayed
Growth, Risk for Disproportionate
Home Maintenance, Impaired
Infant Behavior, Disorganized
Infant Behavior, Readiness for
    Enhanced Organized
Infant Behavior, Risk for Disorganized
Intracranial Adaptive Capacity,
    Decreased
Mobility, Impaired Bed
Mobility, Impaired Physical
Mobility, Impaired Wheelchair
Peripheral Neurovascular Dysfunction,
    Risk for
Self Care Deficit, Bathing/Hygiene
Self Care Deficit, Dressing/Grooming
Self Care Deficit, Feeding
Self Care Deficit, Toileting
Surgical Recovery, Delayed
Tissue Perfusion, Ineffective
Transfer Ability, Impaired
Ventilation, Impaired Spontaneous
Ventilatory Weaning Response,
    Dysfunctional
Walking, Impaired
Wandering

Sleep-Rest Pattern

Sleep Deprivation
Sleep Pattern, Disturbed
Sleep, Readiness for Enhanced

Cognitive-Perceptual Pattern

Confusion, Acute
Confusion, Chronic
Conflict, Decisional
Environmental Interpretation Syndrome,
    Impaired

Knowledge, Deficient
Knowledge, Readiness for Enhanced
Memory, Impaired
Neglect, Unilateral
Pain, Acute
Pain, Chronic
Thought Processes, Disturbed

Self-Perception–
Self-Concept Pattern

Anxiety
Anxiety, Death
Body Image, Disturbed
Fear
Hopelessness
Identity, Disturbed Personal
Loneliness, Risk for
Powerlessness
Powerlessness, Risk for
Self-Concept, Readiness for
    Enhanced
Self-Esteem, Chronic Low
Self-Esteem, Risk for Situational Low
Self-Esteem, Situational Low
Violence, Risk for Self-Directed

Role-Relationship Pattern

Attachment, Risk for Impaired Parent/
    Infant/Child

Caregiver Role Strain
Caregiver Role Strain, Risk for
Communication, Impaired Verbal
Communication, Readiness for
    Enhanced
Conflict, Parental Role
Family Processes, Dysfunctional:
    Alcoholism
Family Processes, Interrupted
Family Processes, Readiness for
    Enhanced
Grieving, Anticipatory
Grieving, Dysfunctional
Parenting, Impaired
Parenting, Risk for Impaired
Parenting, Readiness for Enhanced
Relocation Stress Syndrome
Relocation Stress Syndrome, Risk for
Role Performance, Ineffective
Social Interaction, Impaired
Social Isolation
Sorrow, Chronic
Violence, Risk for Other-Directed

Sexuality–Reproductive
Pattern

Rape-Trauma Syndrome
Rape-Trauma Syndrome: Compound
    Reaction

Rape-Trauma Syndrome: Silent
    Reaction
Sexual Dysfunction
Sexuality Patterns, Ineffective

Coping–Stress Tolerance
Pattern

Adjustment, Impaired
Coping, Ineffective
Coping, Ineffective Community
Coping, Readiness for Enhanced
Coping, Readiness for Enhanced
    Community
Coping, Defensive
Coping, Compromised Family
Coping, Disabled Family
Coping, Readiness for Enhanced Family
Denial, Ineffective
Post-Trauma Syndrome
Post-Trauma Syndrome, Risk for
Self-Mutilation
Self-Mutilation, Risk for
Suicide, Risk for

Value–Belief Pattern

Spiritual Distress
Spiritual Distress, Risk for
Spiritual Well-Being, Readiness for
    Enhanced

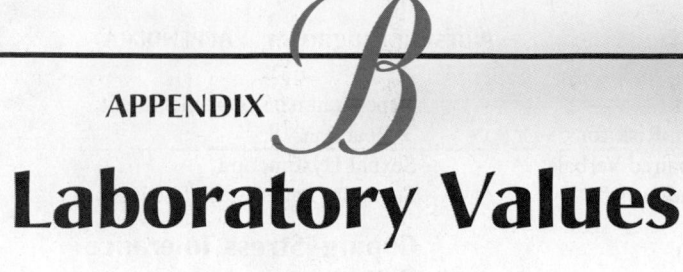

APPENDIX

Laboratory Values

The tables in this appendix list some of the most common tests, their normal values, and possible etiologies of abnormal values. Laboratory values may vary with different techniques or different laboratories. Possible etiologies are presented in alphabetic order. Abbreviations appearing in the tables are defined as follows:

<	=	less than
>	=	greater than
L	=	liter
mEq	=	milliequivalent
ml	=	milliliter
dl	=	deciliter
mm Hg	=	millimeter of mercury
fl	=	femtoliter
mm	=	millimeter

g	=	gram
mg	=	milligram (10^{-3})
μg	=	microgram (one millionth of a gram) (10^{-6})
ng	=	nanogram (one billionth of a gram) (10^{-9})
pg	=	picogram (one trillionth of a gram) (10^{-12})
μU	=	microunit
μl	=	microliter
IU	=	international unit
mOsm	=	milliosmole
U	=	unit
mmol	=	millimole
μmol	=	micromole
nmol	=	nanomole
pmol	=	picomole
kPa	=	kilopascal
μkat	=	microkatal

TABLE B-1 Serum, Plasma, and Whole Blood Chemistries

| | NORMAL VALUES | | POSSIBLE ETIOLOGY | |
TEST	CONVENTIONAL UNITS	SI UNITS	HIGHER	LOWER
Acetone			Diabetic ketoacidosis, high-fat diet, low-carbohydrate diet, starvation	
Quantitative	0.3-2.0 mg/dl	52-344 μmol/L		
Qualitative	Negative	Negative		
Albumin	3.5-5.0 g/dl	35-50 g/L	Dehydration	Chronic liver disease, malabsorption, malnutrition, nephrotic syndrome, pregnancy
Aldolase	1.0-7.5 U/L	0.02-0.13 μkat/L	Skeletal muscle disease	Renal disease
α_1-Antitrypsin	78-200 mg/dl	0.78-2.0 g/L	Acute and chronic inflammation, arthritis, stress syndrome	Chronic lung disease (early onset), malnutrition, nephrotic syndrome
α_1-Fetoprotein	<15 ng/ml	<15 μg/L	Cancer of testes and ovaries, carcinoma of liver	
Ammonia	30-70 μg/dl	17.6-41.1 μmol/L	Severe liver disease	
Amylase	0-130 U/L (method dependent)	0-2.17 μkat/L	Acute and chronic pancreatitis, mumps (salivary gland disease), perforated ulcers	Acute alcoholism, cirrhosis of liver, extensive destruction of pancreas
Ascorbic acid	0.4-1.5 mg/dl	23-85 μmol/L	Excessive ingestion of vitamin C	Connective tissue disorders, hepatic disease, renal disease, rheumatic fever, vitamin C deficiency
Bicarbonate	20-30 mEq/L	20-30 mmol/L	Compensated respiratory acidosis, metabolic alkalosis	Compensated respiratory alkalosis, metabolic acidosis
Bilirubin			Biliary obstruction, impaired liver function, hemolytic anemia, pernicious anemia, prolonged fasting	
Total	0.2-1.3 mg/dl	3.4-22.0 μmol/L		
Indirect	0.1-1.0 mg/dl	1.7-17.0 μmol/L		
Direct	0.1-0.3 mg/dl	1.7-5.1 μmol/L		
Blood gases*				
Arterial pH	7.35-7.45	Same as conventional units	Alkalosis	Acidosis
Venous pH	7.35-7.45	Same as conventional units		
Arterial PCO_2	35-45 mm Hg	4.67-6.00 kPa	Compensated metabolic alkalosis	Compensated metabolic acidosis
Venous PCO_2	42-52 mm Hg	5.60-6.93 kPa	Respiratory acidosis	Respiratory alkalosis
Arterial PO_2	75-100 mm Hg	10.0-13.33 kPa	Administration of high concentration of oxygen	Chronic lung disease, decreased cardiac output
Venous PO_2	30-50 mm Hg	4.0-6.67 kPa		
Calcium	9-11 mg/dl (4.5-5.5 mEq/L)	2.25-2.74 mmol/L	Acute osteoporosis, hyperparathyroidism, vitamin D intoxication, multiple myeloma	Acute pancreatitis, hypoparathyroidism, liver disease, malabsorption syndrome, renal failure, vitamin D deficiency
Calcium, ionized	4-4.6 mg/dl (2-2.3 mEq/L	1.0-1.15 mmol/L		
Carbon dioxide (CO_2 content)	20-30 mEq/L	20-30 mmol/L	Same as bicarbonate	
Carotene	10-85 μg/dl	0.19-1.58 μmol/L	Cystic fibrosis, hypothyroidism, pancreatic insufficiency	Dietary deficiency, malabsorption disorders
Chloride	95-105 mEq/L	95-105 mmol/L	Metabolic acidosis, respiratory alkalosis, corticosteroid therapy, uremia	Addison's disease, diarrhea, metabolic alkalosis, respiratory acidosis, vomiting

*Because arterial blood gases are influenced by altitude, the value for PO_2 decreases as altitude increases. The lower value is normal for an altitude of 1 mile.

Continued

TABLE B-1	Serum, Plasma, and Whole Blood Chemistries—cont'd			
	NORMAL VALUES		POSSIBLE ETIOLOGY	
TEST	CONVENTIONAL UNITS	SI UNITS	HIGHER	LOWER
Cholesterol	140-200 mg/dl (age dependent)	3.6-5.2 mmol/L	Biliary obstruction, hypothyroidism, idiopathic hypercholesterolemia, renal disease, uncontrolled diabetes	Extensive liver disease, hyperthyroidism, malnutrition, corticosteroid therapy
HDL (high-density lipoproteins)				
Male	>45 mg/dl	>1.2 mmol/L		
Female	>55 mg/dl	>1.4 mmol/L		
LDL (low-density lipoproteins)	<130 mg/dl	<3.4 mmol/L		
Cholinesterase (RBC)	0.65-1.00 pH	Same as conventional units	Exercise	Acute infections, insecticide intoxication, liver disease, muscular dystrophy
Pseudocholinesterase (plasma)	5-12 U/ml	Same as conventional units		
Copper	80-150 µg/dl	12.6-23.6 µmol/L	Cirrhosis, female on contraceptives	Wilson's disease
Cortisol	8 AM: 5-25 µg/dl	0.14-0.69 µmol/L	Cushing syndrome, pancreatitis, stress	Adrenal insufficiency, panhypopituitary states
	8 PM: <10 µg/dl	<0.28 µmol/L		
Creatine	0.2-1.0 mg/dl	15.3-76.3 µmol/L	Active rheumatoid arthritis, biliary obstruction, hyperthyroidism, renal disorders, severe muscle disease	Diabetes mellitus
Creatine kinase (CK)			Musculoskeletal injury or disease, myocardial infarction, severe myocarditis, exercise, numerous intramuscular injections, brain damage	
Male	15-105 U/L	0.26-1.79 µkat/L		
Female	10-80 U/L	0.17-1.36 µkat/L		
CK-MB (CK-2)	0-9 U/L	<0.1 µkat/L	Acute myocardial infarction	
Creatinine	0.5-1.5 mg/dl	44-133 µmol/L	Severe renal disease	
Ferritin (serum)			Sideroblastic anemia, anemia of chronic disease (infection, inflammation, liver disease)	Iron-deficiency anemia
Male	20-300 ng/ml	20-300 µg/L		
Female	10-120 ng/ml	10-120 µg/L		
Folic acid (folate)	3-25 ng/ml	7-57 nmol/L	Hypothyroidism	Alcoholism, hemolytic anemia, inadequate diet, malabsorption syndrome, megaloblastic anemia
Gamma-glutamyl transpeptidase (GGT)	0-30 U/L	0-0.5 µkat/L		Liver disease, infectious mononucleosis
Glucose, fasting	70-120 mg/dl	3.89-6.66 mmol/L	Acute stress, cerebral lesions, Cushing's disease, diabetes mellitus, hyperthyroidism, pancreatic insufficiency	Addison's disease, hepatic disease, hypothyroidism, insulin overdosage, pancreatic tumor, pituitary hypofunction, postgastrectomy dumping syndrome
Glucose tolerance (GTT)			Diabetes mellitus	Hyperinsulinism
Fasting	70-120 mg/dl	3.89-6.66 mmol/L		
30 min	30-60 mg/dl above fasting	1.67-3.33 mmol/L		
60 min	20-50 mg/dl above fasting	1.11-2.78 mmol/L		
120 min	5-15 mg/dl above fasting	0.28-0.83 mmol/L		
180 min	Fasting level or lower	Fasting level or lower		

RBC, Red blood cell.

TABLE B-1 **Serum, Plasma, and Whole Blood Chemistries—cont'd**

TEST	NORMAL VALUES CONVENTIONAL UNITS	SI UNITS	POSSIBLE ETIOLOGY HIGHER	LOWER
Haptoglobin	26-185 mg/dl	260-1850 mg/L	Infectious and inflammatory processes, malignant neoplasms	Hemolytic anemia, mononucleosis, toxoplasmosis, chronic liver disease
Insulin	4-24 μU/ml	29-172 pmol/L	Acromegaly, adenoma of islet cells, untreated mild case of type 2 diabetes	Diabetes mellitus, obesity
Iron, total	50-150 μg/dl	9.0-26.9 μmol/L	Excessive RBC destruction	Iron-deficiency anemia, anemia of chronic disease
Iron-binding capacity	250-410 μg/dl	45-73 μmol/L	Iron-deficient state, oral contraceptive use, polycythemia	Cancer, chronic infections, pernicious anemia, uremia
Lactic acid	5-20 μg/dl	0.56-2.2 mmol/L	Acidosis, congestive heart failure, shock	
Lactic dehydrogenase (LDH)	50-150 U/L	0.83-2.5 μkat/L	Congestive heart failure, hemolytic disorders, hepatitis, metastatic cancer of liver, myocardial infarction, pernicious anemia, pulmonary embolus, skeletal muscle damage	
Lactic dehydrogenase isoenzymes				
LDH_1	20%-35%	0.20-0.35	Myocardial infarction, pernicious anemia	
LDH_2	30%-40%	0.30-0.40	Pulmonary embolus, sickle cell crisis	
LDH_3	15%-25%	0.15-0.25	Malignant lymphoma, pulmonary embolus	
LDH_4	0%-10%	0-0.10	Lupus erythematosus, pulmonary infarction	
LDH_5	4%-12%	0.04-0.12	Congestive heart failure, hepatitis, pulmonary embolus and infarction, skeletal muscle damage	
Lipase	0-160 U/L	0-2.66 μkat/L	Acute pancreatitis, hepatic disorders, perforated peptic ulcer	
Magnesium	1.5-2.5 mEq/L	0.62-1.03 mmol/L	Addison's disease, hypothyroidism, renal failure	Chronic alcoholism, hyperparathyroidism, hyperthyroidism, hypoparathyroidism, severe malabsorption
Osmolality	285-295 mOsm/kg	285-295 mmol/kg	Chronic renal disease, diabetes mellitus	Addison's disease, diuretic therapy
Oxygen saturation (arterial)	95%-98%	0.95-0.98 saturated	Polycythemia	Anemia, cardiac decompensation, respiratory disorders
pH	See blood gases			
Phenylalanine	0-2 mg/dl	0-121 μmol/L	Phenylketonuria	
Phosphatase, acid	0-0.6 U/L	0-90 μkat/L	Advanced Paget's disease, cancer of prostate, hyperparathyroidism	
Phosphatase, alkaline	30-120 U/L	0.5-2.0 μkat/L	Bone diseases, marked hyperparathyroidism, obstruction of biliary system, rickets	Excessive vitamin D ingestion, hypothyroidism, milk–alkali syndrome
Phosphorus, inorganic	2.8-4.5 mg/dl	0.90-1.45 mmol/L	Healing fractures, hypoparathyroidism, renal disease, vitamin D intoxication	Diabetes mellitus, hyperparathyroidism, vitamin D deficiency

Continued

TABLE B-1	Serum, Plasma, and Whole Blood Chemistries—cont'd			
	NORMAL VALUES		**POSSIBLE ETIOLOGY**	
TEST	**CONVENTIONAL UNITS**	**SI UNITS**	**HIGHER**	**LOWER**
Potassium	3.5-5.5 mEq/L	3.5-5.5 mmol/L	Addison's disease, diabetic ketosis, massive tissue destruction, renal failure	Cushing syndrome, diarrhea (severe), diuretic therapy, gastrointestinal fistula, pyloric obstruction, starvation, vomiting
Prostate-specific antigen (PSA)	<4 ng/mL	<4 μg/L	Prostate cancer	
Proteins			Burns, cirrhosis (globulin fraction), dehydration	Congenital agammaglobulinemia, liver disease, malabsorption
Total	6.0-8.0 g/dl	60-80 g/L		
Albumin	3.5-5.0 g/dl	35-50 g/L		
Globulin	2.0-3.5 g/dl	20-35 g/L		
Albumin/globulin ratio	1.5:1-2.5:1	Same as conventional units	Multiple myeloma (globulin fraction), shock, vomiting	Malnutrition, nephrotic syndrome, proteinuria, renal disease, severe burns
Renin			Renal hypertension, volume decrease (e.g., hemorrhage)	Increased salt intake, primary aldosteronism
Supine position	1.4-2.9 ng/ml/hr	0.39-0.81 ng/L·sec		
Upright position	0.4-4.5 ng/ml/hr	0.11-1.25 ng/L·sec		
Sodium	135-145 mEq/L	135-145 mmol/L	Dehydration, impaired renal function, primary aldosteronism, corticosteroid therapy	Addison's disease, diabetic ketoacidosis, diuretic therapy, excessive loss from gastrointestinal tract, excessive perspiration, water intoxication
Testosterone				Hypofunction of testes
Male	300-1200 ng/dl	10.4-41.6 nmol/L		
Female	25-90 ng/dl	0.87-3.1 nmol/L	Polycystic ovary, virilizing tumors	
T_4 (thyroxine), total	5-12 μg/dl	64-154 nmol/L	Hyperthyroidism, thyroiditis	Cretinism, hypothyroidism, myxedema
T_4 (thyroxine), free	0.8-2.3 ng/dl	10-30 pmol/L		
T_3 uptake	25%-35%	0.25-0.35	Hyperthyroidism, metastatic neoplasms	Hypothyroidism, pregnancy
T_3 (triiodothyronine)	110-230 ng/dl	1.7-3.5 nmol/L	Hyperthyroidism	Hypothyroidism
Thyroid-stimulating hormone (TSH)	0.3-5.4 μU/ml	0.3-5.4 mU/L	Myxedema, primary hypothyroidism, Graves' disease	Secondary hypothyroidism
Transaminases				
Serum glutamic oxaloacetic (SGOT) or aspartate aminotransferase (AST)	7-40 U/L	0.12-0.67 μkat/L	Liver disease, myocardial infarction, pulmonary infarction, acute hepatitis	
Serum glutamate pyruvate (SGPT) or alanine aminotransferase (ALT)	5-36 U/L	0.08-0.6 μkat/L	Liver disease, shock	
Triglycerides	40-150 mg/dl	0.45-1.69 mmol/L	Diabetes mellitus, hyperlipidemia, hypothyroidism, liver disease	Malnutrition
Urea nitrogen (BUN)	10-30 mg/dl	1.8-7.1 mmol/L	Increase in protein catabolism (fever, stress), renal disease, urinary tract infection	Malnutrition, severe liver damage

TABLE B-1	Serum, Plasma, and Whole Blood Chemistries—cont'd			
	NORMAL VALUES		**POSSIBLE ETIOLOGY**	
TEST	**CONVENTIONAL UNITS**	**SI UNITS**	**HIGHER**	**LOWER**
Uric acid			Gout, gross tissue destruction, high-protein weight reduction diet, leukemia, renal failure, eclampsia	Administration of uricosuric drugs
Male	4.5-6.5 mg/dl	149-327 μmol/L		
Female	2.5-5.5 mg/dl	268-387 μmol/L		
Vitamin A	15-60 μg/dl	0.52-2.09 μmol/L	Excess ingestion of vitamin A	Vitamin A deficiency
Vitamin B$_{12}$	200-1000 pg/ml	148-738 pmol/L	Chronic myeloid leukemia	Strict vegetarianism, malabsorption syndrome, pernicious anemia, total or partial gastrectomy
Zinc	50-150 μg/dl	7.6-22.9 μmol/L		Alcoholic cirrhosis

TABLE B-2	Hematology			
	NORMAL VALUES		**POSSIBLE ETIOLOGY**	
TEST	**CONVENTIONAL UNITS**	**SI UNITS**	**HIGHER**	**LOWER**
Bleeding time (Simplate)	3.0-9.5 min	180-570 sec	Defective platelet function, thrombocytopenia, von Willebrand's disease, aspirin ingestion, vascular disease	
Activated partial thromboplastin time (APTT)	24-36 sec*	Same as conventional units	Deficiency of factors I, II, V, VIII, IX and X, XI, XII; hemophilia; liver disease; heparin therapy	
Prothrombin time (Protime, PT)	10-14 sec*	Same as conventional units	Warfarin therapy; deficiency of factors I, II, V, VII, and X; vitamin K deficiency; liver disease	
Fibrinogen	200-400 mg/dl	2.0-4.0 g/L	Burns (after first 36 hr), inflammatory disease	Burns (during first 36 hr), DIC, severe liver disease
Fibrin split (degradation) products	<10 μg/ml	Same as conventional units	Acute DIC, massive hemorrhage, primary fibrinolysis	
D-Dimer	Negative	Negative	DIC, myocardial infarction, deep vein thrombosis, unstable angina	
Erythrocyte count† (altitude dependent)			Dehydration, high altitudes, polycythemia vera, severe diarrhea	Anemia, leukemia, posthemorrhage
Male	4.5-6.0 × 10^6/μL	4.5-6.0 × 10^{12}/L		
Female	4.0-5.0 × 10^6/μL	4.0-5.0 × 10^{12}/L		
Mean corpuscular volume (MCV)	82-98 fl	Same as conventional units	Macrocytic anemia	Microcytic anemia
Mean corpuscular hemoglobin (MCH)	27-33 pg	Same as conventional units	Macrocytic anemia	Microcytic anemia
Mean corpuscular hemoglobin concentration (MCHC)	32%-36%	0.32-0.36	Spherocytosis	Hypochromic anemia

*Values depend on reagent and instrumentation used.
†Components of complete blood count (CBC).
COPD, Chronic obstructive pulmonary disease; DIC, disseminated intravascular coagulation; WBC, white blood cell.

Continued

| TABLE B-2 | Hematology—cont'd |

| | NORMAL VALUES | | POSSIBLE ETIOLOGY | |
TEST	CONVENTIONAL UNITS	SI UNITS	HIGHER	LOWER
Erythrocyte sedimentation rate (ESR), Westergren			*Moderate increase:* acute hepatitis, myocardial infarction; rheumatoid arthritis	Malaria, severe liver disease, sickle cell anemia
Male <50 yr	<15 mm/hr	Same as conventional units	*Marked increase:* acute and severe bacterial infections, malignancies, pelvic inflammatory disease	
>50 yr	<20 mm/hr			
Female <50 yr	<20 mm/hr	Same as conventional units		
>50 yr	<30 mm/hr			
Hematocrit (altitude dependent)[†]			Dehydration, high altitudes, polycythemia	Anemia, hemorrhage, overhydration
Male	40%–54%	0.40–0.54		
Female	38%–47%	0.38–0.47		
Hemoglobin (altitude dependent)[†]			COPD, high altitudes, polycythemia	Anemia, hemorrhage
Male	13.5–18.0 g/dl	135–180 g/L		
Female	12.0–16.0 g/dl	120–160 g/L		
Hemoglobin, glycosylated	4.0%–6.0%	Same as conventional units	Poorly controlled diabetes mellitus	Sickle cell anemia, chronic renal failure, pregnancy
Red cell distribution width (RDW)	10.2%–14.5%	Same as conventional therapy		Anisocytosis, macrocytic anemia, microcytic anemia
Platelet count (thrombocytes)	150–400 × 10³/μl	150–400 × 10⁹/L	Acute infections, chronic granulocytic leukemia, chronic pancreatitis, cirrhosis, collagen disorders, polycythemia, postsplenectomy	Acute leukemia, DIC, thrombocytopenic purpura
Reticulocyte count (manual)	0.5%–1.5% of RBC	Same	Hemolytic anemia, polycythemia vera	Hypoproliferative anemia, macrocytic anemia, microcytic anemia
White blood cell count[†]	4.0–11.0 × 10³/μl	4.0–11.0 × 10⁹/L	Inflammatory and infectious processes, leukemia	Aplastic anemia, side effects of chemotherapy and irradiation
WBC differential				
Segmented neutrophils	50%–70%	0.50–0.70	Bacterial infections, collagen diseases, Hodgkin's disease	Aplastic anemia, viral infections
Band neutrophils	0%–8%	0–0.08	Acute infections	
Lymphocytes	20%–40%	0.20–0.40	Chronic infections, lymphocytic leukemia, mononucleosis, viral infections	Corticosteroid therapy, whole body irradiation
Monocytes	4%–8%	0.04–0.08	Chronic inflammatory disorders, malaria, monocytic leukemia, acute infections, Hodgkin's disease	
Eosinophils	0%–4%	0–0.04	Allergic reactions, eosinophilic and chronic granulocytic leukemia, parasitic disorders, Hodgkin's disease	Corticosteroid therapy
Basophils	0%–2%	0–0.02	Hypothyroidism, ulcerative colitis, myeloproliferative diseases	Hyperthyroidism, stress
Sickle cell solubility test	Negative	Negative	Sickle cell anemia	

TABLE B-3   Serology-Immunology

TEST	NORMAL VALUES		POSSIBLE ETIOLOGY	
	CONVENTIONAL UNITS	SI UNITS	HIGHER	LOWER
Antinuclear antibody (ANA)	Negative or titer <1:10	Same as conventional units	Chronic hepatitis, rheumatoid arthritis, scleroderma, systemic lupus erythematosus	
Anti-DNA antibody	Negative or titer <1:10 or <20% binding	Same as conventional units	Systemic lupus erythematosus	
Anti-RNP	Negative	Negative	Mixed connective-tissue disease, rheumatoid arthritis, systemic lupus erythematosus, Sjögren syndrome, scleroderma	
Anti-Sm (Smith)	Negative	Negative	Systemic lupus erythematosus	
Antistreptolysin-O (ASO)	≤166 Todd units or ≤1:85	Same as conventional units	Acute glomerulonephritis, rheumatic fever, streptococcal infection	
C-reactive protein (CRP)	Negative or ≤1.2 mg/dl	Same as conventional units	Acute infections, any inflammatory condition, widespread malignancy	
Carcinoembryonic antigen (CEA)	≤2.5 ng/ml	≤2.5 µg/L	Carcinoma of colon, liver, pancreas; chronic cigarette smoking; inflammatory bowel disease; other cancers	
Complement components				Acute glomerulonephritis, systemic lupus erythematosus, rheumatoid arthritis, subacute bacterial endocarditis, serum sickness
C1q	11-21 mg/dl	0.11-0.21 g/L		
C3	80-180 mg/dl	0.8-1.8 g/L		
C4	15-50 mg/dl	0.15-0.5 g/L		
Direct antihuman globulin test (DAT) or direct Coombs	Negative	Negative	Acquired hemolytic anemia, hemolytic disease of the newborn, drug reactions, transfusion reactions	
Fluorescent treponemal antibody absorption (FTAAbs)	Nonreactive	Negative	Syphilis	
Hepatitis A antibody	Negative	Negative	Hepatitis A	
Hepatitis B surface antigen (HBₛAg)	Negative	Negative	Hepatitis B	
Hepatitis C antibody	Negative	Negative	Hepatitis C	
Immunoglobulins				
IgA	90-400 mg/dl	0.9-4.0 g/L	IgA myeloma, chronic liver disease, chronic infection, rheumatoid arthritis, autoimmune disorders	Burns, hereditary telangiectasia, malabsorption syndromes
IgD	0.5-12.0 mg/dl	5-120 mg/L	Chronic infection, connective tissue disease	
IgE	<1.0 mg/dl	<10 mg/L	Anaphylactic shock, atopic disease (allergies), parasite infections	
IgG	650-1800 mg/dl	6.5-18.0 g/L	Infections—acute and chronic, hepatitis, IgG monoclonal gammopathy, systemic lupus erythematosus	Congenital deficiencies, acquired deficiencies, nephrotic syndromes, burns, immunosuppression
IgM	55-300 mg/dl	0.5-3.0 g/L	Acute infections, rheumatoid arthritis, liver disease	Congenital and acquired antibody deficiencies, lymphocytic leukemia, protein-losing enteropathies

Continued

TABLE B-3   Serology-Immunology—cont'd

| | NORMAL VALUES | | POSSIBLE ETIOLOGY | |
| | CONVENTIONAL | | | |
TEST	UNITS	SI UNITS	HIGHER	LOWER
Monospot or monotest	Negative	Negative	Infectious mononucleosis	
Rheumatoid factor (RA factor)	Negative or titer <1:20	Same as conventional units	Rheumatoid arthritis, Sjögren syndrome, systemic lupus erythematosus	
RPR	Nonreactive	Same as conventional units	Syphilis, systemic lupus erythematosus, rheumatoid arthritis, leprosy, malaria, febrile diseases, IV drug abuse	
VDRL	Nonreactive	Same as conventional units	Syphilis	
Thyroid antibodies	≤1:10 titer	Same as conventional units	Hashimoto's thyroiditis, thyroid carcinoma, early hypothyroidism, pernicious anemia, systemic lupus erythematosus, Graves' disease	

CSF, Colony-stimulating factor; *RNP*, ribonuclear protein; *RPR*, rapid plasma reagin test; *VDRL*, Venereal Disease Research Laboratory test.

TABLE B-4   Urine Chemistry

| | | NORMAL VALUES | | POSSIBLE ETIOLOGY | |
| | | CONVENTIONAL | | | |
TEST	SPECIMEN	UNITS	SI UNITS	HIGHER	LOWER
Acetone	Random	Negative	Negative	Diabetes mellitus, high-fat and low-carbohydrate diets, starvation states	
Aldosterone	24 hr	1-80 µg/day (depends on urinary sodium)	2.7-222 nmol/day	*Primary aldosteronism:* adrenocortical tumors *Secondary aldosteronism:* cardiac failure, cirrhosis, large dose of ACTH, salt depletion	ACTH deficiency, Addison's disease, corticosteroid therapy
Amylase	24 hr	1-17 U/hr	Same as conventional units	Acute pancreatitis	
Bence Jones protein	Random	Negative	Negative	Multiple myeloma, biliary duct obstruction	
Bilirubin	Random	Negative	Negative	Hepatitis	
Calcium	24 hr	100-250 mg/day	2.5-6.3 mmol/day	Bone tumor, hyperparathyroidism, milk-alkali syndrome	Hypoparathyroidism, malabsorption of calcium and vitamin D
Catecholamines	24 hr			Pheochromocytoma, progressive muscular dystrophy, heart failure	
Epinephrine		<20 µg/day	<118 nmol/day		
Norepinephrine		<100 µg/day	<591 nmol/day		
Chloride	24 hr	110-250 mEq/day	110-250 mmol/day	Addison's disease	Burns, excess perspiration, vomiting, diarrhea, menstruation
Copper	24 hr	<30 µg/day	<0.5 µmol/day	Cirrhosis, Wilson's disease	

| TABLE B-4 | Urine Chemistry—cont'd |

TEST	SPECIMEN	NORMAL VALUES CONVENTIONAL UNITS	SI UNITS	POSSIBLE ETIOLOGY HIGHER	LOWER
Coproporphyrin	24 hr	50-200 µg/day	76-305 nmol/day	Lead poisoning, oral contraceptive use, poliomyelitis	
Creatine	24 hr	<100 mg/day	<763 µmol/day	Carcinoma of liver, hyperthyroidism, diabetes, Addison's disease, infections, burns, muscular dystrophy, skeletal muscle atrophy	Hypothyroidism
Creatinine	24 hr	0.8-2.0 g/day	7.1-17.7 mmol/day	Anemia, leukemia, muscular atrophy, salmonellae	Renal disease
Creatinine clearance	24 hr	85-135 ml/min	1.42-2.25 ml/sec		Renal disease
Estrogens	24 hr				
Female				Gonadal or adrenal tumor	Agenesis of ovaries, endocrine disturbance, ovarian dysfunction, menopause
Ovulation peak		28-100 µg/day	104-370 nmol/day		
Luteal peak		22-80 µg/day	81-296 nmol/day		
Pregnancy		Up to 45,000 µg/day	Up to 166,455 nmol/day		
Menopause		1.4-19.6 µg/day	5.2-72.5 nmol/day		
Male		5-18 µg/day	18-67 nmol/day		
Glucose	Random	Negative	Negative	Diabetes mellitus, low renal threshold for glucose resorption, physiologic stress, pituitary disorders	
Hemoglobin	Random	Negative	Negative	Extensive burns, glomerulonephritis, hemolytic anemias, hemolytic transfusion reaction	
5-Hydroxyindole-acetic acid (5-HIAA)	24 hr	2-9 mg/day	10.5-47.1 µmol/day	Malignant carcinoid syndrome	
Ketone bodies	24 hr	20-50 mg/day	0.34-0.86 mmol/day	Marked ketonuria	
Lead	24 hr	<100 µg/day	<0.48 µmol/day	Lead poisoning	
Metanephrine	24 hr	<1.3 mg/day	<7.1 µmol/day	Pheochromocytoma	
Myoglobin	Random	Negative	Negative	Crushing injuries, electric injuries, extreme physical exertion	
pH	Random	4.0-8.0	Same as conventional units	Chronic renal failure, compensatory phase of alkalosis, salicylate intoxication, vegetarian diet	Compensatory phase of acidosis, dehydration, emphysema
Phenylpyruvic acid	Random	Negative	Negative	Phenylketonuria	
Phosphorus, inorganic	24 hr	0.9-1.3 g/day	29-42 mmol/day	Fever, hypoparathyroidism, nervous exhaustion, rickets, tuberculosis	Acute infections, nephritis

Continued

TABLE B-4   Urine Chemistry—cont'd

| | | NORMAL VALUES | | POSSIBLE ETIOLOGY | |
| | | CONVENTIONAL | | | |
TEST	SPECIMEN	UNITS	SI UNITS	HIGHER	LOWER
Porphobilinogen	Random 24 hr	Negative <2.0 mg/day	Negative <9 μmol/day	Acute intermittent por- phyria, liver disorders	
Protein (dipstick)	Random	Negative	Negative	Congestive heart failure, nephritis, nephrosis, physiologic stress	
Protein (quantitative)	24 hr	<150 mg/day	<0.15 g/day	Cardiac failure, inflam- matory processes of urinary tract, nephritis, nephrosis, toxemia of pregnancy	
Sodium	24 hr	40-250 mEq/day	40-250 mmol/day	Acute tubular necrosis	Hyponatremia
Specific gravity	Random	1.003-1.030	Same as conventional units	Albuminuria, dehydra- tion, glycosuria	Diabetes insipidus
Titratable acidity	24 hr	20-50 mEq/day	Same as conventional units	Metabolic acidosis	Metabolic alkalosis
Uric acid	24 hr	250-750 mg/day	1.5-4.5 mmol/day	Gout, leukemia	Nephritis
Urobilinogen	24 hr	0.5-4.0 EU/day	Same as conventional units	Hemolytic disease, he- patic parenchymal cell damage, liver disease	Complete obstruction of bile duct
	Random	<1.0 Erhlich unit	Same as conventional units		
Uroporphyrins	Random	Random	Same as conventional units	Porphyria	
Vanillylmandelic acid	24 hr	1-8 mg/day 1.5-7.0 μg/mg creatine	5-40 μmol/day	Pheochromocytoma	

ACTH, Adrenocorticotropic hormone; EU, Ehrlich unit.

TABLE B-5   Gastric Analysis

| | NORMAL VALUES | | POSSIBLE ETIOLOGY | |
| | CONVENTIONAL | | | |
TEST	UNITS	SI UNITS	HIGHER	LOWER
Basal				
Free hydrochloric acid	0.30 mEq/L	Same as conventional units	Hypermotility of stomach	Pernicious anemia
Total acidity	15-45 mEq/L	Same as conventional units	Gastric and duodenal ulcers, Zollinger-Ellison syndrome	Gastric carcinoma, severe gastritis
Poststimulation				
Free hydrochloric acid	10-130 mEq/L	Same as conventional units		
Total acidity	20-150 mEq/L	Same as conventional units		

TABLE B-6	Fecal Analysis			
	NORMAL VALUES		**POSSIBLE ETIOLOGY**	
TEST	**CONVENTIONAL UNITS**	**SI UNITS**	**HIGHER**	**LOWER**
Fecal fat	<6 g/24 hr	Same as conventional units	Chronic pancreatic disease, obstruction of common bile duct, malabsorption syndrome	
Urobilinogen	30-220 mg/100 g of stool	51-372 μmol/100 g of stool	Hemolytic anemias	Complete biliary obstruction
Mucus	Negative	Negative	Mucous colitis, spastic constipation	
Pus	Negative	Negative	Chronic bacillary dysentery, chronic ulcerative colitis, localized abscesses	
Blood*	Negative	Negative	Anal fissures, hemorrhoids, malignant tumor, peptic ulcer, inflammatory bowel disease	
Color				
Brown			Various color depending on diet	
Clay			Biliary obstruction or presence of barium sulfate	
Tarry			More than 100 ml of blood in gastrointestinal tract	
Red			Blood in large intestine	
Black			Blood in upper gastrointestinal tract or iron medication	

*Ingestion of meat may produce false-positive results. Patient may be placed on a meat-free diet for 3 days before the test.

TABLE B-7	Cerebrospinal Fluid Analysis			
	NORMAL VALUES		**POSSIBLE ETIOLOGY**	
TEST	**CONVENTIONAL UNITS**	**SI UNITS**	**HIGHER**	**LOWER**
Pressure	60-150 mm H_2O	Same as conventional units	Hemorrhage, intracranial tumor, meningitis	Head injury, spinal tumor, subdural hematoma
Blood	Negative	Negative	Intracranial hemorrhage	
Cell count (age dependent)				
WBC	0-5 cells/μl	0.5×10^6/L	Inflammation or infections of CNS	
RBC	0	0×10^6/L		
Chloride	100-130 mEq/L	100-130 mmol/L	Uremia	Bacterial infections of CNS (meningitis, encephalitis)
Glucose	40-75 mg/dl	2.5-4.2 mmol/L	Diabetes mellitus, viral infections of CNS	Bacterial infections and tuberculosis of CNS
Protein				
Lumbar	15-45 mg/dl	0.15-0.45 g/L	Guillain-Barré syndrome, poliomyelitis, traumatic tap	
Cisternal	15-25 mg/dl	0.15-0.25 g/L	Syphilis of CNS	
Ventricular	5-15 mg/dl	0.05-0.15 g/L	Acute meningitis, brain tumor, chronic CNS infections, multiple sclerosis	

CNS, Central nervous system.

TABLE B-8	Toxicology of Common Drugs			
	THERAPEUTIC LEVEL		TOXIC LEVEL	
DRUG	CONVENTIONAL UNITS	SI UNITS	CONVENTIONAL UNITS	SI UNITS
acetaminophen (Tylenol)	0.2-0.6 mg/dl	13-40 μmol/L	>5 mg/dl	>330 μmol/L
Barbiturates				
Short acting	1-2 mg/dl	Dependent on composition of mixture	>5 mg/dl	
Intermediate acting	1-5 mg/dl		>10 mg/dl	
Long acting	15-35 mg/dl		>40 mg/dl	
Carbon monoxide (carboxyhemoglobin)				
Normal values	<5% saturation of hemoglobin	<0.05	Symptoms with >20% saturation	>0.20
Urban nonsmokers	<5% saturation of hemoglobin	<0.05		
Rural nonsmokers	0.5%-2.0% saturation of hemoglobin	0.005-0.02		
Smokers	5%-9% saturation of hemoglobin	0.05-0.09		
Heavy smokers	>9% saturation of hemoglobin	>0.09		
chlordiazepoxide (Librium)	0.05-5.0 mg/L	2-17 μmol/L	>10 mg/L	>33 μmol/L
chlorpromazine (Thorazine)	0.5 μg/ml	1.6 μmol/L	>2.0 μg/ml	>6.3 μmol/L
diazepam (Valium)	0.10-0.25 mg/L	0.35-0.88 μmol/L	>1.0 mg/L $\geq$2.0 mg/L (lethal)	>3.5 μmol/L
Digitalis preparations				
digoxin	0.8-2.4 ng/ml	1.0-3.1 nmol/L	>2.5 ng/ml	>2.6 nmol/L
digitoxin	14-30 ng/ml	18-39 nmol/L	>30 ng/ml	>39 nmol/L
Dilantin	10-20 mg/L	40-80 μmol/L	>30 mg/L	>120 μmol/L
gentamicin (Garamycin)				
Peak	4-10 mg/L	9-22 μmol/L	>10 mg/L	>22 μmol/L
Trough	<2 mg/L	<4 mmol/L	>2 mg/L	>4 μmol/L
propranolol (Inderal)	50-100 ng/ml	192-386 nmol/L	>200 ng/ml	>771 nmol/L
Salicylates	10-20 mg/dl	0.724-1.45 mmol/L	>20 mg/dl	>1.45 mmol/L
Alcohol (ethanol)*			>60 mg/dl (lethal)	>4.34 mmol/L

*See Table 10-10.

APPENDIX 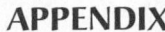 C

Answer Key to Review Questions

Chapter 1
1. d
2. c
3. a
4. c
5. c
6. d
7. c
8. c
9. b
10. d
11. c

Chapter 2
1. d
2. d
3. a
4. b
5. b
6. c
7. a

Chapter 3
1. d
2. a
3. a
4. a
5. c
6. b

Chapter 4
1. d
2. c
3. a
4. a
5. b
6. a
7. b
8. d
9. b
10. a

Chapter 5
1. a
2. c
3. c
4. c
5. d
6. d
7. c
8. c
9. a
10. b
11. a
12. c

Chapter 6
1. d
2. c

3. d
4. d

Chapter 7
1. a
2. b
3. d
4. d
5. b
6. d
7. c
8. b
9. c

Chapter 8
1. b
2. b
3. a
4. c
5. d
6. b
7. a
8. a
9. d

Chapter 9
1. b
2. d
3. d
4. c
5. c
6. b
7. b
8. c
9. d
10. d

Chapter 10
1. b
2. a
3. d
4. c
5. c
6. d
7. d
8. a
9. c

Chapter 11
1. d
2. c
3. a
4. b
5. d
6. b
7. b
8. b
9. b
10. b

Chapter 12
1. b
2. a
3. b
4. d
5. b
6. b
7. d
8. d
9. a
10. b
11. a
12. b
13. c

Chapter 13
1. d
2. c
3. d
4. c
5. a
6. d
7. a
8. d
9. c
10. d
11. a
12. c
13. a

Chapter 14
1. a
2. b
3. d
4. a
5. c
6. c
7. c
8. a
9. a
10. c

Chapter 15
1. d
2. d
3. d
4. d
5. d
6. b
7. c
8. b
9. d
10. c
11. a
12. c
13. a
14. d
15. a

Chapter 16
1. c
2. a
3a. d
3b. a
3c. c
3d. c
3e. a
3f. b
4. a
5. d
6. b

Chapter 17
1. d
2. c
3. c
4. a
5. b
6. c
7. a
8. d

Chapter 18
1. b
2. c
3. c
4. c
5. a
6. d
7. d
8. c
9. c
10. b

Chapter 19
1. d
2. b
3. d
4. a
5. c
6. a

Chapter 20
1. c
2. d
3. c
4. a
5. b
6. d
7. d

Chapter 21
1. b
2. d
3. c
4. b
5. d
6. b

7. a
8. a
9. b
10. a
11. d

Chapter 22
1. b
2. b
3. d
4. c
5. d
6. c
7. d
8. a
9. b

Chapter 23
1. b
2. b
3. d
4. a
5. b
6. a
7. c
8. b
9. a
10. a

Chapter 24
1. c
2. a
3. c
4. d
5. c
6. c
7. b
8. b
9. a
10. b
11. b

Chapter 25
1. c
2. d
3. a
4. a
5. c
6. b
7. d
8. a
9. a
10. a
11. a

Chapter 26
1. d
2. d
3. a
4. c
5. b
6. d
7. a
8. c

Chapter 27
1. a
2. d
3. d
4. a
5. c
6. d

7. c
8. c
9. a
10. c
11. d
12. c
13. b

Chapter 28
1. a
2. a
3. b
4. d
5. d
6. c
7. d

Chapter 29
1. b
2. c
3. b
4. a
5. a
6. c
7. a
8. b

Chapter 30
1. a
2. b
3. d
4. c
5. a
6. a
7. d
8. c
9. d
10. d
11. c
12. c
13. b
14. c
15. d
16. d

Chapter 31
1. c
2. c
3. c
4. d
5. c
6. d
7. b
8. a
9. c
10. a
11. b

Chapter 32
1. d
2. b
3. d
4. b
5. d
6. d
7. a
8. b

Chapter 33
1. c
2. a
3. a

4. d
5. c
6. c
7. c
8. b
9. c

Chapter 34
1. b
2. c
3. a
4. a
5. c
6. c

Chapter 35
1. d
2. b
3. d
4. a
5. b
6. c
7. d
8. d

Chapter 36
1. a
2. b
3. a
4. a
5. c
6. c
7. b
8. c
9. c
10. c

Chapter 37
1. c
2. c
3. b
4. d
5. c
6. b
7. a
8. d
9. b
10. c
11. b
12. d
13. c
14. d

Chapter 38
1. d
2. b
3. b
4. a
5. b
6. c
7. b
8. a
9. b

Chapter 39
1. c
2. d
3. a
4. c
5. b
6. a
7. d

8. d
9. c

Chapter 40
1. b
2. d
3. c
4. d
5. c
6. c
7. a
8. d
9. d
10. b

Chapter 41
1. a
2. d
3. b
4. c
5. a
6. c
7. a
8. b
9. d
10. a
11. d

Chapter 42
1. a
2. b
3. b
4. b
5. d
6. a
7. d
8. d
9. c
10. a

Chapter 43
1. d
2. b
3. d
4. b
5. a
6. a
7. b
8. d

Chapter 44
1. d
2. a
3. b
4. a
5. d
6. a
7. d
8. d
9. b
10. a
11. b
12. d

Chapter 45
1. a
2. b
3. b
4. c
5. d
6. c
7. d

8. c
9. a
10. d
11. b

Chapter 46
1. b
2. c
3. a
4. d
5. a
6. c
7. a
8. c
9. a

Chapter 47
1. b
2. d
3. d
4. d
5. d
6. c
7. c
8. a

Chapter 48
1. b
2. b
3. c
4. a
5. d
6. d
7. a
8. c

Chapter 49
1. c
2. c
3. d
4. c
5. c
6. a
7. a
8. d

Chapter 50
1. d
2. d
3. d
4. a
5. c
6. c
7. d
8. a

Chapter 51
1. b
2. a
3. c
4. d
5. c
6. c
7. a

Chapter 52
1. b
2. d
3. d
4. d
5. c
6. a
7. b
8. c
9. d
10. b
11. b
12. c
13. a

Chapter 53
1. b
2. d
3. c
4. a
5. c
6. c
7. c

Chapter 54
1. c
2. d
3. d
4. c
5. b
6. b
7. d
8. a
9. c
10. a

Chapter 55
1. b
2. d
3. b
4. c
5. a
6. a
7. c
8. d
9. b

Chapter 56
1. d
2. c
3. d
4. c
5. d
6. c
7. b
8. c
9. b

Chapter 57
1. a
2. b
3. c
4. c
5. d

Chapter 58
1. d
2. d
3. c
4. c
5. b
6. a
7. b

Chapter 59
1. d
2. d
3. d
4. c
5. b
6. c
7. a
8. b

Chapter 60
1. c
2. b
3. d
4. d
5. c
6. d
7. c
8. d
9. a

Chapter 61
1. d
2. a
3. c
4. c
5. d
6. b

7. b
8. d
9. b

Chapter 62
1. b
2. d
3. a
4. d
5. c
6. a
7. b

Chapter 63
1. c
2. c
3. a
4. b
5. a
6. c
7. c

Chapter 64
1. d
2. b
3. c
4. d
5. a
6. b
7. a
8. c

Chapter 65
1. c
2. d
3. a
4. b
5. a
6. d

Chapter 66
1. b
2. c
3. d
4. a
5. c
6. c

Chapter 67
1. a
2. b
3. d
4. c
5. a
6. d

Illustration Credits

Chapter 1
1-1, From Potter PA, Perry AG: *Fundamentals of nursing: concepts, process, and practice,* ed 4, St Louis, 1997, Mosby; **1-4, 1-5,** from Rick Brady, Riva, MD.

Chapter 2
2-1, 2-2, 2-3, 2-4, From Rick Brady, Riva, MD.

Chapter 3
3-1, From Wilson SF, Giddens JF: *Health assessment for nursing practice,* ed 2, St Louis, 2001, Mosby.

Chapter 4
4-2, Reprinted from *Patient Educ Couns,* vol. 27, Boise L et al: Facing chronic illness: the family support model and its benefits, p. 76, 1996, with permission from Elsevier Science; **4-3, 4-5,** From Rick Brady, Riva, MD; **4-6,** from Wilson SF, Giddens JF: *Health assessment for nursing practice,* ed 2, St Louis, 2001, Mosby.

Chapter 5
5-1, From US Bureau of Census; **5-2, 5-3, 5-4, 5-6, 5-7, 5-8,** from Rick Brady, Riva, MD; **5-5,** redrawn from Benzon J: Approaching drug regimens with a therapeutic dose of suspicion, *Geriatr Nurs* 12(4):1813, 1991.

Chapter 6
6-1, From Potter PA, Perry AG: *Basic nursing: a critical thinking approach,* ed 4, St Louis, 1999, Mosby; **6-2, 6-3,** from Potter PA, Perry AG: *Fundamentals of nursing: concepts, process, and practice,* ed 4, St Louis, 1997, Mosby; **6-4,** from Rick Brady, Riva, MD.

Chapter 7
7-1, 7-2, 7-3, 7-5, 7-8, From Rick Brady, Riva, MD; **7-7,** from Blake S: *Alternative remedies CD-ROM,* St Louis, 1999, Mosby.

Chapter 8
8-7, From Rick Brady, Riva, MD.

Chapter 9
9-2, Developed by McCaffery M, Pasero C, Paice JA. From McCaffery M, Pasero C: *Pain: clinical manual,* ed 2, St Louis, 1999, Mosby; **9-6,** from McCaffery M, Pasero C: *Pain: clinical manual,* ed 2, St Louis, 1999, Mosby; **9-7,** from Acute Pain Management Guideline Panel, 1992; **9-12,** from Salerno E, Willens J: *Pain management handbook,* St Louis, 1996, Mosby; **9-14,** from Rick Brady, Riva, MD.

Chapter 10
10-1, 10-5, 10-6, Courtesy Kathleen A. Pollard, RN, MSN, CHPN, Phoenix, Ariz; **10-2, 10-4, 10-7,** from Rick Brady, Riva, MD; **10-3,** from Potter PA, Perry AG: *Fundamentals of nursing: concepts, process, and practice,* ed 4, St Louis, 1997, Mosby.

Chapter 11
11-1, 11-2, From Rick Brady, Riva, MD.

Chapter 12
12-2, Courtesy Cameron Bangs, MD. From Auerbach PS, Donner HJ, Weiss EA: *Field guide to wilderness medicine,* St Louis, 1999, Mosby;
12-10, courtesy Molnlyche Health Care, Eddystone, Pa. In Potter PA, Perry AG: *Fundamentals of nursing,* ed 5, St Louis, 2001, Mosby; **12-11A,** from Habif TP: *Clinical dermatology: a color guide to diagnosis and therapy,* ed 2, St Louis, 1992, Mosby; **12-11B,** from Lemmi FO, Lemmi CAE: *Physical assessment findings CD-ROM,* Philadelphia, 2000, Saunders; **12-12,** from Potter PA, Perry AG: *Fundamentals of nursing,* ed 5, St Louis, 2001, Mosby.

Chapter 13
13-1, From Thibodeau GA, Patton KT: *The human body in health and disease,* ed 3, St Louis, 2002, Mosby; **13-12,** from Cerio R, Jackson WF: *A colour atlas of allergic skin disorders,* London, 1992, Wolfe Publishing.

Chapter 14
14-6, 14-7, From Grimes DE, Grimes RM: *AIDS and HIV infection,* St Louis, 1994, Mosby; **14-8,** from the Centers for Disease Control and Prevention. Courtesy Jonathan WM Gold, MD, New York, NY; **14-9,** from Seidel HM et al: *Mosby's guide to physical examination,* ed 5, St Louis, 2003, Mosby. Courtesy Douglas A. Jabs, MD, the Wilmer Ophthalmological Institute, The Johns Hopkins University and Hospital, Baltimore.

Chapter 15
15-4, From Stevens A, Lowe J: *Pathology: illustrated review in color,* ed 2, London, 2000, Mosby; **15-5,** adapted from DeVita VT, Helman S, Rosenberg SA, editors: *Cancer: principles and practice of oncology,* Philadelphia, 1997, Lippincott-Raven; **15-9,** modified from Krakoff IH: Systemic treatment of cancer, *CA Cancer J Clin* 46:134, 1996; **15-18A,** courtesy Pharmacia Deltec, Inc, St Paul, Minn; **15-19,** courtesy Strato/Infusaid, Inc, Norwood, Mass; **15-20,** data from The World Health Organization, 1990.

Chapter 16
16-14, From McCance KL, Huether SE: *Pathophysiology: the biologic basis for disease in adults and children,* ed 4, St Louis, 2002, Mosby.

Chapter 17
17-1, Courtesy St Joseph Hospital, Albuquerque.

Chapter 18
18-1, Courtesy Greg McVicar; **18-2,** courtesy Joseph T. Rothrock, III. From Meeker MH, Rothrock JC: *Alexander's care of the patient in surgery,* ed 11, St Louis, 1999, Mosby; **18-4,** courtesy of The Methodist Hospital, Houston, Tex. Photograph by Donna Dahms, RN, CNOR; **18-5,** from Meeker MH, Rothrock JC: *Alexander's care of the patient in surgery,* ed 11, St Louis, 1999, Mosby.

Chapter 20
20-1, 20-8, From Thibodeau GA, Patton KT: *The human body in health and disease,* ed 3, St Louis, 2002, Mosby; **20-3,** from Thibodeau GA, Patton KT: *Anatomy and physiology,* ed 5, St Louis, 2003, Mosby; **20-7,** courtesy Eye Institute, Department of Ophthalmology and Visual Sciences, University of Iowa Health Care, Iowa City, Iowa; **20-9,** from Seidel HM et al: *Mosby's guide to physical examination,* ed 5, St Louis, 2003, Mosby.

Chapter 21
21-9, From Lemmi FO, Lemmi CAE: *Physical assessment findings CD-ROM,* Philadelphia, 2000, Saunders; **21-10,** courtesy Siemens Hearing Solutions, Piscataway, NJ; **21-11,** courtesy Advanced Bionics Corp., Valencia, Calif.

Chapter 22
Photos in **Table 22-4** (macule, papule, vesicle, plaque, wheal, pustule, fissure, ulcer, atrophy, excoriation), from Thibodeau GA, Patton KT: *The human body in health and disease,* ed 3, St Louis, 2002, Mosby; photos in **Table 22-4** (scale, scar, and atrophy), from Thompson JM, Wilson SF: *Health assessment for nursing practice,* St Louis, 1996, Mosby; **22-1,** from Jarvis C: *Physical examination and health assessment,* ed 4, Philadelphia, 2003, Saunders; **22-3, 22-4,** from Habif TP: *Clinical dermatology: a color guide to diagnosis and therapy,* ed 3, St Louis, 1996, Mosby.

Chapter 23
23-1, From Hooper BJ, Goldman NP: *Primary dermatologic care,* St Louis, 1999, Mosby; **23-2,** from Goldstein BG, Goldstein AO: *Practical dermatology,* ed 2, St Louis, 1997, Mosby. Courtesy Department of Dermatology, Medical College of Georgia, Augusta, Ga; **23-3, 23-4, 23-6, 23-7, 23-10, 23-11,** from Habif TP: *Clinical dermatology: a color guide to diagnosis and therapy,* ed 3, St Louis, 1996, Mosby; **23-5, 23-12,** from Lemmi FO, Lemmi CAE: *Physical assessment findings CD-ROM,* Philadelphia, 2000, Saunders; **23-8,** from Cox N, Lawrence C: *Diagnostic problems in dermatology,* St Louis, 1998, Mosby; **23-13, 23-14,** from Fortunato N, McCullough SM: *Plastic and reconstructive surgery,* St Louis, 1998, Mosby.

Chapter 25
21-1, Redrawn from Price SA, Wilson LM: *Pathophysiology: clinical concepts of disease processes,* ed 6, St Louis, 2003, Mosby; **25-2, 25-3,** from Thompson JM et al: *Mosby's clinical nursing,* ed 5, St Louis, 2002, Mosby; **25-4A,** from Bone RC et al, editors: *Pulmonary and critical care medicine,* vol 1, St Louis, 1993, Mosby; **25-4B,** from Staub NC, Albertine KH: *Anatomy of the lungs.* In Murray JF, Nadel JA, editors: *Textbook of respiratory medicine,* ed 2, Philadelphia, 1994, Saunders; **25-8A,** redrawn from *Principles of pulse oximetry,* Nellcor, Inc, Haywood, Calif; **25-8B,** from Potter PA, Perry AG: *Fundamentals of nursing: concepts, process, and practice,* ed 4, St Louis, 1997, Mosby; **25-10,** redrawn from Wilkins RL et al: *Clinical assessment in respiratory care,* ed 3, St Louis, 1995, Mosby; **25-12, 25-13,** modified from Thompson JM et al: *Mosby's clinical nursing,* ed 5, St Louis, 2002, Mosby; **25-14,** from Beare PG, Myers JL: *Adult health nursing,* ed 3, St Louis, 1998, Mosby; **25-15A,** courtesy Olympus America, Melville, NY; **25-15B,** from Meduri GU et al: Protected bronchoalveolar lavage, *Am Respir Dis* 143:855, 1991; **25-16,** redrawn from Du Bois RM, Clarke SW: *Fiberoptic bronchoscopy in diagnosis and management,* Orlando, Fla, 1987, Grune & Stratton.

Chapter 26
26-4, Courtesy Robert Margulies, Miami. From Smolley LA: How to help patients with obstructive sleep apnea, *J Respir Dis* 11:723, 1990; **26-5,** courtesy Respironics, Inc, Murrysville, Pa; **26-11,** courtesy Passy-Muir, Inc, Irvine, Calif; **26-13,** from the American Cancer Society; **26-16,** courtesy CLG Photographics, Inc, St Louis.

Chapter 27
27-4, From Damjanov I, Linder J: *Anderson's pathology,* ed 10, St Louis, 1996, Mosby; **27-10,** courtesy of Deknatel, Inc, Fall River, Mass.

Chapter 28
28-3, Redrawn from Price SA, Wilson LM: *Pathophysiology: clinical concepts of disease processes,* ed 6, St Louis, 2003, Mosby; **28-5,** from Togger DA, Breener PS: Metered dose inhalers, *Am J Nurs* 101(10):26-32, 2001; **28-11,** from Potter PA, Perry AG: *Fundamentals of nursing,* ed 5, St Louis, 2001, Mosby; **28-14,** courtesy Nellcor Puritan Bennett, Inc; **28-17,** courtesy Axcan Scandipharm, Inc., Birmingham, Ala.

Chapter 29
29-2, From Thibodeau GA, Patton KT: *The human body in health and disease,* ed 3, St Louis, 2002, Mosby; **29-3,** copyright Dennis Kunkel Microscopy, Inc., Kailua, Hawaii; **29-6,** from Seidel HM et al: *Mosby's guide to physical examination,* ed 5, St Louis, 2003, Mosby; **29-8,** from Herlihy B, Maebius N: *The human body in health and illness,* ed 2, Philadelphia, 2003, Saunders.

Chapter 30
30-2, Redrawn from Raven PH, Johnson GB: *Biology,* ed 2, St Louis, 1991, Mosby; **30-3,** redrawn from McCance KL, Huether SE: *Pathophysiology: the biologic basis for disease in adults and children,* ed 4, St Louis, 2002, Mosby; **30-6,** from Bingham BJG, Hawke M, Kwok P: *Atlas of clinical otolaryngology,* St Louis, 1992, Mosby; **30-10, 30-11, 30-14,** from Skarin AT: *Atlas of diagnostic oncology,* ed 2, London, 1996, Mosby-Wolfe; **30-13,** from Cotran RS, Kumar V, Collins T: *Robbins pathologic basis of disease,* ed 6, Philadelphia, 1999, Saunders.

Chapter 31
31-1, 31-3, Modified from Price SA, Wilson LM: *Pathophysiology: clinical concepts of disease processes,* ed 6, St Louis, 2003, Mosby; **31-5, 31-9, 31-12,** modified from Kinney M et al: *Comprehensive cardiac care,* ed 8, St Louis, 1996, Mosby; **31-14,** modified from Kinney M et al: *Comprehensive cardiac care,* ed 7, St Louis, 1991, Mosby.

Chapter 32
32-1, Redrawn from West JB: *Physiological basis of medical practice,* ed 12, Baltimore, 1991, Williams & Wilkins; **32-3,** from Kissane JM: *Anderson's pathology,* ed 9, St Louis, 1990, Mosby; **32-4, 32-5,** from US Department of Health and Human Services: *The sixth report of the Joint National Committee on Detection, Evaluation, and Treatment of High Blood Pressure (JNC-VI),* Washington, DC, 1997, National Institutes of Health.

Chapter 33
33-1, 33-2, From *2002 Heart and stroke statistical update,* American Heart Association; **33-9,** modified and reprinted with permission from Matrisciano L, Alspach JG: Unstable angina: an overview, *Critical Care Nurses* 12:31, 1992; **33-10, 33-11,** courtesy of Mayo Clinic, Rochester, Minn; **33-17,** from *Heart Disease and Stroke* 2:201, 1993, copyright American Heart Association.

Chapter 34
34-1, Redrawn from McCance KL, Huether SE: *Pathophysiology: the biologic basis for disease in adults and children,* ed 4, St Louis, 2002, Mosby; **34-2, 34-4,** redrawn from Urden LD, Stacy KM, Lough ME: *Thelan's critical care nursing: diagnosis and management,* ed 4, St Louis, 2002, Mosby; **34-3, 34-5,** from Cotran RS, Kumar V, Collins T: *Robbins pathologic basis of disease,* ed 6, Philadelphia, 1999, Saunders.

Chapter 35
35-1, 35-5, 35-6, 35-7, 35-8, 35-9, 35-11, 35-12, 35-13, 35-14, 35-15, 35-16, 35-17, 35-18, 35-19, From Huszar RJ: *Basic dysrhythmias: interpretation and management,* ed 3, St Louis, 2002, Mosby; **35-2,** from Goldberger AL, Goldberger E: *Clinical electrocardiography: a simplified approach,* ed 6, St Louis, 1999, Mosby; **35-4, 35-10,** from Urden LD, Stacy KM, Lough ME: *Thelan's critical care nursing: diagnosis and management,* ed 4, St Louis, 2002, Mosby; **35-20, 35-26,** courtesy Medtronic Physio-Control, Redmond, Wash; **35-22A, 35-23A, 35-24,** courtesy Medtronic, Inc., Minneapolis.

Chapter 36
36-2, From Kissane JM: *Anderson's pathology,* ed 9, St Louis, 1990, Mosby; **36-4,** from Cotran RS, Kumar V, Collins T: *Robbins pathologic basis of disease,* ed 6, Philadelphia, 1999, Saunders; **36-5,** from Guzetta CE, Dossey BM: *Cardiovascular nursing: holistic practice,* St Louis, 1992, Mosby; **36-6,** redrawn from Lorell BH, Braunwald E: *Pericardial disease in heart disease: a textbook of cardiovascular medicine,* ed 3, Philadelphia, 1998, Saunders; **36-7, 36-10, 36-11B,** from Stevens A, Lowe J: *Pathology: illustrated review in color,* ed 2, St Louis, 2000, Mosby; **36-9, 36-11A,** from McCance KL, Huether SE: *Pathophysiology: the biologic basis for disease in adults and children,* ed 4, St Louis, 2002, Mosby; **36-12,** redrawn from Block PC: Balloon valvuloplasty, *Cardiol Consult* 9:4, 1988; **36-13A,** courtesy St Jude Medical, Inc, St Paul. All rights reserved; **36-13B,** courtesy Medtronic, Inc, Minneapolis; **35-13C,** courtesy American Red Cross Tissue Services and Baxter Healthcare Corporation, CardioVascular Group, Santa Ana, Calif.

Chapter 37
37-2, Courtesy Jo Menzoian, Boston, Mass; **37-5,** from Damjanov I, Linder J: *Anderson's pathology,* ed 10, St Louis, 1996, Mosby; **37-6,** courtesy FW LoGerfo, Boston; **37-7, 37-8, 37-12,** from Kamal A, Brockelhurst JC: *Color atlas of geriatric medicine,* ed 2, 1991, Mosby–Year Book–Europe; **37-10,** from Lofgren KA: Varicose veins. In Haimovici H, editor: *Vascular surgery: principles and techniques,* New York, 1976, McGraw-Hill.

Chapter 38
38-1, 38-3, From Thibodeau GA, Patton KT: *Anatomy and physiology,* ed 4, St Louis, 1999, Mosby; **38-9,** from Doughty DB, Jackson DB: *Gastrointestinal disorders,* St Louis, 1993, Mosby.

Chapter 39

39-1A, From *Human nutrition information service: making health food choices,* Washington, DC, 1993, US Department of Agriculture; **39-1B,** courtesy The Health Connection, Hagerstown, Md; **39-2,** from Morgan SL, Weiniser RL: *Fundamentals of clinical nutrition,* ed 2, St Louis, 1998, Mosby; **39-3,** redrawn from Mahan LK, Arlin M: *Krause's food, nutrition, and diet therapy,* ed 4, 1992, Saunders; **39-7,** copyright 1978, George A. Bray, MD.

Chapter 40

40-1, From McKenry LM, Salerno E: *Mosby's pharmacology in nursing,* ed 21, St Louis, 2001, Mosby; **40-2,** courtesy University of Washington, Division of Gastroenterology; **40-3,** from Doughty DB, Jackson DB: *Gastrointestinal disorders,* St Louis, 1993, Mosby; **40-5,** from Curon Medical, Inc., Sunnyvale, Calif; **40-6, 40-8, 40-11, 40-15,** redrawn from Price SA, Wilson LM: *Pathophysiology: clinical concepts of disease processes,* ed 6, St Louis, 2003, Mosby; **40-10,** from Stevens A, Lowe J: *Pathology: illustrated review in color,* ed 2, London, 2000, Mosby; **40-12,** from Damjanov I, Linder J: *Anderson's pathology,* ed 10, St Louis, 1996, Mosby.

Chapter 41

41-2, From Damjanov I, Linder J: *Anderson's pathology,* ed 10, St Louis, 1996, Mosby; **41-5, 41-15,** from Stevens A, Lowe J: *Pathology: illustrated review in color,* ed 2, London, 2000, Mosby; **41-8,** from McCance KL, Huether SE: *Pathophysiology: the biologic basis for disease in adults and children,* ed 4, St Louis, 2002, Mosby. Courtesy David Bjorkman, MD, University of Utah School of Medicine, Department of Gastroenterology; **41-10,** from McCance KL, Huether SE: *Pathophysiology: the biologic basis for disease in adults and children,* ed 4, St Louis, 2002, Mosby; **41-12,** redrawn from Meeker MH, Rothrock JC: *Alexander's care of the patient in surgery,* ed 9, St Louis, 1991, Mosby; **41-13,** redrawn from Hampton BG, Bryant RA: *Ostomies and continent diversions,* St Louis, 1992, Mosby; **41-17B,** from Swartz MH: *Textbook of physical diagnosis: history and examination,* ed 4, Philadelphia, 2002, Saunders.

Chapter 42

42-1, From Kamal A, Brockelhurst JC: *Color atlas of geriatric medicine,* ed 2, St Louis, 1991, Mosby–Year Book–Europe; **42-4,** from Damjanov I, Linder J: *Anderson's pathology,* ed 10, St Louis, 1996, Mosby; **42-6,** adapted from Doughty DB, Jackson DB: *Gastrointestinal disorders,* St Louis, 1993, Mosby; **42-10,** from LaBerge JM et al: Transjugular intrahepatic portosystemic shunts: preliminary results in 25 patients, *J Vasc Surg* 16:258, 1992; **42-12, 42-14, 42-16,** from Stevens A, Lowe J: *Pathology: illustrated review in color,* ed 2, London, 2000, Mosby.

Chapter 43

43-1A, 43-2, 43-3, 43-5, From Thibodeau GA, Patton KT: *Anatomy and physiology,* ed 4, St Louis, 1999, Mosby; **43-4,** adapted from Herlihy B, Maebius N: *The human body in health and illness,* ed 2, Philadelphia, 2003, Saunders; **43-6,** from Brundage DJ: *Renal disorders,* St Louis, 1992, Mosby; **43-7,** from Price S, Wilson L: *Pathophysiology: clinical concepts of disease processes,* ed 6, St Louis, 2003, Mosby; **43-9,** courtesy Circon Corp, Santa Barbara, Calif.

Chapter 44

44-4A, From Stevens A, Lowe J: *Pathology: illustrated review in color,* ed 2, London, 2000, Mosby; **44-6,** from Brundage DJ: *Renal disorders,* St Louis, 1992, Mosby; **44-7,** from Lemmi FO, Lemmi CAE: *Physical assessment findings CD-ROM,* Philadelphia, 2000, Saunders; **44-10, 44-12, 44-13,** courtesy Lynda Brubacher, Virginia Mason Hospital, Seattle.

Chapter 45

45-2, From United States Renal Data System, Minneapolis; **45-7, 45-10,** copyright 1994 Baxter Healthcare Corp; **45-12A,** courtesy Quinton Instrument Co, Seattle.

Chapter 46

46-2, Modified from Thibodeau GA, Patton KT: *Anatomy and physiology,* ed 5, St Louis, 2003, Mosby; **46-3, 46-4,** from Herlihy B, Maebius N: *The human body in health and illness,* ed 2, Philadelphia, 2003, Saunders; **46-6,** from McCance KL, Huether SE: *Pathophysiology: the biologic basis for disease in adults and children,* ed 4, St Louis, 2002, Mosby; **46-8, 46-9, 46-10,** from Thibodeau GA, Patton KT: *The human body in health and disease,* ed 3, St Louis, 2002, Mosby; **46-11,** from Thompson JM, Wilson SF: *Health assessment for nursing practice,* St Louis, 1996, Mosby.

Chapter 47

47-6, Courtesy Novo Nordisk Pharmaceuticals, Inc., Princeton, NJ; **47-7,** courtesy Medtronic MiniMed, Northridge, Calif; **47-8, 47-11,** redrawn from McCance KL, Huether SE: *Pathophysiology: the biologic basis for disease in adults and children,* ed 4, St Louis, 2002, Mosby; **47-12,** from Urden LD, Stacy KM, Lough ME: *Thelan's critical care nursing: diagnosis and management,* ed 4, St Louis, 2002, Mosby.

Chapter 48

48-1, Courtesy Linda Haas, Seattle; **48-3, 48-4,** redrawn from Urden LD, Stacy KM, Lough ME: *Thelan's critical care nursing: diagnosis and management,* ed 4, St Louis, 2002, Mosby; **48-5,** from Lemmi FO, Lemmi CAE: *Physical assessment findings CD-ROM,* Philadelphia, 2000, Saunders; **48-6,** courtesy Paul W. Ladenson, MD, The Johns Hopkins University and Hospital, Baltimore. From Seidel HM et al: *Mosby's guide to physical examination,* ed 5, St Louis, 2003, Mosby; **48-7,** from Seidel HM et al: *Mosby's guide to physical examination,* ed 5, St Louis, 2003, Mosby.

Chapter 49

49-1, 49-2, 49-9, From Thibodeau GA, Patton KT: *The human body in health and disease,* ed 3, St Louis, 2002, Mosby; **49-3, 49-4,** from Seidel HM et al: *Mosby's guide to physical examination,* ed 5, St Louis, 2003, Mosby; **49-5,** from Thibodeau GA, Patton KT: *Anatomy and physiology,* ed 4, St Louis, 1999, Mosby; **49-6,** modified from Thibodeau GA, Patton KT: *Anatomy and physiology,* ed 5, St Louis, 2003, Mosby.

Chapter 50

50-2, From Powell DE, Stelling CB: *The diagnosis and detection of breast diseases,* St Louis, 1993, Mosby; **50-3,** from Evans A et al: *Atlas of breast disease management,* Philadelphia, 1998, Saunders; **50-5,** courtesy Proxima Therapeutics, Inc., Alpharetta, Ga; **50-7, 50-8B,** from Fortunato N, McCullough SM: *Plastic and reconstructive surgery,* St Louis, 1998, Mosby. Courtesy Brian W. Davies, MD; **50-8A,** from Cameron J: *Current surgical therapy,* ed 5, St Louis, 1995, Mosby; **50-9,** modified from Beare PG, Myers JL: *Adult health nursing,* ed 3, St Louis, 1998, Mosby, and Fortunato N, McCullough SM: *Plastic and reconstructive surgery,* St Louis, 1998, Mosby.

Chapter 51

51-1, 51-2, 51-3, 51-6, 51-7, 51-9, From Morse S, Moreland A, Holmes K, editors: *Atlas of sexually transmitted diseases and AIDS,* London, 1996, Mosby-Wolfe; **51-4,** courtesy US Public Health Service, Washington, DC; **51-5,** from Habif T: *Clinical dermatology: a color guide to diagnosis and therapy,* ed 3, St Louis, 1996, Mosby; **51-8, 51-10,** reproduced with permission of GlaxoSmithKline, Research Triangle Park, NC.

Chapter 52

52-2, Courtesy Ethicon, Inc., Cornelia, Ga; **52-3,** from Seidel HM et al: *Mosby's guide to physical examination,* ed 5, St Louis, 2003, Mosby; **52-4,** from Lowdermilk DL, Perry SE, Bobak IM: *Maternity and women's health care,* ed 7, St Louis, 2000, Mosby; **52-6,** from Mishell DR et al: *Comprehensive gynecology,* ed 3, St Louis, 1997, Mosby; **52-7,** redrawn from Novak ER, Woodruff JD, editors: *Novak's gynecologic and obstetric pathology,* ed 6, Philadelphia, 1967, Saunders. In McCance KL, Huether SE: *Pathophysiology: the biologic basis for disease in adults and children,* ed 4, St Louis, 2002, Mosby; **52-8, 52-9,** from Symonds EM, MacPherson MBA: *Color atlas of obstetrics and gynecology,* London, 1994, Mosby-Wolfe; **52-10,** from Phipps WJ, Sands JK, Marek JF: *Medical-surgical nursing: concepts and clinical practice,* ed 6, St Louis, 1999, Mosby; **52-12,** redrawn from Seidel HM et al: *Mosby's guide to physical examination,* ed 5, St Louis, 2003, Mosby; **52-13,** from Seidel HM et al: *Mosby's guide to physical examination,* ed 4, St Louis, 1999, Mosby.

Chapter 53

53-5, From Iwamoto RR, Maher KE: Radiation therapy for prostate cancer, *Semin Oncol Nurs* 17(2):90-100, 2001; **53-7, 53-8,** from Swartz MH: *Textbook of physical diagnosis: history and examination,* ed 4, Philadelphia, 2002, Saunders; **53-9,** from Seidel HM et al: *Mosby's guide to physical examination,* ed 5, St Louis, 2003, Mosby.

Chapter 54

54-1, 54-10, 54-11, 54-13, 54-14, 54-15, 54-20, From Thibodeau GA, Patton KT: *Anatomy and physiology,* ed 5, St Louis, 2003, Mosby; **54-4,** from Herlihy B, Maebius N: *The human body in health and illness,* ed 2, Philadelphia, 2003, Saunders; **54-5, 54-6,** adapted from Thibodeau GA, Patton KT:

Anatomy and physiology, ed 5, St Louis, 2003; **54-12,** from McCance KL, Huether SE: *Pathophysiology: the biologic basis for disease in adults and children,* ed 4, St Louis, 2002, Mosby; **54-19A,** courtesy Hitachi Medical Systems America, Inc., Twinsburg, Ohio; **54-19B,** from Chipps E, Clanin N, Campbell V: *Neurologic disorders,* St Louis, 1992, Mosby.

Chapter 55
55-4, Redrawn from McCance KL, Huether SE: *Pathophysiology: the biologic basis for disease in adults and children,* ed 4, St Louis, 2002, Mosby; **55-6,** redrawn from Urden LD, Stacy KM, Lough ME: *Thelan's critical care nursing: diagnosis and management,* ed 4, St Louis, 2002, Mosby; **55-7,** from Clochesy JM et al: *Critical care nursing,* ed 2, Philadelphia, 1996, Saunders; **55-9,** redrawn from Barker E: *Neuroscience nursing: a spectrum of care,* ed 2, St Louis, 2002, Mosby; **55-10,** from Wong J, Wong S, Dempster JK: Care of the unconscious patient: a problem-oriented approach, *Am Assoc Neurosci Nurses* 16:145, 1984; **55-13,** from Bingham BJG, Hawke M, Kwok P: *Clinical atlas of otolaryngology,* St Louis, 1992, Mosby; **55-14,** redrawn from Barker E: *Neuroscience nursing: a spectrum of care,* ed 2, St Louis, 2002, Mosby; **55-15,** from Price SA, Wilson LM: *Pathophysiology: clinical concepts of disease processes,* ed 6, St Louis, 2003, Mosby; **55-16,** from Stevens A, Lowe J: *Pathology: illustrated review in color,* ed 2, London, 2000, Mosby; **55-18,** courtesy Department of Neurological Surgery, Vanderbilt University Medical Center, Nashville, TN.

Chapter 56
56-5, Courtesy Joseph C. Maroon, MD; **56-8,** modified from Hoeman SP: *Rehabilitation nursing,* ed 2, St Louis, 1995, Mosby; **56-9,** courtesy Sammons Preston, Bolingbrook, Ill.

Chapter 57
57-2, From Stevens A, Lowe J: *Pathology: illustrated review in color,* ed 2, London, 2000, Mosby; **57-5,** from McCance KL, Huether SE: *Pathophysiology: the biologic basis for disease in adults and children,* ed 4, St Louis, 2002, Mosby; **57-6,** from Perkin DG: *Mosby's color atlas and text of neurology,* London, 1998, Mosby-Wolfe; **57-7,** redrawn from Rudy E: *Advanced neurological and neurosurgical nursing,* St Louis, 1984, Mosby; **56-8,** redrawn from Barker E: *Neuroscience nursing: a spectrum of care,* ed 2, St Louis, 2002, Mosby.

Chapter 58
58-1A, From Damjanov I, Linder J: *Anderson's pathology,* ed 10, St Louis, 1996, Mosby; **58-2,** from Stevens A, Lowe J: *Pathology: illustrated review in color,* ed 2, London, 2000, Mosby.

Chapter 59
59-1, From Thibodeau GA, Patton KT: *Anatomy and physiology,* ed 5, St Louis, 2003, Mosby; **59-2,** courtesy Joe Rothrock, Media, Pa; 59-3, redrawn from Chipps E, Clanin N, Campbell V: *Neurologic disorders,* St Louis, 1992, Mosby; **59-4,** redrawn from Marciano FF et al: *BNI Quarterly* 11(2):6, 1995. In McCance KL, Huether SE: *Pathophysiology: the biologic basis for disease in adults and children,* ed 4, St Louis, 2002, Mosby; **59-8, 59-9,** from American Spinal Injury Association/International Medical Society of Paraplegic (ASIA/IMOSP): *International standards for neurological functional classification of spinal cord injury patients* (revised), Chicago, 2002, American Spinal Cord Injury Assn; **59-10, 59-13,** courtesy Michael S Clement, MD, Mesa, Ariz; **59-12,** courtesy Acromed Corp, Cleveland; **59-14,** from Barker E: *Neuroscience nursing: a spectrum of care,* ed 2, St Louis, 2002, Mosby.

Chapter 60
60-1, From Herlihy B, Maebius N: *The human body in health and illness,* ed 2, Philadelphia, 2003, Saunders; **60-3, 60-5,** from Thibodeau GA, Patton KT: *Anatomy and physiology,* ed 5, St Louis, 2003, Mosby; **60-6, 60-8,** from Mourad LA: *Orthopedic disorders,* St Louis, 1991, Mosby; **60-7,** from Lemmi FO, Lemmi CAE: *Physical assessment findings CD-ROM,* Philadelphia, 2000, Saunders.

Chapter 61
61-1, Redrawn from Price SA, Wilson LM: *Pathophysiology: clinical concepts of disease processes,* ed 6, St Louis, 2003, Mosby; **61-2,** from Thompson JM et al: *Mosby's clinical nursing,* ed 5, St Louis, 2002, Mosby; **61-3,** from Thibodeau GA, Patton KT: *Anatomy and physiology,* ed 5, St Louis, 2003, Mosby; **61-7,** redrawn from Long BC, Phipps WJ, Cassmeyer VL: *Medical-surgical nursing: a nursing process approach,* St Louis, 1993, Mosby;

61-10, courtesy Howmedica, Inc; **61-11,** from Ryan DW, Park GR: *Color atlas of critical and intensive care: diagnosis and investigation,* London, 1995, Mosby-Wolfe; **61-14,** from Thompson JM et al: *Mosby's clinical nursing,* ed 4, St Louis, 1998, Mosby; **61-15,** courtesy RA Weinstein, Denver, Colo; **61-17,** from Macklin EJ et al: *Hunter, Macklin, and Callahan's rehabilitation of the hand and upper extremity,* vol. 2, ed 5, St Louis, 2002, Mosby; **61-19,** from Maher A, Salmond S, Pellino T: *Orthopedic nursing,* ed 3, Philadelphia, 2002, Saunders; **61-20,** courtesy Zimmer, Inc., Warsaw, Ind.

Chapter 62
62-1, Redrawn from Mourad L: *Orthopedic disorders,* St Louis, 1992, Mosby; **62-2,** from Gartland J: *Fundamentals of orthopaedics,* Philadelphia, 1987, Saunders; **62-3, 62-4,** from Damjanov I, Linder J: *Anderson's pathology,* ed 10, St Louis, 1996, Mosby; **62-6,** from Mercier LR: *Practical orthopedics,* ed 4, St Louis, 1996, Mosby; **62-7,** from Maher A et al: *Orthopedic nursing,* ed 3, Philadelphia, 2002, Saunders.

Chapter 63
63-1, 63-3, From Stevens A, Lowe J: *Pathology: illustrated review in color,* ed 2, London, 2000, Mosby; **63-6, 63-9,** from Habif TP: *Clinical dermatology: a color guide to diagnosis and therapy,* ed 3, St Louis, 1996, Mosby; **63-7,** reprinted from the Clinical Slide Collection on the Rheumatic Diseases, copyright 1991, 1995, 1997. Used by permission of the American College of Rheumatology; **63-11,** from Zitelli BJ, Davis HW: *Atlas of pediatric physical diagnosis,* ed 4, St Louis, 2002, Mosby; **63-12,** redrawn from Freundlich B, Leventhal L: The fibromyalgia syndrome. In Schumacher HR Jr, Klippel JH, Koopman WJ, editors: *Primer on the rheumatic diseases,* ed 11, Atlanta, 1997, Arthritis Foundation. Reprinted with permission from The Arthritis Foundation, 1330 W. Peachtree St., Atlanta, GA 30309.

Chapter 64
64-1, 64-20, Courtesy Spacelabs Medical, Redmond, Wash; **64-2,** redrawn from Gardner PE: *Hemodynamic pressure monitoring,* Redmond, Wash, 1994, Spacelabs Medical; **64-3,** redrawn from Flynn JBM, Bruce NP: *Introduction to critical care skills,* St Louis, 1993, Mosby; **64-4,** from Darovic GO: *Hemodynamic monitoring,* ed 2, Philadelphia, 1995, Saunders; **64-5, 64-7, 64-10,** from Urden LD, Stacy KM, Lough ME: *Thelan's critical care nursing: diagnosis and management,* ed 4, St Louis, 2002, Mosby; **64-6,** courtesy Edwards Critical Care Division, Baxter Healthcare Corporation, Santa Ana, Calif; **64-8, 64-9,** from Lynn-McHale DJ, Carlson KK: *AACN procedure manual for critical care,* ed 4, Philadelphia, 2001, Saunders; **64-12, 64-14,** courtesy Datascope Corporation, Montvale, NJ; **64-15,** redrawn from Thelan LA et al: *Critical care nursing: diagnosis and management,* ed 3, St Louis, 1998, Mosby; **64-16A,** from Beare PG, Myers JL: *Adult health nursing,* ed 3, St Louis, 1998, Mosby; **64-17,** from Sills JR: *Respiratory care certification guide: the complete review resource for the entry level exam,* ed 3, St Louis, 1998, Mosby. In Urden LD, Stacy KM, Lough ME: *Thelan's critical care nursing: diagnosis and management,* ed 4, St Louis, 2002, Mosby; **64-18,** from Henneman E, Ellstrom K, St. John RE: *AACN protocols for practice: care of the mechanically ventilated patient series,* Aliso Viejo, Calif, 1999, American Association of Critical Care Nurses; **64-19,** courtesy Lifecare, Westminster, Colo; **64-21,** courtesy Mallinckrodt, Inc, Carlsbad, Calif.

Chapter 65
65-2, 65-3, 65-4, 65-5, From Urden LD, Stacy KM, Lough ME: *Thelan's critical care nursing: diagnosis and management,* ed 4, St Louis, 2002, Mosby.

Chapter 66
66-6, From Richmond TS: A critical care challenge: the patient with a cervical spinal cord injury, *Focus Crit Care* 12:27, 1985; **66-7,** courtesy Respironics, Inc, Pittsburgh; **66-10,** courtesy Hill-Rom, Inc, Batesville, Ind; **66-11,** courtesy Kinetic Concepts, Inc, San Antonio, Tex.

Chapter 67
67-2, 67-3, Courtesy Cameron Bangs, MD. From Auerbach PS, Donner HJ, Weiss EA: *Field guide to wilderness medicine,* St Louis, 1999, Mosby; **67-5,** from Auerbach PS, Donner HJ, Weiss EA: *Field guide to wilderness medicine,* St Louis, 1999, Mosby; **67-6,** courtesy Sherman Minton, MD. From Auerbach PS, Donner HJ, Weiss EA: *Field guide to wilderness medicine,* St Louis, 1999, Mosby; **67-7,** redrawn from Rosen P et al: *Emergency medicine,* vol 1, ed 2, St Louis, 1988, Mosby; **67-8,** photo used with the permission of the American Red Cross.

Index

Note: Disorder names are in **bold face.** Entries in **bold face** indicate main discussions. Page numbers followed by *f*, *t*, and *b* indicate figures, tables, or boxed material, respectively.

Note: Disorder names are in **bold face.** Entries in **bold
face** indicate main discussions. Page numbers followed
by *f, t,* and *b* indicate figures, tables, or boxed material,
respectively.

Note: Disorder names are in **bold face**. Entries in **bold face** indicate main discussions. Page numbers followed by *f, t,* and *b* indicate figures, tables, or boxed material, respectively.

Note: Disorder names are in **bold face.** Entries in **bold face** indicate main discussions. Page numbers followed by *f, t,* and *b* indicate figures, tables, or boxed material, respectively.

Note: Disorder names are in **bold face.** Entries in **bold
face** indicate main discussions. Page numbers followed
by *f, t,* and *b* indicate figures, tables, or boxed material,
respectively.

Note: Disorder names are in **bold face**. Entries in **bold
face** indicate main discussions. Page numbers followed
by *f, t,* and *b* indicate figures, tables, or boxed material,
respectively.

Note: Disorder names are in **bold face**. Entries in **bold face** indicate main discussions. Page numbers followed by *f*, *t*, and *b* indicate figures, tables, or boxed material, respectively.

Note: Disorder names are in **bold face**. Entries in **bold face** indicate main discussions. Page numbers followed by *f*, *t*, and *b* indicate figures, tables, or boxed material, respectively.

Note: Disorder names are in **bold face.** Entries in **bold face** indicate main discussions. Page numbers followed by *f, t,* and *b* indicate figures, tables, or boxed material, respectively.

Note: Disorder names are in **bold face.** Entries in **bold face** indicate main discussions. Page numbers followed by f, t, and b indicate figures, tables, or boxed material, respectively.

Note: Disorder names are in **bold face.** Entries in **bold face** indicate main discussions. Page numbers followed by *f, t,* and *b* indicate figures, tables, or boxed material, respectively.

Note: Disorder names are in **bold face.** Entries in **bold
face** indicate main discussions. Page numbers followed
by *f*, *t*, and *b* indicate figures, tables, or boxed material,
respectively.

Note: Disorder names are in **bold face**. Entries in **bold face** indicate main discussions. Page numbers followed by f, t, and b indicate figures, tables, or boxed material, respectively.

Note: Disorder names are in **bold face.** Entries in **bold face** indicate main discussions. Page numbers followed by *f, t,* and *b* indicate figures, tables, or boxed material, respectively.

Note: Disorder names are in **bold face.** Entries in **bold face** indicate main discussions. Page numbers followed by *f*, *t*, and *b* indicate figures, tables, or boxed material, respectively.

Note: Disorder names are in **bold face**. Entries in **bold face** indicate main discussions. Page numbers followed by *f*, *t*, and *b* indicate figures, tables, or boxed material, respectively.

Note: Disorder names are in **bold face.** Entries in **bold face** indicate main discussions. Page numbers followed by *f, t,* and *b* indicate figures, tables, or boxed material, respectively.

Note: Disorder names are in **bold face.** Entries in **bold face** indicate main discussions. Page numbers followed by *f, t,* and *b* indicate figures, tables, or boxed material, respectively.

Note: Disorder names are in **bold face.** Entries in **bold face** indicate main discussions. Page numbers followed by *f, t,* and *b* indicate figures, tables, or boxed material, respectively.

*Nursing Care Plan that incorporates NANDA nursing diagnoses, Nursing Outcomes Classification, and Nursing Interventions Classification.